Diseases of Swine 7TH EDITION

7TH EDITION

DISEASES OF SWINE

EDITED BY

Allen D. Leman
Swine Graphics

Barbara E. Straw
University of Nebraska, Lincoln

William L. Mengeling
National Animal Disease Center

Sylvie D'Allaire
University of Montreal

David J. Taylor
University of Glasgow

with 120 authoritative contributors selected for their recognized leadership in this field

 IOWA STATE UNIVERSITY PRESS / AMES, IOWA U.S.A.

First, second, and third editions, 1958 (second printing, 1959), 1964 (second printing, 1965), and 1970 (second printing, 1971; third printing, 1974), edited by Howard W. Dunne. Fourth edition, 1975 (second printing, 1978), edited by Howard W. Dunne and Allen D. Leman. Fifth edition, 1981 (second printing, 1984), edited by Allen D. Leman et al. Sixth edition, 1986 (second printing, 1991), edited by Allen D. Leman et al.

Seventh edition, 1992
Second printing, 1993

Library of Congress Cataloging-in-Publication Data

Diseases of swine / edited by Allen D. Leman . . . [et al.]; with 120 authoritative contributors selected for their recognized leadership in this field. — 7th ed.
     p.   cm.
  Includes bibliographical references and index.
  ISBN 0-8138-0442-6
  1. Swine—Diseases. I. Leman, Allen D.
  [DNLM: 1. Swine Diseases.   SF 971 D611]
SF971.D57   1992
636.4′089′6—dc20
DNLM/DLC
for Library of Congress   91–35402

Contents

v

SECTION **3** Bacterial Diseases

D. J. Taylor, *Editor*

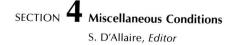

SECTION **4** Miscellaneous Conditions

S. D'Allaire, *Editor*

Foreword

WELCOME to the seventh edition of *Diseases of Swine*. The editorial committee's decisions and efforts were designed to meet the following objectives:

1. Present the most current knowledge available on today's rapidly changing technology and information explosion in the fields of swine diseases and production.
2. Select the best possible authors to achieve the first objective.
3. Make this large book more user friendly.
4. Continue the tradition of excellence established in 1958 by Professor Howard Dunne, of Pennsylvania State University. Dr. Dunne's editiorial direction in the first four editions provides the basis for our continuing efforts.

The seventh edition contains 12 new chapters, numerous new authors, and some major chapter revisions. Theses changes represent the editors' attempts to meet the above objectives and reflect the increasing scope and worldwide responsibility of veterinary science and practice.

The greatest challenge for any editorial group is selecting authors. As new information is added and new experts arise there are some inevitably tough decisions about changing authorship. In some instances this meant dropping highly esteemed pioneers in their fields for less well-known scientists and practitioners, who are on the cutting edge of research and expertise.

You will notice that flow charts, tables, and guidelines for differential diagnoses are no longer presented in a separate chapter, but have been included in the appropriate systems chapters in Section 1. Because the systems chapters provide basic knowledge about the anatomy, physiology, and pathology of each system, they are the most appropriate place to include differential diagnoses of the various diseases affecting that system. We encourage readers to use the first section of the book more aggressively.

Locating information in a book this size can be time consuming. Chapters in Sections 1, 2, 3, and 4 have been alphabetized by topic to allow users to quickly find main chapters without having to refer to the table of contents or index. However, to locate other references on a main topic, we encourage the reader to use the index.

Section 5 has seven new chapters that reflect the changing technology of veterinary practice. This section is designed to help practitioners deliver profitable veterinary service.

A special thanks goes to all the authors who met numerous deadlines and produced what we think is excellent material. Without their unselfish efforts this book would not exist. Their only compensation is the satisfaction of being a part of an internationally recognized resource book.

The Iowa State University Press staff deserve acknowledgement for their part in this publication. They used advanced editing, printing, and publishing technology that facilitated the rapid and accurate production of this text.

Users of *Diseases of Swine* are invited to submit comments and suggestions about improving future editions. Previous comments from students, researchers, practitioners, and reviewers have become part of the evolving ob.ectives of the editorial committee.

The editorial board acknowledges the new genus *Serpulina* for both *Treponema hyodysenteriae* and *Treponema innocens*. These organisms are referred to as *Serpulina hyodysenteriae* and *Serpulina innocens* throughout this edition.

Professor Dunne was a man of courage and vision. We hope that this book would meet his high standards for discipline and excellence.

Authors

Numbers in parentheses beside names refer to chapters.

T. J. L. Alexander (66)
Department of Clinical Veterinary Medicine
University of Cambridge
Cambridge, CB3 OES
England

K. Andries (19)
Department of Life Sciences
Janssen Pharmaceutica
Beerse B-2340
Belgium

L. Backstrom (71, 79)
School of Veterinary Medicine
University of Wisconsin
Madison, WI 53706

D. P. Bane (76)
College of Veterinary Medicine
University of Illinois
Urbana, IL 61801

H. N. Becker (77)
The Upjohn Co.
18520 CR6N
Plymouth, MN 55447

D. H. Beerman (73)
Department of Animal Science
Cornell University
Ithaca, NY 14851

D. A. Benfield (61)
South Dakota State Universtiy
Department of Veterinary Science
P.O. Box 2175
Brookings, SD 57007–1396

G. W. Beran (24)
Department of Microbiology and Preventive
    Medicine
College of Veterinary Medicine
Iowa State University
Ames, IA 50011

M. E. Bergeland (36)
Department of Veterinary Diagnostic Medicine
College of Veterinary Medicine
University of Minnesota
St. Paul, MN 55108

H. U. Bertschinger (39)
Institute of Veterinary Bacteriology
University of Zurich
8057 Zurich 11
Switzerland

A. Bisaillon (4)
Department of Animal Anatomy and Physiology
Faculty of Veterinary Medicine
University of Montreal
C. P. 5000 Saint-Hyacinthe
Quebec J2S 7C6
Canada

B. L. Blagburn (53)
Department of Pathobiology
College of Veterinary Medicine
Auburn University
Auburn, AL 36489–5519

S. R. Bolin (15, 76)
Virology Cattle Research Unit
USDA National Animal Disease Center
Ames, IA 50010

W. Bollwahn (78)
Hannover School of Veterinary Medicine
Bischofsholer Damm 15
D-3000 Hannover
Germany

R. D. Boyd (73)
Department of Animal Science
Cornell University
Ithaca, NY 14851

R. Bradley (5)
Department of Pathology
Central Veterinary Laboratory
Ministry of Agriculture Fisheries and Food
New Has, Weybridge KT15 3NB
England

T. L. Carson (64)
Veterinary Diagnostic Laboratory
College of Veterinary Medicine
Iowa State University
Ames, IA 50011

G. Christensen   (7)
Royal Dane-Quality A/S
Danmarksgade 22
P. O. Box 510
DK-7400 Herning
Denmark

L. L. Christian   (62)
Department of Animal Science
College of Agriculture
225 Kildee Hall
Iowa State University
Ames, IA 50011

R. M. Chu   (21)
Pig Research Institute
P. O. Box 23
Chunan, Miaoli
Taiwan 350

L. K. Clark   (75)
School of Veterinary Medicine
Purdue University
SCC-A
West Lafayette, IN 47907

J. E. Collins   (61)
Department of Veterinary Diagnostic Medicine
College of Veterinary Medicine
University of Minnesota
St. Paul, MN 55108

R. M. Corwin   (58)
Department of Veterinary Microbiology
College of Veterinary Medicine
University of Missouri-Columbia
Columbia, MO 65211

S. E. Curtis   (71)
Department of Dairy and Animal Science
Pennsylvania State University
University Park, PA 16802

R. S. Cutler   (68)
Bendigo Agricultural and Veterinary Centre
Box 125
Bendigo, Victoria 3550
Australia

S. D'Allaire   (69)
Department of Medicine
Faculty of Veterinary Medicine
University of Montreal
C. P. 5000 Saint-Hyacinthe
Quebec J2S 7C6
Canada

P. R. Davies   (54)
Department of Agriculture
Northfield Research Laboratories and Research
     Center
G.P.O. Box 1671
Adelaide, South Australia 5001
Australia

M. F. De Jong   (33)
Animal Health Institute
P.O. Box 13
8000 AA Zwolle
Netherlands

J. B. Derbyshire   (11, 18)
Department of Veterinary Microbiology and
     Immunology
Ontario Veterinary College
University of Guelph
Guelph, Ontario N1G 2w1
Canada

G. D. Dial   (6, 79)
Department of Large Animal Clinical Sciences
College of Veterinary Medicine
University of Minnesota
St. Paul, MN 55108

K. J. Dobson   (54)
6 Reynell Road
Rostrevor, South Australia 5073
Australia

J. T. Done   (5)
3 The Oaks West Byfleet
Surrey KT14 6RL
England

R. Drolet   (69)
Department of Pathology and Microbiology
Faculty of Veterinary Medicine
University of Montreal
C. P. 5000 Saint-Hyacinthe
Quebec J2S 7C6
Canada

B. C. Easterday   (27)
School of Veterinary Medicine
University of Wisconsin
Madison, WI 53706

N. Edington   (16)
Department of Microbiology and Parasitology
Royal Veterinary College
Royal College Street
London M21 OTU
England

M. J. Edwards   (56)
Department of Veterinary Clinical Sciences
Faculty of Veterinary Science
University of Sydney
Sydney, New South Wales 2006
Australia

S. A. Edwards   (72)
Scottish Agricultural College
School of Agriculture
581 King Street
Aberdeen AB9 1UD
Scotland

W. A. Ellis (42)
Veterinary Research Laboratories
Stoney Road
Stormont
Belfast BT4 3SD
Northern Ireland

P. R. English (72)
School of Agriculture
University of Aberdeen
581 King Street
Aberdeen AB9 1UD
Scotland

V. A. Fahy (68)
Bendigo Agricultural and Veterinary Centre
Box 125
Bendigo, Victoria 3550
Australia

J. M. Fairbrother (39)
Faculty of Veterinary Medicine
University of Montreal
C. P. 5000 Saint-Hyacinthe
Quebec, J2S 7C6
Canada

R. M. Friendship (1)
Department of Clinical Studies
University of Guelph
Guelph, Ontario N1G 2W1
Canada

C. J. Giles (34)
Animal Health Product Development Department
Pfizer Central Research
Sandwich, Kent CT13 9NJ
England

D. L. Harris (49, 66)
Pig Improvement Company
P. O. Box 348
Highway 31W South
Franklin, KY 42134

P. H. Hemsworth (52)
Department of Agriculture and Rural Affairs
Animal Research Institute
Werribee, Victoria 3030
Australia

S. C. Henry (1, 60, 67)
Abilene Animal Hospital, P.A.
320 N.E. 14th Street
Abilene, KS 67410

R. Higgins (48)
Faculty of Veterinary Medicine
University of Montreal
C.P. 5000 Saint-Hyacinthe
Quebec J2S 7C6
Canada

H. T. Hill (24)
Veterinary Diagnostic Laboratory
College of Veterinary Medicine
Iowa State University
Ames, IA 50011

M. A. Hill (7)
Large Animal Clinics
School of Veterinary Medicine
Purdue University
West Lafayette, IN 47907

V. S. Hinshaw (27)
School of Veterinary Medicine
University of Wisconsin
Madison, WI 53706

C. A. House (28, 30)
Foreign Animal Disease Diagnostic Laboratory
USDA, APHIS, S & T
P. O. Box 848
Greenport, NY 11944

J. A. House (28, 30)
Foreign Animal Disease Diagnostic Laboratory
USDA, APHIS, S & T
P.O. Box 848
Greenport, NY 11944

A. L. Jenny (61)
Pathobiology Laboratory
National Veterinary Services Laboratories
Ames, IA 50010

J. E. T. Jones (10, 51)
Royal Veterinary College
Boltons Park
Hawkshead Road, Potters Bar
Hertfordshire, EN6 1NB
England

H. S. Joo (17, 21)
Department of Large Animal Clinical Sciences
College of Veterinary Medicine
University of Minnesota
St. Paul, MN 55108

J. P. Kluge (24)
Department of Pathology
College of Veterinary Medicine
Iowa State University
Ames, IA 50011

G. H. K. Lawson (45)
Department of Veterinary Pathology
Edinburgh University Veterinary Field Station
Easter Bush
Roslin
Midlothian EH25 9RG
England

Y. Leforban (14)
Porcine Pathology Station
BP 9
22440 Ploufragan
France

A. D. Leman   (Coordinating Editor)
Swine Graphics
1620 Superior Street
Webster City, IA 50595

E. M. Liebler   (2)
Hannover School of Veterinary Medicine
Bischofsholer Damm 15
D-3000 Hannover
Germany

D. S. Lindsay   (53)
Department of Pathobiology
College of Veterinary Medicine
Auburn University
Auburn, AL 36489–5519

T. J. Loula   (61)
Swine Veterinary Center
1608 South Minnesota Avenue
St. Peter, MN 56082

K. Lundstrom   (62)
Department of Animal Breeding and Genetics
Swedish University of Agricultural Sciences
Uppsala S-750-07
Sweden

R. J. Lysons   (49)
Institute of Animal Health
Compton
Berkshire RG16 0NN
England

A. P. MacMillan   (35)
Central Veterinary Laboratory
Woodham Lane
Weybridge, Surrey KT 3NB
England

W. E. Marsh   (6)
Department of Large Animal Clinical Science
College of Veterinary Medicine
University of Minnesota
St. Paul, MN 55108

G. Martineau   (4)
Department of Medicine
Faculty of Veterinary Medicine
University of Montreal
C. P. 5000 Saint-Hyacinthe
Quebec J2S 7C6
Canada

W. L. Mengeling   (23)
Virology Swine Research Unit
USDA, National Animal Disease Center
Ames, IA 50010

A. R. Mercy   (79)
Department of Agriculture
Baron Hay Court
South Perth
Western Australia 6151
Australia

D. J. Meuten   (65)
School of Veterinary Medicine
North Carolina State University
Raleigh, NC 27606

E. R. Miller   (60)
Department of Animal Science
Michigan State University
East Lansing, MI 48824

L. G. Morehouse   (25)
916 Danforth Drive
Columbia, MO 65201

R. B. Morrison   (70)
College of Veterinary Medicine
385 Animal Science/Veterinary Medicine
University of Minnesota
St. Paul, MN 55108

J. Mousing   (7)
Danske Slagterier
Veterinaerafdelingen
Axeltorv 3
1609 Copenhagen V.
Denmark

R. C. Mulley   (56)
Department of Animal Health
Faculty of Veterinary Science
University of Sydney
Camden, New South Wales 2570
Australia

J. L. Nelssen   (60)
Department of Animal Science
Kansas State University
Manhattan, KS 66506

J. Nicolet   (31, 41)
Institute of Veterinary Bacteriology
University of Berne
P.O. Box 8466
CH-3001 Berne
Switzerland

N. O. Nielsen   (39)
Ontario Veterinary College
University of Guelph
Guelph, Ontario N1G 2W1
Canada

J. J. O'Brien   (55)
Department of Agriculture
Divisional Veterinary Office for Northern Ireland
9 Robert Street
Newtownards Co. Down BT23 4DN
Northern Ireland

G. D. Osweiler   (59)
Veterinary Diagnostic Laboratory
College of Veterinary Medicine
Iowa State University
Ames, IA 50011

P. S. Paul (26)
Veterinary Medical Research Institute
College of Veterinary Medicine
Iowa State University
Ames, IA 50011

M. B. Pensaert (19, 22)
Laboratory of Virology
Faculty of Veterinary Medicine
State University of Ghent
Casinoplein 24
B-9000 Ghent
Belgium

C. Pijoan (44)
Department of Large Animal Clinical Sciences
College of Veterinary Medicine
University of Minnesota
St. Paul, MN 55108

K. B. Platt (24)
Department of Veterinary Microbiology and
    Preventive Medicine
College of Veterinary Medicine
Iowa State University
Ames, IA 50011

J. F. Pohlenz (2, 39)
Institute of Pathology
Hannover School of Veterinary Medicine
Bischofsholer Damm 15
D-3000 Hannover
Germany

A. M. Pointon (79)
Veterinary Laboratory
G.P.O. Box 1671
Adelaide, South Australia 5001
Australia

D. D. Polson (6)
Department of Large Animal Clinical Science
College of Veterinary Medicine
University of Minnesota
St. Paul, MN 55108

M. M. Pullen (74)
University of Minnesota
136-C, ABLMS
1354 Eckles Avenue
St. Paul, MN 55108

D. C. Roberts (80)
Faculty of Veterinary Science
University of Pretoria
Private Bag X04 0110
Onderstepoort
Republic of South Africa

R. F. Ross (43)
Veterinary Medical Research Institute
College of Veterinary Medicine
Iowa State University
Ames, IA 50011

J. A. Roth (3)
Department of Veterinary Microbiology and
    Preventive Medicine
College of Veterinary Medicine
Iowa State University
Ames, IA 50011

M. F. Rothschild (57)
Department of Animal Science
College of Agriculture
Iowa State University
Ames, IA 50011

A. C. Rowland (45)
Department of Veterinary Pathology
Edinburgh University Veterinary Field Station
Easter Bush
Roslin
Midlothian EH25 9RG
England

L. J. Runnels (75, 76)
1501 Ravinia Road
West Lafayette, IN 47906

L. J. Saif (29)
Food Animal Health Research Program
Ohio Agricultural Research and Development
    Center
Ohio State University
Wooster, OH 44691

J. M. Sanchez-Vizcaino (12)
Department of Animal Virology
National Institute of Investigation Agricultural
Embajadores 68
28012 Madrid
Spain

S. E. Sanford (48, 51)
Veterinary Laboratory Services Branch
Ontario Ministry of Agriculture and Food
Huron Park, Ontario, NOM 1YO
Canada

K. J. Schwartz (46)
Veterinary Diagonstic Laboratory
College of Veterinary Medicine
Iowa State University
Ames, IA 5001

A. R. Smith (37)
Department of Veterinary Pathology and Hygeine
College of Veterinary Medicine
University of Illinois
Urbana, IL 61801

B. B. Smith (4)
College of Veterinary Medicine
Oregon State University
Corvallis, OR 97331

W. J. Smith   (63)
Veterinary Investigation Service
Scottish Agricultural College
Mill of Craibstone
Bucksburn, Aberdeen AB2 9TS
Scotland

E. M. Spicer   (68)
Bendigo Agricultural and Veterinary Centre
Box 125
Bendigo, Victoria 3550
Australia

A. H. Stephano   (13)
Villa de Guadelupe 234
Villa del Campestre
Leon, Guanajuato
C.P. 37150
Mexico

G. W. Stevenson   (26)
Animal Disease Diagnostic Laboratory
Purdue University
West Lafayette, IN 47906

T. B. Stewart   (58)
Veterinary Microbiology and Parasitology
School of Veterinary Medicine
Louisiana State University
Baton Rouge, LA 70803–8416

B. E. Straw   (9, 57, 65)
Veterinary Science Department
111 VBS, East Campus
University of Nebraska
Lincln, NE 68583–0905

B. P. Stuart   (53)
Mobay Chemical Corporation
Stanley Research Center
17745 South Metcalf
Stilwell, KS 66085–9104

D. J. Taylor   (36, 40, 47, 51)
Glasgow University Veterinary School
Bearsden Road
Bearsden, Glasgow G61 1QH
Scotland

C. O. Thoen   (50)
Department of Microbiology, Immunology
   and Preventive Medicine
Iowa State University
Ames, IA 50011

D. W. Upson   (67)
College of Veterinary Medicine
Kansas State University
Manhattan, KS 66502

J.-P. Vaillancourt   (6)
Department of Clinical Studies
University of Guelph
Guelph, Ontario N1G 2W1
Canada

P. Vannier   (14)
Central Veterinary Institute
Department of Virology
P.O. Box 365
8200 AJ Lelystad
Netherlands

J. T. Van Oirschot   (20)
Department of Virology
Central Veterinary Institute
P.O. Box 365
8200 AJ Lelystad
The Netherlands

R. A. Vinson   (81)
Box K
Oneida, IL 61467

J. R. Walton   (32)
University of Liverpool Veterinary Field Station
Department of Veterinary Clinical Science
Leahurst
Neston, South Wirral L64 7TE
England

R. D. Wesley   (29)
Virology Swine Research Unit
USDA, National Animal Disease Center
Ames, IA 50010

S. C. Whipp   (2)
Physiology Laboratory
USDA, National Animal Disease Center
Ames, IA 50010

B. P. Wilcock   (46)
Department of Pathology
Ontario Veterinary College
Guelph, Ontario N1G 2W1
Canada

R. L. Wood   (38)
USDA, National Animal Disease Center
Ames, IA 50010

J. A. Yager   (51)
Department of Pathology
University of Guelph
Guelph, Ontario N1G 2W1
Canada

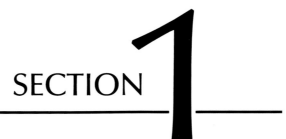

SECTION 1

Anatomy, Physiology, and Systemic Pathology

B. E. Straw, EDITOR

1 Cardiovascular System, Hematology, and Clinical Chemistry

R. M. FRIENDSHIP

S. C. HENRY

Cardiovascular System

THE PIG is used extensively in cardiovascular research as a model for human disease, particularly atherosclerosis (Lee 1986); therefore, a great deal of information is available concerning the morphologic, biochemic, and metabolic functioning of the pig heart. The scope of this chapter will be limited, however, to information relevant to the veterinary practitioner, including an overview of anatomic and physiologic features that might be used in clinical examination, as well as discussion of the differential diagnosis of cardiovascular disease.

ANATOMY AND PHYSIOLOGY. Pigs have a relatively small heart and small blood volume and a rather unstable circulatory physiology with low cardiac output compared with other domestic mammals. The weight of the heart in the suckling piglet is approximately 0.8% of the total body weight, which is similar to other species. However, this heart-to-body ratio decreases with age. A 100-kg pig has a heart that weighs only 0.3% or less of the total body weight (Engelhardt 1966). Selective breeding for fast growth rate has been suggested as an explanation of why the modern domestic pig possesses such a uniquely small heart. In 1800, pigs required 2–3 years to reach a body weight of 40 kg, but today, pigs grow to a weight of 100 kg in 5–6 months (Sack 1982).

The pig heart is broad and short. The blunt apex is positioned almost median, overlying the last sternebra about 2.5 cm from the sternal part of the diaphragm. The heart lies in a more horizontal plane than in other domestic animals and occupies slightly more than the ventral half of the available thoracic space. The anterior vena cava passes cranially from the base of the heart ventral to the trachea. At the level of the first rib, it gives rise to 6 veins: the paired subclavian, internal, and external jugular veins. At the origin of these veins, a large pool of blood is formed. The object of anterior vena cava sampling is to place a needle in this pool or in any of the large veins surrounding it. Thus, despite the procedure's name, the cranial vena cava may not be the vein that is punctured. The external jugular vein, at the point of deepest depression midway on the ventral surface of the neck, is preferred as the site for venipuncture, both in consideration for safety of the pig and for the quality of the sample.

The heart is surrounded by a fibrous pericardium, which is attached to the sternum from a point opposite the third rib to the xiphoid cartilage and to the sternal part of the diaphragm. The pericardium has extensive contact with the chest wall, pushing the mediastinal pleura against the costal pleura at the cardiac notches.

The heart rate in resting pigs decreases exponentially with age. Heart rate of newborn piglets is as high as 200 beats per minute, but this rate declines to 70–100 beats per minute by the time pigs reach 100-kg body weight. Auscultation is helpful in monitoring heart rate and identifying murmurs caused by valvular disease or septal defects. In small pigs, surface palpation of the chest may detect the holosystolic murmur characteristic of valvular endocarditis. This clinical examination technique is most helpful as a large number of animals can be examined rapidly. Auscultation of the apex beat is performed in larger pigs by placing the palm of the hand on the left chest wall with the side of the hand touching the elbow of the pig. The pulse can often be detected either at the anterior rim of the ear or by palpating the underside of the tail. The coarse hair coat, the subcutaneous fat layer, and especially the pig's excitable temperament make examination of the cardiovascular system difficult. Excitement from handling and restraint can cause a rapid increase in heart rate of 50% or more.

Researchers also have recorded sudden, marked increases in blood pressure of pigs as a result of the pig reacting to restraint (Wade et al. 1986). The arterial blood pressure in the systemic circulation in resting swine is within the same range as other domestic animals. The arterial systolic pressure of suckling piglets is about 60 mm Hg, while in market weight animals (100 kg) it is about 140 mm Hg. Clinically, blood pressure is not measured under practical field conditions, but in the case of white breeds, a marked elevation of blood pressure is accompanied by an obvious erythemic change of skin color and also by distension of peripheral veins.

Venous distension in the pig is difficult to appreciate and requires careful visual examination. The auricular veins at the base of the ear and the cephalic, mammary, and recurrent tarsal veins are the most obvious blood vessels to examine for distension if one suspects phlebitis or a cardiac lesion restricting blood flow.

The lymphatic system of pigs is unremarkable. The large thoracic duct divides near its termination into two branches that unite to form an ampulla. This contracts and opens into the terminal part of the left jugular vein. Occasionally the thoracic duct is accidentally punctured during attempts at obtaining blood from the jugular vein. Lymph glands are embedded in fat and many are dark red resembling haemal nodes (which are not present in pigs).

CARDIOVASCULAR DISEASE. Lesions of the endocardium, heart valves, myocardium, and pericardium can lead to chronic or acute heart failure. Early signs of chronic or congestive heart failure include listless behavior, loss of body condition, and respiratory distress after mild exertion. Clinical examination of a pig suffering congestive heart failure might reveal an increased heart rate, peripheral and pulmonary edema, and an enlarged heart. Acute heart failure is relatively more common than chronic heart disease. Whenever sudden death occurs, particularly after mixing or transporting pigs, acute heart failure should be a major consideration (Gary 1989). Clinical signs if observed are short in duration and characterized by a sudden onset of dyspnea, trembling, and then collapse and death. Differential diagnosis is primarily based on postmortem findings and history.

There is scant information regarding the incidence of cardiac disease in the commercial swine population. It has been reported that heart failure is the most important cause of death loss in sows (D'Allaire et al. 1990) and in pigs being transported (Bergmann et al. 1988).

It should be noted that cardiovascular disease can be a problem on a well-managed minimal disease herd. Possibly, as infectious disease is controlled and productivity improved through the institution of good health management programs and sound husbandry practices, cardiovascular problems will become proportionally more important than they have been in the past. The following is a list of the more important agents associated with cardiovascular disease (Gary 1989; and Else 1980):

Diseases of Myocardium

Bacteria – *Streptococcus* spp. and other bacteria following bacteremia

Viruses – Encephalomyocarditis virus, foot-and-mouth, swine vesicular disease

Nutritional – Vitamin E/selenium, iron deficiency

Toxicity – Gossypol, selenium, inorganic ionophores

Inherited conditions – Malignant hyperthermia (porcine stress syndrome)

Diseases of Endocardium and Heart Valves

Bacteria – *Erysipelothrix rhusiopathiae, Streptococcus* spp., and *Escherichia coli*

Congenital defects

Diseases of the Pericardium

Bacterial fibrinous pericarditis – *Pasteurella multocida, Pasteurella hemolytica, Mycoplasma* spp., especially *M. hyorhinis, Hemophilus parasuis, Actinobacillus pleuropneumoniae, Streptococcus* spp., and *Salmonella* spp.

Hydropericardium – mulberry heart disease, edema disease

Diseases of Blood Vessels

Viral vasculitis – African swine fever, hog cholera

Bacterial vasculitis – Erysipelas, *Actinobacillus pleuropneumoniae,* Glasser's disease (*H. parasuis*), and salmonellosis

Vasoconstrictive Agents – ergot poisoning

Hemorrhagic Conditions

Coagulation defects – Prothrombin deficiency (e.g., warfarin poisoning), factor VIII deficiency (simple autosomal recessive inherited disorder), fungal toxins (e.g., aflatoxin, *Fusarium*)

Platelet disorders – Thrombocytopenia purpura, megakaryocytic infection (hog cholera, African swine fever)

Navel bleeding

Gastric ulceration

Hemorrhagic bowel syndrome

Enteric diseases with hemorrhagic component – swine dysentery, salmonellosis, trichuriasis, ileitis

More detailed discussions of these particular conditions are presented elsewhere in this text.

Mulberry heart disease, a peroxidative disorder caused by insufficiency of vitamin E and/or selenium, continues to be a problem on certain farms although the cause of this disorder has been known for many years. Inadequate vitamin E uptake and assimilation from colostrum is associated with lowered biochemical antioxidant status in piglets during the nursing period (Loudenslager et al. 1986). The increased use of oils and fats in starter diets may be another reason that routine dietary supplementation of vitamin E and selenium has proven inadequate at times.

Congenital heart defects remain a common cause of heart failure in young pigs; ventricular septal defects and aortic and subaortic stenosis are reported as the most common of these defects (Else 1980).

Streptococcal and erysipelas infections occur on almost all farms regardless of health status, and these diseases are the cause of the vast majority of the cases of vegetative valvular endocarditis (Taylor 1989). Most valvular lesions are of the left heart and emboli, and if they occur, lead to splenic and kidney infarcts. Congestive right heart failure is rare in pigs and is limited to older adult animals.

Hemorrhagic disorders occur sporadically and can involve large numbers of animals on a particular farm and are therefore of economic significance when they occur. Navel bleeding for example can involve entire litters and persist for months or years on particular farms. The navel cords of affected piglets appear large and fleshy and tend to ooze blood for several hours after birth, causing mild to severe anemia in the newborn. Blood clotting time has been shown to be normal in these animals and it has been suggested that the disorder may be caused by a collagen immaturity. Generally, cases of navel bleeding are associated with the practice of using wood shavings as bedding, prior to and during parturition; when the shavings have been removed from the farrowing area, the problem has stopped. Other treatments have included supplementation with ascorbic acid (Sandholm et al. 1979), folic acid, and vitamin K but with varying degrees of success.

In addition to navel bleeding, a considerable number of infrequently documented disorders are associated with blood loss including conditions affecting blood clotting and diseases causing vascular damage. Pigs also are prone to disseminated intravascular coagulation, initiated by a variety of mechanisms such as extensive tissue necrosis, endotoxicosis, excessive iron administration, or hepatic damage. Shock, as in other animal species, is a consequence of rapid blood loss. Treatment is by restoration of body fluid levels; however, this is seldom of practical application in the pig except possibly as treatment for valuable breeding-stock animals.

Hematology

INTRODUCTION. Hematologic examination is seldom used as a diagnostic tool in swine practice. The low economic value of the individual animal usually does not allow the veterinarian the opportunity to perform an extensive clinical examination of the live pig. There is, however, great potential for hematology and clinical chemistry to be applied on a herd basis as part of a health monitoring program. If a truly representative sample of animals is routinely tested and compared with a well-established data base of reference values, it is possible that early signs of disease or nutritional deficiencies could be detected.

LIMITATIONS. The anatomic features and uncooperative temperament of the pig pose certain challenges in obtaining a good blood sample. Blood sampling sites and techniques are presented elsewhere in this text. It is important to note that the method of collection and the skill of the investigator might alter the values of the constituents being analyzed. Stress for a short duration can result in adrenal corticosteroid elevation, which will influence the cellular picture of blood. Numbers of circulating neutrophils will increase in response to stress while lymphocytes and eosinophils decrease. Excitement caused by handling and restraint can induce splenic contraction and an increase in the packed-cell volume of 10% or more (Brenner and Gurtler 1981). The porcine erythrocyte is relatively fragile and therefore hemolysis is a potential problem. Samples need to be collected in such a manner that excessive turbulence or agitation is avoided. Samples must not contact hypotonic solutions and must be handled carefully to ensure that exposure to excessive heat or cold is avoided. Researchers (Fontaine et al. 1987) have shown that porcine blood samples taken into ethylenediaminetetraacetic acid (EDTA) and stored at room temperature or at 4°C provided stable hemogram values for at least 36 hours with the exception of the differential count, which presented significant variability as early as 12 hours after sampling.

Coagulation of swine blood is rapid, and only through collection into vials containing anticoagulant can unwanted aggregation of cells be avoided. This feature of swine blood may lead to obstruction of the bore of needles and make repeated use of a single needle for sampling unwise. Even saline-flushing between animals fails to adequately remove clots and jeopardizes sample quality. Clean needles should be used for each animal to be sampled.

An additional limitation for the use of hematology in herd medicine is in the selection of an appropriate number of animals to be tested to be representative of the population. For certain hematological values, the variation in normal values is quite large; therefore, the number of animals that need to be sampled to show that the mean of the sampled group is different from the mean of a normal population may be very great. Insufficient numbers sampled or an inappropriate representative group (such as only the smallest pigs in each pen) might lead the practitioner to draw an incorrect conclusion from the hematological information and thus limits its value as a diagnostic tool (Lumsden and Mullen 1978).

REFERENCE VALUES. Hematologic reference values are presented in Table 1.1 (Friendship et al. 1984). The purpose of including reference values in this chapter is to provide a baseline to as-

Table 1.1. Porcine hematology reference intervals

Variable	Units	Weaner Pigs	Feeder Pigs	Gilts	Sows
B-Hemoglobin	g/L	90–140	100–150	120–170	100–170
B-Hematocrit	L/L	0.26–0.41	0.29–0.42	0.33–0.45	0.29–0.46
B-Erythrocytes	x10^{12}/L	5.3–8.0	5.7–8.3	5.9–8.7	5.1–8.0
(B)Erc-MCV	fL	42–62	44–56	48–62	52–63
(B)Erc-MCH	pg	14–21	15–20	17–22	18–22
(B)Erc-MCHC	g/L	320–360	320–380	340–380	340–380
B-Leukocytes	x10^9/L	8.7–37.9	11.6–32.9	11.2–28.8	10.6–24.0
B-Neutrophils segmented	x10^9/L	2.5–23.0	0.3–15.2	1.4–11.6	1.9–10.1
	%	16.6–73.1	4.4–62.1	11.1–53.6	15.1–59.5
Bands	x10^9/L	0.0–3.1	0.0–0.7	0.0–0.7	0.0–0.6
	%	0.0–13.0	0.0–8.0	0.0–2.8	0.0–3.3
B-Lymphocytes	x10^9/L	2.2–16.0	3.6–18.5	3.9–16.8	3.7–14.7
	%	12.5–70.1	22.1–78.0	30.4–74.5	25.5–71.1
B-Monocytes	x10^9/L	0.001–5.000	0.0–4.9	0.0–4.0	0.0–2.4
	%	0.0–17.0	0.1–20.1	0.2–20.8	1.0–14.0
B-Eosinophils	x10^9/L	0.0–1.8	0.0–2.5	0.3–3.3	0.0–2.4
	%	0.0–6.0	0.0–11.1	0.0–16.9	1.0–13.0
B-Basophils	x10^9/L	0.0–0.5	0.0–0.7	0.0–0.7	0.0–0.5
	%	0.0–2.0	0.0–3.6	0.0–3.8	0.0–3.0
B-Rubricytes	x10^9/L	0.0–0.2	0.0–0.3	0.0–0.3	0.0–0.2
	%	0.0–1.0	0.0–1.0	0.0–1.8	0.0–1.0
Disintegrated	x10^9/L	0.0–1.7	0.0–3.3	0.0–1.7	0.0–1.5
	%	0.0–7.4	0.0–14.2	0.0–5.9	0.0–9.3

Source: Friendship et al. (1984).
Note: B = blood; fL = femtoliter; g = gram; L = liter; pg = picogram.

sist veterinarians in interpreting results from individual sick pigs or from herds with suspected subclinical disease or borderline nutritional deficiency or toxicity. The usefulness of such reference values are restricted by biologic variations between animals and by analytical differences between laboratories. Some of the most important causes of variation are listed below with a brief explanation. Greater detail and description of hematological values are provided in reference texts.

INFLUENCING FACTORS

Age. The packed-cell volume of the newborn pig is high. However, there is a 30% reduction in red blood cell (RBC) count and about a 38% decrease in red cell mass during the first week of life, as a consequence of plasma volume expansion from absorption of colostrum. Blood volume is greatest in the young pig and decreases with age (Pond and Houpt 1978). RBC production is very active during the suckling stage; therefore, immature cells appear in the circulation at this time. For the young pig it is important that the white blood cell (WBC) count be corrected for nucleated erythrocytes (Schmidt 1986).

At birth, the neutrophils represent about 70% of the white cells and lymphocytes about 20%. Neutrophils decrease and lymphocytes increase so that within 10 days of birth the proportion of the two cell types is reversed. The overall leukocyte count decreases from 1 to 9 months of age, due almost entirely to a decline in lymphocytes (Burks et al. 1977).

Pregnancy, Parturition, and Lactation. Red cell parameters change during pregnancy and lactation primarily as a result of changes in blood volume, which decreases during the first 8 weeks of gestation. Within the last 2 weeks before parturition, erythrocyte parameters decline and continue to decrease until the end of lactation. The proportion of neutrophils suddenly increases at the time of parturition relative to the number of lymphocytes, but this ratio generally reverses to normal within 12 hours of farrowing (Nachreiner and Ginther 1972a).

Stress and Disease. The blood parameters of pigs respond to stress and inflammatory conditions in a similar manner to other species. Stress results in a leukocytosis characterized by a neutrophilia and reduced numbers of lymphocytes and eosinophils. Pigs reared under minimal disease conditions tend to have lower leukocyte counts than conventionally reared pigs (McTaggert and Rowntree 1969). In an experiment examining specific-pathogen-free (SPF) pigs derived by hysterectomy, it was shown that erythrocyte counts, hematocrits, and leukocyte counts were lower in SPF piglets until 2 months of age. At 3 months of age, leukocyte counts were still lower in SPF pigs and gamma globulin levels were half the level of controls (Kaneko et al. 1987).

A recent study (Odink et al. 1990) examined the hematologic and clinicochemical profiles of healthy swine and swine with inflammatory processes. For most variables examined, significant differences were noted between animals with inflammatory lesions such as abscesses, pleuritis, or pericarditis and healthy pigs. The hematologic parameters that were affected most significantly were erythrocyte sedimentation rate (ESR), hemoglobin, and hematocrit. The implications of this work are that blood analyses may be useful in herd health monitoring and in addition as a technique to assist meat inspectors in the detection of abscesses and inflammatory disease.

Total WBC counts have a wide normal range in the pig. Clinically, the study of Wright-Giemsa–stained blood smears for differential cell appreciation provides a much better indication of infectious disease processes than does the WBC count alone. Absolute neutrophilia with lymphopenia often occurs in early bacterial infections, yet total WBC values may appear to be in the normal range. Eosinophilia, as in other species, is noted with parasitism such as ascariasis and, to a lesser extent, sarcoptic mange. Eosinophilia is not a specific sign of parasitism, however, and may result from many forms of antigenic stimulation.

DISEASES OF BLOOD

Anemia. Anemia is defined as a reduction to below normal in the number of erythrocytes, the quantity of hemoglobin, or the volume of packed red cells that occurs when the equilibrium between blood loss and blood production is disturbed. The best determinant of anemia, with the laboratory equipment available in most clinical settings, is the packed-cell volume or hematocrit (Perman et al. 1989). For general comparison, hemoglobin levels in g/dL are approximately one-third the numeric value of the hematocrit percentage.

The three most common pathologic mechanisms are (1) failure to form hemoglobin due to insufficient substrate (most notably iron); (2) the loss of blood and hemoglobin via hemorrhage and hemolysis, as in navel bleeding or gastric ulceration; and (3) bone marrow suppression and ineffective hematopoiesis due to chronic infectious disease, neoplasia, or toxicosis. The most common causes of anemia in pigs are listed in Tables 1.2 and 1.3. (Straw and Wilson 1985).

Calculation of red cell indices relating cell size and hemoglobin status is an accepted method to objectively quantify anemia and to classify the type and cause. For the practicing swine clinician, such methodology is often unavailable. Examination of Wright-Giemsa–stained blood smears allows conclusion as to red cell size, shape, and color without need for RBC indices. In conjunction with physical examination and history, red cell morphology on stained smears may well provide the information needed for clinical classification of anemia in swine. Normocytic-normochromic cells stain uniformly and are similar in size. Normocytic-normochromic anemia occurs in animals suffering from chronic inflammatory disease or neoplasia. Microcytic-hypochromic cells are indicative of iron deficiency. The macrocytic anemias, with anisocytosis or cell size variation, represent an increased demand for RBCs due to hemorrhage or hemolysis. Such conditions are considered responsive, and immature red cells (reticulocytes and rubricytes) are frequently present. RBC response is a positive prognostic sign.

Iron deficiency anemia in suckling pigs is a combined result of minimal fetal iron storage, the low iron content of sow's milk, and the hygienic standards in accommodations for nursing pigs

Table 1.2. Conditions that cause anemia in unweaned pigs

Cause	Pigs Affected	Signs	Hematologic Findings	Diagnosis
Iron deficiency anemia	Normal at birth; anemia becomes severe as age increases	Rough hair coat, rapid respiration, uneven growth; necropsy—heart dilated, excess pericardial fluid, pulmonary edema, enlarged spleen	Microcytic, hypochromic red cells	History that the pigs did not receive an appropriate iron injection
Eperythrozoonosis	Especially under 5 days of age, but anytime from birth to weaning	Icterus, rough hair coat, uneven growth, listless, swollen yellow-brown liver, enlarged spleen	Organisms seen in red blood cells	Wright-Giemsa stain of blood from febrile pig, titer of 80 or more with indirect hemagglutination test from the sow
Umbilical hemorrhage	Death within a few hours of birth, may be associated with use of wood shavings	Cord remains large and fleshy, fails to shrivel; blood-stained skin	Normal	Clinical signs

Source: Straw and Wilson (1985).

Table 1.3. Conditions that cause anemia in weaned pigs to adults

Cause	Ages Affected	Other Signs	Appearance of Feces	Associated Factors	Diagnosis
Gastric ulcers	Older growing-finishing pigs and adults	Reduced appetite; weight loss; occasional tooth grinding	Normal or firm, dark tarry feces	Finely ground feed	Ulcer observed at necropsy
Iron deficiency	Nursery pigs	Reduced growth; rough hair coat	Normal	Failure to give sufficient iron	History and absence of other
Trichuris suis	Usually in 2- to 6-month-old pigs	Anorexia; diarrhea with mucus; wasting	Dark mucoid diarrhea	Lack of parasite control program, pigs on dirt lot	Lesions in intestine, favorable response to treatment
Eperythrozoonosis	Nursery to adult	Lethargy; reduced growth; occasional icterus; acute episode in sows at farrowing or weaning with mammary and vulvar edema; depression	Normal	Poor mange and lice control	Stained blood smear to demonstrate organisms; indirect hemagglutination titer of 1:80 or higher
Sarcoptes suis	Nursery to adult, anemia severe in younger pigs	Scratching; weight loss; rough hair coat; keratinization of skin	Normal	Poor mange control	Skin scraping to demonstrate mites
Proliferative enteritis	Nursery to adult, anemia most prominent in 2- to 5-month-old pigs	Varying degrees of anorexia, weight loss	Black tarry feces to frank blood	More common in pigs of Landrace breeding	Necropsy—lesions primarily in small intestine; histopathology—mucosal hyperplasia
Mycotoxins: Aflatoxin	All ages, signs severer in younger pigs	Depression; anorexia; ascites; elevated liver enzymes; occasional icterus	Usually normal	Moldy feed, esp. grains raised in the South and Southeastern U.S.A.	Liver lesion of fatty change to necrosis and cirrhosis; feed analysis for toxin
Tricothecenes		Gastroenteritis			Feed analysis for toxin
Zearalenone		Swollen vulva; enlarged mammary glands			
Warfarin toxicity	Any age	Lameness, stiffness; lethargy	Dark tarry feces	Access to rat bait	Prolonged clotting time; elevated prothrombin time (PT), partial PT; demonstrate toxin in blood and liver

Source: Straw and Wilson (1985).

that prevent contact with manure and soil. The rapid growth of nursing pigs results in a significant need for supplemental iron to maintain total body iron at normal levels. While hemoglobin is an obvious and easily measured indication of body iron it is important to realize that iron is also necessary in numerous non-heme enzyme systems. Iron is preferentially shunted to hemoglobin formation, so anemia is an endpoint indicator of iron deficiency in the pig. The measurement of serum iron is the preferred method for iron status determination (Smith et al. 1984). Piglets require 100–

300 mg of supplemental iron between birth and the time they begin to consume solid food. Generally, this is supplied through injections of iron dextran or gleptoferran soon after birth. Oral powdered iron or water soluble iron is also effective but may enhance enteric bacterial growth and cannot be administered with the certainty of dosage possible with parenteral injection. Swine diets generally provide iron and other nutrients essential for hematopoiesis; thus, nutritionally induced anemia is uncommon except for the suckling pig.

Clinical Chemistry

INTRODUCTION. Serum biochemistry is not frequently utilized as a clinical diagnostic tool with swine for many of the same reasons that were noted for hematology. However, it is an important part of research investigations. Controlled studies in nutrition, toxicology, pharmacology, and physiology often include biochemical testing as a means of measuring subclinical effects. Reference values are presented in Table 1.4 as a guideline, but it must be noted that biochemical values may be affected by a wide range of factors, including age, sex, season, laboratory, diet, environment, and stress. Therefore, care is needed in the interpretation and clinical application of blood biochemical analyses in swine practice.

INFLUENCING FACTORS

Method of Collection. The site of blood collection can influence certain values. It has been shown that the amount of muscle that lodges in the bore of a needle during jugular venipuncture significantly elevates creatine kinase levels (Bruss and Becker 1981; Dubreuil et al. 1990). The stress of restraint can cause elevated levels of cortisol, adrenocorticotrophic hormone (ACTH), lactate, glucose, hemoglobin, and packed-cell volume (Brenner et al. 1981). When biochemical analysis was performed on blood obtained by an experienced experimenter versus an inexperienced person, 18 of 22 variables examined were significantly different, suggesting that sampling

Table 1.4. Porcine biochemistry reference intervals

Variable	Units	Weaner Pigs	Feeder Pigs	Gilts	Sows
S-Calcium	mmol/L	2.02–3.21	2.16–2.92	2.22–2.91	1.98–2.87
S-Phosphorous	mmol/L	1.46–3.45	2.25–3.44	8.88–2.78	1.49–2.76
S-Urea Nitrogen	mmol/L	2.90–8.89	2.57–8.57	7.70–9.60	2.10–8.50
S-Creatinine	mmol/L	67–172	77–165	106–225	110–260
S-Glucose	mmol/L	3.5–7.4	4.0–8.1	3.0–6.3	2.9–5.9
S-Cholesterol	mmol/L	1.06–3.32	1.37–3.18	1.37–2.70	1.23–2.74
S-Bilirubin	mmol/L	0.9–3.4	0.0–3.4	0.0–3.0	0.0–3.4
S-Conj. Bilirubin	mmol/L	0.9–3.4	0.0–1.7	0.1–1.7	0.0–1.7
S-Free Bilirubin	mmol/L	0.0–3.4	0.0–3.4	0.0–3.4	0.0–3.4
S-Iron	mmol/L	3–38	39–43	11–35	9–34
S-UIBC	mmol/L	43–96	48–101	57–106	54–99
S-AST	U/L	21–94	16–67	12–65	36–272
S-ALT	U/L	8–46	15–46	17–56	19–76
S-Alk. Phos.	U/L	142–891	180–813	115–434	36–272
S-CK	U/L	81–1586	61–1251	89–886	120–10,990
S-Amylase	U/L	528–2616	913–4626	643–4668	432–2170
S-Protein	g/L	44–74	52–83	65–81	65–90
S-Albumin	g/L	19–39	19–42	32–44	31–43
S-A/G	g/g	0.5–2.2	0.4–1.5	0.7–1.5	0.6–1.3
B-GSHPx	U/gHb	30–137	40–141	44–127	48–135

Source: Friendship et al. (1984).
Note: g = gram; U/gHb = units per gram of hemoglobin; L = liter; mmol = millimole; S = serum; U = international unit.

procedure will have a marked influence on the values obtained (Dubreuil et al. 1990).

Hemolysis may interfere with the analyses of creatinine, protein, phosphorus, calcium, potassium, and certain enzymes. It is suggested that if serum is cherry red, the sample should be rejected (Dorner et al. 1983). For biochemical analysis, serum is the preferred blood component. Plasma is unacceptable because anticoagulants such as EDTA will remove some of the ions for which analyses are required and will remove some of the cofactors needed for enzyme action (Tumbleson and Schmidt 1986).

Serum glucose levels fall rapidly after collection if serum remains in contact with red cells. Collection media that inactivates red cell glycolysis is required for accurate assessment. Studies have shown that most parameters measured by biochemical analysis are stable for at least 12 hours at room temperature and 24 hours at 4°C, but not glucose, creatinine, magnesium, potassium, and inorganic phosphorus (Fontaine et al. 1987).

Age. Total serum protein increases with age, whereas the serum phosphorus and cholesterol concentrations and the alkaline phosphatase activity are lower in older pigs (Friendship et al. 1984). At birth piglets experience marked increases in concentration of serum total protein, urea nitrogen, and total bilirubin as well as increased activities of certain enzymes and decreases in serum sodium, chloride, and potassium following colostrum ingestion.

Estrus, Pregnancy, and Lactation. Plasma protein levels are highest at the time of ovulation and lowest at the luteal phase of the cycle. Blood glucose is lowest during the luteal phase and increases rapidly following luteolysis and decreases during the heat period (Tewes et al. 1977).

Serum albumin, total protein, and total bilirubin concentrations are lower in early pregnancy, whereas aspartate aminotransferase (AST) and lactic dehydrogenase (LDH) are higher at this time (Nachreiner and Ginther 1972b). Serum AST and creatine kinase (CK) activities increase immediately after parturition and remain elevated for the next 24 hours. During lactation, Tewes et al. (1979) reported that plasma protein, blood glucose, inorganic phosphorus concentrations, and LDH activity decrease.

SERUM CHEMICAL CHANGES IN RESPONSE TO DISEASE. Total serum proteins, albumin and globulin, reflect synthesis and catabolism, and in swine remain quite stable. Total serum solids are a good estimate of total serum protein levels and are easily measured clinically. Plasma, harvested from a microhematocrit tube, is viewed through a hand-held refractometer. Results are read in g %. In addition, estimates of

fibrinogen can be made. A second previously centrifuged capillary tube is heated to 55°C for 3 minutes. After recentrifugation, the fluid above the precipitated material is evaluated using a refractometer. The difference between plasma serum solids and the heat-precipitated plasma is a rough prediction of fibrinogen levels. Fibrinogen values greater than 500 mg/dL suggest tissue destruction or inflammatory lesions in body cavities.

In a trial comparing the chemical profiles of healthy swine and swine with inflammatory disease, Odink et al. (1990) illustrated a significant difference between the two groups in a number of parameters, including total protein and fibrogen levels, which were both higher in pigs with abscesses and other inflammatory lesions. Other values that were markedly altered by the inflammatory processes were alkaline phosphatase activity and concentrations of iron, phosphorus, and albumin, which were all reduced.

Blood urea nitrogen and serum creatinine as indictors of glomerular function may be elevated with renal damage due to ochratoxin or other nephrotoxic agents. Most renal disease in swine is due to ascending bacterial infection. It is only late in the course of pyelonephritis that sufficient glomerular change results in azotemia.

Serum enzymes can be used as indicators of hepatic or muscle cell damage. Creatine kinase levels elevate rapidly in response to bruising, intramuscular injection, handling trauma, and when the venipuncture needle traverses muscle. While useful in studies on porcine stress syndrome, the diagnostic value of CK elevation is limited in clinical settings. Simplified tests are commercially available as an aid in the detection of carriers of the stress syndrome genotype. Liver enzymes may become elevated as a result of hepatic damage from toxins or inflammation.

The incidence of cystitis in sows increases with age. While pH of swine urine may be acid or alkaline depending on diet, strongly alkaline urine and pyuria indicate cystitis. Pyelonephritis is an important cause of sow mortality and urinalysis is useful in identifying at-risk individuals as well as in assessment of a group.

SERUM CHEMICAL CHANGES IN RESPONSE TO NUTRITIONAL DEFICIENCY. Serum calcium and phosphorus levels are relatively insensitive indicators of skeletal ossification. Osteoporosis commonly occurs in the heavily lactating sow and may culminate in fracture and dislocation. Serum mineral homeostasis is usually maintained during demineralization with serum calcium and phosphorus, offering poor predictive value in either occurrence or extent.

The detection of trace element deficiencies can be facilitated by measuring the activity of dependent enzyme systems. For example, glutathione peroxidase (GSH-Px) (Chavez 1979) and alkaline phosphatase have been used as diagnostic aids in diagnosing selenium and zinc deficiencies respectively. Caution is needed in the interpretation of reduced enzyme activity in that more than one element can influence a particular enzyme system. Low dietary levels of phosphorus have been shown experimentally to cause a reduction in alkaline phosphatase activity in addition to low zinc levels (Boyd et al. 1982).

Serum iron and iron-binding capacity are useful parameters to examine when evaluating an iron supplementation program in that these values reflect an iron deficiency before a reduction in hemoglobin synthesis occurs.

REFERENCES

BERGMANN, V.; GRAFE, A.; AND SPREMBERG, F. 1988. Transportbedingte herz-kreislauf-insuffezrenz and myokardveranderungen beim schwein. Monatsh Veterinaermed 43:472–474.

BOYD, R. D.; HALL, D.; AND WU, J. F. 1982. Plasma alkaline phosphatase as a criterion for determining biologically available phosphorus for swine. J Anim Sci [suppl 1] 55:263.

BRENNER, K. V., AND GURTLER, H. 1981. Westere untersuchungen zur reaktion von schweinen auf eine fixation miltels oberkieferschlinge anhand metabolischer und hamatologischer parameter arch. Exp Vet Med 35:401–407.

BRUSS, M. L., AND BECKER, H. N. 1980. Effect of method of sampling on serum creatine kinase concentrations in swine. Am J Vet Res 42:528–531.

BURKS, M. F.; TUMBLESON, M. E.; KICKLIN, K. W.; HUTCHESON, D. P.; AND MIDDLETON, C. C. 1977. Age and sex related changes of hematological parameters in Sinclair (S-1) miniature swine. Growth 41:51–62.

CHAVEZ, F. R. 1979. The effect of dietary selenium on glutathione peroxidase activity in piglets. Can J Anim Sci 59:67–75.

D'ALLAIRE, S.; DROLET, R.; AND CHAGNON, M. 1990. The causes of sow mortality. A retrospective study. Proc Am Assoc Swine Pract, p. 159–160.

DORNER, J. L.; HOFFMANN, W. E.; AND FILIPOV, M. M. 1983. Effect of in vitro hemolysis on values for certain porcine serum constituents. Vet Clin Pathol 12:15–19.

DUBREUIL, P.; COUTURE, Y.; TREMBLAY, A.; AND MARTINEAU, G. P. 1990. Effects of experimenters and different blood sampling procedures on blood metabolite values in growing pigs. Can J Vet Res 54:379–382.

ELSE, R. W. 1980. Clinico-pathology of some heart diseases in domestic animals. In Scientific Foundations of Veterinary Medicine. London: W. Heinemann Medical Books, pp. 328–349.

ENGELHARDT, W. V. 1966. Swine cardiovascular physiology – a review. In Swine Biomedical Research. Seattle: Frayn, pp. 307–329.

FONTAINE, M.; HAMELIN, N.; AND MARTINEAU, G. P. 1987. Stabilite des parametres sanguins en fonction du temps, des conditions d'entreposage et de transport chez de porc. Med Vet Quebec 17:15–21.

FRIENDSHIP, R. M.; LUMSDEN, J. H.; MCMILLAN, I.; AND WILSON, M. R. 1984. Hematology and biochemistry reference values for Ontario swine. Can J Comp Med 48:390–393.

GARY, C. C. 1989. Diseases of the Cardiovascular System. In Veterinary Medicine. A text book of the Diseases of Cattle, Sheep, Pigs, Goats, and Horses, 7th ed. London: Bailliere Tindall, pp. 299–340.

KANEKO, H.; SAITO, Y.; AND HONJO, A. 1987. Growth and blood properties of primary SPF piglets. Jpn J Swine Sci 24:212–217.

LEE, K.T. 1986. Swine as animal models in cardiovascular research. In Swine in Biomedical Research. New York: Plenum Press, pp. 1481–1496.

LOUDENSLAGER, M. J.; KU, P. K.; WHETTER, P. A.; ULLREY, D. E.; WHITEHAIR, C. K.; STOWE, H. D.; AND MILLER, E. R. 1986. Importance of diet of dam and colostrum to the biological antioxidant status and parenteral iron tolerance of the pig. J Anim Sci 63:1905–1914.

LUMSDEN, J. H., AND MULLEN, K. 1978. On establishing reference values. Can J Comp Med 42:293–301.

McTAGGERT, H. S., AND ROWNTREE, P. G. M. 1969. The hematology of "minimal disease" bacon pigs: A comparison with genetically-related conventionally-reared pigs. Br Vet J 125:240–247.

NACHREINER, R. F., AND GINTHER, O. J. 1972a. Gestational and periparturient periods of sows: Serum chemical and hematological changes during the periparturient period. Am J Vet Res 33:2233–2238.

_____. 1972b. Gestational and periparturient periods of sows: Serum chemical and hematologic changes during gestation. Am J Vet Res 33:2215–2219.

ODINK, J.; SMEETS, J. F. M.; VISSER, I. J. R.; SANDMAN, H.; AND SNIJDERS, J. M. A. 1990. Hematological and clinicochemical profiles of healthy swine and swine with inflammatory processes. J Anim Sci 68:163–170.

PERMAN, V.; CHRISTIANSON, W.; MURPHY, M.; SCHWARTZ, S.; AND RUTH, G. 1989. Hematology for swine practice and its application in a case study. Proc Minn Swine Herd Health Program Conf, pp. 326–365.

POND, W. G., AND HOUPT, K. A. 1978. The Biology of the Pig. Ithaca: Cornell Univ Press, pp. 244–276.

SACK, W. O. 1982. Essentials of Pig Anatomy. Ithaca: Veterinary Textbooks, p. 3, 21.

SANDHOLM, M.; HONKANEN-BUZALSKI, T.; AND RASI, V. 1979. Prevention of navel bleeding in piglets by preparturient administration of ascorbic acid. Vet Rec 104:337–338.

SCHMIDT, D. A. 1986. Swine hematology. In Swine in Biomedical Research. New York: Plenum Press, pp. 767–782.

SMITH, J. E.; MOORE, K.; BOYINGTON, D.; POLLMAN, D. S.; AND SCHONEWEIS, D. 1984. Serum ferritin and total iron-binding capacity to estimate iron storage in pigs. Vet Pathol 21:597–600.

STRAW, B. E., AND WILSON, M. R. 1985. Diagnosis of Swine Diseases. St. Paul: Pig World Inc.

TAYLOR, D. J. 1989. Pig Diseases, 5th ed. Cambridge, Mass.: Burlington Press, pp. 153–163.

TEWES, H.; STEINBACH, J.; AND SMIDT, D. 1977. Investigations on the blood composition of sows during the reproductive cycle. I. Blood changes during the oestrus cycle. Zuchthyg 12:117–124.

_____. 1979. Investigations on the blood composition of sows during the reproductive cycle. III. Blood changes during lactation. Zuchthyg 14:159–164.

TUMBLESON, M. E., AND SCHMIDT, D. A. 1986. Swine clinical chemistry. In Swine in Biomedical Research. New York: Plenum Press, pp. 783–807.

WADE, C. E.; HANNON, J. P.; BOSSONE, C. A.; HUNT, M. M.; AND RODKEY, W. G. 1986. Cardiovascular and hormonal responses of conscious pigs during physical restraint. In Swine in Biomedical Research. New York: Plenum Press, pp. 1395–1404.

2 Digestive System

E. M. Liebler

J. F. Pohlenz

S. C. Whipp

THE ABILITY OF pigs to convert plant material and some animal by-products into high-quality, palatable human food is widely recognized. The initial step in the conversion process involves uptake and digestion of food by the digestive tract. While guaranteeing an efficient absorption and processing of nutrients, fluid, and electrolytes, the digestive tract also has to maintain a protective barrier and prevent uncontrolled passage of macromolecules and infectious agents. Abnormalities in the digestive system frequently cause financial losses through reduced efficiency or, less frequently, death. Further financial losses arise from treatment and prophylaxis against enteric diseases.

This chapter will deal in a general way with pathophysiological mechanisms involved in disease processes. References to other chapters will be essential to an understanding of specific diseases. The reader is also referred to other texts for more complete coverage of the digestive anatomy (Kidder and Manners 1978; Nickel et al. 1979), physiology (Kidder and Manners 1978; Argenzio 1980; Johnson 1987) and special pathology (Moon 1983; Barker and Van Dreumel 1985). The liver and pancreas are part of the digestive system but will not be included in this discussion.

The digestive system should not be considered isolated from other organ systems. It interacts with the nervous system, circulatory system, endocrine system, and immune system. Before discussing anatomy, physiology, and special pathology of different parts of the digestive tract, an overview about these interactions and the function of the gastrointestinal barrier will be given.

CONTROL OF GASTROINTESTINAL FUNCTIONS.

The gastrointestinal tract is a living barrier, adapting its structures and functions to the circumstances to which it is exposed (Levin 1982). The smallest most responsive unit is the enterocyte, a short-lived cell that is constantly shed and renewed. The complex regulatory mechanisms that ensure quick response to changing conditions during the passage of food through the digestive tract have not all been examined in detail in pigs. The general physiological mechanisms of interaction are summarized in Figure 2.1.

Luminal factors influence various parts of the gastric and intestinal wall. Nutrients have trophic effects on enterocytes. Pancreatic secretions and bile are essential for the turnover of enterocytes. Indigenous microflora and nutritional antigens provide a continuous stimulus for the gut-associated immune system.

The central nervous system regulates appetite and food intake. Sensory impulses from the intestinal tract, e.g., distension of the wall by bulky food, are transformed into motor signals for motility by the autonomous nervous system (vagal, sympathetic, and intrinsic innervation). Sympathetic innervation of blood vessels in the submucosa regulates the blood flow. High perfusion of blood vessels in the intestinal wall transports oxygen to enterocytes and provides energy for active transport of nutrients and electrolytes. At the same time removal of nutrients by blood and lymph maintains a diffusion gradient.

Endocrine regulation of the intestinal functions involves, as in neural regulation, both the systemic endocrine system and the enteroendocrine system. Aldosterone, which is regulated over the hypothalamic-hypophyseal-adrenal pathway, controls water reabsorption in the caudal part of the large intestine. Enteroendocrine cells in the intestinal wall transform chemical stimuli into hormonal stimuli by releasing polypeptide hormones into circulation. These hormones bind to receptors on the cytoplasmic membrane of cells and activate protein kinases over adenylate cyclase and thus may lead to a variety of effects on any given target cell. The physiological actions of the most renown enzymes, gastrin, secretin, cholecystokinin, and enteroglucagon, are discussed later.

The regulatory effect of the immune system has been especially studied in infections. T cell–mediated mucus release has been observed following acute parasite infestation. Mediators released by mast cells serve as transmitters for gastrointestinal secretions. The cytokine PGE, a derivate of the arachidonic acid pathway, was reported to have trophic influence on the mucosa.

GASTROINTESTINAL BARRIER.

The gastrointestinal wall maintains a barrier between the environment, consisting of luminal antigens, and the

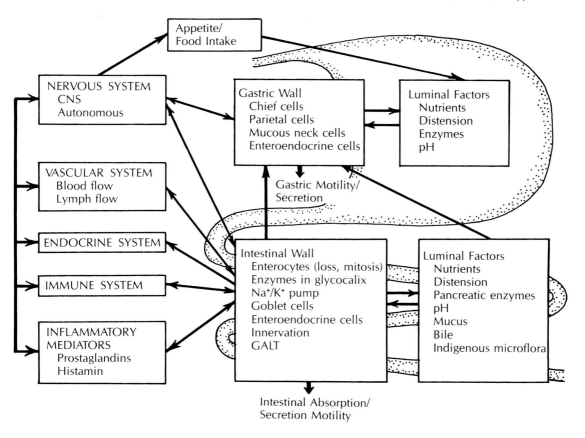

2.1. Factors influencing intestinal function: complex interactions of digestive system with nervous, vascular, endocrine, and immune systems.

host. This barrier includes immunological and nonimmunological elements and can be subdivided into three morphological components (Mouwen et al. 1983): mucous layer, epithelial layer, lymphoid and mononuclear phagocytic system of the mucosa including gut-associated lymphoid system.

Mucus is secreted by goblet cells and is a gel of glycoproteins. It lubricates the mucosal surface, mechanically entraps macromolecules and microorganisms, and passes them along the intestine. Pathogens may be bound by immunoglobulins (IgA and IgM) and digested by enzymes present in the mucous layer. Mucus is also important to maintain the indigenous microflora, which in turn provides protection against attachment of pathogens as will be discussed in more detail later.

The epithelial layer is characterized by enterocytes connected by tight junctions, which are permeable to small ions, but not to macromolecules. Enterocytes are attached to the basement membrane. Macromolecules are digested by the enzymes in the glycocalix and lysosomes of the enterocytes.

The lymphoid and mononuclear phagocytic system of the mucosa can be subdivided into or-

ganized lymphoid aggregates, Peyer's patches (PP) in small intestine and lymphoglandular complexes (LGC) in large intestine; intraepithelial lymphocytes; and leukocytes in the lamina propria (Pabst 1987). In the pig about 20–30 small PP are found in the jejunum and one continuous, long PP in the ileum. The number of LGC in the colon increases from about 500 at birth to 1,500 in adult pigs.

In the epithelium associated with PP and LGC, specialized enterocytes (M cells) can internalize macromolecules and pass them to the underlying lymphoid tissue; thus, they allow contact between luminal antigens and the immune system. They provide potential channels of entrance for pathogens in the epithelial barrier. PP and LGC, which consist of lymphoid follicles and T cell–dependent interfollicular areas, are the sites of initiation for specific humoral and cell-mediated immune responses. IgA precursors from PP lymphoid follicles recirculate and localize in the lamina propria by homing mechanisms. In the lamina propria they mature to IgA-secreting plasma cells under the influence of CD4 + lymphocytes. IgA is selectively transported into the intestinal lumen by enterocytes, where it may protect the mucosal surface by binding antigens. Cytokines released from macrophages and mast cells in the lamina propria may modulate lymphocyte functions besides their regulatory effect on the intestinal wall. Intraepithelial cells are mainly T lymphocytes of the CD8+ subtype. They probably have regulatory functions recognizing and destroying infected epithelial cells and suppressing systemic immune responses to luminal antigens.

ORAL CAVITY. All food ingested has to pass the oral cavity. The oral cavity is lined by a simple stratified squamous epithelium. Predigestion in the oral cavity is facilitated by secretory products of the *salivary glands* (parotis, submandibularis, sublingualis). These glands secrete a mixture of water, mucus, and α-amylase. The enzyme α-amylase breaks down starch into maltose, maltotriose, and dextrins; the mucus lubricates the oral cavity and the esophagus. Chewing and secretory function of the glands in the oral cavity are regulated by central nervous, hormonal, and vagal control. Psychic influences as well as the type of food, e.g., dryness, influence the secretory function. Saliva may also protect against diseases since it contains unspecific factors (lysozyme) and immunoglobulins (especially IgA).

Pigs are omnivorous animals and have a very well developed dentition, which supports the mechanical breakdown of food by grinding. Malformations of teeth as well as incomplete development or lesions of the oral mucosa will impede normal food uptake. Imperfect epitheliogenesis or developmental abnormalities like clefts in lips or palate may impede suckling in newborn animals. If the needle teeth of newborns are clipped too close to the gums, they may shatter and the sharp edges may cause pulpitis, osteomyelitis, gingivitis, cheilitis, and glossitis.

Erosions and ulcerations of the oral mucosa are frequently signs of systemic viral diseases (swine vesicular disease, vesicular stomatitis, vesicular exanthema, foot-and-mouth disease). Clinically these diseases will cause salivation and decreased food intake because of pain. Fast diagnosis is important because some of these diseases are highly contagious and have to be reported. Ulcerative glossitis is found in about one-third of the animals suffering from exudative epidermitis. Differential diagnosis must include lesions caused by exogenous influences, e.g., contact with disinfectants or heated food.

TONSILS. In the porcine species tonsils are concentrated in symmetrical plates at the posterior soft palate. Because of their sentry position at the oropharynx, tonsils are constantly exposed to antigenic stimuli and may serve as entrance for infectious agents. Some bacteria native to the oropharynx may inhabit the tonsils resulting in subclinical carriers, e.g., of *Erysipelothrix rhusiopathiae,* salmonellae, or some groups of strep-

tococci. Primary multiplication of viruses frequently leads to necrosis and lymphoid depletion. For diagnostic purposes, tonsils are collected to detect pseudorabies and hog cholera antigen by immunohistochemistry.

PHARYNX AND ESOPHAGUS. The pharynx and esophagus are infrequently involved in significant disease processes. They are part of the neurally regulated upper digestive system and need to be investigated if nutritive deficiencies or caustic lesions are suspected.

STOMACH. Pigs are monogastric animals. The functions of the stomach are storage and successive release of small portions of ingesta to the intestine, carbohydrate digestion and fermentation, and enzymatic and hydrolytic degradation of proteins as preparation for intestinal digestion and absorption. It is also a barrier (by low pH) to microbial passage into the intestine.

The porcine stomach forms one morphological unit, which is compartmentalized for its different functions by different types of mucosa. These mucosal areas are morphologically distinct and release different secretory products. Although food is mixed in the stomach, layers of distinct pH and specific enzymatic conditions are maintained. The nonglandular, esophageal region, which is covered by squamous epithelium, and the cardiac gland zone together may represent 50% of the stomach. Saliva and cardiac gland secretions maintain a pH above 5 in this compartment; thus permitting a continued activity of salivary α-amylase and bacterial fermentation of carbohydrates. In the fundic and pyloric gland zone, acid is secreted by parietal cells and pepsinogen by chief cells. Pepsin, which is the hydrolytic product of pepsinogen, develops its most potent proteolytic activity at pH 3.5 and lower.

The rate of protein digestion varies depending on types of proteins in the diet. The mucosa of the glandular zone is protected against self-digestion by a thick layer of mucus produced by the mucous neck cells. Bicarbonate secreted by parietal cells is retained in the unstirred layer of mucus, causing a steep pH gradient and preventing damage to the mucosa by pepsin.

Secretory Functions. The secretory functions of the gastric mucosa are regulated by several mechanisms. The most powerful immediate stimulus of acid and fluid secretion is histamine, which is released from mast cells in response to neural, hormonal, and immunological stimuli. After food intake, the first step of secretory stimulation is iniated by the vagus nerve during the cephalic phase. During the gastric phase, food components in the stomach induce the release of gastrin from enteroendocrine cells in the pylorus, resulting in the secretion of fluid and acid. As soon as food passes into the duodenum (intestinal phase), secretin and cholecystokinin are released from enteroendocrine cells in the duodenum and stimulate pepsin secretion in the stomach.

Gastric Functions. Inappropriate diet, inadequate feeding patterns, or abrupt changes in food easily disturb the gastric functions and may cause lesions. The pars esophagea of the stomach is known to be a site of high vulnerability. Ulcers at this site are the most common type of porcine gastric ulceration. One of several factors contributing to their development is feeding of finely ground food, which induces increased secretion and increased mixing of the gastric contents. If the pH gradient between the different gastric compartments is not maintained, the pH in the pars esophagea may drop and cause epithelial damage.

Extremely bulky food given in large portions will distend the stomach and result in the fast release of small portions of stomach contents into the duodenum; thus, the pH will not drop sufficiently to have bactericidal effects. Bacterial overgrowth and multiplication of pathogens in the intestine may result.

Gastric functions of piglets are different from those of adult pigs. During the first hours of life there is no gastric acid production. This allows colostral immunoglobulins and bacteria to pass through the stomach into the intestine. Piglets suckling from sows in a conventional farm environment usually acquire a gastric population of lactobacilli, which produces lactic acid and inhibits the multiplication of other bacteria by lowering the pH. Lactic acid substitutes for as well as suppresses hydrochloric acid secretion until about 3 weeks of age. In early weaned pigs lactobacilli disappear. Until the adult secretory capacity for hydrochloric acid is developed at about 5 weeks of age, bacteria will pass through the stomach into the intestine. Feeding of high-protein diets, which are commonly used for early-weaned pigs, will further postweaning diarrhea by their high buffering capacity.

In vomiting and wasting disease intramural ganglia are altered by infection with a coronavirus. Since neural control of muscular contraction is impeded, ingesta are not transported from stomach to intestine and the stomach becomes distended. Infection with *Hyostrongylus rubidus* may cause mucosal lesions and impair the function of the gastric mucosa. Acute gastric dilatation and volvulus have been observed in adult pigs. Gastric dilatation may occur as a significant cause of death when housed, pregnant sows are fed only once a day.

INTESTINE. The intestine is divided into the small intestine (SI) and large intestine (LI). Each of them consists of three different sections: the duodenum, jejunum, and ileum of the SI and the cecum, colon, and rectum of the LI. The length of the tubelike intestine depends on the age of the animal and the type of food digested; the length increases more rapidly in late gestation and early life than later. Increased development of the large intestine occurs after 3 weeks of life. Common diarrheal diseases of swine grouped by age or dominant clinical signs are summarized in Table 2.1.

Small Intestine. The essential events of digestion and absorption of nutrients take place in the small intestinal mucosa. Microscopically the intestinal wall is composed of three layers: the muscle layer covered by serosa, the submucosa, and the mucosa. The duodenum is characterized by Brunner's glands in the submucosa; the ileum by a continuous Peyer's patch. Typical features of the small intestinal mucosa are tall villi, increasing in length from duodenum to midjejunum. These villi increase the absorptive and digestive capacity of the small intestine.

HISTOLOGY. There are different types of epithelial cells in the intestinal mucosa: mature enteroabsorptive cells, goblet cells, and enteroendocrine cells. They all originate from one type of stem cell in the crypts. Mature cylindrical enterocytes at the surface of the villi are continuously renewed in a turnover process originating from the crypts. With this renewal process older cells are sloughed into the lumen at the tips of the villi. Thus, mature cells in regular arrangement are covering the villi; immature cells in irregular arrangement are in the crypts.

The most important cell of the epithelial barrier is the mature enterocyte on the mucosal surface. Microvilli, which are multiple, long, luminal projections that increase the absorptive surface, are special features of these cells. Most of the cellular digestive enzymes are located in the microvillous glycocalix. The glycocalix also facilitates the adherence of the unstirred layer of mucus to the mucosal surface. The cytoplasm of enteroabsorptive cells is rich in mitochondria and rough endoplasmic reticulum and contains multiple vesicles and lysosomes.

An easily discernible cell is the goblet cell. Large granules of mucus are contained within these cells, which are more frequent in crypts than on villi. The number of goblet cells present in the mucosa varies depending on type of food, age of animal, and area of gut. The mucus secreted by goblet cells is part of the intestinal barrier system. Mucus covers the epithelial layer and protects against adhesion of pathogenic microorganisms.

Within the crypts there are enteroendocrine granulated cells, which release hormones that contribute to the regulatory processes of the renewal system. Currently there are more than 12 different intestinal hormones known to be involved in intestinal endocrine processes called the

Table 2.1. Differential diagnosis of some enteric diseases of swine

Cause	Age	Diarrhea	Gross Lesions	Microlesions	Diagnosis
Escherichia coli (ETEC, EPEC, edema disease, depending on age)	1 day to post-weaning	Watery, white or yellow	Fluid ingesta, white lacteals	None	Culture: interpretation difficult, eliminate other causes
Coronaviruses (TGE-virus, EVD-virus, CV777)	1 day to adult	Watery[a]	Thin-walled SI, clear lacteals	Marked villous atrophy	FAT: of frozen sections, direct electron microscopy; culture: high populations
Rotavirus, pararotavirus	1 day to post-weaning	Variable, watery to pasty	Fluid ingesta, variable lacteals	Moderate villous atrophy	FAT: of frozen sections, direct electron microscopy; culture: high populations
Isospora suis	5–15 days (sometimes older)	Watery, white or yellow	Fluid ingesta, areas of fibrin in SI	Fibrinonecrotic, variable severity	Stained mucosal smear: identify coccidia; histopathology: identify coccidia
Clostridium perfringens	1–14 days (rarely older)	Bloodstained	Necrohemorrhagic with gas bubbles	Mucosal necrosis, hemorrhage	Stained mucosal smear: gram-positive rods, histopathology; culture: interpretation difficult
Serpulina hyodysenteriae	7 days to adult	Mucohemorrhagic	Mucohemorrhagic, diffuse only in LI	Diffuse, mucosal swelling and erosion	Culture, stained smear: presumptive only; darkfield smear: presumptive only
Salmonella spp.	Postweaning (rarely preweaning)	Mucohemorrhagic-variable	Mucohemorrhagic, SI or LI systemic lesions	Diffuse or focal with ulcers and neutrophils, systemic lesions	Culture
Trichuris suis	Postweaning	Mucohemorrhagic	Mucohemorrhagic, diffuse, only in LI	Diffuse, mucosal swelling and erosion	Gross lesions: observe parasites
Campylobacter-related enteritis	Postweaning	Watery, mucohemorrhagic, dark blood	Mucosal hyperplasia, variable hemorrhage, SI or LI	Mucosal hyperplasia, silver stain of *Campylobacter*	Histopathology, stained sections: identify *Campylobacter*

Note: ETEC = enterotoxigenic *E. coli;* EPEC = enteropathogenic *E. coli;* EVD = epizootic viral diarrhea; FAT = fluorescent antibody technique; LI = large intestine; SI = small intestine; TGE = transmissible gastroenteritis.
[a]Usually vomiting also.

amine precursor uptake and decarboxylation (APUD) system (Grube 1986). Porcine enteroglucagon is one of the most important hormones involved in cellular turnover (Bloom and Polak 1982). Other regulatory mechanisms result from immunologically related reactions such as degranulation of mucosal mast cells, attraction of eosinophils, and migration and infiltration of intraepithelial lymphocytes.

DIGESTION

Carbohydrates. Carbohydrates are predominantly degraded by small intestinal digestion. Luminal digestion is mediated by disaccharidases secreted from the exocrine pancreas. At least six different enzymes for carbohydrate digestion are located in the glycocalix of mature absorptive cells. In newborn piglets enzyme activities for lactose digestion are higher in the upper small intestine than in the ileum. During the first 4 weeks of life, lactase activity decreases continuously to less than one-half the value. By 8 weeks of life, lactase activity in the small intestine is not at all detectable. In contrast sucrase activity does not develop before the first week of life. Its activity is continuously increasing; thus, piglets fed with an undigestible sugar will not be able to digest their diet and will develop diarrhea.

Digestion of cellulose does not occur in the small intestine. It depends on bacterial fermentation, which occurs in large intestine only. Hemicellulose is in part predigested in the stomach.

Protein. Protein digestion is initiated in the stomach where proteins are broken down to large peptides. Ingesta entering the small intestine are mixed with duodenal and pancreatic secretions to raise the pH. In contrast to pepsin, pancreatic and brush border–associated peptidases are activated at neutral pH. Intestinal protein digestion depends on the availability of pancreatic juice containing endopeptidases and carboxypeptidases, and aminopeptidases associated with the brush border or contained in the cytoplasm of mature enteroabsorptive cells.

Fat. Digestion of fat is mediated predominantly by pancreatic lipase and colipase. For absorption, micellar dispersion, which depends on a neutral pH and the presence of bile salts, is necessary.

Fluids. All absorptive and digestive processes occur in a fluid phase of ingesta. Fluids are secreted by crypt cells into the lumen and absorbed by enterocytes on the villi; fluid movement is continuous from the lumen to the vascular system. Most of the fluid transport in the small intestine is carried out by passive diffusion across the epithelial membrane and the vascular wall through pores, following the pressure gradient of colloidosmotic pressure versus hydrostatic pressure. Little fluid is actively transported via epithelial cells. In the neonate, fluid and electrolytes are predominantly absorbed in the small intestine, while very little absorption occurs in the large intestine.

PATHOPHYSIOLOGY. Malfunction of intestinal mucosa results in intestinal diseases, most of which are associated with diarrhea (Argenzio and Whipp 1980; Moon 1983; Barker and Van Dreumel 1985). Diarrhea is a condition in which soft, sometimes watery feces are passed more frequently than normal. Feces also may contain increased amounts of fat, mucus, fibrin, or blood clots, all of which indicate different types of mucosal lesions. Diarrhea may be related to enteritis or it may be a consequence of dysfunction of the intestinal secretory system. In both conditions loss of fluids will cause dehydration. Fluid transport and digestion may be disturbed by several mechanisms.

Enterotoxigenic strains of *E. coli* (ETEC) adhere to the epithelial surface. Toxins released from *E. coli* into the gut lumen will activate the adenylate cyclase system and increase fluid secretion up to 10-fold. The fluids passing from the small intestine into the colon will exceed its absorption capacity especially in the neonate, and diarrhea results. In this case there is no primary inflammatory lesion in the intestinal wall present.

Enteropathogenic strains of *E. coli* (EPEC) and *Cryptosporidium* sp. will settle within the microvillous brush border and release toxic substances and/or induce immunologically related reactions. In EPEC infection a shigella-like syndrome occurs. In cryptosporidiosis digestive functions are decreased since the brush border of epithelial cells is destroyed. Along with cellular destruction, the length of villi is reduced. Crypts are activated to replace cells lost at the surface. Immunologically induced release of mediator substances will stimulate secretory function; thus, secretion exceeds villous absorption capacity and increased amounts of fluid and undigested nutrients are passed into the colon.

Several viruses, coronaviruses (transmissible gastroenteritis, epizootic viral diarrhea of pigs), pararotavirus, rotavirus, and adenovirus, have a tropism for enterocytes. Predominantly mature epithelial cells of villi are destroyed resulting in villus atrophy and crypt hyperplasia. Decreased digestion and absorption cause maldigestion and malabsorption. Undigested hygroscopic substances in small intestinal ingesta will draw fluids into the small intestinal lumen. When transported into the large intestine, partly digested or undigested ingesta will contribute to osmotic diarrhea.

There is some evidence that combined infections with viruses, *E. coli* and *Cryptosporidium* sp., are frequent. Not much is known about the significance of the individual pathogens in combined infections. Infection with *Cryptosporidium* sp., which is generally a self-limiting disease will aggravate a mild rotavirus infection and result in loss of animals. Pathogenetic mechanisms may involve suppression of the immune system, for immunosuppressive conditions are known to promote cryptosporidiosis.

In some bacterial diseases (e.g., clostridiosis) cytotoxins destroy the surface epithelium, the basement membrane, and stromal tissue resulting in severe necrosis. Hemorrhagic enteritis causes the peracute death of piglets.

In infections with *Isospora suis,* different developmental stages of coccidia destroy the epithelial cells on villi, and necrotic cells are sloughed into the intestinal lumen. Transudation from capillaries immediately contributes to fluid loss and along with inflammatory response exudation results. Fibrinous enteritis is a common reaction to both isospora infection and acute clostridiosis.

Campylobacter spp. infect the epithelium and replicate in crypt cells. Goblet cells disappear in these areas and crypt cells are converted to a population of highly mitotic cells. Coagulation necrosis of the affected mucosa by anaerobic large bowel flora may result in necrotic enteritis.

Salmonellosis often is a systemic disease that may affect liver and lung as well as the small and large intestine. Enteric lesions vary from catarrhal to fibrinous or hemorrhagic. Pathogenetic mechanisms are discussed under Large Intestine.

Large Intestine. The main functions of the large intestine are absorption of fluids and electrolytes and digestion by microbial fermentation. Resection experiments demonstrated, however, that pigs without a large intestine can survive and have only modest growth retardation (Wilkinson and McCane 1971). In case of small intestinal infections and malfunctions, the large intestine is a functional reserve and will frequently be able to compensate and mask the effects.

The large intestine of adult pigs is between 3.5 and 6 m in length depending on the type of diet. The capacity of the colon in adult pigs is similar to the small intestine although it is only 25% of its length. The largest part, the colon ascendens, is wound up as a double coil. The cecum and part of the colon ascendens are easy to distinguish from the small intestine by their longitudinal taeniae. The internal surface is enhanced by permanent folds. Numerous lymphoid follicles are seen as white flat nodules in the intestinal wall. They are concentrated at the central flexure of the colon ascendens and in the colon descendens.

HISTOLOGY. Histologically, large intestinal mucosa is characterized by the absence of villi and the presence of long straight glands. This appears to be a functional adaptation since villi or remnants of villi are found in fetal and neonatal pigs only. Goblet cells are more numerous than in the small intestine. The epithelial turnover rate of colonic mucosa is 4–8 days, which is slower than that of small intestinal mucosa.

Morphological adaptations of the epithelium to its specific functions can be observed. Junctional complexes between enterocytes consist of several highly intermeshed strands, making the paracellular pathway rather impermeable to solutes, and rediffusion into the intestinal lumen is inhibited. This allows absorption of electrolytes from hypoosmolar fluids in large intestine. Microvilli of colonic enterocytes are fewer, less regular, and do not contain digestive enzymes as found in the brush border and glycocalix of small intestinal enterocytes.

ABSORPTION. Since microorganisms necessary for fermentative processing of digesta require a highly buffered fluid environment, the colon of a pig is presented with large fluid volumes. Within the first one-third of the colon, the dry matter of digesta increases from 13% to 20% and within the remaining two-thirds up to 25%. The colon has a reserve capacity of three to four times the amount of fluid that it is presented with.

Absorption of water is a passive process that follows active electrolyte transport. The colonic epithelium absorbs Na^+ and Cl^- ions and secretes K^+ and $HCO3^-$. The mechanisms of electrolyte transport are different in proximal and distal colon. In the proximal colon, electrically neutral Na^+ and Cl^- absorption occurs either by NaCl cotransport or Na^+/H^+ and $Cl^-/HCO3^-$ countertransport. It is predominantly regulated by the local nervous and paracrine system, especially vasointestinal peptide and enteroglucagon. In the distal colon electrogenic transport, regulated by aldosterone concentration in peripheral blood, takes place. The efficiency of Na^+ uptake by the luminal membrane is dependent on the luminal concentration being more efficient at low Na^+ concentrations. Na^+ is shifted from the enterocytes to the intercellular spaces by Na^+/K^+ ATPase pumps in the basolateral cell membranes. This creates an osmotic pressure gradient within the enterocyte. Passive movement of water depends on the "leakiness" of the epithelium and especially of the type and condition of tight junctions. As mentioned before, the colonic epithelium is very tight, restricting the passive movements of water and water soluble substances; therefore, absorption of electrolytes against an osmolar gradient is possible. Alterations of junctional complexes by pathogens will increase the leakiness.

DIGESTION. The porcine colon also has a digestive function based on bacterial fermentation. If a diet containing carbohydrates of low digestibility is fed or alterations of the small intestine result in maldigestion, significant amounts of carbohydrates may reach the colon. The colon is the only place in the pig where digestion of cellulose is possible. The digestibility of crude fiber in the diet increases with age and is influenced by the presence of easily accessible alternative carbohydrates. Carbohydrates and cellulose are converted to volatile fatty acids, acetic acid, propionic acid, and butyric acid. The relative proportions of volatile fatty acids are influenced by the diet; they are, however, similar in the cecum and along the whole large intestine. The colonic mucosa has a high transport capacity for volatile fatty acids, the rate of which is dependent on the colonic pH.

Proteins and amino acids that reach the colon may be deaminated by bacteria; the absorbed dietary nitrogen is lost with the urine. Application of oral antibiotics may suppress deamination by bacteria and thereby reduce the loss of dietary nitrogens. The nutritional use or fate of the microbial proteins of the colonic indigenous microflora are unknown. No digestion of fat occurs in the large intestine; however, long-chain fatty acids may be converted into unhydrated fatty acids, and depending on their concentration may play a role in the pathogenesis of diarrhea.

INDIGENOUS MICROFLORA. The indigenous microflora of the intestine has several functions besides fermentation (Hirsh et al. 1980). It has a trophic effect on the epithelium and causes a faster turnover rate. It also provides a continuous stimulus to the local lymphoid tissue and protects against pathogenic bacterial species, which have to compete with the indigenous microflora for nutrition. Metabolic by-products of the indigenous microflora create an environment most favorable for the pathogenic bacteria. The action of most of the pathogens is dependent on binding to enterocytes. As the microflora occupies these binding sites, target cells are unavailable. Alterations of the indigenous microflora, e.g., by fasting or rapid change of diet or oral antibiotics, may allow opportunistic pathogenic bacteria to proliferate.

PATHOPHYSIOLOGY. Malfunctions are recognized clinically as diarrhea, which may be caused by alterations and dysfunction of the small intestine, the large intestine, or both.

Infections with ETEC in the small intestine cause high amounts of fluid secretion. Colonic mucosa has a reserve capacity and can absorb about three to four times the amount of fluid presented under normal conditions. If this reserve capacity is exceeded, diarrhea will result. Currently, it is discussed whether certain strains of *E. coli* can also induce secretion in the colon by activating the colonic cyclic adenosine monophosphate (cAMP) and cyclic guanidine monophosphate. In the proximal colon, activation of these systems leads to the loss of neutral Na^+ absorption and to the stimulation of electrogenic Cl^- secretion. In the distal colon, Na^+ absorption is unaffected by cAMP; however, Cl^- secretion is induced. Therefore, the colon may augment these bacterial diarrheas.

In small bowel diseases (viral infections or cryptosporidiosis), which cause maldigestion and malabsorption, an increased amount of fluid with a high concentration of carbohydrates and, therefore, high osmotic pressure will reach the colon. The colon may compensate for some of the small intestinal maldigestion by bacterial fermentation. In neonatal pigs in which the indigenous microflora are not well developed, lactose cannot be fermented in the colon but will cause additional fluid loss into the large intestine by high osmotic pressure. If the amount of carbohydrates in the large intestine is very high, bacterial fermentation exceeds the bicarbonate buffering system and volatile fatty acid transport capacity, resulting in acidification of the contents. The decreased pH may damage the mucosa directly or alter the microflora, leading to a predominant growth of lactobacilli and lactic acid production. This may affect the fluid reabsorption in two ways. Since volatile fatty acids are responsible for concurrent water transport, their reduced production will lead to decreased water absorption. Lactic acid in contrast to other volatile fatty acids is absorbed at a lower rate and increases the intraluminal osmotic load, thereby causing osmotic secretion.

Lesions in the ileum may lead to decreased reabsorption of bile salts. Bile salts converted by the microflora to secondary bile acids and long-chain fatty acids of incomplete fat digestion may alter mucosal permeability and damage the mucosal epithelium. They both stimulate cAMP-mediated secretion most likely by release of prostaglandins, and cause net fluid secretion.

Infectious agents may damage colonic epithelium. They usually cause diarrhea in animals of 3 weeks and older, when the colon is functionally developed. *Cryptosporidia* spp. attach to the superficial surface and reduce the absorptive capacity. *Campylobacter* spp. and *Serpulina hyodysenteriae* infect the epithelium but do not enter further. They invade epithelial cells, especially goblet cells, and cause erosions that increase the turnover rate. Functionally they interfere with fluid and electrolyte absorption. *Serpulina hyodysenteriae* also causes hypersecretion of mucus. The parasite *Trichuris suis* has a similar effect. In salmonellosis, lesions vary depending on the strain of bacteria and the infectious dose. In *Salmonella typhimurium* infection, lesions are mainly confined to the cecum, colon, and rectum. Bacteria invade beneath the epithelial layer into the deeper layers of the intestinal wall and cause a pronounced inflammatory response. Inflammatory reactions will release mediators, which might in turn provoke diarrhea. Mediators may be derived from the arachidonic acid cascade, e.g., prostaglandins and leucotrienes; or from inflammatory cells, e.g., mast cells or neutrophils. In chronic infections, button ulcers as seen in hog cholera may occur. *Salmonella typhimurium* also causes vascular thrombosis, which may result in rectal stricture.

REFERENCES

ARGENZIO, R. A. 1980. Comparative physiology of the gastrointestinal system. In Veterinary Gastroenterology. Ed. N. V. Anderson. Philadelphia: Lea & Febiger, pp. 172–198.

ARGENZIO, R. A., AND WHIPP, S. C. 1980. Pathophysiology of diarrhea. In Veterinary Gastroenterology. Ed. N. V. Anderson. Philadelphia: Lea & Febiger, pp. 220–232.

BARKER, I. K., AND VAN DREUMEL, A. A. 1985. The alimentary system. In Pathology of Domestic Animals, 3d ed., vol. 2. Ed. K. V. F. Jubb, P. C. Kennedy, and N. Palmer. Orlando: Academic Press, pp. 2–239.

BLOOM, S. R., AND POLAK, J. M. 1982. The hormonal pattern of intestinal adaptation. A major role of enteroglucagon. Scan J Gastroenterol [Suppl 74] 17:93–103.

GRUBE, D. 1986. The endocrine cells of the digestive system: Amines, peptides, and mode of action. Anat Embryol 175:151–161.

HIRSH, D. C. 1980. Microflora, mucosa, and immunity. In Veterinary Gastroenterology. Ed. N. V. Anderson. Philadelphia: Lea & Febiger, pp. 199–219.

JOHNSON, L. R., ed. 1987. Physiology of the gastrointestinal tract, 2d ed. New York: Raven Press.

KIDDER, D. E., AND MANNERS, M. J. 1978. Digestion in the pig. Bath, Engl.: Kingston Press.

LEVIN, R. J. 1982. Assessing intestinal function in health and disease in vivo and in vitro. Scan J Gastroenterol [Suppl 74] 17:31–53.

MOON, H. W. 1983. Intestine. In Cell Pathology. 2d ed. Ed. N. F. Cheville. Ames: Iowa State Univ Press, pp. 503–529.

MOUWEN, J. M. V. M.; EGBERTS, H. J. A.; AND KONINKX, J. F. J. G. 1983. The outermost barrier of the mammalian small intestine. Dtsch Tieraerztl Wochenschr 90:477–482.

NICKEL, R.; SCHUMMER, A; AND SEIFERLE, E. 1979. The Viscera of the Domestic Mammals, 2d ed. Berlin and Hamburg: Verlag Paul Parey.

PABST, R. 1987. The anatomical basis for the immune function of the gut. Anat Embryol 176:135–144.

WILKINSON, A. W., AND McCANE, R. A. 1971. The subsequent effects of removing large intestine from newborn pigs. Proc Nutr Soc 30:26A.

3 Immune System

J. A. Roth

THE IMMUNE SYSTEM comprises a variety of components that cooperate to defend the host against infectious agents. These components generally can be divided into nonspecific (or native) immune defense mechanisms and specific (or acquired) immune defense mechanisms. The nonspecific defense mechanisms are not antigen specific. They are present in a normal animal without previous exposure to antigen, and they are capable of responding almost immediately to an infectious agent. The major components of the nonspecific immune system are complement, phagocytic cells (macrophages, neutrophils, and eosinophils), natural killer (NK) cells, and some types of interferon. These components are very important in controlling an infection during the first few days of an initial exposure to an agent, when the specific immune response system is gearing up to produce antibody and a cell-mediated immune response.

B and T lymphocytes and their products are the components of the specific immune response system. This antigen-driven system requires 2–3 weeks to reach optimal functional capacity after the first exposure to antigen. Upon second exposure to antigen, the specific immune response system reaches optimal activity much more rapidly due to the anamnestic, or memory, response. A major mechanism by which B and T lymphocytes enhance resistance to disease is by activating the nonspecific defense mechanisms (phagocytic cells, NK cells, and complement) to be more efficient. The immune response in mammals has been shown to be influenced by genes in the major histocompatibility complex. Immunogenetics and the major histocompatibility complex of the pig are discussed in Chapter 56 of this book.

Providing immunity at mucosal surfaces and to newborn piglets are especially difficult challenges for the immune system and for the swine producer. The nature of these special problems will be discussed as well as generalities about vaccination to improve immunity at mucosal surfaces and in newborn pigs.

If an animal is immunosuppressed due to stress, preexisting viral infection, immunotoxicants, or nutritional factors, the nonspecific defense mechanisms may not be functioning optimally. In addition, the specific immune response may be slow to develop or inadequate, which can result in clinical disease due to an infectious agent that would otherwise be controlled by a nonimpaired immune system.

The immune system has potent mechanisms for protecting the pig from infectious and neoplastic diseases. If the immune system is overstimulated or is not appropriately regulated, it may cause hypersensitivity reactions in response to infection, vaccination, environmental or dietary antigens, or even against normal host tissues.

PHYSIOLOGY OF THE IMMUNE SYSTEM

Native Defense Mechanisms

PHYSICAL, CHEMICAL, AND MICROBIAL BARRIERS. Physical, chemical, and microbial barriers to infection at body surfaces are a very important part of resistance to disease. These factors include squamous epithelium, bactericidal fatty acids, normal flora, the mucous layer and the flow of mucus, low pH, bile, and numerous enzymes. More detailed information on these barriers to infection can be found in chapters dealing with specific organ systems.

COMPLEMENT. The complement system is an enzyme cascade system similar to the coagulation system and is composed of at least 20 serum proteins. In a cascade system something activates the first component, which in turn activates the next component which in turn activates the next component, etc., until the reaction is completed. The components of the mammalian complement system can be divided into different groups: classical pathway, alternative pathway, membrane attack pathway, and regulatory proteins. All nine components of the classical and membrane attack pathways have been individually titrated in swine sera (Barta and Hubbert 1978). The complement system is very important in mediating the inflammatory response and controlling bacterial infection. It also plays a prominent role in many types of allergies and hypersensitivity diseases. The classical pathway is triggered primarily by antigen antibody complexes (IgG and IgM); the alternative pathway may also be activated by antigen antibody complexes (IgA and IgE) and by certain bacterial products, such as endotoxin, and by proteases released by damaged tissue. Both the classical and alternative pathways end in the splitting of the third component of complement (C3) and start the formation of the membrane attack complex.

The complement system has many important biologic activities. Activation of either complement pathway causes vasodilation and increased vascular permeability, resulting in serum components (including antibody and complement) entering the tissues to help control infection. Complement components produced during activation are chemotactic and attract phagocytic cells to the site of infection; they also coat infectious agents so they can be more easily phagocytized. A very important function of the membrane attack pathway of complement is the destruction of cell membranes including some bacterial cell membranes.

The complement system is important for mediating inflammation and controlling bacterial infection. However, since it is so potent it is also capable of causing serious and even life-threatening damage if it is activated in an unregulated fashion. Therefore, numerous regulators of complement, which help to control and stop the complement reaction once it has started, are present in the serum.

PHAGOCYTIC CELLS. Phagocytic cells are responsible for engulfing, killing, and digesting invading bacteria. They also play an important role in controlling viral and fungal infections and in killing cancer cells. There are two main types of phagocytic cells: granulocytes, or polymorphonuclear leukocytes, which include the neutrophils and the eosinophils; and the mononuclear phagocytes, which include the circulating monocytes in the blood and the tissue macrophages. All these cell types are phagocytic and are capable of all the reactions described below for neutrophils. In addition, macrophages play a very important role in processing antigens and presenting them to lymphocytes to initiate and facilitate the cell-mediated and humoral immune responses.

Granulocytes. Neutrophils are produced in the bone marrow and are released into the blood. The half-life of neutrophils in the bloodstream is approximately 8 hours; they then enter the tissues. In healthy individuals the neutrophils are lost primarily into the intestinal tract and lung. Neutrophils migrate into the intestinal tract very rapidly in response to *E. coli* infection in the pig (Sellwood et al. 1986). Neutrophils in the circulation tend to marginate in the capillaries by loosely associating with the endothelial cells. In swine, neutrophils seem to have a high affinity for margination in the capillaries of the lung (Ohgami et al. 1989).

The principal function of neutrophils is to phagocytose and destroy invading microorganisms. Neutrophils are well-equipped with several mechanisms to perform this function. To be effec-

tive, neutrophils must first come into the vicinity of the invading microorganism by the chemotactic attraction to the site. Chemotactic factors may be produced directly by certain microorganisms, generated by the cleavage of certain complement components, or released by sensitized lymphocytes at the site of infection or inflammation. Chemotactic factors will diffuse away from the site to form a gradient, and when they reach a capillary, they cause the endothelial cell membrane and the neutrophil membrane to increase the expression of adhesion proteins. Neutrophils then adhere to the endothelial cells and leave the capillary by diapedesis. Once in the tissues, the neutrophils migrate along the chemotactic factor gradient toward the source of the chemotactic factor and thus arrive at the site of infection; they may begin to ingest the microorganisms if those agents are susceptible to phagocytic activity. Most pathogenic microorganisms must be opsonized before they can be ingested; bacteria are opsonized by the attachment of specific antibody and/or complement to their surface. The opsonization process facilitates ingestion. When a neutrophil comes into contact with an opsonized particle, it attempts to surround the particle with pseudopodia and ingests it by phagocytosis. The ingested particle will be within a membrane-bound vesicle called a phagosome.

The neutrophil cytoplasm contains two main types of membrane-bound lysosomes or granules: primary (or azurophilic) granules and secondary (or specific) granules. These lysosomes contain numerous hydrolytic enzymes and other substances that are important to the bactericidal activity of the neutrophil. After a particle is ingested and is inside a phagosome, the neutrophil "degranulates"; some of the lysosomes will fuse with the phagosome and release their contents into the phagosome with the ingested particle. Hydrolytic enzymes function under both aerobic or anaerobic conditions in an attempt to destroy the ingested microorganisms. Neutrophils die after a short time at sites of inflammation. Hydrolytic enzymes are released and contribute to the inflammatory response and tissue destruction.

In addition to having hydrolytic enzymes in its granules, the neutrophil has potent bactericidal mechanisms that can function under aerobic conditions only. These mechanisms are related to the oxidative metabolism of the neutrophil. When a neutrophil is stimulated by an opsonized particle, oxygen usage increases rapidly. This burst of oxidative metabolism results in the production of some highly reactive short-lived oxygen species, specifically hydrogen peroxide (H_2O_2), superoxide anion (O_2^-), the hydroxyl radical (OH^-), and perhaps singlet oxygen ($^1O_2$). All of these components can damage microbial organisms. The H_2O_2 formed after phagocytosis may also react with halide ions in a reaction catalyzed by a myeloperoxidase enzyme that is released from the primary granules. This reaction is one of the most potent bactericidal mechanisms of the neutrophil and is also potentially fungicidal and virucidal.

In addition to its important role in the phagocytosis and destruction of pathogenic bacteria, the neutrophil may also be important in controlling certain viral infections via a mechanism referred to as antibody-dependent cell-mediated cytotoxicity. As the name implies, this mechanism requires antibody, which presumably forms a bridge between the neutrophil and the virus-infected target cell. The neutrophil will then attempt to destroy the target cell. The mechanism of this cell destruction is not known but is thought to involve a direct membrane-to-membrane interaction. Porcine neutrophils have a high level of antibody-dependent cell-mediated cytotoxicity, even in the fetus and newborn (Zarkower et al. 1982; Yang and Schultz 1986). They are the only cell type capable of antibody-dependent cell-mediated cytotoxicity against African swine fever virus (Norley and Wardley 1983b).

Neutrophils therefore undergo several steps in attempting to control invading microorganisms: (1) adherence to vascular epithelium and exit from blood vessels via diapedesis, (2) random and directed migration along a chemotactic gradient, (3) the engulfment of opsonized microorganisms, (4) degranulation, (5) generation of oxygen-free radicals and H_2O_2, (6) myeloperoxidase-catalyzed reaction, and (7) antibody-dependent cell-mediated cytotoxicity. Assays can be conducted for each of these processes. If any of these processes are impaired in the neutrophil, one would expect that the neutrophil would not be able to perform its function of controlling microbial infection as efficiently, which would make the animal more susceptible to microbial infection. Depression of neutrophil function has been associated with increased susceptibility to experimentally induced *E. coli* mastitis in sows (Lofstedt et al. 1983).

The eosinophil is capable of the same phagocytic and metabolic functions as the neutrophil, but to a different extent. The eosinophil is not as active as the neutrophil in destroying bacteria but is important in the host's defense against the tissue phase of certain parasitic infections. The eosinophil is geared more toward exocytosis than phagocytosis; that is, rather than ingesting and killing small particles like bacteria, it can efficiently attach to and kill migrating parasites that are too large to be ingested. Eosinophils are also important in helping to control certain types of allergic responses.

Mononuclear Phagocytes. Mononuclear phagocytes comprise circulating monocytes, fixed macrophages, and wandering macrophages (histiocytes). Monocytes are produced in the bone marrow and released into the blood stream where they circulate before migrating into tissues to become macrophages. Fixed macrophages are found lining the endothelium of capillaries and sinuses of organs such as the spleen, bone marrow, and lymph nodes. Fixed macrophages are important for trapping and removing foreign antigens from the blood stream and lymph. Wandering macrophages are derived from blood monocytes and are found throughout the tissues of the body. In certain locations, they differentiate into specialized types of macrophages such as the glial cells in the nervous system, Langerhans cells in the skin, and Kupffer cells in the liver.

Macrophages are capable of all the activities described above for neutrophils. Macrophages are said to be the second line of defense but are slower to arrive at sites of inflammation and are not as aggressive as neutrophils in the first few minutes of contact with microorganisms. However, macrophages are capable of much more sustained activity against pathogens than are neutrophils, and thus are able to kill certain types of bacteria that are resistent to killing by neutrophils. This is especially true if the macrophages have been activated by lymphokines secreted by T lymphocytes.

A very important function of macrophages is the processing of antigen and presentation of antigen to T lymphocytes. This is an essential step in the initiation of a cell-mediated immune response and for facilitating an efficient antibody response by B lymphocytes. The interaction of macrophages with antigen and T and B lymphocytes is described below.

NATURAL KILLER CELLS. Natural killer (NK) cells are lymphoid cells capable of "natural" cytotoxicity; that is they can kill a variety of nucleated cells without previous antigenic stimulation. They are part of the native immune system and can kill some (but not all) tumor cells and some (but not all) virus-infected cells. NK cells in most species are also called large granular lymphocytes because of the presence of granules in their cytoplasm. NK cells in most species are part of the null cell population because they are distinct from B cells, T cells, and macrophages. In most species, NK cells have Fc receptors for IgG and can mediate antibody-dependent cell-mediated cytotoxicity (ADCC) against most antibody-coated mammalian cells. When mediating ADCC these cells have been called killer (K) cells.

Natural killer cells in the pig differ markedly from NK cells found in other species. NK activity in swine is mediated by small granular lymphocytes that have the cluster of differentiation (CD)2 T-cell marker (Ferguson et al. 1986; Duncan et al. 1989) and are, therefore, not null cells (Duncan et al. 1989). Swine NK cells initiate the lytic process against typical target cells (YAC-1 lymphoma or K-562 myeloid leukemia cells) more slowly than cells responsible for NK activity in other species (Ferguson et al. 1986). In swine there is evidence that the NK-cell activity and the K-cell activity are from two distinct populations of lymphocytes (Kim and Ichimura 1986; Yang and Schultz 1986).

The activity of NK cells in many species is increased in the presence of gamma interferon and interleukin-2. Swine NK cells have been shown to respond to an interferon inducer (poly I:C) with enhanced NK activity (Lesnick and Derbyshire 1988). Therefore, NK cells are an important part of the native defense mechanisms and also participate in a cell-mediated immune response by enhanced activity through lymphokine activation.

Humoral and Cell-mediated Immunity

CLONAL SELECTION AND EXPANSION. An important concept that is basic to understanding the immune response is the clonal selection process. Each mature T or B lymphocyte in the body is capable of recognizing only one specific antigen. All of the lymphocytes that recognize exactly the same antigen make up a "clone," all of which arise from the same ancestor cell. There are millions of clones of T and B lymphocytes; each clone may contain from a few hundred to a few million cells. The lymphocytes are in a resting stage as they circulate through blood, enter the lymph nodes through the postcapillary venules, percolate through the lymph nodes, and reenter the bloodstream. In the lymph nodes (or other secondary lymphatic tissues), lymphocytes come in contact with antigens that arrive through the afferent lymphatics and are trapped by macrophages. Each lymphocyte can respond only to the one specific antigen that it can recognize through its antigen receptors. Therefore, the vast majority of lymphocytes that contact an antigen in the lymph node cannot respond to it. In an animal that never has been exposed to a particular infectious agent before, there are relatively few lymphocytes in each clone that can recognize a particular antigen. The first step, therefore, in producing an effective primary immune response is to expand the clone of lymphocytes that recognize the antigen. The T and B lymphocytes that contact the antigen are stimulated to undergo a series of cell divisions so that within a few days there will be enough lymphocytes in the clone to mount an effective humoral and/or cell-mediated immune response. If the animal has been exposed to the antigen previously, the clone of lymphocytes has already been expanded, so not nearly as many cycles of cell division are needed to produce enough lymphocytes to mount an immune response. This can result in a degree of protection from vaccination or exposure, even if there is no remaining detectable antibody. The cells present in the expanded clone are called memory cells. If the previous exposure has been relatively recent, there still will be circulating antibody and effector T lymphocytes that can act immediately to begin to control the infection.

CELLULAR INTERACTIONS IN THE INDUCTION OF THE IMMUNE RESPONSE. The induction of clonal expansion and the immune response requires a complex interaction of macrophages, T lymphocytes, and B lymphocytes to phagocytize and destroy infectious agents. After the infectious agent is partially degraded by the macrophage, antigenic fragments appear on the macrophage surface where they can easily be contacted by B and T lymphocytes. Macrophages (and other specialized antigen-presenting cells) have a high density of class II major histocompatibility complex (MHC) molecules on their surface. T helper (T_H) cells are needed to help initiate the immune response. They can only recognize efficiently foreign antigens that are on a cell surface bound to a class II MHC molecule. Therefore, T_H cells cannot respond to free soluble antigen or to whole bacteria or viruses.

In addition to contacting the antigen and a class II MHC molecule, the T_H cell requires a third signal to be fully activated: interleukin-1 (IL-1). IL-1 is a protein molecule (formerly referred to as lymphocyte-activating factor and endogenous pyrogen) that is released by macrophages while they are processing antigens. IL-1 is a key mediator of the host response to infection through its ability to induce fever and neutrophilia, among other things. A very important function of macrophage-produced IL-1 is its action on T_H cells to cause them to secrete interleukin-2 (IL-2). IL-2 is a protein molecule (formerly called T-cell growth factor) secreted by activated T_H cells. The IL-2 is needed for T cells to undergo mitosis and produce more cells in the clone.

T_H cells also secrete other factors that are very important in initiating the B-cell response resulting in antibody production. B cells contact antigen through immunoglobulins, which act as receptors, bound to their surface. Antigens do not have to be presented on MHC class II molecules by macrophages for a B cell to recognize them. An optimal B-cell response to antigen requires the help of soluble factors released by T_H cells. These factors are needed for B-cell mitosis and clonal expansion and for switching the class of antibody produced from IgM to IgG, IgA, or IgE.

LYMPHOCYTE SUBPOPULATIONS. Lymphocyte subpopulations in the peripheral blood of pigs are markedly different from other species. Young pigs have high blood lymphocyte counts compared to most other mammals (approximately 10^7/ml). Up to 50% of these lymphocytes are null cells, which lack all surface markers specific for B or T lymphocytes (Duncan et al. 1989). These null cells do not recirculate between the blood and lymphatic tissues, and they differ from null cells in other species in that they do not have NK cell activity. The functional role and fate of this large population of null lymphocytes is unknown (Duncan et al. 1989).

Swine T lymphocytes have at least three unusual properties compared with other species (Lunney and Pescovitz 1987): (1) Approximately 25% of swine peripheral blood T cells express both the CD4 and CD8 antigens on their surface. (2) The ratio of CD4+/CD8+ T cells is normally approximately 0.6 in pigs, which is a reversal of the expected ratio in other species. A normal ratio of CD4+/CD8+ in humans is 1.5–2.0. Both of these properties are very unusual in other species and only occur in pathological conditions in humans. (3) Resting CD8+ cells in swine preferentially express class II MHC antigens. Since swine have relatively normal antibody production and cell-mediated immune responses, these unique properties of swine lymphocytes do not seem to have a negative impact on resistance to disease.

LYMPHOCYTE CIRCULATION. Lymph node structure and lymphocyte circulation are markedly different in the pig compared with humans or other domestic species. Recirculation of lymphocytes from blood to lymphoid tissues is very important for bringing antigen into contact with the rare lymphocytes that are able to recognize it. Circulation of B cells, T cells, and macrophages through lymph nodes is also important for facilitating cellular interactions needed for the induction of the immune response as described above. Lymphocytes are produced in the bone marrow as well as in the thymus and in all secondary lymphoid tissues in the pig. Lymphocytes are released from the site of production into the bloodstream. T and B lymphocytes circulate in the blood for an average of approximately 30 minutes before entering the tissues. Null cells in the pig apparently remain in the bloodstream and do not recirculate between blood and lymphoid tissues. Porcine lymph nodes are structurally inverted compared with other domestic species. Lymphatics enter the node through the hilus and the lymph passes through the node with the lymph leaving through the periphery. The lymph node has a dense medulla, which lacks sinuses and cords. The germinal centers are located in the interior of the node. Other lymphoid organs such as the Peyer's patches, tonsils, and spleen are similar to those found in other species (Binns et al. 1986; Pabst and Binns 1986). Lymphocytes in swine and other species enter the lymph node through two routes. Lymphocytes leaving the bloodstream and entering the subcutaneous tissues are carried to the lymph node in the afferent lymphatics. Lymphocytes may enter the lymph node directly by adhering to high endothelial cells in the venules of the lymph node and then traversing the endothelial barrier. In other species, the lymphocytes exit the lymph node in the efferent lymphatics and are carried through the thoracic duct back to the circulatory system. In swine, the efferent lymph contains very few lymphocytes; the lymphocytes in the lymph node directly reenter the circulation

(Binns et al. 1986). The emigration of lymphocytes from blood into lymph nodes can be increased by antigenic stimulation. In addition to migrating from blood to lymphoid tissues, lymphocytes in swine migrate into most other tissues as well (Binns et al. 1986). Lymphocyte subpopulations in swine show a distinct preference for circulation to either gut-associated lymphoid tissues or surface nodes (Binns et al. 1986). For instance, mesenteric lymph node cells (both T and B lymphocytes) preferentially home to the gut (Salmon 1986). In rodents the majority of the lymphocytes found in the mammary gland also come from gut-associated lymphoid tissue, whereas in swine approximately equal numbers of lymphocytes in the mammary gland come from gut-associated lymphoid tissue and from peripheral lymph nodes. The dual origin of mammary lymphocytes in swine suggests that the local mammary immune response may not depend solely on oral immunization (Salmon 1986, 1987).

Acquired Immune Defense Mechanisms. An important component of lymphocyte activity in host defense is mediated by soluble products released by stimulated lymphocytes. T lymphocytes secrete a variety of lymphokines, and B lymphocytes differentiate into plasma cells that secrete antibody (B lymphocytes may also be able to secrete some lymphokines). Antibodies are specific for the antigens that induced them, whereas lymphokines are not. These soluble products produced during the immune response play an important role in orchestrating host defense against pathogens partially through their direct activities and partially by enhancing the activity of the nonspecific defense mechanisms (i.e., complement, phagocytic cells, and NK cells).

The cytotoxic T lymphocytes (T_C cells) are an important part of the cell-mediated immune response to virus infection and tumors. Most T_C cells have the CD8 marker on their surface and only recognize antigen associated with MHC class I molecules on a cell surface. They directly attack host cells that have foreign antigen (e.g., viral antigen or tumor antigen) on their surface. These cells do not attack free bacteria or viruses.

IMMUNOGLOBULINS

Production of Immunoglobulins. B lymphocytes from clones that have never been stimulated by antigen have surface monomeric IgM antibody molecules that act as antigen receptors. All of the IgM molecules on one B cell are specific for the same antigen. When a B cell is appropriately stimulated by the antigen it recognizes (along with soluble products from a T_H cell) it begins to undergo mitosis. This results in the formation of many more B cells with IgM receptors that also recognize the same antigen. Some of these newly formed B cells differentiate into plasma cells that secrete IgM antibody. As the antigen-specific IgM antibody concentration begins to increase in the blood, it signals the T_H cell to in turn signal some of the B cells to switch from IgM production to IgG, IgA, or IgE production. These B cells then rearrange their genetic material that codes for antibody production and produce antibody molecules with the same antigenic specificity (i.e., the same light-chain structure and variable portion of the heavy chain) but of a different antibody class (i.e., the constant heavy portion of the antibody molecule is changed). Changing the antibody class gives the antibody molecules different properties. The class of antibody that the T_H cells cause the B cells to switch to depends to a large extent upon the nature of the antigen and where in the body the antigen was trapped. T_H cells located in lymph nodes and the spleen tend to induce B cells to switch to IgG production. T_H cells located in Peyer's patches or under other mucosal surfaces tend to induce B cells to switch to IgA and/or IgE production, depending on the nature of the antigen and the genetic predisposition of the individual.

Antibody molecules have a variety of activities in host defense. Although antibody alone cannot kill infectious agents, it has a very important function to mark such agents for destruction by complement, phagocytic cells, and/or cytotoxic cells. Antibody molecules can coat infectious agents to prevent them from attaching to or penetrating host cells, they can agglutinate infectious agents to reduce their infectivity, and they can directly bind to and neutralize toxins.

Classes of Immunoglobulins. Characteristics of the various classes of porcine immunoglobulin were thoroughly reviewed in the previous edition of this book (Porter 1986).

The predominant Ig class in the pig and other species is IgG. It accounts for more than 80% of the Ig in serum and colostrum (Table 3.1). The two main subclasses of IgG are IgG_1 and IgG_2 (Metzger and Fougereau 1968), with IgG_1 predominating in serum and colostrum. IgG_3 and IgG_4 subclasses are found in lesser concentrations. An 18S Ig has been described that is antigenically similar to IgG_2 and is found in low levels in normal serum and colostrum (Kim et al. 1966). Newborn piglets also possess a 5S IgG, which may not have light chains and may not be functional (Stertzl et al. 1960; Franek and Riha 1964).

IgM accounts for approximately 5–10% of the total Ig in serum and colostrum (Table 3.1). The IgM is a pentamer held together by disulfide bonds and has a sedimentation coefficient of 17.8S (Porter 1969).

IgA is present in swine serum as 6.4S monomers and as 9.3S dimers, which are two monomers bound together with a J chain (Halpern and Koshland 1970; Mestecky et al. 1971; Porter and Allen 1972). IgA at mucosal surfaces is mostly dimeric IgA with a J chain and associated secretory component.

As discussed by Porter (1986), an analog of IgE has apparently not yet been fully defined in the pig. Antibodies against human IgE and bovine IgE have been shown to react with a homocyto-

Table 3.1. Concentration of porcine immunoglobulins (mg/ml) in body fluids

	IgG	IgG_2	IgM	IgA
Adult sow	24.33	14.08	2.92	2.07
	±0.94	±0.49	±0.20	±0.20
Colostrum	61.8	40.3	3.2	9.6
	±2.5	±1.6	±0.2	±0.6
Milk				
(24 hr)	11.8	8.0	1.8	3.8
	±4.8	±3.2	±0.3	±1.0
(48 hr)	8.2	5.0	1.8	2.7
	±3.2	±1.8	±0.4	±0.6
(3–7 days)	1.9	1.3	1.2	3.4
	±0.6	±0.3	±0.2	±1.0
(8–35 days)	1.4	1.00	0.90	3.05
	±0.6	±0.45	±0.25	±0.74
Intestinal fluid				
Piglet	0.002		0.065	0.033
Sow	>0.001		0.001	0.091
Urinary tract	4.7			0.77
Follicle				
Diestrus	18.1			0.7
Estrus	25.1			0.7
Uterine secretions				
Diestrus	0.32			0.20
Estrus	0.34			0.12
Cervicovaginal mucus				
Diestrus	6.7		0.60	1.1
Estrus	2.0		0.06	0.6

Source: Veterinary Clinical Immunology, R. E. W. Halliwell and N. T. Gorman, editors. W. B. Saunders, 1989, with permission.

tropic immunoglobulin in swine serum (Barratt 1972; Nielsen 1977).

Polyclonal and Monoclonal Antibodies. Antibody produced by an animal in response to an infection or vaccination is polyclonal antibody. Infectious agents are complex antigens with many different antigenic specificities on their surface; therefore, they stimulate many clones of B and T lymphocytes to respond. This results in a heterogeneous mixture of antibodies that recognizes a wide variety of surface molecules on the microorganism. This broad spectrum of antibodies that are produced and are present in the serum are most helpful to the animal in overcoming infection. It is sometimes a disadvantage, however, if one wishes to use the serum for developing diagnostic reagents. The polyclonal antibodies produced in response to one infectious agent may cross-react with another infectious agent and thus interfere with the specificity of the assay. The majority of the protein present in a polyclonal antiserum produced against an infectious agent is not antibodies directed against the agent. Therefore, the amount of specific antibody in relation to the amount of protein present is low. This is a disadvantage when attempting to protect an animal from disease by administering antisera.

Monoclonal antibodies are now commonly produced in research laboratories and are used to overcome many of the disadvantages of polyclonal antisera for diagnostic and (less commonly) therapeutic purposes. Monoclonal antibodies are produced by one clone of B lymphocytes and, therefore, are all identical. All of the antibody molecules present in a monoclonal antibody preparation are specific for the same antigenic determinant; thus, the antibody can be present in extremely high concentrations, which reduces the problem of cross-reactivity between microorganisms in diagnostic tests. If monoclonal antibodies can be produced against a protective antigen on a microorganism, the monoclonals can be used in therapy or prevention of disease. Since they can be produced in very high concentration and purity, a much lower volume of monoclonal antibody than polyclonal antibody solution can be used to passively immunize animals. This reduces the risk of serious reaction to the passively administered antibody and its extraneous protein.

LYMPHOKINES. Cell-mediated immunity is mediated through the collective action of the lymphokines and T_c cells (described above). T lymphocytes secrete a variety of lymphokines that are important in regulating the activity of the entire immune system. It is estimated that more than 100 molecules have already been described as lymphokines.

A brief description of some of the more well characterized molecules involved in a cell-mediated immune response is included here.

Interleukin-1. IL-1 is a protein secreted by stimulated macrophages (it was previously known as lymphocyte-activating factor). IL-1 facilitates the production of IL-2 by T_H cells and is, therefore, necessary for lymphocyte proliferation. In addition to its role in triggering lymphocyte proliferation, IL-1 causes fever (it was also known as endogenous pyrogen) and stimulates the liver to secrete acute-phase proteins (an important part of the acute inflammatory response).

Interleukin-2. IL-2 is a glycoprotein secreted by T lymphocytes after antigen and IL-1 stimulation. IL-2 is required for the proliferation of activated T cells, NK cells, and other cytotoxic effector cells.

Interferons. There are three general types of interferon: alpha, beta, and gamma. Alpha interferons are produced by leukocytes and other cells in response to a variety of inducers, such as viruses, bacterial products, polynucleotides, and tumor cells. At least 15 subtypes of human alpha interferon have been described. Even though alpha interferons are secreted by T and B lymphocytes, they are not considered to be lymphokines because their production is not limited to those clones of cells that specifically recognize the antigen. Beta interferon is produced by fibroblasts and epithelial cells (as well as other cell types) in response to the same types of inducers (viruses, bacterial products, polynucleotides) as alpha interferons. Gamma interferon is produced by T lymphocytes in response to antigenic stimulation. It therefore is considered a lymphokine.

All three types of interferon control replication of certain viruses by inhibiting production of viral protein in infected cells. The interferons can also modify a variety of biologic activities and, therefore, have important regulatory functions. Gamma interferon, an especially active biologic response modifier, is one of the lymphokines capable of activating neutrophils and macrophages to be more efficient. Gamma interferon also enhances the activity of NK cells.

Tumor Necrosis Factor. Tumor necrosis factor is a soluble protein secreted by macrophages or lymphocytes that have been appropriately stimulated. It was named for its ability to cause necrosis of subcutaneously transplanted tumors in mice. Tumor necrosis factor is preferentially cytotoxic for transformed cancer cells and is believed to be an important mediator of tumor cell killing. Tumor necrosis factor also may play a role in controlling virus infection and chronic intracellular bacterial infections.

Colony-stimulating Factors. Colony-stimulating factor refers to a group of glycoproteins that stimulate leukocyte production by the bone marrow. Colony-stimulating factors may also enhance the antimicrobial activity of mature neutrophils and macrophages. Many cell types have been shown to produce colony-stimulating factor without an apparent stimulus, including macrophages, fibroblasts, and endothelial cells. Lymphocytes stimulated by antigen also produce various colony-stimulating factors.

Mucosal Immunity. Mucosal surfaces are frequently exposed to infectious agents and providing immunity at mucosal surfaces is a difficult problem. The components of the immune system described previously may not function well in the microenvironment on the mucosal surface. The degree to which the various components of the immune system contribute to protective immunity varies with the mucosal surface. For instance IgG class antibody, complement, and phagocytic cells may function efficiently in the lower respiratory tract and in the uterus but not in the lumen of the gut.

An important component of immunity at mucosal surfaces is the secretory IgA system. Antigen that enters the body through a mucosal surface tends to induce an IgA class antibody response at the mucosal surface. It may also induce secretory IgA at other mucosal surfaces. Specialized epithelial cells called dome cells or M cells are found overlying aggregations of gut- and bronchus-associated lymphoid tissues. These dome cells pinocytose antigen and transport it across the epithelial layer. The antigen may then be processed by antigen-presenting cells and presented to T and B lymphocytes.

Lymphocytes in the bloodstream tend to segregate into two populations: those that circulate between the bloodstream and the systemic lymphoid tissues of the lymph nodes, spleen, and bone marrow; and those that circulate between the bloodstream and lymphoid tissues associated with mucosal surfaces. Because of the nature of the T-helper and T-suppressor cells that home to mucosal surfaces, antigens entering through mucosal surfaces tend to induce an IgA or IgE class antibody. In some cases antigens entering through the intestinal tract may induce oral tolerance, resulting in suppression of IgG class antibody responses.

In the mucosal lymphoid tissues, B cells that have been stimulated by antigen and induced by T-helper cells to switch to IgA class antibody production will leave the submucosal lymphoid tissue and reenter the bloodstream. These lymphocytes exit the bloodstream at submucosal surfaces and locate in the lamina propria where they differentiate into plasma cells that secrete dimeric IgA. Many of these cells return to the same mucosal surface from which they originated, but others can be found at other mucosal surfaces. There is a special affinity for lymphocytes that have been sensitized in the gut of the sow to migrate to the mammary gland to become plasma cells and se-

crete IgA into the milk. The IgA in the milk helps to protect the piglet from intestinal pathogens while it is nursing. This is an important mechanism for transferring immunity from the sow to the piglet for enteric pathogens that the sow has been exposed to.

The dimeric IgA secreted by the plasma cells in the lamina propria binds to secretory component on the basal membrane of mucosal epithelial cells. The dimeric IgA and secretory component are then transported to the mucosal surface of the epithelial cell, and this complex is released onto the mucosal surface. Secretory component is important for protecting the IgA molecule from proteolytic enzymes and also serves to anchor the IgA into the mucous layer so that it forms a protective coating on the mucosal surface.

Secretory IgA plays an important role in immunity at mucosal surfaces by agglutinating infectious agents, preventing attachment of infectious agents to epithelial cells, and neutralizing toxins. Other components of the immune response may also be important in protection against various types of infection at mucosal surfaces. For example, in the pig neutrophils can immigrate into the intestinal lumen in large numbers within a 4-hour period in response to antigen-antibody complexes. The recruitment of neutrophils into the intestinal lumen is dependent upon the presence of antibody, which may be circulating IgG antibody (Bellamy and Nielsen 1974), colostral antibody (Sellwood et al. 1986), or locally induced IgA class antibody (Bhogal et al. 1987). Neutrophils in the lumen have been shown to be actively phagocytic (Bhogal et al. 1987). The immigration of neutrophils into the lumen of the gut and their subsequent destruction has been shown to result in an increased concentration of lactoferrin, lysozyme, and cationic proteins. These substances may also contribute to immunity to bacterial infections in the gut.

T lymphocytes may also be important mediators of immunity at mucosal surfaces. This is especially true for respiratory infections with facultative intracellular bacterial pathogens. T lymphocytes may play a role in immunity in the intestinal tract. Salmon (1987) has shown that a high proportion of the intraepithelial lymphocytes in the intestine are of the T_c phenotype. He speculates that these cytotoxic T cells in contact with intestinal epithelial cells may be important in destroying virus-infected epithelial cells.

More detailed information on aspects of immunity at mucosal surfaces may be found in chapters in this book dealing with specific organ systems or specific pathogens.

Fetal and Neonatal Immunity. All components of the native and acquired immune systems develop in utero and are functional at birth. However, they are generally less efficient than in the adult (Hammerberg et al. 1989). Since the normal newborn piglet has not yet been exposed to antigen, it has not yet developed a humoral or cell-mediated immune response to any infectious agents. After exposure to infectious agents, it will take 7–10 days for a primary antibody or cell-mediated immune response to develop. During this time resistance to infection depends upon the actions of the native defense mechanisms and antibody, which is passively transferred from the sow to the piglet. In the pig there is virtually no transfer of antibody across the placenta. The epitheliochorial placentation of the sow has several epithelial layers between maternal and fetal circulation, which prevents antibody transfer. In the sow, as in other large domestic species, passive transfer of antibody from mother to offspring occurs through the colostrum. The sow concentrates antibody in the colostrum during the last several days of gestation. This antibody is largely transferred intact across the gut epithelial cells into the circulation of the newborn piglet. The passive transfer of antibody from sow to piglet in the colostrum and milk is very important for neonatal survival and is discussed in more detail below.

NATIVE DEFENSE MECHANISMS. The newborn piglet has low levels of hemolytic complement activity at birth, which is related to the birth weight with heavier pigs having significantly higher concentrations of serum complement (Rice and L'Ecuyer 1963). In colostrum-deprived pigs the hemolytic complement activity gradually increases during the first 36 days of life. Piglets allowed to suckle colostrum have higher titers of hemolytic complement than piglets deprived of colostrum during the first 3 weeks of life. This suggests that some of the complement components that are present in limiting amounts are transferred through the colostrum to the piglet (Rice and L'Ecuyer 1963). The third component of complement (C3) plays a central role in complement activity. Newborn piglet serum has approximately 25% of the C3 levels found in adult swine serum. The C3 concentration increases until it reaches adult levels at 14 days of age. The C3 component of complement is apparently not transferred through the colostrum (Tyler et al. 1988, 1989).

Phagocytic cells are present in newborn animals but generally have reduced phagocytic activity when compared with adult animals (Osburn et al. 1982). The phagocytic activity of neutrophils and macrophages from neonatal piglets has apparently not been evaluated. Since phagocytes depend on complement and/or antibody to opsonize many infectious agents, the overall efficiency of phagocytosis may be reduced due to inadequate levels of complement and antibody. Neutrophils from fetal pigs have been shown to have antibody-dependent cell-mediated cytotoxicity activity against chicken red blood cells that is comparable to that of adult pigs. Neutrophils

from neonatal pigs have also been shown to rapidly emigrate into the lumen of the gut in response to the presence of *E. coli* and colostral antibody (Sellwood et al. 1986; Yang and Schultz 1986).

Natural killer cell activity has been shown to be absent in the peripheral blood of fetal pigs and to be low in pigs of less than 2 weeks of age (Yang and Schultz 1986).

PASSIVE TRANSFER IN THE NEONATE. Pigs are born with almost no serum antibody and absorb IgG, IgM, and IgA from sow colostrum, which is enriched for IgG, IgG₂, and IgA when compared with serum. It has approximately the same concentration of IgM as serum (Table 3.1). When the pig suckles, colostrum is replaced with milk that has a much lower immunoglobulin content. From 3 days of age until the end of lactation, IgA is the predominant antibody found in sow milk. The percentage of immunoglobulin in the mammary gland derived from serum and locally produced in the mammary gland is different in colostrum and milk and varies with the immunoglobulin class (Table 3.2).

All three major classes of Ig (IgG, IgA, and IgM) are absorbed from the colostrum into the circulation of newborn pigs (Porter 1969; Curtis and Bourne 1971). IgA, however, is absorbed less efficiently than the other classes of antibody (Porter 1973; Hill and Porter 1974), apparently because much of the IgA in porcine colostrum is dimeric IgA lacking secretory component (Porter 1973). The neonatal colostrum-deprived piglet has been shown to express secretory component in the gut, which tends to localize in the mucus of the crypt areas (Allen and Porter 1973). Because of the affinity of the dimeric IgA and IgM for secretory component, it has been suggested (Butler et al. 1981) that IgA and IgM are bound in association with secretory component and held in the mucus of the crypt areas and are, therefore, less efficiently absorbed from the colostrum. The IgA present in sow's milk throughout the suckling period may also bind to the secretory component in the crypt areas, thereby providing relatively continuous protection against intestinal pathogens.

Table 3.2. Origin of porcine colostral and milk immunoglobulins

	Plasma Derived (%)	Synthesized Locally (%)
Colostrum		
IgM	85	15
IgG	100	0
IgA	40	60
Milk		
IgM	10	90
IgG	30	70
IgA	10	90

Source: Stokes and Bourne (1989).

Intestinal absorption of immunoglobulin from the colostrum normally ceases by 24–36 hours after birth. If pigs suckle normally, the efficiency of absorption decreases with a half-life of about 3 hours (Speer et al. 1959). Lecce et al. (1961) found that the period of time that the intestine could absorb antibodies was extended up to 5 days in starved pigs that were maintained by parental administration of nutrients. Therefore, piglets that have not had an opportunity to eat during the first 24–36 hours may still benefit from colostrum ingestion.

HYPERSENSITIVITIES. Hypersensitivities are conditions in which there is excessive responsiveness to antigen to which the animal has previously been exposed. The clinical signs are due to the immune response to the antigen rather than to a direct action of the antigen. Hypersensitivity conditions can be divided into four types based on their mechanism of action.

Mechanisms of Immune-mediated Hypersensitivity.

Type 1 or immediate-type hypersensitivity involves the synthesis of specific IgE (reaginic or cytotropic) antibodies. The IgE preferentially binds to Fc receptors on the surface of tissue mast cells. When the same antigen is encountered subsequently it will bind to the IgE on the mast cell surface (if there is a sufficiently high concentration of IgE specific for the antigen) and cause the mast cell to release numerous pharmacologically active substances that are responsible for the clinical signs (e.g., histamine, seratonin, kinins, prostaglandins, and others). Type 1 hypersensitivities may be localized in a particular region or organ or may be systemic (anaphylaxis) (Eyre 1980).

Type 2 hypersensitivity (or cytotoxic-type hypersensitivity) involves the presence of antibodies directed against cell membrane antigens. These may be normal tissue antigens in the case of autoimmune diseases or foreign antigens (e.g., drugs or viral or bacterial antigens) that have adhered to the cell surface.

Type 3 hypersensitivity (or immune-complex–type hypersensitivity) involves the presence of antigen-antibody complexes in the circulation or tissue. These immune complexes can fix complement and, therefore, may initiate the inflammatory response, attract neutrophils to the site, and damage cell membranes.

Type 4 hypersensitivity (or delayed-type hypersensitivity) is mediated by sensitized T cells releasing lymphokines and does not involve antibody. The tuberculin skin test is a classic type 4 hypersensitivity reaction.

It is not unusual for clinical hypersensitivity conditions to involve more than one of the four types of hypersensitivity. Hypersensitivity conditions that have been studied in the pig will be briefly reviewed here.

IMMEDIATE-TYPE HYPERSENSITIVITY. Pigs have been shown to develop homocytotropic antibody in response to lungworm (*Metastrongylus* spp.) infection (Barratt 1972). This antibody was demonstrated in the serum of infected pigs using a passive cutaneous anaphylaxis assay. Serum from an infected pig was injected intradermally into a recipient pig. When *Metastrongylus* antigen was injected intravenously 36–48 hours later, an immediate hypersensitivity reaction (wheal and erythema) occurred at the site of serum injection. This reaction was maximal in 30–45 minutes.

Systemic anaphylaxis has been studied experimentally in pigs sensitized to egg albumin (Thomlinson and Buxton 1963). Mild symptoms of anaphylaxis were characterized by heavy and rapid breathing accompanied by coughing and yawning. The animals showed stiffness and incoordination and preferred to lie down. The first signs of severe anaphylactic shock were circling, incoordination, coughing, and intense vascular congestion of the skin, especially of the ears, nose, and periocular area. Convulsions and acute respiratory distress rapidly followed. After a few minutes the pigs began to recover from the severe respiratory distress, then vomiting and defecation occurred; muscular tremors developed 20–40 minutes later. The pigs with severe symptoms of anaphylaxis recovered more rapidly than the pigs with mild symptoms.

It has been suggested that edema disease in swine may be due to an immediate-type hypersensitivity response to *E. coli* antigens (Thomlinson and Buxton 1963).

CYTOTOXIC-TYPE HYPERSENSITIVITY. Type 2 hypersensitivities have been reported in pigs in which autoantibodies have formed against erythrocytes, thrombocytes, or neutrophils (Nordstoga 1965; Lie 1968; Saunders and Kinch 1968; Linklater 1972; Linklater et al. 1973; Dimmock et al. 1982). This results in a depletion of the respective cell type and the associated clinical signs that one would expect (anemia, bleeding diathesis, or increased susceptibility to infection, respectively). These autoantibodies may arise from blood transfusions, from the use of vaccines that contain blood products, or in multiparous sows that develop antibody against the alloantigens shared by the sire and the fetus. In the latter case, one would not expect clinical signs to appear in the sow since she would only produce antibody against cell-surface allotype antigens that are not found on her cells. When a piglet suckles and receives colostral antibody, the passively transferred antibody causes clinical signs if the pig has inherited the sire's alloantigens. Thrombocytopenic purpura in piglets due to passively transferred antiplatelet antibody seems to be rather common. Pigs appear normal at birth. Death usually occurs between 10–20 days of age. The most striking pathologic feature is the presence of hemorrhages in the subcutaneous tissues and internal organs. Castration during the period of thrombocytopenia may greatly increase the death rate.

Antibodies against erythrocytes, thrombocytes, and neutrophils may be present in the same piglet. In one report, 50% of the dams of litters affected with thrombocytopenic purpura had erythrocyte isoantibodies in their serum (Linklater et al. 1973). The concurrent presence of hemolytic disease with thrombocytopenic purpura in the piglets will exacerbate the anemia. The degree of severity of these conditions may vary between piglets in one litter depending on the erythrocyte and platelet isoantigens that they have inherited from the sire and the amount of colostrum ingested.

IMMUNE-COMPLEX-TYPE HYPERSENSITIVITY. Immune-complex-mediated glomerulonephritis is a common sequelae to chronic hog cholera virus infection or African swine fever virus infection (Cheville et al. 1970). The lesion associated with these two infections is moderately severe membranoproliferative glomerulonephritis. The immune complexes found in these diseases may also cause periarteritis nodosa, a systemic vasculitis. Immune-complex deposition in swine kidneys is apparently common. One study evaluated 100 kidneys collected at slaughter that had no gross lesions; 97 of the kidneys had IgG deposits and 98 had C3 deposits as demonstrated by immunocytochemistry. The significance of these immune-complex deposits in the kidney is unknown; however, clinical diagnosis of glomerular disease in swine is rare (Shirota et al. 1986).

FOOD HYPERSENSITIVITY. Food hypersensitivity is thought to be responsible for some cases of postweaning diarrhea in piglets (Stokes et al. 1987; Stokes and Bourne 1989; Li et al. 1990). This is apparently a type 4 or delayed-type hypersensitivity. Following the introduction of a new protein antigen to the diet, a small proportion ($<0.002\%$) of that protein is absorbed intact. This may induce an antibody and/or cell-mediated response. The systemic antibody response (IgG) will be subsequently suppressed (oral tolerance) and a local mucosal antibody will persist. The local antibody prevents further absorption of the intact protein. The oral tolerance that develops is a specifically acquired ability to prevent responses to any of the proteins that may be absorbed. Therefore, following the introduction of new dietary antigen, animals pass through a brief phase of hypersensitivity before the development of a protected state of tolerance.

In pigs that were weaned abruptly and placed on a soya-containing diet, soya protein was detected in the sera of all animals for up to 20 days postweaning. A delayed-type hypersensitivity skin test reaction to soya proteins was transiently positive in the soya-fed group. The changes in gut morphology (crypt hyperplasia and villous atrophy) and the malabsorption associated with early weaning have been characterized. Evidence exists that suggests that these changes occur as a result of a transient hypersensitivity to antigen in the postweaning diet. These intestinal changes can facilitate growth and disease production by *E. coli*. Feeding of large amounts of soya prior to the withdrawal of milk prevented the postweaning malabsorption and diarrhea (Stokes et al. 1987).

IMMUNODEFICIENCY AND IMMUNOSUPPRESSION. Primary or secondary immunodeficiency increases the susceptibility of animals to infectious disease. A primary immunodeficiency is defined as a disorder of the immune system for which a genetic basis is proven or suspected. A secondary immunodeficiency is a disorder in which the animal is genetically capable of normal immune function, but some secondary factor is impairing resistance to disease.

Clinical findings that are associated with immunodeficiency include (a) illness from organisms of normally low pathogenicity or from an attenuated live vaccine, (b) recurrent illnesses that are unusually difficult to control, (c) failure to respond adequately to vaccination, (d) unexplained neonatal illness and death affecting more than one animal in a litter, and (e) a variety of disease syndromes occurring concurrently in a herd. A large number of primary immunodeficiencies have been reported in humans and a few have been reported in other domestic species; however, there are apparently no reports of primary immunodeficiencies in pigs. This is probably due to the relatively low value of the individual piglet and the expense and difficulty associated with diagnosing a primary immunodeficiency. In addition, sows and boars that produce nonvigorous litters are not kept in the breeding herd.

A common cause of secondary immunodeficiency is failure to passively transfer adequate levels of maternal antibody through the colostrum to the piglet, as discussed earlier in this chapter. Other potential causes of secondary immunodeficiency (or immunosuppression) include (a) physical or psychological distress, (b) immunosuppressive infectious agents, (c) inadequate nutrition, and (d) immunotoxic substances. The influence of most of these factors on the porcine immune system has not been adequately studied.

Physical and Psychological Distress. There is ample evidence that both physical and psychological distress can suppress immune function in animals, leading to an increased incidence of infectious disease. Excess heat or cold, crowding, mixing, weaning, limit-feeding, shipping, noise, and restraint are stressors that are often associated with intensive animal production and have been shown to influence immune function in various species (Kelley 1985). Distress-induced alterations in immune function are mediated by interactions between the neuroendocrine and immune systems. The study of these multisystem interactions initially focused on the secretion and influence of glucocorticoids, which suppress several aspects of immune function. It is now recognized that there are many mechanisms by which the neuroendocrine system can alter immune function; in addition, the immune system is capable of altering the activity of the neuroendocrine system (Breazile 1987; Dunn 1988; Kelley 1988).

The neuroendocrine and immune systems communicate in a bidirectional manner via direct neural as well as hormonal signalling systems (Griffin 1989). Neuroendocrine signals that are capable of directly altering the function of cells of the immune system include (a) direct sympathetic innervation to the parenchyma of the thymus, spleen, and bone marrow; (b) glucocorticoids produced by the adrenal cortex after pituitary adrenocorticotrophic hormone (ACTH) stimulation; (c) catecholamines produced by the adrenal medulla; (d) endogenous opiates (endorphin and enkephalins) produced by the pituitary, adrenal medulla, sympathetic terminals, and lymphocytes; (e) vasoactive intestinal peptide released by sympathetic neurons of the intestine and perhaps other sites; and (f) substance P released by sympathetic nerve terminals (Breazile 1987; Dunn 1988; Kelley 1988). Receptors have been detected on lymphocytes and thymocytes for a variety of hormones, including corticosteroids, insulin, testosterone, estrogens, beta-adrenergic agents, histamine, growth hormone, acetylcholine, and metencephalon. Some of these substances have been demonstrated to stimulate lymphocyte differentiation and affect their activity.

Conversely, the immune system can influence the function of the neuroendocrine system. Upon antigenic stimulation, lymphocytes have been shown to produce small amounts of ACTH, beta-endorphin, metencephalon, thyroid-stimulating hormone (TSH), and other classically "neural" peptides (Blalock et al. 1985; Griffin 1989). Activation of the immune system, as during the response to an immunizing antigen, results in a change in neural-firing rates in certain parts of the hypothalamus. Some evidence indicates that certain cytokines (interleukins) can promote hormone release by pituitary cells. Thymic hormones (thymosin alpha 1 in particular) seem to affect the central nervous system (CNS) as well as the immune system and, in turn, are regulated by the CNS. Thus, the interaction between the immune and neuroendocrine systems is reciprocal, and feedback loops have been described.

Weaning is certainly a stressful event for domestic animals. Piglets are usually separated from their sow, handled extensively, regrouped with unfamiliar pigs, and shifted from a liquid to a solid diet. Weaning at 2, 3, or 4 weeks of age (but not at 5 weeks of age) has been shown to decrease the in vivo and in vitro response of porcine lymphocytes to phytohemagglutinin (Blecha et al. 1983). This is considered to be a measure of the pigs ability to mount a cell-mediated immune response. These same parameters were suppressed in artificially reared neonatal piglets compared with their sow-reared littermates (Blecha et al. 1986; Hennessy et al. 1987). Weaning (at 5 weeks of age) 24 hours after the injection of sheep red blood cells (RBCs) decreased the antibody response to the RBCs. Weaning 2 weeks prior to injecting the sheep RBCs did not decrease the antibody response (Blecha and Kelley 1981).

Regrouping of pigs at the time of weaning or at 2 weeks after weaning significantly increased their plasma cortisol concentration. However, there were no measurable changes in lymphocyte blastogenesis or antibody responses at the time of elevated plasma cortisol concentration (Blecha et al. 1985).

Crowding or restraint may also stress pigs sufficiently to decrease their immune responsiveness. Housing eight pigs (11.5–18.0 kg) per group in pens with 0.13 m² of floor space per pig significantly reduced their phytohemagglutinin skin test response as compared with pigs given twice as much space (Yen and Pond 1987). When young pigs were restrained for 2 hours per day over a 3-day period, they had a significantly elevated plasma cortisol concentration, which correlated with a decrease in the size of the thymus gland and with a reduction in the phytohemagglutinin skin test response (Westly and Kelley 1984). Another report indicated that tethering of sows suppressed antibody synthesis to sheep RBCs. It also resulted in a reduction in the amount of antigen-specific antibodies that were transmitted through the colostrum into the blood of the piglets (Kelley 1985).

Immunosuppressive Infectious Agents.   Certain infectious agents are capable of suppressing immune function sufficiently to make the animal more susceptible to secondary infections. For example, infection with *Mycoplasma hyopneumoniae*, virulent or vaccine strains of hog cholera virus, or pseudorabies virus increases the susceptibility of pigs to severe *Pasteurella multocida* pneumonia (Smith et al. 1973; Pijoan and Ochoa 1978; Fuentes and Pijoan 1986, 1987). The mechanism of the immunosuppression induced by these agents has not been completely characterized. The pseudorabies virus has been shown to replicate in alveolar macrophages and to impair their bactericidal functions (Iglesias et al. 1989a,b). Porcine parvovirus replicates in alveolar macrophages, as well as lymphocytes, and has been shown to impair macrophage phagocytosis and lymphocyte blastogenesis (Harding and Molitor 1988). Swine influenza virus also replicates in alveolar macrophages and kills the macrophages (Charley 1983).

The African swine fever virus causes a peripheral lymphopenia and necrosis of lymphoreticular organs (Wardley and Wilkinson 1980). This virus replicates in both lymphocytes and in the mononuclear phagocytic system and presumably impairs their function (Wardley et al. 1979). It has also been shown to strongly reduce NK cell activity by 2 days after infection (Norley and Wardley 1983a).

Nutritional Influences on Immunity. Both malnutrition and overfeeding may result in impairment of immune function and increased susceptibility to disease due to a deficiency or excess of proteins or calories, or a relative imbalance in vitamin or trace mineral content. Animals under intensive production conditions typically have a completely controlled diet. Therefore, it is very important that the diet, especially the vitamin and trace mineral content, be optimally formulated. Key vitamins and minerals for optimal immune function include vitamins A, C, E, and the B-complex vitamins, copper (Cu), zinc (Zn), magnesium (Mg), manganese (Mn), iron (Fe), and selenium (Se). The balance of these constituents is especially important since an excess or deficiency in one component may influence the availability or requirement for another (Tengerdy 1986).

It is difficult to predict the optimal diet for immune function. There is very little research data in this area for swine. The dietary requirements for optimal immune function may differ from the requirements to avoid deficiencies as judged by traditional methods. Relatively slight imbalances of a particular nutrient may suppress immune function, whereas a more severe deficiency must occur before the classical clinical evidence of deficiency of that nutrient is recognized. In addition, stress or the demands of rapid growth may change dietary requirements for optimal immune function.

Dietary and injectable vitamin E and Se have been evaluated for their influence on antibody levels in young pigs. Dietary vitamin E supplementation increased the antibody response to *E. coli* (Ellis and Vorhies 1976). Supplemental (dietary or injectable) vitamin E and/or Se treatment in pigs beginning at 4–5 weeks of age increased their antibody response to sheep RBCs (Peplowski et al. 1981). Dietary vitamin E and Se also increased the blastogenic response of pig lymphocytes to phytohemagglutinin (Larsen and Tollersrud 1981).

Other investigators demonstrated that injection of sows with vitamin E and/or Se at day 100 of gestation resulted in increased serum IgG concentrations in their piglets at 2 weeks postpartum (but not at 20 hours or 4 weeks postpartum) (Hayek et al. 1989). In contrast, other studies found no influence of dietary vitamin E or Se on the im-

mune response of young pigs (Blodgett et al. 1986; Kornegay et al. 1986).

Immunotoxic Substances. In other species, various compounds, including heavy metals, industrial chemicals, pesticides, and mycotoxins, have been shown to be immunosuppressive at very low levels of exposure. These compounds may be detrimental to the immune system and predispose animals to infectious diseases at levels that do not cause other symptoms of toxicity (Koller 1979). Very little immunotoxicology research has been conducted in swine. Aflatoxin in the feed of young pigs has been shown to impair immunity to erysipelas, to enhance the severity of clinical signs due to salmonellosis, and to enhance susceptibility to an oral inoculation with *Serpulina hyodysenteriae* (Cysewski et al. 1978; Miller et al. 1978; Joens et al. 1981).

IMMUNOMODULATION. Immunomodulators are a new form of preventive or therapeutic treatment that show promise for enhancing immune function, thereby increasing resistance to infectious diseases in domestic animals (Blecha 1988). Immunomodulators, also referred to as biologic-response modifiers, can be divided into two categories: endogenous immunomodulators, which are cytokines that are normally produced by the host and are products of the host genome; and exogenous immunomodulators, which are not products of the mammalian genome. The exogenous immunomodulators include bacteria, bacterial derivatives, and pharmacologic compounds, which tend to act either by inducing the release of endogenous immunomodulators or by a direct pharmacologic affect on cells of the immune system.

Advances in protein chemistry and recombinant DNA technology have made possible the production of endogenous immunomodulators in large quantities and of high purity. Endogenous immunomodulators that have been produced in quantities sufficient for in vivo testing include interleukin-2, alpha interferon, gamma interferon, tumor necrosis factor, granulocyte-macrophage colony-stimulating factor, granulocyte colony-stimulating factor, and several peptide hormones from the thymus. There are species differences in these cytokines; however, a cytokine from one species will sometimes work in a different species. The cytokines listed above have all been produced from human and bovine genes. The only porcine recombinant cytokine for which published information is available at the time of this writing is apparently gamma interferon (Charley et al. 1988; Esparza et al. 1988). It has been shown to have antiviral activity in vitro. The technology is readily available to produce the other cytokines if research in other species indicates that they may be useful for therapy or prophylaxis of infectious disease.

Levamisole has been shown to be an immuno-potentiating agent in pigs and other species (Blecha 1988). However, its efficacy is dependent on the physiologic status of the animal, the dosage used, and the time of administration. It has had its greatest activity in stressed or immuno-compromised animals.

Levamisole (1.5 mg/animal, subcutaneously or intramuscularly) given to 5-week-old or 4-month-old pigs at the time of primary and secondary injection with sheep RBCs increased the secondary antibody response to the RBCs. The primary antibody response was not increased (Reyero et al. 1979).

Levamisole and isoprinosine have been evaluated for their ability to reverse the defects observed in lymphocyte blastogenesis and delayed-type hypersensitivity responses in artificially reared piglets (Hennessy et al. 1987). Levamisole (2 mg, subcutaneously) was administered at 5 and 10 days of age. Isoprinosine (75 mg/kg per day) was administered orally from day 0 to day 10 to a different group of pigs. Both levamisole and isoprinosine enhanced the responses in the artificially reared pigs to values comparable to those of sow-reared controls. It has not been demonstrated that the effects observed with either levamisole or isoprinosine would translate into a clinically observable benefit in pigs.

Polyinosinic/polycytidylic acid (poly IC) has been shown to be an effective interferon inducer in swine (Vengris and Mare 1972; Gainer and Guarnieri 1985; Loewen and Derbyshire 1986). Poly IC complexed with poly-L-lysine and carboxymethylcellulose (poly ICLC) was shown to be a more effective interferon inducer than poly IC alone in newborn piglets (Lesnick and Derbyshire 1988). Poly ICLC (0.5 mg/kg, intravenously) given to 2-day-old piglets induced peak serum interferon levels at 6 hours postinjection and enhanced NK cell activity at 24 hours postinjection to the levels normally found in weaned pigs. The poly ICLC delayed the onset of clinical signs from transmissible gastroenteritis (TGE) virus challenge by 24 hours; however, there was no difference in the eventual outcome of the TGE virus infection (Lesnick and Derbyshire 1988). Recombinant bovine alpha-1 interferon, when administered orally to piglets, also failed to influence the course of TGE virus infection (MacLachlan and Anderson 1986).

Recombinant human IL-2 has been shown to be biologically active in pigs (Charley and Fradelizi 1987; Bhagyam et al. 1988). It has been shown to increase the antibody response when administered at the time of vaccination with either an *Actinobacillus pleuropneumoniae* bacterin or a pseudorabies virus subunit vaccine. Upon subsequent infectious challenge the pigs given IL-2 at the time of vaccination had improved resistance to *A. pleuropneumoniae* infection but not to pseudorabies virus infection (Anderson et al. 1987; Kawashima and Platt 1989).

GENERAL PRINCIPLES OF VACCINATION.

For nearly 100 years scientists have known that animals may develop immunity to diseases if exposed to either the killed infectious agent or a live strain of the agent that has been modified so it does not cause disease. This approach led to the development of many successful vaccines in the early 1900s. However, it soon became apparent that for certain diseases this simple approach was not effective. An animal, for example, might produce antibody in response to vaccination but still develop the disease. These are diseases for which circulating antibody alone is not protective or for which the vaccines do not induce antibody against the important antigens of the pathogen. The challenge for these diseases is to understand the basis for successful immunity, then to develop vaccines that induce this type of immunity.

The basic types of immune defense mechanisms against infectious agents (as discussed earlier in this chapter) are (a) native defense mechanisms, the first line of defense and already operational, even in the nonvaccinated animal; (b) humoral immunity, due to the presence of antibodies in the bloodstream; (c) cell-mediated immunity, caused by the action of various types of white blood cells and orchestrated by T lymphocytes; (d) the secretory IgA system, important for resistance to diseases at mucosal surfaces such as the gastrointestinal tract, the respiratory tract, the mammary gland, and the reproductive tract.

It is apparent that different diseases require different types of immunity for protection and the type of vaccine (modified live versus killed), route of administration, and type of adjuvant make a difference in the type of immune response. General principles regarding vaccine efficacy and vaccine failure will be discussed here. It must be remembered that there are exceptions to these general principles for specific vaccines and specific diseases. Information regarding protective immunity and vaccination for specific diseases may be found in later chapters of this book.

Selective Induction of Different Types of Immunity.

It is relatively easy to develop a vaccine that will cause the production of IgG and IgM antibodies in the bloodstream. However, the vaccine may not induce antibodies against the important antigens of the infectious agent. Antibody alone is not capable of killing infectious agents. The presence of circulating IgG and IgM may help to control disease by (a) agglutinating infectious agents, thereby reducing the number of infectious particles (for viruses) and facilitating removal by phagocytosis; (b) binding to and neutralizing toxins; (c) binding to the infectious agent and blocking attachment to cell surfaces; (d) binding to the infectious agent and initiating the classical pathway of complement activation; (e) opsonizing infectious agents and facilitating phagocytosis; (f) mediating attachment of cytotoxic cells to the surface of infected cells so the infected cells may be destroyed by antibody-dependent cell-mediated cytotoxicity. Some disease-causing organisms, however, are resistant to control by these activities of circulating antibody. These organisms must be controlled by the cell-mediated immune system or the secretory IgA system. It is more difficult to develop a safe and effective vaccine that induces these types of immunity.

Protecting the animal from infection at mucosal surfaces such as the intestinal tract, respiratory tract, mammary glands, and reproductive tract is especially difficult for the immune system. The antibodies responsible for humoral immunity and the white blood cells responsible for cell-mediated immunity are found in the bloodstream and in the tissues to some extent but not on some mucosal surfaces. Therefore, they can help to prevent invasion through the mucosal surface; however, they are not very effective at controlling infection on the mucosal surface. Even in the lung and the mammary gland, where IgG and white blood cells are found in relative abundance, they are not able to function as effectively as in the bloodstream and tissues. Protection on mucosal surfaces is due in large part to secretory IgA, which is secreted onto mucosal surfaces where it may bind to mucus and be present in fairly high concentration. Secretory IgA is resistant to destruction by the proteolytic enzymes on mucosal surfaces that are capable of breaking down IgG and IgM.

The nature of the vaccine and the route of administration are important for influencing the type of immunity induced. Subcutaneous or intramuscular injection of a killed vaccine will stimulate the immune system to produce IgM and IgG classes of antibody. However, there is very little production of IgA to protect the mucosal surfaces. In addition, the killed vaccines are not very effective at inducing cell-mediated immunity.

The induction of cell-mediated immunity generally requires a modified live vaccine capable of replicating in the animal or a killed vaccine with a highly effective adjuvant. Adjuvants that have traditionally been used in animal vaccines are not very effective at inducing cell-mediated immunity. New adjuvants are being developed that show promise for inducing cell-mediated immunity using killed vaccines. There are killed vaccines that have been available for many years and have been effective in controlling certain systemic-type diseases, which are generally diseases that can be controlled by the presence of circulating IgG.

The route of vaccine administration is important when attempting to induce mucosal immunity. To get secretory IgA produced at mucosal surfaces, it is best for the vaccine to enter the body through exposure to a mucosal surface. This can be accomplished by feeding the vaccine to the animal, aerosolizing the vaccine so it will be inhaled by the animal, or intramammary exposure. If a sow is exposed to an infectious agent in her intestinal tract, she may respond by producing secretory IgA not only in her own intestinal tract, but also in her mammary gland. The sow passes the IgA against the infectious agent to the piglet when it suckles. Therefore, secretory IgA in the sow's milk can protect the piglet from infectious agents present in the sow's intestine. This protection will only last as long as the piglet continues to suckle. Enteric infections by many organisms are not controlled by the presence of IgG and IgM in the bloodstream or by cell-mediated immunity. If a modified live vaccine is given by injection, but goes to a mucosal surface to replicate, it may also induce a secretory IgA response.

Vaccination Failure. There are many reasons why animals may develop disease even though they have been vaccinated. Disease may occur because (a) the animal may have been incubating the disease when it was vaccinated; (b) something may have happened to the vaccine to make it ineffective; (c) the physiologic status of the host may make it unresponsive or hyporesponsive to the vaccine; or (d) the host may be exposed to an overwhelming challenge dose of infectious agent. By being aware of these factors, veterinarians and producers can help to minimize the occurrence of vaccine failures.

OCCURRENCE OF DISEASE SHORTLY AFTER VACCINATION. The host requires several days after vaccination before an effective immune response will develop. If the animal encounters an infectious agent near the time of vaccination, the vaccine will not have had time to induce immunity. The animal may come down with clinical disease resulting in an apparent vaccination failure. In this situation, disease symptoms will appear shortly after vaccination and may be mistakenly attributed to vaccine virus causing the disease. Modified live vaccine viruses have been attenuated to reduce virulence. The attenuation must be shown to be stable, therefore, reversion to virulence is thought to be a rare event. However, the attenuated vaccine strains may be capable of producing disease in immunosuppressed animals.

ALTERATIONS IN THE VACCINE. Improperly handled and administered vaccines may fail to induce the expected immune response in normal, healthy animals. Modified live bacterial and viral vaccines are effective only if the agent in the vaccine is viable and able to replicate in the vaccinated animal. Observing proper storage conditions and proper methods of administration are very important for maintaining vaccine viability. Failure to store the vaccine at refrigerator temperatures or exposure to light may inactivate the vaccine; even when stored under appropriate conditions, the vaccine loses viability over time. Therefore, vaccines that are past their expiration dates should not be used. Chemical disinfectant residues on syringes and needles can inactivate modified live vaccines. The use of improper diluent or the mixing of vaccines in a single syringe may also inactivate modified live vaccines. Diluent for lyophilized vaccines are formulated specifically for each vaccine. A diluent that is appropriate for one vaccine may inactivate a different vaccine. Some vaccines and diluents contain preservatives that may inactivate other modified live vaccines. For these reasons, multiple vaccines should not be mixed in a single syringe unless that particular combination has been adequately tested to insure there is no interference.

HOST FACTORS CONTRIBUTING TO VACCINE FAILURE. Vaccine failures may occur because a vaccinated animal is not able to respond appropriately to the vaccine. Vaccine failure in young animals may be due to the presence of maternal antibody, which prevents adequate response to vaccination. It can also be due to immunosuppression from a variety of causes.

Maternal antibodies derived from colostrum are a well-known cause of vaccine failure. These antibodies in the piglets' circulation may neutralize or remove the antigen before it can induce an immune response. Typically, virulent infectious agents are capable of breaking through maternal immunity earlier than modified live or killed vaccines. This means that even if young animals are immunized frequently, there still is a period when they are vulnerable to infection. Vulnerability occurs between the time that young animals lose their maternal antibody and before they develop their own active immune response. This period can be shortened by the use of less-attenuated modified live vaccines or the use of killed vaccines with high antigenic mass. A high challenge dose of infectious agents will break through maternal immunity sooner than low exposure to infectious agents; therefore, overcrowding and poor sanitation exacerbate the problem of inducing immunity in young animals before they come down with clinical disease.

Veterinarians commonly recommend that puppies and kittens be vaccinated every 3 weeks between approximately 6 and 18 weeks of age to minimize the period of vulnerability to infectious diseases. However, for large domestic animals, a single vaccination is commonly recommended to induce immunity during the first few weeks or months of life. There is no inherent difference between large and small domestic animals in their response to vaccination in the face of maternal immunity.

Because only one vaccination is commonly recommended for large domestic animals, the timing of the vaccination is important. If the vaccine is administered too soon, it may be ineffective because of the presence of maternal antibody. If the vaccine is administered after all maternal antibodies are gone from animals in the herd, there may be a prolonged period of vulnerability before they develop their own immune response. Most

veterinarians and producers decide that because of time and expense considerations, it is impractical to vaccinate young pigs frequently. However, frequent vaccination may be justified in cases of unusually high incidence of disease.

Immunosuppression due to a variety of factors including stress, malnutrition, concurrent infection, or immaturity or senescence of the immune system may also lead to vaccination failure. If the immunosuppression occurs at the time of vaccination, the vaccine may fail to induce an adequate immune response. If the immunosuppression occurs sometime after vaccination, then disease may occur due to reduced immunity in spite of an adequate response to the original vaccine. This may also occur due to therapy with immunosuppressive drugs (e.g., glucocorticoids).

Another concern is that some modified live vaccines are capable of inducing disease in the immunosuppressed animal. Modified live vaccines are tested for safety in normal, healthy animals and thus are not recommended for use in animals with compromised immune systems. Therefore, these vaccines should not be used in animals that are immunosuppressed for any reason, including animals in the first few weeks of life unless the vaccine has been specifically tested in animals this young. When it is necessary to vaccinate animals under these conditions, killed vaccines should be used.

OVERWHELMING CHALLENGE DOSE. Most vaccines do not produce complete immunity to disease but provide an increased ability to resist challenge by infectious agents. If a high challenge dose of organisms is present due to overcrowding or poor sanitation, the immune system may be overwhelmed, resulting in clinical disease.

Vaccine Efficacy. Vaccines that are licensed by the USDA have been tested to determine that they are safe and effective. However, "effective" is a relative term. It does not mean that the vaccine must be able to induce complete immunity under all conditions that may be found in the field. This would not be realistic since the immune system is not capable of such potent protection under adverse conditions.

To be federally licensed, the vaccine must be tested under controlled experimental conditions. The vaccinated group must have significantly less disease than the nonvaccinated control group. This testing is typically done on healthy, non-stressed animals under good environmental conditions, with a controlled exposure to a single infectious agent. Vaccines may be much less effective when used in animals that are under stress, incubating other infectious diseases, or exposed to a high dose of infectious agents due to overcrowding or poor sanitation.

It is important to remember that for most diseases the relationship between the infectious agent and the host is sufficiently complicated that vaccination cannot be expected to provide complete protection. However, the vaccine can increase the animals resistance to disease, but this resistance can be overwhelmed if good management practices are not followed.

REFERENCES

ALLEN, W. D., AND PORTER, P. 1973. Localization by immunofluorescence of secretory component and IgA in the intestinal mucosa of the young pig. Immunology 24:365.

ANDERSON, G.; URBAN, O.; FEDORKA-CRAY, P.; NEWELL, A.; NUNBERG, J.; AND DOYLE, M. 1987. Interleukin-2 and protective immunity in *Haemophilus pleuropneumoniae:* Preliminary studies. Vaccines 87:22–25.

BARRATT, M. E. J. 1972. Immediate hypersensitivity to *Metastrongylus* spp. infection in the pig. Immunology 22:601–623.

BARTA, O., AND HUBBERT, N. L. 1978. Testing of hemolytic complement components in domestic animals. Am J Vet Res 39(8):1303–1308.

BELLAMY, J. E. C., AND NIELSEN, N. O. 1974. Immune-mediated emigration of neutrophils into the lumen of the small intestine. Infect Immun 9(4):615–619.

BHAGYAM, R. C.; JARRETT-ZACZEK, D.; AND FERGUSON, F. G. 1988. Activation of swine peripheral blood lymphocytes with human recombinant interleukin-2. Immunology 64:607–613.

BHOGAL, B. S.; NAGY, L. K.; AND WALKER, P. D. 1987. Neutrophil mediated and IgA dependent antibacterial immunity against enteropathogenic *Escherichia coli* in the porcine intestinal mucosa. Vet Immunol Immunopathol 14:23–44.

BINNS, R. M.; PABST, R.; AND LICENCE, S. T. 1986. The behavior of pig lymphocyte populations in vivo. Swine Biomed Res 3:1837–1853.

BLALOCK, J. E.; HARBOUR-MCMENAMIN, D.; and SMITH, E. M. 1985. Peptide hormones shared by the neuroendocrine and immunologic systems. J Immunol 135:858–861s.

BLECHA, F. 1988. Immunomodulation: A means of disease prevention in stressed livestock. J Anim Sci 66:2084–2090.

BLECHA, F., AND KELLEY, K. W. 1981. Effects of cold and weaning stressors on the antibody-mediated immune response of pigs. J Anim Sci 53(2):439–447.

BLECHA, F.; POLLMANN, D. S.; AND NICHOLS, D. A. 1983. Weaning pigs at an early age decreases cellular immunity. J Anim Sci 56(2):396–400.

_____. 1985. Immunologic reactions of pigs regrouped at or near weaning. Am J Vet Res 46(9):1934–1937.

BLECHA, F.; POLLMANN, D. S.; AND KLUBER, III, E. F. 1986. Decreased mononuclear cell response to mitogens in artificially reared neonatal pigs. Can J Vet Res 50:522–525.

BLODGETT, D. J.; SCHURIG, G. G.; AND KORNEGAY, E. T. 1986. Immunomodulation in weanling swine with dietary selenium. Am J Vet Res 47:1517–1519.

BREAZILE, J. E. 1987. Physiologic basis and consequences of distress in animals. J Am Vet Med Assoc 191:1212–1215.

BUTLER, J. E.; KLOBASA, F.; AND WERHAHN, E. 1981. The differential localizations of IgA, IgM, and IgG in the gut of suckled neonatal piglets. Vet Immunol Immunopathol 2:53–65.

CHARLEY, B. 1983. Interaction of influenza virus with swine alveolar macrophages: Influence of anti-virus antibodies and cytochalasin B. Ann Virol 134(E):51–59.

CHARLEY, B., AND FRADELIZI, D. 1987. Differential effects of human and porcine interleukin 2 on natural killing (NK) activity of newborn piglets and adult pigs lymphocytes. Ann Rech Vet 18:227–232.

CHARLEY, B.; MCCULLOUGH, K.; AND MARTINOD, S. 1988. Antiviral and antigenic properties of recombinant porcine interferon gamma. Vet Immunol Immunopathol 19:95–103.

CHEVILLE, N. F.; MENGELING, W. L.; AND ZINOBER, M. R. 1970. Ultrastructural and immunofluorescent studies of glomerulonephritis in chronic hog cholera. Lab Invest 22(5):458–467.

CURTIS, J., AND BOURNE, F. J. 1971. Immunoglobulin quantitation in sow serum, colostrum and milk and the serum of young pigs. Biochim Biophys Acta 236:319–332.

CYSEWSKI, S. J.; WOOD, R. L.; PIER, A. C.; AND BAETZ, A. L. 1978. Effects of aflatoxin on the development of acquired immunity to swine erysipelas. Am J Vet Res 39(3):445–448.

DIMMOCK, C. K.; WEBSTER, W. R.; SHIELS, I. A.; AND EDWARDS, C. L. 1982. Isoimmune thrombocytopenic purpura in piglets. Aust Vet J 59:157–159.

DUNCAN, I. A.; BINNS, R. M.; AND DUFFUS, W. P. H. 1989. The null T cell in pig blood is not an NK cell. Immunol 68:392–395.

DUNN, A. J. 1988. Nervous system–immune system interactions: An overview. J Receptor Res 8:589–607.

ELLIS, R. P., AND VORHIES, M. W. 1976. Effect of supplemental dietary vitamin E on the serologic response of swine to an *Escherichia coli* bacterin. J Am Vet Med Assoc 168(3):231–232.

ESPARZA, I.; GONZALEZ, J. C.; AND VINUELA, E. 1988. Effect of interferon alpha, interferon gamma and tumor necrosis factor on African swine fever virus replication in porcine monocytes and macrophages. J Gen Virol 69:2973–2980.

EYRE, P. 1980. Pharmacological aspects of hypersensitivity in domestic animals: A review. Vet Res Commun 4:83–98.

FERGUSON, F. G.; PINTO, A. J.; CONFER, F. L.; AND BOTTICELLI, G. 1986. Characteristics of Yorkshire swine natural killer cells. Swine Biomed Res 3:1915–1924.

FRANEK, F., AND RIHA, I. 1964. Purification and structural characterization of 5S gamma globulin in newborn pigs. Immunochemistry 1:49.

FUENTES, M., AND PIJOAN, C. 1986. Phagocytosis and intracellular killing of *Pasteurella multocida* by porcine alveolar macrophages after infection with pseudorabies virus. Vet Immunol Immunopathol 13:165–172.

_____. 1987. Pneumonia in pigs induced by intranasal challenge exposure with pseudorabies virus and *Pasteurella multocida.* Am J Vet Res 48(10):1446–1448.

GAINER, J. H., AND GUARNIERI, J. 1985. Effects of poly I:C on porcine iron-deficient neutropenia. Cornell Vet 75:454–465.

GRIFFIN, J. F. T. 1989. Stress and immunity: A unifying concept. Vet Immunol Immunopathol 20:263–312.

HALPERN, M. S., AND KOSHLAND, M. E. 1970. Novel subunit in secretory IgA. Nature 228:1276.

HAMMERBERG, C.; SCHURIG, G. G.; AND OCHS, D. L. 1989. Immunodeficiency in young pigs. Am J Vet Res 50(6):868–874.

HARDING, M. J., AND MOLITOR, T. W. 1988. Porcine parvovirus: Replication in and inhibition of selected cellular functions of swine alveolar macrophages and peripheral blood lymphocytes. Arch Virol 101:105–117.

HAYEK, M. G.; MITCHELL, G. E. , JR.; HARMON, R. J.; STAHLY, T S.; CROMWELL, G. L.; TUCKER, R. E.; AND BARKER, K. B. 1989. Porcine immunoglobulin transfer after prepartum treatment with selenium or vitamin E. J Anim Sci 67:1299–1306.

HENNESSY, K. J.; BLECHA, F.; POLLMANN, D. S.; AND KLUBER, E. F. 1987. Isoprinosine and levamisole immunomodulation in artificially reared neonatal pigs. Am J Vet Res 48:477–480.

HILL, I. R., AND PORTER, P. 1974. Studies of bactericidal activity to *Escherichia coli* of porcine serum and colostral immunoglobulins and the role of lysozyme with secretory IgA. Immunol 26:1239–1250.

IGLESIAS, G.; PIJOAN, C.; AND MOLITOR, T. 1989a. Interactions of pseudorabies virus with swine alveolar macrophages I: Virus replication. Arch Virol 104:107–115.

————. 1989b. Interactions of pseudorabies virus with swine alveolar macrophages: Effects of virus infection on cell functions. J Leuk Biol 45:410–415.

JOENS, L. A.; PIER, A. C.; AND CUTLIP, R. C. 1981. Effects of aflatoxin consumption on the clinical course of swine dysentery. Am J Vet Res 42(7):1170–1172.

KAWASHIMA, K., AND PLATT, K. B. 1989. The effect of human recombinant interleukin-2 on the porcine immune response to a pseudorabies virus subunit vaccine. Vet Immunol Immunopathol 22:345–353.

KELLEY, K. W. 1985. Immunological consequences of changing environmental stimuli. In Animal Stress. Ed. G. P. Moberg. Bethesda, Md.: American Physiological Society, pp. 193–223.

————. 1988. Cross-talk between the immune and endocrine systems. J Anim Sci 66:2095–2108.

KIM, Y. B., AND ICHIMURA, O. 1986. Porcine natural killer (NK)/killer (K) cell system. Swine Biomed Res 3:1811–1819.

KIM, Y. B.; BRADLEY, S. G.; AND WATSON, D. W. 1966. Ontogeny of the immune response. I. Development of immunoglobulins in germfree and conventional colostrum-deprived piglets. J Immunol 97:52–63.

KOLLER, L. D. 1979. Effects of environmental contaminants on the immune system. Adv Vet Sci Comp Med 23:267–295.

KORNEGAY, E. T.; MELDRUM, J. B.; SCHURIG, G.; LINDEMANN, M. D.; AND GWAZDAUSKAS, F. C. 1986. Lack of influence of nursery temperature on the response of weanling pigs to supplemental vitamins C and E. J Anim Sci 63:484–491.

LARSEN, H. J., AND TOLLERSRUD, S. 1981. Effect of dietary vitamin E and selenium on the phytohaemagglutinin response of pig lymphocytes. Res Vet Sci 31:301–305.

LECCE, J. G.; MATRONE, G.; AND MORGAN, D. O. 1961. Porcine neonatal nutrition: Absorption of unaltered porcine proteins and polyvinyl pyrrolidone from the gut of piglets. J Nutr 73:158.

LESNICK, C. E., AND DERBYSHIRE, J. B. 1988. Activation of natural killer cells in newborn piglets by interferon induction. Vet Immunol Immunopathol 18:109–117.

LI, D. F.; NELSSEN, J. L.; REDDY, P. G.; BLECHA, F.; HANCOCK, J. D.; ALLEE, G. L.; GOODBAND, R. D.; AND KLEMM, R. D. 1990. Transient hypersensitivity to soybean meal in the early-weaned pig. J Anim Sci 68:1790–1799.

LIE, H. 1968. Thrombocytopenic purpura in baby pigs. Acta Vet Scand 9:285–301.

LINKLATER, K. A. 1972. Iso-antibodies to red cell antigens in pigs' sera 3. The effect of maternal red cell iso-antibodies on the red cells of piglets. Anim Blood Groups Biochem Genet 3:77–84.

LINKLATER, K. A.; McTAGGART, H. S.; and IMLAH, P. 1973. Haemolytic disease of the newborn, thrombocytopenic purpura and neutropenia occurring concurrently in a litter of piglets. Br Vet J 129:36–46.

LOEWEN, K. G., AND DERBYSHIRE, J. B. 1986. Interferon induction with polyinosinic:polycytidylic acid in the newborn piglet. Can J Vet Res 50:232–237.

LOFSTEDT, J.; ROTH, J. A.; ROSS, R. F.; AND WAGNER, W. C. 1983. Depression of polymorphonuclear leukocyte function associated with experimentally induced *Escherichia coli* mastitis in sows. Am J Vet Res 44(7):1224–1228.

LUNNEY, J. K., AND PESCOVITZ, M. D. 1987. Phenotypic and functional characterization of pig lymphocyte populations. Vet Immunol Immunopathol 17:135–144.

MacLACHLAN, N. J., AND ANDERSON, K. P. 1986. Effect of recombinant DNA-derived bovine alpha-1 interferon on transmissible gastroenteritis virus infection in swine. Am J Vet Res 47(5):1149–1152.

MESTECKY, J.; ZIKAN, J.; AND BUTLER, W. T. 1971. Immunoglobulin M and secretory immunoglobulin A: Presence of a common polypeptide chain different from light chains. Science 171:1163.

METZGER, J. J., AND FOUGEREAU, M. 1968. Caracterisations biochimiques des immunoglobulines gamma-G et gamma-M porcines. Rech Vet 1:37.

MILLER, D. M.; STUART, B. P.; AND CROWELL, W. A. 1978. Aflatoxicosis in swine: Its effect on immunity and relationship to salmonellosis. Proc Annu Meet Am Assoc Vet Lab Diagn pp. 135–146.

NIELSEN, K. H. 1977. Bovine reaginic antibody III. Cross-reaction of antihuman IgE and antibovine reaginic immunoglobulin antisera with sera from several species of mammals. Can J Comp Med 41:345–348.

NORDSTOGA, K. 1965. Thrombocytopenic purpura in baby pigs caused by maternal isoimmunization. Pathol Vet 2:601–610.

NORLEY, S. G., AND WARDLEY, R. C. 1983a. Investigation of porcine natural-killer cell activity with reference to African swine fever virus infection. Immunol 49:593–597.

————. 1983b. Effector mechanisms in the pig. Antibody-dependent cellular cytolysis of African swine fever virus infected cells. Res Vet Sci 35:75–79.

OHGAMI, M.; DOERSCHUK, C. M.; ENGLISH, D.; DODEK, P. M.; AND HOGG, J. C. 1989. Kinetics of radiolabeled neutrophils in swine. J Appl Physiol 66:1881–1885.

OSBURN, B. I.; MacLACHLAN, N. J.; AND TERRELL, T. G. 1982. Ontogeny of the immune system. J Am Vet Med Assoc 181(10):1049–1052.

PABST, R., AND BINNS, R. M. 1986. Comparison of lymphocyte production and migration in pig lymph nodes, tonsils, spleen, bone marrow and thymus. Swine Biomed Res 3:1865–1871.

PEPLOWSKI, M. A.; MAHAN, D. C.; MURRAY, F. A.; MOXON, A. L.; CANTOR, A. H.; AND EKSTROM, K. E. 1981. Effect of dietary and injectable vitamin E and selenium in weanling swine antigenically challenged with sheep red blood cells. J Anim Sci 51:344–351.

PIJOAN, C., AND OCHOA, G. 1978. Interaction between a hog cholera vaccine strain and *Pasteurella multocida* in the production of porcine pneumonia. J Comp Pathol 88:167–170.

PORTER, P. 1969. Transfer of immunoglobulins IgG, IgA and IgM to lacteal secretions in the parturient sow and their absorption by the neonatal piglet. Biochim Biophys Acta 181:381–392.

————. 1973. Studies of porcine secretory IgA and its component chains in relation to intestinal absorption of colostral immunoglobulins by the neonatal pig. Immunol 24:163–176.

————. 1986. Immune System. In Diseases of Swine. Ed. A. D. Leman, B. Straw, R. D. Glock, W. L. Mengeling, R. H. C. Penny, and E. Scholl. Ames: The Iowa State Univ Press, p. 44.

PORTER, P., and ALLEN, W. D. 1972. Classes of immunoglobulins related to immunity in the pig. J Am Vet Med Assoc 160:511.

REYERO, C.; STÖCKL, W.; AND THALHAMMER, J. G.

1979. Stimulation of the antibody response to sheep red blood cells in piglets and young pigs by levamisole. Br Vet J 135:17–24.

RICE, C. E., AND L'ECUYER, C. 1963. Complement titres of naturally and artificially raised piglets. Can J Comp Med Vet Sci 27:157–161.

SALMON, H. 1986. Surface markers of swine lymphocytes: Application to the study of local immune system of mammary gland and transplanted gut. Swine Biomed Res 3:1855–1864.

————. 1987. The intestinal and mammary immune system in pigs. Vet Immunol Immunopathol 17:367–388.

SAUNDERS, C. N., AND KINCH, D. A. 1968. Thrombocytopenic purpura of pigs. J Comp Pathol 78:513–523.

SELLWOOD, R.; HALL, G.; AND ANGER, H. 1986. Emigration of polymorphonuclear leukocytes into the intestinal lumen of the neonatal piglet in response to challenge with K88-positive *Escherichia coli.* Res Vet Sci 40:128–135.

SHIROTA, K.; KOYAMA, R.; AND NOMURA, Y. 1986. Glomerulopathy in swine: Microscopic lesions and IgG or C3 deposition in 100 pigs. Jpn J Vet Sci 48(1):15–21.

SMITH, I. M.; HODGES, R. T.; BETTS, A. O.; AND HAYWARD, A. H. S. 1973. Experimental infections of gnotobiotic piglets with *Pasteurella septica* (sero-group A) alone or with *Mycoplasma hyopneumoniae.* J Comp Pathol 83:307–321.

SPEER, V. C.; BROWN, H.; QUINN, L.; AND CATRON, D. V. 1959. The cessation of antibody absorption in the young pig. Immunol 83:632.

STERTZL, J.; KOSTKA, J.; RIHA, I.; AND MANDEL, I. 1960. Attempts to determine the formation and character of globulin and of natural and immune antibodies in young pigs reared without colostrum. Folia Microbiol 5:29.

STOKES, C., AND BOURNE, J. F. 1989. Mucosal immunity. In Veterinary Clinical Immunology. Ed. R. E. W. Halliwell and N. T. Gorman. Philadelphia: W. B. Saunders, p. 164.

STOKES, C. R.; MILLER, B. G.; BAILEY, M.; WILSON, A. D.; AND BOURNE, F. J. 1987. The immune response to dietary antigens and its influence on disease susceptibility in farm animals. Vet Immunol Immunopathol 17:413–423.

TENGERDY, R. P. 1986. Nutrition, immunity and disease resistance. (Proc 6th Int Conf Prod Dis in Farm Anim, Sept. 1986, Belfast, Northern Ireland), p. 175.

THOMLINSON, J. R., AND BUXTON, A. 1963. Anaphylaxis in pigs and its relationship to the pathogenesis of oedema disease and gastro-enteritis associated with *Escherichia coli.* Immunology 6:126–139.

TYLER, J. W.; CULLOR, J. S.; OSBURN, B. I.; AND PARKER, K. 1988. Age-related variations in serum concentrations of the third component of complement in swine. Am J Vet Res 49(7):1104–1106.

TYLER, J. W.; CULLOR, J. S.; DOUGLAS, V. L.; PARKER, K. M.; AND SMITH, W. L. 1989. Ontogeny of the third component of complement in neonatal swine. Am J Vet Res 50(7):1141–1144.

VENGRIS, V. E., AND MARE, C. J. 1972. Swine interferon. II. Induction in pigs with viral and synthetic inducers. Can J Comp Med 36:288–293.

WARDLEY, R. C., AND WILKINSON, P. J. 1980. Lymphocyte responses to African swine fever virus infection. Res Vet Sci 28:185–189.

WARDLEY, R. C.; HAMILTON, F.; AND WILKINSON, P. J. 1979. The replication of virulent and attenuated strains of African swine fever virus in porcine macrophages. Arch Virol 61:217–225.

WESTLY, H. J., AND KELLEY, K. W. 1984. Physiologic concentrations of cortisol suppress cell-mediated immune events in the domestic pig (41926). Proc Soc Exp Biol Med 177:156–164.

YANG, W. C., AND SCHULTZ, R. D. 1986. Ontogeny of natural killer cell activity and antibody-dependent cell-mediated cytotoxicity in pigs. Dev Comp Immunol 10:405–418.

YEN, J. T., AND POND, W. G. 1987. Effect of dietary supplementation with vitamin C or carbadox on weanling pigs subjected to crowding stress. J Anim Sci 64:1672–1681.

ZARKOWER, A.; ESKEW, M. L.; SCHEUCHENZUBER, W. J.; FERGUSON, F. G.; AND CONFER, F. 1982. Antibody-dependent cell-mediated cytotoxicity in pigs. Am J Vet Res 43(9):1590–1593.

4 Mammary Glands and Lactation Problems

B. B. Smith

G. Martineau

A. Bisaillon

INADEQUATE milk production in the postpartum sow is the result of an ill-defined complex of problems. Due to the multiple etiologies associated with insufficient lactation in the sow, clinical evaluation and therapeutic management of these problems necessitate an understanding of the normal anatomy and physiology of lactation, topics covered in the first portion of this chapter. The second section of the chapter discusses the varied clinical presentations associated with lactation problems, examines the etiologies that have been associated with decreased milk production, and outlines prevention and treatment options.

ANATOMY OF THE MAMMARY GLANDS. The mammary glands of swine are located in two parallel rows along the ventral body wall, from the thoracic region to the inguinal area. The nonlactating glands are much smaller than the lactating ones (Schummer et al. 1981). The glands are attached to the ventral body wall by adipose and connective tissue arising from the abdominal fascia. Elastic and connective tissue sheets envelop each glandular complex and form the basic framework in which the glandular parenchyma is embedded. There are usually 1 or 2 pairs of thoracic, 4 pairs of abdominal, and 1 pair of inguinal glands, a total of 6 or 7 mammary glands per side. The most cranial pair of glands lies slightly caudal to the thoracic limbs, while the most caudal pair is located between the pelvic limbs. Schmidt (1971) stated that over 95% of the pigs examined possessed 10–14 glands, while Turner (1952) discussed the variation in number and symmetry of gland placement in pigs.

Each mammary gland normally has one slightly wrinkled teat (papilla) or nipple. Depending on the functional status of the glands, the teats are low, blunt-conical, or cylindrical elevations between 2.0 and 3.5 cm in length and located on the ventral body of the glands. With the exception of the last pair of teats, the space between adjacent teats decreases progressively from cranial to caudal. The teats of the cranial glands also tend to be longer and more slender than caudal teats (English et al. 1982). The teats are hairless and lack sebaceous and apocrine tubular glands. Su-

pernumerary teats may occur in swine, are usually smaller than normal, and are most frequently found between the third and fourth pairs of glands, less frequently between the fourth and fifth pairs, and only occasionally between the other mammary units. Paired vestigial accessory teats not connected to glandular tissue may also occur, usually at the caudal end of the mammary chain between the thighs. In the boar they may occur on the lower cranial part of the scrotum.

Allen et al. (1959) examined the heritability of nipple numbers in Landrace, Poland, and Duroc inbred lines, and in crossbred Landrace × Poland swine and found an overall heritability of approximately 39%. A low, but significant, intrabreed correlation between nipple numbers and the size and weight of litters at farrowing and weaning was observed. In most cases, however, the significance was lost when heritability was calculated on an interbreed basis. The results indicate that, while sows can be selected for increased numbers of nipples, the improvement in litter performance will usually be slight.

The underlines of all gilts and boars should be examined during the selection of breeding stock. Boars and gilts should be retained for breeding only if they have 12–14 well-placed normal nipples. Animals with poorly defined or inverted nipples should be avoided.

Internal Structure. The microscopic and macroscopic anatomy of the mammary gland were described by Barone (1978), Schummer et al. (1981), and Calhoun and Stinson (1987) (Fig. 4.1, 4.2). In the nulliparous sow the mammary gland consists of cell buds distributed among fat and connective tissue, while in the lactating gland, the connective tissue is largely displaced by glandular parenchyma. The mammary gland is a compound tubuloalveolar gland with the secretory units comprising alveoli or acini and alveolar ducts. The alveoli develop as blunt, irregular spherical outgrowths from the side or end of the alveolar ducts. The milk-secreting units are lined by a single layer of cuboidal or low columnar epithelial cells, lactocytes, resting on a basement membrane. Myoepithelial cells are located between the basement membrane and the lactocytes of the secretory units. Lactocytes vary in height during various stages of secretory activity. The myoepithelial cells contract when stimulated by oxytocin released by the neurohypophysis and cause milk ejection into the lumen of the secretory units and into the duct system. Lobules are a group of tubuloalveolar secretory units surrounded by connective tissue. Multiple lobules and the surrounding connective tissue form lobes. Each mammary gland comprises several lobules and lobes. The connective tissue of the gland provides support for the secretory units and the duct system and contains the nerves and the blood and lymph vessels.

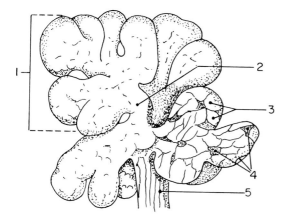

4.1. Glandular secretory units. *1.* alveolus, *2.* alveolar duct, *3.* lactocytes, *4.* myoepithelial cells, *5.* intralobular duct. (Barone 1978, with permission.)

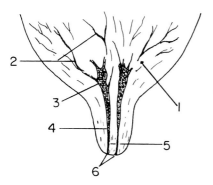

4.2. Sagittal section of one mammary gland. *1.* glandular parenchyma, *2.* lactiferous ducts, *3.* gland sinus, *4.* papillary sinus, *5.* papillary duct, *6.* papillary ostia. (Barone 1978, with permission.)

The duct system begins within a lobule as several alveolar ducts that merge into an intralobular duct, which is lined with single-layered cuboidal epithelium without secretory activity. Fusiform myoepithelial cells may be associated with intralobular ducts. In the interlobular connective tissue, the intralobular duct becomes lined with double-layered cuboidal epithelium. Smooth muscle fibers are found in the walls of these ducts. The interlobular ducts merge with other interlobular ducts to form a large lactiferous duct. The epithelial lining of the interlobular ducts continues in the large lactiferous ducts, and the smooth muscle fibers become more prominent. Several lactiferous ducts finally empty into a lactiferous sinus.

Each lactiferous sinus of the sow comprises two narrow, continuous but poorly demarcated cavities, the gland sinus (gland cistern) lying above the base of the teat, and the papillary sinus (teat sinus or teat cistern) located in the teat. Although the term cistern is used in homology to the cow, the cavities in the sow are much less capacious than in the cow. The papillary sinus opens into the 3- to 4-mm-long papillary duct (teat canal or streak canal) leading to the external surface of the teat at the papillary ostium (teat orifice). The papillary canal and sinus are not distinctly demarcated. The lactiferous sinus is lined by a double-layered cuboidal epithelium, the same as the interlobular and lactiferous ducts. Smooth muscle and elastic fibers are found in the wall of the sinus. In addition, the wall of the teat sinus contains several accessory glands. The papillary duct is lined with a stratified squamous epithelium that is continuous at the papillary ostium with the epidermis of the teat. The papillary duct is tightly closed by longitudinal folds that originate from the sinus. There is no muscular sphincter around the papillary ostium, and its closure is brought about by circularly oriented bundles of elastic fibers.

There are usually two complete gland systems within each mammary gland of the pig. Each system comprises a papillary ostium, papillary duct, papillary sinus, gland sinus, duct system, and the appurtenant glandular parenchyma. The glandular tissue of one system usually interdigitates with the other, although the other components of the two systems are independent. Sometimes three papillary sinuses and an equal number of papillary ducts and ostia are present on the apex of the teat. In these animals, one sinus ends blindly at the base of the teat and does not have glandular tissue.

Blood Circulation. The arterial and venous circulation of the mammary glands have been described by Barone (1978), Ghoshal et al. (1981), and Schummer et al. (1981). The arterial supply to the mammary glands in swine is furnished on each side of the ventral midline by a deep and a superficial network that extends longitudinally from the axillary to the inguinal regions (Fig. 4.3). The deep arterial network is formed by the internal thoracic artery; one of its terminal branches, the cranial epigastric artery; and the caudal epigastric artery. The internal thoracic artery leaves the subclavian artery and runs on the floor of the thorax in a subpleural position. Along its course, it gives off small perforating mammary branches to the thoracic mammary glands. At the level of the sixth intercostal space, the internal thoracic artery gives off the cranial epigastric artery that runs in a paramedian course toward the inguinal area. The cranial epigastric artery runs on the deep face or within the rectus abdominis muscle and ramifies in the ventral abdominal wall. Along its course, it sends several mammary branches that perforate the abdominal muscle layers and vascularize the caudal thoracic and the cranial two abdominal glands. The caudal epigastric artery originates from the pudendoepigastric trunk of the deep femoral artery. It runs cranially toward the umbilicus on the deep face of the rectus abdominis muscle. Along its course, it gives off several mammary branches to the inguinal and caudal abdominal glands. At the level of the umbilicus, the terminal branches of the caudal epigastric artery anastomose with corresponding branches of the cranial epigastric artery.

The superficial arterial network to the mammary glands is formed cranially by the lateral thoracic artery, and caudally by the caudal superficial epigastric artery. The lateral thoracic artery leaves the small external thoracic vessel, a branch of the axillary artery, and reaches a superficial position in the axillary space where it sends numerous branches to the thoracic mammary glands. The caudal superficial epigastric artery originates from the external pudendal artery as this vessel emerges from the inguinal canal. The caudal superficial epigastric artery courses toward the umbilicus where it is situated superficially on the ventral abdominal wall. It supplies the skin, the cutaneous muscles, and the superficial inguinal lymph nodes. Along its course, it also gives off several branches to the inguinal and the four abdominal mammary glands. The cranial terminal branches of the caudal superficial epigas-

tric artery may anastomose with corresponding branches of the lateral thoracic artery.

The venous drainage of the mammary complex is provided by a deep and a superficial network similar to the arterial networks. In addition to the deep and superficial satellite veins, the cranial superficial epigastric vein also returns blood from the thoracic and abdominal mammary glands. The cranial superficial epigastric vein follows a flexuous course subcutaneously along the ventrolateral abdominal wall. It passes through the abdominal muscles to join either the internal thoracic or the cranial epigastric vein and anastomoses in the inguinal area with the caudal superficial epigastric vein.

Within the mammary glands, the blood vessels are located in connective tissue septa between the lobes and lobules. Their terminal ramifications surround the alveoli of the glands, forming rich, dense capillary plexuses. Other vascular branches follow the lactiferous ducts to the lactiferous sinuses. Anastomosing rich vascular networks are also found in the walls of the teats.

Lymphatic Drainage. The lymphatic drainage of the mammary glands is bilaterally symmetrical (Fig. 4.4), as reported by Saar and Getty (1975) and by Schummer et al. (1981). The skin, excretory ducts, and parenchyma of each gland unit are drained by different but interconnected lymphatic networks. The lymphatic vessels of the skin form a superficial and a deep network. The vessels of these two coarse networks are joined together at the base of the teat, forming an annular papillary plexus. The lymphatics of the excretory duct system join the cutaneous lymphatic vessels at the base of the teat. The lymphatic vessels of the glandular parenchyma proceed from intralobular and perilobular networks, course in the connective tissue septa, and reach the base of the teat where many of these vessels join the papillary plexus. Other vessels pass directly to the base of the gland where they join large subcutaneous lymphatic channels. These channels course in company of the superficial abdominal blood vessels to their respective lymph nodes.

There are three groups of lymph nodes that receive lymph from the mammary glands of the sow: the superficial inguinal lymph nodes, the cranial sternal lymph nodes, and the ventral superficial cervical lymph nodes. The superficial inguinal lymph nodes of the female are referred to as the mammary lymph nodes, while in the male they are called the scrotal lymph nodes. In the male, these nodes are located lateral to the penis, while in the female they lie close to the caudolateral border of the inguinal mammary gland and along the caudal superficial epigastric vessels. In both sexes these lymph nodes represent an elongated group of two to six nodes, 3–8 cm in length, although rarely there is only a single main node. The superficial inguinal lymph nodes of the sow

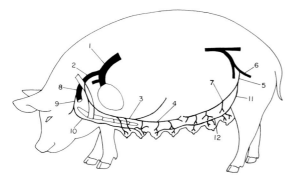

4.3. Arterial blood supply to the mammary glands. *1.* aortic arch, *2.* left subclavian a., *3.* internal thoracic a., *4.* cranial epigastric a., *5.* pudendoepigastric trunk, *6.* deep femoral a., *7.* caudal epigastric a., *8.* axillary a., *9.* external thoracic a., *10.* lateral thoracic a., *11.* external pudendal a., *12.* caudal superficial epigastric a.

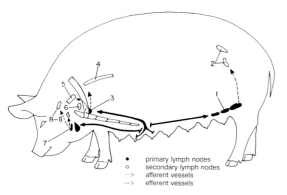

4.4. Lymph drainage of the mammary glands.
1. superficial inguinal lymph nodes (lnn) *2.* iliofemoral
and lateral and medial iliac lnn, *3.* cranial sternal lnn,
4. thoracic duct, *5.* venous system, *6.* axillary lnn of
first rib, *7.* ventral superficial cervical lnn, *8.* dorsal
and middle superficial cervical lnn.

drain the caudal four or five mammary glands.
Their efferent lymph vessels pass into the inguinal canal to the iliofemoral and lateral and medial iliac lymph nodes. The cranial sternal lymph
nodes consist of one to four small nodes that lie
against the manubrium of the sternum in the adipose tissue of the cranial mediastinum. The group
as a whole is 3–5 cm in length. These nodes receive lymph from the cranial two or three mammary glands. Their efferent vessels enter the terminal part of the thoracic duct or right lymphatic
duct or directly into the venous system. Occasionally the efferents may go to the axillary nodes
of the first rib or to the caudal deep cervical
lymph nodes. The ventral superficial cervical
lymph nodes represent a group of six to nine
nodes forming a row between the shoulder joint
and the caudal border of the parotid gland along
the ventrolateral border of the m. cleido-occipita-
lis and on the lateral side of the m. cleidomas-
toideus. The most caudal node is the largest of
the group ranging from 0.5 to 3 cm in length.
This group of nodes receives the efferent lymph
vessels from the cranial two or three mammary
glands. The ventral superficial cervical lymph
nodes are interconnected and their efferent vessels pass to the dorsal and middle superficial cervical lymph nodes. There is considerable variation in the pattern by which the lymph from the
dorsal and middle superficial cervical nodes emp-
ties into the collecting ducts. The efferent vessels
of these two groups of nodes terminate either into
the thoracic duct, the jugular vein, the right tracheal lymphatic duct, or directly into the venous
system.

Nerve Supply. The nerve distribution to the
mammary glands of the pig was described by
Gandhi and Getty (1969a,b) and by Ghoshal
(1975). Each row of mammary glands receives its
innervation from the lateral and ventral cutane-

ous branches of the ventral branches of the last
eight or nine thoracic nerves and the first four
lumbar nerves. The inguinal mammary gland also
receives its innervation from the mammary
branch of the pudendal nerve. These branches
carry somatic sensory fibers and are connected by
rami communicantes with sympathetic fibers
from sympathetic chain ganglia. Parasympathetic
innervation of the mammary glands has not been
demonstrated. The sensory fibers course in the
connective tissue septa and surround the secretory units of each mammary gland. They also
form rich nervous plexuses in the teat wall. The
sympathetic nerves, in general, are distributed in
association with the blood vessels.

MAMMOGENESIS AND LACTOGENESIS.
Throughout the reproductive life span of the sow,
the mammary glands repeatedly go through a cycle of tissue development, lactation, and involution. The process of mammary development is referred to as mammogenesis while the period of
milk production is subdivided into periods of lactogenesis and galactopoiesis. Mammogenesis occurs almost exclusively during the last half of gestation (Hacker and Hill 1972) with secretion into
the alveolar lumen starting by day 75 of gestation
(Pond and Houpt 1978). By day 90 postconcep-
tion, enlargement of the mammary glands can be
seen. During mammogenesis, there is a significant increase in the mammary concentrations of
RNA and DNA reflecting an increase in protein
synthesis (RNA) and total cell numbers (DNA)
(Elmore and Martin 1986).

Mammogenesis is under hormone regulation;
as a prerequisite, the sow requires permissive
concentrations of insulin, thyroxine (T_4), triiodothyronine (T_3), growth hormone, and cortisol to
be present. Mammogenesis will not occur if basal
concentrations of these hormones are not present.
Progesterone concentrations are relatively constant from approximately 30 days of gestation until approximately day 100 when they begin to
decline. In contrast, serum estradiol-17β concentrations are relatively low until approximately
day 70 of gestation when they begin to increase
significantly (Elmore and Martin 1986) until de-
clining abruptly immediately prior to parturition.
Relaxin concentrations increase slowly from approximately day 20 of gestation until approximately day 100 when they also begin to decline.
Prolactin concentrations are very low until approximately day 100 when they begin to increase,
reaching peak concentrations immediately prior
to parturition (Vale and Wagner 1981).

Lactogenesis, the initiation of lactation, occurs
during the periparturient period and is primarily
stimulated by the shift in the progesterone to estrogen ratio immediately prior to delivery. The
increasing estrogen concentrations are also probably the primary stimulus for the periparturient
rise in prolactin concentrations. The mammary

glands have large numbers of prolactin receptors (Sakai et al. 1985; Plaut et al. 1989), and it has previously been demonstrated that a decline in circulating prolactin concentrations will cause an abrupt decrease in milk production (Smith and Wagner 1985a).

Milk Composition. Although pig milk contains protein, fat, lactose, ions, vitamins, and water, the relative concentrations of the components vary according to the stage of lactation, diet, environmental factors, and perhaps genetics (Elmore and Martin 1986). This variability in the composition of swine milk has been reviewed by Pond and Houpt (1978) (Table 4.1).

Nursing Behavior. Piglets will usually start moving about the farrowing crate searching for the mammary glands within a few minutes following birth. An unpublished study of 284 piglets (D'Allaire et al.) examined the correlation between birth weight, direction of movement (toward the mammary glands or the heat lamp), and the time from birth until the piglets found a teat and started to nurse. Although it is generally accepted that most piglets will have started to nurse within 20 minutes of birth, the study reported that only 62% of the animals had started to nurse by this time. It was also noted that 15% of the animals had not started to nurse by 60 minutes following delivery. Of the animals not nursing by 1 hour postpartum, 54% of the piglets weighed less than 1.2 kg.

Normal nursing behavior has previously been described (Fraser 1980; Rushen and Fraser 1989) and involves a sequence of distinct phases occurring over a total of 2–3 minutes with the majority of milk ejection occurring during a 10- to 20-second interval. Most sows will usually nurse at approximately hourly intervals. In one study of 43 Yorkshire-Landrace × Duroc sows, the average interval between nursings was 52.4 minutes, although the nursing frequency declined significantly during the fourth week of lactation (Hernandez et al. 1987). Sow parity, time of day, and season did not influence nursing frequency. Milk production in the sow also occurs at a constant rate throughout the day with milk production during each of four consecutive 6-hour periods varying from 22.1% to 27.5% of the total daily production (Berge and Indrebø 1954; Barber et al. 1955; Salmon-Legagneur 1956; Mahan et al. 1971).

FACTORS INFLUENCING MILK PRODUCTION AND VOLUME. Although numerous factors can influence the quantitative and qualitative aspects of milk production, nutrition is the most important overriding factor in regulating overall milk production. Inadequate feed availability will decrease overall milk production and decrease the relative importance of the factors discussed in this section. It is assumed in the clinical evaluation of lactation problems that the sows have access to a nutritionally balanced food source.

Lactation Number (Parity). The parity status of the sow influences milk production with lower milk production normally observed in primiparous animals. Elsley (1971) demonstrated that milk production in the first and sixth lactation periods was 85% of the sow's overall average productivity. Milk production in the second and the third lactation was 115% of the overall average, while milk production in the fourth and fifth lactation was equivalent to the average milk yield over the five cycles. Speer and Cox (1984) reported that milk production in primiparous sows was even lower, only approximately 60% of that measured in multiparous sows.

Duration of Lactation. Although there is substantial sow-to-sow variability in milk production, the greatest differences are seen after the fourth week of lactation (Salmon-Legagneur 1965; Elsley 1971). Peak milk production usually occurs during the third and fourth weeks of lactation (Table 4.2).

Litter Size. Milk production will vary as a function of litter size (Table 4.3). While total milk production increases with an increase in the number of piglets, the relative milk production per piglet declines (Berge and Indrebø 1954; Salmon-Legagneur 1965). Food consumption increases, however, when the lactational demand on the sow increases.

Table 4.1. Changes in gross composition of swine colostrum and milk with time following parturition

| | Time after Parturition | | | | | | | | |
| | Hours | | | | | | | | Weeks |
Constituent	0	3	6	9	12	15–24	27–48	72–120	2–8
Total solids (%)	30.20	28.70	26.60	23.60	20.80	19.60	21.20	21.80	21.20
Fat (%)	7.20	7.30	7.80	7.80	7.20	7.70	9.50	10.40	9.30
Protein (%)	18.90	17.50	15.20	11.70	10.20	7.20	6.90	6.80	6.20
Lactose (%)	2.50	2.70	2.90	3.00	3.40	3.70	4.00	4.60	4.80
Ash (%)	0.63	0.62	0.62	0.63	0.63	0.66	0.72	0.77	0.95
Calcium (%)	0.05	0.04	0.05	0.05	0.06	0.07	0.11	0.16	0.25
Phosphorus (%)	0.11	0.11	0.11	0.11	0.11	0.12	0.13	0.14	0.15

Source: Pond and Houpt (1978), The Biology of the Pig, © Cornell Univ Press, with permission.

Table 4.2. Changes in daily milk production as a function of the duration of lactation in weeks

	Week of Lactation					
	1	2	3	4	5	6
Milk production (kg/day)	5.10	6.51	7.12	7.18	6.95	6.59

Source: Adapted from Elsley (1971).

Table 4.3. Effect of litter size on daily milk production

Milk Production	Litter Size (# of piglets)								
	4	5	6	7	8	9	10	11	12
kg/litter	4.0	4.8	5.2	5.8	6.6	7.0	7.6	8.2	8.6
kg/piglet	1.0	1.0	0.9	0.9	0.9	0.8	0.8	0.7	0.7

Source: Compiled from Berge and Indrebø (1954); Salmon-Legagneur (1965).

Body Condition. Body condition also influences milk production; sows in good condition produce significantly greater quantities of milk than those in poor condition (O'Grady et al. 1973). Sows in poor condition at parturition did not respond with an increase in milk production when provided additional feed. The milk from poorly conditioned sows also had a lower fat content than milk samples collected from sows on an adequate plane of nutrition.

Although there is a correlation between energy intake and milk production, a significant decrease in food intake usually results in only a moderate decline in milk production (Noblet and Etienne 1986). In one study comparing the effects of high and low energy diets on milk production in sows of the same body condition at farrowing, the relative volume of milk produced in the low-energy group declined (Hovell et al. 1977; Noblet and Etienne 1987). Surprisingly, however, the percentage of fat and dry matter in milk from the low-energy group increased significantly, and the total energy produced in the milk per sow per day was approximately equal in the two groups. The most dramatic effect of limited feed availability during lactation was greater sow weight loss.

Immunoglobulins. Immunoglobulin production varies as a function of both parity and stage of lactation. The interlitter variation, however, is very high, being >70% in some sows of the same parity (Klobasa and Butler 1987). Total milk IgG and IgM concentrations at all stages of lactation increase slightly with increasing numbers of litters (Klobasa and Butler 1987). In contrast, the IgA concentrations increase more dramatically with increasing parity. Although the intersow variability in relative IgG, IgM, and IgA concentrations was high, total immunoglobulin concentrations are relatively constant in colostrum samples collected immediately postpartum (120–130 mg/ml). During the first 24 hours following parturition, immunoglobulin concentrations decline rapidly, at an estimated rate of 3.4% per hour (Klobasa and Butler 1987). Based on an examination of 14 samples collected from each of 80 sows, it has also been demonstrated that the relative

immunoglobulin (IgG, IgM, IgA) composition of milk varies significantly during lactation (Klobasa and Butler 1987) (Fig. 4.5). IgG represents 68–87% of the total colostrum immunoglobulins, while IgA and IgM concentrations vary between 8 and 22% and between 5 and 9%, respectively, during the early stage of milk production. Further complicating our understanding of immunoglobulin production in the sow is the large variation in immunoglobulin concentrations in milk samples collected from adjacent glands (Klobasa and Butler 1987). In general, however, higher Ig concentrations are measured in the caudal rather than in the cranial glands. This variability in Ig production between mammary glands can be sufficiently great to obfuscate differences between sows in total immunoglobulin production.

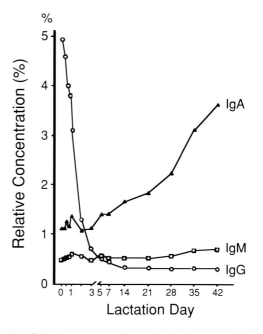

4.5. Relative concentrations of swine immunoglobulins, IgG, IgA, and IgM in lacteal secretions throughout lactation. Relative concentration = (mg of Ig/ml)/(mg of albumin/ml) • 100. (Modified from Klobasa and Butler 1987, with permission.)

There are also differences in the ability of piglets to absorb Igs. Svendsen et al. (1990) demonstrated that immature (<1 kg) or debilitated (splaylegs) piglets had a higher rate of Ig absorption than their heavier litter mates. While the immature group surprisingly had better Ig absorption, their survival rate depended on husbandry practices.

NORMAL PIGLET GROWTH. Piglet growth during the first month postpartum is extremely rapid, with most piglets nearly doubling their birth weight by the end of the first week (Table 4.4). By 4 weeks of age, most animals will have had approximately a fourfold increase in body weight. These rapid growth rates also point out the need for supplemental iron injections, since there is inadequate iron in the sow's milk to meet piglets' metabolic needs for hemoglobin synthesis. Once piglets' basic nutritional needs are met, further increases in milk production produce only a marginal increase in weaning weight. In one study, increasing milk production by more than 40% produced only a 10% increase in piglets' growth rates (Martineau et al. 1991b).

Although birth weight, choice of teat, behavior, and litter size have all been shown to influence the growth variation within a litter, the relative contribution of each factor has not been established. While there appears to be a preference for the cranial mammary glands, teat selection does not appear to be associated with greater milk production by the gland. Fraser and Lin (1984) demonstrated that milk production per gland was approximately equal in all glands, but the quantity of colostrum manually expressed from the cranial glands was approximately four times greater than colostrum from the caudal glands. Closer proximity to vocalization by the sow may also encourage use of the most cranial glands. Fighting for teats is lower for piglets using the most cranial and most caudal teats than for piglets using the middle teats. A high level of teat fidelity is an advantage for piglets, since it reduces teat disputes and the resultant chance of missing a nursing (De Pasillé et al. 1988).

MEASURING MILK PRODUCTION. A valid quantitative measurement of milk production in the sow is difficult to obtain because of the frequency of milk ejection, the short duration of action by oxytocin, and the necessity of the piglets' presence for continued milk production. Five approaches related either to (a) milking of the sow, (b) weight loss of the sow during nursing episodes, (c) litter weight gain during suckling bouts (weigh-suckle-weigh method), (d) piglet growth, or (e) measurement of piglet body water turnover rate (water intake) have been developed to provide an estimation of milk production (Martineau et al. 1991a.).

Milking of the Sow. This method was most intensively studied following discovery of the role of oxytocin in milk ejection and the development and refinement of a suitable milking machine for the pig. Despite its inherent simplicity, this approach does not provide a reliable estimate of milk production due to the variable effects of oxytocin on the volume of milk ejected (Salmon-Legagneur 1959) and individual variability among sows in their responses to milking machines (Van Spaendonck 1972).

Although not universally accepted, this technique is useful for some studies of milk composition (Pond et al. 1962). In comparison with samples collected following "natural" milking, identified changes in milk composition following oxytocin administration include qualitative differences in dry matter, fat, and lactose content (Den Hartog et al. 1984). Milk composition obtained following oxytocin administration also varies from the beginning to the end of the nursing period (McLaughlin et al. 1983). This variation is partially attributable to the difference in endogenous and exogenous oxytocin dosages. During normal nursing, total release of oxytocin from the posterior pituitary is only approximately 25 milliunits (mUI), and dosage of as little as 10 mUI of oxytocin stimulates contraction of the myoepithelial cells of the mammary glands (Ellendorf et al. 1982). These dosages are approximately 1000 times less than the quantities of oxytocin usually administered to stimulate milk ejection.

Sow Weight Loss during Suckling Periods. Weighing the sow before and after a suckling period is another recognized but seldom used ap-

Table 4.4. Average weight, cumulative average weight gain, and weekly average weight gain of 803 piglets from 99 primiparous sows

Age (weeks)	Weight (kg)	Weight Gain (kg) Cumulative	Weekly	Change from the beginning of the week (%)
Birth	1.4			
1	2.7	1.3	1.3	93.0
2	4.2	2.8	1.6	59.0
3	5.7	4.3	1.5	35.0
4 (weaning)	6.9	5.6	1.2	22.0
8	14.0	12.6	7.0	102.0

Source: Adapted from Martineau et al. (1991b). © 1991 Med Vet (Quebec) 22:56–61, with permission.

proach for measuring milk production (Clausen et al. 1952 as cited by Salmon-Legagneur 1965). Its greatest drawback is the lack of precision afforded, since the weight ratio of milk ejected during each nursing period to body weight is approximately 1:1000. The comparative data of Salmon-Legagneur (1956) corroborated the overestimation of milk production with this approach and the associated lack of precision.

Weigh-Suckle-Weigh.   The weigh-suckle-weigh (WSW) method has been used extensively during the past few years and involves repeated weighing of piglets, preceding and following nursing, a predetermined number of times. Apart from suckling periods, the piglets do not have access to the teats. One approach is to remove the piglets from the sow 1 hour prior to the first suckling period. The other nursing periods occur at intervals of 45–70 minutes, and last, on average, 4–5 minutes. Before each suckling period, the piglets are placed on a cold surface to induce urination and defecation.

The piglets can be weighed individually, half the litter at a time, or as a litter (Barber et al. 1955; Lodge and McDonald 1959; Mahan et al. 1971; Lewis et al. 1978). Large flat-topped electronic balances are particularly effective for weighing individual piglets of up to 5 kg. Balances with integration features permit an average animal weight to be determined over a preset period of time (usually 5 seconds) and compensate for animal movement. Piglets rapidly adapt to quiet and careful handling and usually will stand quietly if placed in a lightweight box set atop the balance. Repeated weighings should produce variations of no more than 5 g. The greatest variability in results between methods is associated with the time necessary to complete the measurements. Weighing the entire litter at once is faster, but less accurate, than determining individual weights. The faster technique decreases metabolic losses from the end of the nursing period to the time of weighing. A minimum of five consecutive suckle period measurements is usually required to accurately estimate milk production. The first two sets of measurements have the greatest variability and should be discarded (Speer and Cox 1984).

One problem with the WSW method is that certain normal social interactions between the sow and her litter are precluded, and the piglets do not have an "on-demand" access to the teats. Grouping piglets for a mass suckle may stress the sow and inhibit her milk let-down reflex, which decreases the piglets' capacity to induce this reflex.

Although milk production is relatively constant during a 24-hour interval, there is no consensus as to the minimum sampling frequency necessary to accurately estimate mean daily milk production. Salmon-Legagneur (1965) and Mahan et al. (1971) reported that extrapolation of the results of seven to eight measurements at frequent intervals to 24 hours, provided a good estimate of total daily milk production.

Another problem in measuring daily milk production is to adjust for piglet urinary, fecal, and metabolic losses. Although ignored by some researchers (Lewis et al. 1978), these losses can result in underestimation of milk production by approximately 10%. To compensate for these losses, some researchers have reported only the quantity of milk consumed by piglets that did not urinate during the nursing period (Barber et al. 1955; Lodge and McDonald 1959). Another approach has been to collect the urine with an absorbent material and add the absorbent weight gain to the change in piglet weight (Van Spaendonck and Vanschoubroek 1964), while other researchers have assumed a constant piglet weight loss of 10 g per micturition.

Weight loss due to metabolic loss was reported by Klaver et al. (1981) and Noblet and Etienne (1986) to be proportional to metabolic body size and averaged 30 mg $\cdot$ kg$^{-.75}$ $\cdot$ min^{-1} in sleeping piglets and 60 mg $\cdot$ kg$^{-.75}$ $\cdot$ min^{-1} in moving piglets. In the case of unsuccessful sucklings, there was an additional average piglet weight loss of 150 mg $\cdot$ kg$^{-.75}$ $\cdot$ min^{-1} attributable to their higher activity and the loss of saliva during stimulation of the mammary gland.

Piglet Growth.   Although conceptually simple, measuring piglet growth generally has not been considered sufficiently precise for lactational studies. Lewis et al. (1978) compared piglet growth from birth to 3 weeks of age at weekly intervals with milk yields measured at 14 and 20 days of lactation with the WSW method. At 3 weeks of age, only 34% of the variation in weight gain could be ascribed to differences in milk production. When the percentage of dry matter in the feed was included in the model, 44% of the variation in piglet weight could be ascribed to differences in milk production. This emphasizes the importance of individual weight variation from one animal to another and the impact this has on estimating milk production. The study reported a mean daily weight gain of 164 g (range: 83–233 g, standard deviation: 31 g) during the first 20 days of lactation. Other workers found different correlations between milk production and weight gain varying from 18% to 76%, indicating the inherent weakness of the method for estimating milk production.

Noblet and Etienne (1989) recently have demonstrated that the changes in piglet weight can be a better means for estimating milk production when initial piglet weight, the stage of lactation, and the average daily gain (ADG) are concurrently evaluated. Using this approach, the correlation coefficients (R^2) between milk production and piglet weight varied between 0.91 and 0.96. (Table 4.5). Milk dry matter, energy, and nitrogen

Table 4.5. Estimation of daily milk production for primiparous sows via the average daily growth and the initial body weight

Lactation Period (days)	Formula	Correlation Coefficient (R^2)
1–21	MP = $2.50(\pm0.26) \times$ ADG + $80.2(\pm7.8) \times$ Wi + 7	0.91
1–5	MP = $2.64(\pm0.39) \times$ ADG + 80.2	0.96
5–21	MP = $1.83(\pm0.31) \times$ ADG + $72.9(\pm8.1) \times$ Wi + 176	0.91

Source: Noblet and Etienne (1989) © 1989 J Anim Sci 67:3352, with permission.
Note: MP = daily milk production (g of milk per piglet); ADG = average daily gain (g • day⁻¹); Wi = initial body weight in kg.

output over the entire lactation were predicted from piglets' ADG. Based on these and other observations, a conversion efficiency of approximately 4.5 g of milk per 1 g of growth has been estimated (Lucas and Lodge 1965; Lewis et al. 1978; Noblet and Etienne 1986).

Body Water Turnover. Milk production can also be estimated by measuring water turnover in the piglet. The method, first developed for use in calves (MacFarlane et al. 1969), measures the dilution of endogenous water by water absorbed from nursing. To measure this dilution, each piglet receives a known quantity of deuterium-labelled water prior to nursing by parenteral injection. The difference in isotope concentration preceding and following nursing represents the dilution effect of milk absorption and is directly related to sow milk production. This isotope dilution method permits an estimation of water turnover by measuring differences in milk composition. Differences in analytical techniques for measuring the exact quantity of deuterium injected, as well as the deuterium concentration in the water extracted from the blood (Pettigrew et al. 1987), represent the greatest source of error. The correlation between the measurement of water turnover and changes in piglet weight, as methods for measuring milk production, have been estimated at 0.72 (Pettigrew et al. 1985). Although the technical difficulties of the methodology limit its applications, the approach permits maintenance of more normal sow and litter interactions.

LACTATION INSUFFICIENCY. There is good evidence that insufficient milk production in the sow can result from numerous causes (Smith 1985). This multiplicity of etiologies is reflected in the names that have been associated with this disease complex: coliform mastitis, periparturient hypogalactia syndrome (PHS), agalactia toxemia, puerperal mastitis, dysgalactia, mastitis-metritis-agalactia (MMA), and puerperal toxemia (Penny 1970; Thurman and Simon 1970; Bertschinger and Pohlenz 1980; Ross 1981; Smith 1985). Although the term MMA has been used most extensively in the older literature, it is a misnomer. While most sows have a decrease in milk production, only infrequently is there true agalactia.

Likewise, metritis is rarely part of the syndrome; PHS more accurately describes the problem.

Clinical Presentation. The primary clinical signs of PHS refer to the sow's inability to produce a sufficient volume of milk (Ringarp 1960; Penny 1970; Hermansson et al. 1978a; Martin and Elmore 1980) to meet the nutritional requirements of the piglets. PHS is observed almost exclusively within the first 3 days postpartum, with more than 50% of affected sows showing clinical signs of insufficient milk production within the first 24 hours postpartum (Hermansson et al. 1978a). Rarely is PHS initially observed more than 72 hours postpartum (Ringarp 1960; Penny 1970; Hermansson et al. 1978a). In the normal sow, milk ejection usually starts within <30 seconds following the initiation of nursing behavior and is of short duration (<30 seconds). At the end of milk ejection, the piglets settle down and often sleep, and milk is frequently seen around the piglets' mouths. In contrast, milk ejection in PHS sows is either absent or of brief duration. The piglets will continue their efforts at nursing, frequently resulting in trauma to the nipples (Bertschinger and Pohlenz 1980). Affected sows will commonly roll onto their sternum and not permit the piglets to nurse. During the initial stages of PHS, the activity level of the piglets at nursing time will increase as they fight and jostle for position. Face biting may be seen in severely affected litters. Piglets have a high metabolic rate (Klaver et al. 1981), and as the piglets' energy reserves are depleted, attempts at nursing decrease and the animals often migrate to the warmest portions of the farrowing crate (Penny 1970). As a result, careful observation of nursing behavior is one of the best methods of identifying PHS animals (Whittemore and Fraser 1974; Wagner 1982). The debilitated piglets also are not able to move as rapidly as well-nourished animals, and there may be a resultant increase in the number of crushed piglets.

An increase in rectal temperature of 1.0–1.5°C (2–3°F) is observed in over 50% of affected animals (Ringarp 1960; Martin et al. 1967; Hermansson et al. 1978a; Wagner 1982). It is important to note, however, that the rectal temperature of clinically normal sows will also increase slightly during the first 1–2 days following parturition.

Furniss (1987) measured daily rectal temperatures of normal sows and those that subsequently developed either slight or severe cases of lactation insufficiency from the day preceding until 2 days following parturition. Rectal temperatures of <39.4°C on the afternoon of parturition or at approximately 18 hours following parturition were a good predictor of which animals would develop PHS. Furniss (1987) also reported no difference in the rectal temperatures of normal and PHS sows 1 day prior to parturition, while others (Goransson 1989a,b; Persson et al. 1989) have reported an increase in rectal temperatures of subsequently affected sows when examined 1 day prior to parturition.

The mammary glands of PHS animals may vary in appearance from normal or firm and locally warm to the touch to grossly swollen with a blotched appearance (Jones 1971). The mammary glands of some animals may appear normal due to excess subcutaneous fat, subclinical localized mammary infections, or non-mastitis-related causes of PHS. Milk samples collected from affected sows will vary from normal to serous or creamy and can contain fibrin or blood (Penny 1970; Bertschinger and Pohlenz 1980; Ross et al. 1981). Somatic cell counts and pH may also be elevated in affected sows (Ross et al. 1981). Elevated somatic cell counts can, however, be misleading in the diagnosis of PHS, since it was shown in one study (Bertschinger and Buhlmann 1990) that the somatic cell counts in milk samples collected from adjacent glands of clinically normal sows varied from $<1 \cdot 10^6$ and $<10\%$ neutrophils to $>8 \cdot 10^6$ total cells/ml and 90% neutrophils. Bacterial cultures of the samples were negative. The somatic cell counts per gland are also affected by the time postpartum of sample collection. Pedersen and Persson (1983) and Weber and Ferguson (1982) demonstrated that the somatic cell count from healthy sows increased significantly from day 1 to day 3 postpartum. Milk samples from sows with subclinical PHS also had an increase in somatic cell counts between days 1 and 3 postpartum followed by a significant decline until day 8 postpartum. When both the somatic cell count and the milk pH were evaluated, healthy and PHS sows could be clearly differentiated (Pedersen and Persson 1983).

Classically, affected sows were often anorectic, constipated, or depressed (Ringarp 1960; Penny 1970; Ross et al. 1975; Hermansson et al. 1978a; Bertschinger and Pohlenz 1980). De Passillé and Rushen (1989a) have demonstrated, however, that in some cases the clinical presentation may be different, with only the piglets being affected. The sow is clinically normal, yet the piglets do not grow at the expected rate due to excessive teat fighting or neonatal diarrheas. Although metritis was originally felt to be a significant component of the disease complex (Penny 1970; Thurman and Simon 1970), examinations of the reproductive tracts of normal and affected animals have generally not supported this conclusion (Ringarp 1960; Swarbrick 1968; Ross et al. 1969; Nachreiner et al. 1972; Jones 1976). It is also important not to confuse the normal postpartum vaginal discharge with metritis. Additional work has indicated that urinary tract infections may be a relatively common occurrence in herds with PHS (Madec and David 1982; Berner 1984; Berner and Jöchle 1986b; Madec 1987a). Hematologic changes consistently observed in hypogalactic sows include a decrease in the packed-cell volume and hemoglobin concentration (Ringarp 1960; Hermansson et al. 1978b). An initial leukopenia has been reported within the first 24 hours postpartum although normal leukocyte numbers are commonly measured by 48 hours postpartum (Ringarp 1960; Nachreiner and Ginther 1972b; Ross et al. 1975; Hermansson et al. 1978b). Other reported changes include a decrease in serum calcium (Ringarp 1960; Hermansson et al. 1978b) magnesium and glucose concentrations (Hermansson et al. 1978b), and an increase in serum phosphorous (Cotrut et al. 1980) and aminotransferase concentrations (Nachreiner and Ginther 1972b; Hermansson et al. 1978b) at 1 day postpartum in affected sows.

Consistent changes in hormone concentrations are less well characterized. Cortisol concentrations may be elevated (Nachreiner et al. 1972; Hermansson et al. 1978b), while thyroxin concentrations have been reported to be decreased (Cotrut et al. 1976; Martin and McDowell 1980). The lower thyroxin concentrations may be similar to the "euthyroid sick" syndrome described in humans (Wartofsky and Burman 1982), a condition observed in association with a wide range of diseases. Several studies have also reported a decrease in prolactin concentrations in affected sows (Threlfall et al. 1974).

Studies in the cow (Mattila and Sandholm 1985) and sheep (Maisi et al. 1987) have indicated that N-acetyl-β-D-glucosaminidase (NAGase) concentrations, a lysosomal enzyme released into milk during cellular damage, is a good indicator of mammary infections in these species. Similar work in the pig (Raekallio 1987) has demonstrated that basal NAGase concentrations are extremely high in the sow and NAGase concentrations are not a good indicator of mammary infections in this species. In comparison to normal animals, milk from affected sows also has elevated sodium and decreased potassium and lactose concentrations. Gooneratne et al. (1982) reported that lactose concentrations in the colostrum of sows that subsequently became agalactic were higher than in normal sows. They suggested that the altered lactose concentrations may be associated with the premature initiation of lactation, an interesting theory that has yet to be confirmed.

Incidence. Accurately estimating the incidence of PHS has been difficult due to the wide range of management practices, definitions, and geographic locations reported in studies conducted over the past 30 years. Even when studies have examined herds of approximately similar size, genetic composition, and management in a single region, the incidence of PHS has varied dramatically from herd to herd and has been reported to vary from 0% to 100% (Hermansson et al. 1978a). A 1972 study of 21,536 farrowings in Illinois reported that insufficient milk production was the primary cause of 17.6% of preweaning deaths (Leman et al. 1972). The study also reported that insufficient milk production was the major cause in 30.9% of the piglets killed by crushing and almost 15% of the deaths of "weak pigs." Kertiles and Anderson (1979) reported that 50% of all preweaning deaths were related to insufficient milk production, and Backstrom et al. (1982) indicated that 6.0% to 9.9% of 16,295 sows had insufficient milk production. Studies in Norway and Finland have reported an incidence of insufficient milk production in sows of 20% and 23.3%, respectively (Aass 1987; Lampinen 1987).

The disease incidence also varies with definition. One French study classified all sows (28% of the group) with rectal temperatures exceeding 39.8°C (Madec 1987b) as having a lactation insufficiency, yet reported only 5% having symptoms of clinical mastitis. Unfortunately, none of these studies has adequately defined and estimated the incidence of subclinical mastitis. While the incidence of lactation insufficiency appears to be higher in primiparous and second-litter sows than in older animals, the occurrence of PHS does not appear to predispose a sow to having lactational problems during subsequent lactations. Different results have been reported by Zyczko et al. (1986), however, who indicated a higher incidence of PHS with advancing lactations. The incidence of PHS in the Northern Hemisphere has also been reported to be higher during the third quarter of the year and may be associated with heat stress (Backstrom et al. 1984).

Etiology. Lactation insufficiency in the sow is an extremely complex syndrome, and over 30 different etiologies have been associated with the problem. Elmore and Martin (1986) separated the etiologies into five general categories: infectious diseases, endocrine dysfunction, heredity, management and environment, and nutrition. In recent years, the distinction between some of these categories has blurred and the etiologies causing PHS will be reclassified as (a) noninfectious, (b) infectious, (c) management and environment, and (d) nutritional. Endocrine dysfunction has been deleted as a separate classification, since with the exception of ergot intoxication, the hormonal changes seen in association with PHS are just one manifestation of a larger problem.

Heredity has also been grouped with other noninfectious causes of PHS. It should be noted that these classifications are somewhat arbitrary and that PHS may also be caused by the interaction of multiple factors.

NONINFECTIOUS

Teat Malformation. Piglets cannot nurse from an inverted nipple and will usually move to an adjacent teat. Only in a sow with a large litter and a significant number of inverted nipples will availability of milk be reduced. Since inverted nipples appear to be a genetically based condition, culling animals with inverted nipples is advised. The condition is usually limited to only a few animals within a herd.

Ergot Toxicity. Grain contamination with ergot derivatives produced by *Claviceps purpurea* has been reported to cause lactation failure in the sow (Penny 1970; Anderson and Werdin 1977). In one study (Coitihno et al. 1984), ergot contamination of 0.67% by weight of feed resulted in a 55% piglet mortality by day 21 of lactation. Affected sows were reported to have flaccid mammary glands, normal rectal temperatures, increased excitability, and carpal erosions (Penny, 1970; Anderson and Werdin 1977). Ergot derivatives are known to suppress prolactin release from the anterior pituitary, an absolute hormone requirement for normal lactation in the pig (Whitacre and Threlfall 1981; Bevers et al. 1983; Smith and Wagner 1985b). The incidence of the problem appears to be low.

Infrequently, sows may have hypoplastic mammary glands of unknown etiology. While the sow may deliver a full-term litter, the mammary glands fail to develop during the last weeks of gestation, and the glands will not become engorged prior to parturition. The sows usually will permit the piglets to nurse, although little colostrum or milk can be expressed. It is not known if ergot toxicity is a factor in these animals. Inadequate hormone stimulation of the mammary glands during gestation is another untested possibility.

Psychogenic Agalactia. A few sows may be aggressive toward the piglets and attempt to bite or crush them. Other sows, particularly first-litter gilts, may appear nervous and refuse to permit the piglets to nurse. When palpated, the mammary glands will feel full, and it is usually possible to express a small amount of milk. Mild tranquilization usually will cause the sow to relax and permit nursing. Although a single treatment is generally effective, administration of tranquilizer may need to be repeated for up to 24–48 hours in a few animals, until bonding of the sow and piglets has occurred.

Failure of Milk Ejection. For reasons that are not fully understood, a few sows will fail to have a normal release of oxytocin during nursing. The animals usually will appear bright and alert, and no significant changes will be found on examination of the animal, although some sows may be slightly nervous. Intramuscular treatment with oxytocin (5 IU/sow) will usually cause milk ejection. Repeated treatment is rarely necessary.

Mammary Gland Edema. A poorly characterized aspect of PHS in some sows is mammary edema. While not commonly observed, for unknown reasons some sows will develop substantial mammary edema shortly before parturition. Administration of a diuretic is usually effective in decreasing the edema. Initiation of parturition with F series prostaglandins will also decrease the incidence of mammary edema.

Miscellaneous. Ketosis has occasionally been reported as a cause of lactation insufficiency in sows 2–3 weeks postpartum (Ringarp 1960; Penny 1970). Clinical signs have included weight loss, anorexia, hypoglycemia, generalized weakness, and ketonemia. Hypocalcemia has also been infrequently recognized as a cause of insufficient milk production with signs including restlessness, incoordination, a reluctance to rise, and, rarely, coma. Treatment for both conditions is similar to that used in other species. Overheating of the mammary glands can also occasionally cause a decrease in milk production. Muirhead (1981) reported that placement of heat lamps too close to the glands resulted in localized burning of the glands.

INFECTIOUS

Coliform Mastitis. Gram-negative mastitis is identified in a high percentage of PHS animals and is the most important cause of lactation insufficiency in the sow. To better describe this group of animals, Bertschinger et al. (1986) introduced the term coliform mastitis (CM) to describe gram-negative coliform mammary infections in the periparturient sow caused by bacteria of the genera *Escherichia, Klebsiella, Enterobacter,* and *Citrobacter.* While numerous *Streptococcus* spp. and *Staphylococcus* spp. have been isolated from mammary glands (Pejsak et al. 1990), they rarely have been associated with pathologic changes in tissues. Although an occasional sow may develop a gram-positive mastitis (Ross 1981; Ross et al. 1981), the incidence is relatively low, and will not be further considered.

Coliform bacteria have been cultured from mammary glands in numerous studies (Ringarp 1960; Ross et al. 1975, 1981; Bertschinger et al. 1986). The reported incidence of coliform mastitis has been variable but is usually in excess of 50% of all sows reported to have inadequate milk

production. (Ross et al. 1981) reported that of 72 sows necropsied due to insufficient milk production, gross evidence of mastitis was found in 59 animals. All glands do not have to be affected, however, for milk production to decline. (Middleton-Williams et al. (1977) examined the distribution of histologic lesions in the mammary glands of nine sows with mastitis. In one sow, only one-half of one gland had a low grade CM, while in another, one-half of a gland had an acute to necrotizing mastitis. In both animals, however, milk production was significantly reduced, illustrating the need for careful examination of all glands. Experimental intramammary inoculations with field strains of *E. coli* (Ross et al. 1983) and *Klebsiella pneumoniae* (Lake and Jones 1970) have produced cases of PHS that closely mimic naturally occurring cases of hypogalactia. There does not appear to be a dominant serotype(s) of *E. coli* collected from field cases of PHS. There does, however, appear to be significant differences in strain pathogenicity (Ross et al. 1983).

The milk composition also appears to influence the growth characteristics of *E. coli*. Several coliform strains grew significantly better in whey collected on the day of farrowing than in samples collected later during lactation. Likewise, bacterial growth was better in whey samples collected from sows with elevated temperatures with or without signs of PHS (Raekallio 1987). Similar observations have been reported for the cow, comparing bacterial growth in normal and mastitic milk (Mattila et al. 1984).

It appears that most of the systemic changes observed in CM are the result of endotoxin production within the mammary glands. Lipopolysaccharide (LPS) endotoxins are a normal cell wall component of all gram-negative bacteria and are released during both bacterial replication and death. Intramammary injections of LPS are absorbed rapidly from the glands (Elmore et al. 1978) and produce clinical changes within 1 hour of administration. Infusion of an *E. coli* broth originally isolated from hypogalactic sows into the lactiferous sinus produced an acute mastitis and a concurrent increase in serum LPS concentrations (Smith et al. 1988). The duration of elevated serum LPS concentrations was extremely variable, however, and it has been suggested in other studies that the systemic changes observed following LPS administration are the result of inflammatory endogenous mediators (De Ruijter et al. 1988), perhaps interleukin-1 (IL-1). Although it has not been examined in the pig, work in other species has shown that LPS produces a rapid and significant increase in IL-1. Once absorbed, LPS is removed extremely rapidly from the circulation with a half-life of <10 minutes (Youngberg et al. 1988), probably by the macrophages.

Supporting the role of endotoxins in the development of PHS, experimental administration of LPS to periparturient sows has produced clinical and hematologic changes that closely mimic field cases of hypogalactia (Nachreiner et al. 1972; Nachreiner and Ginther 1974). An interesting study by Morkoç et al. (1983), determined the incidence of detectable LPS concentrations in normal and agalactic sows that were matched for age and parity. The study reported a significantly higher incidence of endotoxemia in hypogalactic animals than in control animals. More recently Trusczynski et al. (1990) found similar results; approximately 33% of the 46 sows with symptoms of CM had detectable endotoxin concentrations. These reports all indicate that bacterial endotoxins play a role in the pathogenesis of PHS.

Once absorbed, endotoxins exert profound effects on the immune, cardiovascular, and endocrine systems. Because of common metabolic pathways associated with some of these effects, it is not possible, however, to evaluate the relative importance of changes to each system on milk production. The primary cardiovascular changes have been previously reviewed (Smith 1985), and include depressed myocardial function, splanchnic blood pooling, decreased systolic and diastolic pressures, peripheral hypotension, pulmonary hypertension, and decreased renal blood flow. Other changes included a decline in the number of circulating platelets, lactic acidosis, and endothelial damage. Immune-mediated changes associated with endotoxemia have included activation of the Hageman factor, stimulation of microthrombi formation, and complement activation.

LPS-stimulated hormonal changes in the pig and other species have included an increase in cortisol (Nachreiner et al. 1972; Nachreiner and Ginther 1974), elevated beta-endorphin (Carr et al. 1982), an initial increase followed by a decline in insulin (Spitzer et al. 1980; Wilson et al. 1982; Cornell 1983), an increase in glucagon and pancreatic polypeptide (Cornell 1983), and a decline in thyroxine concentrations (Smith and Wagner 1985b). While previous research has reported low thyroxine concentrations as a factor in PHS (Elmore and Martin 1986), these observations may be the result of low serum LPS concentrations. A similar decline in thyroid function in concurrence with a wide range of disease conditions has been described in humans (Wartofsky and Burman 1982).

Prolactin (PRL), an anterior pituitary hormone, is involved in the initiation and maintenance of lactation in numerous species and under normal conditions is primarily under inhibitory control by dopamine, released from the medial basal hypothalamus. Threlfall et al. (1974) reported that prolactin concentrations were suppressed in hypogalactic sows. The interaction between LPS and PRL concentrations was further clarified in another study that demonstrated a concurrent decline in PRL concentrations and milk production following LPS administration (Smith and Wagner 1984). The absolute requirement of PRL during lactation was established by administering ergocryptine, a specific dopamine antagonist, and demonstrating a concurrent decline in PRL concentrations and milk production (Bevers et al. 1983). As PRL concentrations returned to normal, milk production showed a similar increase. Additional work has demonstrated the presence of PRL receptors on porcine mammary glands (Sakai et al. 1985; Plaut et al. 1989). The proposed effects of LPS on PRL production and the resultant decline in milk production are summarized in Figure 4.6. Endotoxins or mediators absorbed from an infected mammary gland stimulate the release of IL-1 or other factors that alter hypothalamic function. Resultant hormonal changes that likely influence milk production include decreased thyroxine, triiodothyronine, and PRL and increased cortisol concentrations. Other possible endotoxin sources include the urogenital system and/or the intestines.

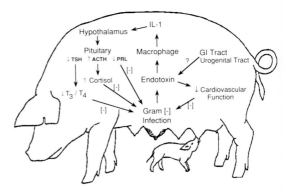

4.6. Proposed pathogenesis of lactation failure due to coliform mastitis. (Modified from Smith 1985a.)

Urinary Tract Infections. Several studies have reported a high incidence of urinary tract infections (UTI), another potentially important source of endotoxemia (Berner 1984; Berner and Jöchle 1986a,b). In a study involving 346 litters, a positive correlation was established between bacteriuria and albuminuria prepartum and the subsequent development of a lactation insufficiency (Petersen 1982). If both gram-negative bacteria and protein were detected in urine samples prepartum, there was a 97% probability of the sow developing PHS postpartum. Likewise, if both prepartum tests were negative, there was a 74% probability of the sow not developing lactation problems.

Based on clinical observations, it appears that there also may be a correlation between low water consumption, the fat sow syndrome, and the development of UTI in the sow. Low consumption may be due to inadequate water supply, lameness, excessive weight, or any other factor limiting normal water consumption. It is hypothesized that in contaminated environments, with less water consumption and subsequent urination, ascending infections can more easily develop. The presence of UTI and the subsequent development of PHS is unclear but may involve UTI seeding the vagina and uterus during the postpartum period. Although vaginal LPS absorption is low, endotoxin absorption from the uterus is high, making this a possible route of endotoxin exposure.

Adding indirect support to the role of UTI in the development of PHS, Pejsak et al. (1990) tested a polyvalent vaccine (Urovac, SOLCO, Ltd, Basel) developed against UTI in humans. The inactivated vaccine contained six strains of *E. coli, Proteus mirabilis, Proteus morganii, Klebsiella pneumoniae,* and *Streptococcus faecalis.* The vaccine was tested on about 40 multiparous Landrace sows randomly selected from a herd with approximately a 40% incidence of PHS. When administered 4 and 2 weeks prepartum, the incidence of PHS was reduced by more than 60%, piglet mortality during the first 10 days of life declined by greater than 50%, and mean piglet weight increased by 24.3% in treated animals during the same period. In a different study, infertile and near-term sows with chronic UTI were treated with various dosages of the same vaccine (Berner et al. 1990). The vaccine was ineffective in reducing the number of pathogens found in urine samples collected from sows at parturition. In contrast, while the vaccine did not eliminate UTI in the chronic nonpregnant animals, it did eliminate bacterial contamination in the genital tract in 5 of 12 pregnant animals. Although the sample size in both studies was not sufficient to adequately evaluate the efficacy of UTI vaccinations, the work does support the concept of UTI playing a significant role in the development of PHS.

Viruses and Mycoplasmas. The role of viral and mycoplasma agents in the development of PHS is unclear. Although *Mycoplasma hyogenitalium* was reported to be the cause of lactation insufficiency (Moore et al. 1966), this observation was not confirmed in a more extensive study that attempted to culture *Mycoplasma* spp. in samples collected from the oviducts, uterus, and cervix of normal and agalactic animals (Ross et al. 1981). The results suggest that *Mycoplasma* spp. are probably not significant factors in the development of PHS.

Decreased milk production can also be a secondary result of any debilitating viral disease in the pig. Sows clinically affected with transmissible gastroenteritis and pseudorabies are known to have decreased milk production. As the infection resolves, milk production usually increases if the piglets are not so debilitated that they are unable to nurse.

MANAGEMENT AND ENVIRONMENT. Although differences in management style appear to play a role in the development of PHS (Backstrom et al.

1984), identifying the specific contributing factors has been difficult. It has been speculated that decreased water availability might be a contributory factor to the development of UTI. Likewise, there is some suggestion that high summer temperatures may also decrease milk production.

Poor sanitation has been implicated in the development of PHS (Bertschinger et al. 1988). In a study by Wegmann et al. (1990), two groups of 12 sows were either individually housed in conventional farrowing crates bedded with straw and wood shavings, or given access to outdoor runs for defecation and urination. Median viable coliform counts were then determined from the teat ends and the farrowing crate floor. The floor and teat end bacterial counts for animals housed in the conventional farrowing crates were approximately 150 and 300 times greater, respectively, than in animals with outside access. The incidence of coliform mastitis was 20% in the sows with outside access and 57% in the sows kept in bedded farrowing crates. This study offers one explanation for the results of an earlier study (Backstrom et al. 1982) in which it was found that the incidence of PHS was significantly lower in sows farrowing in the field than in animals delivering in conventional farrowing facilities. There is not, surprisingly, a positive correlation between sanitation and the development of PHS. Clinical observations suggest that the incidence of PHS is higher in herds with a good health program and clean facilities than in poorer-quality facilities (Martineau 1990).

NUTRITION. Although nutritional disorders are clearly a significant factor in the development of PHS, prior to 1980 there was relatively little research examining the correlation between nutrition and PHS. A major exception was the work of Ringarp (1960), who demonstrated that it was possible to produce agalactia toxemia by making drastic dietary changes during the last week of gestation. He produced PHS by feeding poor-quality feed during the last week of gestation, by administering an antiperistaltic during the same time period, or by feeding large quantities of skim milk during this time. Ringarp (1960) also reported a high incidence of constipation in agalactic sows and indicated that wheat bran in the diet reduced the incidence of PHS by functioning as a laxative, an approach widely used by many producers. Following this approach, Wallace et al. (1974a) reported a decline in the incidence of PHS from 57% to 37% with the inclusion of 15% alfalfa meal in the diet. However, the same group was not able to demonstrate a reduction in the incidence of PHS when 15% alfalfa meal was added to a herd with a "normal" incidence of PHS (Wallace et al. 1974b).

Aherne (1983) examined the effect of wheat bran on altering the incidence of lactation insufficiency, but was unable to evaluate its efficacy, since neither the control nor the experimental groups had symptoms of PHS. Likewise, Nachreiner and Ginther (1972b) were unable to reduce the 12% incidence of PHS in their study with the inclusion of up to 50% wheat bran in the diet. The high-bran diet did, however, increase the fecal water content of treated sows. In both the experimental and control groups, the total fecal volume was decreased on the day of farrowing and the first 2 days postpartum before increasing to prefarrowing amounts.

One of the major difficulties in interpreting the conflicting results of various dietary studies is the different chemical definitions of fiber used and the fact that inclusion of a high-fiber feedstuff also resulted in changes in the relative amounts of other components (Sandstedt et al. 1979; Jensen 1981; Sandstedt and Sjogren 1982; Goransson 1989a, b). Sandstedt and Sjogren (1982) reported that a very low feed allowance in combination with free access to straw during the last 3 weeks prior to parturition significantly reduced the incidence of PHS, a conclusion supported by Jensen (1981) in a similar experiment. With increased dietary fiber content, there is also a concurrent decrease in the incidence of constipation, a problem reported in 22% of the sows classified as PHS (Hermansson et al. 1978a). In contrast, only 5% of the non-PHS sows in the same study were reported to be constipated during the same period. In an experiment designed to estimate the effect of fiber concentration on digestive transit time and the incidence of constipation, Palisse et al. (1979) examined the effects of 3.2% and 6.1% dietary cellulose on the incidence of constipation. Sows receiving the low-fiber diet during gestation had a markedly higher incidence of constipation and an approximately 40% slower intestinal transit time than did the high-fiber group.

Other researchers have suggested that the dietary protein concentration, and not the fiber content, is a critical factor in the development of PHS. Sandstedt (1983) concluded that a high dietary protein content was the most common cause of PHS, a conclusion that differs from Thurmon (1967) who suggested that as long as the dietary protein content was between 10% and 18%, it did not effect the development of PHS. Although the interaction of dietary protein concentration and the development of PHS is unresolved, increasing dietary fiber content usually results in a lower protein concentration, an approach widely used under field conditions to reduce the incidence of PHS.

The type of protein may also influence the incidence of PHS. In a herd with a 50% incidence of PHS, Goransson (1989a) reported that switching to a 100% vegetable diet reduced the incidence of PHS and the mean number of medical treatments required. The effect of drastic feed reduction during the last 2 weeks of gestation was also examined in a related study involving 369 litters

(Goransson 1989b). Reducing the daily feed allowance from 3.4 kg/day to 1.0 kg/day, reduced the incidence of PHS with only a slight decrease in mean piglet birth weight (0.04 kg/piglet) in the restricted feed group.

The interaction of high- and low-energy feeding regimes on the development of PHS was addressed in a study involving 14 pairs of full siblings and a total of 49 litters (Goransson 1989a). The low-energy diet (9.9 megajoules of metabolizable energy [MJ ME]/kg, 15.6% crude protein and 10.6% crude fiber) was compared to a normal diet (11.5 MJ ME/kg, 15.1% crude protein, and 5.8% crude fiber). During the first 80 days of gestation, the normal and low-energy groups received 2.4 and 2.6 kg/day of feed, respectively. Although the dry matter and fat content in the low-energy group was somewhat lower than in the control group, piglet performance was similar between groups, and the incidence of PHS was decreased. While the number of animals examined was relatively small, the results suggest that total dietary energy is probably a more important factor than the protein concentration in the development of PHS.

Vitamin E and Selenium. A growing body of research has suggested a relationship between selenium and vitamin E deficiencies and lactation insufficiency in the sow (Trapp et al. 1970; Whitehair and Miller 1986). In several studies, sows on a selenium and/or vitamin E–deficient diet had a significantly higher incidence of PHS than control animals. The addition of 20,000 IU of vitamin E per ton was reported to decrease the incidence of PHS and increase the 3-week survival rate for piglets (Ullrey 1969). In another study (Whitehair et al. 1983), the addition of selenium to the diet reduced the incidence of PHS. Unfortunately, the studies examining both vitamin E/selenium supplementation and deficiencies have involved relatively small numbers of animals. The mechanism of vitamin E/selenium–induced lactation deficiency has not been established, although it has been shown that both play a role in normal leukocyte function (Elmore and Martin 1986). A decrease in leukocyte numbers has been reported in sows with insufficient milk production, although vitamin E and selenium concentrations have not been concurrently evaluated (Hermansson et al. 1978b). It is unclear whether increasing concentrations of either vitamin E or selenium above generally accepted dietary concentrations will either prevent or reduce the incidence of PHS.

Treatment.   Due to the multiple etiologies that have been associated with PHS, there is no treatment that will be effective for all animals. If a definitive etiology or common cause can be identified, appropriate treatment can be initiated. Unfortunately, identifying the specific cause is usually difficult, and treatment is frequently symptomatic; following are treatments that have been used with variable levels of success. At the end of this section, a general conceptual approach to the clinical management of the problem is suggested.

BABY PIGS. If a relatively small percentage of the sows are affected, it may be possible to cross-foster the piglets. Early identification of affected sows and the rapid transfer of at least part of the litter to other sows at the same stage of lactation is important. It usually is not necessary, however, to move the entire litter, since only occasionally will the sow have a true agalactia. Leaving some piglets on the sow will maintain teat stimulation and encourage the sow to continue lactating. In sows with coliform mastitis, nursing also effectively strips the contaminated milk and may speed the sow's recovery. In cases of true agalactia, the entire litter should be removed. With a cessation of milk production, the piglets rapidly lose weight and frequently will eat small amounts of fecal material, resulting in diarrhea and dehydration. Recent observations (Fraser et al. 1988) suggest that piglets will drink appreciable amounts of tap water on the first day after birth, particularly if milk intake is limited. These authors speculated that under these conditions, water intake may help prevent dehydration and promote the survival of piglets with low early milk intake.

Although labor-intensive and expensive, piglets can also be fed with a commercial milk replacement formula. While feeding intervals can be increased to every 3–4 hours for newborn piglets, for most producers this interval is still impractical. Whether the piglets are cross-fostered or given milk replacer, a relatively high mortality should be anticipated.

OXYTOCIN. While failure of milk ejection is only rarely a cause of PHS, it can be effectively treated with administration of small dosages of oxytocin. The previously recommended dosages of oxytocin (30–50 U.S. Pharmacopeia [USP] units) (Martin and Elmore 1981) are clearly excessive and can be dangerous. Dosages of 5 USP units are adequate to initiate milk ejection and produce circulating oxytocin concentrations higher than those normally produced by suckling. A single intramuscular injection is usually effective, although repeated dosages can safely be given at hourly intervals for at least 6 hours, if necessary. Minimizing stress during the postpartum period will also increase the effectiveness of oxytocin, since stress-induced release of epinephrine has been shown to block oxytocin-induced milk ejection. (Bostedt and Rudloff 1983).

PROSTAGLANDINS. In herds in which a significant percentage of the gilts and sows have PHS, induction of labor with F series prostaglandins

(PGF) has proven effective in reducing the incidence of PHS (Cerne and Jöchle 1981; Diehl and Leman 1982; Holtz et al. 1983). If PGF is administered after day 111 of pregnancy, the duration of birth is shorter, the number of live births is increased, and the incidence of PHS is decreased. The mechanism by which PGF-induced parturition reduces PHS is unknown, although it has been speculated that premature mammary engorgement is prevented. With less engorgement, the incidence of mastitis due to contamination of dilated teats and the subsequent development of PHS is reduced. Not all researchers have reported success using F series prostaglandins to reduce the incidence of PHS. Ehnvall et al. (1977) and Hansen (1979) reported that PGF administration had no effect on the incidence of PHS.

Some studies have also indicated that combining PGF administration with oxytocin injections (10 IU) 15–25 hours later will result in further control over the timing of parturition (Blaisot and Steffan 1984; Lens and Goovaerts 1984; Wilson 1984). In these studies, piglet survival from sows treated with PGF was higher than from untreated control animals. It should be noted, however, that PGF or PGF in combination with oxytocin is still a controversial approach and is not universally accepted.

PROSTAGLANDIN SYNTHETASE INHIBITORS. Flunixin meglumine, a prostaglandin synthetase inhibitor, has been shown to be effective in the treatment of some established cases of PHS. Treatment of the sow with 2.2 mg/kg of flunixin meglumine resulted in a decrease in mammary edema and anorexia and an improvement in piglet weight at 7 days following treatment (Cerne et al. 1984). The prostaglandin synthetase inhibitors are effective in the treatment of endotoxemia in a wide range of species and probably function in a similar manner in the sow with PHS.

BETA-BLOCKING AGENTS. One of the more interesting developments in the past few years has been the use of the β-blocking agents to speed the onset of parturition. The myometrium contains substantial numbers of α and β_2 receptors, the latter being numerically predominant during pregnancy. Stimulation of the α receptors usually results in increased myometrial activity while β_2 stimulation causes myometrial relaxation. Although epinephrine has a differential effect on α and β_2 receptors, its predominant effect is the stimulation of the β_2 receptors resulting in uterine inertia and a delay in parturition. As a result, with stress there will be an increase in β_2 stimulation and a delay in parturition.

Administration of the β_2-blocking agent carazolol (Busse 1990) has been shown to effectively decrease the incidence of PHS. In a double-blind study of 1066 sows, carazolol reduced the incidence of PHS in primiparous sows from 20.5% to

9.9% and from 19.1% to 17.4% in multiparous sows (Bostedt and Rudloff 1983). In one study, Busse (1990) noted an increased frequency of urination and defecation following drug administration and speculated that this might explain the decline in PHS. Another explanation is that by speeding the onset and duration of parturition, the potential for fecal contamination of the engorged mammary glands is decreased.

ANTIBIOTICS. Since most of the bacterial isolates from both the mammary glands and the urinary system of PHS animals are coliforms, a broad-spectrum aminoglycoside or a trimethoprim-sulfa combination is a good initial choice. If multiple animals are affected and/or the problem is of a chronic nature, culture multiple milk samples and determine the antibiotic sensitivity of the bacteria. Prophylactic antibiotic therapy has been largely ineffective in decreasing the incidence of PHS.

GLUCOCORTICOIDS. The efficacy of glucocorticoid usage for the management of PHS has not been clearly demonstrated (Wagner 1982), although early work by Ringarp (1960) reported a moderate improvement (7.6%) in piglet survival following treatment of the sow with prednisolone. In comparison with the nonpregnant, nonlactating sow, glucocorticoid concentrations are normally elevated in the periparturient sow and further increased in PHS animals. Glucocorticoid administration may be effective in the treatment of mammary gland edema but should be used with caution in the treatment of sows with coliform mastitis.

PROLACTIN STIMULATORS. In theory, treatment of PHS animals with drugs that stimulate the synthesis and/or the release of prolactin from the anterior pituitary or purified porcine prolactin would be appropriate. Since purified porcine prolactin is only available in minute amounts, most research has focused on stimulating PRL release. While administration of various phenothiazine and butyrophenone tranquilizers (e.g., chlorpromazine, acetylpromazine, haloperidol, and azaperone) will significantly increase PRL concentrations in various species, they generally have not been effective in stimulating PRL release in the pig (Smith and Wagner 1985a) for reasons that are not clear. Administration of low dosages of these tranquilizers can, however, be effective in quieting the nervous and/or belligerent sow and permitting the piglets to nurse. Thyrotropin-releasing hormone (TRH) has been shown to be effective in increasing PRL concentrations, but was of such short duration (<45 minutes) that it is unlikely to be clinically useful (Smith and Wagner 1985b).

VACCINATIONS. The use of autogenous or mixed bacterins for PHS has produced conflicting results. In one study (Ross et al. 1983), a bacterin was produced from a strain of *E. coli* used to experimentally induce mastitis. In the first experiment, piglet mortality at 14 days of age was reduced from 83% in the untreated control sows to 40% in the vaccinated sows. In subsequent experiments, however, the protective effects of the vaccine could not be repeated. While it has not been carefully documented, some field veterinarians have also reported success using autogenous vaccines.

Based on a recent study by Bertschinger and Buhlmann (1990), it does not appear that mammary glands develop resistance to subsequent infections. In the study, sows were given intramammary injections of the same strain of *E. coli* on subsequent lactations. Although the number of animals was small, the initial infection did not protect the gland from proliferation of the same organism during the following lactation. These results suggest that eventual development of a vaccine for the prevention of coliform mastitis is unlikely. In contrast, the work by Pejsak et al. (1990) suggests that development of vaccines against specific UTI may provide an effective management tool for reducing the incidence of PHS.

MANAGEMENT. Although management practices are rarely the sole cause of PHS, they are important contributory factors, and good sanitation and decreasing animal stress may be effective in decreasing the incidence of PHS. Decreasing fecal contamination of the mammary glands has been clearly shown to decrease the incidence of PHS and can be accomplished by washing the sow prior to movement into the farrowing room and by the regular removal of fecal material.

While limited feeding during the last 1–2 weeks of gestation has been demonstrated to decrease the incidence of PHS in some herds, it is not known if this is due to a decrease in total energy, a decline in protein concentration, or an increase in fiber content. Increasing the dietary fiber content does decrease the incidence of constipation in the periparturient sow. However, the increased fiber content will also result in a larger fecal volume and a greater potential for mammary contamination, necessitating more frequent manure removal. Decreasing food consumption during late gestation appears to be most effective in herds with a high incidence of PHS ($>35\%$). In herds with a relatively low incidence of lactational insufficiency (<10–15%), this approach is less likely to be effective.

THERAPEUTIC APPROACH. In sporadic cases of PHS in which the etiology is uncertain, the most likely cause of PHS is coliform mastitis. Antibiotic administration following an initial oxytocin injection is most likely to be the effective treatment. Selection of an antibiotic should be based on its spectrum of activity against gram-negative organisms and previous experience on that farm. If mammary edema is a problem, a low dose of a diuretic (e.g., furosemide) or glucocorticoid may be effective. Treatment with flunixin meglumine is frequently beneficial.

If PHS is a problem for a significant percentage of the sows (>10–15%), prevention becomes more important than just treatment. Sanitation, particularly during the last few days of gestation, is particularly important, since fecal contamination of the mammary glands appears to be part of the problem. Cleaning the environment may also decrease the incidence of UTI in these animals. While sometimes overlooked, an easily accessible source of fresh water is also extremely important. Although still controversial, timed induction of parturition with an F series prostaglandin or a beta-blocking agent, with or without oxytocin administration, does appear to be effective. It is not clear that treatment with either the prostaglandins or with the beta-blocking agents is clearly superior to the other.

REFERENCES

AASS, R. 1987. Mastitt-Metritt-Agalkti syndromet hos purke (MMA)–En oversikt. Norsk Veterinaertidskr 99:553–557.

AHERNE, F. X. 1983. Dietary laxatives for sows during gestation and lactation. 62nd Annu. Feeders Day Report. Dep Anim Sci, Univ Alberta, Can.

ALLEN, A. D.; TRIBBLE, L. F.; AND LASLEY, J. F. 1959. Inheritance of nipple numbers in swine and the relationship to performance. Univ Missouri Res Bull 694:1–16.

ANDERSON, J. F., AND WERDIN, R. E. 1977. Ergotism manifested as agalactia and gangrene in sows. J Am Vet Med Assoc 170:1089–1091.

BACKSTROM, L.; CONNORS, J.; PRICE, W.; LARSON, R.; AND MORKOÇ, A. 1982. Mastitis-metritis-agalactia (MMA) in the sow: A field survey of MMA and other farrowing disorders under different gestation and farrowing housing conditions. Proc 7th Int Congr Pig Vet Soc, Mexico City, p. 175.

BACKSTROM, L.; MORKOÇ, A. C.; CONNOR, J.; LARSON. R.; AND PRICE, W. 1984. Clinical study of mastitis-metritis-agalactia in sows in Illinois. J Am Vet Med Assoc 185:70–73.

BARBER, R. S.; BRAUDE, R.; AND MITCHELL, K. G. 1955. Studies on milk production of large white pigs. J Agric Sci 46:97–118.

BARONE, R. 1978. Anatomie comparée des mammifères domestiques. Tome troisième; Splanchnologie, foetus et ses annexes. Fasc. 2. Appareil uro-génital, foetus et ses annexes, péritoine et topographie abdominale. Lyon: Ecole nationale vétérinaire.

BERGE, S., AND INDREBØ, T. 1954. Milk production by sows. Meld Nor Landbrukhogsk 33:389–424.

BERNER, H. 1984. Importance of urinary tract infections in development of puerperal endometritis in the sow. Tierærztl Umsch 39:450–458.

BERNER, H., AND JÖCHLE, W. 1986a. Cytological examinations of smears from vagina, cervix and uterus in periparturient sows, with or without endometritis. Proc 9th Int Congr Pig Vet Soc, Barcelona, p. 100.

_____. 1986b. Influence of induction of parturition in the sow with a PGF analog (alfaprostol) on bacterial

ascendance into and colonization of the puerperal uterus. Proc 9th Int Congr Pig Vet Soc, Barcelona, p. 103.

BERNER, H.; BOSSART, W.; AND JÖCHLE, W. 1990. Immunotherapy in infertile sows with urogenital infections and effects on MMA. Proc 11th Int Congr Pig Vet Soc, Lausanne, p. 308.

BERTSCHINGER, H. U., AND POHLENZ, J. 1980. Coliform mastitis. In Diseases of Swine, 5th ed. Ed. A. D. Leman, R. D. Glock, W. L. Mengeling, R. H. C. Penny, E. Scholl, and B. Straw. Ames: Iowa State Univ Press.

BERTSCHINGER, H. U.; POHLENZ, J.; AND ROSS, R. F. 1986. Coliform mastitis. In Diseases of Swine, 6th ed. Ed. A. D. Leman, B. Straw, R. D. Glock, W. L. Mengeling, R. H. C. Penny, and E. Scholl. Ames: Iowa State Univ Press.

BERTSCHINGER, H. U.; ENG, V.; AND WEGMANN, P. 1988. Relationship between coliform contamination of floor and teats and the incidence of puerperal mastitis in two types of farrowing accommodations. Proc 6th Int Congr Anim Hyg, pp. 86–88.

BERTSCHINGER, H. U., AND BUHLMANN, A. 1990. Absence of protective immunity in mammary glands after experimentally induced coliform mastitis. Proc 11th Int Congr Pig Vet Soc, Lausanne, p. 175.

BEVERS, M. M.; WILLEMSE, A. H.; AND KRUIP, T. A. M. 1983. The effect of bromocryptine on luteinizing hormone levels in the lactating sow: Evidence for a suppressive action by prolactin and the suckling stimulus. Acta Endocr 104:261–265.

BLAISOT, S., AND STEFFAN, J. 1984. Induction of parturition in sows, comparison between prostaglandin and prostaglandin + oxytocin programs. Proc 8th Int Congr Pig Vet Soc, Ghent, p. 280.

BOSTEDT, H., AND RUDLOFF, P. R. 1983. Prophylactic administration of the beta-blocker carazolol to influence the duration of parturition in sows. Therio 20:191–196.

BUSSE, F. W. 1990. A study about I.M. injection of Il-irene and Suacron to induce farrowing and to influence the MMA syndrome. Proc 11th Int Congr Pig Vet Soc, Lausanne, p. 176.

CALHOUN, M. L., AND STINSON, A. W. 1987. Integument. Textbook of Veterinary Histology, 3d ed. Philadelphia: Lea & Febiger.

CARR, D. B.; BERGLAND, R.; HAMILTON, A.; BLUME, H.; KASTING, N.; ARNOLD, M.; MARTIN, J. B.; AND ROSENBLATT, M. 1982. Endotoxin-stimulated opiod peptide secretion: Two secretory pools and feedback control in vivo. Science 217:845–848.

CERNE, F., AND JÖCHLE, W. 1981. Clinical evaluations of a new prostaglandin analog in pigs. 1. Control of parturition and of the MMA-syndrome. Therio 16:459–467.

CERNE, F.; JERKOVIC, I.; AND DEBELJAK, C. 1984. Influence of Finadyne on some clinical signs of MMA. Proc 8th Int Congr Pig Vet Soc, Ghent, p. 290.

COITIHNO, H.; FEIPPE, A.; AND RIET, F. 1984. Agalactia en cerdas asociada al hongo, *Claviceps purpurea*. Invest Agron 5:7–8.

CORNELL, R. P. 1983. Role of the liver in endotoxin-induced hyperinsulinemia and hyperglucagonemia in rats. Hepatology 3:188–192.

COTRUT, M.; MARCU, E.; PAPP, E.; COTRUT, M.; COSMULESCV, E.; AND BINTU, V. 1976. Contributions to the study of puerperal agalactia in sows. Proc 4th Int Congr Pig Vet Soc, Ames, p. E1.

COTRUT, M.; MARCU, E.; BINTU, V.; AND BREZULEANU, I. 1980. Changes of some blood haematological and biochemical indicators in agalactic sows. Proc 6th Int Congr Pig Vet Soc, Copenhagen, p. 31.

DEN HARTOG, L. A.; VERSTEGEN, M. W. A.; HERMANS,

H. A. T. M.; Noordewier, G. J.; and Van Kempen, G. J. M. 1984. Some factors associated with determination of milk production in sows by weighing of piglets. Z Tierphysiol Tierernaehr Futtermittelkd 51:148–157.

De Pasillé, A.-M. B., and Rushen J. 1989a. Using early suckling behavior and weight gain to identify piglets at risk. Can J Anim Sci 69:535–544.

———. 1989b. Suckling and teat disputes by neonatal piglets. Appl Anim Behav Sci 22:23–38.

De Pasillé, A.-M. B.; Rushen, J.; and Hartsock, T. G. 1988. Ontogeny of teat fidelity in pigs and its relation to competition at suckling. Can J Anim Sci 68:325–338.

De Ruijter, K.; Verheijden, J. H. M.; Pijpers, A.; and Berends, J. 1988. The role of endotoxin in the pathogenesis of coliform mastitis in sows. Vet Q 10:186–190.

Diehl, J. R., and Leman, A. D. 1982. Effect of PGF2a and neostigmine on induction of parturition, farrowing interval and litter survival in swine. Therio 18:727–732.

Edward, S. A., and Furniss, S. J. 1988. The effects of straw in crated farrowing systems on peripartal behaviour of sows and piglets. Br Vet J 144:139–146.

Ehnvall, R.; Einarsson, S.; and Larson, K. 1977. Prostaglandin-induced parturition in swine. A field study on its accuracy after treatment with different amounts of PGF2α. Nord Vet Med 29:376–378.

Ellendorf, F.; Forsling, M. L.; and Poulain, D. A. 1982. The milk ejection reflex in the pig. J Physiol (London) 333:577–579.

Elmore, R. G., and Martin, C. E. 1986. Mammary glands. In Diseases of Swine, 6th ed. Ed. A. D. Leman, B. Straw, R. D. Glock, W. L. Mengeling, R. H. C. Penny, and E. Scholl. Ames: Iowa State Univ Press.

Elmore, R. G.; Martin, C. E.; and Berg, J. N. 1978. Absorption of *Escherichia coli* endotoxin from the mammary glands and uteri of early post-partum sows and gilts. Therio 10:439–446.

Elsley, F. W. H. 1971. Nutrition and lactation in the sow. In Lactation. Ed. I. R. Flaconer. London: Butterworth.

English, P. R. Smith, W. J.; and MacLean, A. 1982. The sow improving her efficiency. Ipswich, England: Farming Press Ltd.

Fraser, D. 1980. A review of the behavioral mechanism of milk ejection of the domestic pig. Appl Anim Behav Sci. 6:247–255.

Fraser, D., and Lin, C. S. 1984. An attempt to estimate teat quality of sows by hand milking during farrowing. Can J Anim Sci 64:165–170.

Fraser, D.; Phillips, P. A.; Thompson, B. K.; and Peters, W. B. 1988. Use of water by piglets in the first days after birth. Can J Anim Sci 68:603–610.

Furniss, S. J. 1987. Measurement of rectal temperature to predict 'Mastitis, metritis and agalactia' (MMA) in sows after farrowing. Prev Vet Med 5:133–139.

Gandhi, S. S., and Getty, R. 1969a. Cutaneous nerves of the trunk of the domestic pig with special reference to the spinal nerves. Pt 2. Cutaneous nerves of the thoracic region. Iowa State J Sci 44:15–30.

———. 1969b. Cutaneous nerves of the trunk of the domestic pig with special reference to the spinal nerves. Pt 3. Cutaneous nerves of the lumbar, sacral, and coccygeal regions. Iowa State J Sci 44:31–43.

Ghoshal, N. G. 1975. Porcine nervous system. Spinal nerves. In Sisson and Grossman's The Anatomy of the Domestic Animals, 5th ed., vol. 2. Ed. R. Getty. Toronto: W. B. Saunders, pp. 1383–1396.

Ghoshal, N. G.; Koch, T.; and Popesko, P. 1981. The Venous Drainage of the Domestic Animals. Toronto: W. B. Saunders, pp. 130–136.

Gooneratne, A. D.; Hartmann, P. E.; and Nottage, H. M. 1982. The initiation of lactation in sows and the mastitis-metritis-agalactia syndrome. Anim Reprod Sci 5:135–140.

Goransson, L. 1989a. The effect of dietary crude fibre content on the frequency of postpartum agalactia in the sow. J Vet Med Assoc 36:474–479.

———. 1989b. The effect of feed allowance in late pregnancy on the occurrence of agalactia post-partum in the sow. J Vet Med Assoc 36:505–513.

Hacker, R. R., and Hill, D. L. 1972. Nucleic acid content of mammary glands of virgin and pregnant gilts. J Dairy Sci 55:1295–1299.

Hansen, L. H. 1979. Reproductive efficiency and incidence of MMA after controlled farrowing using a prostaglandin analogue, cloprostenol. Nord Vet Med 31:122–128.

Hermansson, I.; Einarsson, S.; Larson, K.; and Backstrom, L. 1978a. On the agalactia post partum in the sow: A clinical study. Nord Vet Med 30:465–473.

Hermansson, I.; Einarsson, S.; Ekman, L.; and Larsson, K. 1978b. On the agalactia postpartum in the sow: A hematological and blood chemical study in affected and healthy sows. Nord Vet Med 30:474–481.

Hernandez, A.; Diaz, J.; Avila, A.; and Cama, M. 1987. A note on the natural suckling frequency of piglets. Cuban J Agric Sci 21:292–294.

Holtz, W.; Hartmann, J. F.; and Welp, C. 1983. Induction of parturition in swine with prostaglandin analogs and oxytocin. Therio 19:583–592.

Hovell, F. D. de B; MacPherson, R. M.; Crofts, R. M. J.; and Smart, R. I. 1977. The effect of pregnancy, energy intake and mating weight on protein deposition and energy retention of female pigs. Anim Prod 25:281–290.

Jensen, H. M. 1981. Forebyggelse af farefeber (MMA) komplekset ved reduktion af fodret til den draektige sode sidste 3 uger før faring. Dansk Vet Tidskr 64:659–662.

Jones, J. E. T. 1971. Reflections on post-parturient diseases associated with lactational failure in sows. Vet Res 89:72–77.

Jones, J. E. T. 1976. Bacterial mastitis and endometritis in sows. Proc 4th Int Congr Pig Vet Soc, Ames, p. E6.

Kertiles, L. P., and Anderson, L. L. 1979. Effect of relaxin on cervical dilatation parturition and lactation in the pig. Biol Reprod 21:57–68.

Klaver, J.; van Kempen, G. J. M.; deLange, P. G. B.; Verstegen, M. W. A.; and Boer, H. 1981. Milk composition and daily yield of different milk components as affected by sow condition and lactation/feeding regimen. J Anim Sci 52:1091–1097.

Klobasa, F., and Butler, J. E. 1987. Absolute and relative concentrations of immunoglobulins G, M, and A, and albumin in the lacteal secretions of sows of different lactation numbers. Am J Vet Res 48:176–182.

Lake, S. G., and Jones, J. E. T. 1970. Postparturient disease in sows associated with *Klebsiella* infection. Vet Res 87:484–485.

Lampinen, A. 1987. Sikojen terveystarkkailu. Sika (Finland) 3:13–14.

Leman, A. D.; Knudson, C.; Rodeffer, H. E.; and Mueller, A. G. 1972. Reproductive performance of swine on 76 Illinois farms. J Am Vet Med Assoc 161:1248–1250.

Lens, S., and Goovaerts, K. 1984. A field evaluation of partus induction by a dinolytic-oxytocin combination. Proc 8th Int Congr Pig Vet Soc, Ghent, p. 281.

Lewis, A. J.; Speer, V. C.; and Haught, D. G. 1978.

Relationship between yield and composition of sows' milk and weight gains of nursing pigs. J Anim Sci 47:634–638.

LODGE, G. A., AND McDONALD, I. 1959. The relative influence of birth weight, milk consumption and supplementary food consumption upon the growth rates of suckling piglets. Anim Prod 1:139–144.

LUCAS, I. A. M., AND LODGE, G. A. 1965. The nutrition of the young pig: A review. Commonw Bur Anim Nutr Tech Commun No. 22, Rowett Inst, Aberdeen, Scot.

MacFARLANE, W. V.; HOWARD, B.; AND SIEBERT, B. D. 1969. Tritiated water in the measurement of milk intake and tissue growth of ruminants in the field. Nature 221:578–579.

McLAUGHLIN, T. L.; PETTIGREW, J. E.; CORNELIUS, S. G; AND MOSER, R. L. 1983. Compositional changes in sows milk during letdown. J Anim Sci [Suppl 1] 57:256. Abstr #304.

MADEC, F. 1987a. Abreuvement des truies en élevage confiné intensif: observations épidémiologiques. Le point Vet 19:611–617.

_____. 1987b. Quelques observations épidémiologiques à propos des métrites chez la truie en élevage intensif. Rec Med Vet 163:171–175.

MADEC, F., AND DAVID, F. 1982. Les troubles urinaires des troupeaux de truie: Diagnostic, incidence et circonstances d'apparition. Rech Porc Fr 14:413–422.

MAHAN, D. C.; BECKER, D. E.; NORTON, H. W.; AND JENSEN, A. H. 1971. Milk production in lactating sows and time lengths used in evaluating milk production. J Anim Sci 33:35–37.

MAISI, P.; JUNTTILA, J.; AND SEPPANEN, J. 1987. Detection of subclinical mastitis in ewes. Br Vet J 143:402–409.

MARTIN, C. E., AND ELMORE, R. G. 1980. Agalactia in Current Therapy in Theriogenology. Ed. D. A. Morrow. Philadelphia: W. B. Saunders, pp. 1083–1086.

_____. 1981. Mammary glands. In Diseases of Swine, 5th ed. Ed. A. D. Leman, R. D. Glock, W. L. Mengeling, R. H. C. Penny, E. Scholl, and B. Straw. Ames: Iowa State Univ Press.

MARTIN, C. E., AND McDOWELL, W. S. 1975. Lactation failure (mastitis-metritis-agalactia). In Diseases of Swine, 4th ed. Ed. H. W. Dunne and A. D. Leman. Ames: Iowa State Univ Press.

MARTIN, C. E.; HOOPER, B. E.; ARMSTRONG, C. H.; AND AMSTUTZ, H. E. 1967. A clinical and pathologic study of the mastitis-metritis-agalactia syndrome of sows. J Am Vet Med Assoc 151:1629–1634.

MARTINEAU, G. P. 1990. Body-building syndrome in sows. Proc Am Assoc Swine Pract, pp. 345–348.

MARTINEAU, G. P.; MATTE, J. J.; DUMAS, G.; AND ROBERT, S. 1991a. Production lactée et croissance chez le porcelet. I. Les méthodes d'évaluation. Méd Vét Québec 21:29–33.

_____. 1991b. Production lactée et croissance chez le porcelet. II. Quelques criteres de variation et croissance du porcelet. Méd Vét Québec 21:56–61.

MATTILA, T., AND SANDHOLM, M. 1985. Antitrypsin and N-acetyl-β-D-glucosaminidase as markers of mastitis in a herd of Ayrshire cows. Am J Vet Res 46:2453–2456.

MATTILA, T.; SYVÄJÄRVI, J.; AND SANDHOLM M. 1984. Bacterial growth in whey from mastitic and nonmastic quarters. Am J Vet Res 45:2504–2506.

MIDDLETON-WILLIAMS, D. M.; POHLENZ, J.; LOTT-STOLZ, G.; AND BERTSCHINGER, H. U. 1977. Untersuchungen ueber dâs Mastitis-Metritis-Agalktie-Syndrome (Milchfieber) der Sau.1. Pathologische Befunde bein Spontanfallen. Schweiz Arch Tierheilkd 119:213–222.

MOORE, R. W.; REDMOND, H. E.; AND LIVINGSTON, C.

W. 1966. Mycoplasma as the etiology of a mastitis-mastitis syndrome in sows. Vet Med Small Anim Clin 61:883–887.

MORKOÇ, A.; BACKSTROM, L.; LUND, L.; AND SMITH, A. R. 1983. Bacterial endotoxin in blood of dysgalactic sow in relation to microbial status of uterus, milk and intestine. Am Vet Med Assoc 183:786–789.

MUIRHEAD, M. 1981. Mastitis: How to deal with a problem. 1. Recognition and definition. Int Piglett 1:1–3.

NACHREINER, R. F., AND GINTHER, O. J. 1972a. Porcine agalactia: Hematologic, serum chemical and clinical changes during the preceding gestation. Am J Vet Res 33:799–809.

_____. 1972b. Gestational and periparturient periods of sows: Effects of altered environment, withholding of bran feeding and induced mastitis on serum chemical, hematologic and clinical variables. Am J Vet Res 33:2221–2231.

_____. 1974. Induction of agalactia by administration of endotoxin (Escherichia coli) in swine. Am J Vet Res 35:619–622.

NACHREINER, R. F.; GARCIA, M. C.; AND GINTHER, O. J. 1972. Clinical, hematologic and blood chemical changes in swine given endotoxin (Escherichia coli) during the immediate postpartum period. Am J Vet Res 33:2489–2499.

NOBLET, J., AND ETIENNE, M. 1986. Effect of energy level in lactating sows on yield and composition of milk and nutrient balance of piglets. J Anim Sci 63:1888–1896.

_____. 1987. Metabolic utilization of energy and maintenance requirements in lactating sows. J Anim Sci 64:774–781.

_____. 1989. Estimation of sow milk nutrient output. J Anim Sci 67:3352–3359.

O'GRADY, J. F.; ELSLEY, F. W. H.; MacPHERSON, R. M.; AND McDONALD, I. 1973. The response of lactating sows and their litters to different dietary energy allowances. 1. Milk yield and composition, reproductive performance of sows and growth of litters. Anim Prod 17:65–74.

PALISSE, M.; COLIN, M.; AND MAURY, Y. 1979. Etudes de quelques aspects du transit digestif chez la truie gestante: Variation avec le taux de cellulose en relation avec le taux de constipation. J Rech Porc Fr 11:217–222.

PEDERSEN, A., AND PERSSON, A. 1983. Udder status during the post-partum period in sows. Proc 5th Int Conf Prod Dis Farm Anim, pp. 217–219.

PEJSAK, Z.; TARASUIK, K.; AND JÖCHLE, W. 1990. Immunoprophylaxis against MMA and/or CM in sows with a vaccine against urinary tract infections (Urovac). Proc 11th Int Congr Pig Vet Soc, Lausanne, p. 307.

PENNY, R. H. C. 1970. The agalactia complex in the sow: A review. Aust Vet J 46:153–159.

PERSSON, A.; PEDERSEN, E.; GORENSEN, L.; AND KUHL, W. 1989. A long term study on the health status and performance of sows on different feed allowances during late pregnancy. 1. Clinical observations with special reference to agalactia post partum. Acta Vet Scan 30:9–17.

PETERSEN, B. 1982. Value of methods of early recognition of puerperal and fertility disorders in the sow. Proc 7th Int Congr Pig Vet, Mexico City, p. 231.

PETTIGREW, J. E.; SOWER, A. F.; CORNELIUS, S. G.; AND MOSER, R. L. 1985. A comparison of isotope dilution and weigh-suckle-weigh methods for estimating milk intake by pigs. Can J Anim Sci 65:989–992.

PETTIGREW, J. E.; CORNELIUS, S. G.; MOSER, R. L.; AND SOWER, A. F. 1987. A refinement and evaluation of the isotope dilution method for estimating milk intake by piglets. Livest Prod Sci 17:163–174.

PLAUT, K. I.; KENSINGER, R. S.; GRIEL, L. C.; AND KAVANAUGH, J. F. 1989. Relationship among prolactin binding, prolactin concentrations in plasma and metabolic activity of the porcine mammary gland. J Anim Sci 67:1509–1519.

POND, W. G., AND HOUPT, K. A. 1978. Lactation and the mammary gland. In The Biology of the Pig. Ithaca, N.Y.: Cornell Univ Press, p. 183.

POND, W. G.; VAN FLECK, L. D.; AND HARTMAN, D. A. 1962. Parameters for milk yield and for percents of ash, dry matter, fat and protein in sows. J Anim Sci 21:293–297.

RAEKALLIO, M. 1987. N-acetyl-β-D-glucosaminidase (NAGase) in porcine milk. Acta Vet Scand 28:173–176.

RINGARP, N. 1960. Clinical and experimental investigation into a postparturient syndrome with agalactia in sows. Acta Agric Scand [Suppl 7].

ROSS, R. F. 1981. Agalactia syndrome of sows. In Current Veterinary Therapy, Food Animal Practice. Ed. J. L. Howard, Philadelphia: W. B. Saunders, pp. 962–965.

ROSS, R. F.; CHRISTIAN, L. L.; AND SPEAR, M. L. 1969. Role of certain bacteria in mastitis-metritis-agalactia of sows. J Am Vet Med Assoc 155:1844–1852.

ROSS, R. F.; ZIMMERMANN, B. J.; WAGNER, W. C.; AND COX, D. F. 1975. A field study of coliform mastitis in sows. J Am Vet Med Assoc 167:231–235.

ROSS, R. F.; ORNING, A. P.; WOODS, R. D.; ZIMMERMAN, B. J.; COX, D. F.; AND HARRIS, D. L. 1981. Bacteriologic study of sow agalactia. Am J Vet Res 42:949–955.

ROSS, R. F.; HARMON, R. L.; ZIMMERMAN, B. J.; AND YOUNG, T. F. 1983. Susceptibility of sows to experimentally induced *Escherichia coli* mastitis. Am J Vet Res 44:949–954.

RUSHEN F., AND FRASER D. 1989. Nutritive and nonnutritive sucking and the temporal organization of the suckling behavior of domestic piglets. Dev Psychobiol 22:789–801.

SAAR, L. I., AND GETTY, R. 1975. Porcine lymphatic system. In Sisson and Grossman's The Anatomy of the Domestic Animals, 5th ed., vol. 2. Ed. R. Getty. Toronto: W. B. Saunders.

SAKAI, S.; KATOH, M.; BERTHON, P.; AND KELLY, P. A. 1985. Characterization of prolactin receptors in pig mammary gland. Biochem J 224:911–922.

SALMON-LEGAGNEUR, E. 1956. La mesure de la production laitière de la truie. Ann Zootech 2:95–110.

_____. 1959. Description et utilisation d'une machine à traire les truies. Ann Zootech 4:345–352.

_____. 1965. Quelques aspects des relations nutritionnelles entre la gestation et la lactation chez la truie. Thèse de doctorat, Université de Paris.

SANDSTEDT, H. 1983. Agalakti hos sugga. Medlemsbl Sver Vet Forb 5:103.

SANDSTEDT, H., AND SJOGREN, U. 1982. Forebuggande atgarder vid hog frekvens av MMA i suggbesattningar. Svensk Veterinartidn 34:487–490.

SANDSTEDT, H.; SJOGREN, U.; AND SWAHN, O. 1979. Foreguggande atgarder mot MMA (agalakti) hos sugga. Svensk Veterinartidn 31:193–196.

SCHMIDT, G. H. 1971. Biology of Lactation. San Francisco: W. H. Freeman.

SCHUMMER, A.; WILKENS, H.; VOLLMERHAUS, B.; AND HABERMEHL, K. H. 1981. The Circulatory System, the Skin, and the Cutaneous Organs of the Domestic Mammals. Trans. W. B. Siller and P. A. L. Wight. Hamburg: Verlag Paul Parey.

SMITH, B. B. 1985. Pathogenesis and therapeutic management of lactation failure in the periparturient sow. Comp Cont Ed Prac Vet 7:S523–S534.

SMITH, B. B., AND WAGNER, W. C. 1984. Suppression of

prolactin in pigs by *Escherichia coli* endotoxin. Science 224:605–607.

_____. 1985a. Effect of dopamine agonists or antagonists, TRH, stress and piglet removal on plasma concentrations of prolactin in lactating sows. Therio 3:283–296.

_____. 1985b. Effect of *Escherichia coli* endotoxin and TRH on prolactin in lactating sows. Am J Vet Res 46:175–180.

SMITH, B. B.; LASSEN, E. D.; MULROONEY, D. 1988. Hematologic changes associated with E. coli endotoxin induced lactation failure in the periparturient sow. Proc 11th Int Congr Repro Artif Insemin, Dublin, Ireland, p. 525.

SPEER, V. C., AND COX, D. F. 1984. Estimating milk yield of sows. J Anim Sci 59:1281–1285.

SPITZER, J. J.; FERGUSON, J. L.; HIRSCH, H. J.; LOO, S.; AND GABBAY, K. H. 1980. Effects of E. coli endotoxin on pancreatic hormones and blood flow. Circ Shock 7:353–360.

SVENDSEN, L. S.; NESTRÖM, B. R.; SVENDSEN, J.; OLSSON, A. C. H.; AND KARLSSON, B. W. 1990. Intestinal macromolecular transmission in underprivileged and unaffected newborn pigs: Implication of survival of underprivileged pigs. Res Vet Sci 48:184–189.

SWARBRICK, O. 1968. The porcine agalactia syndrome: Clinical and histological observations. Vet Res 3:241–251.

THRELFALL, W. R.; DALE, H.; AND MARTIN, C. E. 1974. Serum and adenohypophyseal concentrations of prolactin in sows affected with agalactia. Am J Vet Res 35:313–315.

THURMON, J. C. 1967. The metritis-agalactia-mastitis syndrome of sows. Ph.D. diss., Univ of Illinois.

THURMAN, J. C., AND SIMON, J. 1970. A field study of twelve sows affected with the MMA syndrome. Vet Med Small Anim Clin 65:263–272.

TRAPP, A. L.; KEAHY, K. K.; WHITENACK, D. C.; AND WHITEHAIR, C. K. 1970. Vitamin E-selenium deficiency in swine: Differential diagnosis and nature of field problems. J Am Vet Med Assoc 157:289–300.

TRUSCZYNSKI, M.; PEJSAK, Z.; AND TARASIUK, K. 1990. Role of endotoxin, measured with the LAL test, in coliform mastitis of sows. Proc 11th Int Congr Pig Vet Soc, Lausanne, p. 303.

TUBBS, R. C. 1988a. Sow lactation failure with emphasis on nutritional factors. Agric Pract 9:9–13.

_____. 1988b. The role of vitamin E and selenium in sow lactation failure. Miss Vet J, pp. 7–10.

TURNER, C. W. 1952. The Mammary Gland. Columbia, Mo.: Lucas Brothers, pp. 279–314.

ULLREY, D. E. 1969. Vitamine E and MMA. Mich Agric Exp Stn Res Rep 99.

VALE, G., AND WAGNER, W. C. 1981. Plasma prolactin in the periparturient sow. Therio 15:537–546.

VAN SPAENDONCK, R. A. F. 1972. Bijdrage tot de studie van de energiebehoeften van zeugen tijdens de dracht. Thesis, Universiteit van Gent, Bel.

VAN SPAENDONCK, R. A. F., AND VANSCHOUBROEK, F. 1964. Determination of the milk yield of sows and correction for loss of weight due to metabolic processes of piglets during suckling. Anim Prod 6:119–123.

WAGNER, W. C. 1982. Mastitis-Metritis-Agalactia. Symposium on diagnosis and treatment of swine diseases. Veterinary Clinics of North America: Large Animal Practice. Philadelphia: W. B. Saunders, 4:333–341.

WALLACE, H. D.; THIEU, D. D.; AND COMBS, G. E. 1974a. Alfalfa meal as a special bulky ingredient in the sow diet at farrowing and during lactation. Res Rep Dep Anim Sci. Gainesville, Fla.

_____. 1974b. Wheat bran as a sow ration ingredient

during the farrowing and lactation period. Res Rep Dep Anim Sci, Gainesville, Fla.

WARTOFSKY, L., AND BURMAN, K. D. 1982. Alterations in thyroid function in patients with systemic illness: The "euthyroid sick syndrome." Endocrinol Rev 3:164–217.

WEBER, J. A., AND FERGUSON, F. G. 1982. Analysis of the cellular components of swine colostrum and milk. Proc 7th Int Congr Pig Vet Soc, Mexico City, p. 169.

WEGMANN, P.; BERTSCHINGER, H. U.; AND ENG, V. 1990. Relationship between contamination of the teat ends with coliform bacteria and incidence of coliform mastitis. Proc 11th Int Congr Pig Vet Soc, Lausanne, p. 302.

WHITACRE, M. D., AND THRELFALL, W. R. 1981. Effects of ergocryptine on plasma prolactin, luteinizing hormone and progesterone in the periparturient sow. Am J Vet Res 42:1538–1541.

WHITEHAIR, C. K., AND MILLER, E. R. 1986. Nutritional deficiencies. In Diseases of Swine, 6th ed. Ed. A. D. Leman, B. Straw, R. D. Glock, W. L. Mengeling, R. H. C. Penny, and E. Scholl. Ames: Iowa State Univ Press.

WHITEHAIR, C. K.; VALE, O. E.; LOUDENSLAGER, M.; AND MILLER, E. R. 1983. MMA in sows – A vitamin E-selenium deficiency. Agric Rep (AS-SW-8302). Mich State Univ, pp. 9–15.

WHITTEMORE, C. T., AND FRASER, D. 1974. The nursing and suckling behavior of pigs. 2. Vocalization of the sow in relation to suckling behavior and milk ejection. Br Vet J 130:346–356.

WILSON, M. F.; BRACKETT, D. J.; ARCHER, L. T.; BELLER-TODD, B. K.; TOMPKINS, P.; AND HINSHAW, L. B. 1982. Survival characteristics during septic shock in 39 baboons. Adv Shock Res 7:13–23.

WILSON, M. R. 1984. Synchronization of farrowing using a combination of oxytocin and prostaglandin administration: An aid to piglet survival rates. Proc 7th Int Congr Vet Pig Soc, Ghent, p. 279.

YOUNGBERG, J. A.; SMITH, B. B.; AND REED, P. J. 1988. Clearance characteristics of *Escherichia coli* lipopolysaccharide in the pig. Proc Conf Res Workers Anim Dis, p. 79.

ZYCZKO, K.; KUREMAN, B.; AND GIEREJ, W. 1986. Secretion disorders of mammary glands in sows. Zootechnica 29:45–56.

5 Nervous and Muscular Systems

R. Bradley

J. T. Done

STRUCTURE, DEVELOPMENT, AND FUNCTION. The nervous and muscular organs constitute a completely integrated interreactive system for effecting perception, locomotion, and reflex and voluntary movement; they are also responsible for homeostasis and emergency responses of body functions not under voluntary control.

The Nervous System. Anatomically and functionally the nervous system can be divided into the central nervous system (CNS), wholly protected by the bony skeleton of the cranium and vertebral column; the peripheral nervous system (PNS), which is almost entirely extraskeletal; and the autonomic nervous system (ANS), composed of both central and peripheral elements.

Sensory function is effected through specialized receptors (e.g., in skin, muscle, and retina) that convert environmental stimuli into electrical impulses. These in turn are transmitted by the afferent branches of the cranial and peripheral nerves via ganglionic relays to the spinal cord and brain. Relatively simple semiautomatic activities are mediated by spinal reflex arcs; but fine, coordinated movements and responses to perceived stimuli depend on the highly specialized functions of neurons anatomically located in the brain. Automatic involuntary control of bodily functions is mediated by the ANS, which is also concerned with behavior and the animal's response to environmental and psychic stimuli.

THE CENTRAL NERVOUS SYSTEM. The anatomy of the brain and spinal cord of the pig is generally similar to that of other domestic mammals; see Sack (1982) and Dyce et al. (1987) for gross anatomy; Yoshikawa (1968) for detailed architecture of the brain; and Palmer (1976), King (1978), and De Lahunta (1983) regarding functional anatomy. Approximate weights of the brain and spinal cord are 35 and 4 g in the newborn and 110–120 and 30–40 g in the adult respectively. However, pigs of modern domestic breeds may have brains as much as 34% smaller than wild pigs of comparable body weight; even at full adult size the brain of the domestic pig may weigh some 20% less than that of the wild pig (Röhrs and Kruska 1969).

There are normally 32 or 33 spinal nerves – C8 (cervical), T14–15 (thoracic), L6–7 (lumbar), and S4 (sacral). The brain and cord are physically lubricated and cushioned by the cerebrospinal fluid (CSF), a lymphlike secretion that filters out from the capillary network and drains back via the subarachnoid spaces and the ventricular system to the cysternae at the base of the brain and thence back to the venous circulation.

The general morphologic development of the porcine nervous system is covered by standard embryology texts, e.g., Marrable (1971); the differentiation and growth of the cerebellum by Larsell (1954) and Done and Hebert (1968) respectively; and the dynamics of CNS development by Dickerson and Dobbing (1966–67). The patterns and dynamics of CNS growth and differentiation are important insofar as they contribute to developmental locomotor disorders (Done 1976a), and considerable attention has been given to morphologic and neurochemical parameters since the 1960s.

Histologically, the nervous system is composed of ectodermal and mesodermal elements. The neuroectoderm gives rise to the neurons, myelin-producing glia (oligodendrocytes and Schwann cells), supportive astrocytes (fibrous and protoplasmic), and ependyma. The mesoderm is represented by the vascular network, choroid plexuses, and phagocytic microglia. See Ham (1979) for detailed histology of the nervous system.

The most important single element in the nervous system is the neuron (sensory, motor, or intercalated), including its specialized processes synapsing with its functional coadjutors. Its main process, the axon, is variably invested in a laminated myelin sheath laid down and maintained by oligodendrocytes (CNS) or Schwann cells (PNS), each of which myelinates internodes of one or more axons. The neuronal pattern characteristic of maturity is produced by proliferation, migration, and differentiation of neuroblasts and is virtually complete by some 6 weeks after birth; contrary to earlier views, some degree of neuroblastic activity seems to persist at least into early adult life.

Myelin is a complex, lipid-rich lamellated structure surrounding and apparently responsible for the functional integrity of all but the slenderest axons. Myelination of the CNS in the pig begins at about 55–60 days gestation and rises to a peak around birth. There is a further minor surge some 3 weeks after birth, and myelination of developing axons continues throughout the period of CNS growth; but thereafter myelin metabolism in the normal pig is restricted to a certain amount of turnover of the constituent lipids. For further neurochemical information see Dickerson and Dobbing (1966–67), Sweasey et al. (1976), and Patterson (1977).

THE PERIPHERAL NERVOUS SYSTEM. The PNS is composed of sensory neurons and motor neurons. Sensory neurons have cell bodies located in the cranial or spinal ganglia and specialized receptors at the end of their terminal axons. Motor neurons have cell bodies in the brain or ventral horns of the spinal cord and axons terminating as motor end plates on the surface of muscle cells.

As in the CNS, all but the finest axons are myelinated, the myelin being produced by Schwann cells, each of which myelinates only one internode. Although superficially similar to that of the CNS, the myelin of the PNS differs structurally and chemically, and it can be differentially stained in histologic preparations. It is also under different genetic control and behaves differently when damaged.

THE AUTONOMIC NERVOUS SYSTEM. The ANS is concerned with emergency mechanisms and the homeostasis and rehabilitation of the animal's internal economy. Peripherally, the ANS comprises afferent pathways from the body organs together with pre- and postganglionic lower motor neurons that innervate the muscles of the heart and the smooth muscle of blood vessels, viscera, and glands. Its higher centers are in the hypothalamus, midbrain, pons, and medulla, with the hypothalamus acting as the primary functional integrator. Physiologically and anatomically, it has two distinct component parts: a sympathetic (thoracolumbar) division, which releases the neurotransmitter noradrenaline, and a parasympathetic (craniosacral) system, which utilizes acetylcholine as its terminal neurotransmitter. For more detailed information see Swenson (1977) and De Lahunta (1983).

Behavior patterns are also mediated by the ANS but they are outside the scope of this chapter. The interested reader is referred to Signoret et al. (1975).

The Muscular System

STRUCTURE. Muscles consist principally of muscle cells bound together by connective tissue in fascicles of several orders of size. The endomysium is a thin membrane of glycoprotein—appearing as the basal lamina in the electron microscope (EM)—and reticular fibers, which clothes each multinucleated, cylindrical muscle cell like a nylon stocking around a leg. The perimysium is thicker and sheaths the fascicles; the complete muscle is surrounded by epimysium, which in turn is continuous with the connective tissue of tendons that connects the muscle to its origin and insertion, principally on bones. The blood vessels and nerves are located in these connective tissue sheaths. Lymphatics are difficult to demonstrate in the muscle itself and appear to be confined to the epimysium and tendons. The myelinated axons of lower motor neurons (LMN) or ventral horn cells enter the muscle as the peripheral nerve. Within the muscle the component axons split into solitary fibers and divide near the termination. Each terminal axon loses its myelin sheath and ends on a solitary muscle cell at a motor end plate. Thus each LMN innervates a number of muscle cells, a group of which is called a motor unit. This operates on the all-or-none principle. For any particular muscle, motor end plates are grouped anatomically at specific sites known as motor points. To sample such areas for histologic examination, it is necessary to identify the motor point with electrophysiologic apparatus.

Muscle cells exist as three different types, which can be classified anatomically, physiologically, biochemically, histochemically, or by a combination of these methods (Table 5.1). All cells within a motor unit are of the same histochemical type. The proportions of cells of the three types vary in different muscles, and this is related to the function of the muscle. Type 1 cells are slow-contracting, fatigue-resistant, and red in color because of a high myoglobin content; they have a predominantly aerobic metabolism for obtaining energy; and they occur in high proportion in red muscles in constant work such as those concerned with respiration and posture. Type 2 cells are fast-contracting and susceptible to fatigue and have an anaerobic metabolism for obtaining energy and thus a low myoglobin content and a paler color. Such cells can achieve greater size than type 1 cells because of their lower requirements for oxygen and are said to form a higher proportion of the total population of cells in white muscles of stress-susceptible animals. Intermediate cells have similarities to both type 1 and type 2 cells. Cell-type proportions are probably determined genetically. Differentiation of cells into different types occurs in the fetus and continues after birth. Thus cell type proportion in any muscle can vary with age. Some muscles (e.g., the semitendinosus) consist of red (type 1 cell–rich) and white (type 2 cell–rich) parts, so muscle structure is not necessarily uniform throughout. The means of obtaining energy for contraction in type 2 and intermediate cells can be influenced by muscle training. Muscle cell numbers are under genetic control and maximums are achieved at or close to birth. Thereafter, muscle growth is dependent upon increase in length and girth of preexisting cells. Muscle cells increase in length by adding sarcomeres at their ends. Muscle length determines the range of possible movement about a joint. Muscle cell girth increases because of an increase in myofibrillar number brought about by a process of longitudinal splitting and growth of existing myofibrils. Girth of type 2 cells can be artificially increased still further by isometric training, but this is of little practical value in pig management. Muscle girth determines the strength of a muscle. The main factor in the determination of muscle size is the total number of constituent muscle cells, whereas the ultimate size of each cell is influenced by exercise and nutrition (Luff and Goldspink 1967).

In most animal species with muscles composed of mixed cell types, type 1 cells are scattered in a checkerboard pattern within the fascicles; but in the pig, type 1 cells tend to occur in island groups within fascicles (Fig. 5.1).

Muscle spindles are cigar-shaped encapsulated structures containing 5–13 intrafusal muscle cells bathed in lymphlike fluid. They are arranged in parallel with the contractile extrafusal cells; have a complex, multiple sensory and motor nerve supply; and are the origin of afferent impulses to the CNS. They play a part in the subconscious nervous control of muscular contraction (Simpson 1972). Golgi tendon organs and Golgi-Mazzoni corpuscles are small, encapsulated afferent endings responding to mechanical deformation and are located in tendon and connective tissue sheaths respectively.

Further general information on muscle anatomy can be found in any standard textbook, e.g., Sack (1982). The histology and ultrastructure of muscle are well described and illustrated by Rhodin (1975) and Ham (1979) and the histochemistry by Dubowitz and Brooke (1973).

DEVELOPMENT. In the embryo, mononuclear myoblasts are produced from mesodermal cells. These multiply and fuse to form multinucleate myotubes. Actin and myosin myofilaments are synthesized and organized into sarcomeres along with Z discs, the sarcoplasmic reticulum, and

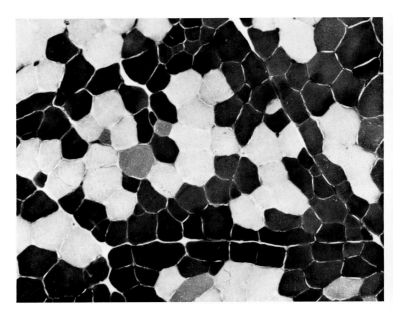

5.1. Cranial tibial muscle of a 12-week-old pig. Type 1 cells (light) occur in island groups. Type 2 cells (dark) predominate. There are some intermediate cells. Myosin ATPase pH 10.4. (British Crown copyright.)

Table 5.1. Relationship between physiologic, biochemical, and histochemical characteristics and three systems of muscle cell-type nomenclature

Contraction Speed	ATPase pH 10.4 Reaction	Energy Method	NADH-TR Reaction or Hemoglobin Content	Cell-type Nomenclature 1	2	3
Slow	Low	Oxidative (aerobic)	High	SO	I	β red
Fast	Int	Oxidative/ glycolytic (combined)	Int	FOG	Int	α red
Fast	High	Glycolytic (anaerobic)	Low	FG	II	α white

Note: SO = slow contraction, oxidative; FOG = fast contraction, oxidative/glycolytic; FG = fast contraction, glycolytic; Int = intermediate.

transverse tubular systems. The central nuclei migrate peripherally to lie under the sarcolemma. The muscle cells are innervated before birth, and this is essential for differentiation, growth, and maintenance of normal function. Some myoblasts remain dormant as solitary satellite cells under the basal lamina (basement membrane) of muscle cells. These, which can be detected readily under the EM, are thought to have a functional capability for differentiation into muscle cells following myodegeneration.

FUNCTION. The brain is connected with the foot, and vice versa (Fig. 5.2). The upper motor neuron (UMN) in the motor area of the cerebral cortex is responsible for the volitional control of the musculature. Operating via interneurons in the spinal cord, these synapse with the LMN. In the case of muscles with a cranial nerve supply, the equivalent neuron is located in specific nuclei (e.g., the facial nucleus) within the brain. Also synapsing with the LMN are the afferent nerves from the muscular spindles, so that the LMN is the final common pathway for the two systems. The circuit from spindle through the dorsal root ganglion (DRG), LMN cell body, peripheral nerve, and end plate to motor unit is called the spinal reflex arc. The patellar reflex is an example of the operation of this arc.

Muscles often share work (e.g., the digital extensors) and are known as synergists. There are also antagonists (e.g., the digital flexors). These are not always passive but assist in the accurate placing of a limb and in the maintenance of posture, which is controlled centrally.

It is important also to recognize that some muscles have a multiple nerve supply (e.g., biceps of the thigh). Thus injury to one particular nerve may not produce exactly the expected pathologic change in such a dually innervated muscle.

The maintenance of muscle stretch is called muscle tone. This fatigue-resistant mechanism is effected by controlled contraction of motor units composed of type 1 muscle cells in the antigravity muscles, and it enables the animal to maintain an erect posture. The muscle spindles play a part in the subconscious nervous control of muscular contraction via stretch reflexes. The efferent, slow motor fibers that innervate the intrafusal cells are under spinocerebellar influence. The spindles control the rate of shortening of the muscle and damp reflex responses. The Golgi tendon organs are deformed when tension develops in tendons, the information is relayed to the CNS by afferent nerves, and they are involved principally as inhibitors in the reflex control of muscle contraction. For further information see Simpson (1972) and Palmer (1976).

It has long been known that muscles do not change in volume when they contract. By analogy it is presumed that the same is true of muscle cells. Thus in transverse section, contracted cells are more rounded and have a larger caliber than when relaxed. The degree of contraction can only be assessed by measurement of sarcomere lengths in longitudinal sections. Muscle cell caliber variation is an important feature of some muscle diseases and must be distinguished from contraction artifacts that can occur if muscles are not clamped in situ at rest length when collected for pathologic examination.

Normal muscle function is dependent on the presence and availability of a number of enzymes. If these are absent or deficient, muscle function can be seriously upset. Normal muscle growth and function is also dependent upon the endocrine system. Growth hormone, thyroxine, insulin, sex hormones, corticosteroids, and adrenaline all have effects on the muscle. Standard veterinary physiology and biochemistry texts should be consulted for more information. Adrenaline is important in the porcine stress syndrome (see Chapter 61). Neuromuscular function in health and disease is well documented by McComas (1977).

PATHOLOGIC PROCESSES AND SIGNS OF SYSTEM DYSFUNCTION

Patterns and Determinants of Disease. Basically, we can envisage three alternative pathologies: (1) organic lesions with resultant functional deficits, as in the viral polioencephalomyelitides;

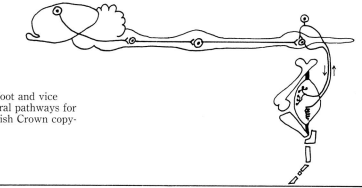

5.2. The brain is connected to the foot and vice versa. Simplified diagram of the neural pathways for muscle innervation and control. (British Crown copyright.)

(2) organic damage or dysgenesis without overt functional disorder, as in piglets with clinically silent cerebellar hypoplasia or myofibrillar hypoplasia; and (3) functional abnormality without readily detectable organic disease of the systems involved, as in Landrace trembles or tetanus.

In relation to the first two of these, and possibly to the third as well, the main determinants of clinical disease and its seriousness and eventual outcome are: (1) the tissues involved and the site(s) of the damage or other abnormality; (2) the nature of the defect; (3) the extent of the damage and/or deficit; (4) the duration of the pathologic process; (5) the timing of the insult relative to age, and especially to the stage of development; and (6) the possibilities for repair and recovery.

The organic lesions themselves may be (1) absent or at least undetectable by simple methods, as in tetanus or edema disease; (2) malformations, gross and/or microscopic, as in type A congenital tremor; (3) degenerative, as in arsanilic acid poisoning, mulberry heart disease, and iron-induced myodegeneration; (4) inflammatory and/or proliferative, as in the acute viral encephalomyelitides; (5) atrophic, as in cerebellar cortical sclerosis and the neurogenic muscle atrophies; or (6) any combination of the above.

The diagnostic significance of these reaction patterns will be discussed further under **Neuropathology.** For more detailed information on pathologic reactions of nervous and muscular tissues the interested reader is referred to Innes and Saunders (1962), Fankhauser and Luginbühl (1968), Jubb and Kennedy (1970), and Blackwood and Corsellis (1976).

Clinically, the responses to impairment of the neuromuscular system may be characterized as either negative or positive, though an individual pig may show both types. Negative signs (e.g., paralysis or other functional loss) are the direct results of the injury; while positive signs are generally ascribable to release from inhibitory control (as in muscle spasticity), increased irritability (as in the fits of pseudorabies or salt poisoning), or functional compensation (as in the broad-based stance characteristic of Talfan disease or the hypermetria of pantothenic acid deficiency).

Assuming that the disease is not itself fatal, the clinical outcome may be an apparently full or at least partial recovery once the causal agent has been removed. Such clinical remission is generally assisted by compensatory activity of undamaged elements in the system. On the other hand, but fortunately more rarely, what starts as a limited functional deficit may progress to a state in which it is uneconomic and/or inhumane to prolong life further. The progressive developmental disorders fall into this latter category, the severity of the locomotor disability being exacerbated by the rapid increase in body weight characteristic of the modern domestic pig.

ABNORMAL DEVELOPMENT. Developmental disorders form a special category in that they mostly represent the results of deviations from normal patterns of tissue differentiation and growth rather than damage to preformed tissues. Done (1976b) has classified the patterns of abnormal nervous development as follows: (1) Dysmorphogenesis—this includes a failure or disorder of morphologic development of varying severity from subcellular to gross organ malformation. (2) Metabolic defects—this includes the failure to synthesize nuclear proteins in sufficient amounts to sustain full-scale cell replication, the synthesis of abnormal compounds, and the partial or complete failure to produce enzymes required for catabolism or excretion of normal body constituents (the so-called lysosomal storage diseases). (3) Dysmaturity (as distinct from immaturity)—this connotes a discrepancy between chronologic and developmental age (e.g., in which a piglet may be born with a deficit in spinal myelin equal to or greater than 40%). Myofibrillar hypoplasia (MFH) may likewise be interpreted as a transient muscle dysmaturity. (4) Dysfunction—though frequently a result of dysmorphogenesis and/or dysmaturity, abnormal function may be evident in the absence of any demonstrable morphologic or biochemical abnormality (e.g., congenital splayleg or hereditary motor defect). (5) Instability—neoplasia, abiotrophy, and premature aging can be included in this category.

Developmental diseases are not limited to those present at birth; and congenital disorders include developmental accidents and teratogen-induced phenocopies as well as simple Mendelian and additive hereditary defects (Done 1968, 1976a,b; WHO 1977). Since, whatever their origin, the causes of developmental defects must operate via the same metabolic pathways, it is not surprising that apparently similar disorders may have quite different causes (see also Chapter 56).

Applied Neurology

NERVOUS SYSTEM. It is important to recognize that neurons are very large cells consisting of cell body, dendrites (receivers of information), and axons (transmitters of information), which may be very long. If neuron cell bodies die, they are not replaced, but there are possibilities for the repair of damaged axons. Axonal damage is followed by myelin breakdown and removal (Wallerian degeneration) and, if the axon is repaired, by remyelination. The myelin can also be destroyed segmentally without damage to the axon, as in lead poisoning.

It is common to find that agents causing damage to axons and/or myelin do so in the CNS and PNS simultaneously, but the distribution of lesions varies with each disease. Because of the different symptoms produced, this assists the clinician and the pathologist to make a diagnosis.

Except for some cranial nerves that contain only afferent sensory fibers, all spinal and most cranial nerves contain both sensory and efferent motor fibers. Close to the spinal cord the peripheral nerve divides into a ventral (motor) root, which contains axons originating from LMNs and a sensory dorsal root. The corresponding sensory neuron is bipolar and is located in the DRG.

Descending axons from the UMN pass down the spinal cord in the corticospinal tracts, which in the lumbar region (though not well defined) occupy the ventral and centromedial white matter. Axons from spinal neurons and dorsal roots ascend to the brain in tracts, which in the cervical cord are located in the dorsal and centrolateral white matter. This simplified description takes no account of Renshaw loops, interneurons, and the like, and the reader is referred to Palmer (1976) and De Lahunta (1983) for further detail.

It is convenient to consider clinical manifestations that occur in disease on the basis of the anatomical distribution of lesions. It is, however, important to recognize that boundaries of lesions and hence clinical signs vary.

Peripheral Nerves. Direct damage to the peripheral nerve alone is rarely seen in the pig. Traumatic injury is nondiscriminatory, so both sensory and motor fibers will be affected. Onset is sudden and commonly is seen as a distal sensory and motor loss.

Degenerative changes of predominantly sensory nerves occur in pantothenic acid deficiency, and this results in hypermetria (goose-stepping gait) from loss of proprioceptive impulses from the hind limbs. There is interference with the normal function of the reflex arc.

Degenerative changes, which predominantly affect motor but also sensory fibers and in which there is a CNS (spinal) component, occur in arsanilic acid toxicity and delayed haloxon neurotoxicity (Wells 1977). In the latter condition the hind limbs sway, and there is knuckling of fetlocks and, in severe cases, paralysis.

Dorsal and Ventral Nerve Roots. Maternal vitamin A deficiency during pregnancy, by its effect on vertebral growth in fetuses, causes herniation and constriction of dorsal and ventral nerve roots and results in a generalized flaccid congenital paralysis of all four limbs.

Irritative lesions of the DRG cell as in Teschen and/or Talfan disease cause hyperesthesia, paresthesia, and increased consciousness of pain in those areas innervated by the affected nerve roots. There is increased sensitivity of spinal reflexes.

Damage resulting in loss of function of dorsal root neurons will produce local anesthesia, diminution, or loss of spinal reflex activity, and

abnormal proprioceptive response such as abnormal gait and stance and decreased muscle tone.

Lower Motor Neuron. Loss of LMN function shows clinically as loss of voluntary and reflex motor activity and flaccid paralysis (lack of resistance to passive movement). It is also characterized by muscular fibrillation detectable by electromyography and after a period of days or weeks by atrophy of the muscles innervated by affected nerves. Muscle atrophy results from atrophy of the denervated motor units.

Reflex Arcs. For practical purposes the only reflexes of the pig that can be easily and profitably tested by the clinician are the pupilloconstriction, eye-preservation, and eye-fixating reflexes (see **Vision** below) and the limb withdrawal (pedal) reflex. The limb withdrawal reflex can be elicited by pinching the interdigital skin or pricking the skin above the claws. The segments of the cord involved in these reflexes in the pig are not precisely known but are likely to be about C6–T2 (forelimb) and L4–S2 (hind limb).

Loss of either the sensory or the motor component or both will result in loss of reflex activity, with flaccid paresis or paralysis. If only the motor component is affected, the animal can react at the cerebral level to painful local stimuli and indicates this by attempting to escape, grunting or groaning, or turning the head quickly to the side affected. If only the sensory component is damaged, voluntary movement is possible, though the withdrawal reflex is lost and proprioception is abnormal.

Upper Motor Neuron. Because the corticospinal fibers in the ventral cord are proximate to the vertebral centers, they are vulnerable to injury following vertebral fracture or dislocation, protrusion of vertebral discs, spondylitis, or pressure from space-occupying lesions such as tumors and abscesses.

Irritative damage to the UMN produces symptoms of motor excitement, which will be dealt with more fully under **Cerebral Function.** Examples of diseases affecting UMNs are pseudorabies (Chapter 24), lead poisoning (Chapter 64), and the salt poisoning–water deprivation syndrome (Chapter 64). Loss of UMN function results in a spastic type paralysis, with limitation of voluntary movement and increase in muscle tone; local reflexes are intact and may be exaggerated or otherwise abnormal. If the lesion is in the thoracic or lumbar regions, only the hind limbs will be affected; but if it is in or anterior to the cranial enlargement, both fore and hind legs will be involved. Pigs with UMN lesions may be able to stand if helped to their feet but fall down if pushed gently backward. In the longer term, UMN loss may lead to slow neurogenic atrophy of muscle through disuse even though the spinal reflex arcs are intact.

Cerebellum. The cerebellum is largely concerned with maintenance of posture and balance (labyrinthine organs), coordination (afferent impulses from ipsilateral proprioceptive tracts in the spinal cord and from the cerebral cortex on the opposite side; efferent impulses to motor and premotor cortex), and the regulation of fine muscular movement (anterior lobe).

Apart from specifically vestibular symptoms, damage to the cerebellar cortex is characterized by ataxia (with compensatory wide-based stance), dysmetria (imprecise movements in any direction), nystagmus, and tremor. Typically, tremors in the pig are at the rate of 2–4/seconds, as in congenital tremor, or 4–8/seconds, as in cerebellar cortical sclerosis. The muscle "weakness" commonly seen in cerebellar ataxias probably results from loss of impulses from the cerebellum to the muscle spindles via the gamma efferent fibers.

The cerebellum is a particularly vulnerable part of the pig's nervous system. In the fetus it is the part of the brain most liable to malformation. Postnatally, it is subject to specific attack (as in Teschen disease and pseudorabies); extension of suppurative processes from the fourth ventricle, meninges, and middle ear in bacterial infections; herniation through the foramen magnum by increased intracranial pressure as a result of internal hydrocephalus or cranial constriction (as in vitamin A deficiency); and hypoxic atrophy by interference with its blood supply (as in cerebellar cortical sclerosis).

Vestibular Syndrome. The vestibular apparatus concerned with posture and balance is composed of the sensory end organ (the labyrinth) in the inner ear, the vestibular ganglion and vestibular division of the auditory nerve, and the flocculonodular lobe of the cerebellum and the vestibular nuclei in the medulla and cerebellum. By virtue of its position, the system is vulnerable to extension of inflammatory processes from the middle ear; pressure from exudate in the lateral meninges or fourth ventricle; and abscesses, tumors, or other space-occupying lesions in the cerebellopontine angle.

Signs of vestibular involvement are rotation and turning of the head to the affected side, with a tendency to circle in the same direction. The pig may fall either to the side to which the head is turned or in the opposite direction. Unilateral nystagmus on the affected side is indicative of damage to the cerebellar part of the system.

Vision. Vision is mediated by afferent impulses from the photoreceptors (rod and cone cells) in the retina by way of the optic nerve, optic tract, lateral geniculate body, and optic radiation to the visual cortex in the occipital lobe of the cerebrum. Voluntary control of eye movements is effected by cranial nerves III, IV, and VI. Control of eyelid movement is effected by the facial nerve (VII), and sensory stimuli are received via the ophthalmic division of the trigeminal nerve (V). Autonomic control of pupil size is maintained via the oculomotor nerve and ciliary ganglion.

Although ophthalmoscopic examination is a laudable procedure in cases of suspected blindness, its performance in the fully conscious pig is extremely difficult; critical descriptions of abnormal conditions of the fundus and even of the lens, cornea, and conjunctiva are scanty or lacking. The availability of such ataractic drugs as azaperone and of efficient and easily portable fundus cameras may help to remedy this deficit.

Assessment of visual function is in practice confined to observation of behavioral signs of blindness (e.g., falling over or colliding with objects in poor light) and to testing for reflex activity. The eye-preservation (blink) reflex and the fixating reflex are both dependent on the integrity of afferent pathways from the retina to the visual cortex. They will be lost in conditions like meningoencephalitis eosinophilia and pseudorabies, which affect the cerebrum, and also in arsanilic acid poisoning, which damages the optic nerve and optic tract. The blink reflex is tested by threatening the eye with a hand or other light-colored object; a sheet of transparent plastic held in front of the pig's eye will obviate reflex closure of the eye because of stimulation of the cornea by moving air. The eye-fixating reflex causes an involuntary turning of the head and eyes toward an object moving across the field of vision. It is readily evoked by dropping tufts of cotton or wool in front of but some distance away from each eye in turn.

Reflex constriction of the pupil when a bright light is shone into the eye depends on the integrity of the autonomic centers in the midbrain but is independent of the visual cortex. Thus in the purely cortical blindness of salt poisoning, the pupilloconstriction reflex is retained; though it is lost in arsanilic acid poisoning, it may be present or absent in pseudorabies and cerebrospinal angiopathy, depending on the extent of the damage to the midbrain and/or optic tract.

It will be recalled that the optic field on one side is represented on the cerebrocortex of the opposite side. Because of the decussation of the great majority of optic nerve fibers in the pig, unilateral lesions in the visual pathways behind the optic chiasma will cause the most severe loss of vision in the opposite eye.

Cerebral Function. Apart from visual function (occipital lobe) the cerebrum is also responsible for voluntary movement, consciousness, and behavior. The motor cortex occupies an area in the superior longitudinal gyrus between the coronal sulcus laterally and the cruciate sulcus medially, but the location of other functions are less well defined. Consciousness and general sensory perception are distributed over the cortex of the frontal, parietal, and temporal lobes, with personality and behavior probably associated with the anterior frontal lobe.

Irritative lesions of the motor cortex are associated with epileptiform fits; compulsive aimless walking and circling; or if the animal is recumbent, periodic or continuous struggling, galloping, or paddling movements of the legs. The causes of fits are traditionally classified as central if the lesion is in the CNS or as peripheral when it is not, as in hypoglycemia or hypoxia resulting from anemia. Fits are always the immediate result of abnormal activity of the cerebral cortex. They may occur spontaneously or be precipitated by suddenly increasing external stimuli such as sudden noise or handling.

The seizures of salt poisoning take a characteristic form, with the pig at first standing or sitting tensely and apprehensively, ears pricked, staring ahead and slightly upward as though seeing some object invisible to the observer. Then the nose starts to twitch, the head nods, the eyes close, and rhythmic chomping of the jaws produces a froth of saliva. As the clonic movements increase in strength and amplitude, the head is forced up and the pig moves backward. The body becomes increasingly rigid until the seizure reaches its climax and the animal falls down in apnea, often preceded by a hoarse cry. After an attack the pig lies quietly in a coma until normal respiration is restored; then it resumes the same behavior as before the fit.

Irritative lesions of the sensory cortex associated with sensation of pain are manifested by grinding the teeth, closing the eyes tightly, and pressing the head hard against a wall or other fixed object. There is also photophobia and increased sensitivity to noise and handling. Disturbance of consciousness may be seen as excitement, depression, or coma.

Loss of UMN activity usually occurs at the same time as irritative symptoms but can be seen alone (e.g., with lesions of the striate body or midbrain in cerebrospinal angiopathy).

Changes in personality and behavior may not be very important in the individual pig but certainly occur. Pigs with granulomatous lesions of visceral larva migrans (larval worms) in the anterior cerebrum became friendly and unapprehensive when handled (Done et al. 1960), and a state of positive euphoria was a distinctive feature of pigs poisoned with arsanilic acid (Harding et al. 1968).

Meningismus. Because the meninges cover the whole brain and spinal cord and are in communication at the cisterna magna with the ventricular system, diffuse meningitis produces a wide-ranging clinical syndrome. By pressure on or exten-

sion to the cerebral cortex there is trismus, opisthotonos, or orthotonos, with rigidity or tonic spasms of the muscles of the head and back. By investing the roots of cranial or spinal nerves, there is disturbance of sensory and motor function. Interference with drainage of cerebrospinal fluid from the cisterna magna, as in streptococcal choriomeningitis, results in increased intracranial pressure. This in turn may cause further pressure on the cerebral cortex and cranial nerves, herniation of the cerebellum with traumatic damage to the posterior vermis, and stenosis or occlusion of arteries in vulnerable positions (e.g., the anterior cerebellar artery).

The animal may vomit because of irritation of the nucleus solitarius, induced by pressure on the upper surface of the medulla.

MUSCULAR SYSTEM. A simplistic view of neuromuscular disease can include possibilities for structural or functional abnormality of the UMN and/or LMN; dorsal root neurons and their myelin sheaths; end plates, spindles, and their central motor neurons; and muscle cells and/or associated structures within the muscle. It is, however, convenient and important to distinguish between neurogenic myopathies, which are secondary, and the primary myopathies. In the former the disease process originates in the nervous system and in the latter in the muscle cells.

Neurogenic Myopathy. Destruction of all UMNs would result in loss of volitional control of the muscle and development of spasticity, which includes increased muscle tone and abnormal reflexes. The spinal reflex (e.g., knee jerk) would remain intact. Total destruction of the LMN would abolish the spinal reflex arc, and the now denervated muscle would exhibit flaccid paralysis. It is irrelevant to the muscle whether the neuronal cell body dies (and hence its axon) or whether there is total axon destruction, as in severing, at least in the acute stage. Subsequently, however, there is a difference. In the former case the muscle cells in the motor unit can only be innervated by a different motoneuron, since dead neurons cannot regenerate. In the latter case the cells in the denervated unit may be reinnervated by the same or different motoneurons. Histochemically, reinnervation of a motor unit by different motoneurons is seen as type grouping. Primary injury to myelin sheaths (segmental demyelination) as distinct from that following axonal injury (Wallerian degeneration) is rare, as is injury or malfunction of the motor end plates (as in myasthenia gravis).

In practice, though most nervous diseases produce lesions in particular areas of the CNS or PNS, they are rarely selective to the UMN or LMN alone. Furthermore, neurons may not be totally destroyed (dead); they may have reduced function (sick), or some in the locality with similar functions may remain healthy. Dead and sick neurons will cause degenerative processes in the muscle. The converse, namely primary muscle disease having an effect on the motoneuron, is a possibility for which there is evidence (McComas 1977).

Primary Myopathy. Symptoms of primary muscle disease depend on the groups of muscles affected. Thus diseases of the tongue, cheek, and pharyngeal muscles are seen as difficulties in eating and swallowing; disease of the diaphragm or intercostal muscles is seen as a respiratory disease not unlike pneumonia. By far the most common signs are muscular weakness, trembling while standing, pain, swelling, or wasting – all being manifested as locomotor and/or postural disorders. With the exception of acute back muscle necrosis, primary myopathies are unaccompanied by sensory dysfunction.

Acute (primary) muscle disorders usually involve myodegenerative change, and this is accompanied by a rise in plasma creatine kinase (CK) activity. If severe, there may also be transient myoglobinuria resulting from release of myoglobin from damaged muscle cells first into the plasma and then the urine. Myodegeneration, as in the selenium-responsive myopathies, can be severe and fatal.

Porcine Stress Syndrome (PSS) and Related Postmortem Defects of Pig Meat. Since skeletal and cardiac muscle is the target tissue in PSS, it is briefly reviewed here for completeness. The reader is also referred to Chapter 61, Swatland (1974), Bradley and Wells (1978), and Bradley and Fell (1981).

PSS is a naturally occurring, acute-onset condition of certain well-muscled strains or breeds (e.g., Pietrain) of pig that have been improved by selection for low-fat, high-lean carcass composition. The initial requirement is a pig with a hereditary liability to the condition. To convert a susceptible animal to a diseased one, a stress is required. Under natural conditions this usually takes the form of any one or more of the following factors: transportation; excitement (especially preslaughter); and exposure to high environmental temperature, to certain depolarizing agents such as succinylcholine, or to anesthetics, of which halothane is the most frequently reported. Use is also made of a sublethal dose of halothane to detect pigs liable to the condition in genetic improvement programs. In clinically positive halothane tests the name given to the condition that develops is malignant hyperthermia (MH), which is analogous to the condition of the same name that occurs in some human patients during halothane anesthesia.

Clinically, pigs show respiratory distress, the skin may show rapidly varying blotches, blood and muscle show increased lactate, and eventually the pig enters premature rigor with pyrexia that persists for an hour or so after death. In pigs with adequate supplies of muscle glycogen, the meat (particularly the loin and to a lesser degree the ham) takes on a pale, soft, and exudative (PSE) appearance. This is most obvious on the days following slaughter. Unacceptable amounts of drip and paleness detract from the sale value of the meat, especially in vacuum packs on days subsequent to the first day of display. In animals in which the muscle glycogen is depleted before slaughter, the meat ends up as dark, firm, and dry (DFD); it has a high pH (from low lactate) and thus poor keeping quality. This affects a much smaller proportion of animals than the PSE condition.

The biochemical mechanism is such that in susceptible animals with adequate glycogen reserves, stress induces an accelerated glycolysis and increase in muscle lactate, while the muscle temperature is high. Denaturation of muscle proteins follows, with a loss of water-binding capacity of the tissue. These changes result in drip and pallor caused by altered surface reflectance.

A number of techniques, of which the halothane test is most common, can be used to detect susceptible individuals. To detect carcasses that are likely to end up as PSE or DFD, muscle pH can be measured in the m. longissimus dorsi at the last rib and/or in the m. semitendinosus 45 minutes (pH_1) and 24 hours (pH_2) postmortem. The critical values, which may vary among authors, are pH_1 pH 6.0 for PSE and pH_2 >pH 6.5 for DFD. Identification at an early stage of a potential PSE carcass enables a decision to be made as to its fate, e.g., for manufacturing as distinct from fresh meat sale. These techniques also enable abattoir managers to monitor the problem and take necessary action to improve preslaughter handling and if necessary to identify herds that are sources of trouble. One has also to take account of the desirable high-lean carcass associated with the condition; therefore, a balanced view must be taken.

Diagnosis is not simple. The clinical signs, particularly in agonal stages, are helpful pointers. If postmortem examination is carried out within 1 hour of death, the high rectal and muscle temperatures and early rigor are useful features. Measurement of pH of the m. longissimus dorsi at the last rib is also a helpful guide. The gross postmortem findings are not specific. It is helpful to note that back muscle necrosis is a component of PSS (see **BACK MUSCLE NECROSIS**).

Histologically in transverse section, muscle cells are shrunken and widely separated, with the occurrence of so-called giant fibers (large, rounded, and supercontracted muscle cells).

In longitudinal sections of the m. longissimus dorsi, multiple contraction bands are usually seen. None of these lesions is pathognomonic but may, with other factors in the history, assist in reaching a tentative diagnosis that would lead to further investigation in the herd of origin, assessment of the economic effects, and establishment of control measures if necessary. These will be a combination of efforts to reduce stress (environmental control) and the liability to stress by halothane or other testing and selection of resistant animals for breeding (genetic control).

Special Pathology. The following aspects are particularly relevant because they influence the genesis and progress of disease, the immediate response to treatment, and the progress in the longer term.

NERVOUS SYSTEM

Permeability of the Blood-Brain Barrier. In the healthy pig, physiologic mechanisms prevent the passage of large molecules such as immunoglobulins and antibiotics into the CSF in more than minute amounts. In practice this limits the access of serum antibodies to viruses replicating intracellularly and spreading within the CNS in the early (prodromal) stages of disease. Once tissue destruction has occurred, with activation of the reticuloendothelial system and increase in vascular permeability, antibodies can pass freely, but by that time extensive invasion and functional loss of susceptible cells may have taken place. The presence of antibody contributes to the reactive process (see below) but may effectively neutralize most or all of the extracellular virus; this explains why it is difficult or impossible to isolate virus from the CNS in Teschen and/or Talfan disease by the time a well-marked encephalomyelitis has developed. In purulent meningitis, vascular permeability is soon increased, and with the involvement of the choroid plexus, the blood-brain barrier offers little impediment to the passage of antibiotics. Thus in streptococcal choriomeningitis, blanket treatment of a litter with penicillin can be expected to build up an effective drug concentration in the CSF of piglets in which subclinical invasion of the CNS has occurred.

Sequelae of Reactive Processes. The direct effects of the primary pathogen, whether toxic, metabolic, or infectious, are responsible for only part of the total damage to nervous tissue. The brain reacts to local damage by cellular exudation and to the presence of necrotic tissue by phagocytosis followed by scar formation. Necrotic areas and foreign material are at first walled off by granulation tissue and subsequently (over 3 weeks) are surrounded by astroglial fibrosis. Some of the necrotic or exogenous material that provokes scar formation originates from the brain's own reaction to stimuli. In this way the CNS tends to overreact and thus to produce further nervous damage during the process of repair. For example, minimal symptoms and lesions are seen while larvae of *Toxocara canis* are actively migrating through the brain, but when the larvae become static and the brain invests them in granulomas, extensive losses of tissue and function may result.

Regeneration and Repair. The full neuronal complement of the CNS of the pig is present by about 6 weeks of age, and neurons lost thereafter are not replaced. However, the normally developed pig has a generous reserve of nervous capacity and, if the pathologic process is stabilized, can usually cope with quite extensive loss or deficiency by education and/or adaptation of its remaining capacity.

It was formerly believed that demyelination within the CNS was irreversible, but more recent observations indicate that in so-called "partial demyelination," myelin sheaths may be involved in degenerative and regenerative processes at the same time (e.g., as in congenital tremor A1). Furthermore, a limited amount of remyelination of the CNS may be effected by Schwann cells that have migrated.

The axons and myelin sheaths of peripheral nerves can regenerate quite readily if the damage is limited to the part of the nerve covered by the sheath of Schwann and the damaged ends are fairly close together. Repair, if it occurs, will probably never exceed a rate of about 0.5 cm/day.

MUSCLE. The remote effects of nervous disease on the muscle are atrophy of cells within an affected motor unit together with slowly developing degenerative changes such as target and motheaten cells. These take days, weeks, or months to become obvious. Atrophy is most easily detected by outlining cell boundaries with a reticulin stain (Fig. 5.3). The degenerative changes are clearly revealed with NADH-tetrazolium reductase (Fig. 5.4).

After myodegeneration, animals can recover completely, particularly if the causal deficiencies are corrected. The degree of recovery, however, depends partly on the extent of initial damage. If this is severe, death can occur in the acute phase. If mild, the degenerated cells undergo phagocytosis, and regeneration of muscle cells occurs, probably by differentiation of satellite cells. In severely damaged parts of muscles, replacement fibrosis occurs, presumably because no, or not enough, satellite cells remain.

Following denervation, muscle cells atrophy; but if they become reinnervated reasonably quickly, they respond by growth to normal or near normal size, though fiber-type distribution may be altered. If reinnervation does not occur, the end result is fibrosis and fatty replacement.

In slowly progressive muscle disorders such as the Pietrain creeper syndrome, changes are progressive and irreversible. Myodegeneration, atrophy, and abnormal cell structure occur together with fibrosis and fatty replacement. However, this end stage is seldom reached, since pigs are

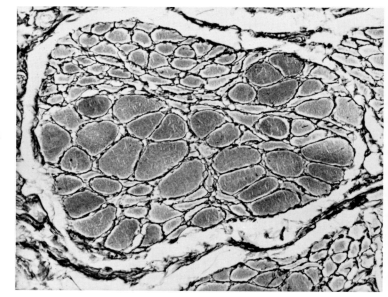

5.3. Ventricularis muscle of a 12-week-old pig with delayed haloxon neurotoxicity. Cell boundaries are well defined and show neurogenic group atrophy. Gomori reticulin stain. (British Crown copyright.)

usually destroyed on humane grounds beforehand.

DIAGNOSTIC PROCEDURES

Clinical Neurology. Diagnosis is essentially a matter of detecting and defining a deviation from normality and attempting to assign physiologic and anatomic bases for them.

Though the pig is not a very cooperative subject for neurologic examination, this aspect of diagnosis should not be neglected. Systematic recording of a relatively small number of clinical variables such as posture, gait, mental state, reflex activity, sensory perception, and occurrence of involuntary movement can provide much useful information as to the possible location of lesions, though there is rarely a simple relationship between symptoms and lesions in naturally occurring nervous disease. Several parts of the nervous system may be affected, with differing and interacting disturbances of function. Palmer (1976) and De Lahunta (1983) are very handy books of reference in this field and should be studied by all clinicians who seriously intend to investigate nervous and muscular disorders of individual pigs.

A general clinical and epidemiologic investigation will probably also contribute significantly to the diagnosis, e.g., Wells (1984).

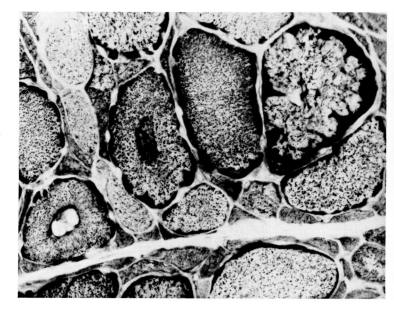

5.4. Diaphragm muscle of a 12-week-old pig with delayed haloxon neurotoxicity. Target, moth-eaten, and atrophic cells can be identified. NADH-TR. (British Crown copyright.)

CLINICAL PATHOLOGY

Cerebrospinal Fluid. The commercial value of an individual pig will rarely justify diagnostic examination of the CSF as an adjunct or alternative to other action, especially since there is a dearth of criteria in the pig for differentiation of nervous diseases by this method. The spinal cord of the pig continues as far as S2–3, so lumbar puncture involves some risk of damage to the cord. However, CSF can be obtained fairly easily and safely from the cisterna magna by the introduction of a graduated needle vertically along the posterior surface of the cranium with the animal under general anesthesia and the neck flexed.

Fankhauser (1962) has summarized most of the available information on the subject. The changes that occur in nonsuppurative polioencephalomyelitis are given in Table 5.2.

Electroencephalography. Electroencephalography is not likely to be generally available for diagnostic use in the field within the foreseeable future, but it is potentially useful in the identification at laboratory level of functional disorders with no known morphologic lesions (see **CONGENITAL MOTOR DEFECT** below). In the pig the electrical activity of the brain has taken on the adult pattern by the end of the first month of postnatal life.

Serology. Serology can be a very useful epidemiologic tool in the investigation of infectious diseases, especially those caused by viruses, but does not supersede effective neurologic and pathologic examination for the diagnosis of nervous disease in an individual pig. Samples of serum taken from identified pigs at 14-day intervals can be expected to show rising titers to the causal organism in acute disease and static or falling titers in chronic or convalescent cases. However, association is not synonymous with causation, and the investigator should be wary of interpreting a rising titer to, say, Talfan virus in recently mixed pigs with abnormal gait as confirmation that the nervous symptoms presented are those of Talfan disease. They may be suffering from hog cholera, pantothenic acid deficiency, or organic arsenical poisoning, and the raised antibody titers may only reflect recent exposure to infection of pigs with a waning passive immunity.

Muscle Biopsy. The general principles and techniques involved in muscle biopsy have been described by Bradley (1978); Dubowitz and Brooke (1973) may also usefully be consulted. A square-wave stimulator is a valuable additional tool for location of motor end plates in exposed muscle prior to surgical sampling.

Clinical Biochemistry. Blood examination is a valuable means of detecting elevated activities of enzymes in disease states. If muscle cells are damaged so that their cell membrane (sarcolemma) is broken or leaky, enzymes normally within the cell are released and enter the bloodstream, where they can be detected and measured. It is important to collect samples in such a way that muscle tissue is not penetrated or allowed to contaminate the sample. CK is specific to skeletal and cardiac muscle and to the CNS, but it occurs in highest concentration in muscle. The source of excess enzyme in blood can be detected by differential estimation of the three isoenzymes, though this is seldom required. Elevated CK activity indicates recent muscle cell damage. Another enzyme, glutathione peroxidase (GSH-PX), contains selenium in its molecular structure and is important in protecting cells from oxidative damage. It is relatively easy and inexpensive to measure the blood GSH-PX activity (compared with assay for selenium itself), and this gives a valuable indication of the selenium status of the animal. Its pathologic importance lies in the fact that dietary selenium deficiency is associated with a number of disease entities, including cardiac and skeletal myodegeneration.

Neuropathology and Muscle Pathology.
The person performing the necropsy may not be carrying out the more specialized parts of a neuropathologic examination but should have sufficient knowledge of the relevant techniques to ensure that the nervous tissues are handled in a way that will give optimal results from the pathologic study as a whole. Even when distinctive symptoms have pointed to a particular part of the nervous or muscular system as the probable seat of trouble, it is wise to carry out a standard "minimum-methods" pathologic examination of the system as a whole, remembering that the brain is connected to the foot, etc. This would be supplemented by closer attention to areas of special interest and using appropriate techniques to demonstrate specific changes.

BASIC PATHOLOGIC TECHNIQUES

Nervous System. The following routine procedure is recommended for examination of the nervous system:

Table 5.2. Characteristics of the CSF in Teschen disease compared with normality

Characteristic	Normal	Teschen Disease
Cells/ml	0.20	140 (5–1,000)
Sugar (mg%)	45–87	92–113 (45–180)
Albumin (mg%)	17–24	19.2–108
Globulin	5–10	9.6–84
Total protein (mg%)	24–40	36–67 (36–192)
Protein quotient	0–49	0.36–1.2
Nonne-Apelt	Negative	+ (inconstant)
Pandy	Negative	+ (inconstant)

Source: Fankhauser (1962).

1. Expose the brain aseptically as far back as the foramen magnum, noting the presence of pus in the meninges or gross brain malformation if present.
2. Remove the choroid plexus of the fourth ventricle aseptically for bacteriologic examination and making impression smears.
3. Remove the brain from the skull, weigh it, and fix it by immersion, normally in phosphate-buffered, normal, 10% formalin.
4. Recover, aseptically, for virologic examination (e.g., for pseudorabies virus) the hypothalamus and the portions of the olfactory bulbs remaining in the cranium.
5. Cut through the vertebral arches and remove the spinal cord with dorsal root ganglia attached. If appropriate, weigh the cord before fixation.
6. Remove and fix 1-cm-long blocks of spinal cord, with ganglia attached, at approximately C3, T1, T8, and L5. If only simple neurochemistry is required, the spinal cord may be fixed entire at this stage.
7. In baby pigs in which myelin dysgenesis is suspected, the remainder of the spinal cord is frozen for neurochemical examination (Patterson and Done 1977). However, simple lipid estimations can be carried out even on fixed tissue.
8. Prepare paraffin sections, stained by hematoxylin and eosin, from a standard set of blocks:
   (a) Brain–coronal sections of cerebrum at the olfactory tubercle; midbrain, through the anterior quadrigeminal bodies; medulla, through the obex; and cerebellum, by a median vertical sagittal section through the vermis.
   (b) Spinal cord–transverse sections at C3, T1, T8, and L5 including spinal nerve roots and dorsal root ganglia.
9. If electron microscopy is contemplated, very thin slices or dices of very fresh tissue should be fixed in an appropriate fixative after consultation with a laboratory specialist.
10. The remainder of the CNS is retained wet-fixed for subsequent examination if required.
11. The middle ear may conveniently be exposed by a vertical saw cut at right angles to the long axis of the skull after removal of the external ear.
12. For critical histologic examination of the ocular structures, the eyeball should be removed as for surgical enucleation, trimmed, and fixed intact by immersion in appropriate fixatives. Suitable techniques and fixatives are given in the publications of Saunders and Jubb (1961) and Saunders and Rubin (1975).

Fixation of nervous tissues after removal from the body is recommended if infectious or toxic conditions are suspected or if the etiology is unknown, as this allows fresh material to be taken for microbiologic or chemical examination. But when abnormal cytoarchitecture or degenerative lesions of neurons and their processes are likely to be involved, fixation in situ, particularly by perfusion, is the method of choice to minimize artifacts. If appropriate fixatives are used (e.g., 10% formol calcium acetate), fairly extensive neurochemical examination of myelin lipids is possible as well as purely morphologic and histochemical examination.

Ideally, the diagnostician would wish to demonstrate the causal agent in significant association with the lesions. For example, isolation of a virus from the CNS would demonstrate that it was present and hence putatively the cause of the disease. Fluorescent antibody techniques can relate virus antigen more specifically to individual cells, but they usually require frozen sections, which are generally inferior for histologic purposes. However, the advent of immunohistochemical methods using enzymes or colloidal gold as markers raises hopes for the detection of antigens in fixed and embedded tissues, which would additionally enable the retrospective investigation of tissues already filed away.

Muscular System. In sampling muscles for histologic examination, it is essential that (1) they be identified and named (see Nomina Anatomica Veterinaria 1983); (2) the site within the muscle is known and specified; (3) the muscle block is clamped in situ at rest length and parallel to the long axis of the muscle cells (Bradley 1978), enabling exact longitudinal and transverse sections to be prepared to allow simple visual comparisons or precise automated measurement of cross-sectional area or sarcomere length without distortion from obliquity or contraction artifacts; (4) it is fixed or frozen appropriately for the procedures to be undertaken.

For paraffin-embedding and light microscopy, the clamped sample is placed in normal saline at 25°C for 20 minutes before fixation in phosphate-buffered, neutral 10% formalin. In addition to the standard morphologic stains, Gomori's reticulin method is recommended to outline cell boundaries and allow detection of cell caliber variation (Fig. 5.3).

For epoxy resin–embedding and electron microscopy, place a small clamped sample directly into phosphate-buffered 3% glutaraldehyde, pH 7.4, at 4°C. After initial fixation, wash in buffer and postfix in buffered osmium tetroxide.

For histochemistry, cover the muscle block with cornstarch, plunge rapidly into liquid nitrogen for 15 seconds, and transfer to the cryostat at below −20°C. React serial frozen sections or acid- and alkali-stable myosin ATPase for cell typing, NADH tetrazolium reductase for determination of aerobic capacity, alpha-glucan phosphorylase for determination of the anaerobic capacity, periodic acid–Schiff for glycogen, and Sudan black B for fat (Dubowitz and Brooke 1973).

PATHOLOGIC INTERPRETATION

Nervous System. From the type and distribution of the morphologic lesions and from the types and proportions of cells and other structures therein, the experienced pathologist can generally get a fairly good idea of the nature of the causal agent, or even its actual identity, as well as the duration and likely progress of the pathologic process.

Space precludes an exhaustive treatise on this subject here, and neuropathologic taxonomies have been produced for the pig by Done (1957, 1968) and O'Hara and Shortridge (1966). However, two or three immediately useful examples will serve to illustrate the potential of this approach. First, Table 5.3 shows how the nonsuppurative encephalomyelitides of viral origin may be separated according to whether the condition is primarily neuronopathic, according to the distribution and relative severity of lesions in standard CNS sections, and according to whether inclusion bodies are present in nucleus or cytoplasm of affected cells.

Second, Figure 5.5 indicates how the distribution of degenerating nerve fibers varies in a number of diseases of different etiology. The usefulness of the method is enhanced by examining sections of spinal cord at several, preferably standard, levels (cervical, thoracic, lumbar).

Whereas the patterns depicted in Table 5.3 essentially represent acute tissue responses to virus invasion, those in Figure 5.5 are characteristic of a later stage in neuronal necrobiosis, probably at least 10 days after the onset of the process. Finally, Table 5.4 illustrates how morphologic information may be combined with neurochemical and epidemiologic data to provide a much sharper separation of entities than could be achieved by any single discipline.

Muscular System. Until quite recently, muscle disorders of farm animals were a rather neglected field. There is still much semantic confusion in this area, so a schematic taxonomy of skeletal myopathies is shown in Figure 5.6.

Muscle Pigmentation. Pathologic pigmentations can be endogenous or exogenous. Endogenous pigmentations that can affect muscle are melanosis (rare), those produced by the breakdown of blood (not uncommon), and lipofuscinosis or wear-and-tear pigmentation that occurs in old age and is therefore not common in pigs. Exogenous pigmentations are only likely following intramuscular injections. Some meat processing plants have reported a yellowish brown pigmentation of hams. Though claims have been made that the pigmentation is from injections of iron to the young pigs, none has been in fact substantiated, and the cause remains a mystery.

Muscle Atrophy. Muscle atrophy is a natural response to disuse, senility, undernutrition, and denervation. It is not a disease and the causes can only be elucidated by a careful examination of the history and microscopic examination of the muscle to determine the nature of the lesion, e.g., whether type 1 or type 2 cells are involved, there is fatty replacement and fibrosis, and there are structural alterations to muscle cells (target, targetoid, and moth-eaten cells) and features such as fiber-type grouping.

DISEASES OF THE NERVOUS AND MUSCULAR SYSTEMS.

Instead of attempting to exhaustively catalog all diseases affecting the nervous and muscular systems, we have presented the most important ones in tabular form in Table 5.5, emphasizing the earliest age of onset, main initial signs, and anatomical location of functional deficits and/or organic damage. For each entry we have referred the reader to an appropriate chap-

Table 5.3. CNS tissue reaction patterns in virus diseases

Disease	Primary Lesions[a]	Inflammatory Reaction[b]						Inclusion Bodies[c]
		Fore-brain	Mid-brain	Hind-brain	Cere-bellum	Spinal Cord	Spinal Ganglia	
Hog cholera	M	+	+ +	+ +	+	+	+	. . .
African swine fever	M	+	+	+	+	≈	≈	. . .
Rabies	E	+ +	+	+ +	+ +	+	+	I/C
Pseudorabies	E	+ +	+	+	+ +	≈	≈	I/N
Teschen/Talfan	E	+	+	+	+ +	+ +	+ +	. . .
Swine vesicular disease	M	+ +	+	+	≈	+	≈	I/N
Enterovirus T52/T80	E	≈	≈	+	≈	+	+	. . .
Hemagglutinating encephalitis virus	E	+	+ +	+ +	≈	≈	≈	. . .
Cytomegalovirus	E	+	+	+	≈	≈	≈	I/N + I/C
Adenovirus	E	+	+	+	≈	≈	≈	I/N

[a]Primary damage to ectodermal tissues (E); primary damage to mesodermal tissues (M).
[b]≈ = mild reaction; + = moderate reaction; + + = severe reaction.
[c]Inclusion bodies in nucleus (I/N); inclusion bodies in cytoplasm (I/C).

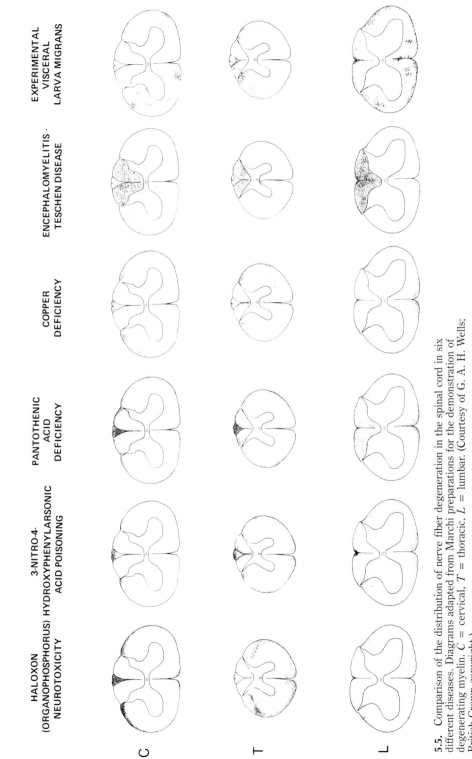

5.5. Comparison of the distribution of nerve fiber degeneration in the spinal cord in six different diseases. Diagrams adapted from Marchi preparations for the demonstration of degenerating myelin. C = cervical, T = thoracic, L = lumbar. (Courtesy of G. A. H. Wells; British Crown copyright.)

Table 5.4. Congenital tremor of pigs—diagnostic taxonomy

	Type[a]					
	AI	AII	AIII	AIV	AV	B
Cause	Virus, hog cholera	Virus, unknown	Genetic, S-L recessive	Genetic, autosomal recessive	Chemical, trichlor-fon	Unknown
Field observations						
Proportion of litters affected	High	High	Low	Low	High	Variable
Proportion of pigs affected within litter (approx.)	≥40%	≥80%	25%	25%	≥90%	Variable
Mortality among affected pigs	Medium-high	Low	High	High	High	Variable
Sex of affected pigs	Both	Both	Male	Both	Both	Any
Breed of dam (pure or crossbred)	Any	Any	Landrace	Saddleback	Any	Any
Recurrence in successive litters of same parents	No	No	Yes	Yes	Yes[b]	?
Duration of outbreak	≤4 mo	≤4 mo	Indefinite	Indefinite	≤1 mo	?
Laboratory observations						
Macroscopic						?
Cerebellum:whole brain ratio (≤ 8% = abnormal)	↓	~	~	~	↓	↓ ~
Spinal cord size (weight)	↓	~	↓	↓	↓	
Microscopic (CNS)						?
Myelin deficiency	+	+	+	+	+	
Myelin aplasia (partial)	−	−	+	−	−	
Oligodendrocytes swollen	+	+	−	−	−	
Oligodendrocytes reduced in number	~	~	+	~	~	
Neurochemistry (spinal cord)						?
Total DNA	↓	~	↓	↓	↓	
Whole lipid/g	↓	↓	↓	↓	↓	↓ ~
Cerebrosides/g	↓	↓	↓	↓	↓	↓ ~
Lipid hexose:phosphorus ratio	↓	↓	↓	↓	~	↓ ~
Cholesterol esters characteristic of demyelination	+	+	−	+	−	− −
Serology						?
Maternal antibodies to hog cholera	+	−	−	−	−	− −

Note: + = present; − = absent; ~ = not significantly changed; ↓ = decreased.

[a]Type A = a form of congenital tremor with defined pathological characters and known etiology; Type B = a form of congenital tremor as yet inadequately characterized and/or of unknown etiology.

[b]Provides similar temporal exposure to teratogen.

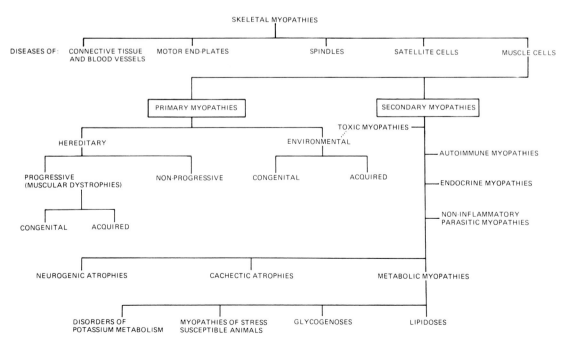

5.6. Classification of skeletal myopathies. (British Crown copyright.)

77

Table 5.5. Disorders of the nervous and muscular systems

Name/cause	Age at Onset	Motor excitement	Paresis/ paralysis	Ataxia	Tremor	Vestibular syndrome	Vision defect	Brain	Spinal cord	PNS	Muscle	Other	Dis. Swine Chap.	Consult Ref.
Arthrogryposis	Birth	-/+	+	+/-	+/-	+/-	+/-	+	+	+	(+)	Joints	56	Swatland (1974)
Brain malformation	Birth		≈	+	-/+			+		(+)	(+)	Eye	56	Done (1968)
Congenital motor defect	Birth		(+)	+	+			+					5	
Congenital tremor	Birth		-/+	+	+		-/+	+	+	+/-			56	Done (1976a)
Spinal malformation	Birth			+/-	-/+			+	+		(+/-)		56, 15	Done (1968)
Congenital muscle hypertrophy	Birth	-		≈				-	?	?	+		5	Done (1990)
Splayleg	Birth		+	+/-				?	?	?	?		56	Ward (1978)
Vitamin A deficiency (maternal)	Birth		+	+	+/-	-/+	+	+	?	(+)	(+)	Eye	56, 60	Palludan (1961)
Blue eye	≤2 wk	-/+	+	+	-/+	-/+	+	+	?			Eye	13	Stephano et al. (1982)
Hemagglutinating encephalomyelitis virus	≤2 wk		+	+	-/+	-/+		+	?				20	Alexander et al. (1959)
Iron toxicity	≤2 wk		+/-						≈		+	Heart	64	Patterson et al. (1971)
Pseudorabies	≤2 wk	+	+	+	+/-	-/+	+/-	+	≈	≈	+	Respiratory	24	
African swine fever	≤2 wk	-/+	+/-	+	-/+	-/+		+	≈	≈		L-R[a] system	12	
Bacterial meningitis	≤2 wk	-/+	-/+	+	-/+	+/-	+/-	+	+	+	+	Joints, heart	41, 43, 60	Fankhauser and Luginbühl (1968); Jubb and Kennedy (1970)
Copper deficiency		+	+	+	+/-			+	+	+	(+)		60	McGavin et al. (1962)
Enterovirus — Teschen/Talfan	≥2 wk	+/-	+	+	+/-	-/+	-/+	+	+	(+)	(+)		18	Mills and Nielsen (1968)
Enterovirus — Other	≥2 wk	-/≈	+	+	+/-	-/+	-/+	+	+	(≈)	?		18	Mills and Nielsen (1968)
Hog cholera	≥2 wk	-/+	+	+	-/+	-/+	-/+	≈	≈	?	?	L-R[a] system	21	Bradley and Wells (1978, 1980)
Pietrain creeper syndrome	≥2 wk			≈/+	+/-		(+)	+	+	+	+		5	
Tetanus	≥2 wk	-/+	-/+	≈/+	-/+	+/-	?	+	+	?	+		36	Done (1962)
Cerebellar cortical sclerosis	≥2 wk		-/+	+	-/+	+/-	(+)	+					5	
Cerebrospinal angiopathy	≥2 wk	+/-	-/+	+/-	+/-	+/-	?	+	≈				5	Harding (1966)
Edema disease	≥2 wk		+	+	+/-	+/-	+	+	+	≈		Bowel, vasculature	39	
Encephalomalacia	≥2 wk	-/+	+	+/-	+/-		-/+	+	≈				39	
Middle ear disease	≥2 wk			+		+		+		+			48	Jubb and Kennedy (1970)
Organic arsenic toxicity	≥2 wk	-/+	+	+	+		+	+	≈	+	(?)		64	Harding et al. (1968); Rice et al. (1980)
Organic mercury toxicity	≥2 wk		+	+	-/+	-/+	+	+	≈	+	(+)		64	Charlton (1974)
Organophosphorus neurotoxicity	≥6 wk		-/+	+			+/-	+	+	+	(+)		64	Wells (1977, 1984)
Pantothenic acid deficiency	≥6 wk		-/+	+	-/+	-/+		+	≈	+			60	
Rabies	≥6 wk	+	+	+	-/+	-/+	-/+	+	+				25	
Salt poisoning/water deprivation	≥6 wk	+	+/-	+	+/-	+	+/-	+				Skin	64	Lenghaus et al. (1976)
Swine vesicular disease	≥6 wk	+/-	-/+	+	+/-	-/+	-/+	+	+		+		30	Done et al. (1960)
Visceral larva migrans	≥6 wk	-/+	-/+	+/-	-/+	-/+	-/+	+			+	Viscera	58	
Vitamin A deficiency	≥6 wk	-/+	-/+	-/+		+	-/+	+	+	+	+		60	Done et al. (1975); Bradley and Wells (1978)
Asymmetric hindquarter syndrome	≥3 mo		+	-/+					+		+	Fat, bone	5	Bradley et al. (1979); Bradley and Wells (1978)
Back muscle necrosis	≥3 mo		+	-/+	+						+		5	
Landrace trembles			-/+	-/+	+			?		(+)			5	Gedde-Dahl and Standahl (1970)
Nutritional myopathy			+	+					+	+	+	Heart	60	Lannek and Lindberg (1975)
Vertebral trauma or disease			+						+	+		Bone, joints	5	Jubb and Kennedy (1970)
Clostridial myonecrosis	Any	?	≈	?	?			?	?	?	+		36	Hulland (1970)
Neoplasia	Any	?	?	?	?	?	?	?	?	?	+		56	
Porcine stress syndrome			≈					?	?	?	+	Heart	61	
Subacute spongiform encephalopathy	Adult only							?	?				5	Prusiner and Hadlow (1979)

Note: + = regularly present; -/+ = inconstantly present; +/- = occasionally present; ≈ = mild/minimal; ? = doubtful/equivocal; () = secondary.

a L-R = lymphoreticular.

ter elsewhere in this book and/or to key references. Of necessity this has involved some simplistic generalizations as well as the exclusion of some rare, protean, or equivocal disorders; but we trust that the reader will find the table generally useful.

Some important disorders not specifically dealt with elsewhere in this book are described below. The WHO Bibliography of Comparative Neuropathology (1966) provides an ongoing guide to new and emerging diseases in this field.

Nervous Disorders

CONGENITAL MOTOR DEFECT. Transmitted by a fully penetrant autosomal recessive gene present in both Large White and British Saddleback pigs,

congenital motor defect is interesting for two reasons. First, it presents primarily a severe functional disorder with ataxia, dysmetria, and perverse movements but with no morphologic lesions in the CNS, though a cerebellar cortical abiotrophy may be demonstrated later in pigs that survive.

Second, it exemplifies the potential usefulness of electroencephalography in the pig (Fig. 5.7). Affected piglets show significantly less electrical activity over the cerebrum, and juvenile brain patterns persist longer than in their clinically normal littermates.

As with other simply inherited defects, the incidence of affected piglets may reach some 6% in closely bred herds that have not selected against it. However, bearing in mind the precept that no

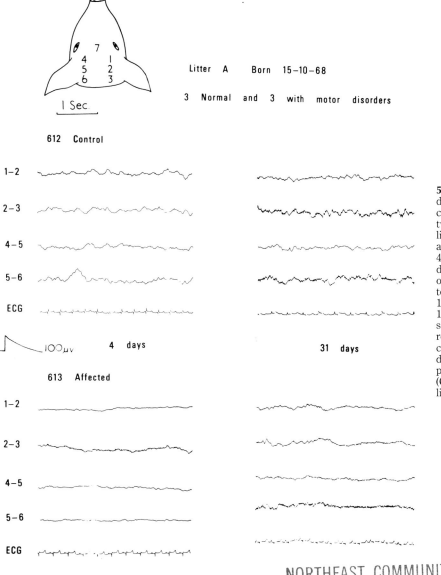

Litter A Born 15-10-68

3 Normal and 3 with motor disorders

612 Control

1-2

2-3

4-5

5-6

ECG

100 µV   4 days   31 days

613 Affected

1-2

2-3

4-5

5-6

ECG

5.7. Congenital motor defect. Electroencephalograms (EEG) of two littermates from litter A, control above and affected below, at 4 (left) and 31 (right) days of age. Numbers on the pig's head refer to recording channels; 1 sec to time scale and 100 µV to amplitude scale. The EEGs are recorded in the fifth channel and show differences between pigs at both ages. (Courtesy G. Pampiglione.)

simply inherited disease is economically important and no economically important disease is simply inherited, this condition is chiefly of interest to neurologists and comparative neuropathologists. To control it, noncarrier boars should be used.

LANDRACE TREMBLES. As its name implies, Landrace trembles is most frequently seen in Landrace pigs (Gedde-Dahl and Standal 1970). Generally, only occasional cases come to light in breeding stock sold for high prices, but prevalence may be as high as 20% of young adults in herds in which its insidious advance is not checked. No diagnostically useful morphologic lesions have so far been found in any part of the locomotor system; i.e., the disorder is idiopathic and apparently purely functional. It is characterized by a postural tremor particularly affecting the tail and the tips of the ears, though in severely affected cases it may involve much of the body as well. The tremor is readily elicited by forcing the pig to walk backward.

The disorder is not ascribable to any single cause, but its heritability is obviously fairly high. It is quite unrelated to the congenital tremor syndrome in which the tremor is a postural one.

No pigs die of this disease, and it constitutes at worst a clinical unsoundness likely to generate sales resistance. However, all but the hardiest or least observant purchaser might be deterred from buying breeding stock from a herd in which a high proportion of the adult pigs twitch violently when approached. In a herd in which the condition is a problem, its incidence may be reduced by genetic selection against "liability to Landrace trembles" (Done and Wijeratne 1972), using explicit standard criteria (e.g., unequivocal tremor of ears and tail of pigs 6 months old or older when forced to walk backward).

CEREBELLAR CORTICAL SCLEROSIS. The symptoms and lesions in cerebellar cortical sclerosis result essentially from hypoxia and intermittent ischemia of the parts of the cerebellum supplied by the anterior (superior) cerebellar artery (Fig. 5.8). It is postulated that the causal restriction of the blood supply to the affected part occurs when the artery, which follows a tortuous course around the tentorium cerebelli, is kinked or occluded as a result of mechanical pressure from organizing exudate and/or interference with intracranial fluid flow (Done 1962). Antecedent diseases that may give rise to cerebellar cortical sclerosis include streptococcal meningitis, toxoplasmosis, pseudorabies, and vitamin A deficiency.

The symptoms are those to be expected of a cerebellar disorder—ataxia with a wide-based stance and often a fine tremor—but they may be confounded with those of the antecedent disease. Though several pigs in a herd may be affected with cerebellar cortical sclerosis at the same time,

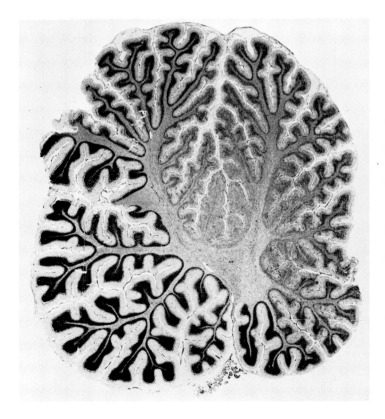

5.8. Cerebellar cortical sclerosis. Sagittal section through the vermis showing atrophic changes in the area supplied by the anterior (superior) cerebellar artery. Chromalum-gallocyanin. (British Crown copyright.)

control measures should be primarily directed at the underlying causes.

CEREBROSPINAL ANGIOPATHY. Originally described by Harding (1966), cerebrospinal angiopathy (CSA) occurs in the 5 weeks following weaning. It is characterized by degenerative changes in the media of medium to small arteries, mainly in the CNS but also in the abdominal viscera. Affected arteries are excessively permeable, leading to accumulations of protein-rich exudate around the vessels and edema or frank malacia of the surrounding tissue. Lesions are particularly prevalent in the cerebrum, midbrain, and brain stem, causing amaurosis, abnormal head carriage, and circling, sometimes for hours at a time. Differential diagnoses included meningoencephalitis eosinophilica, laminar cortical necrosis, polioencephalomalacia, mulberry heart disease, middle ear disease, and arsanilic acid poisoning.

It is believed that CSA represents a subacute form of edema disease and part of a continuous series that may be traced from increased vascular permeability through CSA to polyarteritis nodosa. Hence, regimens suitable for control of edema disease on a herd basis are appropriate to CSA also.

SUBACUTE TRANSMISSIBLE SPONGIFORM ENCEPHALOPATHY. The group of diseases known as subacute transmissible spongiform encephalopathies (STSE) and caused by unconventional agents or viruses (Prusiner and Hadlow 1979) has recently received great prominence because of the epidemic of bovine spongiform encephalopathy (BSE) in Britain (Wells et al. 1987; Wilesmith et al. 1988). BSE, the latest member of the group, has been confirmed by brain histopathology in over 23,000 confirmed cases on over 10,000 farms between November 1986, when it was discovered, and February 1991. The epidemic is expected to peak in 1991–92 and then decline rapidly to extinction by the end of the century as a result of the imposition of a ban, in July 1988, on feeding of ruminant protein to ruminant animals. At the time of writing such food contaminated with scrapie/BSE agent is believed to be the only source of infection for cattle.

The archetype of this disease group is scrapie of sheep and goats. The group also includes transmissible mink encephalopathy, chronic wasting disease of mule deer and elk, and in humans kuru, Creutzfeldt Jakob disease, and Gerstmann Sträussler Scheinker syndrome. The diseases all present clinically as progressive neurological disorders, are fatal, and have characteristic neuropathology.

There is no evidence for naturally occurring STSE in the pig. Pigs in close association with kuru patients did not develop clinical signs of disease. Pigs inoculated intracerebrally with kuru-infected brain developed neither clinical signs of disease nor neuropathological lesions of spongiform encephalopathy (Gibbs et al. 1979).

Experimental studies in Britain are currently in progress to determine whether or not the pig is susceptible to BSE by parenteral or by oral exposure, and also to determine if tissues from such pigs contain detectable agent at slaughter.

In February/March 1989, 10 weaned, 1- to 2-week-old pigs were simultaneously exposed to high levels of infectivity (1 g each) by multiple parenteral routes (intracerebral, intravenous, and intraperitoneal). The inoculum consisted of a 10% saline suspension of pooled homogenized brainstem prepared from four natural BSE cases used for previous primary parenteral transmissions. Eleven control pigs were similarly inoculated with saline; 2 control (by 3 weeks) and 2 challenged pigs (by 11 months) succumbed to intercurrent disease. After 69 weeks, a time by which most pigs reared for food are long since dead, 1 challenged pig showed mild aggressive behavior to animal attendants. The pig was intermittently inappetant and depressed. After a week, aimless biting activity was noted. There was a mild symmetrical pelvic limb ataxia, which subsequently progressed over 4 weeks when the pig was killed. Neuropathological examination revealed lesions of spongiform encephalopathy, and detergent extracts of unfixed medulla oblongata and cervical spinal cord showed fibrils characteristically found in scrapielike diseases (Merz et al. 1984). To date (February 1991) no further cases of clinical disease that can be related to subacute spongiform encephalopathy have occurred in either challenged or control pigs.

In 1990, 10 pigs were orally exposed to large doses of untreated brain from cattle with confirmed BSE. All these were healthy after at least 10 months following exposure, as are controls. Final results from this experiment are not expected until the end of 1992 at the earliest, by which time some pigs will have been killed for pathological study.

The parenteral exposure study reported by Dawson et al. (1990) shows that the porcine species is susceptible to STSE but, so far, at a low incidence after a long incubation period and following multiple parenteral exposure of a high-dose inoculum. Oral exposure to the agents causing STSE is relatively inefficient (by a factor of about 10^5, based on mouse studies), so occurrence of disease via food under natural conditions is most unlikely. In Britain it is now forbidden to use for human consumption animals (including pigs), poultry or other birds, or any of the specified bovine offals or protein derived from them.

These offals are brain, spinal cord, thymus, tonsil, spleen, and intestine and are those that, in an infected subclinical or preclinical cow, would be most likely to harbor the infective agent. Cattle clinically suspected to have BSE are destroyed and no part enters any food chain. The origin of the cattle disease (BSE) appears to have been proprietary cattle feed or protein supplements prepared with meat and bone meal, derived either from sheep or cattle and containing the infectious agent, which was incompletely inactivated by the rendering process (Wilesmith et al. 1988, 1991). Exposure is believed to have increased in the period 1981–82 as a result of the interaction of several factors, including an increase in the sheep population and changes in the British rendering industry, resulting in disease in 1985–86 (i.e., after an incubation period of 4–5 years). Pigs in Britain during this period, and subsequently, have also been exposed to the same potentially infected food source, often at higher inclusion rates without any detectable clinical or pathological effects. Such food from indigenous sources in other countries or even from exported British meat and bone meal is used for pig feed in a number of European and other countries, also with no detectable, detrimental effect. If pigs had been susceptible, the disease would have been expected to manifest itself in them rather than in cattle.

All the evidence therefore points to the pig not being susceptible under natural conditions to the agents that cause scrapie, BSE, or kuru. Nevertheless, veterinarians should be on their guard to detect unexplained progressive neurologic disease in adult pigs and to submit appropriate tissues (brain and spinal cord fixed in formalin and unfixed, deep-frozen upper cervical spinal cord) to a qualified specialist laboratory for pathological and molecular biological examination.

Muscular Disorders

CONGENITAL MUSCLE HYPERTROPHY. Congenital muscle hypertrophy (Done et al. 1990) is a recently recognized condition that affected over 200 piglets. About 50% of each litter of three consecutive batches of sows mated to a single boar by artificial insemination were affected. The ham muscles were rounded and bulging, resulting from muscle hypertrophy.

The clinical signs included two separate elements: stiffness and weakness immediately after farrowing, possibly due to minor abnormalities concerning tendon, muscle, and bone length; and secondarily, excessive bruising of the feet, abscesses, and subsequent further superficial limb and foot injury. These secondary signs developed when the pigs were put into "flat-deck" accommodation but were so severe that they had to be removed a few days later because of severe lameness.

At birth, piglets had no control of their legs and were unable to place their feet on the ground. When walking was possible, the forelimbs were stiff as if joints could not be flexed. The pelvic ilium on each side was prominent. The hind limbs were abducted with stifles angled outward at 45° to the body. The m. quadriceps in the young animal exhibited spasm, leading to hyperextension of the digital joints and tiptoe walking. The defects of posture and gait decreased with increasing age.

Necropsy revealed the secondary lesions of bruising, inflammation, and abscessation of limbs, particularly the feet. The m.'s vastus group, m. gluteobiceps, and m. gastrocnemius weighed significantly more and were volumetrically larger than those from age-matched controls. At 3 weeks of age the muscle hypertrophy collectively added up to a maximum of 3.5 kg more body weight than age-matched controls.

There were no lesions in the central or peripheral nervous system. Muscles had a normal structure, but there was myocyte hypertrophy in affected pigs compared with controls and possibly a degree of myocyte hyperplasia.

The boar used to sire the affected piglets died from severe progressive heart failure but had no detectable gross or microscopic skeletal muscle lesions.

PIETRAIN CREEPER SYNDROME. Pietrain creeper syndrome (Bradley and Wells 1978, 1980) is a familial disease of progressive muscular weakness beginning at 3 weeks of age and ending in permanent recumbency by about 12 weeks of age. Usually, about a quarter of a litter is affected and it is likely though not proved that the disease is inherited as an autosomal recessive trait. Initially, there is tremor when standing, followed by a sudden collapse to sternal recumbency, and then the tremor stops. Progressively, there is an increased reluctance to stand, muscular weakness, and loss of condition; finally, the pigs develop a creeping type of gait using the flexed limbs. There are no significant nervous lesions; myopathic changes, though widespread, are most severe in the proximal muscles of the limbs. Beginning as an extension of the range of muscle cell caliber variation (CCV) and atrophy of type 1 and intermediate cells, the lesions progress to severe CCV, with atrophy, hypertrophy, and an altered pattern of distribution of histochemical cell types (Fig. 5.9). Internal nuclei, focal myodegeneration, targetoid, and moth-eaten cells are additional features. So far this disease has been reported in only two herds of purebred Pietrain pigs.

ASYMMETRIC HINDQUARTER SYNDROME. Asymmetric hindquarter syndrome (AHQS) (Done et al. 1975; Bradley and Wells 1978) is a disease of slaughter-weight pigs, though it can be recognized as early as 2–3 months. When viewed from behind, there is a volumetric asymmetry of the hindquarters (Fig. 5.10). This results from a relative increase of subcutaneous fat on the larger side and a relative decrease in weight and volume of the adductor and posterior thigh muscles on the smaller side (Fig. 5.11). The asymmetry of the individual muscles is principally caused by a

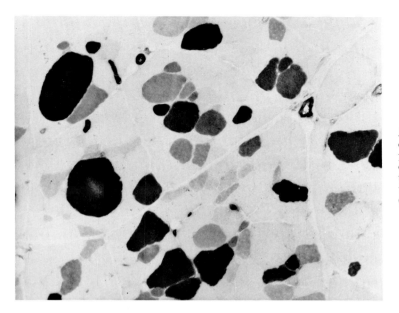

5.9. Deep part of the semitendinosus muscle in a 12-week-old pig with Pietrain creeper syndrome. Severe cell caliber variation and maldistribution of cell types. Myosin ATPase pH 4.35. (British Crown copyright.)

reduction in the number of muscle cells in the smaller limb. The disease appears to arise spontaneously, affecting a high proportion of individual pigs, and then subsides for no apparent reason. Diagnosis can be made clinically or postmortem. At necropsy, weighing of individually dissected adductor and posterior thigh muscles from both sides of an affected and normal pig of the same age and body weight together with subcutaneous fat thickness measurements over the rump are simple and effective diagnostic methods.

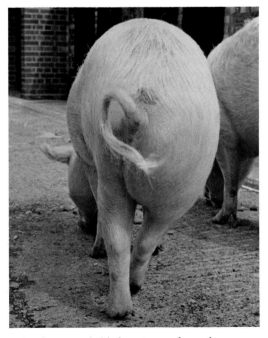

5.10. Asymmetric hindquarter syndrome in a severely affected pig. (British Crown copyright.)

BACK MUSCLE NECROSIS. Back muscle necrosis (Bradley et al. 1979) appears to be a special manifestation of the porcine stress syndrome (see Chapter 60). The condition is sporadic and sudden in onset, affecting pigs over 50 kg body weight. The acute phase is characterized by pain, difficulty in movement, pyrexia, and unilateral or bilateral swelling and heat in the back. Back swelling coincides with the anatomical position of the longissimus dorsi and multifidi muscles. There is loss of skin sensation to needle pricking over the affected area. Bilateral cases may be found dead. Unilateral cases, when standing, have the convexity of the body curvature toward the affected side. There is a reluctance to stand, and a dog-sitting position may be adopted. If the pig is able to stand, there is locomotor difficulty, with knuckling of the lower limb joints and an increased rate of respiration. Because there is massive muscle necrosis, the plasma CK activity is dramatically increased, but the blood selenium level is within the normal range. Postmortem diagnosis is best made by sawing through the carcass transversely at the level of the last rib and observing the cut surfaces of the eye muscle, which are pale with hemorrhages in the affected parts (Fig. 5.12). It is also valuable to cut the longissimus muscle longitudinally through its center to establish the extent of the lesions. Microscopically, the lesion is one of necrosis and hemorrhage.

MUSCULAR STEATOSIS. Muscular steatosis (Bradley and Wells 1978) is found incidentally postmortem in pigs slaughtered for food. The architecture of the muscle is normal, but there are fat cells in place of muscle cells. In severe cases the density of the muscle is reduced sufficiently to allow it to float in water or formalin. There is no degenera-

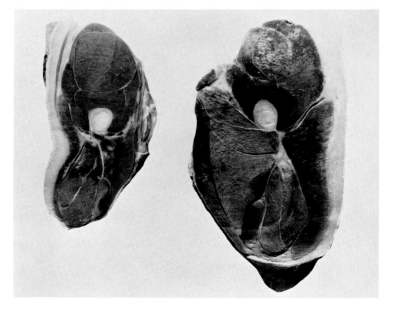

5.11. Midfemur level sections of thighs from the pig in Figure 5.10. There is increased subcutaneous fat on the larger side and reduced volume of adductor and posterior thigh muscles on the smaller side. (British Crown copyright.)

tive or inflammatory change, and the cause is obscure.

MYOSITIS OSSIFICANS. Myositis ossificans (Hulland 1970) is a generalized familial disease in which bony lesions develop in muscles adjacent to the spinal column, ribs, and tarsal bones at 2–6 months of age. The muscle cells atrophy in the vicinity of the lesion. The etiology is obscure.

FOCAL MYOPATHY. Focal myopathy (Bradley and Wells 1978), in which less than 1% of muscle cells show myodegenerative change, can be found incidentally in muscle from pigs that show no locomotor or postural disorders clinically. Muir (1970)

found these changes in stress-susceptible Pietrain pig muscle, but they also occur in stress-resistant individuals. The significance and cause is not known.

TREATMENT. The general principles and practice of disease control at the herd level are dealt with in Chapter 66. We shall restrict ourselves to the individual pig.

The immediate prognosis will depend not only on the location, extent, and severity of the damage already sustained but also on its amenability to treatment and the animal's capacity for repair and compensation.

The continuation of tissue damage into the

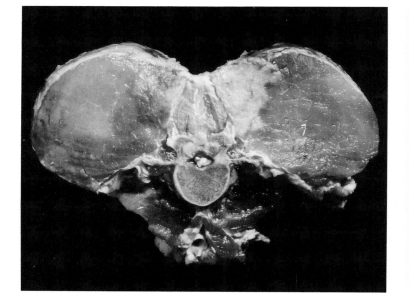

5.12. Section through the loin showing bilateral acute back muscle necrosis. Pale areas of necrosis are seen in the multifidi and longissimus dorsi muscles. (British Crown copyright.)

stage of repair would be less serious in an organ capable of regeneration of its functional units and in which spatial relationships between its parts and its nonflexible container were less critical; but in disease of the CNS it is a process that the clinician should have constantly in mind. Specific therapy for infectious diseases should be supplemented where appropriate by the use of corticosteroids to reduce the vigor of the inflammatory response. Raised intracranial pressure is a sequel to many inflammatory conditions and itself causes further hypoxic damage by mechanical interference with the blood supply. In addition to corticosteroids, diuretics may be useful for lowering fluid pressure.

The permanence of neuronal loss has also been emphasized, as have the limited capacities for regeneration of peripheral nerves and their sheaths and muscle cells. As far as the PNS is concerned, the time required for clinical recovery will obviously depend on the length of the damaged portion of the nerve. However, as a crude generalization, it may be said that whatever return or adaptation of function can be achieved in regard to the neuromuscular system as a whole is likely to be qualitatively apparent by about 6 weeks after the cessation of the acute destructive process.

Apart from muscle weakness, pigs with neuromuscular disorders may suffer cramps, the pain and distress of which should not be underestimated. Depolarizing compounds and analgesics might be used to relieve these symptoms. Where, as in congenital splayleg, the disorder is essentially transient (unless death supervenes from other causes), physical support and protection may be all that is required.

However, as a contributing member of an economically oriented enterprise, there can be no long-term future for any pig that has suffered significant nervous or muscle damage. The stage at which it will be salvaged will be decided by its size, the severity of the condition, and the number of similarly affected pigs in the herd. Small pigs severely affected with conditions of unknown or poor prognosis should be killed as soon as possible on humanitarian as well as economic grounds. When a number of pigs of similar age are similarly affected and the prognosis is reasonably good (as in pantothenic acid deficiency) or when it can be foreseen that a number of further cases will occur before the outbreak has run its course (as in Talfan disease), it may be advisable to house affected animals together in "hospital units" to avoid bullying. Such pigs should be salvaged in batches as soon as they reach a suitable size.

REFERENCES

ALEXANDER, T. J. L.; RICHARDS, W. P. C.; AND ROE, C. K. 1959. An encephalomyelitis of suckling pigs in Ontario. Can J Comp Med 23:316–319.

BLACKWOOD, W., AND CORSELLIS, J. A. N., eds. 1976. Greenfield's Neuropathology, 3d ed. London: Edward Arnold.

BRADLEY, R. 1978. Skeletal muscle biopsy techniques in animals for histochemical and ultrastructural examination and especially for the diagnosis of myodegeneration in cattle. Br Vet J 134:434–444.

BRADLEY, R., AND FELL, B. F. 1981. Myopathies in animals. In Disorders of Voluntary Muscle, 4th ed. Ed. J. Walton. London: Churchill-Livingstone, pp. 824–872.

BRADLEY, R., AND WELLS, G. A. H. 1978. Developmental muscle disorders in the pig. Vet Annu 18:144–157.

———. 1980. The Pietrain creeper pig–a primary myopathy. In Animal Models of Neurological Disease Symposium. London: Pitmans.

BRADLEY, R.; WELLS, G. A. H.; AND GRAY, L. J. 1979. Back muscle necrosis of pigs. Vet Rec 104:183–187.

CHARLTON, K. M. 1974. Experimental alkylmercurial poisoning in swine. Lesions in the peripheral and central nervous systems. Can J Comp Med 38:75–81.

DAWSON, M.; WELLS, G. A. H.; PARKER, B. N. J.; AND SCOTT, A. C. 1990. Primary parenteral transmission of bovine spongiform encephalopathy to the pig. Vet Rec 127:338.

DE LAHUNTA, A. 1983. Veterinary Neuroanatomy and Clinical Neurology, 2d ed. Philadelphia: W. B. Saunders.

DICKERSON, J. W. T., AND DOBBING, J. 1966–67. Prenatal and postnatal growth and development of the central nervous system of the pig. Proc R Soc Lond [Biol] 166:384–395.

DONE, J. T. 1957. The pathological differentiation of diseases of the central nervous system of the pig. Vet Rec 69:1341–1349.

———. 1962. Some cases of cerebellar cortical sclerosis in pigs. Acta Neuropathol [Suppl] (Berl) 1:33–38.

———. 1968. Congenital nervous diseases of pigs: A review. Lab Anim 2:207–217.

———. 1976a. The congenital tremor syndrome in pigs. Vet Annu 16:98–102.

———. 1976b. Developmental disorders of the nervous system in animals. Adv Vet Sci Comp Med 20:69–114.

DONE, J. T., AND HEBERT, C. N. 1968. The growth of the cerebellum in the fetal pig. Res Vet Sci 9:143–148.

DONE, J. T., AND WIJERATNE, W. V. S. 1972. Genetic diseases of pigs. In Pig Production: Proceedings of the 18th Easter School in Agricultural Science, University of Nottingham, 1971. Ed. D. J. A. Cole. London: Butterworth, pp. 53–67.

DONE, J. T.; RICHARDSON, M.; AND GIBSON, T. E. 1960. Experimental visceral larva migrans in the pig. Res Vet Sci 1:133–151.

DONE, J. T.; ALLEN, W. M.; BAILEY, J.; DE GRUCHY, P. H.; AND CURRAN, M. K. 1975. Asymmetric hindquarter syndrome (AHQS) in the pig. Vet Rec 96:482–485.

DONE, S. H.; WALTON, J. R.; CARR, J.; AND HOWARTH, J. 1990. Case Presentation–an unusual disorder of gait and conformation in neonatal piglets. Proc 11th Int Congr Pig Vet Soc, Lausanne, p. 282.

DUBOWITZ, V., AND BROOKE, M. H. 1973. Muscle Biopsy: A Modern Approach. Philadelphia: W. B. Saunders, pp. 77–101.

DYCE, K. M.; SACK, W. O.; AND WENSING, C. J. D. 1987. Textbook of Veterinary Anatomy. London: W. B. Saunders.

FANKHAUSER, R. 1962. The cerebrospinal fluid. In J. R. M. Innes, and L. Z. Saunders. Comparative Neuropathology. New York: Academic Press, pp. 21–54.

FANKHAUSER, R., AND LUGINBÜHL, H. 1968. Pathological Anatomy of the Central and Peripheral Nervous Systems of Domestic Animals. Berlin, Hamburg: Paul Parey.

GEDDE-DAHL, T. W., AND STANDAHL, N. 1970. A note

on a tremor condition in adolescent pigs. Anim Prod 12:665–668.

GETTY, R. 1975. Sisson and Grossman's The Anatomy of the Domestic Animals, 5th ed., vol. 2. Philadelphia: W. B. Saunders.

GIBBS, C. J., JR.; GAJDUSEK, D. C.; AND AMYX, H. 1979. Strain variation in the viruses of Creutzfeldt-Jakob disease and kuru. In Slow Transmissible Diseases of the Nervous System. Ed. S. B. Prusiner and W. J. Hadlow. London: Academic Press, pp. 87–110.

HADLOW, W. J.; KENNEDY, R. C.; AND RACE, R. E. 1982. Natural infection of Suffolk sheep with scrapie virus. J Inf Dis 146:657–664.

HAM, A. W. 1979. Histology, 8th ed. Philadelphia: Lippincott.

HARDING, J. D. J. 1966. A cerebrospinal angiopathy in pigs. Pathol Vet 3:83–88.

HARDING, J. D. J.; LEWIS, G.; AND DONE, J. T. 1968. Experimental arsanilic acid poisoning in pigs. Vet Rec 83:560–564.

HULLAND, T. J. 1970. Muscle. In K. V. F. Jubb, and P. C. Kennedy. Pathology of Domestic Animals, 2d ed. New York: Academic Press, pp. 453–494.

INNES, J. R. M., AND SAUNDERS, L. Z. 1962. Comparative Neuropathology. New York: Academic Press.

JUBB, K. V. F., AND KENNEDY, P. C. 1970. Pathology of Domestic Animals, 2d ed., vol. 2. New York: Academic Press.

KING, A. S. 1978. A Guide to the Physical and Clinical Anatomy of the Nervous System, 6th ed. Liverpool: Univ of Liverpool.

LANNEK, N., AND LINDBERG, P. 1975. Vitamin E and selenium deficiencies (VESD) of domestic animals. Adv Vet Sci Comp Med 19:127–164.

LARSELL, O. 1954. Development of the cerebellum of the pig. Anat Rec 118:73–107.

LENGHAUS, C.; MANN, J. A.; DONE, J. T.; AND BRADLEY, R. 1976. Neuropathology of experimental swine vesicular disease in pigs. Res Vet Sci 21:19–27.

LUFF, A. R., AND GOLDSPINK, G. 1967. Large and small muscles. Life Sci 6:1821–1826.

McCOMAS, A. J. 1977. Neuromuscular Function and Disorders. London: Butterworth.

McGAVIN, M. D.; RANBY, P. D.; AND TAMMEMAGI, L. 1962. Demyelination associated with low copper levels in pigs. Aust Vet J 38:8–14.

MARRABLE, A. W. 1971. The Embryonic Pig. A Chronological Account. London: Pitman Medical.

MERZ, P. A.; ROHWER, R. C.; KASCSAK, R.; WISNIEWSKI, H. M.; SOMERVILLE, R. A.; GIBBS, C. J., JR.; AND GAJDUSEK, D. C. 1984. Infection-specific particle from unconventional slow virus disease. Science 225:437–440.

MILLS, J. H. L., AND NIELSEN, S. W. 1968. Porcine polioencephalomyelitides. Adv Vet Sci 12:33–104.

MUIR, A. R. 1970. Normal and regenerating skeletal muscle fibres in Pietrain pigs. J Comp Pathol 80:137–143.

NOMINA ANATOMICA VETERINARIA, 3D ED. 1983. In Nomina Anatomica Veterinaria, 3d ed. and Nomina Histologica, 2d ed. Eds. R. E. Habel, W. O. Sack, and T. Frewein. Ithaca, N.Y.: International Committee on Veterinary Gross Anatomical Nomenclature, pp. A40–A48.

O'HARA, P. J., AND SHORTRIDGE, E. H. 1966. I. Some diseases of the porcine central nervous system. II. Congenital anomalies of the porcine central nervous system. NZ Vet J 14:1–12, 13–18.

PALLUDAN, B. 1961. The teratogenic effect of vitamin A deficiency in pigs. Acta Vet Scand 2:32–59.

PALMER, A. C. 1976. Introduction to Animal Neurology, 2d ed. Oxford, London, Edinburgh, Melbourne: Blackwell Scientific Publications.

PATTERSON, D. S. P. 1977. Biochemical changes in the developing central nervous system following infection in pregnancy. In C. R. Coid. Infections and Pregnancy. New York: Academic Press, pp. 307–342.

PATTERSON, D. S. P., AND DONE, J. R. 1977. Neurochemistry as a diagnostic aid in the congenital tremor syndrome in piglets. Br Vet J 133:111–119.

PATTERSON, D. S. P.; ALLEN, W. M.; BERRETT, S.; SWEASEY, D.; AND DONE, J. T. 1971. The toxicity of parenteral iron preparations in the rabbit and pig with a comparison of the biochemical responses in 2 days old and 8 days old piglets. Zentralbl Veterinaermed [A] 18:453–464.

PRUSINER, S. B., AND HADLOW, W. J. 1979. Slow Transmissible Diseases of the Nervous System, vols. 1 and 2. London: Academic Press.

RHODIN, J. A. G. 1975. Histology: A Text and Atlas. Oxford, England: Oxford Univ Press.

RICE, D. A.; McMURRAY, C. H.; McCRACKEN, R. M.; BRYSON, D. G.; AND MAYBIN, R. 1980. A field case of poisoning caused by 3-nitro-4-hydroxy phenylarsonic acid in pigs. Vet Rec 106:312–313.

RÖHRS, M., AND KRUSKA, D. 1969. Influence of domestication on the central nervous system and behaviours of pigs. DTW 76:514–518.

SACK, W. O. 1982. Horowitz/Kramer Atlas of musculoskeletal anatomy of the pig. In Pig Anatomy and Atlas. Ed. W. O. Sack. Ithaca: Veterinary Textbooks, pp. 61–187.

SAUNDERS, L. Z., AND JUBB, K. V. 1961. Notes on techniques for postmortem examination. Can Vet J 2:123–129.

SAUNDERS, L. Z., AND RUBUN, L. F. 1975. Ophthalmic Pathology of Animals, an Atlas and Reference Book. London: Karger, pp. 244–253.

SIGNORET, J. P.; BALDWIN, B. A.; FRASER, D.; AND HAFEZ, E. S. 1975. The behaviour of swine. In The Behaviour of Domestic Animals, 3d ed. Ed. E. S. E. Hafez. London: Baillière Tindall, pp. 295–329.

SIMPSON, J. A. 1972. Muscle. In Scientific Foundations of Neurology. Ed. M. Chritchly, J. L. O'Leary, and B. Jennett. London: William Heinemann Medical Books, pp. 44–58.

STEPHANO, H. A., AND GAY, M. 1984. Experimental studies on a new virus syndrome in pigs called "Blue eye," characterized by encephalitis and corneal opacity. Proc 8th Int Congr Pig Vet, Ghent, p. 71.

STEPHANO, H. A.; GAY, M.; RAMIREZ TABCHE, C.; AND MAQUEDA, A. J. 1982. An outbreak of encephalitis in piglets produced by an haemagglutinating virus. Proc 7th Int Congr Pig Vet Soc, Mexico City, p. 153.

SWATLAND, H. J. 1974. Developmental disorders of skeletal muscle in cattle, pigs and sheep. Vet Bull 44:179–202.

SWEASEY, D.; PATTERSON, D. S. P.; AND GLANCY, E. M. 1976. Biphasic myelination and the fatty acid composition of cerebrosides and cholesterol esters in the developing central nervous system of the domestic pig. J Neurochem 27:375–380.

SWENSON, M. J., ED. 1977. Dukes' Physiology of Domestic Animals, 9th ed. Ithaca: Cornell Univ. Press.

WARD, P. S. 1978. The splayleg syndrome in new-born pigs: A review. I, II. Vet Bull 48:279–295, 381–399.

WELLS, G. A. H. 1977. Haloxon neurotoxicity. Pig Farming 25(10):73–76.

———. 1984. Locomotor disorders of the pig. In Pract 6:43–53.

WELLS, G. A. H.; SCOTT, A. C.; JOHNSON, C. T.; GUNNING, R. F.; HANCOCK, R. D.; JEFFREY, M.; DAWSON, M.; AND BRADLEY, R. 1987. A novel progressive spongiform encephalopathy in cattle. Vet Rec 121:419–420.

WILESMITH, J. W.; WELLS, G. A. H.; CRANWELL, M. P.;

AND RYAN, J. B. M. 1988. Bovine spongiform enceph-alopathy: Epidemiological studies. Vet Rec 123:638–644.

WILESMITH, J. W.; RYAN, J. B. M.; AND ATKINSON, M. J. 1991. Bovine spongiform encephalopathy: Epidemi-ological studies on the origin. Vet Rec 128:199–203.

WORLD HEALTH ORGANIZATION (WHO). 1966. Bibliog-raphy of Comparative Neuropathology from 1960 (with 13 supplements 1968–80). Geneva: World Health Organization.

_____. 1977. Non-Mendelian developmental defects: Animal models and implications for research into hu-man disease. Bull WHO 55:475–487.

YOSHIKAWA, T. 1968. Atlas of the Brains of Domestic Animals. Tokyo: Univ of Tokyo Press.

6 Reproductive Failure: Differential Diagnosis

G. D. Dial

W. E. Marsh

D. D. Polson

J.-P. Vaillancourt

TO EFFECTIVELY PRIORITIZE action on production problems, swine producers and practicing veterinarians must, first and foremost, develop an understanding of the relative impact of various measures of herd performance on overall biological and financial productivity. Without an understanding of how various production parameters relate to a herd's productivity, strategies designed to optimize performance will be misdirected, at best, leading to no or modest change in productivity, a waste of effort, and lost opportunities for profit. At worst, misdirected strategies can, and often, cause reduced performance, frustration for the producer, and embarrassment for the veterinary advisor.

There are several ways in which the productivity of the female herd can be assessed, including the number of piglets weaned and number of feeder pigs produced annually by each female.

Less traditional, but in some cases more applicable, measures include piglets weaned/farrowing crate/year, pounds of pork sold/female/year, number of female days/piglet produced, number of piglets weaned/female life, production cost/ weaned piglet, and net return over feed cost/female. While piglets weaned/female/year likely is not the most accurate or even the most appropriate measure of breeding herd productivity for most farms, it is a parameter that is commonly understood and, therefore, frequently used to relate the reproductive performance of one farm to that of another.

It can be easily debated that piglets weaned/ female/year is not the best measure of the financial well-being of the breeding herd. However, increased production efficiency of the female usually results in less expensive piglets at weaning (Fig. 6.1), indicating that biological efficiency

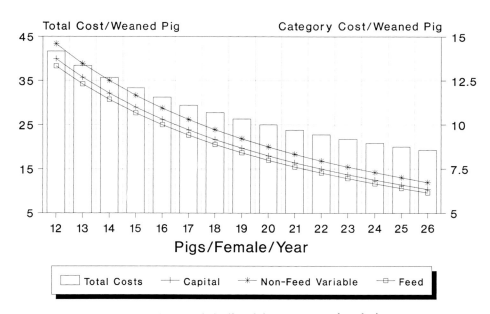

6.1. Schematic representation of the influence of pigs/female/year on costs of producing weaned pigs. Capital costs = depreciation, interest, and breeding; nonfeed variable = labor, utilities, and other.

and financial success often go together. The major costs of producing a weaned piglet are breeding herd feed costs, breeding costs (replacement animal costs minus salvage value of culled stock), capital costs (facility depreciation, interest), utilities, and labor (Fig. 6.2). In general, the fixed costs associated with producing a weaned piglet (e.g., facility depreciation, interest, and utilities), as well as most variable costs (e.g., female feed costs, breeding costs, manure handling, etc.), are reduced as piglets weaned/female/year are increased. In fact, only a few of the variable costs of production, such as piglet medication and vaccination costs and creep feed, increase as female productivity rises. In general, the more piglets weaned/female annually, the less expensive her piglets. Thus, piglets/female/year not only may be one of the most easily measured and broadly understood endpoints of productivity, but also may reflect, to some extent, financial as well as biological efficiency on most farms.

Piglets/female/year is the product of two easily measured components: the number of litters the average inventoried female farrows each year (litters/female/year) and the number of piglets she weans from each litter (pigs weaned/litter) (Fig. 6.3). The number of litters/female/year is highly and positively correlated (r = 0.83) with number of piglets weaned/female/year (Bichard 1983). Similarly, litter size at weaning is highly correlated (r = 0.82) to piglets produced/female/year. Because the correlations are statistically the same, it can be concluded that both contribute

equally to female productivity, and neither can be ignored when troubleshooting problems of herd productivity. Improvements in pigs/female/year can be made either by manipulating either litters/female/year or piglets weaned/litter. Numerous management and environmental factors and many infectious diseases influence female output (i.e., piglets weaned/litter) and/or female throughput (i.e., litters/female/year). This review presents and interrelates the causes and risk factors associated with suboptimal litters/female/year and number of piglets weaned/litter. It will also suggest strategies for troubleshooting suboptimal reproductive performance on commercial swine herds.

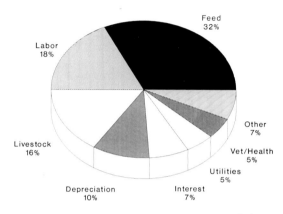

6.2. Breakdown of costs for producing weaned pigs. (Swine Graphics, unpublished guidelines, 1988.)

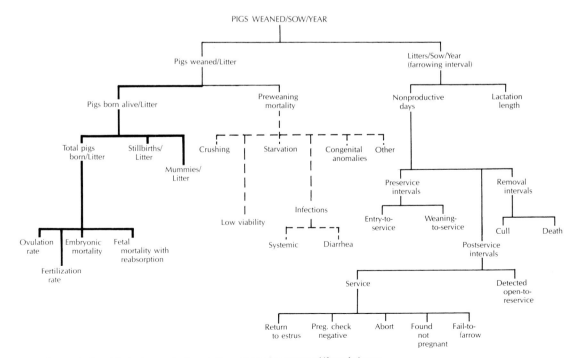

6.3. Interrelationship between factors influencing pigs weaned/female/year.

Litters/Female/Year

WHEN THE YEARLY productivity of a female herd is suboptimal, the number of piglets born alive/litter (born-alive litter size) is often the first thing examined. However, as shown in Table 6.1, litters/female/year dramaticly influence piglets produced per female annually. At 9 piglets weaned/litter, which is not uncommon for commercial farms in North America, there are 0.9 additional piglets produced per female annually for every 0.1 increase in the number of litters/female/year.

Litters inventoried/female/year (L/F/Y) are dependent upon average gestation length, average lactation length, and average number of days that inventoried females are nonproductive (NPD) by the formula:

$$\text{Litters/Female/Year} = \frac{(365 - \text{Nonproductive Days})}{(\text{Gestation Days} + \text{Lactation Days})}$$

Gestation length can be reduced by only a few days, through rigorously implemented induced farrowing programs in which a large proportion of females are induced to farrow using prostaglandin compounds. In retrospective studies in which the large majority of females have not been induced to farrow, gestation length was not related significantly to litters/female/year or piglets weaned/female/year. It appears, therefore, that gestation length apparently cannot be practically manipulated to substantially influence litters/female/year and that controlling lactation length and NPD may be the most promising tools for improving litters/female/year.

LACTATION LENGTH. In recent years, shorter lactation lengths of 3 or 4 weeks have become increasingly common (Dial and BeVier 1987). This seemingly has been based upon the premises that shorter lactations allow females to farrow more times annually and also allows improved facility utilization by increasing the number of farrowings/farrowing space/year. Studies have shown that shorter lactations, in fact, are accompanied by increased litters/female/year and in-

creased piglets weaned/female/year (Pay 1973; Walker et al. 1979). These improvements in female performance with shorter lactations occur even though, as discussed in more detail below, there may be increases in the subsequent weaning-to-estrus interval (Self and Grummer 1958; Svajgr et al. 1974; Cole et al. 1975; Varley et al. 1981), decreases in the farrowing rates of females bred at the subsequent estrus (Pay 1973; Svajgr et al. 1974), and decreases in litter size at the subsequent farrowing (Svajgr et al. 1974; Cole et al. 1975; Aumaitre and Dagorn 1982). Also, shorter lactations may be accompanied by decreased postweaning survival and slower postweaning weight gains of piglets (Self and Grummer 1958). Even though lactation length is potentially one of the most important factors influencing both litters/female/year and piglets weaned/farrowing space/year, it does not have much influence on piglets weaned/female/year through the range of lactations typically seen on intensively managed farms (e.g., 3–4 week lactation lengths). In fact, improvements in subsequent litter size that accompany increases in lactation length are typically negated by corresponding reductions in litters/female/year, such that piglets weaned/female/year remains unchanged. Since gestation length is not easily changed and lactation length is generally fixed by facility type, this leaves the NPD as the most sensitive indicator and, perhaps, one of the best measures of female throughput.

NONPRODUCTIVE DAYS. Recent studies have shown that lactation length and the two principle components of piglets weaned/litter, liveborn litter size, and percent preweaning mortality, relate highly to female productivity, but not as well as the NPD (Leman et al. 1990; Polson et al. 1990a). Further, the farm-to-farm variation in NPD is considerably higher than it is for either litter size or preweaning mortality (Polson et al. 1990b), suggesting that improvements in piglets weaned/female/year might be more easily made through improvements in NPD. Of the common measures of herd productivity, including pre-

Table 6.1.   Influence of litters/sow/year and pigs weaned/litter on pigs weaned/sow/year

Pigs/Litter	Litters/Sow/Year									
	1.6	1.7	1.8	1.9	2.0	2.1	2.2	2.3	2.4	2.5
7.5	12.0	12.8	13.5	14.3	15.0	15.8	16.5	17.3	18.0	18.8
8.0	12.8	13.6	14.4	15.2	16.0	16.8	17.6	18.4	19.2	20.0
8.5	13.6	14.5	15.3	16.2	17.0	17.9	18.7	19.6	20.4	21.3
9.0	14.4	15.3	16.2	17.1	18.0	18.9	19.8	20.7	21.6	22.5
9.5	15.2	16.2	17.1	18.1	19.0	20.0	20.9	21.9	22.8	23.8
10.0	16.0	17.0	18.0	19.0	20.0	21.0	22.0	23.0	24.0	24.0
10.5	16.8	17.9	18.9	20.0	21.0	22.1	23.1	24.2	25.2	26.3
11.0	17.6	18.7	19.8	20.9	22.0	23.1	24.2	25.3	26.4	27.5

weaning mortality, live-born litter size, and lactation length, NPD most accurately predict efficiency of female utilization.

NPD comprises all the days that a female or gilt are not productive while part of an inventoried herd; traditionally, these are days in which the female is neither lactating nor gestating. NPD includes several commonly measured production parameters, such as farrowing rate and weaning-to-reserve interval. As long as you remain within one of the two main branches of litter/female/year or piglets weaned/litter, the accuracy of the prediction of piglets weaned/sow/year is determined by the placement of the parameters on the piglets weaned/ female/year productivity tree. The lower the parameters on the productivity tree, the less accurate the prediction. Thus, NPD relates better to piglets weaned/female/year than to farrowing rate, weaning-to-reserve interval, or any other components of NPD.

Besides farrowing rate, NPD includes several types of females having reproductive or health problems: postweaning anestrous females, repeat breeders, pregnancy-check-negative females, fail-to-farrow females, females to be culled, and weaned females dying before farrowing. In addition, gilts inventoried in the herd but not yet mated and gilts experiencing delayed puberty accumulate NPD. In general, NPD can be broken down into three major categories:

(1) Days that accumulate as an inventoried female waits to be mated; for example, the entry-to-service interval for gilts and the weaning-to-service interval for females. These intervals are called the *preservice intervals.*

(2) Days between the time a female is mated and when she is detected as not being pregnant, such as by returning to estrus, ultrasound, or visual observations. These intervals can be grouped together into the major category *postservice intervals.*

(3) Days prior to a female being removed from the herd, either by culling or after death. NPD associated with removal occur after entry, weaning, service, and detected open events. These intervals can be grouped into the major category *removal intervals.*

Several management practices potentially influence NPD, thereby making farm-to-farm comparisons difficult, if not misleading. Some of the more common practices interfering with these comparisons include intentionally skipping the first postweaning estrus following weaning of primiparous females in order to enhance second parity litter size (21-day skip program), delivering gilts into the breeding herd but not including them in the herd inventory of their record system until they are mated, and removing culled females from the record inventory as soon as the decision is made to cull the female, even if she remains in the herd. Because of these and other differences in recording practices, it is essential that the components of NPD be used, not only the total NPD, if comparisons among farms are to have merit.

There are several schemes by which commercial record systems have broken NPD into its components. One of the more common methods, together with targets is given in Table 6.2. While these intervals are accepted mathematical components of NPD, their use in troubleshooting is limited because they do not describe the female's reproductive failure in terms commonly understood. For example, the interval from weaning to reserve does not discriminate between females returning to estrus following unsuccessful mating from females found nonpregnant by ultrasound, females aborting, and bred females failing to farrow. For this reason, an alternative system has been developed for use by the swine industry. The proposed components, averages for the North American swine industry, and level of significance in influencing NPD are given in Table 6.3.

Table 6.2. Components of nonproductive days and target values

Component[a]	Target (days)
Gilts	
Entry to first service	10–21
Entry to removal (no service)	<3
First service to conception	<3
First service to removal	<3
Females	
Wean to first service	10–15
Wean to removal	<4
First service to conception	<4
First service to removal	<4
TOTAL NONPRODUCTIVE DAYS	30–50

Source: Polson et al. (1990a).
[a]Component of NPD used in the swine production information system, PigCHAMP, Version 2.2.

There are only a few commercial computerized record systems that currently compute NPD and its components. Some systems report NPD and its components in terms of the average number of days that inventoried sows and replacement gilts are nonproductive during a year. Other systems report NPD in terms of the percentage of days in a year that females are either not lactating or gestating. Some computations of NPD are time-driven calculations, wherein females accumulate NPD until a specified date is reached. Other computations of NPD are event-driven calculations, where NPD accumulate between an initiating event, such as weaning, and a subsequent event, such as service. For valid farm-to-farm comparisons to be made, the calculation method must be understood. However, even if a herd utilizes a record system that does not compute NPD, it can be estimated according to the formula:

Table 6.3. Biologically meaningful components for NPD, mean values, and statistical influence of components on NPD

Component[a]	Means	Significance[b]
Entry to first service	32	high
Entry to cull	54	none
Entry to death	14	low
Wean to first service	8	high
Wean to cull	16	high
Wean to death	5	none
Service to return	36	high
Service to preg check negative	47	none
Service to abort	84	none
Service to found nonpregnant	101	none
Service to fail-to-farrow	118	low
Service to cull	72	low
Service to death	68	none
Detected open to service	0.03	none
Detected open to cull	21	none
Detected open to death	8	none

Source: Polson et al. (1990a).

[a]Component of NPD used in the swine production information system, PigCHAMP, Version 2.2.

[b]High significance: $p < .001$; moderate: $p = .02 < x < .001$; low: $p = .05 < x < .02$.

$$NPD = 365 - [(\text{Lactation Length} + \text{Gestation Length}) \times \text{Litters/Female/Year}]$$

where litters/female/year are computed by dividing the total number of litters farrowed in a year by the average female inventory. Computerized information systems programs typically compute NPD using the formula:

$$NPD = \frac{\text{Total NPD in a Given Period}}{\text{Total Female-days in the Period}} \times 365 \text{ days}$$

In general, 1 NPD equates approximately 0.05 pigs/female/year and 0.007 litters/female/year. Thus, an improvement of NPD by 10 days results in an additional 0.5 pigs from each female annually and a jump in the herd's litters/female/year of about 70 points.

To most effectively use NPD in improving litters/female/year, the overall average NPD must be broken into its components. In turn, NPD components must be examined for how much they deviate from industry norms and, also, for what their relative potential is for being improved (i.e., the degree to which they statistically relate to either litters/female/year or piglets weaned/female/year). Those components that deviate the most from target values while being more highly related to female utilization efficiency are most likely to be useful in troubleshooting herd productivity.

Postservice Intervals. The interval from when a female is served until she is detected as not being pregnant, or postservice interval, is one of the leading indicators of NPD, which is influenced largely by the proportion of bred females that farrow to a service (farrowing rate) and the interval from service until females are detected as not pregnant (pregnancy detection). A female may be determined as nonpregnant if she (1) returns to estrus, (2) is found negative by ultrasound pregnancy determinations, (3) is observed to have aborted, (4) is observed visually to not show physical indications of pregnancy, or (5) fails to farrow at the anticipated time (Table 6.3). Of these five intervals, only the service-to-return and service-to-fail-to-farrow intervals are significantly related to NPD (Polson et al. 1990b). The impact of both intervals on NPD are dependent upon a herd's farrowing rate and timeliness and accuracy of pregnancy detection.

A common misconception is that farrowing rate by itself is a leading indicator of herd productivity. However, since it is a component of NPD, and as shown in Figure 6.3 it is one of several, farrowing rate is much less important than NPD in determining piglets weaned/female/year. NPD gives a quantitative measure to farrowing rate. By itself, farrowing rate does not indicate in quantifiable terms herd performance and, thus, cannot be converted into financially meaningful terms, either for days of female inventory or number of pigs. By converting farrowing rate to days of lost productivity, farrowing rate can be interpreted relative to its biological and financial costs. In general, farrowing rates only significantly affect piglets weaned/female/year in herds with substantially depressed farrowing rates and in herds with poor pregnancy detection, where nonconceiving females accumulate NPD as they await detection of their nonpregnancy status. The interval from service until a female is detected as not being pregnant (service-to-detected open interval) is a measure of the accuracy and promptness of pregnancy detection.

PREGNANCY DETECTION. To improve herd productivity through pregnancy detection, both timeliness and accuracy of detection must be considered. Return to estrus following mating and ultrasound (amplitude-depth and doppler) are the most commonly used pregnancy detection procedures used in commercial swine herds. Estrous detection has the advantage of being approximately 98% accurate and is unique among commonly used techniques in that pregnancy status is determined soon after conception has either failed to occur or after the litter has died (Almond and Dial 1986b). It has the disadvantages of potentially being more labor intensive and often requires special facilities and/or management skills. Though easy to use, ultrasound is less accurate (typically <90%) and cannot be conducted with satisfactory accuracy until the fourth week of gestation or later (Holtz 1981/1982; Almond and Dial 1986a).

There are several ways in which poor pregnancy detection on commercial swine herds leads to decreased litters/female/year. Dependence on ultrasound without estrous detection results in females being bred at the second or later estrus following conception failure. Thus, nonconceiving females are allowed to remain unproductive for 40 days or longer. The number of NPD attributable to a delayed detection of estrus can become quite large on farms where conception rates are low. When pregnancy checks are not done periodically throughout gestation, especially when estrous detection is not done daily, females that lose their litters after the last test will be assumed pregnant until failing to farrow. Furthermore, the wide variation in the accuracy of different models of mechanical pregnancy detectors (range: 65–95%; Holtz 1981/1982; Almond and Dial 1986a) often result in nonpregnant females being falsely considered as pregnant for long periods of time. Amplitude-depth and doppler ultrasound devices are based upon different principles and, thus, have complementary accuracies. The use of both types of devices increases the overall accuracy of pregnancy detection to greater than 95% (Almond and Dial 1986b), but neither can be used in advance of approximately 4 weeks.

The regimen that a farm uses for pregnancy detection has a significant influence on the percentage of bred females mistakenly thought to be pregnant and, subsequently, on the NPD. A pregnancy detection program that minimizes NPD and, thereby, optimizes litters/female/year is as follows. In the presence of a boar, females are observed daily throughout gestation for return to estrus, especially during the period of 18–24 days postbreeding. Routine pregnancy determinations, using either one of the amplitude-depth or doppler ultrasound devices, are then conducted at least twice during gestation at approximately 28–35 days and then again at 56–63 days. The first ultrasound pregnancy determination is timed to allow served females to be checked as early as possible with acceptable accuracy. The first and second pregnancy determinations are conducted just in advance of the second and third regular return to estrus after service, respectively, to enable females to be reserviced following an unsuccessful mating in as short an interval as possible. Amplitude-depth machines lose sensitivity at greater than approximately 80 days of gestation, whereas doppler machines are useful from approximately 4 weeks until farrowing (Almond and Dial 1986b). Thus, a third ultrasound test is not reliable in advance of the fourth postservice period of regular return to estrus, unless doppler ultrasound is used. Observations for estrus in the presence of a trained boar should continue daily throughout gestation to compensate for the inaccuracies of ultrasound machines and to ensure that females are served as soon as possible after they are observed as not being pregnant.

FARROWING RATE. Farrowing rate is the second component of the NPD service-to-conception interval, and represents the proportion of served females that farrow, regardless of whether or not they have had an opportunity to farrow. Females that are removed from the herd, either because of culling or mortality, will be included in the denominator of the farrowing-rate calculation, but will be lost from the numerator. In herds with elevated female mortality or culling rates, farrowing rates will be artificially depressed. Thus, low farrowing rates do not consistently reflect a fertility problem. For the farrowing rate to be a consistently useful measure of fertility, the denominator should not include served females that are removed from the herd for reasons not relating to failure to conceive or maintain pregnancy. At least one of the commercially available computerized information systems (PigCHAMP, Version 3.0) computes an "adjusted farrowing rate" that takes into consideration served females not having an opportunity to farrow.

$$\text{Farrowing Rate} = \frac{\text{No. Females Farrowing}}{\text{No. Females Served}}$$

$$\text{Adjusted Farrowing Rate} = \frac{\substack{\text{No. Females in a}\\ \text{Service Group that Farrow}}}{\substack{(\text{No. Females Served}) -\\ (\text{No. Removed for Reasons}\\ \text{not Relating to Fertility})}}$$

The difference between adjusted farrowing rate and farrowing rate reflects the magnitude of sow removal after service (Fig. 6.4).

CONCEPTION RATE. Reduced fertility can be due to reductions in the proportion of females that conceive or to the proportion of females maintaining pregnancy (Fig. 6.5). While implicitly referring to the proportion of bred females having fertilized ova, conception rate can be estimated from

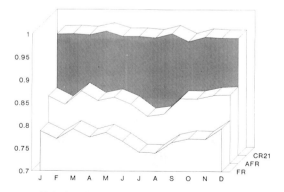

6.4. Relationship between farrowing rate (*FR*), adjusted farrowing rate (*AFR*), and proportion of females failing to return to estrus between 18 and 24 days after service (*CR21*). Data include over 2037 services from 42 farms using PigCHAMP at each data point.

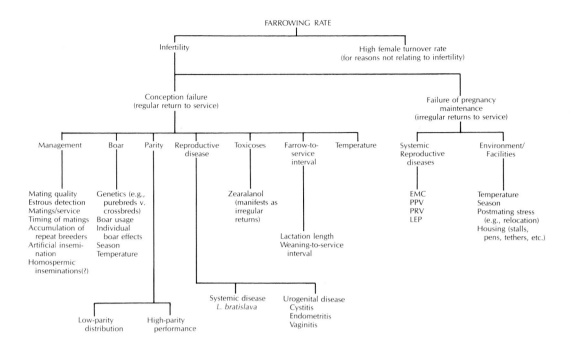

6.5.   Interrelationships between factors influencing farrowing rate. EMC = encephalomyo-carditis; PPV = porcine parvovirus; PRV = pseudorabies virus; LEP = leptospirosis.

the proportion that fail to show estrus during the anticipated time of regular return to estrus (approximately 18–24 days postbreeding). Included with pregnant females and females thought to be pregnant because they failed to return to estrus following unsuccessful service are females that become anestrus following service and females that lose their litters after initiating implantation. Decreased conception rates, as reflected by an increased number of females having regular returns to estrus, occur when an entire crop of ova fail to be fertilized, when all embryos die prior to the initiation of implantation at 12–15 days postcoitus, or when an insufficient number of blastocysts (approximately four embryos) survive until the initiation of implantation (Hunter 1977).

In the absence of vigorous and accurate checks for return to estrus, it is tempting to estimate conception rates from the proportion of bred females found pregnant by ultrasound, typically at 28–35 days postbreeding. Such groups include females that initially conceived but subsequently lost their pregnancies prior to the 30-day pregnancy check. Farrowing rate refers to the proportion of bred females that farrow and, thus, includes females that not only conceive but also maintain their pregnancies until term. Since pregnancies are commonly terminated after conception, conception rate is reflected in farrowing rate, but remains a distinct measure of reproductive performance.

The factors that contribute to decreases in conception rates are different from those that affect the capacity of the female to maintain pregnancy. Consequently, when evaluating fertility problems in commercial swine operations, it is essential, to initially determine if suboptimal farrowing rates are due to reduced conception or to reductions in the proportion of females maintaining pregnancy. A pregnancy loss chart kept throughout gestation for all served groups (Fig. 6.6) may be helpful in differentiating between conception failure and failure of pregnancy maintenance. Females returning to estrus and aborting females should be identified separately on the chart from all other females lost from a group after service in order to (1) minimize the impact on farrowing rate of females removed after service for reasons not relating to fertility and (2) to eliminate the influence of females detected nonpregnant by ultrasound and by visual observations, where time of pregnancy loss is not known.

The risk factors and causes of reductions in conception rates can be generally classified into management, facilities, environment, and disease categories.

Estrous Detection.   The onset of the preovulatory luteinizing hormone (LH) surge, which culminates follicular growth and precipitates ovulation, varies among females, occurring from 8 hours before to 12 hours after the onset of estrus (Tilton et

FARROWING RATE REPORT
22 APR 90 - 30 JUN 90
FARM:

PigCHAMP 3.0
(C) 1985,87,88 Univ of Minn
Printed: 29 JAN 91

| | | | | | | | WEEK: SOWS FOUND NOT PREGNANT | | | | | | | | | | | | | | FARROW | TARGET=48 LONG/ | CUM | EXPECTED |
SERVICE DATES	S	1	2	3	4	5	6	7	8	9	10	11	12	13	14	15	16	F	RATE	SHORT	FARROW	FARROW DATES
22APR-28APR90	63	0	1	4	5	0	0	0	0	0	0	0	0	0	0	0	0	0	53	84.1	5	53	15AUG-21AUG90
29APR- 5MAY90	63	0	1	0	6	0	1	0	0	1	0	0	0	0	0	0	0	0	50	79.4	2	103	22AUG-28AUG90
6MAY9-12MAY90	61	0	0	1	0	0	0	0	0	0	0	0	0	0	0	0	0	0	30	49.2	-18	133	29AUG- 4SEP90

| | | | | | DAYS: SOWS PRESUMED PREGNANT | | | | | | | | | | FARROW | TARGET=48 LONG/ | CUM | EXPECTED |
SERVICE DATES	S	10	17	24	32	39	47	54	71	78	85	92	105	106+	F	RATE	SHORT	FARROW	FARROW DATES
22APR-28APR90	63	63	63	63	60	56	53	53	53	53	53	53	53	53	53	84.1	5	53	15AUG-21AUG90
29APR- 5MAY90	63	63	63	63	62	61	54	53	53	51	51	51	51	51	50	79.4	2	103	22AUG-28AUG90
6MAY9-12MAY90	61	61	61	61	60	59	59	58	58	58	58	58	58	58	30	49.2	-18	133	29AUG- 4SEP90

| | | | | | DAYS: SOWS RETURNED TO ESTRUS | | | | | | | | | | FARROW | TARGET=48 LONG/ | CUM | EXPECTED |
SERVICE DATES	S	10	17	24	32	39	47	54	71	78	85	92	105	106+	F	RATE	SHORT	FARROW	FARROW DATES
22APR-28APR90	63	0	0	3	2	0	0	0	0	0	0	0	0	0	53	84.1	5	53	15AUG-21AUG90
29APR- 5MAY90	63	0	0	1	0	1	1	0	0	0	0	0	0	0	50	79.4	2	103	22AUG-28AUG90
6MAY9-12MAY90	61	0	0	1	0	0	0	0	0	0	0	0	0	0	30	49.2	-18	133	29AUG- 4SEP90

6.6. Pregnancy loss charts showing breakdown of times during pregnancy that females are found nonpregnant relative to weeks after service (upper figure); breakdown number of females presumed pregnant with females being grouped at weekly intervals relative to week of regular return to estrus (18 to 24 days) (middle figure); breakdown of times that females return to estrus following an unsuccessful service with females being grouped at weekly intervals relative to week of regular return to estrus (bottom figure).

al. 1982). The interval between the LH surge and ovulation is relatively constant and is assumed to be approximately 40 hours (Foxcroft and Van de Wiel 1982). It would be expected that the highly variable interval between the onset of estrus and the LH surge would result in a corresponding variation in the interval between onset of estrus and ovulation. In fact, in some females ovulation has been observed prior to 30 hours after the onset of estrus, while in others it was not completed by 45 hours (Signoret et al. 1972). Estrus may extend in some females for greater than a day after ovulation has occurred (Signoret et al. 1972; Hunter 1977). The viable lifespan of porcine ova has been estimated to be approximately 8–10 hours (Hunter 1977). Optimal fertility occurs when insemination takes place approximately 12–16 hours prior to ovulation (Hunter 1977). The synchrony between breeding and ovulation, resulting in reduced fertility, is the adverse consequence of inadequate heat detection. Females commence estrus throughout the day, with a majority show-ing first estrus during the late evening to early morning hours (Clark et al. 1986). The asynchrony between onset of estrus and time of ovulation is potentially compounded by an inability to accurately determine the onset of estrus.

Asynchronous breeding commonly occurs when (1) estrus detection is initiated too late following weaning, (2) when it is done too infrequently, (3) when behavioral signs of estrus are evaluated in the absence of a mature boar, (4) when visual and manual methods of estrous detection are replaced by reliance on the boar to identify an estrous female (rather than a human detecting estrus), (5) when group sizes are too large to allow accurate identification of estrous females, and (6) when submissive females are housed with dominant females. Beside reduced conception rates, manifestations of asynchronous breeding include increased fertilization failures and increased embryonic mortality, which potentially result in decreased litter sizes (Hunter 1977).

Timing of Matings. Only a minority of females ovulate prior to 30 hours after the onset of estrus (Signoret 1971; Signoret et al. 1972). Optimal conception results when matings occur at approximately 28 hours after the onset of estrus (Dziuk 1970). In herds with accurate and frequent estrous detection (<12-hour intervals), the onset of estrus can be estimated, which optimizes the chance that a mating will occur just prior to ovulation. Because estrous detection rarely is conducted more than once daily on most commercial farms, it usually is not possible to obtain sufficiently accurate estimates of the time of ovulation. Single matings, therefore, potentially result in asynchrony between service and ovulation. Thus, conception rates and/or litter sizes may be suboptimal.

Matings/Estrus. It is a common perception that multiple matings during estrus will increase the likelihood that one or more breedings will occur near the time of optimal fertility. In fact, both retrospective and prospective studies have demonstrated that females mated once per estrus have reduced farrowing rates relative to those mated multiple times (Rasbech 1969; Sweistra and Rahnfeld 1972; Eleftheriou 1980; Liptrap et al. 1983; Hilley et al. 1986a; Clark et al. 1989). While some retrospective studies have not demonstrated a significant influence of two versus three matings on farrowing rate (Hilley et al. 1986), other prospective investigations have shown a numerical, but nonsignificant, increase in fertility when females were mated or artificially inseminated three times per estrus rather than twice (O'Grady et al. 1983; Silva and Paz-Gomes-da-Silva 1989). The interval between multiple matings during an estrous period has been shown to have a numerical but nonsignificant influence on farrowing rate (Silva and Paz-Gomes-da-Silva 1989) and litter size (Tilton and Cole 1982).

Retrospective studies examining the relationship between number of matings/service and fertility can be faulted for at least two reasons: (1) less fertile animals would be expected to be in estrus for a shorter duration than more fertile females and, thus, would be more likely to be mated fewer times, and (2) weaned females that return to estrus more slowly are less fertile and in estrus for a shorter duration than those returning within 7 days postweaning (Tarocco 1989). For these reasons, retrospective research may be confounded, and the results should be interpreted with caution.

Type of Service. Both heterospermic (crossmating) and homospermic (straight) mating programs are used in commercial swine operations. Homospermic matings commonly are used in purebred operations and on commercial farms where producers are either attempting to identify subfertile boars or are unable to easily rotate boars during a service period because of facility design restraints. Even though potentially allowing the relative fertilities of boars to be estimated, homospermic matings are often perceived as resulting in lower conception rates than heterospermic matings. The results of some studies indicate that mixed semen from different boars improves conception rates in both females and gilts (Pacova and Dupal 1980; Thorton, 1987). However, in other trials, no differences were observed in either the farrowing rates or litter sizes between females mated multiple times to the same boar during an estrus and those bred to more than one boar (Liptrap 1983; Hilley et al., 1986c). Additional research may be warranted before complete confidence in recommendations is assured. Nonetheless, even though fertility may not be improved through the use of heterospermic services, crossmating may allow a boar having normal fertility to compensate for a subfertile boar.

Boar Usage. It is generally accepted that overuse of boars will result in reduced fertility. However, there is still considerable controversy over the optimal interval of usage. When semen was collected once daily for 5 days, total sperm per ejaculate decreased linearly but remained above the estimated daily sperm production (Paquignon et al. 1984). Farrowing rates remained unaffected by daily boar usage during the 5-day trial, but decreased when boars were used more than once per day. Similar results were obtained in another study that demonstrated no differences in the 7-week pregnancy rate for boars used six times per week versus boars used only twice per week (Hemsworth et al. 1983). In a retrospective study, farrowing rates were found to decrease when boars were used for six or more consecutive days (Leman et al. 1984). In sum, these studies suggest that overuse of boars remains a risk factor for reduced fertility. Overly frequent usage of boars is not common on commercial farms of North America utilizing hand-mating; however, penmating may allow for boars to serve females several times during a day for several days. While there is a controversial influence of duration of sexual rest on litter size, there is no evidence that conception rates are improved when boars are not used for several days prior to breeding (Rasbech 1969; Sweistra and Dyck 1976).

Sperm production increases from puberty to about 18 months of age, indicating that younger boars might require a lower frequency of use than older boars (Sweistra 1973). There are seasonal changes in seminal characteristics and circulating androgens (Claus et al. 1985). As discussed in more detail below, elevated ambient temperatures detrimentally influence boar fertility, and susceptibility to temperature varies among boars (Wetteman et al. 1976; 1979). Thus, while published studies appear to indicate that mature boars can be used for up to 6 consecutive days without detrimentally affecting conception rates, it appears that age, season, and ambient temperature may influence the frequency at which boars may be used. In fact, there may be an advantage to decreasing the frequency of usage of young boars and the usage frequency of all boars during the summer months.

Quality of Mating. Beside requiring a fertile receptive female, conception is dependent upon a sexually aggressive boar identifying an estrous female, being able to mount and copulate, and being capable of ejaculating a sufficient number of fertile spermatozoa in an adequate seminal volume. Matings of poor quality can result from a failure in any of these areas and can potentially occur with all breeding systems, including pen-mating and hand-mating systems. Pen-mating frequently results in lower conception rates than hand-mating. This may be associated with several factors, including too-frequent matings by sexually aggressive dominant boars, less-than-optimal matings/service, inadequate estrous detection by boars resulting in asynchrony between ovulation and breeding, and incomplete ejaculation. On the other hand, conception failures with hand-mating can occur when a producer fails to assure that intromission has been successful and that ejaculation has been completed before the boar withdraws from the female. Suboptimal conception rates may occur when producers attempt to expose too many females to boars at the same time and are, therefore, unable to confirm that matings have been successful. Suboptimal breeding environments (e.g., high ambient temperature, slippery breeding surfaces, breeding in a foreign environment) can cause unsuccessful copulation or incomplete ejaculation and subsequently result in low conception rates. In addition, health problems of either the boar or female (e.g., lameness, osteochondrosis) and behavioral vices (e.g., timidity, overly aggressive behavior, abhorrent sexual behavior) can interfere with successful matings.

Individual Boar Differences. Swine producers have long tried to identify boars having either suboptimal conception rates or inadequate litter sizes. It is generally accepted that differences in fertility exist between boars, and in fact, several studies have shown that boars significantly affect farrowing rates and/or litter sizes (Rasbech 1969; Rahnefeld and Sweistra 1970; Uzu 1979; Egbunike 1982). The prevalence of subfertile boars in commercial operations is not known, nor is it clear how much variation exists within groups of boars on commercial farms. Variations in the farrowing rates of individual boars from 60 to 83% (Rasbech 1969), from 50 to 88% (Uzu 1979), and from 55 to 100% (Egbunike 1982) have been reported following natural matings. Only about 4% of the boars in one study were found to

have <60% farrowing rates, whereas 87.5% had farrowing rates >80% (Egbunike 1982). The farrowing rate of the initial service is not a reliable estimate of the farrowing rate for subsequent services (Clark et al. 1989). Thus, it would appear that an evaluation of a boar's fertility cannot reliably be used to identify boars of suboptimal fertility for subsequent culling.

In contrast to other farm mammal species, regular semen evaluations on large numbers of boars in commercial swine operations are not always practical, being time consuming, requiring an estrous female or boars trained to mount a dummy, and being dependent upon all boars tolerating manual manipulation of their penises. In addition, semen evaluations typically are not sufficiently accurate in determining differences in the relative fertilities of groups of boars where there may not be much variation. As a result, herd records are more often used to evaluate relative boar fertility. When there are large variations in the fertilities of a group, records will potentially allow the identification of boars of suspect fertility, and may help rank boars according to relative fertility. However, if there is only a modest variation in fertility, as may exist on many commercial farms, variations by chance alone will often disguise any differences.

It has been suggested that when normal variation exists in a group of boars, as many as 50 mated females may be needed before records can be used to appraise an individual's fertility (Levis 1986). Thus, when boars mate only one to three females per week, as occurs commonly on commercial farms, it may take 6 months or longer to evaluate the fertility of a boar with an acceptable degree of accuracy. Since semen quality fluctuates with ambient temperature and/or season (Egbunike 1982; Claus et al. 1985; Trudeau and Sanford 1986), there is a risk of culling boars that are transiently subfertile or are immature and have not yet reached peak fertility.

Infectious Systemic Reproductive Diseases. Several systemically borne reproductive pathogens, including porcine parvovirus (PPV), pseudorabies virus (PRV), leptospirosis (LEP), and encephalomyocarditis virus (EMCV) cause a variety of reproductive failures (Thacker and Gonzalez 1988; Christianson et al. 1990). Among other manifestations, transplacental passage of viral pathogens has been associated with reduced litter sizes (Kluge and Mare 1974; Mengeling 1979; Mengeling et al. 1980) when not all the fetuses in a litter are killed, and abortion (Kluge and Mare 1974; Wohlgemuth et al. 1978) or fetal resorption (Mengeling 1979; Mengeling et al. 1980) with delayed return to estrus if all fetuses are destroyed. Exposure of the female near the time of conception to viral pathogens results in early embryonic death (Mengeling et al. 1980).

The clinical sequelae to transuterine infections

of a litter depends upon the time of exposure during gestation (Fig. 6.7). When the entire litter dies prior to the time of initiation of implantation (days 12–23 postcoitus), the female is likely to return to estrus at a regular interval (i.e., 18–24 days postservice). If at least four embryos remain at the time of implantation initiation, the female will remain pregnant, farrowing a reduced litter size. Death of the litter after the initiation of implantation but prior to the onset of skeletal calcification (approximately 30–40 days postcoitus) results in females having a delayed or irregular return to service. Litter death after the onset of fetal skeletal calcification results in fetal remnants being incompletely reabsorbed leaving only inspissated, necrotic tissue (i.e., mummies). Females having entire litters mummified may fail to return to estrus for prolonged periods of time, and some may appear pseudopregnant. Abortion can occur throughout gestation and be followed by estrus within 5–10 days or a period of prolonged anovulatory anestrus. Death of the entire litter during the last days of pregnancy can result in premature farrowing or piglets being stillborn.

Urogenital Infections. Genital tract infections are associated primarily with regular returns to estrus (Muirhead 1986; Dial and MacLachlan 1988a). Presumably, endometritis at the time of breeding reduces the viability of gametes and/or interferes with fertilization. In addition, chronic infections of the genital tract can cause persistent lesions in the oviduct or uterus (Anon. 1975; Dial and MacLachlan 1988b), resulting in the disruption of gamete or zygote transport or interference with implantation. The consequence is often repeat-breeder females and gilts (Karlberg et al. 1981; Dial and MacLachlan 1988a). Urinary tract infections and vaginitis can cause transient ascending uterine infections that interfere with fertility (Von Both et al. 1980; Moller et al. 1981; Dial and MacLachlan 1988a). Isolates from infected genital tracts commonly include facultative pathogenic bacteria such as streptococci, coliform, and corynebacterium species (Dial and MacLachlan 1988b).

In addition to facultative pathogens, there is evidence that uterine infections result from infections with specific microbes more commonly associated with systemic reproductive disease. For example, in addition to the more common irregular returns to estrus caused by systemically borne infections of the fetus, PRV causes placental lesions (Hsu et al. 1980) and, thus, potentially conception failure with regular returns by disrupting nidation and/or placentation. Leptospiral infections of the female pig typically are infections of the fetus and the kidney (Hathaway 1985). However, *Leptospira bratislava* infects the uterus (Ellis et al. 1985; 1986a,b), and thus, is associated with

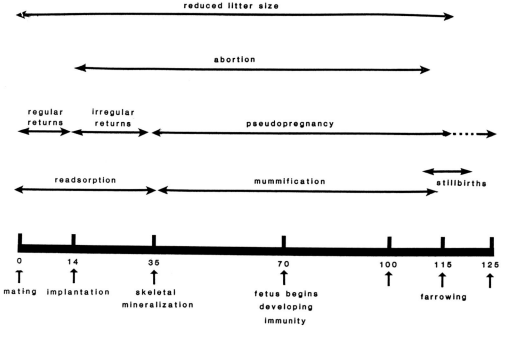

6.7. Effect of embryonic or fetal mortality during different stages of gestation on reproductive activity of females.

reduced conception and regular returns to estrus, as well as fetal death and loss of pregnancy, as observed with other *Leptospira* serovars.

Elevated Ambient Temperature. The exposure of females to increased ambient temperatures (>32°C) after mating is associated with decreased conception and farrowing rates (Edwards et al. 1968; Teague et al. 1968) and increased embryonic mortality (Warnick et al. 1965; Tompkins et al. 1967; Edwards et al. 1968; Omtvedt et al. 1968; Teague et al. 1968). In one study, elevated temperatures caused the greatest reduction in embryonic survival when applied at the time of breeding (Tompkins et al. 1967); in another study, temperature had its most pronounced detrimental effect before day 15 postbreeding (Edwards et al. 1968). A third study revealed greatest embryonic mortality between 8 and 16 days postcoitus (Omtvedt et al. 1968). Implantation commences between 12 and 15 days postbreeding, and fertilization occurs within a few hours postcoitus (Hunter 1977). Conception losses appear to be highest when females are heat stressed around the time of conception and nidation. The inability of a female to acclimate to temperature stress, therefore, is likely manifested as decreased conception rates with regular returns to estrus if all the litter is killed, or smaller litter sizes if embryonic mortality is limited.

Elevated ambient temperatures have similar detrimental effects on the boar. Increases in ambient temperature (>32°C) for as few as 3 days are followed by decreases in both the motility and quantity of sperm and increases in the proportion of abnormal sperm (McNitt and First 1970; Christenson et al. 1972). Long-term exposure of boars to heat stress causes similar reductions in reproductive performance, which persist for at least the duration of temperature elevation and may persist for up to 5–8 weeks after removal of the temperature insult (Wetteman et al. 1976; 1979). When breeding boars are exposed to elevated temperatures, there is a decrease in the conception rates of females bred either naturally or by artificial insemination (Christenson et al. 1972). Individual boars do not appear to be uniformly susceptible to heat stress; some males show a pronounced decrease in fertility after exposure to high ambient temperatures, while others present no change in mean conception rates (Wetteman et al. 1976). Because he is typically involved in several matings each week, an individual boar's infertility affects herd reproductive performance much more than does that of an individual female.

Genetics. There are differences in conception rates in both purebred lines and in crossbred female lines (Quintana and Robison 1983). Estimates of the heterosis of conception rate varies considerably with breeds used in a cross; for example, Yorkshires are associated with a heterosis of approximately 9.7%, whereas Hampshires have a conception rate heterosis of about 1.7%. The average individual heterosis for conception rates across all breeds, which does not account for heterosis in the parents, is approximately 3.5%, indicating crossbreeding heterosis can be used to improve the trait by an average of approximately 2.8% (Johnson 1981). Conception rates tend to be higher when young crossbred boars are used rather than young purebred boars (Johnson 1981b); however, the difference disappears as boars get older. Apparently, crossbred boars mature at a younger age and, thus, are more fertile than purebred boars.

Artificial Insemination. It is generally accepted that artificial insemination results in lower conception rates than natural service. The observation that approximately 40% of herds (n = 172) using artificial insemination had >80% conception rates, suggests that on some herds fertility may be similar to that obtained with natural service (Reed 1982). On farms in which there is an insufficient boar inventory to allow multiple matings per estrus, natural mating followed in 18–30 hours by artificial insemination with extended fresh semen results in farrowing rates that are comparable to that obtained when females are mated naturally multiple times (Henry 1984). Farrowing rates following insemination with frozen semen are commonly less than that obtained with a fresh ejaculate (Reed 1982).

PREGNANCY MAINTENANCE. At or prior to implantation, maternal recognition of pregnancy occurs (Flint et al. 1982). As discussed earlier, death of all the embryos in a litter prior to this time is likely to result in regular returns to estrus (Fig. 6.7). Within the initial 25 days of gestation, embryonic/fetal mortality is higher than at any other time during gestation (Stone 1987); partial loss of a litter is manifested as reduced litter size, while complete litter mortality is followed by return to estrus at an irregular interval (e.g., >25 days postcoitus). Complete resorption of a fetus can occur up to approximately 30 days of gestation, but fetal death after this time, when osteogenesis commences, results in fetal maceration and mummification (Mengeling 1986). The immune system begins to develop at approximately 55 days, and immune competence occurs at about 70 days. However, transplacental exposure to a fetotropic pathogen commonly leads to death, if the fetuses are unable to respond rapidly with protective active immune responses.

In addition to those that influence the capacity of the female to conceive, there are several other factors that adversely affect farrowing rates by influencing the ability of the female to maintain pregnancy. Failure of pregnancy maintenance can be manifested as irregular returns to estrus, abortions, females failing to farrow (not-in-pig females), and pseudopregnancy.

Nutrition. The influences that nutrition, especially the effects of nutrient intake during lactation and the return to estrus following weaning, have been well investigated. Although it has been suggested that thin females and those having the greatest lactational weight losses have reduced fertility (MacLean 1969), the influence that lactational feed intake has on farrowing rates remains unclear. The starvation of gilts for periods exceeding 1 month during pregnancy had no influence on either pregnancy rates or embryonic development, indicating that feed consumption during gestation has no obvious detrimental effects on the ability of the female to maintain pregnancy (Anderson 1975). High-level feeding of gilts (Den Hartog and Van Kempen 1980) and increased feed intake by primiparous (Brooks and Cole 1972) and biparous females (Kirkwood et al. 1987), but not older parity females (Brooks et al. 1975), during the interval from weaning to breeding improved farrowing rates. Thus, there is evidence that flushing may be useful in improving the conception rates of low-parity females, but evidence is lacking that it will be beneficial to older females.

Complete feed and/or water deprivation during the rebreeding period is a common practice used by swine producers to shorten the interval between weaning and rebreeding. It is not uncommon for females to dramatically reduce their feed intakes following weaning. In females housed in groups following weaning, subservient females may have substantially reduced feed intake than more dominant females. Thus, there is reason to question the effect of reduced nutrient intake on reproductive performance during the postweaning period. Feed and/or water deprivation has been found to not influence conception rate or farrowing rate, but may increase the weaning-to-rebreeding interval in primiparous females (Knabe et al. 1986).

The influence of micronutrients on fertility remains unclear. The addition of supplemental choline (Miller and Kornegay 1983) and biotin (Brooks et al. 1977; Penny et al. 1981) to lactation and gestation rations have been suggested to improve conception rates, as well as to decrease the weaning-to-remating interval and to increase the number of live-born pigs. The addition of folic acid to the diets of pregnant and lactating females improves farrowing rate as well as litter size (Lindemann and Kornegay 1987).

Infectious Reproductive Diseases. Pathogens of the fetoplacental unit and the uterus cause decreases in farrowing rate with irregular returns to estrus by killing all the fetuses in a litter. If two or more fetuses remain alive after siblings have died, delivery will occur at the normal time (Stryker and Dziuk 1975). Death of an entire litter prior to skeletal ossification, but after nidation, is followed by resorption of fetal remnants (Mengeling

1986) and, in most cases, by irregular returns to estrus. Some females fail to resume normal ovarian activity following litter resorption and remain anestrus for varying periods (Meredith 1984). Females that are initially diagnosed as pregnant, lose their litters, but either remain in anovulatory anestrus or are simply not observed when in estrus, are commonly called fail-to-farrow females. Another sequelae to reproductive disease is pseudopregnancy, in which the fetuses are destroyed, often after skeletal mineralization has commenced, but the female fails to return to normal ovarian cyclicity due to the persistence of the corpora lutea of pregnancy (Anon. 1975). Abortion is a common manifestation of systemic pathogens of the female and may occur following invasion of the fetoplacental unit by any of several bacterial or viral pathogens (Anon. 1975).

Systemically borne pathogens of the female pig typically cause epidemics of pregnancy failure where farrowing rates are dramatically, but only transiently, reduced. Epidemics of PRV, PPV, LEP, and EMCV can cause abrupt reductions in farrowing rates, typically characterized by increased irregular returns to estrus (Thacker and Gonzalez 1988; Christianson et al. 1990). The clinical pattern of reproductive failure that accompanies reductions in pregnancy maintenance can be used to distinguish the reproductive diseases from each other and from noninfectious causes. For example, in addition to increased irregular returns to estrus and increased proportions of fail-to-farrow and pseudopregnant females, outbreaks of PPV commonly occur in low-parity females causing increased regular returns to estrus (i.e., reduced conception rates) and reduced live-born litter sizes with increased mummy rates (Mengeling 1986). Epidemics of PRV can cause increased abortion rates, increased occurrence of pseudopregnant and fail-to-farrow females of all parities, and reduced live-born litter sizes associated with increased stillbirth and mummy rates (Gustafson 1986). In addition to decreased farrowing rates, LEP epidemics are commonly associated with increased abortion rates and reduced live-born litter size accompanying increased stillbirth rates (Hathaway 1985).

Endemic reproductive disease associated with infectious reproductive pathogens typically present the same clinical pattern in individual animals as disease epidemics, except that clinical signs are restricted to a smaller proportion of susceptible, immunologically naive females. For example, while PPV may be present as an epidemic in a start-up herd containing a large proportion of naive, low-parity females, it most commonly occurs in the endemic form in established herds where only a small proportion of low-parity females are affected. Endemic PRV will present as reproductive failure (e.g., increased mummy rates, abortion, pregnancy failure) involving only a minority of females in a herd as they are exposed to the pathogen during gestation.

Infectious agents not commonly thought to be reproductive pathogens can also cause failure of pregnancy maintenance either through their general systemic effects on the dam or by infecting the fetuses. For example, immunologically naive females infected with erysipelas may abort and subsequently return to estrus at an irregular interval following service.

Season. Numerous retrospective studies have documented decreased farrowing rates of females, especially low-parity females, mated during the summer months (Hurtgen and Leman 1980; Martinat-Botte et al. 1984; Dial et al. 1987). The near pathognomonic sign for seasonal influences on reproduction is a temporal depression in fertility characterized by increased percentages of females returning to estrus at irregular intervals following breeding (Paterson et al. 1978; Love 1981). There appears to be no or only a slight increase during the summer in the proportion of females returning to estrus at regular intervals (Paterson et al. 1978). It has been suggested that some of the females returning to estrus at irregular intervals conceive and initiate their pregnancies but lose their litters after the luteotrophic signal for pregnancy has been given by the blastocyst (Benjaminson and Karlberg 1981). Others that are bred at the postweaning estrus during the summer either fail to conceive or lose their pregnancies and have delayed reinitiation of ovarian cyclicity. Summer decreases in farrowing rates are greater in lower-parity females than in higher-parity females (Hurtgen and Leman 1980). During summer-to-early-fall, there are also increases in the prevalence of abortions and females failing to farrow (Stork 1979; Wrathall et al. 1986).

While the summer decrease in farrowing rates is often blamed on the high ambient temperatures characteristic of this period, it should be remembered that elevated temperatures are characterized by increased conception failures and increased embryonic mortality (Warnick et al. 1965; Tompkins et al. 1967; Edwards et al. 1968; Omtvedt et al. 1968; Teague et al. 1968). The highest rate of embryonic mortality appears to occur when females are heat stressed around the time of nidation, and the exposure of females to elevated ambient temperature during midgestation does not appear to influence fetal survival (Omtvedt et al. 1968). When females are exposed to high ambient temperatures during late gestation, fewer piglets are born alive, preweaning mortality is greater, and average weaning weights tend to be lighter (Omtvedt et al. 1968). Abortion and pregnancy failure has not been observed with gestation females exposed to high ambient temperatures (Warnick et al. 1965; Tompkins et al. 1967; Edwards et al. 1968; Omtvedt et al. 1968). It has been suggested that when females are ex-

posed to elevated ambient temperatures, death of the female is more likely than death of the litter (Edwards et al. 1968). Thus, temperature stress would more likely be associated with reductions in conception than reductions in pregnancy maintenance. In contrast to temperature, seasonal infertility is associated with irregular returns to estrus (Paterson et al. 1978; Love 1981) in accompaniment with no or only a modest change in litter size (Hilley et al. 1986a,b).

Photoperiod has been found in some studies to influence the age of gilts at puberty (Diekman and Hoagland 1983; Diekman and Grieger 1988) and the interval from weaning to estrus (Mabry et al. 1982b; Stevenson et al. 1983). There is growing experimental evidence that decreasing and increasing daylength influence the reproductive performance of both the adult female and boar (Claus et al. 1985). The gradual increase in daylength toward summer solstice is temporally associated with the reduced fertility of females mated during the summer months (Dial 1984). Several weeks later gradual reductions in daylength are followed by improvements in the fertility of females mated during periods of decreasing photoperiod, suggesting that seasonal changes in fertility are mediated, at least in part, by reductions in daylength.

Housing. There is a controversial influence of female housing during the postweaning breeding period and/or during gestation on farrowing rates. While one study demonstrated no significant influence of housing on fertility (Hemsworth et al. 1982), another indicated that females housed in groups following breeding had decreased early pregnancy losses and, subsequently, increased farrowing rates relative to females housed in stalls (Schmidt et al. 1985). Other studies indicate that fertility is higher (Hurtgen and Leman 1980) and rebreeding intervals are shorter (Fahmy and Dufour 1976) when females are placed in individual stalls following breeding. It has been suggested that social stimulation benefits grouped females, and that the detrimental effects of individually housed females are mediated through a stress response (Petherick and Blackshaw 1986). Because of farm-to-farm variations in management, environment, and facilities, the fertility of individually housed females may be acceptable on some farms, but may be persistently low in others. Conversely, the low farrowing rates that commonly occur on farms in which poor attention is paid to individual females housed in groups might be improved by converting gestation facilities to individual stalls.

Female housing also appears to influence the female's reproductive responses to changes in season. Females housed in completely enclosed facilities had less seasonal fluctuations in fertility than those housed in open-front buildings (Martinat-Botte et al. 1984).

Parity. It is commonly known and has been clearly demonstrated that lower-parity females, especially gilts, have lower farrowing rates than higher-parity females (Hurtgen and Leman 1980; Martinat-Botte et al. 1984). Furthermore, as demonstrated in Figure 6.8, older females often have reduced farrowing rates relative to midparity females (parities 3–5) (Leman et al. 1988). Differences among parities are more pronounced during the summer months than during the other seasons (Hurtgen and Leman 1980; Martinat-Botte et al. 1984). The percentage of females returning to estrus within 30 days after breeding, reflecting conception rate, as well as the percentage of females farrowing, was greater for low-parity females than for high-parity females

(Maurer et al. 1985). Thus, it appears that parity influences the ability of swine to conceive, as well as to maintain pregnancy.

Because of the profound influence of parity on fertility, a herd's parity distribution potentially has a significant influence on the herd's farrowing rate. It is not uncommon for start-up herds and herds having a high inventory turnover, and thus, having a large proportion of gilts farrowing, to have a low overall farrowing rate. Similarly, established herds having a high proportion of older females (>30% of females ≥ fifth parity) may have reduced farrowing rates.

Farrowing-to-Service Interval. While lactation length has a significant influence on total-born lit-

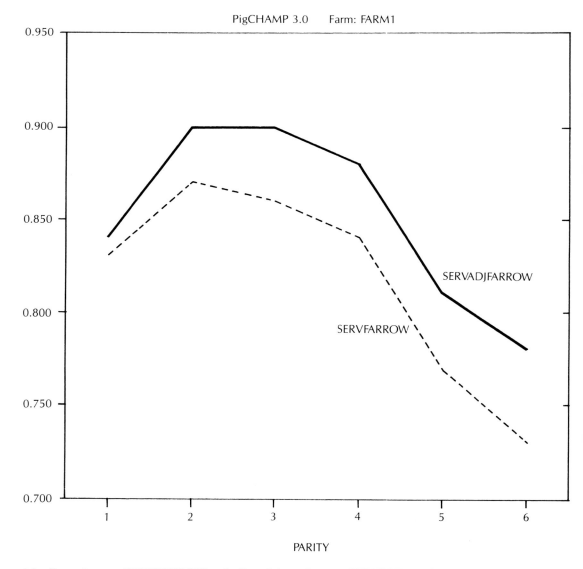

6.8. Farrowing rate (SERVFARROW) and adjusted farrowing rate (SERVADJFARROW) in a 1150-female commercial herd using PigCHAMP. Means for each parity represent from 414 females (parity 6) to 1545 females (parity 1) at each data point.

ter size and weaning-to-reserve interval, as discussed below, there is a controversial influence of lactation length on fertility (Varley 1982). Some studies have demonstrated no difference in farrowing rates as lactation length is shortened (Cole et al. 1975; Varley and Cole 1976a,b; Martinat-Botte et al. 1984); other studies have shown that lactation lengths of 2–10 days are associated with significantly reduced farrowing rates relative to longer lactations (Aumaitre 1972; Te Brake 1972; Svajgr et al. 1974). In a study of a large commercial confinement herd, females lactating approximately 21 days had lower subsequent farrowing rates and litter sizes than those lactating 28 days (Clark and Leman 1984).

It is not clear whether reduced farrowing rates associated with shorter lactations is caused by reduced conception or lower rates of pregnancy maintenance. It has been suggested that the smaller litters observed with short lactations are due to a reduction in the number of ova fertilized (Svajgr et al. 1974) and reduced number of embryos surviving through implantation (Varley and Cole 1978). Thus, it is possible that both conception and pregnancy maintenance are reduced with shorter lactations.

Similar to lactation length, weaning-to-service interval has been found to influence farrowing rate. In one study, females mated after day 9 postmating had reduced farrowing rates relative to those mated on days 3–9 (Martinat-Botte et al. 1984). The results of other retrospective studies indicate that females mated on days 7–9 had reduced fertility relative to those mated prior to or after that interval (Ishii 1981; Leman et al. 1988; Tarocco 1989).

Endocrine Dysfunction. Repeat breeder females are common in commercial swine operations. Some of these females have regular ovarian cyclicity while failing to conceive at repeated matings, while others exhibit irregular estrous cycles (Karlberg et al. 1981). A minority of chronically infertile females that have estrous cycles at regular intervals are subsequently found to have urogenital infections (Karlberg et al. 1981). The majority of females failing to farrow show no evidence of urogenital infections (Karlberg et al. 1981) and either fail to conceive, returning to estrus at a regular interval, or fail to maintain pregnancy, returning at irregular intervals following breeding (Dial and MacLachlan 1988a). The inability to maintain pregnancy, especially during the summer months, has been attributed to insufficient progesterone levels (Wrathall et al. 1986). While remaining to be demonstrated, it is likely that endocrine dysfunction may also be a cause of the failure of pregnancy maintenance in the pig; there may be insufficient hypothalamo-hypophyseal support of the luteal progesterone synthesis to allow maintenance of pregnancy of some females, especially during the summer season.

Mycotoxicosis. Contamination of feed grains with the mycotoxins zearalenone and zearalenol results in a reproductive failure syndrome. Among the multiple manifestations of females fed zearalenone following mating are dramatically reduced farrowing rates with irregular returns to estrus following breeding (Chang et al. 1979; Long et al. 1983; Young and King 1986a,b). While females exposed to zearalenone during lactation had prolonged weaning-to-reserve intervals, subsequent fertility was not impaired when mated at the first postweaning estrus (Edwards et al. 1987). It appears that while zearalenol interferes with conception and disrupts normal ovarian cyclicity, it promotes artificial maintenance of corpora lutea for highly variable lengths of time (Long et al. 1982; Young and King 1986a,b). Zearalenol may also influence farrowing rate through its detrimental affects on sperm production and semen quality (Young and King 1986a,b). Thus, the estrogenic mycotoxins apparently cause reductions in conception rates, which may be manifested in prolonged, irregular returns to service. Other manifestations of zearalenol toxicosis include reduced litter sizes and delayed puberty (Chang et al. 1979; Long et al. 1982).

Preservice Intervals. The weaning-to-service interval and gilt entry-to-service interval are both highly related to NPD (Table 6.3). While over 85% of females on most commercial farms return to estrus within 7 days postweaning, nearly all farrowing females are weaned and accumulate several NPD as they await reservice. Since nearly all females accumulate a few NPD after weaning, weaning-to-service intervals are an important parameter affecting herd productivity. When one considers that the weaning-to-reserve interval also potentially affects a female's fertility (Leman et al. 1988), the interval takes on added importance. Similar to weaned females, all replacement gilts accumulate NPD after they are delivered into the herd. The average days from entry to first service typically exceeds 30 days (Table 6.3). Thus, it is not uncommon for replacement gilts to be a major source of NPD on some herds. In fact, the entry-to-first-service interval is often greater than one-third of the total NPD.

WEANING-TO-SERVICE INTERVAL. While there is only modest follicular development prior to weaning, the removal of piglets from the female at weaning causes an abrupt acceleration in follicular growth and a corresponding increased production of ovarian estrogens (Britt et al. 1985). This appears to be in response to the removal at weaning of inhibitory feedback influences that are present during lactation, resulting in increased pulsatile release of pituitary gonadotropins, particularly LH. Gradually increasing circulating levels of estradiol following weaning eventually precipitate the onset of estrus and trigger the preovulatory discharge of LH that initiates the ovulatory process. In most commercial herds, >85% of the females return to estrus <7 days following weaning (Hurtgen et al. 1980). However, several factors influence the ability of the female to return to estrus following weaning (Fig. 6.9).

Parity. Lower-parity females, especially primiparous females, have a longer mean interval from weaning to estrus and a lower proportion of females returning to estrus within 7 days following weaning than higher-parity females (Hurtgen et al. 1980; Britt et al. 1983). In herds that have uniform and low annual herd turnover (e.g., <35% females culled annually), the influence of parity on NPD may be minimal. However, the reduction in herd productivity due to delayed returns to estrus may be pronounced in herds with high culling and mortality rates and in herds recently populated with gilts (i.e., start-up herds).

Season. During the summer months, there is a decrease in the percentage of females returning to estrus within 7 days following weaning and an increase in the proportion of females remaining persistently anestrus (Hurtgen et al. 1980; Britt et al. 1983). A higher proportion of lower-parity females shows this seasonal delay in estrus return than higher-parity females. As with fertility, the seasonal retardation in returns to estrus appears to be more pronounced in females housed in com-

pletely enclosed buildings versus those housed in open-front buildings (Martinat-Botte et al. 1984).

Both photoperiod and ambient temperature change with season and, thus, potentially may independently or collectively mediate seasonal patterns in weaning-to-service intervals. The artificial supplementation of daylength with unchanging lighting has been found to increase the proportion of females mated by 5 days postweaning in one study (Stevenson et al. 1983), but had no influence in other investigations (Greenberg and Mahone 1982; Mabry et al. 1982a). Gradual increases in an artificial photoperiod reduced the proportion of females having cyclic estrous activity, whereas females on a gradually decreasing daylength had a higher proportion of cyclic estrous activity (Claus et al. 1984). These findings indicate that seasonal changes in the weaning-to-service intervals might be mediated, in part, by photoperiod, and that the female responds positively to gradual increases in daylength. The hot ambient temperatures of the summer months may also mediate seasonal influences on weaning-to-service intervals through direct effects on the hypothalamo-hypophyseal-ovarian axis. In fact, gilts exposed to high ambient temperatures have irregular estrous cycles (Edwards et al. 1968; Teague et al. 1968). Furthermore, females maintained in cooled buildings after weaning returned to estrus more quickly than those housed in naturally ventilated buildings (Kornegay and Thomas

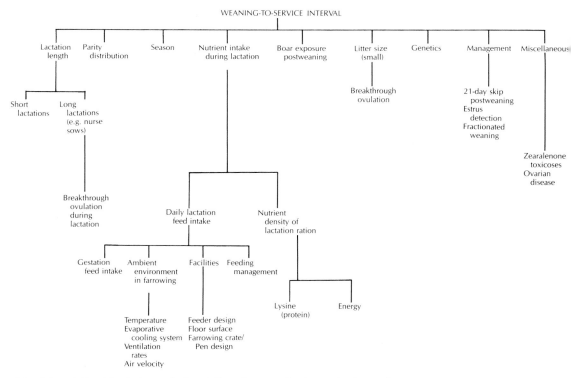

6.9. Interrelationships between factors influencing weaning-to-service interval.

1983). Effective environmental temperature during lactation also might affect weaning-to-reservice interval through effects on feed consumption. However, neither cool farrowing-room temperatures (Stansbury et al. 1987) or the use of drip cooling (McGlone et al. 1988) improved weaning-to-service intervals, even though female feed intakes, body weight and backfat losses, and litter weaning weights were heavier when females were cooled. Farrowing floor, which would be expected to affect conductive heat losses by the female, also had no influence on weaning-to-service interval, even though females housed on concrete lost less weight than those housed on plastic floors (McGlone et al. 1988).

Lactation Length. There is an inverse relationship between the length of time that a female is allowed to lactate and the interval between weaning and return to estrus (Self and Grummer 1958; Svajgr et al. 1974; Cole et al. 1975). The relationship is curvilinear (Cole et al. 1975) with increases in lactation length up to at least 6 weeks, resulting in shorter intervals from weaning to rebreeding. It has been estimated that for each 10-day reduction in lactation length, there is an increase of about 1 day in the weaning-to-conception interval (Clark and Leman 1986).

Because of differences in breeding day and gestation length, it is common for the females comprising a group to have lactation lengths that vary by several days, even though they are weaned on the same day. This may result in females that are weaned at shorter lactations than their groupmates subsequently having longer intervals from weaning to estrus and/or smaller subsequent litter sizes. There is a potential, therefore, that intervention to increase the mean and mode lactation length of farrowing groups will in many farms result in the improvement of litters farrowed annually by each female and, perhaps, pigs weaned/female/year. The average lactation length of a group of females can be increased by split-weaning the group; that is, weaning the older litters followed in a few days by weaning the younger litters in a group. Fractionated weaning, in which the heavier pigs in a litter are weaned followed in a few days by the weaning of the lighter pigs, will also decrease the return interval from weaning to estrus (Cox et al. 1983; Kunavongkrit et al. 1985). Prostaglandin-induced farrowing can be used to synchronize the onset of farrowing of a group of females, and thereby allows synchronous weaning and increased lactation lengths (Dial 1986).

Nutrition. It is well documented that feed and/or caloric intake during lactation is related to weaning-to-estrus interval (King 1987; Hughes 1989). Although the daily caloric intake that results in the shortest average weaning-to-estrus interval is not known, it appears that intakes of at least 16 megacalories (Mcal)/female/day is needed to minimize the prevalence of females having delayed postweaning returns to estrus (Reese et al. 1982). Protein intake during lactation has been suggested to influence the postweaning performance of females in an independent but additive fashion (Brendemuhl et al. 1987; King 1987). A greater proportion of females consuming relatively high levels of both energy and protein during lactation exhibit estrus within 8 days of weaning relative to females having lower intakes of either nutrient (King 1987). Thus, the approach to nutritional management of the female during lactation to optimize weaning-to-service interval is twofold: maintaining feed consumption and ensuring optimal ration formulation to ensure that daily intake during lactation meets daily nutrient needs.

Females having a lower daily caloric intake during lactation lose more weight and backfat than females fed at higher levels (Reese et al. 1982, 1984). However, when females were fed ad libitum during lactation, no relationship was observed between weaning-to-estrus interval and backfat, body condition scores, or heart girth (Esbenshade et al. 1986). Neither backfat at weaning or loss of backfat during lactation are accurate predictors of weaning-to-service intervals, even though both are related to reserve intervals (Johnston et al. 1989). Thus, body condition and back fat may not be consistently useful in predicting females that are destined to have delayed returns to estrus or in determining why females have failed to show estrus following weaning.

Daily caloric and feed intakes during lactation have been improved by increasing the energy density of the lactation diet, as through the addition of fat, and by stimulating increased feed consumption during lactation through environmental and facility management (McGlone et al. 1988), as discussed below. Other factors known to influence feed consumption during lactation include feeding practices, such as liquid versus dry feeding; availability of water; breed; parity; and gestational weight gain (Lynch 1989; Cole 1990). There is the potential that the design of the farrow crate feeder and stray voltage to farrowing crate, feeder, or waterer may interfere with feed consumption. Failure to frequently provide fresh feed in ad libitum amounts may restrict daily feed intake. Systemic diseases, such as bacteremia or toxemia, may also result in suboptimal feed intake during lactation.

Postweaning nutrition has a controversial influence on the weaning-to-estrus interval. Some studies report no influence of feed level or caloric intake on rebreeding interval of multiparous females (Brooks and Cole 1973; Brooks et al. 1975), while others have found that primiparous females fed higher levels had a shorter average interval to return (Brooks and Cole 1972; King and Williams 1984a,b).

Environment. During the summer when ambient temperatures are elevated, the weaning-to-estrus interval is increased. Similarly, lactating females exposed to elevated ambient temperatures (>30°C) have reduced intake, consume more feed, and lose less body weight and backfat relative to females housed at temperatures below the upper critical temperature for adult swine (25°C) (Stansbury et al. 1987). Females housed in airconditioned buildings have shorter weaning-to-estrus intervals than those housed in curtain-sided facilities (Kornegay and Thomas 1983). These observations suggest that variations in ambient temperature influence the ability of the female to return to estrus following weaning, and that high temperatures mediate their effects on postweaning reproductive performance through influences on feed consumption.

Feed consumption during lactation is inversely related to ambient temperature. Females decrease their feed intakes from 0.1 to 0.2 kg/day^{-1} for each 1°C increase in ambient temperature above thermoneutrality (18–22°C) (Lynch 1979). The detrimental effects of high ambient temperatures apparently can be partially alleviated by effective use of evaporative cooling of females during lactation, as through the use of drip sprinkling, which increases the feed intake and decreases weight loss during lactation (Stansbury et al. 1987; McGlone et al. 1988). Furthermore, females housed in farrowing crates having snout coolers in addition to drip coolers eat more feed and return to estrus in a shorter interval than females housed in crates without evaporative cooling or crates having only one of the cooling devices (McGlone et al. 1988). Effective evaporative cooling appears to be dependent not only upon water dripping on the skin of the back neck and back but also upon air moving with sufficient velocity across the skin surface to efficiently evaporate the dripped water. Thus, effective evaporative cooling appears to have two essential components: drip cooling and augmented air movement. It is estimated that the female and her litter needs at least 500 ft³/minute (cfm) during the hot summer months (Midwest Planning Service 1983) for feed consumption to be optimized and the occurrence of delayed returns to estrus following weaning and weaning weights of piglets optimized.

Lactating females housed on concrete floors consume more feed, lose less body weight, and wean heavier piglets than those housed on plastic-coated expanded metal floors (McGlone et al. 1988). Presumably, the superior conductive properties of materials such as concrete facilitate the dissipation of heat and may also increase the radiant heat losses by lactating females. Thus, facility design potentially influences conductive and radiant heat losses of the female as well as her evaporative losses. Water intake as well as feed consumption may be depressed at elevated ambient temperatures.

Genetics. There is a variation in the weaning-to-estrus interval between different purebreeds and between different crossbred lines (Fahmy et al. 1979; Maurer et al. 1985). Furthermore, some breeds have a higher proportion of females that remain persistently anestrus following weaning than others (Fahmy et al. 1979). The heritability of weaning-to-conception interval is low (h² = 0.24) (Irgang and Robinson 1984), indicating that genetic selection for shorter rebreeding intervals would be slow. The F1 crossbreed heterosis for reproductive traits are highly variable, with conception rates, litter size at 21 days of age, and 21-day litter weights being highest (Johnson 1981a).

ENTRY-TO-SERVICE INTERVAL. The interval between the addition of a replacement gilt to a herd and conception is often prolonged in many commercial herds. This may be the result of endocrine dysfunction, as when gilts experience delayed puberty, or may be intentional, as when herd replacements are inventoried into the herd but purposely are not mated for variable lengths of time. Increasing the age at first conception (Omtvedt et al. 1965) or the number of estrous cycles prior to conception (Pay and Davies 1973; MacPherson et al. 1977; Archibong et al. 1987; Vermeer and Slijkhuis 1989) is associated with increased litter size at the first farrowing. Age at farrowing affects total-born litter size of gilts inseminated at their first pubertal estrus, but had no influence on the litter size of gilts inseminated at their second estrus (Vermeer and Slijkhuis 1989). In terms of litter size, there appears to be no added advantage for breeding gilts at ages greater than approximately 210–220 days (Clark et al. 1988; Vermeer and Slijkhuis 1989). In one study, age at mating influenced farrowing rate (Pay and Davies 1973), whereas another investigation failed to show that farrowing rate improved with advancing age (Leman et al. 1988). To take advantage of these potential benefits, producers often intentionally delay mating gilts until they reach optimal chronological and/or physiological age or until they surpass a threshold weight.

Typically, gilts are included in the herd inventory prior to service and, therefore, accumulate NPD. Because of the per diem costs of maintaining gilts in the breeding herd, producers attempt to offset a gilt's NPD while optimizing the potential gains in reproductive performance offered by delayed service. Nonetheless, early puberty allows producers the opportunity to take advantage of the benefits of physiological maturation on subsequent litter size and allows earlier service of gilts. Boar exposure, age, and genetics appear to be the most important factors limiting age at puberty; however, climatic environment (including season, temperature, and photoperiod), housing, nutrition, and various management factors may also influence age at puberty and, thus, time after entry of first service (Fig. 6.10) (Dial et al. 1986; Dyck 1988). It should be remembered that because of the high annualized turnover rate of breeding stock on most confinement swine farms, often between 45–60%, the gilt typically comprises the largest parity group. Thus, the gilt usually has the greatest effect of any parity on herd reproductive performance.

Boar Exposure. The most important stimulus for initiating the onset of puberty in gilts appears to be boar exposure. Stimuli from the boar precipitate the pubertal onset of estrous and ovarian activity after gilts reach a threshold age (Brooks and Cole 1969, 1970; Hughes and Cole 1976; Thompson and Savage 1978). Olfactory stimuli such as the pheromones present in the boar's salivary and genitourinary secretions are the most important sensory cues for puberty initiation (Kirkwood et al. 1983; Pearce et al. 1988), but other sensory stimuli such as visual, tactile, and auditory cues and relocation contribute in a small but additive fashion to the precipitation of puberty (Bourn et al. 1974; Zimmerman et al. 1974; Hughes 1982; Eastham and Cole 1987). While boars as young as 8–9 months of age are effective in inducing puberty (Zimmerman et al. 1986), there appears to be a beneficial effect of using boars at least 11 months of age to induce puberty (Kirkwood and Hughes 1980, 1981). Libido may be an important determinant of interval from first boar exposure to puberty, if the boar is used to detect heat. However, pheromone production, not libido, is the more important factor if the boar is used only for sensory stimuli, and estrus is determined by human observation. Gilts being checked for estrus should not be housed continuously next to a boar for they may be in a period of refractoriness, having been receptive to the boar within the previous few hours (Hemsworth et al. 1987, 1988).

Gilts gradually become habituated to continuous exposure to the same boar during rearing (Kirkwood and Hughes 1980), indicating that boars used to induce puberty should be rotated periodically. The provision of novel boar exposure improves the mean interval from boar exposure to estrus and the proportion of gilts reaching puberty by 210 days of age (Brooks and Cole 1970). Exposure to many different boars also decreases interval from first exposure to estrus (Brooks and Cole 1970). At least 10–15 minutes of daily boar exposure is needed to minimize the mean age of puberty (Kirkwood and Hughes 1980; Caton et al. 1986). Relative to age of first observed estrus, there is no added advantage of exposing gilts continuously to boars beyond that obtained with 10–15 minutes of daily exposure (Caton et al. 1986). In fact, gilts become habituated more quickly when housed continuously with a boar (Hemsworth et al. 1988), and because they only show estrus intensely for brief periods of approximately 7–10 minutes, estrus may be more difficult to detect (Levis 1988). Gilts exposed each day of the week until first estrus have a shorter interval from initial exposure to puberty and a higher proportion responding than those exposed for 10 consecutive days or those exposed five times per week or less prior to puberty (Paterson et al. 1989a,b).

To optimize estrous synchrony, gilts either should be provided with continuous fenceline contact with mature boars that are rotated or should be exposed for at least 15 minutes per day to different mature boars. The initiation of continuous boar exposure can be supplemented with pen relocation to facilitate the synchronous onset of puberty by gilts. When gilts are to be bred, continuous boar exposure must be discontinued for gilts to reliably show heat in response to the boar. Gilts commonly show intense estrus, allowing boars to mount for periods of about 7 minutes, and fe-

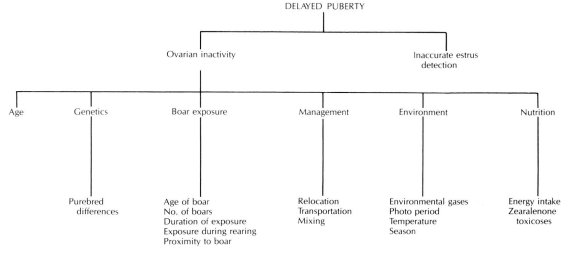

6.10. Interrelationships between factors influencing entry-to-service interval.

males may be highly receptive to the boar for approximately 10 minutes. After these short bouts of lordosis, females enter an extended period of 1–2 hours when they are unable to respond to the boar with estrus or may show only a weak response. Thus, when the ages of puberty are to be accurately determined, gilts should be distantly segregated from all sensory contact with the boar, preferably in a different room or barn or pen. At estrous determinations, gilts can be moved individually or in small groups of less than six gilts to pens next to boars or to pens containing a boar.

Age. The age at which gilts are initially exposed to a boar influences both the rapidity and the synchrony of the gilt's response to initial boar exposure (Kirkwood and Hughes 1979). The presence of a mature boar during rearing apparently has little effect on the time from boar introduction to puberty or the mean age of puberty, although it does improve mating rate (Hemsworth et al. 1982). Providing gilts with exposure to mature boars at approximately 150–165 days stimulates gilts to reach puberty at the shortest interval following boar exposure, the youngest age, and with the highest synchrony (Brooks and Cole 1972; Kirkwood and Hughes 1979). Exposure of gilts at older ages may lead to a less synchronous response, as some gilts begin cycling spontaneously. Exposing gilts at younger ages allows gilts to become acclimated to the boar and may result in retarded puberty. Both situations result in additional NPD and hinder the ability of the producer to integrate new additions into breeding groups in the herd. The number of females bred into each group may not reach targets, and consequently, facility utilization may be compromised.

Genetics. Some purebreds reach puberty earlier than others (Christenson and Ford 1979; Allrich et al. 1985), as do some crossbreds. The heterosis of age at puberty is low (Quintana and Robison 1983).

Relocation. Although results have been inconsistent, transport or periodic relocation of gilts to a different pen at the time of boar exposure moderately improves the synchrony and age of first estrus and the proportion of gilts showing estrus over those kept in the same pen with or without boar exposure (Bourn et al. 1974; Zimmerman et al. 1974; Eastham and Cole 1987).

Rearing Environment. Both social and facility/environmental factors to which gilts are exposed during the maturation phase influence their subsequent reproductive performance. Groups of gilts reared in the presence of mature boars show a stronger first estrus and have a higher proportion of females mated than groups reared in isolation from boars (Hemsworth et al. 1982). When given approximately 0.76–1.14 m²/pig from 4–5

months of age, gilts reared in groups of three or less have a delayed onset of puberty relative to gilts raised in larger groups (Christenson and Hruska 1984). Group size up to at least 30 gilts per pen during rearing apparently has no effect on age at puberty (Christianson and Ford 1979; Christianson and Hruska 1984; Barnett et al. 1986). As long as gilts are given floor space allowance meeting or exceeding that recommended by the Midwest Planning Service (1983) for market hogs, it appears that there is little effect on age at puberty (Ford and Teague 1978). Gilts reared in confinement tend to reach puberty at the same age as those raised outside (Christenson 1981; Rampacek et al. 1981).

Season. As with the female and the boar, there is seasonal variation in the reproductive activity and efficiency of the replacement gilt (Dial 1984). Gilts born during the fall reach puberty earlier and with more synchrony than those born during the spring (Mavrogenis and Robinson 1976; Christenson 1981). Both photoperiod (Dieckman and Hoagland 1983; Diekman and Grieger 1988) and ambient temperature (Flowers et al. 1989) influence age at puberty and, therefore, may mediate seasonal patterns in puberty.

Estrous Detection. The entry-to-service interval is not only influenced by the ability to initiate puberty soon after a gilt arrives in a herd but also by the capacity of the producer to detect estrus. Housing gilts across an aisle approximately 1 m from a boar allows more effective estrous detection than housing gilts in a pen adjacent to a boar (Hemsworth et al. 1984). Additionally, there is a higher percentage of gilts detected in estrus when gilts are housed in 1.9 m² or greater than when housed in 0.95 m² (Hemsworth et al. 1986). In general, group size apparently has no influence on the percentage of gilts detected in estrus as long as there are less than 8 gilts per pen (Christenson and Ford 1979; Christenson and Hruska 1984; Barnett et al. 1986). However, estrous detection is usually problematic in small groups of 2–3 gilts and may be particularly ineffective in groups greater than 30 (Mavrogenis and Robison 1976; Christenson and Hruska 1984). A higher proportion of gilts will be detected in estrus and mated when gilts and a heat-check boar are moved to a mating pen than when breeding is done in either the gilts' or boar's pen (Hemsworth et al. 1984, 1989). Periodic movement of gilts to different pens in combination with exposure to a novel boar will increase the proportion showing estrus (Eastham and Cole 1987).

Removal Intervals. All females inventoried in a herd accumulate NPD prior to being removed from the herd, either by culling or after death. NPD associated with either culling or mortality occur with a minority of gilts after they enter the herd and some females after they are weaned. Both gilts and females accumulate NPD associated with removal after being served and after being detected nonpregnant. Since female mortality rates are low on most commercial farms, typically <4%, most intervals relating to mortality are not significantly related to NPD (Table 6.3). In fact, only the entry-to-death interval of gilts has been found to contribute significantly to NPD. Three culling intervals contribute significantly to NPD. The weaning-to-cull interval is highly related to NPD (P<.0001), and the service-to-cull and entry-to-cull intervals are significantly, but lowly (P = 0.05), related to NPD. No other culling intervals contribute significantly to NPD.

Annual culling rates on commercial swine farms commonly range from 25% to 40%, and often exceed 50% on some farms (Svendson et al. 1975b). Reasons for culling females are numerous and include both voluntary removal, where the producer elects to remove females from a herd, and involuntary removal, where the producer removes females that are incapable of reproducing. In intensively managed confinement operations, the number of females culled involuntarily for reasons such as infertility, anestrus, and health problems are typically greater than the number culled voluntarily for reasons such as small litter sizes, abortion, temperament, and old age (Svendson et al. 1975b; Dagorn and Aumaitre 1979). There are numerous causes for the prolonged intervals between when a female fails in health or fails to reproduce and when she is actually removed by involuntary culling from a herd: lack of early acknowledgment of reproductive or health failure, failure to establish and/or follow guidelines for deciding when to cull a female, waiting for clinical improvement in females having a medical problem, inadvertent culling of potentially productive females. In most cases, NPD can be minimized, but not eliminated, when females are culled voluntarily if producers follow strict guidelines for when to cull following weaning or service. However, it is difficult to limit the number of NPD in herds where involuntary culling dominates. The culling intervals include intervals from entry, weaning, service, and detected open to female death (Table 6.3).

In a recent prospective study of female mortality, the major causes of mortality were, in order, cardiac failure, gastrointestinal problems, uterine problems, cystitis/pyelonephritis, respiratory disease, and downer female syndrome (Chagnon et al. 1990). In herds having high annualized mortality rates (<7%), there is a potential for mortality intervals to significantly influence NPD, even though mortality intervals do not have a significant influence on NPD in most herds. Strategies to improve NPD should, in these cases, place an initial emphasis on developing an understanding of the primary causes of mortality, and then on determining the risk factors predisposing females to health problems.

Pigs Weaned/Litter

THE TOTAL NUMBER of pigs born/litter sets the upper limit for pigs weaned/litter, while preweaning mortality and peripartum deaths dictate the lower extreme (Fig. 6.3). By convention, the total number of piglets born/litter reflects the number of piglets born alive plus the number of stillborn and mummified fetuses. Improvements in the average number of pigs weaned/litter can theoretically be made by increasing the total-born litter size, reducing the proportions of stillbirths and mummies, or improving the number of piglets born alive that survive until weaning. In fact, the total-born litter size, stillbirth rate, and percent preweaning mortality, but not mummy rate, have been found to be significantly associated with pigs weaned/female/year (Polson et al. 1990a).

LIVE-BORN/LITTER.
The causes and risk factors associated with reduced total-born litter size are different, in most cases, from those affecting live-born litter size. While live-born litter size is significantly related to pigs weaned/litter (Fig. 6.3) (Polson et al. 1990a), suboptimal live-born litter size reflects total-born litter size, stillbirth rates, and percent mummies.

Total Pigs Born/Litter.   Many, but not all, of the factors influencing fertility have similar effects on total-born litter size. Improvements in fertility, as commonly estimated using farrowing rate, may be accompanied by increased fecundity. Nonetheless, it should be remembered that clinical problems of reduced litter size will often require the examination of a set of factors (Fig. 6.11) that is distinctly different from those evaluated when other measures of reproductive performance are suboptimal.

Parity.   As with many other reproductive parameters, parity also influences litter size. The results of numerous studies have indicated that litter size is usually smallest at the first parity, rises to a maximum between the third and sixth to seventh parity, and then remains constant or declines slightly with additional parity increases (Clark and Leman 1986; Yen et al. 1987; Clark et al.

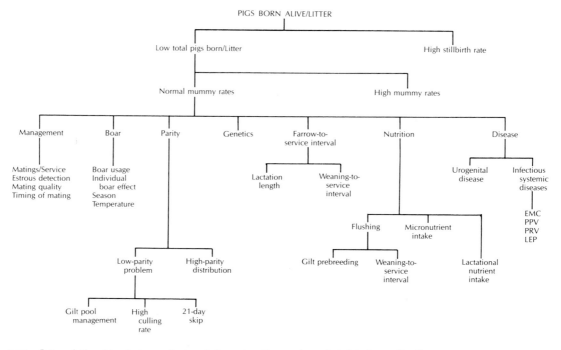

6.11.   Interrelationships between factors influencing the number of piglets born alive/litter. EMC = encephalomyocarditis; PPV = porcine parvovirus; PRV = pseudorabies virus; LEP = leptospirosis.

1988). Increases in the number of intrapartum deaths (stillbirths) commonly occur at higher parities, especially at the fifth or greater parities. One study has indicated that age of the dam rather than parity is associated with litter size (French et al. 1979). As exemplified in Figure 6.12, reductions in pigs weaned/litter in older parity sows may be associated with reduced total-born litter size and increased stillbirth rates with no measurable change in percent preweaning mortality.

Herd parity distributions that are skewed toward the herd being composed of a relatively high proportion of low-parity females, often have suboptimal mean litter sizes. On the other hand, mature female herds, in which there is a high proportion of advanced-parity females (Fig. 6.13), frequently have reduced litter sizes, which may be attributed to either a reduction in the total pigs born or to an increased rate of peripartum deaths. The relationship between parity and litter size is likely to vary with genetic line. Further, there is a large variation, even within the same genetic line, in the parity–litter size relationship (Hilley et al. 1986b). Thus, improvements in herd litter sizes through the manipulation of parity distribution will necessitate a farm-by-farm analysis of the relationship between parity and litter size. That is, the ideal parity distribution that optimizes litter size on one farm, with one type of facilities and husbandry skills, may vary from that of another farm.

Farrowing-to-Conception Interval. The two components of farrowing-to-conception interval, lactation length and weaning-to-service interval, have been found to influence the litter size that females have at subsequent farrowings. There is a negative relationship between lactation length and rebreeding interval, and length of lactation is related positively to litter size (Self and Grummer 1958; Svajgr et al. 1974; Cole et al. 1975; Walker et al. 1979). That is, reductions in weaning age from approximately 6 weeks are accompanied by concomitant litter size reductions. As demonstrated by the curvilinear relationship between lactation length and litter size (Fig. 6.14), reductions in litter size become progressively more pronounced at lactations of less than 4 weeks. It has been estimated that there is a reduction of 0.1 pig/day for each 1-day decrease in lactation length below 28 days (Clark and Leman 1986).

The cause of the reduced litter sizes that accompany short lactations is not clear. Ovulation rate is not influenced by previous lactation length (Varley and Cole 1976a,b). The number of embryos surviving until implantation is insignificantly reduced as lactation length is decreased; whereas there is a significant reduction in the number of embryos present at 3 weeks postbreeding with decreases in lactation length (Varley and Cole 1976a,b, 1978). In sum, these studies suggest that while preimplantation losses and perhaps fertilization failure contribute to the reduced litter

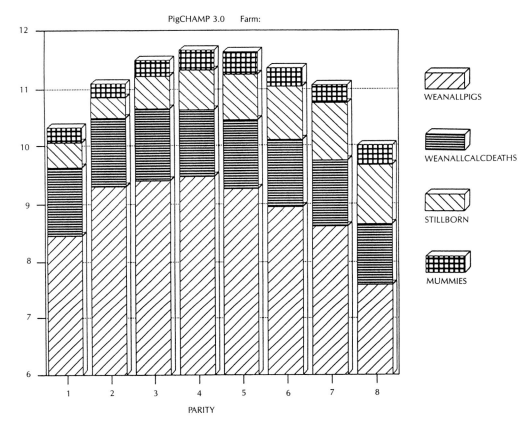

6.12. Parity-related changes in average number of pigs weaned/litter (WEANALLPIGS), percent preweaning mortality (WEANALLCALCDEATHS), percent stillborn piglets (STILLBORN), and percent mummified piglets (MUMMIES) in an 850-female commercial herd using PigCHAMP. There were from 94 females (parity 8) to 1554 females (parity 1) at each data point.

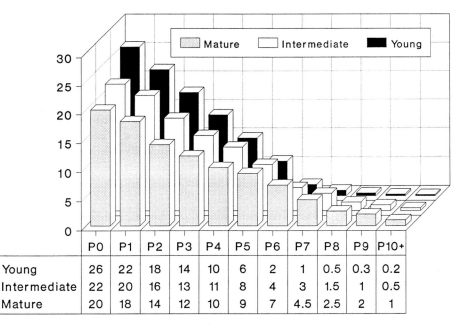

	P0	P1	P2	P3	P4	P5	P6	P7	P8	P9	P10+
Young	26	22	18	14	10	6	2	1	0.5	0.3	0.2
Intermediate	22	20	16	13	11	8	4	3	1.5	1	0.5
Mature	20	18	14	12	10	9	7	4.5	2.5	2	1

6.13. Schematic demonstration of parity distributions for young, intermediate, and mature herds.

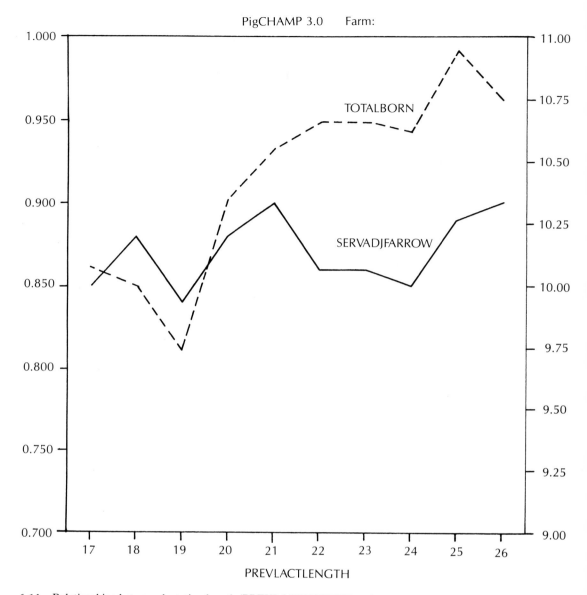

6.14. Relationships between lactation length (PREVLACTLENGTH) and subsequent adjusted farrowing rate (SERVADJFAR) and between lactation length and subsequent total-born litter size (TOTALBORN) in a 1150-female commercial herd using PigCHAMP. There are at least 194 farrowings represented at each data point.

sizes associated with short lactations, litter size reductions may be more attributable to embryonic mortality around the time of implantation.

As mentioned previously, several studies have shown that weaning-to-estrus interval influences fertility (Ishii 1981; Leman et al. 1988; Tarocco 1989); however, its influence on litter size remains less clear. One study demonstrated that reservice interval had no affect on subsequent litter size (Kosztolich and Mayrhofer 1983). In another study, females not mated at their initial postweaning estrus had larger total-born and live-born litter sizes at their subsequent farrowings than those mated at their first postweaning estrus (Morrow et al. 1989).

Breeding Management. Optimal fertilization rates occur when gilts are inseminated 12 hours prior to ovulation (Dziuk 1970). As indicated earlier, the interval between onset of estrus and ovulation is not consistent between females. Further, there are no outward indications and no practical means for routinely determining when females ovulate. Consequently, multiple matings per estrus have been used to optimize the chance that fertile sperm are deposited when optimal fertilization rates and, subsequently, litter sizes and conception rates will occur. Similar to conception rates, litter sizes increase when females are bred twice per estrus, rather than once (Rasbech 1969; Eleftheriou 1980; Liptrap et al. 1983; O'Grady et al. 1983; Hilley et al. 1986a; Clark et al. 1988). In addition, females mated three times per estrus at 24-hour intervals had larger litters than those mated twice (Tilton and Cole 1982). The litter size of females mated three times within 2 days did not differ significantly from females mated twice within 2 days (Tilton and Cole 1982). Results from artificial insemination apparently mirror those of natural matings. Females mated artificially three times had a higher number of pigs born than those inseminated twice (Reed 1982). There appears to be a farm-to-farm variation in the influence that number of matings per estrus has on litter size. On some farms, there is no difference in the litter sizes of females mated once, twice, or three times during an estrus; on others, there is an advantage of multiple matings over single matings (Hilley et al. 1986a,b; Clark and Leman 1987).

When attempts are made to increase litter size through manipulations of matings per estrus, it is not always possible with some genetic lines to get a majority of females mated on 3 consecutive days. Furthermore, multiple matings per day cannot be instituted on some farms because of labor constraints or insufficient boar inventories. Thus, while potentially useful on some commercial operations, increasing the number of matings per estrus either may not be effective or may not be applicable on others.

As with conception rate, there is a controversial influence of type of service on litter size. One study indicated that litter size is greater with heterospermic than homospermic matings (Thorton 1987); others found no advantage for cross-mating (Pacova and Dupal 1980; Liptrap 1983; Hilley et al. 1986c). Since there are no reports indicating that homospermic matings result in larger litters than heterospermic, it may be advisable to utilize cross-mating programs on commercial farms, unless breeding records are being used to evaluate the relative fertilities of boars.

Boar usage appears to have similar influence on litter size as on conception rate. However, there appears to be no influence of boar usage on litter size when boars are used six times or less per week (Hemsworth et al. 1983; Leman et al. 1984). In fact, one retrospective study has demonstrated that litter size remains constant up to eight matings per week before being detrimentally affected (Leman et al. 1984). It has been suggested that litter size is less sensitive to boar overuse than farrowing rate (Leman et al. 1984).

Boar Influence. Numerous studies have demonstrated that boars influence the total number of pigs born, the number of pigs born alive, and/or the number of pigs weaned (Rahnefeld and Sweistra 1970; Singleton and Shelby 1972; Uzu 1979); others have reported no influence of the boar on fecundity (Egbunike 1982). It has also been suggested that differences in litter size are associated with differences in semen quality (Rahnefeld and Sweistra 1970). Perhaps, some boars have ejaculates with higher frequencies of defective sperm than others and, consequently, are associated with increased rates of embryonic mortality. Although not yet demonstrated, it cannot be ruled out that qualitative differences in sperm production also contribute to differences in litter size. Also, chromosomal aberrations of the boar have been found to substantially reduce litter size (Willeke and Richter 1980).

Infectious Reproductive Diseases. Reproductive pathogens that commonly affect litter size include porcine parvovirus, pseudorabies virus, leptospira, and occasionally, enterovirus (Thacker and Gonzalez 1988). Depending upon gestational stage of infection, prenatal exposure to pathogens of the fetus or the placenta can manifest as decreases in total pigs born, with or without increased mummies. Increases in intrapartum deaths and higher prevalence of weak pigs can cause further decreases in the number of live-born pigs.

Genetics. Litter size potential can be improved by either genetic selection or by using crossbreeding heterosis. The heritability of litter size is low (approximately $h^2 = 0.1$) (Strang and King 1970), and selection experiments generally have not been very successful in improving litter size (Bichard and David 1986). Nonetheless, it has been suggested that genetic selection at the commercial farm level should improve litter size at a small but significant rate of approximately 1–3% of the mean, annually (Bichard and David 1986).

There are considerable variations in the prolificacy between purebreds and among crossbred lines (Quintana and Robison 1983). As with other reproductive traits, crossbreeding has been used to improve the fecundity of commercial swine. The heterosis resulting from crossbreeding varies with the crossbreeding program used (e.g., 3-breed rotation, 4-way terminal, etc.) and also with the breeds used in making the cross (Quintana and Robison 1983). The average maternal heterosis for litter size at birth is approximately 2.4%, which relates to an improvement of about 0.23 pig per litter (Johnson 1981a). There appears to be no improvement in litter size by using crossbred over purebred boars (Buchanan 1987).

Maternal effects or rearing environment of gilts appears to affect future fecundity. Gilts reared in small litters (6 piglets) had larger litter sizes (0.5–1.0 piglet) than those reared in normally sized or larger litters (12 piglets) (Nelson and Robison 1976; Rutledge 1980). These improvements in litter size with smaller litters are associated with increased embryonic/fetal survival, not with enhanced ovulation rate (Martin and Crenshaw 1989).

Nutrition. The nutrition of the female can potentially influence litter size through feed or nutrient intake either during lactation or prior to service of both the gilt and the weaned female.

The influence of calory and feed intake during lactation on the weaning-to-service interval of females, especially primiparous females, has been well documented, but the effects on subsequent litter size remain less consistent. Females fed ad libitum high-energy rations (3729 kcal/kg) during lactation had greater litter sizes at the subsequent farrowing than those given lower energy diets (3774 kcal/kg) (Kirkwood et al. 1988). Voluntary female feed intake during lactation is related to subsequent litter size as well as weaning-to-estrus interval (O'Grady et al. 1985; Lynch and Kearney 1987). Lactation nutrition has been suggested to influence embryonic mortality but not ovulation rate (Kirkwood and Thacker 1988). Although lactation calorie intake affected subsequent litter size, subsequent weaning-to-service interval and farrowing rate were not affected (Kirkwood et al. 1988). However, several studies have reported that the weaning-to-service interval was affected by lactation nutrition (Reese et al. 1982; King and Williams 1984a,b; Shurson et al. 1986), with no effect on ovulation rate, embryonic mortality, or litter size at the subsequent farrowing.

Primiparous females fed at a high rate (>3.5 kg/day) during the interval between weaning and remating had higher ovulation rates and greater litter sizes than those fed lower amounts of feed (<2.0 kg/day) (Brooks and Cole 1972; King and Williams 1984a,b). There appears to be no influence of rebreeding feed level on the litter sizes of multiparous females (Brooks et al. 1975).

The influence of dietary energy intake during the prepubertal growth period and prior to breeding has been well reviewed (Den Hartog and Van Kempen 1980). It appears that increasing energy intake during rearing or prior to breeding (flushing) does not consistently improve litter size, since increases in ovulation rate are accompanied by increased embryonic mortality. A program of high-energy feeding followed consecutively by periods of low-energy and high-energy intakes, called a high:low:high flush, may result in a greater number of ovulations than observed with high:high:high or low:low:low flush programs (Den Hartog and Van Kempen 1980). To accomplish a high:low:high flush, gilts on ad libitum feed can be brought from the finishing floor (maturation phase) into the prebreeding phase and held for several weeks on a restricted energy intake of less than 2.7kg/day. Gilts are then allowed ad libitum feed intakes for at least 10–14 days prior to being bred, the switch often being made

as the gilts are moved into the breeding phase. Following flushing, feed level and caloric intake should be reduced to reduce the chance of increased embryonic mortality.

Several micronutrients have been suggested to influence total-born litter size. Injection, but not oral administration, of retinol (vitamin A) and/or beta-carotene (vitamin A precursor) to gilts fed deficient diets resulted in improved litter size (Brief and Chew 1985). The addition of supplemental folic acid to the diets of weaned females resulted in increased litter sizes, associated with reduced embryonic mortality, in females that had been flushed to increase ovulation rates (Tremblay et al. 1989). Similarly, pregnant and lactating females fed supplemental folic acid showed improvements in both litter size and in farrowing rates (Lindemann and Kornegay 1987). As reviewed previously, the supplementation of corn/soybean meal rations with biotin (Kornegay 1986) and with choline (Miller and Kornegay 1983) improves litter size as well as conception rate. An influence of the trace minerals zinc, manganese, copper, and iodine on litter size and embryonic mortality has also been suggested (Kirkwood and Thacker 1988).

Mycotoxins. The reproductive manifestations of mycotoxicoses in swine vary with the stage of reproductive cycle in which females are exposed. When gilts are exposed to zearalenone during early pregnancy, all or part of the litter may be killed, resulting in failure to farrow or reduced litter size, respectively (Chang et al. 1979; Long et al. 1982).

Season. In contrast to other manifestations of season, there is considerable controversy over the influence of season on litter size. Seasonal variations in total pigs born and/or live-born pigs have been observed (Tomes and Nielson 1979; Doboa et al. 1983; Martinat-Botte et al. 1984), but not in others (Kennedy and Moxley 1978; Paterson et al. 1978; Hilley et al. 1986b; Von Lutter and Huhn 1980). When seasonal fluctuations in litter size occur, decreases not only have been observed during the summer months, but also have been noted during other seasons (Tomes and Nielson 1979; Von Keindorf and Plescher 1981; Hilley et al. 1986a). Seasonal changes in litter size occur with females mated artificially, as well as those mated naturally. It appears that, as with other manifestations of swine seasonality, there is a farm-to-farm variation in the influence of season on litter size.

Ambient Temperature. High ambient temperatures (>23°C) can potentially have multiple influences on the female. Besides its detrimental effects on estrous cyclicity and on conception rates (Edwards et al. 1968; Teague et al. 1968), it may also affect litter size (Warnick et al. 1965;

Tompkins et al. 1967; Edwards et al. 1968; Omtvedt et al. 1968; Teague et al. 1968). Some studies have demonstrated that elevated temperatures significantly decrease ovulation rate (Teague et al. 1968; D'Arce et al. 1970), while others revealed no effect (Warnick et al. 1965; Tompkins et al. 1967). Increased embryonic mortality was observed when females were exposed within the first 3 weeks of pregnancy (Warnick et al. 1965; Tompkins et al. 1967; Edwards et al. 1968; Teague et al. 1968), but no effect of temperature was noted during mid- to late gestation (Omtvedt et al. 1968). Peak litter size reductions appeared to occur when temperatures were elevated around the time of conception and near the time of implantation (Tompkins et al. 1967; Edwards et al. 1968; Omtvedt et al. 1968). High temperatures near the onset of farrowing caused a decrease in the number of pigs born alive, and was also associated with decreased postnatal survival (Omtvedt et al. 1968).

Stillbirths. As with live-born litter size, the number of stillbirths per litter is related significantly to pigs weaned/female/year. Stillbirths have been suggested to be the second most costly condition behind pneumonia and ahead of the various causes of preweaning mortality (Miller and Dorn 1987). Stillbirths followed by crushing mortality, starvation, and weak pigs are the major causes of mortality in pigs (Grondalen et al. 1986; Dyck and Sweistra 1987).

Stillborn piglets are those piglets that are alive at the initiation of farrowing but die intrapartum. In the absence of obvious autolytic changes, piglets that die antepartum are also commonly determined by producers as being stillborn. Similarly, piglets classified by producers at birth as being stillborn often have died following delivery. Studies in which piglets classified as being stillborn were examined pathologically to ascertain cause of death have demonstrated that producers are relatively unable to discriminate piglets found dead around farrowing as being stillborn or as dying after farrowing (Vaillancourt and Martineau 1988). In fact, categorization of dead piglets as stillborn and postmortem results varies considerably among producers, the percentage of misclassification may be as high as 40% on some farms (Vaillancourt and Martineau 1988). Misclassification rates of 2–20% have been observed in one study (Vaillancourt 1990) and 12% in another study (Randall and Penny 1968). Preweaning mortality and stillbirth rates are correlated positively (Friendship et al. 1986), indicating, perhaps, that across farms producers are unable to differentiate stillborn pigs from postnatal deaths.

Because misclassifications of stillborn piglets are common, the first step in investigating a herd problem of elevated stillbirth rates is to determine the percentage of stillborn piglets that, in-stead of dying intrapartum, actually died either prior to the initiation of parturition or died after delivery. Once this is done, the proportions of prepartum and postpartum deaths incorrectly classified should be subtracted from the total number of piglets determined as being stillborn. Elevations in prepartum and postpartum deaths should be treated as elevations in mummy and preweaning mortality rates, respectively. When stillbirth rates exceed established interference levels (Table 6.4), there are several risk factors to consider (Fig. 6.15).

Female, Pig, and Litter Factors. Across studies it appears that, in general, as total-born litter size increases with advancing parities up to approximately parities 5–7, the proportion of piglets stillborn similarly increases, such that smallest live-born litter sizes are observed at low (1, 2) and advanced parities (>6), and highest live-born litter sizes are found at the midparities (3–5) (Adilovic and Gvozdenovic 1984; Badouard et al. 1984; Schoeps and Huhn 1986; Blackwell 1987; Fonseca et al. 1988; Petherick and Blackshaw 1989). The proportion of stillborn piglets increases linearly with parity from parity 1 to greater than parity 8 (Bille et al. 1974a; Petherick and Blackshaw 1989). Parity-associated increases in stillbirth are due, at least in part, to the increased durations of farrowing and placental expulsion with advancing parity (Kaczmarczyk et al. 1987). There appears to be some repetition of stillbirths at consecutive farrowings, since females previously having stillbirths are more likely to have elevations in stillbirth rates than those not previously having stillbirths (Blackwell 1987).

Increased litter size is associated with decreased birth weights and increases in stillbirth and mummy rates (Spicer et al. 1986). Live-born litter size is correlated (r = 0.31) with incidence of stillbirths (Horugel et al. 1986). Both small and large litters appear to have a higher stillbirth rates than normal-sized litters, as demonstrated by the observation that stillbirth rates declined gradually from small litters (2 piglets) to litters numbering approximately 9 piglets, then increased gradually to 16 piglets/litter (Stolic 1987). It appears that females having greater than 12 piglets are more likely to have a higher incidence of stillbirths than those having fewer piglets (Chhabra et al. 1983; Blackwell 1987). In fact, stillbirth rates were increased from 54 to 68% in females farrowing 12 piglets or more (Bae and Park 1985).

The number of stillborn piglets is inversely related (r = −0.24) to piglet birth weight (Vidovic et al. 1986). The proportion of stillborn piglets decreases as piglet birth weight increases up to 1 kg and remains relatively stable at higher weights (Edwards et al. 1986). Increases in the variability of piglet birth weight within a litter are associated with an increase in the percentages of stillbirths

Table 6.4. Targets for the biological performance of the breeding herd

Biological Performance	Target
Breeding	
% females bred by <7 days postweaning	> 88.0
% multiple matings	> 90.0
Farrowing rate	> 85.0
% regular returns	< 6.0
% irregular returns	< 3.0
% negative preg test	< 3.0
% abortions	< 0.5
% found not pregnant	< 1.5
% fail-to-farrow	< 1.0
Adjusted farrowing rate	> 92.0
Farrowing	
Total pigs born/litter	> 11.5
Pigs born alive/litter	> 10.5
Mummies	
%	< 1.5
No./litter	< 0.2
Stillbirths	
%	< 7.0
No./litter	< 0.8
Birth weight	
litter, kg	> 16.0
piglet, kg	> 1.5
Weaning	
Number pigs weaned/female farrowed	> 9.5
Number pigs weaned/litter weaned	> 10.0
% total-born weaned	> 83.5
% born-alive weaned (% preweaning mortality)	> 92.0
Trauma deaths	
%	35
No.	0.35
Low viability deaths	
%	20
No.	0.20
Starvation deaths	
%	15
No.	0.15
Diarrhea deaths	
%	10
No.	0.10
Disease deaths	
%	5
No.	0.05
Congenital anomalies	
%	5
No.	0.05
Other deaths	
%	10
No.	0.10
Adjusted 21-day litter weight	> 60.0
Average piglet weaning weight at 21 days, kg	> 6.0
Female Utilization	
Litters/inventoried female/year	
3-week lactation	> 2.35
4-week lactation	> 2.25
Pigs weaned/inventoried female/year	> 21.5
Pigs weaned/bred female/year	> 23.5
Farrowing interval	
3-week lactation	<147.0
4-week lactation	<154.0
Nonproductive days	
%	< 12.0
Days	< 45.0
Entry-to-service interval	< 30.0
Weaning-to-service interval	< 7.0
Weaning-to-cull interval	< 14.0
Service-to-detected open interval	< 50.0
Population Characteristics	
Average gilt pool inventory	
% replacement rate	< 40.0
% culling rate	< 35.0
% mortality	< 5.0
Average parity	> 3.0
Female:boar ratio	> 25:1

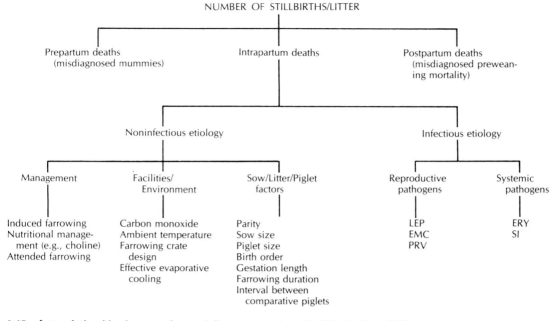

6.15. Interrelationships between factors influencing number of stillbirths/litter. LEP = leptosporosis; EMC = encephalomyocarditis; PRV = pseudorabies virus; ERY = erysipelas; SI = swine influenza.

and preweaning deaths (Pettigrew et al. 1986).

Stillborn piglets tend to be born later during farrowing and after a prolonged interval since the previous piglet (Randall 1972; Spicer et al. 1986). Females experiencing dystocia have at least three times the stillbirth rates as those having normal deliveries (Jackson 1975). Approximately 82% of intrapartum deaths occurred in the last third of the litter farrowed (Randall 1972). Intervals longer than 4 hours between the delivery of the first and last piglet is associated with an increase in the number of stillbirths/litter (Elze 1985). It has been suggested that the majority of stillbirths have died from hypoxia following premature rupture of the umbilical cord or early placental detachment (Kuhn and Wesemeier 1987). Histomorphological studies of the perinatal piglet, in fact, confirm that stillbirth piglets die primarily from anoxia during delivery (Bjorklund et al. 1987). These observations are reinforced by findings that lactate levels are four to five times higher in stillborn piglets than in live-borns (Lauterbach et al. 1987).

Gestation length also influences incidence of stillbirths. Females having both short (<112 days) and long gestations (>117 days) have higher rates of stillborn piglets than those with intermediate gestations (Bille et al. 1974a). While little can be done to prevent spontaneous early farrowing and subsequent increased stillbirth rates, increased stillbirth rates associated with prolonged gestations can potentially be reduced through induced farrowing. In several studies,

the induction of farrowing reduced the incidence of stillbirths (Silva-Filho et al. 1984; Chantaraprateep et al. 1986; Kalashnik and Grutseva 1988); others reported no beneficial influence (Fraser and Connor 1984; Martin et al. 1985; Stone et al. 1987; Stephens and Boland 1988; Ko et al. 1989). Some studies, in fact, have demonstrated that induced farrowing increases stillbirth rates (Cavalcanti et al. 1986). It is possible that continuous attendance of the female following induction of farrowing, along with manual intervention during prolonged deliveries and resuscitation of hypoxic pigs, might explain cited differences in the influence of induced farrowing on stillbirth rates. However, in one study, the supervision of induced farrowings did not reduce stillbirth rates, while improving neonatal survival (Jiken and Too 1988). These observations are somewhat in contrast with those in which farrowings were attended and piglets were artificially resuscitated, where approximately 30% of stillborn piglets were revived (Milosavljevic et al. 1972).

Several studies have tried to synchronize the onset of farrowing and prevent premature farrowing initiation through the administration of exogenous progestogens. Females treated with an orally active progestogen (allyl trenbolone) from day 111 to days 114, 115, or 116 or from day 111 to day 118 had increased stillbirth rates (Varley et al. 1985). In contrast, treatment with progestogen from day 110 to 116 in another study resulted in a longer parturition and a longer interval between successive piglets, but no affect on stillbirth rates

(Kirkwood et al. 1985). Females induced to farrow too early (<113 days) had higher rates of stillbirths than those left untreated or those induced later in gestation (Welp and Holtz 1985; Dial et al. 1990). In sum, these studies appear to indicate that stillbirth rates are potentially elevated in females allowed to gestate too long or in those induced to farrow too early.

Purebreeds and crossbreeds differ in stillbirth rates, with purebreeds having, on average, a higher rate than crossbreeds (Bae and Park 1985; Park et al. 1988). The heritability of number of stillborn piglets/litter was estimated to be from 0.2 to 0.11 (Nesetrilova 1987), 0.15 (Petrovic 1983), and 0.26 (Toelle and Robison 1985).

Feed and Nutrition. It has been suggested that both overweight and underweight females have increased perinatal mortality (Elze 1985). Body weight on day 90 of gestation was significantly correlated to incidence of stillbirths in females of first and second parities; specifically, females having weights averaging 220 kg had higher stillbirth rates than those with body weights of approximately 190 kg or less (Schoeps and Huhn 1986).

During rearing and lactation, females are commonly fed ad libitum, whereas during gestation, feed is typically restricted in most commercial operations. There is the potential that, with malformulated rations, females may not get sufficient micro- and macronutrients during gestation for optimal litter size. Levels of several vitamins in the gestation ration have been suggested to influence the incidence of stillborn piglets. Supplementation of cereal grain and soybean gestation rations with vitamin B_{12} improved stillbirth rates (Reinisch and Gebhardt 1989). Deficiencies of vitamin A are associated with increased stillbirth rates, premature farrowing, weak piglets at birth, and hypogalactia (Pavlov 1987).

Dietary levels of microminerals also have been found to affect stillbirth rates. Gilts fed zinc-deficient diets during pregnancy had increased stillbirth rates associated with prolonged deliveries and reduced postnatal piglet survival during the initial week after birth (Kalinowski and Chavez 1986). Females appear to be relatively resistant to iron deficiency, even though fetal hemopoiesis increases the requirement for iron during pregnancy (Mahan 1990). However, in investigations involving five herds, females having elevated stillbirth rates were found to have subnormal hemoglobin levels, and stillbirth rates were reduced by the oral or injectable administration of supplemental iron (Moore et al. 1965). Copper is essential for enzyme systems involved in musculoskeletal development and hemoglobin synthesis in the fetus; deficiencies result in an increased number of stillborn piglets (Kirchgessner et al. 1980). While gilts fed corn–soybean meal rations without supplemental selenium had normal total-born litter sizes and stillbirth rates at their first

parities, litter sizes were reduced in subsequent parities (Mahan et al. 1974). Females fed diets containing selenium and vitamin E in levels similar to NRC standards but injected with selenium and vitamin E during gestation had higher live-born litter sizes and lower stillbirth rates than noninjected females (Chavez and Patton 1986). These studies suggest that primiparous females have sufficient tissue reserves for optimal reproductive performance, but as parities advance, selenium and vitamin E depletion may occur (Mahan 1990). Piglets born to females fed iodine-deficient rations have piglets that are born weak or dead with a hypertrophic thyroid (Slatter 1955).

The macrominerals calcium and phosphorus have also been suggested to influence stillbirth rates. Gestating females fed low dietary levels of calcium and phosphorus have reduced live-born litter sizes (Kornegay et al. 1973; Mahan and Fetter 1982). However, numerous studies have demonstrated that as long as dietary levels of calcium and phosphorus meet or exceed NRC standards, neither total-born litter size or stillbirth rates are affected by levels of the two macrominerals in the diet (Kornegay et al. 1973; Mahan and Fetter 1982; Kornegay and Kite, 1983). Experimentally induced hypocalcemia has been found to have no influence on stillbirth rates, but there was a delay in the expulsion of piglets in hypocalcemic females (Ayliffe et al. 1984).

Toxicoses also increase intrapartum deaths. Contamination of gestation rations with the mycotoxins zearalenone and ochratoxin is associated with increased incidence of stillbirths (Barnikol and Thalmann 1988). The supplementation of gestation feed with sulfadimethoxine and ormetoprim during late gestation results in increased gestation length and elevated incidence of stillborn and weak piglets (Blackwell et al. 1989).

Environment and Management. In two separate investigations of two clinical cases each, the use of gas heaters in underventilated farrowing facilities was found to cause acute increases in stillbirth rates associated with carbon monoxide toxicoses (Wood 1979; Van Alstine et al. 1985). While one study recorded a significant linear relationship between stillbirth rates and atmospheric carbon monoxide between 150 and 400 ppm (Dominick and Carson 1983), another prospective investigation failed to show an influence on stillbirth rates as carbon monoxide levels were increased to 200–250 ppm, even though postnatal vitality of piglets was reduced (Morris et al. 1985).

Exposure of females to high ambient temperatures during late gestation results in an increased rate of intrapartum deaths. Consequently, the finding that that month of farrowing also influences incidence of stillbirths (Bae and Park 1985) is not surprising. Stillbirth rates were highest in litters farrowing during the summer months relative to the other seasons (Singh et al. 1989).

There is a controversial influence of female housing and management during gestation on perinatal survival of piglets. Females transferred to farrowing sheds at 102 days of gestation had lower stillbirth rates than those transferred at 112 days, and there were fewer females having still-births (Kocwin-Podsiadla et al. 1988). Females housed in pens prior to being tethered at farrowing required more manual assistance during farrowing and had higher stillbirth rates than females continuously tethered, those tethered during pregnancy then farrowed in pens, and those loose-housed at all times (Hansen et al. 1986). Females that were forced to exercise during gestation had reduced farrowing durations and shorter average intervals between successive piglets; however, while neonatal survival of piglets was improved, stillbirth rates remained unchanged (Ferket and Hacker 1985). In contrast to these observations, several studies reported no influence of housing on ease of farrowing or on intrapartum mortality. Housing females in either pens or tethers during late gestation followed by housing in either pens or farrowing crates around farrowing and during lactation did not influence farrowing duration, interval between births, or number of stillborn piglets (Parry 1986). There were no differences in stillbirth rates of females tethered during farrowing or housed in farrowing crates (Lynch et al. 1984). Similarly, neither differences in stillbirth rates nor litter size at birth were observed between tethered females and females housed in stalls during gestation (Lynch et al. 1984). Also, no differences were observed in the incidence of stillbirths between females housed during either gestation or farrowing in groups versus those tethered (Hansen and Vestergaard 1984).

Disease. While numerous facultative and opportunistic pathogens have been isolated from stillborn piglets, there are several primary pathogens of swine causing increased stillbirth rates. Epizootics of leptospirosis, especially *Leptospira interrogans* serovar *pomona* and *L. bratislava* (Kingscote 1986; Ellis et al. 1986a), are frequently associated with increased stillbirth rates and elevated rates of abortions and neonatal deaths. While porcine parvovirus more commonly causes elevated mummy rates, gilts that develop antibody during the middle third of pregnancy also have higher stillbirth rates in addition to elevated mummy rates and reduced live-born litters (Too and Love 1986). Swine influenza, specifically H1N1 and H3N2, has been isolated from aborted and stillborn fetuses in association with respiratory disease in breeding herds (Gourreau et al. 1985). Encephalomyocarditis virus (EMCV) causes increased intrapartum and prepartum deaths as well as increased neonatal mortality (Littlejohns

1984; Links et al. 1986; Joo et al. 1988; Mercy et al. 1988). Epizootics of pseudorabies virus are associated with transient increases in stillbirths as well as increased abortions and mummy rates (Gustafson 1986).

There are several less commonly observed pathogens also associated with increased intrapartum deaths. Similar to EMCV, cytomegalovirus causes increased preweaning mortality and elevations in both stillbirth and mummies, but females also experience fevers, anorexia, coughing, and nasal discharge (Orr et al. 1988). Chlamydia has been isolated from both weak and stillborn piglets (Stellmacher et al. 1983). Paramyxovirus causes increased prepartum and intrapartum deaths in association with encephalomyelitis and corneal opacity in neonates (Stephan et al. 1988). Japanese encephalitis virus causes abortions and increased stillbirths (Ouchi 1987; Takashima et al. 1988). Females experimentally exposed to sporulated oocysts of *Toxoplasma gondii* aborted and delivered an increased number of stillbirths (Vidotto et al. 1987).

Mummies. Mummified fetuses are the inspissated remains of fetal tissues after the maternal uterus has removed bodily fluids leaving only the nonabsorbable components of the fetuses, including the partially calcified skeletons. Mummies are created when death of the fetus occurs after the onset of skeletal calcification, approximately 30–40 days of gestation (Fig. 6.7) (Mengeling 1986). Prior to that prenatal age, fetuses that die prior to birth will be completely reabsorbed. Dead fetuses become mummies up to the time of the initiation of parturition. Piglets dying just prior to the initiation of delivery are generally classified as mummies even though they may not appear to be obviously inspissated. In fact, antepartum deaths typically have subcutaneous edema, excessive amounts of serous fluids, visceral congestion and hemorrhage, discoloration of skin (indicative of subcutaneous hemorrhage), sunken eyes, and friable tissues (Glastonbury 1977a,b,c). Fetuses dying after the onset of delivery are no longer classified as mummies, being called stillborn piglets.

Unlike stillbirths/litter and live-born litter size, the number of mummies in each litter is not related to pigs/female/year under endemic conditions (Polson et al. 1990a). Nonetheless, it is likely that during epidemics of reproductive disease mummy rates frequently become elevated, thereby limiting live-born litter size and pigs/female/year. There are several infectious as well as noninfectious causes of mummified fetuses (Fig. 6.16).

Infectious Disease. Fetal pathogens commonly cited as causing elevated mummy rates include parvovirus (Too and Love 1986; Choi et al. 1987), pseudorabies (Morrison and Joo 1985; Iglesias

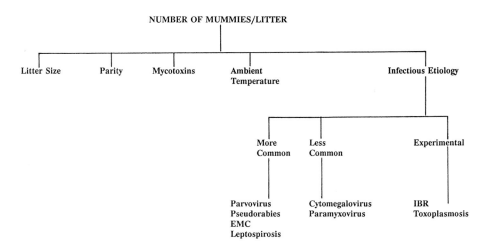

6.16. Interrelationships between factors influencing number of mummies/litter. EMC = encephalomyocarditis; IBR = infectious bovine rhinotracheitis.

and Harkness 1988), encephalomyocarditis virus (Littlejohns 1984; Links et al. 1986; Joo et al. 1988; Mercy et al. 1988; Christianson et al. 1990), and leptospirosis (Hathaway et al. 1983; Desmecht and Castryck 1984). Infectious etiologies of prenatal death with mummification cytomegalovirus (Orr et al. 1988) and paramyxovirus are observed less frequently. Some agents have been shown experimentally to cause fetal mummification, including infectious bovine rhinotracheitis (Joo et al. 1984) and toxoplasmosis (Vidotto et al. 1987). The clinical presentation typically differentiates the infectious agents from each other and from noninfectious causes of elevated mummy rates. For example, parvovirus primarily affects lower-parity females in endemically infected herds. Encephalomyocarditis virus causes neonatal deaths in accompaniment with increased mummy and stillbirth rates. Pseudorabies, leptospirosis, and toxoplasmosis infections may be associated with abortion.

Litter Size. Mummy rates increase as total-born litter sizes increase (Spicer et al. 1986). Females with mummified fetuses have more ovulations, more fetuses, and fewer live-born fetuses than those with no mummies (Wu et al. 1988). As gestation progresses, there is an increase in the proportion of mummified fetuses in larger litters (Wu et al. 1988). It has been suggested that the increase in mummies associated with larger litters is associated with insufficient uterine space for development and survival (Wu et al. 1988). Intrauterine crowding causes reduced endometrial surface area per fetus, thereby inhibiting placental development and causing increased fetal mortality (Knight et al. 1977).

Parity. Under endemic conditions, lower-parity females, especially primiparous females, have higher mummy rates than advanced-parity females. This may be due, at least in part, to the immunological naivete of lower-parity females that have not been inventoried in the herd sufficiently long to be exposed to pathogens endemic in the herd.

Mycotoxins. Occasionally, an observed etiology of prenatal death with mummification is mycotoxicoses. Mycotoxins associated with increased mummy rates include zearalenone (Young and King 1986a; Barnikol and Thalmann 1988), ochratoxin (Barnikol and Thalmann 1988), and trichothecenes (Gadek 1984).

PREWEANING MORTALITY. Preweaning mortality varies widely among herds. During epidemics of some diseases, such as with pseudorabies virus and transmissible gastroenteritis, mortality rates of suckling piglets can exceed 80%. Preweaning mortality in most herds is endemic in nature, being only occasionally dominated by epidemics of disease. In the absence of disease epidemics, preweaning mortality rates commonly exceed 15% (Vaillancourt 1990). Despite its impact on pigs weaned/female/year, suckling piglet mortality has remained relatively stable over recent decades. In fact, preweaning mortality has remained unchanged even though confinement production systems for swine have brought substantial improvements in facility, environment, and management technologies (Vaillancourt 1990). This suggests that many producers either do not understand the causes and risk factors associated with preweaning mortality or are unable to manipulate them to the advantage of piglet survival.

The advent and application of computerized information systems potentially allows the specific causes of preweaning mortality and their associated risk factors to be easily identified (Fig. 6.17). However, even though piglet mortality information is commonly recorded by progressive producers, it is difficult for them to accurately differentiate moribund piglets according to specific cause of mortality (Vaillancourt et al. 1990). Piglets dying from a primary etiology are frequently classified incorrectly as dying from a secondary cause. For example, piglets dying after being born lowly viable, being born with lethal congenital anomalies, and those becoming debilitated by diarrhea or another infectious disease (primary causes) may be recorded by the producer as dying from starvation (secondary cause). Alternatively, because starvation (primary cause) causes piglets to be weak and less active, starved piglets may be incorrectly classified as dying from trauma (secondary cause). When making a decision on how to classify a dead piglet into a category of mortality, producers should sequentially consider the causes of mortality that they may determine, with high statistical specificity and sensitivity, as the specific cause of death (Fig. 6.18). Decisions about mortality causes in which the producer has little specificity in categorizing a dead piglet should be left to the end of a decision tree. Also, primary health conditions that predispose piglets to dying from a secondary cause should be considered first. Developing confidence in accurate and consistent recording of causes of mortality is necessary to troubleshoot herd problems of elevated preweaning mortality.

Highest mortality rates typically occur within the initial 3–4 days of life, representing 55–75% of the total preweaning mortality (Nielson et al. 1974; Glastonbury 1976; Vaillancourt et al. 1990). Approximately 15% of the total mortality occurred during the interval 4–7 days after farrowing; an additional 15% occurred after the first week of age (Vaillancourt et al. 1990). In endemic herds, the principal causes of preweaning mortality vary with piglet age. For example, the majority of piglets (>75%) dying during the initial 3 days of life die from trauma, low viability, and starvation. The other major categories of mortality, including diarrhea, other infectious diseases (such as infectious arthritis), and congenital anomalies, are relatively minor causes of mortality during the immediate postnatal period, except when epizootics occur. As piglets get older, scours and other infectious diseases become increasingly important causes of mortality (Vaillancourt et al. 1990). Thus, strategies to improve overall preweaning mortality must not only focus on identifying the specific etiologies of mortality but also on age-related changes in the principal sources of mortality.

While there is an abundance of published findings on the factors influencing preweaning mortality, there is a paucity of research investigating the impact of risk factors on specific types of piglet mortality. For example, total-born and live-born litter size are known to have strong influences on preweaning mortality (Fahmy and Bernard 1971; Bille et al. 1974a; Simenson and Karlberg 1980), but it is not clear to what extent

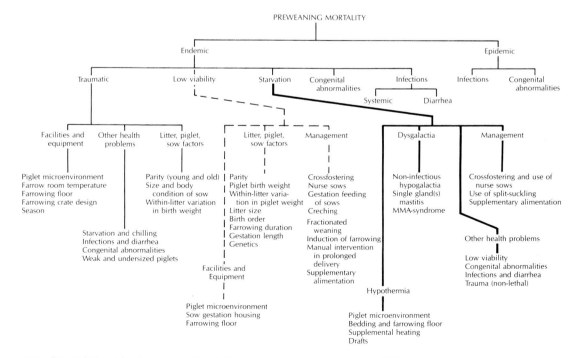

6.17.   Interrelationships between factors influencing number of pigs weaned/litter.

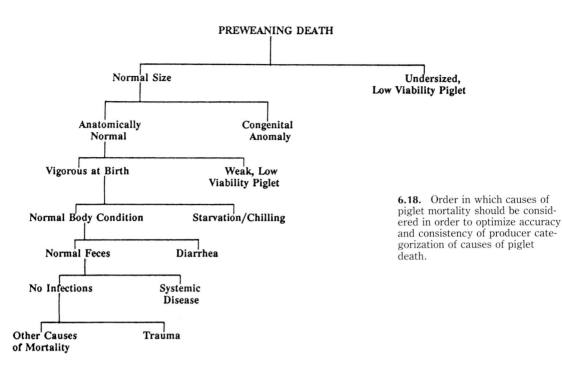

6.18. Order in which causes of piglet mortality should be considered in order to optimize accuracy and consistency of producer categorization of causes of piglet death.

the various types of piglet mortality are affected by litter size. Live-born litter size influences the proportion of piglets dying from traumatic injuries (Bille et al. 1974b), and it can be assumed that litter size also predisposes piglets to mortality due to low viability and starvation, but it is not known. The relationship between litter size and piglet mortality is curvilinear with the highest mortality occurring with the largest and smallest litters (Fahmy and Bernard 1971; Bolet and Etienne 1982).

Similar to litter size, female parity influences overall preweaning mortality (Nielsen et al. 1974; Simensen and Karlberg 1980). Parity also affects the proportion of piglets dying after being laid upon or stepped upon by the female (Bille et al. 1974b; Svendsen et al. 1986). Lower-parity females have smaller litter and individual piglet weights (Lynch et al. 1982), suggesting that parity may influence the proportion of low-viability piglets. Parity is positively associated with metritis-mastitis-agalactia syndrome. Thus, the proportion of piglets dying from starvation may be influenced by parity. Similarly, it is not uncommon for lower-parity females to have a higher prevalence of diarrhea and systemic diseases (such as arthritis) in their litters than older females, presumably because of a time-related acquisition in immunity. Nonetheless, it remains unclear to what degree parity influences many of the causes of piglet mortality.

Season is a third risk factor that may be common to more than one mortality type. The influence of season on preweaning mortality has become well recognized. Several studies have reported that mortality is highest during the fall and winter months and lowest during the spring season (Nielson et al. 1974; Bolet and Etienne 1982), suggesting that season mediates its effect on preweaning mortality, at least in part, through ambient temperature. In fact, the high susceptibility of the neonatal piglet to cold stress, relative to neonates of other species, has been well documented (English and Morrison 1984). Hypothermia and its subsequent suppressive influence on colostrum and milk intake, thereby, predispose the piglet to mortality due to systemic infection, diarrhea, traumatic injury, and low viability.

Piglet environment, including facility and equipment design, also potentially influences several types of preweaning mortality. Farrowing pens using bedding have reduced proportions of piglets with diarrhea, lameness, and hypoglycemia and fewer weak piglets than pens having either partially concrete slats or solid floors (Vellenga et al. 1983; Aumaitre and LeDividich 1984). Bedding also reduces the prevalence of teat and leg damage (Bengtsson et al. 1982) and, thereby, may affect rates of mortality due to starvation and crushing. While bedding reduces conductive heat losses and the lower critical temperature of piglets (Bruce and Clark 1979; Vellenga et al. 1983), there may be no advantage, in terms of preweaning mortality, for the use of bedding in farrowing crates (Edwards and Furniss 1988). Perforated floors without bedding have become increasingly commonplace in the swine industry, in part, because producers consider them easier to maintain hygienically and more simple to manage. Piglets farrowed onto perforated floors have a higher survival rate than those delivered onto concrete floors in some studies (Mabry et al. 1982b), but not in others (Kornegay and Lindemann 1984; Christison et al. 1987). Piglets farrowed onto perforated floors, especially plastic-coated wire or metal floors, also potentially have reduced abrasions and injuries (Kornegay and Lindemann 1984) and less diarrhea (Phuah and Soo 1980). Although mortality from crushing did not vary with floor type, the prevalence of death due to splayleg may increase with some perforated floor surfaces such as fiberglass and metal slats (Christison et al. 1987). In sum, these studies indicate that some perforated floor surfaces may have advantages with some types of mortalities but not with others.

As discussed below, there are other risk factors that are common to more than one cause of mortality. After developing an understanding about the relative contributions of each type of mortality to a herd's overall mortality, specific strategies can then be developed to manipulate those risk factors affecting the major cause(s) of piglet mortality.

Trauma. Trauma includes piglets that suffer lethal injuries or are suffocated when laid on, stepped on, or savaged by the female. Typically, the female crushes piglets as she rises from a lying position and when she lies down again (Svendsen et al. 1986). Less commonly, the female steps on piglets when she is standing or walking, savages the piglet, or crushes the piglet against the farrowing equipment. The most serious injuries and the greatest number of crushing deaths occur with the hindquarters and rear legs (Svendsen et al. 1986).

While there are debilitating illnesses (e.g., diarrhea, arthritis) and conditions (such as myofibrillar hypoplasia, anemia, starvation) that predispose piglets to crushing mortality, the large majority (>70%) of crushing mortality involves healthy, potentially viable piglets (Spicer et al. 1986). Nonlethal injuries can also predispose the piglet to other causes of mortality (English and Morrison 1984). For example, about 30–40% of piglets less than 2 days of age that die from traumatic injuries or suffocation had been debilitated by starvation, as evidenced by empty gastrointestinal tracts (Glastonbury 1977a). Concomitant illnesses of either the female or piglet (Spicer et al. 1986), congenital abnormalities, such as myofibrillar hypoplasia, small piglet size, and low hardiness at birth also predispose piglets to being laid upon or stepped on by the female. While trauma can occur throughout lactation, over 85% of all mortality due to trauma occurs during the initial 3 days after farrowing (Svendsen et al. 1986; Vaillancourt et al. 1990). Trauma accounts for approximately 20–45% of the total mortality (Vaillancourt 1990).

There are several litter, piglet, and female factors predisposing piglets to mortality. While overall mortality rates were higher for first-parity females and those greater than four parities (Nielsen et al. 1974), primiparous females had a lower prevalence of piglets crushed than multiparous females, and crushing rates increased with parity (Bille et al. 1974b; Svendsen et al. 1986). The parity-associated increase in crushing may be related to the larger sizes of higher-parity females, their reduced ambulatory capacity, or poorer mothering ability. Rates of mortality due to trauma also increases with litter size (Bille et al. 1974b). Crushed piglets tend to be smaller than those remaining alive (Svendson et al. 1986).

Mortality has been found in some studies to be highest during the fall and winter months and lowest during the spring seasons (Nielson et al. 1974; Bolet and Etienne 1982), but not all farms show a seasonal pattern in preweaning mortality (Vaillancourt 1990); Some herds have increased mortality during the warmer months, some have higher mortality during the cooler seasons (Vaillancourt 1990). Facilities and management have been suggested to be responsible for the seasonal variation in suckling mortality (Fahmy et al. 1978). In herds with a higher mortality during the cooler months, inadequate piglet microenvironments may encourage piglets to seek the female for warmth and subsequently spend more time in the areas of the farrowing crate or pen occupied by the females. Alternatively, piglets may get chilled and become less active and less able to get from beneath a female as she lies down. In herds having higher mortality during the warmer months, such as evidenced by Bille et al. (1974b), piglets may lie away from zones where supplemental heating is available in areas where the female will have a greater opportunity to step on or lay upon them. During warmer months, increased ventilation rates in confinement farrowing facilities also may cause piglets to lie near the female in an effort to get away from drafts.

The ambient temperature of farrowing facilities should be maintained from 15 to 22°C (Reyns and De Donnea 1974; De la Farge 1981). The optimal temperature for facilities can vary from about 18°C for facilities using bedding to 22°C for those using totally slatted floors (Reyns and De Donnea 1974). Air temperatures at pig level should be 30°C at birth, 27.5°C at the end of the first week, and 22–25°C at weaning (Reyns and De Donnea 1974; De la Farge 1981). Because of convective heat losses, air flows of less than 0.2 m/sec during the winter and less than 1 m/sec during the summer have been recommended (De la Farge and Chosson 1979; DeChamps and Nicks 1984). There is the equivalent of a 4°C drop in temperature when air speed increases from 0.1 to 0.6 m/second (Mount 1968). However, piglets tend to lay near the female during the initial 3 days of life, regardless of heat location or air temperature (English and Morrison 1984). Nonetheless, heat lamp arrangement has been found to influence preweaning mortality (English and Morrison 1984).

Farrowing facilities and equipment influence preweaning mortality, at least in part, through their effects on traumatic injuries to piglets. Rates of crushing mortality, and thus, overall preweaning mortality, are lower in farrowing crates than in pens (Glastonbury 1976; Aumaitre and LeDividich 1984; Hansen and Vestergaard 1984). In one study, the proportion of piglets dying from trauma varied with farrowing crate design (Svendsen et al. 1986). The crate with the lowest crushing mortality had fingerlike projections from the bottom bar, well-insulated side panels, movable heat lamps, and a totally perforated flooring without straw bedding. Farrowing crates fitted with cradles (anticrush bars) that restrict the female as she lies down have a lower rate of crushing mortality than standard crates (English et al. 1982). Varying the width of the female area of the farrowing crate, the length, and the height of the bottom bar of the side panel of the farrowing crate had no influence on preweaning mortality (Curtis et al. 1989). Farrowing crates commonly used in the commercial swine industry include designs having side panels with straight bottom bars, bottom bars that are bowed away from the female (flared or bow-bar crates), and bottom bars with fingerlike projections (finger crates). There is no evidence that bottom bar design influences preweaning mortality (Fraser and Thompson 1986; Fraser et al. 1988).

Although not well investigated, floor types of farrowing equipment also potentially influence rates of trauma mortality. Piglets farrowed onto plastic-coated metal floors have heavier weaning weights but similar preweaning mortality to those housed on concrete slats (Christison et al. 1987; Stansbury et al. 1987). Females consumed more feed and lost less body weight on concrete floors relative to plastic floors (Stansbury et al. 1987). Multisurfaced floors have been developed in recent years to meet the different thermal needs of the suckling piglet and the dam (Svendsen et al. 1986). Neonatal piglets prefer to lie on plastic floors followed, in turn, by perforated metal floors, fiberglass slats, and woven-wire floors (Farmer and Christison 1982). Thus, multisurfaced floors potentially influence where piglets lie, and thus, their risk of being crushed.

Low Viability. The low-viability category includes piglets that are judged by the producer to be incapable of surviving under standard husbandry procedures, because they were born either undersized or weak and therefore are more prone to dying from such things as starvation, hypothermia, and crushing. The birth weight of a piglet can be viewed in terms of its absolute weight or in terms of its relationship to those of the other piglets in the litter. Piglets born into litters with

high variation in birth weight have higher mortality rates than those born into litters with small variation (Perry and Rowell 1969; Fahmy et al. 1978). In fact, variation in birth weight within the litter may be just as important, or perhaps more important, than individual birth weight in influencing survival (Fahmy and Bernard 1971; English and Smith 1975; English and Wilkinson 1982). Smaller piglets that are within approximately 20% of the mean birth weight of their litter have greater survival than those piglets with a higher deviation from the average birth weight (Blackwell 1988).

Birth weight is inversely related to preweaning mortality (Hartsock and Graves 1976; Fraser and Lin 1984; Friendship and Wilson 1985). Piglets have been classified as small when they are less than 900 gm (Bille et al. 1974a) and less than 1000 gm (England 1986). However, recent studies reveal that preweaning mortality falls in a near-linear fashion as birth weight increases up to approximately 1 kg (Blackwell 1988). While preweaning mortality continues to improve as average birth weight increases to over 2 kg, the increase is not as great over 1.1 kg as it is for 1 kg or less (Blackwell 1988). These observations suggest that average piglet birth weights of 1.1 kg and within-litter variations of less than 20% will minimize the proportion of piglets dying from low viability. Heavier piglets are more likely to suckle successfully, whereas lighter piglets take longer to suckle the first time and thus ingest less colostrum and milk (Hartsock et al. 1977; Hendrix et al. 1978; Spicer et al. 1986; Svendson et al. 1986). Thus, birth weight might be expected to not only be associated with mortality due to being born lowly viable, but also may predispose the piglet to being crushed by the female or dying from starvation.

Besides being undersized, low-viability piglets can also be weak. Common causes of piglets being weak after birth are intrauterine asphyxia (Randall and Penny 1968; Randall 1971; DeRoth and Downie 1976) and anemia (Connaughton et al. 1985; Spicer et al. 1986). Asphyxia is common with premature rupture of the umbilical cord and with prolonged deliveries (Randall 1972). Anemia typically results from excessive blood loss from the umbilical cord soon after delivery (Connaughton et al. 1985), but can be a sequelae to exposure of the female to toxins or to vitamin deficiencies (Penny 1980; Svendsen et al. 1986).

Of those piglets recorded as dying because they were born lowly viable, approximately 85% died within the initial 3 days after delivery (Vaillancourt et al. 1990). Low viability constitutes from approximately 20–60% of the total preweaning mortality (Vaillancourt 1990).

There are several management techniques that have been used in commercial herds to reduce the number of low-viability piglets born into each litter (Fig. 6.17). *Crossfostering* is a procedure wherein piglets are transferred from one litter to another to improve the competitive advantage of vulnerable piglets through the standardization of number of piglets per litter and/or improving the uniformity of piglet size within a litter (Hosman 1971; English and Wilkinson 1982; Marcatti et al. 1986). *Nurse females* commonly have their own litters weaned and receive piglets from one or more other females in an attempt to improve the growth performance and/or survival of the lowly viable or undernourished piglets of the donor females. *Creching* is a technique wherein piglets are removed temporarily from the female (Friend and Elliot 1981). In some cases, vulnerable piglets are removed and provided an improved microenvironment and other supplementary care for a brief period. Alternatively, the more vigorous piglets may be creched, allowing more vulnerable piglets unrestricted access to suckling. In *fractionated weaning*, the larger piglets are removed from a litter a few days in advance of the normal time of weaning, allowing undersized piglets and more vulnerable piglets additional days to nurse in a less competitive environment (Cox et al. 1983; Stevenson and Davis 1984).

Survival of piglets born weak or undersized potentially improves with *induced farrowing* when coupled with observed farrowing and intensive care (Bille et al. 1974a; Simensen and Karlberg 1980). While the prevalence of low-viability piglets is elevated at both short and long gestation lengths (Aumaitre et al. 1979), only prolonged gestations can be manipulated, through induced farrowing, to improve postnatal survival. Piglets born after prolonged labor are more likely to have reduced viability due to anoxia (Randall 1971). Thus, *manual intervention* during prolonged farrowings potentially can be used to reduce the occurrence of asphyxia and thereby the proportion of weak piglets. Birth order and perinatal mortality is highly and positively related (Harsock and Graves 1976), such that pigs born earlier during farrowing are more likely to survive. Furthermore, piglets having lighter weights are more likely to be born later in the birth order (Hartsock and Graves 1976). Thus, attendance of females, especially during the later stages of delivery, might be expected to improve postnatal survival of piglets.

Another technique used to improve survival of weak and undersized piglets is *supplementary alimentation* with colostrum, milk, and immunoglobulin-fortified milk (Moody et al. 1966; Kennelly et al. 1979; Whiting et al. 1983; England 1986). The supplementation of lactation rations and rations fed late in gestation with fat increases piglet viability (Pettigrew 1981; Moser 1983) by increasing the amount of milk fat available to suckling piglets (Pettigrew 1981) and by increasing the amount of glucose available to the fetus because of reduced maternal tissue glucose clearance (Seerly and Martin 1983). Apparently, only

herds having an elevated rate of preweaning mortality consistently benefit from added fat rations (Pettigrew 1981). While lactation feed and nutrient intake has been found to influence weaning weights and weaning-to-service intervals, especially in primiparous females, lactation feeding programs have no apparent effect on preweaning survival (Reese et al. 1982; King and Williams 1984a,b).

In addition to birth order, gestation length, and farrowing duration, as discussed above, there are other litter, piglet, and female factors influencing piglet survival. Piglet birth weight increases with female parity (Lynch et al. 1982), and within-litter variation in birth weight varies with parity (English and Brampton 1978). Thus, the proportion of piglets dying from being born lowly viable may change as the parity distribution of the herd changes. Even though the heritability of progeny survival is low ($h^2 < 20\%$) (Fergurson et al. 1985) heterosis has been shown to influence postnatal survival (England 1974; Fahmy et al. 1978). Crossbred piglets are more vigorous at birth and thus have a greater chance of survival than purebred piglets (Fahmy et al. 1978), which suggests that commercial farms utilizing crossbred females may have an advantage in terms of preweaning mortality than those females using purebred lines.

Facilities and equipment may predispose weak and undersized low-viability piglets to mortality. Both types of piglets commonly die from hypothermia and/or starvation (English and Morrison 1984). Thus, improving the piglet microenvironment, such as by the effective use of zone heating, bedding, and appropriate floor surfaces, might be expected to improve the proportion of weak and undersized piglets surviving (Vaillancourt et al. 1990). The piglets from females housed in groups during gestation tend to be heavier than those housed individually (England and Spur 1969). Furthermore, females housed individually have a longer farrowing duration (Svendsen and Andreasson 1980) and require more manual intervention during farrowing than females housed in groups (Hansen and Vestergaard 1984). Thus, gestational environment, as well as farrowing environment, potentially influence the prevalence of lowly viable piglets on some farms.

Starvation. Neonatal piglets of all sizes are highly susceptible to hypoglycemia if starved for only short periods of time after delivery (Nielsen et al. 1974). Blood glucose levels fall to hypoglycemic levels within 36–48 hours of onset of milk deprivation because of deficient hepatic gluconeogenesis (Nielsen et al. 1975a; Svendsen et al. 1975a; Vandenbooren et al. 1986). Mortality due to starvation is typically spread out over several weeks during lactation (Bolet 1982; Dyck and Sweistra 1987). Death due to starvation was highest on days 4 and 5 of age and remained relatively elevated through the second week of lactation, indicating that starvation is gradual (Dyck and Sweistra 1987). Starvation generally constitutes approximately 10% of mortality (Nielsen et al. 1974), but in at least one investigation starvation accounted for approximately 43% of postnatal deaths with 18% and 15% attributed to crushing and weakness, respectively (English and Smith 1975). Piglets with poor body condition and having no milk in their digestive tracts are included in the starvation category (Glastonbury 1977a). Starved piglets may have an antemortem history of failing to suckle regularly following birth.

Other health problems, such as being born lowly viable, congenital abnormalities, diseases, and trauma by the female, can predispose the piglet to dying from starvation, and these should be considered as primary causes of piglet mortality. Additional factors that predispose piglets to starvation include chilling (Kelley et al. 1982; English and Morrison 1984) and female hypogalactia (Tubbs 1988). The effective environmental temperature below which the neonatal piglet must increase its metabolic rate in order to maintain its body temperature is 34°C. Hypothermia and the depressive effects of continuous prolonged exposure to cold ambient temperatures results in reduced colostral and milk intake by piglets, leading ultimately to death by starvation. Death due to secondary lethal factors, such as diarrhea and trauma, are a common sequelae to hypothermia (Curtis 1970, 1974; English and Morrison 1984).

Dysgalactia involving one or more glands of a mammary chain may cause starvation of individual piglets in a litter while the remaining piglets grow normally, or dysgalactia of the entire mammary chain may be associated with starvation of all or a high proportion of piglets in a litter. Mastitis can present as infections of one or more individual glands of the mammary chain or infections/inflammation of the entire mammary chain, commonly called metritis-mastitis-agalactia syndrome (MMA). Piglet mortality may be over 50% in litters of females affected with MMA (Backstrom et al. 1984), and piglet deaths may be spread over several weeks of lactation (Bolet and Etienne 1982; Dyck and Sweistra 1987). Noninfectious lactation failure, as associated with parity, genetics, and nutrition, may also cause increased mortality due to starvation (Tubbs 1988).

Management techniques potentially useful for reducing starvation include procedures that are also helpful for reducing deaths due to low viability. These include cross-fostering, nurse females, fractionated weaning, and supplementary alimentation. Split suckling, wherein the larger piglets in a litter are removed temporarily allowing the starving piglets to suckle without competition, may also reduce starvation rates.

Diarrhea. Scouring typically accounts for 5–15% of the total mortality under endemic conditions (Fahmy and Bernard 1971; Nielsen et al. 1974; Spicer et al. 1986; Vaillancourt et al. 1990). Whereas the greatest proportion of fatal cases of preweaning mortality due to diarrhea occurs during the first week of life (Svendsen et al. 1975a), the proportion of total mortality attributable to diarrhea increases with age (Vaillancourt et al. 1990).

There is an interplay between a piglet's immunity and exposure burden to enteric pathogens that determines whether the piglet will develop diarrhea. Piglets suckling hypogalactic females may have reduced enteric immunity and, therefore, be more susceptible to enteric pathogens. Thus, infectious diseases of the female, such as MMA (Backstrom et al. 1984), and noninfectious processes, for example, the reduced feed intake that accompanies elevated farrowing room temperatures (Tubbs 1988), potentially compromise a litter's capacity to ward off enteric pathogens. The depressive effects of hypothermia are associated with reduced colostral and milk intake, resulting in increased mortality due to diarrhea, as well as other causes (English and Morrison 1984). Seasonal changes in ambient temperature may explain the increased prevalence of gastrointestinal diseases during the cooler months in the litters of all parities of females, as observed by Svendsen et al. (1975a,b). Diarrhea was increased fivefold and its severity doubled in litters exposed to temperatures below the lower critical temperature for the neonatal piglet (Kelley et al. 1982). The occurrence of diarrhea is temporally associated with daily fluctuations in temperatures within farrowing units (Madec et al. 1984).

Elevations in preweaning mortality associated with elevated ambient temperatures can be ameliorated, at least in part, through the use of evaporative drip cooling systems (Stansbury et al. 1987; McGlone et al. 1988). Preweaning mortality is lower when farrowing room temperatures are maintained at 25°C than when they are held at either 20°C or 30°C (Stansbury et al. 1987). Perhaps, the cold-stress at lower temperatures increases piglet mortality due to diarrhea and other infectious diseases, such as pneumonia, and increased crushing as piglets approach the female for warmth. Elevated ambient temperatures may interfere with the female's lactation performance, leading to increased mortality due to diarrhea and infectious disease, as well as increased crushing rates as piglets become less inclined to lie in heated areas.

The thermal and hygienic advantage of bedding would be expected to improve preweaning survival, in part, by reducing the prevalence of diarrhea and other infectious diseases. In fact, the incidence of diarrhea is higher in pigs farrowed on concrete slats than those reared on bedding (Hunneman 1978). By improving hygiene and using some floor types to improve thermal comfort (e.g., plastic-coated expanded metal floors and perforated floors) there is the potential to reduce the prevalence of mortality due to diarrhea. However, while piglets farrowed on perforated floors have a higher mortality rate than those on solid floors (Mabry et al. 1982a), no differences were observed in the incidence of diarrhea among different perforated floor types (metal slats, fiberglass slats, and perforated metal sheet floors) and concrete floors (Christison et al. 1987).

Infections.   The infection category includes piglets having either systemic (bacteremia) or localized infections (polyarthritis, pneumonia). It is not uncommon for piglets to have more than one infection with the same organism. For example, polyarthritis has been found concurrently with pneumonia and endocarditis (Bille et al. 1975; Nielson et al. 1975b). Infections are typically only a small proportion (<2%) of the total piglets dying during the initial days after birth (Vaillancourt 1990). Even though the total number of piglets dying decreases with age, the proportion of piglets dying from infections increases with age until weaning, when infectious diseases become one of the primary causes of mortality (Aumaitre 1971; Glastonbury 1977b). Of piglets dying at 1 week of age or later, approximately 40% of piglets die from infections and over 30% die from diarrhea (Vaillancourt 1990). The overall preweaning mortality throughout the suckling period due to infectious diseases may be as high as 25% (Nielsen et al. 1974).

Acute septicemia and pneumonia are more common during cooler than warmer seasons (Nielson et al. 1975a). It is likely that piglet microenvironment, including hygiene, bedding, floor surface, ambient temperature, and air movement, influences the prevalence of piglets dying due to infections, similar to diarrheas. While the tonsils and upper digestive tract are main portals for entry (Williams et al. 1973; Nielson et al. 1975), skin abrasions, lacerations of the knees and claws, and the umbilical cord are additional entry sites.

Deformities.   The deformed category of preweaning mortality includes piglets with genetically acquired abnormalities and those with congenital lesions having no genetic component. The most common deformities are myofibrillar hypoplasia (splayleg) and hernias of the inguinal ring and umbilicus. Less frequently observed deformities include atresia ani and cleft palate. Nearly all deaths due to lethal deformities occur within the first week of life (Glastonbury 1977b), and approximately 85% of piglets with lethal developmental anomalies die within the first 3 days after birth (Vaillancourt 1990).

Depending upon the severity of the lesion, piglets having birth deformities may survive, as commonly occurs with splayleg and hernias. Alternatively, the lesions either may be lethal or predispose the piglet to another type of mortality (e.g., starvation). Genetic inheritance is one of the most common causes of developmental deformities; however, toxins and nutrient deficiencies may also influence the incidence of deformities. Floor type and physical environment may affect the survival of piglets born with congenital anomalies such as splayleg (Christison et al. 1987).

Minor Causes of Endemic Mortality.   Producers typically have from 10 to 15% of the total mortality classified either outside the six major categories or as undiagnosed (Vaillancourt et al. 1990). Depending upon the producer's diligence, the proportion of piglets classified in the "other" category may exceed 15% (Nielsen et al. 1974; Dyck et al. 1987) and be as high as 40% (Sharpe 1966). The proportion of total piglet mortality classified as dying from other causes remains relatively stable throughout the suckling period (Vaillancourt 1990); included are skin conditions (exudative epidermitis), nervous problems (myoclonia congenital), and nutritional and metabolic conditions (mulberry heart disease).

REFERENCES

ADILOVIC, S., AND GVOZDENOVIC, M. 1984. The effect of parity on litter size of pigs. Anim Breed Abst 052-00765.

ALLRICH, R. D.; CHRISTENSON, R. K.; AND FORD, J. J. 1985. Age at puberty and estrous activity of straightbred and reciprocal crossbred gilts. Anim Reprod Sci 8:281–286.

ALMOND, G. W., AND DIAL, G. D. 1986a. Pregnancy diagnosis in swine: A comparison of the accuracies of mechanical and endocrine test with return to estrus. J Am Vet Med Assoc 189:1567–1571.

——. 1986b. Pregnancy diagnosis in swine: Principles, application, and accuracy of available techniques. J Am Vet Med Assoc 191:858–870.

ANDERSON, L. L. 1975. Embryonic and placental development during prolonged inanition in the pig. Am J Physiol 229:1687.

ANONYMOUS. 1975. Porcine reproductive inefficiency. Vet Rec 96:506–509.

ARCHIBONG, A. E.; ENGLAND, D. C.; AND STORMSHAK, F. 1987. Factors contributing to early embryonic mortality in gilts bred at first estrus. J. Anim Sci 64:474–478.

AUMAITRE, A. 1971. Mortlite des jeunes dans l'espece porcine. Bull Tech Inf 257:1–5.

——. 1972. Influence de mode de sevrage sur la productivite des truies. 23d Annu Meet EAAP Pig Comm.

AUMAITRE, A., AND DAGORN, J. 1982. Influence of lactation length on reproductive performance of the sow. Ann Zootech 31:431–444.

AUMAITRE, A., AND LEDIVIDICH, J. 1984. Improvement of piglet survival rate in relation to farrowing systems and conditions. Ann Recher Vet 15:173–179.

AUMAITRE, A.; DEGLAIRE, B.; AND LEBOST, J. 1979. Prematurite de la mise bas chez la truie et signification du poids a la naissance du porcelet. Ann Biol Anim Biochem Biophys 19:267–275.

AYLIFFE, T. R.; NOAKES, D. E.; AND SILVA, J. R. 1984.

The effect of experimental induced hypocalcaemia on uterine activity in the sow during parturition and postpartum. Therio 21(5):803–822.

BACKSTROM, L.; MORCKOC, A. C.; CONNOR, J.; et al. 1984. Clinical study of mastitis-metritis-agalactia in sows in Illinois. J Am Ved Med Assoc 185:70–73.

BADOUARD, B.; DAGORN, J.; AND SALAUN, Y. 1984. Performance in 1983. Pt 1. Tech Porc 7(2):27–40.

BAE, G. H., AND PARK, Y. I. 1985. The rate of stillbirths in purebred and crossbred swine in relation to the litter size at birth. Korean J Anim Sci 27(5):253–256.

BARNETT, J. L.; HEMSWORTH, P. H.; WINFIELD, C. G.; AND HANSEN, C. 1986. Effects of social environment on welfare status and sexual behavior of female pigs. I. Effects of group size. Appl Anim Behav Sci 16:249–257.

BARNIKOL, H., AND THALMANN, A. 1988. Clinical observations in swine in association with the mycotoxins ochratoxin A and zearalenone. Tieraerztl Umsch 43(2):74–82.

BENGTSSON, A. C.; FAJERSOON, P.; AND SVENDSEN, J. 1982. Leg injuries of piglets. A comparative study of three types of flooring. Dep Farm Bldg Swedish Univ Agric Sci Rep No 26.

BENJAMINSON, E., AND KARLBERG, K. 1981. Postweaning oestrus and luteal function in primiparous and pluriparous sows. Res Vet Sci 30:318–322.

BICHARD, M. 1983. Litter size and sow productivity. In New Developments in Scientific Breeding, No. 3, Pig Improve Suppl (April) pp. 2–6.

BICHARD, M., AND DAVID, P. J. 1986. Producing more pigs per sow per year – genetic contributions. J Anim Sci 63:1275–1279.

BILLE, N.; NIELSEN, N. C.; LARSEN, J. L.; et al. 1974a. Preweaning mortality in pigs. 2. The perinatal period. Nord Vet Med 26:294–313.

BILLE, N.; NIELSEN, N. C.; AND SVENDSEN, J. 1974b. Preweaning mortality in pigs. 3. Traumatic injuries. Nord Vet Med 26:617–625.

BILLE, N.; LARSEN, J. L.; SVENDSEN, J.; et al. 1975. Preweaning mortality in pigs. 6. Incidence and causes of pneumonia. Nord Vet Med 27:482–495.

BJORKLUND, N. E.; SVENDSEN, J.; AND SVENDSEN, L. S. 1987. Histomorphological studies of the perinatal pig. I. The unaffected pig. Acta Vet Scand 28(1):93–104.

BLACKWELL, T. E. 1987. Predicting stillbirth problems. Compend Cont Educ Pract Vet 9(11):F371–F372, F374.

_____. 1988. Studies on the birthweights of pigs. Ph.D. diss., Univ. of Minnesota.

BLACKWELL, T. E.; WERDIN, R. E.; EISENMENGER, M. C.; AND FITZSIMMONS, M. A. 1989. Goitrogenic effects in offspring of swine fed sulfadimethoxine and ormetoprim in late gestation. J Am Vet Med Assoc 194(4):519–523.

BOLET, G., AND ETIENNE, M. 1982. Relations entre les caracteristiques ponderales et numeriques de la portee et la mortlite du porcelet de la naissance au sevrage. Physiologie et pathologie perinatales chez les animaux de ferme. Proc 14th Journ Grenier Theix, pp. 15–17.

BOURN, P.; CARLSON, R.; LANTZ, B.; AND ZIMMERMAN, D. R. 1974. Age at puberty in gilts as influenced by age at boar exposure and transport. J Anim Sci 39:987.

BRENDEMUHL, J. H.; LEWIS, A. J.; AND PEO, E. R., JR. 1987. Effect of protein and energy intake by primiparous sows during lactation on sow and litter performance and sow serum thyroxine and urea concentrations. J Anim Sci 64:1060–1069.

BRIEF, S., AND CHEW, B. P. 1985. Effects of vitamin A and β-carotene on reproductive performance in gilts. J

Anim Sci 60:998–1004.

BRITT, J. H.; SZAREK, V. E.; AND LEVIS, D. G. 1983. Characterization of summer infertility of sows in large confinement units. Therio 20:133–140.

BRITT, J. H.; ARMSTRONG, J. D.; AND COX, N. M.; et al. 1985. Control of follicular development during and after lactation in sows. J Reprod Fertil [Suppl] 33:37–54.

BROOKS, P. H., AND COLE, D. J. A. 1969. The effect of boar presence on the age at puberty of gilts. Rep Sch Agric Univ Nott 69:74–77.

_____. 1970. The effect of the presence of a boar on the attainment of puberty in gilts. J Reprod Fertil 23:435–440.

_____. 1972. Studies in sow reproduction. 1. The effect of nutrition between weaning and remating on the reproductive performance of primiparous sows. Anim Prod 15:259–264.

_____. 1973. The effect of feed pattern in lactation and fasting following weaning on reproductive phenomena in the sow. Vet Rec 93:276–280.

BROOKS, P. H.; COLE, D. J. A.; ROWLINSON, P.; et al. 1975. Studies in sow reproduction. 3. The effect of nutrition between weaning and remating on the reproductive performance of multiparous sows. Anim Prod 20:407–412.

BROOKS, P. H.; SMITH, D. A.; AND IRWIN, V. C. R. 1977. Biotin-supplementation of diets; the incidence of foot lesions, and the reproductive performance of sows. Vet Rec 101:46–50.

BRUCE, J. M., AND CLARK, J. J. 1979. Models of heat production and critical temperature for growing pigs. Anim Prod 28:353–369.

BUCHANAN, D. S. 1987. The crossbred sire: Experimental results for swine. J Anim Sci 65:117–127.

CATON, J. S.; JESSE, G. W.; DAY, B. N.; AND ELLERSIECK, M. R. 1986. The effect of duration of boar exposure on the frequency of gilts reaching first estrus. J Anim Sci 62:1210–1214.

CAVALCANTI, S., DE S.; MARCHATTI NETO, A.; MOURA, J. C., DE A.; SAMPAIO, I. B. M.; SOUZA CAVALCANTI, S. DE; ANDRADE MOURA, J. C. DE; AND MACHADO SAMPAIO, I. B. 1986. Effects of cloprostenol in association with oxytocin on the induction of parturition in sows. Anim Breed Abst 054-03104.

CHAGNON, M.; DROLET, R.; AND D'ALLAIRE, S. D. 1990. A prospective study of sow mortality in commercial breeding herds. Proc Int Congr Pig Vet Soc, Lausanne, p. 383.

CHANG, K.; KURTZ, H. J.; AND MIROCHA, C. J. 1979. Effects of the mycotoxin Zearalenone on swine reproduction. Am J Vet Res 40:1260–1267.

CHANTARAPRATEEP, P.; PRATEEP, P.; LOHACHIT, C.; POOMSUWAN, P.; AND KUNAVONGKRIT, A. 1986. Investigation into the use of prostaglandin F2 alpha (PGF2 alpha) and oxytocin for the induction of farrowing. Aust Vet J 63(8):254–256.

CHAVEZ, E. R., AND PATTON, K. L. 1986. Response to injectable selenium and Vitamin E on reproductive performance of sows receiving a standard commercial diet. Can J Anim Sci 66:1065.

CHHABRA, A. K.; NIELSEN, H. E.; AND JENSEN, P. 1983. A study on the incidence of stillbirths and abnormalities in Large White Yorkshire litters. Indian Vet J 60(5):405–416.

CHOI, S. A.; MOLITOR, T. W.; JOO, H. S.; AND GUNTHER, R. 1987. Pathogenicity of a skin isolate of porcine parvovirus in swine fetuses. Vet Microbiol 15(1/2):19–29.

CHRISTENSON, R. K. 1981. Influence of confinement and season of the year on puberty and estrous activity of gilts. J Anim Sci 52:821–830.

CHRISTENSON, R. K., AND FORD, J. J. 1979. Puberty and estrus in confinement-reared gilts. J Anim Sci 49:743–751.

CHRISTENSON, R. K., AND HRUSKA, R. L. 1984. Influence of number of gilts per pen on estrous traits in confinement-reared gilts. Therio 22:323–330.

CHRISTENSON, R. K.; TEAGUE, H. S.; AND GRIFO, A. P.; et al. 1972. The effect of high environmental temperature on the boar. Ohio Swine Res Inf Rep RS61–4:19–23.

CHRISTIANSON, W. T.; KIM, H. S.; JOO, H. S.; AND BARNES, D. M. 1990. Reproductive and neonatal losses associated with possible encephalomyocarditis virus infection in swine. Vet Rec 126(3):54–57.

CHRISTISON, G. I.; LEWIS, N. J.; AND BAYNE, G. R. 1987. Effects of farrowing crate floors on health and performance of piglets and sows. Vet Rec 121:37.

CLARK, J. R.; KIMKOV, A.; WIGINTON, L. W.; AND TRIBBLE, L. F. 1986. Time of onset of estrus in gilts. Therio 26(5):639–642.

CLARK, L. K., AND LEMAN, A. D. 1984. The effects of weaning age on subsequent litter size and farrowing rate in a large US confinement herd. Proc Int Congr Pig Vet Soc, Ghent, pp. 357.

_____. 1986. Factors that influence litter size in pigs: Pt 1. Pig News & Inf 7:303–310.

_____. 1987. Factors that influence litter size in swine: Parity 3 through 7 females. J Am Vet Med Assoc 9(1):49–58.

CLARK, L. K.; LEMAN, A. D.; AND MORRIS, R. 1988. Factors influencing litter size in swine: Parity-one females. J Am Vet Med Assoc 192(2):187–194.

CLARK, L. K.; SCHINCKEL, A. P.; SINGLETON, W. L.; EINSTEIN, M. E.; AND TECLAW, R. F. 1989. Use of farrowing rate as a measure of fertility of boars. J Am Vet Med Assoc 194(2):239–242.

CLAUS, R.; SCHELKLE, G.; AND WEILER, U. 1984. Erste Versuche zur Verbesserung der Fruchtbarkeitslage von Sauen im Sommer durch ein Lichtprogramm. Zuchthyg 19:49–56.

CLAUS, R.; WEILER, U.; AND WAGNER, H.-G. 1985. Photoperiodic influences on reproduction of domestic boars. II. Light influences on semen characteristics and libido. Zentralbl Vet Med [A] 32:99–109.

COLE, D. J. A. 1990. Nutritional strategies to optimize reproduction in pigs. J Reprod Fertil [Suppl] 40:67–82.

COLE, D. J. A.; VARLEY, M. A.; AND HUGHES, P. E. 1975. Studies in sow reproduction. 2. The effect of lactation length on the subsequent reproductive performance of the sow. Anim Prod 20:401–406.

CONNAUGHTON, I. D.; DRIESEN, S. J.; WILLIAMSON, P. L.; et al. 1985. The pale pig syndrome. Aust Adv Vet Sci 120–121.

COX, N. M.; BRITT, J. H.; ARMSTRONG, W. D.; et al. 1983. Effect of feeding fat and altered weaning schedule on rebreeding in primiparous sows. J Anim Sci 56:21–29.

CURTIS, S. E. 1970. Environmental thermoregulatory interactions and neonatal piglet survival. J Anim Sci 31:576–587.

_____. 1974. Responses of the piglet to perinatal stressors. J Anim Sci 38:1031–1036.

CURTIS, S. E.; HURST, R. J.; WIDOWSKI, T. M.; et al. 1989. Effects of sow-crate design on health and performance of sows and piglets. J Anim Sci 67:80–93.

DAGORN, J., AND AUMAITRE, A. 1979. Sow culling: Reasons for and effect on productivity. Livest Prod Sci 6:167–177.

D'ARCE, R. D.; TEAGUE, H. S.; ROLLER, W. L.; et al. 1970. Effect of short-term elevated dry-bulb and dew-point temperature on the cycling gilt. J Anim Sci 30:374–377.

DASILVA-FILHO, J. M., AND MONTEIRO DASILVA-FILHO, J. 1984. A comparative study of induction of parturition by means of PGF2 alpha and cloprostenol administered by different routes in different doses. Effects on piglet performance at weaning and on sow performance at the subsequent farrowing. Arq Bras Med Vet Zootec 38(1):83–90.

DECHAMPS, P., AND NICKS, B. 1984. Influence de parametres non-infecteux et plus particulierement du confort thermique sur la viabilite et la vitalite des porcelets en maternite. Ann Med Vet 128:261–283.

DE LA FARGE, B. 1981. Climatisation des porcheries. Troisieme partie: Le chauffage. Tech Porc 4:44.

DE LA FARGE, B., AND CHOSSON, B. 1979. La climatisation des porcheries. Deuxieme partie: Le chauffage et la ventilation. Tech Porc 2:4.

DEN HARTOG, L. A., AND VAN KEMPEN, G. J. M. 1980. Relationship between nutrition and fertility in pigs. Neth J Agric Sci 28:211–227.

DEROTH, L., AND DOWNIE, H. G. 1976. Evaluation of viability of neonatal swine. Can Vet J 17:275–279.

DESA, W. F.; PLEUMSAMRAN, P.; MORCOM, C. B.; et al. 1981. Exogenous steroid effects on litter size and early embryonic survival in swine. Therio 15:245–255.

DESMECHT, M., AND CASTRYCK, F. 1984. A case of Leptospira interrogans serovar pomona infection in pigs. Vlaam Diergeneeskd Tijdschr 53(4):335–342.

DIAL, G. D. 1984. Seasonal and environmental influences on swine reproduction. Comp Cont Educ Pract Vet 6(9):528–534.

_____. 1986. Parturition induction of swine: Practical application and relative efficacies of pharmaceuticals for induced farrowing in commercial herds. Proc Upjohn Symp Swine Herd Health, Stratford, Ontario, pp. 1–13.

DIAL, G. D., AND BEVIER, G. W. 1987. Noninfectious causes of reproductive failure in the female pig. In Fertility and Infertility in Veterinary Practice. London: Bailliere-Tindall, pp. 120–139.

DIAL G. D., AND MACLACHLAN, N. J. 1988a. Urogenital infections of swine. Pt I. Clinical manifestations and pathogenesis. Compend Cont Educ Pract Vet 10(1):63–69.

_____. 1988b. Urogenital infections of swine. Part II. Pathology and medical management. Compend Cont Educ Pract Vet 10(4):529–538.

DIAL, G. D.; HILLEY, H. D.; AND ESBENSHADE, K. L. 1986. Sexual development and initiation of puberty in the pig. In Current Therapy in Therio 2. Ed. D. A. Morrow. Philadelphia: Saunders, pp. 901–905.

DIAL, G. D.; MATTIOLI, M.; AND SEREN, E. 1987. Pathophysiology of the seasonal reproduction of domestic swine. Zootech Nutr Anim 13:399–406.

DIAL, G. D.; BUTLER, W. R.; GARCIA, M. C.; MARTIN, P. A.; KEISTER, D. M.; MEO, N. J.; AND GATHEIL, R. F. 1990. Relationship between farrowing parameters and piglet survival. Proc Int Congr Pig Vet Soc, Lausanne, p. 445.

DIEKMAN, M. A., AND GRIEGER, D. M. 1988. Influence of varying intensities of supplemental lighting during decreasing daylengths on puberty in gilts. Anim Reprod Sci 16:295–301.

DIEKMAN, M. A., AND HOAGLAND, T. A. 1983. Influence of supplemental lighting during periods of increasing or decreasing daylength on the onset of puberty in gilts. J Anim Sci 57:1235–1242.

DOBOA, M. T.; RODRIGANEA, J.; AND SILIO, L. 1983. Seasonal influence on fecundity and litter performance characteristics in Iberian pigs. Livest Prod Sci 10:601–610.

DOMINICK, M. A., AND CARSON, T. L. 1983. Effects of carbon monoxide exposure on pregnant sows and their fetuses. Am J Vet Res 44:35–40.

DYCK, G. W. 1988. Factors influencing sexual maturation, puberty and reproductive efficiency in the gilt. Can J Anim Sci 68(1):1–13.

DYCK, G. W., AND SWEISTRA, E. E. 1987. Causes of piglet death from birth to weaning. Can J Anim Sci 67(2):543–547.

DZIUK, P. J. 1970. Estimation of the optimum time for insemination of gilts and ewes by double-mating at certain times relative to ovulation. J Reprod Fertil 22:277–282.

EASTHAM, P. R., AND COLE, D. J. A. 1987. Reproduction in the gilt. 7. Exposure of young gilts to the same mature boar and relocation: Effects on the attainment of puberty. Anim Prod 44:435–441.

EDWARDS, R. L.; OMTVEDT, I. T.; TURMAN, E. J.; AND STEPHENS, D. F.; et al. 1968. Reproductive performance of gilts following heat stress prior to breeding and in early gestation. J Anim Sci 27:1634–1637.

EDWARDS, S.; CANTLEY, T. C.; AND DAY, B. N. 1987. The effects of zearalenone on reproduction in swine. II. The effect on puberty attainment and postweaning rebreeding performance. Therio 28(1)51–58.

EDWARDS, S. A., AND FURNISS, S. J. 1988. The effects of straw in crated farrowing systems on peripartal behaviour of sows and piglets. Br Vet J 144:139–146.

EDWARDS, S. A.; MALKIN, S. J.; AND SPECHTER, H. H. 1986. An analysis of piglet mortality with behavioural observations. Br Soc Anim Prod, Paper No. 126.

EGBUNIKE, G. N. 1982. Sire effect on conception rate and litter size in a hot humid environment. Z Tierz Zuchtungsbiol 99:18–25.

ELEFTHERIOU, E. S. 1980. Researches in the artificial insemination of pigs, farrowing rate of pigs inseminated once or twice in the same oestrus. Center of Artificial Insemination and Diseases of Reproduction.

ELLIS, W. A.; MCPARLAND, P. J.; BRYSON, G.; AND MCNULTY, M. S. 1985. Leptospires in pig urogenital tracts and fetuses. Vet Rec 117:66–67.

ELLIS, W. A.; MCPARLAND, P. J.; BRYSON, G.; THIERMANN, A. B.; AND MONTGOMERY, J. 1986a. Isolation of leptospires from the genital tract and kidneys of aborted sows. Vet Rec 118:294–295.

ELLIS, W. A.; MCPARLAND, P. J.; BRYSON, D. G.; AND CASSELLS, J. A. 1986b. Prevalence of *Leptospira* infection in aborted pigs in Northern Ireland. Vet Rec 118(3):63–65.

ELZE, K. 1985. Correlation between perinatal piglet losses and parturition and puerperium. Monatsh Veterinarmed 40(23):811–814.

ENGLAND, D. C. 1974. Husbandry components in prenatal and perintal development in swine. J Anim Sci 38:1045–1049.

———. 1986. Improving sow efficiency by management to enhance opportunity for nutritional intake by neonatal piglets. J Anim Sci 63:1297–1306.

ENGLAND, D. C., AND SPURR, D. T. 1969. Litter size of swine confined during gestation. J Anim Sci 28:220–223.

ENGLISH, P. R., AND BRAMPTON, P. R. 1978. The importance of within-litter variation in piglet birthweight in relation to piglet survival and the influence of cross-fostering simultaneously farrowed litter so as to achieve more uniform birthweights within litters. Proc Int Congr Pig Vet Soc, Zagreb, p. 248.

ENGLISH, P. R., AND MORRISON, V. 1984. Causes and prevention of piglet mortality. Pig News & Inf 5:369–375.

ENGLISH, P. R., AND SMITH, W. J. 1975. Some causes of death in neonatal piglets. Vet Annu 15:95–104.

ENGLISH, P. R., AND WILKINSON, V. 1982. Management of the sow and litter in later pregnancy and lactation in relation to piglet survival and growth. In Control of Pig Reproduction. Ed. D. J. A. Cole and G. R. Foxcroft. London: Butterworth Scientific, pp. 479–506.

ENGLISH, P. R.; DIAS, M. F. M.; AND BAMPTON, P. R. 1982. Evaluation of an improved design of farrowing crate, incorporating a farrowing cradle, designed to reduce the incidence of overlying of newly born piglets. Proc 7th Int Congr Pig Vet Soc, Mexico City, p. 308.

FAHMY, M. H., AND BERNARD, C. 1971. Causes of mortality in Yorkshire pigs from birth to 20 weeks of age. Can J Anim Sci 51:351–359.

FAHMY, M. H., AND DUFOUR, J. J. 1976. Effects of postweaning stress and feeding management on return to estrus and reproductive traits during early pregnancy in swine. Anim Prod 23:103–110.

FAHMY, M. H.; HOLTMANN, W. B.; MACINTYRE, M.; et al. 1978. Evaluation of piglet mortality in 28 two-breed crosses among eight breeds of pigs. Anim Prod 26:277–285.

FAHMY, M. H.; HOLTMANN, W. B.; AND BAKER, R. D. 1979. Failure to recycle after weaning, and weaning to oestrus interval in crossbred sows. Anim Prod 29:193–202.

FARMER, C., AND CHRISTISON, G. 1982. Selection of perforated floors by newborn and weanling pigs. Can J Anim Sci 62:1229–1236.

FERGURSON, P. W.; HARVEY, W. R.; AND INVIN, K. M. 1985. Genetic phenotypic and environmental relationship between sow body weight and sow productivity traits. J Anim Sci 60:375–384.

FERKET, S. L., AND HACKER, R. R. 1985. Effect of forced exercise during gestation on reproductive performance of sows. Can J Anim Sci 65(4):851–859.

FLINT, A. P. F.; SAUNDERS, P. T. K.; AND ZIECIK, A. J. 1982. Blastocyst-endometrium interactions and their significance in embryonic mortality. In Control of Pig Reproduction. Ed. D. J. A. Cole and G. R. Foxcroft. London: Butterworth Scientific, pp. 253–275.

FLOWERS, B.; CANTLEY, T. C.; MARTIN; M. J.; DAY, B. N. 1989. Effect of elevated ambient temperatures on puberty in gilts. J Anim Sci 67:779–784.

FONSECA, N. A. N.; MILAGRES, J. C.; MELLO, H. V., DE; LUDWIG, A.; VAZ-DE-MELLO, H. 1988. Productivity of crossbred sows in a commercial herd at Jequeri, Minas Gerais. 4. Mortality. Rev Soc Bras Zootec 17(1):92–99.

FORD, J. J., AND TEAGUE, H. S. 1978. Effect of floor space restriction on age at puberty in gilts and on performance of barrows and gilts. J Anim Sci 47:828–832.

FOXCROFT, G. R., AND VAN DE WIEL, D. F. M. 1982. Endocrine control of the oestrous cycle. In Control of Pig Reproduction. Ed. D. J. A. Cole and G. R. Foxcroft. London: Butterworth Scientific, pp. 161–178.

FRANTZ, J. C. 1987. Historical review of *Leptospira bratislava* and association to disease. Annu Meet Am Assoc Swine Pract 77–84.

FRANTZ, J. C.; HANSON, L. E.; AND BROWN, A. L. 1979. Effect of vaccination with a bacterin containing *Leptospira interrogans* serovar *bratislava* on the breeding performance of swine herds. Am J Vet Res 50(7):1044–1047.

FRASER, D., AND CONNOR, M. L. 1984. Effect of dosage of cloprostenol on induction of farrowing and body temperature of sows. Can Vet J 25(11):421–423.

FRASER, D., AND LIN, C. S. 1984. An attempt to estimate teat quality of sows by hand milking during farrowing. Can J Anim Sci 64:165–170.

FRASER, D., AND THOMPSON, B. K. 1986. Variation in

piglet weight: Relationship to suckling behavior, parity number and farrowing crate design. Can J Anim Sci 66:31–46.

FRASER, D.; PHILLIPS, P. A.; AND THOMPSON, B. K. 1988. Initial test of a farrowing crate with inward-sloping sides. Livest Prod Sci 20(3):249–256.

FRENCH, L. R.; RUTLEDGE, J. J.; AND FIRST, N. L. 1979. Effect of age and parity on litter size in pigs. J Reprod Fertil 57:59–60.

FRIEND, D. W., AND ELLIOT, J. I. 1981. Drop farrowing as an aid to sow management. Can J Anim Sci 61:1071–1074.

FRIENDSHIP, R. M., AND WILSON, M. R. 1985. Piglet blood glutathione peroxidase levels and preweaning mortality. Can J Comp Med 49:311–314.

FRIENDSHIP, R. M.; WILSON, M. R.; AND McMILLAN, I. 1986. Management and housing factors associated with piglet preweaning mortality. Can Vet J 27(8):307–311.

GADEK, B. 1984. Influence of mycotoxins on pregnancy and lactation in the sow. Tieraerztl Umsch 39(6):461–469.

GLASTONBURY, J. R. W. 1976. A survey of preweaning mortality in pigs. Aust Vet J 52:272–276.

———. 1977a. Preweaning mortality in the pig. Pathological findings in piglets dying between birth and weaning. Aust Vet J 53:310–314.

———. 1977b. Preweaning mortality in the pig. The prevalence of various causes of preweaning mortality and the importance of some contributory factors. Aust Vet J 53:315–318.

———. 1977c. Preweaning mortality in the pig: Pathological findings in piglets dying before and during parturition. Aust Vet J 53:282–286.

GOURREAU, J. M.; KAISER, C.; MADEC, F.; LABIE, J.; VANNIER, P.; AYMARD, M.; VIGOUROUX, A.; AND SALINGARDES, F. 1985. Transplacental passage of influenza virus in the sow under natural conditions. Pig News & Inf 006–01725.

GREENBERG, L. G., AND MAHONE, J. P. 1982. Failure of a 15 h L:8 h D or an 8 h L:16 h D photoperiod to influence lactation or reproductive efficiency in sows. Can J Anim Sci 62:141–145.

GRONDALEN, T.; LIVEN, E.; DJONNE, B. K.; GJESTVANG, M. S.; JAEGER, G.; AND UTKLEV, H. E. 1986. Piglet production and mortality in thirteen Norwegian herds. Nor Veterinaertidskr 98(9):611–622.

GUSTAFSON, D. P. 1986. Pseudorabies. In Diseases of Swine, 6th ed. Ed. A. D. Leman, B. Straw, R. D. Glock, W. L. Mengeling, R. H. C. Penny, and E. Scholl. Ames: Iowa State Univ Press, pp. 274–289.

HANSEN, L. L., AND VESTERGAARD, K. 1984. Tethered versus loose sows: Ethological observations and measures of productivity. II. Production results. Ann Rech Vet 15(2):185–191.

HANSEN, L. L., VESTERGAARD, K., LYDEHOF-HANSEN, L. 1986. Behaviour and production of tethered and loose-housed sows. 2. Productivity and health. Dansk Veterinaertidsskr 69(6):319–331.

HARTSOCK, T. G., AND GRAVES, H. B. 1976. Neonatal behavior and nutrition-related mortality in domestic swine. J Anim Sci 42:235–241.

HARTSOCK, T. G.; GRAVES, H. B.; AND BAUMGARDT, B. R. 1977. Agonistic behavior and the nursing order in suckling piglets: Relationships with survival, growth and body composition. J Anim Sci 44:320–330.

HATHAWAY, S. C. 1985. Porcine leptospirosis. Pig News & Inf 6(1):31–34.

HATHAWAY, S. C.; LITTLE, T. W. A.; AND WRATHALL, A. E. 1983. Experimental infection of pregnant gilts with leptospires isolated from British wildlife. I. Sero-

logical response to infection. II. Clinical, bacteriological and pathological aspects of infection. British Vet J 139(5):393–414.

HEMSWORTH, P. H.; SALDEN, N. T. C. J.; AND HOOGERBRUGGE, A. 1982. The influence of the postweaning social environment on the weaning to mating interval of the sow. Anim Prod 35:41–48.

HEMSWORTH, P. H.; WINFIELD, C. G.; AND HANSEN, C. 1983. High mating frequency for boars: Predicting the effects on sexual behavior, fertility and fecundity. Anim Prod 37:409–413.

HEMSWORTH, P. H.; CRONIN, G. M.; HANSEN, C.; AND WINFIELD, C. G. 1984. The effects of two oestrus detection procedures and intense boar stimulation near the time of oestrus on mating efficiency of the female pig. Appl Anim Behav Sci 12:339–347.

HEMSWORTH, P. H.; BARNETT, J. L.; HANSEN, C.; AND WINFIELD, C. G. 1986. Effects of social environment on welfare status and sexual behaviour of female pigs. II. Effects of space allowance. Appl Anim Behav Sci 16:259–267.

HEMSWORTH, P. H.; WINFIELD, C. G.; BARNETT, J. L.; HANSEN, C.; SCHIRMER, B.; AND FOOTE, M. 1987. The efficiency of boars to detect oestrous females housed adjacent to boars. Appl Anim Behav Sci 19:81–87.

HEMSWORTH, P. H.; WINFIELD, C. G.; TILBROOK, A. J.; HANSEN, C.; AND BARNETT, J. L. 1988. Habituation to boar stimuli: Possible mechanism responsible for the reduced detection rate of oestrous gilts housed adjacent to boars. Appl Anim Behav Sci 19:255–264.

HEMSWORTH, P. H.; HANSEN, C.; AND WINFIELD, C. G. 1989. The influence of mating conditions on the sexual behaviour of male and female pigs. Appl Anim Behav Sci 23:207–214.

HENDRIX, W. F.; KELLEY, K. W.; GASKINS, C. T.; et al. 1978. Porcine neonatal survival and serum gammaglobulins. J Anim Sci 47:1281–1286.

HENRY, S. C. 1984. Use of A. I. in double mating – a farm experience. Proc Am Assoc Swine Pract, Kansas City, Missouri, p. 173.

HILLEY, H. D.; DIAL, G. D.; HAGAN, J.; et al. 1986a. Influence of the number of services and season on the litter size and farrowing rate of primiparous sows. Proc Int Congr Pig Vet Soc, Barcelona, p. 23.

HILLEY, H. D.; DIAL, G. D.; HAGAN, J.; et al. 1986b. The influence of parity, season of the year, number of matings, and previous lactation length on the number of pigs born alive to multiparous sows. Proc Int Congr Pig Vet Soc, Barcelona, p. 24.

HILLEY, H. D.; DIAL, G. D.; HAGAN, J.; AND ALMOND, G. W. 1986c. Influence of breeding practices on litter sizes and farrowing rate. Proc Am Assoc Swine Pract, Minneapolis, p. 303.

HOLTZ, W. 1981/1982. Pregnancy detection in swine by pulse mode ultrasound. Anim Reprod Sci 4:219–226.

HORUGEL, K.; GARNTER, H.; AND SCHLEGEL, W. 1986. Effect of selected endogenous factors on piglet birth weight and their interactions. Monatsh Veterinarmed 41(4):121–126.

HOSMAN, L. 1971. Prispevek ke studiu chovnai prasnic pri starbe hnizda. Sb Vys Sk Zemed 484:87–208.

HSU, F. S.; CHU, R. M.; LEE, R. C. T.; AND CHU, S. H. J. 1980. Placental lesions by pseudorabies virus in pregnant sows. J Am Vet Med Assoc 177:636–641.

HUGHES, P. E. 1982. Factors affecting the natural attainment of puberty in the gilt. In Control of Pig Reproduction. Ed. D. J. A. Cole and G. R. Foxcroft. London: Butterworth Scientific, pp. 117–138.

———. 1989. A symposium – nutrition, reproduction interactions in the breeding sow. Manipulating Pig Prod II, pp. 277–280.

HUGHES, P. E., AND COLE, D. J. A. 1976. Reproduction in the gilt. 2. The influence of gilt age at boar introduction on the attainment of puberty. Anim Prod 23:89–94.

HUNNEMAN, W. A. 1978. Diarrhee bij biggen in de eerste 4 levensweken. De Trogge 19:3–6.

HUNTER, R. H. F. 1977. Physiological factors influencing ovulation, fertilization, early embryonic development and establishment of pregnancy in pigs. Br Vet J 133:461–468.

HURTGEN, J. P., AND LEMAN, A. D. 1980. Seasonal influence on the fertility of sows and gilts. J Am Vet Med Assoc 177:631–635.

HURTGEN, J. P.; LEMAN, A. D.; AND CRABO, B. 1980. Seasonal influence on estrous activity in sows and gilts. J Am Vet Med Assoc 176:119–123.

IGLESIAS, J. G., AND HARKNESS, J. W. 1988. Studies of transplacental and perinatal infection with two clones of a single Aujeszky's disease (pseudorabies) virus isolate. Vet Microbiol 16:243–254.

IRGANG, R., AND ROBINSON, O. W. 1984. Heritability estimates for ages at farrowing, rebreeding interval and litter traits in swine. J Anim Sci 59:67–73.

ISHII, Y. 1981. Lactation and ovulation in the pig. Jpn J Anim Reprod 27(5):44–48.

JACKSON, P. G. G. 1975. The incidence of stillbirth in cases of dystocia in sows. Vet Rec 97:411–412.

JIKEN, J. R., AND TOO, H. L. 1988. The influence of induced and supervised parturitions on neonatal piglet survival. Am Breeding Abst 056–03795.

JOHNSON, R. K. 1981a. Crossbreeding in swine: Experimental results. J Anim Sci 52:906–923.

_____. 1981b. Effect of crossbred boars on reproductive efficiency. Proc Am Pork Congr, Kansas City, Missouri, pp. 5–7.

JOHNSTON, L. J.; FOGWELL, R. L.; WELDON, W. C.; AMES, N. K.; ULLREY, D. E.; AND MILLER, E. R. 1989. Relationship between body fat and postweaning interval to estrus in primiparous sows. J Anim Sci 67:943–950.

JOO, H. S.; DEE, S. A.; MOLITOR, T. W.; AND THACKER, B. J. 1984. In utero infection of swine fetuses with infectious bovine rhinotracheitis virus (bovine herpesvirus-1). Am J Vet Res 45(10):1924–1927.

JOO, H. S.; KIM, H. S.; AND LEMAN, A. D. 1988. Detection of antibody to encephalomyocarditis virus in mummified or stillborn pigs. Arch Virol 100(1–2):131–134.

KACZMARCZYK, J.; KLOCEK, C.; AND MIGDAL, W. 1987. Course of parturition in sows kept in farrowing pens of three types: Meprozet, Ml-K Technirol and Olszanicki. Zesz Nauk Akad Roln Hug Kollat Krakow Zootechn 25:57–75.

KALASHNIK, B. A., AND GRUTSEVA, O. I. 1988. Natural and Induced Parturition in Sows. 1989 Anim Breed Abstr 057–07356.

KALINOWSKI, J., AND CHAVEZ, E. R. 1986. Low dietary zinc intake during pregnancy and lactation of gilts. 2. Effects on offspring. Can J Anim Sci 66(1):217–227.

KARLBERG, K.; REIN, K. A.; AND NORDSTOGA, K. 1981. Histological and bacteriological examination of uterus from the repeat breeder gilt and sow. Nord Vet Med 33:359–365.

KELLEY, K. W.; BLECHA, F.; AND REGNIER, J. A. 1982. Cold exposure and absorption of colostral immunoglobulins by neonatal pigs. J Anim Sci 55:363–368.

KENNEDY, B. W., AND MOXLEY, J. E. 1978. Genetic and environmental factors influencing litter size, sex ratio and gestational length in the pig. Anim Prod 27:35–42.

KENNELLY, J. J.; BALL, R. O.; AND AHERNE, F. X. 1979. Influence of porcine immunoglobulin administration

on survival and growth of pigs weaned at two and three weeks of age. Can J Anim Sci 59:693–698.

KING, R. H. 1987. Nutritional anoestrus in young sows. Pig News & Inf 8:1.

KING, R. H., AND WILLIAMS, I. H. 1984a. The effect of nutrition on the reproductive performance of first-litter sows. 1. Feeding level during lactation, and between weaning and remating. Anim Prod 36:241–247.

_____. 1984b. The effect of nutrition on the reproductive performance of first-litter sows 2. Protein and energy intakes during lactation. Anim Prod 38:249–256.

KINGSCOTE, B. F. 1986. Leptospirosis outbreak in a piggery in southern Alberta. Can Vet J 27(4):188–190.

KIRCHGESSNER, M.; MADER, H.; AND GRASSMAN, E. 1980. Zur Fruchtbarkeitsleistung von Saven bei unterschiedlicher Cu-Versorgung. Zuechtungskd 52:46.

KIRKWOOD, R. N.; AND HUGHES, P. E. 1979. The influence of age at first boar contact on puberty attainment in the gilt. Anim Prod 29:231–238.

_____. 1980. A note on the efficacy of continuous v. limited boar exposure on puberty attainment in the gilt. Anim Prod 31:205–207.

_____. 1981. A note on the influence of boar age on its ability to advance puberty in the gilt. Anim Prod 32:211–213.

KIRKWOOD, R. N., AND THACKER, P. A. 1988. Nutritional factors affecting embryo survival in pigs (results and speculations). Pig News & Inf 9:1.

KIRKWOOD, R. N.; HUGHES, P. E.; AND BOOTH, W. D. 1983. The influence of boar-related odours on puberty attainment in gilts. Anim Prod 36:131–136.

KIRKWOOD, R. N.; MOLLER, K.; SMITH, W. C.; LAPWOOD, K. R.; AND GARRICK, D. J. 1985. The influence of allyl trenbolone (Regumate) on the timing, duration and endocrinology of parturition in sows. Anim Reprod Sci 9(2):163–171.

KIRKWOOD, R. N.; BAIDOO, S. K.; AHERNE, F. X.; AND SATHER, A. P. 1987. The influence of feeding level during lactation on the occurrence and endocrinology of the postweaning estrus in sows. Can J Anim Sci 67:405–415.

KIRKWOOD, R. N.; MITARU, B. N.; GOONERATNE, A. D.; BLAIR, R.; AND THACKER, P. A. 1988. The influence of dietry energy intake during successive lactations on sow prolificacy. Can J Anim Sci 68(1):283–290.

KLUGE, J. P., AND MARE, C. J. 1974. Swine pseudorabies: Abortion, clinical disease, and lesions in pregnant gilts infected with pseudorabies virus (Aujeszky's Disease). Am J Vet Res 35:911–915.

KNABE, D. A.; PRINCE, T. J.; AND ORR, D. E. 1986. Effect of feed and(or) water deprivation prior to weaning on reproductive performance of sows: A cooperative study. J Anim Sci 62:1–8.

KNIGHT, J. W.; BAZER, F. W.; THATCHER, W. W.; FRANKE, D. E.; AND WALLACE, H. D. 1977. Conceptus development in intact and unilaterally hysterectomized gilts: Interrelationship among hormonal status, placental development, fetal fluids and fetal growth. J Anim Sci 44:620–627.

KO, J. C. H.; EVANS, L. E.; HSU, W. H.; AND HOPKINS, S. M. 1989. Farrowing induction with cloprostenol-xylazine combination. Therio 31(4):795–800.

KOCWIN-PODSIADLA, M.; PIECH, H.; CHRZANOWSKA, M.; POLAKOWSKA, E.; AND PALKA, B. 1988. Time of transfer to a farrowing shed of pregnant sows and their biochemical and physiological response. Anim Breed Abst 056–00898.

KORNEGAY, E. T. 1986. Biotin in swine nutrition: A review. Livest Prod Sci 14:65–89.

KORNEGAY, E. T., AND KITE, B. 1983. Phosphorus in

swine. IV. Utilization of nitrgoen, calcium, and phosphorus and reproductive performance of gravid gilts fed two dietary phosphorus levels for five parities. J Anim Sci 57:1463-1469.

KORNEGAY, E. T., AND LINDEMANN, M. D. 1984. Floor surface and flooring materials for pigs. Pig News & Inf 5:351-357.

KORNEGAY, E. T., AND THOMAS, H. R. 1983. Effects of air-conditioned versus naturally ventilated housing during hot weather on the reproductive efficiency of gilts or sows. Livest Prod Sci 10:387-395.

KORNEGAY, E. T.; THOMAS, H. R.; AND MEACHAM, T. N. 1973. Evaluation of dietary calcium and phosphorus for reproducing sows housed in total confinement on concrete or in dirt lots. J Anim Sci 37:493.

KOSZTOLICH, O., AND MAYRHOFER, G. 1983. Zusammenhange zwischen Ostruseintritt und Fruchtbarkeit beim Folgewurf in der Schweinezucht. Wien Tieraerztl Monatsschr 70(11):358-360.

KUHN, M., AND WESEMEIER, H. 1987. Morphology of the liver of retarded and stillborn piglets. 3. Causes of intrauterine growth retardation and fetal death. Arch Exp Veterinarmed 41(2):271-275.

KUNAVONGKRIT, A.; ROJANASTHIEN, S.; AND OGLE, R. B. 1985. Effect of fractionated weaning on hormonal patterns and weaning to oestrus interval in sows. Swed J Agric Res 15:39-44.

LAUTERBACH, K.; KOLB, E.; GERISCH, V.; GRUNDEL, G.; SCHINEFF, C.; AND SCHMIDT, U. 1987. Content of haemoglobin in blood and glucose, lactate and free fatty acids in blood plasma of stillborn piglets of varying birth weights. Arch Exp Veterinarmed, 41(4):522-530.

LEMAN, A. D.; GREENLEY, W.; AND BARRICK, E. R. 1984. Observations on boar fertility. Proc Am Assoc Swine Pract, Kansas City, p. 161.

LEMAN, A. D.; FRASER, D.; AND GREENLEY, W. 1988. Factors influencing farrowing rate in confined Large White × Landrace sows. Proc Int Congr Pig Vet Soc, Rio de Janeiro, p. 288.

LEMAN, A.; FRASER, D.; AND GREENLEY, W. 1990. Factor affecting non-productive sow days. Proc Int Congr Pig Vet Soc, Lausanne, p. 378.

LEVIS, D. G. 1986. Reproductive management of the boar. Proc George A. Young Swine Conf, pp. 1-13.

———. 1988. Designing an efficient breeding area. Proc George A. Young Swine Conf, pp. 79-90.

LINDEMANN, M. D., AND KORNEGAY, E. T. 1987. Folic acid supplementation to diets of gestating/lactating swine. Va Tech Livest Res Rep, pp. 35-37.

LINKS, I. J.; WHITTINGTON, R. J.; KENNEDY, D. J.; GREWAL, A.; AND SHARROCK, A. J. 1986. An association between encephalomyocarditis virus infection and reproductive failure in pigs. Aust Vet J 63(5):150-152.

LIPTRAP, D. O.; ZAVOS, P. M.; AND REESE, D. E. 1983. The influence of the boar on farrowing rate and litter size. Univ Kentucky Swine Res Prog Rep 274:52-53.

LITTLEJOHNS, I. R. 1984. Encephalomyocarditis virus from stillborn pigs. Aust Vet J 61(3):93.

LONG, G. G.; DIEKMAN, M. A.; TUITE, J. F.; et al. 1982. Effect of Fusarium roseum corn culture containing zearalenone on early pregnancy in swine. Am J Vet Res 43:1599-1603.

LONG, G. G.; DIEKMAN, M. A.; TUITE, J. F.; SHANNON, G. M.; AND VESONDER, R. F. 1983. Effect of *Fusarium roseum* (*Gibberella zea*) on pregnancy and the estrous cycle in gilts fed molded corn on days 7-17 post-estrus. Vet Res Comm 6:199-204.

LOVE, R. J. 1981. Seasonal infertility in pigs. Vet Rec 109:407-409.

LYNCH, P. B. 1989. Voluntary food intake of sows and

gilts. Brit Soc Anim Prod 71-77.

LYNCH, P. B., AND KEARNEY, P. A. 1987. Seasonal patterns of sow fertility in Ireland. Anim Breed Abstr 055-07756.

LYNCH, P. B.; KEARNEY, P. A.; AND O'GRADY, J. F. 1982. What influences birth weight of piglets? Anim Breed Abstr 50:6428.

LYNCH, P. B.; O'GRADY, J. F.; AND KEARNEY, P. A. 1984. Effect of housing system on sow productivity. Ann Rech Vet 15(2):181-184.

MABRY, J. W.; JONES, R. D.; AND SEERLEY, W. 1982a. Effect of adaptation of a solid-floor farrowing facility utilizing elevated farrowing crates. J Anim Sci 55:484-488.

MABRY, J. W.; CUNNINGHAM, F. L.; KRAELING, R. R.; AND RAMPACEK, G. B. 1982b. The effect of artificially extended photoperiod during lactation on maternal performance of the Sow. J Anim Sci 54(5):918-921.

MCGLONE, J. J.; STANSBURY, W. F.; AND TRIBBLE, L. F. 1988. Management of lactating sows during heat stress: Effects of water drip, snout coolers, floor type and a high energy-density diet. J Anim Sci 66:885-891.

MACLEAN, C. W. 1969. Observations on noninfectious infertility in swine. Vet Rec 85:675-682.

MCNITT, J. I., AND FIRST, N. L. 1970. Effects of 72-hour heat stress on semen quality in boars. Int J Biometeorol 14:373-380.

MACPHERSON, R. M.; HOVELL, F. D. DEB; JONES, A. S. 1977. Performance of sows first mated at puberty or second or third oestrus, and carcass assessment of once-bred gilts. Anim Prod 24:333-342.

MADEC, F.; JOSSE, J.; AND CHARIOLET, R. 1984. Influence des conditions de milieu sur la sante et les performances du porcelet sous la mere. Physiol Pathol 439-448.

MAHAN, D. C. 1990. Mineral nutrition of the sow: A review. J Anim Sci 68:573-582.

MAHAN, D. C., AND FETTER, A. W. 1982. Dietary calcium and phosphorus levels for reproducing sows. J Anim Sci 54:285-291.

MAHAN, D. C.; PENHALE, L. H.; CLINE, J. H.; MOXON, A. L.; FETTER, A. W.; AND YARRINGTON, J. T. 1974. Efficacy of supplemental selenium in reproductive diets on sow and progeny performance. J Anim Sci 39:536.

MARCATTI, A.; BARBOSA, A. S.; SILVA, I. J.; et al. 1986. Cross-fostered effects on the performance of suckling piglets. Proc Int Congr Pig Vet Soc, Barcelona, p. 61.

MARTIN, M. J.; MEISINGER, T. C.; FLOWERS, W. L.; CANTLEY, T. C.; AND DAY, B. N. 1985. Parturition control in sows with a prostaglandin analogue (alfaprostol). Therio 24(1):13-19.

MARTIN, R. E., AND CRENSHAW, T. D. 1989. Effect of postnatal nutrition status on subsequent growth and reproductive performance of gilts. J Anim Sci 67:975-982.

MARTINAT-BOTTE, F.; DAGORN, J.; TERQUI, M.; et al. 1984. Effect of confinement, climatic conditions and litter parity on the seasonal variations of the fertility rate and prolificacy. Ann Rech Vet 15:165-172.

MAURER, R. R.; FORD, J. J.; AND CHRISTIANSON, R. K. 1985. Interval to first postweaning estrus and causes for leaving the breeding herd in Large White, Landrace, Yorkshire, and Chester White females after three parities. J Anim Sci 61:1327-1334.

MAVROGENIS, A. P., AND ROBISON, O. W. 1976. Factors affecting puberty in swine. J Anim Sci 42:1251-1255.

MENGELING, W. L. 1979. Prenatal infection following maternal exposure to porcine parvovirus on either the seventh or fourteenth day of gestation. Can J Comp Med 43:106-109.

_____. 1986. Porcine parvovirus. In Diseases of Swine. Ed. A. D. Leman, B. Straw, R. D. Glock, W. L. Mengeling, R. H. C. Penny; and E. Scholl. Ames: Iowa State Univ Press, pp. 411–424.

MENGELING, W. L.; PAUL, P. S.; AND BROWN, T. T. 1980. Transplacental infection and embryonic death following maternal exposure to porcine parvovirus near the time of conception. Arch Virol 65:55–62.

MERCY, A. R.; PEET, R. L.; ELLIS, T. M.; AND PARKINSON, J. 1988. Encephalomyocarditis virus infection in pigs. Aust Vet J 65(11):355.

MEREDITH, M. J. 1984. Anoestrus in the pig. Pig News & Inf 5:213–218.

MIDWEST PLANNING SERVICE. 1983. Swine Housing and Equipment Handbook, 4th ed. Ed. D. B. Geiser. Ames: MWPS, Iowa State Univ, p. 20.

MILLER, E. R., AND KORNEGAY, E. T. 1983. Mineral and vitamin nutrition of swine. J Anim Sci 57 [Suppl 2]:315–329.

MILLER, G., AND DORN, C. R. 1987. An economic summary of the National Animal Health Monitoring System data in Ohio, 1986–87. Proc US Anim Health Assoc 91:154–172.

MILOSAVLJEVIC, S.; MILJKOVIC, V.; SOVLJANSKI, B.; RADOVIC, B.; TRBOJEVIC, G.; AND STANKOV, M. 1972. The revival of apparently stillborn piglets. Acta Vet Beograd 22(2):71–76.

MOLLER, K.; BUSSE, F. W.; AND VON BOTH, G. 1981. Zur Frage der Beziehungen zwischen Fruchtbarkeitsstorungen und Harnwegsinfektionen beim Schwein. 2. Mitteilung: Einfluss des Alters und der Aufstallungsart. Tieraerztl Umsch 36:624–631.

MOODY, N. W.; SPEER, V. C.; AND HAYS, V. W. 1966. Effects of supplemental milk on growth and survival of suckling pigs. Midwest Sect Am Soc Anim Sci 25:1250.

MOORE, R. W.; REDMOND, H. E.; AND LIVINGSTON, C. W. 1965. Iron deficiency anemia as a cause of stillbirths in swine. J Am Vet Med Assoc 147(7):746–748.

MORRIS, G. L.; CURTIS, S. E.; AND SIMON, J. 1985. Perinatal piglets under sublethal concentrations of atmospheric carbon monoxide. J Anim Sci 61(5):1070–1079.

MORRISON, R. B., AND JOO, H. S. 1985. Prenatal and preweaning deaths caused by pseudorabies virus and porcine parvovirus in a swine herd. J Am Vet Med Assoc 187(5):481–483.

MORROW, W. E. M.; LEMAN, A. D.; WILLIAMSON, N. B.; et al. 1989. Improving parity-two litter size in swine. J Anim Sci 67:1707–1713.

MOSER, B. D. 1983. The use of fat in sow diets. In Recent Advances in Animal Nutrition. Ed. W. Haresign. London: Butterworth, pp. 71–80.

MOUNT, L. E. 1968. Energy metabolism. In The Young Pig and Its Physical Environment. Ed. K. L. Blaxter. London: Academic Press, p. 379.

MUIRHEAD, M. R. 1986. Epidemiology and control of vaginal discharges in the sow after service. Vet Rec 119:233–235.

NELSON, R. E., AND ROBISON, O. W. 1976. Effects of postnatal maternal environment on reproduction of gilts. J Anim Sci 43:71–77.

NELSSON, J. L.; LEWIS, A. J.; PEO, E. R.; et al. 1985. Effect of dietary energy during lactation on performance of primiparous sows and their litters. J Anim Sci 61:1164–1171.

NESETRILOVA, H. 1987. Methods of estimation of heritability of all-or-none traits and their use in estimating heritability of perinatal and postnatal mortality in pigs. Anim Breed Abst 055–00331.

NIELSEN, N. C.; CHRISTENSEN, K.; BILLE, N.; et al. 1974. Preweaning mortality in pigs. 1. Herd Investigations. Nord Vet Med 26:137–150.

NIELSEN, N. C.; RIISING, H. J.; LARSEN, J. L.; et al. 1975a. Preweaning mortality in pigs. 5. Acute septicaemias. Nord Vet Med 27:129–139.

NIELSEN, N. C.; BILLE, N.; LARSON, J. L.; et al. 1975b. Preweaning mortality in pigs. 7. Polyarthritis. Nord Vet Med 27:529–543.

O'GRADY, J. F.; LYNCH, P. B.; AND KEARNEY, P. A. 1983. Mating management of sows. Irish J Agric Res 22:11–19.

_____. 1985. Voluntary feed intake by lactating sows. Livest Prod Sci 12:355–365.

OMTVEDT, I. T.; STANISLAW, C. M.; AND WHATLEY, J. A. 1965. Relationship of gestation length, age, and weight at breeding, and gestation gain to sow productivity at farrowing. J Anim Sci 24:531–535.

OMTVEDT, I. T.; NELSON, R. E.; EDWARDS, R. L.; et al. 1968. Influence of heat stress during early, mid and late pregnancy of gilts. J Anim Sci 32:312–317.

ORR, J. P.; ALTHOUSE, E.; DULAC, G. C.; AND DURHAM, P. J. K. 1988. Epizootic infection of a minimal disease swine herd with a herpesvirus. Can Vet J 29(1):45–50.

OUCHI, N. 1987. Epidemiological survey of outbreaks of stillbirth in swine due to Japanese encephalitis virus in Hokkaido. Jpn J Vet Res 35(2):143.

PACOVA, J., AND DUPAL, J. 1980. The effect of heterospermy on conception rate and fertility of inseminated sows and gilts. Cited in Anim Breed Abst 2191:374.

PAQUIGNON, M.; NOWAK, R.; KUO, Y. H.; et al. 1984. Sperm production in the boar under intensive ejaculation rhythm. 10th Int Congr Anim Reprod Artif Insemination 2:61–63.

PARK, Y. I.; KIM, J. B.; AND CHUNG, H. W. 1988. Effect of crossbreeding on the incidence of stillbirths in swine. Proc World Conf Anim Prod, p. 503.

PARRY, M. A. 1986. The effect of confinement on behaviour and reproductive performance in the sow. Agric Prog 61:46–54.

PATERSON, A. M.; BARKER, I.; AND LINDSAY, D. R. 1978. Summer infertility in pigs: Its incidence and characteristics in an Australian commercial piggery. Aust J Exp Agric Anim Husb 18:698–701.

PATERSON, A. M.; HUGHES, P. E.; AND PEARCE, G. P. 1989a. The effect of limiting the number of days of contact with boars, season and herd of origin on the attainment of puberty in gilts. Anim Reprod Sci 18:293–301.

_____. 1989b. The effect of season, frequency and duration of contact with boars on the attainment of puberty in gilts. Anim Reprod Sci 21:115–124.

PAVLOV, V. N. 1987. Vitamin A deficiency in pigs. Pig News & Inf 008–01150.

PAY, M. G. 1973. The effect of short lactations on the productivity of sows. Vet Rec 92:255–259.

PAY, M. G., AND DAVIES, T. E. 1973. Growth, food consumption and litter production of female pigs mated at puberty and at low body weights. Anim Prod 17:85–91.

PEARCE, G. P.; HUGHES, P. E.; AND BOOTH, W. D. 1988. The involvement of boar submaxillary salivary gland secretions in boar-induced precocious puberty attainment in the gilt. Anim Reprod Sci 16:125–134.

PENNY, R. H. 1980. Navel bleeding in piglets and the pale piglet syndrome. Vet Ann 10:281–290.

PENNY, R. H. C.; CAMERON, R. D. A.; JOHNSON, S.; et al. 1981. Influence of biotin supplementation on sow reproductive efficiency. Vet Rec 109:80–81.

PERRY, J. S., AND ROWELL, J. G. 1969. Variations in foetal weight and vacular supply along the uterine horn of the pig. J Reprod Fertil 19:527–534.

PETHERICK, J. C., AND BLACKSHAW, J. D. 1986. A review of housing systems for nonlactating sows. Pig News & Inf 7:33–38.

_____. 1989. A note on the effect of feeding regime on

the performance of sows housed in a novel group-housing system. Anim Prod 49(3):523–526.

PETROVIC, M. 1983. The variability and inheritance of fertility in Swedish Landrace pigs. Arh Poljopr Nauk 44(156):387–404.

_____. 1986. The variability and inheritance of fertility in Swedish Landrace pigs. Anim Breed Abst 054–04577.

PETTIGREW, J. E. 1981. Supplemental dietary fat for peripartal sows: A review. J Anim Sci 53:107–117.

PETTIGREW, J. E.; CORNELIUS, S. G.; MOSER, R. L.; HEEG, T. R.; HANKE, H. E.; MILLER, K. P.; AND HAGEN, C. D. 1986. Effects of oral doses of corn oil and other factors on preweaning survival and growth of piglets. J Anim Sci 62:601–612.

PHUAH, C. H., AND SOO, S. P. 1980. Farrowing crates with partially slatted floors for sows. Mal Agric 52:14–19.

POLSON, D.; DIAL, G.; AND MARSH, W. 1990a. A biological and financial characterization of nonproductive days. Proc Int Congr Pig Vet Soc, Lausanne, p. 372.

POLSON, D. D.; DIAL, G. D.; MARSH, W. E.; et al. 1990b. Relative contributions of commonly used measures of reproductive performance on herd productivity. Proc Minn Swine Health Prog Conf, pp. 74–85.

QUINTANA, F. G., AND ROBISON, O. W. 1983. Systems of crossbreeding in swine. I. Estimation of genetic parameters. Sonderdr Z Tierz Zuchtungbiol 4:271–279.

RAHNEFELD, G. W., AND SWEISTRA, E. E. 1970. Influence of the sire on litter size in swine. Can J Anim Sci 50:671–675.

RAMPACEK, G. B.; KRAELING, R. R.; AND KISER, T. E. 1981. Delayed puberty in gilts in total confinement. Therio 15:491–499.

RANDALL, G. C. 1971. The relationship of arterial blood pH and pCO$_2$ to the viability of the newborn piglet. Can J Comp Med 35:41–146.

_____. 1972. Observations on parturition in the sow. I. Factors associated with the delivery of the piglets and their subsequent behaviour. Vet Rec 90:178–182.

RANDALL, G. C., AND PENNY, R. H. 1968. Stillbirths in pigs: Observations on blood lactic acid levels. Vet Rec 83:57.

RASBECH, N. O. 1969. A review of the causes of reproductive failure in swine. Br Vet J 125:599–614.

REED, H. C. B. 1982. Artificial insemination. In Control of Pig Reproduction. Ed. D. J. A. Cole and G. R. Foxcroft. London: Butterworth Scientific, pp. 65–90.

REESE, D. E.; MOSER, B. D.; PEO, E. R.; et al. 1982. Influence of energy intake during lactation on the interval from weaning to first estrus in sows. J Anim Sci 55:590–598.

REESE, D. E.; PEO, E. R.; AND LEWIS, A. J. 1984. Relationship of lactation energy intake and occurrence of postweaning estrus to body and backfat composition in sows. J Anim Sci 58:1236–1244.

REINISCH, F., AND GEBHARDT, G. 1989. Effect of vitamin B12 on fertility in sows. Anim Breed Abst 057–02550.

REVELLE, T. J., AND ROBISON, O. W. 1973. An explanation for the low heritability of litter size in swine. J Anim Sci 37(3):668–675.

REYNS, L., AND DE DONNEA, R. 1974. Construction et amenagement des porcheries. Rev Agric 27: 35–41.

RUTLEDGE, J. J. 1980. Fraternity size and swine reproduction. 1. Effect on fecundity of gilts. J Anim Sci 51:868–874.

SCHMIDT, W. E.; STEVENSON, J. S.; AND DAVIS, D. L. 1985. Reproductive traits of sows penned individually or in groups until 35 days after breeding. J Anim Sci 60:755–759.

SCHOEPS, S., AND HUHN, U. 1986. Relationships between body weight gain of sows in advanced preg-

nancy and litter size. Monatsh Veterinarmed 41(22):767–769.

SELF, H. L., AND GRUMMER, R. H. 1958. The rate and economy of pig gains and the reproductive behavior in sows when litters are weaned at 10 days, 21 days, or 56 days of age. J Anim Sci 17:862–868.

SEERLEY, R. W., AND MARTIN, R. J. 1983. Baby pig survival: Feeding animal fat to sows and the effect on baby pig energy storage and milk yield of sows. In Pork Prod Res Inves Report NPPC. Ed. D. Meisinger. Iowa, pp. 25–26.

SHARPE, H. B. 1966. Preweaning mortality in a herd of large white pigs. Br Vet J 122:99–111.

SHURSON, G. C.; HOGBERG, M. G.; DEFEVER, N.; RADECKI, S. V.; AND MILLER, E. R. 1986. Effects of adding fat to the sow lactation diet on lactation and rebreeding performance. J Anim Sci 62(3):672–680.

SIGNORET, J. P. 1971. The mating behavior of the sow. In Pig Production. Ed. D. J. A. Cole. University Park: Pennsylvania State Univ Press, pp. 295–313.

SIGNORET, J. P.; DU MESNIL DU BUISSON, F.; AND MAULEON, P. 1972. Effect of mating on the onset and duration of ovulation in the sow. J Reprod Fertil 31:327–330.

SIMENSEN, E., AND KALBERG, K. A survey of preweaning mortality in pigs. Nord Vet Med 32:194–200.

SINGH, B. K.; SINGH, B. K.; AND DUBEY, C. B. 1989. Studies on certain economic traits of exotic breeds of pigs under tropical climate. Ind Vet J 66(4):322–328.

SINGLETON, W. L., AND SHELBY, D. R. 1972. Variation among boars in semen characteristics and fertility. J Anim Sci 34:762–766.

SLATTER, E. E. 1955. Milk iodine deficiency and losses of newborn pigs. J Am Vet Med Assoc 127:149.

SPICER, E. M.; DRIESEN, S. J.; FAHY, V. A.; et al. 1986. Causes of preweaning mortality on a large intensive piggery. Aust Vet J 63(3):71–75.

STANSBURY, W. F.; MCGLONE, J. J.; AND TRIBBLE, L. F. 1987. Effects of season, floor type, air temperature and snout coolers on sow and litter performance. J Anim Sci 65:1507–1513.

STELLMACHER, H.; KIELSTEIN, P.; HORSCH, F.; AND MARTIN, J. 1983. Importance of *Chlamydia* infection in pigs, with reference to pneumonia. Monatsh Veterinarmed 38(16):601–606.

STEPHAN, H. A.; GAY, G. M.; AND RAMIREZ, T. C. 1988. Encephalomyelitis, reproductive failure and corneal opacity (blue eye) in pigs, associated with a paramyxovirus infection. Vet Rec 122(1):6–10.

STEPHENS, S., AND BOLAND, M. P. 1988. Farrowing induction by a long-acting prostaglandin. Anim Breed Abst 056–02878.

STEVENSON, J. S., AND DAVIS, D. L. 1984. Infuence of reduced litter size and daily litter separation on fertility of sows at 2 to 5 weeks of age postpartum. J Anim Sci 59:284–293.

STEVENSON, J. S.; POLLMANN, D. S.; DAVIS, D. L.; AND MURPHY, J. P. 1983. Influence of supplemental light on sow performance during and after lactation. J Anim Sci 56(6):1282–1286.

STOLIC, N. 1987. The effect of litter size on the incidence of stillbirths in Swedish Landrace gilts. Anim Breed Abst 055–03771.

STONE, B. A. 1987. Determinants of embryonic mortality in the pig. Pig News & Inf 8(3):279–284.

STONE, B. A.; HEAP, P. A.; AND GODFREY, B. M. 1987. Induction of farrowing in sows with prostaglandin F2-alpha, alone or in combination with a parasympathomimetic or oxytocic. Aust Vet J 64(8):254–256.

STORK, M. G. 1979. Seasonal reproductive efficiency in large pig breeding units in Britain. Vet Rec 104:49–52.

STRANG, G. S., AND KING, J. W. B. 1970. Litter productivity in Large White pigs. 2. Heritability and repeatability estimates. Anim Prod 12:235–243.

STRAW, B. 1984. Causes and control of sow deaths. Mod Vet Pract (May): 349–353.

STRYKER, J. L., AND DZIUK, P. J. 1975. Effects of fetal decapitation on fetal development, parturition and lactation in pigs. J Anim Sci 40:282–287.

SVAJGR, A. J.; HAYS, V. W.; CROMWELL, G. L.; et al. 1974. Effect of lactation duration on reproductive performance of sows. J Anim Sci 38:100–105.

SVENDSEN, J., AND ANDREASSON, B. 1980. Perinatal mortality in pigs: Influence of housing. Proc Int Congr Pig Vet Soc, Copenhagen, p. 83.

SVENDSEN, J.; BILLE, N.; NIELSEN, N. C. et al. 1975a. Preweaning mortality in pigs. 4. Diseases of the gastrointestinal tract in pigs. Nord Vet Med 27:85–101.

SVENDSEN, J.; NIELSON, N. C.; BILLE, N.; et al. 1975b. Causes of culling and death in sows. Nord Vet Med 27:604–615.

SVENDSEN, J.; SVENDSEN, L. S.; AND BENGTSSON, A. C. 1986. Reducing perinatal mortality in pigs. In Diseases of Swine, 6th ed. Ed. A. D. Leman, B. Straw, R. D. Glock, W. L. Mengeling, R. H. C. Penny, and E. Scholl. Ames: Iowa State Univ Press, pp. 813–825.

SWEISTRA, E. E. 1973. Influence of breed, age, and ejaculation frequency on boar semen composition. Can J Anim Sci 53:43–53.

SWEISTRA, E. E., AND DYCK, G. W. 1976. Influence of the boar and ejaculation frequency on pregnancy rate and embryonic survival in swine. J Anim Sci 42:455–460.

SWEISTRA, E. E., AND RAHNFELD, G. W. 1972. Effects of cold stress and repeat mating on reproductive performance of swine. Can J Anim Sci 52:309–316.

TAKASHIMA, I.; WATANABE, T.; OUCHI, N.; AND HASHIMOTO, N. 1988. Ecological studies of Japanese encephalitis virus in Hokkaido: Interepidemic outbreaks of swine abortion and evidence for the virus to overwinter locally. Am J Trop Med Hyg 38(2):420–427.

TAROCCO, C. 1989. The farm fertility profile. Sel Vet 30(4):653–659.

TEAGUE, H. S.; ROLLER, W. L.; AND GRIFO, A. P., JR. 1968. Influence of high temperature and humidity on the reproductive performance of swine. J Anim Sci 27:408–411.

TE BRAKE, J. H. A. 1972. Pig rearing in cages – the extra early weaning of piglets and the fertility of sows. 23d Annu Meet, E.A.A.P. Comm Pig Prod.

THACKER, B. J., AND GONZALEZ, P. L. 1988. Infectious reproductive diseases in swine. Comp Cont Ed Pract Vet 10(5):669–679.

THOMPSON, L. H., AND SAVAGE, J. S. 1978. Age at puberty and ovulation rate in gilts in confinement as influenced by exposure to a boar. J Anim Sci 47:1141–1144.

THORTON, K. 1987. Management techniques for survival in the breeding herd. PIC Pig Improver 6(2):2–6.

TILTON, J. E., AND COLE, D. J. A. 1982. Effect of triple versus double mating on sow productivity. Anim Prod 334:279–282.

TILTON, J. E.; FOXCROFT, G. R.; ZIECIK, A. J.; et al. 1982. Time of the preovulatory LH surge in the gilt and sow relative to the onset of behavioral estrus. Therio 18:227–236.

TODD, J. N.; WELLS, G. A. H.; AND DAVIE, J. 1985. Mycotic abortion in the pig. Vet Rec 116(13):350.

TOELLE, V. D., AND ROBISON, O. W. 1985. Estimates of genetic relationship between testes measurements and female reproductive traits in swine. Z Tierz Zuchtungsbiol 102(2):125–132.

TOMES, G. J., AND NIELSON, H. E. 1979. Seasonal variations in the reproductive performance in sows under different climatic conditions. World Rev Nim Prod 15(1):9–19.

TOMPKINS, E. C.; HEIDENREICH, C. J.; AND STOB, M. 1967. Effect of post-breeding thermal stress on embryonic mortality in swine. J Anim Sci 26:377–380.

TOO, H. L., AND LOVE, R. J. 1986. Some epidemiological features and effects on reproductive performance of endemic porcine parvovirus infection. Aust Vet J 63(2):50–53.

TREMBLAY, G. F.; MATTE, J. J.; AND DUFOUR, J. J. 1989. Survival rate and development of fetuses during the first 30 days of gestation after folic acid addition to a swine diet. J Anim Sci 67:724–732.

TRUDEAU, V., AND SANFORD, L. M. 1986. Effect of season and social environment on testes size and semen quality of the adult Landrace boar. J Anim Sci 63:1211–1219.

TUBBS, R. C. 1988. Sow lactation failure with emphasis on nutritional factors. Agric Pract 9:9–13.

UZU, G. 1979. Influence of the boar on the main pregnancy parameters of the herd and on the pregnancy rate. Ann Zootech 28:315–323.

VAILLANCOURT, J.-P.; 1990. Validation of a swine production data base and its use in a study of temporal patterns in preweaning mortality. Ph.D. diss., Univ Minnesota.

VAILLANCOURT, J.-P., AND MARTINEAU, G.-P. 1988. La congelation: Un outil dans l'investigation des mortalites pre-sevrage en medecine porcine. Med Vet Quebec 18:139–144.

VAILLANCOURT, J.-P.; STEIN, T. E.; MARSH, W. E.; et al. 1990. Validation of producer-recorded causes of preweaning mortality in swine. Prev Vet Med. In press.

VAN ALSTINE, W.; COOK, W. O.; AND CARLSON, T. L. 1985. Carbon monoxide-induced fetal death in swine: Diagnosis and prevention. Vet Med 68–73.

VANDENBOOREN, J. C.; NIEWOLD, T. A.; VAN LITH, P. M.; et al. 1986. Fasting newborn piglets: Changes in plasma glucogen contents of biopsies taken from liver and skeletal muscle. Proc Int Congr Pig Vet Soc, Barcelona, p. 470.

VARLEY, M. A. 1982. The time of weaning and its effects on reproductive function. In Control of Pig Reproduction. London: Butterworth Scientific, pp. 459–478.

VARLEY, M. A., AND COLE, D. J. A. 1976a. Studies in sow reproduction. 4. The effect of level of feeding in lactation and during the interval from weaning to remating on the subsequent reproductive performance of the early weaned sow. Anim Prod 22:71–77.

_____. 1976b. Studies in sow reproduction. 5. The effect of lactation length of the sow on the subsequent embryonic development. Anim Prod 22:79–85.

_____. 1978. Studies in sow reproduction. 6. The effect of lactation length on preimplantation losses. Anim Prod 27:209–214.

VARLEY, M. A.; ATKINSON, T.; AND ROSS, L. N. 1981. The effect of lactation length on the circulating concentrations of progesterone and oestradiol in the early weaned sow. Therio 16:179–184.

VARLEY, M. A.; BROOKING, P.; AND McINTYRE, K. A. 1985. Attempt to control parturition in the sow using an oral progestogen. Vet Rec 117(20):515–518.

VELLENGA, L.; VAN VEEN, H. M.; AND HOOGERBRUGGE, A. 1983. Mortality, morbidity, and external injuries in piglets housed in two different housing systems. I. Farrowing house. Vet Q 5:101–106.

VERMEER, H. M., AND SLIJKHUIS, A. 1989. Inseminatie van opfokzeugen bij eerste of tweede bronst. Proef, Proefstn Varkensh, P1.36–1.56.

VIDOTTO, O.; COSTA, A. J.; REIS, A. C. F.; AND VIOTTI, N. M. A. 1984. Experimental toxoplasmosis in pregnant sows. III. Pathological changes. 1st Vet Res

Meet, State Univ of Londrina, Brazil.

VIDOTTO, O.; DA COSTA, A. J.; BALARIN, M. R. S.; AND DA ROCHA, M. A. 1987. Experimental toxoplasmosis in pregnant sows. I. Clinical and haematological observations. Arq Bras Med Vet Zootec 39(4):623–639.

VIDOVIC, V.; SRECKOVIC, A.; STANCIC, B.; AND HAJDU, B. 1986. Povezanost starosti prilikom fertilnog pripusta i plodnosti u nazimica meleza razlicitih genotipova. Anim Breed Abst 054–01793.

VON BOTH, G.; MOLLER, K.; AND BUSSE, F. W. 1980. Zur Frage der Beziehungen zwischen Fruchtbarkeitsstorungen und Harnwegsinfektionen beim Schwein. 1. Mittelung: Untersuchung an Harnproben mittels bacteriologischer Teststreifen. Tieraerztl Umsch 35:468–473.

VON KEINDORF, A., AND PLESCHER, W. 1981. Der Jahreszeiteneinfluss auf die Fruchtbarksleistungen der Schweine unter besonderer Berucksichtigung der Sommermonate. Monatsh Vet Med 36:324–330.

VON LUTTER, K., HUHN, U. 1980. Untersuchungen uber jahreszeitliche Schwankungen der Sauenfruchtbarkeit. Monatsh Vet Med 35:819–822.

WALKER, N.; WATT, D.; MACLEOD, A. S.; et al. 1979. The effect of weaning at 10, 25, or 40 days on the reproductive performance of sows from the first to the fifth parity. J Agric Sci Camb 92:449–456.

WARNICK, A. C.; WALLACE, H. D.; PALMER, A. Z.; et al. 1965. Effect of temperature on early embryo survival in gilts. J Anim Sci 24:89–92.

WELP, C., AND HOLTZ, W. 1985. Induction of parturition with prostaglandin analogs under field conditions. Anim Reprod Sci 8(1/2):171–179.

WETTEMAN, R. P.; WELLS, M.; OMTVEDT, I. T.; et al. 1976. Influence of elevated ambient temperature on reproductive performance of boars. J Anim Sci 42:664–669.

WETTEMAN, R. P.; WELLS, M.; JOHNSON, R. K. 1979. Reproductive characteristics of boars during and after exposure to increased ambient temperature. J Anim Sci 49:1501–1505.

WHITING, R.; OWEN, B. D.; ELLIOTT, J. I.; et al. 1983. Porcine immunoglobulin-fortified milk replacers for newborn low-birth-weight pigs. Can J Anim Sci 63:993–996.

WILLEKE, VON H., AND RICHTER, L. 1980. Der Einflub des Ebers auf die Wurfgrobe beim Schwein – Genetisch-statistiche Auswertungen von Fruchtbarkeitsdaten einer Besamungs Population. Zuchtungskd 52(6):438–443.

WILLIAMS, D. M.; LAWSON, G. H.; AND ROWLANDS, A. C. 1973. Streptococcal infection in piglets: The pelantive tonsils as portal of entry for *Streptococcus suis*. Res Vet Sci 15:352–362.

WISE, M. E.; ALLRICH, R. D.; JONES, A.; KITTOK, R. J.; AND ZIMMERMAN, D. R. 1981. Influence of photoperiod (16L:8D) and size of rearing group (10 vs 30) on age at puberty in confinement-reared gilts. J Anim Sci 53:104.

WOHLGEMUTH, K.; LESLIE, P. F.; REED, D. E.; et al. 1978. Pseudorabies virus associated with abortion in swine. J Am Vet Med Assoc 172:478–479.

WOOD, E. N. 1979. Increased incidence of stillbirth in piglets associated with high levels of atmospheric carbon monoxide. Vet Rec 104:283–284.

WRATHALL, A. E.; WELLS, D. E.; JONES, P. C.; et al. 1986. Seasonal variations in serum progesterone levels in pregnant sows. Vet Rec 118:685–687.

WU, M. C.; HENTZEL, M. D.; AND DZIUK, P. J. 1988. Effect of stage of gestation, litter size and uterine space on the incidence of mummified fetuses in pigs. J Anim Sci 66(12):3203–3207.

YEN, H. F.; ISLER, G. A.; HARVEY, W. R.; AND IRVIN, K. M. 1987. Factors affecting reproductive performance in swine. J Anim Sci 64:1340–1348.

YOUNG, L. G., AND KING, G. J. 1986a. Low concentrations of zearalenone in diets of mature gilts. J Anim Sci 63:1191–1196.

———. 1986b. Low concentrations of zearalenone in diets of boars for a prolonged period of time. J Anim Sci 63:1197–1200.

ZIMMERMAN, D. R., AND KOPF, J. D. 1986. Age at puberty in gilts as affected by boar maturity, type of boar exposure and age of gilts when boar exposure is initiated. J Anim Sci 63 [Suppl] 1:355.

ZIMMERMAN, D. R.; CARLSON, R.; AND LANTZ, B. 1974. The influence of exposure to the boar and movement on pubertal development in the gilt. J Anim Sci 39:230.

7 Respiratory System

G. Christensen

J. Mousing

THE STRUCTURE of swine production in industrialized countries has changed substantially in recent years; large groups of animals are housed under intensive conditions, often in regions with an extremely dense pig population. High stocking density in closed environments facilitates transmission of airborne pathogens inside the herd, and current investigations (Henningsen et al. 1988; Jorsal and Thomsen 1988) as well as experience in the field have revealed that several pathogens are able to infect herds over considerable distances suspended in aerosols from other herds.

Consequently, respiratory disorders as well as systemic airborne diseases are today regarded as the most serious disease problem in modern swine production.

STRUCTURE AND FUNCTION OF THE NORMAL RESPIRATORY SYSTEM

Structure. The respiratory tract develops from the anterior part of the embryonic gut as a tree-structured tubular organ. The mature respiratory apparatus comprises the nasal cavity, pharynx, larynx, trachea, and lungs with bronchi, bronchioli, and alveoli. The lungs are embedded in the pleural sac.

There are two separate blood-conducting systems in the lungs. The arteria pulmonalis system vascularizes the capillary plexus surrounding the alveoli with venous blood from the right ventricle. The close structural and functional parallelism between this bloodstream and the tubular airway system is important to realize when possible infection routes in the lungs have to be interpreted. The supporting structures around the trachea, bronchi, bronchioli, and even the wall of the arteria pulmonalis are vascularized with blood from the arteria bronchialis tree.

TUBULAR TRACT SYSTEM

Nasal Cavity. The nasal cavity of Landrace breeds and in particular of the wild boar is long and narrow. The nose of most other breeds, for example the Yorkshire, is somewhat shorter; some Asiatic breeds have extremely short noses.

The nasal cavity is divided longitudinally by a wall (septum nasi). Two turbinate bones divide each of the two halves of the cavity into three meatuses–dorsal, middle, and ventral (Fig 7.1). The vestibular region of the nasal cavity is lined with stratified squamous epithelium. Posteriorly, the epithelium changes through stratified columnar into ciliated pseudostratified epithelium with goblet cells (respiratory epithelium). This epithelium is covered by a mucous film produced by the goblet cells.

Trachea, Bronchi, Bronchioli, and Alveoli. The trachea is short and divides posteriorly into two principal bronchi, one for the left lung and one for the right lung (Fig. 7.2). A special stembronchus branches from the trachea leading to the apical lobe of the right lung. The right principal bronchus sends a stembronchus to the right cardiac lobe and another to the intermediate lobe and then continues until it ramifies into the diaphragmatic lobe. The left principal bronchus

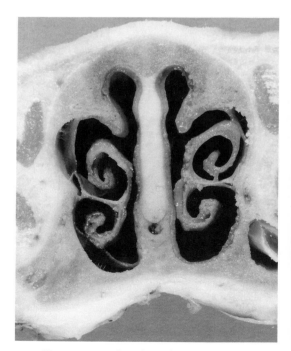

7.1. Transverse section of nasal structures.

gives off a stembronchus that divides into one branch for the apical lobe and one for the cardiac lobe. The principal bronchus then continues posteriorly in the diaphragmatic lobe. The finest branches of the tubular system are the bronchioli, each dividing into alveolar ducts and alveoli.

The larynx, trachea, and bronchi are, as the respiratory section of the pharynx, lined with ciliated pseudostratified epithelium with goblet cells. As the bronchioli approach the alveoli, the epithelium is reduced in height, becoming squamuous. Sections of the bronchioli (called respiratory bronchioli) and the walls of the alveoli are formed entirely of very flat, single-layered epithelium. Here, the alveolic wall is very intimately attached to the capillary plexus of the pulmonary blood circulation.

GROSS APPEARANCE OF THE LUNG. In the pig the lungs are divided with deep fissures into seven lobes: the right lung comprises the apical, cardiac, diaphragmatic, and intermediate lobes; the left lung comprises the apical, cardiac, and diaphragmatic lobes (Fig. 7.2). The left apical and cardiac lobes are not separated by a fissure but only by the cardiac notch. The lobes are subdivided by solid interlobular septa into lobuli. Pathological processes, therefore, often will be retained within lobular structures, typically seen in catarrhal pneumonia as sharp demarcated limits between normal and affected tissue.

When assessing the extent of lung lesions it is necessary to know the relative size or weight of each lobe. Table 7.1 shows the relative weight of the lung lobi as percentage of the total lung weight, as determined in three different studies. The right lung contributes more than half of the total lung weight with small differences between the investigations. The variations might be caused partly by different average live weights of the animals examined. The animals in the last study (C) had a lower average live weight (90 kg) than in the first (A) (100 kg) and in the second (B). We found a tendency of higher weight difference between the two lung halves in animals of lower slaughter weight.

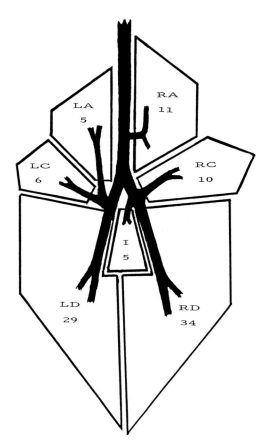

7.2. Schematic outline of lung lobulation and branching of the bronchus tree. *LA, RA:* left and right apical lobes; *LC, RC:* left and right cardiac lobes; *LD, RD:* left and right diaphragmatic lobes; *I:* intermediate lobe. Numbers = relative lobe weight as percent of total lung weight based on a study of Christensen (1990).

Function. The vital gaseous exchange between inhaled air and venous blood from the pulmonary artery takes place at the alveolar level. Only a minor part of the total alveolar air volume is renewed with each breath. In the resting pig 10–15% of the alveolar air is exchanged per inspiration. The normal respiratory rate (breaths/min) varies according to age of the animal (piglets and growing pigs, 25–40; finishing pigs, 25–35; sows in gestation, 15–20).

DEFENSE MECHANISMS OF THE RESPIRATORY SYSTEM. The mucosal surface of the respiratory tract provides a critical interface between the pig and its environment. While the skin of the pig is

Table 7.1.   Relative weights of lung lobes as percent of total lung weight

| Study | Left Lung Lobes | | | Right Lung Lobes | | | | |
	Apical	Cardiac	Diaphr.	Apical	Cardiac	Diaphr.	Interm.	N[a]
A	7	7	32	12	8	30	5	11
B	5	7	32	6	9	36	5	20
C	5	6	29	11	10	34	5	13

Note: A = Morrison et al. 1985; B = Heilmann et al. 1988; C = Christensen 1990. Rounding of numbers may cause total percentages to equal more than 100.
[a]N = number of pigs examined in each study.

well adapted to prevent invasion of potentially harmful agents and has a limited surface area (about 1.8 m² in humans), the epithelial surface of the respiratory tract primarily serves as a diffusion membrane. The gaseous exchange requires a very large surface (in humans more than 100 m²). Thus, it is understandable that the respiratory tract must be equipped with a potent and specialized defense apparatus. The most important components of the respiratory defense are listed in Table 7.2.

The nasal cavity is designed to remove large particles trapped by hairs in the nostrils and deposited by gravity in the mucus by the eddy currents around the conchal structures. Another function of the nasal cavity with its immense venous sinusoids and wet surfaces is humidification and warming of the air before it reaches the lower airways.

Most inspired particles are trapped in the epithelial mucus of the nasal, pharyngeal, laryngeal, and tracheal cavities. From many experiments it is known that only particles below an aerodynamic diameter of 5 μm (the respirable fraction) are able to reach and settle at the alveolar level. Particles of an aerodynamic diameter greater than 10 μm almost entirely settle before reaching the branches of the bronchial tree (Baskerville 1981).

Mucociliary Defense. Particles trapped in the epithelial mucus are handled by the mucociliary clearance mechanism. The ciliary carpet in the bronchi and bronchioli gives rise to a continuous flow of mucus toward the pharynx. The rhythmic beating of cilia results in a mucous flow of about 4–15 mm/minute (Done 1988). Like mucus from the nasal cavity, it is delivered to the pharyngeal cavity and subsequently swallowed.

Phagocytes. Alveolar macrophages neutralize foreign material that escapes the mucociliary defense mechanism. Nonpathogen particles and microbes are handled by simple phagocytic activity and are removed in the mucous flow or by the lymphatic system. Pathogenic microorganisms are neutralized with the aid of secretions such as lysozymes, interferons, opsonins, lactoferrins,

complement factors, and specific immunoglobulins in the mucus. If the invading agents are not neutralized by the alveolar macrophages, inflammation will occur. Neutrophils from the blood will then invade the alveolus and assist the macrophages in the phagocytic activity. In healthy pigs the normal ratio between the cellular elements in the bronchoalveolar mucus is 70–80% alveolar macrophages, 11–18% lymphocytes, 8–12% neutrophils, and up to 5% eosinophilic granulocytes (Neumann et al. 1985). The phagocytic cell system also comprises intravascular macrophages, which in the pig are particularly numerous (Bertram 1985; Ohgami et al. 1989) in the lung, and histiocytes with phagocytic properties in the connective tissue.

The activity of the phagocytes is highly accelerated if introduced pathogens are not eliminated quickly or if pathogens are recognized from a previous attack. Then a complex immune response is activated with production of specific immunoglobulins affected by B lymphocyte–derived plasma cells under the direction of T lymphocytes.

Immunoglobulins. The production of specific immunoglobulins is of crucial importance in the respiratory immune defense. Their biological function consists of neutralization of antigens by generating non pathogenic antigen-antibody complexes.

The predominant immunoglobulins in mucus are of IgA type. A secretory component takes part in the secretion of IgA and probably also of IgM. IgM globulins are potent proteins released in the early immune response, particularly in the newborn pig. IgG originating from blood serum forms the greater part of the immunoglobulins in mucus of the lower respiratory tract near the alveoli. Immunoglobulins in the mucous carpet act primarily in preventing the initial establishment and penetration of pathogens. IgE globulins are generated in the immune response against parasites; e.g., lungworm (*Metastrongylus* spp.) and migrating ascarid larvae.

Cell-mediated Immune Response. Traditionally, immunity is divided into a humoral immune response in which the immunoglobulins play an es-

Table 7.2. Respiratory system defense components

Physical/Chemical
  Hairs in nostrils
  Structure of the nasal cavity
  Structure of mucosa
  Properties of mucus (physical and chemical; e.g., adhesiveness, nonspecific lysozymes, interferon, opsonins, lactoferrin, complement factors, specific immunoglobulins)
  Humoral components (as mucus contents + multiple types of immune modulators; e.g., lymphokines)
Cellular
  Phagocytes (alveolar macrophages, vascular macrophages, histiocytes, monocytes, neutrophils, eosinophils)
  Bone marrow–derived B lymphocytes (plasma cells)
  Thymus-derived T lymphocytes (helper lymphocytes, suppressor lymphocytes, cytotoxic lymphocytes [natural killer cells])

sential role and a cell-mediated immune response based on antibody-independent components. Today it is realized that the immunity cannot be distinctly separated into these two parts for many mechanisms and elements are shared, including cells and antibodies.

Generally cell-mediated immunity is identified with the effector arm of the cellular immune response: cytotoxic T cells, natural killer cells, activated macrophages, and cells mediating antibody-dependant cytotoxicity. The cell-mediated immune response is assumed to be of special importance in viral respiratory infections such as influenza and Aujeszky's disease.

Surface proteins belonging to the swine lymphocyte-antigen (SLA) gene complex (major histocompatibility gene complex [MHC]) play a significant role in the cellular as well as the humoral immune response. Rothschild et al. (1984) demonstrated that the SLA complex was associated with immune response following vaccination with *Bordetella bronchiseptica*. Genetic variability of the SLA complex has been demonstrated in European breeds of pigs (Vaiman et al. 1979).

The newborn piglet is capable of absorbing intact lymphocytes from the colostrum. These cells might confer an active cellular immunity from the sow to the piglets (Tuboly et al. 1988). Future possibilities in aerosol vaccines are indicated by the fact that transepithelial passage from the lumen of the respiratory tract into the blood of antigenically intact macromolecules can take place during the first days of life and also to a considerable degree in older pigs (Folkesson et al. 1990).

Vaccination experiments with Aujeszky's disease in young piglets with passively acquired antibodies indicate that the systemic immune mechanism can be bypassed and a local immune response obtained by application of antigen on the respiratory epithelium (Schlesinger et al. 1990). Nielsen et al. (1990b) obtained good immunological protection against *Actinobacillus pleuropneumoniae* with local application of antigens in the respiratory tract.

RESPIRATORY DISORDERS

Pathology. Under commercial conditions no pig can be expected to reach slaughter weight without contracting some sort of respiratory lesion. Pathological alterations can be categorized into three main disease entities: atrophic rhinitis, pneumonia, and pleuritis.

A detailed characterization of microscopic and gross pathology of the individual diseases will be given elsewhere. However, some general features of pathology will be emphasized.

ATROPHIC RHINITIS. Catarrhal inflammation of the nasal mucosa is a common phenomenon in young animals. The cause is often infectious (Aujeszky's disease virus, cytomegalovirus, *Bordetel-*

la bronchiseptica, Mycoplasma hyorhinis), but also ammonia and dust in the air as well as foreign bodies can provoke mild mucosal inflammation of short duration. However, if toxigenic strains of *Pasteurella multocida* are present, even a slightly damaged mucosa might promote adherence and proliferation of the bacteria and subsequently provoke progressive atrophic rhinitis with permanent alteration of the nasal structure and function. The structural changes in atrophic rhinitis are fundamentally induced by an osteoclastic process without inflammation of tissue (Foged et al. 1987).

PNEUMONIA

Catarrhal Bronchopneumonia. Catarrhal bronchopneumonia, located cranioventrally, is a frequent lesion of the lung in all age groups. Since *Mycoplasma hyopneumoniae* almost always is involved, such lesions are often given the term mycoplasmal or mycoplasmallike pneumonia. Noncomplicated mycoplasmal pneumonia typically appears as purple consolidated areas, often more "collapsed" than normal tissue. Early lesions may be somewhat indistinct, but more advanced cases are clearly demarcated from adjacent normal tissue by a sharp line following the interlobular septa. When incised, the consistency is "meaty" but not excessively firm. Catarrhal exudate may be expressed from the airway openings of affected tissue.

Lesions of secondary infections may change to a more grayish color, and the consistency will be firmer due to formation of fibrous tissue. Further, complicated catarrhal bronchopneumonia may be associated with abscess formation. The fissures seen in lobes previously affected with catarrhal bronchopneumonia (Bertschinger 1972) are of diagnostic importance.

Fibrinous/Necrotizing Pneumonia. Another common pathological entity of the lung is fibrinous/necrotizing pneumonia, which chiefly affects the dorsocaudal portions of the organ in contrast to the cranioventrally located catarrhal pneumonia. Affected tissue is frequently raised above the adjacent area and crosses interlobular septae unlike catarrhal pneumonia. Fibrinous/necrotizing pneumonia is often given the term pleuropneumonia for the pleural surface of affected lung tissue is involved in nearly all cases. In the acute stage the inflamed pleural surface is covered with fibrinous exudate. In subacute/chronic cases the associated pleural lesion consists of fibrous tissue, often resulting in firm adherence of the lung to the chest wall.

Embolic Pneumonia. A third common type of lung affection in swine, embolic pneumonia, is caused by hematogenically disseminated agents, mostly pyogenic bacteria from lesions somewhere else in the body. Typically this type of pneumonia starts as minute necrotic foci surrounded by a hemorrhagic zone. Usually suppuration of the centers follows and circumscript abscesses are formed. A secondary bronchopneumonia or a pleuropneumonialike inflammation may develop around the primary process. Verminous migration through lung tissue induces small hemorrhagic foci, small abscesses, or firm granulomas. The verminous processes are mainly located dorsocaudally in the lung.

The healing of catarrhal bronchopneumonia is a rather slow process requiring several weeks or months. However, the healing period depends highly on the agents involved. In specific-pathogen-free (SPF) pigs inoculated with *Mycoplasma hyopneumoniae*, induced pneumonic lesions were healed after 2 months, whereas fissuring of the lung persisted more than 3 months (Bertschinger et al. 1972; Kobisch and Genin 1989). Pattison (1956) still found pneumonic lesions 175 days after inoculation with *Mycoplasma hyopneumoniae*, presumably due to secondary bacterial infection. Contrary to catarrhal pneumonia, the interval between the appearance and disappearance of fibrinous/necrotizing pneumonia may be surprisingly short (2–3 weeks) if not complicated with secondary infections (Christensen 1990).

PLEURITIS. Fibrotic adherence between the visceral and pleural membranes of the pleural sac (chronic pleuritis, pleural scar) is the most frequent pathological alteration seen in slaughter swine. Fibrous pleuritis affecting larger areas is often associated with similar lesions in the pericardial sac (chronic pericarditis). The repairing of such lesions is a long-lasting process with a duration of at least 1 month, more often 2–3 months (Christensen 1984). More serious pleural lesions and particulary pericardial lesions may persist more than a year based on examinations of slaughter sows with known history (Christensen 1990). The resolving of chronic pleuritis may cause younger fatteners to have a higher frequency of this lesion than older pigs (Mousing 1988).

Lesion Distribution Patterns. The cause for catarrhal pneumonic lesions having a distribution in the lung other than pleuropneumonic lesions is not clear. However, fundamentally it must be due to differences in deposition and clearance of the inhaled agents. Experimentally, inhaled aerosolized suspensions of *Bacillus subtilis, Actinobacillus pleuropneumoniae* (Sebunya et al. 1983), and *Staphylococcus aureus* (Kastner and Mehlhorn 1989) are deposited primarily in the caudal lobes. In another investigation (Heilmann et al. 1988), inhalation of aerosolized suspension of radioactively labelled *Pasteurella multocida* resulted in a relatively uniform deposition in the lung lobes. Such experiments could partly explain the typical distribution pattern of pleuropneumonia, but not

of mycoplasmal pneumonia and other catarrhal bronchopneumonias; here, other pathogenetic mechanisms must be involved.

Pneumonic lesions due to hematogenously introduced bacteria have a random distribution pattern, which makes them easily distinguishable from lesions due to bronchogenically disseminated bacteria (Buttenschøn 1989). Verminous lung lesions have a caudodorsal location in spite of the assumption that the larvae are introduced into the bloodstream. However, some extravascular migration through the diaphragm might take place (Buttenschøn 1990).

Since chronic pleuritis almost always is associated with a present or more often a previous inflammation of lung tissue, the localization of pleuritic lesions are of diagnostic value in regard to the type of pneumonia involved.

CAUSAL FACTORS IN RESPIRATORY DISEASE

General Epidemiological Considerations. Respiratory disease must be seen as the result of a complexity of events including infectious, environmental, managemental, and genetic factors. So, due to the fact that the etiology of respiratory diseases is multifactorial, one should be conscious of not just considering some specific infectious agent, as is often done, but regarding other relevant factors as well.

A given pathogen or environmental factor acts by increasing the prevalence (actual frequency) or incidence (accumulated frequency during a defined period) of disease. In quantifying this increase, the ratio between the prevalence or incidence among pigs exposed to the factor and the prevalence or incidence among pigs that are not exposed can be calculated. This ratio is most often referred to as the relative risk. The higher the relative risk, the stronger the association between the disease factor and disease. When two or more risk factors act simultaneously, the total relative risk often will be a multiple of the relative risk of the individual factors (Mousing et al. 1990).

Relative risk factors have to be evaluated with caution, for such associations may be confounded by other factors. Several epidemiological studies have indicated a positive correlation between herd prevalence of pigs with pneumonia and atrophic rhinitis. This association obviously relies on the fact that the two disease entities are provoked by the same external factors, and not that one disease predisposes to the other. In fact, there was no evidence that animals suffering from one of the diseases are more susceptible to the other when correlation studies included individuals in the same herd (Madec and Kobisch 1984; Straw 1986).

Infection. Respiratory infections are common in all swine-producing areas with a high prevalence at herd level (Table 7.3). The spread of respiratory diseases from herd to herd can be based on two distinct mechanisms. First, like other infections, disease may disseminate through infectious contacts (purchase of pigs, incoming and outgoing vehicles, birds, persons, etc.). Second and very importantly, several respiratory diseases also propagate from herd to herd by means of airborne transmission.

AIRBORNE TRANSMISSION OF RESPIRATORY DISEASES BETWEEN HERDS. Respiratory infections in swine with the capability of airborne transmission over distances up to several kilometers include porcine respiratory coronavirus (PRCV) (Henningsen et al.1988) and *Mycoplasma hyopneumoniae* (Goodwin 1985; Jorsal and Thomsen 1988). Systemic infections such as foot-and-mouth disease and Aujeszky's disease (Mortensen et al. 1990) follow this pattern. The typical pattern of influenza outbreaks with the simultaneous appearance of many diseased herds highly suggests that this infection can also be airborne transmitted. In Danish epidemics even though special precautions are taken against introduction of infec-

tious diseases, SPF herds are attacked by influenza just as frequently as conventional neighboring herds. Epidemics in Brittany also seemed to follow an airborne transmission (Madec et al. 1982). Table 7.4 addresses factors affecting the risk of a herd receiving an airborne infection.

Airborne spread of disease between herds is facilitated by several meteorological factors, most significantly, the direction and velocity of the prevailing winds. But also, factors such as cloud cover, turbulence, and topography are important. Overcast skies, night (in which case the turbulence is often low), and relative humidity of more than 90% (Gloster et al. 1981) facilitate airborne transmission.

RESPIRATORY INFECTION IN INDIVIDUALS AND IN HERDS. The upper respiratory tract is the natural habitat for myriads of commensal microorganisms, including viruses, mycoplasmas, chlamydias, and bacteria. The commensal flora may have a favorable competitive effect for its host in outnumbering pathogenic agents. There is no distinct limit between commensals and potentially pathogenic microorganisms. Different studies cat-

Table 7.3. The prevalence of some respiratory infections of swine

Factor	Prevalence	Country
	Prevalence (%) of positive pigs within affected herds	
Actinobacillus pleuropneumoniae		
serotype 2	75 se	Denmark[a]
serotype 6	41 se	Denmark[a]
Swine influenza virus		
H1N1	71–82 se	France[b]
H3N2	29–48 se	France[b]
Toxigenic *Pasteurella multocida*	30–50 cu	United Kingdom[c]
	35 se	Germany[d]
Mycoplasma suipneumoniae	80–90 se	Sweden[e]
	37 cu	Austria[f]
Haemophilus parasuis	55 se	Denmark[a]
	Prevalence (%) of positive herds	
Actinobacillus pleuropneumoniae		
serotype 2	24 se	Norway[g]
serotypes 1–5	69 se	Iowa, USA[h]
serotypes 1, 3, 5, 7, or 9	86 se	Minnesota, USA[i]
	23 cl	Ontario, Canada[j]
Swine influenza virus H1N1	70 se	Denmark[a]
Toxigenic *Pasteurella multocida*	11 cl	Missouri, USA[k]
	7 cl	Australia[l]
Mycoplasma suipneumoniae	85 cl	Australia[l]
Haemophilus parasuis	69 se	Denmark[a]

Note: se = serological method; cu = culturing was employed; cl = clinical signs corresponding to the infection were observed.
  [a]Mousing et al. 1990.
  [b]Madec et al. 1990 (covering 1984, 1985, and 1988).
  [c]Goodwin et al. 1990 (fattening pigs).
  [d]Bechmann and Schöss 1990 (fattening pigs).
  [e]Wallgren et al. 1990 (fattening pigs at slaughter).
  [f]Awad-Masalmeh et al. 1990.
  [g]Falk et al. 1990.
  [h]Schultz et al. 1982.
  [i]Anderson et al. 1990.
  [j]Rosendal and Mitchell 1983.
  [k]Kliebenstein et al. 1982/83.
  [l]Mercy and Brennan 1988.

Table 7.4.   Some important herd-related factors that increase the risk of airborne disease transmission between herds

Factor	Disease
Increasing herd size	Porcine Respiratory Corona Virus (PRCV)[a]
	Aujeszky's disease[b,c]
Forced ventilation	PRCV[a]
Short distance between herds	*Mycoplasma suipneumoniae*[d]
	PRCV[a]
Large size of neighboring herds	*Mycoplasma suipneumoniae*[d]
	PRCV[a]
Herd infected with *Actinobacillus pleuropneumoniae*	Aujeszky's disease[c]

[a]Henningsen et al. 1988.
[b]Mortensen et al. 1990.
[c]Anderson et al. 1990.
[d]Jorsal and Thomsen 1988.

egorize the same microorganism as either commensal or potentially pathogenic; for example, *Mycoplasma flocculare, Mycoplasma hyorhinis,* and *Haemophilus parasuis.* These species belong to a group of microorganisms that can regularly be isolated, not only in the upper respiratory tract but also in the bronchial tree of healthy pigs.

Ganter et al. (1990) examined the bacterial flora in live, healthy, 20–30 kg SPF pigs. The bacteria normally found by alveolar lavage belonged to two or three species, most often streptococci (nonhemolytic, alpha-hemolytic), staphylococci, *Escherichia coli, Klebsiella,* and *Corynebacterium. Haemophilus parasuis* and *Bordetella bronchiseptica* were rarely isolated and, *Pasteurella multocida* was never isolated in the bronchial tree of healthy pigs. In about 40% of conventionally reared healthy pigs, *Haemophilus parasuis* and *Mycoplasma hyorhinis* were detected (Castryck et al. 1990). Møller and Killian (1990) found that the porcine upper respiratory tract harbors a much wider spectrum of V5 factor–dependant Pasteurellaceae species than hitherto recognized, probably with no or low pathogenicity.

Haemophilus parasuis and *Mycoplasma hyorhinis* behave as commensals only as long as their pathogenicity is neutralized by the respiratory defense. In nonimmune individuals *H. parasuis* (Nielsen and Danielsen 1975) and to some extent *M. hyorhinis* may become pathogenic, resulting in severe systemic disease (polyserositis, polysynovitis, meningitis). The fine balance between animal population and pathogens evidently requires that all the pigs are exposed to the pathogens in question. Outbreaks appear under circumstances where this does not happen, e.g., in small herds, in herds with restricted contact between individuals (very early weaning, strict separation between animals of different ages), and in SPF herds established originally from cesarian-derived piglets (Nielsen and Danielsen 1975; Smart et al. 1989).

Actinobacillus pleuropneumoniae and *Mycoplasma hyopneumoniae* can be regarded as representatives of different types of respiratory microorganisms, which may be common at the herd level but which are relatively seldom isolated from healthy individuals (Friis 1974; Castryck et al. 1990; Møller and Killian 1990). Their presence usually will be associated with disease, subclinical more often than clinical, particularly during the critical period when passive immunity in young pigs is normally replaced by active immunity.

The reasons that these two groups of microorganisms behave differently, especially in the immunologically weak state between passive and active immunity, are several. First, *A. pleuropneumoniae* and *M. hyopneumoniae* have a higher pathogenicity than *H. parasuis* and *M. hyorhinis.* However, since *H. parasuis* and to some extent *M. hyorhinis* are capable of causing disease in nonimmune animals, other mechanisms also must be involved.

Second, it is known that *H. parasuis* and *M. hyorhinis* invade the nasal and tracheobronchial epithelium very early in the piglet's life (Ross 1984). This might facilitate a gradual development of active immunity under the cover of humoral colostral antibodies, a situation beneficial to host as well as to pathogen. The host continually is protected against the pathogen, which is on the other hand accepted by the host.

A third aspect is that the sites (pleural, pericardial, peritoneal, meningeal, articular serotic cavities) where the real pathogenic properties of *H. parasuis* and *M. hyorhinis* are affected are outside the respiratory tract. A clear physical barrier exists between the effector site and the residential site in which the active immunity can be generated. In contrast, *A. pleuropneumoniae* and *M. hyopneumoniae* are easily brought to their point of attack with the inhaled air, directly from the environment or from the nasal and tonsillar epithelium.

Finally, the ability of strains with low pathogenicity to generate protecting antibodies against closely related but more pathogenic strains must be considered (Nielsen 1988).

In conclusion, constant presence at the herd level is advantageous for pathogens that cannot permanently be excluded from the herd and that behave as *H. parasuis* and *M. hyorhinis.* However, the presence is not benefical for pathogens behaving as *A. pleuropneumoniae* and *M. hyopneumoniae.*

The group of advantageous/acceptable respiratory microorganisms includes species such as *Haemophilus* "minor group," *Bordetella bronchiseptica,* staphylococci, streptococci, most strains of *Pasteurella multocida,* and some strains of *A. pleuropneumoniae.* In contrast, the most pathogenic strains of *A. pleuropneumoniae* and *P. multocida,* particularly toxigenic strains, are highly disadvantageous as herd infections for they periodically will give rise to respiratory problems.

Even the most pathogenic strains of *P. multocida,* are not capable of infecting a healthy lung, as is *A. pleuropneumoniae.* However, *P. multocida* probably is the most frequent and damaging secondary invader in the debilitated lung. In conventionally reared 7-day-old piglets, *Bordetella bronchiseptica* induces a discrete pneumonia (Lambotte et al. 1990). However, in gnotobiotic piglets the infection causes severe and long-lasting pneumonia (Underdahl et al. 1982). *B. bronchiseptica* is categorized as an acceptable microorganism for like *P. multocida,* it is not easily held out of herds due to the fact that several other animal species, including cats and dogs, are reservoirs.

INTERACTION BETWEEN INFECTIOUS AGENTS. Clinically significant disease seldom is the result of an infection with only one pathogen. As a rule several pathogens are involved. One pathogen acts as the key agent, the "door opener," for secondary invaders by lowering the local and sometimes also the systemic defense mechanisms of the host. In the nasal cavity *B. bronchiseptica* frequently acts as the predisposing key agent facilitating the invasion and replication of toxigenic strains of *P. multocida* (Pedersen and Barfod 1981).

Generally, key agents are viruses or mycoplasmas, while secondary invaders are bacteria. For example, susceptibility in swine to *A. pleuropneumoniae* is increased following an influenza infection (Scatozza and Sidoli 1986) and Aujeszky's disease (Lai et al. 1986). A similar effect was observed in experiments in mice infected first with influenza virus and subsequently with *A. pleuropneumoniae* (Bröring et al. 1989). Pigs infected

with *M. hyopneumoniae* had a decreased resistance against *A. pleuropneumoniae* (Yagihashi et al. 1984).

Lesions caused by key agents themselves are often faint and without clinical significance. It is well known from field experiences that influenza and Aujeszky's disease seldom are followed by severe pneumonic complications in herds where *A. pleuropneumonia* and *M. hyopneumoniae* are not present (e.g., SPF herds), whereas serious respiratory complications regularly ensue these viruses in other herds.

As a rule one pathogen intensifies the proliferation of another, but the reverse effect also can be demonstrated. Mousing et al. (1990) examined in a seroepidemiological study 4800 slaughter pigs for serological evidence of *A. pleuropneumoniae* type 2 and type 6, *Haemophilus parasuis,* and swine influenza virus (type H1N1 with the American and European variants). The interrelationship between these five respiratory infections is illustrated in Table 7.5, demonstrating the increase in chance (relative risk) of confirming a specific infection when a pig also possesses antibodies against another agent. Most infections appear to be positively associated with *A. pleuropneumoniae* serotype 2, except for *A. pleuropneumoniae* serotype 6. The probable explanation is that *A. pleuropneumoniae* species share antigens that provoke generation of cross-protecting antibodies (Nielsen 1988). The reverse effect demonstrated for the two *Influenza* variants is associated with serological cross-reaction.

Further statistical modeling has shown an even more complex pattern when considering two, three, or four infections simultaneously; none of the studied infections could be regarded as independent entities. The effect on prevalence of pleurisy by an increasing number of infections is visualized in Figure 7.3. The prevalence of pleurisy increases from 12.5% in pigs free from any of the five infections to more than 60% in pigs infected with four or five of these.

Environment/Management. Maintaining of good respiratory health at the herd level is fundamentally a question of keeping the balance between the pigs' resistance and the respiratory

Table 7.5. **Interrelationship between some respiratory infections**

| Infection B | Infection A | | | |
	AP$_6$	*H.par.*	H1N1 (A)	H1N1 (B)
AP$_2$	0.4	1.3	1.3	1.5
AP$_6$		(0.9)	(1.0)	0.9
H.par.			1.2	1.3
H1N1 (A)				4.0

Note: AP$_2$ = *Actinobacillus pleuropneumoniae* type 2; AP$_6$ = *A. pleuropneumoniae* type 6; *H.par.* = *Haemophilus parasuis;* H1N1 (A) = swine influenza virus type H1N1/A/SW/New Jersey/8/76; H1N1 (B) = swine influenza virus type H1N1/A/SW/Belgium/2/79. All infections assessed through individual serologic examination of slaughter pigs.

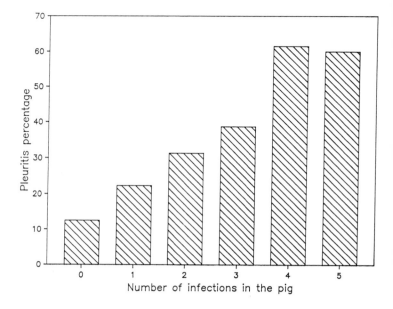

7.3. The prevalence of pleurisy in the presence of an increasing number of infections.

pathogens. Environmental and managemental factors greatly influence this balance. Differences in environmental and managemental conditions explain why the incidence of clinical disease may be low in some herds and high in others even if the herds are exposed to the same microorganisms. Environmental and managemental factors are mutually dependant and thus cannot be separated when analyzing respiratory problems. Nonchangeable environmental conditions (buildings, surroundings) will limit the managemental possibilities of influencing physical and microbial environment; on the other hand, managemental practice determines the physical environment.

SPECIALIZED/MIXED PRODUCTION SYSTEM. In our experience it is by far simpler to control respiratory diseases in breeding herds marketing all growers and feeders than in herds that also finish the pigs. An obvious reason is freedom of the "pathogen generator" effect associated with growing pigs. In mixed herds a periodic transmission of airborne pathogens from growers to the breeding herd is inevitable. Kliebenstein et al. (1982/83) found the largest total animal health expenditures in mixed farrow-to-finish operations, suggesting more health problems in this production system. The advantage of separating the sow herd from the growing/finishing unit, however, does not concern the specialized fattening herd.

ORIGIN OF PIGS. The origin of introduced animals significantly influences the risk of the herd contracting respiratory diseases (Rosendahl and Mitchell 1983). It is evident that respiratory problems can be expected if pigs with low health status are introduced into a healthy herd. However, there also is a risk when introducing animals with

a high health status into herds with a lower health status without taking any precautions to protect the healthy animals against infection. Such animals, insufficiently protected by specific immunity, easily develop clinical disease. Consequently, a sudden rise in excretion of pathogens occurs, and an established herd balance between infection and immunity is jeopardized.

In Danish SPF herds it is clearly illustrated that the chance of a herd catching respiratory problems increases with the number of groups and the number of sources (Jorsal and Thomsen 1988). Castryck et al. (1990) made the same observation in Belgian conventional pig production systems. An examination of 450,000 baconers revealed that pigs born from gilts had a significantly higher prevalence of lung lesions than those born from older sows (Mehlhorn and Hoy 1985).

CONTINUOUS BATCH PRODUCTION. In herds with an inadequate separation between pigs of different ages, there remains a continuous transmission of microbes from older to younger pigs with a subsequently continuous replication of pathogens. Dissimilar climatic demands of different age groups may be a contributing adverse factor. Contrarily, all-in/all-out pig movements on farms with properly separated facilities protect young animals against catching pathogens from groups of older pigs. The benefits of all-in/all-out production compared to continuous production have clearly been revealed in several investigations (Lindqvist 1974; Bäckström and Bremer 1978; Tielen et al. 1978).

NUMBER OF ANIMALS IN HERD/ROOM. Most epidemiological studies have revealed that the risk of contracting respiratory disease increases significantly with increasing herd size (Aalund et al. 1976; Bäckström and Bremer 1976; Flesja and Solberg 1981; Mehlhorn and Hoy 1985). However, a very large herd might have a somewhat lower level of respiratory disease than simply a big herd (Willeberg et al. 1984/85; Martinsson and Lundeheim 1988). The probable explanation is that very large herds are forced to subdivide facilities and move pigs into groups to control infectious diseases. In other herds it is, by more reasons, not cost effective to divide the facilities for an all-in/all-out production. Therefore, the health status of middle-sized and big herds often is surpassed by that of large enterprises. Tielen (1989) found none and Martinsson and Lundeheim (1988) found only a weak relationship between respiratory disease and herd size.

The number of animals placed in the same airspace significantly affects the incidence of disease even in enterprises with all-in/all-out production. Experience from several investigations (Lindqvist 1974; Tielen et al. 1978; Pointon et al. 1985) indicates that respiratory problems are difficult to control if more than 200–300 animals are housed in the same barn; in the Netherlands housing only 80 fatteners together is advised (Tielen 1989). Theoretically, for pigs sharing airspace, the risk of exchanging suspended particles increases substantially ($n^2 - n$, n = the number of animals). The same effect is seen by lowering floor space per pig (Lindqvist 1974; Bäckström and Bremer 1978; Mehlhorn and Hoy 1985; Pointon et al. 1985).

VENTILATION. To avoid massive air pollution and to maintain an acceptable relative humidity, it is necessary to use forced ventilation in confined facilities. The lower the airspace per pig the higher the air exchange is necessary. However, it is difficult to obtain full compensation for overcrowding. For example, if stocking rate is doubled, the ventilation rate should be increased tenfold to maintain the same clearance of air contaminants (Wathes et al. 1983); large air-cleaning equipment is necessary if a significant effect on the dust concentration is to be achieved (Gustafsson 1989).

Ventilation systems often recirculate room air with fresh air. This mixing of air contributes to a spread of respiratory pathogens. Accordingly, the level of the respirable dust is increased in high-speed recirculation systems (Meyer and Manbeck 1986). Hunneman et al. (1986) indicate that respiratory diseases can be better controlled in buildings under pressure ventilation where polluted air is removed and changed by totally fresh air. Nicks et al. (1989) found the aerial ammonia concentration was 21 ppm and 12 ppm in two compartments of a farrowing house. In the former, there was more recirculation of the extracted air.

CLIMATE. Bille et al. (1975) found a significantly higher incidence of pneumonia in piglets during the winter season than during the summer months. This indicates that climatic factors are included in the etiology of pneumonia. Data from the Danish abattoirs confirm the climatic influence on respiratory diseases at slaughter. The maximum prevalence of pleurisy occurs in summer, being 25% higher than minimum, which occurs in winter. The maximum prevalence of atrophic rhinitis occurs in autumn, being 75% higher than minimum, which occurs in spring.

A high exchange rate of air often causes local draught and chilling of animals. It is a common experience in pigs as in humans that a sudden chilling by draft predisposes to respiratory infections. Flesja et al. (1982) found that solid-sided pens were associated with a reduction in incidence of pneumonia, presumably by preventing draught. According to Kelley (1980), cold draughts and wide temperature differentials stress the immune mechanisms thus increasing susceptibility to disease. This is confirmed in weaner pigs, where exposure to cold draughts significantly reduced immune response (Scheepens et al. 1988). Prolonged cold stress in sucking piglets experimentally infected with *P. multocida* resulted in lowered levels of serum IgG, lowered phagocytic activity of the polymorphonuclear granulocytes, and delayed local cellular reaction in the lungs of some of the piglets compared with controls. However, there were no differences in the course of infection, the clinical response, and postmortem findings (Rafai et al. 1987).

AIR POLLUTION. High concentrations of ammonia in the air may be detrimental to respiratory health. Ammonia in concentrations of 50–100 ppm particularly interferes with normal mucociliary function (Curtis et al. 1975a; Johannsen et al. 1987; Neumann et al. 1987). Under ordinary conditions the ammonia concentration in pig pens does not exceed 20 ppm. Nevertheless, epidemiological studies have revealed the highest incidence of respiratory disease in herds with the highest ammonia concentrations in the air (Pointon et al. 1985).

Investigations have failed to demonstrate any significant relationship between dust and respiratory disease (Martin and Willoughby 1972; Curtis et al. 1975b). In young pigs, the rate of clearance of *P. multocida* from the lung was not affected by inhalation of TiO_2 dust for 2 weeks prior to exposure to bacteria (Gilmour 1989). However, dust particles could play a role as a vehicle for pathogens (Donham et al. 1986).

ENTERITIS. Digestive disorders reduce the resistance against pneumonia. A high prevalence of respiratory lesions at slaughter was found in pigs with previous enteritis (Aalund et al. 1976). A highly significant correlation was found between pigs that needed treatment for enteritis and pigs that were treated for pneumonia (Jørgensen

1988). Litters that shed rotavirus during the preweaning period had higher incidence rates of respiratory diseases than virus-free litters (Svensmark et al. 1989). Marois et al. (1989) demonstrated aggravation of experimentally induced mycoplasmal pneumonia in piglets also infected with transmissible gastroenteritis (TGE) virus.

CASTRATION. From surveillance of slaughter swine at Danish abattoirs, it has continuously been revealed that the prevalence of pneumonia and pleuritis in castrated males is 10% higher than in females. In the Netherlands lesions in lungs, pleura, and pericardium were also more prevalent in castrated males than in females (Kruijf et al. 1988). Castration may have been responsible for the differences through stress and hormonal changes.

Heredity. Several investigations indicate that respiratory disorders are to some extent influenced by heredity. In genetically selected obese swine, the phagocytic functions of pulmonary alveolar macrophages were found to be significantly more effective than those from genetically selected lean swine. The difference was most pronounced during winter and spring months (Caruso and Jeska 1990). Clinical observations in a herd having purebred Hampshires and Yorkshires revealed a much lower level of respiratory diseases in Hampshire than Yorkshire pigs (Lundeheim and Tafvelin 1986). The same investigators examined 45,000 slaughter pigs consisting of Hampshire, Landrace, and Yorkshire crosses. The Hampshire crossings had a significantly lower incidence of pneumonia as well as

of pleuritis than the other crosses. Susceptibility to atrophic rhinitis is greater in Yorkshire pigs than in Landrace pigs (Lundeheim 1979; Smith 1983; Straw et al. 1983).

DIAGNOSIS AND DIFFERENTIAL DIAGNOSIS OF RESPIRATORY DISEASE. Definitive diagnoses of respiratory diseases are based upon a combination of history, clinical observation, laboratory tests, and autopsy, including slaughter checks. A clinical diagnosis can only be tentative, since visible signs from the respiratory system may be the result of dysfunction of other organs. Also, pathological disorders of the respiratory system such as acute/subacute pleuropneumonia, chronic pneumonias, and pleuritis will often be without clinical signs or signs typical for respiratory disorders. Acute pleuropneumonia may be widespread in a herd before the disease is revealed at slaughter. Therefore, signs of laziness and decreased appetite in fatteners, often misinterpreted and attributed to bad feed, should remind the observer of the possibility of an outbreak of acute pleuropneumonia.

Table 7.6 summarizes some principal respiratory disorders. The basic elements in the table are typical pathological-anatomical disease entities. Useful differential diagnostic facts concerning gross pathology, clinical signs, and agents involved are given for every disease entity leading to the diagnosis. Additionally, in Tables 7.7 and 7.8 differential diagnostic information can be found concerning disease entities usually associated with the important respiratory signs such as sneezing and coughing.

Table 7.6.   Principal respiratory disorders, clinical signs, causative agents, and diagnosis

Disease Based on Pathology	Important Clinical Signs	Causative Agents	Diagnosis
01 Rhinitis: Possibly slight but reversible turbinate atrophy (*B. bronchiseptica*)	Sneeze; nasal discharge; conjuctivitis	*Bordetella bronchiseptica; cytomegalovirus*	Nasal swabs; culture; virus isolation; histology
02 Progressive atrophic rhinitis: Varying turbinate atrophy and nasal wall alteration	Sneeze; nasal discharge; tear tracks below eyes; occasional nasal bleeding; no or varying brachygnathia and snout deviation	Toxigenic *Pasteurella multocida*; predisposing: *Bordetella bronchiseptica*, aerial ammonia, dry air	Nasal swabs; culture; serology; ELISA; slaughter checks; clinical signs
03 Catarrhal pneumonia (mycoplasmalike pneumonia): Cranioventrally located; lobular; plum; meaty structure	Hard nonproductive cough, particularly when pigs are forced to move; slight fever; slightly decreased appetite	*Mycoplasma hyopneumoniae;* also *Mycoplasma hyorhinis* + streptococci and other bacteria in piglets	Culture; immunofluorescence; serology; clinical signs; necropsy; slaughter checks
04 Complicated catarrhal pneumonia (enzootic pneumonia): Located as 03; mostly lobular; purulent exudate; eventual formation of abscesses; red to gray; firm, fibrous structure; often associated with pleuritis	Productive cough, particularly when pigs are forced to move; abdominal "thumping" respiration; periodically high fever; decreased appetite	As 03 + *Pasteurella multocida, Bordetella bronchiseptica,* streptococci, staphylococci, *Corynebacterium,* and others; *Salmonella choleraesuis,* Aujeszky's virus may act as primary agents	As 03; virus isolation; clinical course: prolonged; frequent recidives; decreased weight gain

Table 7.6. (*Continued*)

Disease Based on Pathology	Important Clinical Signs	Causative Agents	Diagnosis
05 Disseminated catarrhal pneumonia: Spread, lobular distribution; red to gray colored; firm, fibrous structure	Occasional cough	*Bordetella bronchiseptica*	Necropsy; culture
06 Acute disseminated lobular pneumonia: Dark purple; bleeding from cuts; lobular emphysema	Varying degrees of depression; from no to hard cough; rapid, superficial respiration; fever; prostration; complete anorexia	Swine influenza virus	Virus isolation from nasal swabs or affected lung tissue; clinical signs: sudden onset; adults, slaughter sw. most severely affected, abortions
07 Peracute fibrinous/ necrotizing pneumonia (pleuropneumonia): Extensive dissemination; associated with blood-tinged fluid in the pleural cavity	Depression; prostration; high fever; severe dyspnea, open-mouth breathing; occasional blood-tinged foam from nose and mouth; dogsitting or sternal recumbency	*Actinobacillus pleuropneumoniae* (pathogenic strains)	Culture; necropsy; clinical signs; history: nonimmune herd
08 Acute/subacute fibrinous/necrotizing pneumonia (pleuropneumonia): Predominatly caudodorsally located; associated with a local fibrineous pleuritis	Varying depression, often none; respiration normal to superficial; depressed productive coughing or no cough; temperature: normal-high; decreased appetite	*Actinobacillus pleuropneumoniae;* occasionally *Haemophilus* "minor group"	Culture; necropsy; clinical signs; history: non- to low-immune herd
09 Chronic fibrinous/ necrotizing pneumonia (pleuropneumonia): Located as 08; firm, capsulated processes with necroses and abscesses	Slight depression; cough and decreased appetite if secondary infection occurs	*Actinobacillus pleuropneumoniae; Haemophilus* "minor group"; eventual secondary infection with pyogenic bacteria	Necropsy; culture; serology; history: previous acute pleuropneumonia
10 Embolic pneumonia: Randomly distributed abscesses in the lungs	Usually no clinical signs from the respiratory system	Pyogenic bacteria; streptococci, staphylococci, *Corynebacterium,* and others from the bloodstream	Necropsy; slaughter checks; primary conditions causing septicemia
11 Verminous pneumonia: Small focal areas with hemorrhage, later granulomas or capsulated abscesses	Cough with minimal other signs	*Ascaris suum* and other ascarids	Necropsy; slaughter checks; white spots in the liver
12 Verminous bronchitis: Bronchitis, bronchiolitis in caudoventventrally margins of diaphragmatic lobes, atelectatic areas	Cough with minimal other signs	*Metastrongylus* spp.	Necropsy; history: access to dirt
13 Hemorrhagic pleuritis: Associated with 07	As 07; No or depressed cough	As 07	Necropsy
14 Fibrinous pleuritis: Associated with 08 or 04, occasionally with 06 and 10; also associated with Glässer's disease; also the same localization if associated with 08 or 04	As 08	As 08, occasionally staphylococci released from pyemic processes; in piglets: *Haemophilus suis, Mycoplasma hyorhinis,* occasionally rare types of *E. coli;* seldom *Pasteurella multocida*	Necropsy; culture; infection with *H. parasuis:* lameness, central nervous signs; lesion often located dorsocaudally if induced by *A. pleuropneumoniae,* ventrocranially if associated with *P. multocida*
15 Fibrous pleuritis: Association with and located as 14	None	As 14; seldom *H. parasuis* and *M. hyopneumoniae*	Necropsy; slaughter checks; serology
16 Fibrous pericarditis: Associated with 15	None	As 15	Necropsy; slaughter checks

Table 7.7.   Respiratory disease entities and agents associated with sneezing

Age Group	Disease	Agent
Unweaned piglets	01 Rhinitis	*Bordetella bronchiseptica; Cytomegalovirus*
	02 Atrophic rhinitis	*B. bronchiseptica* and toxigenic *Pasteurella multocida* strains
	Aujeszky's disease	Aujeszky's disease virus
	Acute HEV infection	Hemagglutinating encephalomyelitis virus; dust, ammonia
Other pigs	02 Atrophic rhinitis	Late effect of *B. bronchiseptica* and toxigenic *P. multocida* (decreased mucosal clearance)
	Aujeszky's disease	Aujeszky's disease virus
	Swine fever	Swine fever virus; dust; ammonia

Table 7.8.   Respiratory disease entities and agents associated with coughing

Age Group	Disease	Agent
Unweaned piglets	03 Mycoplasmalike pleuropneumonia	*M. hyopneumoniae, B. bronchiseptica, P. multocida,* and other species
	04 Enzootic pneumonia	(nonproductive coughing in 03 and 05)
	05 Disseminated catarrhal pneumonia	
Weaners, growers	03 Mycoplasmalike pneumonia	*M. hyopneumoniae, B. bronchiseptica, P. multocida,* and other species
	04 Enzootic pneumonia	(nonproductive coughing in 03 and 05)
	05 Disseminated catarrhal pneumonia	
	06 Acute disseminated lobular pneumonia	Influenza virus (initially nonproductive coughing)
	09 Chronic pleuropneumonia	*A. pleuropneumoniae* in combination with other infections
	Glässer's disease	*Haemophilus parasuis* (nonproductive coughing)
	Swine fever	Swine fever virus
	Aujeszky's disease	Aujeszky's disease virus
Feeders, adults	03 Mycoplasmalike pneumonia	*M. hyopneumoniae, B. bronchiseptica, P. multocida,* and other species
	04 Enzootic pneumonia	(nonproductive coughing in 03)
	06 Acute disseminated lobular pneumonia	Influenza virus (initially nonproductive coughing)
	09 Chronic pleuropneumonia	*A. pleuropneumoniae* in combination with other infections
All ages	Cardiac insufficiency	

MONITORING RESPIRATORY DISEASE.

The purpose of monitoring respiratory diseases is to transform observed phenomena in a swine population into numeric values suitable for analysis. A reliable assessment of the level of disease and the effect of therapeutic or preventive measures can only be obtained by monitoring disease levels at a fixed time (prevalences) or during periods (incidences). Results of monitoring diseases of the respiratory tract comprise data collected in the herd and from laboratory tests and slaughter examinations. Large-scale data on the respiratory health of slaughter swine is routinely carried out in some countries: Denmark (Willeberg et al. 1984/85; Mousing 1986), Netherlands (Van der Valk et al. 1984), and Sweden (Bäckström and Bremer 1976).

Examinations in the Herd.   Clinical observations and postmortem examination of dead or euthanatized animals are traditionally the basis on which the consulting veterinarian estimates type and herd level of respiratory disease. The clinical examination is of greatest value in acute outbreaks when fever and specific signs from the respiratory tract may be observed. Conditions such as pleuropneumonia, chronic enzootic pneumonia, and pleuritis will often be without clinical signs; thus, a diagnosis based upon clinical observations always will be tentative.

The value of monitoring at the herd level naturally increases with the amount of objective data recorded. In many situations valuable data can be obtained by staff recordings during a defined period. Relevant data are number of deaths and treatments associated with respiratory problems, age or weight of affected animals, and performance records, e.g., days to market (Pijoan and Leman 1986).

Clinical signs are difficult parameters to handle in quantifying a disease problem. A model for assessment of pneumonia levels through measurement of the amount of coughing has been proposed (Straw et al. 1986).

Laboratory Tests.   In recent years tremendous progress in biotechnology has accelerated the development of new, highly specific laboratory tests on respiratory diseases. Useful diagnostic data may be obtained from laboratory examinations made on serum, secretions, and tissue. Particularly, it is advantageous to combine clinical examinations with laboratory tests in monitoring the health status of specific-pathogen-free (SPF) herds. Recently, it has been possible to detect antibodies against toxigenic *Pasteurella multocida* by enzyme-linked immunosorbent assay (ELISA) technique (Foged et al. 1989). This test will probably be a valuable tool in future monitoring of atrophic rhinitis at the herd level. Recent investigations have indicated that antibodies in colostrum instead of in serum could improve the diagnostic value of laboratory tests in monitoring for pleuropneumonia (Zimmerman et al. 1990) and mycoplasmal pneumonia (Zimmerman et al. 1988).

Examinations on Slaughter Swine.

As mentioned, national herd health monitoring programs by means of slaughter inspection data are used in several countries. Such programs are designed for long-term surveillance of herd health and cannot fulfill the need for current and specified examinations (slaughter checks) on selected groups of slaughter swine. Slaughter checks can be a profitable supplementary tool in handling respiratory problems (Pijoan and Leman 1986; Schulz 1986) and are used routinely in the surveillance of the health state of SPF herds (Keller 1988). Slaughter checks also have been devised to calculate the economic impact of pneumonia in herds. From different studies on the association between the severeness of pneumonia and the decrease in weight gain, Straw et al. (1989) deduced that (on the average) for every 10% of the lung with pneumonic lesions, the mean daily gain is reduced by 37 g. Based upon their own results Scheidt et al. (1990), however, states that there may be no basis for using data from slaughter checks to assess the economic effect of pneumonia and atrophic rhinitis, especially if the pigs examined are from different age groups.

EXAMINING THE SNOUT FOR ATROPHIC RHINITIS. Slaughter checks for atrophic rhinitis are usually performed by examining a transverse section of the snout. Optimal results are obtained if the cut is placed between premolar 1 and 2 (Martineau-Doizé 1990). Several methods of scoring athrophic rhinitis have been used (Bendixen 1971; Straw et al. 1983; Bäckström et al. 1985). These methods are based on subjective and visual assessments of structures. Results from different slaughter checks should be compared with caution as demonstrated by D'Allaire et al. (1988). Valid comparisons should be performed by the same experienced observer using the same scoring system.

A morphometric technique described by Collins et al. (1989) produced highly reproducible results. The method is rather time consuming and therefore of particular interest in experimental work.

A rapid method using inspection of longitudinal snout sections could be performed at slaughter (Visser et al. 1988). However, a drawback of this method was an unreliable estimation of the severity of mild cases of atrophic rhinitis.

EXAMINING THORACIC ORGANS (PLUCKS). Retrospective evaluations of the respiratory health by means of slaughter checks is based on the presence of chronic lesions. Slowly regressing lesions make long retrospects possible. As demonstrated by Noyes et al. (1988), the progressing and regressing of pneumonia in growing pigs is a dynamic process. The rate of which highly depends on the type of pneumonia involved as previously described. Another long-term lesion worth noticing in slaughter examinations is fissures in lung tissue that has previously been infected with catarrhal/catarrhal-purulent pneumonia (Bertschinger et al. 1972). Thus, if all significant pathological conditions of the thoracic organs are included, a reasonable long history of respiratory health can be revealed by means of slaughter check.

Several investigators have described methods of scoring the extent of "enzootic" pneumonia (Morrison et al. 1985) whereas little interest has been given to scoring and recording other types of lesions. However, examinations on plucks may be of minor diagnostic value if only the presence of pneumonia (percentage of animals with pneumonia and extent of pneumonic tissue) is considered. All macroscopic lesions in thoracic organs should be categorized according to type and assessed quantitatively by means of an appropriate scoring technique.

Careful slaughter checks of thoracic organs cannot normally be performed at the slaughter line. The material has to be transferred to an appropriate place for a thorough examination. Christensen (1990) devised a method by which 50–100 plucks can be examined per examiner per hour. The extent of all lesions detected are sketched on a special form with two schematic drawings of the lung (Fig. 7.4, left side). Lesions of the lung tissue are marked on the upper drawing and pleuritis on the lower drawing. The types of lesions are marked by a number indicating lesion category, other than mycoplasmal pneumonia or chronic pleuritis, which is prevalent in almost 90% of all cases. Following macroscopic examination and sketching, the extent of the lesions are quantified and recorded using marked lobe measures as guidelines. The recording form illustrated in Figure 7.4, right side, is used when experimental studies require further data collection.

The result of a slaughter check is presented in Figure 7.5. Specially programmed personal computer software automatically executes the calculations and printing.

Pleuritis is categorized as dorsocaudal or ventrocranial according to localization. The bor-

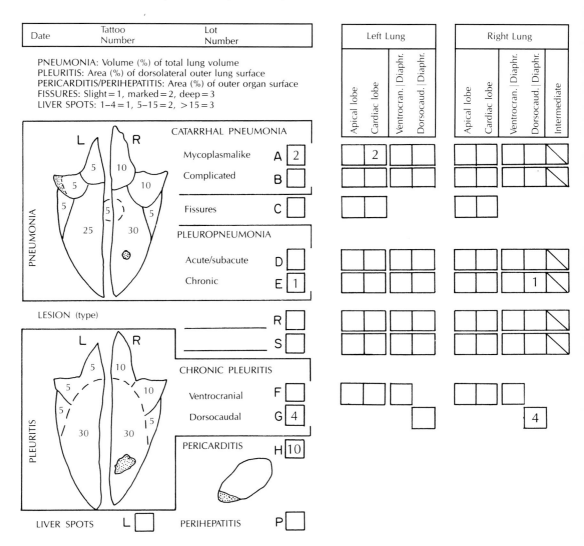

7.4. Form for recording findings on plucks at slaughter check (left). Form for recording experimental data in slaughter check (right).

derline is drawn through the dorsal endpoints of the interlobular fissures. The dorsal areas of the apical and cardiac lobes are regarded as belonging to the dorsocaudal lung surface area. We consider dorsocaudal localized pleuritis as nearly pathognomonic for a previous pleuropneumonic lesion.

Only using a scoring technique, describing the percentage of affected respiratory tissue, ensures that unbiased and repeatable results can be obtained. In most situations slaughter checks should be performed on at least 30 pigs (with similar or known age if possible) to get a sufficient sample and thus a reliable picture of the herd problem (Morrison et al. 1985; Straw et al. 1989).

CONTROL OF RESPIRATORY DISEASE.
Pathogenic microorganisms are involved in all im-

portant respiratory disorders. In practice it is impossible to protect pig herds from every pathogenic microorganism, and the development of respiratory disease fundamentally depends on the current balance between pressure from pathogenic microorganisms and the pigs' ability to resist them. This balance is very fragile and highly affected by a lot of herd factors (Fig. 7.6).

Control of respiratory diseases at the herd level must be based on two principles: to eliminate certain pathogens present in the environment; to sustain the herd's defense mechanisms (nonspecific, immunological, and inherited) and diminish the infection pressure in the herd. Elimination of certain pathogens is by far the most effective remedy in controlling many respiratory disorders. However, this can only be accomplished if the agent in question can be surely identified, transmission

SLAUGHTER CHECK–PLUCKS

Producer:_____

Slaughter date: 07/03/90

_____

_____

_____

Tattoo number: 11947

Clinic: _____

_____

_____

Number of pigs examined:
39

Type of lesion		Pigs with lesion		Average extension/intensity of lesion
		number	%	
Catarrhal pneumonia, mycoplasmalike	A	30	76.9	5.4
Catarrhal pneumonia, complicated	B	1	2.6	3.0
Fissures in apical and cardiac lobes	C	4	10.3	0.5
Pleuropneumonia, acute/subacute	D	1	2.6	3.0
Pleuropneumonia, chronic	E	0	0.0	0.0
Chronic pleuritis, ventrocranial	F	3	7.7	10.7
Chronic pleuritis, dorsocaudal	G	4	10.3	8.7
Embolic pneumonia	R	1	2.6	1.0
	S	0	0.0	0.0
Chronic pericarditis	H	3	7.7	83.3
Chronic perihepatitis	P	0	0.0	0.0
Liver spots	L	0	0.0	0.0

Average extension of pneumonia: % of total lung vol
Average intensity of fissures: slight = 1, marked = 2, deep = 3
Average extension of pleuritis: area % of outer lung surface
Average extension of pericarditis: area % of heart surface
Average intensity of liverspot: 1–4 = 1, 5–15 = 2, > 15 = 3

ABC: lesions are often caused by *Mycoplasma hyopneumoniae*
DEG: lesions are often caused by *Actinobacillus pleuropneumoniae*

7.5. Sample report of results of plucks examination at slaughter check.

routes effectively cut off, sufficient diagnostic capacity is available, and the owner is highly motivated (Nielsen 1972).

Elimination of Pathogens from the Herd.
Specific-pathogen-free production has been used successfully in Denmark and Switzerland in the control of economic important diseases such as mycoplasmal pneumonia, pleuropneumonia, and progressive atrophic rhinitis. To prevent reinfection of SPF herds with respiratory pathogens, a strict control over introduced pigs, vehicles, etc., must be maintained. The role of the upper respiratory tract of humans as a temporary reservoir of swine pathogens has generally been overestimated. However, the risk of transmission of *Mycoplasma hyopneumoniae* by human carriers cannot be totally neglected for other mycoplasmas are

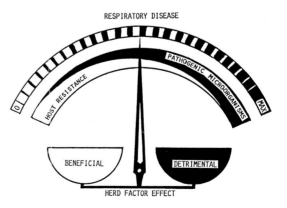

7.6. The influence of herd factors on the host/pathogen balance and the subsequent respiratory health status.

able to propagate in both species (Erickson et al. 1988). Nielsen and Frederiksen (1990) recently have demonstrated that human isolates of toxigenic *Pasteurella multocida* can induce progressive atrophic rhinitis in pigs, indicating that humans may act as carriers of swine pathogenic *Pasteurella* strains between herds.

Other detrimental herd factors (crowding, housing of differently aged pigs in the same barn, infection with influenza or Aujeszky's disease virus, enteric disorders) that regularly cause respiratory problems in conventional herds are to a great extent tolerated in SPF herds free from *M. hyopneumoniae* and *P. multocida.*

In practice it is not possible to eliminate more respiratory pathogens simultaneously from herds without total repopulation with hysterotomy-derived SPF pigs or their offspring. However, it is shown that *Actinobacillus pleuropneumoniae* may be eliminated from piglets by medicated early weaning (Larsen et al. 1990a) and sometimes from infected herds by means of heavy medication and culling of seropositive animals (Larivière

et al. 1990). Atrophic rhinitis seems to be impossible to eliminate by medication programs (Larsen et al. 1990b).

Sustaining Herd Defense Mechanisms and Infection Pressure. As illustrated in Figure 7.6, the influence of herd factors is decisive in sustaining herd resistance against respiratory pathogens and in reducing the amount of such pathogens in the herd. A catalog of herd factors influencing the host/pathogen balance is long. In Table 7.9 factors with a detrimental effect are listed and weighted in accordance to their importance. As can be seen short-term measures against respiratory disease predominantly comprise correcting managerial factors such as strategic medication procedures, vaccination, immediate treatment of sick animals, isolation arrangements, etc. Permanent improvement of respiratory health requires more radical and expensive changes in production systems and housing. Important long-acting herd factors to take in consideration are stocking rate; flow of animals to the herd and internal flow of

Table 7.9. Herd factors with detrimental effects on respiratory disease

Factors	Degree of Effect
Production System	
Large herd size	+ + +
High stocking density	+ + +
Conventional health system (not SPF or minimal disease production system)	+ + +
Introduction of animals from herds with unknown/low health status	+ + +
Continuous flow of animals through facilities (no movement of pigs in batches)	+ + +
Low average age of sows	+ + +
Average age of piglets at weaning	
very low	+ +
medium	+
high	+ +
Use of inherit disposed breeds	+
Use of purebreeds instead of crossings	+
Housing	
Badly insulated and ventilated facilities (causing improper temperature regulation and air exchange, draught)	+ + +
Insufficiently divided facilities combined with housing of differently aged animals in same airspace	+ + +
Pens divided without solid separations	+ + +
Large grower/finishing apartments (containing more than 200–300 pigs)	+ +
Nutrition	
Insufficient caloric intake	+
Improper content of macro/micro elements in feed	+
Feed not supplemented with fat (increases dust from feed)	+
Presence of Nonrespiratory Pathogens	
Colibacillosis	+ +
Dysentery	+ +
Mange	+
Ascarids	+
Management Deficiencies	
Insufficient control of climate	+ + +
Poor monitoring of signs of disease	+ +
Lacking/incorrect treatment of sick animals	+ +
Lacking/incorrect preventive measures (vaccinations, strategic medications)	+ +
Poor caretaking of sick animals (isolation, handling)	+
Poor hygiene	+ +

animals through the facilities; separation of age groups in the nonbreeding units; and improvement, insulation, and ventilation of buildings and separation of large barns.

MANAGEMENT. Management remains the most central factor in controlling respiratory problems. A constant and competent supervision of installations and animal behavior ensures that immediate and appropriate intervention can occur in case of arising problems. In this context it has to be recognized that respiratory diseases are not always associated with obvious clinical signs. In fact, most cases of respiratory disease occur subclinically or with only vague symptoms. Even outbreaks of acute pleuropneumonia may occur without clear respiratory symptoms (see DIAGNOSIS).

INTRODUCTION OF ANIMALS. The risk of introducing disease through purchase of traditionally reared animals can be avoided if a necessary supply of genetic material is ensured (artificial insemination, embryonated eggs, or cesarian-derived piglets. However, under commercial conditions a more practicable alternative will be to introduce breeding animals in batches from a breeding herd with the same or better health status as the buyer's. Prior to introduction into the herd, the animals shall be quarantined for at least 6 weeks, blood tested, and medicated. Animals determined for culling are placed in quarantine to transmit endemic microbes to the newly introduced breeding animals.

STOCKING DENSITY. In spite of the fact that crowding highly increases the incidence of respiratory diseases, it may be difficult to motivate managers to decrease stocking rate for calculations do not convincingly reveal an economic profit caused by this remedy. In case of only moderate respiratory problems, the profit due to better health often will be counterbalanced by the loss due to decreased utilization of herd facilities. Nevertheless, lowering stock density remains one of the most effective remedies against serious respiratory problems.

BARRIERS BETWEEN DIFFERENTLY AGED ANIMALS. To limit a continuous multiplication of pathogens in younger animals due to infections transmitted from older pigs, it is of crucial importance in larger herds to build barriers between groups of differently aged animals, and to move pigs in batches. The facilities should be adapted to all-in/all-out production, with rooms containing not more than 200–300 individuals. Ideally, the age difference in weaner batches should not exceed 2 weeks.

Generally, replication of pathogens and subsequent respiratory disease is most intense in growing animals. Thus, a safe barrier between the grower/finishing apartments and the breeding herd should always be maintained.

Weaning at about 4 weeks of age is preferable to weaning at an older age. This ensures the presence of an adequate level of colostral antibodies, and thus prevents infection of piglets from the sow with respiratory pathogens (in particular, toxigenic *P. multocida* and *A. pleuropneumoniae*).

CLIMATE. Respiratory problems often arise in cold and humid barns with no artificial heating. Frequently, the choice is whether the humidity shall be reduced by means of high air exchange rate, resulting in a lower room temperature, or the room has to be warmed by means of a lower air exchange rate. The first alternative is advisable according to experience. Cold, clean, dry air is by far superior to warm, polluted, humid air. Besides, the microclimate in a cold barn can be improved and protected against draught by straw bedding or by some sort of covering of resting places (Feenstra 1985) and by establishing solid separations between pens; pen separations should be solid to a height of 60 cm.

NUTRITION. In practice, malnutrition is rarely of importance in creating respiratory problems. Nevertheless, the relevance of vitamin E and selenium in immunity (Hayek et al. 1989) has to be considered. A major part of the dust particles in the air in swine barns arises from the feed. The addition of fat or wet feeding systems significantly reduces the dust problem.

NONRESPIRATORY PATHOGENS. There is a well-documented association between enteric disorders and respiratory problems. Therefore, solving respiratory problems is not possible if concurrent enteric problems are neglected. Mange and ascarids also have to be considered. Severe attacks of mange weaken the general resistance while migrating ascarids cause lung lesions, increasing the susceptibility to respiratory pathogens.

MEDICATION. The chance of quickly combatting outbreaks of respiratory disease depends on immediately medicating diseased individuals and penmates. Pigs with signs of pneumonia should be treated parenterally for their consumption of water and feed is significantly decreased (Goovaerts et al. 1986; Pijpers et al. 1990). Medicating for 2–3 days would in most cases be appropriate. Jørgensen (1988) found that pigs receiving immediate and intensive parenteral treatment against clinical pneumonia had a better weight gain than pigs receiving a less-intensive treatment. In outbreaks of pneumonia, pigs in contact with clinically diseased individuals should receive medication in food or water for 4–7 days.

In many herds pneumonia regularly occurs about 1 week after pigs are transferred to the grower/finishing unit. To prevent clinical disease in such herds, a reasonable strategic measure would be to medicate introduced animals for a period of 4–7 days, beginning just before signs of disease are expected. The pigs should, however, initially receive sufficient exposure to the current infections to develop immunity. Preventing this exposure will only delay the pneumonia problem, as demonstrated by Burch et al. (1986). These investigators obtained an improved weight gain and feed efficiency in fatteners by providing medicated feed for 7 days to a herd with complicated enzootic pneumonia. However, during the following 3 weeks most of the initial gains were lost, owing to reinfection.

Instead of protecting growers and feeders against pneumonia by means of long-term or permanent application of antimicrobials, it could be more profitable to apply pulse medication. Heard (1986) used medication for 5 days, repeated every 2–3 weeks, and Kavanagh (1990) medicated 2 days every week. The favorable effect obtained in these medication trials probably can be explained by a periodic low-level exposure of the pigs to the current infections and a subsequent development of immunity.

In outbreaks of pleuropneumonia in finishing units, Desrosiers (1986) found parenteral treatments early in the course of clinical disease much more cost effective than adding high levels of antimicrobials in feed and water.

VACCINATION. New effective vaccines have recently been developed against atrophic rhinitis. Vaccines against Aujeszky's disease and Glasser's disease have also shown a satisfactory effect in most cases, whereas existing vaccines against pleuropneumonia, enzootic pneumonia, and influenza still are not generally accepted.

HYGIENE. In preventing the transmission of respiratory pathogens between herds, particularly in production systems where certain respiratory pathogens are totally prohibited (SPF), it is important to clean, wash, and disinfect possible outside transmitters such as vehicles, delivery rooms, entrance rooms, tools, etc. However, cleaning the herd inside is of minor significance for the prevention of spread of respiratory pathogens. Too much washing may even in some cases aggravate a situation by cooling and humidifying the rooms. Generally speaking, respiratory diseases cannot be "washed out" of herds, as enteric diseases sometimes can.

ECONOMIC IMPORTANCE OF RESPIRATORY DISEASE.

Respiratory disorders are the cause of substantial losses to the swine industry. In a survey of swine health expenditures in Missouri, pneumonia and rhinitis were the two disease categories with the highest impact on total disease expenses (14% and 10% respectively) (Kliebenstein et al. 1982/83). Data from the National Animal Health Monitoring System in Ohio, 1986–87, revealed that pneumonia was by far the most costly disease in swine, accounting for $5.42 per pig per year out of total costs of $21.34 per pig due to diseases (Miller and Dorn 1987). Respiratory disease expenditures for the swine production of then East Germany were estimated at M 700 million per year. This reduction in returns was allocated to damaged lungs, 3%; destroyed and disposed of diseased animals, 37%; and reduced growth rate, 60% (Hoy et al. 1987).

Losses associated with respiratory disease vary considerably between herds (Lindqvist 1974; Wilson et al. 1986) but also between seasons. Boessen et al. (1988) reported a seasonal variation in the losses due to pneumonia at more than 30% (from $1.31 per hog in the winter of 1986, to $.89 in the following summer, and back to $1.26 in the winter of 1987). Similarly, the variation in losses due to rhinitis were more than 60% (from $.54 per hog in the winter of 1986, to $1.37 in the following summer, and back to $.50 in the winter of 1987). At the herd level the total cost of respiratory disease is the sum of output losses, namely, increased mortality, decreased weight gain, increased feed consumption, and decreased meat quality or payment, and of control expenditures, namely, treatments, vaccination programs, hygiene procedures, and extra labor (Schepers 1990).

In practical situations, the estimated economic impact of respiratory disorders in a herd must be based on slaughterhouse information and data on productivity and disease recordings in the herd: current weight gain or days to slaughter, feed efficiency, incidence of clinical respiratory disease and other diseases, mortality rate, results of necropsies, prevalence and severeness of lesions detected at slaughter, and finally the costs of current treatment and prophylaxis strategy.

OUTPUT LOSSES DUE TO ENZOOTIC PNEUMONIA. Most investigations on the economic effect of enzootic pneumonia are based on the prevalence of pneumonia at slaughter. However, in herds where pneumonia predominantly occurs in young pigs, the lesions may be resolved at the time of slaughter (Wallgren et al. 1990). This is, without doubt, a main reason for the great variability in estimates on the economic effect of enzootic pneumonia (Table 7.10).

In a clinical trial, Baekbo and Szancer (1990) reported a reduction in growth rate associated with enzootic pneumonia in medicated postweaning pigs, but no effect of pneumonia in nonmedicated animals. Pigs with no apparent pneumonic symptoms but with enzootic pneumonia demonstrable at slaughter did not have significant reduction in daily gain, whereas clinical pneumonic cases presented a 9–17% lowering in weight gain (Done 1990). Lundeheim (1979) and Wallgren et al. (1990) suggested that pneumonia possesses its greatest influence on total weight gain when it occurs in young pigs. Contrarily, Dijk et al. (1984), Hartley et al. (1988), and Jørgensen (1988) proposed that pneumonia in older pigs is more damaging to the weight gain.

OUTPUT LOSSES DUE TO PLEUROPNEUMONIA. The cost of pleuropneumonia is highly variable (Tables 7.11, 7.12). All the results presented refer to infection with pathogenic types of *Actinobacillus pleuropneumoniae*. Generally, the disease has become gradually milder since its occurrence, probably due to the establishment of a widespread herd immunity, which to a great extent may be generated by strains with low pathogenicity.

Total losses due to pleuropneumonia were assessed at 2% of the value of produced slaughter swine, estimated in three pleuropneumonia-in-fected herds with 10–20% pleuritis at slaughter (Christensen 1981b). Occasionally, 10–20% or more of individuals in batches of slaughter swine from newly infected herds are totally condemned at slaughter due to acute pleuropneumonia. The risk of condemnation highly increases if pigs are stored alive at the slaughterhouse for more than 24 hours (Christensen 1986). Slaughter pigs from nonimmune herds, in particular pigs from SPF herds, also are at risk of contracting acute pleuropneumonia if housed more than 24 hours together with infected pigs.

OUTPUT LOSSES DUE TO CHRONIC PLEURITIS. A high frequency of chronic pleuritis at slaughter is a typical symptom of the herd that is infected with *Actinobacillus pleuropneumoniae* (Christensen 1981b), but several infections may participate in increasing the frequency of the disease.

Table 7.10. Effect of enzootic pneumonia on weight gain and feed efficiency

Reference	Effect	
Weibel et al. 1983	−6%	fe
Hoy et al. 1985	−	wg
Wilson et al. 1986	−	wg (one herd)
Le Foll et al. 1988	−	wg (up to −19% in swine 110–115 days of age; less marked decrease in younger swine)
Cowart et al. 1990	−13%	wg (severe enzootic pneumonia)
Bäckström et al. 1975	0	wg
Christensen 1984	0	wg
Love et al. 1985	0	wg
Wilson et al. 1986	+	wg (one herd)
Straw et al. 1989	−17%	wg (more studies, great variation)
Straw et al. 1989	−14%	fe (more studies, great variation)

Note: wg = weight gain; fe = feed efficiency; − = decrease; + = increase; 0 = no adverse effect.

Table 7.11. Effect of pleuropneumonia on weight gain and feed efficiency

Reference	Effect	
Saunders et al. 1981	−	wg (considerable)
Christensen 1982	−20%	wg (recently infected SPF herd)
Hunneman 1983	0	wg
Rosendal and Mitchell 1983	−	wg (considerable)
Weibel et al. 1983	−7%	wg
Desrosiers 1986	−6%	wg
Desrosiers 1986	0	fe
Wilson et al. 1986	−	wg (considerable)
Straw et al. 1989	−33%	wg (more studies, great variation)
Straw et al. 1989	−25%	fe (more studies, great variation)

Note: wg = weight gain; fe = feed efficiency; − = decrease; + = increase; 0 = no adverse effect.

Table 7.12. Effect of pleuropneumonia on mortality in infected herds

Reference	Effect	
Saunders et al. 1981	+	(high mortality; loss was 1.5% of herd's total income in 4 months after outbreak)
Christensen 1982	0	(two conventional herds)
Christensen 1982	+0.5%	(newly infected SPF herd)
Hunneman 1983	+1.0%	
Rosendal and Mitchell 1983	+2–10%	(considerable)
Desrosiers 1986	+0.4%	
Wilson et al. 1986	0	

Note: + = increase; 0 = no adverse effect.

Several studies have been conducted describing the economic implications of pleuritis: in several herds, chronic pleuritis resulted in 7–12 extra days to attain slaughter weight (Christensen 1982, 1984). Following a clinical outbreak of respiratory disease in a large integrated herd, pigs with chronic pleuritis grew slower than pigs without this lesion (requiring 8 extra days to attain market weight), but prior to the outbreak there was no apparent association between chronic pleuritis and days to market (Hartley et al. 1988). Results from several other studies indicate that pigs with chronic pleuritis have a reduced rate of weight gain (Bäckström et al 1975; Rasmussen 1984; Hoy et al. 1985; Love et al. 1985). On the other hand, Le Foll et al. (1988) reported no effect of chronic pleuritis on growth rate.

OUTPUT LOSSES DUE TO ATROPHIC RHINITIS. As is the case for pneumonia, the output losses reported for atrophic rhinitis vary from one study to another (Table 7.13). Not only have results differed between surveys, but researchers often have found a varying effect between herds in a given survey. In a study of two herds, a decreased rate of weight gain could only be attributed to atrophic rhinitis in one of them (Wilson et al. 1986), while Scheidt et al. (1990) could demonstrate a negative effect of atrophic rhinitis in only one out of three herds.

It is understandable that disease effects on mortality and performance vary considerably between studies due to the fact that respiratory diseases always will be the result of numerous interacting microbial and physical insults, different in type and grade as well. Therefore, of any two examined disease situations, each will always be unique. Data from an investigation actually can only be assessed by an observer with an in-detail knowledge of the situation in question.

REFERENCES

AALUND, O.; WILLEBERG, P.; MANDRUP, M.; AND RIEMANN, H. P. 1976. Lung lesions at slaughter: Associations to factors in the pig herd. Nord Vet Med 28:487–495.

ANDERSON, P. L.; MORRISON, R. B.; MOLITOR, T. W.; AND THAWLEY, D. G. 1990. Factors associated with circulation of pseudorabies virus within swine herds. J Am Vet Med Assoc 196:877–880.

AWAD-MASALMEH, M.; KÖFER, J.; AND SCHUH, M. 1990. On the occurrence of chronic respiratory disease at swine herds in Austria. Bacteriological findings, efficacy of autogenous vaccines. Proc Int Pig Vet Soc, Lausanne, p. 107.

BÄCKSTRÖM, L.; AND BREMER, H. 1976. Sjukdomsregistreringar på Svin vid Slaktbesiktning-Ett Hjälpmedel i Förebyggande Svinhälsovard. Svensk Vet Tidn 28:312–336.

_____. 1978. The relationship between disease environmental factors in herds. Nord Vet Med 30:526–533.

BÄCKSTRÖM, L.; BREMER, H.; DYRENDAHL, I.; AND OLSSON, H. 1975. Sambandsstudier av produktions- och sjukdomsdata på slaktsvin i en integreret besättning med hög frekvens av atrofisk rhinit, enzootisk pneumoni ock pleurit. Svensk Vet Tidn 27:1028–1040.

BÄCKSTRÖM, L. R.; HOEFLING, D. C.; AND MORKOC, A. C. 1985. Effect of atrophic rhinitis on growth rate in Illinois swine herds. J Am Vet Med Assoc 187:712–715.

BAEKBO, P., AND SZANCER J. 1990. Strategisk medicinering af fravænnede grise mod *Actinobaccillus* (*Haemophilus*) infektion. [Prophylactic treatment of weaned pigs against *Actinobacillus pleuropneumoniae*]. Dansk Vet Tidskr 73:804–811.

BASKERVILLE, A. 1981. Mechanisms of infection in the respiratory tract. NZ Vet J 29:235–238.

BECHMANN, G. AND SCHÖSS, P. 1990. Neutralizing activity against *Pasteurella multocida* toxin in sera of pigs with atrophic rhinitis. Proc Int Pig Vet Soc, Lausanne, p. 50.

BENDIXEN, H. C. 1971. Om nysesyge hos svinet. Nord Vet Med [Suppl] 23:1.

BERTRAM, T. A. 1985. Quantitative morphology of peracute pulmonary lesions in swine induced by *Haemophilus pleuropneumoniae*. Vet Pathol 22:598–609.

BERTSCHINGER, H. U.; KELLER, H.; LÖHRER, A.; AND WEGMANN, W. 1972. Der zeitliche Verlauf der experimentellen enzootischen Pneumonie beim SPF-Schwein. Schweiz Arch Tierheilkd 114:107–118.

BILLE, N.; LARSEN, J. L.; SVENDSEN, J.; AND NIELSEN, N. C. 1975. Preweaning mortality in pigs. 6. Incidense and causes of pneumonia. Nord Vet Med 27:482–495.

BOESSEN, C. R.; KLIEBENSTEIN, J. B.; COWART, R. P.; MOORE, K. C.; AND BRURBEE, C. R. 1988. Effective use of slaughter checks to determine economic loss from morbidity in swine. Proc 5th Int Symp Vet Epidemial Econ, Acta Vet Scand [Suppl] 84:436–438.

BRÖRING, S.; MÜLLER, E.; PETZOLDT, K.; SCHOON, H. A.; AND BERGMANN, K. C. 1989. Das Zusammenwirken von *Actinobacillus pleuropneumoniae* und influenza A-virus bei experimentell infizierten Mäusen. J Vet Med [B] 36:681–690.

BURCH, D. G. S.; JONES, G. T.; HEARD, T. W.; AND TUCK, R. E. 1986. The synergistic activity of tiamulin and chlortetracycline: In-feed treatment of bacterially

Table 7.13. Effect of atrophic rhinitis on weight gain

Reference		Effect
Love et al. 1985	−	
Straw and Ralston 1986	−5–10%	(10 out of 19 studies)
Straw and Ralston 1986	0	(9 out of 19 studies)
Nielsen et al. 1990	−13%	(experimentally, individual)
Cowart et al. 1990	−9%	
Lieschke et al. 1989	−	(−9, 4 kg in equally aged slaughter swine)
Dumas et al. 1990	0	(four herds)
Love et al. 1985	0	
Le Foll et al. 1988	0	

complicated enzootic pneumonia in fattening pigs. Vet Rec 119:108–112.

BUTTENSCHØN, J. 1989. Differentiation between five types of pneumonia distribution pattern in pigs. J Vet Med [A] 36:494–504.

_____. 1990. Kvantitativ og kvalitativ karakterisering af pneumonier hos kvæg og svin. Thesis, Institut for veterinær Mikrobiologi, Den kgl. Veterinær-og Landbohøjskole, København.

CARUSO, J. P., AND JESKA, E. L. 1990. Phagocytic functions of pulmonary alveolar macrophages in genetically selected lean and obese swine and effects of exogenous linolenic acid upon cell function. Vet Immunol Immunolopathol 24:27–36.

CASTRYCK, F.; DEVRIESE, L. A.; HOMMEZ, J.; CASSIMON, P.; AND MIRY, C. 1990. Bacterial agents associated with respiratory disease in young feeder pigs. Proc Int Pig Vet Soc, Lausanne, p. 112.

CHRISTENSEN, G. 1981a. Ondartet lungesyge (Schweizisk lungesyge). Hyologisk Tidskr Svinet 3(8):25–28.

_____. 1981b. Pleuropneumoni hos svin fremkaldt af *Haemophilus pleuropneumoniae*. II. Undersøgelser vedrørende epidemilogi samt relation til kronisk pleuritis (brysthindear) hos slagtesvin. [Pleuropneumonia in swine due to *Haemophilus pleuropneumoniae*. II. Studies on the epidemiology and the relation to chronic pleuritis (pleural scars) in baconers]. Nord Vet Med 33:236–249.

_____. 1982. Pleuropneumoni hos svin fremkaldt af *Haemophilus pleuropneumoniae*. III. Observationer vedrørende klinisk manifestation på besætningsplan samt terapeutiske og immunprofylaktiske muligheder. [Pleuropneumonia in swine due to *Haemophilus pleuropneumoniae*. III. Studies on clinical manifestation in herds, treatment and control by vaccination]. Nord Vet Med 34:113–123.

_____. 1984. Brysthindear (kronisk fibrøs pleuritis) hos slagtesvin. En undersøgelse vedrørende brysthindearrenes ætiologi og udviklingsforløb i en lukket, konventionel svinebesætning med høj frekvens af brysthindear. Dansk Vet Tidskr 67:1067–1075.

_____. 1986. Ondartet lungesyge (pleuropneumoni) hos slagtesvin. Betragtninger vedrørende sygdommens natur, udbredelse, kødkontrolmæssige forhold og dens indflydelse på produktionsøkonomi. Hyologisk Tidskr Svinet 8(6):3–8.

_____. 1990. Unpublished results.

COLLINS, M. T.; BÄCKSTRÖM, L. R.; AND BRIM, T. A. 1989. Turbinate perimeter ratio as an indicator of conchal atrophy for diagnosis of atrophic rhinitis in pigs. Am J Vet Res 50:421–424.

COWART, R. P.; LIPSEY, R. J.; AND HEDRICK, H. B. 1990. Measurements of conchal atrophy and their association with growth rate in commingled feeder pigs. J Am Vet Med Assoc 196: 1262–1264.

CURTIS, S. E.; ANDERSON, C. R.; SIMON, J., JENSEN, A. H.; DAY, D. L.; AND KELLEY, K. W. 1975a. Effects of aireal ammonia, hydrogen sulfide and swine-house dust on rate of gain and respiratory tract structure in swine. J Anim Sci 41:735–739.

CURTIS, S. E.; DRUMMOND, J. G.; GRUNLOH, D. J.; BRENDAN LYNCH, P.; AND JENSEN, A. H. 1975b. Relative and qualitative aspects of aerial bacteria and dust in swine houses. J Anim Sci 41:1512–1521.

D'ALLAIRE, S.; BIGRAS-POULIN, M.; PARADIS, M. A.; AND MARTINEAU, G.-P. 1988. Evaluation of atrophic rhinitis: Are the results repeatable? Proc Int Pig Vet Soc, Rio De Janeiro, p. 38.

DESROSIERS, R. 1986. Therapeutic control and economic aspects of porcine pleuropneumonia in finishing units. Vet Rec 119:89–90.

DIJK, W. P. J. VAN; KLAVER, J.; AND VERSTEGEN, M. W. A. 1984. Frequentie van enkele aandoeningen bij schlachtvarkens en de effecten op groei en schlachtkwaliteit. Tijdschr Diergeneeskd 109:539–548.

DONE, S. H. 1988. Some aspects of respiratory defence with special reference to immunity. Proc Int Pig Vet Soc, Rio de Janeiro, pp. 31–60.

_____. 1990. Relationship between clinical respiratory disease and production parameters in pigs. Proc Int Pig Vet Soc, Lausanne, p. 391.

DONHAM, K. J.; SCALLON, L. J.; POPENDORPH, W.; TREUHAFT, M. W.; AND ROBERTS, R. C. 1986. Characterization of dust collected from swine confinement buildings. Am Ind Hyg Assoc J 47:404–410.

DUMAS, G.; DENICOURT, M.; D'ALLAIRE, S.; BIGRAS-POULIN, M.; AND MARTINEAU, G.-P. 1990. Atrophic rhinitis and growth rate: A potential confounding effect related to slaughter weight. Proc Int Pig Vet Soc, Lausanne, p. 385.

ERICKSON, B. Z.; ROSS, R. F.; AND BOVE, J. M. 1988. Isolation of *Mycoplasma salivarium* from swine. Vet Microbiol 16:385–390.

FALK, K.; LIUM, B. M.; ØDEGAARD, Ø. 1990. Occurrence of lung lesions and antibodies to serotypes 2 and 6 of *Actinobacillus pleuropneumoniae* and to *Haemophilus parasuis* in 5176 slaughter weight pigs from 113 elite herds in Norway. Proc Int Pig Vet Soc, Lausanne, p. 31.

FEENSTRA, A. 1985. Effects of air temperatures on weaned piglets. Pig News Inf 6:295–299.

FLESJA, K. I., AND SOLBERG, I. 1981. Pathological lesions in swine at slaughter. Acta Vet Scand 22:272–282.

FLESJA, K. I.; FORUS, I. B.; AND SOLBERG, I. 1982. Pathological lesions in swine at slaughter. V. Pathological lesions in relation to some environmental factors in the herds. Acta Vet Scand 23:169–183.

FOGED, N. T.; PEDERSEN, K. B.; AND ELLING, F. 1987. Characterization and biological effects of the *Pasteurella multocida* toxin. FEMS Microbiol Lett 43:45–51.

FOGED, N. T.; NIELSEN, J. P.; AND JORSAL, S. E. 1989. Protection against progressive atrophic rhinitis by vaccination with *Pasteurella multocida* toxin purified by monoclonal antibodies. Vet Rec 125:7–11.

FOLKESSON, H. G.; WESTSTRÖM, B. R.; PIERZYNOWSKI, S. G.; SVENDSEN, J.; LUNDIN, S.; AND KARLSSON, B. W. 1990. Lung permeability to different-sized macromolecules in developing pigs. Proc Int Pig Vet Soc, Lausanne, p. 430.

FRIIS, N. F. 1974. *Mycoplasma suipneumoniae* and *Mycoplasma flocculare* in comparative pathogenicity studies. Acta Vet Scand 15:507–518.

GANTER, M.; KIPPER, S.; AND HENSEL, A. 1990. Bronchoscopy and bronchoalveolar lavage of live anaesthetized pigs. Proc Int Pig Vet Soc, Lausanne, p. 109.

GILMOUR, M. I. 1989. Airborne pollution and respiratory disease in animal houses. Diss Abstr Int [B] 49 (7):2521.

GLOSTER, J.; BLACKALL, R. M.; SELLERS, R. F.; AND DONALDSON, A. I. 1981. Forecasting the airborne spread of foot-and-mouth disease. Vet Rec 108:370–374.

GOODWIN, R. F. W. 1985. Apparent reinfection of enzootic pneumonia-free pig herds: Search for possible causes. Vet Rec 116:690–694.

GOODWIN, R. F. W.; CHANTER, N.; AND RUTTER, J. M. 1990. Detection and distribution of toxigenic *Pasteurella multocida* in pig herds with different degree of atrophic rhinitis. Vet Rec 126:452–456.

GOOVAERTS, K.; JANSEGERS, L.; AND LENS, S. 1986. The effect of the water-consumption of fattening pigs. Proc Int Pig Vet Soc, Barcelona, p. 283.

GUSTAFSSON, G. 1989. Mass balances of dust in houses

for pigs. In Agricultural Engineering. Proc 11th Int Congr Agric Eng [CIGR], Dublin, Ire, 4–8 September 1989. Ed. V. A. Dod and P. M. Grace, p. 1465–1470.

HARTLEY, P. E.; WILESMITH, J. W.; AND BRADLEY, R. 1988. The influence of pleural lesions in the pig at slaughter on the duration of the fattening period: An on-farm study. Vet Rec 123:208.

HAYEK, M. G.; MITCHELL, G. E., JR.; HARMON, R. J.; STAHLY, T. S.; CROMWELL, G. L.; TUCKER, R. E.; AND BARKER, K. B. 1989. Porcine immunoglobulin transfer after prepartum treatment with selenium or vitamin E. J Anim Sci 67:1299–1306.

HEARD, T. W. 1986. The control of some pneumonia problems in pigs by strategic medication procedures. Proc Int Pig Vet Soc, Barcelona, p. 284.

HEILMANN, P.; MÜLLER, G.; AND FINSTERBUSCH, L. 1988. Lobäre Deposition radioaktiv markierter *Pasteurella-multocida* Aerosole in den Lungen von Ferkeln und Kälbern. Arch Exp Vet Med 42:490–501.

HENNINGSEN, D.; MOUSING, J.; AND AALUND, O. 1988. Porcint corona virus (PCV) i Danmark. En epidemiologisk tvaersnitsanlyse baseret på screeningsområde spørgeskema data. Dansk Vet Tidskr 71:1168–1177.

HOY, S.; MEHLHORN, G.; EULENBERGER, K.-H.; ERWERTH, W.; JOHANNSEN, U.; DORN, W.; AND HÖRÜGEL, K. 1985. Zum Einfluss entzündlicher Lungenveränderungen auf ausgewählte Parameter der Schlachtleistung beim Schwein. Monatsh Veterinaermed 40:584–587.

HOY, S.; MEHLHORN, G.; AND LIESCKHE, B. 1987. Zur ökonomische Bedeutung von Atemwegskrankungen der Schweine. [The economic importance of respiratory diseases of pigs.] Tierzucht 41:334–336.

HUNNEMAN, W. A. 1983. Vóórkomen, ekonomische betekenis en bestrijding van *Haemophilus pleuropneumoniae*–infektes bij varkens. Ph.D. diss., Government Univ of Utrecht, Netherlands.

HUNNEMAN, W. A.; VOETS, M. T.; SCHOOL, A. C. M.; AND VERHAGEN, F. A. P. 1986. *Haemophilus pleuropneumoniae* infections in fattening pigs. Effect of subclinically infected breeding herds and different ventilation systems. Proc Int Pig Vet Soc, Barcelona, p. 276.

JOHANNSEN, U.; ERWERTH, W.; MENGER, S.; NEUMANN, R.; MEHLHORN, G.; AND SCHIMMEL, D. 1987. Experimentelle Untersuchung zur Wirkung einer chronischen aerogenen Schadgasbelastung des Saugferkels mit Ammoniak unterschiedlicher Konzentrationen. J Vet Med [B] 34:260–273.

JØRGENSEN, B. 1988. Epidemiologiske analyser af sygdomsdata fra svineavlens forsøgsstationer. II. Dansk Vet Tidskr 71:9–23.

JORSAL, S. E., AND THOMSEN, B. L. 1988. A Cox regression analysis of risk factors related to *Mycoplasma suipneumoniae* reinfection in Danish SPF-herds. Acta Vet Scand [Suppl] 84:436–437.

KASTNER, P., AND MEHLHORN, G. 1989. Untersuchungen zur Deposition und Clearance inhalierter Bakterien (*Staphylococcus aureus*) in der Lunge von Ferkeln. Arch Exp Vet Med 43:379–389.

KAVANAGH, N. 1990. The effect of pulse medication with a combination of tiamulin and oxytetracycline on the performance of fattening pigs infected with enzootic pneumonia. Proc Int Pig Vet Soc, Lausanne, p. 351.

KELLER, H. 1988. The Swiss health service (PHS). Proc Int Pig Vet Soc, Rio De Janeiro, p. 334.

KELLEY, K. W. 1980. Stress and immune function: A bibliographic review. Ann Vet Res 11:445–478.

KLIEBENSTEIN, J. B.; KIRTLEY, C. L.; SELBY, L. A. 1982/83. A survey of swine production health problems and health maintenance expenditures. Prev Vet Med 1:357–369.

KOBISCH, M., AND GENIN, F. 1989. Les modeles experimentaux dans la pathologie pulmonaire du porc: Leur interet pour evaluer l'activite des molecules. J Rech Porc Fr 21:187–192.

KRUIJF, J. M. DE, AND WELLING, A. A. W. M. 1988. Het voorkommen van chronische ontstekingen bij gelten en borgen. [Occurrence of chronic inflammatory conditions in gilts and castrated male pigs.] Tijdschr Diergeneeskd 113:415–417.

LAI, S.-S.; HO, W.-C.; AND CHANG, W.-M. 1986. Persistent infection of pseudorabies virus resulted in concurrent infections with Haemophilus SPP in pigs. Proc Int Pig Vet Soc, Barcelona, p. 335.

LAMBOTTE, J. L.; PECHEUR, M.; CHARLIER; COIGNOUL, F.; AND DEWALE, A. 1990. Aerosol infection with *Bordetella bronchiseptica* – morphological alterations in the respiratory tract – and in the lung of piglets. Proc Int Pig Vet Soc, Lausanne, p. 106.

LARIVIÈRE, S.; D'ALLAIRE, S.; DELASALLE, F.; NADEAU, M.; MOORE, C.; AND ETHIER, R. 1990. Eradication of *Actinobacillus pleuropneumoniae* serotypes 1 and 5 infections in four herds. Proc Int Pig Vet Soc, Lausanne, p. 17.

LARSEN, S. H.; HØGEDAHL JØRGENSEN, P.; AND SZANCER, J. 1990a. Eradication of *Actinobacillus pleuropneumoniae* from a breeding herd. Proc Int Pig Vet Soc, Lausanne, p. 18.

LARSEN, S. H.; JØRGENSEN, P. H.; NIELSEN, P. A. 1990b. Elimination of specific pathogens in 3 to 4 week piglets by use of strategic medication. Proc Int Pig Vet Soc, Lausanne, p. 387.

LE FOLL, P.; AMARA, N.; GIRAL, B.; AND SOLIGNAC, T. 1988. Influence de la pathologie sur la croissance des porcs entre le sevrage et l'abattage. J Rech Porc Fr 20:95–100.

LIESCHKE, B.; HOY, S.; MEHLHORN, G.; AND WARNECKE, H.-W. 1989. Auswirkungen der Rhinitis atrophicans suum auf die Schlachtleistung gleichaltriger Mastswheine unter Berücksichtigung entzündlicher Lungenveränderungen. [Effects of rhinitis atrophicans suum on slaughter yield of equally aged fattening pigs with reference to inflammatory pulmonary alterations.] Menatsh Veterinaermed 44:11–16.

LINDQVIST, J. O. 1974. Animal health and environment in the production of fattening pigs. Acta Vet Scand [Suppl] 51:1–78.

LOVE, R. J.; WILSON, M. R.; AND TASLER, G. 1985. Porcine atrophic rhinitis. Austr Vet J 62:377–378.

LUNDEHEIM, N. 1979. Genetic analysis of respiratory diseases in pigs. Acta Agric Scand 29:209–215.

LUNDEHEIM, N., AND TAFVELIN, B. 1986. Pathological lesions at slaughter in Swedish pig production – Hampshire crosses compared with Landrace and Yorkshire crosses. Proc Int Pig Vet Soc, Barcelona, p. 380.

MADEC, F. AND KOBISCH, M. 1984. État sanitaire du porcellets et évolution des lésions au niveau de l'arbre respiratoires au cours des différentes phases d'élevages. J Rech Porc Fr 16:215–226.

MADEC, F.; GOURREAU, J. M.; AND KAIZER, C. 1982. Epidemiology of swine influenza $H_{sw}1N1$ on farms in Brittany (first outbreak – 1982). Épidemiol Sante Anim 2:56–64.

MADEC, F.; GOURREAU, J. M.; KAIZER, C.; AND AYMARD, M. 1990. A retrospective study about influenza infections in the pig in France. Proc Int Pig Vet Soc, Lausanne, p. 201.

MAROIS, P.; DIFRANCO, E.; BOULAY, G.; AND ASSAF, R. 1989. Enzootic pneumonia in feeder pigs: Association with transmissible gastroenteritis virus infection. Can Vet J 30:328–330.

MARTIN, S. W., AND WILLOUGHBY, R. A. 1972. Organic dusts, sulfur dioxide, and the respiratory tract of swine. Arch Environ Health 25:158–165.

MARTINEAU-DOIZÉ, B.; LAROCHELLE, R.; BOUTIN, J.; AND MARTINEAU, G.-P. 1990. Atrophic rhinitis caused by toxigenic *Pasteurella multocida* type D: Morphometric analysis. Proc Int Pig Vet Soc, Lausanne, p. 63.

MARTINSSON, K., AND LUNDEHEIM, N. 1988. Effekter av driftsform, besättnings-och stallstorlek. Svensk Vet, 40:313-319.

MEHLHORN, G., AND HOY, S. 1985. Influence of endogenic and exogenic factors on the prevalence rate of lung lesions of fattening pigs and sows. Proc 5th Int Congr Anim Hyg, September 1985, Hannover, pp. 391-396.

MERCY, A. R., AND BRENNAN, C. M. 1988. The Western Australia pig health monitoring scheme. Proc 5th Int Symp Vet Epidemiol Econ, Acta Vet Scand [Suppl] 84:212-214.

MEYER, D. J., AND MANBECK, H. B. 1986. Dust levels in mechanically ventilated swine barns. Am Soc Agr Eng Pap No. 86-4042.

MILLER, G., AND DORN, C. R. 1987. An economic summary of the national animal health monitoring system data in Ohio, 1986-87. Proc USA Health Assoc 91:154-172.

MØLLER, K., AND KILIAN, M. 1990. V factor dependant Pasteurellaceae in the porcine upper respiratory tract. R Den Coll, Aarhus, Denmark. To be published.

MORRISON, R. B.; HILLEY, H. D.; AND LEMAN, A. D. 1985. Comparison of methods for assessing the prevalence and extent of pneumonia in market weight swine. Can Vet J 26:381-384.

MORTENSEN, S.; MOUSING, J.; HENRIKSEN, C. A.; AND ANDERSEN, J. B. 1990. Evidence of long distance transmission of Aujeszky's disease virus. II: Epidemiological and meteorological investigations. Proc Int Pig Vet Soc, Lausanne, p. 279.

MOUSING, J. 1986. Slagtesvinesundhedstjenesten. En vurdering af omfang og funktion baseret på opgørelser for 1984. Dansk Vet Tidskr 69:1149-1159.

————. 1988. Chronic pleuritis in pigs: The relationship between weight, age and frequency in 3 conventional herds. Proc 5th Int Symp Vet Epidemiol Econ, Acta Vet Scand [Suppl] 84:253-255.

MOUSING, J.; LYBYE, H.; BARFOD, K.; MEYLING, A.; RØNSHOLT, L.; AND WILLEBERG, P. 1989. Brysthindear hos svin. Serologiske reaktioner for luftvejsinfektioner og disses sammenhæng med brysthindearfrekvensen hos slagtesvin. Dansk Vet Tidskr 72:865-873.

————. 1990. Chronic pleuritis in pigs for slaughter: An epidemiological study of infectious and rearing system-related risk factors. Prev Vet Med 9:107-119.

NEUMANN, R.; LEONHARDT, W.; BALLIN, A.; MEHLHORN, G.; AND DIECKE, S. 1985. Die Methode der intravitalen Lungenspülen beim Schwein–Gewinnung und Differenzierung von Alveolarzellen. Arch Exp Vet Med 39:525-534.

NEUMANN, R.; MEHLHORN, G.; BUCHHOLZ, I.; JOHANNSEN, U.; AND SCHIMMEL, D. 1987. Experimentelle Untersuchung zur Wirkung einer chronischen aerogenen Schadgasbelastung des Saugferkels mit Ammoniak unterschiedlicher Konzentrationen. J Vet Med [B] 34:241-253.

NICKS, B.; DECHAMPS, P.; CANART, B.; BUZITU, S.; AND DEWAELE, A. 1989. Exemple de résultats inattendu lors d'un contrôle de la concentration en ammoniac dans une porcherie. Ann Med Vet 133:613-616.

NIELSEN, J., AND FREDERIKSEN, W. 1990. Atrophic rhinitis in pigs caused by a human isolate of toxigenic *Pasteurella multocida*. Proc Int Pig Vet Soc, Lausanne, p. 75.

NIELSEN, J. P.; FOGED, N. T.; SØRENSEN, V.; BARFOD, K.; JENSEN, A. B.; AND PETERSEN, S. E. 1990a. Protection against progressive atrophic rhinitis with a re-combinant *Pasteurella multocida* toxin derivative. Proc Int Pig Vet Soc, Lausanne, p. 55.

NIELSEN, N. C. 1972. Präventiv medicin på besætningsplan. Medlemsbl Danske Dyrlaegeforen 55:272-281.

NIELSEN, R. 1988. Seroepidemiology of *Actinobacillus pleuropneumoniae*. Can Vet J 29:580-582.

NIELSEN, R., AND DANIELSEN, V. 1975. An outbreak of Glässers disease. Studies of etiology, serology and the effect of vaccination. Nord Vet Med 27:20-25.

NIELSEN, R.; LOFTAGER, M.; AND ERIKSEN, L. 1990b. Mucosal vaccination against *Actinobacillus pleuropneumoniae* infection. Proc Int Pig Vet Soc, Lausanne, p. 13.

NOYES, E. P.; FEENEY, D.; AND PIJOAN, C. 1988. A prospective radiographic study of swine pneumonia. Proc Int Pig Vet Soc, Rio De Janeiro, p. 67.

OHGAMI, M.; DOERSHUK, C. M.; ENGLISH, D.; DODEK, P. M.; AND HOGG, J. C. 1989. Kinetics of radiolabeled neutrophils in swine. J Appl Physiol 66:1881-1885.

PATTISON, I. H. 1956. A histological study of transmissible pneumonia of pigs characterized by extensive lymphoid hyperplasia. Vet Rec 68:490-494.

PEDERSEN, K. B., AND BARFOD, K. 1981. The aetiological significance of *Bordetella bronchiseptica* and *Pasteurella multocida* in atrophic rhinitis of swine. Nord Vet Med 33:513-522.

PIJOAN, C., AND LEMAN, A. D. 1986. Veterinary services to growing and finishing pigs. Proc Int Pig Vet Soc, Barcelona, p. 209-213.

PIJPERS, A.; VERNOOY, J. A. C. M; LEENGOED, L. A. M. G. VAN; AND VERHEIJDEN, J. H. M. 1990. Feed and water consumption in pigs following an *Actinobacillus pleuropneumoniae* challenge. Proc Int Pig Vet Soc, Lausanne, p. 39.

POINTON, A. M.; MCCLOUD, P.; AND HEAP, P. 1985. Enzootic pneumonia of pigs in South Australia–factors relating to incidence of disease. Austr Vet J 62:98-101.

RAFAI, P.; NEUMANN, R.; LEONHARDT, W.; FRENYÓ, L.; RUDAS, P.; FODOR, L.; AND BOROS, G. 1987. Effect of environmental temperature on pigs infected with *Pasteurella multocida* type A. Acta Vet Hung 35:211-223.

RASMUSSEN, J. F. 1984. The economic importance of chronic pleuritis in slaughter pig production. Proc Int Pig Vet Soc, Ghent, p. 347.

ROSENDAL, S., AND MITCHELL, W. R. 1983. Epidemiology of *Haemophilus pleuropneumoniae* infection in pigs: A survey of Ontario pork producers. 1981. Can J Comp Med 47:1-5.

ROSS, R. F. 1984. Chronic pneumonia of swine. Emphasis on mycoplasmal pneumonia. Proc Am Assoc Swine Pract, Kansas City, Mo., p. 79-95.

ROTHSCHILD, M. F. 1985. Selection for disease resistance in the pig. Pig News Inf 6:277-280.

ROTHSCHILD, M. F.; CHEN, H. L.; CHRISTIAN, L. L.; LIE, W. R.; VENIER, L.; COOPER, M.; BRIGGS, C.; AND WARNER, C. M. 1984. Breed and swine lymphocyte antigen haplotype differences in agglutination titers following vaccination with *B. bronchiseptica*. J Anim Sci 59:643-649.

SAUNDERS, J. R.; OSBORNE, A. D.; AND SEBUNYA, T. K. 1981. Pneumonia in Saskatchewan swine: Abattoir incidence of intrathoracic lesions in pigs from a herd infected with *Haemophilus pleuropneumoniae* and from other herds. Can Vet J 22:244-247

SCATOZZA, F., AND SIDOLI, L. 1986. Effects of *Haemophilus pleuropneumonia* infection in piglets recovering from influenza. Proc Int Pig Vet Soc, Barcelona, p. 150.

SCHEEPENS, C. J. M.; TIELEN, M. J. M.; AND HESSING, M. J. C. 1988. Influence of climatic stress on health status of weaner pigs. In Environment and animal health. Proc 6th Int Congr Anim Hyg 14-17 June 1988, Skara, Sweden. Vol. II, ed. Ekesbo, I. Skara,

Sweden, p. 543–547.

SCHEIDT A. B.; MAYROSE, V. B.; HILL, M. A.; CLARK, L. K.; CLINE, T. R.; KNOX, K. E.; RUNNELS, L. J.; FRANTZ, S.; AND EINSTEIN, M. E. 1990. Relationship of growth performance to pneumonia and atrophic rhinitis detected in pigs at slaughter. J Am Vet Med Assoc 196:881–884.

SCHEPERS, J. A. 1990. Data requirements and objectives for economic analysis of diseases in farm livestock. Proc Soc Vet Epidemiol Prev Med, 4–6 June 1990, Belfast, pp. 120–132.

SCHLESINGER, K. J.; WILLIAMS, J. M.; AND WIDEL, P. W. 1990. Intranasal administration of pseudorabies (Bartha K61) vaccine in neonates and grow/finish pigs: Safety and efficacy of vaccination and effects of virulent challenge exposure. Proc Int Pig Vet Soc, Lausanne, p. 260.

SCHULTZ, R. A. 1986. Swine pneumonia: Assessing the problem in individual herds. Vet Med 81:757–762.

SCHULTZ, R. A.; YOUNG, T. F.; ROSS, R. F.; AND JESKE, D. R. 1982. Prevalence of antibodies to *Haemophilus pleuropneumoniae* in Iowa swine. Am J Vet Res 43:1848–1851.

SEBUNYA, T. N. K.; SAUNDERS, J. R.; AND OSBORNE, A. D. 1983. A model aerosol exposure system for induction of porcine *Haemophilus pleuropneumoniae*. Can J Comp Med 47:48–53.

SMART, N. L.; MINIATS, O. P.; ROSENDAL, S.; AND FRIENDSHIP, R. M. 1989. Glasser's disease and prevalence of subclinical infection with *Haemophilus parasuis* in swine in South Ontario. Can Vet J 30:339–434.

SMITH, W. J. 1983. Infectious atrophic rhinitis – Noninfectious determinants. In Atrophic Rhinitis in Pigs. CEC Rep Eur En, Copenhagen, pp. 149–151.

STRAW, B. 1986. A look at the factors that contribute to development of swine pneumonia. Vet Med 81:747–756.

STRAW, B. E., AND RALSTON, N. 1986. Comparative costs and methods for assessing production impact on common swine diseases. Economics of animal diseases. Proceedings of a conference held at Michigan State Univ, 23–25 June 1986, pp. 165–180.

STRAW, B.; BÜRGI, E. J.; HILLEY, H. P.; AND LEMAN, A. D. 1983. Pneumonia and atrophic rhinitis from a test station. J Am Vet Med Assoc 182(6):607–611.

STRAW, B. E.; LEMAN, A. D.; AND ROBINSON, R. A. 1984. Pneumonia and atrophic rhinitis in pigs from a test station – a follow-up study. J Am Vet Med Assoc 185(12):1544–1546.

STRAW, B. E.; HENRY, S. C.; SCHULTZ, R. S.; AND MARSTELLER, T. A. 1986. Clinical assessment of pneumonia levels in swine through measurement of the amount of coughing. Proc Int Pig Vet Soc, Barcelona, p. 275.

STRAW, B. E.; TUOVINEN, V. K.; AND BIGRAS-POULIN, M. 1989. Estimation of the cost of pneumonia in swine herds. J Am Vet Med Assoc 195:1702–1706.

SVENSMARK, B.; NIELSEN, K.; DALSGAARD, K.; AND WILLEBERG, P. 1989. Epidemiological studies of piglet diarrhoea in intensively managed Danish sowherds. III. Rotavirus infection. Acta Vet Scand 30:63–70.

TIELEN, M. J. M. 1989. Integrale Qualitätskontrolle: Garantie für Gesundheit ?, Vortrag am 10. Intensivseminar des Steirischer Schweinegesundheitdienstes vom 2–9. April 1989, Nassfeld, Österreich.

TIELEN, M. J. M.; TRUIJEN, W. T.; VAN DE GROOS, C. A. M.; VERSTEGEN, M. A. W.; DEBRUIN, J. J. M.; AND CONBEY, R. A. P. H. 1978. De invloed van bedrijfsstructuur en stalbouw op varkensmestbedrijven op het voorkomen van long-en leveraandoeneningen bij slachtvarkens. [Conditions of management and the construction of piggeries on pig-fattening farms as factors in the incidence of disease of the lung and liver of slaughtered pigs.] Tijdschr Diergeneeskd 103:1155–1165.

TUBOLY, S.; BERNATH, S.; GLAVITS, R.; AND MEDVECZKY, I. 1988. Intestinal absorption of colostral lymphoid cells in newborn piglets. Vet Immunol Immunopathol 20:75–85.

UNDERDAHL, N. R.; SOCHA, T. E.; AND DORSTER, A. R. 1982. Long-term effect of *Bordetella bronchiseptica* infection in neonatal pigs. Am J Vet Res 43(4):622–625.

VAIMAN, M.; CHARDON, P.; AND RENARD, C. 1979. Genetic organization of the pig SLA complex. Studies on non recombinants and biochemical lysostrip analysis. Immunigenetics 9:353–361.

VAN DER VALK, P. C.; BUURMAN, J.; VANDENBOOREN, J. C. M. A.; VERNOY, J. C. M.; AND WIERDA, A. 1984. Automatic herd health and production control programs for swine farms. Proc Int Pig Vet Soc, Ghent, p. 342.

VISSER, I. J. R.; VAN DEN INGH, T. S. G. A. M.; KRUIJF, J. M.; TIELEN, M. J. M.; URLINGS, H. A. P.; AND GRUYS, E. 1988. Atrofische rhinitis: Beoordeling van de lengtedoorsnede van varkenskoppen aan de slachtlijn ter bepaling van voorkomen en mate van concha-atrofie. [Atrophic rhinitis: The use of longitudinal sections of pig's heads in the diagnosis of atrophy of the turbinate bones at the slaughter line.] Tijdschr Diergeneeskd 113(deel) or 24(afl):1345–1355.

WALLGREN, P.; MATTSSON, S.; ARTURSSON, K.; AND BÖLSKE, G. 1990. The relationship between *Mycoplasma hyopneumoniae* infection, age at slaughter and lung lesions at slaughter. Proc Int Pig Vet Soc, Lausanne, p. 82.

WATHES, C. M. 1983. Ventilation, airhygiene and animal health. Vet Rec 113:554–559.

WEIBEL, W.; BÜHLMANN, J.; AND HÄNI, H., 1983. Vergleichende Untersuchungen über Mortalität, Morbidität und Mastleistung in konventionellen und dem Schweinegesundheitsdienst angeschlossenen Mastbetrieben. III. Morbidität und Mastleistung. Schweiz Arch Tierheilkd 125:861–869.

WILLEBERG, P.; GERBOLA, M.-A.; KIRKEGAARD PETERSEN, B.; ANDERSEN, J. B. 1984/85. The Danish pig health scheme: Nation-wide computerbased abattoir surveillance and follow-up at the herd level. Prev Vet Med 3:79–91.

WILSON, M. R.; TAKOV, R.; FRIENDSHIP, R. M.; MARTIN, S. W.; McMILLAN, I.; HACKER, R. R.; AND SWAMINATHAN, S. 1986. Prevalence of respiratory diseases and their association with growth rate and space in randomly selected swine herds. Can J Vet Res 50:209–216.

YAGIHASHI, T.; NUNOYA, T.; MITUI, T.; AND TAJIMA, M. 1984. Effect of *Mycoplasma hyopneumoniae* infection on development of *Haemophilus pleuropneumoniae* pneumonia in pigs. Jpn J Vet Sci 46:705–713.

ZIMMERMANN, W.; NICOLET, J.; CHASTONAY, M.; AND SCHATZMANN, E. 1988. Recognition of enzootic pneumonia (EP) in acutely and chronically infected pigs: A sero-epidemiological study based on the ELISA in colostrum and blood. Proc Int Pig Vet Soc, Rio de Janeiro, p. 52.

ZIMMERMANN, W.; STAEGER, M.; AND BOMMELI, W. 1990. A sero-epidemiological study on the occurrence of serotypes of *A. pleuropneumoniae* (AAP) on Swiss breeding herds surveyed by the pig health service. Proc Int Pig Vet Soc, Lausanne, p. 32.

8 Skeletal System and Feet

M. A. Hill

BEFORE THE CLINICIAN can embark on a thorough investigation of locomotor disorders, an understanding of underlying principles and unique features of the structural components of the locomotor system is essential. For the skeletal system to function adequately, there is a dependence on the integrity of the nervous system, the muscular system, the articulating surfaces and associated synovial membranes, and the feet, as well as production of optimal amounts of normal synovia in joints. During the lifetime of the majority of commercial pigs, the skeleton does not mature and, therefore, bony components never achieve their potential strength. Because bone and growth cartilages are dynamic tissues, they are subject to the effects of various deficiencies and insults throughout the life of the pig.

Bones provide a strong framework for the body, which accommodates the hemopoietic tissues, protects the brain and abdominal viscera as well as the thoracic viscera, and is integral in respiration. Bone acts as a storehouse for calcium, phosphorus, magnesium, and sodium, and through metabolic processes is intrinsic in the homeostasis of calcium and phosphorus in the fluid compartments of the body.

LOCOMOTOR DISORDERS IN PIGS.
Lameness is an all-encompassing condition with a spectrum of clinical signs that ranges between a slight abnormality in the angulation of a joint or a shortened stride length and an incapacitating ambulation in which a limb does not bear weight; paralysis and prostration are included. Although leg weakness has been investigated for many years as though it were a specific syndrome, it represents no more than the broad concept of lameness. Therefore, a major factor that has limited our understanding of the etiopathogenesis of locomotor disorders, or the effects that dysfunction of one system has on the function of others, has been the paucity of adequate evaluations of definitive diseases or syndromes. Because of the relatively low monetary value of individual pigs, it is rare that isolated cases of lameness are studied in detail. However, given an understanding of the financial impact of an ongoing problem, it becomes apparent that in many herds locomotor disorders are worth investigating. In herds of valuable purebred pigs or in breeding companies that produce premium hybrid pigs, individualized attention to boars, gilts, and sows is economically justified. Only when extensive diagnostic evaluations are conducted on a widespread scale will it be possible to use an epidemiological approach to understanding the distribution of specific diseases.

Economic Impact of Locomotor Diseases.
Unlike the commonplace enteric and respiratory diseases of pigs that increase morbidity and mortality in herds and may quickly affect the condition and growth performance of pigs, locomotor disorders seem to be underrated. In both herds of breeding stock and commercial farrow-to-finish units, locomotor diseases are often insidious in onset and unless morbidity is high, as may be the case with some systemic infections, they do not stimulate sufficient interest to warrant a request for veterinary attention. However, available data and clinical experiences of many practitioners confirm that lameness and associated problems play a major role in financial losses in swine herds. Perceived problems in the swine herd depend on the morbidity, severity of lesions, and intensity of clinical signs of lameness at any particular time.

Information on locomotor diseases is extensive but piecemeal in surveys, either in reports from observation of live pigs and carcasses or from questionnaires, or in findings from a variety of laboratory investigations (Table 8.1). The cost, internationally, of locomotor disorders to the swine industry is unknown. However, an understanding of their economic impact is essential to (1) verify the costs to individual swine units so that investigative, treatment, control, and preventive steps can be justified; (2) continue profitable production of wholesome pork at competitive prices; and (3) justify financial support for specific areas of research.

Losses associated with diseases of the locomotor system accrue from several phases of the production cycle. In neonatal pigs, mortality may be high and subclinical or chronic diseases that affect nursery or grower pigs become established. Svendsen et al. (1979) found a frequency of 3.65% for arthritis in baby pigs in the farrowing house, and foot lesions were a frequent injury in a study by Smith and Mitchell (1977). As well as injuries and local infections associated with environmental conditions, specific infectious arthritides affect

163

Table 8.1. Culling and condemnation data for different categories and sexes of pigs

Reason for Culling or Condemning	Rate (%) of Culls	Rate (%) of Group (annual)	Population Examined	Age, Parity, or Weight	Sex	Country	Author (year)
Locomotor disorder	10.7		PIDA[a] member herds (3306 sows)		F	United Kingdom	(1964) Quoted in Jones (1967)
Lameness and posterior paralysis	34.7	9.4	1 herd (457 sows)	P0–P4	F	United Kingdom	Jones (1967)
Foot and leg injury		13.6–45	4 herds (20–144 sows)		F	United Kingdom	Smith and Robertson (1971)
Lameness (leg weakness)	8.8		5118 commercial herds (52,800 sows)	>210 day (50%, P0–P3)	F	France	Dagorn and Aumaitre (1979)
Lameness	35.0	4.2	60 herds	majority P0–P2	F	United Kingdom	Pattison et al. (1980)
Foot/leg problems	11.03	3.3	40 herds (1460 sows)		F	Alberta, Canada	Stone (1981)
	12.67	4.3	(434 gilts)		F		
Foot and leg problems	11.8	5.2	30 herds (7924 sows)		F	Ontario, Canada	Friendship et al. (1986)
Locomotor problems	9.2	4.4	80 herds (5918 sows)	P0–P10+ (Average parity 2.93, P0–P3)	F	Minn., United States	D'Allaire, et al. (1986)
Locomotor disturbances	[12.5]		(1324 gilts) [Includes associated deaths]				
Lameness	9.1		8 herds (8736 sows)		F	Yugoslavia	Zivkovic et al. (1986)
		22.3	Feeding study (790 gilts) Poor condition		F	France	Gatel et al. (1987)
		24.5	Good condition				
Limb involvement Kovacs (1982)	10		252 farms (60,000 breeding pigs)			?	Hungary
Lameness	11	4.4	Sows from purebred herd + 21 herds it supplied 82 breeding stock farms		F	Ontario, Canada	Dewey et al. (1988) (1990) Personal communication
	6	2.35	(sows)				
	7	0.14	(gilts)				
Leg disorders	12.7	5.33	1 herd (787 sows)		F	United Kingdom	Dunne et al. (1990)
Locomotor diseases		10.03	1 herd (581 sows)		F	Ind., United States	Clark (1990) Personal communication
Leg weakness	30		BTS[b] (450 boars)	81.8 kg	M	United Kingdom	Smith (1965)
Locomotor problems	4.6		AIC[c]	≤1.5 yr	M	United Kingdom	Melrose (1966)
Leg weakness	35.3		AIC[c]	≥1.5 yr	M	Norway	Grondalen (1974)
	12.1		(67 boars)				
Leg weakness	11.0		BTS[b] (362 boars) A further 9% were allowed to recover from leg weakness	25.3 wk	M	Australia	McPhee and Lewis (1976)
Crooked legs, deformed feet, poor conformation	2.71		Breeding company replacing boars		M	Iowa, United States	Nelson (1976)
Lameness	29.2		BTS[b] (82 boars)		M	Minn., United States	Hilley (1980)

Table 8.1. *(Continued)*

Reason for Culling or Condemning	Rate (%) of Culls	Rate (%) of Group (annual)	Population Examined	Age, Parity, or Weight	Sex	Country	Author (year)
Leg weakness		53	(118 boars)	6 mo	M	Poland	Empel (1980)
		51	(139 gilts)		F		
Leg and foot abnormality	24.5		BTS[b]		M	Yugoslavia	Sabec (1980)
Locomotor disorders		30	Breeding company complaints		M	United Kingdom	Walters et al. (1984)
Mild or severe leg weakness		15.43	Progeny test Landrace (1542 pigs)		M & F	Sweden	Lundeheim (1986)
		9.44	Yorkshire (1154 pigs)		M & F		
Locomotor problems	11.8	6.7	84 breeding companies (440 boars)		M	Minn., United States	D'Allaire (1988)

[a]PIDA = Pig Industry Developer Association.
[b]BTS = boar test station.
[c]AIC = Artificial Insemination Center.

growing pigs. Foot lesions seem commonplace; 47.7% of herd managers questioned in a health survey reported pigs with foot injuries (Anon. 1981). Morbidity of specific diseases and availability of effective treatments probably most affect economic losses caused by reduced growth performance and carcass quality. Reports on slaughterhouse condemnations and trimming rates associated with locomotor diseases give an insight into some of the costs of these diseases. Norval (1962) described abscesses, 12% of which involved feet, as a serious cause of condemnation in one UK slaughter plant. In excess of 0.5 million pigs (about 0.87%) slaughtered in the 10 highest hog-producing states in the United States had arthritis in fiscal year 1989 (Anon. 1990a, b). Of these, 9208 were condemned at a conservatively estimated cost exceeding $911,000. Wastage associated with trimming carcasses that passed inspection is unknown. Condemnation rates probably vary from year to year and from country to country. Whereas Evans and Pratt (1978) reported that in the United Kingdom, 0.02% whole and 0.5% part carcasses were condemned because of arthritis, there was a reduction to 0.006% total carcass condemnation by 1984 (Anon. MAFF report cited by Wells 1986). In Hungary, Kovacs and Beer (1979) found foot lesions in 85.15% of 2000 slaughtered porkers. On-farm deaths subsequent to locomotor disorders are poorly understood, but Jones (1968) indicated that 4.94% of pigs that died in 106 herds in the United Kingdom were affected by arthritis, posterior paresis, or epiphyseal separations. Chagnon et al (1990) reported a frequency of 2.2% for downer sow syndrome among 137 sows and gilts from 24 herds in Quebec; the average parity was only 1.3.

The major economic losses in farrow-to-finish and breeding stock herds probably occur in young breeding pigs of both genders. By the time pigs are in the breeding herd, they will have gone through several selection processes and the lost potential in unsound pigs that were culled in the grow-finishing phases cannot be estimated. However, several studies indicate that cull rates for lame sows and boars or the frequency of specific conditions result in considerable losses (Table 8.1). Osteochondrosis (OC) and osteoarthrosis (OA) can cause severe crippling, and the frequency of these conditions has been high in pigs with otherwise ideal growth characteristics (Grondalen 1974a, b; Reiland 1978b, c). The covert costs associated with losses in the breeding herd include reduced prolificacy in replacement gilts, a reduced pool from which to select replacements, increased farrowing house mortality because sows or baby pigs are lame, and reduced feed intake and growth performance in crippled grow-finishing pigs.

Variability in the numbers of pigs or herds examined and the methods of investigating locomotor disorders make it difficult to determine exact losses associated with culling sows and boars. Boar losses include those which failed to enter breeding herds after preliminary selection, as well as those removed from herds. In some studies in which pigs were observed rather than those in which the managers completed questionnaires, the frequency of specific locomotor problems seemed higher.

In the United States between December 1989 and November 1990, the census for breeding pigs was 6,872,000 (Anon. 1990a). At an accepted ratio of 1 boar per 20 sows, this number included 6,544,762 sows and 327,238 boars. Taking estimates of cull rates associated with lameness at 6.0% for gilts and sows and 20% for boars at entry or subsequent to entry into the breeding herd, and losses at the rate of $65 per sow replaced and $345 per boar lost, the minimal cost to the US swine industry was $48,103,933 over 1 year. Replacement costs assume that the entire sow or boar carcass is salvageable.

Examination for Lameness. Effective examination for lameness in the pig is dependent on a consistent methodology. Only when a thorough approach has been developed can it be used regularly and refined. For each examination conducted, all systems involved in locomotion should be considered, i.e., bones and joints, feet, the muscular system, and the nervous system. Only then is the likelihood of reaching a preliminary diagnosis enhanced. Nevertheless, clinical examination of pigs is often difficult because they tend to resist handling or restraint, especially when they are approached in an open area or after attempts to restrain them have failed.

A concise but accurate history is an important starting point for investigating locomotor problems. Morbidity, mortality, the location of affected pigs, duration of lameness, age of affected animals, and sites of any visible lesions all need to be understood. Details concerning the type of housing, the stocking density, feeding routines and movements of livestock also provide a framework for the investigation.

GENERAL ASPECTS OF EXAMINATION OR EVALUATION. For any productivity or disease problems, it is important to consider all the animals within an affected group to determine the frequency of the problem. Logically, an investigator should briefly examine all age groups or categories of pigs and their respective environments to determine whether or not there are clinical signs or lesions in pigs in groups other than those that were identified initially.

Within the groups of pigs examined during a walk-through, it may be appropriate to isolate individuals for a cursory examination. Before any hands-on examination is considered, each pig should be examined from a distance, preferably while they either stand or move about freely in their pen. However, to examine the pig closely, the nature of the animal is such that restraint often is necessary. Minimal restraint that is compatible with humane and safe handling, an efficient examination process, and safety of the handler is required.

Restraint methods fall into three major categories: manual restraint, mechanical restraint (which may possibly involve some manual restraint), chemical restraint. A method of restraint or control of a placid sow is the simple process of stroking the udder while talking softly to her. Lively, fractious, or timid animals will need to be restrained, since this allows a more thorough examination. Sucking and weaned piglets are best held by the hind legs with the head downward to minimize squealing (Fig. 8.1A). Hind feet can be examined easily with the animal held in this position. However, if all four feet are to be considered, it is possible for a person to sit and hold the piglet on the lap in a supine position with a thoracic and pelvic limb in each hand (Fig. 8.1B). Weaned and growing pigs can be restrained in lateral recumbency by firmly grasping the thoracic limb and flexing and slightly adducting the humeroradio-ulnar or carpal joint (Fig 8.1C). Growing and finishing pigs can be cast with a rope and restrained (Fig. 8.1D). Place a loop around the snout; the free end of the rope is then passed around a leg above the tarsus in a half-hitch and pulled so that the snout and tarsus are drawn together as the pig is pulled off balance. A simple slipknot is used to secure the ropes while the pig's feet are examined. Larger finishing pigs, sows, and boars can be restrained using the crisscross or half-hitch methods of casting, comparable with those demonstrated for cattle by Leahy and Barrow (1953). However, the half-hitch method is a less strenuous method for casting a mature pig.

A cable snare (hog snare) placed around the upper jaw behind the tusks can be used to restrain a pig for a short time for examination, palpation, and manipulation of extremities. If the foot is to be examined, it must be picked up to examine the volar aspect; this can be facilitated by a firm manual grip on the tendon of the gastrocnemius or placement of a lariat noose above the tarsus for examination of the hind foot. Usually, at least two people are required to restrain larger pigs.

For pigs ≤50 kg in weight, simple V-shaped cradles consisting of sawhorse frames and a wooden or canvas hammock suffice to hold pigs on their backs (McTaggart 1977, Leahy and Barrow 1953). However, two people are required to lift the pig into the cradle. More sophisticated crates, which can be turned manually or semi-automatically, have been made to hold finishing pigs and even sows and boars (Baker and Andresen 1964; Pugh and Penny 1966). These cradles

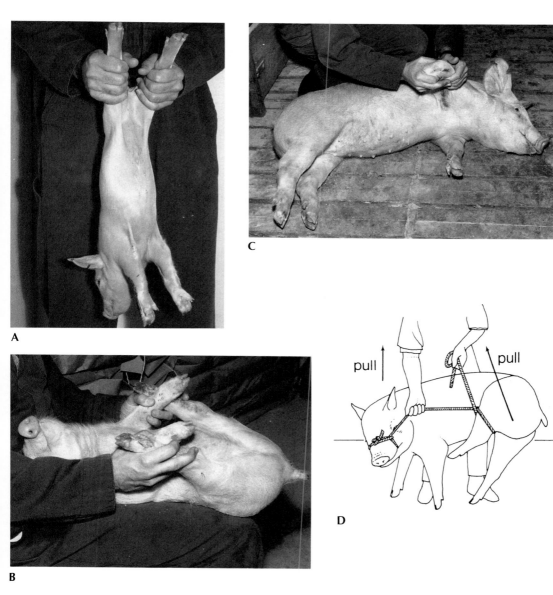

8.1. Restraint techniques. (A) Holding by hind legs for easy examination of hind feet of sucking and weaned pigs. (B) Lap position for examination of all four feet of sucking and weaned pigs. (C) Lateral recumbency for examination of weaned and growing pigs. (D) Casting with a rope for examination of growing and finishing pigs.

and crates can be used for bleeding pigs from the anterior vena cava and jugular vein and simple surgery, as well as for examination and treatment of feet. Areas that are to be scrutinized should be cleansed at this stage. When manual restraint is too difficult, it is as simple, expedient, and humane to use chemical restraints, either in the form of tranquilizers or general anesthetics (see Chapter 76).

Inadequate environmental conditions may initiate locomotor disorders or exacerbate problems. Therefore, while pigs are being observed during the walk-through, an assessment of the environ-

ment should also be made with emphasis on examining floor type, dampness and drainage efficiency, slat design, and roughness and newness of concrete. Although much of the evaluation of floors has been in relation to foot lesions, there have also been concerns about the effect of different types of slats and combinations of solid floors and slats or bedding on the occurrence of leg weakness and OC. Heights of steps should be noted. If bedding is used, the quantity, quality, and condition should be noted. Damp, uninsulated rough concrete floors, particularly during winter, may predispose to foot problems. In floor feeding systems, the accumulation of a rough food cake on concrete may be important in causing lesions. Pigs that were previously running in dirt lots may be particularly susceptible to foot damage. Also, during the walk-through, consideration should be given to the quantity and quality of foodstuffs available to the different age groups of pigs. Absolute quantities of protein will directly affect growth of the pig (Pratt and McCance 1964), but deficiencies of micronutrients are probably more relevant to skeletal development in the context of diseases that occasionally are encountered.

EXAMINATION OF THE INDIVIDUAL PATIENT. As was indicated earlier, each pig should be examined from a distance before it is disturbed to determine the behavior pattern and mental status of the pig in its immediate environment. It is necessary to look for neurological signs such as a head tilt, circling movement, hypermetria (goose-stepping), paresis or paralysis, but it is important for the clinician to develop a consistent approach to evaluating the locomotor system.

At this point in the physical examination there are options for continuation of the process. Ideally, the individual pig should be walked around on a firm, flat surface so that specific observations can be made about its gait. The severity of lameness sometimes may help in predicting a cause and in focusing further inspection. Abnormal ambulation may relate to pain in any of the major joints when young adult sows and boars walk on their carpi (Fig 8.2); to pain in lacerated hind feet, which causes piglets to attempt to shift the weight from pelvic to thoracic limbs; or to myalgia associated with myodegeneration, which causes pigs to tremble and crouch.

If the pig is placid, it may be possible to initiate the hands-on examination and then to walk the pig around its pen. Confined, quiet, adult pigs generally are the easiest to examine by palpation

and manipulation. If, however, the pig is unwilling to be handled after its gait has been evaluated, it is appropriate to apply one of the restraint methods so that the physical examination can progress. The author prefers to continue the examination by considering each of the limbs from the feet upward, usually starting with the thoracic limbs. In addition to using sight and touch, it is equally important to listen for crepitus. There may be cracks in the wall of the hoof, and the wall and heel should be evaluated in terms of whether there has been excessive growth. The foot must be lifted to check the sole for contusions, and clefts in the wall, sole, or heel should be checked to determine how deeply they penetrate. Foreign bodies, wounds, exudates, or blood also should be sought. Vesicles, erosions, or ulcers at the coronary band and in the interdigital space may be associated with viral diseases (see Chapter 30). Regulations relating to notifiable diseases should be kept in mind. Deep-seated infections, such as foot rot, may cause abscesses and sinuses at the coronary band or initiate an ascending cellulitis. Palpation may help in the differentiation of tendinitis, tenosynovitis, and ruptured tendons.

In neonatal pigs, skin erosions and ulcers are commonly seen over the cranial surface of the carpus and at other sites within hours of birth (Fig 8.3).

Calluses and adventitious bursae may develop over bony prominences if pigs spend more time than is usual in a recumbent position; common sites for lesions are over the carpi, olecranon processes, and calcanii. In old animals, severe or prolonged trauma results in the development of ulcers such as those seen over the spine of the scapula or tuber coxae. Crates, stalls, and rough flooring predispose to these lesions. Myositis and osteomyelitis may follow skin ulceration.

Fluctuating swellings in the joint regions usually relate to the presence of pus, blood, or fluid in

8.2. A boar in a typical kneeling position associated with degenerative joint disease of the humeroradio-ulnar joints.

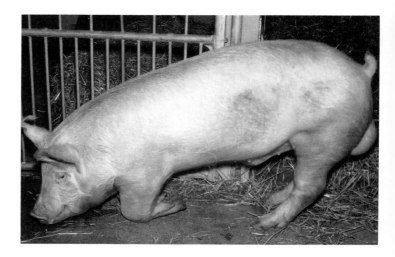

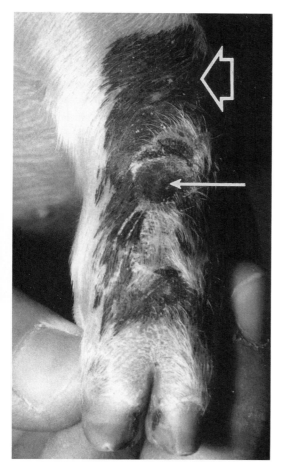

8.3. Carpus of a 2-week-old pig. Note the lesion (small arrow) despite the use of tar (large open arrow) applied soon after birth as a protective covering for the skin.

or around the joint capsule. Edema and inflammation may be localized or involve much of the limb. A comparison between normal and abnormal areas can readily be made by observing other limbs on the same animal or, if necessary, by comparison to limbs of other pigs in the group. Hard swellings around joints usually represent chronic exostoses or periarticular fibrosis.

Manipulation in addition to palpation may be essential for assessment of joints such as the shoulder and hip, which are not readily visualized in muscular or fat pigs. However, because the pig may be distressed by having its limbs manipulated, it is advisable to complete the palpations and other procedures first.

The pelvis should be examined for symmetry and the lumbar region should be subjected to downward pressure. Pain or swelling in the coxofemoral region may be the result of hip dislocation, separation of the proximal epiphysis of the femur, or fractures in the proximal part of the femur. Manipulation of the limb also may reveal crepitation in these regions. Transmission of sound along an intact bone such as the tibia can be useful as a diagnostic aid. If the craniomedial surface of the tibia, which is superficial, is struck with a hemostat or scissors handles while a stethoscope is placed over the femoral head, the sound should be heard in the hip if the bones are intact. Pain over the ischial tuberosity may be associated with separation of the ischial epiphysis from the body of the bone.

Hardness or swelling of muscle masses should also be noted. Atrophy of some muscle groups from disuse may be obvious in chronically lame animals. In the case of lame baby pigs, it is always worthwhile palpating and examining the umbilicus, as well as limbs and joints.

When other elements of the physical examination have been completed, or possibly intermixed with other examinations, the neurological examination should be concluded; if the pig has not been chemically restrained, this is not difficult. Pain withdrawal reflexes, patellar reflexes, and in small pigs, placing reflexes should be considered when attempting to differentiate neurological abnormalities. Neurological examination is of special relevance if proprioceptive dysfunction, dysmetria, hypermetria, paresis, or paraplegia have developed. Details of a neurological examination are given in Chapter 65, and a more specific approach to individual joints and sites was given by Hilley (1982).

DIAGNOSTIC AIDS. If an individual animal is sufficiently valuable or a herd lameness problem is of considerable magnitude, the cost of further investigation is readily justified. If radiologic examination or arthrocentesis is to be performed, the pig will probably have to be anesthetized. Radiographs should be taken with craniocaudal or caudocranial, mediolateral, dorsopalmar, or dorsoplantar views, depending on the joints that are to be evaluated. If such conditions as OC, degenerative joint disease (DJD), or suppurative polyarthritis are suspected, it is advisable to examine the same joints in contralateral limbs. Successfully identifying lesions with radiography will depend on the extent of lesions and the chronicity of any changes that occur.

Arthrocentesis should only be carried out with strict asepsis. Evaluation of synovia can parallel the procedure for synovia from horses (Van Pelt 1974). However, culture of the fluid for bacteria or mycoplasmas may be of more value provided the disease is at an acute or subacute phase and the pig has not been treated with antimicrobial compounds.

Often, it is simpler and less expensive to euthanatize one or more pigs and perform a necropsy to obtain a definitive diagnosis. Acutely affected, untreated pigs should be selected for necropsy, and the different components of the locomotor system should be examined. All major joints should be opened completely and samples of synovial membrane, as well as synovia, should be collected for evaluation by light microscopy. If there is any suspicion of disruption of bones, growth cartilages, or articular surfaces, it may be appropriate to cut the ends of long bones, vertebrae, and costochondral junctions into 5-mm-thick slabs using a coping saw. If possible, specimens from the slaughter plant, whether they are feet or bones and joints, should be collected and examined. Condemnation rates for skeletal lesions may also provide useful information if there is an ongoing herd lameness problem.

STRUCTURE OF BONES AND JOINTS.
Long bones increase in length by the process of endochondral ossification within growth plates (Fig 8.4) at both extremities. Chondrocytes proliferate, the new cells hypertrophy, the matrix

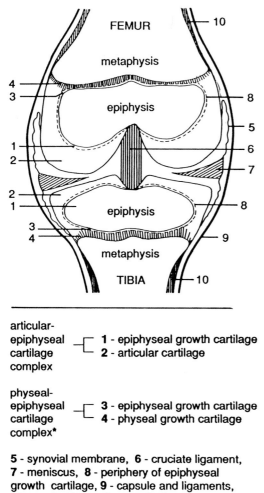

articular-
epiphyseal
cartilage
complex
   1 - epiphyseal growth cartilage
   2 - articular cartilage

physeal-
epiphyseal
cartilage
complex*
   3 - epiphyseal growth cartilage
   4 - physeal growth cartilage

5 - synovial membrane, 6 - cruciate ligament,
7 - meniscus, 8 - periphery of epiphyseal
growth cartilage, 9 - capsule and ligaments,
10 - cortical bone, * - growth plate

8.4. Schematic frontal section through the femorotibial joint of a 4-month-old pig.

undergoes mineralization, and then capillary buds penetrate the chondrocyte lacunae and initiate ossification. Primary spongiosa is laid down on the cartilaginous framework, and eventually remodeling occurs so that a more structurally organized lamellar bone replaces the initial woven bone. The process is repeated until growth plates close. The epiphyseal growth component of the articular-epiphyseal cartilage complex (AECC) (Fig. 8.4) is responsible for the increase in size of the secondary centers of ossification, e.g., head and greater tuberosity of the humerus, by a similar process of ossification. In the pig, skeletal growth is still incomplete at 3–3.5 years of age because growth plates in long bones continue to be functional (Getty 1975). Resorption and deposition of bone is a continual process even when older animals have stopped growing.

Within the developing chondroepiphysis, nutrients and oxygen are considered to be provided by and metabolites removed by capillaries in cartilage canals that penetrate growth cartilages from the perichondrium directly or indirectly after passing through the epiphysis. The AECC becomes thinner as the epiphysis matures and the epiphyseal growth component becomes redundant.

A variety of joints has evolved along with the bones. These joints vary in complexity and, in conjunction with the neuromuscular system, permit movement between two or more bones, thus allowing flexibility of an otherwise rigid skeleton, and hence, locomotion. Generally, in the pig it is the synovial joints that are most frequently affected by disorders. Synovial joints (Fig 8.4) have evolved to allow maximal movement while providing a high level of stability. Each synovial joint consists of two or more adjacent bone extremities (which are partially encapsulated by hyaline cartilage), a synovial membrane, a fibrous capsule, and a sheath of stabilizing ligaments. In specific joints such as that between the femur and tibia, additional intraarticular structures are found in the form of menisci (which enhance congruency between articular cartilages) and ligaments (which provide additional stability to the joint).

The synovial membrane is a folded vascular structure comprising two or three types of cells that form an incomplete barrier between the capillary beds in the synovial connective tissue and the joint cavity (Ghadially 1983). One group of cells, the fibrocytelike cells, secretes synovia, which nourishes and lubricates articular components of the AECC in young pigs and the full depth of cartilage in mature pigs. A second group of macrophagelike cells phagocytoses material from the joint cavity. The third type of cell has morphological features of both the preceding cells and it is possible that cell phenotype changes depending on the needs of the joint. Because of the loose organization of the synovial membrane, the potential for organisms gaining access to the synovial cavity, particularly when an inflammatory reaction has been initiated, is considerable. Enzymes released by bacteria and inflammatory cells also put the integrity of the network of collagen and proteoglycans, which forms the articular cartilage, at risk of being damaged.

Synovial fluid is a transudate to which hyaluronic acid is added. The viscosity associated with the content of hyaluronic acid polymer enhances the lubricating function of the fluid. Nerve receptors in the synovial membrane, capsule, and ligaments respond to pressure or tension stimuli and thus are responsible for perception of pain and joint movement. Further details of the anatomy, biochemistry, immunobiology, physiology, and engineering of joints and synovial fluid are available in the texts of Getty (1975) and Sokoloff (1978).

Noninfectious Diseases of Bones and Joints

DISEASES WITH MULTIPLE OR UNDETERMINED CAUSES

Dyschondroplasia (Osteochondrosis), Degenerative Joint Disease, and Leg Weakness. Osteochondrosis, OA, and leg weakness are worldwide problems that have caused concern in the pig industry for 50 or more years (Duthie and Lancaster 1964; Grondalen 1974a; Pointillart and Gueguen 1978; Reiland 1978a; Rothschild and Christian 1988). Particularly during the last 20 years, the interest aroused by these conditions in pigs has resulted in numerous investigations of possible causes. However, as the knowledge about OC and OA has increased, conflicting findings have resulted in confusion rather than clarification of the initiation and development of these conditions. Confusion has also developed because of the inconsistency between investigative techniques, and because there were few accurate descriptions of lesions in early studies. A plethora of alternative names for OC and OA, e.g., arthropathy, arthritis, polyarthrosis, DJD, and metaphyseal dysplasia, has added to the confusion. Even the names osteochondrosis and osteoarthrosis are inaccurate, because lesions are initiated in growth cartilages and bones are affected only secondarily. Ljunggren and Reiland (1970) gave the name osteochondrosis to a DJD of Swedish pigs. Later, Grondalen (1974a) in Norway was more specific when he defined OC as a primary, noninflammatory disturbance of joint cartilages and growth plates that prevented the progression of endochondral ossification. Because lesions were initiated in cartilage, Olsson (1978) suggested that dyschondroplasia was a more suitable name for lesions affecting growth and articular cartilages of pigs. As the etiopathogeneses of OC and OA have been investigated, particularly with the use of microradiography, light microscopy, and electron microscopy, the commonalities of lesions helped investigators to define typical le-

sions. Thus, the study of OC and OA in different breeds and genetic lines of pigs in different countries has contributed to a better understanding of the development and nature of lesions.

Based on various descriptions (Grondalen 1974a; Reiland 1978b; Nakano et al. 1979a; Farnum et al. 1984; Hill et al. 1984a, 1990; Carlson et al. 1986), the author believes that OC is best used to define a group of syndromes that cause limb deformities or DJD in young, fast-growing pigs of either gender. Other names should be given to different aspects/elements of the syndrome. Dyschondroplasia should be used to identify the majority of lesions affecting growth plates (especially the physeal growth cartilages or physes) and a few lesions involving AECC (particularly the epiphyseal growth cartilage). Foci of hypertrophied chondrocytes persist in the metaphysis or epiphysis, resulting in focal thickening of the growth plate or epiphyseal growth cartilage (Fig. 8.5A, B). Dyschondroplastic foci may undergo calcification and ossification, or alternatively, the chondrocytes die and the necrotic chondrocytes and the denatured matrix surrounding them are replaced by fibrous connective tissue that ossifies. Occasionally, fractures develop at the chondro-osseous interface with the metaphysis or within the calcified portion of the zone of hypertrophying chondrocytes; cysts or clefts that contain blood persist. Secondarily, cysts or clefts appear to inhibit the ossification front. The outcome is a disproportionate thickening of portions of the growth plate and interference with metaphyseal growth, which in turn can result in deformation of bones, joints, and ultimately, limbs. Small, simple dyschondroplastic foci have been observed in pigs as young as 1 day old.

Many of the lesions affecting AECC have been examined at a stage when DJD has become established. The articular surface was breached and subchondral bone often was exposed (Fig. 5C). Again, on the basis of reports in other studies and his own experience, the author believes that the lesions are initiated as microscopic foci of chondrolysis at or near the interface of the articular cartilage and epiphyseal growth cartilage. The lesion may progress at this site and lysed cartilage persists in the deeper layers of the AECC, at the chondro-osseous interface, and within the bone of the epiphysis. Recently replicated cells die and there is either failure of matrix production or formed matrix is disrupted. Clusters of chondrocytes often develop at the periphery of the lesion in an attempt to repair the lesion. The soft, denatured cartilage is probably subject to further damage during joint movement so that fissures, flaps, and ultimately, craters develop (Fig. 8.5A, C). It is believed that when the AECC is breached and subchondral bone is in contact with the joint space, the joint becomes painful and clinical lameness develops. Cartilage flaps and fragments may

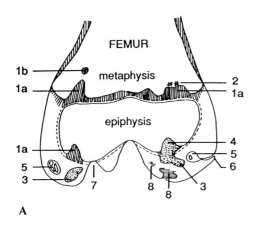

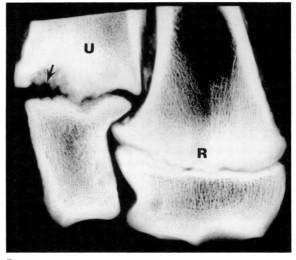

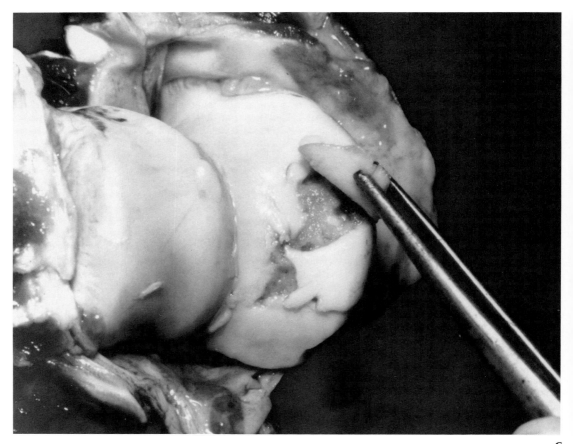

8.5. (A) Schematic frontal section through the distal part of the femur, with different types of lesions that affect the growth plate and articular-epiphyseal cartilage complex. *1a,* dischondroplastic focus; *1b,* island of cartilage; *2,* fracture/fissure at chondro-osseous junction; *3,* focus of chondrolysis; *4,* persistent lysed cartilage; *5,* cysts; *6,* flap; *7,* crater (osteoarthritic area); *8,* focus of fibrocartilage. (B) Radiograph of a slab of cartilage and bone (5 mm thick) from the distal parts of the radius (*R*) and ulna (*U*). Note the irregular and deepened area of radiolucency (compare with *la* in A). (C) Distal part of the humerus of a young boar with DJD. Note the cartilage flap (held in forceps) and the adjacent exposed subchondral bone.

impinge on the synovial membrane or impede movement of the joint, but synovitis is minimal. Although a few lesions have been observed in pigs between 15 and 53 days old, damaged articulating surfaces generally have not been observed in pigs until they were between 4 and 6 months old (Grondalen 1974a; Reiland 1978a). This, typically, is the age range when lameness develops.

Osteochondroses affecting growth cartilages and DJD are generalized conditions. Because the nature of lesions that affect growth plates and AECC and the mechanisms that cause lesions to progress or enable them to heal are incompletely understood, it is difficult to justify the use of subjective scoring systems that quantify the numbers and the severity of lesions. The extent and morphologic features of a lesion depend on the stage of development of that lesion, i.e., a dynamic rather than a static phase. Therefore, information may be used out of context, e.g., lesions may be less advanced in slow-growing pigs, but as pigs reach the same body weight the extent of lesions may be similar for all pigs (Grondalen 1974d). Likewise, the comparison of scores for lesions is probably meaningless for pigs at different ages (Reiland et al. 1978). Major sites utilized for clinical and experimental evaluations were the distal growth plate of the ulna and the AECC of the medial condyles of the humerus and femur. Because predilection sites for DJD were the same as those for OC, Reiland (1978b, c) concluded that DJD was secondary to OC.

Although the nature of lesions associated with OC and DJD is incompletely defined, there is a consensus that vascular injury within cartilage canals is part of the pathogenesis of lesions (Bullough and Heard 1967; Kincaid and Lidvall 1982; Kincaid et al. 1985; Carlson et al. 1986, 1989, 1990; Woodard et al. 1987b; Visco et al. 1991). Hill et al. (1985a, 1990) and Nakano et al. (1986) were unable to conclusively incriminate damaged blood vessels. Nevertheless, anything that increases compressive or traumatic forces across growth cartilages must be considered in any preventive measures to reduce the frequency of crippling lesions.

The names osteochondrosis and osteoarthrosis have become part of common usage for clinical conditions affecting bones and joints, as well as for descriptions of pathologic states. On the other hand, leg weakness has never been used to describe specific diseases or syndromes. Originally, leg weakness was used to describe a condition in boars that were unable to remain mounted and complete coitus. Now, leg weakness applies to any deficit in locomotor ability and any of the systems involved in movement; i.e., bones and joints, muscles, nervous system, or feet could be involved. Signs range from conformational abnormalities and slight deficits in stride to an inability to stand. Although leg weakness is not synonymous with OC or DJD, Reiland (1978b) found that

OC was the commonest cause of leg weakness in adolescent pigs.

Economic Impact of OC and DJD. Osteochondrosis and DJD caused considerable wastage, especially in Scandinavia, where up to 100% of breeding animals culled because of lameness had OC or DJD and 40% of boars in a boar test station were affected by OC (Grondalen 1974a, b; Reiland 1978b). Elsewhere, estimates have varied, but recently in Canada, Dewey (1989, personal communication 1990) demonstrated that 47% of sows culled because of lameness had OC and DJD. The problem was worst in start-up herds. Walker and Aherne (1987) indicated that almost 100% of commercial pigs had lesions in joint cartilages by 6 months of age. Hill (1990) estimated that the cost of OC and DJD to the U.S. pig industry was over $24 million in 1988–89 alone, and covert costs were excluded. Internationally, losses would have been many times higher and there was concern that international trade of affected pigs or lines of pigs may have exacerbated the problem worldwide (Becker et al. 1985; Hill 1990).

Onset of Clinical Problems and Clinical Signs of OC and DJD. Although lesions developed in pigs from birth (Bullough and Heard 1967; Hill et al. 1985b), clinical signs caused by OC or DJD were unapparent until pigs reached between 4 and 8 months old (Reiland 1978a). Frequently, the fastest growing, heaviest pigs became lame, but by 12 months of age, lesions may have partially repaired so that lameness had disappeared. However, extensive, severe, multicentric DJD can progress to an extent that older pigs have to be culled.

Ambulatory difficulties range from a shortened stride to a non-weight-bearing lameness, and from stiffness in the limbs to an inability or unwillingness to stand. Onset of signs can be insidious (e.g., a swaying gait) or acute, and lameness can be episodic. In the breeding barn, sows sometimes are unable to stand or boars unable to mount and complete copulation (Christensen 1953) (Fig. 8.6).

Despite the presence of generalized DJD or angulation deformities, pigs have developed lameness in a single limb. It has been suggested that the pain threshold of an individual determined whether or not a pig was lame at all, but a pig probably "protected" the most painful joints by altering the pattern of weight bearing (Reiland et al. 1978). Thus, weight had been shifted to a contralateral limb, although joints in the limb that took the weight had macroscopically severe lesions. A kyphotic posture may have relieved pressure from intervertebral synovial joints, and a kneeling stance, which enabled pigs to walk on the cranial surface of their carpi, probably alleviated discomfort in humeroradio-ulnar joints (Fig. 8.2).

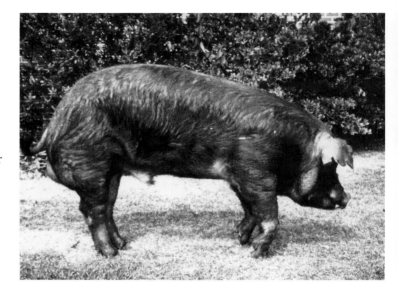

8.6. Duroc boar standing on the tips of his thoracic hooves and the carpi are permanently flexed. Kyphosis of the lumbar region also is apparent.

To date, specific causes of dyschondroplasias, chondrolysis, and DJD are unknown. However, the syndromes appear to have multiple causes, and morphologic changes may represent the limited responses that different populations of chondrocytes are capable of making in response to the various inciting factors.

Hereditary Influences on OC and DJD. Internationally, many lines of pigs that are used in contemporary hog production are affected by OC and DJD (Thomasen 1939; Duthie and Lancaster 1964; Grondalen 1974a; Perrin and Bowland 1977; Reiland 1978b; Kincaid and Lidvall 1982). For different studies in which lesions were examined either macroscopically or microscopically, or by both methods, and then were scored subjectively, there was variation in the frequency of pigs that had lesions, in the frequency of lesions in different pigs, and in the severity of lesions. Between breeds, differences were found in frequency and severity of lesions at many sites, and frequency and severity of lesions at specific sites (Grondalen 1974c; Reiland et al. 1978; Goedegebuure et al. 1980; Hani et al. 1984; Lundeheim 1986). Landrace pigs seemed to be most susceptible to developing OC and DJD, with between 90 and 100% of pigs affected by lesions in at least one site (Grondalen 1974c; Reiland et al. 1978; Hani et al. 1984; Lundeheim 1986). Within the Norwegian Landrace breed, there were line differences for the distribution and severity of lesions; leaner, faster growing pigs had a higher frequency of lesions that, generally, were more severe than those in fatter, slower growing pigs (Grondalen and Vangen 1974). Reiland et al. (1978) demonstrated differences in the frequency and distribution of lesions between offspring of different boars in the same breed and Grondalen (1974c, f) also found litter differences for Norwe-

gian Landrace and Yorkshire pigs.

Smaller, slower growing European wild pigs or crossbred commercial and wild pigs did not develop OC, and Reiland (1978e) considered that a fast growth rate was related to the initiation of lesions. Yucatan, Pitman-Moore, and Gottingen miniature pigs do not appear to develop lesions (Empel 1980; Farnum et al. 1984). However, Fell et al. (1967) found dyschondroplastic foci in distal ulnar growth plates of wild East African pigs.

Crossbreeding programs with commercial pigs have not proved useful as a means of eliminating OC or DJD. Indeed, faster growing muscular hybrids may have been as prone to the syndromes. Although through two- and three-way breeding trials Reiland and Anderson (1979) were able to demonstrate significant differences in the severity of DJD in specific joints of pigs from maternal lines (Landrace and Yorkshire) compared with paternal lines (Hampshire and Welsh), there were no significant differences between crossbred pigs if scores for all joints were considered.

Because the frequency and severity of lesions were associated with fast growth, large hams, and lean carcasses, selection against OC and DJD has been problematical (Grondalen 1974c; Grondalen and Vangen 1974; Reiland et al. 1978). Particularly in the United States, selection for carcass quality and dimensions of muscles has prevailed, rather than consideration of the frequency of pigs with lesions. Various correlations between production indicators or carcass characteristics and scores for lesions in sites that included humeral and femoral condyles, and distal ulnar growth plates have been reported (Reiland et al. 1978, 1980; Hani et al. 1984, 1990; Lundeheim 1986). Heritability estimates determined by Hani et al. (1990) for lesions in humeral and femoral condyles were higher than those estimated by Lundeheim (1987) or Reiland et al. (1978); all concluded that selection against the development of OC and DJD on the basis of certain body or carcass characteristics was feasible. The presence of lesions in pigs ≤15 days old was evidence for dyschondroplasia or chondrolysis being congenital as well as inherited (Bullough and Heard 1967; Bjorklund and Svendsen 1980; Hill et al. 1984a, 1985b, 1990). After a 10-year period (1970–80), Grondalen (1981) remarked that the frequency of severe lesions (DJD) in femora of pigs in Norway had decreased. However, the overall frequency of pigs with cartilage affected by chondrolysis and DJD had increased. Although control of OC and DJD in herds will probably have to be related to genetic selection, the benefit of selection on the basis of conformation was limited in Norway.

Effect of Growth Rate on OC and DJD. Several studies have been conducted to investigate the impact of growth rate on lesions in AECC and growth plates. Equally important considerations were the inherent ability for fast growth and the quantity and quality of rations that were given to enhance growth. Grondalen (1974d) finished pigs at 90 kg liveweight after feeding them different quantities of a balanced ration, and found no difference in the frequency or severity of lesions. Similarly, Perrin et al. (1978) and Nakano et al. (1979b, 1984) found no correlation between the frequency or severity of gross lesions and growth rate in pigs that had reached 120 kg and 90 kg liveweight respectively. Pigs derived from sows that were fed lactation rations, which were low in protein and energy, grew faster than pigs derived from sows that were fed conventionally. Despite the faster (compensatory) growth rate of the former pigs, the frequency of lesions and the composite score for severity of lesions was no different for either group when pigs were slaughtered at ≥ 100 kg liveweight (Walker and Aherne 1987). However, Reiland (1978e), who used relatively small numbers of pigs, concluded that a restriction of feed intake that resulted in a slower growth rate reduced the frequency of lesions. The results of Goedegebuure et al. (1980) were in agreement with those of Reiland because the fastest growing pigs had more severe lesions in AECC of medial femoral condyles and distal ulnar growth plates by the time they were killed (between 96 and 100 kg liveweight). Later, Woodard et al. (1987a) compared lesions in pigs fed rations that contained either 12% or 16% protein. Although pigs on the former ration grew more slowly, it appeared to have no impact on the development of lesions in distal radial growth plates or AECC of femoral or humeral condyles. Carlson et al. (1988a) also compared lesions on femoral and humeral condyles of control pigs fed ad libitum and pigs fed at 70% of the intake of controls. They concluded that in pigs killed at the same weight as the controls, lesions in femoral condyles had time to resolve, but this did not ac-

count for the similarities in lesions affecting humeri in different groups. Because early lesions were found in pigs 15 days old, it is uncertain as to whether growth rate affects the onset of lesions. However, the conformation of commercial pigs has changed dramatically over the past 50 years, and growth cartilages that are subjected to relatively high weights or compressive forces as the pig grows rapidly may be increasingly susceptible to OC and DJD.

In contrast to the hypothesis that faster growing pigs were more likely to develop lesions, Hani et al. (1984) and Lundeheim (1987) found that the pigs with the most severe lesions were in fact the slowest growing ones overall. It was possible that growth rate slowed dramatically only late in the finishing phase, because pigs were extremely uncomfortable and they did not move to the feeder and eat. Lundeheim (1987) speculated that only the scores for lesions at the highest end of the severity scale may have caused clinical signs that precipitated a reduction in growth rate. An early effect of growth rate on the outcome as far as development of lesions was concerned was in agreement with the conclusion of Reiland (1978e), who considered growth rate during the first 4 months of life influenced the frequency of OC. Therefore, the evidence for restricted feed intake, which would slow growth rate, is of debatable value for preventing lesions and clinical signs. Pigs selected for fast growth rate and low backfat had higher levels of growth hormone activity than pigs selected for slow growth rate and thicker backfat and had a higher frequency of OC and DJD (Grondalen and Vangen 1974). Based on preliminary studies, the use of growth hormone may be related to the development of OC in pigs (Chung et al. 1985; Etherton et al. 1986; Carlson et al. 1988b; Evock et al. 1988) and as the use of this hormone becomes widespread, it will be worth monitoring the impact it may have on locomotor disorders.

Nutrition and OC and DJD. Although imbalances or deficiencies of micronutrients have affected growth cartilages and bone, none of them have been specifically implicated in the etiopathogenesis of OC or DJD. Joints were affected in pigs subjected to calcium or vitamin D deficiencies (Kernkamp 1925; Pepper et al. 1978). In various investigations that involved the manipulation of dietary concentrations of calcium, phosphorus, vitamin A, vitamin C, and vitamin D, there were no differences in the frequency or severity of lesions between treated pigs and control pigs that were fed conventional rations (Walker and Jones 1962; Grondalen 1974d; Reiland 1978d; Hilley 1980). Deficiencies of zinc and manganese also may have been associated with DJD (Neher et al. 1956; Hill and Bebiak 1979). It was possible that in the studies in which specific minerals or vitamins were included at concentrations considered to be suboptimal, there were in fact sufficient quantities to meet the physiological needs for growth of cartilage and for endochondral ossification. Therefore, future investigations should not preclude deficiencies of various micronutrients, and evaluation of rations in herds with a high frequency of pigs with OC and DJD is advisable.

Decreased growth rate associated with restricted intakes of nutritionally balanced rations or reduced concentrations of protein had little impact on the frequency or severity of lesions (Grondalen 1974d, Reiland 1978e, Woodard et al. 1987a, Carlson et al. 1988a). Van der Wal et al. (1982, 1986) considered that metabolic acidosis exacerbated lesions, but attempts to alter the acidotic state by administration of $NaHCO_3$ did not result in a lessening in the severity of lesions affecting the AECC of femoral condyles. Nevertheless, ambulatory ability of treated pigs was not as impaired as that of untreated pigs.

Effects of Compression and Overloading of Growth Cartilages on OC and DJD. Excessive compressive forces associated with rapid weight gain or overly developed muscles have been considered to cause abnormal stresses in growth cartilages of pigs. This concern was justified by the alterations in the triplicity of growth curves such that an increasingly immature skeletal system has been expected to carry greater muscle masses, which affect compressive forces across joints (McMeekan 1940). Excessive loading of limbs of pigs has been achieved either by fitting pigs with weighted saddles so that both limbs were overloaded or by immobilizing one limb so that the contralateral limb was weight bearing and overloaded (Walker et al. 1966; Jussila and Paatsama 1972; Grondalen and Grondalen 1974). Radiographic alterations in distal ulnar growth plates were considered to be consistent with a dyschondroplasia, and lesions resolved after excessive loads were removed (Grondalen and Grondalen 1974). Brennan et al. (1986) examined AECC from medial humeral condyles, and although mild changes occurred near the articular surface in pigs that carried an extra 15% of their body weight in saddles, lesions regarded as OC in pigs were from both treated and control groups.

Whereas lesions developed in distal radial growth plates (Woodard et al. 1987a), an absence of lesions in growth plates from non-weight-bearing metacarpi and metatarsi (second and fifth digits) lent support to the hypothesis that loading initiated or exacerbated OC or DJD. Because lesions developed in costochondral junctions and in growth plates of ischial tuberosities, either compressive forces were of no relevance or tensile forces were of equal importance in the initiation of dyschondroplasia (Hill et al. 1984b). Lesions appeared to be initiated in pigs ≤1 month old, an age range when muscle masses were poorly de-

veloped, but at a time when AECC and growth plates were proportionally thicker and possibly susceptible to stress (Hill et al. 1984b, 1990). Because evidence for either absolute weight or excessive compressive forces being initiators of either dyschondroplasia or chondrolysis is conflicting, downgrading carcass characteristics to prevent OC and DJD would be difficult to justify economically.

Nakano and Aherne (1988) subjected commercial pigs of average body weight (29 kg) to either a single traumatic event and transport in a wooden-floored box cart for a distance of 50 m or to walking a similar distance. Pigs were slaughtered at 90 kg liveweight and in 8 of 40 pigs, the AECC of the humeral condyles was disrupted. Scores for changes in the AECC of pigs subjected to transport in the box cart were significantly higher than scores for pigs that walked between buildings. If trauma (or excessive compression) was important in the etiopathogenesis of chondrolysis, either by damage caused to blood vessels in cartilage canals or by a direct effect on chondrocytes, the effects were more likely the result of repeated insults. Therefore, efforts to prevent injury would probably be futile.

Influences of Exercise and Floor Types on OC and DJD. Comparisons have been made between scores for conformational features, locomotor ability, or leg weakness and the use of confinement vs. extensive facilities or exercise protocols for pigs. However, studies that lacked a definitive diagnosis for ambulatory abnormalities have contributed little to our understanding of any relationships between environment or exercise and OC or DJD. A number of investigators have at least examined growth cartilages macroscopically.

Elliot and Doige (1973) found a higher frequency of changes in articular surfaces of pigs housed individually in small pens compared with pigs housed in groups of four in larger pens, but attributed lack of muscular tone to posterior weakness or lameness. Grondalen (1974e) concluded that the severity of joint lesions was unrelated to the amount of exercise the pigs had. Although exercise on a treadmill reduced deformities of thoracic limbs and the degree of lameness, Perrin et al. (1975) and Perrin and Bowland (1977) found no significant differences between mean scores for lesions in pigs in different exercise groups. When comparisons were made between Yorkshire or crossbred boars reared on concrete or deep straw, lesions were most severe on the AECC of distal parts of humeri and proximal parts of femora, and there were no significant differences for frequency or severity of lesions between groups (Perrin et al. 1975, 1978). Sather and Fredeen (1982) found no significant relationship between the severity of joint lesions and leg weakness in pigs reared in confinement, but lesions were more severe and lameness was more pronounced for pigs that were housed individually. In pigs that were held on pasture at the end of the initial study, lesions were considered to have healed by the time the pigs were ≥ 90 kg liveweight. Sather (1980) and Sather and Fredeen (1982) indicated that the amount of damage on articular surfaces of humeroradio-ulnar joints and the degree of leg weakness was greatest in pigs kept in confinement compared with those on dirt lots.

No benefit in terms of severity of lesions or locomotor ability was demonstrated when lame boars were placed on dirt lots at the end of their test period compared with boars in concrete yards (Nakano et al. 1981). Although Sather (1987) only evaluated leg weakness, it was apparent that locomotor ability improved in some Lacombe boars and gilts, while in others it worsened during a 3-month stay on pasture. Dewey et al. (1988, 1990 personal communication) found that the percentage culling rate for pigs kept on solid floors, with or without straw, was less than that for pigs kept on concrete or metal slats. Of 50 sows culled for lameness, approximately 50% had OC or DJD.

Because the degree of lameness and the severity of lesions has been exaggerated in pigs kept individually in confinement, it has been presumed that pigs reared in larger pens and in extensive systems had more exercise either because of group interaction or an innate tendency to use the space for exercising. However, Ewbank (1974) demonstrated that, whatever the housing system, if pigs were adequately fed they only moved around the pen 20% of the time, even on dirt lots. Therefore, conflicting findings concerning softer, bedded floors are not helpful in making clinical judgments as to whether or not the frequency or severity of lesions associated with OC or DJD can be controlled by modifying the environment. Of concern is the fact that different types of flooring may mask an underlying genetic problem and may accelerate the selection of lines of pigs susceptible to OC and DJD with higher pain thresholds.

Dirt lots or deep straw bedding may help reduce the frequency of other problems, e.g., foot lesions. It is logical that exercise increases muscle tone, but if it also increases muscle mass, there may be excessive compressive forces exerted over immature joints, thus exacerbating OC and DJD. In reality, the balance between compressive forces sufficient to maintain normal cartilage and those that may be injurious must be extremely complex.

Infectious Agents and OC and DJD.

Infectious agents have not been associated with OC or DJD in pigs, but attempts to culture organisms have generally been made in pigs that had chronic lesions (Ljunggren and Reiland 1970; Reiland 1978b; Van Sickle et al. 1980). Because infectious agents such as swine fever virus (Thurley 1966) and *Streptococcus equisimilis* (Roberts et al. 1967) affect growth

plates and metaphyses, and because bacteria can initiate thrombi in vessels adjacent to the growth plate (Martens and Auer 1980), infections in young pigs cannot be excluded.

Control and Preventive Measures against OC and OA.

Various investigations to determine the cause or causes of OC and OA have been discussed, and commentaries on control measures have been made. However, to date there is not enough information on the etiopathogenesis of these conditions for specific preventive steps to be taken. The hereditary nature of these conditions needs closer scrutiny because selection characteristics such as overall leanness, and larger muscles are those that seem to be correlated with a higher frequency of lesions, which also tend to be more severe. A deliberate reduction in growth rate, which may only be of clinical benefit, is obviously an additional expense for the herd in terms of lost profit. The degree of lameness or leg weakness has not been closely associated with the extent or severity of lesions in bones or joints. This finding, together with the concern of Reiland et al. (1978) that the degree of lameness exhibited by a pig was related to its pain threshold, meant that selection programs to eliminate pigs with OC or DJD from a herd could not be based on clinical signs alone. Selection of this kind would simply result in retention of pigs with the highest pain thresholds.

The use of drugs, e.g., glycosaminoglycan polysulfate ester (Brennan and Aherne 1986), which may alleviate clinical signs, or the use of more extensive accommodation for increased activity, may mask the underlying problem that is perpetuated by boars and sows retained in the herd. However, at present the best preventive measures that can be offered seem to include adequate exercise on nonslippery floors, the supply of a suitably balanced ration that allows normal skeletal growth, and selection against conformationally poor or lame animals. Future investigations of OC and DJD will have to consider all the potential causes listed, but the lines of pigs retained for breeding programs will need exceptional scrutiny. This may involve necropsy of siblings of selected tested boars and sows for examination of cartilage at the microscopic and molecular level.

Epiphyseolysis.

Epiphyseolysis with separation of the femoral head along the proximal femoral growth plate occurs in sows and boars (Duthie and Lancaster 1964; Grondalen 1974a; Nemeth and Van der Valk 1976; Van Alstine and Toben 1989). A severe, debilitating lameness develops and despite the fact that recovery may occur, the process is slow and the pig develops chronic lameness. If secondary bacterial infections become established, bone and surrounding muscles become necrotic. Separation of the ischial tuberosity was more frequent in sows than in boars

(Grondalen 1974b). Unilateral lesions cause a moderate to severe lameness, but bilateral separation may prevent the sow from rising or walking (Done et al. 1979).

Some researchers consider that OC weakens the growth plate, which ultimately splits in thickened areas, resulting in separation of the epiphyseal center of ossification from the body of the bone. However, trauma during fighting, foreplay, or act of copulation may be sufficient in itself to cause lesions.

Prevention relates to selecting lines free of OC/OA (if possible), providing adequate nutrition for maintenance of the skeleton, and avoiding traumatic incidents when pigs are moved or placed together for breeding, something that is difficult to accomplish in pen-breeding systems.

Ankylosing Spondylosis. Although Grondalen (1974b, c), in Norway, has demonstrated ankylosing spondylosis in culled sows and boars at the slaughterhouse, lesions may start to develop during the first year of life. In the early stages of the disease pigs have a painful lumbar region and may avoid breeding activity. Kyphosis and a waddling gait or dragging of hind feet may develop, and boars that mount a sow or a dummy slip off in a caudal direction before completing ejaculation.

The various causal factors considered to initiate lesions include trauma, abnormal conformation, or chronic DJD of the intervertebral, synovial joints secondary to OC or erysipelas (Grabell et al. 1962; Grondalen 1974b, c; Reiland 1978c). Given time, vertebrae fuse and the pig may regain normal motor function.

Prevention involves selection of lines of pigs free of OC and OA, an adequate vaccination program to prevent erysipelas from occurring in the herd, and improvement of wet, slippery floor surfaces, especially in the breeding area.

Downer Sow Syndrome. This nonspecific syndrome is initiated by any condition that causes a sow to become unable to stand because of weakness, cachexia, or paralysis. Any component of the locomotor system may be affected, but often, it is bone or an element of the nervous system that is affected. In the author's opinion, downer sows rarely are worth treatment because complete recoveries are rare, whatever the injury.

DISEASES ASSOCIATED WITH INADEQUATE NUTRITION AND MANAGEMENT

Rickets. Although unexpected in contemporary hog production, rickets occasionally occurs. Clinical signs include a stunted, unthrifty appearance, lameness, fractured long bones, and paresis. At necropsy, bones are soft (particularly the ribs, which bend rather than snap under pressure) and radiolucent. Joint surfaces may be folded and growth plates are thickened and irregular. Hemorrhages develop in the cartilage or adjacent bone. Rickets develops as a result of (1) inadequate concentrations of calcium (Ca), phosphorus (P), and/or vitamin D in the ration, (2) improperly balanced Ca and P in the ration, resulting in a ratio greatly different from 1.2:1, (3) inadequate concentrations of active vitamin D, (4) the potentially lost opportunity for pigs to adequately metabolize vitamin D in darkened confinement buildings, and (5) a system whereby rations are balanced on paper, rather than by use of periodic ration analysis.

By the time lesions develop and clinical signs occur in pigs ≥ 10 weeks old, rickets is a costly problem because the prognosis is poor. Affected pigs grow slowly and for humane, as well as economic, reasons may have to be euthanatized, even following the use of therapy (Pepper et al. 1978). Accepting that in larger herds the food from a particular batch may be used by the time clinical signs are observed, it is good practice to retain a sample of each batch for future reference. Ration analysis is not prohibitively expensive and should be considered, together with the function of the mix-mill, as part of a quality control program.

Osteomalacia/Osteoporosis Complex, and Skeletal Strength and Integrity. In herds that include many moderate and high-producing sows, downer sows are seen intermittently. Typically, the sow collapses in the farrowing crate, as she is walked from the crate, during movement or transport from the farrowing facilities to the breeding area, or when she is placed with a group of sows in the breeding barn. Sows that become trapped under the rails of a farrowing crate and struggle to free themselves may become paraplegic. Following episodes of fighting or estrus behavior, some sows become extremely lame or are unable to stand, and occasionally, a sow collapses while the boar is mounting her.

Sows that have skeletal injuries are in extreme discomfort, are unwilling or unable to stand, and hold affected limbs rigid if they are manipulated. Most sows become inappetant, lose condition, and ultimately need to be culled. Frequently during the physical examination, crepitus can be felt and heard if limbs are manipulated. However, a limb may be held so rigidly that even extensive damage cannot be detected. At necropsy, the most frequent sites for lesions are the proximal one-third of the humerus and the proximal one-third of the femur. At both sites, comminuted, spiral fractures extend from the metaphysis down into the diaphysis. In pigs that have developed paraplegia, a fracture in one or more of the lumbar vertebrae should be anticipated. If the sow is kept in the herd, a large callus will form at the fracture site. Unfortunately, callus develops around fragments of bone embedded in the surrounding, damaged muscle, and a solid mass of mineralized, fibrous connective tissue eventually replaces muscle as well as blood clots.

Bones of sows fracture as a result of one or more underlying pathological changes. Because the majority of pigs in breeding herds have immature skeletons, precautions to prevent rickets should be followed. Indeed, rickets may be a part of the syndrome and thickened, irregular growth plates may be weak and susceptible to fracturing.

Osteomalacia has been described in sows (Gayle and Schwartz 1980; Doige 1982), and in addition to inadequate amounts of Ca, P, and vitamin D, or an imbalance in the Ca:P ratio, lesions are attributable to the inability of some lactating sows to consume adequate amounts of food to provide the micronutrients. In place of calcified bone, large quantities of unmineralized osteoid develop, thereby weakening the bones. Lactational osteoporosis also has been associated with fractured long bones in sows (Spencer 1979). In order to maintain homeostasis in the fluid compartments of the body, including the milk, Ca and P are mobilized. The net result is bone remodelling and weaker bones that have lower mass, but are structurally normal. Additional factors that may induce osteoporosis include restricted exercise during gestation in association with confinement in small pens, stalls, or tethers, and virtually no exercise during lactation while the sow is in a farrowing crate. If a limb is immobilized, the bones tend to become osteoporotic; if persons or animals are, respectively, subjected to prolonged bed rest or cage rest or to weightlessness in spaceflight, bone mass is lost. Therefore, it is reasonable to presume that the lactating sow, which already is mobilizing bone for milk production, is at greater risk of osteoporosis because of the restricted amount of exercise she is able to get. Suboptimal concentrations of Ca and P or inappropriate ratios of Ca:P have been shown to result in a shorter longevity for sows in the breeding herd (Kornegay et al. 1973), and are not adequate for meeting the needs of sows during their first gestation and lactation, a time when skeletal growth is still very active (Nimmo 1980).

Little can be done to alleviate osteomalacia or osteoporosis once they are established. Culling or euthanasia of the sows is perhaps the most cost-effective and humane approach to dealing with these problems. There may not be salvage value in the carcass. However, preventive measures should include feeding regimens that allow for (1) adequate skeletal development in the gilt and young sow, (2) selection of replacement gilts (and boars) on the basis of the size and structure of bones, (3) feeding sows (and boars) to condition, and (4) consideration of the impact that exercise has on the development and maintenance of a sturdy skeleton. Related to the last measure, interaction of small groups of sows in pens on suitable flooring in confinement may be an ideal from the sow's viewpoint. Transducer/transponder technology has paved the way for efficient individual feeding of sows, provided that condition is regularly evaluated. However, a simple approach to limiting sows without completely restricting their movement in conventional gestation crates or tethers has recently been developed by one U.S. company. The rear portion of each gestation crate is movable, which enables each sow to turn around, thus allowing some increase in exercise and socialization (Hummel and Bernick 1990). Additional costs that may be incurred must be considered with any intensive system and the relevant equipment; however, Clough (1984) has made the point that occupant-oriented design can be used to improve the conditions for farm animals for the benefit of both productivity and welfare.

Infectious Diseases Of Bones and Joints

Neonatal Arthritis and Polyarthritis. A variety of pathogens or facultative pathogens, including streptococci (*Streptococcus suis,* Lancefield group C [*Streptococcus equisimilis*], or group L), staphylococci, *E. coli*, etc., which gain entry to the body via the umbilical stalk and skin wounds in conditions of poor hygiene or via the oropharynx (when the sow is a carrier) (Helms 1962; Sanford and Tilker 1982; Clifton-Hadley 1983), cause arthritis in baby pigs in the farrowing house. Nielsen et al. (1975) found an average preweaning mortality of 3.3% and mortality of 1.5% associated with polyarthritis. Piglets of P1 and P2 sows were most susceptible. Joints are hot, swollen, and painful and the umbilicus may be affected. Lincomycin may be useful in treating these infections (Johnson and Coulson 1986), but if it is to be effective, antimicrobial therapy should be initiated as soon as clinical signs are seen. Control and prevention involve improving hygiene and management in the farrowing house.

Arthritides Occurring in the Nursery and Grow-Finishing Units. A chronic arthritis initiated by *Mycoplasma hyorhinis* can cause problems over a period of 6 months or more. The chronic effects of polyserositis as well as polyarthritis may cause stunting when pigs fail to feed adequately. Organisms are common inhabitants of the oropharynx (Roberts et al. 1963) and antimicrobial therapy is of limited value; therefore, stunted pigs should be culled and pigs from affected litters or rooms in which the problem occurred should not be kept for breeding.

Preventive measures include reducing the levels of stressors in the nursery, reducing the numbers and severity of concomitant diseases (enteric, respiratory), and in extreme cases, considering a depopulation/repopulation program (specific-pathogen-free pigs).

Polyarthritis caused by *M. hyosynoviae* occurs in pigs between 12 and 24 weeks of age and occasionally affects young adults (Ross and Spear

1973). Based on clinical and serological evidence, Burch (1986) demonstrated that lameness in replacement gilts that peaked in frequency between 22–28 weeks was associated with this pathogen. Infection is passed from carrier sows to baby pigs, or from growers to growers (Ross and Spear 1973). Clinical disease is precipitated by stressors such as movement to new pens, transport, changes in ambient temperature, and predisposing lesions typical of OA (Lawrisuk et al. 1987). Sudden onset of lameness that affects one or more limbs usually lasts up to 10 days.

Unlike infection with *M. hyorhinis,* animals infected by *M. hyosynoviae* usually show a rapid response to early parenteral treatment with tylosin or lincomycin. Burch and Goodwin (1984) and Madeiros (1984) indicated that tiamulin also may be effective. Corticosteroids may reduce the inflammatory response and help to alleviate pain. Control measures should be aimed at reducing stress and it may be advisable to treat any new, naive stock with the antimicrobial compounds as soon as they are moved into the herd.

Glasser's disease is a syndrome caused by *Hemophilus parasuis* and can resemble polyserositis and polyarthritis caused by *M. hyorhinis* (Nielsen and Danielsen 1975). Febrile animals become lame and may develop a meningitis. An acute septicemic condition without polyarthritis has been reported (Peet et al. 1983; Desrosiers et al. 1986). Morbidity and mortality (up to 10%) is higher than that occurring with mycoplasmal polyserositis and polyarthritis. Losses tend to be greatest in herds that have had little exposure to the disease or if specific-pathogen-free (SPF) pigs are introduced into conventional herds (Madsen 1984; Miniats et al. 1986). However, *H. parasuis* has been found unexpectedly in SPF herds in Canada (Smart et al. 1986). Because most serious losses occur in SPF herds, as for mycoplasmal polyarthritis it is important to keep the disease out of the herd. To reduce the risk of disease outbreaks, stressors, particularly those during transport of the pigs, must be reduced to a minimum. Stunted pigs should be culled, and it is probably advisable to dispose of all pigs from infected groups when they reach 104.5 kg liveweight. Generally, response to a variety of antimicrobial compounds including penicillin, tetracycline, and sulfa drugs is good. Successful vaccines have been utilized, but there is need for research in terms of cross-immunity between bacterin prepared from different strains of *H. parasuis* (Riising 1981; Miniats and Smart 1988). Vaccination programs for SPF pigs that are to enter conventional herds are important control measures (Miniats and Smart 1988).

Although most herds in which sows are vaccinated to protect them and their offspring against erysipelas have little in the way of problems with erysipelas, occasionally, costly outbreaks occur in the growing-finishing unit. Disease may occur in herds in which growers as well as adults are vaccinated and, therefore, this condition should be included in the differential diagnosis for lameness in grow-finishing pigs. An epidemic of erysipelas in the upper Midwest was reported by Thomson et al. (1990). Predisposing factors included inadequate vaccination programs and lower usage of feed-grade antibiotics.

The acute form of erysipelas is a systemic infection, but unwillingness to stand, stiffness, or lameness are typical clinical signs. Urticarial "diamonds" develop as welts over the skin surface, and eventually the skin lesions may slough. A chronic arthritis develops with fibrous thickening of the synovial membrane and joint capsule, pannus formation, osteophyte formation, and eventually destruction of the articular surfaces (Grabell et al. 1962).

Penicillin, in conjunction with antiserum if it is available, is effective as a treatment, provided animals with acute disease are treated. Corticosteroids may help alleviate acute inflammation, but if arthritis is established, treatment is of little value.

Killed or live-attenuated vaccines generally provide active protection for sows and, provided regular booster doses are used, a strong passive immunity in the baby pigs. However, Tasker (1981) demonstrated variability in vaccinal titer response in commercial herds. It may also be necessary to vaccinate growers between 7 and 10 weeks of age. As with other infectious diseases affecting this age category of pigs, it is important to reduce stress and predisposing factors.

STRUCTURE OF FEET. During the past 30–40 years there have been differing levels of interest in lameness caused by foot diseases in pigs. Initially, efforts were centered on characterizing lesions (often superficial changes on the wall, sole, or heel) and attempting to find infectious agents in deep-seated lesions. The influence of environment, particularly of rough floors, was recognized and nutrition was arbitrarily implicated. However, during the past decade emphasis has shifted to analysis of floor types and to better understanding of micronutrient deficiencies, especially biotin.

The pig is tetradactylous and the third and fourth digits are the largest. Between birth and the end of the grower phase, an estimated 90% of increase in size of the hoof occurs. Also, during this time a disparity between the size of claws develops such that the fourth digit is larger than the third digit. Nordby (1939) examined feet from 30 slaughter hogs and was concerned that in excessively long fourth digits, phalanges were distorted. Strangely, he stated that "almost all hogs have this defect" and noted that Sisson (1938) illustrated this "undesirable trait." If the disparity between digits was so frequent, it might have been logical to have recognized it as a phenotypic characteristic of contemporary hogs. Penny et al. (1963) determined a ratio of 1.11:1 for mean lengths of fourth and third digits in 31 pigs ≥ 3 days, whereas Smith and Mitchell (1977) found no difference in digit length in 1 day old pigs (despite 60% of fourth digits being longer than third digits); at 5 and 14 days fourth digits were significantly longer. In another study, the mean lengths were generally greater for fourth digits compared with third digits in pigs kept on various types of slats, but significant differences were found only for hoof and sole lengths on pelvic feet (Newton et al. 1980). Therefore, it is reasonable to accept that despite Nordby's concern, the longer fourth digit is the current norm, especially on pelvic limbs. Because of their larger size, the fourth digits may take a proportionately larger share of the body weight and be more susceptible to excessive compressive forces. Also, the fourth digits may be at greater risk of traumatic injury because of their size.

Second and fifth digits are the accessory digits (dewclaws); the first digit is absent. The third phalanx and part of the second phalanx are covered by the keratinized hoof, which protects structures within the foot. Each hoof has three distinct areas: the heel, the sole, and the wall. The heel is large and prominent compared with that of other species, and houses the digital cushion, which reduces concussion to the foot. The sole covers a relatively small area. A region of nonpigmented soft horn (white-line) forms a junction between the hoof wall and the sole. The wall is attached to the third phalanx, which has a specialized periosteum, by interdigitation of the soft laminae of the corium and the harder laminae of the white-line material, which is firmly attached to and is a backing for the wall. Epidermal cells at the tips of the laminae of the corium produce keratinized cells that form the white-line material. The corium is highly vascular and nourishes various parts of the hoof, including the periople, sole, and heel. The corium in the periople, coronary band, and heel is supplied with numerous nerves, and injury in any of these areas is, therefore, likely to cause pain and lameness. Numerous tubules of keratinized flat cells interspersed by keratinized "pancake" cells are laid down in a proximodistal direction as the hoof is produced by the coronary band and as the sole and heel are formed by the corium, which is distal and caudal to the third phalanx (Geyer and Tagwerker 1986). The density of tubules and their parallel arrangement determine the hardness of the horn; consequently, the hoof wall has a greater density of tubules per square millimeter than the softer sole, and the resilient heel, which is softest, has the lowest density of tubules. The rate of growth of the hoof wall measured proximodistally parallel with the tubules varies with age; in pigs between 20 and 100 kg, the growth rate is about 10 mm per month, but in sows it is

only 5–6 mm per month (Geyer and Tagwerker 1986). Consequently, if a hoof wall is damaged, the repair time can be prolonged in adult pigs.

Generally, if a pig is to be productive and profitable, it must have eight functional digits, all weight-bearing surfaces must be intact, and the feet must be able to adapt to different surfaces over a period of approximately 6 months for finishing hogs and considerably longer for breeding stock. To maintain integrity of the foot and for the length and vertical angle of the wall to remain constant, there must be a precise balance between growth and wear of both hard and soft tissues of the hoof. The rate of growth of the horn is governed, in part, by the surface of the floor on which the pig is reared (Ledecky et al. 1984). Therefore, during a pig's lifespan the response of the foot to the environment probably varies.

Kovacs and Szilagyi (1973 a, b, 1974) analyzed the mineral content of components of the normal hoof wall of different breeds of pigs at different ages and then collected damaged horn from fattening pigs. The calcium content of damaged horn was disproportionately high, and an inflamed corium produced a more porous horn that was less resistant to damage. Anything that predisposes to breaching the integrity of the wall, sole, or heel puts the pig at risk of developing chronic pododermatitis, cellulitis, osteomyelitis, or arthritis, all of which can precipitate an incapacitating lameness.

Evaluation of Feet.   Only as clinicians acquire a greater understanding of structural characteristics of normal and abnormal feet and the effects of different floor surfaces, degrees of dampness, etc., on feet will they be able to predict outcomes of foot-floor interactions. To date, scant knowledge about and a limited ability to quantify locomotion or conformation of pigs has meant that clinical and research projects have relied on purely subjective evaluations. Techniques such as video-imaging, cinematography, and force-plate analyses have been little used, but these methods potentially would enable the development of objective evaluations of both simple and complex locomotor dysfunctions. Even radiology has been underutilized. In preliminary studies, Webb and Clark (1981) demonstrated by force-plate and pressure-plate analyses that, for at least part of the time, when a pig is standing or moving, much of the weight is carried by the fourth digit. Although the distribution of weight varied or was adjusted over the components of the foot, the toe and the bulb of the heel were principal weight-bearing areas. Force-plate analyses measured three perpendicular forces as the foot impacted on the ground (force plate). The strength and hardness of the wall horn have also been measured (Webb et al. 1984). In other experiments in which the effects of moisture content or viability of the horn might influence the effect of floor surfaces on horn, resin substitutes for horn have been utilized.

If the clinician is to be able to investigate lamenesses associated with feet, it is important to establish a standardized international terminology for lesions and gait abnormalities and to develop practical, objective evaluation techniques. Once evaluation techniques have been established, preventive measures, treatments, and genetic selections can be instituted to eliminate predisposing causes.

Another limiting factor in determining the nature of lesions on pigs' feet is the difficulty encountered in physical examination of the load-bearing extremities. Despite the various restraint methods that can be utilized, physical examination of the pig can be strenuous (Penny et al. 1963). The volar surface of each digit must be examined because specific lesions affect this area. Nevertheless, superficial lesions may not provide a complete answer to the gravity of local damage. It is important to determine how deeply lesions penetrate before they can be implicated in lameness, unless there are obvious signs such as hemorrhage or suppuration. In the case of valuable boars or sows, imaging techniques may be utilized. However, if there is a serious, ongoing problem in a herd, it is as effective to collect feet from a packing plant and to cut them into slabs parallel with the sole of the hoof. Cuts can be made with a coping or lightweight meat saw at 5 mm apart (Hill and Dalrymple 1987). Superficial cracks or black, grey, and brown tracks that pass through damaged keratin may be limited and separated from the deep connective tissue by a focally thickened area of keratinizing epithelium. However, necrotic debris and pus in this area or in the phalangeal bone or interphalangeal joints are indicative of a severe problem. Unfortunately, on the slaughter line some hoof walls are lost in the scald tank or are trimmed off before they can be examined. The softer periople and skin at the coronary band often are destroyed. In these circumstances it is necessary to submit groups of pigs to smaller locker plants so that postmortem examination can be utilized. Unless feet are examined in conjunction with other elements of the locomotor system, concomitant or alternative causes of lameness may be missed.

Influence of Flooring on Foot Integrity. As intensive systems have evolved, the stresses to which feet and legs of pigs are subjected have changed. Pigs have been removed from grass or dirt lots and placed on solid concrete floors or slats or permutations of solid floors and slats. Jensen (1979) believed that the evolution of slatted floors was the single most important influential factor for the transition to confinement production. More pigs could be kept in the same space with less labor input (Smith and Mitchell 1977). However, the transition from one type of floor to another has not been without problems; use of various floor materials and designs preceded research information (Jensen 1979). Therefore, the veterinary and agricultural engineering professions have followed in the wake of this evolution, rather than leading the way.

Current trends are related to analysis of different floor types and their effects on the hooves of pigs. Additionally, comfort levels and welfare of pigs have been considered (Sainsbury 1984; Lindemann et al. 1985; Christison and de Gooijer 1986; Wells 1986). Factors that need to be taken into consideration while devising suitable floors for pigs include the cost of materials and installation, efficiency for self-cleaning, cleanliness of the pigs on the floor, and the durability of the material (Scott 1985). Physical characteristics of the flooring material that have been considered include slipperiness, softness, abrasiveness, resistance to wear, and surface profile (Mitchell 1979; Smith 1982). When feasible, physical characteristics of floor surfaces have been measured (Penny et al. 1965; Kovacs and Beer 1979; Mitchell 1979), and data have been related to subjective assessments. Although expectations for lifespans of flooring materials of over 10–15 years have been expressed (Kovacs and Beer 1979), in light of rapid technicological changes, this projection should probably be modified to shorter periods. Clinician involvement in advising clients on the well-being of pigs on different floor types should increase on the basis of experience with different enterprises and an understanding of foot diseases. For example, the requirements of the sow in terms of surface texture, abrasiveness, heat conductivity, and void:solid ratio of the floor are different from those of the baby pig (Lindemann et al. 1985; Furniss et al. 1986). Although associations of cause and effect are simpler to understand in the relationship of floor surface to feet, it is equally important for the clinician to explain that not all lesions will cause lameness and that the nature of the floor may have ramifications on other elements of the locomotor system. For example, increased length of the hoof wall in finishing pigs that were reared on slats resulted in a more acute angle between the floor and the cranial surface of the hoof (Baumann and Wisser 1972). In turn, this probably affected angulation of other joints in pelvic and thoracic limbs and may have predisposed to DJD (Grondalen 1974e). Slippery floors may result in damage to muscles, joints, or bones as a pig attempts to rise or lie down, or as pigs in a newly comingled group fight to establish a "pecking" order.

Smith and Robertson (1971) described four herd cases in which increased culling rates of up to 45% in sows were associated with foot and leg injuries. Poorly made concrete slats that had worn and chipped edges caused damage to digits and limbs. Some sows stood with hunched backs while others were crippled. The problem was alleviated when old slats were covered by expanded metal or were replaced by new slats with pencil edges, and when sows were placed on deep straw bedding. In another problem the soles, heels, and accessory digits of piglets were damaged in farrowing pens that had expanded metal floors (Smith and Mitchell 1977). A high proportion of second and third digits were injured and sole erosions often led to infection and swelling of the feet. Factors considered to cause or exacerbate lesions were the thrusting action of sucking pigs and the fact that digits probably slipped into the perforations, which had sharp edges. Other studies in which the effects of different floors on the integrity of feet of pigs have been examined are in Table 8.2.

There are many difficulties encountered in attempting to interpret clinical evaluations of feet on different types of flooring. Apart from a spectrum of scoring techniques that was used, the variability in slat widths, slot widths, and surface textures confounded the issue. When slats are narrow, for a given area the length of slat edge is greater than for wide slats. Thus, the length of sharp slat edges, which can lacerate digits, is increased. Unless surface characteristics of floors are defined or measured, it is difficult to assess the amount of damage they might cause. Smith (1982) considered that it was difficult or even dangerous to extrapolate from one study to another or from one floor to another. However, in summary of findings listed in Table 8.2, rough or irregular concrete, concrete slats, and aluminum slats often caused a higher frequency of lesions or more severe lesions in grow-finishing pigs. Plastic slats and plastic coverings were not always ideal; for sows, plastic-covered woven wire and perforated metal sheets have been implicated with higher frequencies of lesions if they are slippery enough to prevent the animal from rising easily or if digits (especially second and fifth) become trapped in the spaces. Geyer and Tagwerker (1986) recommended different slat widths for concrete (≥ 80 mm) and cast iron (30–40 mm) and a range of slot widths between 9 (pigs <8kg) and 22mm (pigs >100 kg) for concrete slats and between 9 and 16 mm for cast-iron slats for the same weight range of pigs. Shaw (1979) emphasized the need for quality control for concrete used in flooring or slats because cost-saving shortcuts invariably shortened the "lifespan" of the floor.

Consideration also has been given to comfort and preferences of pigs in relation to different floor types. Pouteaux et al. (1980, 1983), and Farmer and Christison (1982) demonstrated that young pigs preferred plastic-coated expanded metal over expanded metal, molded plastic, fiberglass slats, or woven wire. Surface friction, void:solid ratio, and surface temperature were probably the factors that most influenced this preference (Farmer and Christison 1982); the fre-quency with which piglets were willing to lie on a particular floor surface was regarded as the best index of preference. Floors of plastic-coated expanded metal or solid concrete with concrete slats at the rear enabled sows to stand with greater ease than did floors of fiberglass or perforated metal slats (Christison and de Gooijer 1986).

Clinicians should contribute to developing and evaluating new management practices, equipment, and flooring. Increasingly, veterinarians should be involved in working with their clients in interpreting codes of practice or welfare recommendations so that the financial impact of diseases associated with foot and locomotor disorders is alleviated (Sainsbury 1984). Bedding may play a greater role in future low-input-sustainable-agriculture projects; Penny et al. (1986) indicated a benefit in hardening-off gilts on straw and Tuovinen et al. (1990) saw a reduction in partial carcass condemnations in pigs reared on average or large amounts of bedding compared with pigs reared with little or no litter. In the future, selection may involve preferences exhibited by the pigs for different environments, flooring materials, and feeding troughs, but it should always be kept in mind that preservation of health and well-being of the pigs must also be directed toward profitability.

Noninfectious Diseases of Feet

Biotin-Responsive Changes in the Hoof. Although biotin has been shown to have an effect on growth rate, reproductive performance, and hoof integrity in pigs, it is uncertain if the majority of rations need to be supplemented with biotin. The relationships between dietary biotin and performance or lameness are poorly understood. In part, doubt has developed because of the variability in content of biotin for basal rations fed to pigs, the quantity of biotin used to supplement rations, the duration of treatment, and the ages of pigs subjected to treatments.

Biotin content of different grains, etc., varies and bioavailability also varies between different components of the ration. Unfortunately, bioavailability of biotin for pigs is unknown, and for practical purposes extrapolations have been made from studies in chickens; this may have led to inaccuracies in formulating rations. In view of disparities between the estimated and real content of biotin of foodstuffs that were evaluated for some of the studies quoted in this text, there is need for information on the bioavailability of biotin to the pig. It is the d-isomer of biotin that is generally regarded as bioavailable, and as such this form has usually been used for supplementing rations.

Biotin is also produced by the gut microflora. Therefore, biotin requirements have been considered to be met by the supply in the rations and by absorption from the hindgut. However, the avail-

Table 8.2. The influence of floor type or combination of floor types on foot lesions and soundness in pigs

Investigator (year)	Floor type	Ratio of Surfaces (solid:perforated)	Slot Width (cm)	Slot Width (cm)	Rank for Effect on Lesions[a] Frequency	Severity	Comments
Fritschen (1973)	Solid concrete:						
	Concrete slats	0:100 75:25				1 2	
Fritschen (1974)	Concrete slats	0:100	12.70	2.54		2	Pigs had shortest toes
	Steel slats	0:100	7.62	1.90		3	
	Aluminum slats	0:100	7.62	1.90		1	
	Dirt lots	100:0				4	
Fritschen and Zoubeck (1974)	Solid concrete: Plastic slats	50:50	12.70	1.90		5	
	Plastic slats	0:100	12.70	1.90		4	Slippery
	Solid concrete: Concrete slats	50:50	10.16	2.54		3	
	Steel slats	0:100	7.62	1.90		2	
	Aluminum slats	0:100	7.62	1.90		1	
Fritschen (1976)	Solid concrete: Plastic slats	50:50	12.70	2.54		1	
	Solid concrete: Concrete slats	50:50	20.32	2.54		2	
Svendsen et al. (1979)	Plain concrete	100:0			3	1	Sawdust then straw bedding
	Smooth ground	100:0			1	3	Injury frequency dropped between day 3 and day 21
	Rubber paint–covered	100:0			4	2	
	Polyurethane with rubber particles–covered	100:0			2	4(3)	
Newton et al. (1980)	Plastic slats on wood support	0:100	12.8	2.54		1	100 days 23–98 kg foot pad lesion
	Porcelainized steel slats	0:100	10.05	2.54		3	
	Concrete slats	0:100	12.7	2.54		2	Concrete with rough edge; volar surface affected by lesion and wall lesions
	Aluminum slats	0:100	10.2	2.54		3	
Lindemann et al. (1985)	Galvanized, expanded metal	0:100				1	Foot pad Scores
	Plastic-coated, expanded metal	0:100				4	
	Perforated galvanized panels	0:100				3	
	Galvanized woven wire	0:100				2	
	Plastic-coated, woven wire	0:100				3	

Table 8.2. *(Continued)*

Investigator (year)	Floor type	Ratio of Surfaces (solid:perforated)	Slot Width (cm)	Slot Width (cm)	Rank for Effect on Lesions[a] Frequency	Rank for Effect on Lesions[a] Severity	Comments
Newton et al. (1985)	Concrete	100:0				1	Foot pad scores and hoof lesions
	Concrete flushing slats	0:100				2	More severe lesions in winter, especially outside toe
Edwards and Lightfoot (1986)	Concrete screed	100:0				5	Rear foot, many with accessory digits injured related to slipping
	Concrete, fibrocen screed	100:0				5	
	Concrete, latex screed	100:0				5	
	Galvanized punched metal	0:100				3	
	Plastic-covered woven wire	0:100				1	
	Concrete:gpm[b]	66.6:33.4				4	
	Concrete:pcww[c]	66.6:33.4				2	
Christison et al. (1987)	Perforated metal slats	0:100				6	
	Fiberglass slats	0:100				3	
	Perforated metal sheet	0:100				1	
	Solid concrete: Plastic-coated metal sheet	77:33				2	
	Solid concrete: Fiberglass sheet	77:33				5	
	Solid concrete: Concrete slats	77:33	100	25 (rear) 10 (side creep)		4	
Brennan and Aherne (1987)	Plastic-coated expanded metal					2	Significantly different at end of starter period
	Woven wire					1	

[a]Ranking of frequency or severity of lesions does not of itself indicate that there were significant differences between values.
[b]gpm = galvanized punched metal
[c]pcww = plastic-covered woven wire

ability of this biotin in terms of the amount that can be absorbed from the hindgut is unknown. Assessments of biotin content in food or blood have not always been performed, and methods of measuring the benefit of biotin supplementation also have been inconsistent.

Although biotin is intimately involved as a cofactor or coenzyme in a variety of reactions, including gluconeogenesis and fatty acid synthesis (Stryer 1988), its effects on different systems have not been clearly defined. Exactly how biotin influences the nature of keratin of the hoof is unknown.

Although they were not pathognomic, typical changes in the skin, hair coat, and the integrity of the hoof wall were described in preliminary studies of biotin deficiencies of pigs by Cunha et al. (1946) and Lindley and Cunha (1946). For 6 weeks postweaning, Cunha et al. (1946) fed a purified diet that included avidin in egg white which complexes with biotin, making biotin unavailable. Two of four pigs were treated with 100 μg biotin daily intramuscularly (IM). After 2 weeks on the ration, untreated pigs developed alopecia and dermatosis, but by 5 weeks, cracked hooves and hind limb spasticity occurred. Because biotin is produced naturally by the gut microflora, Lindley and Cunha (1946) fed sulfathalidine to pigs on purified rations in an attempt to create biotin deficiency. After 6 weeks, two pigs that received no supplemental biotin developed the aforementioned clinical signs. Lehrer et al. (1952) fed a biotin-deficient milk replacer to five pigs that were weaned at 48 hours of age. Within 29 days, unsupplemented pigs developed severe clinical signs, which included dermatitis, brown ocular exudate, skin ulcers, transversely cracked hooves with coronary band and solar hemorrhages, lameness, stomatitis, and diarrhea. Similar biotin-responsive clinical changes were described by Glattli (1975). Alterations in fat metabolism were noted and this author indicated that plasma biotin concentrations were useful in determining the biotin status of pigs. In other studies, Glattli (1976) used injectable biotin to prevent lesions in avidin-induced biotin deficiency. Plasma concentrations of ≤ 40 μg/100 ml were considered to be an indication of deficiency.

Seemingly, clinical and investigatory interest in the biotin status of pigs was revived in a report by Brooks et al. (1977). Lesions in sows resembled those described in experimental pigs. The condition of feet of sows and gilts were noted before and after split-group trials in which the sows received dietary supplements of biotin at 250 μg/kg d-biotin during pregnancy and 150 μg/kg during lactation. Whereas there was no reduction in the number of foot lesions recorded for untreated sows, treated sows had a 28% reduction in the number of lesions over 6 months. Comben (1977) suggested that repair of foot lesions might have been enhanced if higher concentrations of biotin

had been given. Later, Brooks and Comben (1980) described clinical signs of biotin deficiency in a herd in which 50% of 240 sows were lame and 45 severely lame sows were destined to be culled. Hoof horn was soft and rubbery, lesions were severe, and many were infected. Rations were supplemented with 200 μg/kg of d-biotin for 2 months and lameness was no longer a herd problem. After 12 months foot health was excellent. However, Bane et al. (1980) were unable to demonstrate an improvement in foot lesions on sows that received dietary supplements of 440 μg d-biotin daily. There was an improvement in foot lesions of sows housed individually in crates, compared with those housed on concrete. It is unclear whether flooring on which pigs were kept prior to breeding caused lesions, but the initial biotin status of the sows was not indicated, and a single gestation length was probably too little time for lesions induced by marginal biotin status to have responded to treatment.

In a herd of 116 sows that had a high frequency of foot lesions and lameness, Penny et al. (1980a, b) initiated another split-group trial. Sows were on a standard ration that contained an estimated 56 μg/kg available biotin and half of them received biotin supplement of 1160 μg/day during pregnancy and 2320 μg/day during lactation over 12 months. Biotin supplementation was of no benefit to sows already in the herd, but among 44 gilts that were introduced to the study during the trial, biotin significantly reduced the severity and frequency of lesions on the fourth pelvic digits, i.e., those digits that were generally most affected. The only benefit that Grandhi and Strain (1980) were able to demonstrate after supplementing rations of gilts and first-parity sows with biotin (200 or 300 μg/kg) over one or two subsequent reproductive cycles was a slight decrease in severity of lesions. However, levels of supplementation were probably inadequate in view of the small grain ration that was fed.

De Jong and Sytsema (1983) initiated split trials in which the effects of biotin supplementation were determined in a 130 sow herd. Culling rates for gilts with foot lesions and lameness approximated 50%. Replacement pigs at 2.5 months and gilts at 7 months received a basal ration with or without a biotin supplement at 1250 μg/kg, whereas all the sows received a biotin supplement of 500 μg/kg. Plasma biotin concentrations increased by 2.5 to sixfold over initial marginal concentrations of 50 ng/100 ml. Although the claw lesion scores for treated and control pigs rose between 2.5 and 7 months of age, the average score in supplemented pigs was only about 48% of that for controls, i.e., biotin had a preventative effect. For gilts, the average lesions were improved by almost 28% after only 2.5 months. During 11 months of treatment, the culling rate associated with lameness for sows fell from 25 to 14%. In a 3-year evaluation of the effects of supplementary biotin (550 μg/kg) on soundness of feet and legs in a herd of 161 sows, Hamilton and Veum (1984) were unable to demonstrate any benefits. Since the animals were fed a corn-based ration, it is possible that other causes of foot lesions, rather than biotin deficiency, had considerable impact on this study. In a preliminary study, Bryden et al. (1984) also were unable to demonstrate any improvement in hoof scores in pigs in three herds after supplementation with 500 μg/kg biotin for 6 months.

In avidin-induced biotin deficiency, Misir et al. (1986) considered that serum biotin concentrations below 60 ng/100 ml were inadequate. Misir and Blair (1986) assigned four, P1 or P2 biotin-deficient sows to rations of a basal diet or basal diet supplemented with 100, 200, or 400 μg/kg d-biotin. After 9 months, hoof cracks improved, hoof walls were harder, and foot pads were more resilient. The response was dose and time dependent, but all treated sows were sound after 3 months. At lower biotin concentrations, peak serum biotin concentrations took 2.5 months to develop and unsupplemented sows had inadequate serum concentrations. Simmins and Brooks (1988) fed pigs from 25 kg through to the end of the fourth lactation on a basal diet (32 μg/kg available biotin) or supplemented the ration with 350 μg/kg biotin. Feet were examined at 170 days and, subsequently, at each weaning. Defects such as cuts, bruises, and abrasions were limited throughout; however, the frequency of foot lesions increased between 170 days and the first weaning. After this time, treated sows had significantly fewer lesions per sow, and there was considerable improvement in lesions affecting third digits on thoracic limbs and fourth digits on pelvic limbs (fourth digits on both limbs had the highest scores).

Ironically, not until the 1980s were the effects of biotin deficiency on hoof horn scrutinized other than at a macroscopic level. Simmins and Brooks (1980) and Brooks and Simmins (1980a, b) utilized avidin-induced biotin deficiency and biotin supplements of 120 or 720 μg/kg d-biotin in pigs between 25 and 85 kg, but demonstrated no difference in horn strength between groups. Later, Webb et al. (1984) showed that compressive strength and hardness of the midabaxial sidewall was increased in pigs fed a biotin supplement of 1000 μg/kg between 18.4 and 117.8 kg liveweight. Horn strength from the leading edge of the hoof was harder and did not respond to treatment, and these authors concluded that Simmins and Brooks (1980) found no difference because they selected samples from this area. A combination of harder sidewall and a softer heel bulb, which also was found, were considered by Webb et al. (1984) to reduce the susceptibility of the foot to injury and provide a rational basis for biotin therapy. Microscopic changes in the superficial layers of periopic and coronary horn, which

were loosely arranged, and disruption of superficial tubules were observed by Geyer and Tagwerker (1986) in samples from pigs with avidin-induced biotin deficiency. Additionally, the laminae of the heel corium were exposed and hemorrhage occurred. Other changes included disruption of tubules and cracks at the interface of the wall and heel. Kempson et al. (1989) utilized scanning electron microscopy to examine hoof wall, coronary wall, and periople of pigs fed between 18 and 86.4 (mean) kg on rations used by Webb et al. (1984). Tubules were more densely packed and the structure of tubules, intertubular horn, and horn-corium interface was more compact, cohesive, and clearly defined in pigs fed supplemental rations. The horn was also harder in treated pigs. In pigs on unsupplemented rations, Kempson et al. (1989) concluded that keratinization was affected detrimentally so that the wall was weaker or more susceptible to disruption; a conclusion that agreed with findings of Geyer and Tagwerker (1986). Therefore, in terms of involvement in structural integrity and hardness of hoof, the importance of adequate biotin concentrations in rations has been demonstrated.

In the face of an apparent biotin deficiency in pigs, the clinician needs to address several points. The herd should be considered as a whole, and the skin and feet of affected pigs should be examined on all surfaces. Lameness is probably not a feature of biotin-responsive lesions unless septic laminitis has developed. Environmental conditions must be assessed and it should be determined whether pigs can be coprophagic; this may be a means by which biotin from gut microflora is obtained. Likewise, it is important to be aware of ongoing oral medications or enteric diseases that might affect the gut organisms. Hard, rough floors and perforated floors probably exacerbate lesions. The stage of the life cycle of affected pigs should be considered. Young, fast-growing pigs may have a greater biotin requirement. Lactating sows have a greater need, related to biotin output in the milk, than gestating sows or gilts. Because the greatest benefit appears to be from supplementing rations of growing pigs so that resilient, resistant horn is formed, the greatest cost benefit may be achieved by targeting replacement gilts and boars from an early age.

The nature of the ration should be assessed for biotin content of components and the estimated bioavailability of biotin in these components should be considered. Many deficiency problems that were reported appeared to be related to feeding small grains, which have relatively little biotin. If corn-soybean-based rations are already supplemented with biotin, the environment may well be reconsidered. If the problem persists and does not appear to be environmentally induced, the biotin status of the ration should be analyzed, with the assistance of biotin manufacturers. Ideally, the biotin status of the pigs should be determined, but unless the problem is demonstrably economically serious, this may not be practicable. The National Research Council (NRC) of the National Academy of Science (1988) remain fairly noncommittal concerning the need for biotin supplements, but recommend ration contents between 20 μg/kg for young pigs (1–5 kg) and 200 μg/kg for boars and sows. Presumably, this repre sents highly bioavailable biotin as would be provided in a corn-soybean ration. The wide variation in supplementary biotin utilized in field cases and clinical studies listed earlier creates difficulties for recommending specific treatment regimens. If a ration were to be supplemented at full NRC-recommended concentrations (200 μg/kg), at 1991 prices this would represent an added cost of approximately $1.2 per ton for gilt, sow, and boar rations. However, experimental supplements have been at much higher concentrations, as have therapeutic levels and, in the field, additional supplementation may be necessary to alleviate lamenesses in a timely manner. Therefore, a cost benefit of biotin supplements should be determined for individual herds if there is a clinical problem.

Biotin therapy should not be considered in isolation from improving the environment. Because hoof horn grows relatively slowly, following the onset of biotin supplementation, lesions may take 6–9 months to heal in sows. Concurrent parenteral and antibacterial therapy may be essential if septic laminitis has developed; the effect of oral medications on the gut flora should not be forgotten.

Overgrown Hooves. Boars and sows housed in stalls often have overgrown hooves resulting from limited exercise (Retzel 1931; Von Knezevic 1962). Overgrown hooves may also develop in pigs housed on soft, nonabrasive surfaces or loosely packed dirt lots. Arnbjerg (1972) found exostoses and fractures of the end of the third phalanx, which he considered to be from vascular insufficiency. It is possible that painful injury to the toe causes a pig to shift weight to the heel of the foot resulting in overgrowth of the hoof at the toe. Hooves can be trimmed as is done with sheep and cattle. However, as the hoof grows the angle between the cranial surface of the wall and the sole becomes more acute and the sensitive corium remains close to the cranial margin, thus limiting the likelihood of being able to trim the foot to a normal shape. There is also a risk of selecting lines of pigs that have poor foot conformation when pigs can only be retained in the herd if their feet are regularly trimmed.

Miscellaneous Conditions of Feet. A report by Palludan (1966) described congenital malformations such as clubfoot, absence of the fibula, and abnormal appendages resembling hooves. Polydactyly was recorded by Hughes (1935), and syndactyly

was described by Ross et al. (1944) and Leopold and Dennis (1972). Systemic diseases such as mercury toxicity or postparturient fever can be complicated by nonseptic laminitis affecting all four feet (Nilsson 1964; Maclean 1968). Nilsson also thought that laminitis may result from overfeeding. However, the frequency of laminitis associated with systemic illnesses is unknown. Perhaps the most common form is that associated with postparturient fever (fever and agalactia). Although all four feet are usually affected, lameness is primarily observed in the front limbs (Maclean 1968). Heat and pain will be revealed by palpation of the hoof, and a digital pulse may be detected on palpation of the fetlock.

Infectious Diseases of Feet

Foot Rot and Septic Laminitis. A high frequency of hoof lesions is seen in pigs in confinement. Aseptic laminitis may follow trauma to the hoof, but superficial damage is not always visible. Likewise, superficial damage is not always an indication of deep-seated infections. Osborne (1950) in New Zealand characterized foot rot on the basis of clinical and pathological changes that occurred in pigs between 3 and 6 months that were kept on concrete floors. The condition rarely occurred in growers on wooden floors or in adult pigs, and recurred annually in spring and summer seasons. Foot rot was observed in 25 of 63 farms that kept records, with a morbidity averaging 20%, but on five of these units ≥50% of pigs were affected. Single-limb lameness developed in groups of pigs over a 1 week period. All pigs had cracks or faults in the hoof wall and these extended ≤ two-thirds of the distance from the wall and sole interface to the coronary band (false sand cracks). As sepsis developed, the digits became swollen and different changes during the pathogenesis of lesions included (1) deep necrotic ulcers that focally involved horn, laminae, and coronary band; (2) necrotic sinuses that extended from the laminae and formed granulomatous ulcers at the coronary band; (3) necrotic sinuses that penetrated deep into the phalangeal bone, tendons, and joints of the distal part of the extremity and sometimes opened at the coronary band or heel; and (4) a chronic fibrous tissue response surrounding black or grey debris. Some severe lesions progressed to a point where pigs had to be slaughtered, and others resolved, but the feet were chronically swollen and deformed. In smear preparations from lesions, a mixture of spirochetes, gram-negative fusiform organisms and bacilli, and gram-positive bacilli and cocci was found. Spirochetes also were numerous in histologic sections. Foot rot does not kill pigs unless a fulminating pyemia develops (Hoskin 1965); thus, it is difficult to assess the cost of the condition. However, Osborne (1950) found a drop in return of almost 43% in affected pigs.

Shortly after Osborne's report, Hogg (1952) in England described acute, highly infectious foot rot that affected the ability of pigs to walk and prevented boars from completing breeding. Lesions started as an erosion of the sole, which healed to leave a rough, deformed sole or progressed to the extent of the chronic lesions described by Osborne (1950). Edwards (1954) summarized a survey of pigs that were examined for the presence of foot rot or necrotic ulcer disease. Of 254 farms from which survey forms were returned, over 68% had foot rot. Rough concrete aggravated the condition, and the frequency of the problem doubled if these floors were also wet. The frequency of infection was greatest in pigs that had access to both concrete and dirt lots (approximately 19% of pigs affected). An additional predisposing factor appeared to be whey feeding. Control measures included cleaning floors and keeping them dry, covering rough floors with a bituminous screed, and twice weekly using a footbath containing 10% $CuSO4$ solution after the feet had been cleaned.

In further observations of foot rot on 130 farms, Osborne and Ensor (1955) found that approximately 20% of the pigs on 69% of farms utilizing concrete floors had foot rot, whereas only 1.1% of the pigs on 8% of farms that had little or no concrete had pigs with foot rot. Lesions were more frequently on lateral than medial claws and on pelvic feet rather than thoracic feet. Although lesions partially healed in pigs put out on pasture, pigs maintained on concrete became stunted and were in poor condition. Control measures included cleaning and disinfecting buildings or supplementation of vitamin A in the rations, but these steps were ineffective. Penicillin injections of either 200,000 units into the lesion or 600,000 units IM gave variable responses, but local treatment seemed to be most effective.

Penny et al. (1963) carried out surveys in the southwest of England for the frequency of pigs with foot lesions. Of 1036 pigs at one slaughterhouse and 2154 pigs at a second slaughterhouse, 64.1 and 65.0% of pigs, respectively, had problems. A larger percentage of fourth rather than third digits were affected, with approximate ratios of 4:1. Overall ranking of different types of lesions for the two surveys were (highest frequency first) heel erosion, separation of the wall from the sole along the white line, toe erosion, sole erosion, and false sand cracks. Spirochetes and gram-positive cocci were seen in smears and *Fusiformis necrophorus* and *Corynebacterium pyogenes* were isolated from some lesions.

Later, Penny et al. (1965) investigated foot rot in four herds. In the first and second of the herds in which detailed clinical evaluation for all age groups was available, 78.6% and 73.5% of sows and gilts, respectively, had one or more sand cracks; in the second herd in which the volar aspect of hooves was examined, 100% of sows and

gilts had at least one type of lesion. In the first herd, 80% of sows and gilts were lame. Secondary problems included refusal of boars by lame sows and returns to service, reluctance of boars to serve or slow service, and poor condition despite individualized feeding. The high frequency of false sand cracks was different from that in an earlier survey by Penny et al. (1963), but the authors agreed with the conclusions of Osborne (1950) and Osborne and Ensor (1955), that cracks were associated with rough floors, which predisposed the foot to infections. *F. necrophorus* and spirochetes were isolated from lesions. Treatment and control measures included straw or shavings as bedding on concrete floors and use of 5–10% formalin footbaths. In the first and fourth herds, there was a marked improvement in feet in as little as 10 days. In the second herd, which had slatted floors, footbaths alone improved the situation. Attempts were made to improve floors by smoothing the surfaces of solid floors and applying a bitumastic or resin and sawdust surface to slatted floors, but these measures were either too expensive or lacked durability (bitumastic).

Based on the assumption that foot rot in pigs is associated with agents observed in smears, i.e., *F. necrophorus, C. pyogenes,* and spirochetes (*Borellia suilla*) (Osborne 1950; Penny et al. 1963; Penny et al. 1965), crude extracts from necrotic ulcers and foot rot lesions were introduced into the feet of unaffected pigs. Typical lesions developed in some feet in the form of abscesses, ulcers, and sinuses. Wright et al. (1972) initiated lesions in pigs placed on a rough concrete surface until they were 90.9 kg liveweight. Bruising of the heel or heel/sole junction often preceded erosions; heel erosions and white-line lesions predominated. The frequency of pigs with various lesions on third and fourth digits was approximately the same for both thoracic and pelvic limbs, except for pigs on smooth concrete in which 36–40% less pigs had lesions on their third digits. In other words, rough concrete floors affected all digits equally in the same way that smooth floors affected fourth digits. However, whereas approximately 19% of pigs on smooth concrete had no lesions and only 12.5% had moderate or severe lesions, all pigs on rough concrete developed lesions, and in 80% of pigs they were moderate or severe. Dirty conditions underfoot had little effect on the frequency of lesions, and formalin or $CuSO4$ footbaths did little to prevent lesions, but appeared to delay their onset.
appeared to delay their onset.

Although major predisposing factors for foot rot are traumatic lesions caused by rough floors, only when organisms penetrate the hoof do suppurative and necrotizing lesions develop. Underlying nutritional deficiencies have been implicated in causing debilitating changes in the hoof wall, but Osborne and Ensor (1955) found no benefit in supplementing rations with vitamin A.

However, Penny et al. (1980a, b) demonstrated less severe and fewer lesions typical of foot rot in gilts fed biotin supplements through pregnancy and lactation, but seemingly, there was no benefit in older sows.

With the exception of valuable boars or sows, it is probably not economically justifiable to treat foot lesions by idealistically combining curettage, packing and dressing of wounds, local and parenteral antimicrobial therapy, and provision of clean, soft, dry flooring material. Lesser steps for deep-seated infection may be ineffective; therefore, prevention is the most logical approach. Flooring surfaces associated with contemporary husbandry often are injurious to feet that have evolved for softer terrain. The fit between void ratios or dimensions may be unsuitable for differently aged pigs in the same building and should be evaluated. Footbaths containing 10% CuSO4 or formalin solution may be used to prevent or alleviate lesions, but permanent alleys and troughs should be installed for cost-effective use of these. If biotin therapy or supplementation is to be contemplated, young stock must be supplemented so that a tougher, more resilient hoof develops as the pigs grow. A balance between growth and wear of the horn is essential, so that floors should be abrasive without causing trauma that can initiate wounds and precipitate septic laminitis. Pigs' preferences for different types of flooring may be considered more in the future, and bedding may have to be reevaluated in contemporary husbandry systems.

REFERENCES

Anon. 1981. MAFF, Animal Health Division. Injuries caused by flooring: A survey in pig health scheme herds. Proc Pig Vet Soc 8:119–125.
_____. 1990a. Agricultural Statistics Service, Agricultural Statistics Department, Purdue University. Agric Rep 10(2):40.
_____. 1990b. U. S. Dep of Agric Food Safety Insp Serv, Insp Oper. Personal Communication.
Arnjberg, J. 1972. Pathologic changes in the feet of Swedish Landrace pigs: A radiologic study. Acta Radiol (Stockh) [Suppl] 319:117–120.
Baker, L. N., and Andresen, E. 1964. Restraining rack and blood collecting technique for large pigs. Am J Vet Res 25:1559–1560.
Bane, D. P.; Meade, R. J.; Hilley, H. D.; and Leman, A. D. 1980. Influence of d-biotin and housing on hoof lesions. Proc Int Pig Vet Soc, p. 334.
Baumann, G., and Wisser, J. 1972. Effect of slatted flooring on the feet of fattening pigs. Arch Exp Vet 26:569–588.
Becker, H. N.; White, C. E.; Woodard, J. C.; and Poulos, P. 1985. The relationship between osteochondrosis/dyschondroplasia and lameness in purebred boars: Clinical signs and results of preliminary histochemical studies. J Anim Sci [Suppl] 61:57.
Bjorklund, N. E., and Svendsen, J. 1980. Perinatal mortality in pigs: Histological changes in various organs of intrapartal dead and of weak newborn pigs. Proc Int Pig Vet Soc, p. 81.
Brennan, J. J., and Aherne, F. X. 1986. Treatment of boar leg weakness. Univ Alberta 56th Ann Feeders Day Rep, Agric For Bull (1986): 95–97.
Brennan, J. J.; Aherne, F. X.; Thompson, J. R.; and Nakano, T. 1986. Effect of increased weight stress on joint integrity and cathepsin B-like activity of articular cartilage in growing swine. In Swine in Biomedical Research. Ed. M. E. Tumbleson. New York: Plenum Press, pp. 61–70.
Brooks, P. H., and Comben, N. 1980. The effect of biotin supplementation of sow diets on the reproductive performance of sows and the development of foot lesions. Proc Int Pig Vet Soc, p. 333.
Brooks, P. H., and Simmins, P. H. 1980a. Influence of biotin supplementation on foot lesions in sows. Vet Rec 107:430.
_____. 1980b. The effect of supplementing breeding pig diets with biotin on the maintenance of hoof integrity. Proc Int Conf Prod Dis Farm Anim, pp. 174–177.
Brooks, P. H.; Smith, D. A.; and Irwin, V. R. 1977. Biotin-supplementation of diets: Incidence of foot lesions and reproductive performance of sows. Vet Rec 101:46–50.
Bryden, W. L.; Greer, E. B.; Macoun, R. E.; and Leibholz, J. 1984. Foot health of sows and dietary biotin supplementation. Proc Aust Soc Anim Prod 15:657.
Bullough, P. G., and Heard, T. W. 1967. Pathological lesions associated with the "leg weakness" syndrome in pigs. Br Vet J 123:305–310.
Burch, D. G. S. 1986. A comparison of the serological findings of two herds infected with *Mycoplasma hyosynoviae* but with different disease patterns. Proc Int Pig Vet Soc, p. 286.
Burch, D. G. S., and Goodwin, R. F. W. 1984. Use of tiamulin in a herd of pigs seriously affected with *Mycoplasma hyosynoviae* arthritis. Vet Rec 115:594–595.
Carlson, C. S.; Hilley, H. D.; Henrikson, C. K.; and Meuten, D. J. 1986. The ultra-structure of osteochondrosis of the articular-epiphyseal cartilage complex in growing swine. Calcif Tissue Int 38:44–51.
Carlson, C. S.; Hilley, H. D.; Meuten, D. J.; Hagan, J. M.; and Moser, R. L. 1988a. Effect of reduced growth rate on the prevalence and severity of osteochondrosis in gilts. Am J Vet Res 49:396–402.
Carlson, C. S.; Wood, C. M.; Kornegay, E. T.; and Dial, G. D. 1988b. Effect of porcine growth hormone on the severity of lesions of osteochondrosis in swine. Proc Int Pig Vet Soc, p. 235.
Carlson, C. S.; Hilley, H. D.; and Meuten, D. J. 1989. Degeneration of cartilage canal vessels associated with lesions of osteochondrosis in swine. Vet Pathol 26:47–54.
Carlson, C. S.; Meuten, D. J.; and Richardson, D. C. 1990. Ischemic necrosis of cartilage in spontaneous and experimental lesions of osteochondrosis. Proc Orthop Res Soc, p. 347.
Chagnon, M.; Drolet, R.; and D'Allaire, S. 1990. A prospective study of sow mortality in commercial breeding herds. Proc Int Pig Vet Soc, p. 383.
Christensen, N. O. 1953. Impotentia coeundi in boars due to arthrosis deformans. I. Proc 15th Int Vet Congr 2:742–745.
Christison, G. I.; and De Gooijer, J. A. 1986. Foothold of sows on farrowing crate floors. Livest Prod Sci 15:191–200.
Chung, C. S.; Etherton, T. D.; and Wiggins, J. P. 1985. Stimulation of swine growth by porcine growth hormone. J Anim Sci 60:118–130.
Clifton-Hadley, F. A. 1983. *Streptococcus suis* type 2 infections. Br Vet J 139:1–5.
Clough, C. E. 1984. An evaluation of the farrowing crate. Farm Build Prog 76:21–26.
Comben, N. 1977. Biotin for pigs. Vet Rec 101:84.
Cunha, T. J.; Lindley, D. C.; and Ensminger, M. E. 1946. Biotin deficiency syndrome in pigs fed desic-

cated egg white. J Anim Sci 5:219–223.

DE JONG, M. F., AND SYTSEMA, J. R. 1983. Field experience with d-biotin supplementation to gilt and sow feeds. Vet Q 5:58–67.

DESROSIERS, R.; PHANEUF, J. B.; BROES, A.; AND ROBINSON, Y. 1986. An outbreak of atypical Glasser's disease in Quebec. Proc Int Pig Vet Soc, p. 277.

DEWEY, C. E. 1989. Herd Health Memo (Penn State Univ Ext Serv) Dec:7–8.

———. 1990. Univ Guelph, Ontario: Personal communication.

DEWEY, C. E.; WILSON, M. R.; FRIENDSHIP, R. M.; AND PALMER, N. C. 1988. An observational study of lameness in breeding-stock swine in Ontario. Proc Int Pig Vet Soc, p. 238.

DOIGE, C. E. 1982. Pathological findings associated with locomotory disturbances in lactating and recently weaned boars. Can J Comp Med 46:1–6.

DONE, S. H.; MEREDITH, M. J.; AND ASHDOWN, R. R. 1979. Detachment of the ischial tuberosity in sows. Vet Rec 105:520–523.

DUTHIE, I. F., AND LANCASTER, M. C. 1964. Polyarthritis and epiphysiolysis in pigs in England. Vet Rec 76:263–273.

EDWARDS, E. D. 1954. Foot-rot and necrotic ulcer diseases in pigs. NZ J Agric 88:11–14.

EDWARDS, F. A., and Lightfoot, A. L. 1986. The effect of floor type in farrowing pens on pig injury. II. Leg and teat damage of sows. Brit Vet J 142:441–445.

ELLIOT, J. I., AND DOIGE, C. E. 1973. Effects of type of confinement on performance and on the occurrence of locomotory disturbances in market pigs. J Anim Sci 53:211–217.

EMPEL, W. 1980. Incidence of leg weakness syndrome and the frequency of the pathological lesions in the skeleton of growing Polish Large White, Norwegian Landrace and Hampshire pigs. Ann Warsaw Agric Univ 10:51–55.

ETHERTON, T. D.; WIGGINS, J. P.; CHUNG, C. S.; EVOCK, C. M.; REBHUN, J. F.; AND WALTON, P. E. 1986. Stimulation of pig growth performance by porcine growth hormone and growth hormone-releasing factor. J Anim Sci 63:1389–1399.

EVANS, D. G., AND PRATT, J. H. 1978. A critical analysis of condemnation data for cattle, pigs, and sheep, 1969–1975. Br Vet J 134:476–492.

EVOCK, C. M.; ETHERTON, T. D.; CHUNG, C. S.; AND IVY, R. E. 1988. Pituitary porcine growth hormone (pGH) and a recombinant pGH analog stimulate pig growth performance in a similar manner. J Anim Sci 66:1928–1941.

EWBANK, R. 1974. The influence of diet on general activity in fattening pigs. Abstr Commun Int Congr Pig Vet Soc, Lyon (French ed), p. C3.

FARMER, C., AND CHRISTISON, G. I. 1982. Selection of perforated floors by newborn and weanling pigs. Can J Anim Sci 62:1229–1236.

FARNUM, C. E.; WILSMAN, N. J.; AND HILLEY, H. D. 1984. An ultrastructural analysis of osteochondritic growth plate cartilage in growing swine. Vet Pathol 21:141–151.

FELL, B. F.; JONES, A. F.; AND BOYNE, R. 1967. Lesions of distal ulnar epiphysis in wild East African pigs. Vet Rec 81:341.

FURNISS, S. J.; EDWARDS, S. A.; LIGHTFOOT, A. L.; AND SPECHTER, H. H. 1986. The effect of floor type in farrowing pens on pig injury. I. Leg and teat damage of suckling piglets. Br Vet J 142:434.

GAYLE, L. G., AND SCHWARTZ, W. L. 1980. Pathologic fractures in young sows during lactation. Southwest Vet 33:69–71.

GETTY, R. 1975. Sisson and Grossman's The Anatomy of the Domestic Animal. Philadelphia: W. B. Saunders.

GEYER, H., AND TAGWERKER, F. 1986. The pig's hoof: Its structure and alterations. Basel: Hoffmann-La Roche, pp. 1–27.

GHADIALLY, F. N., 1983. Fine Structure of Synovial Joints. London: Butterworth, pp. 1–41.

GLATTLI, H. R. 1975. Zur Klinik des experimentell erzeugten Biotinmangels beim Schwein und Mitteilung erster Ergebnisse aus Feldversuchen. Schweiz Arch Tierheilk 117:135–144.

———. 1976. Experimental biotin deficiencies and biotin responsive conditions in pigs. Proc Int Pig Vet Soc, p. A10.

GOEDEGEBUURE, S. A.; HANI, H. J.; VAN DER VALK, P.C.; AND VAN DER WAL, P. G. 1980. Osteochondrosis in six breeds of slaughter pigs. I. A morphological investigation of the status of osteochondrosis in relation to breed and level of feeding. Vet Q 1:28–41.

GRABELL, I.; HANSEN, H.; AND OLSSON, S. 1962. Discospondylitis and arthritis in swine erysipelas. Acta Vet Scand 3:33–50.

GRANDHI, R. R., AND STRAIN, J. H. 1980. Effect of biotin supplementation on reproductive performance and foot lesions in swine. Can J Anim Sci 60:961–969.

GRONDALEN, T. 1974a. Osteochondrosis and arthrosis in pigs. I. Incidence in animals up to 120 kg liveweight. Acta Vet Scand 15:1–25.

———. 1974b. Osteochondrosis and arthrosis in pigs. II. Incidence in breeding animals. Acta Vet Scand 15:26–42.

———. 1974c. Osteochondrosis and arthrosis in pigs. III. A comparison of the incidence in young animals of the Norwegian Landrace and Yorkshire breeds. Acta Vet Scand 15:43–52.

———. 1974d. Osteochondrosis and arthrosis in pigs. VI. Relationship to feed level and calcium, phosphorus and protein levels in the ration. Acta Vet Scand 15:147–169.

———. 1974e. Leg weakness in pigs. I. Incidence and relationship to skeletal lesions, feed level, protein and mineral supply, exercise and exterior conformation. Acta Vet Scand 15:555–573.

———. 1974f. Leg weakness in pigs. II. Litter differences in leg weakness, skeletal lesions, joint shape and exterior conformation. Acta Vet Scand 15:574–586.

———. 1981. Osteochondrosis and arthrosis in Norwegian slaughter-pigs in 1980 compared to 1970. Nord Vet Med 33:417–422.

GRONDALEN, T., AND GRONDALEN, J. 1974. Osteochondrosis and arthrosis in pigs. IV. Effect of overloading on the distal epiphyseal plate of the ulna. Acta Vet Scand 15:53–60.

GRONDALEN, T., AND VANGEN, O. 1974. Osteochondrosis and arthrosis in pigs. V. A comparison of the incidence in three different lines of the Norwegian Landrace breed. Acta Vet Scand 15:61–79.

HAMILTON, C. R., AND VEUM, T. L. 1984. Response of sows and litters to added dietary biotin in environmentally regulated facilities. J Anim Sci 59(1):151–157.

HANI, H.; SCHWORER, D.; AND BLUM, J. K. 1984. Osteochondrosis (OC) in performance-tested pigs: Incidence in Swiss Landrace (SLR) and Swiss Large White (SLW) breeds, relationships to carcass characteristics, performance traits and leg weakness. Proc Int Pig Vet Soc, p. 266.

HANI, H.; SCHWORER, D.; AND MOREL, P. 1990. Genetic analysis of osteochondrosis (OC) in Swiss Landrace (SLR) and Swiss Large White (SLW) breeds. Proc Int Pig Vet Soc, p. 459.

HELMS, H. T. 1962. Uterine infections in sows and navel infections in pigs. Controlled field study. Ft Dodge Biochem Rev 31:8–27.

HILL, G. M., AND BEBIAK, D. M. 1979. Interactions of

selenium and Vitamin E with high levels of zinc and copper. Michigan Agric Exp Stat Res Rep 386:45–48.

HILL, M. A. 1990. Economic relevance, diagnosis, and countermeasures for degenerative joint disease (osteoarthrosis) and dyschondroplasia (osteochondrosis) in pigs. J Am Vet Med Assoc 197(2):254–259.

HILL, M. A., AND DALRYMPLE, R. H. 1987. Evaluation of feet and skeletons of limbs from pigs treated with a repartitioning agent, Cimaterol. Can J Anim Sci 51:217–223.

HILL, M. A.; HILLEY, H. D.; FEENEY, D. A.; RUTH, G. R.; AND HANSGEN, D. C. 1984a. Dyschondroplasias, including osteochondrosis, in boars between 25 and 169 days of age: Radiologic changes. Am J Vet Res 45:917–925.

HILL, M. A.; RUTH, G. R.; HILLEY, H. D.; AND HANSGEN, D. C. 1984b. Dyschondroplasias, including osteochondrosis, in pigs between 29 and 159 days of age: Histologic changes. Am J Vet Res 45:903–916.

HILL, M. A.; RUTH, G. R.; BAGENT, J. K.; TORRISON, J. L.; AND LEMAN, A. D. 1985a. Angiomicrographic investigation of the vessels associated with physes in young pigs. Res Vet Sci 38:151–159.

HILL, M. A.; RUTH, G. R.; HILLEY, H. D.; TORRISON, J. L.; BAGENT, J. K.; AND LEMAN, A. D. 1985b. Dyschondroplasias of growth cartilages (osteochondrosis) in crossbred commercial pigs at one and 15 days of age: Radiological, angiomicrographical and histological findings. Vet Rec 116:40–47.

HILL, M. A.; KINCAID, S. A.; AND VISCO, D. M. 1990. Use of histochemical techniques in the characterisation of osteochondroses affecting pigs. Vet Rec 127:29–37.

HILLEY, H. D. 1980. Osteoarthrosis and osteochondrosis of the pig Ph.D. diss., Univ of Minnesota.

———. 1982. Skeletal abnormalities in the pig. Vet Clin N Am: Lg Anim Pract 4(2):225–258.

HOGG, A. H. 1952. II. Foot-rot in pigs. Vet Rec 64(3):39–42.

HOSKIN, B. D. 1965. Foot abscesses in pigs. Vet Rec 77:10–48.

HUGHES, E. H. 1935. Polydactyly in swine. J Hered 26:415–418.

HUMMEL, T., AND BERNICK, K. A. 1990 (October). Moorman's News. Quincy, Ill.: Moorman Mfg Co.

JENSEN, A. H. 1979. The effects of environmental factors, floor design and materials on performance and on foot and limb disorders in growing and adult pigs. Proc Pig Vet Soc 5:85–94.

JOHNSON, L. A., AND COULSON, A. 1986. Clinical experiences in the treatment of pneumonia and septic arthritis with a combination of lincomycin plus spectinomycin. Proc Int Pig Vet Soc, p. 362.

JONES, J. E. T. 1968. The cause of death in sows; a one year survey of 106 herds in Essex. Br Vet J 124:45–54.

JUSSILA, J., AND PAATSAMA, S. 1972. Radiological changes in the distal epiphysis, epiphyseal cartilage and metaphysis of the radius and ulna in pigs. Acta Radiol 319:121–126.

KEMPSON, S. A.; CURRIE, R. J. W.; AND JOHNSTON, A. M. 1989. Influence of biotin supplementation on pig claw horn: A scanning electron microscopic study. Vet Rec 124:37–40.

KERNKAMP, H. C. H. 1925. A study of a disease of bones and joints of swine. Univ of Minnesota Agric Exp Sta Tech Bull 31:1–47.

KINCAID, S. A., AND LINDVALL, E. R. 1982. Communicating cartilage canals of the physis of the distal part of the ulna of growing swine and their potential role in healing of metaphyseal dysplasia of osteochondrosis. Am J Vet Res 43:938–944.

KINCAID, S. A.; ALLHANDS, R. V.; AND PIJANOWSKI,

G. J. 1985. Chondrolysis associated with cartilage canals of the epiphyseal cartilage of the distal humerus of growing pigs. Am J Vet Res 46:726–732.

KORNEGAY, E. T.; THOMAS, H. R.; AND MEACHAM, T. N. 1973. Evaluation of dietary calcium and phosphorus for reproducing sows housed in total confinement on concrete or in dirt lots. J Anim Sci 37(2):493–500.

KOVACS, A. B., AND BEER, G. Y. 1979. The mechanical properties and qualities of floors for pigs in relation to limb disorders. Proc Pig Vet Soc 5:99–104.

KOVACS, A. B., AND SZILAGYI, M. 1973a. Data on mineral components of the horny part of the foot of cattle, sheep and swine. Acta Vet Acad Sci Hung 23:187–192.

———. 1973b. Mineral contents of the horn of the foot of swine of different breeds and ages. Acta Vet Acad Sci Hung 23:241–246.

———. 1974. "Ragged claw" defect in pigs and the mineral composition of the abnormal horn. Magy Allatorv Lapja 29:165–167.

LAWRISUK, L. S.; ROTHSCHILD, M. F.; ROSS, R. F.; AND CHRISTIAN, L. L. 1987. Relationship between *Mycoplasma hyosynoviae* infection and front limb weakness in Duroc swine. Am J Vet Res 48(9):1395–1397.

LEAHY, J. R., AND BARROW, P. 1953. Restraint of Animals, 2d ed. Ithaca: Cornell Campus Store, pp. 117–123.

LEDECKY, V.; ORSAG, A.; HUBA, F.; AND SEVCIK, A. 1984. Relationship of some floor surfaces to the growth and abrading of the keratoid wall of ungulae in pigs. Folia Vet 24(1–2):51–58.

LEHRER, W. P.; WEISE, A. C.; AND MOORE, P. R. 1952. Biotin deficiency in suckling pigs. J Nutr 47:203–212.

LEOPOLD, W. H., AND DENNIS, S. M. 1972. Syndactyly in a pig. Cornell Vet 62:269–272.

LINDEMANN, M. D.; KORNEGAY, E. T.; AND COLLINS, E. R. 1985. The effect of various flooring materials on performance and foot health of early-weaned pigs. Livest Prod Sci 13:373–382.

LINDLEY, D. C., AND CUNHA, T. J. 1946. Nutritional significance of inositol and biotin for the pig. J Nutr 32:47–59.

LJUNGGREN, G., AND REILAND, S. 1970. Osteochondrosis in adolescent animals; an endocrine disorder? Calcif Tissue Res [Suppl] 4:150–153.

LUNDEHEIM, N. 1986. Osteochondrosis and growth rate in the Swedish pig progeny testing scheme. Proc Int Pig Vet Soc, p. 434.

———. 1987. Genetic analysis of osteochondrosis and leg weakness in the Swedish pig progeny testing scheme. Acta Agric Scand 37:159–173.

MACLEAN, C. W. 1968. Acute laminitis in sows. Vet Rec 83:71–75.

MCMEEKAN, C. P. 1940. Growth and development in the pig, with special reference to carcass quality characters. J Agric Sci 30:276–347.

MCTAGGART, H. S. 1977. A simple cradle for handling pigs. Vet Rec 101:386–387.

MADEIROS, C. A. 1984. *Mycoplasma hyosynoviae* treatment in pigs. Vet Rec 115(17):446.

MADSEN, P. 1984. Atypical outbreaks of Glasser's disease in Danish pig herds. Proc Int Pig Vet Soc, p. 107.

MARTENS, R. J., AND AUER, J. A. 1980. Hematogenous septic arthritis and osteomyelitis in the foal. Proc Am Assoc Eq Pract, pp. 47–63.

MINIATS, O. P., AND SMART, N. L. 1988. Immunization of primary SPF pigs against Glasser's disease. Proc Int Pig Vet Soc, p. 157.

MINIATS, O. P.; SMART, N. L.; AND METZGER, K. 1986. Glasser's disease in southwestern Ontario. I. A retrospective study. Proc Int Pig Vet Soc, p. 279.

MISIR, R., AND BLAIR, R. 1986. Effect of biotin supplementation of a barley-wheat diet on restoration of healthy feet, legs and skin of biotin deficient sows. Res Vet Sci 40:212–218.

MISIR, R; BLAIR, R; AND DOIGE, C. E. 1986. Development of a system for clinical evaluation of the biotin status of sows. Can Vet J 27:6–12.

MITCHELL, D. 1979. The measurement of surface texture. Proc Pig Vet Soc 5:105–113.

NAKANO, T., AND AHERNE, F. X. 1988. Involvement of trauma in the pathogenesis of Osteochondritis Dissecans in swine. Can J Vet Res 52:154–155.

NAKANO, T.; AHERNE, F. X.; AND THOMPSON, J. R. 1979a. Changes in swine knee articular cartilage during growth. Can J Anim Sci 59:167–169.

——. 1979b. Effects of feed restriction, sex and diethylstilbesterol on the occurence of joint lesions with some histological and biochemical studies of the articular cartilage of growing-finishing swine. Can J Anim Sci 59:491–502.

——. 1981. Effect of housing system on the recovery of boars from leg weakness. Can J Anim Sci 61:335–342.

NAKANO, T.; AHERNE, F. X.; BRENNAN, J. J.; AND THOMPSON, J. R. 1984. Effect of growth rate on the incidence of osteochondrosis in growing swine. Can J Anim Sci 64:139–146.

NAKANO, T.; THOMPSON, J. R.; CHRISTOPHERSON, R. J.; AND AHERNE, F. X. 1986. Blood flow distribution in hind limb bones and joint articular cartilage from young growing pigs. Can J Vet Res 50:96–100.

NATIONAL ACADEMY OF SCIENCES (NAS). 1988. Nutrient Requirements of Swine. Washington, D.C.: NRC, NAS, pp. 38, 47–53.

NEHER, G. M.; DOYLE, L. P.; THRASHER, D. M.; AND PLUMLEE, M. P. 1956. Radiographic and histopathological findings in the bones of swine deficient in manganese. Am J Vet Res 1:121–128.

NEMETH, F., AND VAN DER VALK, P. C. 1976. Vascular lesions in epiphysiolysis capitis femoris in swine. Proc Int Conf Prod Dis Farm Anim, pp. 226–228.

NEWTON, G. L.; BOORAM, C. V.; HALE, O. M.; AND MULLINIX, B. G., Jr. 1980. Effects of four types of floor slats on certain feet characteristics and performances of swine. J Anim Sci 50:7–20.

NIELSEN, N. C.; BILLE, N.; LARSEN, J. L.; AND SVENDSEN, J. 1975. Preweaning mortality in pigs. Nord Vet Med 27:529–543.

NIELSEN, R., AND DANIELSEN, V. 1975. An outbreak of Glasser's Disease. Studies on etiology, serology and the effect of vaccination. Nord Vet Med 27:20–25.

NILSSON, S. A. 1964. Laminitis in pigs. Nord Vet Med 16:128–139.

NIMMO, R. D. 1980. Proc George A. Young Conf and 20th Annu Nebr SPF Conf, pp. 63–72.

NORDBY, J. E. 1939. Inequalities in the digits of swine. J Hered 30:307–310.

NORVAL, J. 1962. Emergency Slaughter. Vet Rec 74:386–392.

OLSSON, S. E. 1978. Introduction: Osteochondrosis in domestic animals. Acta Radiol [Suppl] 358:9–12.

OSBORNE, H. G. 1950. Foot-rot in pigs. Aust Vet J 26:316–317.

OSBORNE, H. G.; AND ENSOR, C. R. 1955. Some aspects of the pathology, etiology, and therapeutics of foot-rot in pigs. NZ Vet J 3:91–99.

PALLUDAN, B. 1966. Swine in teratological studies. In Swine in Biomedical Research. Ed. L. K. Bustad, R. O. McClellan, and M. P. Burns. Richland, Wash.: Pacific Northwest Laboratory, p. 51.

PEET, R. L.; FRY, J.; LLOYD, J.; HENDERSON, J.; CURRAN, J.; AND MOIR, D. 1983. *Haemophilus parasuis* septicaemia in pigs. Aust Vet J 60(6):187.

PENNY, R. H. C.; OSBORNE, A. D.; AND WRIGHT, A. I.

1963. The causes and incidence of lameness in store and adult pigs. Pt I: Review. The causes and incidence of lameness in store and adult pigs. Pt II: Foot lesions in pigs: A slaughterhouse survey. Vet Rec 75(47):1225–1240.

PENNY, R. H. C.; OSBORNE, A. D.; WRIGHT, A. I.; AND STEPHENS, T. K. 1965. Foot-rot in pigs: Observations on the clinical disease. Vet Rec 77(38):1101–1108.

PENNY, R. H. C.; CAMERON, R. D. A.; JOHNSON, S.; KENYON, P. J.; SMITH, H. A.; BELL, A. W. P.; COLE, J. P. L.; AND TAYLOR, J. 1980a. Foot rot of pigs: The influence of biotin supplementation on foot lesions in sows. Vet Rec 107(15):350–351.

PENNY, R. H. C.; CAMERON, R. D. A.; JOHNSON, S.; SMITH, H. A.; COLE, J. P. L.; KENYON, P. J.; AND TAYLOR, J. 1980b. Foot-rot of pigs: The benefits of biotin supplementation of sows. Proc Int Pig Vet Soc, p. 332.

PENNY, R. H. C.; WALTERS, J. R.; AND GRAY, J. 1986. Experiences of a breeding company: The establishment and management of gilt herds. Proc Int Pig Vet Soc, p. 29.

PEPPER, T. A.; BENNETT, D.; BROWN, P. J.; AND TAYLOR, D. J. 1978. Rickets in growing pigs and response to treatment. Vet Rec 103:4–8.

PERRIN, W. R., AND BOWLAND, J. P. 1977. Effect of enforced exercise on the incidence of leg weakness in growing boars. Can J Anim Sci 57:245–253.

PERRIN, W. R.; BOWLAND, J. P.; AND AHERNE, F. X. 1975. Leg weakness studies with growing boars. Annu Feed Day Rep, Alberta Univ, Dep Anim Sci 54:24–26.

PERRIN, W. R.; AHERNE, F. X.; BOWLAND, J. P.; AND HARDIN, R. T. 1978. Effects of age, breed and floor type on the incidence of articular cartilage lesions in pigs. Can J Anim Sci 58:129–138.

POINTILLART, A., AND GUEGUEN, L. 1978. Osteochondrose et faiblesse des pattes chez le porc. Ann Biol Anim Biochem Biophys 18:201–210.

POUTEAUX, V. A.; STRICKLIN, W. R.; AND CHRISTISON, G. I. 1980. Weanling pig preference on perforated floors. Can J Anim Sci 60:1037.

POUTEAUX, V. A.; CHRISTISON, G. I.; AND STRICKLIN, W. R. 1983. Perforated-floor preference of weanling pigs. Appl Anim Ethol 11:19–23.

PRATT, C. W. M., AND McCANCE, R. A. 1964. Severe undernutrition in growing and adult animals. 12. The extremities of the long bones in pigs. Br J Nutr 18:393–406.

PUGH, O. L., AND PENNY, R. H. C. 1966. A crate for the restraint of large pigs. Vet Rec 79:390–392.

REILAND, S. 1978a. Growth and skeletal development of the pig. Acta Radiol [Suppl] 358:14–22.

——. 1978b. Pathology of so called leg weakness. Acta Radiol [Suppl] 358:23–44.

——. 1978c. Morphology of osteochondrosis and sequelae in pigs. Acta Radiol [Suppl] 358:45–90.

——. 1978d. Effects of vitamin D and A, calcium, phosphorus, and protein on frequency and severity of osteochondrosis in pigs. Acta Radiol [Suppl] 358:91–105.

——. 1978e. The effect of decreased growth rate on frequency and severity of osteochondrosis in pigs. Acta Radiol [Suppl] 358:107–122.

REILAND, S., AND ANDERSON, K. 1979. Cross breeding experiments with swine. Influence of different combinations of breed on frequency and severity of osteochondrosis: A preliminary report. Acta Agric Scand [Suppl] 21:486–489.

REILAND, S.; ORDELL, N.; LUNDEHEIM, N.; AND OLSSON, S. E. 1978. Heredity of osteochondrosis, body constitution, and leg weakness in the pig. Acta Pathol [Suppl] 358:123–137.

REILAND, S.; ORDELL-GUSTAFSON, N.; AND LUNDE-HEIM, N. 1980. Heredity of osteochondrosis: A correlative and comparative investigation in different breeds using progeny testing. Proc Int Pig Vet Soc, p. 328.

RETZEL, N. 1931. CITED BY VON KNEZEVIC, P. 1962. Klauenpflege beim Schwein. DTW 60:364–366.

RISING, H. J. 1981. Prevention of Glasser's disease through immunity to *Haemophilus parasuis*. Zentralbl Veterinaermed [B] 28(8):630–638.

ROBERTS, E. D.; SWITZER, W. P.; AND RAMSEY, F. K. 1963. The pathology of *Mycoplasma hyorhinis* arthritis produced experimentally in swine. Am J Vet Res 24:19–31.

ROBERTS, E. D.; RAMSEY, F. K.; SWITZER, W. P.; AND LAYTON, J. M. 1967. Influence of *Streptococcus equisimilis* on sites of endochondral ossification in swine. Am J Vet Res 28:1677–1686.

ROSS, O. B.; PHILLIPS, P. H.; BOHSTEDT, G.; AND CUNHA, T. J. 1944. Congenital malformations, syndactylism, talipes, and paralysis agitans of nutritional origin in swine. J Anim Sci 3:406–414.

ROSS, R. F., AND SPEAR, M. L. 1973. Role of the sow as a reservoir of infection for *Mycoplasma hyosynoviae*. Am J Vet Res 34:373–378.

ROTHSCHILD, M. F., AND CHRISTIAN, L. L. 1988. Genetic control of front-leg weakness in Duroc swine. I. Direct response to five generations of divergent selection. Livest Prod Sci 19:459–471.

SAINSBURY, D. W. B. 1984. Pig housing and welfare. Pig News Inf 5(4):377–381.

SANFORD, S. E., AND TILKER, A. M. E. 1982. *Streptococcus suis* type II-associated diseases in swine. Observations of a one year study. J Am Vet Med Assoc 181:673–676.

SATHER, A. P. 1980. The effect of management upon the incidence of leg weakness in swine. Can J Anim Sci 60:1061–1062.

———. 1987. A note on the changes in leg weakness in pigs after being transferred from confinement housing to pasture lots. Anim Prod 44(3):450–453.

SATHER, A. P., AND FREDEEN, H. T. 1982. The effect of confinement housing upon the incidence of leg weakness in swine. Can J Anim Sci 62:1119–1128.

SCOTT, G. B. 1985. Designing floors for animal's feet: A review of biomechanical 'ground' work at the Scottish Farm Buildings Investigation Unit. Farm Build Prog 82:27–32.

SHAW, J. D. N. 1979. Some thoughts on the use of special materials and finishes for floor surfaces in animal housing. Proc Pig Vet Soc 5:115.

SIMMINS, P. H., AND BROOKS, P. H. 1980. The effect of dietary biotin level on the physical characteristics of pig hoof tissue [abstr]. Anim Prod 30 (3):469.

———. 1988. Supplementary biotin for sows: Effect on claw integrity. Vet Rec 122:435–437.

SISSON, S. 1938. The Anatomy of Domestic Animals, 3d ed. Philadelphia: W. B. Saunders, p. 69.

SMART, N. L.; MINIATS, O. P.; FRIENDSHIP, R.M.; AND MACINNES, J. 1986. Glasser's disease in South Western Ontario. II. Isolation of *Haemophilus parasuis* from SPF and conventional swine herds. Proc Int Pig Vet Soc, p. 280.

SMITH, W. J. 1982. Floor Problems. Proc Pig Vet Soc 9:184–189.

SMITH, W. J., AND MITCHELL, C. D. 1977. Observations on injuries to suckled pigs confined on perforated floors with special reference to expanded metal. Pig Vet Soc Proc 1:91–104.

SMITH, W. J., AND ROBERTSON, A. M. 1971. Observations on injuries to sows confined in part slatted stalls. Vet Rec 89:531–533.

SOKOLOFF, L. 1978. The Joints and Synovial Fluid. New York: Academic Press.

SPENCER, G. R. 1979. Animal model of human disease: Pregnancy and lactational osteoporosis. (Animal model: Porcine lactational osteoporosis). Am J Pathol 95:277–280.

STRYER, L. 1988. Biochemistry, 3d ed. New York: W. H. Freeman and Co., pp. 40–42.

SVENDSEN, J.; OLSSON, O.; AND NILSSON, C. 1979. The occurence of leg injuries on piglets with the various treatment of the floor surface on the farrowing pen. Nord Vet Med 31:49–61.

TASKER, J. 1981. Problems associated with the use of swine *Erysipelas* vaccine. Proc Pig Vet Soc 7:82–86.

THOMASEN, A. 1939. Epiphyseal necrosis of the caput femoris. Acta Ortho Scand 10:331–337.

THOMSON, J. U.; NELSON, D. T.; AND JOHNSON, D. D. 1990. Epidemic of swine *Erysipelas* in the upper Midwest. Proc Am Assoc Swine Pract, p. 341.

THURLEY, D. C. 1966. Disturbance in endochondral ossification associated with acute swine fever infection. Br Vet J 122:177–180.

TUOVINEN, V. K.; GROHN, Y. T.; STRAW, B. E.; AND BOYD, R. D. 1990. Environmental factors in feeder pig finishing units associated with partial carcass condemnations in a slaughterhouse. Proc Int Pig Vet Soc, p. 394.

VAN ALSTINE, W. G., AND TOBEN, C. G. 1989. Detachment of the tuber ischiadicum in swine. Cont Educ 11(7):874–879.

VAN DER WAL, P. G.; GOEDEGEBUURE, S.A.; AND VAN DER VALK, P. C. 1982. Leg weakness, osteochondrosis and blood acid-base parameters in pigs. Proc Int Pig Vet Soc, p. 136.

VAN DER WAL, P. G.; HEMMINGA, H.; GOEDEGEBURRE, S. A.; AND VAN DER VALK, P. C. 1986. The effect of replacement of 0.30% sodium chloride by 0.43% sodium bicarbonate in rations of fattening pigs on leg weakness, osteochondrosis and growth. Vet Q 8:136–144.

VAN PELT, R. W. 1974. Interpretation of synovial fluid findings in the horse. J Am Vet Med Assoc 165:91–95.

VAN SICKLE, D. C.; RUNNELS, L. J.; BLEVINS, W. E.; ARMSTRONG, C. H.; AND LAMAR, C. H. 1980. Radiology, gross, and histopathology of articular lesions from lame boars. Proc Int Pig Vet Soc, p. 330.

VISCO, D. M.; HILL, M. A.; VAN SICKLE, D. C.; AND KINCAID, S. A. 1991. Cartilage canals and lesions typical of osteochondrosis in growth cartilages from the distal part of the humerus of pigs between 1 day and 15 weeks old. Vet Rec. In press.

VON KNEZIVIC, P. 1962. Klauenpflege beim Schwein. DTW 69:364–366.

WALKER, B., AND AHERNE, F. X. 1987. The effects of sow nutrition on leg weaknesses in their offspring. Agric For Bull, Univ Alberta, pp. 18–19.

WALKER, T., AND JONES, A. S. 1962. A study in leg weakness in boars. Anim Prod 4:297.

WALKER, T.; BELL, B. F.; JONES, A. S.; BOYNE, R.; AND ELLIOT, M. 1966. Observations on "leg weakness" in pigs. Vet Rec 79:472–479.

WEBB, N. G., AND CLARK, M. 1981. Livestock foot-floor interactions measured by force and pressure plate. Farm Build Prog 66:23–36.

WEBB, N. G.; PENNY, R. H. C.; AND JOHNSTON, A. M. 1984. Effects of a dietary supplement of biotin on pig hoof horn strength and hardness. Vet Rec 114:185–189.

WELLS, G. A. H. 1986. Locomotor disorders of the pig. Pig News Inf 7(1):17–20.

Woodard, J. C.; Becker, H. N.; and Poulos, P. W., Jr. 1987a. Effect of diet on longitudinal bone growth and osteochondrosis in swine. Vet Pathol 24:109–117.

———. 1987b. Articular cartilage blood vessels in swine osteochondrosis. Vet Pathol 24:118–123.

Wright, A. I.; Osborne, A. D.; Penny, R. H. C.; and Gray, E. 1972. Foot-rot in pigs: Experimental production of the disease. Vet Rec 90:93–99.

9 Skin

B. E. Straw

GROSS FEATURES. The skin is a major organ that provides an enclosing barrier, sense organ, thermoregulation, storage of water and electrolytes, and immunosurveillance for the body. At birth, skin and associated subcutaneous tissue account for about 10–12% of liveweight (Heath 1984). As pigs mature, skin makes up a somewhat smaller percentage of the total body size; at 105 kg, skin was 7.8% of body weight and at 145 kg, it was 6.7% of the body weight of boars (Knudson et al. 1985). When removed by typical slaughter plant skinning techniques, the skin of market swine (100–109 kg) weighs approximately 11 kg.

Skin in different parts of the body varies in thickness, hair covering, vascularity, innervation, and number of glands. Skin of the dorsum is thicker and hairier than skin of the ventrum, the average thickness of adult swine being 2.2 mm (Marcarian and Calhoun 1966). One particularly thick area of boar skin is called the shield. This thick, hard skin of the scapular and costal regions is a normal secondary sex characteristic commonly seen in aged boars. A shield only rarely occurs in barrows, cryptorchids, or sows. Skin in the shield contains a tremendous amount of thick, fibrous connective tissue in the dermis and subcutis and provides protection to boars when engaged in lateral conflict typical of porcine aggression (McCarthy and Howlett 1988).

The number of hair follicles is defined at birth and does not change throughout the pig's life although, due to the relative expansion of the skin surface, the number of hairs/cm² decreases with age. Hair follicles are usually arranged in groups of three. In domestic pigs at birth, pelage population density over the shoulder, back, and flank ranged from 220 to 265 hairs/cm², and skin on the ventral abdomen averaged 116 hairs/cm² (Hansen et al. 1972). The number of hairs/cm² in older pigs was 1 month, 119; 4 months, 29; 6 months, 18; 9–12 months, 14; 15–22 months, 10; 36–60 months, 6. Hair also becomes longer and coarser with development. At 1 month of age, pigs' hair was 11.5 mm long and weighed 0.037 μg/mm compared to a length of 56.7 mm and a weight of 13 μg/mm at 1 year (Cabak et al. 1962). Wild pigs have nearly twice the number of hairs/cm² compared to domestic pigs (Hansen et al. 1972).

Some breeds of swine, such as the Yucatan Miniature pig, the Mexican Hairless pig, and the Large White Ulster, normally exhibit hypotrichosis, which in these breeds is thought to be an autosomal dominant trait. Occasional animals in other breeds may carry the "hairless" gene (Meyer and Drommer 1968). The wooly hair condition is common in certain breeds of Brazilian swine in which woolliness is inherited as autosomal dominant, allelomorphic to normal straight hair (Rhoad 1934).

Wattles are seen infrequently in pigs. These cylindric, teatlike appendages contain a central fibrocartilaginous core covered by dense connective tissue and skin and hang from the ventral mandibular region. They are inherited as an autosomal dominant trait (Roberts and Morrill 1944).

HISTOLOGIC APPEARANCE. The microscopic appearance of pigskin is similar to that of other domestic animals, especially humans. The two major layers, the epidermis and the dermis, rest upon a relatively thick layer of adipose tissue, the hypodermis. In general, for most mammals the greater the density of the hair coat, the thinner the epidermis. Because swine and humans have a relatively sparse hair coat, the epidermis is thicker and associated with a dermis containing rete pegs, which are not found in other domestic species.

Epidermis. The major cell of the epidermis is the keratinocyte, which appears as one layer of cuboidal to columnar cells in the stratum basale, several layers of polyhedral cells in the stratum spinosum, several layers of flattened cells in the stratum granulosum, and varying thicknesses of cornified cells in the stratum corneum. The stratum lucidum is only readily seen in the snout of the pig. Melanocytes are found between the epidermal-dermal junction and the stratum basale, while Langerhans-like cells appear in the strati basale and spinosum (Montiero-Riviere and Stromberg 1985). Merkel cells, specialized mechanoreceptors containing serotonin, are numerous in the epidermis of the snout (Garcia-Caballero et al. 1989). The thickness of the epidermis ranges from 70 to 140 μm (Meyer et al. 1978).

Dermis. The relatively thick dermis is composed of papillary and reticular layers. The papillary layer interdigitates with the epidermis in rete pegs. The dermis consists largely of dense, irregular collagenous fibers and sparse connective tissue cells (Mowafy and Cassens 1975). The dermis is sparsely populated with fibroblasts, melanocytes, and mast cells. An average of 32 mast cells/mm² of skin was seen in parasite-free swine, and the numbers decreased when swine were stressed (Rang 1973).

Hypodermis. The hypodermis consists mainly of fat. In it are found the origins of the hair follicles and the sweat glands. In most other farm animals the hair follicles do not penetrate the hypodermis (Mowafy and Cassens 1975).

Glandular Components. All the epithelial glands are present at birth. The number of glands/cm² decreases with age (1 month, 132; 1 year, 18) due to skin expansion, while the diameter of the acini increases (1 month, 430 μ; 1 year, 949 μ) (Cabak et al. 1962). Pigskin contains relatively few sweat glands (about 25/cm²) compared with other species (e.g., cattle, 800–1600/cm²). Specialized seromucoid glands, the carpal glands, are located behind the carpus, and the mental or mandibular organ is located in the intermandibular space (Montagne and Yung 1964). A relatively small sebaceous gland with a single unbranched alveolus is associated with each hair follicle.

GENERAL FEATURES

Skin Surface. The skin surface and the keratinized cells of the stratum corneum are permeated by sebum, which acts as a physical and chemical barrier. Fatty acids, water soluble substances, sodium chloride, albumin, transferrin, complement, and immunoglobulins in the sebum possess antibacterial and antifungal properties (Noble 1981).

Normal Skin Flora. Bacteria and fungi recovered from the skin of normal swine include *E. coli, Klebsiella pneumoniae, Proteus* sp., *Pseudomonas* sp., various species of staphylococci and streptococci, *Alternaria* sp., *Aspergillus* sp., *Candida* sp., *Cephalosporium, Chaetomium, Mortierella, Mucor, Oospora, Penicillium, Rhizopus, Scopulariopsis,* and *Trichothecium* (Devriese et al. 1985; Scott 1988). Skin microflora exist in an equilibrium determined by the types of organisms present and the degree of hydration of the skin. Increasing moisture at the stratum corneum, due to increased ambient temperature or increased relative humidity, is the major factor fostering microbial growth (Noble 1981). Certain bacteria are able to bar the colonization of other bacteria by the production of diffusible inhibitor substances (Allaker et al. 1989).

Role in Thermal Regulation. Air next to the surface of the skin provides most of the thermal insulation for pigs less than 2 weeks of age. Pelage and piloerection have little insulative value. The pig's sparse hair coat at birth contributes, at most, 15% to its total thermal insulation; hence, its removal does not markedly affect total thermal insulation or thermal stability (Hansen et al. 1972). The pig's tissue insulation is supplied by the skin and subcutaneous fat. Dilation and constriction of vessels in the dermis keeps the microclimate of the dermis relatively constant. The thick subcutaneous fat layer in older animals has a high insulating value in cold conditions when the skin blood vessels external to the fat are constricted (Mount 1964). Skin rids the body of excess heat primarily through evaporative thermolysis. Pigs wallow in mud, a very efficient medium for evaporative thermolysis, to dissipate excess body heat. Heat loss from an area smeared with mud is greater and more sustained than that from a comparable area wetted with water alone. Evaporative flux from a pig's mudded side reaches a high rate of 800 gm/hour/m². A mudded pig has greater evaporative heat flux than a cow sweating maximally. While sweat glands are present in pigskin, they do not respond to heat stress (Curtis 1981).

The skin of the scrotum is well supplied with warm receptors and in boars acts as a thermoregulatory organ. Warming the scrotum depressed operant heat-seeking behavior in pigs exposed to 15°C, while cooling the scrotum did not affect behavior (Swiergiel and Ingram 1987). Changes in scrotal skin temperature also affect feed consumption (Swiergiel 1988). Ambient temperature has been shown to influence the development and relative size of the skin. Pigs weaned at 2 weeks of age and raised at 35°C had a greater mass of skin and subcutaneous fat, better vascularized skin, and larger ears than littermates raised at 10°C (Heath 1984).

Immune Function. Langerhans' cells, keratinocytes, epidermotropic T lymphocytes, and draining peripheral lymph nodes collectively form an integrated system of skin-associated lymphoid tissues (SALT) that mediate cutaneous immunosurveillance. The Langerhans' cells have antigen-processing and alloantigen-stimulating functions. Keratinocytes are phagocytic, produce various cytokines and a substance similar to interleukin 1, and can express immune response gene-associated antigen (Katz 1985).

Economic Importance of Skin Disease. Skin disease may impact economics of production in two areas. Dermatitis has a negative impact on growth and performance of pigs during the fattening period, and skin lesions require extra processing at slaughter.

Economic effects have been reported for a number of skin diseases. Infestation with sarcoptic mange was associated with up to a 10% reduction in growth rate and feed efficiency. Recently weaned pigs affected with exudative epidermitis gained up to 0.07 kg/day less, converted feed 13% less efficiently, and had mortality rates from 1.2 to 80% higher than nonaffected pigs. Fly-infested pigs had daily gains 0.05 kg less and feed efficiencies 0.04 worse than pigs in fly-free pens. Swine affected with abscesses grew 0.11–0.14 kg/day less than unaffected penmates. Other skin diseases, while not decreasing production efficiency, are important because they are highly visible. Gross skin lesions are a source of concern to the swine producer and especially to those who sell breeding stock or feeder pigs (Straw 1985).

Some pigskin is processed into leather. At the time of writing, U.S. buyers were paying $1.00 to $1.25 per skin to be used for leather. While the skin itself is of minor economic value, trimming and skinning of affected carcasses are costly to the meat-processing industry. In the Netherlands, the economic loss resulting from skinning and trimming of pig carcasses was estimated at from 2.5 to 3 million guilders per annum (Smeets et al. 1989).

SKIN AS A DIAGNOSTIC TISSUE FOR OTHER ORGAN SYSTEMS

Reflection of General Health. Normal hair growth and keratinization of skin require 25–30% of the animal's daily protein requirement. Deficiencies of protein and calories, whether due to dietary inadequacy or debilitating disease show up as dry, scaly, thin, inelastic skin (Worden 1965). Undernutrition causes the hair to become dull, dry, and brittle and change in length and thickness. Hair of severely undernourished (runt) pigs was approximately twice as long as hair from normal pigs of a comparable body weight. The thickness of hair from runt pigs was greater than weight-matched but less than age-matched controls (Cabak et al. 1962). The skin also reflects the adequacy of the circulatory system. Blue or purplish extremities are seen with cardiac insufficiency or circulatory impairment, and pale or white skin is seen in anemia or shock.

Interaction with Other Systems/Diseases. Skin disease has been associated with disease in other body systems. Pigs that experienced postweaning diarrhea had a higher relative risk (1.4) of skin disease than did pigs without diarrhea (Svensmark 1989). Outbreaks of diarrhea and coughing were reported in pigs that failed to improve until they were treated for mange (McPherson 1960).

Immune Function. Tests to evaluate immune responsiveness, such as for immediate and delayed-type hypersensitivity, and cellular immunity are performed on the skin. In pigs, intradermal injection of phytohemagglutinin provides a good measure of cellular immunity, while intradermal injection of *Staphylococcus* lysate reflects delayed hypersensitivity to staphylococci (Raszyk and Pillich 1989). Skin tests based on cell-mediated immunity have been used to screen for pseudorabies and tuberculosis (Chaps. 24 and 50).

Mineral Status. Mineral content of swine hair has been examined to monitor general mineral status. The concentration of essential minerals in swine has been reported to be influenced by age, sex, season, breed, color, and body location. Most researchers evaluated copper and zinc levels, and because findings between studies are conflicting, use of hair for monitoring mineral status in swine appears to be of limited value (Kornegay et al. 1981).

Use as a Model for Human Disease. Because of its similarity to human skin, pigskin has been used extensively as a model for human disease in research on radiation injury, burns, wound repair, graft procedures, and impact of high-velocity projectiles.

GENERAL CHANGES IN DISEASE. Head (1970) divides pathologic processes in the skin into regressive-degenerative change (atrophy, hydropic change, and necrosis) and reactive change (hyperplasia, vascular response, inflammation, and healing). Atrophy appears as a thinning of the epidermis and loss of hair. Accumulation of fluid between and within cells is termed status spongiosis. When severe, these hydropic changes lead to vesicle formation, rupture, and erosion. Cell death may be seen as a coagulative necrosis or more commonly as a process that also invokes an inflammatory response. Hyperplasia is seen as an increase in number and size of cells and a thickening of the epidermis. In hyperplastic skin, the easily visualized stratum spinosum is termed acanthosis. Hyperkeratosis, or increase in the stratum corneum, is often a corollary to acanthosis. Normally, the cells in the stratum spinosum and stratum granularum do not retain viable nuclei, but when this occurs in certain disease states it is termed parakeratosis. Erythema is capillary distension (congestion or hyperemia) that is grossly visible at the skin surface. An urticarial weal develops if damaged blood vessels leak fluid into surrounding dermal fibers. Impedance of the lymphatic drainage exacerbates this local reaction. Inflammatory response may be triggered either by an agent's direct damage to the dermis or by its products reaching the dermis from some other site. Complete healing of skin is possible if damage was slight enough to leave an intact stratum basale. More severe lesions resolve by dermal fibroplasia and epithelialization (scarring) (Head 1970).

DIAGNOSTIC TECHNIQUES

History. An accurate history is essential in making a diagnosis. The herd manager should be asked the following questions: What are the ages of affected pigs? What is the progression of signs in an affected pig? How long do the signs persist? In addition to skin lesions, what other signs are observed? Is recovery complete, or do the pigs remain unthrifty? In the group affected, what are the morbidity and the mortality? Has treatment been used and to what effect? What is the course of disease within the herd? Did the disease have a sudden onset, or was it insidious? What animals were originally affected? To what animals did the disease spread? Did the initial picture differ from later signs? Is the disease becoming more or less severe? Is the disease sporadic or enzootic? What is the distribution of affected pigs? What vaccines are routinely used in the herd? How are external parasites controlled? Do pigs have access to pasture or any stored chemicals (Straw 1985)?

Physical Examination. In addition to a general physical examination (Chap. 65), a detailed examination of the skin should be done to determine the distribution of lesions; lesions may be distributed in a symmetric or nonsymmetric pattern. They may be generalized or localized predominantly to the ventrum, on the back, around the face and ears, or on the extremities or points of friction (e.g., elbows, knees, and hocks) (Fig. 9.1). Color changes such as reddening, pallor, jaundice, cyanosis, and gray discoloration are observed most easily on white pigs in natural or incandescent light; fluorescent light tends to make the skin appear paler and more yellowish. Color changes in pigmented pigs may only be observable in the mucous membranes. The skin of a young pig about 2 weeks of age is a good representation of normal skin. Mange is so widespread in the swine population that even people who have a long association with swine may not recognize how smooth, flat, and unblemished the normal pig's skin is. Palpation of lesions will reveal whether they are raised or flat. The edges should be examined to determine whether the boundary between normal and affected skin is discrete or a gradual progression. Lesions may be flat and consist mostly of color changes, or they may show varying degrees of proliferation. The pig should be observed for itching and rubbing and to determine whether it is normally alert or depressed (Straw 1985).

Collection of Diagnostic Samples

SKIN SCRAPINGS. Skin scrapings are made for identification of dermatomycosis and mange. When dermatomycosis is suspected, the edge of the lesion should be scraped with a scalpel blade and the material transferred to a medium that supports fungal growth. Hairs plucked from the area should also be included in the sample. An indicator medium, such as Fungassay (Pitman-Moore), provides a rapid-screening device. Identification of pathogenic fungal organisms is based on the growth rate of the organism; growth pattern; color of the colony; rate, time, and character of the color change in the agar; and microscopic examination of the mature colony. Hairs plucked from the affected area may be covered with a drop of a potassium hydroxide dimethyl sulfoxide (KOH-DMSO) solution (three parts water, two parts DMSO, and one part KOH) and examined microscopically ($\times 40$). Affected hair exhibits gross distortion, loss of architectural detail and symmetry, destruction of the pigmented medullary portion, increase in diameter, and breakage.

In affected herds, mange mites are most readily demonstrated in pigs weighing between 15 and 25 kg. Scrapings should be taken from the ear canal and placed on a slide, covered with a drop of 10% KOH that has been heated gently, covered with a coverslip, and examined under a low-power objective. A better method, because it concentrates the parasites, is to boil the material in a tube with a 10% KOH solution or to bathe the tube in water at 100°C for 10 minutes. The tube is then centrifuged and the sediment examined as before (Straw 1985).

CULTURE. Skin cultures are desirable in suspected cases of staphylococcal acne, pustular dermatitis, and exudative epidermitis. Because of the combination of extensive surface contamination and the deep nature of the infections, surface cultures are seldom diagnostic. The preferred method of culturing skin is to obtain a large piece of affected skin (either by wide-excision biopsy or sacrifice of an animal), remove the subcutaneous tissue, and culture at the junction of the dermis and the epidermis at the level of the base of the hair follicles. Skin specimens for culture should be kept chilled during transport to the laboratory (Straw 1985).

VESICLE COLLECTION. Vesicular diseases may be differentiated by isolation of the virus from fluid collected from vesicles and paired serology from acute and convalescent animals (Straw 1985).

BIOPSY AND ASPIRATION. Skin biopsies or necropsy samples for histopathologic examination should be taken from the edge of lesions. In most cases biopsy of a fully developed primary lesion provides more information than an early or late lesion. However, in the cases of vesicular, bullous, or pustular lesions, early lesions should be selected to avoid secondary changes that obscure the primary lesions. The biopsy site may be cleansed by soaking with 70% alcohol, but iodo-

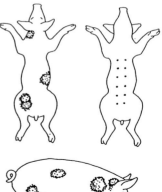

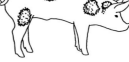

Hyperkeratosis

Ringworm

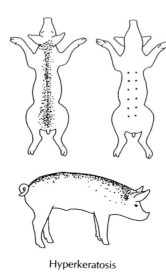

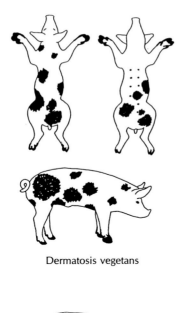

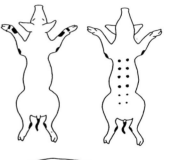

Dermatosis vegetans

Skin necrosis—piglets

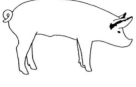

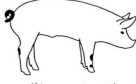

Necrotic ear syndrome

Skin necrosis—sow

9.1. Distribution of lesions in some skin diseases.

200

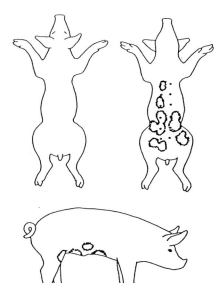

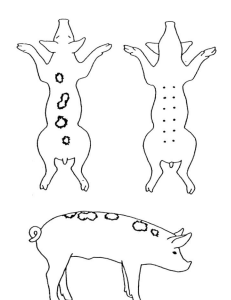

Pityriasis rosea
typical distribution

Pityriasis rosea
atypical distribution

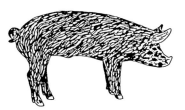

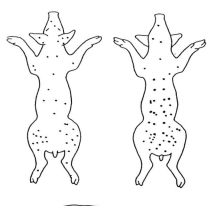

Exudative epidermitis—
generalized acute form

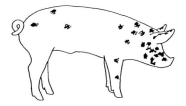

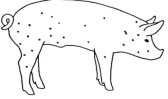

Exudative epidermitis—chronic
localized form

Swine pox

201

phor disinfectants should not be used and the area should not be scrubbed because such processes may remove important surface pathology or create iatrogenic lesions. The specimen may be collected with a 6-mm biopsy punch (Baker's Biopsy Punch, Key Pharmaceuticals), gently blotted to remove artifactual blood, and placed subcutaneous side down on a wooden tongue depressor. This will assure proper anatomic orientation and prevent artifacts that result from folding or curling of the specimen. Biopsy material should be fixed in 10% buffered formalin. Because many laboratories do little work with swine skin, it may be desirable to provide a sample of normal skin for comparison; however, normal skin should be placed in a separate container and labelled as such. When samples that contain both affected tissue and adjacent normal skin are submitted, the clinician runs the risk that during histopatho-

logic processing the lesion may be missed and the normal skin sectioned instead (Scott 1988).

Lumps or swellings in the skin can be aspirated with a 20-gauge needle and a 12-ml sterile syringe. Aspirated material should be cultured both aerobically and anaerobically. A small amount also should be placed on a slide; stained with Gram's stain; and examined microscopically for bacteria, white blood cells, or tumor cells.

Differential Diagnosis. After a history has been collected and a physical examination performed, the clinician should consider differential diagnosis; Tables 9.1 through 9.4 summarize information that is helpful in this process. When one or more diseases are suspected, the clinician should collect the appropriate diagnostic samples to confirm or reject a diagnosis.

Table 9.1. Ages at which certain skin diseases are more frequently seen

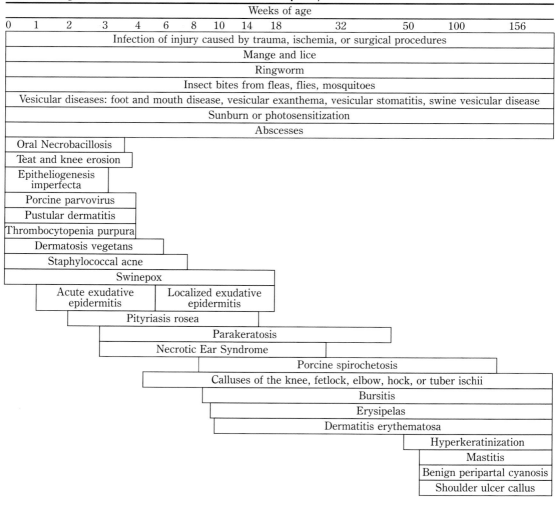

Table 9.2. Diseases affecting the skin of pigs by location and gross appearance of lesions

Location	Relation to Normal Tissue	Proliferative or Nonproliferative	Demarcation of Lesion	Cause
Face	Elevated	. . .	Discrete	Staphylococcal acne
	Flat	Nonproliferative	Discrete	Necrotic stomatitis. Initial lesion of exudative epidermitis
Face and feet	Elevated	. . .	Discrete	Vesicular diseases[a]
Shoulder	Elevated	. . .	Discrete	Callus Hematoma
	Flat	Nonproliferative	Discrete	Ulcer
Knees, elbows, hocks	Flat	Nonproliferative	Discrete	Knee erosions
	Elevated	. . .	Discrete	Callus
			Diffuse	Bursitis
Ear	Elevated	. . .	Discrete	Hematoma
	Flat	Nonproliferative	Diffuse	Greasy spot behind ear
		Proliferative	Discrete	Ear necrosis
			Diffuse	Mange
Ear, eye, udder	Flat	Nonproliferative	Diffuse	Photosensitization
Extremities	Flat	Nonproliferative	Diffuse	Cyanosis or reddening secondary to disease[b]
Dorsal	Elevated	. . .	Discrete	Fleas, flies, mosquitoes
			Diffuse	Lumpy skin disease
	Flat	Proliferative	Diffuse	Hyperkeratinization
		Nonproliferative	Diffuse	Sunburn
			Discrete	Epitheliogenesis imperfecta
Ventral abdomen	Elevated	. . .	Discrete	Pityriasis rosea Eosinophilic dermatitis
			Diffuse	Urticarial mange
	Flat	Nonproliferative	Discrete	Transit erythema Teat necrosis
			Diffuse	Mastitis Benign peripartal cyanosis
Ventral cervical area	Elevated	. . .	Discrete	Jowl abscess Tuberculosis
			Diffuse	Pharyngeal anthrax
Generalized	Elevated	. . .	Discrete	Pustular dermatitis Swine pox Infected injuries Neoplasia Abscess Staphylococcal dermatitis
			Diffuse	Dermatosis vegetans. Porcine spirochetosis
	Flat	Proliferative	Diffuse	Parakeratosis Demodectic mange Lice Sarcoptic mange Exudative epidermitis *Dermatophilus congolensis*

		Nonproliferative	Discrete	Dermatomycosis:
				  Ringworm
				  Dermatophilus
				  Cutaneous candidiasis
				Dermatitis erythematosa
				Thrombocytopenia purpura
				Erysipelas

			Diffuse	Carbon monoxide toxicity Porcine stress syndrome Hypotrichosis Cyanosis or reddening secondary to hog cholera, African swine fever, *Streptococcus*
	Depressed	Nonproliferative	Discrete	Epitheliogensis imperfecta Subcutaneous fat necrosis Porcine cutaneous asthenia

[a]Foot and mouth disease, vesicular exanthema, vesicular stomatitis, swine vesicular disease, San Miguel sea lion virus.

[b]Salmonellosis, *Haemophilus parasuis, H. pleuropneumoniae,* colibacillosis, hemagglutinating encephalomyelitis virus, organophosphate toxicity.

Table 9.3. Discoloration of the skin in the absence of gross skin lesions

Discoloration	Distribution	Pigs Affected	Cause	Associated Factors
Erythema Dilation of capillaries and increased blood flow produce a red color	General	Perinatal pigs	Carbon monoxide toxicity	Seen in winter. Incomplete combustion of fuel in heater
			Actinobacillosis	Petechial hemorrhage, cyanosis and congestion of extremities
		Any age but usually growing pigs	Erysipelas, hog cholera, African swine fever, acute salmonellosis or Strep suis	Seen as a transitory change prior to the onset of typical signs
	Mammary glands	Sows, post-partum	Mastitis, esp. due to *E. coli* or *Klebsiella*	Soiled, wet, or sawdust bedding
	Dorsum	Any age	Sunburn	Exposure to the sun
	Ventrum	Any age	Transit erythema	Wet, urine-soaked or lime bedding in transport truck
	Blotchy distribution	Any age, but especially in 50–150 kg pigs	Porcine stress syndrome	Triggered by physical exercise, excitement, heat, or halothane anesthesia
		Any age	Dermatosis erythematosis	Possible association with clover pasture, but also seen in confinement
Cyanosis Presence of reduced hemoglobin in superficial capillaries appears deep red to bluish	Ears, tail, ventrum, and extremities	Pigs 2–4 mo	Systemic salmonellosis	Continuous flow operation especially after addition of new pigs
		Nursery and grower pigs	*Haemophilus parasuis*	Associated with systemic disease
		Any age	Organophosphate toxicity	Hypoxia develops due to increased respiratory tract secretions and bronchoconstriction. Eratic slow heart beat and neurologic signs
		Growing and finishing pigs	*Actinobacillosis pleuropneumoniae*	Associated with peracute respiratory disease
		Nursing pigs	*E. coli* enteritis and Hemagglutinating encephalomyelitis	Seen in terminal stages of the disease
		Any age, but usually sows	Congestive heart failure, cardiac or pulmonary insufficiency	Other signs of cardiovascular insufficiency
		Laboratory pigs	Thiamine deficiency	Experimental diets
	Udder and hindquarters	Sows around the time of farrowing	Benign peripartal cyanosis	Especially in sows bedded on urine-soaked sawdust
Jaundice Increased amounts of bilirubin appear yellow	General	Neonatal pigs	Isoimmune hemolytic anemia	Incompatable sow and piglet blood types
		Neonatal or nursery pigs	Eperythrozoonosis	Mange infestation
		Growing pigs to adults	Leptospirosis	Occasional finding in infected animals
		Any age	Liver dysfunction	Various toxicities, mycotoxicosis, bile duct obstruction by *Ascaris suum*
		Any age	Copper toxicity	Feed mixing error
Grayish skin Capillary constriction	General	Any age	Cardiovascular shock	Traumatic incident or toxemia
		Growing pigs	Mecadox toxicity	Feed-mixing error
Pale or white	General	Any age	Anemia	See Chapter 2

Table 9.4. Conditions that cause lumps or swellings under the skin of pigs

Location of Lumps or Swelling	Cause	Aspirate Appearance
Submandibular	Jowl abscess *Streptococcus* group E)	Pus with organisms
	Pharyngeal anthrax	Edema
	Tuberculosis	Sulfur granules
Variable distribution	Neoplasia—sarcoma, malignant melanomatoma, cavernous hemangioma, others	Solid tissue, neoplastic cells
	Actinomyces pyogenes, Fusiformis necrophorus, Actinobacillus sp.	Pus with organisms
Over back, shoulders, thigh	Lumpy skin disease	Solid, dermal cells
Neck caudal to the ear or in the ham	Injection reaction	Pus with or without organisms
Epididymis or testicles	Brucellosis	Pus with organisms
Shoulder, flank, over the hindquarters, vulva, or ear	Hematoma	Blood or serum
Posterior aspect of hocks, usually bilateral	Adventitious bursitis of the hocks	Synovial fluid (not recommended)
Base of tail, hindquarters	Infection secondary to tail biting	Pus with organisms
Mammary glands	*Actinomyces suis* infection	"Sulfer granules"; gram-positive filamentous organisms

COLOR CHANGES. Discoloration of the skin in the absence of gross skin lesions is seen with some primary skin diseases but more commonly occurs secondary to disease in another system. Table 9.3 lists causes of skin discoloration in pigs. Various bacterial infections that cause septicemia produce signs in the skin; most are color changes produced by thrombosis, capillary dilatation, or circulatory insufficiency. Diseases that produce cyanosis of extremities include systemic salmonellosis (Chap. 46), *Haemophilus parasuis* (Chap. 41), *Actinobacillus suis* (Chap. 51) and certain forms of erysipelas (Chap. 38). Generalized erythema is seen in streptococcosis (Chap. 48). Mastitis causes a local reddening over the affected glands.

LUMPS AND SWELLINGS. A number of conditions produce swelling of, or under the skin. Table 9.4 provides differentiating features of various causes of skin swellings. Edematous conditions of the skin include urticaria and angioedema. Urticarial reactions have been reported in association with insect stings, erysipelas, *Actinobacillus suis,* edema disease (Chap. 39), anthrax (Chap. 32), malignant edema (Chap. 36), topical and systemic medications (especially parasiticides), feeds, stinging nettle, and biologics. Lesions are most common over the trunk and front legs (Scott 1988).

SKIN DISEASES

Bacterial Skin Diseases

ABSCESSES. Bacteria isolated from abscesses in relative order of their frequency include *Actinomyces pyogenes;* beta-hemolytic streptococci, especially *S. zooepidemicus* and *S. equisimilis; Fusobacterium necrophorum; Bacteroides* sp.; *Staphylococcus* spp., especially *S. hyicus* and *S. epidermidis; E. coli; Flavobacterium; Peptostreptococcus* sp.; *Pseudomonas aeruginosa;* and *Actinobacillus* spp.

Abscesses result from secondary infection of wounds caused by fighting, trauma, or parasites. In one report, cutaneous abscesses developed following an outbreak of swine pox (Miller and Olson 1978). At the site of bacterial invasion, a circumscribed subcutaneous accumulation of purulent material with fibrous capsule develops. Clinically, abscesses appear as well-demarcated enlargements under the skin sometimes with red discoloration of the skin covering the area. The most common locations include the more prominent areas of the body that are most exposed to trauma, such as shoulders, neck, flank, feet, ears, as well as sites of injection. "Jowl abscesses" occur in the mandibular lymph nodes after infection with Lancefield group E streptococci (Chap. 48). Infection causes a mild febrile reaction and is seen as a swelling under the skin of the mandibular area.

Diagnosis is based on clinical signs. It is important to determine the cause of the original injury, whether wounds are caused by fighting, rough floors, protruding points in the pen, damaged feeders, or poor injection technique so that attention can be directed toward eliminating the cause. Well-organized abscesses may be drained and flushed with antibacterials; however, unless the procedure can be carried out in an area far removed from the remaining pigs, drainage may serve to "seed" the environment with additional organisms (Krantz 1965; Amtsberg 1978; Miller and Olson 1978; Jones 1980; Cameron 1984; Straw et al. 1990).

ACTINOBACILLUS EQUULI, A. LIGNIERESII, A. SUIS. *Actinobacillus equuli* or *A. suis* infections are rare in swine and usually take the form of a septicemia in nursing piglets. Cutaneous manifestations in piglets may include diffuse hyperemia and petechial hemorrhages on the ears and abdomen. After death, purpura or skin necrosis may be seen on the carcass. Sows may be anorexic and have skin lesions resembling erysipelas or develop abscesses on the neck, withers, or flanks. A more complete description is given in Chapter 51. *Actinobacillus lignieresii* infection occasionally causes abscesses in the udders of sows (Windsor 1973; Mair 1974).

ACTINOMYCOSIS. *Actinomyces suis* has been associated with suppurative, granulomatous, fibrous enlargement of the udder. Severe lesions may have fistulous draining tracts. Since *Actinomyces* is a normal inhabitant of the oral cavity, the opportunity exists for bacteria to enter skin on the mammary gland that is damaged by the sharp teeth of nursing piglets. Diagnosis is made by direct smears, biopsy, and culture. Material from the granulomatous lesions frequently contains "sulfur granules," which microscopically are seen to be composed of gram-positive filamentous organisms (Magnussen 1928; Franke 1973). Surgical excision and penicillin have both shown value in treatment (Bethke 1971).

EXUDATIVE EPIDERMITIS (GREASY PIG DISEASE) ("MARMITE" DISEASE). Exudative epidermitis is caused by infection with *Staphylococcus hyicus.* It is most common in pigs between 1 and 8 weeks of age. In the acute form pigs are covered with moist, odoriferous, greasy material composed of sebaceous gland secretion and serum (Fig. 9.2). Lesions may start on the face and progress to the entire body. In chronic forms, lesions are smaller and appear as patches of scabby skin usually around the head or shoulders (Fig. 9.3) (Chap. 40).

PORCINE SPIROCHETOSIS (ULCERATIVE GRANULOMA OF SWINE) (ULCERATIVE SPIROCHETOSIS). Porcine spirochetosis is caused by *Borrelia suis,* sometimes in conjunction with *Fusiformis necrophorus.* In well-developed lesions, infection with other secondary invaders such as *Actinomyces pyogenes* and *Streptococcus* is common. Lesions are most often seen in young pigs 2–3 weeks after weaning, although occasionally, the mammary glands of sows are affected. Cutaneous wounds are necessary for infection to develop. The condition is more likely to occur in herds with poor sanitation, mange, and management practices that lead to skin trauma. Outbreaks have been related to excessive fighting after weaning, ear biting, and infection of needle teeth and castration wounds.

In young pigs, lesions appear on the head, ears, gums (after teeth clipping), shoulders, side of body, and scrotum (after castration). Ear lesions start at the base of the pinnae and extend along the ventral margin to the tip of the ear. In sows, lesions have been seen along the underline. Affected areas may become 20–30 cm in diameter and resemble actinomycosis. Initially, affected areas are reddened, swollen, and edematous, with

9.2. Acute generalized exudative epidermitis.

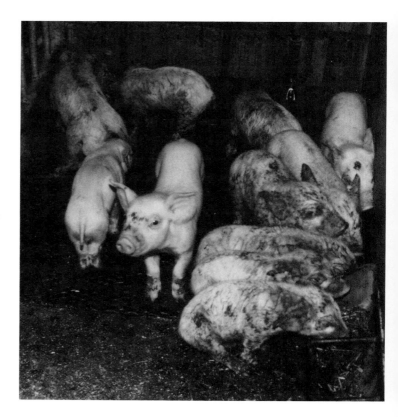

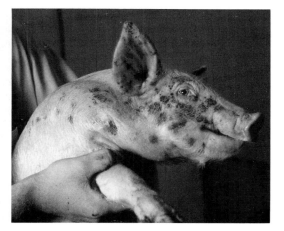

9.3. Localized chronic exudative epidermitis.

discharge of a grayish brown, sticky, pustular discharge. Later, necrosis and ulceration are prominent. Lesions often appear tumorlike and without treatment may continue to enlarge for weeks to months, finally involving deeper tissues of the body. Older lesions exhibit swelling, fistulae formation, and sloughing of the central area.

Diagnosis is based on clinical signs, dark-field examination and histopathologic findings. A direct smear of fresh tissue examined under dark-field illumination reveals numerous motile spirochetes, which can be demonstrated with silver stains. The major pathologic changes seen on histologic examination of biopsy material are necrosis and granulation tissue. Ulceration, granulomatous inflammation, and vasculitis have also been reported.

Various treatments have been reported to be effective, including injections of penicillin for 3 days, injected or oral sulfadimidine for 3–5 days, and oral potassium iodide at 1 gm/35 kg up to 3 gm total. Control measures include improving sanitation and altering management to reduce fighting and traumatic injury (Blanford et al. 1957; Albiston 1965; Harcourt 1973; Beaton et al. 1974; Cameron 1981, 1984).

PORCINE NECROTIC EAR SYNDROME. Massive erosive lesions at the margins of the pinnae have also been seen in pigs in which spirochetes could not be found. Excessive fighting after weaning produced numerous superficial lacerations, which progressed to areas of hyperemia, edema, vesicle formation, and necrosis. *Staphylococcus hyicus* was recovered from early and late lesions and beta-hemolytic streptococci were isolated from more advanced cases that featured thick crusting and ulcerated lesions. One sequelae to infection was bacteremia with suppurative polyarthritis, and pneumonia with multifocal abscesses and necrosis. Another was a diffuse, fulminating cellulitis of the pinna resulting in complete sloughing of the ear (Richardson et al. 1984).

ORAL NECROBACILLOSIS (NECROTIC STOMATITIS) (FACIAL NECROSIS) (FACIAL PYEMIA). The principal infectious agent associated with oral necrobacillosis is *Fusiformis necrophorus,* although sometimes *Borrelia suilla* or *Streptococcus* sp. may be involved. These organisms infect wounds that were inflicted by the sharp needle teeth of other piglets. Lesions typically occur within the first few days of life. Usually the smaller piglets in large litters are affected, but sometimes the disease may affect whole litters. Cases may occur when hygiene is poor, but the disease has also been seen in well-managed herds. Factors that increase competition during suckling, such as a poor-milking sow or very large litter, contribute to fighting and the development of facial wounds that become infected.

Affected piglets have bilateral lesions on their faces between the mouth and eyes, and occasionally on the lips, gums, tongue, legs, and body. Other piglets in the litter may have lacerations over their cheeks. Contaminated wounds undergo necrosis and ulceration, with the development of a thick, adherent brown to black crust. If mucous surfaces are involved there is a fetid odor. More extensive facial lesions may be painful or restrict jaw movement so that nursing is impeded and the piglet becomes listless and emaciated.

Diagnosis is based on a history of fighting or failure to clip needle teeth, clinical signs, direct smears of lesions and identification of typical organisms, and anaerobic culture. Oral necrobacillosis should be differentiated from porcine spirochetosis and exudative epidermitis.

Crusts over lesions should be gently removed and necrotic material debrided. A mild disinfectant or antibiotic ointment can be applied topically. In severe cases, systemic sulfonamides or penicillin-streptomycin combinations may be needed parenterally for 3–4 days. Further cases can be prevented by prompt and careful clipping of needle teeth using sanitized instruments and cross-fostering piglets to even up litter sizes (Simon and Stovall 1969; Hungerford 1970; Golovin 1977; Cameron 1984).

PUSTULAR DERMATITIS (INFECTIOUS DERMATITIS) (CONTAGIOUS PYODERMA). Nursing piglets with pustular dermatitis due to infection with beta-hemolytic Lancefield type C streptococci have been reported. A similar infection has also been seen on the udder of sows. Infection starts with fever and depression in piglets and is then followed by development of cutaneous lesions. First, the skin becomes reddened and occasional petechial hemorrhages may be seen on the ventral abdomen. Pustules appear in the inguinal area, inner thighs, dorsum, and edges of eyes, lips, and ears. The pustules rupture and are then replaced by scabs with dark centers and lighter edges.

Diagnosis is based on clinical signs and isolation and identification of the organism. Usually, infection with streptococci is responsive to treatment with tetracycline or erythromycin. Control centers on removing sources of skin abrasion and improving hygiene (Hare et al. 1942; Cabak et al. 1962; Cameron 1981).

STAPHYLOCOCCAL DERMATITIS (STAPH ACNE) (STAPH FOLLICULITIS). Occasionally, staphylococci have been associated with infection of the hair follicles of pigs less than 8 weeks of age. Pustular dermatitis with erythema occurs over the entire body and especially on the hindquarters, abdomen, and chest. Infection occurs sporadically and individual cases resolve without treatment after a few weeks.

Viral Skin Diseases

PARVOVIRUS. Kresse et al. (1985) described a vesiclelike dermatitis in six herds in the midwest. A porcine parvovirus, (Kresse virus) was isolated from these outbreaks. The involvement of a bacterium in conjunction with the Kresse virus was suspected. Kresse virus was more pathogenic than NADL-8 to late-stage fetuses and also was associated with the deposition of immune complexes in the skin, kidneys, and brain of infected fetal pigs.

The pigs affected were usually between 1–2 weeks of age, but on one farm disease occurred in 4-week-old pigs. On all six farms pigs were maintained outside. Morbidity ranged from 13% to 100%, and mortality from 0% to 58%. Lesions appeared as remnants of vesicles on snout, coronary band, interdigital space, and mouth. Affected areas had fissurelike erosions to large areas of necrosis and sloughing of skin. Some lesions were very severe and led to separation of the hoof wall and sloughing of the hoof. Anorexia, diarrhea, conjunctivitis, and sneezing were also observed in affected pigs.

Diagnosis was made by virus isolation, and finding specific porcine parvovirus direct immunofluorescence in the outer layers of the hair follicles. Because three herds showed improvement after treatment with antibiotics, antimicrobial therapy is probably indicated (Kresse et al. 1985; Choi et al. 1987).

VESICULAR DISEASES OF SWINE. Foot-and-mouth disease (FMD), vesicular stomatitis (VS), vesicular exanthema, and swine vesicular disease (SVD) produce vesicular lesions especially on the snout and coronary band (Chap. 30).

IDIOPATHIC VESICULAR DISEASES. There are several reports of vesicular disease in which an etiologic agent could not be identified. In New Zealand, 28 of 800 pigs had vesicles and erosions on the snout and feet. In an outbreak in Australia, 30% of the pigs in a herd of 600 had vesicles and erosions on the snout and occasionally on the

back, tail, and ears. In both of these outbreaks, feeding pigs marine products was suspected to have been related to the disease. Because of the possibility of an infectious and/or exotic etiology, all pigs on these two farms were slaughtered. In another outbreak in Florida, only 10 of 160 pigs showed lesions. Affected pigs were febrile, lame, and had vesicles only on their feet. FMD, SVD, and VS could not be detected in samples submitted to Plum Island Animal Disease Center (NZ Vet Assoc and Gen News 1981; Munday and Ryan 1982; Gibbs et al. 1983).

Swine that had been fed waste from a potato distillery developed pyrexia, anorexia, vesicular dermatitis on the legs, lameness, and lacrimation (Scott 1988).

SWINE POX. Swine pox lesions start as papules and progress to pustules covered with a hard crust. Lesions often are over the back and sides, but may be distributed over the entire body (Chap. 28). Lice infestation contributes to infection.

Fungal Skin Diseases

CUTANEOUS CANDIDIASIS. Dermatitis, due to infection with *Candida albicans,* was found in pigs that were fed garbage and that laid in their heated food to keep warm. About 40% of growers were affected. Lesions appeared as circular areas (2 cm diameter), covered with loosely adherent moist grey exudate, on the abdomen and lower limbs. On some pigs the posterior hindquarters were most severely affected. Affected skin was thickened, wrinkled, bluish, and hairless and hung in folds. Diagnosis was made by skin scrapings and dark-field exam, which showed budding yeast forms and mycelial fragments. Histologic examination showed great thickening of the stratum corneum, hyperplasia of keratinocytes, and infiltration of neutrophils and hyphae. Improvement of hygiene and provision of bedding lead to resolution of lesions (Reynolds et al. 1966).

***DERMATOPHILUS CONGOLENSIS* INFECTION.** Infection with *Dermatophilus congolensis* is rare in swine. Zoospores of *D. congolensis* penetrate damaged skin, germinate, encapsulate, and produce hyphae in the epidermis. Affected pigs have a generalized exudative, crusting dermatitis. A primary insult such as trauma or infection with *Staphylococcus hyicus* may be necessary for infection with *Dermatophilus* to occur. Diagnosis is based on isolation of the organism and histologic demonstration of hyphae arranged in cuboidal packets of coccoid cells (railroad track appearance) (Stankusheve et al. 1968; Lomax and Cole 1983).

RINGWORM. *Microsporum nanum* and *Trichophyton verrucosum* are the most common agents causing ringworm in swine. *M. canis, M. gypseum,* and *T. mentagrophytes* have also been reported. Ringworm may affect any age pig. Morbidity is usually sporadic, but up to 100% of sows may be affected. Lesions start as small (2 cm), red to brownish circular lesions that spread concentrically (up to 12 cm diameter) and later are covered with a thin, dark crusty scab. Lesions may be single or multiple and may coalesce. Lesions may occur anywhere on the body, especially behind the ears but usually not on the ventral abdomen. Sows sometimes develop chronic infection behind the ears. There is minimal hair loss, and pruritus seldom occurs. Infection does not produce any general debility or affect productivity. The disease is usually self limiting in 2–3 months but occasionally may persist 6 months without treatment. Diagnosis is described in the section on skin scraping above. Histopathologic examination of affected skin shows nonspecific perifolliculitis, folliculitis, and furunculosis. Animals may be treated orally with nystatin or griseofulvin (10 mg/kg), or topically with iodine, captan, or salicylic acid. Ringworm in swine presents a public health hazard to people in contact with them (McPherson 1956; Dodd et al. 1965; Ginther 1965; Ginther and Ajello 1965; Cannole 1966; Ginther and Bubash 1966; Smith and Steffert 1966; Kielstein and Gottschalk 1970; Koehne 1972; Long et al. 1972; Morganti et al. 1976; Mos et al. 1978; Arora et al. 1979; Das et al. 1980; Cameron 1981, 1984).

Parasitic Skin Diseases.

Common parasitic dermatitis in swine includes infestation with sarcoptic mange, demodectic mange, lice, and fleas (Chap. 53).

Percutaneous infection of piglets with cercariae of *Schistosoma japonicum* produced urticaria, a pustular maculopapular rash, and pruritus at the site of invasion. Later, pigs developed anorexia, lethargy, pallor, diarrhea, and progressive weight loss (Yason and Novilla 1984).

Physical and Chemical Agents

SUNBURN. Pigs not previously exposed to sunlight may develop sunburn. It occurs most often in pigs that are housed out-of-doors, but is sometimes seen in pigs kept in modified open-front housing. Lesions consist of erythema and edema of skin especially over the back and behind the ears. The skin is hot and painful. Pigs may show an altered gait as they try to walk without disturbing their affected skin. Later, in severely affected pigs, layers of skin will peal off. Usually no treatment is given except to move pigs to a shaded area.

PHOTOSENSITIZATION (PHOTODYNAMIC DERMATITIS). Photosensitization occurs in pigs exposed to sunlight and a photodynamic agent such

as found in alfalfa, clover, rape, oats, buckwheat, St. John's-wort, lucerne, and various drugs; phenothiazine, tetracycline, or sulfonamides. Lesions occur only in areas of white skin. Initially, there is erythema, edema, and serum exudation. Pigs may walk stiffly or appear lame due to pain associated with movement of the skin. Conjunctivitis may also be present. After a few days the skin is matted with dried serum and becomes dry, hard, fissured, and intensely pruritic. At the end of a week necrotic skin separates from the underlying tissue. Treatment consists primarily of removing animals from pasture and housing them away from sunlight.

PRESSURE SORES (SHOULDER ULCER, SKIN NECROSIS OF SOWS, SKIN NECROSIS OF PIGLETS). Pressure sores are common in swine housed on concrete, wire mesh, and other hard floors. Studies on pigs implanted with monolithic silicon pressure sensors demonstrated that pressure is three to five times higher internally near a bony prominence than it is at the surface of the skin over the prominence. Lesions were found to start near the bone and progress outward. Pressure produced ischemia and subsequent tissue damage and necrosis (Le et al. 1984).

Underweight sows that lack a sufficient fat cushion suffer pressure sores over the scapula, hip, angle of the mandible, hocks, elbows, and carpus. Because circulation to the affected area is compromised, systemic antibacterials are of little benefit in treatment of affected sites. Topical dressings should be applied to the lesion and the lying area of the sow made more comfortable through provision of bedding or rubber mats. Prevention is primarily through maintaining proper body condition of sows.

In decreasing order of frequency, piglets in the first week of life suffer pressure sores on the knees, fetlocks, hocks, elbows, and coronets. Lesions are bilateral, and it is usual for the less common sites to be involved only when the common sites are severely affected. Lesions start as small abraded areas that become covered with a dark reddish brown scab (Fig. 9.4). Unless infection gains entry through the necrotic skin, lesions do not appear to cause much inconvenience to the piglet. Most cases heal without treatment by 5 weeks of age. Necrosis of the teats, vulva, tail, chin, sternum, and rump following pressure and ischemia also occurs (Penny et al. 1971).

HEMATOMA. Hemorrhage under the skin produces a circumscribed area of fluctuant swelling. Blunt trauma may produce a hematoma on the shoulders, dorsum, flanks, or hindquarters, but in pigs, the most common occurrence is for a hematoma to form on an ear after repeated, vigorous head shaking due to mange infestation. Diagnosis is by clinical signs or fine-needle aspirate. Usually, the hematoma is allowed to organize and re-

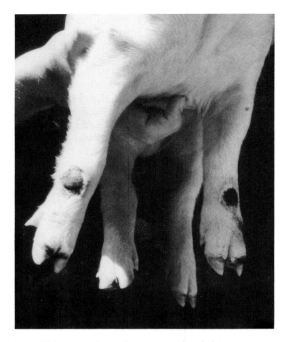

9.4. Skin necrosis on the carpus of a piglet.

solve without intervention. Surgical repair may be complicated by secondary bacterial infection or cannibalism by other pigs.

CONTACT DERMATITIS (EOSINOPHILIC DERMATITIS) (TRANSIT ERYTHEMA). Primary irritants cause dermatitis when they come into contact with skin in a sufficient concentration for a long enough period. Moisture is an important predisposing factor, for it decreases the effectiveness of the normal skin barriers and increases the intimacy of contact between the contactant and the skin surface (Scott 1988). Contact dermatitis typically appears as erythema, edema, and papules. Urine and soiled, wet bedding is associated with dermatitis over the hindquarters. Salt, lime, or disinfectants applied to the floors of trucks used to transport pigs have been reported to produce large irregular areas of erythema and edema on the ventrum and legs (transit erythema). Salt-induced dermatitis produced superficial and deep perivascular inflammation with eosinophilia (Anderson and Petaja 1968; Penny and Muirhead 1986).

CALLUS. A callus is a localized area of hyperkeratosis and epidermal hyperplasia caused by intermittent pressure and friction, resulting in recurring cutaneous ischemia and hyperplasia. Calluses occur most commonly over joints and bony prominences. Chronic lesions contain annular, well-circumscribed plaques of lichenification and hyperkeratosis. Treatment of calluses is not indicated (Scott 1988).

BURSITIS. Lesions of the skin covering the hocks, knees, and feet, and pathologic changes in the bursae around joints are described in Chapter 9.

Neoplasia. Various tumors have been reported in the skin of swine, including melanoma, lymphangioma, rhabdomyoma, multiple acanthoma, fibroma, hemangioma, histiocytoma, sweat gland adenoma, nephroblastoma, squamous cell carcinoma, mast cell tumor, and dermoid choristoma. Papillomatosis rarely occurs in swine. As in other species, warts are probably caused by a virus and tend to be located on the face and genitalia (Nordby 1933; Parish and Done 1962; Case 1964; Hjerpe and Thielen 1964; Teredesai 1974; Fisher and Olander 1978; Moulton 1978; Bundza and Dukes 1982; Brightman et al. 1985; Scott 1988).

Miscellaneous Conditions

PITYRIASIS ROSEA (PORCINE JUVENILE PUSTULAR PSORIAFORM DERMATITIS). The name pityriasis rosea was originally used for this dermatitis in swine because of similarities to pityriasis rosea in humans. Recently, because of greater dissimilarities between the two conditions, the term porcine juvenile pustular psoriaform dermatitis has been suggested as being more appropriate (Dunstan and Rosser 1986). The exact cause of pityriasis rosea is unknown, but a clear hereditary predisposition to the condition, especially among Landrace pigs, exists. One boar was known to have sired 120 litters of which 72 were affected (Corcoran 1964). In another study, pityriasis rosea was only seen in pigs related to others that also had the disorder (Wellman 1963). Efforts to isolate any significant microorganisms or to transmit the disease have been unsuccessful, and pityriasis rosea has occurred in gnotobiotic pigs (Heuner 1957; Wellman 1963; Done 1964; McDermid 1964). Typically the condition is seen in weaned pigs between 4 and 10 weeks of age, but may sometimes occur in suckling pigs.

At first small erythematous papules are seen on the skin of the ventral abdomen and inner thighs (Fig. 9.5). These papules expand centrifugally forming scaly plaques, which later become ring-shaped erythematous lesions when the central area returns to normal. The rings expand and coalesce in a mosaic pattern. Occasionally, lesions are seen on the dorsum of the pig (Fig. 9.6). Diagnosis is made from physical examination and recognition of the characteristic lesions. Histologic findings include superficial perivascular dermatitis with psoriaform epidermal hyperplasia, mucinous degeneration in the dermis, parakeratotic hyperkeratosis, and accumulation of eosinophils and neutrophils (Jubb and Kennedy 1970). It is rare for secondary infection to occur and usually uncomplicated cases resolve without treatment in about 4 weeks.

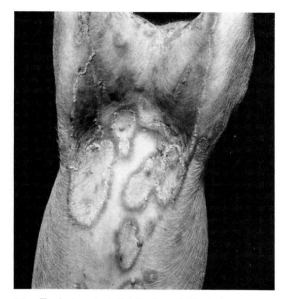

9.5. Typical ventral distribution of pityriasis rosea. (Courtesy of Dr. Alex Hogg.)

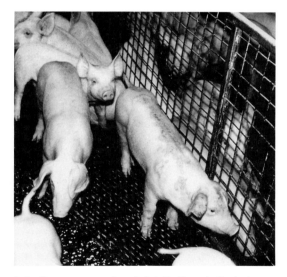

9.6. Less common dorsal distribution of pityriasis rosea.

DERMATOSIS VEGETANS. Dermatosis vegetans is a hereditary defect, inherited as a simple recessive, semilethal factor that originated in the Danish Landrace breed. Piglets show signs at birth that progress rapidly; usually within a few weeks to months, affected animals die from giant cell pneumonitis. The first report of dermatosis vegetans was from Norway (1948), followed by Sweden (1952), Britain (1967), Canada (1967), Switzerland (1980), Austria (1984), and Australia (1987).

At birth affected piglets have marked swelling and erythema in the coronary region of the front feet and to a lesser extent in the hind feet (Fig.

9.7). Surrounding skin is covered with a yellow-brown greasy material. Small reddish papules are seen on the skin in other areas of the body especially the ventral abdomen and inner thighs. These enlarge rapidly to form plaques of thick skin overlaid with a brown brittle material. The hoof wall is thickened and contains ridges and furrows running parallel to the coronary band. Mild respiratory dysfunction is manifested in an increased respiratory rate and prolonged inspiration with forced, rapid irregular expiration. Histologically, the epidermis shows rapid irregular growth, acanthosis, acantholysis, hyperkeratosis, parakeratosis, and numerous keratin pearls and intradermal microabscesses. The dermis shows a massive infiltration of neutrophils, along with a lesser invasion of other white cells. Multinucleate giant cell pneumonitis with epithelialization and fibrosis is seen in the lungs.

Diagnosis is by clinical signs, family history relating to Scandinavian Landrace pigs, and typical histologic appearance of lesions. Treatment of affected individuals is of no value. Parents and littermates of affected animals should be culled (Hjarre et al. 1952; Flatla et al. 1961; Done et al. 1967; Percy and Hulland 1967; Webb and Bourke 1987).

EPITHELIOGENESIS IMPERFECTA (APLASIA CUTIS) (CONGENITAL ECTODERMAL DEFECT). Epitheliogenesis imperfecta is an inherited condition in Yorkshire, Berkshire, Large White, and Wessex pigs that results in areas of abrupt termination of squamous epithelium. It is transmitted as a single autosomal recessive. Affected pigs appear to be missing patches of skin 3–8 cm in diameter over the back, loins, thighs, and sometimes tongue, oral cavity, and coronets. Hydroureter and hydronephrosis are commonly found in pigs with epitheliogenesis imperfecta. Small lesions resolve by scar formation in about 3 weeks. Larger lesions allow bacterial invasion and septicemia (Bentinck-Smith 1951; Parish and Done 1962; Bille and Nielsen 1977; Huston et al. 1978).

SUBCUTANEOUS FAT NECROSIS AND CONGENITAL FOCAL DEFICIENCY OF SUBCUTANEOUS TISSUE. Dimpling of the skin over the flank and shoulder was reported in nine litters of Large White pigs. Affected pigs grew normally, but at slaughter the lesions were even more pronounced with large skin depressions containing small blood vessels at their base. Histologically, there was local fat necrosis and replacement with fibrous tissue. Contraction of the scar tissue produced depressions in the skin. No hereditary, infectious, or nutritional cause was identified (Penny 1957).

Similar gross lesions were observed in a Large White pig at birth. Histologic study revealed no abnormalities of epidermis or dermis, but there was a local deficiency of subcutaneous fat and muscle bundles (Parish and Done 1957).

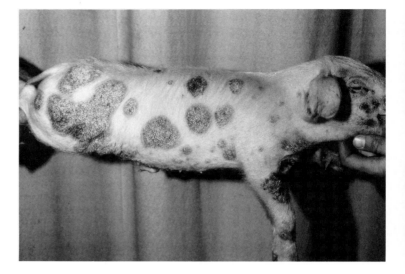

9.7. Dermatosis vegetans. (Courtesy of Dr. Robert Friendship.)

HYPERKERATINIZATION. Intensively housed sows and boars are subject to accumulation of brownish greasy scales, particularly over the dorsum (Fig. 9.8), behind the ears, and sometimes in the axilla (Fig. 9.9). This accumulation is easily cleaned off, leaving normal skin underneath. Pruritus and pain are absent and affected swine are otherwise healthy. Hyperkeratinization routinely occurs in mange-free herds. The condition has been conjectured to be due to a deficiency of essential fatty acids and feeding 1 gallon of cod liver oil per 50 sows per week has been reported to reduce its incidence (Penny and Muirhead 1986).

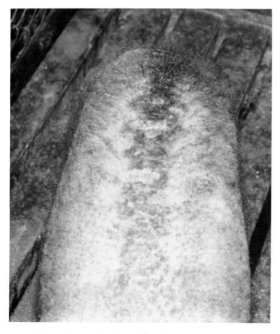

9.8. Hyperkeratosis along the dorsum.

THROMBOCYTOPENIC PURPURA. Neonatal thrombocytopenic purpura occurs when there is an incompatibility between the piglets' platelet antigens inherited from the sire and maternal isoantibodies absorbed from the colostrum. Most cases have involved progeny of Large White boars and multiparous Landrace sows. The resulting thrombocytopenia results in clinical signs of bruising and petechial hemorrhage in the skin, especially the ears and ventrum (Dimmock et al. 1982).

DERMATITIS ERYTHEMATOSIS. Prominent patchy or diffuse erythema over much of the body occasionally is seen in fattening and breeding stock. Outbreaks occur in pigs on pasture and also in pigs housed in total confinement. There are no other signs and affected animals appear otherwise healthy. The condition resolves without treatment in a few days (Gibbon 1962).

BENIGN PERIPARTAL ERYTHEMA. Occasionally, a generalized patchy erythema in seen in sows around the time of farrowing. The sow's general health does not appear to be affected and the condition resolves without treatment in a few days.

PORCINE CUTANEOUS ASTHENIA (CUTIS HYPERELASTICA). Piglets in one litter of Large White–Essex crossbred swine had shallow depressions (3–7 cm diameter) in the skin over the back, flanks, and thighs. Skin was hyperextensible but not fragile. Lesions in other systems were not observed (Parish and Done 1962).

Nutritional Deficiencies. Various nutritional excesses and deficiencies produce skin lesions in swine. However, only a few occur as field problems when pigs are fed typical rations containing soybean plus corn, barley, wheat, or milo. Deficiencies of vitamin A, pantothenic acid, niacin,

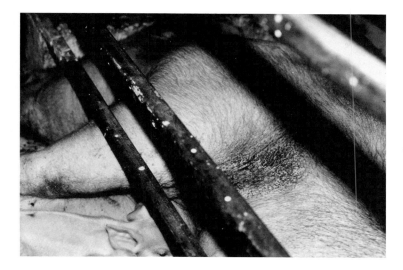

9.9. Hyperkeratosis in the axilla.

and riboflavin produce a dull, dry hair coat and a scaly, dandrufflike dermatitis, along with poor growth and various other signs. Field cases are extremely rare. Iodine deficiency during gestation causes sows to deliver hairless piglets with edema over the head, neck, and shoulders. Vitamin K deficiency produces subcutaneous hemorrhages. Unless an antagonist such as warfarin or mycotoxin was present in the feed, vitamin K deficiency is unlikely (Mullowey and Hall 1984).

Biotin deficiency is not likely in the field because of its wide distribution in traditional feedstuffs. Experimental deficiency following the feeding of a ration containing albumin produced alopecia, hoof cracks, and dermatosis characterized by dryness, roughness, and a brownish exudate (Mullowey and Hall 1984). Conversely, provision of additional biotin was reported to reduce the incidence and severity of heel and sidewall cracks, as well as increase the number of hairs/cm² skin (Bryant et al. 1985).

Fatty-acid deficiency has been produced experimentally in swine using diets that contained 0.06% fat. Skin changes included diffuse scaling, alopecia, and accumulation of brownish exudate on the ears, axillae, and flanks. Fatty-acid deficiency is not likely to occur with conventional rations (Witz and Beeson 1951; Leat 1962).

PARAKERATOSIS. Deficiency of zinc (Zn) produces a generalized dermatitis especially in growing pigs. Initially, there are small, circumscribed, erythematous areas and papules on the ventral abdomen and inner thighs. Later, the area becomes overlaid with scales and keratinous crusts. In severe cases, the crusts fissure and crack; the cracks often contain sticky brown debris composed of sebum and dead cells. Lesions may develop secondary bacterial infections. Because most rations are supplemented with zinc, a primary deficiency (less than 40 mg Zn/kg dry matter) is unusual in the field. More likely is the situation in which high levels of calcium (Ca) in the ration (over 7 gm Ca/kg dry matter) and low levels of essential fatty acids may produce a relative or secondary deficiency. Diagnosis is based on clinical signs, ration analysis, and typical histopathologic findings. Correction includes supplementing the ration with 200 gm zinc carbonate per ton of feed and eliminating excess calcium (Mullowey and Hall 1984).

GENERAL PRINCIPLES OF TREATMENT. After a definitive diagnosis has been made, the practitioner should select a specific treatment regimen and consider preventive measures. When possible, agents responsible for damaging the skin should be removed. These include noxious chemicals, photosensitizing agents, environmental trauma, and parasites. Treatment should be given by injection to animals affected by primary bacterial infections. Antibacterials in the feed or water may be useful in cases of secondary bacterial infection of skin damaged by some other primary agent. Severely affected individuals should be isolated from their healthier penmates to avoid harassment and cannibalism. While treatment is an immediate concern in outbreaks of skin disease, prevention often is more important. Environmental and management procedures should be reviewed and appropriate steps taken to prevent recurrence.

REFERENCES
ALBISTON, H. E. 1965. Spirochetal granuloma of swine. In Diseases of Domestic Animals in Australia II. Ed. T. G. Hungerford. Canberra: Commonwealth Bur Health, p. 5.
ALLAKER, R. P.; LLOYD, D. H.; NOBLE, W. C. 1989. Studies of antagonism between porcine skin bacteria. J Appl Bacteriol 66:507–514.
AMTSBERG, G. 1978. Untersuchungen zum Vorkommen von Staphylocuccus hyicus beim Schein bzw. von Staphylococcus epidermidis Biotyp 2 bei anderen Tierarten. Dtsch Tierærztl Wochenschr 85:385.

ANDERSON, P., AND PETAJA, E. 1968. Profound eosinophilic dermatitis in swine caused by sodium chloride. Nord Vet Med 20:706.

ARORA, B. M.; DAS, S. C.; AND PATGIRI, G. P. 1979. Dermatomycosis in pigs (rubromycosis). Indian Vet J 56:791–793.

BEATON, D.; WATSON, W. A.; AND HARDING, J. D. J. 1974. An outbreak of ulcerative dermatitis in pigs. Vet Rec 94:611.

BENTINCK-SMITH, J. 1951. A congenital epithelial defect in a herd of Berkshire swine. Cornell Vet 41:47.

BETHKE, M. 1971. Mammary actinomycosis of the sow: Comparison of treatment with antibiotics plus enzymes, penicillin plus streptomycin, and surgical treatment. Vet Bull 43:497.

BILLE, N., AND NIELSEN, N. C. 1977. Congenital malformations in pigs in a postmortem material. Nord Vet Med 29:128.

BLANDFORD, T.; BYGRAVE, A. C.; HARDING, J. D. J.; AND LITTLE, T. W. A. 1957. Suspected porcine ulcerative spirochetosis in England. Vet Rec 90:15.

BRIGHTMAN, A. H.; EVERITT, J.; AND BEVIER, G. 1985. Epibulbar solid dermoid choristoma in a pig. Vet Pathol 22:292–294.

BRYANT, K. L.; KORNEGAY, E. T.; KNIGHT, J. W.; VEIT, H. P.; AND NOTTER, D. R. 1985. Supplemental biotin for swine. III. Influence of supplementation to corn and wheat based diets on the incidence and severity of toe lesions, hair and skin characteristics, and structural soundness of sows housed in confinement during parities. J Anim Sci 60:154.

BUNDZA, A., AND DUKES, T. W. 1982. Cutaneous and systemic porcine mastocytosis. Vet Pathol 19:453.

CABAK, V.; GRESHAM, G. A.; AND McCANCE, R. A. 1962. Severe undernutrition in growing and adult animals. 10. The skin and hair of pigs. Br J Nutr 16:635–640.

CAMERON, R. D. A. 1981. Skin diseases of the pig. Univ Sydney Post-Grad Comm Vet Sci Proc 56:445.

————. 1984. Skin diseases of the pig. Univ Sydney Post-Grad Found Vet Sci. Vet Rev No. 23.

CASE, M. T. 1964. Malignant melanoma in a pig. J Am Vet Med Assoc 144:254.

CHOI, C. S.; MOLITOR, T. W.; JOO, H. S.; AND GUNTHER, R. 1987. Pathogenicity of a skin isolate of porcine parvovirus in swine fetuses. Vet Microbiol 15:19–29.

CONNOLE, M. D., AND BAYNES, I. D. 1966. Ringworm caused by *Microsporum nanum* in pigs in Queensland. Aust Vet J 42:19.

CORCORAN, C. J. 1964. Pityriasis rosea in pigs. Vet Rec 76:1407–1409.

CURTIS, S. E. 1981. Environmental Management in Animal Agriculture. Mahomet, Ill.: Anim Environ Serv, pp. 5–8.

DAS, T. K.; ZACHARIAH, K.; AND MATTADO, R. R. 1980. Isolation of *Microsporum nanum* from Northeastern part of India. Indian J Microbiol 20:326.

DEVRIESE, L. A.; SCHLEIFER, K. H.; AND ADEGOKE, G. O. 1985. Identification of coagulase-negative staphylococci from farm animals. J Appl Bacteriol 58:45–55.

DIMMOCK, C. K.; WEBSTER, W. R.; SHIELS, I. A.; AND EDWARDS, C. L. 1982. Isoimmune thrombocytopenic purpura in piglets. Aust Vet J 59:157–158.

DODD, D. C.; NEWLIN, R. W.; AND NIKSH, G. R. 1965. Infection of swine with *Microsporum nanum*. J Am Vet Med Assoc 146:486.

DONE, J. T. 1964. Pityriasis rosea in pig. Vet Rec 76:1507.

DONE, J. T.; LOOSMORE, R. M.; AND SAUNDERS, C. N. 1967. Dermatosis vegetans in pigs. Vet Rec 80:292–297.

DUNSTAN, R. W., AND ROSSER, E. J. 1985. Does a condition like human pityriasis rosea occur in pigs? Am J Dermatolopathol 8:86–89.

FISHER, L. F., AND OLANDER, H. J. 1978. Spontaneous neoplasia of pigs: A study of 31 cases. J Comp Pathol 88:505.

FLATLA, J. L.; HANSEN, M. A.; AND SLAGSVOLD, P. 1961. Dermatosis vegetans in pigs. Symptomatology and genetics. Zentralbl Veterinaermed 8:25–42.

FRANKE, F. 1973. Aetiology of actinomycosis of the mammary gland of the pig. Zentralbl Bakteriol Parasitenkd 223:111.

GARCIA-CABALLERO, T.; GALLEGO, R.; ROSON, E.; BASANTA, G.; MOREL, G.; AND BEIRA, A. 1989. Localization of serotonin-like immunoreactivity in the Merkel cells of pig snout skin. Anat Rec 225:267–271.

GIBBON, W. J. 1962. Skin diseases. Mod Vet Pract 43:76.

GIBBS, E. P. J.; STODDARD H. L.; YEDLOUTCHNIG, R. J.; HOUSE, J. A.; AND LEGGE, M. 1983. A vesicular disease of pigs in Florida of unknown etiology. Fla Vet J 12:25–27.

GINTHER, O. J. 1965. Clinical aspects of *Microsporum nanum* infection in swine. J Am Vet Med Assoc 146:945.

GINTHER, O. J., AND AJELLO, L. 1965. The prevalence of *Microsporum nanum* infection in swine. J Am Vet Med Assoc 146:36.

GINTHER, O. J., AND BUBASH, G. R. 1966. Experimental *Microsporum nanum* infection in swine. J Am Vet Med Assoc 148:1034.

GOLOVIN, V. I. 1977. Outbreak of cutaneous necrobacillosis in swine. Veterinariya (Moscow) 54:56.

HANSEN, W. J.; FOLEY, C. W.; SEERLEY, R. W.; AND CURTIS, S. E. 1972. Pelage traits in neonatal wild, domestic and "crossbred" piglets. J Anim Sci 34:100–102.

HARCOURT, R. A. 1973. Porcine ulcerative spirochetosis. Vet Rec 92:647–648.

HARE, T.; FRY, R. M.; AND ORR, A. B. 1942. First impressions of the beta-hemolitic Strepotococcus infection of swine. Vet Rec 54:267–269.

HEAD, K. W. 1970. Pathology of the skin. Vet Rec 87:460–471.

HEATH, M. E. 1984. The effects of rearing-temperature on body conformation and organ size in young pigs. Comp Biochem Physiol [B] 77:63–72.

HEUNER, F. 1957. Weitere Beobachtungen uber das Auftreten der Bauchflechte (pityriasis rosea) der Ferkel. Tierærztl Umsch 12:354.

HJARRE, A.; EALERS, T. O.; ANDTHAL, E. 1952. Riesenzellenpneumonien bei Tieren. Schweiz Z Pathol Bakteriol 15:566–590.

HJERPE, C. A., AND THEILEN, G. H. 1964. Malignant melanomas in porcine littermates. J Am Vet Med Assoc 144:1129.

HUNGERFORD, T. G. 1970. Diseases of Livestock, vol. 7. Sydney: Angus and Robertson.

HUSTON, R.; SAPERSTEIN, G.; SCHOENEWEIS, D.; AND LEIPOLD, H. W. 1978. Congenital defects in pigs. Vet Bull 48:645.

JONES, J. E. T. 1980. Observations on the bacaterial flora of abscesses in pigs. Br Vet J 146:343.

JUBB, K. V. F., AND KENNEDY, P. C. 1970. Pathology of Domestic Animals, vol. 2. New York, London: Academic Press.

KATZ, S. I. 1985. The skin as an immunologic organ. A tribute to Marion B. Sulzberger. J Am Acad Dermatol 13:530.

KIELSTEIN, P., AND GOTTSCHALK, C. 1970. Eine Trichophyton mentagrophytes Infektion in einem Schweinezuchtbestund. Monatsh Vet Med 25:127.

KNUDSON, B. K.; HOGBERG, M. G.; MERKEL, R. A.; ALLEN, R. E.; AND MAGEE, W. T. 1985. Developmental comparisons of boars and barrows. II. Body composition and bone development. J Anim Sci 61:797–801.

KOEHNE, G. 1972. Microsporum gypseum dermatitis in a pig. J Am Vet Med Assoc 161:168.

KORNEGAY, E. T.; THOMAS, H. R.; AND BARTLETT, H. S. 1981. Phosphorus in swine. III. Influence of dietary calcium and phosphorus levels and growth rate on mineral content of hair from gilts or boars. J Anim Sci 52:1060–1069.

KRANTZ, G. E., AND DUNNE, H. W. 1965. An attempt to classify streptococci isolated from domestic animals. Am J Vet Res 26:951.

KRESSE, J. I.; TAYLOR, W. D.; STEWART, W. W.; AND EERNISSE, K. A. 1985. Parvovirus infection in pigs with necrotic and vesicle-like lesions. Vet Microbiol 10:525–531.

LE, K. M.; MADSEN, B. L.; BARTH, P. W.; KSANDER, G. A.; ANGELL, J. B.; AND VISTNES, L. M. 1984. An in-depth look at pressure sores using monolithic silicon pressure sensors. Plast Reconstr Surg 74:745–756.

LEAT, W. M. F. 1962. Studies on pig diets containing different amounts of linoleic acid. Br J Nutr 16:559.

LOMAX, L. G., AND COLE, J. R. 1983. Porcine epidermitis and dermatitis associated with Staphylococcus hyicus and Dermatophilus congolensis infections. J Am Vet Med Assoc 183:1091–1092.

LONG, J. R.; BRANDENBURG, A. C.; AND OLIVER, P. G. 1972. Microsporum nanum: A cause of porcine ringworm in Ontario. Can Vet J 13:164–166.

McCARTHY, P. H., AND HOWLETT, C. R. 1988. The shield of the domestic boar (Sus scrofa L.): Its gross anatomy, histology and possible function. Anat Histol Embryol 17:232–245.

McDERMID, K. A. 1964. Ontario certified herd policy for swine. Can Vet J 5:95.

McPHERSON, E. A. 1956. Trichophyton mentagrophytes: Natural infection in pigs. Vet Rec 68:710.

_____. 1960. Sarcoptic mange in pigs. Vet Rec 72:869–870.

MAGNUSSEN, H. 1928. The commonest forms of actinomycosis in domestic animals and their etiology. Acta Pathol Microbiol Scand 5:170.

MAIR, N. S. 1974. Actinobacillosis suis infection in pigs: A report of four outbreaks and two sporatic cases. J Comp Pathol 84:113.

MARCARIAN, N. Q., AND CALHOUN, M. L. 1966. Microscopic anatomy of the integument of adult swine. Am J Vet Res 27:765.

MEYER, V. H., AND DROMMER, W. 1968. Erbliche Hypotrichie beim Schein. Dtsch Tierærztl Wochenshcr 75:13.

MEYER, W.; SCHWARTZ, R.; AND NEURAND, K. 1978. The skin of domestic animals as a model for human skin with special reference to the domestic pig. Curr Probl Dermatol 7:39–52.

MILLER, R. B., AND OLSON, L. D. 1978. Epizootic of concurrent cutaneous streptococcal abscesses and swinepox in a herd of swine. J Am Vet Med Assoc 172:676–680.

MONTAGNA, W., AND YUNG, J. S. 1964. The skin of the domestic pig. J Invest Dermatol 42:11.

MONTIERO-RIVIERE, N. A., AND STROMBERG, M. W. 1985. Ultrastructure of the integument of the domestic pig (Sus scrufa) from one through fourteen weeks of age. Zentralbl Veterinaermed [C] Anat Hist Embryol 14:97–115.

MORGANTI, L.; BIANCHEDI, M.; AJELLO, L.; AND PADHYE, A. 1976. First European report of swine infection by Microsporum nanum. Mycopathologia 59:179.

MOS, E.; MACRUZ, R.; AND LENCI, O. 1978. Dermatomycosis caused by Microsporum nanum in a herd of swine. Rec Fac Vet Zootec 15:159.

MOULTON, J. E. 1978. Tumors in Domestic Animals, vol. 2. Berkeley: Univ California Press.

MOUNT, L. E. 1964. The tissue and air components of thermal insulation in the new-born pig. J Physiol 170:286.

MOWAFY, M., AND CASSENS, R. G. 1975. Microscopic structure of pig skin. J Anim Sci 41:1281–1290.

MULLOWEY, P. C., AND HALL, R. F. 1984. Skin diseases of swine. In Veterinary Clinics of North America, Large Animal Practice, vol. 6, no. 1. Philadelphia: W. B. Saunders Co.

MUNDAY, B. L., AND RYAN, F. B. 1982. Vesicular lesions in swine – possible association with the feeding of marine products. Aust Vet J 59:193.

NEW ZEALAND VETERINARY ASSOCIATION AND GENERAL NEWS. 1981. The Temuka incident. NZ Vet J 29:55.

NOBLE, W. C. 1981. Microbiology of the Human Skin, vol. 2. London: Lloyd-Luke.

NORDBY, J. E. 1933. Congenital melanotic skin tumors in swine. J Hered 24:361.

PARISH, W. E., AND DONE, J. T. 1962. Seven apparently congenital non-infectious conditions of the skin resembling congenital defects in man. J Comp Pathol 72:286.

PENNY, R. H. C. 1957. An unusual skin condition in the Pig. Vet Rec: 528–530.

PENNY, R. H. C., AND MUIRHEAD, M. R. 1986. Skin. In Diseases of Swine, 6th ed. Ed. A. D. Leman, B. Straw, R. D. Glock, W. L. Mengling, R. H. C. Penny, and E. Scholl. Ames: Iowa State Univ Press.

PENNY, R. H. C.; EDWARDS, M. J.; AND MULLEY, R. 1971. Clinical observations of necrosis of the skin of suckling piglets. Aust Vet J 47:529–537.

PERCY, D. H., AND HULLAND, T. J. 1967. Dermatosis vegetans (vegetative dermatosis) in Canadian swine. Can Vet J 8:3–9.

RANG, H. 1973. Quantitative und qualitative Untersuchungen an Mastzellen des Schweines. Zentralbl Veterinaermed [A] 20:546.

RASZYK, J., AND PILLICH, J. 1989. Immunologic skin tests in piglets. Vet Med Praha 34:275–286.

REYNOLDS, I. M.; MINER, P. W.; AND SMITH, R. E. 1966. Cutaneous conditions of swine. J Am Vet Med Assoc 152:182–186.

RHOAD, A. O. 1934. Woolly hair in swine. J Hered 18:371–375.

RICHARDSON, J. A.; MORTER, R. L.; REBAR, A. H.; AND OLANDER, H. J. 1984. Lesions of porcine necrotic ear syndrome. Vet Pathol 21:152–157.

ROBERTS, E., AND MORRILL, C. C. 1944. Inheritance and histology of wattles in swine. J Hered 35:14.

SCOTT, D. W. 1988. Large Animal Dermatology. Philadelphia: W. B. Saunders Co.

SIMON, P. C., AND STOVELL, P. L. 1969. Diseases of animals associated with Sphaerophorus necrophorus: Characteristics of the organism. Vet Bull 39:311.

SMEETS, J. F. M.; SNIJDERS, J. M. A.; AND GRUYS, E. 1989. Dermatitis in slaughtered pigs, studies on the prevalence, pathology and economic importance. Tijdschr Diergeneeskd 114:603–610.

SMITH, J. M. B., AND STEFFERT, I. J. 1966. Microsporum nanum in New Zealand pigs. NZ Vet J 14:97.

STANKUSHEVE, K.; SIMOV, I.; DENEV, I.; AND KORNU, M. 1968. Mycotic dermatitis in pigs. Vet Sb 65:3–5.

STRAW, B. E. 1985. Diagnosis of skin disease in swine. Compend Cont Ed 7:S650–S660.

STRAW, B. E.; SHIN, S.; CALLIHAN, D.; AND PETERSEN, M. 1990. Antibody production and tissue irritation in swine vaccinated with *Actinobacillus bacterins* containing various adjuvants. J Am Vet Med Assoc 196:600–604.

SVENSMARK, B.; NIELSEN, K.; WILLEBERG, P.; AND JORSAL, S. E. 1989. Epidemiological studies of piglet diarrhoea in intensively managed Danish sow herds. Acta Vet Scand 30:55–62.

SWIERGIEL, A. H. 1988. Effect of changes in scrotal temperature on food intake in pigs. Comp Biochem Physiol [A] 89:323–327.

SWIERGIEL, A. H., AND INGRAM, D. L. 1987. Effect of localized changes in scrotal and trunk skin temperature on the demand for radiant heat by pigs. Physiol Behav 40:523–526.

TEREDESAI, A. 1974. Kongenitale Histioztyose der Haut beim Ferkel. Berl Munch Tierærtzl Wochenschr 87:253.

WEBB, R. F., AND BOURKE, C. A. 1987. Dermatosis vegetans in pigs. Aust Vet J 64:287–288.

WELLMAN, G. 1963. Weitere Beobachtungen uber die Erblichkeit der Disposition zur Bauchflechte (pityriasis rosea) der Ferkel. Berl Munch Tieraerztl Wochenschr 76:107.

WINDSOR, R. S. 1973. Actinobacillosis equuli infection in a litter of pigs and a review of previous reports of similar infections. Vet Rec 92:178.

WITZ, W. M., AND BEESON, W. M. 1951. The physiological effects of a fat-deficient diet on the pig. J Anim Sci 10:112.

WORDEN, A. 1965. Nutritional influences on the skin of domestic animals. In Comparative Physiology and Pathology of the Skin. Ed. A. J. Rook and G. S. Walton. Oxford: Blackwell Scientific Publications, p. 261.

YASON, C. V., AND NOVILLA, M.N. 1984. Clinical and pathologic features of experimental Schistosoma japonicum infection in pigs. Vet Parasitol 17:47–64.

10 Urinary System

J. E. T. Jones

THE KIDNEYS are brown, bean-shaped, smooth-surfaced organs; they are not lobate, although sometimes there may be some shallow grooves on the surface. They weigh between 0.5 and 0.65% of total body weight. They are located beneath the psoas muscles, ventral to the first four lumbar vertebrae. One, usually the left, is often cranial to the other. In the middle of the medial border is the hilus where the blood vessels, lymphatics, nerves, and ureter enter or leave the kidney; near each hilus is the renal lymph node.

The renal cortex is about 1.5–2 times the thickness of the medulla. The medulla consists of numerous pyramids that form single or aggregate papillae; the latter arise from the fusion of 2–5 pyramids. There are 8–12 papillae, each being related to a minor calyx. There are two major calyces that, with the cavity forming the origin of the ureter, make up the renal pelvis.

The ureter of each side leaves the kidney at the hilus and follows a caudal course, ultimately penetrating the neck of the bladder, passing obliquely through the wall, and opening to the mucosa at the ureteric orifices.

The bladder is capable of considerable distension and, when full, is in the abdomen, resting on the ventral abdominal wall. At the apex of the bladder is scar tissue that is a remnant of the urachus, the tube connecting the fetal bladder to the allantoic sac. The bladder is supported by one median and two lateral ligaments.

In the adult female the urethra is 6–8 cm long and enters the floor of the genital tract at the junction of the vagina and the vestibule at the external urethral orifice; on the floor of this orifice is the suburethral diverticulum. The external urethral orifice in the sow is about 9 cm from the vulva. In the male the short proximal part of the urethra begins at the internal urethral orifice and ends at the entrance of each ductus deferens. The short part of the urethra transports urine only; but the longer part, beginning at the ischiatic arch and incorporated in the shaft of the penis, transports urine and semen. The urethra terminates at the slitlike external orifice at the tip of the penis. The anatomic features of the penis and prepuce are described elsewhere, but it may be noted here that in the dorsal wall of the prepuce is the curious preputial diverticulum. Its function is not known, but it contains a foul-smelling urinelike fluid, epithelial debris, and frequently spermatozoa. It has considerable bacterial flora, some of which may be associated with urinary tract infection.

MORPHOLOGIC FEATURES. The functional unit of the kidney is the uriniferous tubule consisting of a nephron and a collecting tubule. The nephron is concerned with the formation of urine, and the collecting tubule conveys the urine to the renal pelvis. The nephron consists of a renal corpuscle and a tubular component. The corpuscle is formed from a tuft of capillaries, the glomerulus, and a double-walled envelope of squamous epithelium—the capsule; the space between the walls of the capsule is continuous with the lumen of the tubule.

The tubular part of the nephron has three segments, the proximal convoluted tubule, the loop of the tubule, and the distal convoluted tubule. The epithelium of the tubule shows functional differentiation. In the proximal tubule the cells are cuboidal and have a brush border of microvilli. There is an abrupt change from cuboidal to squamous epithelium at the junction of the straight part of the proximal tubule and the descending thin limb. In the ascending thick limb, the height of the epithelium increases. The epithelium of the distal convolution is lower than in the proximal convolution. In the small collecting tubules the epithelium is cuboidal, but as these tubules become larger, it changes to columnar. The mucous membrane of the renal pelvis, ureters, and bladder is covered by transitional epithelium.

PHYSIOLOGY. The kidneys eliminate the end products of metabolism—particularly the nitrogenous products, urea, creatinine, and ammonia—and maintain homeostasis by selective excretion of water and solutes. Excretion of metabolites is achieved by glomerular filtration. Control of the variation in fluid volume and solute concentration is a function of the tubular activity in reabsorbing water and solutes from the glomerular filtrate such as glucose, fixed cations, and amino acids, thus ensuring conservation of these substances. The kidney eliminates excess hydrogen ions and contributes to the maintenance of the correct pH of body fluids; it also excretes complex organic compounds. It produces two endocrine substances—erythropoietin, which plays a part in hematopoiesis, and renin, which is concerned with regulation of aldosterone secreted by the adrenal cortex.

Integration of renal function is achieved by interrelated nervous and endocrine mechanisms. Important endocrine factors include antidiuretic hormone (lysine vasopressin), steroid secretions of the adrenal cortex, and parathyroid hormone. For detailed information on renal function see Gans and Mercer (1977).

Urine. The amount of urine excreted daily varies with body size and particularly with systems of management employed insofar as these determine water intake. For example, sows housed in groups that have free access to water excrete more urine than sows in stalls that may drink only twice a day. According to Ellenberger and Scheunert (1925) the daily output of urine in adult pigs is 2–6 liters, but Green (1944) and Jeffcott et al. (1967) reported higher volumes.

Glomerular filtration rate (GFR) has been estimated as averaging 5 ml/minute/kg body weight in Minnesota miniature pigs (Munsick et al. 1958). In anesthetized, female, Pitman-Moore miniature pigs, Suarez et al. (1968) recorded a value of 3.5 ml/minute/kg body weight for the GFR and estimated the basal urine flow rate at 0.31–0.57 ml/minute. In the same pigs, urine osmolarity ranged between 253 and 994 mOsmol/kg H_2O. The specific gravity of urine is between 1.01 and 1.05; the pH is usually between 5.5 and 7.7, with a mean of 6.4 (the pH of the fluid in the preputial diverticulum is about 8.5–9.0).

A knowledge of urine protein concentrations is of special interest when considering the possible significance of proteinuria in disease. Physiologic proteinuria occurs in piglets and reaches a peak within 20 hours of birth and lasts for 48 hours (Loh et al. 1972). A decrease in protein levels after this period coincides with gut closure to intact proteins. During the period of proteinuria there is a direct relationship between urinary protein output and serum protein levels. In pigs between 1 and 20 weeks of age, urine protein levels are between 22 and 54 mg/100 ml. In the same investigation Loh et al. (1972) found that sows housed in groups with free access to water had urine protein concentrations of 6.2 (±2.1) mg/100 ml, whereas in sows kept in stalls the concentration was twice as much at 12.9 (±2.9) mg/100 ml.

Renal Function Tests. These tests are seldom employed in clinical investigation of disease in pigs. For some purposes, nevertheless, measurement of water ingested and urine volume over a given period could give useful information. Suarez et al. (1968) have investigated renal clearance of inulin, creatinine, and urea and provided data on urinary concentrations of sodium, potassium, nitrate, chlorine, and urea.

A renal-needle biopsy procedure, suitable for

following sequential changes in renal disease in the pig, has been described by Hatfield and Cameron (1975).

GENERAL PATHOLOGY. The urinary tract is subject to the same general pathologic changes as those occurring in other body systems.

Malposition of the kidneys is usually manifested as caudal displacement of one kidney, more often the left, to the pelvic region. Fusion of the anterior or posterior poles may result in the formation of a "horseshoe" kidney. Persistence of fetal lobulation is occasionally seen. Congenital bilateral hypoplasia and agenesis have been recorded in stillborn pigs (Mason and Cooper 1985) in Australia and were thought to be caused by a recessive gene defect inherited in a simple Mendelian manner.

Cystic kidneys occur more frequently in pigs than in other domestic animals. The cysts are located mainly in the cortex. There may be few or many, and they vary greatly in size, some being just visible while others may be several centimeters in diameter. Hydronephrosis is more common in adults than young pigs.

In some herds in which there is a high incidence of renal cysts, affected pigs may be the progeny of a particular boar. Wijeratne and Wells (1980) have shown that 60% of the progeny of matings between a Landrace boar and each of five unrelated Large White sows had renal cysts; such an incidence is compatible with autosomal dominant inheritance. The number of cysts may be determined by polygenic inheritance.

Degenerative changes in the renal parenchyma occur in many systemic infectious diseases and in various forms of poisoning, e.g., mercury and other metallic compounds, gossypol, ochratoxin A, and plants containing pyrrolizidine alkaloids, e.g., *Crotalaria*. In many of these conditions the degenerative changes may be accompanied by inflammatory reactions. Shirota et al. (1986) described glomerular lesions, found at the time of slaughter, in the kidneys of 96 of 100 pigs aged 6 months. The most frequently occurring lesion was mesangial enlargement accompanied by deposits of IgG and C3. The cause of the disorder was not determined.

Degenerative changes in the urinary tract are found in some cases of exudative epidermitis, a generalized dermatitis caused by *Staphylococcus hyicus*. These changes occur in the convoluted tubules and are accompanied by dilation of collecting tubules. There is epithelial hyperplasia in the collecting tubules and the renal pelvis. The epithelial cells undergo ballooning degeneration and desquamation. Uric acid crystals are present in the papillary ducts of the kidneys, renal pelvis, ureters, and bladder. In severely affected pigs, cysts develop in the kidneys, and the ureters become enlarged, possibly to more than twice their normal size; distension of the ureters is caused by mechanical obstruction by cellular debris.

Hemorrhage usually occurs in the form of widespread petechiae, which may be found in any part of the kidney, ureters, bladder, and sometimes the urethra in generalized bacterial infections, especially with salmonellae, streptococci, and *Erysipelothrix rhusiopathiae*. Petechiae are very commonly seen in hog cholera (HC) and African swine fever (ASF).

Infarcts in the kidney may be caused by obstruction of blood vessels by bacterial aggregates but are more especially seen as embolic manifestations of endocarditis. Bilateral cortical necrosis has been seen occasionally in pigs affected with HC; it may also occur as a consequence of endotoxemia.

Perirenal edema may result from the ingestion of poisonous plants (e.g., species of the genus *Amaranthus* and *Crotalaria*) and mycotoxins.

Calcification is rarely seen in pig kidneys but may occur as a result of the ingestion of excessive amounts of vitamin D.

URINARY TRACT DYSFUNCTION. In pigs the principal signs of urinary tract dysfunction are changes in the volume of urine voided, frequency of urination, and presence of abnormal constituents in the urine. Frequency of micturition occurs in cystitis and pyelonephritis; in some cases there is polyuria. Anuria occurs in boars with urethral obstruction, a rare condition.

It is unlikely that changes in the volume of urine voided would be observed under farm conditions. Alterations in the character of the urine are easier to detect, but the opportunity of observing micturition is very much determined by the system of management. Thus it would be relatively easy to observe abnormalities in stalled sows but difficult in pigs housed in groups.

Turbidity of the urine may be due to the presence of cells or tissue debris, indicating an inflammatory reaction. Sometimes, turbidity is due to the precipitation of salts in the bladder, particularly yellow, amorphous phosphate; such material is not usually of clinical significance.

Hematuria is rare in young pigs, but in breeding animals it is one of the most important signs of cystitis and pyelonephritis. The urine may be red or brown and usually contains clots of blood, shreds of fibrin, and necrotic tissue. Blood may be present in the urine of sows because of damage to the urethral meatus during mating. The penis of the boar may be damaged at mating; blood may accumulate in the prepuce and be voided during micturition.

Pus in the urine (pyuria) is nearly always indicative of cystitis or pyelonephritis. Care must be taken to distinguish pyuria from vaginal pus originating in the genital tract, which may be flushed out by urine.

The urine of healthy pigs contains small quantities of protein, but except in newborn pigs, which have high concentrations, this protein is not usually detectable by ordinary tests for proteinuria; e.g., dipstick tests detect protein only when it is in excess of 20 mg/100 ml. Significantly raised levels of protein in urine indicate an inflammatory reaction in the urinary tract. However, care must be taken to ensure that the protein does not originate in the lower genital tract.

URINARY TRACT INFECTION. The urinary tract may become infected in the course of any systemic infectious disease if organisms are present in the bloodstream, e.g., with streptococci, salmonellae, HC, or ASF virus. When infection is confined to the urinary tract, it is usually the result of organisms ascending from the urethra and becoming established in the bladder, giving rise to bacteriuria. Symptomatic and covert bacteriurias are well-known events in humans, and a bacterial count in urine of 10^5 per ml or more is considered to be clinically significant. Very little information is available on quantitative aspects of bacteriuria in the pig.

Berner (1971) found that 10–50% of pregnant sows in three herds in which there was a history of puerperal disease had what he regarded as significant bacteriuria. *Escherichia coli* and enterococci were the organisms mainly involved; in several cases bacteriuria was accompanied by an increase in the number of cells in the urine. During the postpartum period, sows in which bacteriuria had been demonstrated during pregnancy developed puerperal disease; six sows having a history of sterility developed cystitis. Akkermans and Pomper (1980) maintain that there is a relationship between the occurrence of bacteriuria and increasing age, small number of pigs per litter, and infertility. According to Bollwahn et al. (1984) bacteriuria is commonest in the early postpartum period when sows may have endometritis; the endometrial lesions provide a nidus for infection of the bladder, possibly leading to cystitis. Berner and Jochle (1988) claim that genital tract infections, some of which lead to pathologic changes, are preceded by urinary tract infections.

Cystitis and Pyelonephritis. Cystitis and pyelonephritis result from ascending bacterial infection of the urinary tract and occur mainly in adults. Most reported cases have involved sows, but this may be a reflection of the relative number of each sex at risk. Cystitis and pyelonephritis are among the principal causes of death in sows (Biering-Sørensen 1967; Jones 1968).

ETIOLOGY. *E. coli,* klebsiellae, streptococci of various serologic groups, and anaerobic streptococci are often associated with ascending urinary tract infection, but the organism that has received most attention in this respect is *Eubacterium (Corynebacterium) suis* (Soltys and Spratling 1957). *E. (C.) suis* is a gram-positive bacillus that grows on blood agar in 3–4 days when incubated anaerobically. It is a common inhabitant of the preputial diverticulum of male pigs of all ages (Jones and Dagnall 1984). *E. (C.) suis* is found only occasionally in the vestibule of sows, but it may be that presently available cultural techniques are insufficiently sensitive to detect it at that site. The characteristics of *E. (C.) suis* are described in detail in Chapter 51.

Little is known about the conditions that predispose to ascending infection of the urinary tract. Possible factors to be considered include trauma to the urethra of the sow during coitus or at parturition, reduced water intake, infrequent micturition, failure to empty the bladder at micturition, high urinary pH, and change in composition of the urine. The role of water intake as a risk factor in urinary tract infection has been investigated by Madec et al. (1986). In a study of tethered, pregnant sows they found that the average daily consumption of water was 17 L (range 4–40 L). A low water intake resulted in crystalluria, proteinuria, and bacteriuria and therefore may predispose sows to the development of cystitis. They emphasized the effect of restricted movement on behavior and, particularly, on water intake; 20% of tethered sows spent more than 22 hours of a 24-hour period in recumbency, and this may result in decreased water intake. The account that follows deals mainly with disease caused by *E. (C.) suis* infection.

EPIDEMIOLOGY. *E. (C.) suis* cystitis was first reported by Soltys and Spratling in England in 1957. Since that time it has been observed in Australia, Brazil, Canada, Denmark, Finland, Germany, Hong Kong, Malaysia, the Netherlands, Norway, Switzerland, and the United States.

E. (C.) suis is frequently transmitted from the prepuce of the boar to the vestibule of the sow at the time of mating, but it does not usually survive in the vestibule for more than an hour or two. However, under some circumstances that are not understood, *E. (C.) suis* survives and ascends the urethra to reach the bladder where it multiplies and produces an inflammatory reaction. Clinical signs of cystitis may be seen as early as 3–4 days after mating or at any time in the ensuing 2–3 weeks.

PATHOGENESIS. In some cases, lesions are found only in the urethra and bladder, but in those in which infection has spread farther there may be unilateral or bilateral involvement of the ureters and kidneys. Carr et al. (1990) have shown that in acute and chronic pyelonephritis, the intravesicular part of the ureter is shorter than it is in clinically healthy sows. They postulate that this shortening leads to vesicoureteric reflux, which enables bacteria to ascend from the bladder to the kidney. They also consider that damage to the intravesicular ureter may occur suddenly, resulting in large numbers of bacteria and their products reaching the renal pelvis; acute renal failure may then develop. In cystitis the bladder usually contains blood-stained urine in which are suspended blood clots, fibrin, pus, and necrotic debris shed from the damaged mucosa. The presence and quantity of any of these abnormal constituents of urine will depend on the nature and degree of development of mucosal lesions. In recently infected sows, changes in the bladder may be minimal, the mucosa may be covered by mucus, and there may be discrete or diffuse areas of reddening. In more advanced cases most or all the bladder mucosa is involved in a hemorrhagic, fibrinous, or fibrinopurulent inflammatory reaction. Extension of infection results in the development of similar lesions in the ureters and renal pelvis. The ureters become thick walled and dilated, and the mucosa of the ureters and renal pelvis exhibit the same changes as those in the bladder. The disease may progress to involve the renal medulla and cortex. When this occurs, yellow bands of degenerating and necrotic tissue extend to the kidney surface, where they are seen as aggregates of yellow nodules or diffuse yellow foci, particularly prominent at the poles; such changes may indicate long-standing renal damage.

Histologically, the changes in all affected sites are those of degenerative, necrotic, and inflammatory reactions. It is often possible to observe bacterial aggregates adherent to the epithelium at any site in the urinary tract mucosa.

CLINICAL SIGNS. Clinical signs vary according to the severity of the disease. In mild cases appetite, thirst, and general condition may be within the normal range; the only signs may be the presence of some purulent discharge at the vulva and hematuria. In more severe cases there is inappetence, excessive thirst, polyuria, pyuria, hematuria, and rapid loss of body weight. Quite often, because of the difficulty of observing individual sows, the early detection of hematuria may not be possible, and the first sign of illness noted may be loss of body weight. Affected animals are usually afebrile. The most reliable diagnostic sign is the frequent passing of bloodstained, turbid urine.

DIAGNOSIS. In the live animal, diagnosis is based on clinical findings and microscopic examination of urine. In Gram-stained films of pus or necrotic tissue present in urine, large numbers of bacteria are usually seen. In many cases gram-positive cocci, in clusters or chains, are present along with *E. (C.) suis*. Cultural examination should be undertaken to isolate and identify the organisms seen microscopically. It is essential to incubate blood agar, inoculated with appropriate material, aerobically and anaerobically at 37°C. If *E. (C.) suis* is present, colonies will be evident on the medium incubated anaerobically in 3 or 4 days. If the presence of enterobacteria is suspected, the use of MacConkey's agar in addition to blood agar will be helpful. Rapid identification of *E.* (*C.*) *suis* can be achieved by the use of fluorescent antibody techniques (Schällibaum et al. 1976).

In sows affected with acute inflammation of the urinary tract, Stirnimann (1988) found evidence of normocytic, normochromic anemia, neutrophilia, uremia, hypercreatinemia, increased concentrations of alpha and beta globulins, and low concentrations of albumin and gamma globulins. These findings could form the basis of useful and simple diagnostic tests.

TREATMENT AND PREVENTION. If cases are detected early, treatment with an appropriate antibiotic, e.g., penicillin in *E.* (*C.*) *suis* infections, will usually be successful. However, in more advanced cases, although antibiotics may bring about abatement of clinical signs, there is a tendency for relapses to occur. For this reason it is often best to advise immediate slaughter. It is essential to isolate affected animals and to ensure that other animals in the herd are not exposed to the risk of infection.

There are no proven methods of prevention. In an attempt to prevent the establishment of *E.* (*C.*) *suis* in the urinary tract of sows at the time of mating, it may be worthwhile administering penicillin to the sow at this time and for a few days afterward. If the disease is economically serious, it may be desirable to use artificial insemination on a temporary basis. Since boars appear to be the usual source of infection, removal of suspects from the herd has been advocated. However, this does not seem justified because a high proportion of healthy boars are carriers of *E.* (*C.*) *suis*.

Other Infectious Diseases. Embolic purulent nephritis caused by renal localization of infection with corynebacteria, streptococci, staphylococci, or *E. coli* has been described by Weidlich (1954). Interstitial nephritis of infective origin has been reported by Larsen and Tøndering (1954). Neither appears to be of much economic significance.

Leptospirae have an affinity for kidney tissue. They localize in the tubules and interstitial tissue, and pigs may become urinary excretors for as long as 2 years (Mitchell et al. 1966). In the acute stage of infection grayish white focal lesions develop in the kidney. These consist of inflammatory cells that are predominantly lymphocytes, but monocytes and neutrophils are also present. In the tubules there is epithelial degeneration and cast formation. Jones et al. (1987) regard "white spotting" of the kidneys as an indicator of previous leptospiral infection but of limited value in identifying pigs that are shedding or carrying leptospires; some infected pigs do not develop macroscopic lesions in the kidneys. McCormick et al. (1989) have applied a DNA hybridization technique to detect leptospires in kidney tissue.

Kidney lesions in erysipelas include capillary hyperemia with plugging of vessels by inflammatory cells and bacteria, swelling and degeneration of endothelium, and arteritis. There may be embolic glomerulonephritis. Glomerulonephritis may occur as a sequel to chronic infection with the viruses of HC and ASF.

Stephanurus dentatus (kidney worm) is found mainly in tropical and subtropical areas and causes, among other effects, cystic and purulent lesions in the kidneys and ureters. Abscesses may develop in the kidneys. Hydatid cysts and *Cysticercus tenuicollis* may be found in the kidneys, but very rarely.

NONINFECTIOUS DISEASES

Urolithiasis. Occasional examples of urolithiasis are seen in pigs of all ages. In sows irregular small calculi may be present in the renal pelvis in association with pyelonephritis. A yellow amorphous sediment is sometimes found in the bladder of sows at necropsy. The sediment is largely phosphatic and seems to be of no clinical significance. In the live sow the presence of precipitated salts in the urine may give it a cloudy appearance. Microscopic examination of such cloudy urine will usually reveal the cause of turbidity.

In young piglets urolithiasis may give rise to neurologic signs (Windsor 1977). In the cases that Windsor described, newborn piglets were depressed and had splayed legs; they became paralyzed and comatose, then died. At necropsy, macroscopic abnormalities were confined to the kidneys. On section, large amounts of pink and orange deposits were present in the papillary region, and the pelvis and the renal tubules appeared to be blocked. Similar deposits were in the ureters and bladder; these were acid urates and uric acid. Basing his interpretation on earlier reports of uremia and urolithiasis from the United States (Madsen et al. 1944; Djurickovic et al. 1973), Windsor diagnosed acute uremia resulting from urolithiasis; the cause was not established.

Urolithiasis in older pigs, resulting in retention of urine, has been reported from Japan by Inoue et al. (1977). The uroliths consisted of calcium carbonate; associated changes in the bladder wall included degeneration of the mucosa and smooth muscle.

Tumors. In a survey of 3.7 million pigs at the time of slaughter, Anderson et al. (1969) found only 16 urinary tract tumors. Of these, 13 were nephroblastomas and 3 were renal carcinomas. In Japan, Hayashi et al. (1986) found 74 (0.007%) cases of nephroblastoma among 1,063,788 slaughter pigs and classified them as nephroblastic, epithelial, mesenchymal, and miscellaneous types. Two of the nephroblastic types had metastasized. Usually nephroblastomas are benign with no clinical signs.

REFERENCES

AKKERMANS, J. P. S. N., AND POMPER, W. 1980. The significance of bacteriuria with reference to disturbances in fertility. Proc 6th Int Congr Vet Pig Vet Soc, Copenhagen, p. 44.

ANDERSON, L. J.; SANDISON, A. T.; AND JARRETT, W. F. H. 1969. A British abattoir survey of tumours in cattle, sheep and pigs. Vet Rec 84:547–551.

BERNER, H. 1971. Die Bedeutung chronischer Erkrankungen der Harnwege bei der Entstehung von Puerperalstorungen und Mastitiden der Muttersau. DTW 78:233–256.

BERNER, H., AND JOCHLE, W. 1988. The role of urogenital infection on infertility and sterility in sows. Proc 10th Int Congr Pig Vet Soc, Rio de Janeiro, p. 306.

BIERING-SØRENSEN, U. 1967. Om den almindelige forekomst af cystitis og ascenderende pyelonephritis hos søer. Medlemsbl Dan Dyrlaegeforen 50:1103–1107.

BOLLWAHN, W.; V VOPELIUS-FELDT, A.; AND ARNHOFER, G. 1984. The clinical value of bacteriuria in sows. Proc 8th Int Congr Vet Pig Vet Soc, Ghent, p. 149.

CARR, J.; WALTON, J. R.; AND DONE, S. H. 1990. Observations on the intra-vesicular portion of the ureter from healthy pigs and those with urinary tract disease. Proc 11th Congr Int Pig Vet Soc, Lausanne, p. 286.

DJURICKOVIC, S. M.; GANDHI, D.; BROWN, K.; AND YOON, S. 1973. Urolithiasis in baby pigs. Vet Med Small Anim Clin 68:1151–1153.

ELLENBERGER, W., AND SCHEUNERT, A. 1925. Der Harn und seine Absorbderung. In Lehrbuch der Vergleichenden Physiologie der Haussaeugetiere, 3d ed. Berlin: Paul Parey.

GANS, J. H., AND MERCER, P. F. 1977. The kidneys. In Duke's Physiology of Domestic Animals, 9th ed. Ithaca, N.Y.: Comstock, pp. 463–492.

GREEN, W. W. 1944. Urine excretion by boars. Am J Vet Res 5:337–340.

HATFIELD, P. J., AND CAMERON, J. S. 1975. Renal biopsy in the pig. Res Vet Sci 19:88–89.

HAYASHI, M.; TSUDA, H.; OKUMURA, M.; HIROSE, M.; AND ITO, N. 1986. Histopathological classification of nephroblastomas in slaughtered swine. J Comp Pathol 96:35–46.

INOUE, I.; BABA, K.; OGURA, Y.; AND KONNO, S. 1977. Pathology of the urinary bladder in urolithiasis in swine. Bull Natl Inst Anim Health 75, pp. 29–36.

JEFFCOTT, L. B.; BETTS, A. O.; AND HARVEY, D. G. 1967. Nephritis in sows. Vet Rec 123:446–448.

JONES, J. E. T. 1968. The cause of death in sows: A one year survey of 106 herds in Essex. Br Vet J 124:45–55.

JONES, J. E. T., AND DAGNALL, G. J. R. 1984. The carriage of *Corynebacterium suis* in male pigs. J Hyg (Camb) 94:381–388.

JONES, R. T.; MILLAR, B. D.; CHAPPEL, R. J.; AND ADLER, B. 1987. Macroscopic kidney lesions in slaughtered pigs are an inadequate indicator of current leptospiral infection. Aust Vet J 64:258–259.

LARSEN, N. B., AND TØNDERING, E. 1954. Nephritis interstitialis leucolymfocytaria hos svin. Nord Vet Med 6:35–46.

LOH, S. W.; BOURNE, F. J.; AND CURTIS, J. 1972. Urine protein levels in the pig. Anim Prod 15:273–283.

McCORMICK, B. M.; MILLAR, B. D.; MONCKTON, R. P.; AND JONES, R. T. 1989. Detection of leptospires in pig kidney using DNA hybridisation. Res Vet Sci 47:134–135.

MADEC, F.; CARIOLET, R.; AND DANTZER, R. 1986. Relevance of some behavioural criteria concerning the sow (motor activity and water intake) in intensive pig farming and veterinary practice. Ann Rech Vet 17:177–184.

MADSEN, L. L.; EARLE, I. P.; HEEMSTRA, L. C.; AND MILLER, C. O. 1944. Acute uremia associated with "uric acid infarcts" in the kidneys of baby pigs. Am J Vet Res 5:262–273.

MASON, R. W., and COOPER, R. 1985. Congenital bilateral renal hypoplasia in Large White pigs. Aust Vet J 62:413–414.

MITCHELL, D. A.; ROBERTSON, A.; CORNER, A. H.; AND BOULANGER, P. 1966. Some observations on the diagnosis and epidemiology of leptospirosis in swine. Can J Comp Med 30:211–217.

MUNSICK, R. A.; SAWYER, W. H.; AND VAN DYKE, H. B. 1958. The antidiuretic potency of arginine and lysine vasopressins in the pig with observations on porcine renal function. Endocrinology 63:688–693.

SCHÄLLIBAUM, M.; HÄNI, H.; AND NICOLET, J. 1976. Infektion des Harntraktes beim Schwein mit *Corynebacterium suis:* Diagnose mit Immunfluoreszenz. Schweiz Arch Tierheilkd 118:329–334.

SHIROTA, K.; KOYAMA, R.; AND NOMURA, Y. 1986. Glomerulopathy in swine: Microscopic lesions and IgG or C3 deposition in 100 pigs. Jpn J Vet Sci 48:15–22.

SOLTYS, M. A., AND SPRATLING, F. R. 1957. Infectious cystitis and pyelonephritis of pigs: A preliminary communication. Vet Rec 69:500–504.

STIRNIMANN, J. 1988. Ergebnisse einiger Blutuntersuchungen bei Muttersauen mit akuter Harnwegsentzundung. Schweiz Arch Tierheilk 130:599–604.

SUAREZ, C. A.; GUERRERO, A. A.; MUSIL, G.; AND HULET, W. H. 1968. Renal function and nephron structure in the miniature pig. Am J Vet Res 29:995–1007.

WEIDLICH, N. 1954. Zur Kenntnis der embolisch-eitrigen Nierenentzundung des Schweines. Zentralbl Veterinaermed 1:455–468.

WENDT, M., AND AENGENHEISTER, J. 1988. Cystoscopy in sows. Proc 10th Congr Int Pig Vet Soc, Rio de Janeiro, p. 309.

WIJERATNE, W. V. S., AND WELLS, G. A. H. 1980. Inherited renal cysts in pigs: Results of breeding experiments. Vet Rec 107:484–488.

WINDSOR, R. S. 1977. Urolithiasis in piglets. Vet Rec 101:367.

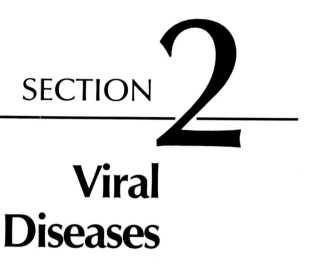

SECTION 2

Viral Diseases

W. L. Mengeling, EDITOR

11 Adenovirus

J. B. Derbyshire

THE FIRST ISOLATION of a porcine adenovirus was made from a rectal swab from a piglet with diarrhea by Haig et al. (1964). A second isolation was made by Kasza (1966) from the brain of a pig with encephalitis. Subsequently, porcine adenoviruses were isolated from a variety of sources, including stocks of hog cholera virus, swine feces, and kidney tissue used for routine cell culture production. Serologic surveys have indicated that adenovirus infections are widespread and probably ubiquitous in swine (Bibrack 1974). Strains of serotype 4 appear to be the most widely distributed, both in Europe and North America. While the majority of infections are asymptomatic, these viruses have been associated with encephalitis, pneumonia, kidney lesions, and diarrhea. Porcine adenoviruses are not known to be infectious for other species, although pigs can be infected with certain human adenoviruses (Betts et al. 1962), and some DNA homology has been demonstrated between porcine and bovine subgroup 1 adenoviruses (Benko et al. 1990).

ETIOLOGY

Physicochemical Characteristics. The basic characteristics of porcine adenoviruses resemble those of other members of the Adenoviridae. The roughly spherical, nonenveloped virions of about 75 nm diameter contain a genome of double-stranded deoxyribonucleic acid (DNA) surrounded by an icosahedral capsid of 252 capsomeres. Strains of porcine adenovirus type 4 hemagglutinate various species of red blood cells. The porcine adenoviruses are stable at pH 4 or when treated with chloroform or ether. They are relatively heat-resistant viruses, surviving for more than 10 days at room temperature (Kasza 1966). Effective chemical disinfectants for porcine adenoviruses include sodium hypochlorite, formaldehyde, phenolic compounds, ethyl alcohol, and sodium hydroxide (Derbyshire and Arkell 1971). In liquid manure, porcine adenoviruses are inactivated by aeration or treatment with calcium hydroxide (Derbyshire and Brown 1979).

Laboratory Cultivation. Porcine adenoviruses can be cultivated fairly readily in primary pig kidney (PK) cell cultures and in certain established porcine cell lines. Relatively high yields were reported from secondary pig thyroid cell cultures by Dea and Elazhary (1984a). In unstained cultures the cytopathic effects (CPE) are characterized by enlargement and rounding of the cells, followed by detachment; in stained monolayers characteristic nuclear inclusion bodies are seen. Ultrastructural studies of infected cells showed that the virus was intranuclear, sometimes in crystalline arrays (Chandler 1965).

Serologic Classification. The porcine adenoviruses contain the mammalian adenovirus group-specific antigen, detectable by immunodiffusion or complement fixation. Virus-neutralization (VN) tests have failed to reveal relationships between porcine adenoviruses and those of other species. Four serotypes of porcine adenovirus are currently recognized (Table 11.1) on the basis of VN tests, and there is evidence that additional serotypes may exist (Derbyshire et al. 1975).

Table 11.1. Serologic classification of porcine adenoviruses

Serotype No.	WHO Reference Strain
1	25R
2	A47
3	6618
4	F618

EPIDEMIOLOGY. Strains of porcine adenovirus type 4 appear to be the most widely distributed infection, with this virus having been identified either serologically or by virus isolation in Australia, Belgium, Bulgaria, Canada, Denmark, Germany, Hungary, Japan, the Netherlands, the United Kingdom, and the United States. Transmission of porcine adenoviruses is probably by the fecal-oral route. Inhalation of infectious aerosols may also occur. Virus is excreted in the feces, most frequently by pigs in the postweaning period (Derbyshire et al. 1966). Adults rarely excrete virus, but they frequently have high serum antibody levels. Nursing piglets are probably protected by antibodies in the milk of the sow.

CLINICAL SIGNS. The reference strain of porcine adenovirus type 4 was isolated from the brain of a pig that showed anorexia, enteritis, incoordination, muscle twitching, and frequent recumbency (Kasza 1966); other strains of the same serotype have been isolated from pigs with respiratory or gastrointestinal disease (Genov and Bodon 1976). Other serotypes have also been isolated from piglets with diarrhea (Coussement et al. 1981), but adenoviruses have also been isolated fairly frequently from the feces of clinically normal piglets. The only consistent clinical sign in piglets infected experimentally with porcine adenovirus type 4 was diarrhea (Shadduck et al. 1967), and infections with other strains have also produced diarrhea experimentally (Coussement et al. 1981). Although experimentally infected piglets may develop lesions in the brain, lungs, and kidneys, clinical signs associated with these lesions have not been described. In a study of two herds with respiratory disease, Watt (1978) concluded that porcine adenovirus type 4 may have been directly associated with the disease, and Kirkbride and McAdaragh (1978) reported the isolation of adenovirus from a small proportion of abortions in swine. Narita et al. (1985) found skin cyanosis and subcutaneous edema in newborn piglets with natural transplacental adenovirus infections.

PATHOGENESIS. Natural infection with porcine adenoviruses is acquired by ingestion or inhalation. Experimentally, intranasal inoculation of virus was the most effective route of infection in terms of the widespread distribution of virus and production of lesions (Shadduck et al. 1967). Experimental pathogenesis studies with various strains of adenovirus (Sharpe and Jessett 1967; Shadduck et al. 1968; Ducatelle et al. 1982) suggest that the primary sites of viral replication are the tonsil and lower small intestine. Spread of the infection to a variety of tissues, including the central nervous system, lung, heart, liver, kidney, and spleen, was recorded. Viremia was detected in one piglet. Viral excretion in the feces continued for several weeks after infection, and there was also evidence of persistence of the virus in the kidney and other tissues. Some limited findings suggest that adenoviruses may play a role in the pathogenesis of bacterial infections of the respiratory tract. Thus Kasza et al. (1969) found that porcine adenovirus type 4 and *Mycoplasma hyopneumoniae* produced a more severe experimental pneumonia when inoculated together than either agent did alone. However, Smith et al. (1973) found that the experimental pneumonia produced by porcine adenovirus type 4 was not enhanced by infection with *Pasteurella septica.*

LESIONS. Although most of the descriptions of lesions associated with porcine adenoviruses are based on experimental infections, there are several reports of adenovirus-associated lesions in field material. Porcine adenovirus type 4 was iso-

lated from the brain of a pig that showed lesions of encephalitis, including perivascular cellular infiltration and microglial nodule formation (Kasza 1966). Rondhuis (1972) isolated a strain of the same serotype from pneumonic lung. Pavlov (1977) described kidney lesions in pigs naturally infected with adenovirus. The lesions involved dystrophy of the kidney tubules and capillary dilatation, which gave the gross appearance of petechiation. Nuclear inclusion bodies have been found in the enterocytes of the terminal jejunum and ileum in natural infections (Ducatelle et al. 1982; Sanford and Hoover 1983). Transplacentally infected piglets showed vascular lesions, with nuclear inclusions in the endothelial cells (Narita et al. 1985).

In experimentally infected piglets gross lesions have been described only in the lungs. These consisted of areas of atelectasis of variable extent (Shadduck et al. 1967). Microscopically, the lungs showed interstitial pneumonia characterized by thickened alveolar septa due to proliferated septal cells, some of which contained inclusion bodies, infiltrating lymphocytes, plasma cells, and histiocytes. The histologic lesion produced most consistently with porcine adenovirus type 4 was a severe peritubular infiltration in the kidney, although meningoencephalitis, characterized by focal accumulations of microglia and oligodendrocytes within the brain substance and perivascular lymphocytic cuffing, was also produced by this virus (Edington et al. 1972). Brack et al. (1969) produced meningoencephalitis experimentally with porcine adenovirus types 1 and 3 and also described chronic inflammatory changes in the liver, heart, pancreas, and adrenal. In a sequential study of the enteric lesions produced by porcine adenovirus type 3, Ducatelle et al. (1982) described stunting of the villi in the lower jejunum and ileum and demonstrated infected enterocytes by histology, immunoperoxidase staining, and electron microscopy.

DIAGNOSIS. Clinical signs and gross lesions are minimal or absent in porcine adenovirus infections. Histologically, nuclear inclusion bodies in the lung, kidney, or intestinal epithelium may be suggestive of adenovirus infection, but they are not diagnostic unless viral antigen is demonstrated by immunofluorescence or immunoperoxidase staining. A virologic diagnosis can best be made by isolation of the virus from infected tissue, which can be fairly readily accomplished in porcine cell cultures. Some strains of the virus require several blind passages in cell culture before CPE are evident. Stained cover slip preparations of the infected cells show nuclear inclusion bodies, and the virions may be demonstrated by negative staining of lysates of the infected cells. The virus can also be identified by specific immunofluorescence of the infected cells (Dea and Elazhary 1984b). Serologic typing of the isolated virus may be attempted by VN if reference antisera are available. Serologic diagnosis of suspected adenovirus infections in swine may be attempted by the demonstration of rising titers of antibody in VN or immunodiffusion tests, or by an indirect fluorescent antibody test (Dea and Elazhary 1984b).

TREATMENT AND PREVENTION. No specific antiviral treatment is available. Porcine adenovirus infections have not been shown to be of sufficient economic importance to justify the development of vaccines, although adenovirus vaccines have been used successfully in other species. Repopulation of herds with specific pathogen-free stock does not appear to be a reliable means of excluding infection with porcine adenoviruses (Derbyshire and Collins 1971).

REFERENCES

Benkö, M.; Harrach, B.; and D'Halluin, J.-C. 1990. Molecular cloning and physical mapping of the DNA of bovine adenovirus serotype 4; study of the DNA homology among bovine, human and porcine adenoviruses. J Gen Virol 71:465–469.

Betts, A. O.; Jennings, A. R.; Lamont, P. H.; and Page, Z. 1962. Inoculation of pigs with adenoviruses of man. Nature 193:45–46.

Bibrack, B. 1974. Vorkommen und Verbreitung von klinisch inapparenten Virusinfektionen beim Schwein in der Bundesrepublik Deutschland. Zentralbl Veterinaermed [B] 20:193–196.

Brack, M.; Bernhardt, D.; Liess, B.; Bahr, H.; Rohde, G.; and Amtsberg, G. 1969. Untersuchungen uber pathogene Eigenschaften von Adenovirustammen des Schweines. Zentralbl Veterinaermed [B] 16:671–688.

Chandler, R. L. 1965. Demonstration of a porcine adenovirus by electron microscopy. Virology 25:143–145.

Coussement, W.; Ducatelle, R.; Charlier, G.; and Hoorens, J. 1981. Adenovirus enteritis in pigs. Am J Vet Res 42:1905–1911.

Dea, S.; and Elazhary, M. A. S. Y. 1984a. Cultivation of a porcine adenovirus in porcine thyroid cell cultures. Cornell Vet 74:208–217.

———. 1984b. Prevalence of antibodies to porcine adenovirus in swine by indirect fluorescent antibody test. Am J Vet Res 45:2109–2112.

Derbyshire, J. B., and Arkell, S. 1971. The activity of some chemical disinfectants against Talfan virus and porcine adenovirus type 2. Br Vet J 127:137–142.

Derbyshire, J. B., and Brown, E. G. 1979. The inactivation of viruses in cattle and pig slurry by aeration or treatment with calcium hydroxide. J Hyg 82:293–299.

Derbyshire, J. B., and Collins, A. P. 1971. Virological studies on an experimental minimal disease herd of pigs. Br Vet J 127:436–441.

Derbyshire, J. B.; Clarke, M. C.; and Jessett, D. M. 1966. Observations on the faecal excretion of adenoviruses and enteroviruses in conventional and "minimal disease" pigs. Vet Rec 79:595–599.

Derbyshire, J. B.; Clarke, M. C.; and Collins, A. P. 1975. Serological and pathogenicity studies with some unclassified porcine adenoviruses. J Comp Pathol 85:437–443.

Ducatelle, R.; Coussement, W.; and Hoorens, J. 1982. Sequential pathological study of porcine adenovirus enteritis. Vet Pathol 19:179–189.

Edington, N.; Kasza, L.; and Christofinis, G. J. 1972. Meningoencephalitis in gnotobiotic pigs inoculated intranasally and orally with porcine adenovirus 4. Res Vet Sci 13:289–291.

Genov, I., and Bodon, L. 1976. Vurkhu tipiziraneto i razprostranenieto na adenovirus i po svine. Vet Med Nauki 13:32–88.

Haig, D. A.; Clarke, M. C.; and Pereira, M. S. 1964. Isolation of an adenovirus from a pig. J Comp Pathol 74:81–84.

Kasza, L. 1966. Isolation of an adenovirus from the brain of a pig. Am J Vet Res 27:751–758.

Kasza, L.; Hodges, R. T.; Betts, A. O.; and Trexler, P. C. 1969. Pneumonia in gnotobiotic pigs produced by simultaneous inoculation of a swine adenovirus and *Mycoplasma hyopneumoniae*. Vet Rec 84:262–267.

Kirkbride, C. A., and McAdaragh, J. P. 1978. Infectious agents associated with fetal and early neonatal death and abortion in swine. J Am Vet Med Assoc 172:480–483.

Narita, M.; Imada, T.; and Fukosho, A. 1985. Pathologic changes caused by transplacental infection with an adenovirus-like agent in pigs. Am J Vet Res 46:1126–1129.

Pavlov, N. 1977. Morfologichni promeni v vuvretsite na praseta pri adenovirusna infektsiya. Vet Med Nauki 14:21–25.

Rondhuis, P. R. 1972. Some physicochemical and biological characteristics of an adenovirus isolated from a pig in The Netherlands. Tijdschr Diergeneeskd 97:841–851.

Sanford, S. E., and Hoover, D. M. 1983. Enteric adenovirus infection in piglets. Can J Comp Med 47:396–400.

Shadduck, J. A.; Koestner, A.; and Kasza, L. 1967. The lesions of porcine adenoviral infection in germfree and pathogen-free pigs. Pathol Vet 4:537–552.

Shadduck, J. A.; Kasza, L.; and Koestner, A. 1968. Distribution of a porcine adenovirus after inoculation of experimental animals. Zentralbl Bakteriol [Orig B] 207:152–157.

Sharpe, H. B. A., and Jessett, D. M. 1967. Experimental infection of pigs with two strains of porcine adenovirus. J Comp Pathol 77:45–50.

Smith, I. M.; Betts, A. O.; Watt, R. G.; and Hayward, A. H. S. 1973. Experimental infections with *Pasteurella septica* (serogroup A) and an adeno- or enterovirus in gnotobiotic piglets. J Comp Pathol 83:1–12.

Watt, R. G. 1978. Virological study of two commercial pig herds with respiratory disease. Res Vet Sci 24:147–153.

12 African Swine Fever

J. M. Sanchez-Vizcaino

AFRICAN swine fever (ASF) is one of the most complex viral animal diseases that affects livestock. It is caused by a DNA virus, classified tentatively into the Iridoviridae family (Matthews 1982). The porcine species are the only species found to be naturally susceptible to this disease. ASF produces clinical signs ranging from an acute form to a subacute and/or a chronic form, characterized by high fever, high mortality (in acute form), extensive hemorrhages in the internal organs, and functional alteration of the respiratory and nervous systems. (DeTray 1957; Sanchez Botija 1982). Clinically, ASF may resemble a variety of other swine hemorrhagic diseases, especially hog cholera (Maurer et al. 1958). Laboratory tests are required to establish a correct diagnosis (Sanchez-Vizcaino 1986). Immunologically, ASF virus infects macrophages, which are the main target cells (Malmquist and Hay 1960; Wardley et al. 1987). Humoral and cell-mediated immunity seems not to be affected, but most of recovered pigs are virus carriers even in the presence of antibodies. No neutralizing antibodies have been reported in animals recovered from natural or experimental infection (DeBoer 1967; DeBoer et al. 1969). However, infection-inhibitory antibodies have been observed in vitro from pigs recovered from experimental ASF virus infection (Ruiz Gonzalvo et al. 1986a). In these last animals, virus isolation from different tissues was negative.

The disease can course as an inapparent infectious form in warthogs, bushpigs, and giant forest hogs that act as reservoir hosts in Africa (DeTray 1957; Heuschele and Coggins 1965). ASF virus is also maintained in nature in ticks of the genus *Ornithodoros moubata* in Africa (Plowright et al. 1969) and *O. erraticus* in the Iberian Peninsula (Sanchez Botija 1963a).

There is no treatment or effective vaccine available against ASF, and the disease control is based on a rapid laboratory diagnosis and the enforcement of strict sanitary measures.

ASF was described for first time in Kenya by Montgomery in 1921, and since then it has been reported as endemic in the African countries of Angola, Zimbabwe, Sudan, Republic of South Africa, Mozambique, and Sao Tome and Principe.

1957 was the first time that ASF occurred outside the African continent, when it appeared in Lisbon as a peracute form with a mortality rate of almost 100%. In 1960 the disease reappeared near Lisbon, apparently as a new outbreak, and spread through the rest of Portugal, reaching Spain the same year (Polo Jover and Sanchez Botija 1961). Since then Portugal and Spain have been endemic until 1989, when most Spanish territories were declared ASF free.

Different outbreaks occurred in France in 1964, 1967, and 1974 (Larenaudie et al. 1964; Gayot et al. 1974) and in Italy in 1968 (Mazzaracchio 1968). In all these cases the disease was eradicated by application of a drastic slaughter program and restriction on movements of swine and pork products. ASF appeared in Cuba in 1971 (Oropesa 1971) and was eradicated in the same year after more than 400,000 pigs were slaughtered.

During 1978, ASF appeared in Malta (Wilkinson et al. 1981), Sardinia (Contini et al. 1982), and Brazil and Dominican Republic (Mebus et al. 1978). In 1979 an outbreak was reported in Haiti and in 1980 it reappeared in Cuba. In all these countries, except Sardinia where the disease became endemic in 1978, ASF was eradicated.

In 1982, ASF virus appeared in Cameroon, an African country where it had never been reported before. In 1983, a new outbreak was reported in northern Italy, and in 1985 in Belgium; in both cases the disease was eradicated.

Due to the lack of neutralizing antibodies in ASF, the correlation between a new outbreak and the possible source of virus strain has been very difficult to establish. Even the use of the hemadsorption inhibition reaction (Malmquist 1963) is not conclusive. New studies on molecular epidemiology, comparing the patterns of DNA from different ASF isolates, appear more promising (Blasco et al. 1989). However, it is epidemiologically well established that in an infected country, the new outbreaks are very much related to the movements of sick or carrier animals; in a noninfected country the appearance of outbreaks is related to the entrance of uncooked pork. International airports and ports where garbage containing uncooked pork can be found and used for pig feeding are clear examples.

ETIOLOGY. ASF virus is an enveloped icosahedral virus, with a double-stranded linear DNA of 170,000 base pairs (Enjuanes et al. 1976) that is terminally cross-linked (Ortin et al. 1979). At one time ASF was classified in the family Iridoviridae (Matthews 1982); however, because of its unique properties, a proposal to classify it as a mono-generic family separate from the Iridoviridae was accepted by the International Committee on Taxonomy of Virus in 1984.

Virus particles have an average diameter of 200 nm (Breese and DeBoer 1966), and are formed by several concentric structures with an external hexagonal membrane that is acquired by budding through the cell membrane (Carrascosa et al. 1984). ASF is a very complex virus; at least 28 structural proteins have been identified in the intracellular particles (Tabares et al. 1980). Recently, more than 100 proteins have been identified in infected cell cultures, and at least 50 of them react with sera from infected or recovered pigs. The identification of these proteins is important to clarify their role in protection. It has also been of great interest to produce more specific antigens for ASF diagnosis as well as to adapt new diagnostic tests (Sanchez-Vizcaino 1986; Pastor et al. 1987).

The presence of neutralizing antibodies has not been demonstrated in sera from naturally or experimentally infected pigs. However, there is evidence that suggests the inability to produce neutralizing antibodies might be due to the nature of the virus rather than to the host immunity, since recovered ASF virus pigs normally respond to foot-and-mouth virus vaccine, producing neutralizing antibodies (DeBoer 1967). Recently, infection-inhibitory antibodies have been observed in sera from pigs recovered from ASF infection (Ruiz Gonzalvo et al. 1986a). The role that these antibodies can play in the protection against ASF

infection has not yet been established.

In infected pigs, ASF virus mainly replicates in monocytes and macrophages (Wardley et al. 1987; Minguez et al. 1988) (Fig. 12.1), as well as in reticuloendothelial cells (Mebus 1988). No infection has been observed in T lymphocytes (Minguez et al. 1988); however, some functional alterations of lymphocytes in vitro have been reported (Sanchez-Vizcaino et al. 1981). In nature, ASF virus also replicates in some soft ticks, *Ornithodoros moubata* (Plowright et al. 1970) and *O. erraticus* (Sanchez Botija 1963a).

ASF virus has been adapted to grow in a large number of stable cell lines, such as Vero, MS, and CV (Hess et al. 1965). This facilitates molecular research as well as the production of a great quantity of diagnostic reagents.

ASF virus is very resistant to inactivation by environmental conditions such as temperature changes and acid pH. The virus can be isolated from sera or blood kept at room temperature for 18 months. However, it is inactivated by heat treatment at 60°C for 30 minutes (Plowright and Parker 1967), many lipid solvents, and many commercial disinfectants.

ASF virus may persist for several weeks or months in frozen or uncooked meat. In cured products, such as Parma ham, viral infectivity was not demonstrated after 300 days of processing and curing (McKercher et al. 1987). In cooked or canned hams, no infected ASF virus was found when it was heated at 70°C.

EPIDEMIOLOGY. ASF is endemic in many countries of Africa that are south of the Sahara. In Europe, the disease has been successfully

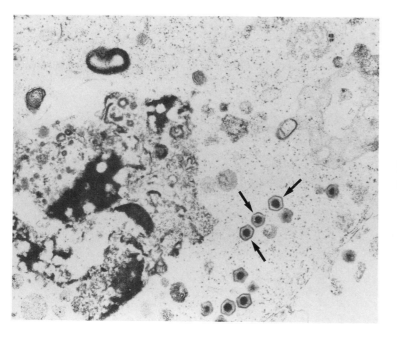

12.1. Swine macrophages infected with African swine fever virus. Several ASF virus particles (arrows) can be seen.

eradicated except where it remains endemic in swine in Portugal, Sardinia (Italy), and southwestern Spain.

Different species of soft ticks have been proved as ASF virus reservoirs and vectors, *Ornithodoros moubata* in Africa (Plowright 1969) and *O. erraticus* in the Iberian Peninsula (Sanchez Botija 1963a). In *O. moubata* a transovarial and transstadial ASF transmission has been described (Plowright et al. 1970). More recently, a number of other tick species widely distributed in North and South America have been found to harbor and transmit ASF virus (Groocock et al. 1980) and a new species in Africa can transmit ASF virus to pigs experimentally (Mellor and Wilkinson 1985).

Pigs are the only domestic animal species naturally infected by ASF virus. Wild boars have been identified as susceptible to ASF infection with clinical symptoms and mortality similar to those observed in domestic pigs in Spain and Portugal (Sanchez Botija 1982) and Sardinia (Italy) (Contini et al. 1982) and in feral pigs in Florida (McVicar et al. 1981). Infected wild and feral pigs can transmit the disease directly to domestic pigs.

In Africa, ASF virus induced an inapparent infection in two species of wild boars, warthogs (*Phacochoerus aethiopicus*) and bushpigs (*Potamochoerus porcus*), but the transmission of the disease from these animals to domestic pigs has not been successfully proved (DeTray 1957). However, ASF virus is maintained in Africa by a cycle of infection between wild boars and soft ticks (Wilkinson 1984). In some of these wild boars the ASF virus infection is characterized by low levels of virus in the tissues and low or undetectable levels of viremia (Plowright 1981), but it is enough for ticks transmission. In Africa, there could be areas with ASF virus but no clinical signs. This disease cycle makes it very difficult to eradicate ASF in Africa.

In European countries, where ASF is still present, no inapparent infection in wild or domestic pigs has ever been observed. Wild pigs are as susceptible as domestic pigs and their role in epidemiology is similar to domestic infected pigs. Recovered ASF-infected animals can be detected in these countries where they play a very important epidemiological role. The serological control of these animals has been very successful in the eradication program of Spain (Arias 1990).

It is generally accepted, from an epidemiological point of view, that the entrance of ASF virus into a free area is related to feeding swine with uncooked infected pork products from international airports and ports. Once ASF is established in domestic swine, infected animals are the most important source for further virus dissemination.

CLINICAL SIGNS. The clinical signs of ASF cannot be differentiated from those of other viral pig diseases, particularly those of hog cholera (Maurer et al. 1958). On the other hand, ASF presents different clinical signs, depending mostly on the virus virulence and route of infection, with clinical forms ranging from acute to subclinical to chronic. In Africa and in the Iberian Peninsula, the beginning of a disease episode appears mostly as an acute form, characterized by loss of appetite; high temperature (40–41°C); leukopenia; petechia and hemorrhages on skin, especially in ears and on flanks; and high mortality (Polo Jover and Sanchez Botija 1961; Mebus et al. 1983). Today, it is still possible to find an acute ASF outbreak; however, outside Africa, outbreaks are more frequently subacute or chronic, characterized by respiratory alteration, abortion, and low mortality (Arias et al. 1986).

Incubation periods for the natural infection vary widely from 4 to 8 days in short incubation periods to 15 to 19 days in the longest periods. In experimental infections, the incubation period is shorter and varies from 2 to 5 days, depending on the virus doses and route of inoculation.

PATHOGENESIS. Generally, ASF virus is spread in domestic pigs by oral or nasal secretions (Plowright et al. 1968; Colgrove et al. 1969). However, it has also been shown that the virus can be transmitted by a number of other routes, including tick bites (Plowright et al. 1969); cutaneous scarification; and intramuscular, intravenous, subcutaneous, and intraperitoneal injection (Kovalenko et al. 1965; McVicar 1984). Airborne spread has been demonstrated only under experimental conditions (Wilkinson et al. 1977). Primary infection usually starts in tonsils and mandibular lymph nodes and spreads via lymph and blood to the blood vessels, other lymph nodes, bone marrow, spleen, lung, and kidney, which are the main sites of secondary replication (Coggins 1974). The viremia in ASF starts between 6 and 8 days postinfection and is maintained for long periods, perhaps due to virus associated with the red blood cell membrane (Quintero et al. 1986).

The main target cells of ASF virus are the monocyte-macrophage phagocytic cells (Wardley et al. 1987; Minguez et al. 1988), but neutrophils (Casals et al. 1984), platelets (Nesser et al. 1986), and endothelial cells (Wilkinson and Wardley 1978) have also been described as target cells to the virus. No viral replication has been observed in T lymphocytes (Minguez et al. 1988).

LESIONS. A wide variety of lesions can be observed in ASF depending on the virulence, from peracute and acute forms, characterized by extensive hemorrhages in internal organs, to subclinical and chronic forms, in which lesions may be minimal or be absent (Mebus et al. 1983).

Peracute and acute ASF gross lesions are characterized by a septicemia with hemorrhages and enlargement of the spleen, hemorrhages in several other internal organs, intensive hydropericardium, hydrothorax, and ascites (Moulton and Coggins 1968). The main gross lesions are found in spleen, lymph nodes, kidneys, and heart (Sanchez Botija 1982).

The spleen may be darkened, enlarged, infarcted, and friable. Sometimes lesions are multiply infarcted on the edge with subcapsular hemorrhages. (Fig. 12.2). The lymph node presents large hemorrhages, edema, and a friable consistency. It often looks like a dark red hematoma, and in some cases, with congestion and subcapsular hemorrhages that in a cut section gives a marmoreal appearance. (Fig. 12.3). Kidneys usually present petechia on the cortical surface (Fig. 12.4) and cut surfaces, as well as in the renal pelvis. In some cases, an intense hydropericardium with serohemorrhagic liquid is observed in heart. Petechial and echymotic hemorrhages can be observed in the epicardium and endocardium.

Other lesions can also be observed in acute ASF, such as serohemorrhagic fluid in the abdominal cavity with edema and hemorrhages through-

out the alimentary tract. Congestion of the liver and gall bladder can be observed, as well as petechiae in the mucosa of the urinary bladder. Hydrothorax and petechiae of the pleura are frequently found in the thoracic cavity, and the lungs are usually edematous. Intense congestion is observed in the meninges, choroid plexus, and encephalon (Arias et al. 1986).

During the last 15 years, the most predominant form of ASF outside Africa has been the subacute form, which is similar to the acute form but with milder lesions. The subacute form is characterized by hemorrhages in lymph nodes and kidney and an enlarged and hemorrhagic spleen. Congestion and edema can be observed in lungs, and in some cases an interstitial pneumonia has been found (Arias et al. 1986).

Histopathologic lesions in the acute form of ASF are seen on vessel walls and in the lymphoreticular cell system. They are characterized by hemorrhages, necrosis and damage of the en-

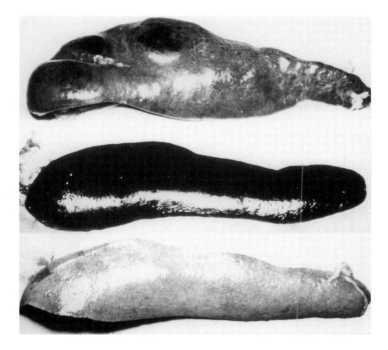

12.2. The top and middle spleens are from an acute and peracute ASF infection. The bottom spleen is from a normal pig.

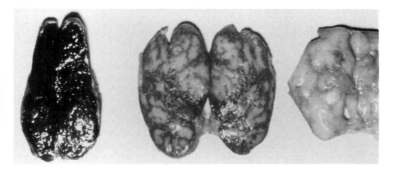

12.3. The lymph node on the left shows typical lesions from peracute or acute ASF; the center node is from an acute or subacute form; the node on the right is from a normal pig.

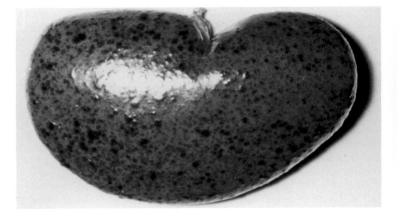

12.4. Kidney from acute ASF with extensive hemorrhages and petechiae on the cortical surface.

dothelial cells, as well as necrosis in the perifollicular, paracortical, and stomach areas of the lymphatic nodes and perifollicular red pulp of spleen and Kupffer cells in liver (Mebus et al. 1983).

The chronic form of ASF is characterized primarily by macroscopic and microscopic lesions of the respiratory tract, lymph nodes, and spleen (Arias et al. 1986). These include fibrous pericarditis and pleuritis, pleural adhesions, pneumonia (Fig. 12.5), and lymphoreticular hyperplasia. Necrotic skin lesions may also be observed (Moulton and Coggins 1968; Arias et al. 1986).

DIAGNOSIS. A fast and definative laboratory diagnosis of ASF is essential for two main reasons: the great similarity of clinical signs and necropsy lesions with those of other hemorragic pig diseases, and the lack of a vaccine. Therefore, control of this disease must be through eradication based on a fast laboratory diagnosis and strict sanitary measures.

As with other virus diseases, the laboratory diagnosis of ASF can be based on the demonstration of infectious virus, viral antigens, or specific antibodies. A wide variety of laboratory tests are

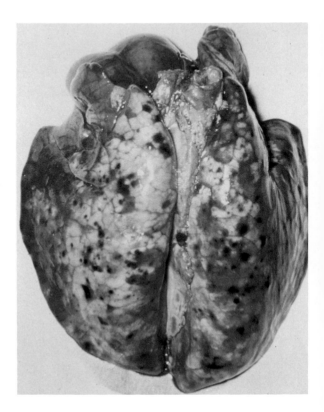

12.5. Lung from chronic ASF with caseous pneumonia.

already available for both ASF virus and antibody detection (Sanchez-Vizcaino 1986). Several techniques have been adapted to identify the ASF virus. Some of them, such as the agar double diffusion test (Coggins and Heuschele 1966), complement fixation (Cowan 1961), immunoperoxidase (Pan et al. 1978), ELISA sandwich (Wardley and Wilkinson 1980), electron microscopy, and more recently DNA-hybridization methods (Pastor and Escribano 1990), for one reason or another are not practical for routine or outbreak diagnosis (Sanchez-Vizcaino 1986). The most convenient, safe, and frequent techniques used at present are direct immunofluorescence (Bool et al. 1969), hemadsorption test (Malmquist and Hay 1960), and in some cases, pig inoculation.

Direct immunofluorescence (DIF) is the first test recommended when a new ASF outbreak is suspected. DIF is based on the use of conjugated immunoglobulin to ASF virus to demonstrate viral antigen in impression smears or frozen tissue sections from spleen, lung, lymphatic nodes, or kidney. It is a very fast and economical test with high sensitivity to the acute form of ASF. For subacute or chronic forms, DIF presents a sensitivity of only 40%. This decrease in sensitivity seems to be related to the formation of antigen-antibody complexes, which do not allow the reaction with the ASF conjugate (Sanchez-Vizcaino 1986).

The hemadsorption test (HA) is a universal technique used for ASF virus identification due to its sensitivity and specificity. This test should be performed to confirm any new outbreak, as well as when other tests have been negative. HA is based on the hemadsorption characteristics of ASF virus, which are induced when the virus infects macrophages and the attachment of the erythrocytes on the infected membrane cells forms a characteristic rosette around the macrophages and before the cytopathic effect appears (Malmquist and Hay 1960). Even though HA is the most sensitive test for ASF virus identification, it is important to point out that a small number of field strains showing only cytopathic effect without producing the hemadsorption phenomenon have been reported (Sanchez Botija 1982). These strains are identified using DIF on the sediments of these cell cultures.

Basically, inoculation is recommended to confirm the first outbreak in an ASF-free area, using two groups of pigs: one unvaccinated group and one vaccinated against hog cholera. After inoculation of both groups with the suspicious samples, the animals should be studied daily with respect to temperature, blood samples collected for HA determination, and sera for antibody detection.

Detection of ASF antibody presents a very special situation for two main reasons: first, the lack of vaccine antibodies and second, specific IgG antibodies are detectable in blood from 7 days postinoculation for long periods of time, even years. That is why ASF antibodies are recommended for the study of subacute and chronic forms, as well as being specially suitable for eradication programs (Sanchez-Vizcaino 1986).

Several techniques have been adapted for ASF antibody detection: complement fixation (Cowan 1961), indirect immunofluorescence (IIF) (Bool et al. 1969), immunoelectroosmophoresis (Pan et al. 1972), enzyme-linked immunosorbent assay (ELISA) (Sanchez-Vizcaino et al. 1979, 1982), radioimmunoassay (Wardley and Wilkinson 1980), and immunoblotting (IB) (Pastor et al. 1987). However, IIF, ELISA, and IB are the most frequently used.

The IIF test is a fast technique with high sensitivity and specificity for the detection of ASF antibodies from either sera or tissue exudates (Sanchez Botija et al. 1970). It is based on the detection of ASF antibodies that bind to a monolayer of cell lines infected with an adapted ASF virus. The antibody-antigen reaction is detected by a fluorescein-labelled protein A (Hortiguela and Sanchez-Vizcaino 1984).

Using both the IIF and IB tests, it is possible to detect from 85% to 95% ASF cases (acute, subacute, and chronic) in less than 3 hours (Sanchez-Vizcaino 1986).

At present, the ELISA is the most useful method for large-scale ASF serological studies. This assay is based on the detection of ASF antibodies bound to viral proteins by the addition of protein A, which is conjugated with an enzyme that produces a visible color reaction when it reacts with the appropriate substrate.

The IB test is a highly specific, sensitive, easy to interpret technique that has been used successfully as an alternative method to IIF for low or doubtful ELISA sera confirmation (Arias 1990).

Lymph nodes, kidneys, spleen, lung, whole blood, and serum should be sampled for ASF laboratory diagnosis. Tissues are used for virus isolation (HA test) and viral antigen detection (DIF test), while whole blood is used for virus isolation and the tissue exudates and serum for antibody detection (IIF, ELISA, IB).

TREATMENT. At present, no treatment or effective vaccine against ASF virus is available. Since 1963 when the first vaccine was used in Portugal, many efforts have been made in this area with unsatisfactory results. Inactivated vaccine is not protective and while live-attenuated vaccine protects some animals against the clinical effects of infection with the homologous virus, most become carriers and develop chronic lesions, especially if vaccination is on a large scale (Sanchez Botija 1963b).

Although pigs develop antibodies that can be detected by different techniques and humoral and cell-mediated immunity does not seem to be affected, virus-neutralizing antibodies have not been convincingly demonstrated (DeBoer 1967).

However, other studies have shown that serum from pigs resistant to homologous and heterologous virulent ASF virus inhibits the infection of different heterologous virus in vitro (Ruiz Gonzalvo et al. 1986a), even after the virus has been adsorbed (Ruiz Gonzalvo et al. 1986b). These antibodies were not considered as neutralizing because the immune serum must be present in the assay cultures during the test period. However, it is important to point out that no ASF virus was isolated from the tissues of recovered pigs where these infection-inhibition antibodies were detected. More work should be done to identify this immune mechanism and the role of different virus proteins involved in it.

PREVENTION. Since no vaccine for ASF is available, control of this disease in ASF-free areas depends on preventing the introduction of the virus. The epizootiological studies have shown that the most frequent source of ASF contamination has been from garbage of international airports or ports. It is clear that all food waste from planes and ships should be incinerated. Also, rapid laboratory diagnosis of any suspicious hemorrhage disease in pigs is recommended. It is important to remember that low-virulence ASF strains do not produce great lesions. Advanced preparation of an eradication program for disease-free areas is suggested.

In Portugal, Sardinia, and southwestern Spain where the disease is enzootic and where mild or inapparent clinical signs can be observed, the most important aspects to ASF prevention include the control of animal movements and to establish an extensive serological survey to detect and slaughter carrier pigs.

In Africa, the most important factor is to control the natural reservoirs (*O. moubata* and the warthog) and prevent its contact with domestic pigs.

REFERENCES

ARIAS, M. L. 1990. Personal communication.

ARIAS, M. L.; ESCRIBANO, J. M.; RUEDA, A.; AND SANCHEZ-VIZCAINO, J. M. 1986. La peste porcina Africana. Med Vet 3:333–350.

BLASCO, R.; AGUERO, M.; ALMENDRAL, J. M.; AND VIÑUELA, E. 1989. Variable and constant region in African swine fever virus DNA. Virology 168:330–338.

BOOL, P. H.; ORDAS, A.; AND SANCHEZ BOTIJA, C. 1969. The diagnosis of African swine fever by immunofluorescence. Bull Off Int Epizoot 72:819–839.

BREESE S. S., AND DEBOER, C. J. 1966. Electron microscope observation of African swine fever virus in tissue culture cells. Virology 28:420–428.

CARRASCOSA, J. L.; CARAZO, J. M.; CARRASCOSA, A. L.; GARCIA, N.; SANTISTEBAN, A.; AND VIÑUELA, E. 1984. General morphology and capsid fine structure of African swine fever virus particles. Virology 132:160–172.

CASALS, I.; ENJUANES, L.; AND VIÑUELA, E. 1984. Porcine leukocyte cellular subsets sensitive to African swine fever virus in vitro. J Virol 52:37–46.

COGGINS, L. 1974. African swine fever. Pathogenesis. Prog Med Virol 18:48–63.

COGGINS, L., AND HEUSCHELE, W. P. 1966. Use of agar gel precipitation test in the diagnosis of African Swine Fever. Am J Vet Res 27:485–488.

COLGROVE, G.; HAELTERMAN, E. O.; AND COGGINS, L. 1969. Pathogenesis of African swine fever virus in young pigs. Am J Vet Res 30:1343–1359.

CONTINI, A.; COSSU, P.; RUTILI, D.; AND FIRINU, A. 1982. African swine fever in Sardinia. In African Swine Fever. Ed. P. J. Wilkinson. EUR 8466 EN, Pro CEC/FAO research seminar, Sardinia, September 1981, pp.1–6.

COWAN, K. M. 1961. Complement fixation test for African swine fever diagnosis. J Immunol 86:465–470.

DEBOER, C. V. 1967. Studies to determine neutralizing antibody in sera from animals recovered from African swine fever and laboratory animals inoculated with African swine fever virus with adjuvants. Arch Gesamte Virusforsch 20:164–179.

DEBOER, C. V.; HESS, W. R.; AND DARDIRI, H. A. 1969. Studies to determine the presence of neutralizing antibody in sera and kidneys from swine recovered from African swine fever. Arch Gesamte Virusforsch 27:44–54.

DETRAY, D. E. 1957. African swine fever in warthogs (*Phacochoperus aethiopicus*). J Am Vet Med Assoc 130:537–540.

ENJUANES, L.; CARRASCOSA, A. L.; AND VIÑUELA, E. 1976. Isolation and properties of DNA of African swine fever (ASF) virus. J Gen Virol 32:479–492.

GAYOT, G.; CARNERO, R.; COSTES, C.; PLATEAU, F.; DECLOS, G.; AND CAZAUBON, P. 1974. Peste porcine Africaine. Isolement et identification en France metropolitaine. Donnees epidemiologiques, cliniques, anatomopathologiques et de laboratoire. Bull Acad Vet Fr 47:91–97.

GROOCOCK, C. M.; HESS, W. R.; AND GLADNEY, W. J. 1980. Experimental transmission of African swine fever virus by *Ornithodoros coriaceus*, an argasid tick indigenous to United States. Am J Vet Res 41:591–594.

HESS, W. R.; COX, B. F.; HEUSCHELE, W. P.; AND STONE, S. S. 1965. Propagation and modification of African swine fever virus in cell cultures. Am J Vet Res 26:141–146.

HEUSCHELE, W. P., AND COGGINS, L. 1965. Isolation of African swine fever virus from a giant forest hog. Bull Epizoot Dis Afr 13:255–256.

HORTIGUELA, O., AND SANCHEZ-VIZCAINO, J. M. 1984. Valoracion epidemiologica de la proteina A marcada con peroxidasa en el enzimoinmunoensayo indirecto para la deteccion de anticuerpos de peste porcina africana. Med Vet 5:269–274.

KOVALENKO, Y. R.; SIDOROV, M. A.; AND BURBA, L. G. 1965. Experimental investigations on African swine fever. Bull Off Int Epizoot 63:169–189.

LARENAUDIE, B.; HAAG, J.; AND LACAZE, B. 1964. Identification en France metropolitaine de la peste porcine africaine ou maladie de Montgomery. Bull Acad Vet Fr 37:257–259.

MCKERCHER, P. D.; YEDLOUTSCHNIG, R. J.; CALLIS, J. J.; MURPHY, R.; PANINA, G.; CIVARDI, A.; BUGNETTI, M.; FONI, E.; LADDOMADA, A.; SCARANO, C.; AND SCATOZZA, F. 1987. Survival of viruses in "Prosciutto di Parma" (Parma ham). Can Inst Food Sci Technol J 20:267–272.

MCVICAR, J. W. 1984. Quantitative aspects of transmission of African swine fever virus. Am J Vet Res 45:1535–1541.

MCVICAR, J. W.; MEBUS, C. A.; BECKER, H. N.; BELDEN, R. C.; AND GIBBS, E. P. J. 1981. Induced African swine fever virus in feral pigs. J Am Vet Med Assoc 179:441–446.

MALMQUIST, W. A. 1963. Serologic and immunologic studies with African swine fever virus. Am J Vet Res 24:450–459.

MALMQUIST, W. A., AND HAY, D. 1960. Hemadsorption and cytophathic effect produced by African swine fever virus in swine bone marrow and buffy coat cultures. Am J Vet Res 21:104–108.

MATTHEWS, R. E. F. 1982. Classification and Nomenclature of Viruses. Basel: Karger.

MAURER, F. D.; GRIESEMER, R. A.; AND JONES, T. C. 1958. The pathology of Africa swine fever. A comparison with hog cholera. Am J Vet Res 19:517–539.

MAZZARACHIO, V. 1968. L episodio di peste suina africane in Italia. Ann Inst Sup San 4:650–673.

MEBUS, C. A. 1988. African swine fever. Adv Virus Res 35:251–269.

MEBUS, C. A.; DARDIRI, A. H.; HAMDY, F. M.; FERRIS, D. H.; HESS, W. R.; AND CALLIS, J. 1978. Some characteristics of African swine fever viruses isolated from Brazil and the Dominican Republic. Proc US Anim Health Assoc 82:232–236.

MEBUS, C. A.; MCVICAR, J. W.; AND DARDIRI, A. H. 1983. Comparison of the pathology of high and low virulence African swine fever infections. In African Swine Fever. Ed. P. J. Wilkinson. EUR 8466 EN, Proc CEC/FAO research seminar, Sardinia, September 1981, pp. 183–194.

MELLOR, P. S., AND WILKINSON, P. 1985. Experimental transmission of African swine fever virus by *Ornithodoros savignyi* (Audouin). Res Vet Sci 39:353–356.

MINGUEZ, I.; RUEDA, A.; DOMINGUEZ, J.; AND SANCHEZ-VIZCAINO, J. M. 1988. Double labeling immunohistological study of African swine fever virus infected spleen and lymph nodes. Vet Pathol 25:193–198.

MONTGOMERY, R. E. 1921. On a form of swine fever occurring in British East Africa (Kenya Colony). J Comp Pathol 34:159–191.

MOULTON, J., AND COGGINS, L. 1968. Comparison of lesions in acute and chronic African swine fever. Cornell Vet 58:364–388.

NESSER, J. A.; PHILIPS, T.; AND THOMSON, G. R. 1986. African swine fever. Morphological changes and virus replication in blood platelets of pigs infected with virulent haemadsorbing and non-haemadsorbing isolates. Onderstepoort J Vet Res 53:133–141.

OROPESA, P. R. 1971. Reporte preliminar del brote de Fiebre porcina africana en Cuba. Inst Med Vet, Havana, Cuba.

ORTIN, J.; ENJUANES, L.; AND VIÑUELA, E. 1979. Crosslinks in African swine fever virus DNA. J Virol 31:579–583.

PAN, I. C.; DEBOER, C. J.; AND HESS, W. R. 1972. African swine fever: Application of immunoelectroosmophoresis for the detection of antibody. Can J Comp Med 36:309–316.

PAN, I. C.; SHIMIZU, M.; AND HESS, W. R. 1978. African swine fever: Microplaque assay by an immunoperoxidase method. Am J Vet Res 39:491–497.

PASTOR, M. J., AND ESCRIBANO, J. M. 1990. Evaluation of sensitivity of different antigen and DNA-hybridization methods in African swine fever virus detection. J Virol Methods 28:67–78.

PASTOR, M. J.; LAVIADA, M. D.; SANCHEZ-VIZCAINO, J. M.; AND ESCRIBANO, J. M. 1987. Detection of African swine fever virus antibodies by immunoblotting assay. Can J Vet Res 53:105–107.

PLOWRIGHT, W. 1981. African swine fever. In Infectious Diseases of Wild Mammals, 2d ed. Ed. J. W. Davis, L. H. Karstand and D. O. Trainer. Ames: Iowa State Univ Press, pp.178–190.

PLOWRIGHT, W., AND PARKER, J. 1967. The stability of African swine fever virus with particular reference to heat and pH inactivation. Arch Gesamte Virusforsch 21:383–402.

PLOWRIGHT, W.; PARKER, J.; AND STAPLE, R. F. G. 1968. The growth of a virulent strain of African swine fever virus in domestic pigs. J Hyg 66:117–134.

PLOWRIGHT, W.; PARKER, J.; AND PEIRCE, M. A. 1969. The epizootiology of African swine fever in Africa. Vet Rec 85:668–674.

PLOWRIGHT, W.; PERRY, C. T.; AND PEIRCE, M. A. 1970. Experimental infection of the Argasid tick, *Ornithodoros moubata porcinus*, with African swine fever virus. Arch Gesamte Virusforsch 31:33–50.

POLO JOVER, F., AND SANCHEZ BOTIJA, C. 1961. La peste porcina africana en España. Bull Off Int Epizoot 55:107–147.

QUINTERO, J.; WESLEY, R. D.; WHYARD, T. C.; GREGG, D.; AND MEBUS, C. A. 1986. In vitro and in vivo association of African swine fever virus with swine erythrocytes. Am J Vet Res 47:1125–1131.

RUIZ GONZALVO, F.; CARNERO, M. E.; AND CABALLERO, C. 1986a. Inhibition of African swine fever infection in the presence of immune sera in vivo and in vitro. Am J Vet Res 47:1249–1252.

RUIZ GONZALVO, F.; CABALLERO, C.; MARTINEZ, J.; AND CARNERO, M. E. 1986b. Neutralization of African swine fever virus by sera from African swine fever resistant pigs. Am J Vet Res 47:1858–1862.

SANCHEZ BOTIJA, C. 1963a. Reservorios del virus de la peste porcina africana. Investigacion del virus de la PPA en los artropodos mediante la prueba de la hemoadsorcion. Bull Off Int Epizoot 60:895–899.

———. 1963b. Modificacion del virus de la peste porcina africana en cultivos celulares. Contribucion al conocimiento de la accion patogena y del poder de proteccion de las estirpes atenuadas. Bull Off Int Epizoot 60:901–919.

———. 1982. African swine fever. New developments. Rev Sci Technol Off Int Epizoot 1:1065–1094.

SANCHEZ BOTIJA, C.; ORDAS, A.; AND GONZALEZ, J. 1970. La inmunofluorescencia indirecta aplicada a la investigacion de anticuerpos de la peste porcina africana. Su valor para el diagnostico. Bull Off Int Epizoot 74:397–417.

SANCHEZ-VIZCAINO, J. M. 1986. Africa swine fever diagnosis. In African Swine Fever. Ed. J. Becker. Boston: Martinus Nijhoff, pp. 63–71.

SANCHEZ-VIZCAINO, J. M.; MARTIN, L.; AND ORDAS, A. 1979. Adaptacion y evaluacion del enzimoinmunoensayo para la deteccion de anticuepos para la peste porcina africana. Laboratorio 67:311–319.

SANCHEZ-VIZCAINO, J. M.; SLAUSON, D.; RUIZ, F.; AND VALERO, F. 1981. Lymphocyte function and cell-mediated immunity in pig infected with experimental African swine fever. Am J Vet Res 42:1335–1341.

SANCHEZ-VIZCAINO, J. M.; TABARES, E.; SALVADOR, E.; AND ORDAS, A. 1982. Comparative studies of two antigens for the use in the indirect ELISA test for the detection of ASF antibodies. In African Swine Fever. Ed. P. J. Wilkinson. EUR 8466 EN Proc CEC/FAO research seminar, Sardinia, September 1981, pp. 195–325.

TABARES, E.; MARCOTEGUI, M. A.; FERNANDEZ, M.; SANCHEZ BOTIJA, C. 1980. Proteins specified by African swine fever virus. I. Analysis of viral structural proteins and antigenic properties. Arch Virol 66:107–117.

WARDLEY, R., AND WILKINSON, P. J. 1980. Detection of African swine fever antigen and antibody by radioimmunoassay. Vet Microbiol 5:169–176.

WARDLEY, R. C.; NORLEY, S. G.; MARTINS, C. V.; AND LAWMAN, M. J. 1987. The host response to African swine fever virus. Prog Med Virol 34:180–192.

WILKINSON, P. J. 1984. The persistence of African swine fever in Africa and the Mediterranean. Prev Vet Med 2:71–82.

WILKINSON, P. J.; DONALDSON, A. I.; GREIG, A.; AND BRUCE, W. 1977. Transmission studies with African swine fever virus. Infections of pigs by airborne virus. J Comp Pathol 87:487–495.

WILKINSON, P. J., AND WARDLEY, R. C. 1978. The replication of ASFV in pig endothelial cells. Br Vet J 134:280–282.

WILKINSON, P. J.; WARDLEY, R. C.; AND WILLIAMS, S. M. 1981. African swine fever (Malta/78) in pigs. J Comp Pathol 91:277–284.

13 Blue Eye Disease

A. H. Stephano

BLUE EYE (BE) is a disease of swine associated with a paramyxovirus infection, characterized by central nervous disorders, reproductive failure, and corneal opacity.

In 1980 the disease was reported in central Mexico with numerous outbreaks of encephalitis and corneal opacity in piglets, from which a hemagglutinating virus was isolated (Stephano et al. 1981). This virus was identified as a member of the genus *Paramyxovirus* (Stephano and Gay 1983, 1984, 1985a) and was shown not to be serologically related to previously described paramyxoviruses (Stephano et al. 1986a). The virus was named the "blue eye paramyxovirus" (BEP).

Members of the *Paramyxovirus* genus have been isolated from pigs in other countries. In Japan (Sasahara et al. 1954) the hemagglutinating virus of Japan or Sendai virus was isolated from pigs with porcine influenza and encephalitis; this virus proved to be pathogenic for pigs, producing central nervous system, respiratory, and reproductive disorders. In Canada (Greig et al. 1971) a paramyxovirus was isolated from the brain of a pig in outbreaks of hemagglutinating encephalomyelitis virus; this virus was not able to produce signs and lesions in experimentally inoculated piglets. In Israel (Lipkind et al. 1986) a paramyxovirus was isolated from nasal swabs of apparently healthy pigs before slaughter.

The first reported outbreak of BE was observed on a commercial farm with 2500 sows located in La Piedad, Michoacan, Mexico. That year similar outbreaks were observed on other farms in the same area, as well as in the states of Jalisco and Guanajuato. Since then, the disease has become economically important in Mexico and has been diagnosed in the states of Nuevo Leon, Hidalgo, Tlaxcala, Estado de Mexico, Federal District, Queretaro, Tamaulipas, Puebla, and Campeche. Pigs with BE lesions were identified in slaughterhouses in the states of Tabasco and Yucatan. These pigs apparently were brought from central Mexico, but no clinical outbreaks have been identified in these states. In the states of Tamaulipas and Campeche, no new cases have been observed since 1984 and 1988 respectively. The main focus of the disease, however, is in central Mexico in the states of Michoacan, Jalisco, and Guanajuato where there is a dense population of pigs (Stephano et al. 1988a).

Differences in clinical signs have become evident. In 1980 mainly piglets were affected. Mortality and nervous system disorders in pigs older than 30 days were uncommon. Since 1983, however, severe outbreaks of encephalitis with high mortality in pigs 15–45 kg of body weight have been observed frequently on badly managed farms with concomitant disease (Stephano and Gay 1985b, 1986a). It was not until 1983 that reproductive failure in sows and transient infertility in boars were identified (Stephano and Gay 1985a). In 1988 severe problems of orchitis, epididymitis, and testiclar atrophy in boars became evident (Campos and Carbajal 1989; Stephano et al. 1990). Differences in strain virulences have been described (Gay and Stephano 1987).

This disease has not been reported elsewhere.

ETIOLOGY. BEP replicates and produces cytopathic effects in a wide variety of cell cultures, and agglutinates erythrocytes of both mammalian and avian origin (Stephano and Gay 1985a; Moreno-Lopez et al. 1986; Stephano et al. 1986a).

Size and Morphology. Electron microscopic examination of BEP has demonstrated particles similar to paramyxovirus, measuring from 135–148 nm to 257–360 nm. The virion is pleomorphic but usually more or less spherical; no filamentous forms have been observed. The envelope is covered with a layer of closely spaced surface projections or spikes. Nucleocapsids from disrupted virus particles are frequently seen as a single entity with a diameter of 20 nm and a length of 1000–1630 nm or more.

Biologic Properties and Replication. The BEP has been grown with cytopathic effect in monolayer cultures of pig kidney (PK), bovine thyroid, bovine embryo, equine dermis, swine testicle, cat kidney, baby hamster kidney-21, and Vero cells. In monolayer cultures of primary PK cells and cells of an established PK cell line (PK-15), the cytopathic effects start between 24 and 48 hours after inoculation and are complete between 5 and 7 days. They consist of individual rounded cells, cytoplasmic vacuoles, and syncytia; dead cells detach, leaving small plaques. In PK-15 cells the virus was seen free in the cytoplasm and within vesicles. Some cells also contained viral inclusion bodies (Stephano and Gay 1985a; Stephano et al. 1986a). Cytopathic effect

237

also has been observed in other types of monolayer cell cultures of porcine origin (turbinate, choroid plexus), as well as in monolayer cell cultures of bovine (turbinate, kidney, testicle, skin, palatine, choroid plexus), monkey (GMK), mink (lung), and human (fetal) origin. Syncytia were observed in BEP-infected monolayer cultures of porcine turbinate cells and of bovine turbinate and kidney cells (Moreno-Lopez 1986). The chick embryo also supports BEP replication.

Hemagglutination has been tested in erythrocytes from chickens, guinea pigs, mice, rats, rabbits, hamsters, horses, pigs, goats, cats, and dogs, as well as in the four groups (A, B, AB, and O) of human erythrocytes. Spontaneous elution at 37°C occurred after 30–60 minutes. The infected PK-15 cells are also positive to hemadsorption with chicken erythrocytes (Stephano and Gay 1985a; Stephano et al. 1986a).

Physicochemical Properties. The infectivity of the virus is abolished by treatment with ether, chloroform, formalin, and beta propiolactone, but it is resistant to actinomycin D. Formalin treatment inactivated both the replication activity and the hemagglutination properties. Virus inactivation is detected at 56°C after 4 hours of heat treatment. The virus has a buoyant density of 1.21 g/ml in sucrose gradients (Stephano and Gay 1985a).

Serology. Antiserum prepared against paramyxovirus 1, 2, 3, 4, 6, and 7 and parainfluenza 1, 2, 3, 4a, 4b, and 5 do not affect BEP infectivity (Stephano et al. 1986a).

EPIDEMIOLOGY. Pigs are the only animals that are known to be affected clinically by BEP when infected under natural conditions. Experimentally, BEP affects mice and chick embryos; rabbits, dogs, and cats do not have clinical signs, but rabbits produce antibodies (Stephano and Gay 1985a; Stephano et al. 1988a).

Subclinically infected pigs are the main reservoirs of BEP. The virus may be disseminated by people and vehicles, and possibly by birds and wind; other sources of infection have not been demonstrated.

The disease is apparently self-limiting in closed herds. Sentinel pigs introduced to the farm 6–12 months after an outbreak remain asymptomatic and do not produce antibodies against BEP (Stephano and Gay 1986b; Stephano et al. 1986b).

Naturally infected animals develop antibodies that usually persist throughout their life. However, the disease can recur in susceptible progeny and when susceptible pigs are added to the herd. Farms with a continuous system of production may have cases periodically.

Blue eye is more common from March to July, which are the driest and hottest months of the year in Mexico, but outbreaks are observed throughout the year.

CLINICAL SIGNS. Blue eye may start in any area of commercial breeding units, but it is usually observed first in the farrowing house, with central nervous system signs and high piglet mortality. At about the same time, the farmer may observe corneal opacity in some weaned or fattened pigs (Stephano and Gay 1985a, 1986a; Stephano et al. 1988a). The mortality rate increases rapidly and then decreases within a short time. Once the initial outbreak is over, no new clinical cases appear unless susceptible pigs are introduced to an infected farm, as has been observed on farms that operate on a continuous-flow pattern.

The clinical signs are variable and depend mainly on the age of the pig. Piglets 2–15 days old are most susceptible, and the clinical signs are sudden in onset. Healthy piglets may suddenly become prostrate generally in lateral recumbency or show nervous system signs. But the disease usually runs a course that starts with fever, a rough-hair coat, and an arched back, sometimes accompanied by constipation or diarrhea. These signs are followed by progressive nervous signs of ataxia, weakness, rigidity (mainly of the hind legs), muscle tremor, and abnormal posture, such as a sitting position. Anorexia does not occur while the piglets can still walk. Some piglets are hyperexcitable, squealing and showing paddling movements when handled. Other signs include lethargy with some involuntary movements, dilated pupils, apparent blindness, and sometimes nystagmus. Some piglets suffer from conjunctivitis with swollen eyelids and lacrimation. Often the eyelids are closed and adherent with exudate. In 1–10% of the affected piglets, either unilateral or bilateral corneal opacity is present. Frequently, corneal opacity can be seen without other signs and is commonly resolved spontaneously. In the first cases observed, piglets usually die within 48 hours of the appearance of clinical signs, but in later cases, death occurs after 4–6 days.

Of the litters farrowed during an outbreak, 20–65% are affected. In these litters piglet morbidity is between 20% and 50% and mortality between 87% and 90%; mortality lasts from 2 to 9 weeks depending mainly on the system of management. Most of the sows of affected litters are clinically normal. Some of them show moderate anorexia 1 or 2 days before the appearance of clinical signs in the piglets, and corneal opacity has also been observed in the farrowing house during outbreaks.

Pigs more than 30 days old show moderate and transient clinical signs such as anorexia, fever, sneezing, and coughing. Nervous system signs are less common and less obvious but when present they consist of listlessness, ataxia, circling, and rarely swaying of the head. As in piglets, unilateral or bilateral corneal opacity and conjunctivitis continue to appear on the farm for another month without other signs. Only 1–4% of pigs older than 30 days are affected and mortality is generally low. Outbreaks with 20% mortality and severe central nervous system manifestations have been observed in 15- to 45-kg pigs; corneal opacity was present in up to 30% of these pigs (Stephano and Gay 1985b).

Gilts and other adult pigs also occasionally develop corneal opacity. In pregnant sows an increase in the number of animals returning to estrus is observed, which lasts 6–8 months. Abortion has been observed in some dams. During outbreaks, there is also an increase in stillbirths and mummified fetuses up to 24% and 12% respectively.

In herds affected by BEP, 14–40% of the boars show a reduction in fertility associated with an increase in the size of the testicle and epididymis. This increase is usually unilateral, and later, the testicle atrophies with hardening of the epididymus (Campos and Carbajal 1989; Stephano et al. 1990).

PATHOGENESIS. It has been presumed that the natural infection with BEP is acquired by inhalation. Experimental intratracheal or intranasal exposure by either instillation or aerosol are effective routes of infection, which result in clinical signs and lesions similar to those observed in natural cases. One-day-old piglets developed a nervous syndrome in 20–66 hours postinoculation; some weaned pigs (21–50 days old) developed a nervous syndrome at 11 days postinoculation, and pregnant sows developed reproductive failure when inoculated during pregnancy. The corneal opacity is also occasionally reproduced in these cases. The disease was also reproduced in susceptible pigs placed in contact with experimentally infected pigs for up to 19 days after experimental infection (Stephano and Gay 1983; Perez et al. 1988; Stephano et al. 1988b).

The initial site of replication has not been established; however, the nasal mucosa and tonsils have been suggested. The virus can be recovered from nasal and tonsillar swabs. Immunofluorescence is easily detected in these tissues in naturally or experimentally infected pigs. Also, the virus has been observed in the axon of neurons. From the initial site of replication, the virus spreads early in the infection to the brain and lung, since histological lesions and central nervous manifestation occurred early in the disease. The brain is the elected tissue for isolation and immunofluorescence.

The interstitial pneumonia observed suggests dissemination through the blood. In experimentally inoculated piglets, the virus could be isolated from the brain, lung, tonsil, liver, turbinate, spleen, kidney, mesenteric lymph node, heart, and blood. Brain, lung, and tonsil are the most common sites for isolation (Stephano et al. 1988a).

It is not clear how the corneal opacity occurs. It is not easily reproduced experimentally, but histologic lesions such as anterior uveitis are commonly observed in the cornea (Stephano and Gay 1986b; Perez et al. 1988). Usually the opacity occurs late in the course of the disease. The histological lesions and signs suggest it is due to an immunologic reaction similar to that produced by canine adenovirus hepatitis. Recent results indicate that the virus replicates in the cornea since intracytoplasmic inclusion body formation in the epithelial cells close to the corneo-scleral angle is observed in acutely infected pigs. The corneal opacity has been observed in pigs otherwise clinically normal and resistant to the infection, and it usually disappears after some period.

It has been suggested that the virus reaches the uterus through the blood. In pregnant sows this produces reproductive failure, with embryonic mortality and return to oestrus in the first one-third of gestation, and stillbirths and mummified fetuses when it occurs late in gestation (Stephano and Gay 1984). The role of the boar has not been experimentally studied, but infertility due to orchitis, epididymitis, and testicle atrophy associated with spermatic granuloma occurred.

The BEP infection has been commonly associated with pneumonia, especially *Actinobacillus pleuropneumoniae,* but experimental inoculation of BEP prior to infection with *Pasteurella multocida* types A and D does not result in colonization of the bacteria in the lung (Garcia et al. 1988).

LESIONS

Gross Lesions. There are no specific gross changes. A mild pneumonia is frequently observed at the ventral tips of the cranial lung lobes. Mild gastric distension with milk (in piglets), distension of the urinary bladder with urine, and small accumulation of fluid with fibrin in the peritoneal cavity are observed. Brain congestion and an increase in the cerebrospinal fluid also occurs. Conjunctivitis, chemosis, and varied degrees of corneal opacity, usually unilateral, have been confirmed. Vesicle formation, ulcers, and "queratocono" have been observed in the cornea as well as exudate in the anterior chamber. Recently pericardial and kidney hemorrages have been observed (Stephano and Gay 1985a, 1986b). In boars, orchitis, epididymitis, and later, testicle atrophy with or without granulomatous formation in the epididymus may be present (Campos and Carbajal 1989; Stephano et al. 1990).

Microscopic Lesions. The main histological changes are located in the brain and spinal cord.

There is a nonsuppurative encephalomyelitis affecting mainly the gray matter of the thalamus, midbrain, and cerebral cortex and characterized by multifocal and diffuse gliosis, perivascular cuffing with lymphocytes, plasma cells and reticular cells, neuronal necrosis, neuronophagia, meningitis, and choroiditis (Ramirez and Stephano 1982). Intracytoplasmic inclusion bodies are found in neurons. There are variations in the severity and extent of these lesions (Stephano and Gay 1986b; Perez et al. 1988; Stephano et al. 1988a).

The lungs have scattered localized areas of interstitial pneumonia characterized by thickened septa with mononuclear cell infiltration.

Changes in the eye are mainly corneal opacity, characterized by corneal edema, and anterior uveitis. Neutrophils, macrophages, or mononuclear cells infiltrate the iridocorneal endothelium, corneo-scleral angle, and cornea. The external sheet of the cornea is often with cytoplasmic vesicles and in some, intracytoplasmic inclusions are observed in the epithelial cells near the corneoscleral angle (Stephano and Gay 1986b; Perez et al. 1988; Stephano et al 1988a).

Many animals showed a mild tonsillitis with desquamated epithelium and inflammatory cells in the crypts.

DIAGNOSIS.   Clinical signs such as encephalitis, corneal opacity, and reproductive failure in the sow and orchitis and epididymitis in the boar are consistent with a diagnosis of BE. Additional diagnostic evidence is provided by histologic lesions such as nonsuppurative encephalitis, anterior uveitis, keratitis, orchitis, and epididymitis, and the presence of intracytoplasmic inclusion bodies in neurons and corneal epithelium confirm diagnosis.

Serological tests such as hemagglutination-inhibition antibodies (HI), virus-neutralization antibodies, and ELISA have been developed to identify positive animals. Until now HI is the most used test, but false-positive titers 1:16 have been detected when chicken erythrocytes are used or when the BEP antigen is grown in chicken embryos; guinea pig erythrocytes are recommended. Also DIF has been performed in tissue sections and monolayers, using a conjugate prepared with rabbit or pig serum (Stephano and Gay 1985a; Stephano et al. 1988a).

Virus is easily isolated by adding a homogenate or triturated suspension of brain or tonsil from infected pigs to the medium of monolayer cultures of PK-15 or primary porcine kidney cells. The virus-induced cytopathic effect is characterized by syncytium formation.

A differential diagnosis must include other causes of encephalitis and reproductive disease; especially Aujeszky's disease virus. Until now, only the BEP produces corneal opacity in up to 30% of pigs (Stephano and Gay 1985b; Stephano 1986; Stephano et al. 1988a).

TREATMENT.   As in most viral diseases of swine, there are no specific treatments for BEP. Antiviral drugs such as amantadine, isathiazone, or monensin have not been used. Once the clinical signs are evident, nothing can be done to modify the course of the disease. Pigs with corneal opacity frequently spontaneously recover while pigs with central nervous disturbances generally follow a fatal course.

Serum from sows of previously affected litters has been administered orally to piglets, apparently without effective results.

Antimicrobial therapy is commonly used to treat and prevent secondary infections. Medication is commonly used for controlling associated respiratory problems. Proper management such as providing a healthy environment and proper housing and nutrition reduce the detrimental effect of the disease in the herd.

PREVENTION AND CONTROL.   Health control programs are the most reliable method of preventing the entrance of BEP on a farm. Swine populations must be established or replaced from a healthy herd. Location is particularly important. Perimeter fencing, separate load-out areas, changing rooms and showers; control of personnel, visitors, and vehicles; control of birds, rats, and mice; waste removal, dead pig disposal, and a quarantine are insurances. Serological analysis should be performed in the replacement animals.

Elimination of BEP from infected herds has been performed by management practices such as closing the herd, cleaning and disinfecting, all-in all-out, elimination of clinically affected animals (pigs with nervous signs or infertile boars), and dead pig disposal. These procedures followed by serological testing, herd performance analyses, and entrance of sentinel BEP seronegative pigs confirm the elimination of the BEP (Stephano et al. 1986b).

To reduce the economic impact of BEP, different measures have to be taken. Infertile boars, with or without orchitis, must be eliminated. Artificial insemination should be performed if necessary. Sows and gilts that are presumed to be pregnant should be carefully observed for signs of estrus and, if possible, examined by sonication to confirm pregnancy. It is unknown whether purposeful, and thus quicker, dissemination of the virus in an infected herd has a tendency to limit the total economic impact of the disease.

The disease has become so economically important in Mexico that the development of vaccines is justified. A killed-virus vaccine, produced in cell monolayer cultures, is being evaluated.

REFERENCES

CAMPOS, H. R., AND CARBAJAL, S. M. 1989. Trastornos reproductivos de los sementales de una granja porcina de ciclo completo ante un brote de ojo azul. Mem 24th Congr Assoc Mex Vet Esp Cerdos, Morelia, Mex, pp. 62–64.

GARCIA, G. J.; CAMACHO, M. J.; MENDOZA, E. S.; CIPRIAN, C. A.; GONZALEZ, G. S.; DIAZ, C.; and STEPHANO, H. A. 1988. Infection experimental con el virus de ojo azul y *Pasteurella multocida* en cerdos convencionales. Mem 23d Congr Assoc Mex Vet Esp Cerdos, Leon, Mex, pp. 88–89.

GAY, G. M., AND STEPHANO, H. A. 1987. Stain analysis of a new Paramyxovirus isolated from 12 outbreaks of encephalitis and corneal opacity in pigs (Blue Eye Syndrome). Proc 23d World Vet Congr, Montreal, p. 161.

GREIG, A. S.; JOHNSON, C. M.; AND BOUILLANT, A. M. P. 1971. Encephalomyelitis of swine caused by a haemagglutinating virus. VI. Morphology of the virus. Res Vet Sci 12:305–307.

LIPKIND, M.; SHOHAM, D.; AND SHIHMANTER, E. 1986. Isolation of a Paramyxovirus from pigs in Israel and its antigenic relationship with avian paramyxoviruses. J gen Virol 67:427–439.

MORENO-LOPEZ, J.; CORREA-GIRON, P.; MARTINEZ, A.; AND ERICSSON, A. 1986. Characterization of a Paramyxovirus isolated from the brain of a piglet in Mexico. Arch Virol 91:221–231.

PEREZ, P. F.; STEPHANO, H. A.; AND GAY, G. M. 1988. Estudio histologico en lechones inoculados experimentalmente con el paramyxovirus de ojo azul. Mem 23d Congr Assoc Mex Vet Esp Cerdos, Leon, Mex, pp. 81–83.

RAMIREZ, T. C. A., AND STEPHANO, H. A. 1982. Histological central nervous system lesions produced by an hemagglutinating virus in naturally infected piglets. Proc 7th Int Congr Pig Vet Soc, Mexico City, p. 154.

SASAHARA, J.; HAYASHI, S.; KUMAGAI, T.; YAMAMOTO, Y.; HIRASAWA, K.; MUNEKATA, K.; OKANIWA, A.; AND KATO, K. 1954. On a swine virus disease newly discovered in Japan. 1. Isolation of the virus. 2. Some properties of the virus. Virus 4:131–139.

STEPHANO, H. A. 1986. Diagnostico diferencial entre Aujeszky y syndrome del ojo azul. Sint Porc 5 (12):41–48.

STEPHANO, H. A., AND GAY, G. M. 1983. El syndrome del ojo azul. Estudio experimental. Mem Reun Inv Pecu Mexico, Mex, D. F. pp. 523–528.

———. 1984. Experimental studies of a new viral syndrome in pigs called "Blue Eye" characterized by encephalitis and corneal opacity. Proc 8th Int Congr Pig Vet Soc, Ghent, p. 71.

———. 1985a. El syndrome del ojo azul en cerdos. Sint Porc 4 (5):42–49.

———. 1985b. El syndrome del ojo azul en granjas engordadoras. Mem 19th Congr Assoc Mex Vet Esp Cerdos. Merida, pp. 71–74.

———. 1986a. El syndrome del ojo azul. Una nueva enfermedad en cerdos asociada a un paramyxovirus. Vet Mex 17:120–122.

———. 1986b. Encefalitis, falla reproductiva y opacidad de la cornea, ojo azul. Sint Porc 5(12):26–39.

STEPHANO, H. A.; GAY, G. M.; RAMIREZ, T. C.; AND Maqueda, A. J. J. 1981. Estudio de un brote de encefalitis en lechones por un virus hemoaglutinante. Mem 17th Congr Assoc Mex Vet Esp Cerdos, Puerto Vallarta, p. 43.

STEPHANO, H. A.; GAY, M.; AND KRESSE, J. 1986a. Properties of a paramyxovirus associated to a new syndrome (blue eye) characterized by encephalitis, productive failure and corneal opacity. Proc 8th Int Congr Pig Vet Soc, Barcelona, p. 455.

STEPHANO, H. A.; DOPORTO, J. M.; AND GAY, M. 1986b. Estudio epidemiologico en dos granjas afectadas por el ojo azul. Proc 9th Int Congr Pig Vet Soc, Barcelona, p. 456.

STEPHANO, H. A.; GAY, G. M.; AND RAMIREZ, T. C. 1988a. Encephalomyelitis, reproductive failure and corneal opacity in pigs, associated with a new paramyxovirus infection (blue eye). Vet Rec 122:6–10.

STEPHANO, H. A.; FUENTES, R. M.; HERNANDEZ, J. P.; HERRADORA, L. M.; AND CARREON, R. 1988b. Encefalitis y opacidad de la cornea en cerdos destetados, inoculados experimentalmente con paramyxovirus de ojo azul. Mem 23d Congr Assoc Mex Vet Esp Cerdos, Leon, Mex, pp. 90–92.

STEPHANO, H. A.; HERNANDEZ, D.; PEREZ, C.; GONZALEZ, C. T.; RAMIREZ, M. H.; AND CERVANTES, A. 1990. Boar infertility and testicle atrophy associated with blue eye paramyxovirus infection. Proc 11th Int Congr Pig Vet Soc, Barcelona, p. 456.

14 Bovine Viral Diarrhea and Border Disease

P. Vannier

Y. Leforban

ONE OF THE best known and most widely studied viral pathogens of the pig is the hog cholera (HC) virus, a pestivirus of the family Togaviridae. There are, however, other pestiviruses to which pigs might be exposed, including bovine viral diarrhea (BVD) virus and border disease (BD) virus.

The discovery of an antigenic relationship between the pestiviruses (Darbyshire 1961) stimulated further investigations into natural and experimental BVD and BD infections of swine. The first report of natural infection of swine with BVD virus came from Australia in 1964, but BVD virus was not isolated from a naturally infected pig until 1973 (Fernelius et al. 1973). The presence of BVD-BD antibodies in pig sera interferes with HC eradication programs. Therefore, it is essential to identify the origin of any pestivirus antibodies encountered in such programs.

In addition, the teratogenic property of pestiviruses has been well established (Terpstra and Wensvoort 1988; Vannier et al. 1988; Wensvoort and Terpstra 1988) and the infection of pregnant sows by BVD and BD viruses induces a pathology partially resembling that of congenital HC.

ETIOLOGY. Together with the HC virus, BVD and BD viruses have been classified in the genus *Pestivirus,* family Togaviridae (Westaway et al. 1985). However, this classification will probably be modified in view of the recent progress in the description of the molecular structure of pestiviruses, which shows that its genome is more related to Flaviviridae than to Togaviridae (Collett et al. 1989). Morphological and structural characteristics of the three pestiviruses are similar (Laude 1979; Collett et al. 1989). They are one-strand positive enveloped RNA viruses of 25–120 nm diameter. This wide range in size is the result of either the entire particle or the core only being measured (Chu and Zee 1984). Their density ranges from 1.09 to 1.16 g/cm^3 and is dependent on the type of host cell used for their propagation (Laude 1979; Horzinek and Van Berlo 1987).

Bovine viral diarrhea was first described in 1946 as an infectious and contagious bovine disease (Olafson 1946) and mucosal disease was reported a few years later in 1953 (Ramsey and Chivers 1953). Further studies showed that the viruses responsible for these two conditions were

similar, and they have been referred to by most authors as BVD virus (Gillespie et al. 1961). Some isolates of BVD virus induced cytopathic changes in cell culture while others were definitely noncytopathic (Gillespie et al. 1960). Investigation of the relationship between the cytopathic effect and the pathogenesis of the disease has established that mucosal disease occurs only in calves persistently infected with a noncytopathic biotype, yet both cytopathic and noncytopathic biotypes sharing the same epitopic pattern can be isolated from these calves (Brownlie et al. 1984, 1987).

The third member of the *Pestivirus* genus is the causative agent of border disease in sheep. This disease, characterized by congenital disorders in lambs, was first described in 1959 in Great Britain along the border between England and Wales (Hughes et al. 1959); however, the immunological relationship of BD virus with BVD virus was discovered later (Hamilton and Timoney 1972).

The terms bovine viral diarrhea virus (BVDV) and border disease virus (BDV) are used to indicate that the virus was isolated from either cattle or sheep respectively, although the two viruses cannot be differentiated morphologically or structurally (Laude 1979). There is also evidence that BVDV can infect sheep and BDV can infect cattle (Barlow et al. 1980; Terlecki et al. 1980). In pigs, pestivirus isolates are usually hog cholera virus (HCV). However, BVDV and BDV can be isolated from naturally infected pigs (Carbrey et al. 1976; Terpstra and Wensvoort 1988). Moreover, it has been demonstrated through cross-neutralization tests and tests using monoclonal antibodies (Wensvoort et al. 1989a,b; Leforban 1990) that, in the past, BVDV may have been isolated from pigs but mislabelled as HCV on the basis of tests with polyclonal antibodies only.

EPIDEMIOLOGY. From HC-free countries like Australia, Ireland, Great Britain, and Denmark, prevalences of BVD antibodies within the pig population have been described as varying from 1.6% to 43.5% depending on the age of the animals and possibly to some extent on the degree of contact with cattle (Holm Jensen 1985). In countries where HC is present, the situation with regard to BVD antibodies seems to be about the same. In the Netherlands, although up to 15% of slaughtered sows had antibodies against BVDV, only 13 naturally occurring infections have been encountered over a 10-year period (Terpstra and Wensvoort 1988). Cattle are usually regarded as the source of BVDV infection in pigs, by feeding whey or milk to sows, a common practice in units with dairy farming (Terpstra and Wensvoort 1988). In some cases, pigs had contact with cattle recently vaccinated with BVDV (Stewart et al. 1971). In other cases, the pigs and cattle were kept in separate lots and buildings, but personnel and equipment moved freely between the different farm units (Carbrey et al. 1976). Nevertheless, pigs can be infected without any contact with cattle and without being fed bovine milk or offal (Terpstra and Wensvoort 1988).

The use of contaminated modified live virus vaccines (HC or Aujeszky's disease) or contaminated biological products can be the source of infection to pigs (Vannier et al. 1988; Wensvoort and Terpstra 1988). In these cases, ovine or bovine contaminants are involved in the disorders.

In all probability, the prolonged presence of a persistently infected litter is responsible for the dissemination of BVDV or BDV in a herd, and the virus could then be transmitted to other susceptible pregnant sows (Terpstra and Wensvoort 1988; Vannier et al. 1988). For example, it has been shown that the persistent BDV infection of litters occurs when sows are infected during early pregnancy; then the fetuses are transplacentally infected and most piglets show persistent infection and immunotolerance (Vannier et al. 1988). The course of the infection is quite similar to the one described after a BVD infection in pregnant cows (Baker 1987). Such congenitally BDV-infected piglets appear to excrete large amounts of virus, because other young animals in contact with them have rapid seroconversion and high antibody titers in their sera. Conversely, when the pigs are infected after birth, spread of infection to in-contact animals under the same experimental conditions is absent, which suggests a low or nil excretion of virus (Vannier et al. 1988).

BVD or BD viruses can be isolated or identified by immunofluorescence from blood, tonsil, spleen, kidney, ileum, and lymph nodes. Isolation of virus from ileum indicates that fecal excretion of the virus is a possibility.

CLINICAL SIGNS

Natural Conditions. Natural infection of pigs with BVDV usually occurs without clinical signs. However, in some cases, natural infection of pig herds with pestiviruses other than HC is associated with breeding problems such as poor conception, small litters, and a few abortions. Hyperthermia and clonic spasms have also been described (Carbrey et al. 1976; Stewart et al. 1977). More recently in the Netherlands and

France, signs resembling those of congenital HC infections were described, namely, an increased death rate in piglets up to 2–5 weeks old that were born to sows vaccinated 4 months earlier against HC or Aujeszky's disease with a batch of vaccines accidentally contaminated with a ruminant pestivirus. The clinical signs included anemia, rough-hair coat, growth retardation, wasting, and congenital tremors. Conjunctivitis, diarrhea, polyarthritis, petechiae in the skin, and blue eartips were also observed (Terpstra and Wensvoort 1988).

Natural infection of sows with BDV often resulted in repeat breeding and, at birth, many litters contained dead and mummified fetuses. Clinical signs of eyelid edema and locomotor disorders, sometimes associated with diarrhea and arthritis, occurred in a high proportion of piglets from these sows. The mortality rate up to 2 days of age varied between 30% and 70% (Vannier et al. 1988).

Experimental Conditions. Several trials of BVDV and BDV inoculation of pigs, mainly pregnant sows, have been done using oral, intranasal, and intramuscular and intrauterine routes with inconsistent results (Fernelius et al. 1973; Wrathall et al. 1978; Stewart et al. 1980; Mengeling 1988; Leforban et al. 1990b).

The result mainly depends on the strain used and on the stage of pregnancy of the sow. Inoculation of pregnant sows with the National Animal Disease Laboratory (NADL) strain of BVDV (Gutekunst and Malmquist 1963) between days 28 and 54 of gestation did not result in transplacental infection of the fetuses (Stewart et al. 1980). Inoculation of 9- to 18-kg piglets with the Singer strain of BVDV (Coria and McClurkin 1978) did not result in disease but the virus could be recovered from blood and tissues of the inoculated pigs, and antibodies were detected in their sera after 3 weeks. When later challenged with a virulent HCV strain, these inoculated piglets developed a severe disease, but six of seven survived (Stewart et al. 1971). The same strain used to inoculate fetuses between 41 and 65 days by transuterine injection caused either death or small-sized fetuses (Mengeling 1988).

Field BDV strains administered to pregnant sows between day 30 and 34 of gestation were able to infect the fetuses and cause disease characterized by low body weights and shorter lengths of newborn piglets (Wrathall et al. 1978). In another experiment (Leforban et al. 1990b), the perinatal death rate increased; elevated rectal temperature, eyelid edema, and anemia were observed in survivors during their second week of life. Subsequent growth retardation associated with respiratory signs and diarrhea developed in some pigs that eventually died within 2 months. Pigs without respiratory and enteric signs survived and had normal growth despite a marked snout deformation, with prognathism observed in one of them. Virus was isolated from blood and organs of all dead piglets but not from those that survived. When 40-day-old new specific-pathogen-free (SPF) pigs were put in contact with these transplacentally infected piglets, they did not show any disease but developed a high level of antibody to BDV that was able to protect them completely against a challenge with a virulent strain of HCV.

PATHOGENESIS. The ability of BVDV and BDV to establish intrauterine infection in swine has been well demonstrated by numerous authors (Wrathall et al. 1978; Stewart et al. 1980; Vannier et al. 1988). These two pestiviruses are embryotoxic but have little or no pathogenicity for the pig infected after birth. The intensity of the symptoms is associated with the stage of gestation of pregnant sows; clinical signs are more serious if the sows are infected during the first third of pregnancy. Indeed, the most spectacular clinical signs or lesions in fetuses or piglets are observed when the sows are infected 25–41 days postbreeding (Mengeling 1988; Leforban et al. 1990b).

In experimental infection of pregnant sows, most of the congenitally infected piglets showed persistent infection and immunotolerance. After the disappearance of the maternal passively acquired antibodies, no active immunity was detected in the serum of the majority of the piglets. The virus could be isolated from slaughtered piglets and was excreted by some of them, as evidenced by the contamination of young animals in contact with them (Vannier et al. 1988).

In some experimental infection with BDV of pregnant sows, for unknown reasons the onset of clinical signs was delayed in the piglets until 13–14 days after birth. It can be assumed that colostral antibodies ingested by the piglets blocked the multiplication of the pestiviruses or delayed disease in transplacentally infected piglets (Vannier et al. 1988; Leforban et al. 1990b). However, the delayed postnatal clinical expression of the infection in piglets when sows are infected during early pregnancy remains unexplained.

The pathogenicity of BVD or BD viruses seems variable depending on strains used in experimental conditions. BDV seems to be more constantly pathogenic for fetuses, whereas variable results were obtained with BVDV strains. The Singer strain, adapted to replicate in porcine cells, can infect and cause death of porcine fetuses, whereas NADL strains do not induce a real disease in the piglet (Mengeling 1988; Leforban et al. 1990b).

LESIONS. When postnatally infected by BVD or BD viruses, no or very mild lesions are observed in pigs: hyperemia of the small intestine was seen in a pig 11 days after being placed in contact with NADL strain–infected calves (Stewart et al. 1971), and transient leukopenia was detected during the first week following experimental infection of pigs with a pig isolate of BVDV (Carbrey et al. 1976).

The prenatal infection of fetuses by diaplacental transmission of the viruses from the infected sow is followed by consistent pathological disorders in fetuses or piglets.

In the 13 naturally occurring BVD outbreaks in Holland, chronic gastroenteritis and septicemia with hemorrhages in lymph nodes, epicardium, and kidneys were the most consistent lesions reported. Inflammation of the digestive tract was frequently characterized by catarrh, hypertrophy, or ulceration of the mucosa. Necrotic tonsillitis, icterus, polyserositis, polyarthritis, and atrophy of the thymus were also noted (Terpstra and Wensvoort 1988).

When a pig isolate of BVDV is given to gilts between 42 and 46 days of pregnancy, significant microscopic lesions are observed in the leptomeninges and choroid plexus of the fetus as collections of lymphocytes and histiocytes and cellular accumulation in the vascular adventitia and perivascular spaces (Stewart et al. 1980).

After experimental inoculation of 34-day pregnant sows with BDV, postmortem dissection of newborn piglets revealed cerebellar hypoplasia in 9 of 19 live-born piglets associated with a small meningocoele in 1 of the 9 (Wrathall et al. 1978). The isolated Aveyron strain of BDV (Chappuis et al. 1984) inoculated into 30-day-pregnant sows was responsible for lesions in lymphoid tissues in some piglets; marked hemorrhages in lymph nodes and other lymphoid tissues were found in stillborn fetuses and in piglets that died in the first few days. The histological examination of lymph nodes, spleen, and tonsil revealed marked subacute inflammatory lesions characterized by accumulations of lymphocytes, plasmocytes and eosinophilic polymorphonuclear leukocytes, numerous secondary follicles, increased populations of reticulocytes, and lymphoid hypoplasia with pyknosis and karyorrhexis. Thymus, liver, and nervous tissues were normal (Leforban et al. 1990b).

DIAGNOSIS. Isolation of the virus may be achieved from tissues that are submitted for HC diagnosis, i.e., tonsil, lymph node, spleen, and heparinized blood. In HC-free countries BVD and BD must be considered as differential diagnoses of HC, and all suspect cases of HC should be tested for BVD and BD viruses.

The diagnosis can be readily achieved using immunofluorescence or immunoenzymatic tests on cryostat sections of tissues. Isolation of the virus in pestivirus-free cell culture can also be used; cells can be either porcine or ruminant in origin. If BVDV or BDV is isolated from pigs it is reported to grow better with a higher titer in cells from ruminant origin than in porcine cells (Wensvoort et al. 1989a). However, the definitive identification of an isolate can only be done by using a panel of monoclonal antibodies able to link specifically to ruminant pestiviruses or to HCV. Three types of monoclonal antibodies are used for this purpose: those that detect all strains of pestivirus including HCV, those that detect HCV only, and those that detect ruminant pestivirus strains only (Peters et al. 1986; Bolin et al. 1988; Edwards et al. 1988; Hess et al. 1988; Wensvoort et al. 1989b).

Because the three pestiviruses share most of their structural proteins, the serological tests for detection of antibodies to HCV also detect antibodies to ruminant pestiviruses. The practical importance of this is that the presence of ruminant pestivirus antibodies in pig sera very often causes false positives in serological surveys for HC (Holm Jensen 1985). These cross reactivities are causing difficulties in eradication programs and in epidemiosurveillance programs for HC. However, the differentiation between antibodies to HCV and antibodies to ruminant pestivirus can be done by the neutralization test (Holm Jensen 1981) or the ELISA test (Leforban et al. 1990a) by comparing the antibody titers to the two viruses; i.e., HCV and ruminant pestivirus, or through a monoclonal-antibody-based hog cholera ELISA that is able to specifically detect antibodies to HC while ignoring antibodies to other pestiviruses (Wensvoort et al. 1988).

PREVENTION. To prevent the infection of pigs by BVD or BD viruses, it is necessary to avoid direct or indirect contact with cattle or sheep. In addition, since natural infection with BVDV often occurs when pigs are fed cow's milk or bovine offal, this practice must cease. The biological risk is also important when live-virus vaccines are used. Indeed, the cells used for multiplication of master-seed virus in the preparation of vaccine batches can be contaminated by BVD or BD viruses. HC and Aujeszky's disease vaccines were contaminated by a pestivirus (probably BDV) because secondary lamb kidney cells were used to multiply the vaccinal strains (Vannier et al. 1988; Wensvoort and Terpstra 1988). Thirty-five of 158 tested bovine kidney or testis primary cells were found contaminated by BVDV (Wellemans and Van Opdenbosch 1987). For this reason, the use of primary or secondary cells to prepare modified live-virus vaccines must be prohibited.

Moreover, both bovine and nonbovine cell lines might be infected and all cell lines must be controlled very carefully in regard to pestiviruses (Wellemans and Van Opdenbosch 1987; Potts et al. 1989). The main source of contamination for cells is the bovine serum, which is added to the nutrient medium. The high prevalence of BVDV in the world and the existence of persistently infected calves or bovine fetuses increases the risk

of contamination of bovine serum. Rossi et al. (1980) reported that up to 62% of examined batches of nonirradiated bovine fetal sera might be found positive for BVDV. Therefore, the systematic testing and treatment of bovine serum and of biological products used for the preparation of vaccines is firmly recommended.

REFERENCES

Baker, J. C. 1987. Bovine viral diarrhoea virus: A review. J Am Vet Med Assoc 190:1449–1458.

Barlow, R. M.; Rennie, J. C.; and Gardiner, A. C. 1980. Infection of pregnant sheep with the NADL strain of bovine virus diarrhoea virus and their subsequent challenge with Border Disease II B pool. J Comp Pathol 90:67–72.

Bolin, S.; Moennig, V.; Kelso Gourley, N. E.; and Ridpath, J. 1988. Monoclonal antibodies with neutralizing activity segregate isolates of bovine viral diarrhoea virus into groups. Arch Virol 99:117–123.

Brownlie, J.; Clarke, M. C.; and Howard, C. J. 1984. Experimental production of fatal mucosal disease in cattle. Vet Rec 114:535–536.

———. 1987. Clinical and experimental mucosal disease defining a hypothesis for pathogenesis. I. Pestivirus Infections of Ruminants. CEC Publication, Eur. 10 238 Luxembourg:147–156.

Carbrey, E. A.; Stewart, W. C.; Kresse, J. I.; and Snyder, M. L. 1976. Natural infection of pigs with bovine viral diarrhoea virus and its differential diagnosis from hog cholera. J Am Vet Med Assoc 169:1217–1219.

Chappuis, G.; Brun, A.; Kato, F.; Dufour, R.; and Durant, M. 1984. Isolement et caractérisation d'un pestivirus dans un foyer d'enterocolite leucopenie chez des moutons de l'Aveyron. Epidemiol. Santé Anim 6:117–118.

Chu, Hsien-Jue, and Zee, Yuan Chung. 1984. Morphology of bovine viral diarrhoea virus. Am J Vet Res 45:845–850.

Collett, M.; Moennig, V.; and Horzinek, M. C. 1989. Recent advances in pestivirus research. J Gen Virol 70:253–266.

Coria, M. F., and McClurkin, A. W. 1978. Duration of active and colostrum-derived passive antibodies to bovine viral diarrhoea virus in calves. Can J Comp Med Vet Sci 42:239–243.

Darbyshire, J. M. 1961. A serological relationship between swine fever and mucosal disease of cattle. Vet Res 72:331.

Edwards, S.; Sand, J. J.; and Harkness, J. W. 1988. The application of monoclonal antibody panels to characterize pestivirus isolates from ruminants in Great Britain. Arch Virol 102 (3.4):197–206.

Fernelius, A. L.; Amtower, W. C.; Lambert, G.; McClurkin, A. W.; and Matthews, P. J. 1973. Bovine viral diarrhoea in swine: Characteristics of virus recovered from naturally and experimentally infected swine. Can J Comp Med 37:13–20.

Gillespie, J. H.; Baker, J. A.; and McEntee, K. 1960. A cytopathic strain of bovine diarrhoea virus. Cornell Vet 50:73–79.

Gillespie, J. H.; Coggins, L.; Thompson, J.; and Baker, J. A. 1961. Comparison by neutralisation tests of strains of virus isolated from virus diarrhoea and mucosal disease. Cornell Vet 51:155–159.

Gutekunst, D. E., and Malmquist, W. A. 1963. Separation of a soluble antigen and infectious particles of bovine virus diarrhoea and their relationship to Hog Cholera. Can J Comp Med Vet Sci 27:121–123.

Hamilton, A., and Timoney, P. J. 1972. BVD virus

and border disease. Vet Rec 91:468.

HESS, R. G.; COULIBALY, C. O. Z.; GREISER-WILKE, I.; MOENNIG, V.; AND LIESS, B. 1988. Identification of hog cholera virus isolates by use of monoclonal antibodies to pestiviruses. Vet Microbiol 16:315–321.

HOLM JENSEN, M. 1981. Detection of antibodies against hog cholera virus and bovine viral diarrhoea virus in porcine serum. A comparative examination using CF, PLA and MLVA assays. Acta Vet Scand 22:85–98.

————. 1985. Screening for neutralizing antibodies against hog cholera and/or bovine viral diarrhoea virus in Danish pigs. Acta Vet Scand 26:72–80.

HORZINEK, M. C., AND VAN BERLO, M. F. 1987. The Pestiviruses: Where do they belong? Ann Rech Vet 18:115–119.

HUGHES, L. E.; KERSHAW, G. F.; AND SHAW, I. G. 1959. "B" or border disease. An undescribed disease of sheep. Vet Rec 71:313–317.

LAUDE, H. 1979. Nonarbo–Togoviridae: Comparative hydrodynamic properties of the pestivirus genus. Arch Virol 62:347–352.

LEFORBAN, Y. 1990. Profils épitopiques comparés de 18 souches de peste porcine classique: Comparaison des souches isolées de formes chroniques et des autres souches. Rec Med Vet 166. In press.

LEFORBAN, Y.; EDWARDS, S.; IBATA, G.; AND VANNIER, P. 1990a. A blocking ELISA to differentiate hog cholera virus antibodies in pig sera from those due to other pestiviruses. Ann Rech Vet 21:119–129.

LEFORBAN, Y.; VANNIER, P.; AND CARIOLET, R. 1990b. Pathogenicity of border disease and bovine viral diarrhoea viruses for pig: Experimental study on the vertical and horizontal transmission of the viruses. Proc 11th Int Congr Pig Vet Soc, Lausanne, p. 204.

MENGELING, W. L. 1988. The possible role of bovine viral diarrhoea virus in maternal reproductive failure of swine. Proc 10th Int Cong Pig Vet Soc, Rio de Janeiro, p. 228.

OLAFSON, P.; MACCALLUM, A. D.; AND FOX, F. H. 1946. An apparently new transmissible disease of cattle. Cornell Vet 36:205–213.

PETERS, W.; GREISER-WILKE, I.; MOENNIG, V.; AND LIESS, B. 1986. Preliminary serological characterisation of bovine viral diarrhoea virus strains using monoclonal antibodies. Vet Microbiol 12:195–200.

POTTS, B. J.; SAWYERS, M.; SHEKARCHI, I. C.; WISMER, T.; AND HUDDLESTON, D. 1989. Peroxidase-labeled primary antibody method for detection of pestivirus contamination in cell cultures. J Virol Methods 26:119–124.

RAMSEY, F. K., AND CHIVERS, W. H. 1953. Mucosal disease of cattle. North Am Vet 34:629–633.

ROSSI, C. R.; BRIDGMAN, C. R.; AND KIESEL, G. K. 1980. Viral contamination of bovine fetal lung cultures and bovine fetal serum. Am J Vet Res 41:1680–1681.

STEWART, W. C.; CARBREY, E. A.; JENNEY, E. W.; BROWN, C. L.; AND KRESSE, J. I. 1971. Bovine viral

diarrhoea infection in pigs. J Am Vet Med Assoc 159:1556–1563.

STEWART, W. C.; CARBREY, E. A.; KRESSE, J. I.; AND SNYDER, M. L. 1977. Experimental and natural-occurring bovine virus diarrhoea infections of pigs. Proceedings, agricultural research seminar on hog cholera/classical swine fever and African swine fever, E.E.C. EUR 5904 EN, p. 262.

STEWART, W. C.; MILLER, C. D.; KRESSE, J. I.; AND SNYDER, M. L. 1980. Bovine viral diarrhoea infection in pregnant swine. Am J Vet Res 41:459–462.

TERLECKI, S.; RICHARDSON, C.; DONE, J. T.; HARKNESS, J. W.; SAND, J. J.; SHAW, I. G.; WINKLER, C. E.; DUFFEL, S. J.; PATTERSON, D. S. P.; AND SWEASEY, D. 1980. Pathogenicity for sheep foetus of bovine virus diarrhoea–mucosal disease virus of bovine origin. Br Vet J 136:602–611.

TERPSTRA, C., AND WENSVOORT, G. 1988. Natural infections of pigs with bovine viral diarrhoea virus associated with signs resembling swine fever. Res Vet Sci 45:137–142.

VANNIER, P.; LEFORBAN, Y.; CARNERO, R.; AND CARIOLET, R. 1988. Contamination of a live virus vaccine against pseudorabies (Aujeszky's disease) by an ovine pestivirus pathogen for the pig. Ann Rech Vet 19:283–290.

WELLEMANS, G., AND VAN OPDENBOSCH, E. 1987. Presence of bovine viral diarrhoea (BVD) virus in several cell lines. Ann Rech Vet 18:99–102.

WENSVOORT, G., AND TERPSTRA, C. 1988. Bovine viral diarrhoea virus infections in piglets born to sows vaccinated against swine fever with contaminated vaccine. Res Vet Sci 45:143–148.

WENSVOORT, G.; BLOEMRAAD, M.; AND TERPSTRA, C. 1988. An enzyme immunoassay employing monoclonal antibodies and detecting specifically antibodies to classical swine fever virus. Vet Microbiol 17:129–140.

WENSVOORT, G.; TERPSTRA, C.; AND DE KLUIJVER, E. P. 1989a. Characterization of porcine and some ruminant pestivirus by cross neutralization. Vet Microbiol 20:291–306.

WENSVOORT, G.; TERPSTRA, C.; DE KLUIJVER, E. P.; KRAGTEN, C.; AND WARNAAR, J. C. 1989b. Antigenic differentiation of pestivirus strains with monoclonal antibodies against hog cholera virus. Vet Microbiol 21:9–20.

WESTAWAY, E. G.; BRINTON, M. A.; GAIDAMOVICH, S. Y. A.; HORZINEK, M. C.; IGARASHI, A.; KAARIAINEN, L.; LVOV, D. K.; PORTERFIELD, J. S.; RUSSELL, P. K.; AND TRENT, D. W. 1985. Togaviridae. Intervirology 24:125–139.

WRATHALL, A. E.; BAILEY, J.; DONE, J. T.; SHAW, I. G.; WINKLER, C. E.; GIBBONS, D. F.; PATTERSON, D. S. P.; AND SWEASEY, D. 1978. Effects of experimental border disease infection in the pregnant sow. Zentralbl Veterinaermed [B] 25:62–69.

15 Congenital Tremors Virus

S. R. Bolin

CONGENITAL TREMORS (myoclonia congenita) is a sporadic disease of neonatal swine that is characterized by clonic contractions of the skeletal muscles. Early reports of the disease were made by Kinsley (1922) in the United States, Payen and Fournier (1934) in France, and Hindmarsh (1937) in Australia. The disease is widely distributed and has been reported in several European countries, Australia, New Zealand, North America, and South America.

The term congenital tremors defines clinical signs that may be observed with inherited disorders (Harding et al. 1973; Patterson et al. 1973); trichlofon toxicity (Knox et al. 1978); and fetal infections with hog cholera virus (Harding et al. 1966), Japanese encephalitis virus (Morimoto 1969), and pseudorabies virus (Maré and Kluge 1974). However, herd histories and diagnostic tests indicate most outbreaks of congenital tremors are induced by an unknown infectious agent, probably a virus. This chapter will discuss this last form of congenital tremors.

ETIOLOGY. The infectious nature of the congenital tremors agent was first indicated by a detailed report of experimental induction of the disease, using filtered nutrient medium from cell cultures derived from affected pigs (Gustafson and Kanitz 1974). The disease also has been induced by intramuscular inoculation of pregnant sows with bacteria-free suspensions of brain and spinal cord from affected pigs (Done et al. 1986; Vandekerckhove et al. 1989). The identity of the congenital tremors agent is not known, but small viruslike particles of 20 nm in diameter were seen with electron microscopy in negatively stained fluids from cell culture materials used to induce the disease (Gustafson and Kanitz 1974). A virus-induced cytopathic effect was not noted in those cell cultures, indicating the virus was noncytopathic. The presence of a noncytopathic virus was further indicated by resistance of those cell cultures to infection with several cytopathic viruses. Other investigators (Vandekerckhove et al. 1989) described a transient cytopathic effect that disappeared after two passages of primary porcine kidney cells that had been inoculated with a suspension of brain and spinal tissue from affected pigs. Electron microscopic examination of cells and fluids from those cell cultures did not reveal viral particles. Other biophysical and bio-

chemical data on the congenital tremors virus are not available.

EPIDEMIOLOGY. The distribution of congenital tremors is probably worldwide, but incidence of the disease is low. Congenital tremors occurs in most, if not all, breeds and crossbreeds of swine, is not seasonally limited, and is more prevalent in litters of gilts than sows (Stromberg and Kitchell 1958). Spread of the disease has been associated with introduction of new breeding stock into a herd, which may indicate latent or asymptomatic chronic infection of mature swine. Experimental and epidemiologic data indicate a fetal infection is necessary for manifestation of clinical signs, which are detected immediately after birth and usually persist for less than 1 month. Morbidity in outbreaks of congenital tremors varies among swine herds; a few pigs in one or two litters or all pigs in several litters may be affected. The disease usually occurs in several litters farrowed over a 1-week to 2-month period, then disappears from the farm. Adjacent farms usually remain free of the disease. After an outbreak, the disease rarely recurs in subsequent litters from a sow and seldom becomes enzootic on a farm (Stromberg and Kitchell 1958; Vandekerckhove et al. 1989). In enzootic congenital tremors, clinical disease is usually sporadic and occurs in litters from gilts on farms that farrow >100 sows and gilts (Vandekerckhove et al. 1989).

CLINICAL SIGNS. The prominent clinical sign of congenital tremors is bilateral, clonic contractions of skeletal muscle. Congenital tremors is usually seen at or shortly after birth; however, some pigs may be several days old before tremors become evident. The intensity and frequency of muscle contractions is variable. The contractions may be mild, with only a fine tremor being evident in the head, flank, or hind leg region. In such cases the pigs may appear to be shivering. In severe cases, the contractions are violent and pigs may appear to be hopping. The pig has difficulty standing and walking and may not be able to hold onto a nipple to nurse. In most pigs, the tremors become milder with time and disappear by 1 month after birth. Sometimes the tremors are mild at birth and become stronger after a few days, then they begin to diminish and disappear. In a few pigs, mild tremors persist for several months or longer. The tremors subside and frequently disappear when the pigs are recumbent and asleep. External stimuli, such as noise, chilling, or a sudden cause of excitement, induce and exacerbate the tremors (Christensen and Christensen 1956; Stromberg 1959).

Other clinical signs associated with congenital tremors are mental dullness and splayleg. Pigs with the splayleg condition assume a sitting position, with hind legs extended in front of them. Death from congenital tremors is dependent on severity of muscle contractions and whether or not splayleg occurs. Half or more of the affected pigs in a litter may be lost, but usually death loss is low. Death is from starvation, attributable to inability to nurse, and from the sow crushing pigs with reduced mobility due to violent tremors or splayleg. After recovery, some pigs have pelvic limb incoordination, and others may have an abnormal, mincing gait (Gustafson and Kanitz 1974). Sows are clinically normal prior to farrowing litters of pigs affected with congenital tremors.

PATHOGENESIS. Congenital tremors occurs after fetal infection with congenital tremors virus. The disease has been induced by inoculation of the sow with infective material from the fourth week of gestation to 14 hours before farrowing (Gustafson and Kanitz 1974; Done et al. 1986; Vandekerckhove et al. 1989). Experiments in which infective material was inoculated into the allantoic cavity of selected fetuses demonstrated viral spread from fetus to fetus within the uterus (Vandekerckhove et al. 1989). Those experiments also indicated some fetal infections may not lead to clinical disease. The stage of development when the fetus is most susceptible to congenital tremors virus and the sequence and extent of viral replication in fetal tissues are not known. The virus appears to affect the developing central nervous system (CNS), causing retarded myelinization (Christensen and Christensen 1956). Although severity of clinical signs does not correlate with the degree of retarded myelinization, surgical ablation experiments locate the mechanism for production of muscle contractions at the spinal cord (Stromberg 1959; Fletcher 1968). The effect of the virus on myelinization is most pronounced in younger pigs and appears to be reversible with age.

LESIONS. There are no gross lesions associated with congenital tremors. The microscopic lesion most frequently observed is hypomyelinization in the CNS, especially in the spinal cord (Christensen and Christensen 1956; Fletcher 1968; Lamar and Van Sickle 1975). Morphometric analysis indicates that, compared with normal pigs, the cross-sectional area of both white and grey matter is reduced at all levels of the spinal cord in pigs with congenital tremors (Done et al.

1986). Hypomyelinization is most evident and reduction in cross-sectional area is greatest in the white matter of the spinal cord. Also in the spinal cord, the concentration of cerebroside, a glycolipid, is reduced and concentrations of cholesterol esters are elevated (Patterson and Done 1977; Sweasey and Patterson 1980). These biochemical alterations are consistent with decreased perinatal myelin synthesis and abnormal myelinization. In skeletal muscle, myofibrillar protein nitrogen concentration is increased compared with normal pigs, and the time course for rigor mortis is reduced (Sink et al. 1966).

DIAGNOSIS. A presumptive diagnosis of congenital tremors may be made on the basis of the clinical signs and history of the case. Serologic tests and viral isolation may be of value to eliminate hog cholera virus as the causal agent. Unfortunately, there are not any serologic tests specific for congenital tremors virus. Because the congenital tremors virus appears to be noncytopathic in cell culture and immunochemical tests are not available, viral isolation is of little diagnostic value. Histopathologic examination of CNS tissues for hypomyelinization may aid in diagnosis, but this lesion is common in neonatal pigs showing clonic muscle contractions, regardless of etiology (Done 1976). Neurochemical examination of the CNS tissues is not practical in most cases.

TREATMENT. At present, there is no specific treatment for disease caused by congenital tremors virus. Because the disease is usually self-limiting, supportive measures may be helpful for reducing losses. Pigs should be kept warm and dry to reduce chilling, and auditory stimuli should be kept to a minimum. Supervision of nursing may help reduce crushing of pigs with impaired mobility.

PREVENTION. Prophylactic biologics or chemicals are not available. Sound management practices, however, may aid in prevention of the disease. Pregnant sows should not be exposed to litters of pigs affected with congenital tremors. Because boars have been suspected of transmitting infection to susceptible females at breeding, newly acquired boars should be introduced into the herd gradually. Boars and gilts from litters affected with congenital tremors should not be kept as breeders because a chronically infected carrier state may exist. Before purchase of new breeding swine, inquiry should be made about previous experience with congenital tremors at the farm of origin.

REFERENCES

CHRISTENSEN, E., AND CHRISTENSEN, N. O. 1956. Studies on "trembling in newborn pigs." Nord Vet Med 8:921–934.

DONE, J. T. 1976. The congenital tremor syndrome in pigs. Vet Annu 16:98–102.

DONE, J. T.; WOOLLEY, J.; UPCOTT, D. H.; AND HEBERT, C. N. 1986. Porcine congenital tremor type AII: Spinal cord morphometry. Br Vet J 142:145–150.

FLETCHER, T. F. 1968. Ablation and histopathologic studies on myoclonia congenita in swine. Am J Vet Res 29:2255–2262.

GUSTAFSON, D. P., AND KANITZ, C. L. 1974. Experimental transmission of congenital tremors in swine. Proc US Anim Health Assoc 78:338–345.

HARDING, J. D. J.; DONE, J. T.; AND DARBYSHIRE, J. H. 1966. Congenital tremors in piglets and their relation to swine fever. Vet Rec 79:388–390.

HARDING, J. D. J.; DONE, J. T.; HARBOURNE, J. F.; RANDALL, C. J.; AND GILBERT, F. R. 1973. Congenital tremors type A III in pigs: An hereditary sex-linked cerebrospinal hypomyelinogenesis. Vet Rec 92:527–529.

HINDMARSH, W. L. 1937. Trembling in young pigs. Aust Vet J 13:249–251.

KINSLEY, A. T. 1922. Dancing pigs? Vet Med 17:123.

KNOX, B.; ASKAA, J.; BASSE, A.; BITSCH, V.; ESKILDSEN, M.; MANDENEP, M.; OTTOSEN, H. E.; OVERBY, E.; PEDERSEN, K. B.; AND RASMUSSEN, F. 1978. Congenital ataxia and tremor with cerebellar hypoplasia in piglets borne by sows treated with Neguvon™ vet. (Metrifonate, trichlorfon) during pregnancy. Nord Vet Med 30:538–545.

LAMAR, C. H., AND VAN SICKLE, D. C. 1975. Evaluation of chromatin clumping and myelination of the spinal cord of pigs with congenital tremor. Vet Pathol 12:1–5.

MARÉ, C. J., AND KLUGE, J. P. 1974. Pseudorabies virus and myoclonia congenita in pigs. J Am Vet Med Assoc 164:309–310.

MORIMOTO, T. 1969. Epizootic swine stillbirth caused by Japanese encephalitis virus. Proceedings, Symposium on Factors Producing Embryonic and Fetal Abnormalities, Deaths, and Abortion in Swine. USDA, Agric Res Ser, 91–73, pp. 137–153.

PATTERSON, D. S. P., AND DONE, J. T. 1977. Neurochemistry as a diagnostic aid in the congenital tremor syndrome of piglets. Br Vet J 133:111–119.

PATTERSON, D. S. P.; SWEASEY, D.; BRUSH, J.; AND HARDING, J. D. J. 1973. Neurochemistry of the spinal cord in British saddleback piglets affected with congenital tremor, type A-IV, a second form of hereditary cerebrospinal hypomyelinogenesis. J Neurochem 21:397–406.

PAYEN, B., AND FOURNIER, P. 1934. Pocelets "trembleurs." Rec Med Vet 110:84–86.

SINK, J. D.; JUDGE, M. D.; CASSENS, R. G.; HOEKSTRA, W. G.; GRUMMER, R. H.; AND BRISKEY, E. J. 1966. Preliminary investigation of certain aspects of myoclonia congenita in swine. Am J Vet Res 27:1494–1497.

STROMBERG, M. W. 1959. Studies on myoclonia congenita. III. Drugs and other factors affecting severity of tremor in pigs. Am J Vet Res 20:319–323.

STROMBERG, M. W., AND KITCHELL, R. L. 1958. Studies on myoclonia congenita. I. Review of literature and field investigations. Am J Vet Res 19:377–382.

SWEASEY, D., AND PATTERSON, D. S. P. 1980. Neurochemical diagnosis of congenital tremor in piglets. In Animal Models of Neurological Disease. Baltimore: Univ Park Press, pp. 306–314.

VANDEKERCKHOVE, P.; MAENHOUT, D.; CURVERS, P.; HOORENS, J.; AND DUCATELLE, R. 1989. Type A_2 congenital tremor in piglets. J Vet Med [A] 36:763–771.

16 Cytomegalovirus

N. Edington

LARGE basophilic intranuclear inclusions in cytomegalic cells were first described in the mucous glands of porcine turbinate mucosa by Done (1955). Their occurrence in pigs with rhinitis led to the designation "inclusion body rhinitis." Experimental transmission aligned with ultrastructural examination (Duncan et al. 1965; Valíček et al. 1970) indicated that herpeslike virions were the causal agent and that infection frequently also involved the lachrymal and salivary glands as well as renal tubular epithelium. Subsequently the characteristic histologic lesions have been described in the turbinates of pigs from countries throughout the world. The nature and distribution of the lesions suggested that the agent belonged to that group of herpesviruses affecting humans and animals described as "salivary gland viruses" (Smith 1959) and then as cytomegaloviruses (Weller et al. 1960; Plummer 1973) and finally as beta herpesvirinae (Matthews 1982). Inasmuch as they form a subgroup of the herpesviruses, they are slow growing and produce cytomegaly with distinctive intranuclear inclusions; they tend to be species-specific; they usually induce a clinically silent infection in the adult but often a fatal, generalized infection in the young animal; and they have the ability to cross the placenta and infect the fetus. Since the virus of "inclusion body rhinitis" shows all these features, it is justifiable to call it porcine cytomegalovirus (PCMV). PCMV also shares with the other herpesviruses the capacity to induce latent infection and to be excreted in the presence of circulating antibody. In susceptible herds the virus may cause fetal and piglet deaths, runting, rhinitis, and pneumonia as well as poor liveweight gain. However, in herds under good management the virus may be endemic without any apparent economic loss.

ETIOLOGY

Size and Structure. PCMV has an electron-dense core 45–70 nm in diameter, a surrounding icosahedral capsid of 80–100 nm, and an outer single, or more rarely double, membrane 120–150 nm across (Duncan et al. 1965; Valíček et al. 1970). The core has a usually elongated, variable outline that is oval, rectangular, or dumbbell in shape. The nuclear nucleocapsids appear to acquire an electron-dense coat, which is separated by a translucent halo from the envelope, while the envelope of extracellular and cytoplasmic virions has external projections and a clear unit-membrane structure (Valíček et al. 1973). As with other herpesviruses, particles without cores or with translucent cores as well as cytoplasmic or extracellular nucleocapsids without envelopes are frequently seen in vivo and in vitro.

Physicochemical Properties. PCMV is sensitive to chloroform or ether (Booth et al. 1967), but other physicochemical properties have not been investigated.

Cultivation. Propagation of PCMV in vitro has been problematic. L'Ecuyer and Corner (1966) passaged an isolate five times in primary pig lung cells, while Watt et al. (1973), investigating the susceptibility of a wide range of tissues, found that only lung macrophages from 3- to 5-week-old pigs were highly sensitive for both primary isolation and the serial propagation of virus. Cytomegaly and the formation of intranuclear and occasional small intracytoplasmic inclusions (Fig. 16.1) were seen 3–14 days postinoculation (DPI), depending on the titer of virus used, with a maximum at 11–14 DPI producing up to 5.5 TCD50/ ml of virus. However, the limitations of lung macrophages are that they do not replicate and therefore demand primary cultures that must be screened for contaminant viruses, including PCMV; also, the absence of an identifiable cytopathic effect (CPE) in unstained preparations necessitates the reading of the macrophages on flying coverslips stained either with Giemsa or immunofluorescent reagents (Watt et al. 1973; Plowright et al. 1976) (Fig. 16.2). Bouillant et al. (1975) reported that a cell line derived from porcine fallopian tube will support viral replication, while Shirai et al. (1985) reported isolation from porcine testis.

Replication. Systematic studies of in vitro replication have not been reported. Infected cells are enlarged about six times that of normal cells, with swelling of the mitochondria, endoplasmic reticulum, and Golgi apparatus (Duncan et al. 1965). The large basophilic intranuclear inclusion is seen to be surrounded by a light halo, separating it from the nuclear membrane in conventional preparations. However, ultrathin sections and ace-

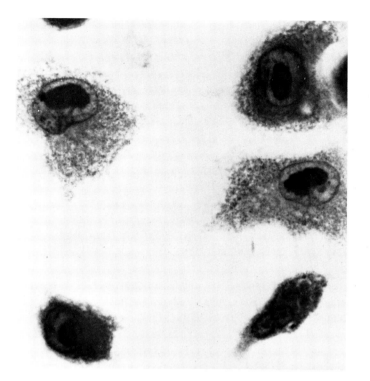

16.1. Cultured pig lung macrophages 11 days after infection with PCMV. The basophilic intranuclear inclusions stand out clearly in the enlarged cells. May-Grünwald-Giemsa. ×720. (Courtesy R. G. Watt.)

tone-fixed smears of nasal scrapings examined by light microscopy indicate that the halo is a fixation artifact. The inclusions stain apple green with acridine orange, and their development is inhibited by 5-iodo-2-deoxy uridine (IUDR), as with other deoxyribonucleic acid (DNA) viruses. Much smaller acidophilic inclusions are seen, sometimes in the nucleus but more often in the cytoplasm.

Ultrathin sections show that the large intranuclear inclusions correlate with the formation of nucleocapsids, often in crystalloid arrays. The capsids acquire an electron-dense coat in the nucleus, and the envelope is taken from the inner nuclear membrane, the virions coming to lie free or within membranous sacs in the cytoplasm. In the late stages of replication, as the cell is disintegrating, crystalloid arrays of virus may also be seen in the cytoplasm (Valiček et al. 1973).

Serology. An indirect immunofluorescence (IIF) test on infected lung macrophages fixed in acetone has been described (Plowright et al. 1976) (Fig. 16.2). Sera, titrated in twofold dilutions onto PCMV-infected macrophages on flying coverslips, were incubated for 1 hour at 37°C, were washed repeatedly in phosphate-buffered saline (PBS), and a commercial antipig gamma globulin–fluorescein isothiocyanate conjugate was added for a further 30 minutes. IIF titers up to 1:64–1:128 were frequent in commercial pig sera, the test being at least eightfold more sensitive than virus-neutralizing assays. There was no evidence of serologic variations between the limited number of U.K. isolates. Assaf et al. (1982) described an ELISA that gave a more sensitive detection system than IIF.

Host Range. PCMV appears to be host-specific both in vivo and in vitro. The virus has failed to replicate in rabbits, mice, hamsters, chick embryos, or cattle.

EPIDEMIOLOGY. The virus has worldwide distribution. Serologic evidence in the United Kingdom indicates that over 90% of herds have been exposed to infection, and the possibility of

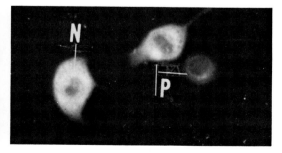

16.2. Lung macrophage cultures showing fluorescence after IIF, using specific PCMV antiserum. The nuclear staining (N) is most intense at the membrane. Cytoplasmic and discrete paranuclear fluorescence (P) can also be seen. ×480.

transplacental infection demands that hysterotomy-derived litters should be carefully monitored.

Virus may be recovered from nasal and ocular secretions, urine, and cervical fluids of pregnant sows exposed to PCMV for the first time; while isolation of virus from the testis and epididymis (Booth et al. 1967; Shirai et al. 1985) indicates that boars should be carefully examined. Dissemination of and infection by PCMV is probably most commonly via the nasal route, with the environment also being contaminated by urine. In a longitudinal survey of winter and summer cohorts of pigs, the majority excreted virus nasally between 3 and 8 weeks of age, correlating with the mixing of stock in the early postweaning period. Immunofluorescent antibody levels decreased during the period of virus excretion but rose again at 8–11 weeks, continuing up to slaughter at 23 weeks (Plowright et al. 1976). The pattern suggests that maternal antibody was replaced by active immunity.

In a smaller number of pigs, virus excretion was predominant at 3 weeks and had terminated at 5 weeks, suggesting that early postnatal or congenital infection had occurred. This has been associated with mummification and stillbirths, neonatal deaths, and runt pigs with rhinitis and/or pneumonia in field situations (Cameron-Stephen 1961; Rac 1961; Corner et al. 1964) and has been confirmed experimentally (L'Ecuyer et al. 1972; Edington et al. 1977).

The reactivation of PCMV excretion after the administration of corticosteroids (Edington et al. 1976a; Narita et al. 1985) points to the possible reactivation of replication when new breeding stock is introduced or when routine is otherwise disturbed. The recovery of virus from the lung macrophages of quiescent pigs indicates that the macrophage is a reservoir of infection. PCMV may also modify the outcome of intercurrent infections by analogy with murine cytomegalovirus, which modifies the host defensive mechanism, particularly inhibiting T-cell function (Booss and Wheelock 1977; Kelsey et al. 1977).

CLINICAL SIGNS. Uncomplicated infection with PCMV is usually a clinically silent event in pigs older than 3 weeks but can be fatal for the fetus or newborn pig. Such a statement is qualified by the observations that some adult animals exposed to PCMV for the first time may develop the lesions of a generalized infection and be anorexic and lethargic without pyrexia during the period of viremia (i.e., 14–21 DPI), while some piglets less than 3 weeks old develop only the lesions of disseminated epithelial infection and survive.

PCMV does not induce atrophic rhinitis but will produce a mild rhinitis in young pigs. In short-term trials no synergystic effect was observed between PCMV and *Bordetella bronchiseptica* (Edington et al. 1976c), but prolonged expo-

sures warrant investigation, as these results contradict field observations (Cameron-Stephen 1961; Corner et al. 1964).

The susceptible pregnant sow is frequently listless and anorexic while viremic but shows no pyrexia or any other clinical abnormality throughout pregnancy. Piglets may be born dead or die soon after birth without clinical symptoms. Others are stunted, pale due to anemia, with a variable edema often most noticeable around the jaw and tarsal joints. Natural outbreaks have included symptoms of shivering, sneezing, and respiratory distress. Up to 25% of the litter may be lost, with the remainder showing poor liveweight gains. The possibility of surviving pigs being persistent excretors must also be considered.

PATHOGENESIS. In experimental intranasal infections the occasional isolation of virus from nasal and conjunctival swabs prior to viremia suggests that the primary site of replication is in the nasal mucous glands or the lachrymal or harderian gland. Viremia was detected 14–16 DPI in 3-week-old pigs inoculated intranasally and over an extended period (5–19 DPI) in neonatal pigs (Edington et al. 1976a). Infectivity was restricted to the leukocytes. Subsequently, virus may be recovered from nasal secretions for up to 32 days, pharyngeal and conjunctival shedding being of shorter duration, while the persistence of viruria has been difficult to determine.

The site of tertiary viral replication varies with age. At an age of 3 weeks or more, when most animals experience infection, the virus disseminates to epithelial sites—particularly the glands of the nasal mucosa, harderian and lachrymal glands, kidney tubules, and more rarely the epididymis and mucous glands of the esophagus—to hepatocytes, and to duodenal epithelium. In the fetal or neonatal pig there is a predilection for reticuloendothelial (RE) cells, particularly capillary endothelium and the sinusoids of lymphoid tissues, thus giving rise to generalized lesions. While there is a tendency for replication to predominate in either RE or epithelial cells, they are not mutually exclusive, some individuals developing inclusions in both groups of cells. Infectivity persists at least in lung macrophages, since virus is recoverable from the cultured lung washings from pigs that were not excreting virus; viral shedding has been restimulated in quiescent animals following administration of corticosteroids (Edington et al. 1976a; Narita et al. 1985).

Experimentally, IIF antibody is detected 3 weeks after exposure to PCMV, rising to a peak at 6 weeks and persisting until slaughter. However, in rearing units in which PCMV is endemic, virus would appear to be released in the presence of circulating maternal antibody (Plowright et al. 1976).

Pregnant sows inoculated with virus were lethargic and anorexic 14–21 DPI, coinciding with the period of viremia, and this was immediately followed by the recovery of virus from nasal swabs. PCMV was isolated from cervical fluids later, at 30–35 DPI, and radiographic assessment of growth arrest indicated that the majority of fetal deaths occurred in this period. This would suggest that the virus takes a further 14–20 days to replicate in the fetus and favors cervical shedding being of fetal rather than maternal origin. Neither virus nor inclusions were detected in the cervix or endometrium at this stage. In a small number of fetuses, virus was detected as late as 60–80 DPI, but it was not clear whether this represented in utero spread by contact infection, delayed replication in these fetuses, or virus crossing the placenta on more than one occasion. The small number of congenitally infected animals that were examined excreted virus persistently and died suddenly with the histologic lesions of generalized infection within 7 days of birth (Edington et al. 1977). Late-term fetuses and congenitally infected neonates were all seronegative. Superinfection of sows with low levels of circulating antibody has been associated with transplacental infection (Edington et al. 1988a). Infection of the embryo shortly after implantation certainly occurred and may result in embryonic deaths. The virus was most commonly found in the meninges, Kuppfer cells, and peritoneal macrophages of these early fetuses (Edington et al. 1988b).

Although inclusion bodies have occasionally been seen in the epididymis, attempts to isolate virus from semen have been unsuccessful. Nor has it been possible to establish infection by preputial inoculation. Nevertheless, boars can excrete virus in urine and nasal secretions.

LESIONS. It is useful to distinguish between disseminated infection of epithelial tissues in the older animal and generalized infection of RE tissues in the fetus or neonate (Edington et al. 1976b).

Epithelial Lesions. No macroscopic changes are seen. Histologically, the characteristic basophilic intranuclear inclusion bodies and cytomegaly are seen in the nasal mucous glands (Fig. 16.3), acinar and duct epithelium of harderian and lachrymal glands, and renal tubular epithelium. In these tissues the number of affected cells may be extensive. Isolated inclusions are more rarely seen in the mucous glands of the esophagus, the epithelial lining of the ductus epididymis, and the seminiferous epithelium as well as the epithelial lining of the duodenum and jejunum. In these minor sites the desquamation of infected cells leaves no trace of infection, but in the major sites lymphocytes, plasma cells, and macrophages accumulate around the affected epithelial tissue and invade the acini as the cells are shed. Where complete acini are lost, there may be

some attempted replacement by a more squamous type of epithelium from the duct; but frequently in the nasal mucosa the remnants of the acinus have the appearance of focal lymphoid hyperplasia (Fig. 16.4). In natural cases the simultaneous infection with *B. bronchiseptica* or possibly *Pasteurella* spp. will produce changes in the ciliated epithelium lining the nasal mucosa and in the lesion of atrophic rhinitis, but these are not seen in pigs that are infected with PCMV only. The reparative lesions in the kidney are those of an interstitial nephritis (Kelly 1967). Sparsely distributed focal gliosis is seen in the central nervous system (CNS), with inclusions occasionally seen in the glial cells.

Generalized Lesions. The salient macroscopic lesions in young pigs are widespread petechiae and edema. The edema most commonly involves the thoracic cavity and subcutaneous tissues. In the thorax, pericardial and pleural effusions are

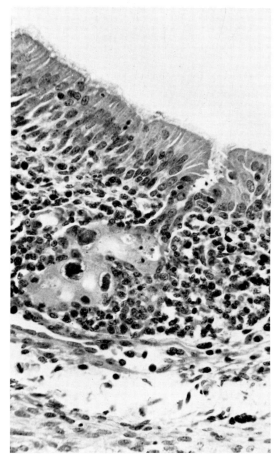

16.3. The basophilic intranuclear inclusion, translucent halo, and defined nuclear membrane are prominent in the enlarged superficial mucous gland epithelium of an animal 18 days after experimental intranasal inoculation. H & E. ×480.

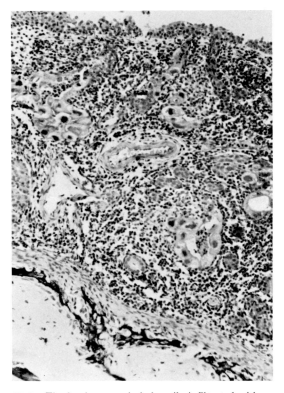

16.4. The lamina propria is heavily infiltrated with lymphocytes and plasma cells 24 days after inoculation of PCMV. Many of the acini of the mucous glands still show cytomegaly and prominent inclusion bodies. H & E. × 120.

seen, while the pulmonary edema occurs throughout the lungs, the interlobular septae being most distended and the ventral tips of the lobes appearing purple and consolidated (Fig. 16.5). The subcutaneous edema was most marked round the throat and tarsal joints. The lymph nodes were all enlarged and edematous and with petechiae. While petechiae were also marked at the other sites of edema they were most extensive in the kidneys, particularly subcapsular, so that the appearance varied from speckling to completely purple or black. In the small intestine, hemorrhages were seen, but rarely, varying from complete involvement to focal areas <1 cm long.

Fetal infection did not result in pathognomonic macroscopic lesions. The mummified fetuses were randomly distributed and sometimes of variable age.

In the acute fatal syndrome most inclusions are seen in capillary endothelial and sinusoidal cells and thus occur in all lymphoid and parenchymatous tissues. The fact that these cells are smaller than the epithelial cells of the disseminated disease means that the cytomegaly and inclusion bodies are not so prominent and may be overlooked (Fig. 16.6). The damaged endothelium is associated with the local edema and/or hemor-

rhage, with macrophages and erythrocytes in the distended extracellular space. Mononuclear cells with inclusions are found in blood vessels and also in the spleen; infected macrophages are prevalent in alveolar tissues. Replication in hepatocytes results in focal necrosis. In the kidney the inclusions are most common in areas of differentiating renal tissue and in glomerular capillary endothelium (Fig. 16.6). Hemorrhage and gliosis occur throughout the CNS, with a predilection for the choroid plexus, cerebellum, and olfactory lobes (Stephano-Hornedo and Edington 1987).

In field outbreaks these lesions may be complicated by intercurrent infections – mucopurulent rhinitis, pneumonia, and enteritis being reported (Cameron-Stephen 1961; Corner et al. 1964).

DIAGNOSIS. The presence of PCMV in a herd of pigs is most easily confirmed using the IIF antibody or ELISA test on random samples of sera from fattening pigs; this is also the most practical way of monitoring hysterotomy-derived litters.

In sows showing reproductive disorders, differentiation must be made from parvovirus and possibly from Aujeszky's disease (although abortion has not been observed with PCMV). Virus may be isolated from affected animals by sampling nasal mucosa, lung, and kidney and making direct cultures of lung macrophages if possible. If the carcass is kept at 4°C, viral antigen can be detected by the IIF test on frozen sections of these tissues at least 24 hours after infectivity has been lost. Alternatively, the pathognomonic inclusions and cytomegaly may be detected in histologic sections.

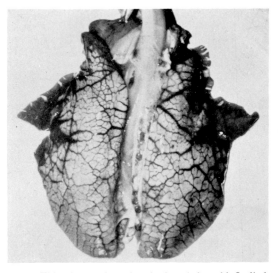

16.5. This pig was inoculated when 1 day old. It died at 16 days of age with widespread petechiae and subcutaneous edema. The interlobular septae of the lungs are distended with transudate, while the tips of apical, cardiac, and diaphragmatic lobes are also consolidated.

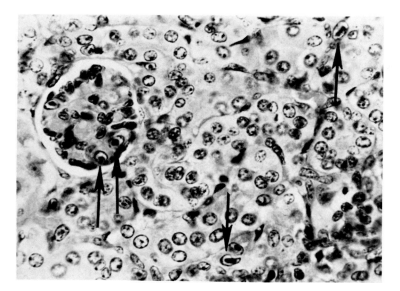

16.6. Section of kidney from a piglet with viral inclusions (arrows) in capillary endothelium both in the glomerulus and interstitial tissue. Infected cells show enlargement but only reach the size of normal tubular epithelium. H & E. ×240.

In determining the presence of PCMV as a component of infectious rhinitis in a herd, virus isolation may be made from nasal swabs or confirmed histologically from nasal scrapings (Done 1958) or fixed sections.

TREATMENT. No specific treatment can be given, although medication against concurrent bacterial infection is used in outbreaks of infectious rhinitis. Where rhinitis and/or reproductive disorders have been associated with the detection of PCMV, the outbreaks have usually been self-limiting (Cameron-Stephen 1961; Corner et al. 1964).

PREVENTION. In populations where PCMV is endemic, it does not appear to be a problem under good management systems. However, the introduction of new stock must always be regarded as hazardous since it may stimulate latent infection in the presence of circulating antibody or give rise to the problems of primary infection in susceptible herds.

Virus-free herds can be established by hysterotomy, but the ability of PCMV to cross the placenta dictates that offspring must be carefully monitored serologically for at least 70 days.

REFERENCES
ASSAF, R.; BOUILLANT, A. M. P.; AND DI FRANCO, E. 1982. Enzyme-linked immunosorbent assay (ELISA) for the detection of antibodies to porcine cytomegalovirus. Can J Comp Med 46:183–185.
BOOSS, J., AND WHEELOCK, E. F. 1977. Role of viraemia in the suppression of T cell function during murine cytomegalovirus infection. Infect Immun 17:378–381.
BOOTH, J. C.; GOODWIN, R. F. W.; AND WHITTLESTONE, P. 1967. Inclusion-body rhinitis of pigs: Attempts to grow the causal agent in tissue cultures. Res Vet Sci 8:338–345.
BOUILLANT, A. M. P.; DULAC, G.; WILLIS, N.; GIRARD, A.; GREIG, A. S.; AND BOULANGER, P. 1975. Viral susceptibility of a cell line derived from the pig oviduct. Can J Comp Med 39:450–456.
CAMERON-STEPHEN, I. D. 1961. Inclusion-body rhinitis of swine. Aust Vet J 37:87–91.
CORNER, A. H.; MITCHELL, D.; JULIAN, R. J.; AND MEADS, E. B. 1964. A generalised disease in piglets associated with the presence of cytomegalic inclusions. J Comp Pathol 74:192–199.
DONE, J. T. 1955. An "inclusion body" rhinitis of pigs. Vet Rec 67:525–527.
———. 1958. Inclusion-body rhinitis of swine, nasal scrapings as an aid to diagnosis. Vet Rec 70:877–878.
DUNCAN, J. R.; RAMSEY, F. K.; AND SWITZER, W. P. 1965. Electron microscopy of cytomegalic inclusion disease of swine (inclusion body rhinitis). Am J Vet Res 26:939–946.
EDINGTON, N. 1985. Unpublished data.
EDINGTON, N.; WATT, R. G.; AND PLOWRIGHT, W. 1976a. Cytomegalovirus excretion in gnotobiotic pigs. J Hyg (Camb) 77:283–290.
EDINGTON, N.; PLOWRIGHT, W.; AND WATT, R. G. 1976b. Generalised cytomegalic inclusion disease: Distribution of cytomegalic cells and virus. J Comp Pathol 86:191–202.
EDINGTON, N.; SMITH, I. M.; PLOWRIGHT, W.; AND WATT, R. G. 1976c. Relationship of porcine cytomegalovirus and *B. bronchiseptica* to atrophic rhinitis in gnotobiotic piglets. Vet Rec 98:42–45.
EDINGTON, N.; WATT, R. G.; PLOWRIGHT, W.; WRATHALL, A. E.; AND DONE, J. T. 1977. Experimental transmission of porcine cytomegalovirus. J Hyg (Camb) 78:243–251.
EDINGTON, N.; BROAD, S. C.; WRATHALL, A. E.; AND DONE, J. T. 1988a. Superinfection with PCMV initiating transplacental infection. Vet Microbiol 16:189–193.
EDINGTON, N.; WRATHALL, A. E.; AND DONE, J. T. 1988b. Porcine cytomegalovirus in early gestation. Vet Microbiol 17:117–128.
KELLY, D. F. 1967. Pathology of extranasal lesions in experimental inclusion body rhinitis of pigs. Res Vet Sci 8:472–478.
KELSEY, D. K.; OLSEN, G. A.; OVERALL, J. C.; AND

GLASGOW, L. A. 1977. Alteration of host defense mechanisms by murine cytomegalovirus. Infect Immun 18:754–760.

L'ECUYER, C., AND CORNER, A. H. 1966. Propagation of porcine cytomegalic inclusion disease virus in cell cultures. Preliminary report. Can J Comp Med 30:321–326.

L'ECUYER, C.; CORNER, A. H.; AND RANDALL, G. C. B. 1972. Porcine cytomegalic inclusion disease: Transplacental transmission. Proc 2d Int Congr Pig Vet Soc, Hannover, Germany, p. 99.

MATTHEWS, R. E. F. 1982. Classification and Nomenclature of Viruses (1982). Basel, London, N.Y.: S. Karger, pp. 49, 50.

NARITA, M.; SHIMIZU, M.; KAWANURA, H.; HARITARI, M.; AND MORIWAKI, M. 1985. Pathologic changes in pigs with prednisolone induced recrudescence of herpesvirus infection. Am J Vet Res 46:1506–1510.

PLOWRIGHT, W.; EDINGTON, N.; AND WATT, R. G. 1976. The behaviour of porcine cytomegalovirus in commercial pig herds. J Hyg (Camb) 75:125–135.

PLUMMER, G. 1973. Cytomegaloviruses of man and animals. Prog Med Virol 15:92–125.

RAC, R. 1961. Infectious rhinitis in pigs: Laboratory aspects. Aust Vet J 37:91–93.

SHIRAI, J.; NARITA, M.; AND IIJIMA, Y. 1985. A cytomegalovirus isolation from swine testicle culture. Jpn J Vet Sci 47:697–703.

SMITH, M. G. 1959. The salivary gland viruses of man and animals. Prog Med Virol 2:171–202.

STEPHANO-HORNEDO, A., AND EDINGTON, N. 1987. Encefalitis experimental por citomegalovirus porcino en cerdos gnotobioticos: Estudio histopatologica. Vet Mex 18:189–202.

VALIČEK, L.; ŠMID, B.; PLEVA, V.; AND MEUŠIK, J. 1970. Porcine cytomegalic inclusion disease virus. Electron microscopic study of the nasal mucosa. Arch Gesamte Virusforsch 32:19–30.

VALIČEK, L.; ŠMID, B.; AND MEUŠIK, J. 1973. Electron microscopy of porcine cytomegalovirus. Arch Gesamte Virusforsch 41:344–353.

WATT, R. G.; PLOWRIGHT, W.; SABØ, A.; AND EDINGTON, N. 1973. A sensitive cell culture system for the virus of porcine inclusion body rhinitis (cytomegalic inclusion disease). Res Vet Sci 14:119–121.

WELLER, T. H.; HANSHAW, J. B.; AND SCOTT, D. E. 1960. Serologic differentiation of viruses responsible for cytomegalic inclusion disease. Virology 12:130–132.

17 Encephalomyocarditis Virus

H. S. Joo

ENCEPHALOMYOCARDITIS virus (EMCV) has been recognized as a swine pathogen since the virus was first isolated during an outbreak of acute disease in Panama (Murnane et al. 1960). Subsequently outbreaks have been reported in many different countries. Major epizootics with high mortality in baby pigs were reported in Florida from 1960–1966 (Gainer 1967), New South Wales, Australia, in 1970 and 1984 (Acland and Littlejohns 1975; Seaman et al. 1986), and Cuba (Ramos et al. 1983). Clinical disease was also reported in New Zealand (Sutherland et al. 1977), South Africa (Williams 1981), Brazil (Roehe et al. 1985), Italy (Sidoli et al. 1988), and Canada (Sanford et al. 1989), while detection of EMCV antibodies without clinical disease was reported in the United Kingdom (Sangar et al. 1977).

Besides baby pig mortality, EMCV has been implicated as a cause of reproductive failure (Littlejohns 1984; Joo et al. 1988). Reproductive problems associated with EMCV infections have been reported in Cuba (Gomez et al. 1982), Australia (Links et al. 1986), Canada (Sanford et al. 1989), and the United States (Kim et al. 1989a; Christianson et al. 1990). Furthermore EMCV has recently received great attention in several U.S. midwestern states because the virus is a potential cause of the so-called "mystery swine disease" (see Chapter 61).

ETIOLOGY. The EMCV group is classified as genus *Cardiovirus* of the family Picornaviridae (Matthews 1979). The first EMCV isolation was made from a chimpanzee with myocarditis in Florida (Helwig and Schmidt 1945), and subsequently the virus has been isolated from a variety of animal species over a wide geographic area (Tesh and Wallace 1977). During the 1940s several virus strains including Columbia-SK, Mengo, and MM were isolated and subsequently found to be antigenically similar and are considered to be in the same group as EMCV. EMCV has been further reported to be antigenically related to the cricket paralysis virus of insects (Tinsley et al. 1984).

Many properties of EMCV are shared by other picornaviruses. The virus is ether resistant and stable over a wide range of pH; is inactivated at 60°C for 30 minutes, although some strains have shown a marked thermal stability; and replicates well in cell cultures originating from several animal species including rodents, swine, and humans. The virus also replicates in mice and chicken embryos and is pathogenic to many laboratory animal hosts. Acute fatal disease is most often produced in mice and hamsters following inoculation by various routes. Neurologic disease due to encephalitis is observed, but myocarditis may also be seen at necropsy. Pathogenicity in rats, guinea pigs, rabbits, and monkeys appears to vary depending on the age of the animals and the virus strains used. The virus has hemagglutinating ability with guinea pig, rat, horse, and sheep erythrocytes, and most EMCV strains require KCl-borate (0.12M KCl; 0.05M H_3BO_3) buffered solution for an optimal hemagglutination reaction. Some differences in hemagglutinating activity between EMCV strains have been reported (Sangar et al. 1977; Kim et al. 1991). The EMCV virions contain a single strand of RNA of molecular weight 2.6×10^6 daltons, which comprises 31% of the virion mass and is enclosed in a protein capsid shell. The viral proteins show four nonidentical polypeptide bands in SDS-polyacrylamide gel electrophoresis. Other molecular characteristics including the nucleotide sequence of the RNA are relatively well understood (Rueckert 1985).

EPIDEMIOLOGY. The epidemiology of EMCV infection is poorly understood because of a lack of experimental data. The EMCV group is generally regarded as a rodent virus, although the virus naturally infects a wide range of vertebrate species. The host range includes chimpanzees, monkeys, elephants, lions, squirrels, mongooses, racoons, and swine, the domestic animal most susceptible to clinical disease by EMCV infection.

Rats and mice are believed to be the principal reservoir of the virus (Tesh and Wallace 1977). EMCV-neutralizing antibodies have been demonstrated in sera from wild rats, *Rattus* spp., trapped in several areas of the United States and Canada. Many rodents are susceptible to experimental infection, showing high levels of virus in their tissues, and infected rodents excrete virus in their feces and urine. The virus has been isolated

The author acknowledges Drs. H. M. Acland and I. R. Littlejohns, the previous authors of the EMCV chapter in the 6th edition of the Diseases of Swine. The present chapter contains some materials by the previous authors.

from dried feces and from intestines of rats or mice captured on farms where swine disease had previously occurred (Gainer 1967; Acland and Littlejohns 1975). Although the virus has been isolated from mosquitoes caught in Africa, Brazil, and the United States, and from ticks in India (Tesh and Wallace 1977), there is no evidence of vector-borne natural EMCV infection in swine.

The most important sources for swine infection appear to be feed or water contaminated with virus by rats, other rodents, or diseased carcasses. Feed contaminated with infected carcasses may contain high doses of virus, since a large amount of virus is found in the carcasses. An episode of lion deaths at a zoo was found to be due to feeding carcasses of African elephants that had died of EMCV infection (Simpson et al. 1977).

The mode of virus transmission is not clear but rodent-to-pig transmission is probably common. Several outbreaks in Australia were found to be closely associated with rat and mouse plagues (Acland and Littlejohns 1975; Seaman et al. 1986). Pig-to-pig transmission has been questioned because sentinel pigs failed to become infected after contact with experimentally infected and sick pigs (Littlejohns and Acland 1975; Horner and Hunter 1979). However, the role of infected pigs in natural transmission, either directly or indirectly, cannot be excluded, since infected pigs have been shown to excrete the virus at least for a short period.

The virulence of EMCV isolates in pigs may vary depending on the virus strains maintained in reservoir hosts within geographical areas. For example, Australian strains were shown to be more virulent in experimental infection of pigs than New Zealand strains (Littlejohns and Acland 1975; Horner and Hunter 1979), and certain isolates in Florida were found to cause only myocarditis without deaths (Gainer et al. 1968).

To date there is no clear evidence to support the role of EMCV as a pathogen in livestock other than swine, although Gainer (1974) reported the isolation of EMCV from dead calves in Florida and the detection of antibodies in Canadian horses. Serologic evidence of EMCV infection has also been reported in cattle and horses in Queensland, Australia (Spradbrow and Chung 1970).

Evidence for human infection with EMCV has been demonstrated by antibody detection in human populations (Tesh 1978), but there are no reports that the virus causes human heart disease. However, EMCV has been utilized in different research models for human diseases, including the investigation of the pathogenesis of myocarditis, vasculitis, and viral-induced diabetes mellitus (Murnane 1981).

CLINICAL SIGNS. EMCV infection in young pigs is characterized most commonly by acute disease with sudden deaths due to myocardial failure. Other clinical signs including anorexia, listlessness, trembling, staggering, paralysis, or dyspnea are also observed. Experimentally infected swine (Craighead et al. 1963; Littlejohns and Acland 1975) have shown temperatures up to 41°C and death between days 2 and 11, usually days 3–5, postinoculation or occasional recovery with chronic myocarditis. Severity of the disease in pigs appears to vary depending on virus strains and age of pigs at the time of infection. Mortality approaching 100% is usually confined to pigs of preweaning age. Infections in pigs from postweaning age to adult are usually subclinical, although some mortality may be observed even in adult pigs.

In breeding females, the first clinical signs noted may be anorexia and fever. Such sows will show near-term abortions (107–111 days of gestation) and low farrowing rates. Following the near-term abortions, the numbers of mummified and stillborn fetuses increase along with preweaning mortality (Christianson et al. 1990). Mummified fetuses are large in size at the initial stage and smaller afterward. These reproductive problems last for 2–3 months and are observed in sows of all parities.

PATHOGENESIS. The natural infection of swine most likely occurs by the oral route. Following experimental oral infection in piglets, viremia was demonstrated as early as 2 days postinoculation and persisted 2–4 days (Craighead et al. 1963). Virus was present in the feces for as long as 9 days following oral administration. The persistence of the virus beyond the viremic period suggests some viral replication in the intestine. Large amounts of virus were found in the spleen and mesenteric lymph nodes indicating that lymphatic tissue was a site of virus replication. The highest virus titers were recovered from heart muscle in both experimental and natural infections, and myocardial lesions were predominant at necropsy. Other tissues such as liver, pancreas, and kidney usually contained virus at a greater concentration than blood. Animals that survive the acute disease produced EMCV antibodies. After antibody formation the virus was no longer recoverable. The course of infection in swine appears to be influenced by virus strain, viral dose, history, and level of viral passage and susceptibility of the individual animal.

The pathogenesis of transplacental infection with EMCV in pregant sows is not well understood. Following intramuscular infection of pregnant sows with EMCV, a transplacental infection with fetal deaths was observed in one of the three sows infected in late gestation, while fetal infection in sows during the early pregnancy was not conclusive (Love and Grewal 1986). Infected and dead fetuses showed myocardial lesions varying from multiple small foci to large diffuse patches. Some difficulty in producing experimental reproductive disease in pregnant sows was also observed with a U.S. isolate; however, transplacental infection was successful when the virus was passaged in young pigs rather than cell culture before inoculation (Christianson et al. 1991). Fetal deaths following infection in sows occur as early as 2 weeks postinfection. At this time it is not known whether all EMCV strains can cause both the typical myocarditis observed in young pigs and reproductive failure.

Pathogenic variability of different EMCV isolates in swine fetuses has been reported (Kim et al. 1989b). Little pathogenicity was observed following infection of swine fetuses in utero with laboratory-passaged strains. Pathogenic effects of field isolates were obvious in fetuses of both mid and late gestational ages. It has been suggested that virulent strains may have been attenuated and lost pathogenicity by prolonged laboratory passages.

Among the laboratory animals, clinical manifestations and the pathogenesis of EMCV infection were variable. Experimental infection has resulted in fatal myocarditis in adult guinea pigs and in some strains of white rats. Owls or night monkeys and marmosets were reported to be highly susceptible to infection. The virus has seldom been pathogenic to rabbits and rhesus monkeys, causing only inapparent infections despite high viremic levels. It is interesting to note that the pathogenicity of EMCV can be modified by laboratory manipulations. The virus appears to be readily adapted with continuous passages by various routes, and EMCV variants that differ in organ tropism and in pathogenicity have been developed. Certain strains cause predominantly fatal encephalomyelitis (encephalotrophism) or widespread myocardial damage (cardiotrophism), or even specific destruction of pancreatic beta cells (pancreotrophism) (Craighead 1966; Cerutis et al. 1989).

LESIONS.   Pigs dying in the acute phase of cardiac failure may show only epicardial hemorrhage or no gross lesions. At necropsy of experimentally infected young pigs, hydropericardium, hydrothorax, pulmonary edema, and ascites are frequently observed, and gross myocardial lesions are prominent. The heart is usually enlarged, soft and pale, with visible yellowish or white necrotic foci (2–15 mm in diameter) or large ill-defined pale areas (Fig. 17.1). The lesions are most commonly observed on the epicardium of the right ventricle and may extend to varying depths within the myocardium. Virus is present in heart muscle in most cases, even when myocardial lesions are minimal or occasionally absent (Gainer et al. 1968; Littlejohns and Acland 1975).

Infected fetuses become mummified in various sizes depending on the stage of infection and may be hemorrhagic, edematous, or apparently normal (Fig. 17.2). The myocardial lesions may be

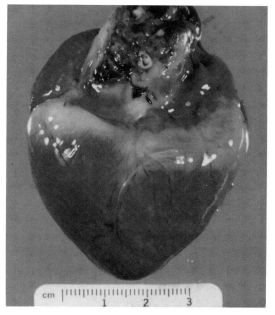

17.1.   Heart of pig with EMCV infection showing multiple white foci in myocardium.

seen in some infected fetuses, but it is difficult to observe under field conditions. The gross abnormalities of the fetuses are not easy to distinguish from those of other viral infections, unless the myocardial lesions are observed.

Histopathologically, the most significant finding in young pigs is myocarditis with focal or diffuse accumulation of mononuclear cells (Fig. 17.3), vascular congestion, edema, and degeneration of the myocardial fibers with necrosis. Mineralization of necrotic heart muscle is common but not always present. Congestion with meningitis, perivascular infiltration with mononuclear cells and some neuronal degeneration may be observed in the brain (Murnane et al. 1960; Gainer et al. 1968; Acland and Littlejohns 1975). Nonsuppurative encephalitis and myocarditis were also observed in swine fetuses with natural EMCV infection (Kim et al. 1989a).

DIAGNOSIS.   The clinical history of reproductive failure along with high preweaning mortality is a useful tip in the diagnosis of EMCV infection. EMCV-induced reproductive problems should be differentiated from those of porcine parvovirus infection. EMCV causes reproductive problems in sows of all parities along with high neonatal mortality, while porcine parvovirus infection is manifested by increased mummified fetuses, mainly in gilt litters without neonatal mortality. Other infections such as pseudorabies virus or *Leptospira* spp. should also be considered.

Dyspnea manifested as rapid abdominal breathing or "thumping" due to heart failure is

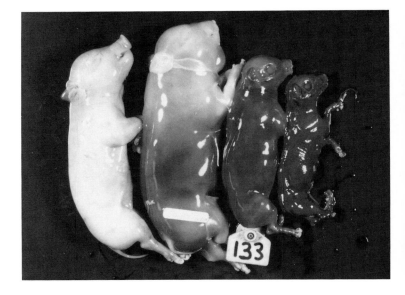

17.2. From right to left, mummified, hemorrhagic, edematous, or normal-appearing swine fetuses from a sow infected intramuscularly with EMCV at 50 days of gestation and examined 28 days after infection.

common among EMCV-infected baby pigs in farrowing houses. Gross lesions of white necrotic areas in the heart muscle are characteristic of EMCV infection, although such lesions resemble those of vitamin E and selenium deficiency and heart infarcts by septic embolism.

A definitive diagnosis should be based on virus isolation and identification. Heart is the best tissue for virus isolation from swine fetuses and young pigs. Tissue samples can be frozen without apparent loss of infectivity. The virus can be isolated by inoculating samples in mice, chicken embryos, or cell cultures. Infected mice or chicken embryos will die in 3–6 days postinoculation. For virus isolation in cell culture, baby hamster kidney (BHK-21), HeLa, or Vero cell cultures are commonly used. For primary cell culture, fetal mouse fibroblasts are suitable. Infected cell monolayers will show a rapid and complete cytolysis, and viral identification can then be made by staining the infected monolayers with EMCV-fluorescent antibody conjugate or by the inhibition of the cytopathic effects by specific immune serum. Virus isolation is usually successful from pigs during the acute phase but is difficult from pigs in the stage after development of circulating antibody.

Histopathologic lesions consistent with EMCV infection may play an important role in making a diagnosis. As described previously, myocarditis of varying stages with infiltration of mononuclear cells along with nonsuppurative encephalitis is in-

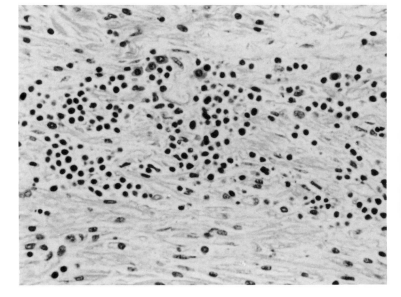

17.3. Focal infiltration of mononuclear cells in myocardium of a stillborn swine fetus with natural EMCV infection.

dicative of EMCV infection. Serologic methods may also help in the diagnosis of EMCV infection. Detection of antibody specific to EMCV from stillborn or large mummified fetuses is particularly significant for fetal infection (Joo et al. 1988), because there is no transmission of maternal immunoglobulins across the placenta in swine. Interpretation of sow serology is often confusing, for positive antibody titers have not always been associated with clinical disease. Both serum-neutralization and hemagglutination-inhibition tests (Joo et al. 1988) can be used to detect EMCV antibody in serum samples. Although the specificity of each test is not well defined, antibody titers of $\geq$ 1:16 appear to be significant.

TREATMENT AND PREVENTION. There is no treatment, but mortality may be minimized by avoiding stress or excitement of the pigs at risk. It is important to control rodents on pig farms or to minimize their contact with pigs, either directly or indirectly via contamination of feed or water. Although pig-to-pig transmission is not clear, introduction of pigs from previously infected farms should be avoided. Basic rules of sanitation and hygiene should be applied. Animals dying of the disease should be promptly and sanitarily disposed of. The virus can be inactivated in water containing 0.5 ppm residual chlorine. For disinfectants, iodine-based preparations or mercuric chloride can be used.

An inactivated adjuvant vaccine has recently been developed and is commercially available in the United States. Although efficacy of the vaccine is yet to be determined, production of humoral immunity in pigs following vaccination appears to be satisfactory.

REFERENCES

ACLAND, H. M., AND LITTLEJOHNS, I. R. 1975. Encephalomyocarditis virus infection of pigs. I. An outbreak in New South Wales. Aust Vet J 51:409–415.

CERUTIS, D. R.; BRUNER, R. H.; THOMAS, D. C.; AND GIRON, D. J. 1989. Tropism and histopathology of the D, B, K, and MM variants of encephalomyocarditis virus. J Med Virol 29:63–69.

CHRISTIANSON, W. T.; KIM, H. S.; JOO, H. S.; AND BARNES, D. M. 1990. Porcine reproductive and neonatal losses associated with possible encephalomyocarditis virus infection. Vet Rec 126:54–57.

CHRISTIANSON, W. T.; KIM, H. S.; YOON, I. J.; AND JOO, H. S. 1991. Transplacental infection of midgestation sows with encephalomyocarditis virus. Am J Vet Res (Submitted for publication).

CRAIGHEAD, J. E. 1966. Pathogenicity of M and E variants of the encephalomyocarditis (EMC) virus. I. Myocardiotropic and neurotropic properties. Am J Pathol 48:333–343.

CRAIGHEAD, J. E.; PERALTA, P. H.; MURNANE, T. G.; AND SHELOKOV, A. 1963. Oral infection of swine with the encephalomyocarditis virus. J Infect Dis 112:205–212.

GAINER, J. H. 1967. Encephalomyocarditis virus infection in Florida, 1960–1966. J Am Vet Med Assoc 151:421–425.

———. 1974. Viral myocarditis in animals. Adv Cardiol 13:94–105.

GAINER, J. H.; SAUDEFUR, J. R.; AND BIGLER, W. J. 1968. High mortality in a Florida swine herd infected with the encephalomyocarditis virus. An accompanying epizootiologic survey. Cornell Vet 58:31–47.

GOMEZ, L.; LORENZO, M.; RAMOS, J. R.; LUYA, M. J.; MAYO, D.; AND GIRAL, T. 1982. Isolation of the encephalomyocarditis virus in a sow and her fetus. Rvta Cub Cienc Vet 13:21–24.

HELWIG, F. C., AND SCHMIDT, E. D. H. 1945. A filter-passing agent producing interstitial myocarditis in anthropoid apes and small animals. Science 102:31–33.

HORNER, G. W., AND HUNTER, R. 1979. Experimental infection in pigs with encephalomyocarditis virus. NZ Vet J 27:202–203.

JOO, H. S.; KIM, H. S.; AND LEMAN, A. D. 1988. Detection of antibody to encephalomyocarditis virus in mummified or stillborn pigs. Arch Virol 100:131–134.

KIM, H. S.; JOO, H. S.; AND BERGELAND, M. E. 1989a. Serologic, virologic and histopathologic observations of encephalomyocarditis virus infection in mummified and stillborn pigs. J Vet Diagn Invest 1:101–104.

KIM, H. S.; CHRISTIANSON, W. T.; AND JOO, H. S. 1989b. Pathogenic properties of encephalomyocarditis virus isolates in swine fetuses. Arch Virol 109:51–57.

———. 1991. Characterization of encephalomyocarditis virus isolated from aborted swine fetuses. Am J Vet Res. In press.

LINKS, I. J.; WHITTINGTON, R. J.; KENNEDY, D. J.; GREWAL, A.; AND SHARROCK, A. J. 1986. An association between encephalomyocarditis virus infection and reproductive failure in pigs. Aust Vet J 63:150–152.

LITTLEJOHNS, I. R. 1984. Encephalomyocarditis virus from stillborn pigs. Aust Vet J 61:93.

LITTLEJOHNS, I. R., AND ACLAND, H. M. 1975. Encephalomyocarditis virus infection in pigs. II. Experimental diseases. Aust Vet J 51:416–422.

LOVE, R. J., AND GREWAL, A. S. 1986. Reproductive failure in pigs caused by encephalomyocarditis virus. Aust Vet J 63:128–129.

MATTHEWS, R. E. F. 1979. Classification and nomenclature of viruses. Intervirology 11:133–135.

MURNANE, T. G. 1981. Encephalomyocarditis. In Viral Zoonoses. Boca Raton, Fla: CRC Press, pp. 137–147.

MURNANE, T. G.; CRAIGHEAD, J. E.; MONDRAGON, H.; AND SHELOKOV, A. 1960. Fetal disease of swine due to encephalomyocarditis virus. Science 131:498–499.

RAMOS, J. R.; GOMEZ, L.; MAYO, M.; AND SANCHEZ, G. 1983. Infection due to encephalomyocarditis virus in swine and other species over the 1975–1981 period. Rvta Cub Cienc Vet 14:71–77.

ROEHE, P. M.; RODRIGUES, N. C.; AND DE OLIVEIRA, S. J. 1985. Encephalomyocarditis virus (EMC) in swine in the state of Rio Grande do Sul, Brazil. Rev Microbiol (Sao Paulo) 16:117–120.

RUECKERT, R. R. 1985. Picornaviruses and their replication. In Virology. New York: Raven Press, pp. 705–738.

SANFORD, S. E.; JOSEPHSON, G. K. A.; REHMTULLA, A. J.; AND CARMAN, P. S. 1989. Antibodies to encephalomyocarditis virus in aborted and stillborn pigs. Can Vet J 30:757.

SANGAR, D. V.; ROWLANDS, D. J.; AND BROWN, F. 1977. Encephalomyocarditis antibodies in sera from apparently normal pigs. Vet Rec 100:240–241.

SEAMAN, J. T.; BOULTON, J. G.; AND CARRIGAN, M. J. 1986. Encephalomyocarditis virus disease of pigs associated with a plague of rodents. Aust Vet J 63:292–294.

SIDOLI, L.; BARIGAZZI, G.; FONI, E.; MARCATO, P. S.; AND BARBIERI, G. 1988. Encephalomyocarditis due to cardiovirus in Po Valley swine. Preliminary observations. Proc Ital Soc Swine Pathol, pp. 249–260.

SIMPSON, C. F.; LEWIS, A. L.; AND GASKIN, J. M. 1977. Encephalomyocarditis virus infection of captive elephants. J Am Vet Med Assoc 171:902–905.

SPRADBROW, P. B., AND CHUNG, Y. S. 1970. Hemagglutination-inhibition antibodies to encephalomyocarditis virus in Queensland cattle. Aust Vet J 46:126–128.

SUTHERLAND, R. J.; HORNER, G. W.; HUNTER, R.; AND FYFE, B. H. 1977. An outbreak of viral encephalomyocarditis in pigs. NZ Vet J 25:225.

TESH, R. B. 1978. The prevalence of encephalomyocarditis virus neutralizing antibodies among various human populations. Am J Trop Med Hyg 27:144–149.

TESH, R. B., AND WALLACE, G. D. 1977. Observations on the natural history of encephalomyocarditis virus. Am J Trop Med Hyg 27:133–143.

TINSLEY, T. W.; MACCALLUM, F. O.; ROBERTSON, J. S.; AND BROWN, F. 1984. Relationship of encephalomyocarditis virus to cricket paralysis virus of insects. Intervirology 21:181–186.

WILLIAMS, M. C. 1981. Encephalomyocarditis virus infection. J S Afr Vet Assoc 52:76.

18 Enterovirus

J. B. Derbyshire

PORCINE ENTEROVIRUSES are ubiquitous, and no conventional herd of pigs has been shown to be free of infection. While the majority of infections are asymptomatic, porcine enteroviruses have been associated with a variety of clinical conditions including polioencephalomyelitis, female reproductive disorders, enteric disease, and pneumonia. They have also been isolated from the male genital tract (Phillips et al. 1972), although the insemination of gilts with contaminated semen did not influence their fertility (De Meurichy and Pensaert 1977). A possible association between porcine enteroviruses and cutaneous lesions resembling swine vesicular disease has been proposed (Knowles 1988).

The first evidence of porcine enterovirus infection to be reported was the occurrence of Teschen disease, a polioencephalomyelitis with high mortality, in Czechoslovakia over 60 years ago. This severe disease has continued to occur sporadically, mainly in central Europe but also in Africa; milder forms of polioencephalomyelitis (Talfan disease, benign enzootic paresis), caused by serologically related but less virulent strains of porcine enterovirus, have been reported in the last 35 years in western Europe, North America, and Australia. In France, the encephalomyelitis is intermediate in severity between Teschen and Talfan diseases (Métianu 1986). The association of porcine enteroviruses with reproductive, enteric, and respiratory disorders in swine is less well established than their role in polioencephalomyelitis. Strains that have not been shown to be pathogenic have been referred to as enteric cytopathogenic swine orphan (ECSO) or enteric cytopathogenic porcine orphan (ECPO) viruses. The only known natural host for porcine enteroviruses is the pig, although experimentally infected pregnant guinea pigs developed placental lesions (Lieu 1976).

ETIOLOGY

Physicochemical Characteristics. Porcine enteroviruses resemble the enteroviruses of other species in their basic properties and are classified within the family Picornaviridae. The virions are spherical, 25–31 nm in diameter, and nonenveloped, with a buoyant density in cesium chloride of 1.34. They contain a core of single-stranded ribonucleic acid (RNA), which is surrounded by a cubic capsid. Lipoprotein is lacking, and the viruses are stable when treated with lipid solvents. Porcine enteroviruses are also relatively stable to heat and pH values between 2 and 9. Hemagglutination has not been demonstrated for porcine enteroviruses. They are relatively resistant to many disinfectants; of 10 commonly used disinfectants tested by Derbyshire and Arkell (1971) against Talfan virus, only sodium hypochlorite or 70% ethanol completely inactivated it. Porcine enteroviruses are also highly resistant to the environment, with Teschen disease virus surviving for more than 168 days at 15°C (Ottis 1976). They survive for long periods in liquid manure, in which they are inactivated more rapidly if the manure is aerated (Lund and Nissen 1983); they are also inactivated in liquid manure by ionizing radiation (Simon et al. 1983), and by anaerobic digestion (Derbyshire et al. 1986).

Laboratory Cultivation. Porcine enteroviruses are readily cultivated in the laboratory in cell cultures of porcine origin. They are most frequently grown in primary or secondary pig kidney (PK) cell cultures or in established kidney cell lines such as IBRS-2, but they may also be cultivated in other cells of porcine origin such as the SST cell line. Some strains can be grown in HeLa, monkey kidney, or baby hamster kidney (BHK) cell lines. Different strains produce one of three kinds of cytopathic effect (CPE) in PK cultures, and this characteristic, together with the cytopathogenicity of the viruses for BHK 21, HeLa and Vero cells, enables strains to be placed in one of four groups (Knowles et al. 1979).

Serologic Classification. The serologic classification of porcine enteroviruses is based upon the virus-neutralization (VN) test; numerous attempts to achieve such a classification have been recorded in the literature. The early work in this area was by Dunne et al. (1971) and extended by Knowles et al. (1979); Table 18.1 is based mainly upon these authors' findings. A complement-fixation test, suitable for the rapid screening and typing of porcine enteroviruses, has also been described (Knowles and Buckley 1980). Subsequent findings (Knowles 1983) suggest that additional serogroups may exist. Some limited cross-reactivity among the existing serogroups is evident, and Hazlett and Derbyshire (1978)

263

Table 18.1. Serologic classification of porcine enteroviruses

Serogroup No.	CPE	Reference Strain	Other Strains
1	I	Teschen	Talfan, PS34 (SMEDI C), PS35, F65, J1, WR1, T1, ECPO-3, E1, PE6
2	I	T80	T52A, O3b, F17, F59, E4, J2, T3
3	I	O2b	PS2-PS13, PS14 (SMEDI B), PS15-PS20, F34, PE1, PE3, PE10
4	I	PS36	PS38, F78, DE8
5	I	F26	F12, J3
6	I	PS37 (SMEDI E)	T4, WR4, F7, ECPO-2, J5
7	I	F43	WR2
8	II	PS27 (SMEDI A)	PS23, PS25, PS26, PS28-PS30, PS32 (SMEDI D), V13, A1, WR3, WR5, WR6, ECPO-1, ECPO-5, CHICO, PE4, PE5, PE7
9	III	UKG410/73	UKG139/3, UKG194/73, UKG298/73(c), UKG380/73, Pd2
10	III	LP54	GF50
11	I	UKG173/74	MV1-76

showed that gastrointestinal antibodies were more broadly specific than serum antibodies.

EPIDEMIOLOGY. The virulent serogroup 1 strains associated with classical Teschen disease appear to be restricted to those areas in which the disease occurs, and they have not been isolated in North America. Less virulent serogroup 1 viruses and representatives of the other serogroups appear to be ubiquitous (Odend'hal 1983). Transmission of porcine enterovirus infection is most frequently by the fecal-oral route, and indirect transmission by fomites is extremely likely to occur since they are relatively resistant viruses. Endemic infection with several serogroups of porcine enteroviruses can always be demonstrated in conventional herds and is probably maintained in groups of weaned piglets. Singh and Bohl (1972) demonstrated waves of infection with six different serotypes over a period of 26 months in a long-term study of enterovirus infection in a single herd. Infection is normally acquired by piglets shortly after weaning when maternally derived antibodies are withdrawn and pigs from several litters are mixed together, and it persists for at least several weeks. Adults rarely excrete virus but have high antibody levels. Pigs of any age are, however, fully susceptible to infection with a porcine enterovirus belonging to a serogroup to which they have not previously been exposed.

CLINICAL SIGNS. While porcine enterovirus infection is most frequently asymptomatic, various clinical syndromes have been associated with certain serogroups, as indicated in Table 18.2 and outlined below.

Table 18.2. Natural or experimental clinical syndromes associated with porcine enterovirus infection

Syndrome	Serogroups
Polioencephalomyelitis	1, 2, 3, 5
Reproductive disorders	1, 3, 6, 8
Diarrhea	1, 2, 3, 5, 8
Pneumonia	1, 2, 3, 8
Pericarditis and myocarditis	2, 3

Polioencephalomyelitis. The most severe form of polioencephalomyelitis is that produced by the highly virulent serogroup 1 strains that cause Teschen disease. This is a disease of high morbidity and high mortality, affecting all ages of swine and associated with major economic losses. The early signs of Teschen disease include fever, anorexia, and listlessness, rapidly followed by locomotor ataxia. In severe cases there may be nystagmus, convulsions, opisthotonus, and coma. Paralysis ensues, and the animal may assume a dog-sitting posture or remain in lateral recumbency. Stimulation by sound or touch may elicit uncoordinated limb movements or opisthotonus. Death is common within 3 or 4 days of the onset of clinical signs. Since the appetite returns after the acute phase, some animals may be kept alive by careful nursing, but these cases show muscle wasting and residual paralysis. The less virulent type 1 strains (Talfan disease, benign enzootic paresis) and the other serogroups associated with polioencephalomyelitis produce a milder disease with relatively low morbidity and mortality. Young piglets are mainly affected, and the disease rarely progresses to complete paralysis.

Reproductive Disorders. The term SMEDI was introduced initially (Dunne et al. 1965) to designate a group of viruses, subsequently shown to be porcine enteroviruses, that had been isolated in assocation with stillbirth (S), mummified fetuses (M), embryonic death (ED), and infertility (I). Subsequent studies by the same group of workers and by others (De Meurichy et al. 1976) indicated that the syndrome could be reproduced experimentally. However, it is now well established that parvovirus infection may also lead to embryonic death and fetal mummification, and this virus may be more frequently associated with these disorders of early and midgestation. Other findings (Cropper et al. 1976) substantiate a role for enteroviruses as well as parvoviruses in these disorders, and experimental (Bielanski and Raeside 1977) and field (Kirkbride and McAdaragh 1978) data confirm an association between enterovirus infection and abortion in swine. These reproductive disorders are not usually accompanied by clinical signs in the sow or gilt.

Diarrhea. The role of porcine enteroviruses as enteric pathogens is uncertain. They have frequently been isolated from the feces of piglets with diarrhea; but since they can be readily isolated from normal piglets, particularly postweaning, and since diarrhea can be caused by a variety of other viral and bacterial agents, their presence may be coincidental. However, diarrhea has been produced experimentally by enteroviruses in piglets believed to be free of other pathogens. The diarrhea is mild and relatively transient, and it seems clear that porcine enteroviruses are considerably less important enteric pathogens than rotaviruses or coronaviruses. When piglets were infected with porcine enteroviruses together with rotaviruses, the disease was less severe than in piglets infected only with the rotavirus (Janke et al. 1988).

Pneumonia, Pericarditis, and Myocarditis. The role of enteroviruses as respiratory pathogens is also uncertain. It is probable that alone they rarely cause clinical signs of respiratory disease, although Pospisil et al. (1971) noted increased respiration, coughing, snorting, reduced appetite, and depression in piglets exposed to an aerosol of porcine enterovirus. While pathogenic studies indicate some degree of tropism of these viruses for the lung, the pneumonia produced is usually subclinical. Two serotypes of porcine enterovirus have been shown experimentally to be capable of producing pericarditis, and in one experiment myocardial involvement occurred (Long et al. 1969). These findings might lead to a suspicion of enterovirus infection in the case of sudden death in piglets, although encephalomyocarditis virus might be a more likely candidate.

PATHOGENESIS. Natural infection occurs by ingestion of the virus, and it is well established (Long 1985) that initial replication occurs in the tonsil and intestinal tract. The large intestine and ileum are infected more frequently than the upper small intestine, and the former tissues contain higher titers of virus. It has not been clearly established which cells in the intestine support viral replication, but by analogy with experiments on poliovirus (Kanamitsu et al. 1967) it is probable that the reticuloendothelial tissue of the lamina propria is involved. Epithelial cell destruction is not a feature of enterovirus infections. Viremia follows regularly in infections with the virulent serogroup 1 viruses, but occurs less regularly with the less virulent strains, leading to infection of the central nervous system (CNS) (Holman et al. 1966). It may be assumed that the pregnant uterus is also infected by viremic spread of the

virus, since embryonic or fetal infections were demonstrated in gilts following nasal or oral inoculation of enterovirus (Huang et al. 1980). Intranasal inoculation of virus may lead experimentally to lung infection (Meyer et al. 1966), but the significance of the natural inhalation of viral aerosols is not known. It has also been clearly demonstrated that when piglets are inoculated parenterally with swine enteroviruses, the virus rapidly infects the intestine. Extraintestinal infections are relatively transient, while the virus persists in the large intestine for several weeks.

LESIONS. No specific changes have been associated with intestinal enterovirus infections. They do not appear to cause villous atrophy, which is characteristic of primary intestinal pathogens such as coronaviruses and rotaviruses. Other than muscle atrophy in chronic cases, no gross lesions are found in polioencephalomyelitis. The histologic lesions associated with the latter are widely distributed in the CNS but are especially numerous in the ventral columns of the spinal cord, the cerebellar cortex, and the brain stem. The changes are more marked and extensive in Teschen disease than in milder encephalomyelitides such as Talfan disease. The neurons show progressive, diffuse chromatolysis (Koestner et al. 1966), and there are focal areas of gliosis and perivascular lymphocytic cuffing. Some meningeal infiltration with lymphocytes, particularly over the cerebellum, may also occur. The SMEDI syndrome is remarkable for the lack of specific lesions in stillborn or neonatal piglets, although mild focal gliosis and perivascular cuffing in the brain stem have been found occasionally. Placental changes are restricted to nonspecific degeneration. Pneumonic lesions have been produced by several investigators. Smith et al. (1973) described areas of grayish red consolidation in the ventral anterior lobes of lungs infected with a serogroup 2 strain. There were exudates in the alveoli and bronchi, slight perivascular and peribronchiolar cuffing, and some hyperplasia of the bronchiolar epithelium. A serogroup 3 strain consistently produced serofibrinous pericarditis experimentally, and the more severely affected piglets showed focal myocardial necrosis (Long and Koestner 1969).

DIAGNOSIS. The occurrence of clinical signs associated with polioencephalomyelitis is suggestive of viral infection, but the differentiation of enteroviral infection from other neurotropic viruses requires isolation of the virus from the CNS or the demonstration of viral antigen by specific immunofluorescence. Virus isolation from the CNS requires the collection of tissues from a piglet showing early nervous signs; animals that have been paralyzed for several days may no longer contain infectious virus in the CNS (Lynch et al. 1984). The virus may be isolated in PK cell cultures from suspensions of spinal cord, brain stem, or cerebellum; it may subsequently be identified on the basis of its physicochemical characteristics, by immunofluorescence (Watanabe 1971), or immunoperoxidase staining (Sulochana and Derbyshire 1978). Serologic identification of the isolate is desirable. The isolation of an enterovirus from the gastrointestinal tract of a piglet with nervous signs does not establish the etiology of the disease, since the enteric infection may be coincidental. An enzyme-linked immunosorbent assay, suitable for mass screening, has been described for the detection of antibodies against Teschen disease virus (Hubschle et al. 1983). In the SMEDI syndrome, mummified fetuses carried to term rarely contain live virus but may contain viral antigen detectable by immunofluorescence. Enterovirus isolation in PK cell culture may be attempted from tissues of aborted or stillborn fetuses. Lung tissue appears to be the most reliable source for the isolation of porcine enteroviruses from fetuses (Huang et al. 1980). VN tests on the body fluids of such fetuses can be carried out against the SMEDI-associated serogroups. Serology on the sow is not of value. In the investigation of pneumonia or diarrhea, virus isolation from the respiratory or intestinal tracts may be attempted, but the virologic findings should be cautiously interpreted, especially in relation to diarrhea, since enteric infections with enteroviruses are common in healthy piglets.

TREATMENT. As in most viral infections, control measures for porcine enteroviruses depend on prevention rather than treatment. Potential antiviral chemotherapeutics for porcine enteroviruses have received little attention. Piglets with mild polioencephalomyelitis may recover if nursing care is provided during the period of transient paresis.

PREVENTION. Vaccination has been practiced in the field only for the control of Teschen disease. The earlier Teschen disease vaccines, containing inactivated virus of pig tissue origin, have been superseded by attenuated or inactivated cell culture vaccines. Mayr and Correns (1959) attenuated Teschen disease virus by cell culture passage and showed that live or formalin-inactivated vaccines prepared from this virus induced similar levels of protection in piglets. Success has been claimed for a Teschen disease eradication program involving ring vaccination and slaughter (Schaupp 1968). Restrictions on the import of swine and pork products from areas in which Teschen disease is endemic seem to be effective in limiting the spread of virulent serogroup 1 viruses. If such strains were introduced into North America, they would be controlled by a policy of quarantine and slaughter.

Vaccination has not been practiced against the milder forms of polioencephalomyelitis nor against the other clinical manifestations of enterovirus infection in swine. Of the latter, only the SMEDI syndrome is of sufficient economic importance to justify specific control measures in the field, but the multiplicity of serogroups that may be involved complicates the development of an effective vaccine. The best current approach to the prevention of reproductive disorders associated with enteroviruses would appear to be the application of management practices that ensure that gilts are exposed to infection with endemic enteroviruses at least 1 month before breeding. This can be achieved naturally if the animals remain in a single building from birth to breeding, with thorough mixing of piglets from different litters at weaning; but if breeding stock is segregated at an early age, they should be contaminated with fecal material from recently weaned piglets. This can be readily accomplished by adding fresh feces to the feed of gilts or by dosing gilts with capsules of feces, which should be a pooled sample collected from weaned piglets in several pens to ensure exposure to as wide a range as possible of the virus present in the herd. The operation of a closed herd system reduces the risk of introducing extraneous viruses, but it is not possible to eliminate this risk, since the relatively resistant enteroviruses can be transmitted by a variety of fomites. If the introduction of fresh stock is essential for breeding purposes, consideration should be given to ensuring exposure, by fecal contamination as described above, of gilts or sows before they are bred, to any virus that may be present or introduced.

Exclusion of porcine enteroviruses by repopulation of herds with specific-pathogen-free (SPF) stock seems to be difficult or impossible to achieve over a prolonged period, since enteroviruses have been isolated from a commercial SPF herd (Derbyshire et al. 1966) and the accidental introduction of Talfan virus into SPF gilts maintained under strict isolation has been described (Parker et al. 1981).

REFERENCES

Bielanski, A., and Raeside, J. I. 1977. Plasma concentration of steroid hormones in sows infected experimentally with *Leptospira pomona* or porcine enterovirus T1 in late gestation. Res Vet Sci 22:28–34.

Cropper, M.; Dunne, H. W.; Leman, A. D.; Starkey, A. L; and Hoefling, D. C. 1976. Prevalence of antibodies to porcine enteroviruses and porcine parvovirus in body fluids of fetal pigs from small vs large litters. J Am Vet Med Assoc 168:233–235.

De Meurichy, W., and Pensaert, M. 1977. Effect of an enterovirus in gilts inseminated with a semen-virus mixture. Zentralbl Veterinaermed [B] 24:97–103.

De Meurichy, W.; Pensaert, M.; and Bonte, P. 1976. Het SMEDI-syndrome bij het varken: Rol van de enterovirussen en het parvovirus. Vlaam Diergeneeskd Tijdschr 45:241–261.

Derbyshire, J. B., and Arkell, S. 1971. The activity of some chemical disinfectants against Talfan virus and porcine adenovirus type 2. Br Vet J 127:137–142.

Derbyshire, J. B.; Clarke, M. C.; and Collins, A. P.

1966. Observations on the faecal excretion of adenoviruses and enteroviruses in conventional and minimal disease pigs. Vet Rec 79:595–599.

DERBYSHIRE, J. B.; MONTEITH, H. D.; AND SHANNON, E. E. 1986. Virological studies on an anaerobic digestion system for liquid manure. Agri Wastes 18:309–312.

DUNNE, H. W.; GOBBLE, J. L.; HOKANSON, J. F.; KRADEL, D. C.; AND BUBASH, G. R. 1965. Porcine reproductive failure associated with a newly identified "SMEDI" group of picorna viruses. Am J Vet Res 26:1284–1297.

DUNNE, H. W.; WANG, J. T.; AND AMMERMAN, E. H. 1971. Classification of North American porcine enteroviruses: A comparison with European and Japanese strains. Infect Immun 4:619–631.

HAZLETT, D. T. G., AND DERBYSHIRE, J. B. 1978. Broad specificity of gastrointestinal antibodies following vaccination of piglets with a porcine enterovirus. J Comp Pathol 88:467–471.

HOLMAN, J. E.; KOESTNER, A.; AND KASZA, L. 1966. Histopathogenesis of porcine polioencephalomyelitis in the germ-free pig. Pathol Vet 3:633–651.

HUANG, J.; GENTRY, R. F.; AND ZARKOWER, A. 1980. Experimental infection of pregnant sows with porcine enteroviruses. Am J Vet Res 41:469–473.

HUBSCHLE, O. J. B.; RAJANARISON, I.; KOKO, E.; RAKOTONDRAMARY, E.; AND RASIOFOMANANA, P. 1983. ELISA zur prufung von schweinseren auf antikorper gegen Teschenvirus. DTW 90:86–88.

JANKE, B. H.; MOREHOUSE, L. G.; AND SOLORZANO, R. F. 1988. Single and mixed infections of rotaviruses and enteroviruses: Clinical signs and microscopic lesions. Can J Vet Res 52:364–369.

KANAMITSU, M.; KASAMAKI, A.; OGAWA, M.; KASAHARA, S.; AND INAMURA, M. 1967. Immunofluorescent study on the pathogenesis of oral infection of poliovirus in monkey. Jpn J Med Sci Biol 20:175–194.

KIRKBRIDE, C. A., AND McADARAGH, J. P. 1978. Infectious agents associated with fetal and early neonatal death and abortion in swine. J Am Vet Med Assoc 172:480–483.

KNOWLES, N. J. 1983. Isolation and identification of porcine enteroviruses in Great Britain, 1979 to 1980. Br Vet J 139:19–22.

————. 1988. The association of group III porcine enteroviruses with epithelial tissues. Vet Rec 122:441–442.

KNOWLES, N. J., AND BUCKLEY, L. S. 1980. Differentiation of porcine enterovirus serotypes by complement fixation. Res Vet Sci 29:113–115.

KNOWLES, N. J.; BUCKLEY, L. S.; AND PEREIRA, H. G. 1979. Classification of porcine enteroviruses by antigenic analysis and cytopathic effects in tissue culture: Description of 3 new serotypes. Arch Virol 62:201–208.

KOESTNER, A.; KASZA, L.; AND HOLMAN, J. E. 1966. Electron microscopic evaluation of the pathogenesis of porcine polioencephalomyelitis. Am J Pathol 49:325–337.

LIEU, C. I. 1976. The experimental infection of pregnant guinea pigs with porcine enterovirus–"SMEDI A" virus. Taiwan J Vet Med Anim Husb 28:1–14.

LONG, J. F. 1985. Pathogenesis of porcine polioencephalomyelitis. In Comparative Pathobiology of Viral Diseases, Vol. 1. Ed. R. A. Olsen, S. Krakowka, and J. R. Blakeslee. Boca Raton, Fla.: CRC Press Inc., pp. 179–197.

LONG, J. F., AND KOESTNER, A. 1969. Pericarditis and myocarditis in germ-free and colostrum-deprived pigs experimentally infected with a porcine polioencephalomyelitis virus. J Infect Dis 120:245–249.

LUND, E., AND NISSEN, B. 1983. The survival of enteroviruses in aerated and unaerated cattle and pig slurry. Agri Wastes 7:221–223.

LYNCH, J. A.; BINNINGTON, B. D.; AND HOOVER, D. M. 1984. Virus isolation studies in an outbreak of porcine encephalomyelitis. Can J Comp Med 48:233–235.

MAYR, A., AND CORRENS, H. 1959. Experimentelle Untersuchungen uber Lebend- und Totimpfstoffe aus einem modifizierten Gewebekulturstamm des Teschenvirus (poliomyelitis suum). Zentralbl Veterinaermed 6:416–428.

MÉTIANU, T. 1986. La maladie de Teschen-Talfan en France. Bull Acad Vet Fr 59:291–302.

MEYER, R. C.; WOODS, G. T.; AND SIMON, J. 1966. Pneumonitis in an enterovirus infection in swine. J Comp Pathol 76:397–405.

ODEND'HAL, S. 1983. The Geographical Distribution of Animal Virus Diseases. New York: Academic Press, p. 415.

OTTIS, K. 1976. Vergleichende Untersuchungen uber die Tenazitat von Viren in Trink- und Oberflachenwasser. Inaug. diss., Munich.

PARKER, B. N. J.; WRATHALL, A. E.; AND CARTWRIGHT, S. F. 1981. Accidental introduction of porcine parvovirus and Talfan virus into a group of minimal disease gilts and their effects on reproduction. Br Vet J 137:262–267.

PHILLIPS, R. M.; FOLEY, C. W.; AND LUKERT, P. D. 1972. Isolation and characterization of viruses from semen and the reproductive tract of male swine. J Am Vet Med Assoc 161:1306–1316.

POSPISIL, Z.; GOIS, M.; VEZNIKOVA, D.; AND CERNY, M. 1971. The pathogenesis of experimental infection of gnotobiotic piglets with enterovirus strain Kr 69TK. Acta Vet Brno 40[Suppl 2]:43–46.

SCHAUPP, W. 1968. Eradication of contagious paralysis (Teschen disease) in Austria. Wien Tieraerztl Wochenschr 55:346–356.

SIMON, J.; MOCSARI, E.; DI GLERIA, M.; AND FELKAI, V. 1983. Effect of radiation on certain animal viruses in liquid swine manure. Int J Appl Radioisot 34:793–795.

SINGH, K. V., AND BOHL, E. H. 1972. The pattern of enteroviral infection in a herd of swine. Can J Comp Med 36:243–248.

SMITH, I. M.; BETTS, A. O.; WATT, R. G.; AND HAYWARD, A. H. S. 1973. Experimental infections with Pasteurella septica (serogroup A) and an adeno- or enterovirus in gnotobiotic piglets. J Comp Pathol 83:1–12.

SULOCHANA, S., AND DERBYSHIRE, J. B. 1978. Use of indirect immunoperoxidase test for detection of porcine enteroviral antigens in infected PK15 cell cultures. Kerala J Vet Sci 9:111–119.

WATANABE, H. 1971. Fluorescent antibody technique in cultured cells infected with porcine enteroviruses. Jpn J Vet Res 19:1–6.

19 Hemagglutinating Encephalomyelitis Virus

M. B. Pensaert

K. Andries

IN CANADA IN 1962, Greig et al. isolated a previously unrecognized viral pathogen of swine from the brain of suckling pigs with encephalomyelitis. The virus responsible for this disease was called hemagglutinating encephalomyelitis virus (HEV) because of its hemagglutinating properties; it was later classified as a coronavirus (Greig et al. 1971; Phillip et al. 1971).

In 1969, an antigenically similar if not identical virus was isolated in England from suckling pigs showing anorexia, depression, and vomiting but without signs clearly associated with encephalomyelitis (Cartwright et al. 1969). Animals that did not die remained stunted in growth; the condition was therefore called vomiting and wasting disease (VWD). Mengeling and Cutlip (1976) were later able to experimentally reproduce both of the major forms of the disease, i.e., the clinically apparent encephalomyelitis and VWD, using the same field isolates. Although epizootiologic studies have revealed that infection of swine with HEV is prevalent, naturally occurring disease is uncommon. Neonatal pigs are usually protected by passively acquired colostral antibody, and they subsequently develop an age-related resistance to the potential clinical effects of the virus.

ETIOLOGY

Virus Structure. HEV has an electron microscopic appearance similar to other coronaviruses. Negatively stained particles have a spherical shape, with an overall diameter of 120 nm (Greig et al. 1971). Club-shaped surface projections arranged as a solar "corona" protrude from the envelope. Lamontagne et al. (1981) showed that the viral particle contains two concentric membranes (an external envelope and an inner membranous bag) encircling a central core.

Studies on the chemical composition revealed that the virus contains five polypeptides, four of which are glycosylated, with molecular weights from 31,000 to 180,000 daltons (Pocock and Garwes 1977; Callebaut and Pensaert 1980). The viral nucleic acid was considered to be of the RNA type since the growth of HEV is not affected by inhibitors of DNA metabolism (Greig and Girard 1969). The buoyant density was 1.21 g/cm³ in cesium chloride (Mengeling and Coria 1972) and 1.18 g/cm³ in potassium tartrate (Greig and Bouillant 1972).

Physicochemical Properties. The virus is stable between pH4 and 10 and moderately sensitive to heat (Chappuis et al. 1975). All viral infectivity is lost after 30 minutes at 56°C, but the infectivity titer is reduced by only $0.8 \log_{10}$ after 7 days at 4°C. HEV was shown by Greig and Girard (1969) to be sensitive to lipid solvents, including sodium desoxycholate. Lipid solvent agents are thus suitable for disinfection. Ultraviolet irradiation also results in a significant reduction of viral infectivity (Pensaert and Callebaut 1974).

Biologic Properties. The natural host of HEV is the pig. The virus also has been adapted experimentally to replicate in mice (Kaye et al. 1977; Yagami et al. 1986). The susceptibility of mice was found to be influenced by age and inoculation routes.

HEV was first isolated in primary cultures of pig kidney (PK) cells by Greig et al. (1962), who described a cytopathic effect (CPE) characterized by the appearance of syncytia. Many of these syncytia degenerated soon after their formation, detached from the cell sheet, and floated in the medium as semiopaque gelatinous masses. The incorporation of a noncytotoxic amount of diethylaminoethyl-dextran may enhance the CPE (Sato et al. 1983).

Using the immunofluorescence (IF) test, HEV was also shown to propagate in several other porcine cell cultures such as adult thyroid gland, embryonic lung, testicle cell line, PK-15 cell line (Pirtle 1974), IBRS₂ cell line (Chappuis et al. 1975), SK cell line (Lucas and Napthine 1971), and SK-K cell line (Hirano et al. 1990). Nonporcine cell cultures were shown to have little susceptibility for growth of HEV.

Virus particles can be seen by electron microscopy in cytoplasmic vesicles of infected cells. Assembly occurs by budding through membranes of the endoplasmic reticulum (Ducatelle et al. 1981).

HEV was demonstrated to possess a virion-associated hemagglutinin. The virus spontaneously agglutinates erythrocytes of mice, rats, chickens, and several other kinds of animals (Girard et al. 1964). Elution of HEV from red blood cells has not been observed. Using the same kinds of erythrocytes, a hemadsorption test can be used to demonstrate viral growth in inoculated cell cultures.

Antigenic Characteristics. Although HEV is known to be the cause of different clinical syndromes, only one serotype of the virus is known to exist. The susceptibility of the infected pigs and strain differences in virulence are probably responsible for the fact that usually only one of the syndromes is seen in a particular outbreak. An antigenic relationship exists between HEV and the neonatal calf diarrhea virus, as shown by seroneutralization (SN), hemagglutination inhibition (HI) (Sato et al. 1980), IF, and immunoelectron microscopy (Pensaert et al. 1981). HEV is also related to human respiratory coronavirus OC 43 (Kaye et al. 1977) and mouse hepatitis virus (Pedersen et al. 1978). Moderate cross-reactivity was observed between HEV and turkey enteric coronavirus (Dea and Tijssen 1989).

EPIDEMIOLOGY. Pigs are the only species known to be naturally susceptible to HEV infection. Most of the infections in this species are subclinical and the economic importance of the disease is low. The spread of HEV in the pig population has been studied in several countries. The HI and SN tests proved to be almost equally sensitive in the demonstration of specific antibodies to HEV in swine sera (Mengeling 1975). Serologic surveys revealed that infection of swine with HEV is very common and probably worldwide. In fattening pigs, 31% of the sera were positive in Canada (Girard et al. 1964), 46% in Northern Ireland (McFerran et al. 1971), 49% in England (Cartwright and Lucas 1970), 52% in Japan (Hirai et al. 1974), 75% in Germany (Hess and Bachmann 1978), and 0–89% in the United States, depending on the region surveyed (Mengeling 1975). The percentage of sows with antibodies at slaughter varied from 43% in Northern Ireland to 98% in the United States. A high number of seropositive animals was also found in Denmark (Sørensen 1975), France (Vannier et al. 1981), Australia (Forman et al. 1979), Belgium (Pensaert et al. 1980), and Austria (Möstl 1990). Conversely, Neuvonen et al. (1982) found 40 Finnish elite breeding pig herds to be free of seropositive animals.

Under experimental conditions, disease has been produced in most instances when nonimmune pigs have been exposed oronasally to HEV sometime during the first few weeks of life (Alexander 1962; Appel et al. 1965). Clinical signs may vary, however, and in a study in which several field isolates of HEV were compared as to virulence, the severity of such signs was related to a difference in host susceptibility (even among littermates) as well as to the apparent virulence of each isolate (Mengeling and Cutlip 1976). In con-

trast, older pigs and neonatal pigs that had received antibody in colostrum were usually clinically unaffected when exposed to HEV under otherwise similar conditions (Appel et al. 1965). These observations are believed to explain why naturally occurring disease is relatively uncommon even though HEV is ubiquitous among swine. In herds where HEV infection is enzootic, most pigs receive protective antibody in colostrum, and circulating maternal antibodies persist for about 4–18 (mean 10.5) weeks (Paul and Mengeling 1984). By the time such antibody wanes, the pigs have already developed an age-related resistance to the disease. Additional support for this concept is provided by a serologic study on two Belgian breeding farms, which showed that passively acquired colostral immunity was replaced by active immunity as a consequence of subclinical infection of pigs between 8 and 16 weeks of age (Pensaert et al. 1980).

CLINICAL SIGNS. Upon infection with HEV, two clinical syndromes are possible: an acute, clinically apparent encephalomyelitis and VWD. Both syndromes are confined almost exclusively to pigs less than 3 weeks of age, although older swine may occasionally vomit and have a brief period of inappetence and listlessness. Thus far the encephalomyelitic form has been described only in Canada (Alexander et al. 1959) and the United States (Werdin et al. 1976). Both syndromes show many signs in common, and between the acute encephalomyelitis and the chronic VWD, all degrees of severity may occur.

At the start of a VWD outbreak, sneezing or coughing may occur. The primary sign seen after an incubation period of 4–7 days is repeated retching and vomiting. Pigs under 4 weeks of age start suckling but soon stop, withdraw from the sow, and vomit the milk they have taken in. They huddle together, look pale and listless, and often have an arched back. Body temperature can be elevated at the beginning of the disease but returns to the normal range within 1–2 days. Affected pigs are often observed to grind their teeth. They dip their mouths into water bowls but drink little, if any at all, indicating a possible pharyngeal paralysis. The persistent vomiting and decreased food intake results in constipation and a rapid decline of condition. The youngest pigs become severely dehydrated after a few days, exhibit dyspnea and cyanosis, fall in coma, and die. Older pigs lose their appetite and rapidly become emaciated. They continue to vomit, although less frequently than in the early stage of the disease. A large distension of the cranial abdomen is developed by some animals. This "wasting" state may persist for several weeks until the pigs die of starvation. Mortality approaches 100% within the same litter, and survivors remain permanently stunted.

An outbreak of the encephalomyelitic form

may start as a VWD outbreak. Some pigs vomit 4–7 days after birth. The vomiting is continued intermittently for 1–2 days but is rarely severe and does not result in dehydration. In other outbreaks, the first sign is acute depression and a tendency to huddle. Pigs may become sick as soon as 2 days after birth. Occasionally, sneezing, coughing, or upper respiratory embarassment is observed. The pigs lose weight rapidly and their hair loses its luster and becomes rough. After 1–3 days, symptoms of a severe encephalomyelitis arise. Younger pigs are most severely affected and exhibit various combinations of nervous signs. Generalized muscle tremors and hyperesthesia are common findings. Pigs that are able to stand usually have a jerky gait, and they tend to walk backwards, often ending in a dog-sitting position. They soon become very weak, are unable to rise, and paddle their limbs. Their noses and feet become cyanotic. Blindness, opisthotonus, and nystagmus can also occur. Finally, the animals become prostrate, lying on their sides, and have dyspnea. In most cases, coma precedes death. Mortality in younger pigs is usually 100%. Older pigs usually suffer a mild transient illness in which posterior paralysis is the most common sign. The paresis in a few cases is accompanied by blindness. The animals are apparently able to recover completely after 3–5 days. The interval for onset of the disease in the first litter to cessation of the disease or its failure to appear in a litter is usually 2–3 weeks (Werdin et al. 1976). Disappearance of the disease coincides with the time it takes sows to develop immunity and to pass this protection on to their offspring. It has been shown that pigs exposed to HEV develop seroneutralizing and hemagglutination-inhibiting antibodies (Pensaert and Callebaut 1974).

PATHOGENESIS. Several observations indicate that HEV is able to replicate in the upper respiratory tract without producing clinical signs. Mengeling et al. (1972) and Pensaert et al. (1980) recorded the isolation of HEV from the nasal cavity of healthy pigs. Clinical disease can be reproduced by oronasal inoculation of colostrum-deprived piglets; the virus is excreted for 6–8 days in oronasal secretions (Pensaert and Callebaut 1974). The mode of transmission is probably through nasal secretions.

In a series of studies on the pathogenesis of the disease, Andries and Pensaert (1980c) inoculated newborn colostrum-deprived pigs oronasally with a HEV strain from pigs showing the VWD syndrome. Anorexia and vomiting were seen after an incubation period of 4 days. Pigs were killed at different times after inoculation; results of the examination by the immunofluorescent antibody technique revealed that the epithelial cells of nasal mucosa, tonsils, lungs, and small intestine served as sites of primary viral replication. After local replication near the sites of entry, the virus spread via the peripheral nervous system to the central nervous system (CNS). At least three pathways appeared to be involved. A first pathway led from the nasal mucosa and tonsils to the trigeminal ganglion and the trigeminal sensory nucleus in the brainstem. A second pathway occurred along the vagal nerves via the vagal sensory ganglion to the vagal sensory nucleus in the brainstem. A third pathway led from the intestinal plexuses to the spinal cord, also after replication in local sensory ganglia. Earlier studies had already shown that viremia is probably of little or no importance in the pathogenesis (Andries and Pensaert 1980b). In the CNS, the infection started in well-defined nuclei of the medulla oblongata but progressed later into the entire brainstem, the spinal cord, and sometimes also the cerebrum and cerebellum. Fluorescence in the brain was always restricted to the perikaryon and processes of neurons (Fig. 19.1). Vomiting was

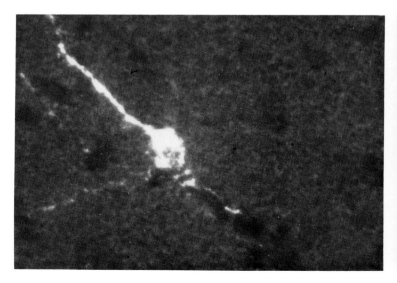

19.1. Viral multiplication in the brainstem of a pig inoculated with HEV. Fluorescence is seen in the axon and the perikaryon of a neuron. ×500.

induced by viral replication in the vagal sensory ganglion (ganglion distale vagi) or by impulses to the vomiting center produced by infected neurons at different sites (Andries 1982).

To elucidate the pathogenesis of the wasting, radiologic studies were performed on chronically infected animals, vagotomized animals, and controls (Andries 1982). The stomach of control pigs was always empty within 10 hours, whereas barium was retained in the stomach for 2–7 days in pigs with HEV. In pigs with a bilateral abdominal vagotomy, the stomach emptying was less disturbed. This indicated that the delayed emptying in pigs with HEV was not due only to earlier viral replication in the vagal ganglion and vagal nuclei in the brain. The virus-induced lesions in the intramural plexi of the stomach were probably also responsible for the gastric stasis. The disturbance of the stomach emptying was considered to play an important role in the pathogenesis of the wasting.

LESIONS.   The only significant gross lesions reported in natural HEV infections are cachexia and a distension of the abdomen, which develops in some chronically affected pigs (Schlenstedt et al. 1969; Hoorens et al. 1977). The stomach of such pigs is dilated and filled with gas.

Microscopic lesions are found in the tonsils, the nervous system, respiratory system, and stomach of acutely diseased pigs. The lesions tend to disappear in animals surviving acute stages of the disease. Tonsillar changes are characterized by epithelial degeneration and lymphatic cell infiltration in the crypts (Narita et al. 1989a). A nonsuppurative encephalomyelitis was reported in 70–100% of pigs with nervous signs and in 20–60% of pigs showing the VWD syndrome. The lesions are characterized by perivascular cuffing, gliosis, and neuronal degeneration (Richards and Savan 1960; Alexander 1962; Hoorens et al. 1977; Narita et al. 1989b). They are most pronounced in the gray matter of the pons Varoli, the medulla oblongata, and the dorsal horns of the upper spinal cord. It was suggested that encephalitic lesions are a specific immune response to HEV following its replication in the CNS (Narita et al. 1989b). Neuritis of peripheral sensory ganglia, particularly the trigeminal ganglia, also occurs.

Microscopic changes in the stomach wall and the lungs were found only in pigs showing the VWD syndrome. Degeneration of the ganglia of the stomach wall and perivascular cuffing were present in 15–85% of diseased animals. The lesions were most pronounced in the pyloric gland area (Steinicke and Nielsen 1959; Schlenstedt et al. 1969; Hoorens et al. 1977). Interstitial peribronchiolar pneumonia, with infiltration of neutrophils and macrophages in the alveoli, was observed in 20% of naturally infected animals (Hoorens et al. 1977) and to a much larger extent in experimentally infected pigs (Cutlip and Mengeling 1972).

DIAGNOSIS.   To effect diagnosis by virus isolation, the tonsils, brain, and lungs are dissected aseptically from young diseased piglets slaughtered as soon as possible after the first signs of infection. It is very difficult to isolate the virus from pigs that have been sick for more than 2 days. Crude suspensions of selected tissues are inoculated into primary PK cells or secondary pig thyroid cells. The presence of HEV is shown by the developing of syncytia, hemadsorption, and hemagglutination (Andries and Pensaert 1980a). A single blind passage with cells and culture fluid is recommended, since clinical specimens from pigs infected with HEV often contain very small amounts of infectious virus.

Antibodies to the virus can be detected by the SN, plaque reduction, or HI test (Mengeling 1975; Sato et al. 1983). Since subclinical infections with the virus are very common, antibody titers must be evaluated very carefully. Moreover, a significant rise in antibody titer can be obtained only if acute sera are taken as soon as possible after the appearance of clinical signs. Pigs that become ill after an incubation period of 6–7 days may indeed have already built up a high antibody titer at that moment, making an interpretation of paired sera very difficult.

Differential diagnosis must be made between HEV infection, Teschen-Talfan disease, and Aujeszky's disease. Clinical signs of encephalomyelitis associated with the latter two diseases are usually more severe than those associated with HEV infection and may appear among older pigs as well as piglets. Respiratory signs in older pigs and abortions in sows are typical for Aujeszky's disease. The viruses can be grown in PK and pig thyroid cells; in PK cells they are distinguishable by their CPE. They can be further differentiated by virus identification tests and the production of hemagglutinin by HEV.

PREVENTION.   On most breeding farms, HEV infection persists enzootically and is maintained through a subclinical infection of the respiratory pathways. Sows usually will have come into contact with the virus before the time of first farrowing. They will protect their offspring against clinical signs by colostral antibodies. When infection occurs in such pigs, it will remain subclinical. Only when through circumstances sows are not immune at the time of farrowing (newly populated farms, small farms in which the virus is not maintained through lack of sufficient litters), an infection of pigs within the first 3 weeks after birth will result in clinical signs. Maintaining the virus on farms to obtain immune sows at the time of their first farrowing creates a favorable situation in avoiding breakthroughs of disease in piglets.

Once clinical signs are evident, the disease will run its course; spontaneous recoveries are rare. Litters born 2–3 weeks after the onset of disease are usually protected by maternal immunity. Before that time, piglets born from nonimmune sows can be protected by specific hyperimmune serum injected at birth. However, the time lapse between diagnosis and cessation of the disease is usually too short to gain much profit from this procedure.

REFERENCES

ALEXANDER, T. J. L. 1962. Viral encephalomyelitis of swine in Ontario. Experimental and natural transmission. Am J Vet Res 32:756–762.

ALEXANDER, T. J. L.; RICHARDS, W. R. C.; AND ROE, C. K. 1959. An encephalomyelitis of suckling pigs in Ontario. Can J Comp Med 23:316–319.

ANDRIES, K. 1982. Pathogenese en epizootiologie van "vomiting and wasting disease," een virale infektie bij het varken. Ph.D. diss., Med Fac Diergeneeskd Rijksuniv, Ghent 24:164.

ANDRIES, K., AND PENSAERT, M. 1980a. Propagation of hemagglutinating encephalomyelitis virus in porcine cell cultures. Zentralbl Veterinaermed [B] 27:280–290.

―――. 1980b. Virus isolation and immunofluorescence in different organs of pigs infected with hemagglutinating encephalomyelitis virus. Am J Vet Res 41:215–218.

―――. 1980c. Immunofluorescence studies on the pathogenesis of hemagglutinating encephalomyelitis virus after oronasal inoculation. Am J Vet Res 41:1372–1378.

APPEL, M.; GREIG, A. S.; AND CORNER, A. H. 1965. Encephalomyelitis of swine caused by a haemagglutinating virus. IV. Transmission studies. Res Vet Sci 6:482–489.

CALLEBAUT, P. E., AND PENSAERT, M. B. 1980. Characterization and isolation of structural polypeptides in haemagglutinating encephalomyelitis virus. J Gen Virol 48:193–204.

CARTWRIGHT, S. E., AND LUCAS, M. 1970. Vomiting and wasting disease in piglets. Vet Rec 86:278–280.

CARTWRIGHT, S. F.; LUCAS, M.; CAVILL, P. J.; GUSH, A. F.; AND BLANDFORD, T. B. 1969. Vomiting and wasting disease of piglets. Vet Rec 84:175–176.

CHAPPUIS, G.; TEKTOFF, J.; AND LETURDU, Y. 1975. Isolement en France et identification du virus de la maladie du vomissement et du deperissement des porcelets (coronalike virus). Rec Med Vet 151:557–566.

CUTLIP, R. C., AND MENGELING, W. L. 1972. Lesions induced by hemagglutinating encephalomyelitis virus strain 67N in pigs. Am J Vet Res 33:2003–2009.

DEA, S., AND TIJSSEN, P. 1989. Detection of turkey enteric coronavirus by enzyme-linked immunosorbent assay and differentiation from other coronaviruses. Am J Vet Res 50:226–231.

DUCATELLE, R.; COUSSEMENT, W.; AND HOORENS, J. 1981. Morphogenesis of hemagglutinating encephalomyelitis in vivo and in vitro. VI. Diergeneeskd Tijdschr 50:326–336.

FORMAN, A. J.; HALE, C. J.; JONES, R. T.; AND CONAUGHTON, I. D. 1979. Haemagglutinating encephalomyelitis virus infection of pigs. Aust Vet J 55:503–504.

GIRARD, A.; GREIG, A. S.; AND MITCHELL, D. 1964. Encephalomyelitis of swine caused by a haemagglutinating virus. III. Serological studies. Res Vet Sci 5:294–302.

GREIG, A. S., AND BOUILLANT, A. M. P. 1972. Studies on the hemagglutination phenomenon of hemagglutinating encephalomyelitis virus (HEV) of pigs. Can J Comp Med 36:366–370.

GREIG, A. S., AND GIRARD, A. 1969. Encephalomyelitis of swine caused by a haemagglutinating virus. V. Re-

sponse to metabolic inhibitors and other chemical compounds. Res Vet Sci 10:509.

GREIG, A. S.; MITCHELL, D.; CORNER, A. H.; BANNISTER, G. L.; MEADS, E. B.; AND JULIAN, R. J. 1962. A hemagglutinating virus producing encephalomyelitis in baby pigs. Can J Comp Med 26:49–56.

GREIG, A. S.; JOHNSON, C. M.; AND BOUILLANT, A. M. P. 1971. Encephalomyelitis of swine caused by a haemagglutinating virus. VI. Morphology of the virus. Res Vet Sci 12:305–307.

HESS, R. G., AND BACHMANN, P. A. 1978. Erbrechen und Kummern der Ferkeln. Vorkommen und Verbreitung in Suddeutschland. Tieraerztl Umschau 33:571–574.

HIRAI, K.; CHANG, C.; AND SHIMAKURA, S. 1974. A serological survey on haemagglutinating encephalomyelitis virus infection in pigs in Japan. Jpn J Vet Sci 36:375–380.

HIRANO, N.; ONO, K.; TAKASAWA, H.; MURAKAMI, T.; AND HAGA, S. 1990. Replication and plaque formation of swine haemagglutinating encephalomyelitis virus (67N) in swine cell line, SK-K culture. J Virol Methods 27:91–100.

HOORENS, J.; THOONEN, H.; GHEYLE, M.; AND VAN BUYTEN, A. 1977. Braakziekte bij biggen. Vlaams Diergeneeskd Tijdschr 46:209–224.

KAYE, H. S.; YARBROUGH, W. B.; REED, C. J.; AND HARRISON, A. K. 1977. Antigenic relationship between human coronavirus strain OC43 and hemagglutinating encephalomyelitis virus strain 67N of swine: Antibody responses in human and animal sera. J Infect Dis 135:201–209.

LAMONTAGNE, L.; MAROIS, P.; MARSOLAIS, G.; DIFRANCO, E.; AND ASSAF, R. 1981. Inner structure of some coronaviruses. Can J Comp Med 45:177–181.

LUCAS, M. H., AND NAPTHINE, P. 1971. Fluorescent antibody technique in the study of three porcine viruses. J Comp Pathol 81:111–117.

McFERRAN, J. B.; CLARKE, J. K.; CONNOR, T. J.; AND KNOX, E. R. 1971. Serological evidence of the presence of haemagglutinating encephalomyelitis virus in Northern Ireland. Vet Rec 88:339.

MENGELING, W. L. 1975. Incidence of antibody for hemagglutinating encephalomyelitis virus in serums from swine in the United States. Am J Vet Res 36:821–823.

MENGELING, W. L., AND CORIA, M. F. 1972. Buoyant density of hemagglutinating encephalomyelitis of swine: Comparison with avian bronchitis virus. Am J Vet Res 33:1359–1363.

MENGELING, W. L. AND CUTLIP, R. C. 1976. Pathogenicity of field isolants of hemagglutinating encephalomyelitis virus for neonatal pigs. J Am Vet Med Assoc 168:236–239.

MENGELING, W. L.; BOOTHE, A. D.; AND RITCHIE, A. E. 1972. Characteristics of a coronavirus (strain 67N) of pigs. Am J Vet Res 33:297–308.

MÖSTL, K. 1990. Erhebungen über Porcine Coronaviren in Österreich. III. Teil: Das hemagglutinating Encephalomyelitis Virus (HEV) der Schweine. Wien Tieraerztl Monatsschr 77(4):117–120.

NARITA, M.; KAWAMURA, H.; TSUBOI, T.; HARITANI, M.; AND KOBAYASHI, M. 1989a. Immunopathological and ultrastructural studies on the tonsil of gnotobiotic pigs infected with strain 67N of haemagglutinating encephalomyelitis virus. J Comp Pathol 100:305–312.

NARITA, M.; KAWAMURA, H.; HARITANI, M.; AND KOBAYASHI, M. 1989b. Demonstration of viral antigen and immunoglobulin (IgG and IgM) in brain tissue of pigs experimentally infected with haemagglutinating encephalomyelitis virus. J Comp Pathol 100:119–128.

NEUVONEN, E.; EK-KOMMONEN, C.; VEIJALAINEN, P.; AND SCHULMAN, A. 1982. Absence of hemagglutinating encephalomyelitis virus in Finnish elite breeding pig herds. Nord Vet Med 34:334–335.

PAUL, P. S., AND MENGELING, W. L. 1984. Persistence of passively acquired antibodies to haemagglutinating encephalomyelitis virus in swine. Am J Vet Res 45:932–934.

PEDERSEN, N. C.; WARD, J.; AND MENGELING, W. L. 1978. Antigenic relationship of the feline infectious peritonitis virus to coronaviruses of other species. Arch Virol 58:45–53.

PENSAERT, M. B., AND CALLEBAUT, P. E. 1974. Characteristics of a coronavirus causing vomiting and wasting in pigs. Arch Gesamte Virusforsch 44:35–50.

PENSAERT, M.; ANDRIES, K.; AND CALLEBAUT, P. 1980. A seroepizootiologic study of vomiting and wasting disease virus in pigs. Vet Q 2:142–148.

PENSAERT, M. B.; DEBOUCK, P.; AND REYNOLDS, D. J. 1981. An immunoelectron microscopic and immunofluorescent study on the antigenic relationship between the coronavirus-like agent CV777 and several coronaviruses. Arch Virol 68:45–52.

PHILLIP, J. I. H.; CARTWRIGHT, S. F.; AND SCOTT, A. C. 1971. The size and morphology of T.G.E. and vomiting and wasting disease viruses of pigs. Vet Rec 88:311–312.

PIRTLE, E. C. 1974. Titration of two porcine respiratory viruses in mammalian cell cultures by direct fluorescent antibody staining. Am J Vet Res 35:249–250.

POCOCK, D. H., AND GARWES, F. J. 1977. The polypeptides of haemagglutinating encephalomyelitis virus and isolated subviral particles. J Gen Virol 37:487–499.

RICHARDS, W. P. C., AND SAVAN, M. 1960. Viral encephalomyelitis of pigs. A preliminary report on the transmissibility and pathology of a disease observed in Ontario. Cornell Vet 50:132–155.

SATO, K.; INABA, Y.; AND MATUMOTO, M. 1980. Serological relation between calf diarrhea coronavirus and hemagglutinating encephalomyelitis virus. Arch Virol 66:157–159.

SATO, K.; INABA, Y.; MIURA, Y.; TOKUHISA, S.; AND MATUMOTO, M. 1983. Inducement of cytopathic changes and plaque formation by porcine hemagglutinating encephalomyelitis virus. Vet Microbiol 8:521–530.

SCHLENSTEDT, V. D.; BARNIKOL, H.; AND PLONAIT, H. 1969. Erbrechen und Kummern bei Saugferkeln. DTW 76:694–695.

SØRENSEN, K. J. 1975. Haemagglutinerende encephalomyelitis virus (HEV) infektioner hos grise. Serologisk indikation for infektionens tilstedevaerelse i Denmark. Nord Vet Med 27:208–212.

STEINICKE, O., AND NIELSEN, A. 1959. Histological changes of the mesenteric plexus of the stomach in "baby pig disease." Nord Vet Med 11:399–429.

VANNIER, P.; CHAPPUIS, G.; LABADIE, J. L.; RENAULT, L.; AND JOSSE, J. 1981. A serological survey of the virus of vomiting and wasting disease in piglets. Ann Zootech 30:379.

WERDIN, R. E.; SORENSEN, D. K.; AND STEWART, W. C. 1976. Porcine encephalomyelitis caused by haemagglutinating encephalomyelitis virus. J Am Vet Med Assoc 168:240–246.

YAGAMI, K.; HIRAI, K.; AND HIRANO, N. 1986. Pathogenesis of haemagglutinating encephalomyelitis virus (HEV) in mice experimentally infected by different routes. J Comp Pathol 96:645–657.

20 Hog Cholera

J. T. Van Oirschot

HOG CHOLERA (HC) (synonym: classical swine fever) is a highly contagious viral disease of swine. The infection can run an acute, subacute, chronic, atypical, or inapparent course. Acute HC is caused by virulent virus and generally results in high morbidity and mortality, whereas infections with low-virulence virus can go unnoticed.

The question of whether HC originated in the United States or elsewhere will probably remain conjectural. According to Hanson (1957), the first description of a choleralike disease was from Tennessee, about 1810. Later outbreaks were reported from Ohio in the early 1830s. HC may possibly have occurred in France in 1822 and in Germany in 1833, but other reports suggest that the disease first appeared in England in 1862 and subsequently spread to the European continent (Fuchs 1968). HC was reported from South America in 1899 and from South Africa in 1900.

At present, HC has a worldwide distribution, but the following countries are free of the disease: Australia, Canada, Great Britain, Iceland, Ireland, New Zealand, the Scandinavian countries, Switzerland, and the United States.

A state-federal HC eradication program was begun in the United States in 1962. The last U.S. outbreak occurred in 1976. Total cost of the effort to eradicate HC amounted to about $140 million.

The European Communities (EC) support a program to eliminate HC virus (HCV) from the member countries. It is based on stamping out and is supported by other veterinary legislative and zoo sanitary measures. In spite of these combined efforts, outbreaks of HC are still reported from the EC countries, causing severe economic losses; for example, in the Netherlands the direct cost of the control program amounted to $93 million in the period 1983–85.

ETIOLOGY. HCV is a member of the family Togaviridae and belongs to the genus *Pestivirus*. Bovine virus diarrhea virus (BVDV), which can infect cattle, sheep, and swine, is another member of the genus *Pestivirus*.

HCV measures 40–50 nm in diameter, with a nucleocapsid of about 29 nm. It is an enveloped RNA virus, the membrane surrounding an isometric core. Fringelike projections of 6–8 nm have been demonstrated on the surface of the virion. The buoyant density, depending on the gradient material and on the cells used to propagate the virus, has been reported between 1.12 and 1.17 g/ml. Sedimentation coefficient values of 140–180 S have been found (Horzinek 1981).

The single-stranded RNA of the virus is infective and is about 12 kb long (Moormann and Hulst 1988). There is a high degree of sequence homology between the genomes of HCV and BVDV (Meyers et al. 1989). HCV possesses two glycoproteins of 55,000 and 46,000 daltons, located in the viral envelope, and a nucleocapsid protein of 36,000 daltons (Enzmann and Weiland 1978).

Inactivation of HCV by physical treatment is partly dependent on the medium containing the virus. Thus cell culture fluid infectivity is lost after 10 minutes at 60°C, whereas in defibrinated blood the virus is not inactivated after 30 minutes at 68°C. HCV is stable at pH 5–10; above and below these pH values, infectivity is rapidly destroyed. Lipid solvents such as ether, chloroform, and deoxycholate quickly inactivate the virus. For disinfection, 2% sodium hydroxide is still considered most suitable. In pens and dung the virus appears to be inactivated in a few days. However, in pork and pork products it can remain infective for months, which is of great epizootiologic importance.

Although HCV can replicate in nonporcine cells, porcine kidney cells are used most frequently for virus growth. Virus replication is restricted to the cytoplasm of the cell and does not result in a cytopathic effect. The first progeny virus is released from the cells at 5–6 hours postinfection. Under single growth cycle conditions, there is an exponential increase in virus titer until 15 hours postinfection, after which virus production continues at a high level for several days. In cell cultures, HCV spreads by means of the medium, by cytoplasmic bridges to neighboring cells, and from mother to daughter cells. HCV can persist in cell culture. The virus seems to mature at intracytoplasmic membranes, which is in accordance with the inability to detect HCV antigens at the surface of the infected cell (Van Oirschot 1980).

A marked antigenic variation is present among strains of HCV (Edwards and Sands 1990). Based on the reaction with monoclonal antibodies (MAbs) raised against HCV, several antigenic groups could be distinguished. Even within some strains of HCV, antigenic heterogeneity was present. No relation was observed between antigenic groups and virulence (Wensvoort et al. 1989a). On the other hand, field isolates that were neutralized more readily by BVDV antibody than by HCV antibody were of reduced virulence (Kamijyo et al. 1977).

There is a close antigenic relationship between HCV and BVDV, as evidenced by cross-reactions in immunodiffusion, immunofluorescence, and to a lower degree in neutralization tests. Certain strains of HCV also induce neutralizing antibody to BVDV, and pigs can be partially immunized against HC with BVDV. Extensive cross-neutralization studies, however, classified HCV strains into another antigenic group of pestiviruses than BVDV strains (Wensvoort et al. 1989b). MAbs produced against HCV react only with HCV strains and not with BVDV strains (Cay et al. 1989). Common antigens of HCV and BVDV seem not to reside on the 55-kD glycoprotein E1, because MAbs reacting with 13 epitopes on this protein did not recognize BVDV strains. With some of these MAbs it is possible to identify field isolates as either HCV or BVDV (Wensvoort 1989).

Field strains of HCV vary widely in virulence. Strains of high virulence induce acute disease and high mortality, whereas moderately virulent strains generally give rise to subacute or chronic infections. Postnatal infection with low-virulence HCV results in mild disease or subclinical infection. However, such low-virulence strains can produce mortality in porcine fetuses and newborn piglets.

The outcome of HCV infections with strains of moderate virulence is partially determined by host factors such as age, immune competence, and nutritional condition, whereas in infections with highly virulent or avirulent HCV, host factors seem to play a minor role.

It has been reported that virulence of HCV may be an unstable property, since enhancement of virulence has been observed after one or more passages in pigs (Dunne 1975).

EPIDEMIOLOGY. The pig is the only natural host and is the significant source of spread of HCV. Direct contact between infected and susceptible pigs is the principal means of viral transmission. Infected pigs may be shedding virus before the onset of disease and continue to do so during the entire disease period. HCV is notably excreted with oronasal and lacrimal secretions, urine, and feces. Pigs that recover from HC generally shed virus until specific antibodies have developed. Thus pigs infected with virulent HCV may shed large amounts of virus during 10–20 days, whereas postnatal infections with low-virulence strains are characterized by short virus-excretion periods. Consequently, virulent HCV will usually spread faster in a herd and induce higher morbidity than low-virulence strains. Chronically infected pigs shed the virus continuously or intermittently till death.

When a pregnant sow is exposed to HCV strains of low virulence, the infection initially will often go unnoticed, but the virus can be transmitted to the fetuses in utero. Such a congenital infection usually results in stillbirth and/or birth of weak pigs, which die shortly after birth. Because HCV persists in fetuses, large quantities of virus may then be disseminated at farrowing. However, if congenitally infected piglets are born healthy and remain so for months, they act as a hardly recognizable and continuous source of viral spread (Van Oirschot and Terpstra 1977). Thus HCV infection may smolder in a herd for months before the eventual diagnosis is made. These persistent congenital infections are therefore of utmost importance in the epidemiology of HC, particularly in regions where viruses of reduced virulence predominate.

The introduction of newly purchased, healthy-looking infected pigs into a herd is the most common cause of HC outbreaks. The infection may originate from breeding farms, or pigs may be exposed to the virus at places where many pigs are assembled or during transport in contaminated vehicles. An important source of infection is virus-containing garbage that has not been properly sterilized. This mode of virus spread was responsible for 22% of the outbreaks of HC in the United States in 1973 (Dunne 1975). The virus can be carried over long distances in pork and pork products, which may lead to the introduction of HC into countries free of the disease.

Mechanical vectors contribute to the spread of HCV between premises. In this respect, farmers, veterinarians, and other personnel with their equipment constitute a great risk, but virus may also be mechanically transmitted by pets, birds, and arthropods (Stewart 1981).

Airborne virus seems of little significance in herd-to-herd transmission.

HCV can circulate in wild pig populations, in some countries posing a threat to domestic pig husbandry.

Several countries, including those of the EC, have eradication programs in force, based on rapid diagnosis and stamping out of infected herds, supplemented by other control measures. Despite these efforts, HC has still not been eliminated in many countries. This may be accounted for by the high density of pigs in certain areas, the movement over long distances of pigs and pork and pork products, and the frequent inability to trace the source of outbreaks. During the 1982–85 epizootic in the Netherlands the source of infection was recorded as "unknown" in 54% of breeding and mixed herds and in 29% of fattening herds (Terpstra 1987). In Europe, the origin of 13 out of 32 outbreaks (42%) in 1988 was unknown (Picard 1989). The emergence of HCV strains of reduced virulence is also a major factor to explain hitherto unsuccessful eradication programs.

Such strains give rise to persistent and inapparent infections that are clinically hard to recognize and therefore may be diagnosed only after the virus has spread to other herds.

CLINICAL SIGNS. When virulent HCV first appears in a herd, only a few pigs will show clinical signs of disease. Initially, the pigs may only appear drowsy or less active. If they are disturbed and made to stand, some will have arched backs and others may appear chilled. Still others may stand with a drooping head and straight tail as if lost in thought. At this time, a reduced appetite is noticed. Later, it progresses to a marked anorexia exemplified by the pig nosing around in the feed for a short while before returning to its resting place.

At the first sign of inactivity, fever can be recorded. Within 6 days of exposure to HCV, the temperature of an affected animal may become higher than 42°C, although values between 41 and 42°C are more common during the course of the disease. Concurrent with the temperature rise is a corresponding drop in the leukocyte count. Total leukocyte counts of 9000 to as low as 3000/mm³ of blood may be found.

Early in the course of the disease, the eyes show a marked discharge associated with conjunctivitis, which may progress until the eyelids are completely adhered. Constipation commonly develops during the period of initial high temperature, followed by a severe, watery, yellowish gray diarrhea. Sick pigs become chilled and will huddle or pile on each other while seeking warmth. It is not uncommon for pigs to vomit a yellowish fluid containing much bile. Convulsions may occur in a few swine, which usually die within hours or at most a few days after the convulsions begin. Hyperemia of the skin may occur concurrently with the initial temperature rise.

As the disease progresses, more pigs become affected, and those that were first sick become gaunt and tucked up in the flank and have a characteristic weaving, staggering gait that appears to be directly related to a weakness in the hindquarters. This is usually followed by a posterior paresis. A purplish discoloration extending over the abdomen, snout, ears, and medial sides of the legs may occur near the terminal stage of the disease (Stewart 1981). Most pigs that suffer from acute HC die between 10 and 20 days postinfection. In subacute HC, pigs show less severe signs of disease and succumb within 30 days (Dunne 1975).

Persistence of HCV in the host can result in different clinical syndromes. Mengeling and Packer (1969) described three phases of chronic HC based on the clinical signs observed. In the first or acute phase of illness, anorexia, depression, elevated temperature, and leukopenia were present. After several weeks, the appetite and

general appearance of the pigs improved markedly and their temperatures decreased to normal or slightly above normal values. Leukopenia usually persisted. This general clinical improvement characterized the second phase of illness. In the third phase, pigs again became anorectic and depressed, with temperatures often elevated until shortly before death. Runt pigs can develop during the course of chronic HC. Such pigs are severely retarded in growth, have skin lesions, and frequently stand with arched backs. Pigs with chronic HC may survive for more than 100 days.

Van Oirschot and Terpstra (1977) reported a "late-onset" disease as a sequel of congenital HCV infection. The syndrome was characterized by an initial, relatively long period during which pigs remained free of disease. Not until a few months after primary exposure did the pigs develop mild anorexia and depression, conjunctivitis, dermatitis, diarrhea, and locomotive disturbances leading to posterior paresis. Body temperatures were normal. Most pigs survived for more than 6 months, but all eventually died (Table 20.1).

Persistent, virtually inapparent infections can also develop after postnatal inoculation with HCV strains of reduced virulence (Carbrey et al. 1977). Leukopenia is a consistent manifestation of persistent HC, but in the terminal stages of disease, leukocytosis may develop. Low-virulence strains of HCV generally induce mild disease or subclinical infections, which can be accompanied with leukopenia.

A congenital HCV infection can result in abortion, fetal mummification, malformations, stillbirth, and the birth of weak pigs with tremors or of healthy-looking yet infected piglets. Among piglets infected in utero, skin hemorrhages are common and neonatal mortality is high. However, piglets can recover from an in utero–acquired HCV infection.

PATHOGENESIS. Under natural conditions, the mode of entry of HCV in the pig is the oronasal route. Occasionally, the virus gains access to the host through conjunctival or genital mucous membranes or skin abrasions. The tonsil is the primary site of virus replication after oral and parenteral infection.

The virus initially infects epithelial cells of the tonsillar crypts and subsequently spreads to the surrounding lymphoreticular tissue. From the tonsil, HCV is transferred via lymphatic vessels to the lymph nodes draining the tonsillar region. The virus replicates in the regional lymph nodes; then reaches the peripheral blood; and from that time grows to high titers in spleen, bone marrow, visceral lymph nodes, and lymphoid structures lining the small intestine. As a result of the growth in lymphoid tissue and in circulating leukocytes and mononuclear cells, the level of viremia is high. The virus probably does not invade

Table 20.1. General features of acute, chronic, and late-onset HC

Feature	Acute	Chronic	Late-onset
Virulence of virus	High	Moderate	Low
Time of infection	Postnatal	Postnatal	Prenatal
Course of illness	Short incubation period, severe depression, high fever, anorexia, conjunctivitis, constipation, diarrhea, convulsions, incoordination, hemorrhages of skin	Short incubation period, three phases of illness: (1) depression, fever, anorexia; (2) clinical improvement; (3) terminal, exacerbation of disease	Late onset of disease, gradually aggravating depression and anorexia, normal to slightly elevated body temperatures, conjunctivitis, dermatitis, locomotion disturbances
Viremia	High level	Temporary reduction or disappearance	Persistent high level
Leukopenia	Develops quickly	Develops quickly, followed by leukocytosis	Develops late during infection
Immune response to HCV	Absent	Present	Absent
Death	10–20 days	1–3 months	2–11 months
Gross lesions	Multiple hemorrhages (especially in lymph nodes and kidney), infarction of spleen	Ulcers of cecum and colon, infarction of spleen, rib lesions	Lymph node swelling, thymic atrophy
Microscopic	Degeneration of endothelial cells, proliferation of reticular cells, encephalitis	Degeneration of endothelial cells, severe lymphocyte depletion, histiocytic hyperplasia, glomerulonephritis	Degeneration of endothelial cells, severe lymphocyte depletion, histiocytic hyperplasia

parenchymatous organs until late in the viremic phase. Generally, HCV titers in lymphoid tissues are higher than in parenchymatous organs. The spread of virulent virus throughout the pig is usually completed in 5–6 days (Ressang 1973).

The multiple hemorrhages seen in acute HC are caused by degeneration of endothelial cells in conjunction with severe thrombocytopenia and disturbance in fibrogen synthesis. Virtually all pigs die from acute HC. The mechanism actually responsible for death is not clear, but severe disturbance of the circulatory system appears to be the most likely cause (Fuchs 1968).

During acute HC, the pig's immune reactivity changes. A depressed secondary antibody response to lysozyme (Charley et al. 1980) and highly abnormal responses of peripheral blood and organ lymphocytes to T- and B-cell mitogens have been reported (Van Oirschot et al. 1981, 1983).

Persistent HCV infections are generally caused by strains of reduced virulence. Arbitrarily, two forms of persistence may be distinguished: chronic and late-onset HC (Table 20.1).

The first phase of chronic HC resembles acute HC, but the virus spreads more slowly and virus titers in serum and organs tend to be lower. In the period of clinical improvement, virus titers in serum are low or absent and viral antigen is usually limited to epithelial cells of tonsil, salivary gland, ileum, and kidney. A specific antibody response and/or decrease in the number of cells producing virus probably account for the temporary disappearance of HCV from the serum. The simultaneous circulation of viral antigens and antibody may result in deposition of antigen-antibody complexes in the kidneys, which eventually can lead to glomerulonephritis. During the exacerbation of acute disease, virus is again distributed throughout the body. Its spread may be promoted by the immune exhaustion that appears to develop in pigs with chronic HC (Cheville and Mengeling 1969).

Late-onset HC initially runs an inapparent course. It may not be until several months after primary contact with the virus that pigs develop signs of disease. These infections are the sequel of exposure to HCV strains of low virulence during fetal life (Van Oirschot and Terpstra 1977). The pigs have a lifelong high level of viremia, which can be transiently decreased after the ingestion of colostral antibody. HCV antigen is widespread throughout epithelial, lymphoidal, and reticuloendothelial tissues. Pigs with congenital persistent HC do not mount a neutralizing antibody response to the virus. However, the antibody response to antigens unrelated to HCV is generally normal, indicating a specific immune tolerance to the virus. The response of peripheral blood lymphocytes to mitogens is only slightly depressed in these persistently infected pigs (Van Oirschot 1979).

The pathogenesis of postnatal infections with low-virulence HCV is not well known. The growth of virus seems to be mainly restricted to tonsil and regional lymph nodes, but the virus can be disseminated via the bloodstream, as evidenced by the frequently occurring transplacental transmission in pregnant sows. HCV appears to grow across the placental barrier at one or more sites and subsequently spreads from fetus to fetus. The developmental age of the fetus and the virulence of the virus strain largely determine the outcome of a congenital infection. Generally, the risk for fetal damage is higher the earlier infection occurs during pregnancy.

Pigs that have recovered from HC possess antibodies to HCV, but neutralizing antibodies can also be produced in subacute fatal cases. Whereas pigs with chronic HC are able to elicit a specific antibody response, pigs with congenital persistent HC appear to be immunotolerant to the virus. Although porcine fetuses gain immunocompetence around midgestation, only some of them may produce antibodies to HCV in the last phase of fetal development. Occasionally, after postnatal infection with certain strains of HCV, neutralizing antibodies are only transiently detectable or completely absent. This may be the consequence of a poor immunogenicity of the virus. Such strains are generally of reduced virulence.

In pigs that do not mount a normal antibody response after a primary contact with HCV, two phenomena have repeatedly been observed. Reexposure of such pigs to HCV can result in a kind of hyperreactivity characterized by a shorter incubation period and a more severe illness than in primarily infected pigs. In contrast with this sensitization phenomenon, an enhanced resistance to virulent HCV has been described. Pigs persistently infected with HCV of reduced virulence have a markedly prolonged survival when inoculated with virulent HCV. It is conceivable that these phenomena play a role under field conditions.

The role of cell-mediated immunity in HC has not yet been elucidated. Corthier (1978) and Remond et al. (1981) detected a transient blastogenic response to HCV antigens in subclinically affected or vaccinated pigs, whereas others failed to show such a response (Van Oirschot et al. 1983).

The precise pathogenic mechanisms of HCV infections are not well understood. Some hypotheses are described in extensive reviews by Fuchs (1968) and Mahnel and Mayr (1974).

LESIONS. In peracute cases of HC, pathologic lesions are often absent. In acute to subacute HC, the pathologic picture is that of a septicemic disease characterized by multiple hemorrhages of various sizes (caused by hydropic degeneration and necrosis of endothelial cells lining the vascular system) in conjunction with defects in the blood coagulation mechanism. In addition, catarrhal, fibrinous, and hemorrhagic inflammatory reactions are present in digestive, respiratory, and urogenital tracts.

Pathologic changes are most frequently observed in lymph nodes and kidney. The lymph nodes become swollen, edematous, and then hemorrhagic. They commonly have peripheral or more diffuse hemorrhages, giving the nodes a marbled or red to near black appearance respectively (Fig. 20.1). Virtually all lymph nodes may be affected. Microscopically, depletion of lymphocytes and reticular hyperplasia are seen.

Hemorrhages of the kidney may vary in size from hardly visible petechiae to ecchymotic hemorrhages. They frequently occur on the surface of the cortex (Fig. 20.2) and are less common in the medullary pyramids and hilus. Petechial to ecchymotic hemorrhages can also be observed in urinary bladder, larynx and epiglottis, heart, intestinal mucosa, serous and mucous membranes, and skin. The skin may also become cyanotic.

Infarction is the result of a disrupted blood flow into a certain area resulting from the occlusion of blood capillaries by thrombi. The thrombi in turn may be caused by the hydropic degeneration of endothelial cells coupled with the tendency of erythrocytes to clump in a manner termed "sludging." Infarction of the spleen (Fig. 20.3) is considered to be almost pathognomonic for HC. Infarctions occur as dark blebs of various sizes, raised slightly above the surrounding surfaces. They may appear singly or as a series of lesions coalescing to form a continuous border of infarcts along the edge of the spleen. Infarction of the gallbladder and tonsil may occur. In the latter organ it causes necrosis, which upon bacterial invasion leads to suppurative tonsillitis.

Pigs with acute to subacute HC can show infarctions and hemorrhages in the lung. Presumably as a consequence of secondary bacterial infections, catarrhal to fibrinous bronchopneumonia and pleuritis may develop. The heart is usually flabby and shows some myocardial congestion. In an animal dying of HC, the stomach is usually empty except for a yellow, bilious fluid and a small amount of feed. The fundus is often markedly congested and hemorrhagic. The mucosal surface may contain petechiae and mild to severe erosions. A mild to moderate catarrhal or necrotic enteritis is found in the intestines. Mesenteric blood vessels are usually markedly engorged. Occasionally, subserous ecchymotic and suffusive hemorrhages occur in the small and large intestines (Stewart 1981).

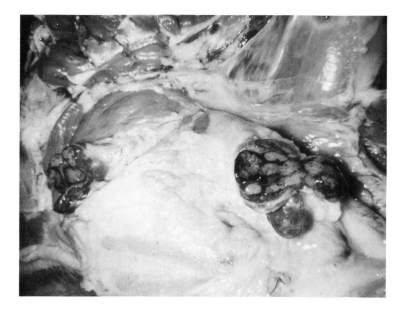

20.1. Peripheral hemorrhage of the mandibular lymph node. (Courtesy W. C. Stewart.)

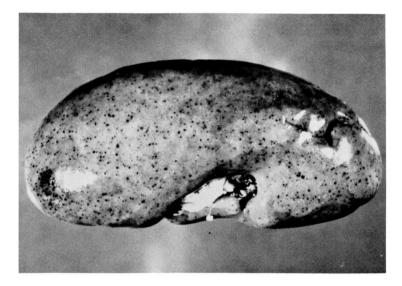

20.2. Kidney showing numerous petechial hemorrhages. (Courtesy W. C. Stewart.)

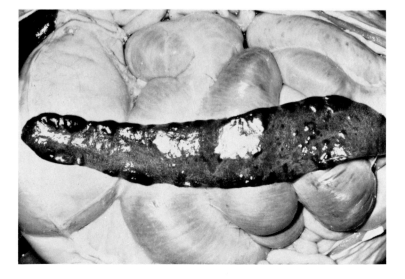

20.3. Infarction of the spleen. (Courtesy L. D. Miller.)

Most HCV-infected swine show an encephalitis at necropsy, of which the principal lesion is perivascular cuffing. Proliferation of endothelial cells, microgliosis, and focal necrosis can also be observed in the brain.

In persistent HC, hemorrhages and infarctions are less pronounced or are completely absent. Although degeneration of endothelial cells is a consistent finding in persistently infected pigs, it does not result in severe circulatory disturbances. The most outstanding lesions in pigs with persistent HC are atrophy of the thymus and severe depletion of lymphocytes and germinal follicles in peripheral lymphoid organs. Histiocytic hyperplasia with phagocytosis of lymphocytic debris is also frequently seen. The plasmacytosis and glomerulonephritis that occur in chronic HC were not present in pigs with late-onset HC. Persistent HCV infections induce adrenal cortical hyperplasia characterized by an increased width of the zona fasciculata and atrophy of the zona glomerulosa and zona reticulata (Cheville and Mengeling 1969; Van der Molen and Van Oirschot 1981). Necrosis and ulcerations, sometimes in the form of button ulcers (Fig. 20.4), in the cecum and colon and rib lesions are common in persistent HC. Chronic rib lesions are caused by a sudden calcification of large numbers of mature cartilage cells and appear as a marked transverse line of semisolid bone structure across the rib proximal from the costochondral junction (Dunne 1975) (Table 20.1).

Congenital HCV infections can result in mummification, stillbirth, and malformations (Fig. 20.5). Generalized subcutaneous edema, hydrops ascites, and hydrothorax are the most pronounced lesions in stillborn pigs. Malformations consist of deformities of head and limbs, hypoplasia of cerebellum and lungs, and hypomyelogenesis. In utero–infected piglets that die shortly after birth often show petechial hemorrhages of skin and internal organs.

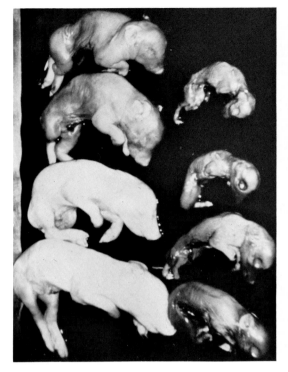

20.5. Mummified fetuses and stillborn pigs of a sow exposed to low-virulence HCV at day 43 of gestation. (Courtesy W. C. Stewart.)

DIAGNOSIS. Outbreaks of typical acute HC can be diagnosed in the field with reasonable certainty on the basis of an accurate anamnesis and a thorough clinical and pathologic investigation. An anamnesis of a HC outbreak often includes one or more of the following: recent purchase of pigs, cases of HC on adjacent or nearby farms, garbage feeding, or a recent visit of persons having close contact with swine. In acute HC there is a rapid

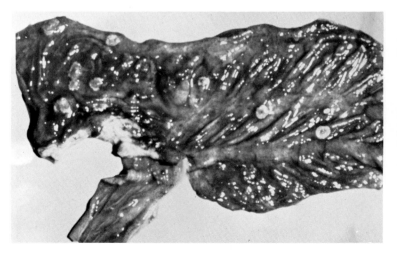

20.4. Button ulcers in the cecum and colon. (Courtesy L. D. Miller.)

spread of the disease among pigs of all ages and high mortality at 1–2 weeks after the onset of clinical signs. Leukopenia is a consistent finding in pigs with HC. At necropsy, lesions of diagnostic significance are hemorrhages in lymph nodes, kidney, and other organs and infarction of the spleen.

Acute HC may be confused on clinical and pathologic grounds with African swine fever, septicemic salmonellosis, pasteurellosis, streptococcosis, erysipelas, or *Haemophilus suis* infections; therefore, it is recommended that clinical diagnosis be confirmed in the laboratory. In many countries where eradication programs with stamping out of positive herds are in force, any tentative field diagnosis has to be confirmed by laboratory investigations.

Unlike in acute HC, it is virtually impossible to make a clinical diagnosis in cases of subacute, chronic, or late-onset HC because of the wide variability of clinical signs and pathologic lesions. Clinical signs are milder than in acute HC; they can occur intermittently, or the infection may go unnoticed for months. In addition, persistent infections may involve only a few pigs in a herd. In such cases, counting of blood leukocytes may prove useful. Finally, infected swine may not have signs indicative of HC because of concurrent infections with other infectious agents. Persistent HCV infections are difficult to recognize, so the

diagnosis is often delayed. Consequently, such an infected herd may act as a source for further dissemination of the virus. Therefore, in countries where HC is present, samples should be submitted to the laboratory when the clinical signs combined with the anamnesis raise even the slightest suspicion of HC. HCV infections by strains of reduced virulence seem to increase in importance, particularly in areas where HC is endemic for a long period and in final stages of eradication programs. In the United States 55% of field isolates in the period 1965–75 were characterized as being of reduced virulence (Carbrey et al. 1977).

Laboratory diagnosis of HC is based on detection of viral antigen, isolation of virus, or demonstration of viral antibody.

The direct fluorescent antibody (FA) test on frozen tissue sections is the method of choice for detecting viral antigen. Samples should be collected from dead or sick pigs and submitted fresh (preferably on ice) and without the addition of any preservatives to the laboratory. Tissues to submit for laboratory diagnosis are tonsil, spleen, kidney, and distal part of the ileum. The tonsil, which is the first tissue to become positive after exposure to HCV, is by far the most important organ for detecting viral antigen (Fig. 20.6). The ileum is frequently found positive in more prolonged cases of HC. An absence of viral antigen in several tissues does not exclude HC as the cause of the out-

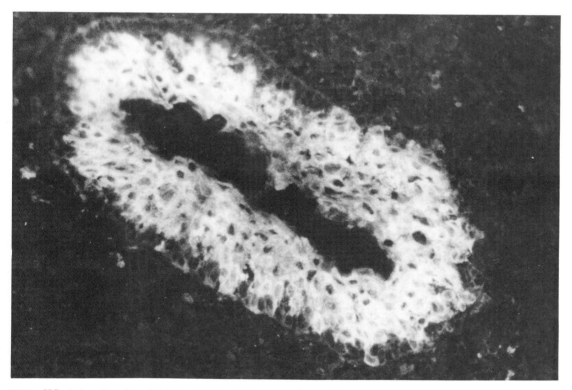

20.6.   HC viral antigen in epithelial cells of tonsillar crypts detected by FA test. (Courtesy C. Terpstra.)

break; where suspicion remains, more pigs should be examined. The FA test on frozen tissue sections is a simple, rapid (can be completed in 2 hours), and reliable technique and has become the official diagnostic test in many HC eradication programs.

HCV and BVDV share common antigens. Therefore, the direct FA test fails to discriminate between HCV and BVDV antigens. Because pigs can become infected with BVDV, the FA test may yield false-positive results. It is crucial to distinguish HCV from BVDV, because a BVDV infection erroneously diagnosed as HC leads, in most countries, to stamping out of the herd and other control measures, and may result in loss of the HC-free status. To differentiate between HCV and BVDV it no longer is necessary to perform time-consuming cross-neutralization tests with sera of in-contact pigs or pigs inoculated with the isolate. A rapid differentiation can be made by staining frozen tissue sections or infected cell cultures with conjugates of MAbs directed against conserved epitopes of HCV. When the selected MAbs react with the isolate, it is HCV and when antigen is not detected, BVDV is involved (Fig. 20.7) (Wensvoort et al. 1986, 1989a). Such nonreactive isolates would need to be confirmed as BVDV.

In pigs vaccinated with the attenuated Chinese (C) strain of HCV, viral antigen can be demonstrated by the direct FA test until about 2 weeks postvaccination (Terpstra 1978). Thus in areas where vaccination is practiced, it may sometimes be necessary to differentiate between field virus and vaccine virus. For this purpose, a pair of conjugated MAbs can be used one of which reacts with a conserved epitope of HCV and the other with most HCV strains, but not with vaccine strains. A positive reaction by the first MAb and a negative by the second indicates that vaccine virus may be present (Fig. 20.7), and warrants further investigation. Lapinized vaccine strains can be distinguished from field strains by their ability to induce fever and antibodies to HCV after intravenous inoculation in rabbits.

HCV may be isolated by inoculation of a porcine kidney (PK-15) cell line with a 2% mixed homogenate of tonsil and spleen of a suspected pig. After 24–72 hours, the cultures are examined for viral antigen by the FA test (Fig. 20.7). The virus isolation procedure is more sensitive than the FA on frozen tissue sections.

Antibody detection can be a useful diagnostic tool for suspected farms where the usual virus detection procedures have failed and in the last phase of an eradication program to detect subclinically infected herds. Serologic tests are imperative if a country desires to become internationally recognized as free from HC.

Several tests are available for the detection of antibodies to HCV. The virus-neutralization test in its various modifications (Holm Jensen 1981; Terpstra et al. 1984) is often used for large-scale serologic investigations. However, it may measure antibodies to BVDV, because low neutralizing antibody titers to HCV can be induced by infections with BVDV (Liess et al. 1977); therefore such sera need to be tested in a BVDV-neutralization test. Higher antibody titers to BVDV than to HCV indicate infection with BVDV, but a concurrent infection with HCV may not be completely excluded. In such cases, more pigs from the herd should be tested. Enyzme-linked immunosorbent assays (ELISAs), which are rapid and simple to perform, have been developed (Wensvoort et al. 1988; Afshar et al. 1989; Moennig et al. 1990). One of these ELISAs differentiates between antibodies to HCV and BVDV; it employs two MAbs directed against different epitopes on glycoprotein E1 of HCV. Because neither MAb recognizes BVDV, the chance that BVDV antibodies are detected is virtually negligible (Wensvoort et al. 1988). This ELISA is routinely used in seroepidemiological surveys in the Netherlands and Belgium.

Because antibodies to field strains of HCV cannot yet be distinguished from antibodies to vaccine virus, vaccination limits the use of serologic tests for diagnostic purposes.

PREVENTION. To prevent the reintroduction of HCV, countries free of HC ban the import of live pigs, pork, and insufficiently heated pork products from countries where HC is present. In addition, swill is generally destroyed or effectively sterilized before being fed to pigs. Should a case of HC arise in countries free of HC, veterinary police and zoo sanitary measures may come into force to eradicate the disease. All pigs in infected herds are destroyed (stamping out), the source of infection and possible contacts are traced, "standstill" restrictions become operative, and infected farms are intensively disinfected. Countries with sporadic outbreaks of the disease usually apply similar control and eradication procedures.

In countries where HC is enzootic, vaccination is often practiced, and in some countries vaccination is supplementary to a stamping-out policy. Vaccination is usually ceased when no more outbreaks occur or when a stage is reached where stamping out alone may eliminate the residual virus.

In the Netherlands, a strict vaccination regime pursued for 1 year and supported by the usual veterinary police and zoo sanitary measures succeeded in eradicating HC from three enzootic areas. The program consisted of a mass vaccination campaign of all pigs over 2 weeks of age and supplementary vaccination of previously unvaccinated 6- to 8-week-old pigs and newly introduced stock at monthly intervals. Vaccination was compulsory, and all vaccinated pigs were identified by ear tagging. The number of outbreaks in the vac-

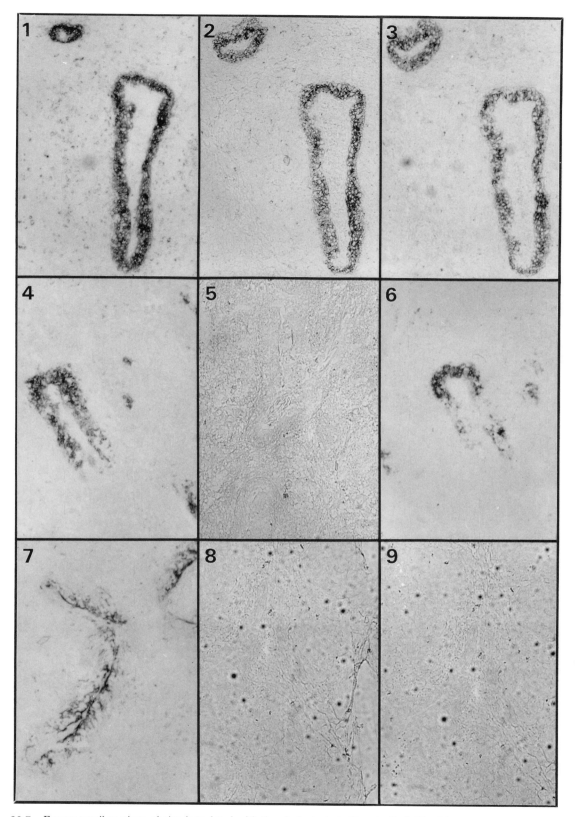

20.7. Frozen tonsil sections of pigs inoculated with the virulent strain Brescia (1, 2, 3), with vaccine strain C (4, 5, 6) or with a BVDV strain (7, 8, 9) and stained with an anti-HCV polyclonal peroxidase conjugate (1, 4, 7), or with HRPO conjugates of MAbs (one MAb 2, 5, 8, the other MAb 3, 6, 9) recognizing two different epitopes. (Courtesy G. Wensvoort.)

cinated areas declined in 2 weeks, and the areas were free of HC from the fifth month after the start of the program (Terpstra and Robijns 1977). In a recent emergency vaccination campaign, supplementary vaccination was conducted in piglets born from vaccinated sows at the age of 7–9 weeks, and breeding gilts born from vaccinated sows were revaccinated when 6–7 months old to boost herd immunity (Terpstra and Wensvoort 1987).

At present, vaccines attenuated by serial passages in rabbits (C strain) or in cell cultures (Japanese GPE-strain, French Thiverval strain) are widely used as an aid in the control of HC. These vaccines are highly efficacious and safe (Aynaud 1988). The simultaneous vaccination method and use of inactivated vaccines have been abandoned in most countries. In addition, the early attenuated HCV vaccines are no longer used because they induced a variety of fetal abnormalities after vaccination of pregnant sows.

The C strain is the most extensively used vaccine. The growth of the C strain appeared to be mainly restricted to lymphoid tissues, especially the tonsil, although C viral antigen has occasionally been detected in kidneys (Terpstra 1978). The C strain can pass the placental barrier of pregnant sows but does not seem to produce any abnormality in infected fetuses (Tesmer et al. 1973). It is innocuous for pregnant sows and newborn piglets. The C strain can be transmitted from vaccinated pigs to nonvaccinated contact pigs (Van Bekkum 1977). However, the chance of reversion to virulence appears to be minimal, because it retained its attenuated characteristics after 20–30 serial passages in pigs (Aynaud 1988) and behaved similarly in pigs treated with corticosteroids as in nontreated pigs (Florent et al. 1969; Kamijyo et al. 1976).

The attenuated vaccines usually confer immunity within 1 week after inoculation, and the immunity persists for at least 2–3 years. Vaccination not only protects against disease, but also highly reduces the replication of virulent HCV upon challenge (Biront et al. 1987) and prevents transmission of challenge virus from pigs with moderate neutralizing antibody titers to in-contact pigs (Terpstra and Wensvoort 1988). Vaccinated sows transmit antibodies to their offspring via colostrum. Because the intestine of the newborn piglet is permeable for immunoglobulins during the first 36–48 hours of life, antibodies to HCV enter directly into the circulation. These maternally derived antibodies have a half-life of approximately 14 days. Piglets born to vaccinated sows are protected for 5–8 weeks against mortality from HC but not against replication and shedding of virulent virus (Terpstra 1977).

Maternally derived antibodies inhibit the development of active immunity after vaccination. Although a high percentage of piglets born to vaccinated sows can effectively be vaccinated around 6

weeks of age, revaccination of such pigs around 5 months will probably increase herd immunity. The suppression by maternally derived antibodies can be reduced by substantially increasing the amount of vaccine virus per dose (Lin et al. 1982).

Aerosol immunization of pigs has yielded varying results with regard to efficacy.

REFERENCES

Afshar, A.; Dulac, G. C.; and Bouffard, A. 1989. Application of peroxidase labelled antibody assays for detection of porcine IgG antibodies to hog cholera and bovine viral diarrhea viruses. J Virol Meth 23:253–262.

Aynaud, J. M. 1988. Principles of vaccination. In Classical Swine Fever and Related Viral Infections. Ed. B. Liess. Boston: Martinus Nijhoff Publishing, pp. 165–180.

Biront, P.; Leunen, J.; and Vandeputte, J. 1987. Inhibition of virus replication in the tonsils of pigs previously vaccinated with a Chinese strain vaccine and challenged oronasally with a virulent strain of classical swine fever virus. Vet Microbiol 14:105–113.

Carbrey, E. A.; Stewart, W. C.; Kresse, J. L.; and Snijder, M. L. 1977. Inapparent hog cholera infection following the inoculation of field isolates. CEC Semin on Hog Cholera/Classical Swine Fever and African Swine Fever, Hannover, EUR 5904, p. 214.

Cay, B.; Chappuis, G.; Coulibaly, C.; Dinter, Z.; Edwards, S.; Greiser-Wilke, I.; Gunn, M.; Have, P.; Hess, G.; Juntti, N.; Liess, B.; Mateo, A.; McHugh, P.; Moennig, V.; Nettleton, P.; and Wensvoort, G. 1989. Comparative analysis of monoclonal antibodies against pestiviruses: Report of an international workshop. Vet Microbiol 20:123–129.

Charley, B.; Corthier, G.; Houdayer, M.; and Rouze, P. 1980. Modifications des reactions immunitaires au cours de la peste porcine classique. Ann Rech Vet 11:27.

Cheville, N. F., and Mengeling, W. L. 1969. The pathogenesis of chronic hog cholera (swine fever). Histologic, immunofluorescent, and electron microscopic studies. Lab Invest 20:261.

Corthier, G. 1978. Cellular and humoral immune response in pigs given vaccinal and chronic hog cholera viruses. Am J Vet Res 39:1841.

Dunne, H. W. 1975. Hog cholera. In Diseases of Swine, 4th ed. Ed. H. W. Dunne and A. D. Leman. Ames: Iowa State Univ Press.

Edwards, S., and Sands, J. J. 1990. Antigenic comparisons of hog cholera virus isolates from Europe, America and Asia using monoclonal antibodies. Dtsch Tieraerztl Wochenschr 97:79–81.

Enzmann, P. J., and Weiland, F. 1978. Structural similarities of hog cholera virus with togaviruses. Arch Virol 57:339.

Florent, A.; Thomas, J.; and Leunen, J. 1969. Controles des vaccins vivants contre la peste porcine. Interet de l'immunodepression pour la mise en evidence de la virulence residuelle. Bull Off Int Epizoot 72:665.

Fuchs, F. 1968. Schweinepest. In Handbuch der Virusinfektionen bei Tieren, Band 3. Ed. H. Röhrer. Jena: Gustav Fischer.

Hanson, R. P. 1957. Origin of hog cholera. J Am Vet Med Assoc 131:211.

Holm Jensen, M. 1981. Detection of antibodies against hog cholera virus and bovine viral diarrhea virus in porcine serum. A comparative examination using CF, PLA and NPLA assays. Acta Vet Scand 22:85.

Horzinek, 1981. Non-Arthropod-Borne Togaviruses. New York: Academic Press.

KAMIJYO, Y.; OHKUMA, S.; SHIMIZU, M.; AND SHIMIZU, Y. 1976. Effect of dexamethasone on the multiplication of attenuated strains of hog cholera virus in pigs. Vet Microbiol 1:475.

_____. 1977. Differences in pathogenicity and antigenicity among hog cholera virus strains. Natl Inst Anim Health Q (Tokyo) 17:133.

LIESS, B.; FREY, H. R.; AND PRAGER, D. 1977. Antibody response of pigs following experimental infections with strains of hog cholera and bovine viral diarrhea virus. CEC Semin on Hog Cholera/Classical Swine Fever and African Swine Fever, Hannover, EUR 5904, p. 200.

LIN, T. T. C.; LAI, S. S.; CHEN, C. S.; AND LEE, R. C. T. 1982. Immune response to different doses of LPC-China virus in pigs with different levels of colostral hog cholera antibody. Proc 7th Int Congr Pig Vet Soc, Mexico City, p. 132.

MAHNEL, H., AND MAYR, A. 1974. Schweinepest. Infektionskrankheiten und ihre Erreger, Band 16 VEB Jena: Gustav Fischer.

MENGELING, W. L., AND PACKER, R. A. 1969. Pathogenesis of chronic hog cholera: Host response. Am J Vet Res 30:409.

MEYERS, G.; RUMENAPF, T.; AND THIEL, H.-J. 1989. Molecular cloning and nucleotide sequence of the genome of hog cholera virus. Virology 171:555–567.

MOENNIG, V.; SCHAGEMANN, G.; DAHLE, J.; GREISER-WILKE, I.; AND LEDER, L. 1990. A new approach for the diagnosis of hog cholera. Dtsch Tieraerztl Wochenschr 97:91–93.

MOORMANN, R. J. M., AND HULST, M. M. 1988. Hog cholera virus: Identification and characterization of the viral RNA and the virus-specific RNA synthesized in infected swine kidney cells. Virus Res 11:281–291.

PICARD, M. 1989. Les pestes porcines en France et en Europe en 1988. Epidémiol Santé Anim 16:27–32.

REMOND, M.; PLATEAU, E.; AND CRUCIERE, C. 1981. In vitro study of the cellular response of pigs vaccinated against classical swine fever. Zentralbl Veterinaermed [B] 28:743.

RESSANG, A. A. 1973. Studies on the pathogenesis of hog cholera. I. Demonstration of hog cholera virus subsequent to oral exposure. Zentralbl Veterinaermed [B] 20:256.

STEWART, W. C. 1981. Hog cholera. In Diseases of Swine, 5th ed. Ed. A. D. Leman, R. D. Glock, W. L. Mengeling, R. H. C. Penny, E. Scholl, and B. Straw. Ames: Iowa State Univ Press.

TERPSTRA, C. 1977. The immunity against challenge with swine fever virus of piglets from sows vaccinated with C-strain virus. Tijdschr Diergeneeskd 102: 1293.

_____. 1978. Detection of C-strain virus in pigs following vaccination against swine fever. Tijdschr Diergeneeskd 103:678.

_____. 1987. Epizootiology of swine fever. Vet Q [Suppl] 9:50–60.

TERPSTRA, C., AND ROBIJNS, K. G. 1977. Experience with regional vaccination against swine fever in enzootic areas for limited periods using C-strain virus. Tijdschr Diergeneeskd 102:106.

TERPSTRA, C., AND WENSVOORT, G. 1987. Influence of the vaccination regime on the herd immune response for swine fever. Vet Microbiol 13:143–151.

_____. 1988. The protective value of vaccine-induced neutralising antibody titres in swine fever. Vet Microbiol 16:123–128.

TERPSTRA, C.; BLOEMRAAD, M.; AND GIELKENS, A. L. J. 1984. The neutralizing peroxidase-linked assay for detection of antibody against swine fever virus. Vet Microbiol 9:113–120.

TESMER, S.; URBANECK, D.; KADEN, V.; WITTMANN, D.; AND HAHNEFELD, H. 1973. Zur Wirkung von Schweinepest-Lebendvirusvakzine aus dem Impfvirusstam "C" bei tragenden Sauen und deren Nachzucht. Monatsh Veterinaermed 28:251.

VAN BEKKUM, J. G. 1977. Experience in the Netherlands with the lapinised, so-called Chinese (C) strain of vaccine. Agric Res Semin on Hog Cholera/Classical Swine Fever and African Swine Fever, Hannover, EUR 5904, p. 379.

VAN DER MOLEN, E. J., AND VAN OIRSCHOT, J. T. 1981. Congenital persistent swine fever (hog cholera). I. Pathomorphological lesions in lymphoid tissues, kidney and adrenal. Zentralbl Veterinaermed [B] 28:89.

VAN OIRSCHOT, J. T. 1979. Experimental production of congenital persistent swine fever infections. II. Effect on functions of the immune system. Vet Microbiol 4: 133.

_____. 1980. Persistent and inapparent infections with swine fever virus of low virulence. Their effects on the immune system. Thesis, State Univ of Utrecht.

VAN OIRSCHOT, J. T., AND TERPSTRA, C. 1977. A congenital persistent swine fever infection. I. Clinical and virological observations. Vet Microbiol 2:121.

VAN OIRSCHOT, J. T.; DE JONG, D.; AND HUFFELS, A. D. N. H. J. 1981. Effect of infections with swine fever virus on immune functions. I. Response of lymphocytes from blood and lymphoid organs from infected and normal pigs to antiimmunoglobulin serum and protein A. Vet Microbiol 6:41–57.

_____. 1983. Effect of infections with swine fever virus on immune functions. II. Lymphocyte response to mitogens and enumeration of lymphocyte subpopulations. Vet Microbiol 8:81.

WENSVOORT, G. 1989. Epitopes on structural proteins of hog cholera (swine fever) virus. Thesis, State Univ of Utrecht.

WENSVOORT, G.; TERPSTRA, C.; BOONSTRA, J.; BLOEMRAAD, M.; AND VAN ZAANE, D. 1986. Production of monoclonal antibodies against swine fever virus and their use in laboratory diagnosis. Vet Microbiol 12:101–108.

WENSVOORT, G.; BLOEMRAAD, M.; AND TERPSTRA, C. 1988. An enzyme immunoassay employing monoclonal antibodies and detecting specifically antibodies to classical swine fever virus. Vet Microbiol 17:129–140.

WENSVOORT, G.; TERPSTRA, C.; DEKLUIJVER, E. P.; KRAGTEN, C.; AND WARNAAR, J. C. 1989a. Antigenic differentiation of pestivirus strains with monoclonal antibodies against hog cholera virus. Vet Microbiol 21:9–20.

WENSVOORT, G.; TERPSTRA, C.; AND DEKLUIJVER, E. P. 1989b. Characterization of porcine and some ruminant pestiviruses by cross-neutralization. Vet Microbiol 20:291–306.

21 Japanese B Encephalitis

R. M. Chu

H. S. Joo

JAPANESE B ENCEPHALITIS, referred to herein simply as Japanese encephalitis, (JE), is a mosquito-borne, infectious viral disease in animals and humans that causes encephalitis and reproductive failures. Most domestic animals are vulnerable to the virus, including horses, cattle, sheep, goats, and pigs. Other animals such as rabbits, rats, pigeons (Chang et al. 1984), dogs, ducks, chickens (Huang 1982), wild birds, and reptiles are also susceptible. Experimental infection has been reported in mice and in a few species of lizards.

The pig is considered the most important natural amplifying animal for JE virus (JEV). The disease is important in pregnant sows, because infection causes stillbirth and other reproductive disturbances; affected boars may have an acute inflammatory reaction in the testes. Horses infected by the virus develop lesions in the central nervous system (CNS), and similar lesions have been found in donkeys and monkeys. In other animals, infection is usually subclinical.

Japanese encephalitis is of primary significance in humans, epidemics having been recorded in Japan (1935), Korea (1949), and India and Nepal (1978). The disease is one of the most common mosquito-borne diseases of the human CNS in Japan, China, and other Western Pacific countries. Isolation and identification of the virus were first described by Fujita (1933) and Taniguchi et al. (1936). Episodes of infection in humans occur annually during mosquito (*Culex tritaeniorhynchus*) season. In most people disease is subclinical or mild, but fatal encephalitis develops in some children, and abortion is reported in pregnant woman (Chaturvedi et al. 1980).

Geographic distribution of the disease is restricted to Southeast Asia (Fig. 21.1); infection has been recognized in Japan, far eastern Soviet Union, Korea, China, Taiwan, the Philippines, Indonesia, Singapore, Malaysia, Hong Kong, Vietnam, Laos, Bangladesh, Nepal, Thailand, Burma, Srilanka, India, and the Pacific islands.

ETIOLOGY

Physicochemical Properties. Japanese encephalitis is caused by a filterable virus, of the genus *Flavivirus,* the only genus in the family

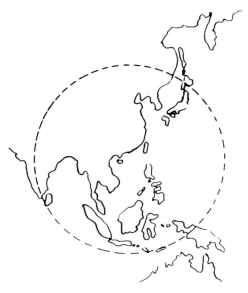

21.1. Geographic distribution of JE. Enzootic infection is shown within the dotted circle.

Flavivirudae, formally grouped in the family Togavirudae. *Flavivirus* has over 60 members; however, only 3 are of significance in veterinary medicine, those causing JE, Louping ill, and Wesselsbron disease. The virus is described as spherical about 40 nm in diameter and enveloped and it contains single-strained ribonucleic acid (RNA) with icosahedral capsid. The complete nucleotide sequence of the JE virus genome RNA contains 10,976 nucleotides corresponding to 3432 amino acid residues (Sumiyoshi et al. 1987). There are three structural and several nonstructural proteins. The structural proteins are envelope glycoprotein E (54 kD), nonglycosylated envelope protein M (8 kD), and capsid protein C (14 kD). Envelope protein E carries epitopes that elicit neutralization antibody. At least eight epitopes are found on protein E, and one of the critical N sites on the protein shows JE virus specificity (Kimura-Kuroda and Yasui 1986). The oligonucleotide fingerprinting technique (Hori et al. 1986) reveals that mutations of JE virus are present in strains that were isolated years apart in Japan and Thailand.

Use of monoclonal antibodies in hemagglutination inhibition, neutralization, enzyme-linked immunosorbent assay (ELISA), and competitive-binding assay has shown that the closest relative of the JE virus is the Murray Valley encephalitis virus; the next closest relative is the West Nile virus; and the St. Louis encephalitis virus is the least closely related (Kimura-Kuroda and Yasui 1986). These relationships are confirmed by comparing the homology of the viruses' nucleotides and amino acids (McAda et al. 1987).

The JEV is unstable in the environment and easily inactivated by disinfectants. The virus is sensitive to ether, chloroform, and sodium desoxycholate, and also to proteolylic or lipolytic enzymes. It is readily inactivated at 56°C after 30 minutes and has an optimal pH stability of 8.5.

Replication.

The JEV replicates well and produces a cytopathic effect in a wide range of host cell culture systems, such as primary cells and cell lines from mammals, including Vero cells, baby monkey kidney (BMK)-21 cells, and L-M mouse fibroblast cells. Cells originating from mosquitoes are also frequently used. In general, mosquito cells are derived from embryonic or larval tissues. Examples include C6/36 cell lines from larval cells of *Aedes albopctus* and *A. aegrpti* cell line from embryonic tissue. Recent studies indicate that leukocyte cultures from various animals are good media for growing the virus (Kadarnath et al. 1987). Hormones such as insulin, adrenocorticotrophic hormone (ACTH), hydrocortisone, and concanavalin A have been shown to enhance JE virus replication in cell culture systems (Kelkar 1985; Kokorev and Kolotvinova 1986).

Like the other flaviviruses, JEV proteins are encoded by a single open reading frame that continues uninterrupted throughout the region that is sequenced (McAda et al. 1987). A short pulse of actinomycin D has no effect on early replication of the virus, but continuous exposure partially inhibits replication. Mitomycin, a DNA-synthesis inhibitor, does not exert any influence on replication of the virus. In addition, the nuclear involvement is apparently not present (Leary and Blair 1983). Latent period of the virus is fairly long, about 12–16 hours postinfection. The virus-specific proteins are synthesized and incorporated into the cytoplasmic membrane system, especially the rough endoplasmic reticulum. The cytoplasmic membrane system of infected cells undergoes hypertrophy and is filled with vesicles, vacuoles, and laminated endoplasmic reticulum. Maturation of the virions takes place within the cisternae of rough endoplasmic reticulum, and transport of the mature virions is by the intracellular secretory system. The virions are released into the medium by cell lysis or by reverse phagocytosis; no virus budding is seen at the host cell membrane. Virions are formed similarly in anthropod cells and on the plasma membrane, but the host cell is not damaged by their release.

EPIDEMIOLOGY.

The epidemiologic features of JE have been described in detail by Konno et al. (1966) and Kono and Kim (1969). In nature, infection with JEV is maintained cyclically, involving vector mosquitoes (mainly *Culex tritaeniorhynchus*) (Self et al. 1973), birds (especially ardeids), and mammals. Other mosquito species may assume the role of main vector according to local ecology.

Japanese encephalitis is of public health concern. A correlation between infection in pigs and infection in humans is apparent, with evidence indicating that swine play an important role in the build-up of the virus within a population. In enzootic zones, pigs are invariably found in high concentration, and are favored feeding sources for mosquitoes. Consistent development of viremia in susceptible pigs ensures a continued supply of infected mosquitoes. In Japan and Korea, the mosquito season starts in late June, varying somewhat according to latitude, and the pig-mosquito cycle becomes evident shortly afterward. At that time, the pig population contains a high proportion of young, susceptible breeding stock in which passive immunity to JEV has waned during the winter (Konno et al. 1966). This build-up of susceptible stock is not as prevalent in tropical areas of Southeast Asia, where the pig-mosquito cycle may continue throughout the year, allowing most young stock to develop an early active immunity. Epidemiologic patterns may differ among areas of Southeast Asia, as vector activity is modified by differing climatic conditions.

Recent data, however, indicate that other animals, different mosquito species, and altered infection cycles are factors involved in the transmission of JE. The disease is a growing threat in India where the pigs are much less numerous compared with other endemic areas. In southern Thailand, 70% of the pigs are infected with JEV, and the JEV vector mosquito is prevalent; however, the encephalitis in humans is rare (Burke et al. 1985).

In temperate zones, JEV survives the winter, but infection of pigs in winter is not an important problem (Takashima et al. 1988). Chickens and wild birds, especially herons and egrets, are able to maintain a positive sera year-round (Hammon et al. 1958; Bhattacharya et al. 1986). The JEV may also be carried by cold-blooded vertebrates throughout the winter; experimentally, the virus survives in two species of lizard (*Takydromus tadydromoides* and *Eumeces latiscutatus*) in hibernation (Doi et al. 1983). The virus can also be isolated naturally from snakes, and bats are possible reservoirs. Multiplication of JEV has been demonstrated in a variety of mosquitos including the species in *Culex, Aedes,* and *Anopheles.* The role of ticks has been described in animals with overwinter infection. Transovarial vertical infection is observed in some mosquitos, such as *Aedes,* which may be another mechanism for the infection. Latent infection, which is demonstrated congenitally in Swiss albino mice and tissue culture systems, may also play a role in overwinter infection.

CLINICAL SIGNS. Although young susceptible piglets may occasionally show clinical signs, clinical illness is not a feature of JEV infection in adults or pregnant pigs. However, various degrees of abnormality in fetuses may be evident when infected pregnant pigs come to term. Litters commonly contain varying numbers of stillborn and mummified fetuses (Fig. 21.2), weak piglets with nervous system signs, and apparently normal piglets. Experimental induction of reproductive failure by infection with JEV causes similarly damaged litters, an additional observation being the presence of subcutaneous edema and hydrocephalus in some stillborn piglets (Shimizu et al. 1954). Experimental infection of susceptible pregnant sows causes no clinical signs in dams, but results in infection of fetuses in utero and subsequent abnormal farrowings: varying numbers of mummified fetuses of different sizes, stillborn, and weak piglets with subcutaneous edema and hydrocephalus (Shimizu et al. 1954). Abortion has not been a feature of intrauterine infection in experimental studies.

Infertility in boars in summer appears to be associated with JEV infection. Hashimura et al. (1976) isolated JEV from testicles of boars with orchitis, and Ogasa et al. (1977) demonstrated that JEV infection of susceptible boars resulted in invasion of the sexual organs and disturbance of spermatogenesis. Such boars developed edematous, congested testicles and hardening of the epi-

didymis, reduced libido, and virus was excreted in the semen, which had significantly depressed total and motile sperm counts, with numerous abnormalities of spermatozoa. In most boars, damage was temporary, with subsequent complete recovery, but occasionally, boars with severe infection became permanently infertile.

PATHOGENESIS. Pigs become infected with JEV via the bites of mosquitoes carrying the virus. Infected pigs develop viremia, which persists for approximately 12 hours to a few days. The multiplication model of the JEV in pigs has not been thoroughly studied; however, some data are available for humans, monkeys, and mice.

After the initial viremia, the virus disseminates to vascular tissues such as the liver, spleen, and muscle, where further replication augments the viremia. The virus enters the CNS via cerebral spinal fluid; endothelial cell, macrophage, or lymphocyte infection; or a hematogenous route. In humans and mice, JEV infects and destroys neurons selectively, mostly in the areas of brain stem, thalamus, basal ganglion, and lower layer of cortex (Johnson 1987).

In mosquitoes, JEV infection is noncytopathic; the virus is multiplied in phagocytic or hemolymph cells of the fat body in 2 days (Johnson 1987). After infection the viral antigens spread widely in many organs, but selective infection in the CNS (Leake and Johnson 1987) is always present 4 days postinfection; 1 or 2 days later the virus can be found in salivary gland.

Macrophages play an important role in the pathogenesis of the disease. After intraperitoneal inoculation in mice, the virus replicates first in the peritoneal macrophages and later, on day 3, in the splenic macrophages of the prefollicular region. Viral productive infection is observed in

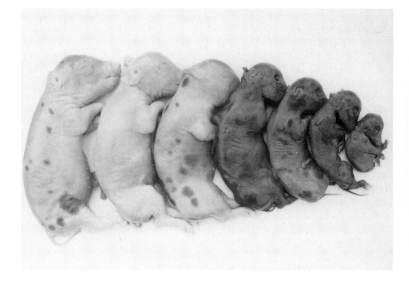

21.2. Mummified and stillborn fetuses from a gilt, associated with natural JEV infection.

macrophages and T cells. Macrophages are also claimed to be involved in the development of latent infection.

Experimentally, JE infection induces the generation of suppressor T cells through the production of a soluble suppressor factor, and suppresses the humoral- and cell-mediated immune responses of the infected animal. This is manifested by depressed activities of plaque-forming cells and delayed hypersensitivities. These suppressions involve at least two generations of suppressor T cells. Infection with JEV initially stimulates the production of first-generation phenotypic Ly 1–2 suppressor cells, which release the suppressor factor having a molecular weight of 12,000 daltons. This factor is nondialyzable and sensitive to hydrocortisone. Suppressor factor adheres to the peritoneal or splenic macrophages and further stimulates the generation of another subpopulation of suppressor T cells, which then exert their suppressor activities on plaque-forming cells and delayed hypersensitivities (Mathur et al. 1986b; Rawat et al. 1986).

Latent infection of pigs in nature has not been well documented. After introperitoneal inoculation of JEV into pregnant Swiss albino mice, latent infection develops in both pregnant mother and their offspring (Mathur et al. 1986a). Reactivation of the virus at 21 weeks of age can be demonstrated by stimulation with allogenic spleen cells in 41% of the offsprings that are congenitally infected. The same is true of pregnant mice. Reactivation of the virus by treatment with cyclophosphamide is more efficient. At the same time, secondary suppressor T cells are produced by memory suppressor cells in mice latently infected by interior or exogenous viruses; this promotes persistance of the virus in animals.

Transplacental infection of JEV has been reported in pigs and mice. In pregnant pigs, fetuses may become infected via this route during the viremic period. Experimentally, after intravenous infection of pregnant pigs with JEV, virus is recoverable from fetuses as early as 7 days postinfection. In some animals, the virus fails to cross the placenta. Shimizu et al. (1954) have suggested that successful transplacental infection may depend on the time of gestation at which the dam was infected or on the strain of virus. When infection of pregnant dams takes place in the mid-third of gestation, transplacental infection and pathogenic effects are more obvious (Shimizu et al. 1954). Field observations show that fetal death and mummification are associated with JEV infection of dams between 40 and 60 days of gestation; fetuses from the gilts infected after 85 days gestation were little affected (Sugimori et al. 1974). Fetal deaths are assumed to be associated with uncontrolled multiplication of the virus and subsequent destruction of vital stem cells in fetuses that have not reached the stage of immuno-

competence. The stage of gestation at which fetuses become immunocompetent for JEV has not yet been determined. The average time of immunocompetence for other viruses such as porcine parvovirus is 70 days of gestation (Joo et al. 1976), and the findings of Sugimori et al. (1974) suggest that there are no pathogenic effects of JEV on the fetus when the virus crosses the placenta after this stage of gestation. Thus, the pathogenesis of JEV for the porcine conceptus seems comparable to that described for porcine parovirus (Joo et al. 1976); i.e., the virus must reach the conceptus before the stage of immunocompetence for pathogenic effects to occur. In mice (Fujisaki et al. 1982), transplacental infection fails to develop unless the virus is inoculated at 4 days of gestation or later; but fetal infection is successful only when the virus is inoculated in between 7 and 10 days of gestation. Infection is rare at any other time of gestation. It is concluded that transplacental infection of JEV depends on the degree of development between placenta and fetal tissues, not on the intensity of viremia.

LESIONS. Major pathologic lesions have not been found in pigs postnatally infected with JEV. However, various abnormalities have been observed in litters from dams infected with the virus during pregnancy. Gross pathologic lesions noted in stillborn or weak neonatal piglets include hydrocephalus, subcutaneous edema, hydrothorax, ascites, petechial hemorrhages on serous membranes, congestion of lymph nodes, necrotic foci in liver and spleen, and congested meninges or spinal cord (Burns 1950). It was further observed that the CNS appeared hypoplastic in areas, the cerebral cortex particularly being extremely thin in some hydrocephalic piglets (Shimizu et al. 1954). Cerebellar hypoplasia and spinal hypomyelinogenesis have also been described (Morimoto 1969).

Histopathologically, significant lesions in affected piglets or stillborn pigs are restricted to the CNS; little data on changes in other tissues were recorded. Most CNS lesions, mainly involving the cortex, basal ganglion, brain stem, and spinal cord, occur in pigs up to 6 months of age. Diffuse nonsuppurative encephalitis and spondylitis are also reported. The highly selective damage to neurons found in humans is not well described in pigs; however, scattered neuronal degeneration and necrosis are found in the cerebrum and cerebellum in pigs. Neuronal degeneration is prominant in the gray matter and Purkinje layers. Most cells in perivascular cuffs in humans are T-helper/inducer cells; however, one-fourth of the cells are T-suppressor/cytotoxic cells. The data is similar in mice, in which suppressor T cells proliferate during JEV infection. Involvement of visceral organs including lung, liver, kidney, and spleen is documented in humans and experimentally in monkeys and horses. Pathologic changes are seen mostly in the reticuloendothelial system, such as focal hyperplasia of germinal centers in the spleen, and interstitial pneumonia (Rawat et al. 1986; Johnson 1987; Chu and Liao 1990).

Pathologic changes in the testes in association with JEV infection are not well described. In naturally affected pigs, a large amount of mucous fluid is observed in the cavity of the tunica vaginalis, as well as fibrous thickening along the edge of the epididymis and the visceral layer of the tunica vaginalis. Microscopically, such testicles show edema and inflammatory changes, with cellular infiltrations in the interstitial tissue of the epididymis and tunica vaginalis. Cell infiltration and hemorrhage are also evident in the interstitial tissue of the testes. Degenerative changes are often seen in the seminiferous epithelium (Hashimura et al. 1976; Ogasa et al. 1977).

DIAGNOSIS. The definitive diagnosis of JEV infection is based upon isolation of the virus from fetuses and infected pigs. A differential diagnosis must include parvovirus infection, Aujeszky's disease, toxoplasmosis, and hog cholera. Other infections associated with reproductive failure such as cytomegalovirus, leptospirosis, and enterovirus infections are also considered. Lack of clinical signs in sows and piglets with JE infection is useful in excluding many diseases. Seasonal distribution also indicates JEV infection.

Several serologic tests are available that detect antibody titers of JEV infection in pig serum, such as the hemagglutination inhibition test, ELISA, antigen biotin-labelled ELISA, single radial hemolysin, and SN techique. Newly developed epitope-blocking immunoassay (Burke et al. 1987) and detection of cerebral spinal fluid–IgM, using ELISA diagnostic kits are used in humans. However, in an area where vaccination is routine, the diagnostic value of the serologic tests is challenged, and paired serum samples should be considered. Presence of the antibody in fetuses is also of diagnostic value.

Although isolation of the virus from suitable specimens is essential to make a definitive diagnosis, detecting viral antigens in infected tissues such as brains, placenta and mummified fetuses is also diagnostically important. Methods such as avidin-biotin staining and flourescent antibody staining have been used to detect JE viral antigen in formalin-fixed tissues following treatment of such tissues with trypsin or other proteolytic enzyme (Kurata et al. 1983; Iwasaki et al. 1986).

Isolation of the virus can be performed by intracerebral inoculation of brain extracts into suckling mice between 1 and 5 days of age. Signs of CNS disturbance or death follow between 4 and 14 days postinoculation, and virus in mouse brain tissue can readily be identified by in vivo neutralization tests in suckling mice or in cell culture. However, it must be noted that the multiple blind passages of brains in mice may inactivate the latent infectious agents in the brain. The commonly used cell cultures are derived from hamster, pig kidney, and mosquito, in all of which the virus causes a cytopathic effect; the mosquito cell line from *A. albopictus* clone C6/36 is the most efficient. It should be recognized that tissue suspected of being infected with JEV must be handled with care, because the virus is not only heat labile but also pathogenic to humans.

PREVENTION. The treatment of JE in humans with human recombinant interferon-alpha A gives clinically satisfactory results. This treatment of JE in swine is not available. Breaking the infectious cycle in this anthropod-borne disease is usually a good step toward management; however, JEV multiplies in a variety of species of mosquitoes, and the infectious patterns vary according to local ecology. It is impractical to control the insect; therefore, immunizing the breeders with JEV vaccine is widely applied as an applicable control and preventive measure.

A variety of mostly live-attenuated vaccines have been developed for the prevention of JE in pigs and are being used successfully in the field (Hsu et al. 1972; Fujisaki et al. 1975; Kwon et al. 1976). Inactivated vaccines have proved to be less efficient and have become less popular. It is recommended that attenuated vaccines be given to young gilts or boars twice at an interval of 2–3 weeks before the start of the mosquito season. As an extra precaution, it is advisable that during the mosquito season, young gilts or boars selected for breeding be vaccinated before mating. The vaccine may be used simultaneously with other viral vaccines such as hog cholera vaccine or porcine parvovirus vaccine.

Attempts have also been made to develop a genetically engineered vaccine, but no commercial product is available. Some studies have demonstrated that monoclonal antibodies to epitopes on the E envelope of JEV prevent mice from JEV infection (Kimura-Kuroda and Yasui 1988). However, application of this to the pigs needs further investigation.

REFERENCES

BHATTACHARYA, S.; CHAKRABORTY, S. K.; CHAKRABORTY, S.; GHOSH, K. K.; PALIT, A.; MUKHERJEE, K. K.; CHAKRABORTY, M. S.; TANDON, N.; AND HATI, A. K. 1986. Density of Culex vishnui and appearance of JE antibody in sentinel chicks and wild birds in relation to Japanese encephalitis cases. Trop Geogr Med 38(1):46–50.

BURKE, D. S.; TINGPALAPONG, M.; WARD, G. S.; ANDRE, R.; AND LEAKE, L. J. 1985. Intense transmission of Japanese encephalitis virus to pigs in a region free of epidemic encephalitis. Southeast Asian J Trop Med Public Health 16(2):199–206.

BURKE, D. S.; NISALAK, A.; AND GENTRY, M. K. 1987. Detection of flavivirus antibodies in human serum by epitope-blocking immuno assay. J Med Virol 23(2):165–173.

BURNS, K. F. 1950. Congenital Japanese B encephalitis infection of swine. Proc Soc Exp Biol Med 75:621–625.

CHANG, H. C.; TAKESHIMA, I.; ARIKAWA, J.; AND HASHIMOTA, M. 1984. Biotin-labeled antigen sandwich enzyme-linked immunosorbent assay (BLAS-ELISA) for the detection of Japanese encephalitis antibody in human and a variety of animal sera. J Immunol Methods 72(2):401–409.

CHATURVEDI, U. C.; MATHUR, A.; CHANDRA, A.; DAS, S. K.; TANDON, H. O.; AND SINGH, U. K. 1980. Transplacental infection with Japanese encephalitis virus. J Infect Dis 141:712–714.

CHU, R. M., AND LIAO, M. Y. 1990. Unpublished data.

DOI, R.; OYA, A.; SHIRASAKA, A.; YABE, S.; AND SASA, M. 1983. Studies on Japanese encephalitis virus infection of reptiles. II. Role of lizards on hibernation of Japanese encephalitis virus. Jpn J Exp Med 53(2):125–134.

FUJISAKI, Y.; SUGIMORI, T.; MORIMOTO, T.; MIURA, Y.; KAWAKAMI, Y.; AND NAKANO, K. 1975. Immunization of pigs with the attenuated S strain of Japanese encephalitis virus. Natl Inst Anim Health Q (Tokyo) 15:55–60.

FUJISAKI, Y.; MIUYA, Y.; SUGIMORI, T.; MURAKAMI, Y.; INO, T.; AND MIURA, K. 1982. Experimental studies on vertical infection of mice with Japanese encephalitis virus. III. Effect of gestation days at the time of inoculation on placental and fetal infection. Natl Inst Anim Health Q 22(3):95–101.

FUJITA, T. 1933. Studies on the causative agent for epidemic encephalitis. Jpn J Exp Med 17:1441–1501.

HAMMON, W. McD.; SATHER, G. E.; AND McCLURE, H. E. 1958. Serological survey of Japanese B encephalitis virus infection in birds in Japan. Am J Hyg 67:118–134.

HASHIMURA, K.; UEMIYADA, S.; KOMEMURA, S.; FUKUMOTO, S.; OKUDA, G.; MIURA, K.; AND HAYASHI, S. 1976. Isolation of Japanese encephalitis virus from orchitis in pigs. Summ 81st Meet Jpn Soc Vet Sci, p. 136.

HORI, H.; IGARASHI, A.; YOSHIDA, I.; AND TAKAGI, M. 1986. Oligonucleotide fingerprint analysis on Japanese encephalitis virus strains after passage histories. Acta Virol 30(5):428–431.

HSU, S. T.; CHANG, L. C.; LIN, S. Y.; CHUANG, T. Y.; MA, C. H.; INOUE, Y. K.; AND OKUNO, T. 1972. The effect of vaccination with a live attenuated strain of Japanese encephalitis virus on stillbirths in swine in Taiwan. Bull WHO 46:465–471.

HUANG, C. H. 1982. Studies of Japanese encephalitis in China. Adv Virus Res 27:71–101.

IWASAKI, Y.; ZHAO, J. X.; YAMAMOTA, T.; AND KOUUO, H. 1986. Immunohistochemical demonstration of viral antigens in Japanese encephalitis. Acta Neuropathol 70(1):79–81.

JOHNSON, R. T. 1987. The pathogenesis of acute viral encephalitis and postinfectious encephalomyelitis. J infect Dis 155(3):359–364.

JOO, H. S.; DONALDSON-WOOD, C. R.; AND JOHNSON, R. H. 1976. Observations on the pathogenesis of porcine parvovirus infection. Arch Virol 51:123–129.

KADARNATH, N.; DAYARAJ, C.; GOVERDHAN, M. K.; AND GHOSH, S. N. 1987. Replication of Japanese encephalitis virus in monkey, pig and chick leucocyte cultures. Trans R Soc Trop Med Hyg 81(5):829–832.

KELKAR, S. D. 1985. Enhancement of Japanese encephalitis virus growth in vitro by concanavalin A. Indian J Med Res 81:437–440.

KIMURA-KURODA, J., AND YASUI, K. 1986. Antigenic comparison of envelope protein E between Japanese encephalitis virus and some other flaviviruses during monoclonal antibodies. J Gen Virol 67:2663–2672.

———. 1988. Protection of mice against Japanese encephalitis virus by passive administration with monoclonal antibodies. J Immunol 141(10):3606–3611.

KOKOREV, V. S., AND KOLOTVINOVA, E. G. 1986. Stimulation of arbovirus reproduction in cell cultures by hormones. Vopr Virusol 31(5):623–629.

KONNO, J.; ENDO, K.; AGATSUMA, H.; AND ISHIDA, N. 1966. Cyclic outbreaks of Japanese encephalitis among pigs and humans. Am J Epidemiol 84:292–300.

KONO, R., AND KIM, K. H. 1969. Comparative epidemiological features of Japanese encephalitis in the Republic of Korea, China (Taiwan) and Japan. Bull WHO 40:263–277.

KURATA, T.; HONDO, R.; SATO, S.; ODA; A.; AOYAMA, Y.; McCORMICK, J. B. 1983. Detection of viral antigens in formalin-fixed specimens by enzyme treatment. Ann NY Acad Sci 420:192–207.

KWON, H. J.; KANG, B. J.; LIM, Y. M.; LEE, C. K.; KWON, Y. B.; HUR, W.; AND JEON, Y. S. 1976. Studies on Japanese encephalitis live virus vaccine. III. Pathogenicity of tissue culture attenuated strain of virus (Anyang strain). Res Rep Off Rural Dev (Korea) 18:21–28.

LEAKE, C. J., AND JOHNSON, R. T. 1987. The pathogenesis of Japanese encephalitis virus in Culex tritaeniorhynchus mosquitos. Trans R Soc Trop Med Hyg 81(4):681–685.

LEARY, K. R., AND BLAIR, C. D. 1983. Japanese encephalitis virus replication: Studies on host cell nuclear involvement. Exp Mol Pathol 38(2):264–270.

McADA, P. C.; MASON, P. W.; SCHIMALJOHN, C. S.; DALRYMPLE, J. M.; MASON, T. L.; AND FOURNIER, M. J. 1987. Partial nucleotide sequence of the Japanese encephalitis virus genome. Virology 158(2):348–360.

MATHUR, A.; ARORTA, K. L.; RAWAT, S.; AND CHATURVEDI, U. C. 1986a. Persistence, latency and reactivation of Japanese encephalitis virus infection in mice. J Gen Virol 67:381–385.

MATHUR, A.; RAWAT, S.; CHATURVEDI, U. C.; AND MISRA, V. S. 1986b. Macrophage transmission of suppressor signal for suppression of delayed hypersensitivity and humoral response in JEV-infected mice. Br J Exp Pathol 67(2):171–179.

MORIMOTO, T. 1969. Epizootic swine stillbirth caused by Japanese encephalitis virus. Proceedings of a symposium on factors producing embryonic and fetal abnormalities, death, and abortion in swine. US ARS 91–73:137–153.

OGASA, A.; YOKOKI, Y.; FUJISAKI, Y.; AND HABU, A. 1977. Reproductive disorders in boars infected experimentally with Japanese encephalitis virus. Jpn J Anim Reprod 23:171–175.

RAWAT, S.; MATHUR, A.; AND CHATURVEDI, U. C. 1986. Characterization of Japanese encephalitis virus-specific suppressor T cells and their product in suppression of the humoral immune response in mice. Ann Inst Pasteur Immunol 1370(3):391–401.

SELF, L. S.; SHIN, H. K.; KIM, K. H.; LEE, K. W.; CHOW, C. Y.; AND HONG, H. K. 1973. Ecologic studies on Culex tritaeniorhynchus as a vector of Japanese encephalitis. Bull WHO 49:41–47.

SHIMIZU, T.; KAWAKAMI, Y.; FUKUHARA, S.; AND MATSUMOTO, M. 1954. Experimental stillbirth in pregnant swine infected with Japanese encephalitis virus. Jpn J Exp Med 24:363–375.

SUGIMORI, T.; MORIMOTO, T.; FUJISAKI, Y.; SUGAWARA, S.; TOMISHIMA, S.; AND OGATA, M. 1974. A status quo survey on stillbirth and abortion in swine. III. Relationship between the day of pregnancy at the time of outbreak of Japanese encephalitis and the occurrence of stillbirth and abortion. J Jpn Vet Med Assoc 27:282–285.

SUMIYOSHI, H.; MORI, C.; FUKE, I.; MORITA, K.; KUHARA, S.; KONDOU, J.; KIKUCHI, Y.; NAGAMATU, H.; AND IGARASHI, A. 1987. Complete nucleotide sequence of the Japanese encephalitis virus genome RNA. Virology 16(2):497–510.

TAKASHIMA, I.; WATANABE, T.; OUCHI, N.; AND HASHIMOTO, N. 1988. Ecological studies of Japanese encephalitis virus in Hokkaido: Interepidemic outbreaks of swine abortion and evidence for the virus to overwinter locally. Am J Trop Med Hyg 38(2):420–427.

TANIGUCHI, T.; HOSOKAWA, M.; AND KUGA, S. 1936. A virus isolated in 1935 epidemic of summer encephalitis of Japan. Jpn J Exp Med 14:185–196.

22 Porcine Epidemic Diarrhea

M. B. Pensaert

IN 1971, previously unrecognized acute outbreaks of diarrhea were observed in feeder pigs and fattening swine in England (Oldham 1972). The clinical appearance was similar to that of an infection with transmissible gastroenteritis (TGE) virus except for the important difference that suckling pigs (under 4–5 weeks of age) did not become sick. TGE virus (TGEV) or other known enteropathogenic infectious agents were ruled out, but a viral etiology of unknown identity was suspected. The name epidemic viral diarrhea (EVD) was adopted. During the early 1970s, a similar type of infectious diarrhea was also observed in certain continental European countries such as Belgium.

In 1976, TGE-like outbreaks of acute diarrhea in swine of all ages, including suckling pigs, were observed (Wood 1977), but TGEV was ruled out as the cause. Again, these outbreaks could not be attributed to known enteropathogenic agents. The name EVD type 2 was used to differentiate them from the outbreaks described in the earlier 1970s (designated type 1). The difference between types 1 and 2 was that only in type 2 outbreaks were baby piglets involved.

In 1978, a coronaviruslike agent was found to be associated with the type 2 outbreaks (Chasey and Cartwright 1978; Pensaert and DeBouck 1978). Experimental inoculations with an isolate revealed its enteropathogenic character not only for piglets (DeBouck and Pensaert 1980) but for fattening swine. More recently, it was demonstrated that outbreaks of types 1 and 2 EVD are caused by the same coronavirus; the name porcine epidemic diarrhea (PED) was proposed and is still being used (Pensaert et al. 1982).

ETIOLOGY. On a morphologic basis, PED virus (PEDV) particles show characteristics similar to those of the species of the family Coronaviridae (Chasey and Cartwright 1978; Pensaert and DeBouck 1978). The particles detected in fecal material are pleomorphic, with a tendency to a spherical shape. Their mean diameter, projections included, is 130 nm, with a range of 95–190 nm. Many particles have an electron-opaque central area. The club-shaped projections measure 18–23 nm and are radially spaced from the core. An internal structure cannot be recognized. The morphogenesis of PEDV in intestinal epithelial cells was found to be identical to that of other coronaviruses. Assembly of the virus occurs by budding through intracytoplasmic membranes (Ducatelle et al. 1981a).

Physicochemical and biological characterization studies have confirmed the classification of PEDV as a member of the Coronaviridae family. The virus is ether and chloroform sensitive. Its density in sucrose is 1.18 g/ml. Concentrated and purified virus containing intestinal perfusate from infected piglets fails to agglutinate erythrocytes of 12 different animal species (Callebaut and De-Bouck 1981, Witte et al. 1981). Cell culture–adapted PEDV loses its infectivity when heated $\geq 60°C$ for 30 minutes, but is moderately stable at 50°C. The virus is stable between pH 5.0 and 9.0 at 4°C and between pH 6.5 and 7.5 at 37°C. Viral infectivity is not impaired by ultrasonication or by multiple freezing and thawing. Replication is not inhibited by 5-iodo-2'-deoxyuridine, indicating that the viral nucleic acid is RNA (Hofmann and Wyler 1989).

The pattern of the structural proteins of PEDV is similar to that of other coronaviruses. The virus possesses a glycosylated peplomer protein with a molecular weight of 85,000 to 135,000 daltons, a glycosylated envelope protein of 20,000 to 32,000 daltons, and an unglycosylated RNA-binding nucleocapsid protein of 58,000 daltons (Egberink et al. 1988).

Using direct immunofluorescence (IF) and immunoelectron microscopy, PEDV was found to be antigenically distinct from the two known porcine coronaviruses (TGEV and hemagglutinating encephalomyelitis virus) and canine coronavirus, neonatal calf diarrhea virus, infectious bronchitis virus, and feline infectious peritonitis virus (Pensaert et al. 1981; Witte et al. 1981). However, examination with the aid of more sensitive techniques such as immunoblotting and immunoprecipitation showed that PEDV has antigenic determinants in common with feline infectious peritonitis virus. These determinants are located on the nucleocapsid protein. This provides a firm argument in favor of the classification of PEDV as a coronavirus (Yaling et al. 1988).

Cultivation of the virus has been accomplished by orally inoculating piglets and subsequently collecting the small intestine and its contents during the early stages of diarrhea. However, virus stocks of higher purity have been prepared by orally inoculating hysterectomy-derived piglets and washing out the small intestinal lumen through surgical procedures, starting at the onset of diarrhea. This perfusion may continue for 12 hours; a virus stock of 1500 ml containing 10^4–10^5 pig infectious doses per ml can be obtained (De-Bouck and Pensaert 1980).

The adaptation of PEDV to grow in an artificial host under laboratory conditions has been fastidious. Attempts with different virus isolates were unsuccessful in intestinal or tracheal explants from swine fetuses or newborn pigs. Also, numerous cell types have been employed with or without treatments with trypsin and pancreatin, but were nonpermissive for PEDV replication (Hess et al. 1980; Callebaut and DeBouck 1981; Witte et al. 1981). However, Vero (African green monkey kidney) cells were recently found to support the serial propagation of PEDV. Viral growth depends on the presence of trypsin in the cell culture medium. Cytopathic effects consist of vacuolation and formation of syncytia. The syncytia may contain over 100 nuclei. Growth kinetics show peak titers of $10^{5.5}$ plaque-forming units per ml 15 hours after inoculation (Hofmann and Wyler 1988, 1989).

PEDV or viral antigens have until now been detected in fecal material by electron microscopy (EM) and enzyme-linked immunosorbent assay (ELISA). The sensitivity of the ELISA test is much higher than that of EM (Callebaut et al. 1982). With ELISA, PED viral antigens were demonstrated in feces of pigs until at least 7 days postinoculation.

Specific antibodies have been detected in sera from swine after natural or experimental infection with PEDV. They can be demonstrated by immunoelectron microscopy, ELISA, ELISA blocking, indirect IF, IF blocking, and seroneutralization in piglets and in Vero cell cultures (Pensaert et al. 1981; Prager and Witte 1981a, b; Callebaut et al. 1982; Witte and Prager 1987; Hofmann and Wyler 1989, 1990). By ELISA, antibodies against the viral peplomer protein are easier to detect than antibodies against the nucleocapsid protein (Knuchel et al. 1990).

There are no indications that different serotypes of PEDV exist. Isolates from Germany and France are serologically identical to the prototype CV777 strain (Hess et al. 1980; Witte et al. 1981; Vannier and DeBouck 1983).

EPIDEMIOLOGY. Using the ELISA-blocking test, serologic surveys have been carried out in 1982 and antibodies have then been detected in swine sera from Belgium, England, Germany, France, the Netherlands, Switzerland, Bulgaria, and Taiwan but not from Sweden, Northern Ireland, the United States, Australia, or Hungary (DeBouck et al. 1982). The presence of PEDV antibodies in sera from pigs in Switzerland has recently been confirmed using the indirect IF test (Hofmann and Wyler 1987). In 1990, antibodies

against PEDV still were not found using the ELISA-blocking test in swine sera collected in four states of the United States (Ohio, Missouri, Kansas, and Minnesota) as well as in Austria (Möstl et al. 1990).

The agent itself has been isolated in Belgium, France, England, Germany, and China.

A disease syndrome similar to PED and caused by an unidentified coronaviruslike agent has been described in Hungary and East Germany (Horvath and Moscari 1981; Leopoldt et al. 1981).

Serologic surveys carried out in Belgium on sow sera collected between 1969 and 1984 revealed no antibodies in 1969 but up to 19% in 1984 (Table 22.1). A serosurvey carried out on fattening farms showed that on 33% of the farms, animals had antibodies to PEDV.

Table 22.1. Antibodies to PEDV in Belgian sow sera collected in abattoirs, using the ELISA-blocking test

Year	Number Tested	Number Positive (%)
1969	80	none (0)
1971	63	7 (11)
1975	107	45 (42)
1980	210	68 (32)
1984	265	51 (19)

The first clinical outbreaks of PED were described in 1971–72, which coincides with the appearance of positive sera. No information is available on the possible origin of PEDV.

PEDV is transmitted mainly if not only by feces from infected animals. The natural infection starts after oral uptake. The feces-oral route of transmission is probably the main if not the only one.

Outbreaks of PED on a farm often occur within 4–5 days after sale or purchase of animals. Entrance of the virus probably occurs by infected animals by way of transport trucks, virus contaminated boots, or other virus-carrying fomites. After an outbreak has occurred on a breeding farm, the virus may either disappear or may become enzootic. The enzootic status can be established when sufficient litters of pigs are produced and weaned so that the virus is maintained through continuous presence of pigs that have lost their lactogenic immunity at weaning. PEDV has been diagnosed as the cause of persistent weaning diarrhea on such breeding farms.

Little information is available on the exact number of PED outbreaks in a particular country. In Germany, blood samples collected from 158 farms with a history of recent outbreaks of diarrhea revealed that 28% had antibodies against PEDV. PED viral antigens were detected by IF in animals from 12% of the diarrheic outbreaks on breeding farms and 19% on fattening farms (Prager and Witte 1983).

During the early 1980s, about 7% of the diarrheic outbreaks with deaths in baby pigs were found to be caused by PEDV in Belgium. In recent years, however, acute diarrheic outbreaks with sow and baby pig involvment due to PEDV have become very rare, probably as a consequence of the enzootic status. PEDV is now regularly the cause of outbreaks of acute diarrhea in fattening units and should be considered as an agent that can be associated with weaning diarrhea on some breeding farms and with diarrhea in feeder pigs in some situations. Detection of PEDV in 13 out of 16 groups of feeder pigs that developed diarrhea after arrival on the fattening farms (Callebaut et al. 1986) shows that the virus must be carried on some breeding farms by pigs after weaning. In each group, the feeder pigs were brought together from several breeding farms and diarrhea was observed within a few days after transport to and entrance into the fattening unit.

CLINICAL SIGNS.

The main and often the only obvious clinical sign of PED is watery diarrhea. Acute outbreaks on breeding farms are rare in regions or countries where the virus has become widespread and where the sow population is largely immune. Outbreaks in susceptible breeding herds may show much variation in morbidity and mortality.

On some farms, animals of all ages become sick, with morbidity approaching 100%. The disease is then very similar to TGE, except for a slower spread and a lower mortality in baby piglets. Piglets up to 1 week of age may die from dehydration after the diarrhea has lasted 3–4 days. Mortality rates average 50% but may be as high as 90%. Older animals recover after about 1 week. On other farms, however, weaned pigs and even adult animals are severely affected, while suckling pigs have no or only mild diarrhea. Morbidity in baby pigs is then low. No explanation can be given for this variation in clinical picture in the absence of immunity.

Much less variation is observed when an acute PED outbreak occurs in a fattening unit. All the pigs in the unit will show diarrhea within a week. The animals are anorectic, depressed, and their feces are watery (no blood). Clinically, PEDV-affected animals are more severely sick than TGE-affected ones. They appear to have more abdominal pain. Recovery occurs as a rule after 7–10 days. A mortality rate of 1–3% may be seen in fattening pigs infected toward the end of the fattening period. They die acutely, usually in the early stages of diarrhea or even prior to the appearance of diarrhea. A common necropsy finding in these animals is acute back muscle necrosis. The highest mortality rate is found on farms with stress-sensitive pig breeds.

No explanation can be given at this time for the high variation in clinical signs observed on breeding farms. Several isolates have been tested for variation in virulence for piglets, but such variation has not been found. In general, PEDV replication starts more easily in the intestine of feeder and fattening pigs than in baby pigs. Consequently, fattening animals are more susceptible to the virus, and 100% morbidity during an outbreak is common.

PEDV spreads more slowly throughout the premises of closed-breeding farms and also within and between fattening units than TGEV. On breeding farms that have several separate units, it may take 4–5 weeks before the virus has infected different age groups. Some units may even remain free of infection.

PATHOGENESIS.

The pathogenesis of PED has been studied in hysterectomy-derived, colostrum-deprived piglets inoculated with the CV777 isolate. Piglets were orally inoculated at the age of 3 days (DeBouck et al. 1981b). Upon inoculation, the pigs became sick after 22–36 hours. Viral replication, as demonstrated by IF and transmission EM, occurred in the cytoplasm of villous epithelial cells throughout the small intestine and in the colon. A few fluorescent foci were also observed in the crypts and mesenteric lymph nodes, but the infection at these sites always remained scattered and was possibly nonproductive.

Infected epithelial cells were observed as early as 12–18 hours postinoculation, and a maximum was reached between 24 and 36 hours. Viral replication in the small intestine resulted in cell degeneration leading to villous shortening. A reduction of villous height:crypt depth ratio from the normal 7:1 value to 3:1 was observed. No cell degeneration was seen in the colonic epithelial cells. Fluorescent cells were detectable until 5 days postinoculation.

The pathogenetic features of PEDV in the small intestine of piglets are very similar to those of TGEV. However, the events with TGEV are of a more rapid and drastic nature, leading to a villous shortening that is more extensive and occurs within 18–24 hours postinoculation. Since viral replication and progress of the infection in the small intestine with PEDV occurs at a slower rate, a longer incubation period is observed. PEDV replication in piglets has not been detected in cells outside the intestinal tract.

The pathogenesis of PEDV in older swine has not been studied in much detail, but fluorescence was found in the epithelial cells of the small intestinal and colonic villi of conventional fattening swine after experimental as well as natural infection. Such observation was not made by Witte et al. (1981), who found the colon positive only in 1-day-old piglets and not in older specific-pathogen-free swine.

It is not clear how much the colonic infection adds to the severity of clinical signs. Also, no pathogenetic explanation can be given for the sudden death accompanied by acute back muscle necrosis often observed in finishing pigs and adult animals. A recent study proved that halothane-positive fattening swine of 40–70 kg showed markedly increased concentrations of the skeletal muscle enzymes creatine phosphokinase and lactate dehydrogenase in their blood, starting 3 days after inoculation with PEDV.

Using direct EM, virus particles were detected in feces of experimentally inoculated piglets until 4 days postinoculation. With the ELISA test, feces were positive until 7 days.

LESIONS. Macroscopic lesions have been described in experimentally and naturally infected piglets (Pospischil et al. 1981; Ducatelle et al. 1982b). They are confined to the small intestine, which is distended with yellow fluid. Microscopically, vacuolation and exfoliation of enterocytes on the small intestinal villi were observed starting at 24 hours postinoculation, which coincided with the onset of diarrhea. From that time on, shortening of the villi occurred. Those findings were confirmed in scanning EM studies (Ducatelle et al. 1981a). Histochemically, the enzymatic activity in the small intestine was found to be markedly reduced. All these events are very similar to those described with TGEV (Pospischil et al. 1981). No histopathologic changes have been observed in the colon.

Ultrastructural changes occurred mainly in the cytoplasm of enterocytes (Horvath and Moscari 1981; Pospischil et al. 1981) in which cell organelles had decreased, leaving electron translucent areas. Later, the microvilli and terminal web disappeared, and parts of the cytoplasm protruded into the intestinal lumen. The cells became flattened, the tight junction was lost, and cell release occurred into the gut lumen. Intracellular virus formation was seen by budding through membranes of the endoplasmic reticulum (Ducatelle et al. 1981b). In the colon, some cellular changes were observed in enterocytes containing virus particles, but no exfoliation was seen.

DIAGNOSIS. A diagnosis of PED cannot be made on a clinical basis only. Acute PED outbreaks in which diarrhea is observed in animals of all ages, baby pigs included, cannot be clinically differentiated from TGE. Acute diarrhea in weaned pigs and older animals on a breeding farm, with no or only slight clinical signs in baby piglets, points toward PED. Since diarrhea is always present in adult animals, rotavirus and *Escherichia coli* infections are not to be considered.

An etiologic diagnosis can be made in the laboratory by direct demonstration of PEDV and/or its antigens or by detection of antibodies.

The direct IF test applied on cryostat sections of the small intestine of pigs with diarrhea is the most sensitive, rapid, and reliable method. It can only be used on the intestine of pigs killed during the acute phase of diarrhea, preferably within 48 hours after the onset. The results of this technique are not reliable on pigs that die naturally (DeBouck et al. 1981b).

PEDV particles can be demonstrated in the feces of pigs with diarrhea by direct EM. Examination of feces for coronavirus is often difficult because the virus particles are not easy to detect if the spikes are lost or not clearly visible. The highest percentage of positive fecal samples obtained in experimentally inoculated piglets was 73% in feces collected the first day after the onset of diarrhea. Furthermore, immunoelectron microscopy has to be applied to make a differentiation with TGEV, since both viruses have the same morphology.

A sensitive and reliable method for diagnosis in older animals as well as in piglets is the ELISA test on fecal material or intestinal contents. The test is more sensitive and reliable than EM. Fecal material should be collected from several animals, preferably during the acute phase of diarrhea. In experimentally inoculated pigs, PED viral antigens were consistently detected between 2 and 5 days after infection but inconsistently between 6 and 8 days (Callebaut et al. 1982).

Recently, a method has been described for the isolation in Vero cell cultures of cytopathogenic PEDV from intestinal homogenate and contents. No data are available on the sensitivity and reliability of this technique as a diagnostic tool (Hofmann and Wyler 1988).

A serologic diagnosis can be made by demonstration of PEDV antibodies. Several methods have been reported: the indirect IF test and the IF-blocking test on PEDV-positive cryostat sections of pig intestine, the ELISA and the ELISA-blocking test. With all tests, paired serum samples should be examined. The second (convalescent) serum sample should be collected not sooner than 4 weeks after the onset of diarrhea, since in experimentally inoculated animals, antibodies were only detectable after 15 days postinoculation.

The antibodies demonstrated with the indirect IF technique are reported to be temperature labile, which appears to make the use of this method difficult under practical diagnostic circumstances (Prager and Witte 1981a,b). The indirect IF test has also been found to be less sensitive than the IF-blocking test and the ELISA (Prager and Witte 1981a,b; Witte and Prager 1987; Hofmann and Wyler 1990).

PEDV antibodies demonstrated in the serum with the ELISA-blocking and IF-blocking tests have been shown to persist for at least 1 year. Reinfection of the intestine, with development of diarrhea, may occur in seropositive animals that have recovered from a first infection 5 months previously. However, such animals will show a rapid booster reaction (DeBouck and Pensaert 1984; Witte and Prager 1987).

TREATMENT AND PREVENTION. Definite

recommendations with regard to measures to be taken during a PED outbreak cannot be given at this time. Antibiotic treatments are of no help. Animals with diarrhea should have free access to water to diminish dehydration. It is advisable to withhold feed, particularly in fattening swine. Since PEDV does not spread very quickly, preventive measures to temporarily avoid virus entrance into farrowing units with newly born piglets may be of help to postpone the infection of these piglets until a later age, resulting in less deaths. In the meantime, artificial spread of the virus to pregnant sows will stimulate a rapid lactogenic immunity and thus shorten the disease on the farm. This artificial exposure can be accomplished by use of fecal material from animals with watery diarrhea or of intestinal contents from sick piglets. This approach is similar to that used with TGEV.

Sanitary measures should prevent introduction of the virus into the farm. Present epizootiologic knowledge indicates that virus introduction occurs mainly (if not only) by animal and human traffic (Bollwahn 1983).

REFERENCES

BOLLWAHN, W. 1983. Epizootic viral diarrhoea of pigs. Pig News Inf 4:141–144.
CALLEBAUT, P., AND DEBOUCK, P. 1981. Some characteristics of a new porcine coronavirus and detection of antigen and antibody by ELISA. Proc 5th Int Congr Virol, Strasbourg, p. 420.
CALLEBAUT, P.; DEBOUCK, P.; AND PENSAERT, M. 1982. Enzyme-linked immunosorbent assay for the detection of the coronavirus-like agent and its antibodies in pigs with porcine epidemic diarrhea. Vet Microbiol 7:295–306.
CALLEBAUT, P.; PENSAERT, M.; MIRY, C.; HAESEBROUCK, F.; AND VERGOTE, J. 1986. Prevalence of influenza-Aujeszky, transmissible gastroenteritis- and porcine epizootic diarrhea virus infections in feeder pigs. Proc 9th Int Congr Pig Vet Soc, Barcelona, p. 213.
CHASEY, D., AND CARTWRIGHT, S. F. 1978. Virus-like particles associated with porcine epidemic diarrhoea. Res Vet Sci 25:255–256.
DEBOUCK, P., AND PENSAERT, M. 1980. Experimental infection of pigs with a new porcine enteric coronavirus CV777. Am J Vet Res 41:219–223.
———. 1984. Porcine epidemic diarrhea: Kinetics of actively and passively acquired serum antibodies and the effect of reinfection. Proc 8th Int Congr Pig Vet Soc, Ghent, p. 53.
DEBOUCK, P.; PENSAERT, M.; AND COUSSEMENT, W. 1981a. The pathogenesis of an enteric infection in pigs experimentally induced by the coronavirus-like agent CV777. Vet Microbiol 6:157–165.
DEBOUCK, P.; CALLEBAUT, P.; AND PENSAERT, M. 1981b. The diagnosis of coronavirus-like agent (CVLA) diarrhea in suckling pigs. Curr Top Vet Med Anim Sci 13:59–61.

———. 1982. Prevalence of the porcine epidemic diarrhea (PED) virus in the pig population of different countries. Proc 7th Int Congr Pig Vet Soc, Mexico City, p. 53.
DUCATELLE, R.; COUSSEMENT, W.; CHARLIER, G.; DEBOUCK, P.; AND HOORENS, J. 1981a. Three-dimensional sequential study of the intestinal surface in experimental porcine CV777 coronavirus enteritis. Zentralbl Veterinaermed [B] 28:483–493.
DUCATELLE, R.; COUSSEMENT, W.; PENSAERT, M. B.; DEBOUCK, P.; AND HOORENS, J. 1981b. In vivo morphogenesis of a new porcine enteric coronavirus, CV777. Arch Virol 68:35–44.
DUCATELLE, R.; COUSSEMENT, W.; DEBOUCK, P.; AND HOORENS, J. 1982a. Pathology of experimental CV777 coronavirus enteritis in piglets. I. Histological and histochemical study. Vet Pathol 19:46–56.
DUCATELLE, R.; COUSSEMENT, W.; CHARLIER, G.; DEBOUCK, P.; AND HOORENS, J. 1982b. Pathology of experimental CV777 coronavirus enteritis in piglets. II. Electron microscopic study. Vet Pathol 19:57–66.
EGBERINK, H. F.; EDERVEEN, J.; CALLEBAUT, P.; AND HORZINEK, M. C. 1988. Characterization of the structural proteins of porcine epizootic diarrhea virus, strain CV777. Am J Vet Res 49:1320–1324.
HESS, R. G.; BOLLWAHN, W.; POSPISCHIL, A.; HEINRITZI, K.; AND BACHMANN, P. A. 1980. Neue Aspekte der Virusaetiologie bei Durchfallerkrankungen des Schweines: Vorkommen von Infektionen mit dem Epizootischen Virusdiarrhoe-(EVD-) Virus. Berl Muench Tieraertzl Wochenschr 93:445–449.
HOFMANN, M., AND WYLER, R. 1987. Serologische Untersuchung über das Vorkommen der Epizootischen Virusdiarrhoe der Schweine (EVD) in der Schweiz. Schweiz Arch Tierheilkd 129:437–442.
———. 1988. Propagation of the virus of porcine epidemic diarrhea in cell culture. J Clin Microbiol 26:2235–2239.
———. 1989. Quantitation, biological and physiochemical properties of cell culture–adapted porcine epidemic diarrhea coronavirus (PEDV). Vet Microbiol 20:131–142.
———. 1990. Enzyme-linked immunosorbent assay for the detection of porcine epidemic diarrhea coronavirus antibodies in swine sera. Vet Microbiol 21:263–273.
HORVATH, I., AND MOSCARI, E. 1981. Ultrastructural changes in the small intestinal epithelium of suckling pigs affected with a transmissible gastroenteritis (TGE)-like disease. Arch Virol 68:103–113.
KNUCHEL, M.; ACKERMANN, M.; MÜLLER, H. K.; AND KIHM, U. 1990. Characterization of the E2-glycoprotein and nucleoprotein of porcine epidemic diarrhoea virus (PEDV) and application of their physico-chemical properties for the detection of anti PEDV antibodies by ELISA. Proc 11th Int Congr Pig Vet, Lausanne, p. 214.
LEOPOLDT, D.; LEHNERT, C.; KOITZSCH, R.; TESMER, S.; GRANZOW, H.; AND HEINRICH, H. W. 1981. Neue virusbedingte Durchfallerkrankungen des Schweiner (TGE-aehnliche Erkrankungen). Monatsh Veterinaermed 36:411–415.
MÖSTL, K.; HORVATH, E.; BÜRKI, F. 1990. Erhebungen über porcine Coronaviren in Österreich. II. Teil: Porcine epidemic diarrhea virus (PEDV) der Schweine. Wien Tieraerztl Monatsschr. 77:10–18.
OLDHAM, J. 1972. Pig Farming [Oct suppl]:72–73.
PENSAERT, M. B., AND DEBOUCK, P. 1978. A new coronavirus-like particle associated with diarrhea in swine. Arch Virol 58:243–247.
PENSAERT, M. B.; DEBOUCK, P.; AND REYNOLDS, D. J. 1981. An immunoelectron microscopic and immuno-

fluorescent study on the antigenic relationship between the coronavirus-like agent CV777 and several coronaviruses. Arch Virol 68:45–52.

PENSAERT, M.; CALLEBAUT, P.; AND DEBOUCK, P. 1982. Porcine epidemic diarrhea (PED) caused by a coronavirus: Present knowledge. Proc 7th Int Congr Pig Vet Soc, Mexico City, p. 52.

POSPISCHIL, A.; HESS, R. G.; AND BACHMANN, P. A. 1981. Light microscopy and ultrahistology of intestinal changes in pigs infected with enzootic diarrhoea virus (EVD): Comparison with transmissible gastroenteritis (TGE) virus and porcine rotavirus infections. Zentralbl Veterinaermed [B] 28:564–577.

PRAGER, D., AND WITTE, K. 1981a. Die serologische Diagnose der Epizootischen Virusdiarrhoe (EVD) des Schweines mit Hilfe der indirekten Immunofluoreszenztechnik (IIFT). Tieraerztl Umsch 36:404–414.

——. 1981b. Die serologische Diagnose der Epizootischen Virusdiarrhoe (EVD) des Schweines mit Hilfe der indirekten Immunofluoreszenztechnik (IIFT). II. Antikorper-Antwort nach experimenteller Infektion. Tieraerztl Umsch 36:477–480.

——. 1983. Die Haufigkeit von Transmissible Gastroenteritis (TGE) und Epizootische Virusdiarrhoe (EVD)-Virusinfektionen als Ursachen seuchenhafter Durchfaelle in westfaelischen Schweinenzucht-und-mastbestaenden. Tieraerztl Umsch 38:155–158.

VANNIER, P., AND DEBOUCK, P. 1983. Identification de la diarrhee epidemique porcine (DEP) en Bretagne. Rec Med Vet 159:19–24.

WITTE, K. H., AND PRAGER, D. 1987. Der Nachweis von Antikörpern gegen das Virus der Epizootischen Virusdiarrhoe (EVD) des Schweines mit dem Immunofluoreszenz-blockadetest (IFBT). Tieraerztl Umsch, 42:817–820.

WITTE, K. H.; PRAGER, D.; ERNST, H.; AND NEUHOFF, H. 1981. Die Epizootische Virusdiarrhoe (EVD). Tieraerztl Umsch 36:235–250.

WOOD, E. N. 1977. An apparently new syndrome of porcine epidemic diarrhoea. Vet Rec 100:243–244.

YALING, Z.; EDERVEEN, K.; EGBERINK, H.; PENSAERT, M.; AND HORZINEK, M. C. 1988. Porcine epidemic diarrhea virus (CV777) and feline infectious peritonitis virus (FIPV) are antigenically related. Arch Virol 102:63–71.

23 Porcine Parvovirus

W. L. Mengeling

PORCINE PARVOVIRUS (PPV) causes reproductive failure of swine characterized by embryonic and fetal infection and death, usually in the absence of outward maternal clinical signs. The disease develops mainly when seronegative dams are exposed oronasally to the virus anytime during about the first half of gestation, and conceptuses are subsequently infected transplacentally before they become immunocompetent. There is no definitive evidence that infection of swine other than during gestation is of any clinical or economic significance. The virus is ubiquitous among swine throughout the world and is enzootic in most herds that have been tested. Diagnostic surveys have indicated that PPV is the major infectious cause of embryonic and fetal death (Cartwright and Huck 1967; Mengeling 1978b; Thacker and Leman 1978; Vannier and Tillon 1979; Mengeling et al. 1991).

ETIOLOGY. PPV (Latin parvus = small) is classified in the genus *Parvovirus* of the family Parvoviridae (Siegl 1976; Bachmann et al. 1979). All isolates of PPV that have been compared have been found antigenically similar if not identical (Cartwright et al. 1969; Johnson and Collings 1969; Morimoto et al. 1972a; Johnson et al. 1976; Ruckerbauer et al. 1978). PPV is also antigenically related to several other members of the genus (Cotmore et al. 1983; Mengeling et al. 1986, 1988). However, its identity can be established by relatively stringent serologic tests such as serum neutralization (SN) and hemagglutination inhibition (HI).

Biophysical and Biochemical Properties. The biophysical and biochemical properties of PPV have been extensively studied (Siegl 1976; Molitor et al. 1983; Berns 1984) and are summarized as follows. A mature virion has cubic symmetry, two or three capsid proteins, a diameter of approximately 20 nm, 32 capsomeres, no envelope or essential lipids, and a weight of 5.3×10^6 daltons. The viral genome is single-stranded deoxyribonucleic acid (DNA) with a molecular weight of 1.4×10^6, i.e., about 26.5% of the weight of the complete virion. Buoyant densities (g/ml in cesium chloride) of complete infectious virions, incomplete "empty" virions, and extracted virion DNA are 1.38–1.395, 1.30–1.315, and 1.724 respectively. Viral infectivity, hemag-glutinating activity, and antigenicity are remarkably resistant to heat, a wide range of hydrogen ion concentrations, and enzymes.

Replication. Replication of PPV in vitro is cytocidal and characterized by "rounding up," pyknosis, and lysis of cells (Fig. 23.1A). Many of the cell fragments often remain attached, eventually giving the affected culture a ragged appearance. Intranuclear inclusions develop (Cartwright et al. 1969) but they are often sparsely distributed (Rondhuis and Straver 1972). Infected cultures may hemadsorb slightly (Cartwright et al. 1969) (Fig. 23.1B). Cytopathic changes are extensive when cell culture–adapted virus is propagated under appropriate conditions. However, on initial isolation several serial passages of the virus (Cartwright et al. 1969), or better, the infected culture, may be necessary before the effects are recognized. The use of immunofluorescence (IF) microscopy greatly increases the likelihood of detecting minimally infected cultures (Lucas and Napthine 1971; Mengeling 1975).

Primary and secondary cultures of fetal or neonatal porcine kidney cells are most often used for propagation and titration of PPV, although other kinds of cultures are also susceptible (Pirtle 1974). Replication is enhanced by infection of mitotically active cultures (Mayr et al. 1968; Cartwright et al. 1969; Bachmann 1972; Hallauer et al. 1972). Many cells in such cultures are in the S phase, i.e., the DNA synthesis phase, of their cell cycle, wherein the DNA polymerases of cell origin needed for viral replication are available (Tennant 1971; Siegl and Gautschi 1973a,b).

If either fetal or adult bovine serum is incorporated in the nutrient medium of cell cultures used to propagate PPV, it should be pretested for viral inhibitors (Coackley and Smith 1972; Johnson 1973; Pini 1975). The same may apply to sera of several other species (Joo et al. 1976d). Because replication of PPV is affected by mitotic activity, the effect of the serum on the cells is also especially important. In addition, cultures should be pretested for PPV contamination (Lucas and Napthine 1971; Mengeling 1975). Cultures are sometimes unknowingly prepared from infected tissues of fetal (Mengeling 1975) and postnatal (Huygelen and Peetermans 1967; Bachmann 1969; Cartwright et al. 1969; Hafez and Liess 1979) pigs. Moreover, PPV can be accidentally

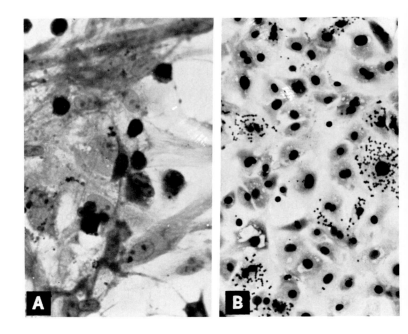

23.1. Cell cultures infected with PPV. (A) Cytopathic effect, secondary fetal porcine kidney cells, 120 hours after infection. ×250. (Mengeling 1972). (B) Hemadsorption, secondary adult porcine thyroid cells, guinea pig erythrocytes, 22 hours after thyroid cells were infected and then subcultured. May-Grünwald-Giemsa. ×100.

introduced into cultures in several ways (Hallauer et al. 1971), including the use of contaminated trypsin (Croghan and Matchett 1973; Croghan et al. 1973). If contamination is detected before all cells are infected, the virus can be eliminated by repeatedly subculturing the cells in the presence of nutrient medium containing PPV antiserum (Mengeling 1978a).

Several investigators have used IF microscopy to follow the development of PPV in cell culture (Cartwright et al. 1969; Lucas and Napthine 1971; Mengeling 1972; Siegl et al. 1972; Bachmann and Danner 1976). In general, the sequence of events is as follows. Viral antigen is detected in the cytoplasm of cells soon after infection if the inoculum contains a high titer of virus and viral antigen. Most if not all of this early cytoplasmic fluorescence is the result of antigen phagocytized from the inoculum (Mengeling 1972; Mengeling and Cutlip 1975). By sequential examinations, such antigen can be demonstrated first on the external surface of the cytoplasmic membrane and later within the cytoplasm, often relatively concentrated in a juxtanuclear location. The first unequivocal evidence of viral replication is the appearance of nascent viral antigen in the nucleus (Fig. 23.2A). In at least some infected cells, nascent antigen next appears in the cytoplasm in sufficient quantity so that both cytoplasm and nucleus are brightly fluorescent. Infected cells commonly seen in the lung of fetuses that develop a high titer of antibody for PPV probably represent this stage of replication (see Fig. 23.8C). Affected cells subsequently round up, become pyknotic, and disintegrate with release of virus and viral antigen (Fig. 23.2B). Other cells in the culture that are not at the appropriate stage to

support viral replication continue to phagocytize and accumulate viral antigen in their cytoplasm (Fig. 23.2C). A second wave of viral replication can be induced if these cells are stimulated to enter the S phase of the cell cycle as, e.g., by the addition of fresh culture medium.

Hemagglutination. PPV agglutinates human, monkey, guinea pig, cat, chicken, rat, and mouse erythrocytes. Erythrocytes of other kinds of animals that have been tested are relatively or completely insensitive, or the results have been equivocal (Darbyshire and Roberts 1968; Mayr et al. 1968; Cartwright et al. 1969; Hallauer et al. 1972; Mengeling 1972; Morimoto et al. 1972a). Several parameters of the hemagglutination (HA) test, such as the temperature of incubation (Mayr et al. 1968; Mengeling 1972), the species of erythrocyte used, and in the case of chicken erythrocytes the genetic composition (Cartwright et al. 1969; Pini 1975; Ruckerbauer et al. 1978) and age (Morimoto et al. 1972a) of the donor may quantitatively affect results. The HA test is most commonly conducted at room temperature, at approximately neutral pH, and with guinea pig erythrocytes. Higher HA titers have been recorded when the diluent used in the test was veronal buffer rather than phosphate-buffered saline (Ruckerbauer et al. 1978). Elution of virus (the hemagglutinin is part of the virion) can be induced by suspending erythrocytes in alkaline buffer, pH 9 (Hallauer et al. 1972).

Infectivity Titrations. Infectivity titrations are conducted in a standard manner except that, because cytopathic changes at terminal dilutions are often vague, endpoints of infectivity are often de-

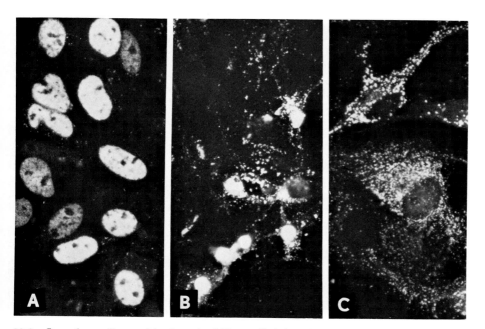

23.2. Secondary cultures of fetal porcine kidney cells infected with PPV and examined by immunofluorescence microscopy. × 500. (A) 14 hours after infection, culture fixed and then reacted with fluorescent antibodies (FA). (B) 24 hours after infection, culture reacted with FA and then fixed; only extracellular antigen and antigen in cells with disrupted cytoplasmic and nuclear membranes are identified. (C) 48 hours after infection, culture fixed and then reacted with FA.

termined either by examining cell cultures for intranuclear inclusions after appropriate staining or by examining cell culture medium for viral hemagglutinin (Cartwright et al. 1969). A titration procedure wherein infected cells are made evident by IF microscopy (Mengeling 1972) and a plaque assay (Kawamura et al. 1988) also have been described.

Serologic Tests. The HI test is frequently used for detection and quantitation of humoral antibody for PPV. Antibody sometimes can be detected as early as 5 days after swine are exposed to live virus, and it may persist for years (Johnson et al. 1976). Sera examined by the HI test are usually pretreated by heat inactivation (56°C, 30 minutes) and by adsorption with erythrocytes (to remove naturally occurring hemagglutinins) and kaolin (to remove or reduce nonantibody inhibitors of HA) (Mengeling 1972; Morimoto et al. 1972a). Trypsin also has been used to remove nonantibody inhibitors of HA (Cartwright et al. 1969). Parameters of the HI test have been studied in detail (Kim 1974; Joo et al. 1976c).

The SN test is occasionally used for detection and quantitation of humoral antibody for PPV. Neutralization of infectivity is usually confirmed by the absence or reduction either of intranuclear inclusions or fluorescent cells in cultures or of viral hemagglutinin in the culture medium (Mengeling 1972; Johnson 1973; Joo et al. 1975).

The SN test has been reported to be more sensitive than the HI test (Johnson and Collings 1971; Joo et al. 1975). A microtechnique for application of the SN test has been described (Joo et al. 1975).

Immunodiffusion (Joo et al. 1978), a modified direct complement-fixation test (Ruckerbauer et al. 1978), and enzyme-linked immunosorbent assay (Hohdatsu et al. 1988; Westenbrink et al. 1989) also have been used successfully to detect antibody for PPV.

EPIDEMIOLOGY. Porcine parvovirus is ubiquitous among swine throughout the world. In major swine-producing areas such as the midwestern United States, infection is enzootic in most herds, and with few exceptions sows are immune. In addition, a large proportion of gilts are naturally infected with PPV before they conceive, and as a result they develop an active immunity that probably persists throughout life. Collectively, the seroepidemiologic data indicate that exposure to PPV is common. They also emphasize the high risk of infection and reproductive disease among gilts that have not developed immunity before conception. The most common routes of infection for postnatal and prenatal pigs are oronasal and transplacental respectively.

Pigs nursing immune dams absorb a high titer of antibody for PPV from colostrum. These titers decrease progressively with time by dilution as pigs grow as well as by biological degradation. They usually reach subdetectable levels in 3–6 months if sera are examined by the HI test (Etoh et al. 1979; Paul et al. 1982). Sometimes passively acquired antibody persists for a longer interval. Moreover, levels of antibody too low to be detected by the HI test may be detected by the SN test (Johnson et al. 1976). The primary significance of passively acquired antibody is that it interferes with the development of active immunity. High levels of such antibody can prevent infection, and lower levels can minimize dissemination from infected pigs (Suzuki and Fujisaki 1976; Paul et al. 1980). Consequently, some groups of gilts are not fully susceptible to infection and dissemination of virus until either shortly before conception or during early gestation.

Contaminated premises are probably major reservoirs of PPV. The virus is thermostable, resistant to many common disinfectants (Brown 1981), and may remain infectious for months in secretions and excretions from acutely infected pigs. It was shown experimentally that although pigs transmitted PPV for only about 2 weeks after exposure, the pens in which they were initially kept remained infectious for at least 4 months (Mengeling and Paul 1986). The ubiquity of PPV also raises the possibility that some pigs are persistently infected and at least periodically shed virus. However, shedding beyond the interval of acute infection has not been demonstrated (Johnson et al. 1976). The possibility of immunotolerant carriers of PPV as a result of early in utero infection has been suggested (Johnson 1973). When gilts were infected with PPV before day 55 of gestation, their pigs were born infected but without antibody. Virus was isolated from kidneys, testicles, and seminal fluid of such pigs killed at various times after birth up to the time they were 8 months of age; at which time the experiment was terminated (Johnson and Collings 1971). Results of another study, wherein dams were infected early in gestation and their pigs were born infected but without antibody, also suggest an acquired immunotolerance (Cartwright et al. 1971). A possible example of an infected, immunotolerant, sexually active boar was reported (Johnson et al. 1976).

Boars may play a significant role in dissemination of PPV at a critical time. During acute infection the virus is shed by various routes, including semen, and the isolation of PPV from semen of naturally infected boars has been reported (Cartwright and Huck 1967; Cartwright et al. 1969; McAdaragh and Anderson 1975). Semen may be contaminated externally, as for example with virus-containing feces, or within the male reproductive tract. Virus was isolated from a testicle of a boar 5 days after it was injected into the boar's prepuce (Lucas et al. 1974) and from testicles of boars killed 5 and 8 days after they were infected oronasally (Mengeling 1976). Virus was also isolated from scrotal lymph nodes of boars killed 5, 8, 15, 21, and 35 days after oronasal exposure. After day 8, isolation was accomplished by cocultivating lymph node fragments with fetal porcine kidney cells (Mengeling 1976). Irrespective of their immune status, boars can also function as a vehicle for mechanical dissemination of PPV among susceptible females.

CLINICAL SIGNS. Acute infection of postnatal pigs, including pregnant dams that subsequently develop reproductive failure, is usually subclinical (Johnson and Collings 1969; Cutlip and Mengeling 1975a; Fujisaki et al. 1975; Johnson et al. 1976; Joo et al. 1976a; Mengeling and Cutlip 1976). However, in young pigs and probably in older breeding stock as well, the virus replicates extensively and is found in many tissues and organs with a high mitotic index. Viral antigen is especially concentrated in lymphoid tissues (Cutlip and Mengeling 1975a; Fujisaki et al. 1975) (Fig. 23.3A, B). Many pigs, irrespective of age or sex, have a transient, usually mild, leukopenia sometime within 10 days after initial exposure to the virus (Johnson and Collings 1969, 1971; Joo et al. 1976a; Mengeling and Cutlip 1976). PPV and other structurally similar viruses have been identified in the feces of pigs with diarrhea (Dea et al. 1985; Yasuhara et al. 1989). However, there is no experimental evidence to suggest that PPV either replicates extensively in the intestinal crypt epithelium or causes enteric disease as do parvoviruses of several other species (Cutlip and Mengeling 1975a; Brown et al. 1980). PPV also has been isolated from pigs with lesions described as vesiclelike. The etiologic role of PPV in such lesions has not been clearly defined (Kresse et al. 1985).

The major and usually only clinical response to infection with PPV is maternal reproductive failure. Pathologic sequelae depend mainly on when exposure occurs during gestation. Dams may return to estrus, fail to farrow despite being anestrus, farrow few pigs per litter, or farrow a large proportion of mummified fetuses. All can reflect embryonic or fetal death or both. The only outward sign may be a decrease in maternal abdominal girth when fetuses die at midgestation or later and their associated fluids are resorbed. Other manifestations of maternal reproductive failure, namely, infertility, abortion, stillbirth, neonatal death, and reduced neonatal vitality, also have been ascribed to infection with PPV (Cartwright and Huck 1967; Johnson 1969; Morimoto et al. 1972b; Narita et al. 1975; Forman et al. 1977). These are normally only a minor component of the disease. The presence of mummified fetuses in a litter can prolong both gestation (Narita et al. 1975) and the farrowing interval (Mengeling et al. 1975). Either may result in stillbirth of apparently normal littermates, whether or not they are infected.

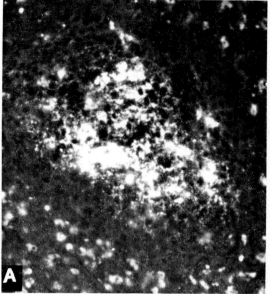

23.3. Cryostat-microtome sections of tissues from PPV-infected 8-week-old pigs, examined by immunofluorescence microscopy. × 312.5. (A) Viral antigen in germinal center, tonsil. (B) Viral antigen in osteogenic layer of periosteum, rib: *a* = connective tissue, *b* = cortical bone, *c* = marrow cavity.

There is no evidence that either fertility or libido of boars is altered by infection with PPV (Biront and Bonte 1983; Thacker et al. 1987).

PATHOGENESIS. Dams are susceptible to PPV-induced reproductive failure if infected anytime during about the first half of gestation. This interval of maternal susceptibility is indicated by the collective results of several experimental studies (Joo et al. 1976a; Mengeling and Cutlip 1976; Mengeling 1979; Mengeling et al. 1980a), by in-depth epidemiologic investigations (Donaldson-Wood et al. 1977; Gillick 1977), and by estimates of the time of death of fetuses collected during epidemiologic surveys (Mengeling 1978b; Mengeling et al. 1991). Consequences of maternal infection during this interval are embryonic and fetal death followed by resorption and mummification respectively. Transplacental infection also follows maternal exposure after midgestation, but fetuses usually survive without obvious clinical effects in utero. The likely reason is that transplacental infection often requires 10–14 days (Mengeling et al. 1978, 1980a) or longer (Joo et al. 1976a), and by 70 days of gestation most fetuses are able to develop a protective immunologic response to the virus. In general, fetuses experimentally infected by transuterine inoculation of virus have died when infected before day 70 of gestation, but they have survived and produced antibody when infected later in gestation (Redman et al. 1974; Bachmann et al. 1975; Cutlip and Mengeling 1975b; Mengeling and Cutlip 1975). A strain of PPV of slightly greater virulence also has been reported (Choi et al. 1987). The usual consequences of infection at different stages of gestation are summarized in Table 23.1.

When only part of a litter is infected transpla-

centally, as is often the case, one or more littermates are frequently infected by subsequent intrauterine spread of virus. The same would apply if initial infection were through contaminated semen. As a result, any combination or all of the sequelae indicated in Table 23.1 can develop in the same litter. Intrauterine dissemination is probably less common when early embryos are infected because they are quickly resorbed after death, effectively removing the intrauterine reservoir of virus (Mengeling et al. 1980a). In such cases there is no evidence at farrowing for the cause of fewer pigs per litter.

The effect, if any, of PPV on the ovum before ovulation is unknown. Virus adheres tenaciously to the external surface of the zona pellucida of the fertilized porcine ovum (Wrathall and Mengeling 1979a,b) and although it apparently cannot penetrate this layer, speculation is that it could pose a

Table 23.1.   Consequences of infection with PPV at different intervals of gestation

Interval of Gestation (days)[a]		Description of Conceptus	Consequences of Infection
Infection of Dam	Infection of Conceptus[b]		
≤56	10–30	Embryo	Death and resorption
	30–70	Fetus	Death and mummification
>56	70–term	Fetus	Immune response and usually survival in utero

[a]Intervals are approximations.
[b]Assuming transplacental infection 10–14 days after maternal exposure.

threat to the embryo after hatching (Wrathall and Mengeling 1979a).

Despite strong circumstantial evidence (Cartwright et al. 1971), a direct causal role of PPV-contaminated semen in reproductive failure has not been established unequivocally (Lucas et al. 1974). The zona pellucida could protect the early embryo while local immunity is developing. Conversely, virus may cause uterine changes incompatible with gestation (Wrathall and Mengeling 1979c). In any event, a female infected through semen provides a focus of infection for others.

With the possible exception of the uterine changes alluded to in the preceding paragraph, PPV-induced reproductive failure is caused by the direct effect of virus on the conceptus. In the absence of an immune response, virus replicates extensively throughout these tissues. By the time the conceptus dies, most of its cells contain large quantities of intracytoplasmic viral antigen that can be demonstrated by IF microscopy. The relative lack of nuclear fluorescence at the time of death, compared to earlier stages of the disease, indicates that when the conceptus is severely affected, mitotic activity and the associated conditions necessary for viral replication are suppressed more than phagocytic activity.

Death of the conceptus probably results from the collective damage by the virus to a variety of tissues and organs, including the placenta (Cutlip and Mengeling 1975b). However, in the absence of an immune response, changes in almost any vital organ are probably sufficient to eventually cause death. One of the most striking features of viral distribution is the extensive involvement of endothelium. This seems to preclude further development of the vascular network of the conceptus. Preparation for cellular mitosis, i.e., the S phase, results in concomitant viral replication and cell death. Damage to the fetal circulatory system is indicated by edema, hemorrhage, and the accumulation of large amounts of serosanguineous fluids in body cavities. Necrosis of the endothelium is microscopically evident (Lenghaus et al. 1978).

The mechanism of transplacental infection has been investigated by using IF microscopy to identify infected cells in maternal and fetal tissues at progressively longer intervals after maternal oronasal exposure (Mengeling et al. 1978). Examination of tissues contiguous with the maternal-fetal junction revealed viral antigen in endothelial and mesenchymal cells of the chorion, with increasing involvement of these tissues at progressively later stages of gestation. Viral antigen was never detected unequivocally in either uterine epithelium or trophectoderm. Consequently, there was no evidence for maternal-fetal transfer of virus by replicating through these tissues. However, this route cannot be excluded, since only a small part of the total area of contact was examined. Transfer of virus within macrophages has been considered (Paul et al. 1979). Whatever the route, maternal viremia seems a likely prerequisite for transplacental infection (Joo et al. 1976a; Mengeling and Cutlip 1976).

LESIONS. Neither macroscopic nor microscopic lesions have been reported for nonpregnant pigs (Cutlip and Mengeling 1975a; Brown et al. 1980). It is conceivable that cellular infiltrations subsequently described for fetuses could be induced by infection during the perinatal interval.

Macroscopic lesions have not been reported in pregnant dams; however, microscopic lesions have been seen in tissues of gilts killed after their fetuses were infected by transuterine inoculation of virus. Gilts that were seronegative when their fetuses were infected at 70 days of gestation had focal accumulations of mononuclear cells adjacent to the endometrium and in deeper layers of the lamina propria when they were killed 12 and 21 days later. In addition, there were perivascular cuffs of plasma cells and lymphocytes in the brain, spinal cord, and choroid of the eye (Hogg et al. 1977). When fetuses were infected earlier in gestation (35, 50, and 60 days) and their dams were killed 7 and 11 days later, the lesions were similar. However, uterine lesions were more severe and also included extensive cuffing of myometrial and endometrial vessels with mononuclear cells (Lenghaus et al. 1978). Only focal accumulations of lymphocytes were seen in uteruses of gilts that were seropositive when their fetuses were infected (Cutlip and Mengeling 1975b).

Macroscopic changes of embryos are death followed by resorption of fluids (Fig. 23.4) and then soft tissues (Fig. 23.5). Virus and viral antigen are widely distributed in tissues of infected embryos and their placentas (Mengeling et al. 1980a), and it is probable that microscopic lesions of necrosis and vascular damage, subsequently described for fetuses, also develop in advanced embryos.

There are numerous macroscopic changes in fetuses infected before they become immunocompetent (Fig. 23.6). These include a variable degree of stunting and sometimes an obvious loss of condition before other external changes are apparent; occasionally, an increased prominence of blood vessels over the surface of the fetus due to congestion and leakage of blood into contiguous tissues; congestion, edema, and hemorrhage with accumulation of serosanguineous fluids in body cavities; hemorrhagic discoloration becoming progressively darker after death; and dehydration (mummification). Many of these changes also apply to the placenta. Microscopic lesions consist primarily of extensive cellular necrosis in a wide variety of tissues and organs (Joo et al. 1977; Lenghaus et al. 1978) (Fig. 23.7A). Inflammation (Joo et al. 1977) and intranuclear inclusions (Lenghaus et al. 1978) also have been described.

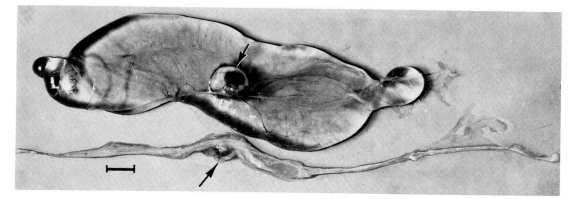

23.4. Embryos from a gilt experimentally infected oronasally immediately after breeding and killed 22 days later. Bar = 1 cm. (Top) Noninfected, clinically normal embryo (arrow) and associated extraembryonic membranes; (bottom) PPV-infected, dead littermate embryo (arrow) and associated extraembryonic membranes, recent death, no obvious resorption of soft tissues. (Mengeling et al. 1980a.)

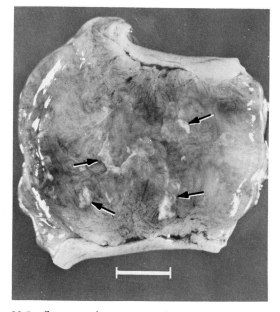

23.5. Segment of uterus opened to show necrotic remnants of a partially resorbed PPV-infected embryo (arrows) and associated extraembryonic membranes of a gilt experimentally infected oronasally immediately after breeding and killed 22 days later; remnants laden with virus and viral antigen. Bar = 1 cm. (Mengeling et al. 1980a.)

In contrast, macroscopic changes have not been reported for fetuses infected after they become immunocompetent for PPV. Microscopic lesions are primarily endothelial hypertrophy (Hogg et al. 1977) and mononuclear cell infiltrations consistent with an immune response (Hogg et al. 1977; Joo et al. 1977). Meningoencephalitis characterized by perivascular cuffing with proliferating adventitial cells, histiocytes, and a few plasma cells was seen in the gray and white mat-

ter of the cerebrum and in the leptomeninges of PPV-infected stillborn pigs. These lesions were believed to be pathognomonic for PPV infection (Narita et al. 1975). Similar lesions have been observed in PPV-infected, live fetuses collected late in gestation (Hogg et al. 1977; Joo et al. 1977) (Fig. 23.7B).

Both general types of microscopic lesions, i.e., necrosis and mononuclear cell infiltration, may develop in fetuses infected near midgestation (Lenghaus et al. 1978) when the immune response is insufficient to provide protection.

DIAGNOSIS. PPV should be considered in a differential diagnosis of reproductive failure of swine whenever there is evidence of embryonic or fetal death or both. The pathologic sequelae of maternal infection during gestation have been described (see **CLINICAL SIGNS**). If gilts but not sows are affected, maternal illness is not seen during gestation, there are few or no abortions or fetal developmental anomalies, and other evidence suggests an infectious disease, then a tentative diagnosis of PPV-induced reproductive failure can be made. The relative lack of maternal illness, abortions, and fetal developmental anomalies differentiates PPV from most other infectious causes of reproductive failure. However, a definitive diagnosis requires laboratory support.

Several mummified fetuses (<16 cm in length) or lungs from such fetuses, if sufficiently developed, should be submitted to the diagnostic laboratory. Larger mummified fetuses, i.e., more than about 70 days of gestational age (Marrable and Ashdown 1967), stillborn pigs, and neonatal pigs are not recommended for submission unless they are the only samples available. If infected, their tissues will usually contain antibody that interferes with laboratory tests for either virus or viral antigen.

If females fail to farrow despite being anestrus

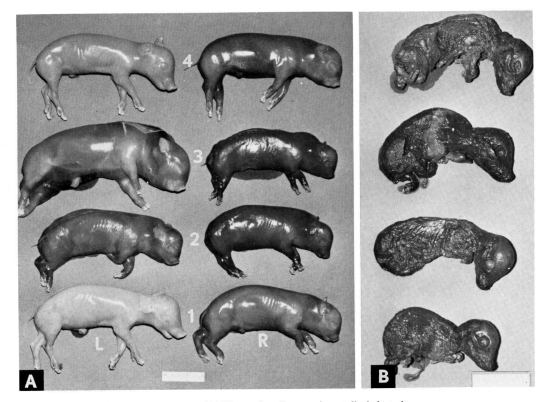

23.6. PPV-infected fetuses. Bars = ~5 cm. (A) Litter of a gilt experimentally infected oronasally day 47 of gestation and killed 34 days later; fetuses from left (*L*) and right (*R*) horn of uterus, numbered *1–4* from cervix toward ovary; fetuses *L1* and *L4* stunted but alive at necropsy, fetus *L3* recent death, others later stages. (B) Fetuses from litter of a naturally infected gilt, collected at about 114 days of gestation, advanced stage of dehydration (mummification). (Mengeling et al. 1975.)

and are sent to an abattoir, their uteruses should be collected and examined for affected fetuses. Sometimes only remnants of fetal tissues remain when fetuses die early in the middle third of gestation. Nevertheless, these are adequate samples if tested for viral antigen by IF microscopy (Mengeling and Cutlip 1975; Mengeling 1978b). The absence of affected fetuses or fetal remnants does not exclude PPV-induced reproductive failure. When all embryos of a litter die and are completely resorbed after the first few weeks of gestation, the dam may remain endocrinologically pregnant and not return to estrus until after the expected time of farrowing (Rodeffer et al. 1975).

Identification of viral antigen by IF microscopy is a reliable and sensitive diagnostic procedure. Sections of fetal tissues are prepared with a cryostat microtome and are then reacted with standardized reagents (Mengeling et al. 1975; Mengeling 1978b). The test can be completed within a few hours. In the absence of a fetal antibody response, antigen is seen throughout fetal tissues (Fig. 23.8A, B); even when antibody is present, infected cells usually can be detected in fetal lung (Fig. 23.8C).

Detection of viral hemagglutinin also has been

recommended as a diagnostic technique (Joo et al. 1976b; Joo and Johnson 1977a). Tissues are triturated in diluent and then sedimented by centrifugation. The supernatant fluid is tested for agglutinating activity for guinea pig erythrocytes. This test requires a minimum of laboratory equipment and is effective in the absence of antibody.

Virus isolation is less suitable as a routine diagnostic procedure than either of the aforementioned tests. Infectivity is slowly but progressively lost after fetal death (Mengeling and Cutlip 1975); as a result, isolation of virus from mummified fetuses that have died as a result of infection is sometimes unsuccessful (Mengeling 1978b). Moreover, the procedure is time consuming, and contamination is a constant threat because of the stability of PPV in the laboratory (Cartwright et al. 1969) and because cell cultures are sometimes unknowingly prepared from infected tissues (Huygelen and Peetermans 1967; Bachmann 1969; Cartwright et al. 1969; Mengeling 1975; Hafez and Liess 1979). IF microscopy is often used to determine whether PPV has been isolated in cell culture (Cartwright 1970; Johnson 1973; Mengeling 1978b).

In general, serologic procedures are recom-

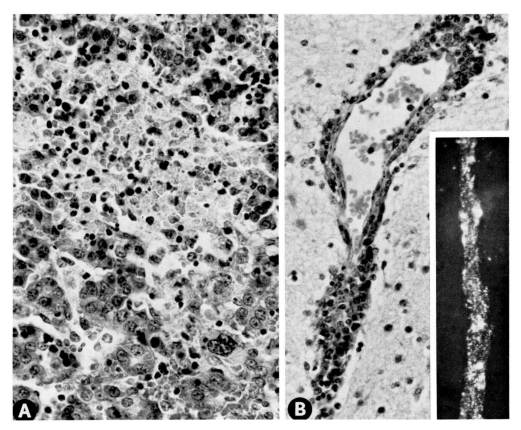

23.7. Tissues of PPV-infected fetuses of gilts experimentally infected oronasally. (A) Necrotic focus in liver of live fetus of a gilt infected day 40 of gestation and killed 42 days later; fetus had numerous macroscopic lesions. ×400. H & E. (B) Perivascular cuffing with mononuclear cells in cerebrum of live fetus, littermate of A; fetus had no macroscopic lesions. ×320. H & E. (Insert) Viral antigen associated with endothelium of cerebral vessel of fetus of a gilt infected day 46 of gestation and killed 25 days later, immunofluorescence microscopy. ×312.5. All fetuses were probably infected by intrauterine spread of PPV from transplacentally infected littermates. (Photographs A and B courtesy of T. T. Brown, Jr., National Animal Disease Center.)

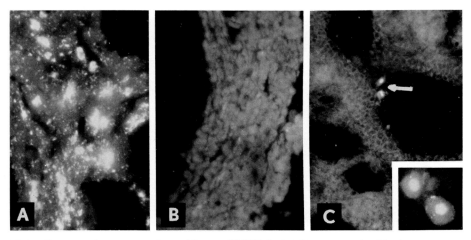

23.8. Cryostat-microtome sections of lungs of PPV-infected fetuses examined by immuno-fluorescence microscopy. (A) Lung of mummified fetus reacted with FA plus nonimmune serum. ×312.5. (B) Replicate section reacted with FA plus PPV-immune serum, i.e., blocking control. ×312.5. (C) Lung of live fetus with HI antibody titer of 640 reacted with FA plus nonimmune serum, two infected cells (arrow). ×162.5. (Insert) Two similar infected cells in the same section as C. ×500. (Mengeling 1978b.)

mended for diagnosis only when tissues from mummified fetuses are not available for testing as previously described. Results with maternal sera are of value if antibody is not detected, thus excluding PPV as a cause, and if samples collected at intervals reveal seroconversion for PPV coincident with reproductive failure (Morimoto et al. 1972b; Mengeling et al. 1975; Rodeffer et al. 1975). Because PPV is ubiquitous, the presence of antibody in a single sample is otherwise meaningless. However, a determination of relative amounts of antibody present as immunoglobulin M and G can indicate recency of infection (Kim 1974; Joo et al. 1978). Detection of antibody in sera of fetuses and stillborn pigs and in sera collected from neonatal pigs before they nurse is evidence of in utero infection, since maternal antibody does not cross the maternal-fetal junction (Johnson and Collings 1969; Cartwright et al. 1971; Johnson and Collings 1971; Mengeling 1972; Chaniago et al. 1978). When serum is not available, body fluids collected from fetuses or their viscera that have been kept in a plastic bag overnight at 4°C have been used successfully to demonstrate antibody (Cropper et al. 1976; Joo et al. 1976b).

TREATMENT AND PREVENTION. There is no treatment for PPV-induced reproductive failure.

Gilts should be either naturally infected with PPV or vaccinated for PPV before they are bred. To promote natural infection, a common practice is to arrange contact between seronegative gilts and seropositive sows with the expectation that one or more of the sows will be shedding virus. Moving gilts to a potentially contaminated area, either currently or recently inhabited by seropositive swine, also can be recommended. Once infection is started the virus spreads rapidly among fully susceptible swine. Just how effective these procedures are in increasing the incidence of natural infection is unknown. For whatever reasons, infection is common, and probably well over one-half of all gilts in areas where PPV is enzootic are infected before they are bred for the first time (Mengeling 1972).

The use of vaccine is the only way to assure that gilts develop active immunity before conception. Both inactivated (Suzuki and Fujisaki 1976; Ide et al. 1977; Joo and Johnson 1977b; Mengeling 1977; Fujisaki 1978; Fujisaki et al. 1978b; Mengeling et al. 1979, 1980b) and modified live-virus (MLV) vaccines (Paul and Mengeling 1980; Fujisaki and Murakami 1982) have been developed. An inactivated vaccine has been tested under field conditions (Fujisaki 1978; Fujisaki et al. 1978a), and both types of vaccines were effective when tested under controlled laboratory conditions (Mengeling et al. 1979, 1980b; Paul and Mengeling 1980).

Vaccines should be administered several weeks before conception to provide immunity throughout the susceptible period of gestation, but after the disappearance of passively acquired colostral antibody that could interfere with the development of active immunity (Paul and Mengeling 1986). These limits may define a very brief interval for effective vaccination of gilts that are bred before 7 months of age. Although inactivated vaccine provides maximum safety, there is experimental evidence that PPV can be sufficiently attenuated so that it is unlikely to cause reproductive failure even if inadvertently administered during gestation (Paul and Mengeling 1980). The apparent safety of MLV vaccine may be due to its reduced ability to replicate in tissues of the intact host and cause the level of viremia needed for transplacental infection (Paul and Mengeling 1984). Moreover, it has been shown by transuterine inoculation of both virulent and attenuated virus that a much larger dose of attenuated virus is required to establish infection of fetuses (Mengeling et al. 1984). Duration of immunity following vaccination is unknown; however, in one study antibody titers were maintained for at least 4 months after administration of an inactivated vaccine (Joo and Johnson 1977b). Low levels of antibody found to be protective allow speculation that, once the immune system has been primed with PPV, subsequent exposure to virulent virus during gestation is unlikely to result in transplacental infection even if antibody from vaccination is no longer detected (Mengeling et al. 1979).

Vaccination is recommended also for seronegative sows and boars. Seronegative sows would usually be found only in PPV-free herds; in such cases, inactivated vaccine is indicated. Experience has indicated that few herds can be expected to remain free of PPV even if access is carefully controlled. Introduction of PPV into a totally susceptible herd can be disastrous (Donaldson-Wood et al. 1977). Vaccination of boars should reduce their involvement in dissemination of virus.

Vaccines are used extensively in the United States and in several other countries where PPV has been recognized as an economically important cause of reproductive failure. All federally licensed vaccines marketed in the United States are inactivated.

REFERENCES

BACHMANN, P. A. 1969. Vorkommen und Verbreitung von Picodna (Parvo)-Virus beim Schwein. Zentralbl Veterinaermed [B] 16:341–345.

———. 1972. Porcine parvovirus infection in vitro: A study model for the replication of parvoviruses. I. Replication at different temperatures. Proc Soc Exp Biol Med 140:1369–1374.

BACHMANN, P. A., AND DANNER, K. 1976. Porcine parvovirus infection in vitro: A study model for the replication of parvoviruses. II. Kinetics of virus and antigen production. Zentralbl Veterinaermed [B] 23:355–363.

BACHMANN, P. A.; SHEFFY, B. E.; AND VAUGHAN, J. T.

1975. Experimental in utero infection of fetal pigs with a porcine parvovirus. Infect Immun 12:455–460.

BACHMANN, P. A.; HOGGAN, M. D.; KURSTAK, E.; MELNICK, J. L.; PEREIRA, H. G.; TATTERSALL, P.; AND VAGO, C. 1979. Parvoviridae: Second report. Intervirology 11:248–254.

BERNS, K. I. 1984. The Parvoviruses. New York: Plenum.

BIRONT, P., AND BONTE, P. 1983. Porcine parvovirus (P.P.V.) infection in boars. I. Possibility of a genital localization in the boar after oronasal infection. Zentralbl Veterinaermed 30:541–545.

BROWN, T. T., JR. 1981. Laboratory evaluation of selected disinfectants as virucidal agents against porcine parvovirus, pseudorabies virus, and transmissible gastroenteritis virus. Am J Vet Res 42:1033–1036.

BROWN, T. T., JR.; PAUL, P. S.; AND MENGELING, W. L. 1980. Response of conventionally raised weanling pigs to experimental infection with a virulent strain of porcine parvovirus. Am J Vet Res 41:1221–1224.

CARTWRIGHT, S. F. 1970. Tests available for the detection of some virus infections of pigs and their interpretation. Vet Annu 11:77–82.

CARTWRIGHT, S. F., AND HUCK, R. A. 1967. Viruses isolated in association with herd infertility, abortions and stillbirths in pigs. Vet Rec 81:196–197.

CARTWRIGHT, S. F.; LUCAS, M.; AND HUCK, R. A. 1969. A small haemagglutinating porcine DNA virus. I. Isolation and properties. J Comp Pathol 79:371–377.

_____. 1971. A small haemagglutinating porcine DNA virus. II. Biological and serological studies. J Comp Pathol 81:145–155.

CHANIAGO, T. D.; WATSON, D. L.; OWEN, R. A.; AND JOHNSON, R. H. 1978. Immunoglobulins in blood serum of foetal pigs. Aust Vet J 54:30–33.

CHOI, C. S.; MOLITOR, T. W.; JOO, H. S.; AND GUNTHER, R. 1987. Pathogenicity of a skin isolate of porcine parvovirus in swine fetuses. Vet Microbiol 15:19–29.

COACKLEY, W., AND SMITH, V. W. 1972. Porcine parvoviruses in Western Australia. Aust Vet J 48:536.

COTMORE, S. F.; STURZENBECKER, L. J.; AND TATTERSALL, P. 1983. The autonomous parvovirus MVM encodes two nonstructural proteins in addition to its capsid polypeptides. Virology 129:333–343.

CROGHAN, D. L., AND MATCHETT, A. 1973. β-propiolactone sterilization of commercial trypsin. Appl Microbiol 26:832.

CROGHAN, D. L.; MATCHETT, A.; AND KOSKI, T. A. 1973. Isolation of porcine parvovirus from commercial trypsin. Appl Microbiol 26:431–433.

CROPPER, M.; DUNNE, H. W.; LEMAN, A. D.; STARKEY, A. L.; AND HOEFLING, D. C. 1976. Prevalence of antibodies to porcine enteroviruses and porcine parvovirus in body fluids of fetal pigs from small vs large litters. J Am Vet Med Assoc 168:233–235.

CUTLIP, R. C., AND MENGELING, W. L. 1975a. Experimentally induced infection of neonatal swine with porcine parvovirus. Am J Vet Res 36:1179–1182.

_____. 1975b. Pathogenesis of in utero infection of eight- and ten-week-old porcine fetuses with porcine parvovirus. Am J Vet Res 36:1751–1754.

DARBYSHIRE, J. H., AND ROBERTS, D. H. 1968. Some respiratory virus and mycoplasma infections of animals. J Clin Pathol 21 [Suppl 2]:61–92.

DEA, S.; ELAZHARY, M. A. S. Y.; MARTINEAU, G. P.; AND VAILLANCOURT, J. 1985. Parvovirus-like particles associated with diarrhea in unweaned piglets. Can J Comp Med 49:343–345.

DONALDSON-WOOD, C. R.; JOO, H. S.; AND JOHNSON, R. H. 1977. The effect on reproductive performance of porcine parvovirus infection in a susceptible pig herd. Vet Rec 100:237–239.

ETOH, M.; MORISHITA, E.; AND WATANABE, Y. 1979. Transitional antibodies and spontaneous infection in porcine parvovirus infection. Jpn J Swine Husb Res 16:237–239.

FORMAN, A. J.; LENGHAUS, C.; HOGG, G. G.; AND HALE, C. J. 1977. Association of a parvovirus with an outbreak of foetal death and mummification in pigs. Aust Vet J 53:326–329.

FUJISAKI, Y. 1978. Incidence and control of stillbirth caused by porcine parvovirus in Japan. Proc 5th Int Congr Pig Vet Soc, Zagreb, p. KA 14.

FUJISAKI, Y., AND MURIKAMI, Y. 1982. Immunity to infection with porcine parvovirus in pigs inoculated with attenuated HT-strain. Natl Inst Anim Health (Tokyo) 22:36–37.

FUJISAKI, Y.; MORIMOTO, T.; SUGIMORI, T.; AND SUZUKI, H. 1975. Experimental infection of pigs with porcine parvovirus. Natl Inst Anim Health Q (Tokyo) 22:205–206.

FUJISAKI, Y.; ICHIHARA, T.; SASAKI, N.; SHIMIZU, F.; MURAKAMI, Y.; SUGIMORI, T.; AND SASAHARA, J. 1978a. Field trials on inactivated porcine parvovirus vaccine for prevention of viral stillbirth among swine. Natl Inst Anim Health Q (Tokyo) 18:184–185.

FUJISAKI, Y.; WATANABE, Y.; KODAMA, K.; HAMADA, H.; MURAKAMI, Y.; SUGIMORI, T.; AND SASAHARA, J. 1978b. Protection of swine with inactivated porcine parvovirus vaccine from fetal infection. Natl Inst Anim Health Q (Tokyo) 18:185.

GILLICK, J. C. 1977. An outbreak of swine foetal mummification associated with porcine parvovirus. Aust Vet J 53:105–106.

HAFEZ, S. M., AND LIESS, B. 1979. Isolation of parvovirus from kidney cell cultures of gnotobiotic piglets. Zentralbl Veterinaermed [B] 26:820–827.

HALLAUER, C.; KRONAUER, G.; AND SIEGL, G. 1971. Parvovirus as contaminants of permanent human cell lines. I. Virus isolations from 1960–1970. Arch Gesamte Virusforsch 35:80–90.

HALLAUER, C.; SIEGL, G.; AND KRONAUER, G. 1972. Parvoviruses as contaminants of permanent human cell lines. III. Biological properties of the isolated viruses. Arch Gesamte Virusforsch 38:369–382.

HOGG, G. G.; LENGHAUS, C.; AND FORMAN, A. J. 1977. Experimental porcine parvovirus infection of foetal pigs resulting in abortion, histological lesions and antibody formation. J Comp Pathol 87:539–549.

HOHDATSU, T.; BABA, K.; IDE, S.; TSUCHIMOTO, M.; NAGANO, H.; YAMAGAMI, T.; YAMAGISHI, H.; FUJISAKI, Y.; AND MATUMOTO, M. 1988. Detection of antibodies against porcine parvovirus in swine sera by enzyme-linked immunosorbent assay. Vet Microbiol 17:11–19.

HUYGELEN, C., AND PEETERMANS, J. 1967. Isolation of a hemagglutinating picornavirus from a primary swine kidney cell culture. Arch Gesamte Virusforsch 20:260–262.

IDE, S.; YAMAGISHI, K.; YOSHIMURA, M.; MANIWA, E.; YASUDA, H.; AND IGARASHI, J. 1977. Reaction of pigs to injection with a bivalent vaccine of Japanese B encephalitis virus and porcine parvovirus. J Jpn Vet Med Assoc 30:322–325.

JOHNSON, R. H. 1969. A search for Parvoviridae (Picornaviridae). Vet Rec 84:19–20.

_____. 1973. Isolation of swine parvovirus in Queensland. Aust Vet J 49:257–259.

JOHNSON, R. H., AND COLLINGS, D. F. 1969. Experimental infection of piglets and pregnant gilts with a parvovirus. Vet Rec 85:446–447.

_____. 1971. Transplacental infection of piglets with a porcine parvovirus. Res Vet Sci 12:570–572.

JOHNSON, R. H.; DONALDSON-WOOD, C. R.; JOO, H. S.; AND ALLENDER, U. 1976. Observations on the epidemiology of porcine parvovirus. Aust Vet J 52:80–84.

Joo, H. S., AND JOHNSON, R. H. 1977a. Observations on rapid diagnosis of porcine parvovirus in mummified foetuses. Aust Vet J 53:106–107.

_____. 1977b. Serological responses in pigs vaccinated with inactivated porcine parvovirus. Aust Vet J 53:550–552.

Joo, H. S.; DONALDSON-WOOD, C. R.; AND JOHNSON, R. H. 1975. A microneutralization test for the assay of porcine parvovirus antibody. Arch Virol 47:337–341.

_____. 1976a. Observations on the pathogenesis of porcine parvovirus infection. Arch Virol 51:123–129.

_____. 1976b. Rapid diagnostic techniques for detection of porcine parvovirus infection in mummified foetuses. Aust Vet J 52:51.

_____. 1976c. A standardised haemagglutination inhibition test for porcine parvovirus antibody. Aust Vet J 52:422–424.

Joo, H. S.; DONALDSON-WOOD, C. R.; JOHNSON, R. H.; AND WATSON, D. L. 1976d. Antibody to porcine, feline and rat parvoviruses in various animal species. Res Vet Sci 21:112–113.

Joo, H. S.; DONALDSON-WOOD, C. R.; JOHNSON, R. H.; AND CAMPBELL, R. S. F. 1977. Pathogenesis of porcine parvovirus infection: Pathology and immunofluorescence in the foetus. J Comp Pathol 87:383–391.

Joo, H. S.; JOHNSON, R. H.; AND WATSON, D. L. 1978. Serological procedures to determine time of infection of pigs with porcine parvovirus. Aust Vet J 54:125–127.

KAWAMURA, H.; FUJITA, T.; AND IMADA, T. 1988. Plaque formation and replication of porcine parvovirus in embryonic swine kidney cell line, ESK cells. Jpn J Vet Sci 50:803–808.

KIM, Y. H. 1974. Studies on hemagglutination and hemagglutination-inhibition reaction of porcine parvovirus. Bull AZABU Vet Coll 27:61–65.

KRESSE, J. I.; TAYLOR, W. D.; STEWART, W. C.; AND EERNISSE, K. A. 1985. Parvovirus infection in pigs with necrotic and vesicle-like lesions. Vet Microbiol 10:525–531.

LENGHAUS, C.; FORMAN, A. J.; AND HALE, C. J. 1978. Experimental infection of 35, 50 and 60 day old pig foetuses with porcine parvovirus. Aust Vet J 54:418–422.

LUCAS, M. H., AND NAPTHINE, P. 1971. Fluorescent antibody technique in the study of three porcine viruses. Transmissible gastroenteritis virus, vomiting and wasting disease virus, and the parvovirus 59e/63. J Comp Pathol 81:111–117.

LUCAS, M. H.; CARTWRIGHT, S. F.; AND WRATHALL, A. E. 1974. Genital infection of pigs with porcine parvovirus. J Comp Pathol 84:347–350.

MCADARAGH, J. P., AND ANDERSON, G. A. 1975. Transmission of viruses through boar semen. Proc 18th Annu Meet Am Assoc Vet Lab Diagn, pp. 69–76.

MARRABLE, A. W., AND ASHDOWN, R. R. 1967. Quantitative observations on pig embryos of known ages. J Agric Sci 69:443–447.

MAYR, A.; BACHMANN, P. A.; SIEGL, G.; MAHNEL, H.; AND SHEFFY, B. E. 1968. Characterization of a small porcine DNA virus. Arch Gesamte Virusforsch 25:38–51.

MENGELING, W. L. 1972. Porcine parvovirus: Properties and prevalence of a strain isolated in the United States. Am J Vet Res 33:2239–2248.

_____. 1975. Porcine parvovirus: Frequency of naturally occurring transplacental infection and viral contamination of fetal porcine kidney cell cultures. Am J Vet Res 36:41–44.

_____. 1976. Unpublished data.

_____. 1977. Diagnosing porcine parvovirus-induced reproductive failure. Proc 20th Annu Meet Am Assoc

Vet Lab Diagn, pp. 237–244.

_____. 1978a. Elimination of porcine parvovirus from infected cell cultures by inclusion of homologous antiserum in the nutrient medium. Am J Vet Res 39:323–324.

_____. 1978b. Prevalence of porcine parvovirus-induced reproductive failure: An abattoir study. J Am Vet Med Assoc 172:1291–1294.

_____. 1979. Prenatal infection following maternal exposure to porcine parvovirus on either the seventh or fourteenth day of gestation. Can J Comp Med 43:106–109.

MENGELING, W. L., AND CUTLIP, R. C. 1975. Pathogenesis of in utero infection: Experimental infection of 5-week-old porcine fetuses with porcine parvovirus. Am J Vet Res 36:1173–1177.

_____. 1976. Reproductive disease experimentally induced by exposing pregnant gilts to porcine parvovirus. Am J Vet Res 37:1393–1400.

MENGELING, W. L., AND PAUL, P. S. 1986. The relative importance of swine and contaminated premises as reservoirs of porcine parvovirus. J Am Vet Med Assoc 188:1293–1295.

MENGELING, W. L.; CUTLIP, R. C.; WILSON, R. A.; PARKS, J. B.; AND MARSHALL, R. F. 1975. Fetal mummification associated with porcine parvovirus infection. J Am Vet Med Assoc 166:993–995.

MENGELING, W. L.; CUTLIP, R. C.; AND BARNETT, D. 1978. Porcine parvovirus: Pathogenesis, prevalence, and prophylaxis. Proc 5th Int Congr Pig Vet Soc, Zagreb, p. KA 15.

MENGELING, W. L.; BROWN, T. T., JR.; PAUL, P. S.; AND GUNTEKUNST, D. E. 1979. Efficacy of an inactivated virus vaccine for prevention of porcine parvovirus-induced reproductive failure. Am J Vet Res 40:204–207.

MENGELING, W. L.; PAUL, P. S.; AND BROWN, T. T., Jr. 1980a. Transplacental infection and embryonic death following maternal exposure to porcine parvovirus near the time of conception. Arch Virol 65:55–62.

MENGELING, W. L.; PAUL, P. S.; GUTEKUNST, D. E.; PIRTLE, E. C.; AND BROWN, T. T., JR. 1980b. Vaccination for reproductive failure caused by porcine parvovirus. Proc 6th Int Congr Pig Vet Soc, Copenhagen.

MENGELING, W. L.; PEJSAK, Z.; AND PAUL, P. S. 1984. Biological assay of attenuated strain NADL-2 and virulent strain NADL-8 of porcine parvovirus. Am J Vet Res 45:2403–2407.

MENGELING, W. L.; PAUL, P. S.; BUNN, T. O.; AND RIDPATH, J. F. 1986. Antigenic relationships among autonomous parvoviruses. J Gen Virol 67:2839–2844.

MENGELING, W. L.; RIDPATH, J. F.; AND VORWALD, A. C. 1988. Size and antigenic comparisons among the structural proteins of selected autonomous parvoviruses. J Gen Virol 69:825–837.

MENGELING, W. L.; LAGER, K. M.; ZIMMERMAN, J. K.; SAMARIKERMANI, N.; AND BERAN, G. W. 1991. A current assessment of the relative role of porcine parvovirus as a cause of fetal porcine death. J Vet Diagn Invest 3:33–35.

MOLITOR, T. W.; JOO, H. S.; AND COLLECT, M. S. 1983. Porcine parvovirus: Virus purification and structural and antigenic properties of virion polypeptides. J Virol 45:842–854.

MORIMOTO, T.; FUJISAKI, Y.; ITO, Y.; AND TANAKA, Y. 1972a. Biological and physiochemical properties of porcine parvovirus recovered from stillborn piglets. Natl Inst Anim Health Q (Tokyo) 12:137–144.

MORIMOTO, T.; KUROGI, H.; MIURA, Y.; SUGIMORI, T.; AND FUJISAKI, Y. 1972b. Isolation of Japanese encephalitis virus and a hemagglutinating DNA virus from the brain of stillborn piglets. Natl Inst Anim Health Q (Tokyo) 12:127–136.

NARITA, M.; INUI, S.; KAWAKAMI, Y.; KITAMURA, K.;

AND MAEDA, A. 1975. Histopathological changes of the brain in swine fetuses naturally infected with porcine parvovirus. Natl Inst Anim Health Q (Tokyo) 15:24–28.

PAUL, P. S., AND MENGELING, W. L. 1980. Evaluation of a modified live virus vaccine for the prevention of porcine parvovirus-induced reproductive disease in pigs. Am J Vet Res 41:2007–2011.

_____. 1984. Oronasal and intramuscular vaccination of swine with a modified live porcine parvovirus vaccine: Multiplication and transmission of vaccine virus. Am J Vet Res 45:2481–2485.

_____. 1986. Vaccination of swine with inactivated porcine parvovirus vaccine in the presence of passive immunity. J Am Vet Med Assoc 188:410–413.

PAUL, P. S.; MENGELING, W. L.; AND BROWN, T. T., JR. 1979. Replication of porcine parvovirus in peripheral blood lymphocytes, monocytes, and peritoneal macrophages. Infect Immun 25:1003–1007.

_____. 1980. Effect of vaccinal and passive immunity on experimental infection of pigs with porcine parvovirus. Am J Vet Res 41:1368–1371.

PAUL, P. S.; MENGELING, W. L.; AND PIRTLE, E. C. 1982. Duration and biological half-life of passively acquired colostral antibodies to porcine parvovirus. Am J Vet Res 43:1376–1379.

PINI, A. 1975. Porcine parvovirus in pig herds in southern Africa. J S Afr Vet Assoc 46:241–244.

PIRTLE, E. C. 1974. Titration of two porcine respiratory viruses in mammalian cell cultures by direct fluorescent antibody staining. Am J Vet Res 35:249–250.

REDMAN, D. R.; BOHL, E. H.; AND FERGUSON, L. C. 1974. Porcine parvovirus: Natural and experimental infections of the porcine fetus and prevalence in mature swine. Infect Immun 10:718–723.

RODEFFER, H. E.; LEMAN, A. D.; DUNNE, H. W.; CROPPER, M.; AND SPRECHER, D. J. 1975. Reproductive failure in swine associated with maternal seroconversion for porcine parvovirus. J Am Vet Med Assoc 166:991–995.

RONDHUIS, P. R., AND STRAVER, P. J. 1972. Enige kenmerken van een klien, hemagglutinerend DNA-virus, geisoleer uit een verworpen varkensfoetus. Tijdschr Diergeneeskd 97:1257–1267.

RUCKERBAUER, G. M.; DULAC, G. C.; AND BOULANGER, P. 1978. Demonstration of parvovirus in Canadian swine and antigenic relationships with isolates from other countries. Can J Comp Med 42:278–285.

SIEGL, G. 1976. The Parvoviruses, 1st ed. Vienna, Austria: Springer-Verlag.

SIEGL, G., AND GAUTSCHI, M. 1973a. The multiplication of parvovirus Lu III in a synchronized culture system. I. Optimum conditions for virus replication. Arch Gesamte Virusforsch 40:105–118.

_____. 1973b. The multiplication of parvovirus Lu III in a synchronized culture system. II. Biochemical characteristics of virus replication. Arch Gesamte Virusforsch 40:119–127.

SIEGL, G.; HALLAUER, C.; AND NOVAK, A. 1972. Parvoviruses as contaminants of permanent human cell lines. IV. Multiplication of KBSH-virus in KB-cells. Arch Gesamte Virusforsch 36:351.

SUZUKI, H., AND FUJISAKI, Y. 1976. Immunizing effects of inactivated porcine parvovirus vaccine on piglets. Natl Inst Anim Health Q (Tokyo) 16:81.

TENNANT, R. W. 1971. Inhibition of mitosis and macromolecular synthesis in rat embryo cells by Kilhan rat virus. J Virol 8:402–408.

THACKER, B., AND LEMAN, A. D. 1978. Evaluation of gravid uteri at slaughter for porcine parvovirus infection. Proc 5th Int Congr Pig Vet Soc, Zagreb, p. M-49.

THACKER, B. J.; JOO, H. S.; WINKELMAN, N. L.; LEMAN, A. D.; AND BARNES, D. M. 1987. Clinical, virologic, and histopathologic observations of induced porcine parvovirus infection in boars. Am J Vet Res 48:763–767.

VANNIER, P., AND TILLON, J. P. 1979. Diagnostic de certitude de l'infection a parvovirus dans les trouble de la reproduction de l'espece porcine. Rec Med Vet 155:151–158.

WESTENBRINK, F.; VELDIUS, M. A.; AND BRINKHOF, J. M. A. 1989. An enzyme-linked assay for detection of antibodies to porcine parvovirus. J Virol Methods 23:169–180.

WRATHALL, A. E., AND MENGELING, W. L. 1979a. Effect of porcine parvovirus on development of fertilized pig eggs in vitro. Br Vet J 135:249–254.

_____. 1979b. Effect of transferring parvovirus-infected fertilized pig eggs into seronegative gilts. B Vet J 135:255–261.

_____. 1979c. Effect of inseminating seropositive gilts with semen containing porcine parvovirus. Br Vet J 135:420–425.

YASUHARA, H.; MATSUI, O.; HIRAHARA, T.; OHGTANI, T.; TANAKA, M. L.; KODAMA, K.; NAKAI, M; AND SASAKI, N. 1989. Characterization of parvovirus isolated from diarrheic feces of a pig. Jpn J Vet Sci 51:337–344.

24 Pseudorabies (Aujeszky's Disease)

J. P. Kluge

G. W. Beran

H. T. Hill

K. B. Platt

THE HISTORY OF pseudorabies (PR) has been summarized by Baskerville et al. (1973) and more recently by Wittmann and Rziha (1989). The disease was first described in the United States in 1813 in cattle. The cattle suffered from extreme pruritus and eventually died, consequently the disease was termed "mad itch." The term "pseudorabies" was first used in Switzerland in 1849 because the clinical signs in cattle were similar to those of rabies. In 1902 Aujeszky established the etiologic agent as nonbacterial and subsequently in 1910 Schmiedhofer confirmed that the agent was viral by filtration experiments. In 1934 Sabin and Wright identified the virus as a herpesvirus that was immunologically related to herpes simplex and herpes B viruses.

Prior to the 1960s the disease was important in Eastern Europe but not considered of economic importance in the United States. Subsequently, pseudorabies has emerged as an important disease in the United States and most areas of the world where swine are raised. Several reasons have been postulated for the apparent increase in disease severity, prevelance, and worldwide distribution. First, new and more virulent viral strains may have emerged. Another possible reason is the decline of hog cholera and the development of effective hog cholera vaccines and specific diagnostic tests. Prior to fluorescent antibody techniques, cases of pseudorabies may have been misdiagnosed as hog cholera. Porcine hyperimmune serum was often used in conjunction with virulent hog cholera virus as part of the vaccination regimen. Shope demonstrated that most of the serum contained both pseudorabies and hog cholera viral antibodies, which provided some passive immunity to both diseases. The third reason commonly cited is the dramatic change in swine management systems during the past 20 years. The advent of total confinement systems with large numbers of animals and the incorporation of continuous farrowing has created an environment that facilitates the maintenance and spread of a virus within herds.

ETIOLOGY. Pseudorabies virus belongs to the alphavirus subfamily of the Herpesviridae. Alpha herpesviruses include viruses with both broad, as in the case of PR virus, and narrow host ranges. Other biological characteristics of the alpha herpesviruses include lytic replication cycles of less than 24 hours and the ability to establish latent infections, particularly in sensory ganglia of the nervous system.

The pig is the only natural host for PR virus, which accounts for its ability to be subclinically and latently infected. Other common farm animals that the virus infects include cattle, sheep, goats, dogs, cats, and on rare occasions the horse. Infection of these animals is lethal although there is one report that documents the survival of an infected cow. Several wild animal species are also susceptible to lethal PR virus infection. The most common of these species include the raccoon, opossum, rat, and mouse, all of which are commonly found around farmsteads. Experimental studies in nonhuman primates have shown chimpanzees and Barbary apes to be refractory to PR virus infection but rhesus monkeys and marmosets to be susceptible. Reports of human infection have been limited and are inadequately documented. None of these reports have been based on virus isolation. The most recent report, in 1987, described three patients in Denmark and France who developed low-level transient seroconversion to PR virus following an illness that was possibly transmitted by cats. The possibility that the transient seroconversions were due to a serological cross-reaction induced by another herpesvirus was not considered.

Pseudorabies virus consists of an enveloped nucleocapsid that surrounds a linear genome of about 145 kb of DNA. The PRV genome is about 30 times the size of the smallest known DNA-containing viral pathogen of swine (i.e., porcine parvovirus) and is large enough to code for about 100 proteins. The overall dimension of the virus ranges from 150 to 180 nm in diameter. The size of the nucleocapsid is reported to be 105–110 nm in diameter. The nucleocapsid is composed of at least eight proteins ranging in size from 22.5 to 142 kD. Proteins with molecular weights of 142, 34, and 32 kD are the most prominent (Stevely 1975). The viral envelope contains at least nine structural proteins with molecular weights ranging from 50 to 130 kD (Hampl et al. 1984; Wittmann and Rhiza 1989). Eight of these proteins have sugar residues attached to them and are referred to as glycoproteins. These glycoproteins include gI; gII, which is a complex of three proteins referred to as IIa, IIb, and IIc; gIII; gIV; gp 50; gp 63. The remaining protein is nonglycosylated and has a molecular weight of 115 kD. Other important proteins that are encoded by the viral genome include gX and thymidine kinase (TK). Genes that code for many of the above proteins are not essential for viral replication. For example, vaccine strains of PR virus have been genetically engineered to be deficient in one or more of the following proteins: gI, gIII, gX, and TK.

The role that individual PR viral proteins play in virulence and in the induction of immunity has been partially characterized. Virulence of PR virus is controlled synergistically by several genes, most notably the genes encoding glycoproteins gI, gIII, gp 63, and TK (Wittmann and Rziha 1989); gII, gIII, and gp 50 appear to be the most important with respect to the induction of immunity. This conclusion is based on observations that monoclonal antibodies that represent multiple epitopes of gII neutralize PR virus in vitro and are also active in antibody-dependent cell-mediated cytotoxicity. Specific gII monoclonal antibodies also confer protective immunity to mice that are experimentally infected with PR virus. Monoclonal antibodies to gIII also neutralize PR virus in vitro and confer protective immunity to both mice and pigs. Protective immunity has also been conferred to both mice and swine injected with gp 50–specific monoclonal antibody (Marchioli et al. 1988) or immunized with recombinant-derived gp 50 and gp 63 (Marchioli et al. 1987; Kost et al. 1989).

Only one serotype of PR virus is recognized although distinct differences between some strains can be demonstrated by panels of monoclonal antibodies. Pseudorabies virus strains can also be differentiated with a high degree of certainty by biological and physical markers. Vaccine as well as field strains of PR virus have been reliably differentiated by using the heat and trypsin inactivation markers in combination with the mouse and rabbit virulence markers. Genomic differences, as revealed by restriction endonuclease analysis can also be used to reliably differentiate PR virus strains. All of these characteristics have been shown to be stable in several PR virus strains after serial passage in pigs (Platt 1981; Mengeling et al. 1983), which makes them useful in epidemiological studies. Differentiation of virus strains may also help resolve questions of liability. However, in this respect it must be remembered that although it is possible to say with a high degree of certainty that strains are different, it is not possible to say with the same certainty that virus strains with genomic similarities and identical biological markers are one and the same.

EPIDEMIOLOGY. After a primary outbreak of PR has been resolved, transmission becomes effectively limited to the breeding herd, and depending on their access to exposure, the finishing swine. Suckling, nursery, and grower pigs usually escape infection, which in the breeding herd may be maintained by introduction of actively shedding gilts or boars, or may occur at irregular intervals following stress-induced viral recrudescence in latently infected breeding animals. Frequently this is observed at first farrowing of latently infected gilts, or following temperature stress in inadequately ventilated breeding/gestation houses during winter (Davies and Beran 1980; Howarth 1969). A characteristic pattern of infection in a breeding herd follows a sigmoid curve, showing a high prevalence that declines with turnover of the breeding herd, followed by a rise as viral transmission is reinitiated, followed again by a decline in prevalence. Under most fortuitous conditions, especially in herds of <100 breeding swine with turnover within 2 years, the prevalence of infection may continue to decline and PR virus may be eliminated. In herds in which finishing swine have been infected, PR virus may continue to cycle in swine older than 3–4 months of age. Where all-in/all-out production is practiced in finishing units, PR virus may be eliminated (Thawley et al. 1982).

Spread of PR virus within a herd may be by direct nose-to-nose contact, during insemination either from infected vaginal mucosa or semen, or by transplacental transmission. Indirect transmission is more common by inhalation of aerosolized virus or drinking of water contaminated with PR virus. Infective levels of virus can persist for up to 7 hours in air with a relative humidity of 55% and higher (Schoenbaum et al. 1990). Infectious virus also has been shown to exist in unchlorinated farm well water and in anaerobic lagoon effluent for periods of up to 7 hours and up to 2 days respectively (Beran 1982).

Pseudorabies virus–contaminated fomites common to swine units have been an area of considerable interest as potential sources of PR virus for oral exposure of susceptible swine, although under farm conditions the role of fomite-mediated transmission is always difficult to prove. Pseudorabies virus generally has a low survivability in the environment. It is most stable between pH 6 and 8, in moist environments at cool nonfluctuating temperatures. The virus is inactivated in 1–7 days at pH 4.3 or 9.7 between 37°C and 4°C (Davies and Beran 1981). Inactivation is nearly instantaneous when virus is exposed to drying conditions especially in the presence of direct sunlight. Table 24.1 summarizes the times required for infectious levels of PR virus to drop to noninfectious levels at 25°C when virus is suspended in porcine saliva, nasal washings, or glucose-saline and placed on fomites. A number of reports have identified much longer survival times, frequently in months, for PR virus on fomites at winter temperatures, usually below 4°C (Beran 1982).

Dogs, cats, raccoons, rats, and mice, all of which are dead-end hosts, can also play a role in the spread of PR within herds. The infection in these animals is initially acquired through direct or indirect contact with infected pigs. Disease is generally of short duration, and most infected animals die within 2–3 days after the appearance of clinical signs, which commonly appear within 3 days of infection. Consequently, transmission by these species to pigs is generally restricted to a single farmstead. The presence of virus in nasal and oral secretions of these animals provides a means by which virus can be transmitted either directly or indirectly to pigs. Infective levels of virus are also present in the tissue of dead animals. Consumption of infective carcasses or feed that has been inadvertently contaminated during the milling process is a means by which PR virus is transmitted.

There is not sufficient evidence to suggest that avian species play an important role in the epidemiology of PR. Some species of birds have been infected with PR virus when the virus was given parenterally. Attempts to establish infection by the oral route have not been successful. It has been suggested that birds may transport the virus on their feathers or feet; however, PR virus rapidly loses its infectivity when experimentally placed on the feet of birds (Schoenbaum and Beran 1988).

The role of insects in the transmission of PR virus has not been adequately assessed. Houseflies experimentally fed PR virus in sugar solution at 5 days postemergence from pupae were not shown to be infected. However, the half-life of virus infectivity in the gut varied from 13 hours when flies were maintained at 10°C to 3 hours at 30°C. Attempts to experimentally transmit PR virus by flies to cornea, mucous membranes, or abraded skin of susceptible swine have produced variable results (Zimmerman et al. 1989).

Among the multiple mechanisms by which PR virus may be transmitted from one farm to another, movement of actively shedding or latently infected swine is the most frequent single source. Epidemiological investigation was reported on 1154 of the nearly 2000 herd outbreaks recorded in the United States during 1989, with reports providing data on source of transmission to 631 of these newly infected herds. Among these herds, 45.8% of the herds were exposed through movement of domestic swine, 18.8% by purchase of breeding swine, 17.2% by purchase of feeder pigs, 9.8% by division and dispersal of swine from infected herds, and 2.8% through contact with feral swine. Contact with contaminated fomites or infected swine carcasses were reported as sources of exposure in 1.2% of the herd outbreaks and 4.4% from other identified sources. Area spread, undifferentiated as to mechanisms, includes interherd movement of companion and wild animals, houseflies, people, vehicles, and air or water movement (Beran and Yang 1990). Evidence is emerging, especially from England, Denmark, and the United States, that airborne transmission of aerosolized virus may occur over 2 km or more from infected foci to uninfected areas.

CLINICAL SIGNS. The clinical signs associated with PR are primarily dependent on the strain of virus, the infectious dose, and more im-

Table 24.1. Survival of pseudorabies virus in contact with fomites

Fomites (at 25°)	Survival at Infectious Levels (Days)		
	In glucose saline	In saline	In nasal washings
Nonfomite-Control test	58	4	2
Steel	18	4	2
Concrete	<1	4	<1
Plastic	8	3	3
Rubber	7	2	2
Denim cloth	<1	<1	<1
Loam soil	4	7	2
Green grass	<1	2	<1
Shelled corn	36	4	2
Pelleted hog feed	3	3	3
Meat and bone meal	5	2	2
Alfalfa hay	<1	<1	<1
Straw bedding	3	4	4
Sawdust bedding	<1	2	<1
Swine feces	2	2	2
Swine skeletal muscle (4°C)	19	ND	ND

portantly, the age of the swine affected. Like herpesvirus of other animal species, younger swine are the most severely affected by PR virus. The virus has a predilection for respiratory and nervous tissue, thus the majority of clinical signs are associated with dysfunction of these two organ systems. Generally, nervous signs are more commonly observed in suckling and weaned pigs, while respiratory signs are observed in finishing pigs and adult swine.

The response to a PR viral infection within herds can be markedly different. The disease may manifest itself as a rapidly spreading disease affecting all ages of swine on the farm, or it may be a completely inapparent infection being detected only when a serological evaluation of the herd is made. Pseudorabies is more often inapparent when the infection occurs while neonatal pigs are not present, as in a period between farrowing groups in a group-type farrowing operation. Inapparent herd infections rarely occur when PR virus is introduced into a herd for the first time where neonatal pigs are present, because this age pig is so highly susceptible. Inapparent infection in breeding herds or separate finishing barns may actually be mild PR respiratory infections that are ignored or misdiagnosed as some other disease, such as swine influenza.

The first clinical signs observed in a farrow-to-finish herd will vary depending on the age group first infected. Typically, the first clinical signs will be a few gilts or sows aborting; or finishing pigs coughing and becoming listless and anorectic; or rough-haired suckling pigs that become listless, anorectic, and within 24 hours ataxic and convulsive. If any of these scenarios occurs, immediate diagnosis is imperative, because early vaccination in the face of an outbreak can limit losses.

Neonatal Pigs. The incubation period in suckling pigs is usually quite short, ranging from 2 to 4 days. Before aggressive clinical signs are noted, suckling pigs will become listless, anorectic, and febrile (41°C). Some pigs will develop central nervous signs within 24 hours of the onset of clinical signs, which progress from trembling, hypersalivation, incoordination, ataxia and nystagmus to opisthotonos, to severe epileptiformlike seizures. Affected pigs may sit like dogs because of posterior paralysis, while others will circle or become recumbent and paddle. Vomiting and diarrhea may also occur, but neither of these clinical signs are consistent. Pigs with central nervous system (CNS) signs usually die within 24–36 hours of onset. Mortality in suckling pigs is quite high, often approaching 100%. In herds with dams of varying immune status to PR virus, clinical signs may be seen in some litters, or pigs within a litter, while neighboring litters or littermates remain normal. If susceptible sows or gilts are infected close to term, pigs may be born weak and show clinical signs immediately and die within the first day or two of life.

Weaned Pigs (3–9 weeks). Younger pigs in this age group tend to have clinical signs similar to those described for suckling pigs. However, the clinical signs are less severe and fewer pigs develop the severe CNS involvement, which invariably leads to coma and death. Mortality in 3- to 4-week-old pigs may approach 50% in severe outbreaks. Older pigs in this age group become listless, anorectic, and febrile (41–42°C) within 3–6 days of exposure. Often, respiratory signs are present, characterized by sneezing, nasal discharge, and dyspnea and progress to a severe cough. Pigs displaying these clinical signs will lose significant body condition and weight. Duration of clinical signs is usually only 5–10 days; most pigs make a rapid full recovery once the fever and anorexia disappear. Pigs that develop CNS signs often die, as do pigs with a PR viral respiratory infection that develop a secondary or concurrent bacterial infection such as *Pasteurella multocida* or *Actinobacillus pleuropneumonia*. However, the mortality rate in pigs 5–9 weeks of age, if cared for properly and treated for secondary infections, will usually not exceed 10%, and is often lower. The more severely affected pigs that survive, especially those developing CNS signs, will often be stunted and sometimes show lasting signs, such as head tilt. These pigs reach market weight 1–2 months after the rest of the group.

Grower/Finishing Swine. Respiratory signs have become the hallmark of PR in grower/finishing pigs. The morbidity rate is usually very high, approaching 100%, but in uncomplicated cases mortality is low, 1–2%. CNS signs do occur, but only sporadically, and they may vary from mild muscle tremors to violent convulsions. Typically, clinical signs appear in 3–6 days and are characterized by a febrile response (41–42°C), depression, anorexia, and mild to severe respiratory signs. A rhinitis develops causing sneezing and a nasal discharge that progress to pneumonia, resulting in a harsh cough and labored breathing, especially when the pigs are forced to move about. These pigs become gaunt and lose considerable body weight. The duration of clinical signs is usually 6–10 days, and recovery is rapid once the fever disappears and the appetite returns. Although compensatory gain negates some of the lost body weight, grower/finishing pigs will lose at least a week in the production cycle. Losses may be dramatically increased if a PR virus infection is superimposed on an *A. pleuropneumonia* infection. It has been reported that PR virus inhibits the function of alveolar macrophages (Iglesias et al. 1989), thus reducing the capacity of the these defense cells to process and destroy bacteria.

Adult Swine. Sows and boars develop clinical signs, primarily respiratory in nature, very similar to those described above for grower/finishing pigs. Pregnant gilts often abort, and in a farrow-to-finish operation this may be the first clinical sign observed. Pregnant females infected with PR virus in the first trimester may resorb the fetuses and return to estrus. Reproductive failure due to PR in the second or third trimester is usually manifested by abortion or stillborn or weak pigs if the infection is close to term. If the gilt or sow is very close to farrowing when infected, pigs may be born with PR, in which case they die within a day or two. The PR virus can cross the placenta and infect and kill fetuses in utero, resulting in abortion. Fortunately, reproductive failure usually has a low incidence, occurring in 20% or less of the pregnant females on a farm. Mortality in gilts, sows, and boars infected with PR virus rarely exceeds 2%.

PATHOGENESIS. The pathogenesis is variable depending on viral strain, age of the pig, size of inoculum, and route of infection.

There is an increased resistance to development of clinical signs with age; strains of low virulence may not produce clinical signs in adult animals and the viral replication may be limited locally to the site of introduction.

To produce clinical disease experimentally, a minimum dose is required; however, under field conditions very low quantities of virus may cause pigs to seroconvert and even become latent carriers although no clinical signs can be detected in the herd. Experimental infection by intranasal inoculation requires ≥ 10 TCID50 in pigs under 2 weeks of age, $\geq 10^3$ TCID50 in 6-week-old pigs, and $\geq 10^4$ TCID50 in swine 4 months of age or older (McCullough 1989).

Experimentally, pigs develop infection after inoculation via the following routes: intramuscular, -venous, -cerebral, -gastric, -nasal, -tracheal, -conjunctival, -uterine, and -testicular, and oral. Intranasal inoculation results in clinical signs and lesions similar to the natural disease, and under field conditions the oral-nasal routes are the most common.

Under natural conditions the primary site of replication is epithelium in the nasopharynx and tonsil (Masic et al. 1965). From these sites there is lymphatic spread to regional lymph nodes and replication in the nodes. Virus also spreads via nerves from the primary site of infection to the CNS. Examples of this are spread within axoplasm of the trigeminal nerve to the medulla and pons and spread along olfactory nerves and the glossopharyngeal nerve to the medulla. After replication in neurons in the medulla and pons, there may be spread to other portions of the brain. As noted earlier with low-virulence strains and moderate-virulence strains in older animals, viral spread may be limited to those locations.

Strains of higher virulence will follow a course similar to the above, but in addition there is widespread virus distribution in the body and older swine will have clinical signs and may have gross lesions (McFerran and Dow 1965; Sabó et al. 1968, 1969; Wittmann et al. 1980). Probably all strains have a tropism for the upper respiratory tract and the CNS. Strains of higher virulence produce a brief viremia and virus can be demonstrated in the serum and also associated with buffy-coat cells. High-virulence strains can be isolated from alveolar macrophages, epithelium of terminal bronchioles, hepatocytes, lymphoid cells of the spleen and lymph nodes, adrenal cortical cells, trophoblasts and embryos from the gravid uterus, and luteal cells of the ovary. Virus has been isolated from semen but probably originated from preputial lesions, since attempts to isolate virus from the testes and accessary sex glands have failed (Gueguen and Aynaud 1980, Medveczky and Szabó 1981). The observed decrease in sperm quality is probably the result of fever and systemic disease. Embryos are resistant to infection as long as the zona pellucida is intact, thus associated virus can be washed from embryos and embryo transplantation can be used as a method of salvaging genetic material from an infected herd (Bolin et al. 1983; Bolin and Bolin 1984).

Virus excretion precedes or coincides with the onset of clinical disease, or in clinically inapparent infection, excretion begins after an incubation period of 2–5 days. PR virus may be recovered from nasal exudate or secretions at levels from 10^7 to $\geq 10^8$ TCID50 per swab for 1 to more than 2 weeks and for similar periods but in lesser quantities from tonsillar scrapings, vaginal secretions, prepuce, milk, and occasionally urine (Wittmann and Rziha 1989). Active immunity from vaccination or prior infection decreases the period of viral shedding. As with other herpesviruses, infection with PR virus results in a high percentage of latent infections in host pigs (Rziha et al. 1982). The virus persists in ganglia such as the trigeminal ganglia. Latently infected pigs often have detectable viral recrudescence during times of stress, such as farrowing, crowding, and transport. Experimentally, corticosteroid injection results in subsequent viral recrudescence and nasal shed of virus. This should be considered when administering steroids to animals in an infected herd that is in the midst of an eradication program. Vaccination with live or killed vaccines appears to have little or no effect in preventing the development of latency in postvaccination exposed swine.

LESIONS

Gross Lesions. Gross lesions are often absent or are minimal and undetected. When they are present they aid in arriving at a tentative diagnosis when combined with herd history and clinical signs.

Serous to fibrinonecrotic rhinitis is common but may be missed unless the head is split to expose the entire nasal cavity (Csontos and Széky 1966; Olander et al. 1966). The lesions may extend to the larynx and even down the trachea. Necrotic tonsillitis is frequently seen along with swollen and hemorrhagic lymph nodes of the oral cavity and upper respiratory tract (Narita et al. 1984a). When present, lesions in the lower respiratory tract range from pulmonary edema to scattered small foci of necrosis, hemorrhage, and/or pneumonia (Becker 1964; Corner 1965).

Keratoconjunctivitis is common and often more obvious in white breeds because of the discoloration caused by excessive lacrimation and periocular deposits of exudate (Schneider and Howarth 1973).

Typical herpetic yellow-white foci (2–3 mm) of necrosis may be scattered through the liver and spleen and may be seen just beneath the serosal surface.

Sows that have recently aborted may have a mild endometritis and the wall of the uterus is often thickened and edematous (Kluge and Maré 1978; Hsu et al. 1980). If the placenta is available for examination a necrotic placentitis is often observed. Aborted fetuses may appear fresh, macerated, or occasionally mummified. Some pigs in an affected litter may be normal and others weak or dead at birth. Infected fetuses or neonatal pigs frequently have the previously described necrotic foci (Csontos et al. 1962; Kluge and Maré 1976; Wohlgemuth et al. 1978) in liver and spleen as well as hemorrhagic necrotic foci in lungs and tonsils. A history of abortion along with the presence of necrotic foci is strongly suggestive of a tentative diagnosis of PR. The only gross lesion reported in the male reproductive tract is scrotal edema.

Necrotic enteritis in the lower jejunum and ileum has been reported in young pigs (Narita et al. 1984c).

Microscopic Lesions. Microscopic lesions are most frequently reported in the CNS and persist for many weeks (12–24 weeks postinfection) (Olander et al. 1976). They may also be present in pigs that failed to develop clinical signs, but they are often absent in aborted fetuses. Nonsuppurative meningoencephalitis and ganglioneuritis are the characteristic lesions (Dow and McFerran 1962; Sabó et al. 1969; Baskerville 1972). Lesions are present in both the gray and white matter and the distribution is dependent on the route of entry into the CNS. Affected areas are characterized by predominately mononuclear cell perivascular cuffing and glial nodules. A few granulocytes may be mixed with the mononuclear cells and pyknosis and karyorrhexis of the latter cells is often prominent. The endothelium of affected vessels ap-

pears normal. Neuronal necrosis may be focal and the neurons surrounded by mononuclear cells or affected neurons may be diffusely scattered. Similar lesions may be present in the spinal cord, especially in the cervical and thoracic regions. Meninges over affected areas of brain and cord may be thickened because of infiltrates of mononuclear cells. Similar lesions have been reported in ganglia and ganglia cells (cerebrospinal, cardiac and celiac ganglia, Meissner's and Auerbach's plexi and ganglion cell layer of the retina). Intranuclear inclusion bodies may be present in neurons, astrocytes, and oligodendroglia, but in our experience are much more common in lesions outside the nervous system.

In tonsils, necrosis begins in the subepithelial area and then spreads to the epithelium and deeper into the lymphoid tissue (Narita et al. 1984c). Intranuclear inclusion bodies are common in crypt epithelial cells adjacent to necrotic foci. The upper respiratory tract lesions consist of mucosal epithelial necrosis and submucosal infiltrations of mononuclear cells (Baskerville 1971, 1973). Lung lesions consist of necrotic bronchitis, bronchiolitis, and alveolitis. Peribronchial mucous gland epithelium may be necrotic. There is often hemorrhage and fibrin exudation because of involvement of connective tissue and endothelium. Lesions often are patchy in major airways and healing by fibrosis is often observed in areas adjacent to acute lesions. Intranuclear inclusion bodies are frequently present in the epithelial lining of the airways, connective tissue cells, and cells sloughed into alveolar spaces.

Focal necrotic lesions are similar regardless of the tissue involved. They are most frequently found in spleen, liver, lymph nodes, and adrenal glands. Necrotic foci are randomly distributed and surrounded by a few inflammatory cells, or the latter may be absent. Parenchymal cells at the margins of necrosis commonly contain intranuclear inclusion bodies. In macerated fetuses microscopic necrotic foci often are visible even though cellular detail can not be discerned since the pyknotic nuclei stain with hematoxylin.

Uterine infection is characterized by multifocal to diffuse lymphohistiocytic endometritis and vaginitis and necrotic placentitis with coagulative necrosis of chorionic fossae (Bolin et al. 1985). Intranuclear inclusion bodies are present in degenerate trophoblasts associated with the necrotic lesions (Kluge and Maré 1978a; Hsu et al. 1980). Depending upon the stage of infection, corpora lutea may be necrotic and contain neutrophils, lymphocytes, plasma cells, and macrophages (Bolin et al. 1985).

In the male reproductive tract there may be degeneration of seminiferous tubules and necrotic foci in the tunica albuginea of the testicles (Corner 1965; Larson et al. 1980; Hall et al. 1984). Boars with exudative periorchitis have necrotic and inflammatory lesions in the serosa covering the genital organs. Spermatozoa abnormalities include tail abnormalities, retained distal cytoplasmic droplets, knobbed cystic acrosomes, double heads, and detached heads. These changes may be the result of pyrexia and not the result of viral infection of spermatogenic epithelium.

Enteric lesions consist of focal necrosis of the mucosal epithelium and may involve the underlying muscularis mucosa and tunica muscularis (Narita et al. 1984b). Intranuclear inclusion bodies may be present in degenerate crypt epithelial cells.

There may be necrotizing vasculitis of arterioles, venules, and lymphatic vessels around tonsils and submaxillary lymph nodes (Narita et al. 1984a). Endothelial nuclei are pyknotic and karyorrhectic and the vessel walls are infiltrated by neutrophils. Intranuclear inclusion bodies often are present in affected endothelial cells.

Two types of intranuclear inclusion bodies may be observed (Corner 1965): a homogenous basophilic body that fills the entire nucleus and an eosinophilic body that has a definite halo between it and the marginated chromatin. In either case, specificity of the inclusion must be determined by demonstrating viral particles or antigen by electron microscopy or immunohistochemistry.

DIAGNOSIS. The diagnosis of PR is usually made on a herd basis using a combination of herd history, clinical signs, gross lesions, microscopic lesions, serology, and virus detection by either the fluorescent antibody tissue section (FATS) test or virus isolation. Classical clinical signs will often lead to a presumptive diagnosis that is often supported if gross lesions (focal hepatic and splenic necrosis and necrotic tonsillitis) are observed in neonatal pigs. PR is more difficult to diagnose if only grower/finishing pigs or adult swine are involved. A PR outbreak in these age groups can easily be misdiagnosed as swine influenza if the disease is manifested only by respiratory signs. If, however, a few individuals develop CNS signs, it is easier to make a presumptive diagnosis of PR. PR virus is relatively easy to demonstrate in infected swine if samples are taken at the right time and handled properly. Serology is not the test of choice when trying to diagnose an acute PR virus infection because of the delay required for humoral antibodies to develop. Microscopic lesions can confirm a viral etiology and are helpful in finalizing the diagnosis (see **Microscopic Lesions**).

Virus Isolation. Brain, spleen, and lung are the organs of choice for virus isolation (VI). The tissues should be collected from two or three acutely affected pigs. Tissues should be refrigerated, preferably not frozen unless dry ice is used, and transported to the laboratory as soon as possible. If only grower/finishing and/or adult swine are affected and none have died, nasal swabs collected in cold cell culture media with antibiotics may be utilized. If cell culture fluid or a balanced salt solution is not available, a cold sterile saline solution may be used. The sample is inoculated onto cell cultures and the cultures observed for the presence of characteristic cytopathic effect. The suspected isolate can be confirmed utilizing a fluorescent antibody test. For most cases, PR virus will be isolated within 2–5 days. However, most laboratories will conduct two blind passages 1 week apart before reporting the specimen as negative. Tissues from aborted fetuses can also be submitted for VI; however, if the abortion was due to a febrile response in the dam rather than a direct effect of the virus on the fetuses, VI results would be negative. Caution needs to be taken when interpreting these results, and additional diagnostic tests may be required to confirm a diagnosis of a PR virus–induced abortion.

In developing countries or in remote areas where diagnostic laboratories are not available, the supernatant fluid of a 20% brain suspension can be injected intramuscularly into the hind leg of a rabbit. Typical signs of intense pruritus and self-mutilation at the site of injection within 48–96 hours will confirm the diagnosis of PR. This method should only be used as a last resort due to concern for the experimental animal.

Fluorescent Antibody Tissue Section Test. The FATS test is a rapid, reliable method of detecting PR virus in tissue. The tissue of choice is tonsil, but brain or pharyngeal smears may also be used. In the pig, the tonsil is easily identified for it is in the dorsal area of the anterior pharynx and it has visible crypts. The advantage of the FATS test is that it can be completed in 1 hour and the results in neonatal pigs with typical clinical signs is comparable to VI results. In grower/finishing pigs and in adults the FATS test is not as sensitive as VI. If clinical signs and history are suggestive of PR, a negative FATS test result in older animals must be confirmed by VI.

Serodiagnosis. Numerous serological tests have been developed to assay serum for PR antibodies. Currently the most widely utilized tests are microtitration serum virus neutralization (SVN) test, enzyme-linking immunosorbent assay (ELISA), and latex agglutination (LA). Other serologic tests have been developed, such as complement-fixation, immunodiffusion, countercurrent immunoelectrophoresis, indirect immunofluorescence; all have limitations of sensitivity, require considerable time to conduct the test, or are difficult to perform. Consequently, they have received limited acceptance. The SVN test is a reliable yet time-consuming test and requires 48 hours to perform. The SVN test is considered the standard and is the test used to compare new test procedures. It can be used to titrate PR viral antibody in serum, and it is still the most widely used test for this purpose. The ELISA has replaced the SVN test in laboratories that test large numbers of serums for PR viral antibody, primarily because of the short time required to conduct the test. Several commercial ELISA kits are available worldwide that allow large numbers of serums to be tested in 3–4 hours. The LA test is the simplest of these three tests to perform, and it is commercially available on a worldwide basis. The LA test can be performed on a single serum sample in 10 minutes. Some problems of specificity have been noted with this test; however, it is quite sensitive, making it an excellent test for quick screening of serums for PR viral antibodies. Generally, the LA test will detect seroconversion in 6–7 days, while the ELISA requires 7–8 days; the SVN requires 8–10 days.

Interpretation of serological results can be difficult, especially in young pigs. Maternal antibodies can be present for up to 4 months of age. The half-life of the maternal antibodies that pigs received in the colostrum of PR immune sows is approximately 18 days. It takes 18 days for the antibody titer to be divided in half; i.e., be reduced from 1:16 to 1:8. If pigs from an immune sow are tested too early, they could be identified as being infected when the antibody is only passive and not the result of exposure and active infection.

If serology is used to diagnose an active infection, it is necessary to use paired serum samples collected at a 2-week interval, and to demonstrate a fourfold rise in the antibody titer. A single, positive serological test indicates infection, but it does not indicate when the infection occurred. High antibody titers versus low titers may only indicate a superior immunological response in a particular individual rather than a recent exposure.

The most important technological breakthroughs in PR control and eradication programs have been the development of the gene-deleted PR vaccines and the accompanying differential ELISA serology tests. These tests detect a specific antibody produced by one of the viral glycoproteins. There are vaccines and companion diagnostic serology tests for gI, gIII, and gX. Animals vaccinated with a gene-deleted vaccine will lack antibody against the specific protein coded for by the deleted gene, allowing a vaccinated pig to be differentiated from an infected pig. Once the pig is infected, it will develop antibody against all of the PR viral proteins and be positive on all differential serology tests. Some countries have restricted commercial companies as to which gene can be deleted from the vaccine, but in other countries there are vaccines, each with a different deletion. These vaccines would not be compatible in a single herd because a pig vaccinated with two different gene-deleted vaccines would have antibodies to all the glycoproteins and be falsely identified as a PR virus–infected pig. Therefore, it is important to know which vaccine is used and to not vaccinate a pig with vaccines with different deletions. In countries with a PR eradication program there eventually will be a need to conduct slaughter-plant surveillance once the prevalence of PR is low. The surveillance will be possible only if a universal gene deletion is used in all vaccines.

TREATMENT

Vaccines. Modified live (virus, MLV), inactivated, and gene-deleted vaccines have been developed for PR control. The use of vaccines has been controversial, and opinions have varied based on the desire to control or eradicate the disease. The PR vaccines presently available effectively protect pigs against clinical signs and have therefore reduced the economic loss to producers that have vaccinated in endemic areas.

Vaccinated swine that become subsequently infected have more limited invasion of tissues, usually limited to the lower respiratory system; do not transmit virus intrauterine; shed lesser amounts of virus, in most studies at least 1000-fold less; and experience shorter duration of shedding, in most studies reduced 4- to 7-fold. However, latent infections are not prevented in swine infected subsequent to vaccination, and are not eliminated if pre-existing at the time of vaccination. Only a small number of studies have indicated that formation of latency may be inhibited by certain MLV vaccines.

The role of vaccination in reducing reactivation of latent PR virus subsequent to environmental stresses remains undetermined. The laboratory immunosuppression experiments through which such reactivation can be demonstrated are more drastic than simulated field conditions; however, transmission of PR virus does occasionally occur from latently infected, fully vaccinated swine within a herd.

The MLV vaccines replicate principally at the site of injection and regional lymph nodes; they have been shown to be shed in nasal secretions and tonsillar mucus, but at too low levels to be any practical risk of transmission to swine or any other animals. These vaccines vary in virulence in animal species other than swine. Appropriate precautions must be taken when using MLV vaccines in species other than swine, and extreme care must be taken that syringes, needles, or wash solutions used with MLV vaccines are not then used when vaccinating other animals with other vaccines. This hazard, and the concern for the potential for reversion of MLV vaccines has led to the improvement of killed PR vaccines. The employment of new adjuvants has made efficacy of some of these killed vaccines quite competitive with MLV vaccines, especially when multiple doses are used.

There are numerous MLV and killed PR vaccines available throughout the world. The killed vaccines have been developed from wild-type strains or from the Bucharest or Bartha MLV vaccine strains. Genetically engineered PR vaccines and some of the conventionally attenuated vaccines have deletions in nonessential glycoprotein genes such as gI, gIII, gX, and gp 63. The absence of these glycoproteins makes them useful as negative immunological markers and has been utilized in serological tests designed to identify virus-infected vaccinated swine.

The TK gene has also been deleted from genetically engineered PR vaccines. TK facilitates PR infections of neurons, permitting viral replication. Since the natural endogenous level of TK in differentiated neural tissue is low, the virulence of a PR vaccine can be reduced by removing the TK gene so that the virus can no longer encode for the production of this enzyme.

The recombination of gene-deleted vaccines that might lead to a virulent virus that still contains a negative immunological marker is a concern (Henderson et al. 1990). A recent study has demonstrated that when pigs were inoculated with two different gene-deleted vaccines, recombination did occur; recombination might be possible in the field if pigs were vaccinated with more than one gene-deleted vaccine. It is therefore imperative that only one type of gene-deleted vaccine be used in a single animal. Recombination potentially could also occur when gene-deleted MLV vaccines are used in the face of an outbreak with field PR virus, resulting in a gene-deleted virulent virus as a result of recombination between the field strain and the gene-deleted vaccine strain. This apparently does not occur or occurs very infrequently, for gene-deleted MLV vaccines have been widely used in the face of PR outbreaks and, as yet, there are no reports of a virulent PR virus with a deletion of a gene for one of the glycoproteins.

CONTROL AND ERADICATION. Forty-three countries reported the occurrence of PR in 1989 (FAO, WHO, OIE 1990). England, Denmark, and German Democratic Republic reported successful eradication programs. The program in England was started in 1983 and was financed by a check-off of 30 p (about $0.55) per hog slaughtered. Identification was based on clinical and laboratory reporting with traceback and 2-km (1.2-mile) circle testing of all infected herds. Infected herds were depopulated and owners indemnified. Culled-sow surveys were used at packing plants from 1984–88 to monitor the national swine population. Three clinical herd outbreaks were identified in March 1988 and promptly eliminated by depopulation (Taylor 1989).

In Denmark eradication measures were instituted in 1980 and based on serological testing of all swine herds, strict regulatory measures on swine movement, and indemnified cleanup of infected herds by depopulation or test and removal

of seropositive swine. Funds were generated by an industry two-tiered checkoff. A higher levy was assessed for slaughter swine from infected herds than from uninfected herds. Eradication was reported in 1986 but occasional outbreaks have occurred along the southern border with Germany. Virus isolated from these outbreaks was shown by restriction endonuclease patterns to belong to Central European genomic types not previously found in Denmark (Anderson et al. 1989). Surveillance is continuing and is based on sentry monitoring of breeding boars.

In the German Democratic Republic, PR control measures were instituted in 1966 and an active eradication program was conducted between 1981 and 1985. All swine herds in the nation were tested, swine movements were severely restricted, and intensive vaccination and phased depopulation were used in cleaning up infected herds. Since 1985, four outbreaks that occurred along the border with the Federal Republic of Germany have been eliminated by depopulation. One of these outbreaks was introduced by infected rats; PR virus was recovered both from swine and rats (Kretzchmar 1989).

Thirteen countries report active eradication programs at this time: Bulgaria, Cuba, Czechoslovakia, Jamaica, Japan, Mexico, Netherlands, Norway, Romania, the United States, the U.S.S.R., Vietnam, and Yugoslavia (FAO, WHO, OIE 1990). In addition, active planning for control is reported by Germany, France, and Hungary.

Major components of PR control and eradication programs include

1. A national or strategic area plan. Elimination of infection must be carried out comprehensively by region or transmission will reoccur. In areas of dense swine populations and in the absence of areawide control measures, PR moves in successive waves, maintaining endemicity following initial epidemic invasion.

2. Organization and education. The swine-production managers of control areas must be knowledgeable of the entire program, and participants in program planning and implementation.

3. Guidelines and regulations. Standard procedures for development and monitoring the entire program and for regulating sales and movement of swine must be organized and swine producer compliance achieved.

4. Scheduling and budgeting. Goals must be set and time schedules for achieving program objectives developed to achieve control and then eradication of PR. Budgets for anticipated costs must be prepared.

5. Sources of funding. Most programs at this time have been jointly funded by industry through levies on swine slaughtered and government appropriations for surveillance, regulation of swine movement, monitoring of infected-herd cleanup, and program assessment. Indemnifica-

tion of producers for swine depopulation or subsidization of market payments for uninfected swine are paid by some governments. It is essential that funding be continuous so that costly halts with spreading of intraherd and interherd infections do not occur.

6. Surveillance plan. Case finding must be organized and comprehensive. Prompt, effective reporting of serologic tests for sale or movement and of diagnostic laboratory findings is essential. In countries or areas of low PR prevalence, slaughter sampling of culled breeding swine or market testing of sale swine followed by traceback of seropositive animals and circle testing of herds within 1- to 2-km (0.6–1.2 miles) radius of infected herds are being applied effectively. In countries or areas with over 10% prevalence of herd infections, on-farm area testing of herds is most effective.

7. Herd testing. Statistical sampling based on 95 or 99% probability of detecting infection in herds in which at least 10, 20, or 30% of swine are seropositive is most cost efficient. Testing is commonly limited to breeding and finishing swine sampled as separate herds; separated groups of swine under single management must also be sampled as separate herds. A brief guide for statistical sampling is shown as Table 24.2.

8. Certification of clean herds. Many countries utilize systems of regular sample testing and certification of uninfected herds, emphasizing seed stock producer herds, feeder pig producer herds, and breeding herds dispersing grower pigs to multiple premises. Area cleanup of infected herds and controlled movement of infected swine are needed to help protect certified herds from reinfection.

9. Herd cleanup methods. Three basic approaches, each of which must be adapted to individual infected herds, are commonly used. Depopulation of infected herds, followed by cleaning and disinfecting of premises and repopulation with clean stock is effective but generally costly, and is most applicable in areas of low and sporadic incidence of infection. Total testing and removal of seropositive breeding swine are effective in herds in which infection is stable and involves not over 10–20% of mature swine, with immature swine being uninfected. Offspring segregation is carried out by segregating uninfected gilt progeny of infected breeding swine, rearing them as replacement gilts in facilities separated from infected swine, and then progressively depopulating, cleaning and disinfecting production units, and repopulating with the clean replacement stock.

10. Cleaning and disinfection. After emptying entire units or premises of swine and removing feed and water from common feeders or troughs and manure from pits, thorough cleaning to remove all foreign material from floors, walls and ceilings, partitions, ventilation systems and fans, heaters, feeders, troughs, and other furnishings must be carried out, followed by disinfection. Surfaced feeding floors should be cleaned, or dirt lots scraped down and soil tilled to expose it to sunlight. Disinfection should be thorough with disinfectants selected for greatest effectivity in the presence of organic matter; sodium hydroxide, phenolic compounds, iodine compounds, or chlorhexadine are examples. Greater assurance of effectivity is achieved in two cleaning and disinfecting actions with at least 1 week drying time between them; a total 30-day empty time is strongly recommended.

11. Use of vaccine in herd cleanup. Intensive areawide vaccination of infected herds can help to stabilize infection in these herds and reduce area transmission prior to extensive implementation of cleanup of infected herds, as was effectively carried out in the German Democratic Republic. Herd vaccination with differentiable vaccines by test and removal can be effective preceding and during cleanup. Vaccination of breeding swine, especially with differentiable vaccine, is an asset in offspring segregation to reduce transmission of PR virus to progeny, and thus to select uninfected weanling gilts to be reared in segregation. Repeated vaccination of segregated gilts during maturation and gestation enhances resistance, but does not ensure protection from infection as the segregated clean gilts and their progeny are rotated into the production facilities. Differentiable vaccines are most applicable in ensuring that replacement swine are free of infection.

12. Program evaluation. Monitoring of individual herd cleanup and of infection status of area herds is necessary. As eradication is approached

Table 24.2. Size of sample required to detect reactor animals by population size for 95% and 99% certainty of detection

| Population Size | Number of Reactor Animals in the Population | | | | | |
| | ≥10% | | ≥20% | | ≥30% | |
	95%	99%	95%	99%	95%	99%
≤100	25	36	13	19	9	13
101–200	27	40	13	20	9	13
201–300	28	41	14	20	9	13
301–500	28	42	14	21	9	13
501–1000	29	43	14	21	9	13
>1000	29	44	14	21	9	13

or achieved, a system of population sampling must be maintained, usually with special intensity in high-risk areas, as along borders with infected areas. Most countries use slaughter sampling of cull breeding swine in monitoring, but Denmark is utilizing total breeding boar population surveillance (Thawley et al. 1957).

REFERENCES

ANDERSON, J. B.; BITSCH, V.; CHRISTENSEN, L. S.; HOFF-JORGENSEN, R.; AND KIRKEGAARD PETERSEN, B. 1989. The control and eradication of Aujeszky's disease in Denmark: Epidemiological aspects. In Vaccination and Control of Aujeszky's Disease. Ed. J. T. Van Oirschot. Brussels, Luxembourg: ECSC, EEC, EAEC, pp. 175–183.

BASKERVILLE, A. 1971. The histopathology of pneumonia by aerosol infection of pigs with a strain of Aujeszky's disease virus. Res Vet Sci 12:590–592.

———. 1972. Aujeszky's disease encephalitis in pigs produced by different modes of infection. Res Vet Sci 14:223–228.

———. 1973. The histopathology of experimental pneumonia in pigs produced by Aujeszky's disease virus. Res Vet Sci 14:223–228.

BASKERVILLE, A.; McFERRAN, J. B.; AND DOW, C. 1973. Aujeszky's disease in pigs. Vet Bull (London) 43:465–480.

BECKER, C. H. 1964. Zur Bedeutung der Lunge für die pathologisch-anatomische Diagnose der Aujeszkyschen Krankheit des Schweines. Monatsh Veterinaermed 19:5–11.

BERAN, G. W. 1982. The epidemiology of pseudorabies. Proceedings. Pork Producers Day, Iowa State Univ, Ames. AS 535-G:1–9.

BERAN, G. W., AND YANG, P.-C. 1990. Proc U.S. Anim Health Assoc, Denver.

BOLIN, S. R., AND BOLIN, C. A. 1984. Pseudorabies virus infection of six-and ten-day-old porcine embryos. Theriogenology 22:101–106.

BOLIN, S. R.; TUREK, J. J.; RUNNELS, L. J.; AND GUSTAFSON, D. P. 1983. Pseudorabies virus, porcine parvovirus, and porcine enterovirus interactions with the zona pellucida of the porcine embryo. Am J Vet Res 44(6):1036–1039.

BOLIN, C. A.; BOLIN, S. R.; KLUGE, J. P.; AND MENGELING, W. L. 1985. Pathologic effects of intrauterine deposition of pseudorabies virus on the reproductive tract of swine in early pregnancy. Am J Vet Res 46:1039–1042.

CORNER, A. H. 1965. Pathology of experimental Aujeszky's disease in piglets. Res Vet Sci 6:337–343.

CSONTOS, L., AND SZÉKY, A. 1966. Gross and microscopic lesions in the nasopharynx of pigs with Aujeszky's disease. Acta Vet Acad Sci Hung 16:175–186.

CSONTOS, L.; HEJJ, L.; AND SZABÓ, I. 1962. A contribution to the aetiology of Aujeszky's disease in the pig. Foetal damage and abortion due to the virus. Acta Vet Acad Sci Hung 12:17–23.

DAVIES, E. B., AND BERAN, G. W. 1980. Spontaneous shedding of pseudorabies virus from a clinically recovered post parturient sow. J Am Vet Med Assoc 176:1345–1347.

———. 1981. Influence of environmental factors upon the survival of Aujeszky's disease virus. Res Vet Sci 31:32–36.

DOW, C., AND McFERRAN, J. B. 1962. The neuropathology of Aujeszky's disease in the pig. Res Vet Sci 3:436–442.

FAO, WHO, OIE. 1990. Animal Health Yearbook.

GUEGUEN, B., AND AYNAUD, J. M. 1980. Étude de l'excrétion du virus de la maladie d'Aujeszky par les voies génitales du porc. Rec Méd Vét 156:307–312.

HALL, L. B.; KLUGE, J. P.; EVANS, L. E.; AND HILL, H. T. 1984. The effect of pseudorabies (Aujeszky's) virus infection on young mature boars and boar fertility. Can J Comp Med 48:192–197.

HAMPL, H.; BEN-PORAT, T.; EHRLICHER, L.; HABERMEHL, K. O.; AND KAPLAN, A. S. 1984. Characterization of the envelope proteins of pseudorabies virus. J Virol 52:583–590.

HENDERSON, L. M.; LEVINGS, R. L.; DAVIS, A. J.; KATZ, J. B.; STRUTZ, D. R.; AND MAYFIELD, J. E. 1990. Vaccine strains of fluid herpesvirus I recombine in swine to produce virulent progeny virus. 15th Int Herpesvirus Workshop (Abstr). Washington, D.C., p. 433.

HOWARTH, J. A. 1969. A serologic study of pseudorabies in swine. J Am Vet Med Assoc 154:1583–1589.

HSU, F. S.; CHU, R. M.; LEE, R. C.; AND CHU, S. H. 1980. Placental lesions caused by pseudorabies virus in pregnant sows. J Am Vet Med Assoc 177:636–641.

IGLESIAS, G.; PIJOAN, C.; AND MOLITOR, T. 1989. Interactions of pseudorabies virus with swine alveolar macrophages: Effects of virus infection on cell functions. J Leukocyte Biol 45:410–415.

KLUGE, J. P., AND MARÉ, C. J. 1976. Gross and microscopic lesions of prenatal and neonatal pseudorabies (Aujeszky's disease) in swine. Proc 4th Int Congr Pig Vet Soc, Ames, p. G3.

———. 1978. Natural and experimental in utero infection of piglets with Aujeszky's disease (pseudorabies) virus. Am Assoc Vet Lab Diagn 21:15–24.

KOST, T. A.; JONES, E. V.; SMITH, K. M.; REED, A. I.; BROWN, A. L.; AND MILLER, T. J. 1989. Biological evaluation of glycoprotein mapping to two distinct mRNAs within the BamHI fragment 7 of pseudorabies virus: Expression of the coding regions by vaccinia virus. Virology 171(2):365–376.

KRETZCHMAR, C. 1989. Eradication and control of Aujeszky's disease in the German Democratic Republic. In Vaccination and Control of Aujeszky's Disease. Ed. J. T. Van Oirschot. Brussels, Luxembourg: ECSC, EEC, EAEC, pp. 239–247.

LARSEN, R. E.; SHOPE, R. E.; LEMAN, L. D.; AND KURTZ, H. J. 1980. Semen changes in boars after experimental infections with pseudorabies virus. Am J Vet Res 41:733–739.

McCULLOUGH, S. J. 1989. Vaccination and control of Aujeszky's disease in Northern Ireland. In Vaccination and Control of Aujeszky's Disease. Ed. J. T. Van Oirschot. Boston: Kluwer Academic Publishers, pp. 231–238.

McFERRAN, J. B., AND DOW, C. 1965. The distribution of the virus of Aujeszky's disease (pseudorabies virus) in experimentally infected swine. Br Vet J 126:173–179.

MARCHIOLI, C. C.; YANCEY, R. J., Jr.; PETROVSKIS, E. A.; TIMMINS, J. G.; AND POST, L. E. 1987. Evaluation of pseudorabies virus glycoprotein gp50 as a vaccine for Aujeszky's disease in mice and swine: Expression by vaccinia virus and Chinese hamster ovary cells. J Virol 61:3977–3982.

MARCHIOLI, C. C.; YANCEY, R. J., Jr.; TIMMINS, J. G.; POST, L. E.; YOUNG, B. R.; AND POVENDO, D. A. 1988. Protection of mice and swine from pseudorabies virus–induced mortality by administration of pseudorabies virus–specific mouse monoclonal antibodies. Am J Vet Res 49:860–864.

MASIC, M.; ERCEGAN, M.; AND PETROVIC, M. 1965. Die Bedeutung der Tonsillen für die Pathogenese und Diagnose der Aujeszkyschen Krankheit bei Schweinen. Zentralbl Veterinaermed 12:389–405.

MEDVECZKY, I., AND SZABÓ, I. 1981. Isolation of Aujeszky's disease virus from boar semen. Acta Vet

Acad Sci Hung 29:29–35.

MENGELING, W. L.; PAUL, P. S.; PIRTLE, E. C.; AND WATHEN, M. W. 1983. Restriction endonuclease analysis of the pseudorabies (Aujeszky's disease) virus before and after serial passage in-vivo and in-vitro. Arch Virol 78:213–220.

NARITA, M.; HARITANI, M.; AND MORIWALI, M. 1984a. Necrotizing vasculitis in piglets infected orally with the virus of Aujeszky's disease. Jpn J Vet Sci 46:119–122.

NARITA, M.; KUBO, M.; FUKUSHO, A.; HARITANI, M.; AND MORIWAKI, M. 1984b. Necrotizing enteritis in piglets associated with the virus of Aujeszky's disease. Vet Pathol 21:450–452.

NARITA, M.; INUI, S.; AND SHIMIZU, Y. 1984c. Tonsillar changes in pigs given pseudorabies (Aujeszky's disease) virus. Am J Vet Res 45:247–251.

OLANDER, H. J.; SAUNDERS, J. R.; GUSTAFSON, D. P.; AND JONES, R. K. 1966. Pathologic findings in swine affected with a virulent strain of Aujeszky's virus. Pathol Vet 3:64–82.

OLANDER H. J.; GUSTAFSON, D. P.; AND QURESHI, S. R. 1976. Residual lesions in swine convalescent from pseudorabies virus infection. Proc 4th Int Congr Pig Vet Soc, Ames, p. G13.

PLATT, K. B. 1981. Genetic stability of the thermal, trypsin, rabbit and mouse markers of Aujeszky's disease (pseudorabies) virus in the pig. Vet Microbiol 6:225–232.

RZIHA, H. J.; DÖLLER, P. C.; AND WITTMANN, G. 1982. Detection of Aujeszky's disease virus and viral DNA in tissues of latently infected pigs. In Current Topics in Veterinary Medicine and Animal Science. Ed. G. Wittmann and S. A. Hall, 17–205–211.

SABÓ, A.; RAJCANI, J.; AND BLÅSKOVIČ, D. 1968. Studies on the pathogenesis of Aujeszky's disease. I. Distribution of the virulent virus in piglets after peroral infection. Acta Virol 12:214–221.

———. 1969. Studies on the pathogenesis of Aujeszky's disease. III. The distribution of virulent virus in piglets after intranasal infection. Acta Virol 13:407–414.

SCHNEIDER, W. J., AND HOWARTH, J. A. 1973. Clinical course and histopathologic features of pseudorabies virus–induced keratoconjunctivitis in pigs. Am J Vet Res 34:393–401.

SCHOENBAUM, M. A., AND BERAN, G. W. 1988. Laboratory data, Iowa State Univ.

SCHOENBAUM, M. A.; ZIMMERMAN, J. J.; BERAN, G. W.; AND MURPHY, D. P. 1990. Survival of pseudorabies virus in aerosol. Am J Vet Res 51:331–333.

STEVELY, W. S. 1975. Virus induced proteins in pseudorabies infected cells. II. Proteins of the virion and nucleocapsid. J Virol 16:944–950.

TAYLOR, K. C. 1989. Epidemiological aspects of Aujeszky's disease control in Great Britain. In Vaccination and Control of Aujeszky's Disease. Ed. J. T. Van Oirschot. Brussels, Luxembourg: ECSC, EEC, EAEC, pp. 185–196.

THAWLEY, D. G.; GUSTAFSON, D. P.; AND BERAN, G. W. 1982. Swine pseudorabies eradication guidelines. Livest Conserv Inst, South St. Paul, Minn., pp. 1–11.

WITTMANN, G., AND RZIHA, H. J. 1989. Herpesvirus diseases of cattle, horses, and pigs. In Developments in Veterinary Virology. Boston: Klower Academic Publishers, pp. 230–325.

WITTMANN, G.; JAKUBIK, J.; AND AHL, R. 1980. Multiplication and distribution of Aujeszky's disease (pseudorabies) virus in vaccinated and non-vaccinated pigs after intranasal infection. Arch Virol 66:227–240.

WOHLGEMUTH, K.; LESLIE, P. F.; REED, D. E.; AND SMIDT, D. K. 1978. Pseudorabies virus associated with abortion in swine. J Am Vet Med Assoc 172:478–479.

ZIMMERMAN, J. J.; BERRY, W. J.; BERAN, G. W.; AND MURPHY, D. P. 1989. Influence of temperatures and age on the recovery of pseudorabies (Aujeszky's disease) virus from house flies, *Musca domestica*. Am J Vet Res 50:1471–1474.

25 Rabies

L. G. Morehouse

RABIES is a highly infectious viral disease of humans and animals, which dates to antiquity. Reports of the dramatic clinical signs of this disease were described in the writings of Plutarch and Celsus in A.D. 100 (Kelser 1947). Tierkel (1971) lists the earliest reference to the disease in Asia as one that occurs in the pre-Mosaic Eshnunna Code, predating the code of Hammurabi of ancient Babylon in the twenty-third century B.C.

In spite of the ancient history of the disease, many aspects of rabies are not clearly understood. Although almost all warm-blooded animals are susceptible, it is not well defined that long-held concepts of the fatal termination of the disease in humans is so for all species. There is, in fact, record of recovery from human rabies (U.S. Dep. HEW 1970) and recovery of dogs from experimental rabies infection (Nillson and Cortes 1975; Blenden 1979; Fekadu et al. 1983). Evidence also indicates that some animal species are more resistant to the infection than others (Bisseru 1972; Botros et al. 1979); discussion in this chapter suggests that swine fall in this category. Nonetheless, the overwhelming mortality associated with rabies infection makes it one of the most feared diseases of humans and animals.

ETIOLOGY. Rabies is caused by a filterable virus of the rhabdovirus group (Melnick and McCombs 1966). The external dimensions of the rabies particle are 75 × 180 nm. Its surface has a honeycomb appearance with projections 6–7 nm long (Witkor 1971). The particle is cylindrical, with one round or conical end and one planar or concave end (Murphy 1975). The virus is classified as a ribonucleic acid (RNA)-containing virus. The RNA is a single-stranded molecule with a molecular weight of 4.6×10^6 daltons per nucleocapsid (Witkor 1971). Sokol et al. (1969) have separated the different components of rabies virions from the purified virus. By treatment with sodium deoxycholate and combined velocity and equilibrium gradient centrifugation, the viral coat and the nucleocapsid are separated. The latter

contains all the RNA and is made up of 96% protein and 4% RNA. The five structural proteins and conclusions regarding their function and arrangement within the virion have been reviewed (Cox 1982).

EPIDEMIOLOGY. Traditionally, the disease has been said to exist in two epidemiologic forms: the urban type, spread mainly by dogs; and the wildlife type, seen principally in skunks, foxes, wolves, jackals, coyotes, weasels, and bats (Bisseru 1972). There was a marked shift to wildlife rabies in the United States during the 1960s and 1970s. By 1964, 75% of the rabies in the United States was in wildlife, and less than 10% was reported from dogs (U.S. Dep. HEW 1964). A more recent report confirms this trend with 88.4% of recorded cases in wildlife and only 2.7% in dogs (U.S. Dep. HHS 1989).

With this increased percentage of rabies occurring in wild animals, farm animals have been placed at greater risk to exposure. The true incidence of rabies in swine is difficult to assess. In the United States 854 cases were reported over the 17-year period of 1938–55 (Schoening 1956), representing 6.6% of cases reported in all farm animals. Cases of rabies on record in swine in the United States dropped to 3–8 annually and from 10 to 21 cases on an annual basis in Canada and Mexico (U.S. Dep. HEW 1969–83). This trend has continued through 1988 (U.S. Dep. HHS 1989). In a review of the global rabies situation, however, specific reference has been made to confirmed cases of porcine rabies in 25 different countries on five continents (Bisseru 1972). Yates et al. (1983) describe rabies outbreaks in 15 swine herds in western Canada over a 14-year period. Epidemiologic studies are now aided by monoclonal antibody analysis of various strains of rabies virus from different animals and geographic regions (Smith et al. 1984). Major antigenic groups of rabies virus in Canada have been determined by antinucleocapsid monoclonal antibodies allowing classification of antigenic groups by geographic area (Webster et al. 1986).

CLINICAL SIGNS. The typical course of the disease is one of sudden onset, loss of coordination, dullness, and later prostration. Death will likely ensue within 72 hours from the appearance of clinical signs (Merrimann 1966; Morehouse et

Some of the material presented in this chapter is based on experience encountered in an outbreak of rabies in a herd of Missouri swine. The author acknowledges contributions of his colleagues, Dr. L. D. Kintner, Dr. S. L. Nelson, and Dr. B. L. Moseley of the University of Missouri; the Veterinary Public Health Unit, Jefferson City, Mo.; and Veterinary Services Laboratories, APHIS, USDA, Ames, Iowa.

al. 1968). Peculiar twitching and preoccupation with the nose, similar to that observed in swine with rings recently placed in their noses, has been noted. This may be followed by prostration, rapid chewing movements, excessive salivation, and generalized clonic muscular spasms, which become less marked as the disease progresses until muscular activity is manifested only by fine tremors. Affected swine may be unable to squeal, and elevation of body temperature may be absent (Morehouse et al. 1968).

Oldenberger (1963) reported a paralytic form of rabies in swine in the U.S.S.R., with a duration of illness of 5–6 days. Gigstad (1971) reported clinical signs of rabies in experimentally infected swine that included an intermittent weakness in the rear legs, weakness in the shoulders, incoordination, posterior paralysis, prostration, paddling, and death. Merrimann (1966) documented one case of the furious form of rabies in a pig, but this pattern of behavior was observed in only 1 of 17 affected pigs. Hazlett and Keller (1986) reported an outbreak of porcine rabies in a closed feeder barn where clinical signs were not observed.

Although most reports suggest that swine die within 72–96 hours following development of clinical signs, there is indication of a wide variation in the incubation period. The report of Merrimann (1966) suggests an incubation period of approximately 70 days for one group of swine. Morehouse et al. (1968) reported that, since there was a progression of rabies cases in a drove of swine over a 2-month period, the incubation period would have been extremely variable if the disease resulted from a simultaneous exposure of a number of swine. Reichel and Möckelmann (1963) reported an outbreak of rabies in swine where the exposure time from rabid foxes was documented. Incubation periods of 9, 56, and 123 days were reported for the affected swine. Gigstad (1971) reported incubation periods in experimentally infected swine that varied from 12 days when exposed intracerebrally to 98 days when exposed intramuscularly.

PATHOGENESIS. The spread of rabies virus along peripheral or cranial nerves appears to be the major avenue of access to the central nervous system (CNS) following intramuscular or subcutaneous exposure to the virus. Dean et al. (1963) published convincing evidence that fixed and street rabies virus are ordinarily transmitted from the site of inoculation to the CNS by way of the peripheral nerves. Johnson (1971) emphasized that integrity of the nerve is necessary for CNS invasion, thus confirming the case for a neural pathway for the virus.

Rabies virus may enter the host via many routes, but the importance of oral and respiratory transmission is uncertain (Johnson 1971). Kucera et al. (1985) report three routes of entry from the eye to the brain: the oculomotor parasympathetic nerve, the preopticoretinal pathway, and the ophthalmic nerve. The mechanism by which virus gains access to the CNS has been studied by a number of workers. A progression of rabies infections in hamsters has been demonstrated, starting in striated muscle cells near the site of inoculation, with infection of myocytes and shedding of virus into extracellular spaces. A working hypothesis was proposed that the route of passive centripetal passage of rabies virus to the CNS is via peripheral nerve axoplasm from invasion at unmyelinated distal end organs to progeny release at synaptic junctions in the spinal cord (Murphy et al. 1973a). An infection of myocytes at the site of inoculation with rabies virus in skunks has been reported (Charlton and Casey 1979). Immunofluorescence in muscle fibers remote from the inoculation site occurred only after infection of lumbar cord and dorsal root ganglia, suggesting infection as a result of centrifugal neural migration of virus.

In the development of infection within the CNS, neurons of spinal cord, brain stem, hippocampus, septal nuclei, and limbic cortex appear especially vulnerable. Meningeal, ependymal, vascular endothelial, and glial cells show no antigen (Johnson 1971). However, Jackson and Reimer (1989) later reported infection of ependymal cells lining lateral ventricles in mice following intracerebral exposure and postulate that virus entry occurs at least in part by a cerebrospinal fluid pathway. Murphy et al. (1973b) proposed a mechanism of viral spread to include ascending infection within the CNS and centrifugal peripheral neural spread, with passive intraneuronal movement of subviral entities interspersed with active viral replication at cell surfaces, such that progeny virus might invade contiguous neurons or move within intercellular spaces to involve neural elements elsewhere. Charlton and Casey (1979) suggested direct transneuronal transfer of virus from perikarya and dendrites to adjacent axon terminals as a mechanism in dissemination of rabies in the CNS of striped skunks.

Whether or not factors such as the mechanism of virus spread via the nerves, significance of oral and respiratory transmission, selective cellular vulnerability, and host cell–virus relationships that might allow for latent infection can result in a variability in species susceptibility remains an unanswered question in the pathogenesis of rabies. This is particularly true in the case of swine, where the lack of detailed case reports or experimental studies and the relatively low reported number of cases in this species compound the problem.

LESIONS. Necropsy examination of rabid swine will likely fail to reveal gross changes (Merrimann 1966; Morehouse et al. 1968; Hazlett and Koller 1986). Histopathologic changes may be observed in the brain and spinal cord but may be variable. This is true for many species where changes may range from indiscernible, except for early necrosis of neurons and specific cytoplasmic inclusions in affected nerve cells, to a diffuse encephalitis (Smith et al. 1972).

The variability in neuropathologic response in other species affected with rabies seems true also for swine. In one text the authors indicate that neuronal degeneration may be very slight in pigs (Jubb et al. 1985). Merrimann (1966) reported the presence of Negri bodies in only one of three brains from rabid swine, although they were positive to the fluorescent rabies antibody test and had shown clinical signs of the disease. Gigstad (1971) reported an extensive nonsuppurative encephalitis in four pigs that had died following experimental inoculation with rabies virus. One animal had been inoculated intramuscularly and died 42 days postinoculation (PDI), while the other three had been inoculated intracerebrally and died 12–18 days PDI. Negri bodies were not observed. Hazlett and Koller (1986) reported only one Negri body in 10 sections of brain from a rabid pig.

Neuropathologic changes were observed in pigs dying from rabies, varying from a mild reaction in the brain consisting primarily of a mild vasculitis and focal gliosis to marked changes throughout the brain and spinal cord. Negri bodies were not observed (Morehouse et al. 1968). The changes included a diffuse meningitis of the brain and spinal cord, which was most severe in the leptomeninges covering the folia of the cerebellum (Fig. 25.1). The inflammatory response in the brain and spinal cord was characterized by perivascular cuffing that involved a high percentage of the larger vessels in both gray and

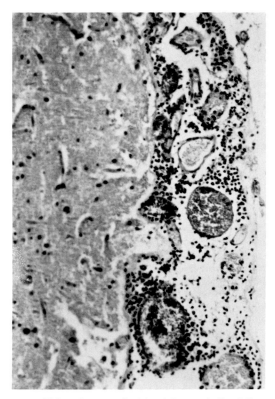

25.1. Diffuse leptomeningitis of the cerebellar folia. H & E. ×135.

white matter. Figure 25.2 shows marked perivascular cuffing of a vessel in the medulla.

Neuronal destruction observed throughout the brain and spinal cord was manifested by degeneration of neurons in the Purkinje cell layer of

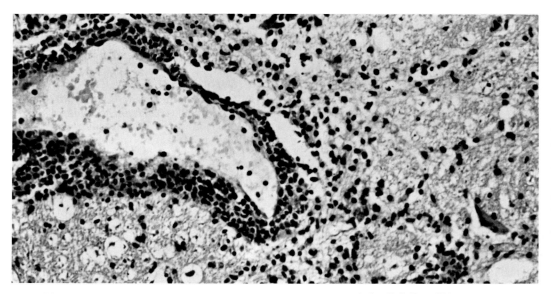

25.2. Marked perivascular cuffing and neuronal degeneration in the medulla. H & E. ×100.

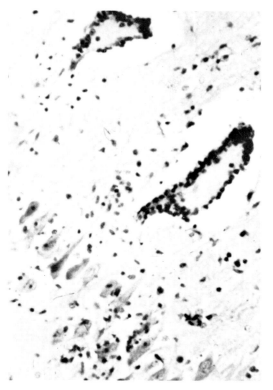

25.3. Neuronal degeneration in the pyramidal cell layer of the hippocampus. H & E. ×100.

the cerebellum. Phagocytosis of pyramidal cells was apparent (Fig. 25.3). The inflammatory change associated with the vessels in Figure 25.3 was primarily intramural in nature, with the Virchow-Robin space appearing clear. Degenerating neurons in other areas of the hippocampus were shrunken and stained heavily with eosin (Fig. 25.4). There was necrosis of neurons in the pons with accompanying satellitosis (Fig. 25.5) and neuronophagia (Fig. 25.6). Large motor neurons in the ventral horn of some segments of the spinal cord were undergoing degeneration (Fig. 25.7).

DIAGNOSIS

Animal Inoculation Test. The intracerebral inoculation of laboratory animals with brain material from animals suspected of being rabid is the oldest method of diagnosing rabies. Symptoms in weanling mice may be observed within 6–14 days, and the diagnosis of rabies is confirmed by the fluorescent antibody (FA) test (or the demonstration of Negri bodies in the mouse brains). For a negative result it is common to wait at least 21 days, although some workers have reported at least a 27-day incubation period in mice receiving brain material from rabid swine (Morehouse et al. 1968; Dillman 1973; Keiffer 1973). Additional confirmation includes a neutralization test in mice, using specific rabies immune serum.

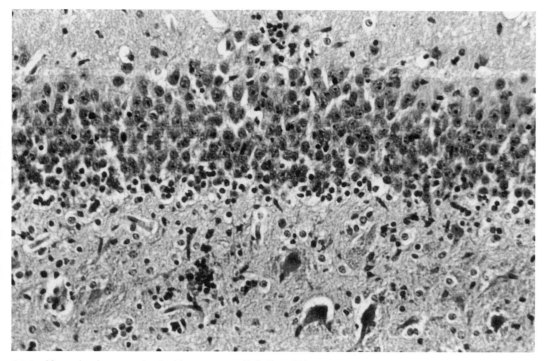

25.4. Necrosis of neurons in the hippocampus. H & E. ×100.

Histopathologic Examination. Negri (1903) established the first definitive pathologic diagnosis of rabies when he described the eosinophilic cytoplasmic inclusions in nerve cells and dendrites. A number of stains are available for demonstrating these inclusion bodies (Gradwohl 1943). Bosch (1966) described the use of acidified phenolphloxine for staining Negri bodies in paraffin sections. Negri bodies, however, are not found in all rabid animals. Runnells et al. (1965) stated that Negri bodies are not present in about 25% of rabid animals, and in many of the remaining 75% they are so few in number as to be overlooked. Lennette et al. (1965) reported that in a series of 365 rabies-positive specimens, only 239 (65.8%) were detected by the presence of Negri bodies; variability of their presence in swine rabies has been reported by Merrimann (1966), Morehouse et al. (1968), Gigstad (1971), Dhillon and Dhingra (1973), and Hazlett and Koller (1986).

Fluorescent Antibody Test. Goldwasser and Kissling (1958) were the first to apply the FA technique to the diagnosis of rabies. It has proved to be a rapid and accurate test. McQueen et al. (1960) demonstrated its dependability for diagnosing rabies in brain tissue that was Negri-body negative. Lennette and Emmons (1971) have emphasized that fluorescent antigen will be present and detectable in the brain at any stage of the disease in which the animal could possibly

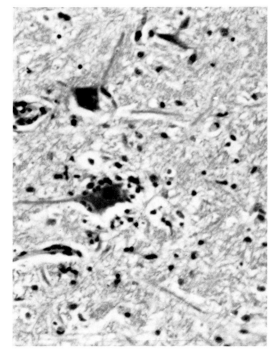

25.5. Satellitosis of a neuron in the pons. H & E. × 100.

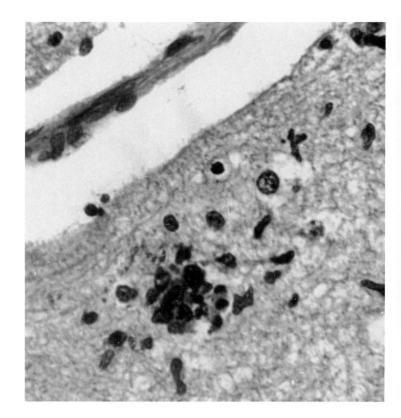

25.6. Phagocytosis of a dying neuron in the pons. H & E. × 400.

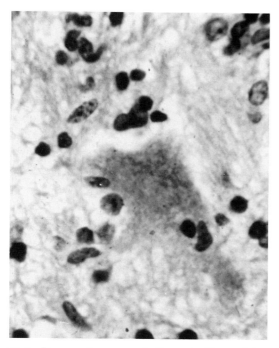

25.7. Degenerating neuron in the ventral horn of the spinal cord. H & E.

have transmitted rabies. Blenden (1978) described FA identification of rabies virus antigen in the skin of mice before clinical signs developed; he later reported its value for early detection of rabies virus antigen (Blenden et al. 1983). Several authors, however, have found swine specimens negative on FA in cases later diagnosed positive by mouse inoculation (Beauregard et al. 1965; Morehouse et al. 1968; Dhillon 1973).

Other Methods. Bourgon and Charlton (1987) demonstrated rabies antigen in paraffin-embedded tissue by the peroxidase-antiperoxidase method and found it superior to the FA technique for detection of antigen and preservation of morphologic detail. Perrin and Sureau (1987) described an experimental kit for rapid rabies enzyme immunodiagnosis (RREID). They found it to be specific, convenient, and a useful tool for epidemiologic studies and for laboratories without ultraviolet microscopes; it was not as sensitive as the FA technique.

Comment. Gigstad (1971) concluded from experimental studies that swine may have a relatively high natural resistance to the rabies virus and this might be responsible for unpredictable behavior of the disease when it occurs as a herd problem. Blenden (1979) inoculated two weanling pigs by the intramuscular route with street rabies virus. No clinical signs were observed, although high titers of antibody were found in cerebrospinal fluid and blood. Whether natural resistance

of swine to rabies results in aberrant clinical signs, thus confusing the diagnosis, remains open to question.

These observations do emphasize problems that may be encountered in the clinical and laboratory diagnosis of rabies in swine, and they point to the value of careful neuropathologic examination and other laboratory procedures in differentiating rabies from other encephalitides of swine described in this volume.

TREATMENT AND PREVENTION. The extremely limited literature and experience with rabies in swine give no indication of effective treatment for this disease, nor is there any indication of vaccine development for this species. However, producers and veterinarians should be aware of the unpredictable behavior of swine affected with this disease when it occurs as a herd problem. Preventive measures consist principally of limiting exposure, particularly where rabies is endemic in wildlife populations adjacent to areas where swine are maintained.

REFERENCES

BEAUREGARD, M.; BOULANGER, P.; AND WEBSTER, W. A. 1965. The use of fluorescent antibody staining in the diagnosis of rabies. Can J Comp Med 29:141–147.
BISSERU, B. 1972. Rabies. London: William Heinemann Medical Books, p. 17.
BLENDEN, D. C. 1978. Identification of rabies virus antigen in the skin by immunofluorescent staining. Zoonoses 1, PAHO/WHO Zoonoses Center, pp. 7–11.
_____. 1979. Personal communication.
BLENDEN, D. C.; BELL, J. L.; TSAO, A. L.; AND USNOK, O. U. 1983. Immunofluorescent examination of skin of rabies infected animals as a means of early detection of rabies antigen. J Clin Microbiol 18:631–636.
BOSCH, R. 1966. Acidified phenol-phloxine for staining Negri bodies in paraffin section. Stain Technol 41(4):250.
BOTROS, B. A. M.; LEWIS, J. C.; AND KERKOR, M. 1979. A study to evaluate nonfatal rabies in animals. J Trop Med Hyg 82:137–141.
BOURGON, A. R., AND CHARLTON, K. M. 1987. The demonstration of rabies antigen in paraffin-embedded tissues using a peroxidase anti-peroxidase method. Can J Vet Res 51(1):117–120.
CHARLTON, K. M., AND CASEY, G. A. 1979. Experimental rabies in skunks—immunofluorescence light and electron microscope studies. Lab Invest 41:36–44.
COX, J. H. 1982. The structural proteins of rabies virus. Comp Immun Microbiol Infect Dis 5:21–25.
DEAN, D. J.; EVANS, W. M.; AND McCLURE, R. C. 1963. Pathogenesis of rabies. Bull WHO 29:803.
DHILLON, S. S., AND DHINGRA, P. N. 1973. Rabies in swine. Vet Med Small Anim Clin 68:1044.
DILLMAN, R. 1973. Personal communication.
FEKADU, M.; SHADDUCK, J. H.; CHANDLER, T. W.; AND BAER, G. M. 1983. Rabies virus in the tonsils of a carrier dog. Arch Virol 78:37–47.
GIGSTAD, D. C. 1971. Experimental rabies in swine. Dev Stud Lab Invest, APHIS, USDA, p. 20.
GOLDWASSER, R. A., AND KISSLING, R. E. 1958. Fluorescent antibody staining of street and fixed rabies virus antigens. Proc Soc Exp Biol Med 98:219.

GRADWOHL, R. B. H. 1943. Clinical Laboratory Methods and Diagnosis, 3d ed., vol. 1. St. Louis: C. Y. Mosby.

HAXLETT, M. F., AND KELLER, M. A. 1986. Porcine rabies in a closed feeder barn. Can Vet J 27:116–118.

JACKSON, A. C., AND REIMER, D. L. 1989. Pathogenesis of experimental rabies in mice: An immunohistochemical study. Acta Neuropathol 78(2):159–165.

JOHNSON, R. T. 1971. The pathogenesis of experimental rabies. In Rabies. Ed. Y. Nagano and F. Davenport. Baltimore, London, Tokyo: University Park Press, pp. 59–72.

JUBB, K. F. V.; KENNEDY, P. C.; AND PALMER, N. 1985. Pathology of Domestic Animals, vol. 1. New York: Academic Press, p. 295.

KEIFFER, M. 1973. Personal communication.

KELSER, R. A. 1947. Rabies. In Diseases Transmitted from Animals to Man, 3d ed. Ed. T. G. Hull. Springfield, Ill.: Charles C Thomas, p. 338.

KUCERA, P.; DOLIVO, M.; COULON, P.; AND FLAMAND, A. 1985. Pathways of the early propagation of virulent and avirulent rabies strains from the eye to the brain. J Virol 55:158–162.

LENNETTE, E. H., AND EMMONS, R. W. 1971. The laboratory diagnosis of rabies: Review and perspective. In Rabies. Ed. Y. Nagano and F. Davenport. Baltimore, London, Tokyo: University Park Press, p. 77.

LENNETTE, E. H.; WOODIE, J. D.; NAKAMURA, K.; AND MAGOFFIN, R. L. 1965. The diagnosis of rabies by fluorescent antibody method (FRA) employing immune hamster serum. Health Lab Sci 2(12):24.

McQUEEN, J. L.; LEWIS, A. L.; AND SCHNEIDER, N. J. 1960. Diagnosis by fluorescent antibody. I. Its evaluation in a public health laboratory. Am J Public Health 50:1743.

MELNICK, J. L., AND McCOMBS, R. M. 1966. Classification and nomenclature of animal viruses. Prog Med Virol 8:400.

MERRIMANN, G. M. 1966. Rabies in Tennessee swine. J Am Vet Med Assoc 148:809.

MOREHOUSE, L. G.; KINTNER, L. D.; AND NELSON, S. L. 1968. Rabies in swine. J Am Vet Med Assoc 153:56.

MURPHY, F. A. 1975. Rabies virus. Morphology and morphogenesis. In The Natural History of Rabies. Ed. G. M. Baer. New York, London: Academic Press, p. 33.

MURPHY, F. A.; BAUER, S. P.; HARRISON, A. K.; AND WINN, W. C. 1973a. Comparative pathogenesis of rabies and rabies-like viruses – viral infection and transit from inoculation site to the central nervous system. Lab Invest 28:361–376.

MURPHY, F. A.; HARRISON, A. K.; WINN, W. C.; AND BAUER, S. P. 1973b. Comparative pathogenesis of rabies and rabies-like viruses – Infection of the central nervous system and centrifugal spread of virus to peripheral tissues. Lab Invest 29:1–16.

NEGRI, A. 1903. Beitrag zum Studium der Aetiologie der Zollswith. Z Hyg Infektionskr 43:507. Cited in Infectious Diseases of Domestic Animals, 3d ed. Ed.

W. A. Hagan and D. W. Bruner. Ithaca, N.Y.: Comstock, p. 735.

NILLSON, M. R., AND CORTES, J. DE A. 1975. Spontaneous recovery from rabies of a dog infected experimentally. Rev Fac Med Vet Zootech Univ Sao Paulo 12:229–233.

OLDENBERGER, A. A. 1963. Peculiarities in the trend of rabies in swine. Veterinariia 40:30.

PERRIN, P., AND SUREAU, P. 1987. A collaborative study of an experimental kit for rapid rabies enzyme immunodiagnosis (RREID). Bull WHO 65(4):489–493.

REICHEL, K., AND MÖCKELMANN. 1963. Tollwut bein Schwein. Tieraerztl Umsch 18:445. Abstr Vet Bull 34 (189):143. 1964.

RUNNELLS, R. A.; MONLUX, W. S.; AND MONLUX, A. W. 1965. Principles of Veterinary Pathology, 7th ed. Ames: Iowa State Univ Press.

SCHOENING, H. 1956. Rabies. In Animal Diseases. Yearbook of Agriculture. Washington, D.C.: USDA, p. 199.

SMITH, H. A.; JONES, T. C.; AND HUNT, R. D. 1972. Veterinary Pathology, 4th ed. Philadelphia: Lea & Febiger, p. 353.

SMITH, J. S.; SUMNER, J. W.; ROUMILLAT, L. F.; BAER, G. M.; AND WINKLER, W. G. 1984. Antigenic characteristics of isolates associated with a new epizootic of racoon rabies in the United States. J Infect Dis 149:769–774.

SOKOL, F.; SCHLUMBERGER, D.; WITKOR, T. J.; KOPROWSKI, H.; AND HUMMELER, K. 1969. Biochemical and biological studies on the nucleocapsid and RNA of rabies virus. Virology 38:651.

TIERKEL, E. S. 1971. In Rabies. Ed. Y. Nagano and F. M. Davenport. Baltimore, London, Tokyo: University Park Press, p. 3.

U.S. DEPARTMENT OF HEALTH, EDUCATION AND WELFARE (HEW). 1964. Communicable Disease Center Zoonoses Surveillance, Annual Rabies Summary. Public Health Serv, Washington, D.C.

_____. 1970. Communicable Disease Center Zoonoses Surveillance. Annual Rabies Summary. Public Health Serv, Washington, D.C.

_____. 1969–83. Communicable Disease Center Zoonoses Surveillance. Annual Rabies Summary. Public Health Serv, Washington, D.C.

U.S. DEPARTMENT OF HEALTH AND HUMAN SERVICES (HHS). 1989. Rabies Surveillance Annual Summary for 1988. Atlanta: Centers for Disease Control.

WEBSTER, W. A.; CASEY, G. A.; AND CHARLTON, K. M. 1986. Major antigenic groups of rabies virus in Canada determined by antinucleocapsid monoclonal antibodies. Comp Immunol Microbiol Infect Dis 9(1):59–69.

WITKOR, T. J. 1971. Nature and properties of the rabies virus in rabies. In Rabies. Ed. Y. Nagano and F. M. Davenport. Baltimore, London, Tokyo: University Park Press, p. 37.

YATES, W. D. H.; REHMTULLA, A. J.; AND McINTOSH, D. W. 1983. Porcine rabies in western Canada. Can Vet J 24:162–163.

26 Rotavirus and Reovirus

P. S. PAUL

G. W. STEVENSON

Porcine Rotavirus

ROTAVIRUSES ARE important enteric pathogens in neonates of many species, including pigs. The enteropathogenicity of porcine rotavirus has been demonstrated by their ability to produce severe gastroenteritis and villous atrophy under experimental conditions in gnotobiotic and colostrum-deprived pigs in the absence of other pathogens. They are also frequently detected in pigs with diarrhea. Subclinical infections with porcine rotavirus are equally common and suggest that other factors such as host, agent, and environment may be important in the pathogenesis of disease by porcine rotavirus.

Rotaviruses were first detected in calves (Mebus et al. 1969) and were subsequently identified in humans and other animals (Estes et al. 1983). Serologic evidence for rotavirus infection in pigs was first shown using bovine rotavirus as an antigen (Woode and Bridger 1975). Subsequently, porcine rotavirus was detected by other researchers (Rodger et al. 1975; Lecce et al. 1976; McNulty et al. 1976; Woode et al. 1976; Chasey and Lucas 1977; Bohl et al. 1978; Tzipori and Williams 1978). Porcine rotaviruses have now been detected in many of the swine-producing countries (Lecce et al. 1976; McNulty et al. 1976; Woode et al. 1976; Bohl et al. 1978; Bridger 1980; Corthier et al. 1980; Saif et al. 1980; Bohl et al. 1982; Askaa et al. 1983; Nilsson et al. 1984; Utrera et al. 1984; Theil et al. 1985; Dea et al. 1986; Ferrari et al. 1986; Fu and Hampson 1987; Kim et al. 1987; Nagesha and Holmes 1988; Paul et al. 1988a). Rotaviruses, regardless of species of origin, were initially shown to share a common group antigen (Woode et al. 1976; Thouless et al. 1977; Estes et al. 1983). It was later shown that rotaviruses are quite diverse serologically (Bridger 1980; Saif et al. 1980; Askaa and Bloch 1981; McNulty et al. 1981). To date seven distinct serogroups of rotavirus have been described (Pedley et al. 1986; Bridger 1987). Group A rotavirus appears to be the most common and best studied group of rotaviruses. Therefore, the majority of the information presented here pertains to porcine group A rotavirus. Information on other rotavirus groups is covered where appropriate.

ETIOLOGY

Virus Morphology. Rotavirus particles are nonenveloped and have a distinctive wheellike appearance when examined by negative-staining electron microscopy. *Rota* is wheel in Latin, hence, they were classified as rotavirus. Complete rotavirus particles have a well-defined outer rim, a feature that distinguishes them from the other two genus members, reovirus and orbivirus, of family Reoviridae. Three forms of virus particles are visible by negative-staining electron microscopy. The double-capsid virus particles have an outer capsid layer, an inner capsid layer, and an icosahedral core and measure approximately 75 nm in diameter (Fig. 26.1A). The single-capsid virus particles are approximately 60 nm in diameter and lack the outer capsid layer (Fig. 26.1B). Cores are approximately 52 nm in diameter and contain viral genome and RNA-dependent RNA polymerase. Only double-capsid virus particles are infectious.

Classification. Rotaviruses are classified in the family Reoviridae under the genus *Rotavirus*. Early studies demonstrated that all rotaviruses, regardless of species of origin, were antigenically related (Woode et al. 1976; Thouless et al. 1977; Estes et al. 1983). The common group antigen is contained in viral structural protein VP6 on the inner capsid (Estes and Cohen 1989). It became clear that rotaviruses are quite diverse antigenically, for rotaviruses that resembled classical rotaviruses but lacked common group antigen were detected (Bridger 1980; Saif et al. 1980; Askaa and Bloch 1981; McNulty et al. 1981; Bridger et al. 1982). Such rotaviruses have been termed novel rotavirus, rotaviruslike virus, pararotavirus, atypical rotavirus, and antigenically distinct rotavirus (Bridger 1980; Saif et al. 1980; Bohl et al. 1982; Bridger et al. 1982; Pedley et al. 1983; Snodgrass et al. 1984; Theil et al. 1985; Pedley et

331

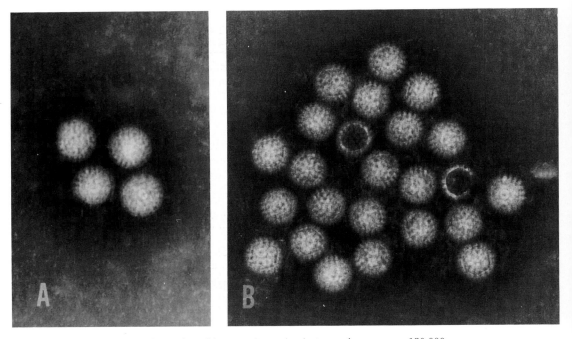

26.1. Rotavirus particles in feces viewed by negative-stain electron microscopy. × 130,000. (A) Double-shelled virus particles with intact outer capsids have characteristic smooth outlines. (B) Single-shelled particles lack outer capsids and have spiked outlines.

al. 1986; Bridger 1987). Serogroups with common group antigen on inner capsid were identified by serologic tests such as immunofluorescence, enzyme-linked immunosorbent assay (ELISA), or immune electron microscopy (Bridger 1980; Saif et al. 1980; Pedley et al. 1983; Theil and Saif 1985; Chasey et al. 1986; Pedley et al. 1986). Seven antigenically distinct groups (A–G) of rotavirus have now been reported, four (A, B, C, and E) of which affect pigs (Bridger 1980; Saif et al. 1980; Bohl et al. 1982; Pedley et al. 1983; Chasey et al. 1986; Pedley et al. 1986). Group A rotaviruses represent the earliest recognized rotaviruses, which appear to be most commonly associated with gastroenteritis and are best characterized. Group B rotaviruses, also referred to as atypical rotaviruses or rotaviruslike virus, have been detected in pigs, cattle, and humans (Bridger 1980; Bridger et al. 1982; Pedley et al. 1983; Theil et al. 1985). Group C rotaviruses, also designated as pararotavirus, have been detected in pigs and humans (Saif et al. 1980; Bohl et al. 1982; Pedley et al. 1983; Espejo et al. 1984; Bridger et al. 1986). Group E rotaviruses have only been detected in pigs in the United Kingdom (Chasey et al. 1986), whereas, rotavirus of groups D, F, and G have been detected in chickens and turkeys (Pedley et al. 1986; Bridger 1987). Genome of rotavirus when subjected to electrophoresis in polyacrylamide gel yields a characteristic electrophoretic migration commonly referred to as an electropherotype. Rotaviruses of serogroups identified thus far have unique elec-

tropherotypes, which have been used to differentiate rotaviruses into groups (Pedley et al. 1986). RNA segments cluster in four regions, I–IV (Fig. 26.2). Group A rotaviruses have 4:2:3:2 segments in regions I, II, III, and IV respectively. This pattern is 4:2:2:3 for group B rotavirus, and 4:3:2:2 for group C rotavirus. In group E rotavirus, the pattern is similar to that seen with group B rotavirus except segments 7–11 migrate equidistance from each other (Pedley et al. 1986). There appears to be a correlation between electropherotype and serogroups, however, it is emphasized that serological assays are more reliable.

Rotaviruses within group A have been further divided into subgroups and serotypes. Two subgroups, S_I and S_{II}, within group A rotavirus have been reported (Greenberg et al. 1983a). Recent evidence indicates that viruses of additional subgroups may be prevalent in nature (Svensson et al. 1988). Serotypes within a serogroup are defined by plaque reduction or fluorescent focus-reduction assays using hyperimmune serum (Bohl et al. 1984; Hoshino et al. 1984; Paul et al. 1988a). A minimum of twentyfold difference in the neutralization titer between the homologous and heterologous rotavirus is required for a virus to be considered as a different serotype. A total of 11 serotypes have been described (Estes and Cohen 1989).

Serotyping is complex and sometimes gives ambiguous results, due to involvement of two surface proteins, VP4 and VP7, which induce neutralizing antibodies (Greenberg et al. 1983b). The

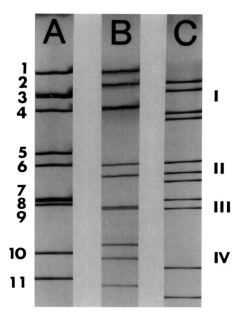

26.2. Electrophoretic patterns (electropherotypes) of A/OSU, B/IA1146, and C/Cowden strains of group A, B, and C rotavirus in polyacrylamide gel stained with silver. Each rotavirus group has a distinct electropherotype. Double-stranded RNA segments cluster in four regions, I–IV. Numbers of bands in the four regions are 4:2:3:2, 4:2:2:3, and 4:3:2:2 for rotavirus groups A, B, and C respectively.

genes coding for these surface proteins segregate independently (Hoshino et al. 1985). A majority of hyperimmune antisera prepared against the purified virions contain antibodies to VP7, therefore, classical neutralization assays using hyperimmune antisera recognize serotypes based on VP7. A new classification scheme has been proposed that takes into account typing of both VP4 and VP7 surface proteins (Estes and Cohen 1989). VP7 types are designated as G types for glycoprotein, whereas VP4 types are designated as P types for protease sensitive protein.

Virus is designated by group/strain/subgroup/G type/P type. At least five G (VP7) serotypes of porcine rotavirus have been described (Bohl et al. 1984; Hoshino et al. 1984; Nagesha and Holmes 1988; Paul et al. 1988a; Ruiz et al. 1988; Paul et al. 1990a,b, 1991). Information on G type and other serotype designations of selected porcine rotavirus strains is presented in Table 26.1. At least two P (VP4) types have been detected among porcine rotaviruses, however, information on P type on most porcine strains is not available at this time. Monoclonal antibodies (Kang et al. 1989; Nagesha et al. 1989) and nucleic acid probes (Johnson et al. 1990; Paul et al. 1990a,c; Rosen et al. 1990) are becoming available, which will allow typing of porcine rotaviruses by G and P types in the near future.

Physicochemical and Biologic Properties. Rotavirus is extremely stable and is resistant to environmental conditions such as temperature, pH, chemicals, and disinfectants. Rotavirus is stable at pH 3–9. In fecal preparations rotavirus are resistant to temperatures of 60°C for 30 minutes and for at least 7–9 months at 18–20°C (Woode 1986). Cell culture–adapted rotavirus vary in susceptibility to heat. Strains A/OSU and C/Cowden were inactivated by heat at 56°C for 30 minutes, whereas, A/Gottfried strain was resistant to heat at 56°C (Terrett et al. 1987). Rotavirus in the presence of organic material is inactivated by 2% acid glutaraldehyde, 70% ethanol, 3.7% formaldehyde, 10% povidone-iodine, 67% chloramine T, and 0.5% triclosan (Sattar et al. 1983; Woode 1986). Rotavirus is resistant to treatments by ether, chloroform, and genetron. Calcium chloride but not magnesium chloride stabilizes infectivity. Calcium ion chelators such as ethylenediamine tetraacetic acid (EDTA) at 5 mM concentration remove the outer layer and destroy infectivity.

The rotavirus genome is double-stranded RNA and has 11 segments. The total molecular size of rotavirus is estimated at approximately 18,522 base pairs by nucleic acid–sequence analysis and

Table 26.1.   **Serogroup and serotype designations of selected porcine rotavirus isolates**

Sero-group	Strain	Serotype VP7 (G)[a]	Serotype VP4 (P)[a]	Other Serotype Designations	Reference
A	OSU	5	7	Porcine serotype 1	Bohl et al. 1984; Hoshino et al. 1984
	Gottfried	4	6	Porcine serotype 2	Bohl et al. 1984; Hoshino et al. 1984
	SB-1A	4	7	Natural reassortant	Hoshino et al. 1984, 1988
	CRW-8	3	?		Nagesha and Holmes 1988
	ISU-64	9-like	7		Paul et al. 1988a, 1991a
	ISU-65	3	7		Paul et al. 1988a, 1990a
	YM	11	?		Ruiz et al. 1988
B	Ohio				Theil et al. 1985
	NIRD-I				Pedley et al. 1983
	IA1146				Paul 1990
C	Cowden				Bohl et al. 1982
	IA850				Proescholdt and Paul 1990
E	DC-9				Pedley et al. 1986

[a]Based on classification scheme proposed by Estes and Cohen (1989).

electron microscopy (Rixon et al. 1984; Estes and Cohen 1989). The inner capsid is composed of two major structural proteins, VP2 and VP6. The VP6 protein contains the group and subgroup antigens. Recent evidence shows that subgroup-specific epitopes may also be located on VP2 (Greenberg et al. 1983a; Svensson et al. 1990). The outer capsid has two surface proteins, VP4 and VP7 (Estes and Cohen 1989). The VP4 protein, also referred to as VP3 prior to 1987 (Liu et al. 1988), is nonglycosylated, contains hemagglutinin, and is important for infectivity and virulence (Greenberg et al. 1983a; Kalica et al. 1983; Offit et al. 1986a). Proteolytic cleavage of VP4 into VP5 and VP8 is important for viral infectivity. It is coded in gene segment 4. The VP7 is the second most abundant viral structural protein of 37 kD, is glycosylated, and is coded in either gene segment 8 or 9 depending upon strain of virus. Both VP4 and VP7 induce neutralizing antibodies (Greenberg et al. 1983b; Offit and Blavat 1986), are important in induction of immunity (Offit et al. 1986b), and segregate independently (Hoshino et al. 1985). Thus, theoretically reassortant rotavirus strains containing any combination of P and G types are possible. One such strain, SB-1A, with a G4 and P7 type has been described (Hoshino et al. 1984; Midthun et al. 1987). The buoyant density of the double-shelled, single-shelled, and core particles in cesium chloride is 1.36 g/ml, 1.38 g/ml, and 1.44 g/ml respectively (Bridger and Woode 1976; Bican et al. 1982). Some strains of porcine rotavirus possess a hemagglutinin (Eiguchi et al. 1987; Paul 1990) and hemagglutinate human type O, guinea pig, and rat erythrocytes.

Cultivation. Rotaviruses have been difficult to cultivate in cell cultures. Porcine rotavirus was first adapted to grow in porcine primary kidney cell cultures by pretreatment of virions with trypsin or pancreatin (Theil et al. 1977). Virus was later successfully propagated in African monkey kidney cell line MA-104 (Bohl et al. 1984). Use of roller cultures of MA-104 and addition of proteolytic enzymes, trypsin or pancreatin, was essential in isolation of rotavirus. Trypsin enhances growth of bovine rotavirus by as much as 1000-fold (Almeida and Hall 1978). Many strains of group A porcine rotavirus have now been cultivated in roller cultures of MA-104 cell line by pretreatment of virions with trypsin (10 μg/ml for 30 minutes) or pancreatin before infection. Alternatively, trypsin or pancreatin (0.5–1.0 μg/ml) is added in serum-free culture medium after virus adsorption. Cell culture–adapted rotavirus strains produce cytopathic effect characterized by rounding of cells followed by removal of cells from the surface. Viral antigen can be demonstrated in cytoplasm of virus-infected cells by immunofluorescence (Fig. 26.3) or immunochemical methods.

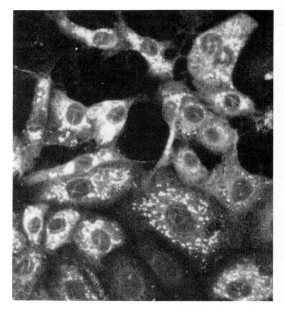

26.3. Immunofluorescent staining of MA-104 cell line infected with group A porcine rotavirus showing cytoplasmic accumulation of rotaviral antigens. × 400.

Rotavirus form plaques under agarose in the presence of neutral red.

One strain of group C rotavirus has been propagated in porcine primary kidney cell cultures (Terrett and Saif 1987). Roller cultures and incorporation of high concentrations of pancreatin in culture medium were essential for virus propagation (Terrett and Saif 1987). After nine passages in primary kidney cells, group C rotavirus was adapted to grow in MA-104 cell line (Saif et al. 1988). Recently, a porcine intestinal cell line has been successfully used to propagate C/Cowden and an Iowa strain C/IA850 of group C rotavirus (Proescholdt and Paul 1991). Roller cultures and addition of high concentrations of pancreatin were required for virus growth. Groups B and E rotavirus and some strains of group A rotavirus still cannot be serially propagated in cell cultures. Group B porcine rotavirus produces syncytia in monolayers of MA-104 following centrifugation of virus (Theil and Saif 1985). Viral antigen is present in inoculated cells without evidence for productive infection. Such cultures with cytoplasmic viral antigen have proven useful in a cell culture immunofluorescent assay (CCIF) for the detection of antibodies (Theil and Saif 1985).

EPIDEMIOLOGY. Porcine rotavirus is ubiquitous in swine herds wherever swine are raised. Serologic surveys show that high percentage (77–100%) of the adult swine are seropositive for porcine groups A, B, and C rotavirus (Bridger and Brown 1985; Terrett et al. 1987). Antibodies to group E rotavirus are also common in the United

Kingdom (Chasey et al. 1986). It is difficult to raise pigs free of rotavirus under normal husbandry conditions.

There appears to be an age-related variation in serologic incidence, for antibodies to group B and C were lowest in pigs 3–8 weeks of age, whereas all pigs of this age had antibodies to the group A rotavirus (Bridger and Brown 1985). Similarly, antibodies to group C rotavirus were detected in 100% of adults, 59% of weanlings, and 86% of nursing pigs tested from Ohio (Terrett et al. 1987).

Infection with porcine rotavirus is enzootic in swine herds. Virus spreads among pigs via fecal-oral route. Following natural infection with rotavirus, pigs develop circulating and secretory antibodies and are immune to infection with homologous rotavirus. Antibodies are transferred to newborns through colostrum and milk; duration of persistence of these passively acquired antibodies varies with the initial antibody level acquired and appears to last 3–5 weeks (Tzipori et al. 1980a). Piglets born to gilts are more susceptible to rotavirus infection than those born to sows (Askaa et al. 1983; Svensmark et al. 1989a). Pigs usually become infected between 7 and 41 days of age, and infrequently infected at less than 7 days of age (Bohl et al. 1978). In one cohort study (Fu and Hampson 1987), pigs became infected at an average age of 19 days with a range of 13–39 days. Virus is shed in feces and is the major source of infection; highest amount of virus is shed during the acute stages of infection. The duration of group A porcine rotavirus shedding in feces is about 7.4 days with a range of 1–14 days. Virus shedding is affected by the level of passive immunity and serogroup of porcine rotavirus. In group B rotavirus infections, lower amounts of rotavirus are shed for a shorter duration (Bridger 1980; Theil et al. 1985).

Recurrent infections with porcine rotavirus have been detected with intermittent virus shedding (Debouck and Pensaert 1983). These possibly represent infections of different serogroup or serotype. Adult animals do not generally shed rotavirus (Debouck and Pensaert 1983; Fu and Hampson 1987); however, occasionally they may shed rotavirus near farrowing (Benfield et al. 1982) and may serve as source of infection for susceptible pigs.

Limited data is available on the relative prevalence of rotaviruses, especially of different serogroups and serotypes. Rotavirus infections account for about 14% of diarrheas in pigs (Janke et al. 1989, 1990; Paul et al. 1990c). Group A rotavirus is by far the predominant porcine rotavirus detected in diarrheic pigs (Janke et al. 1989; Paul et al. 1990c). Out of 90 rotavirus samples 67% were group A, 10% group B, 12% C, and 11% mixed rotavirus infections (Janke et al. 1989). In nursing pigs the majority were group A;

whereas, in weaned pigs 38% were group A, 19% were group B, and 24% were group C. Similarly, 89% of the samples that were positive for rotavirus were group A rotavirus (Paul et al. 1990c). Groups B and C accounted for 8% and 3% respectively. Additional studies are needed to fully determine the relative prevalence of rotavirus serogroups and serotypes.

Contaminated environment plays an important role in maintenance of rotavirus in swine herds. Porcine rotavirus is stable at extreme environmental conditions and is resistant to commonly used disinfectants. Porcine rotavirus can be detected in dry feces, dust, and sewage of farrowing and weaner barns (Fu et al. 1989). Porcine rotavirus survived in swine barns kept empty for 3 months (Fu et al. 1989).

CLINICAL SIGNS. Numerous rotavirus inoculation studies in nonimmune gnotobiotic or colostrum-deprived pigs fed a liquid diet have resulted in consistent production of clinical disease. Disease is most severe in pigs inoculated when 1–5 days of age (Woode et al. 1976; Pearson and McNulty 1977; Tzipori and Williams 1978; Debouck and Pensaert 1979; McAdaragh et al. 1980; Narita et al. 1982a). After an incubation period of 12–24 hours, pigs become anorexic and listless and occasionally vomit. Severe, profuse diarrhea begins 1–4 hours later. Feces are watery, yellow to white, and contain variable amounts of flocculent material. Diarrhea continues for 3–5 days, then feces progressively return to normal in 7–14 days. Pigs become dehydrated and may die 2–5 days following the onset of diarrhea; mortality may reach 50–100%. Diarrhea and dehydration are less severe in pigs inoculated when 7–21 days old (Crouch and Woode 1978; Theil et al. 1978; Shaw et al. 1989a). Disease is limited to transient diarrhea of 1–1.5 days duration in pigs inoculated when 28 days old (Tzipori et al. 1980b; Lecce et al. 1982). Mortality rates decrease as the age of inoculation increases; death is unusual in pigs older than 14 days. No clinical disease results when 21- to 28-day-old pigs that have consumed a dry diet for more than 3 days are inoculated with rotavirus (Tzipori et al. 1980b; Stevenson 1990; Stevenson et al. 1990).

Rotavirus inoculation studies conducted in nonimmune pigs likely represent the more severe limits of rotavirus-induced clinical disease. Naturally occurring rotavirus infection in pigs often results in less severe clinical disease or is subclinical. Rotavirus is endemic in most swine herds, i.e., nearly all gilts and sows are to some degree immune. A commensurate degree of immunity is passed to suckling pigs via colostrum and milk (Askaa et al. 1983). Levels of specific rotavirus antibodies in colostrum and milk decline dramatically in the first few days of lactation and rotavirus replication occurs in pigs when the oral challenge level of virus exceeds the consumed milk-borne passive immunity. Management practices that impact either the level of passive immunity or the level of oral virus challenge differ between swine herds and may result in consistent yet differing patterns of rotavirus-associated disease.

Naturally occurring rotavirus-associated diarrheal disease is most often reported in 7- to 41-day-old suckling pigs (Bohl et al. 1978; Roberts et al. 1980; Askaa et al. 1983; Debouck and Pensaert 1983; Svensmark et al. 1989b) or within 7 days following weaning (Woode et al. 1976; Bohl et al. 1978; Lecce and King 1978; Tzipori et al. 1980a). The age of onset is often consistent in a given herd. Where rotavirus is not complicated by concurrent infection with other enteric pathogens, diarrhea in suckling pigs is usually mild and limited to 2–3 days duration. Feces are yellow or white, watery to creamy, and variably flocculant. Dehydration is usually mild and mortality is less than 15% of clinically ill pigs. Morbidity is variable, but is often 10–20%. Diarrhea sometimes progresses to younger pigs in a farrowing room as more pigs are affected. Dehydration is more severe in the younger pigs. Gilt litters may be affected at a younger age with more severe disease than are sow litters. Diarrheic suckling pigs frequently shed rotavirus along with other enteric pathogens such as transmissible gastroenteritis (TGE) virus (Bohl et al. 1978), coccidia (Roberts et al. 1980), or enterotoxigenic *E. coli* (Bohl et al. 1978). Diarrhea is generally more severe and morbidity and mortality are greater in combined infections.

The role of rotaviruses in diarrheic syndromes in recently weaned pigs is unclear. Rotaviruses have been implicated as a primary cause of severe diarrhea in recently weaned pigs resulting in 10–50% mortality (Woode 1986); however, rotavirus inoculation studies in weaned pigs do not support such conclusions. Where rotavirus shedding has been associated with severe diarrhea in weaned pigs, it has been in combination with TGE virus (Bohl et al. 1978) or with hemolytic colony types of enterotoxigenic *E. coli* (Bohl et al. 1978; Tzipori et al. 1980a; Lecce et al. 1982). Inoculation studies in weaned pigs with rotavirus and hemolytic colony types of enterotoxigenic *E. coli* suggest a subservient yet potentially important role for rotaviruses in severe diarrheic postweaning syndromes in pigs (Tzipori et al. 1980b; Lecce et al. 1982). Inoculation of weaned pigs with rotavirus or hemolytic *E. coli* alone results in mild transient diarrhea or no clinical disease; whereas, inoculation of weaned pigs with rotavirus followed by hemolytic *E. coli* results in efficient hemolytic *E. coli* colonization and severe protracted diarrhea typical of that reported in natural outbreaks.

Differences in virulence between group A rotavirus strains have been reported in humans (Ka-

pikian and Chanock 1990) and calves (Bridger and Pocock 1986). Differences in the outer capsid protein VP4 have been implicated as the cause of the differing virulence between human group A rotavirus strains (Kapikian and Chanock 1990). It is not clear whether there are differences in virulence between serotypes or strains of swine group A rotaviruses. Inoculation studies in pigs with serotype 4 (Bohl et al. 1984; Benfield et al. 1988), serotype 5 (Theil et al. 1978; Janke et al. 1988), and a new serotype represented by strain ISU64 (Stevenson 1990; Stevenson et al. 1990) have resulted in similar clinical disease and similar lesions. One inoculation study suggested a difference in virulence between two strains of group A rotavirus in pigs (Woode et al. 1976); whereas, other studies have shown no difference in virulence between group A rotavirus strains (Debouck and Pensaert 1979; Collins et al. 1989).

Little is known regarding natural disease in swine caused by groups B, C, and E rotaviruses. Inoculation studies in gnotobiotic pigs with group C rotaviruses resulted in clinical disease typical of group A rotaviruses (Bohl et al. 1982; Snodgrass et al. 1984). In contrast, inoculation studies in gnotobiotic pigs with group B rotaviruses (Bridger et al. 1982; Theil et al. 1985) and group E rotaviruses (Chasey et al. 1986) resulted in less severe diarrhea of shorter duration than that observed with groups A or C.

PATHOGENESIS. Rotaviruses replicate predominately in the cytoplasm of differentiated small intestinal villous epithelial cells and to a lesser extent in the cytoplasm of M cells overlying Peyer's patches (Buller and Moxley 1988) and in cecal or colonic epithelial cells (Theil et al. 1978; Collins et al. 1989). Rotavirus replication results in small intestinal villous epithelial cell dysfunction and death; lysis or desquamation of infected cells leads to villous atrophy. The degree of villous atrophy and the distribution of atrophic villi in the small intestine varies relative to the age of the pig and is a primary factor determining the severity of clinical disease. In general, villous atrophy is more severe and extensive in younger pigs.

Numerous rotavirus inoculation studies in 1- to 7-day-old pigs have demonstrated that virus replication is usually most extensive in the distal one-half to two-thirds of the small intestine (Pearson and McNulty 1977; Theil et al. 1978; Narita et al. 1982a; Collins et al. 1989; Stevenson 1990). Rotaviral antigen may be demonstrated in the cytoplasm in a few epithelial cells on villous tips in the duodenum and in nearly all villous epithelial cells in the jejunum and ileum by 12–48 hours postinoculation (Fig. 26.4). Villous atrophy is most severe by 24–72 hours postinoculation when villi may be as short as one-tenth normal length in the jejunum and ileum. In contrast, rotavirus inoculation studies in 21- to 24-day-old pigs revealed the

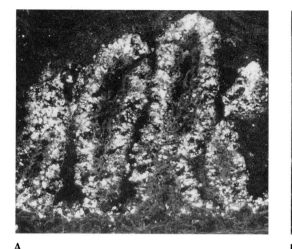
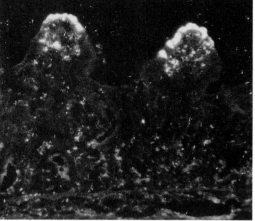

A   B

26.4. Rotavirus antigen in the cytoplasm of vilous epithelial cells as viewed by indirect fluorescent antibody method. ×90. (A) Ileum from a 1-day-old gnotobiotic pig 16 hours postinoculation with porcine rotavirus. Nearly all villous epithelial cells contain viral antigen. (B) Mid-jejunum from a 27-day-old weaned conventional pig 3 days postinoculation. Viral antigen is in epithelial cells on villous tips.

most extensive virus replication in the proximal one-half to two-thirds of the small intestine (Shaw et al. 1989a; Stevenson 1990). Virus-infected epithelial cells were most often on the distal half of villi (Fig. 26.4) resulting in moderate villous atrophy. The most atrophic villi were one-third normal length.

Diarrhea begins slightly before or concurrent with villous atrophy and has been attributed to multiple pathogenic mechanisms. Most proven mechanisms are related to decreased small intestinal digestive and absorptive functions caused by the loss of differentiated enterocytes. Decreased small intestinal disaccharidase activities (primarily lactase) results in the retention of disaccharides (primarily lactose) in the lumen of the small intestine. The excess disaccharides result in hyperosmolarity of the intestinal contents, which causes an osmotic diarrhea (Davidson et al. 1977; Graham et al. 1984). Decreased small intestinal Na^+K^+-ATPase activity and glucose-coupled Na^+ absorption results in decreased Na^+ absorption at villous tips. The normal secretion of Na^+ and water from crypts into the small intestinal lumen is not balanced by adequate absorption at villous tips and may result in net Na^+ and water flux toward the small intestinal lumen (Davidson et al. 1977; Graham et al. 1984). Recent studies in children have also suggested that prostaglandins, which are produced as a result of rotavirus-induced enteric inflammation, may enhance the severity of rotavirus-associated diarrhea (Yamashiro et al. 1989). Children with rotavirus-associated diarrhea had higher serum and fecal levels of two prostaglandins than did clinically normal children. Furthermore, oral aspirin therapy, which decreased serum and fecal prostaglan-

din levels, also shortened the duration of diarrhea. Similar studies in pigs have not been reported.

Several interrelated factors may be involved in causing death in rotavirus-inoculated pigs. Diarrhea causes dehydration and electrolyte imbalances and may lead to exhaustion of extracellular fluid reserves. Malabsorption results in malnutrition and may lead to energy deficiency and hypothermia. Observed higher mortality in neonatal pigs is most likely related to more severe and extensive villous atrophy, coupled with decreased extracellular fluid and energy reserves as compared to slightly older pigs. Suboptimal ambient temperatures have been shown to increase mortality rates in rotavirus-infected pigs. Inoculation of newborn pigs with a human strain of group A rotavirus resulted in no mortality when pigs were maintained at 35°C and resulted in 70–90% mortality when pigs were maintained at 26°C (Steel and Torres-Medina 1984). Differences in mortality were attributed to increased energy demands at lower ambient temperatures combined with rotavirus-induced malnutrition. Mortality rates may also be affected by virus dose. The minimum infective dose of two strains of porcine group A rotavirus has been shown to be as low as 1 plaque-forming unit of virus (Graham et al. 1987; Shaw et al. 1989b). Virus titration studies using a porcine group A rotavirus strain done in a limited number of neonatal colostrum-deprived pigs suggested higher mortality rates in pigs inoculated with lower dilutions (higher virus dose) of inoculum (Shaw et al. 1989b).

The duration of rotavirus-induced diarrhea is determined by the time needed for the restoration of an adequate number of differentiated villous epithelial cells in the small intestine. Complete restoration of morphologically normal villi in 3-day-old pigs requires 6–10 days; whereas, only 2–4 days are required in 21-day-old pigs. Recovery is slower in younger pigs owing to more severe villous atrophy and to sluggish crypt epithelial cell turnover. Complete replacement of villous epithelial cells requires 8–10 days in newborn pigs and 2–3 days in 21-day-old pigs (Moon 1971).

The pathogenesis of groups B, C, and E rotaviruses in pigs has been studied much less extensively than that of group A rotaviruses. The limited information gained through inoculation studies in pigs with group B rotaviruses (Pedley et al. 1983; Theil et al. 1985), group C rotaviruses (Bohl et al. 1982; Snodgrass et al. 1984), and group E rotaviruses (Chasey et al. 1986) suggests a pathogenesis similar to that described for group A rotaviruses. Virus replication was most extensive in the distal small intestine for all rotavirus groups; however, villous atrophy was more severe with groups A and C than with groups B and E.

The pathogenesis of combined infections of rotavirus and other commonly recognized enteropathogens has been examined in a limited number of studies. Inoculation of 3-day-old germ-free pigs with group A rotavirus followed 24 hours later by K99 pilus-producing enterotoxigenic *E. coli* caused more severe diarrheal disease than did inoculation of pigs with either agent separately. Villous atrophy was no more severe in pigs infected with both agents than in pigs inoculated with rotavirus alone (Benfield et al. 1988). Inoculation of 28-day-old pigs with rotavirus followed by hemolytic strains of enterotoxigenic *E. coli* resulted in more severe diarrheal disease than was seen in pigs inoculated with either agent separately (Tzipori and Williams 1978; Lecce et al. 1982). It was concluded that rotavirus infection enhances colonization of the small intestine by hemolytic strains of enterotoxigenic *E. coli*. Inoculation of 7-day-old germ-free pigs with rotavirus and TGE virus resulted in more severe diarrheal disease than in pigs inoculated with rotavirus alone (Woode and Crouch 1978). In contrast, simultaneous inoculation of 1-day-old pigs with rotavirus and enterovirus resulted in less severe diarrheal disease and less severe villous atrophy than was seen in pigs inoculated with rotavirus alone (Janke et al. 1988). It was concluded that nonlethal enterovirus infection of villous epithelial cells interfered with subsequent rotavirus infection.

LESIONS. The lesions caused by rotaviruses in pigs are limited to the small intestines and are the sum of the degenerative and functional consequences of rotavirus-induced villous epithelial cell destruction and the adaptive and regenerative responses of the small intestine.

Gross lesions are visible slightly before or concurrent with the onset of diarrhea and are most severe in 1- to 14-day-old pigs (Pearson and McNulty 1977; Theil et al. 1978; Benfield et al. 1988; Janke et al. 1988; Collins et al. 1989; Stevenson 1990). The stomachs usually contain food and the distal one-half to two-thirds of the small intestine is thin walled, flaccid, and dilated with a large volume of watery, flocculent, yellow or gray fluid. Following 24 hours of diarrhea, increased small intestinal motility may result in less distention and a less thin-walled, more nearly normal appearance. The lacteals in the distal two-thirds of the intestine contain no chyle, and the associated mesenteric lymph nodes are small and tan. The cecum and colon are likewise dilated with similar contents. Gross lesions are less severe or are absent in pigs that are 21 days of age or older (Shaw et al. 1989a; Stevenson 1990).

Light microscopic lesions have been described in numerous rotavirus inoculation studies in suckling pigs (Woode et al. 1976; Pearson and McNulty 1977; Crouch and Woode 1978; Theil et al. 1978; McAdaragh et al. 1980; Benfield et al. 1988; Janke et al. 1988; Collins et al. 1989; Stevenson 1990). Villous epithelial cell degeneration begins in cells on villous tips and in groups of cells on lateral villi by 16–18 hours postinoculation. Degenerative cells are swollen and have rarified cytoplasm, swollen nuclei, and irregular brush borders. Degenerative cells are frequently partially detached from adjacent cells or from the basement membrane. By 16–24 hours postinoculation, sloughing of degenerative villous epithelial cells results in significant villous atrophy, which is most severe by 24–72 hours postinoculation (Fig. 26.5). The tips of atrophic villi may be eroded or may be covered by attenuated, nearly squamous epithelial cells, and there is a variable amount of cellular debris in the lamina propria. Contact of the exposed lamina propria of adjacent villi results in villous fusion, which may be observed for 24–168 hours postinoculation. Crypt epithelial cell hyperplasia results in significantly deeper crypts beginning 48–72 hours postinoculation. Villi are completely covered by differentiated columnar epithelial cells by 72–128 hours postinoculation. The time required for complete regeneration of normal villi depends on the age of pig.

Scanning electron microscopy has allowed detailed study of the surface topography of affected small intestinal mucosa in numerous rotavirus inoculation studies (McAdaragh et al. 1980; Torres-Medina et al. 1980; Collins et al. 1989; Stevenson 1990). Degenerate villous epithelial cells lyse and/or detach, resulting in villous erosion and shortening (Fig. 26.6A, B). Within a few hours, eroded villous tips are covered with a continuous layer of epithelial cells and there are few remaining swollen and degenerate epithelial cells (Fig. 26.6C).

Ultrastructural studies in rotavirus-inoculated or naturally infected pigs have revealed lesions in the cytoplasm of virus-infected villous epithelial

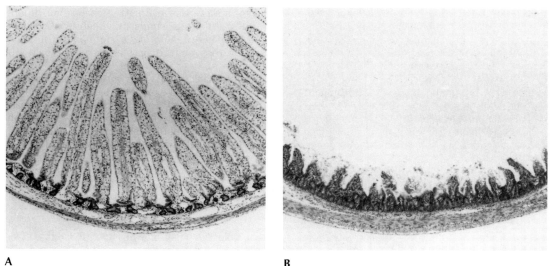

26.5.   Ileum from 3-day-old gnotobiotic pigs. H & E. ×35. (A) Normal villi in an uninoculated control pig. (B) Severe villous atrophy present 18 hours postinoculation.

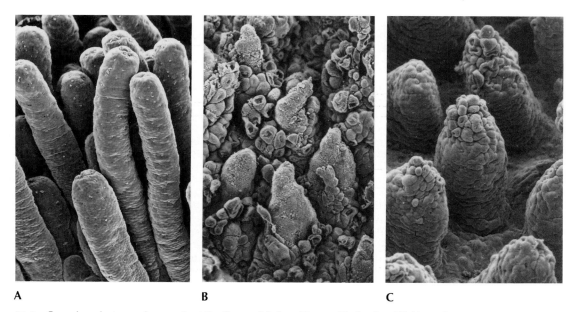

26.6.   Scanning electron micrograph of the ileum of 3-day-old gnotobiotic pigs. (A) Normal villi in an uninoculated control pig. ×70. (B) Sloughing, degenerate, villous epithelial cells and exposed lamina propria on severely atrophic villi, 18 hours postinoculation. ×165. (C) The tips of atrophic villi are covered by a continuous layer of sometimes swollen and degenerate epithelial cells, 24 hours postinoculation. ×230.

cells that are typical of those also described for rotaviruses in many other mammalian and avian species (Chasey 1977; Saif et al. 1978; Pearson and McNulty 1979; Narita et al. 1982b). Virus-infected cells contain within their cytoplasm multiple, variably sized, electron-dense granular viroplasms that often have dense subviral cores, or single-shelled particles on the periphery. Single-shelled viral particles obtain the outer capsid by budding through the membranes of the rough endoplasmic reticulum (Fig. 26.7). Mature, 75- to 78-nm double-shelled virus particles accumulate in the cysternae of the endoplasmic reticulum and are released by cell lysis. Other degenerative changes in virus-infected cells include cell swelling, mitochondrial swelling, nuclear swelling, dilatation of the cytocavitary network, and fragmentation of microvilli. Macrophages in

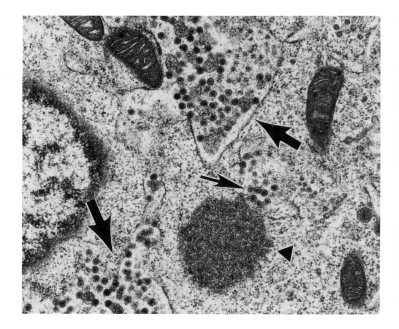

26.7. Ultrastructure of a swollen and degenerate rotavirus-infected villous epithelial cell containing dense granular viroplasm (arrow head). Virus particles form and obtain outer capsids through budding into the rough endoplasmic reticulum (small arrow). Many double-shelled virus particles are within the cysternae of the endoplasmic reticulum (large arrows). ×23,800.

the lamina propria contain cellular membrane profiles, virus particles, viroplasm, and other cellular debris in phagosomes.

DIAGNOSIS. Rotavirus should be considered as a cause of diarrhea in neonatal pigs 1–8 weeks of age. Fecal samples or intestinal contents should be collected in acute phases of disease and submitted for diagnosis. Highest concentrations of porcine rotavirus are shed during the first 12–24 hours from start of diarrhea. This is especially critical for the detection of certain groups of rotaviruses, for the amount of virus shed is lower and the duration of virus shedding is shorter in pigs infected with group B rotavirus infection (Bridger 1980; Theil et al. 1985; Paul 1990).

A number of methods have been employed for the detection of rotavirus, including electron microscopy, immune electron microscopy, ELISA, CCIF, virus isolation, latex agglutination, dot blot hybridization, and RNA electropherotyping. Electron microscopy has been extensively used for the detection of rotaviruses and remains a reference method for the detection of rotaviruses. This methods allows detection of different serogroups of rotaviruses. The morphology and type of virus particles detected by negative-staining electron microscopy is affected by staining methodology utilized and serogroup of rotavirus. Negative staining with phosphotungstic acid (PTA) of neutral pH results in predominantly single-shelled capsids; whereas, PTA of pH 4.5 or uranyl acetate gave double-shelled particles (Nakata et al. 1987; Suzuki et al. 1987). Core particles have been detected in group B rotavirus (Bridger et al. 1982; Theil et al. 1985). Immune electron microscopy allows their differentiation into serogroups.

ELISA is frequently used for the detection of rotaviral antigens in fecal samples or intestinal contents, and is more sensitive than latex agglutination test (Goyal et al. 1987) but less sensitive than electron microscopy (Benfield et al. 1984; Benfield 1990). Human-based diagnostic kits may be used for the detection of porcine group A rotaviruses.

Electropherotyping of viral RNA is often used for the detection and differentiation of rotavirus groups. Rotaviruses of different serogroups have distinct electropherotypes (Fig. 26.2), which only provide a tentative diagnosis of a serogroup and should be confirmed serologically. For electropherotyping, viral RNA can be isolated in a crude form directly from feces and analyzed by polyacrylamide gel electrophoresis (Paul et al. 1988b) or purified by CF-11 cellulose chromatography (Theil et al. 1981). RNA bands in gels are visualized by ethidium bromide or silver-staining methods.

Terminal oligonucleotide fingerprinting has been used in differentiating porcine rotavirus and is useful in molecular epidemiological studies (Clarke and McCrae 1981). Nucleic acid probes offer an attractive alternative for the detection and differentiation of rotavirus groups and serotypes (Dimitrov et al. 1985 ; Johnson et al. 1990; Paul et al. 1990a,c; Rosen et al. 1990).

Serologic evidence of rotavirus infection is of little significance in the diagnosis of rotavirus infection, for antibodies are common in swine herds; however, antibody titers and isotypes shed light on immune status of animals. Antibodies to rotavirus can be detected by a number of serologic tests. Indirect immunofluorescence test commonly has been used to detect antibodies to porcine rotavirus (Theil and Saif 1985; Chasey et al. 1986). Monolayers of MA-104 cells are inoculated with group A, B, or C rotavirus. Virus is allowed to adsorb onto cells in case of group A rotavirus or is centrifuged onto cells in case of group B or C rotavirus. Cells are fixed with acetone-methanol mixture and used as antigen in an indirect immunofluorescence test. Alternatively, cryostat intestinal sections from pigs infected with noncultivable rotaviruses may be used as antigens. Antibodies to serogroups B, C, and E have been detected by this method. Indirect ELISA has also been used to detect antibodies to rotavirus. Antibodies detected by the above methods are usually directed against the common group antigen. ELISA combined with isotype-specific monoclonal antibodies (Paul et al. 1985, 1989) have been used to detect classes of antibodies to rotavirus (Paul et al. 1986). Plaque-reduction and fluorescent focus-reduction neutralization assays have been used to detect neutralizing antibodies (Hoshino et al. 1984; Paul et al. 1988a). Hemagglutination inhibition test has also been developed for the detection of antibodies to porcine rotavirus (Eiguchi et al. 1987).

TREATMENT. No known therapeutic agents are available for the specific treatment of porcine rotavirus infections. General supportive therapy, management procedures, and antibiotics are recommended to minimize mortality due to rotavirus and secondary bacterial infections. Electrolyte solutions containing glucose-glycine fed ad libitum minimize dehydration and weight loss induced by rotavirus infection (Bywater and Woode 1980; Bywater 1983). Ambient environment should be optimized, minimizing draft and temperature fluctuations. Antibiotic therapy may be used to reduce losses from secondary bacterial infections. In herds with a persistent problem of postweaning diarrhea with high mortality, a change in weaner diet and weaning procedure should be considered. Scheduled feeding of a high-energy weaner diet has been successfully used to reduce morbidity and mortality rates (Tzipori et al. 1980a; Hampson and Beban 1985).

PREVENTION

Management. Rotavirus infection persists enzootically in most swine herds. Rotavirus survives in dust and organic matter and may persist as subclinical infections in adult swine (Benfield et al. 1982). It is therefore difficult, if not impossible, to eliminate. Studies have shown that increasing concentrations of rotavirus in the environment cause more severe disease at a younger age (Lecce et al. 1978). Thus, management practices should be directed at reducing the virus load for susceptible pigs and boosting passive immunity. Virus load may be reduced by sanitation and limiting contact between young

susceptible pigs and older pigs more likely to be shedding virus. The floors in farrowing and nursing houses should be constructed to minimize feces buildup during use and to facilitate cleaning. All-in/all-out management practices should be followed and rooms should be thoroughly cleaned and disinfected between groups. Recommended disinfectants include formaldehyde and chlorine-based disinfectants such as chlorox or chloramine T (Multichlor). Farrowing interval should be minimized to prevent virus buildup and infection of later-farrowed litters. Mixing animals of different ages should be discouraged for it promotes virus transmission from older to younger pigs. To enhance passive immunity, replacement gilts should be exposed to the feces of older sows. Attention to lactation diet, feed intake, sow comfort, and farrowing-crate design are all important to ensure adequate milk supply and effective suckling necessary for successful passive immunity.

Immunoprophylaxis. Pigs recovered from a natural infection with rotavirus are immune to infection with homologous rotavirus for at least a short time; the duration of immunity is unknown. The mechanisms of immunity have not been completely elucidated. Protection is generally correlated with the presence of antibodies in secretions. Antibodies in the intestinal lumen bathe susceptible villous epithelial cells and protect them from infection. Secretory IgA (sIgA) is more effective than IgG and IgM for sIgA is more resistant than IgG and IgM to proteolytic degradation in the intestinal tract and sIgA is the predominant immunoglobulin (Ig) in secretions. Circulating serum antibodies do not provide protection against rotavirus infections (Offit and Clark 1985). Recent studies in mice indicate that cellular immunity may also be important in protection against rotavirus infections (Offit and Dudzik 1988, 1989).

Piglets suckling immune sows are protected from rotavirus gastroenteritis during the nursing period. This passive immunity is related to the continuous presence of specific virus-neutralizing antibodies in the gastrointestinal tract of suckling pigs. Secretory IgA is the predominant Ig in milk of lactating sows and is the primary Ig providing passive protection.

The route of immunization of sows influences the classes of Igs produced. Primary immunization by the oral route is the best method known to date for induction of sIgA in milk. Parenteral routes, however, may be used to booster sIgA in animals previously primed by oral immunization. Levels of virus attenuation also influence its ability to induce lactogenic immunity. Inactivated viral immunogens are not as good as immunogens of the live virus. Induction of active immunity against postweaning diarrhea in the presence of passive milk antibodies is problematic. Oral immunization is required for optimal priming of sI-gA response, yet passively acquired milk antibodies will likely interfere in replication of immunizing rotavirus. Immunization by the parenteral route is not as apt to result in protective immunity. Immunity to rotavirus, in general, is serotype specific (Bohl et al. 1982; Losonsky et al. 1986). Pigs orally immunized with the A/OSU strain were resistant to infection and were protected from gastroenteritis following challenge with the A/OSU strain but not from challenge with the A/Gottfried strain (Bohl et al. 1982). Similarly, pigs immunized with the A/Gottfried strain were protected from challenge with A/Gottfried but not from the A/OSU strain. This study demonstrated feasibility for the development of a modified live rotavirus vaccine. Two surface proteins, VP4 and VP7, are important in induction of neutralizing antibodies and in protection (Greenberg et al. 1983b; Offit et al. 1986b; Hoshino et al. 1988). In addition to serotype-specific epitopes, these proteins also possess heterotypic epitopes, which are conserved among different serotypes. Heterotypic immunity is not as effective as that induced by homotypic strains. Reassortant rotaviruses containing the VP4 and VP7 genes from two different serotypes may be used to induce immunity to both serotypes (Offit et al. 1986b; Hoshino et al. 1988). The reassortant rotavirus 11-1, containing VP4 gene from the A/OSU strain and the VP7 gene from the A/Gottfried strain, induced neutralizing antibodies to both the OSU and Gottfried strains and protected orally immunized pigs from challenge with either the OSU or Gottfried strain (Hoshino et al. 1988). Protection, however, was greater against the Gottfried strain than the OSU strain.

Modified live and inactivated virus vaccines are commercially available for immunization of sows as well as nursing pigs. Modified live virus vaccines are administered orally, orally and intramuscularly, or intramuscularly. Inactivated virus vaccines are administered intramuscularly in sows and intraperitoneally in nursing pigs. Some of the commercially available vaccines have not been evaluated by independent investigators. Two separate studies of a modified live rotavirus vaccine for postweaning diarrhea resulted in conflicting data. In one study, immunization of nursing pigs improved the weight gain and reduced the severity of disease (Westercamp 1986). In the second study, neither improvement in weight gain nor curtailment of virus shedding was observed (Hoblet et al. 1986). Bovine rotavirus vaccine is not effective in preventing rotaviral diarrhea in pigs (Lecce and King 1979). Recent identification of new porcine rotavirus serotypes (Nagesha and Holmes 1988; Paul et al. 1988a, 1991) may require their incorporation into vaccines if they are found to be a significant cause of gastroenteritis in swine. Both VP4 and VP7 genes of porcine rotavirus have been cloned and sequenced (Gorziglia et al. 1986, 1988, 1990; Nishikawa and Gorziglia 1988), and VP4 of one strain has been expressed in baculovirus vector (Nishikawa et al. 1989). The recombinant VP4 protein induced neutralizing antibodies, but its efficacy against rotavirus gastroenteritis has not been examined. Recombinant proteins and reassortant rotaviruses offer potential alternatives as immunogens for rotavirus gastroenteritis.

Porcine Reovirus

REOVIRUSES HAVE been detected from healthy pigs as well as from pigs with respiratory and reproductive disease (Kasza 1970; Kirkbride and McAdaragh 1978; McFerran 1986). Their role in these swine diseases is unclear. Reoviruses are associated with tenosynovitis in chickens (Van der Heide 1977; Robertson and Wilcox 1986) and systemic illness affecting the majority of organs in rodents (Tyler and Fields 1990), and thus have the potential to be significant pathogens in swine.

ETIOLOGY

Virus Morphology. Reovirus was the first genus identified in the family Reoviridae. The other two genuses of importance to animals are *Rotavirus* and *Orbivirus*. Reo is an acronym for respiratory and enteric orphan virus. Reovirus particles are nonenveloped, icosahedral shaped with a fuzzy outer rim, and measure 75 nm in diameter (Fig. 26.8). The inner capsid is about 45–50 nm in diameter. Reovirus replicates in the cytoplasm.

Physicochemical and Biological Properties. Reovirus has a double-stranded RNA genome and 10 segments. The density in cesium chloride is 1.36 g/cm³. Porcine reovirus is resistant to ether, chloroform, and trypsin; is stable at acidic pH 3, and is sensitive to 0.1% sodium deoxycholate (Hirahara et al. 1988). Porcine reovirus is susceptible to heat at 50°C for 1 hour; it was stabilized by the presence of 1 M MgCl². Virus possesses a hemagglutinin that agglutinates human group O and porcine erythrocytes at 4°C, 22°C, and 37°C, but not erythrocytes from guinea pig, rat, hamster, cattle, dog, cat, or chicken. Mammalian reoviruses share a group antigen that can be detected by complement fixation, immunofluorescence, and immunodiffusion (Sabin 1959). Avian

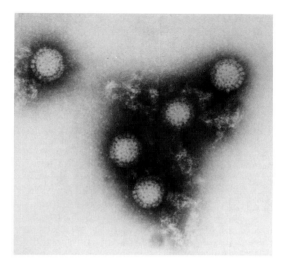

26.8. Electron micrograph of reovirus particles viewed by negative-staining electron microscopy. ×115,000.

reoviruses are not antigenically related to mammalian reoviruses but possess a group antigen that is shared by avian reoviruses. All mammalian isolates can be divided serologically into three types: types 1, 2, and 3. Reoviruses of different types can be distinguished by serum neutralization and hemagglutination inhibition tests.

Cultivation.   Reoviruses can be cultivated in a wide variety of cell cultures from many species: pig, bovine, cat, African monkey kidney cell lines Vero and MA-104; HeLa; and canine thyroid adenocarcinoma cell line (Kasza 1970; Hirahara et al. 1988; Paul 1990). Reovirus replication is slow and the majority of reovirus is cell associated, 20% virus being extracellular (McFerran 1986).

The cytopathic effect of reovirus varies somewhat, depending on the cell line used. In general, cells round up, become granular, and slough off the surface. Eosinophilic intracytoplasmic inclusion bodies can easily be seen in cultures stained with May-Greenwald-Giemsa stain.

EPIDEMIOLOGY.   Porcine reovirus infections appear to be widespread in swine herds, and antibodies to all three types have been detected in pigs (Harkness et al. 1971; Zindel et al. 1980). In a study by Zindel et al. (1980), pigs in 54% of the swine herds surveyed were seropositive for all three reovirus types. Passively acquired antibodies to reovirus persist in neonatal pigs for about 11 weeks, at which time pigs become susceptible to infection (Watt 1978). Reovirus is spread via fecal-oral and respiratory routes. Following experimental infection, virus is shed in nasal secretions and feces for 6 and 14 days respectively. Virus is spread by contact exposure (McFerran et al. 1971).

CLINICAL SIGNS.   Reovirus has been isolated from clinically healthy pigs as well as pigs with respiratory or enteric disease (Kasza 1970; McFerran and Connor 1970; Elazhary et al. 1978; McFerran 1986) and from aborted fetuses (Kirkbride and McAdaragh 1978).

Experimental studies have not consistently resulted in reproduction of disease. In a majority of the studies, intranasal, intraperitoneal, or intracerebral inoculation of conventional and gnotobiotic pigs of 1–6 weeks of age with porcine reovirus type 1 or human reovirus type 1 did not result in clinical disease except for a transient febrile reaction (Kasza 1970; McFerran and Connor 1970; Baskerville et al. 1971; McFerran et al. 1971; Watt 1978). Virus could be isolated from respiratory and alimentary tracts for up to 2 weeks postinfection. In one study, rise in body temperature and diarrhea was detected in cesarean-derived colostrum-deprived 1-week-old pigs inoculated orally with type 1 reovirus, however, no clinical disease was detected in gnotobiotic pigs (Elazhary et al. 1978). Mild respiratory disease characterized by pyrexia, sneezing, inappetance, and listlessness was reproduced in cesarean-derived colostrum-deprived pigs and conventional pigs inoculated intranasally or exposed via aerosol to reovirus type 1 (Hirahara et al. 1988). Intravenous or intramuscular inoculation of seronegative sows between 40 and 85 days of gestation with reovirus resulted in term litters containing a mixture of mummified, stillborn, weak, and normal pigs.

PATHOGENESIS.   Reovirus replicates mainly in intestinal and respiratory tracts and can be isolated from nasal and fecal swabs. Virus is excreted in nasal secretions and feces as early as 24 hours postinfection and may last for 14 days. Virus can also be isolated from boar semen (McAdaragh and Anderson 1975). Virus was isolated from fetal tissues and placenta of sows inoculated intravenously or intramuscularly with type 3 reovirus. Virus was recovered only from fetal tissues of sows inoculated at 30–60 days of gestation, from both placental and fetal tissues of sows inoculated at 50–70 days of gestation, and only placenta of sows inoculated after 70 days of gestation (McAdaragh and Robl 1976). Hemagglutination-inhibiting antibodies may be detected at 7 days postinfection and reach peak titers between 11 and 21 days postinfection (McFerran 1986).

LESIONS.   A limited number of reovirus inoculation studies in swine have revealed few gross lesions and only mild microscopic lesions. Although intravenous or intramuscular inoculation of sows between 40 and 85 days of gestation with reovirus resulted in litters containing a mixture of mummified fetuses, stillborn pigs, small weak pigs, and normal pigs, no specific gross or histologic lesions were reported (McAdaragh and Robl 1976). Oral inoculation of 1-week-old cesarean-derived colostrum-deprived pigs with enteric origin reovirus resulted in focal villous atrophy in the jejunum and ileum (Elazhary et al. 1978). Aerosol exposure of 4-week-old specific-pathogen-free (SPF) pigs to porcine origin type 1 reovirus resulted in no gross lesions; however, there were consistant microscopic lesions in the lungs consisting of multifocal aggregates of lymphocytes and macrophages in alveoli and alveolar septae and mild peribronchiolar nodular lymphocytic hyperplasia (Baskerville et al. 1971). Intranasal inoculation of 70-kg SPF pigs with a porcine respiratory isolate of type 3 reovirus resulted in lobular atalectasis and vessicular emphysema in the apical portions of lung lobes (Robl et al. 1971). Microscopic examination revealed mild interstitial pneumonia, alveolar emphysema, and peribronchiolar nodular lymphocytic hyperplasia, which varied in intensity between lobules. Additional studies are needed to clearly characterize the clinical disease and lesions in swine caused by porcine reovirus.

DIAGNOSIS. A number of methods may be employed for the detection of reovirus, including electron microscopy, immune electron microscopy, virus isolation, and RNA electropherotyping. Virus isolation has commonly been used for diagnosis. A wide variety of cells may be used; primary swine kidney cells and African monkey kidney cell lines such as MA-104 are extremely susceptible and are commonly available. Electron microscopy, immunofluorescence, or RNA electropherotyping may be used to detect reovirus. Typing of reovirus is achieved by virus neutralization and hemagglutination inhibition tests with reference antisera to three reovirus types.

TREATMENT AND PREVENTION. No methods are available for treatment or prevention of porcine reovirus infections and possibly none are warranted until clinical significance of reovirus infections in swine is documented.

REFERENCES

ALMEIDA, J. D., AND HALL, T. 1978. The effect of trypsin on the growth of rotavirus. J Gen Virol 40:213–218.

ASKAA, J., AND BLOCH, B. 1981. Detection of porcine rotavirus by EM, ELISA and CIET. Acta Vet Scand 22:32–38.

ASKAA, J.; BLOCH, B.; BERTELSEN, G.; AND RASMUSSEN, K. O. 1983. Rotavirus-associated diarrhea in nursing piglets and detection of antibody against rotavirus in colostrum, milk, and serum. Nord Vet Med 35:441–447.

BASKERVILLE, A.; McFERRAN, J. B.; AND CONNOR, T. 1971. The pathology of experimental infection of pigs with type 1 reovirus of porcine origin. Res Vet Sci 12:172–174.

BENFIELD, D. A. 1990. Diagnosis of rotavirus infections in food animals. Proc Commer Diagn Technol Anim

Health Monit. Natl Vet Serv Lab and Iowa State Univ Vet Diagn Lab, Ames, pp. 181–193.

BENFIELD, D. A.; STOTZ, I.; MOORE, R.; AND McDARAGH, J. P. 1982. Shedding of rotavirus in feces of sows before and after farrowing. J Clin Microbiol 16:186–190.

BENFIELD, D. A.; STOTZ, I. J.; NELSON, E. A.; AND GROON, K. S. 1984. Comparison of a commercial enzyme-linked immunosorbent assay with electron microscopy, fluorescent antibody, and virus isolation for the detection of bovine and porcine rotavirus. Am J Vet Res 45:1998–2002.

BENFIELD, D. A.; FRANCIS, D. H.; McADARAGH, J. P.; JOHNSON, D. D.; BERGELAND, M. E.; ROSSOW, K.; AND MOORE, R. 1988. Combined rotavirus and K99 Escherichia coli infection in gnotobiotic pigs. Am J Vet Res 49:330–337.

BICAN, P.; COHEN, J.; CHARPILIENNE, A.; AND SCHERRER, R. 1982. Purification and characterization of bovine rotavirus cores. J Virol 43:1113–1117.

BOHL, E. H.; KOHLER, E. M.; SAIF, L. J.; CROSS, R. F.; AGNES, A. G.; AND THEIL, K. W. 1978. Rotavirus as a cause of diarrhea in pigs. J Am Vet Med Assoc 172:458–463.

BOHL, E. H.; SAIF, L. J.; THEIL, K. W.; AGNES, A. G.; AND CROSS, R. F. 1982. Porcine pararotavirus: Detection, differentiation from rotavirus, and pathogenesis in gnotobiotic pigs. J Clin Microbiol 15:312–319.

BOHL, E. H.; THEIL, K. W.; AND SAIF, L. J. 1984. Isolation and serotyping of porcine rotaviruses and antigenic comparison with other rotaviruses. J Clin Microbiol 19:105–111.

BRIDGER, J. C. 1980. Detection by electron microscopy of caliciviruses, astroviruses, and rotavirus-like particles in the faeces of piglets with diarrhoea. Vet Rec 107:532–533.

———. 1987. Novel rotaviruses in animals and man. In Novel Diarrhea Viruses. Chichester: Wiley, CIBA Found Symp 128:6–23.

BRIDGER, J. C., AND BROWN, J. F. 1985. Prevalence of antibody to typical and atypical rotaviruses in pigs. Vet Rec 116:50.

BRIDGER, J. C., AND POCOCK, D. H. 1986. Variation of virulence of bovine rotaviruses. J Hyg 96:257–264.

BRIDGER, J. C., AND WOODE, G. N. 1976. Characterization of two particle types of calf rotavirus. J Gen Virol 31:245–250.

BRIDGER, J. C.; CLARKE, I. N.; AND McCRAE, M. A. 1982. Characterization of an antigenically distinct porcine rotavirus. Infect Immun 35:1058–1062.

BRIDGER, J. C.; PEDLEY, S.; AND McCRAE, M. A. 1986. Group C rotaviruses in humans. J Clin Microbiol 23:760–763.

BULLER, C. R., AND MOXLEY, R. A. 1988. Natural infection of porcine ileal dome M cells with rotavirus and enteric adenovirus. Vet Pathol 25:516–517.

BYWATER, R. J. 1983. Diarrhea treatments-fluid replacement and alternatives. Ann Rech Vet 14:556–560.

BYWATER, R. J., AND WOODE, G. N. 1980. Oral fluid replacement by a glucose glycine electrolyte formulation in E. coli and rotavirus diarrhea in pigs. Vet Rec 106:75–78.

CHASEY, D. 1977. Different particle types in tissue culture and intestinal epithelium infected with rotavirus. J Gen Virol 37:443–451.

CHASEY, D., AND LUCAS, M. 1977. Detection of rotavirus in experimentally infected piglets. Res Vet Sci 22:124–125.

CHASEY, D.; BRIDGER, J. C.; AND McCRAE, M. A. 1986. A new type of atypical rotavirus in pigs. Arch Virol 89:235–243.

CLARKE, I. N., AND McCRAE, M. A. 1981. A sensitive method for the production of diagnostic fingerprints of the genome segments of field isolates of rotavirus. J Virol Methods 3:261–269.

COLLINS, J. E.; BENFIELD, D. A.; AND DUIMSTRA, J. R. 1989. Comparative virulence of two porcine group-A rotavirus isolates in gnotobiotic pigs. Am J Vet Res 50:827–835.

CORTHIER, G.; COHEN, J.; AND SCHERRER, R. 1980. Isolation of pig rotavirus in France: Identification and experimental infections. Ann Rech Vet 11:45–48.

CROUCH, C. F., AND WOODE, G. N. 1978. Serial studies of virus multiplication and intestinal damage in gnotobiotic piglets infected with rotavirus. J Med Microbiol 11:325–334.

DAVIDSON, G. P.; GALL, D. G.; PETRIC, M.; BUTLER, D. G.; AND HAMILTON, J. R. 1977. Human rotavirus enteritis induced in conventional piglets. J Clin Invest 60:1402–1409.

DEA, S.; ELAZHARY, M. A. S. Y.; AND ROY, R. S. 1986. Distinct serotypes of porcine rotavirus associated with diarrhea in suckling piglets in Southern Quebec. Can J Vet Res 50:130–132.

DEBOUCK, P., AND PENSAERT, M. 1979. Experimental infection of pigs with Belgian isolates of the porcine rotavirus. Zentralbl Veterinaermed [B] 26:517–526.

———. 1983. Rotavirus excretion in suckling pigs followed under field circumstances. Ann Rech Vet 14:447–448.

DIMITROV, D. H.; GRAHAM, D. Y.; AND ESTES, M. K. 1985. Detection of rotaviruses by nucleic acid hybridization with cloned DNA of simian rotavirus SA11 genes. J Infect Dis 152:293–300.

EIGUCHI, Y.; YAMAGISHI, H.; FUKUSHO, A.; SHIMIZU, Y.; AND MATUMOTO, M. 1987. Hemagglutination and hemagglutination-inhibition tests with porcine rotavirus. Kitasato Arch Exp Med 60:167–172.

ELAZHARY, M. A. S. Y.; MORIN, M.; DERBYSHIRE, J. B.; LAGACE, A.; BERTHIAUME, L.; AND CORBEIL, M. 1978. The experimental infection of piglets with porcine reovirus. Res Vet Sci 25:16–20.

ESPEJO, R. T.; PUERTO, F.; SOLER, C.; AND GONZALEZ, N. 1984. Characterization of a human pararotavirus. Infect Immun 44:112–116.

ESTES, M. K., AND COHEN, J. 1989. Rotavirus gene structure and function. Microbiol Rev 53:410–449.

ESTES, M. K.; PALMER, E. L.; AND OBIJESKI, J. F. 1983. Rotaviruses: A review. Curr Top Microbiol Immunol 105:123–184.

FERRARI, M.; GUALANDI, G. L.; AND GELMETTI, D. 1986. Isolation of cytopathic strains of rotavirus from pigs. Microbiologica (Bologna) 9:287–294.

FU, Z. F., AND HAMPSON, D. J. 1987. Group A rotavirus excretion patterns in naturally infected pigs. Res Vet Sci 43:297–300.

FU, Z. F.; HAMPSON, D. J.; AND BLACKMORE, D. K. 1989. Detection and survival of group A rotavirus in a piggery. Vet Rec 125:576–578.

GORZIGLIA, M.; AGUIRRE, Y.; HOSHINO, Y.; ESPARZA, J.; BLUMENTALS, I.; ASKAA, J.; THOMPSON, M.; GLASS, R. I.; KAPIKIAN, A. Z.; AND CHANOCK, R. M. 1986. VP7 serotype-specific glycoprotein of OSU porcine rotavirus: Coding assignment and gene sequence. J Gen Virol 67:2445–2454.

GORZIGLIA, M.; NISHIKAWA, K.; GREEN, K.; AND TANIGUCHI, K. 1988. Gene sequence of the VP7 serotype specific glycoprotein of Gottfried porcine rotavirus. Nucleic Acids Res 16:775.

GORZIGLIA, M.; NISHIKAWA, K.; HOSHINO, Y.; AND TANIGUCHI, K. 1990. Similarity of the outer capsid protein VP4 of the Gottfried strain of porcine rotavirus to that of asymptomatic human rotavirus strains. J Virol 64:414–418.

GOYAL, S. M.; RADEMACHER, R. A.; AND POMEROY, K. A. 1987. Comparison of electron microscopy with

three commercial tests for the detection of rotavirus in animal feces. Diagn Microbiol Infect Dis 6:249–254.

GRAHAM, D. Y.; SACKMAN, J. W.; AND ESTES, M. K. 1984. Pathogenesis of rotavirus-induced diarrhea. Preliminary studies in miniature swine piglets. Dig Dis Sci 29:1028–1035.

GRAHAM, D. Y.; DUFOUR, G. R.; AND ESTES, M. K. 1987. Minimal infective dose of rotavirus. Arch Virol 92:261–271.

GREENBERG, H. B.; FLORES, J.; KALICA, A. R.; WYATT, R. G.; AND JONES, R. 1983a. Gene coding assignments for growth restriction, neutralization and subgroup specificities of the W and DS-1 strains on human rotavirus. J Gen Virol 64:313–320.

GREENBERG, H. B.; VALDESUSO, J.; VAN WYKE, K.; MIDTHUN, K.; WALSH, M.; MCAULIFFE, V.; WYATT, R. G.; KALICA, A. R.; FLORES, J.; AND HOSHINO, Y. 1983b. Production and preliminary characterization of monoclonal antibodies directed at two surface proteins of Rhesus rotavirus. J Virol 47:267–275.

HAMPSON, D. J., AND BEBAN, R. L. G. 1985. Diet and control of porcine post-weaning diarrhea. NZ Vet J 33:190.

HARKNESS, J. W.; CHAPMAN, M. S.; AND DERBYSHIRE, J. H. 1971. A survey of antibodies to some respiratory viruses in the sera of pigs. Vet Rec 88:441–447.

HIRAHARA, T.; YASUHARA, H.; MATSUI, O.; KODAMA, K.; NAKAI, M.; AND SASAKI, N. 1988. Characteristics of reovirus type 1 from the respiratory tract of pigs in Japan. Jpn J Vet Sci 50:353–361.

HOBLET, K. H.; SAIF, L. J.; KOHLER, E. M.; THEIL, K. W.; BECH-NIELSON, S.; AND STITZLEIN, G. A. 1986. Efficacy of an orally administered modified-live porcine-origin rotavirus vaccine against postweaning diarrhea in pigs. Am J Vet Res 47:1697–1703.

HOSHINO, Y.; WYATT, R. G.; GREENBERG, H. B.; FLORES, J.; AND KAPIKIAN, A. Z. 1984. Serotype similarity and diversity of rotaviruses of mammalian and avian origin as studied by plaque-reduction neutralization. J Infect Dis 149:694–702.

HOSHINO, Y.; SERENO, M. M.; MIDTHUN, K.; FLORES, J.; KAPIKIAN, A. Z.; AND CHANOCK, R. M. 1985. Independent segregation of two antigenic specificities (VP3 and VP7) involved in neutralization of rotavirus infectivity. Proc Natl Acad Sci (USA) 82:8701–8704.

HOSHINO, Y.; SAIF, L. J.; SERENO, M. M.; CHANOCK, R. M.; AND KAPIKIAN, A. Z. 1988. Infection immunity of piglets to either VP3 or VP7 outer capsid protein confers resistance to challenge with a virulent rotavirus bearing the corresponding antigen. J Virol 62:744–748.

JANKE, B. H.; MOREHOUSE, L. G.; AND SOLORZANO, R. F. 1988. Single and mixed infections of neonatal pigs with rotaviruses and enteroviruses: Clinical signs and microscopic lesions. Can J Vet Res 52:364–369.

JANKE, B. H.; NELSON, J. K.; BENFIELD, D. A.; AND NELSON, E. A. 1989. Relative prevalence of typical and atypical strains among rotaviruses from diarrheic pigs in conventional swine herds. Proc 32d Annu Meet Am Assoc Vet Lab Diagn, Las Vegas, p. 24.

———. 1990. Relative prevalence of typical and atypical strains among rotaviruses from diarrheic pigs in conventional swine herds. J Diagn Invest 2:308–311.

JOHNSON, M. E.; PAUL, P. S.; GORZIGLIA, M.; AND ROSENBUSCH, R. 1990. Development of specific nucleic acid probes for the differentiation of porcine rotavirus serotypes. Vet Microbiol 24:307–326.

KALICA, A. R.; FLORES, J.; AND GREENBERG, H. B. 1983. Identification of the rotaviral gene that codes for the hemagglutinin and protease-enhanced plaque formation. Virology 125:194–205.

KANG, S.; SAIF, L. J.; AND MILLER, K. L. 1989. Reactivity of VP4–specific monoclonal antibodies to a serotype 4 porcine rotavirus with distinct serotypes of human (symptomatic and asymptomatic) and animal rotaviruses. J Clin Microbiol 27:2744–2750.

KAPIKIAN, A. Z., AND CHANOCK, R. M. 1990. Rotaviruses. In Virology, 2d ed. N.Y.: Raven Press, pp. 1353–1404.

KASZA, L. 1970. Isolation and characterization of a reovirus from pigs. Vet Rec 87:681–686.

KIM, Y. H.; LEE, O. S.; CHOI, C. U.; AND AN, S. H. 1987. Epidemiological studies on porcine rotavirus infection in piglets. Res Rep Rural Div Adm 29:129–133.

KIRKBRIDE, C. A., AND McADARAGH, J. P. 1978. Infectious agents associated with fetal and early neonatal death and abortion in swine. J Am Vet Med Assoc 172:480–483.

LECCE, J. G., AND KING, M. W. 1978. Role of rotavirus (reo-like) in weanling diarrhea of pigs. J Clin Microbiol 8:454–458.

_____. 1979. The calf reo-like virus (rotavirus) vaccine: An ineffective immunization agent for rotaviral diarrhea of piglets. Can J Comp Med 43:90–93.

LECCE, J. G.; KING, M. W.; AND MOCK, R. 1976. Reovirus-like agent associated with fatal diarrhea in neonatal pigs. Infect Immun 14:816–825.

LECCE, J. G.; KING, M. W.; AND DORSEY, W. E. 1978. Rearing regimen producing piglet diarrhea (rotavirus) and its relevance to acute infantile diarrhea. Science 199:776–778.

LECCE, J. G.; BALSBAUGH, R. K.; AND CLARE, D. A. 1982. Rotavirus and hemolytic enteropathogenic *Escherichia coli* in weanling diarrhea in pigs. J Clin Microbiol 16:715–723.

LIU, M.; OFFIT, P. A.; AND ESTES, M. A. 1988. Identification of the simian rotavirus SA11 genome segment 3 product. Virology 163:26–32.

LOSONSKY, G. A.; VONDERFECHT, S. L.; EIDEN, J.; WEE, S.; AND YOLKEN, R. H. 1986. Homotypic and heterotypic antibodies for prevention of experimental rotavirus gastroenteritis. J Clin Microbiol 24:1041–1044.

McADARAGH, J. P., AND ANDERSON, G. A. 1975. Transmission of viruses through boar semen. Proc 18th Annu Meet Am Assoc Vet Lab Diagn, p. 69–76.

McADARAGH, J. P., AND ROBL, M. G. 1976. Experimental reovirus infections of pregnant sows. Proc 4th Int Congr Pig Vet Soc, Iowa State Univ, p. DD1.

McADARAGH, J. P.; BERGELAND, M. E.; MEYER, R. C.; JOHNSHOY, M. W.; STOTZ, I. J.; BENFIELD, D. A.; AND HAMMER, R. 1980. Pathogenesis of rotaviral enteritis in gnotobiotic pigs: A microscopic study. Am J Vet Res 41:1572–1581.

McFERRAN, J. B. 1986. Reovirus infection. In Diseases of Swine, 6th ed. Ames: Iowa State Univ Press, pp. 390–394.

McFERRAN, J. B., AND CONNOR, T. 1970. A reovirus isolated from a pig. Res Vet Sci 11:388–390.

McFERRAN, J. B.; BASKERVILLE, A.; AND CONNOR, T. 1971. Experimental infection of pigs with a human strain of type 1 reovirus. Res Vet Sci 12:174–175.

McNULTY, M. S.; PEARSON, G. R.; McFERRAN, J. B.; COLLINS, D. S.; AND ALLAN, G. M. 1976. A reovirus-like agent (rotavirus) associated with diarrhea in neonatal pigs. Vet Microbiol 1:55–63.

McNULTY, M. S.; ALLAN, G. M.; TODD, D.; McFERRAN, J. B.; AND McCRACKEN, R. M. 1981. Isolation from chickens of a rotavirus lacking the rotavirus group antigen. J Gen Virol 55:405–413.

MEBUS, C. A.; UNDERDAHL, N. R.; RHODES, M. B.; AND TWIEHAUS, M. J. 1969. Calf diarrhea (scours): Reproduced with a virus from a field outbreak. Univ Nebraska Agric Exp Stn Res Bull 233.

MIDTHUN, K.; VALDESUSO, J.; HOSHINO, Y.; FLORES, J.; KAPIKIAN, A. Z.; AND CHANOCK, R. M. 1987. Analysis by RNA-RNA hybridization assay of intertypic rotaviruses suggests that the gene reassortment occurs in vivo. J Clin Microbiol 25:295–320.

MOON, H. W. 1971. Epithelial cell migration in the alimentary mucosa of the suckling pig. Proc Soc Exp Biol Med 137:151–154.

NAGESHA, H. S., AND HOLMES, I. H. 1988. New porcine rotavirus serotype antigenically related to human rotavirus serotype 3. J Clin Microbiol 26:171–174.

NAGESHA, H. S.; BROWN, L. E.; AND HOLMES, I. A. 1989. Neutralizing monoclonal antibodies against three serotypes of porcine rotavirus. J Virol 63:3545–3549.

NAKATA, S.; PETRIE, B. L.; CALOMENI, E. P.; AND ESTES, M. K. 1987. Electron microscopy procedure influences detection of rotaviruses. J Clin Microbiol 25:1902–1906.

NARITA, M.; FUKUSHO, A.; KONNO, S.; AND SHIMIZU, Y. 1982a. Intestinal changes in gnotobiotic piglets experimentally inoculated with porcine rotavirus. Natl Inst Anim Health Q (Tokyo) 22:54–60.

NARITA, M.; FUKUSHO, A.; AND SHIMIZU, Y. 1982b. Electron microscopy of the intestine of gnotobiotic piglets infected with porcine rotavirus. J Comp Pathol 92:589–597.

NILSSON, O.; MARTINSSON, K.; AND PERSSON, E. 1984. Epidemiology of porcine neonatal steatorrhea in Sweden. I. Prevalence and clinical significance of coccidial and rotavirus infections. Nord Vet Med 36:103–110.

NISHIKAWA, K., AND GORZIGLIA, M. 1988. The nucleotide sequence of the VP3 gene of porcine rotavirus OSU. Nucleic Acids Res 16:11847.

NISHIKAWA, K.; FUKUHARA, N.; LIPRANDI, F.; GREEN, K.; KAPIKIAN, A. Z.; CHANOCK, R. M.; AND GORZIGLIA, M. 1989. VP4 protein of porcine rotavirus strain OSU expressed by a baculovirus recombinant induces neutralizing antibodies. Virology 173:631–637.

OFFIT, P. A., AND BLAVAT, G. 1986. Identification of the two rotavirus genes determining neutralization specificities. J Virol 57:376–378.

OFFIT, P. A., AND CLARK, H. F. 1985. Protection against rotavirus-induced gastroenteritis in a murine model by passively acquired gastrointestinal but not circulating antibodies. J Virol 54:58–64.

OFFIT, P. A., AND DUDZIK, K. I. 1988. Rotavirus-specific cytotoxic T lymphocytes cross-react with target cells infected with different rotavirus serotypes. J Virol 62:127–131.

_____. 1989. Rotavirus-specific cytotoxic T lymphocytes appear at the intestinal mucosal surface after rotavirus infection. J Virol 63:3507–3512.

OFFIT, P. A.; BLAVAT, G.; GREENBERG, H. B.; AND CLARK, H. F. 1986a. Molecular basis of rotavirus virulence: Role of gene segment 4. J Virol 57:46–49.

OFFIT, P. A.; CLARK, H. F.; BLAVAT, G.; AND GREENBERG, H. B. 1986b. Reassortant rotaviruses containing structural proteins vp3 and vp7 from different parents induce antibodies protective against each parental serotype. J Virol 60:491–496.

PAUL, P. S. 1990. Unpublished data.

PAUL, P. S.; VAN DEUSEN, R. A.; AND MENGELING, W. L. 1985. Monoclonal precipitating antibodies to porcine immunoglobulin M. Vet Immunol Immunopathol 8:311–328.

PAUL, P. S.; MENGELING, W. L.; SAIF, L. J.; AND VAN DEUSEN, R. A. 1986. Detection of classes of antibodies to transmissible gastroenteritis virus and rotavirus of swine using monoclonal antibodies to porcine immunoglobulins. Proc 9th Int Congr Pig Vet Soc, Barcelona, p. 190.

PAUL, P. S.; LYOO, Y. S.; ANDREWS, J. J.; AND HILL, H. T. 1988a. Isolation of two new serotypes of porcine rotavirus from pigs with diarrhea. Arch Virol 100:139–143.

PAUL, P. S.; LYOO, Y. S.; WOODE, G. N.; ZHENG, S.; GREENBERG, H. B.; MATSUI, S.; SCHWARTZ, K. J.; AND HILL, H. T. 1988b. Isolation of a bovine rotavirus with a "super-short" RNA electrophoretic pattern from a calf with diarrhea. J Clin Microbiol 26:2139–2143.

PAUL, P. S.; MENGELING, W. L.; MALSTROM, C. E.; AND VAN DEUSEN, R. A. 1989. Production and characterization of monoclonal antibodies to porcine immunoglobulin gamma, alpha, and light chains. Am J Vet Res 50:471–479.

PAUL, P. S.; BROOKS, M. A.; AND LYOO, Y. S. 1990a. Characterization of serotypic and genetic diversity among porcine rotaviruses. Proc 11th Int Congr Pig Vet Soc, Lausanne, p. 276.

PAUL, P. S.; JOHNSON, M. E.; AND GORZIGLIA, M. 1990b. Nucleic acid probes for the detection and differentiation of rotavirus serotypes. Proc 11th Int Congr Pig Vet Soc, Lausanne, p. 212.

PAUL, P.; PROESCHOLDT, T.; AND HILL, H. 1990c. The prevalence of rotavirus groups in pigs with diarrhea. Proc Commer Diagn Technol in Anim Health Monit. Natl Vet Serv Lab and Iowa State Univ Vet Diagn Lab, Ames, p. 236.

PAUL, P. S.; GORZIGLIA, M.; AND JOHNSON, M. 1991. Antigenic and genetic characterization of ISU-64 strain of porcine rotavirus. In preparation.

PEARSON, G. R., AND MCNULTY, M. S. 1977. Pathological changes in the small intestine of neonatal pigs infected with a pig reovirus-like agent (rotavirus). J Comp Pathol 87:363–375.

––––––. 1979. Ultrastructural changes in small intestinal epithelium of neonatal pigs infected with pig rotavirus. Arch Virol 59:127–136.

PEDLEY, S.; BRIDGER, J. C.; BROWN, J. F.; AND MC-CRAE, M. A. 1983. Molecular characterization of rotaviruses with distinct group antigens. J Gen Virol 64:2093–2101.

PEDLEY, S.; BRIDGER, J. C.; CHASEY, D.; AND MCCRAE, M. A. 1986. Definition of two new groups of atypical rotaviruses. J Gen Virol 67:131–137.

PROESCHOLDT, T., AND PAUL, P. S. 1991. Cultivation of porcine group C rotavirus in porcine intestinal cell line. In preparation.

RIXON, F. P.; TAYLOR, P.; AND DESSELBERGER, U. 1984. Rotavirus RNA segments sized by electron microscopy. J Gen Virol 65:233–239.

ROBERTS, L.; WALKER, E. J.; SNODGRASS, D. R.; AND ANGUS, K. W. 1980. Diarrhea in unweaned piglets associated with rotavirus and coccidial infections. Vet Rec 107:156–157.

ROBERTSON, M. D., AND WILCOX, G. E. 1986. Avian reovirus. Vet Bull 56:155–174.

ROBL, M. G.; MCADARAGH, J. P.; PHILLIPS, C. S.; AND BICKNELL, E. J. 1971. Experimental swine pneumonia caused by reovirus type III. Vet Med 66:903–904.

RODGER, S. M.; CRAVEN, J. A.; AND WILLIAMS, I. 1975. Demonstration of reovirus-like particles in intestinal contents of piglets with diarrhoea. Aust Vet J 51:536.

ROSEN, B. I.; SAIF, L. J.; JACKWOOD, D. J.; AND GORZIGLIA, M. 1990. Hybridization probes for the detection and differentiation of two serotypes of porcine rotavirus. Vet Microbiol 24:327–339.

RUIZ, A. M.; LOPEZ, I. V.; LOPEZ, S.; ESPEJO, R. T.; AND ARIAS, C. F. 1988. Molecular and antigenic characterization of porcine rotavirus YM, a possible new rotavirus serotype. J Virol 62:4331–4336.

SABIN, A. B. 1959. Reoviruses. A new group of respiratory and enteric viruses formerly classified as ECHO type 10 is described. Science 130:1387–1389.

SAIF, L. J.; THEIL, K. W.; AND BOHL, E. H. 1978. Morphogenesis of porcine rotavirus in porcine kidney cell cultures and intestinal epithelial cells. J Gen Virol 39:205–217.

SAIF, L. J.; BOHL, E. H.; THEIL, K. W.; CROSS, R. F.; AND HOUSE, J. A. 1980. Rotavirus-like, calicivirus-like, and 23-nm virus-like particles associated with diarrhea in young pigs. J Clin Microbiol 12:105–111.

SAIF, L. J.; TERRETT, L. A.; MILLER, K. L.; AND CROSS, R. F. 1988. Serial propagation of porcine group C rotavirus (pararotavirus) in a continuous cell line and characterization of the passaged virus. J Clin Microbiol 26:1277–1282.

SATTAR, S. A.; RAPHAEL, R. A.; LOCHNAN, H.; AND SPRINGTHORPE, V. S. 1983. Rotavirus inactivation by chemical disinfectants and antiseptics used in hospitals. Can J Microbiol 19:1464–1469.

SHAW, D. P.; MOREHOUSE, L. G.; AND SOLORZANO, R. F. 1989a. Experimental rotavirus infection in three-week-old pigs. Am J Vet Res 50:1961–1965.

––––––. 1989b. Rotavirus replication in colostrum-fed and colostrum-deprived pigs. Am J Vet Res 50:1966–1970.

SNODGRASS, D. R.; HERRING, A. J.; CAMPBELL, I.; INGLIS, J. M.; AND HARGREAVES, F. D. 1984. Comparison of atypical rotaviruses from calves, piglets, lambs, and man. J Gen Virol 65:909–914.

STEEL, R. B., AND TORRES-MEDINA, A. 1984. Effects of environmental and dietary factors on human rotavirus infection in gnotobiotic piglets. Infect Immun 43:906–911.

STEVENSON, G. W. 1990. Pathogenesis of a new porcine serotype of group A rotavirus in neonatal gnotobiotic and weaned conventional pigs. Ph.D. diss., Iowa State Univ.

STEVENSON, G. W.; PAUL, P. S.; AND ANDREWS, J. J. 1990. Pathogenesis of a new serotype of porcine group A rotavirus in the small intestine mucosa of neonatal gnotobiotic and weaned conventional pigs. Proc Am Assoc Vet Lab Diagn, p. 12.

SUZUKI, H.; CHEN, G. M.; HUNG, T.; BEARDS, G. M.; BROWN, D. W. G.; AND FLEWETT, T. H. 1987. Effects of two negative staining methods on the Chinese atypical rotavirus. Arch Virol 94:305–308.

SVENSMARK, B.; JORSAL, S. E.; NIELSEN, K.; AND WILLEBERG, P. 1989a. Epidemiological studies of piglet diarrhoea in intensively managed Danish sow herds. I. Pre-weaning diarrhoea. Acta Vet Scand 30:43–53.

SVENSMARK, B.; NIELSEN, K.; DALSGAARD, K.; AND WILLEBERG, P. 1989b. Epidemiological studies of piglet diarrhoea in intensively managed Danish sow herds. III. Rotavirus infection. Acta Vet Scand 30:63–70.

SVENSSON, L.; GRAHNQUIST, L.; PETTERSON, C.; GRANDIEN, M.; STINTZING, G.; AND GREENBERG, H. B. 1988. Detection of human rotaviruses which do not react with subgroup I and II specific monoclonal antibodies. J Clin Microbiol 26:1238–1240.

SVENSSON, L.; PADILLA-NORIEGA, L.; TANIGUCHI, K.; AND GREENBERG, H. B. 1990. Lack of cosegregation of the subgroup II antigens on genes 2 and 6 in porcine rotaviruses. J Virol 64:411–413.

TERRETT, L. A., AND SAIF, L. J. 1987. Serial propagation of porcine group C rotavirus (pararotavirus) in primary porcine kidney cell cultures. J Clin Microbiol 25:1316–1319.

TERRETT, L. A.; SAIF, L. J.; THEIL, K. W.; AND KOHLER, E. M. 1987. Physicochemical characterization of porcine pararotavirus and detection of virus and viral antibodies using cell culture immunofluorescence. J Clin Microbiol 25:268–272.

THEIL, K. W., AND SAIF, L. J. 1985. In vitro detection of

porcine rotavirus-like virus (group B rotavirus) and its antibody. J Clin Microbiol 21:844–846.

THEIL, K. W.; BOHL, E. H.; AND AGNES, A. G. 1977. Cell culture propagation of porcine rotavirus (reovirus-like agent). Am J Vet Res 38:1765–1768.

THEIL, K. W.; BOHL, E. H.; CROSS, R. F.; KOHLER, E. M.; AND AGNES, A. G. 1978. Pathogenesis of porcine rotaviral infection in experimentally inoculated gnotobiotic pigs. Am J Vet Res 39:213–220.

THEIL, K. W.; McCLOSKEY, C. M.; SAIF, L. J.; REDMAN, D. R.; BOHL, E. H.; HANCOCK, D. D.; KOHLER, E. M.; AND MOORHEAD, P. D. 1981. Rapid, simple method of preparing rotaviral double-stranded ribonucleic acid for analysis by polyacrylamide gel electrophoresis. J Clin Microbiol 14:273–280.

THEIL, K. W.; SAIF, L. J.; MOORHEAD, P. D.; AND WHITMOYER, R. E. 1985. Porcine rotavirus-like virus (group B rotavirus): Characterization and pathogenicity for gnotobiotic pigs. J Clin Microbiol 21:340–345.

THOULESS, M. E.; BRYDEN, A. S.; FLEWETT, T. H.; WOODE, G. N.; BRIDGER, J. C.; SNODGRASS, D. R.; AND HERRING, J. A. 1977. Serological relationships between rotaviruses from different species as studied by complement fixation and neutralization. Arch Virol 53:287–294.

TORRES-MEDINA, A., AND UNDERDAHL, N. R. 1980. Scanning electron microscopy of intestine of gnotobiotic piglets infected with porcine rotavirus. Can J Comp Med 44:403–411.

TYLER, K. L., AND FIELDS, B. N. 1990. Reoviruses in Virology, 2d ed. N.Y.: Raven Press, pp. 1307–1328.

TZIPORI, S., AND WILLIAMS, I. H. 1978. Diarrhea in piglets inoculated with rotavirus. Aust Vet J 54:188–192.

TZIPORI, S.; CHANDLER, D.; SMITH, M.; MAKIN, T.; AND HENNESSY, D. 1980a. Factors contributing to postweaning diarrhea in a large intensive piggery. Aust Vet J 56:274–278.

TZIPORI, S.; CHANDLER, D.; MAKIN, T.; AND SMITH, M. 1980b. *Escherichia coli* and rotavirus infections in four-week-old gnotobiotic piglets fed milk of dry food. Aust Vet J 56:279–284.

UTRERA, V.; MAZZALI DE ILJA, R.; GORZIGLIA, M.; AND ESPARZA, J. 1984. Epidemiological aspects of porcine rotavirus infection in Venezuela. Res Vet Sci 36:310–315.

VAN DER HEIDE, L. 1977. Viral arthritis/tenosynovitis: A review. Avian Pathol 6:271–284.

WATT, R. G. 1978. Virological study of two commercial pig herds with respiratory disease. Res Vet Sci 24:147–153.

WESTERCAMP, D. H. 1986. Field trial of porcine rotavirus vaccine to combat postweaning scours in baby pigs. Mod Vet Pract (January):17–18.

WOODE, G. N. 1986. Porcine rotavirus infection. In Diseases of Swine, 6th ed. Ed. A. D. Leman, B. Straw, R. D. Glock, W. L. Mengeling, R. H. C. Penny, and E. Scholl. Ames: Iowa State Univ Press, pp. 368–382.

WOODE, G. N., AND BRIDGER, J. C. 1975. Viral enteritis of calves. Vet Rec 96:85–88.

WOODE, G. N., AND CROUCH, C. F. 1978. Naturally occurring and experimentally induced rotaviral infections of domestic and laboratory animals. J Am Vet Med Assoc 173:522–526.

WOODE, G. N.; BRIDGER, J.; HALL, G. A.; JONES, J. M.; AND JACKSON, G. 1976. The isolation of reovirus-like agents (rotaviruses) from acute gastroenteritis of piglets. Med Microbiol 9:203–209.

YAMASHIRO, Y.; SHIMIZU, T.; OGUCHI, S.; AND SATO, M. 1989. Prostaglandins in the plasma and stool of children with rotavirus gastroenteritis. J Pediatr Gastroenterol Nutr 9:322–327.

ZINDEL, F.; BOMMELI, W.; AND KIHM, U. 1980. A survey of neutralizing antibodies against some porcine viruses in Swiss pig herds. Proc Int Congr Pig Vet Soc, Copenhagen, p. 65.

27 Swine Influenza

B. C. Easterday

V. S. Hinshaw

SWINE INFLUENZA (SI)—also known as swine flu, hog flu, and pig flu—is a specific acute, infectious, respiratory disease of swine caused by type A influenza viruses. The disease is characterized by sudden onset, coughing, dyspnea, fever, prostration, and rapid recovery. Lesions develop rapidly in the respiratory tract and regress quickly except in a few cases where severe viral pneumonia may be followed by death. The course, nature, and severity of the disease is likely to vary with the strain of the virus, the age and immune status of the pig, and the presence of concurrent infections.

SI has received considerable attention since the disease was first described in 1918. In the late summer of that year an epizootic disease, having many clinical and pathologic similarities to influenza in humans, appeared among swine in the north central United States. The appearance of the disease in swine was coincidental with the 1918 influenza pandemic that was responsible for the death of an estimated 20 million people throughout the world. The exact date or locality of its initial occurrence is unknown, but observers stated that cases were seen in August 1918 on farms in western Illinois (Shope 1964). While the infection and disease may have existed among swine populations before that time, it is unlikely that a disease with such distinctive characteristics would have gone unnoticed and unreported.

According to Dorset et al. (1922), Dr. J. S. Koen, an inspector in the division of hog cholera control of the USDA Bureau of Animal Industry, was the first to recognize the disease as being different from any previously encountered. He was impressed by the coincidental prevalence of epidemic human influenza and the similarity of signs and symptoms seen in humans to those occurring in swine. He was convinced that the two diseases were the same and he was the first to apply the name "flu" to this new disease of hogs. His opinion that the condition represented a new epizootic disease of swine and that swine had been infected from humans was shared by veterinarians and farmers in the area.

Various aspects of the disease, signs, lesions, and course were described by Dorset et al. (1922) and McBryde (1927) during the decade following the first report. It was not until 1930 that the SI virus (SIV) was isolated and identified by Shope (1931b). For the next 25 years Shope expanded his work to include studies of immunity, transmission, adaptation of the virus to laboratory hosts, antigenic relationships with other influenza viruses, and maintenance of the disease in nature. Few other investigators reported studies on SI during that time. From all accounts, the infection and disease in swine has not changed significantly in the north central United States since it was first observed in 1918. However, as will be described later, the infection and disease may be caused by type A influenza viruses with different antigenic and/or biologic characteristics.

Prior to 1975, swine influenza was considered to be unique to the United States. However, since that time, clinical SI and various type A viruses and their antibodies have been observed and reported in most parts of the world where swine are found.

While SI has continued to be a common endemic disease in north central United States for more than 70 years, it is clear, based on clinical observations and serologic and virologic surveillance studies, that the infection and disease are found throughout the United States. About 25–33% of all pigs (6–7 months old) slaughtered in the United States have SIV antibody; the rate is higher (about 45%) among older swine (2 or more years) that are slaughtered, i.e., those animals that have been used for breeding purposes (Woods 1975; Pirtle et al. 1976; Hinshaw et al. 1978; Chambers et al. 1990). There is little seasonal variation in the rate of infection based on the presence of antibodies in serum of slaughter swine. However, SIV has been most readily recovered in the late fall and early winter in virus surveillance studies conducted on slaughter swine.

ETIOLOGY. SI is caused by influenza A viruses, which belong to the family Orthomyxoviridae. There is an enormous amount of information available on antigenic, genetic, structural, and biologic characteristics of influenza A viruses (for review, see Murphy and Webster 1990). SIV are pleomorphic, medium-sized, enveloped virions with glycoproteins, commonly called "spikes," extending from their surface. These glycoproteins are the major surface antigens and are of two distinct kinds, hemagglutinin (H) and neuraminidase (N), an enzyme. Hemagglutinin is responsible for attachment of viruses to cells and causes agglutination of erythrocytes. Neuraminidase is responsible for elution of virus from erythrocytes, and it may play a role in the release of virus from infected cells. Antibodies to the hemagglutinin are responsible for preventing infection with an influenza virus containing the same hemagglutinin, whereas antibodies against the neuraminidase restrict the spread of virus from infected cells. The antigenic characteristics of these two surface glycoproteins are the bases for dividing the viruses into subtypes. Recent antigenic comparison of H1N1 viruses (Sherrar et al. 1989) have indicated that the hemagglutinins of H1N1 swine viruses have not changed extensively during the last 50 years, which is in contrast to the marked antigenic variation (or drift) seen with human strains. The reason for this is not yet clear but it seems likely that there is little immune pressure on swine viruses because pigs are short-lived and their viruses are continually transmitted to nonimmune, susceptible pigs.

The H and N spikes are embedded in a lipid envelope that surrounds the core of the virus particle. Matrix protein molecules line the underside of the envelope and surround the core, inside of which is a helical complex of molecules consisting of ribonucleic acid (RNA) in association with nucleoprotein (NP) and polymerases (enzymes that initiate replication). Influenza viruses are classified as A, B, or C, based on the antigenic relatedness of the NP and M proteins, which are closely related among influenza A viruses. The viral genome consists of 8 single-stranded RNA segments and codes for 10 viral proteins. Because the viral RNA is segmented, genetic exchange or reassortment between different influenza A viruses can occur during mixed infections. Genetic reassortant between human and nonhuman viruses is considered a likely mechanism for the origin of new human pandemic strains. At least one reassortment virus, A/swine/Kanagawa/2/78 (H1N2), was isolated from swine in Japan (Sugimura et al. 1980). The hemagglutinin of that virus was indistinguishable from the current swine H1N1 virus, but the neuraminidase was similar to that of earlier H3N2 human viruses.

So far, 13 hemagglutinins and 9 neuraminidases have been identified among all influenza A viruses (WHO 1980). The current system of nomenclature of influenza viruses introduced in 1980 designates the type, host, place, year of origin, and antigenic subtype. For example, a SIV isolated in Wisconsin in 1984 would be designated A/swine/Wis/1/84(H1N1). The first character, A, identifies the type, followed by the host of origin (except human), geographic origin, strain number (if any), the year of isolation, and the antigenic subtype of the H and N in parentheses.

Prior to 1980, the influenza viruses of swine origin were designated as Hsw1N1. Most SI is caused by H1N1 viruses; H3N2 viruses are responsible to a lesser extent, but significant disease due to this strain among pigs has been reported in England and Europe (Haesebrouk et al. 1985; Pritchard et al. 1987; Castro et al. 1988).

Laboratory Cultivation. SIV grows readily when injected into chicken eggs embryonated 9–12 days. It may be inoculated by either the intraallantoic or intraamniotic routes. The temperature of incubation ranges from 33 to 37°C. The embryos usually do not die, and presence of the virus is demonstrated after 72–96 hours of incubation by hemagglutination tests on the allantoic and/or amniotic fluids. With the diversity of influenza viruses that have been recovered from swine, it is reasonable to expect cultural differences, e.g., temperature of incubation for optimal growth, time of incubation, and embryo death.

Although the embryonated chicken egg is the culture system most commonly used, various cell culture systems have been used for the growth and assay of SIV. These include calf kidney cells, fetal pig lung cells, canine kidney cells, pig kidney cells, chicken embryo fibroblasts, human diploid cells, and Chang conjunctival cells (Easterday 1975). Other cell culture systems include a pig oviduct cell line (Bouillant et al. 1975) and a swine testicle cell line (Potgeiter et al. 1977). Fetal pig trachea, lung, and nasal epithelial organ cultures and tracheal organ cultures from chickens, horses, and ferrets also support the growth of SIV (Nakamura and Easterday 1970; Schmidt et al. 1974).

EPIDEMIOLOGY. At least three major aspects to consider in any discussion of the epidemiology of SI are the epidemic characteristics of classical SI, interspecies transmission of influenza viruses, and public health aspects.

Acute Swine Influenza. The first appearance of SI in a swine population is commonly associated with the movement of animals, e.g., the introduction of breeding stock, introduction of feeder pigs, or return of show stock to the farm. Once the infection has appeared in a swine-breeding operation or any situation where there is no complete depopulation, it is likely to be maintained in the herd with at least annual episodes of acute disease.

It is common for many outbreaks to appear simultaneously on several farms within an area. Such multicentric outbreaks are not necessarily the result of recent movement of infected animals but rather are due to the wide distribution of the virus among herds in an area. Many outbreaks are clearly related to the movement of animals from infected to susceptible herds. It is generally reported that outbreaks are explosive, with all of the pigs in the herd becoming ill at the same time. However, owners who observe their herds closely are often aware of one to a few pigs with signs of the disease 2–5 days before the whole herd is involved. The primary route of transmission is presumed to be direct pig-to-pig transmission by the nasopharyngeal route. Nasal secretions are laden with virus during the acute febrile stages of infection, providing an abundant source of infectious materials for susceptible animals. Swine are readily infected under experimental procedures by instillation of virus suspensions into the nostrils or by exposure to small-particle aerosols. Contact transmission is easily demonstrated under experimental conditions.

Episodes of acute SI in the north central United States have commonly occurred from the late summer into the winter. The appearance of these outbreaks often coincides with the mixing of swine at shows such as county fairs and with the onset of marked fluctuations of outdoor temperatures from moderate daytime temperatures to below freezing at night and cold autumn rains. Swine held in confinement housing are not subjected to those environmental stresses, and as more swine are held in confinement housing, the seasonal nature and severity of the disease may change.

While outbreaks of SI generally have been seasonal, especially in the north central United States, the infection and disease are present throughout the year. Acute typical disease has been reported in early summer (Potgeiter et al. 1977). SIV has been recovered from pigs with respiratory disease without the typical signs of influenza (Nakamura et al. 1972), and SIV has been recovered from swine with no signs of disease (Hinshaw et al. 1978).

During one period of 14 months, Hinshaw et al. (1978) conducted extensive virologic and serologic surveillance on slaughter swine in the north central and south central United States. They recovered 478 influenza viruses from approximately 9400 swine tested (about 5% infectivity rate). Antibodies against SIV(H1N1) were found in 21% of those swine. Studies in both areas revealed the presence of viruses in the pigs throughout the year, but the frequency of virus isolation was much higher in the northern states. The north central states showed peak virus activity from October to December, whereas the southern states did not have a marked peak other than a slight increase in the spring months. These results are in agreement with those of Nakamura et al. (1972) and Pirtle et al. (1976), who reported a similar prevalence and presence throughout the year. A recent serologic survey (Chambers et al. 1990) on U.S. pigs in 1988–89, indicated that 51% of pigs in the north central United States had antibodies to H1N1 viruses, emphasizing the continued circulation of this virus at high frequency.

The seasonal occurrence of the disease was a phenomenon reported during the first 10 years after its appearance in 1918 (Dorset et al. 1922; McBryde et al. 1928). There was a general opinion that the annual outbreaks were due to stress related to meteorologic factors and related management procedures. Dr. R. E. Shope became intrigued by the seasonal occurrence of the disease and investigated the mechanism(s) by which the virus was maintained between epidemic seasons. It was assumed at that time (late 1930s) that the virus disappeared after an epidemic episode and that a recovered animal would not harbor the virus. His interesting studies led him to offer the hypothesis that SIV survived during the epidemic period in the adult or larval stages of swine lungworms (*Metastrongylus*) or their intermediate hosts, the earthworm (family Lumbricidae) (Shope 1964). Shope, as well as other investigators, could not demonstrate the virus in any stage of the lungworm or the earthworm by direct means; thus, there is really no evidence at this time that the virus is maintained in worms. The widespread occurrence of the virus in pigs indicates that the pigs themselves maintain the virus by continual passage to young, susceptible pigs.

Over the years there has been speculation about a carrier state that would provide for the interepidemic survival of SIV. Several investigators have made observations and/or conducted experiments that suggested a persistent infection or carrier state (Scott 1939, 1941; Nakamura 1967; Blaskovic et al. 1970; Nakamura et al. 1972). In an experimental infection of 22 specific-pathogen-free pigs with an H1N1 virus, Vannier et al. (1985) reported the recovery of virus from nasal swabs collected from one pig 29 days after initial infection. There was no contact infection detected when susceptible pigs were placed with the previously infected pigs 30–45 days and 60 days post-infection. The widespread occurrence of SI in the United States and other parts of the world at all times of the year supports the probability that the virus is constantly circulating. There are no clear data to support or reject the existence of a long-term true-carrier state of influenza viruses in swine.

There seems to be no unique pattern of occurrence of the infection or disease in other parts of the world, except in those cases where human origin influenza virus such as H3N2 is transmitted to swine populations during an epidemic among humans. Nardelli et al. (1978) reported SI in northern Italy during the fall and early winter of 1976 and indicated that the clinical signs and epizootiology coincided with those of the classical SI as it occurred in North America. Hsu et al. (1976) reported classical SI for the first time in Taiwan in March and April 1975. In neither case was the origin of the virus determined. An epidemic of SI that began in December 1981 in Brittany (France) involved about 70% of the herds (4 million pigs) in the province by September 1982. The rapid spread was attributed to the contagiousness of the disease, high density of swine, and high rate of movement of swine among farms. Some spread was attributed to the wind (Madec et al. 1982). There was no mention of association with season or time of year in outbreaks reported in Great Britain and Belgium in more recent years.

Interspecies Transmission. Influenza A viruses exist in many different species in nature, including humans, lower mammals, and birds. An important aspect regarding this situation is that interspecies transmission occurs and pigs are certainly involved in this natural exchange of viruses. Based on studies of viruses isolated from pigs in Europe since 1980 (Hinshaw et al. 1984), there is convincing evidence that recent epidemics in pigs have been caused by H1N1 viruses most closely related to avian H1N1 strains. This indicates that avian viruses are capable of infecting and causing disease in pigs in the natural setting.

During the last decade, swine H1N1 virus have also been responsible for disease outbreaks in turkeys (Hinshaw et al. 1983), which experienced respiratory disease and diminished egg production (Mohan et al. 1981; Andral et al. 1985). This was the first indication that a mammalian virus could be responsible for infection and disease in birds. It is thought that the viruses were introduced into turkeys by contact with infected pigs or people. Thus, evidence accumulated in recent years indicates that H1N1 viruses have the capacity to move among species, particularly swine, ducks, turkeys, and humans; pigs can be infected with viruses from birds and humans. This has stimulated Scholtissek and Naylor (1988) to propose pigs as a "mixing vessel" for viruses from avian and mammalian species. These findings underline the significance of pig influenza viruses in the ecology of all influenza viruses.

Infection of swine with human H3N2 viruses (the Hong Kong influenza of 1968 and its many antigenic relatives) was described soon after it appeared in the human population (Kundin 1970; Romvary and Tanyi 1975; Tumova et al. 1976). Typically, H3N2 virus in pigs occurred during epidemics in humans and did not appear to be established and maintained in swine. However, more recently, there is evidence that the H3N2 viruses are established in swine (Chapman et al. 1978; Shortridge and Webster 1979; Haesebrouk et al. 1985; Pritchard et al. 1987; Castro et al. 1988) and cause significant disease (Pensaert 1984) in areas outside the United States, whereas the H3N2 viruses appear in U.S. swine infrequently.

Public Health Aspects. In 1976, it was clearly demonstrated that SIV was transmitted from pigs to humans in the natural setting and caused acute respiratory disease in humans. Prior to that time, there was serological evidence that people, particularly those in close contact with pigs, were infected with SIV.

A major milestone in the chronology of zoonotic influenza came in January 1976 with the isolation of an influenza virus, A/NJ/8/76(H1N1), closely related to swine influenza viruses, from sick military recruits at Fort Dix, N.J. (Goldfield et al. 1977; Kendal et al. 1977). There were many cases of acute respiratory disease, and serologic investigations revealed that several hundred recruits had been infected. Epidemiologic investigations could not identify infected or sick pigs that might have been the source of the virus for that outbreak.

There was speculation and concern that the virus would be the new epidemic strain of influenza for humans—perhaps a return of the virus that was responsible for the 1918 pandemic. There followed a national program to vaccinate humans against A/NJ/8/76(H1N1) virus; a surveillance program was also initiated to investigate pigs and their human contacts.

All speculation about the zoonotic nature of influenza came to an end in November 1976 when SIV (H1N1) was isolated from pigs and their caretaker on a farm in southern Wisconsin (Easterday et al. 1976; Hinshaw et al. 1978). In November 1976, pigs on a farm near Brodhead, Wis., had been sick 2 or 3 days when one of the caretakers also became ill and had moderate to severe signs of influenza requiring bed rest for 2 days. Nasal swabs from the pigs and throat washings from the man were collected on the same day. The virus was recovered from six of eight pigs sampled and from three throat washings collected from the young man over a period of approximately 18 hours. There was no evidence that the virus spread from the caretaker to any of his family or other human contacts. The characterization of the viruses from the man and the pigs indicated they were identical (Palese and Ritchey 1977; Hinshaw et al. 1978).

Two weeks later an almost identical case occurred in a 14-year-old boy on another farm approximately 100 km away. In that case the virus was isolated from one of five pigs and from one throat washing taken from the boy. Further testing indicated that the virus had spread from that boy to at least one and probably three of his close schoolmates.

Dasco et al. (1980) reported the isolation of an H1N1 virus from a young man who had worked in a large swine show. Patriarca et al. (1984) recovered an H1N1 virus similar to contemporary strains isolated from swine in the United States following a fatal infection in an immunocompromised child. Extensive epidemiologic investigation did not reveal a probable animal source of the virus. Most recently, a swine H1N1 virus was recovered from a Wisconsin woman who died of primary viral pneumonia. She had attended a fair where sick pigs were present. The more recent isolations of H1N1 viruses from avian species (especially turkeys) and the recovery of one such virus from a human signal concern about species other than swine serving as a source of swine H1N1 viruses for humans (Hinshaw et al. 1983).

These documented cases of transmission of SIV resulting in acute respiratory disease in humans in contact with swine have been young people under 30 years of age. In the United States there is a plentiful source of virus in the pig populations, and there are thousands of contacts between humans and pigs every day. Such exposure constitutes an occupational hazard and a potential public health problem of undetermined magnitude and significance.

CLINICAL SIGNS AND PATHOGENESIS.

Classical SI is a herd disease. The signs of the disease currently observed are essentially as they were described in the 1920s (Dorset et al. 1922; McBryde 1927; Shope 1931a).

The onset is sudden after an incubation period of 1–3 days. Most of the animals in the herd appear affected at the same time. There is anorexia, inactivity, prostration, huddling, and piling. One can walk among the inactive animals and they will not move, even with vigorous prodding. There is open-mouthed, labored, jerking, and abdominal breathing, especially when the animals are forced to move.

Movement will also be accompanied by severe paroxysms of coughing that may sound like a herd of barking dogs. Fever is usually in the range of 40.5–41.7°C. One may observe conjunctivitis, rhinitis, nasal discharge, and sneezing. There is obvious loss of weight and weakness related to the anorexia and inactivity. Morbidity is high (near 100%) but mortality is low (generally less than 1%) unless there are intercurrent infections and/or the pigs are very young. Generally, recovery begins 5–7 days after onset and it is as sudden and remarkable as the onset.

Virus isolation and or the detection of specific antibody are necessary for a definitive diagnosis. The clinical signs may be influenced by intercurrent infections and low levels of immunity.

It is not uncommon for producers and veterinarians to report reproductive, farrowing, and neonatal problems associated with outbreaks of SI. Abortions, stillbirths, infertility, and small and weak litters have been reported in association with acute SI. Limited studies of these conditions have concluded that the virus was not directly responsible (Walker 1971; Renshaw 1975; Brown et al. 1982). However, Madec et al. (1989) reported that of 13 sows infected less than 1 week before an outbreak of SI, only 3 farrowed normal pigs. Of the other 10, 7 returned to estrus and 3 were not "with pigs" and did not return to estrus.

Sows more than 1 month into pregnancy were minimally affected. SIV was isolated from one aborted fetus. Their observations are consistent with the results of studies by Young and Underdahl (1949a,b; 1950a,b). They reported that pigs farrowed by dams inoculated during gestation had a higher mortality rate than those from control dams. This influence was found to be most pronounced among pigs farrowed by dams inoculated during the first month of pregnancy.

The clinical signs described in the European outbreaks are similar to those observed in the United States, e.g., fever, anorexia, inactivity, pneumonia, respiratory disease, cough, high morbidity, low mortality, rapid onset, rapid recovery, and abortion in some sows late in pregnancy (Muller et al. 1981).

LESIONS

Gross Lesions. The gross lesions found in uncomplicated SI are mainly those of a viral pneumonia. The changes are most likely to be limited to the apical and cardiac lobes of the lungs, although in severe cases more than half of the lung may be affected. Generally, there is a sharp line of demarcation between the affected and normal lung tissue. The involved areas will be purple and firm. Some interlobular edema may be evident. The airways are likely to be filled with blood-tinged, fibrinous exudate. The associated bronchial and mediastinal lymph nodes are usually enlarged. In severe cases there may be fibrinous pleuritis (Shope 1931a; Nayak et al. 1965; Nakamura 1967).

Brown et al. (1980) described pulmonary hypoplasia in swine fetuses inoculated with H1N1 virus about day 55 of gestation. Within 3–7 days there was epithelial necrosis in the bronchial buds and the more fully differentiated major bronchi. By 28 days postinoculation the lungs were about half the normal size.

Microscopic Lesions. As with the gross lesions, the microscopic lesions in uncomplicated cases are consistent with viral pneumonia. Bachmann (1989) has provided a concise summary of the microscopic lesions of SI: "Histologically, a widespread degeneration and necrosis of the epithelium in bronchi and bronchioli, can be observed. The lumen of bronchi, bronchioli, and alveoli are filled with exudate containing desquamated cells and neutrophils, later mostly monocytes. Furthermore, variable hyperemia with dilatation of the capillaries and infiltration of the alveolar septae with lymphocytes, histiocytes, and plasma cells occurs. Widespread alveolar atelectasis, interstitial pneumonia, and emphysema accompany these lesions. There is also peribronchial and perivascular cellular infiltration (Shope 1931a; Urman et al. 1958; Witte et al. 1981)."

Nayak et al. (1965) describe the detection of

SIV antigen in many cells of the respiratory tract using immunocytologic techniques in experimental pathogenesis studies. Viral antigen was detected in bronchial epithelial cells within 2 hours postinfection. By 16 hours there were large fluorescent areas of bronchial epithelium. Staining was intense through 72 hours postinfection and then diminished, disappearing from the bronchial mucosa by day 9. Antigen was also detected in the alveolar septa within 4 hours after infection, and at 24 hours there were numerous fluorescent cells in the alveoli and alveolar ducts. The fluorescent staining in the alveoli also disappeared by day 9. Antigen was detected in the lower portion of the trachea near the bifurcation and it was most evident 48 hours postinfection. Antigen was not detected in the trachea after day 4. Occasional fluorescence was observed in the epithelium of the turbinates and mediastinal lymph nodes. Fluorescent cells were not detected in the tonsil, larynx, liver, or kidney.

DIAGNOSIS. SI may be suspected when there is an outbreak of acute respiratory disease involving most or all of the pigs in a herd in the fall or early winter. Although signs of the classical disease have been described in some detail above, a clinical diagnosis is presumptive. Nakamura et al. (1972) described conditions clinically identical to classical SI but not caused by SIV and respiratory disease not typical for SI from which SIV was isolated. SI must be differentiated from enzootic pneumonia of pigs and other acute and chronic respiratory diseases.

A definitive diagnosis of SI can be made only by the isolation of SIV or demonstration of specific antibodies. The best sample for virus isolation is nasal mucus obtained by swabbing the nasal passages. The swab is suspended in a suitable transport medium such as glycerol saline; it is important to keep the sample moist and cold (4°C, refrigerator temperatures) during transport to the laboratory. In very small pigs, where it is difficult to swab the nasal passages, pharyngeal mucus may be obtained by swabbing. If the samples for virus isolation can be tested within 48 hours after collection, they should be kept at 4°C. If the samples must be held longer, storage at −70°C is recommended. Freezing at −20°C is not usually recommended, but dry ice or liquid nitrogen storage is appropriate. Filtration of the samples should be avoided to conserve small amounts of virus that might be in the transport medium. Adventitious bacterial and fungal agents may be controlled with the addition of appropriate antimicrobial agents to the transport medium. Virus is more likely to be found in nasal secretion during the febrile period than after the fever has subsided. It may also be isolated from lung tissue from pigs killed during the acute stage of the disease. The lung tissue is ground, suspended in saline, and injected into 10-day embryonated chicken eggs.

The inoculated eggs are generally incubated at 35°C. Since SIV usually does not kill the chick embryo, the allantoic fluids are collected after 72–96 hours incubation and tested for hemagglutination of chicken red blood cells, which is presumptive evidence for the presence of an influenza virus. The hemagglutinin subtype is determined by the hemagglutination-inhibition (HI) test and that of the neuraminidase with the neuraminidase-inhibition test (Centers for Disease Control 1982).

Serologic diagnosis of SI requires the use of paired serum samples (one obtained during the acute phase of the disease and the second, 3–4 weeks later) to demonstrate an increase in the amount of antibody. The most common test for antibody is the HI test as described in Centers for Disease Control (1982). A single radial hemolysis (SRH) technique has been described for the detection and measurement of SIV antibody in swine serum (Ogawa et al. 1978, 1982); however, the HI test is more widely used. The diagnostician must be aware of the possibility of the presence of nonspecific inhibition of hemagglutination and nonspecific agglutinins that may occur in swine serum. Appropriate treatment, e.g., receptor-destroying enzyme (RDE) to destroy the inhibitors or adsorption of serum with erythrocytes from the same source used for the test, may be necessary to remove the inhibitors and agglutinins.

Positive diagnosis of the disease by serologic and virologic means among suckling or weanling pigs from dams with antibody to the virus may be complicated. Maternal antibody persists 2–4 months, depending on the initial level. It has been shown that weanling pigs with maternal antibody may be infected and may shed virus (Easterday 1971, 1972; Renshaw 1975). Depending on the level of antibody, it may be very difficult to isolate virus. It has been shown that pigs with maternal antibody against SIV did not produce active antibody against that virus (Easterday 1971, 1972; Renshaw 1975). In these cases, even though virus may be isolated, the level of antibody in the convalescent-phase serum will be lower than in the acute-phase serum.

The inhibition of active antibody production by maternal antibody has been described (Mensik 1960, 1963, 1966; Easterday 1971; Renshaw 1975). The maternal antibody does not prevent infection, but active antibody production does not follow. The rate of virus recovery and severity of signs of disease are inversely related to level of antibody. After the maternal antibody is depleted, pigs may be infected again, shed virus, have signs of disease, and have a typical primary antibody response.

TREATMENT. There is no specific therapy for SI. Careful nursing is important, with the provision of comfortable, draft-free shelter. Clean, dry, dust-free bedding should be provided. Pigs should not be moved or transported during the acute stages of the disease to avoid additional stress to the respiratory system.

Fresh, clean water should be accessible at all times, because most animals will be febrile. There is a marked loss of appetite during the course of the disease, but it returns quickly with clinical improvement.

Expectorants are commonly used as a herd treatment and are administered in the drinking water. Antibiotics and other antimicrobial treatments have been used on a herd basis to control concurrent or secondary bacterial infections. Individuals may require additional supportive and antibacterial treatment in severe cases.

Amantadine (1-adamantanamine) is licensed in the United States for treatment and prevention of influenza in humans, but not pigs. It has been shown to be effective in reducing the febrile response and shedding of virus in experimentally infected pigs (McGregor and Easterday 1979).

PREVENTION AND CONTROL. Standard sanitary measures to prevent susceptible animals from contacting infected animals are appropriate to prevent the introduction of SI into a herd. Influenza A viruses are inactivated by soap, heat, sodium hypochlorite, formalin, or one-stroke Environ (FADR 1987). Because of the known occurrences of H1N1 viruses in turkeys and migratory waterfowl, producers should employ measures to prevent contact with those species. The possibility of introduction of type A influenza viruses from infected humans should not be ignored. Animals recovered from SI develop hemagglutination-inhibiting, virus-neutralizing, complement-fixing, and neuraminidase-inhibiting antibody. The degree and duration of resistance to subsequent infection in swine recovered from influenza have not been precisely determined. Substantial levels of antibody are found for at least 6 months after infection. As with many other infections, the relationship of the amount of antibody in the serum or respiratory secretions to the degree of resistance has not been defined. There is considerable variation in the antibody response of individual pigs following exposure. Antibodies have been detected in secretions and serum 8 days postinfection (Charley 1977). Cell-mediated immune responses were detected during the second week postinfection.

There are no licensed vaccines available in the United States for the prevention of SI. Inactivated-virus vaccines have been developed and/or tested by several investigators (Woods and Mansfield 1976, 1978, 1980; Easterday et al. 1977; Pirtle 1977). There is considerable variation in antibody response and protection from infection following vaccination. A live temperature-sensitive strain of SIV has been shown to provide some protection against disease (Easterday et al. 1977). Other studies have shown that nonvaccinated, experimentally infected pigs required 2 weeks

longer to reach market weight than their vaccinated exposed cohorts. (Easterday et al. 1977).

Gourreau et al. (1980) described an inactivated adjuvant vaccine against SIV (H1N1) that was superior to an aqueous inactivated vaccine. Antibodies were detected 15 days after vaccination and remained at a "satisfactory level" until the second month after vaccination. With a second inoculation (booster) "immunity" persisted until the eighth month.

There is widespread use of vaccine in Europe against SIV. In view of the extensive circulation of H1N1 virus in pigs and the antigenic conservation of these viruses, it seems quite possible that vaccines are a viable option for control. 1401H

REFERENCES

ANDRAL, B.; TOQUIN, D.; MADEC, F.; AYMARD, M.; GOURREAU, J. M.; KAISER, C.; FONTAINE, M.; AND METZ, M. H. 1985. Disease in turkeys associated with H1N1 influenza virus following an outbreak of the disease in pigs. Vet Rec 116:617–618.

BACHMANN, P. A. 1989. Swine influenza virus. In Virus Infections of Porcines. Ed. M. B. PENSAERT. Amsterdam: Elsevier Science, pp. 193–207.

BLASKOVIC, D.; JAMRICHOVA, O.; RATHOVA, V.; KOCISKOVA, D.; AND KAPLAN, M. M. 1970. Experimental infection of weanling pigs with A/swine influenza. II. The shedding of virus by infected animals. Bull WHO 42:767–770.

BOUILLANT, A. M.; DULAC, G. C.; WILLIS, N.; GIRARD, A.; GRIEG, A. S.; AND BOULANGER, P. 1975. Viral susceptibility of a cell line derived from the pig oviduct. Can J Comp Med 39:450–456.

BROWN, T. T.; MENGELING, W. L.; PAUL, P. S.; AND PIRTLE, E. C. 1980. Porcine fetuses with pulmonary hypoplasia resulting from experimental swine influenza virus infection. Vet Pathol 17:455–468.

BROWN, T. T., Jr.; MENGELING, W. L.; AND PIRTLE, E. C. 1982. Failure of swine influenza virus to cause transplacental infection of porcine fetuses. Am J Vet Res 43:817–819.

CASTRO, J. M.; DEL POZO, M.; SIMARRO, I. 1988. Identification of H3N2 influenza virus isolated from pigs with respiratory problems in Spain. Vet Rec 122(17):418–419.

Centers for Disease Control. 1982. Concepts and procedures for laboratory-based influenza surveillance. Centers for Disease Control, U.S. Dep of Health and Human Serv, Washington, D.C.

CHAMBERS, T. M.; HINSHAW, V. S.; KAWAOKA, Y.; EASTERDAY, B. C.; AND WEBSTER, R. G. 1990. Influenza viral infection of swine in the United States 1988–89. Arch Virol. In press.

CHAPMAN, M. S.; LAMONT, P. H.; AND HARKNESS, J. W. 1978. Serological evidence of continuing infection of swine in Great Britain with an influenza A virus (H3N2). J Hyg (Camb) 80:415–422.

CHARLEY, B. 1977. Local immunity in the pig respiratory tract. I. Cellular and humoral immune responses following swine influenza infection. Ann Microbiol 128B:95–107.

DASCO, C. C.; COUCH, R. B.; AND QUARLES, J. M. 1980. Sporadic occurrence of swine influenza in man. Abstr Annu Meet Am Soc Microbiol 80:288.

DORSET, M.; McBRYDE, C. N.; AND NILES, W. B. 1922. Remarks on "hog flu." J Am Vet Med Assoc 62:162–171.

EASTERDAY, B. C. 1971. Influenza virus infection of the suckling pig. Acta Vet [Suppl]2:33–42.

———. 1972. Immunologic considerations in swine influenza. J Am Vet Med Assoc 160:645–648.

———. 1975. Swine influenza. In Diseases of Swine, 4th ed. Ed. H. W. Dunne and A. D. Leman. Ames: Iowa State Univ Press, pp. 141–167.

EASTERDAY, B. C.; MURPHY, B. R.; AND MCGREGOR, S. 1977. Infection and vaccination of pigs with influenza A/New Jersey/8/76 (Hsw1N1) virus. J Infect Dis 136 [Suppl]:699–702.

Foreign Animal Disease Report. 1987. Approved disinfectants. Washington, D.C.: U.S. Dep Agric, p. 143.

GOLDFIELD, M.; NOBLE, G.; AND DOWDLE, W. R. 1977. Identification and preliminary antigenic analysis of swine influenza-like viruses isolated during an influenza outbreak at Fort Dix, New Jersey. J Infect Dis 136 [Suppl]:381–385.

GOURREAU, J. M.; HANNOUN, C.; AND KAISER, C. 1980. Evaluation of an inactivated, adjuvant vaccine against swine influenza. Comp Immunol Microbiol Infect Dis 3:147–153.

HAESEBROUCK, F.; BIRONT, P.; PENSAERT, M. B.; AND LEUNEN, J. 1985. Epizootics of respiratory tract disease in swine in Belgium due to H3N2 influenza virus and experimental reproduction of disease. Am J Vet Res 46(9):1926–1928.

HINSHAW, V. S.; BEAN, W. J., Jr.; WEBSTER, R. G.; AND EASTERDAY, B. C. 1978. The prevalence of influenza viruses in swine and the antigenic and genetic relatedness of influenza viruses from man and swine. Virology 84:51–62.

HINSHAW, V. S.; WEBSTER, R. G.; BEAM, W. J.; DOWNIE, J.; AND SENNE, D. A. 1983. Swine influenza-like viruses in turkeys: Potential source of virus in humans? Science 220:206–208.

HINSHAW, V. S.; ALEXANDER, D. J.; AYMARD, M.; BACHMANN, P. A.; EASTERDAY, B. C.; HANNOUN, C.; KIDA, H.; LIPKIND, M.; MACKENZIE, J. S.; NEROME, K.; SCHILD, G. C.; SCHOLTISSEK, C.; SENNE, D. A.; SHORTRIDGE, K. F.; SKEHEL, J. J.; AND WEBSTER, R. G. 1984. Antigenic comparisons of swine-influenza-like H1N1 isolates from pigs, birds and humans: An international collaborative study. Bull WHO 62:871–878.

HSU, F. S.; JOSEPH, P. L.; CHANG, C. P.; CHEN, W. F.; AND CHOU, N. Y. 1976. An epizootic of swine in Taiwan. Proc 4th Int Congr Pig Vet Soc, Ames, p. 16.

KENDAL, A. P.; GOLDFIELD, M.; NOBLE, G. R.; AND DOWDLE, W. R. 1977. Identification and preliminary antigenic analysis of swine influenzalike viruses isolated during an influenza outbreak at Fort Dix, New Jersey. J Infect Dis 136 [Suppl]:381–385.

KUNDIN, W. D. 1970. Hong Kong A₂ influenza virus infection among swine during a human epidemic in Taiwan. Nature 228:857.

MCBRYDE, C. N. 1927. Some observations on "hog flu" and its seasonal prevalence in Iowa. J Am Vet Med Assoc 71:368–377.

MCBRYDE, C. N.; NILES, W. B.; AND MOSKEY, H. E. 1928. Investigations on the transmission and etiology of hog flu. J Am Vet Med Assoc 73:331–346.

MCGREGOR, S.; AND EASTERDAY, B. C. 1979. Unpublished data.

MADEC, F.; GOURREAU, J. M.; AND KAISER, C. 1982. Epidemiology of swine influenza Hsw1N1 on farms in Brittany (first outbreak-1982). Epidemiol Sante Anim 2:56–64.

MADEC, F.; KAISER, C.; GOURREAU, J. M.; MARTINAT BOTTE, F.; and KERANFLECH, A. 1989. Pathological consequences of a severe outbreak of swine influenza (H1N1 virus) in the nonimmune sow at the beginning of pregnancy, under natural conditions. Comp Immun Microbiol Infect Dis 12(1/2):17–27.

MENSIK, J. 1960. Production and behavior of swine influenza antibodies. I. Influence of colostral antibodies on immunity in piglets during early life. Sb Cesk Akad Zemed Ved 5:599–619. Vet Bull 31, Abstr 127.

———. 1963. Formation of antibodies in swine influenza. III. Colostrol immunity and inhibition of antibody formation. Ved Pr Ustav Vet 3:141–149.

———. J. 1966. The formation and dynamism of antibodies in swine influenza. V. A long-term depression of the antibody formation in the progeny of hyperimmune mothers. Vet Med (Prague) 11:589–595.

MOHAN, R.; SAIF, Y. M.; ERICKSON, G. A.; GUSTAFSON, G. A.; AND EASTERDAY, B. C. 1981. Serologic and epidemiologic evidence of infection in turkeys with an agent related to the swine influenza virus. Avian Dis 25:11–16.

MULLER, E.; KNOCKE, K. W.; WILLERS, H.; AND JOCHIMS, R. 1981. Occurrence of swine influenza in northern Germany. Prakt Tieraerztl 62:669–672.

MURPHY, B. R., AND WEBSTER, R. G. 1990. Influenza viruses. In Virology. Ed. B. Fields. New York: Raven Press, pp. 1091–1154.

NAKAMURA, R. M. 1967. In vivo and in vitro studies of swine influenza: A hypothesis on the interepizootic survival of virus. Ph.D. diss.; Univ of Wisconsin.

NAKAMURA, R. M., AND EASTERDAY, B. C. 1970. Studies on swine influenza. III. Propagation of swine influenza virus in explants of respiratory tract tissues from fetal pigs. Cornell Vet 60:28–35.

NAKAMURA, R. M.; EASTERDAY, B. C.; PAWLISCH, R.; AND WALKER, G. L. 1972. Swine influenza: Epizootiological and serological studies. Bull WHO 47:481–487.

NARDELLI, L.; PASCUCCI, S.; GUALANDI, G. R.; AND LODA, P. 1978. Outbreaks of classical swine influenza in Italy in 1976. Zentralbl Veterinaermed [B] 25:853–857.

NAYAK, D. P.; TWIEHAUS, M. T.; KELLEY, G. W.; AND UNDERDAHL, N. R. 1965. Immunocytologic and histopathologic development of experimental swine influenza infection in pigs. Am J Vet Res 26:1271–1282.

OGAWA, T.; SUGIMURA, T.; TANAKA, Y.; AND KUMAGAI, T. 1978. A single radial hemolysis technique for the measurement of influenza virus antibody in swine serum. Natl Inst Anim Health (Tokyo) 18:58–62.

OGAWA, T.; SUGIMURA, T.; AND TANAKA, Y. 1982. Statistical analysis of results of a pig survey on antibody against swine influenza virus in pigs by single radial hemolysis and hemagglutination-inhibition tests. Natl Inst Anim Health (Tokyo) 22:32–33.

PALESE, P., AND RITCHEY, M. B. 1977. Polyacrylamide gel electrophoresis of the RNAs of new influenza virus strains: An epidemiological tool. Dev Biol Stand 39:411–415.

PATRIARCA, P. A.; KENDAL, A. P.; ZAKOWSKI, P. C.; COX, N. J.; TRAUTMAN, M. S.; CHERRY, J. D.; AUERVACH, D. M.; MCCUSKER, J.; BELLIVEAU, R. R.; AND KAPPUS, K. D. 1984. Lack of significant person-to-person spread of swine influenza-like virus following fatal infection in an immunocompromised child. Am J Epidemiol 119:152–158.

PENSAERT, M. 1984. Personal communication.

PIRTLE, E. C. 1977. Evaluation of A/New Jersey/76 influenza whole-virus vaccine in hysterectomy-deprived pigs. J Infect Dis [Suppl]136:703–705.

PIRTLE, E. C.; HILL, H. R.; SWANSON, M. R.; AND VAN DEUSEN, R. A. 1976. Hemagglutination-inhibiting antibodies against swine influenza and Hong Kong influenza viruses in swine sera in the U.S.A. Bull WHO 53:7–11.

POTGEITER, L. N. D.; STAIR, E. L.; MORTON, R. J.; AND WHITENACK, D. L. 1977. Isolation of swine influenza virus in Oklahoma. J Am Vet Med Assoc 171:758–760.

PRITCHARD, G. C.; DICK, I. G. C.; ROBERTS, D. H.; AND

WIBBERLEY, G. 1987. Porcine influenza outbreak in East Anglia due to influenza A virus (H3N2). Vet Rec 121:548.

RENSHAW, H. W. 1975. Influence of antibody-mediated immune suppression on clinical, viral, and immune responses to swine influenza infection. Am J Vet Res 36:5–13.

ROMVARY, J., AND TANYI, J. 1975. Hong Kong Influenza virus infections in animals in Hungary. Proc 20th World Vet Congr, pp. 1455–1456.

SCHMIDT, R. C.; MAASAB, H. F.; AND DAVENPORT, F. M. 1974. Infection by influenza A viruses of tracheal organ cultures derived from homologous and heterologous hosts. J Infect Dis 129:28–36.

SCHOLTISSEK, C., AND NAYLOR, E. 1988. Fish farming and influenza pandemics. Nature 331:215.

SCOTT, J. P. 1939. Swine influenza. Rep 13th Int Vet Congr, 1938, pp. 479–490.

———. 1941. Swine influenza experiments. Proc 45th Annu Meet US Livest Sanit Assoc, pp. 28–37.

SHERRAR, M. G.; EASTERDAY, B. C.; HINSHAW, V. S. 1989. Antigenic conservation of H1N1 swine influenza viruses. J Gen Virol 70:3297–3303.

SHOPE, R. E. 1931a. Swine influenza. I. Experimental transmission and pathology. J Exp Med 54:349–359.

———. 1931b. Swine influenza. III. Filtration experiments and etiology. J Exp Med 54:373–385.

———. 1964. Swine influenza. In Diseases of Swine, 2d ed. Ed. H. W. Dunne. Ames: Iowa State Univ Press, p. 109.

SHORTRIDGE, K. F., AND WEBSTER, R. G. 1979. Geographical distribution of swine (Hsw1N1) and Hong Kong (N3N2) influenza virus variants in pigs in Southeast Asia. Intervirology 11:9–15.

SUGIMURA, T.; YONEMOCHI, H.; OGAWA, T.; TANAKA, Y.; AND KUMAGAI, T. 1980. Isolation of a recombinant influenza virus (Hsw1N2) from swine in Japan. Arch Virol 66:271–274.

TUMOVA, B.; MENSIK, J.; STUMPA, A.; FEDOVA, D.; AND POSPISIL, Z. 1976. Serological evidence and isolation of a virus closely related to the human A/Hong Kong/68 (H3N2) strain in swine populations in Czechoslovakia in 1969–1972. Zentralbl Veterinaermed [B] 23:590–603.

URMAN, H. K.; UNDERDAHL, N. R.; AND YOUNG, G. A. 1958. Comparative histopathology of experimental swine influenza and virus pneumonia of pigs in disease-free, antibody-devoid pigs. Am J Vet Res 19:913–917.

VANNIER, P.; GOURREAU, J. M.; AND KAISER, C. 1985. Infection experimentale de porcs exempts d'organismes pathogenes specifiques avec une souche du virus de la grippe porcine (HSW1N1) et etude de la duree d'excretion virale. Can Vet J 26:138–143.

WALKER, G. L. 1971. Experimental infections of swine fetuses with swine influenza virus. M.S. thesis, Univ of Wisconsin.

WITTE, K. H.; NIENHOFF, H.; ERNST, H.; SCHMIDT, U.; AND PRAGER, D. 1981. First outbreak of swine influenza in pig herds in the Federal Republic of Germany. Tieraerztl Umsch 36:591–606.

WOODS, G. T. 1975. Prevalence of hemagglutination-inhibition (HI) antibodies to influenza viruses A/swine/IV/63 and A/swine/Taiwan/7310/70 (H3N2) in Illinois swine herds, 1971–1973. Res Commun Chem Pathol Pharmacol 10:573–57.

WOODS, G. T., AND MANSFIELD, M. E. 1976. Antigenicity of inactivated swine influenza virus concentrated by centrifugation. Res Commun Chem Pathol Pharmacol 13:129–132.

———. 1978. Serologic response of gilts of breeding age to human influenza vaccines containing A/New Jersey/76 (Hsw1N1) antigen. Res Commun Chem Pathol Pharmacol 19:177–180.

———. 1980. Experimental challenge of pregnant gilts after vaccination with vaccine prepared for the national vaccination program in the United States. Bovine Pract 1:41–44.

World Health Organization (WHO). 1980. Memorandum: A revision of the system of nomenclature for influenza virus. Bull WHO 58:585–591.

YOUNG, G. A., AND UNDERDAHL, N. A. 1949a. Swine influenza as a possible factor in suckling pig mortalities. I. Seasonal occurrence in adult swine as indicated by hemagglutinin inhibitors in serum. Cornell Vet 39:105–119.

———. 1949b. Swine influenza as a possible factor in suckling pig mortalities. II. Colostral transfer of hemagglutinin inhibitors for swine influenza virus from dam to offspring. Cornell Vet 39:120–128.

———. 1950a. Swine influenza as a possible factor in suckling pig mortalities. III. Effect of live virus vaccination of the dam against swine influenza on suckling pig mortalities. Cornell Vet 40:24–33.

———. 1950b. Swine influenza as a possible factor in suckling pig mortalities. IV. Relationship of passive swine influenzal immunity in suckling pigs to rate of weight gain. Cornell Vet 40:201–205.

28 Swine Pox

J. A. House
C. A. House

SWINE POX (SwP) was first reported in 1842 by Spinola in Europe and in North America by McNutt et al. in 1929. The clinical signs of pox infection may be caused by either vaccinia virus (VV) or SwP virus (SwPV) (Manninger et al. 1940; Shope 1940). Since the eradication of small pox (variola) and the cessation of vaccination with VV, infection of swine with VV has essentially disappeared (Meyer and Conroy 1972). This chapter will address the disease caused by SwPV. Worldwide in distribution, SwP is usually associated with operations that have poor sanitation and/or intensive breeding with open herd management. SwP causes little economic loss and can usually be differentiated from vesicular and other diseases by its clinical signs and epidemiology; therefore, its elimination has not been a high priority objective.

ETIOLOGY. Swine pox virus is classified in the family Poxviridae and is the only member of the genus *Suipoxvirus* (Matthews 1979). The large virion (300–450 nm × 176–260 nm) contains double-stranded DNA in a characteristic core or nucleoid bordered by lateral bodies and surrounded by an outer coat of numerous proteins typical of poxviruses.

The SwPV is ether sensitive (Cheville 1966a) and not readily neutralized by serum from recovered swine (Shope 1940). Primary isolation of the SwPV may require up to five passages in swine cell cultures, but once adapted, it grows readily to high titers and maintains its pathogenicity for swine (Kasza et al. 1960; Kasza and Griesemer 1962).

EPIDEMIOLOGY. Worldwide, SwP is typically found in herds with poor sanitation. There may be differences in susceptibility to infection resulting from age, breed, and management conditions. The virus is host-restricted and does not infect cattle, horses, sheep, dogs, cats, domestic fowl, rabbits, guinea pigs, rats, mice, or humans (Shope 1940; Schwarte and Biester 1941; Datt 1964). The source of SwPV is infected swine, which represent the reservoir, the source of contamination for mechanical, in contrast to biological, vector, wherein the virus replicates (multiplies) and is then transmitted to the higher animal host, and

the primary means of spread from herd to herd. SwPV is particularly resistant to inactivation when contained in dry scabs produced in the later stages of infection; it may persist for up to a year in this desiccated condition and may play a role in the persistence of SwPV in affected herds.

The pig louse (*Haematopinus suis*) serves as a mechanical vector and is considered the primary means of transmission of SwPV (Shope 1940). The ventral distribution of pox lesions on swine can be correlated to the habitat of *H. suis*. Flies and mosquitoes have been incriminated as mechanical vectors and, in this situation, pox lesions were distributed on the backs and sides of affected pigs (Schwarte and Biester 1941). Occasionally, horizontal transmission may occur in the absence of insects, since SwPV is shed from nasal and oral excretions and is present in contaminated debris from pox lesions. Infection may occur following introduction of SwPV into skin abrasions.

The morbidity of SwP may approach 100% in young stock up to 3–4 months of age, where poor hygiene occurs. The disease may have a seasonal incidence related to the prevalence of insects. Mortality is usually less than 5%.

The main factors accounting for long-term infection of herds include poor sanitation, poor insect control, and the introduction of new susceptible stock.

CLINICAL SIGNS. Swine pox is a typical pox disease, with the development of the lesions progressing through the classical stages of macule (reddening), papule (reddening with edema), vesicle (fluid exuding from the pox lesion), and pustule or crust formation (drying of the lesion with scab formation) (Fig. 28.1). The vesicular stage is not readily observed in SwP. The time from macule formation to scabbing and resolution of the lesion is 3–4 weeks. A lymphadenitis may occur. Complication with bacterial infection prolongs the resolution of the lesion (Miller and Olson 1978, 1980).

Young animals are more severely affected than adults. Suckling piglets may have a generalized disease with lesions all over the body. Pigs up to 3–4 months of age have lesions that are more prominent on the hairless parts of the skin. The

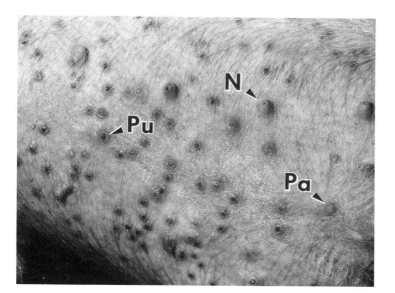

28.1. Swine pox lesions on the belly of a pig. *Pa* = papule; *Pu* = pustule; *N* = nipple.

pig louse has a predilection for the lower parts of the body and mechanically transmits the virus as it feeds. Flies and mosquitoes feed predominantly over the top of the body and may account for lesions in these locations. Adults generally develop a mild form of the disease, with lesions distributed ventrally on the hairless skin, the udder, ears, snout, and vulva.

Sporadic congenital infection was recently reported, with only one piglet affected per litter on four farms that had no other cases of SwP. One piglet was stillborn, two died shortly after birth, and the fourth was severly affected and was sacrificed (Borst et al. 1990).

The incubation period following experimental intradermal inoculation is 2–5 days. The incubation period following intravenous inoculation is 10–14 days (Shope 1940), but can be as short as 5 days (Kasza and Griesemer 1962), the range likely being related to the inoculation dosage. Incubation under field conditions may be up to 10–14 days.

PATHOGENESIS. Swine pox is initiated by SwPV entering a break in the skin, perhaps by a louse bite. SwPV replicates in the cytoplasm of the cells of the stratum spinosum. Viral lesions in local lymph nodes are not extensive, and virus is not readily isolated from them. Secondary lesions are believed to result exclusively from spread of the virus from an existing lesion, not by a cell-associated viremia as in most other pox infections. Virus has not been recovered from the blood (Kasza and Griesemer 1962; Shope 1940), but this may be due to the fact that the SwPV is difficult to isolate, especially when in low concentrations. Viremia must occur to account for congenital infection in piglets.

Following intravenous inoculation, gnotobiotic piglets developed skin lesions uniformly over the entire body but not in internal organs (Meyer and Conroy 1972), confirming the propensity of SwPV to infect the integument. In gnotobiotic pigs, the macular stage was not observed; therefore, the early reddening may be the combined effect of opportunistic bacteria and SwPV.

LESIONS. The gross lesions of SwP are described under clinical signs.

The histopathological changes caused by SwPV are similar to those of other poxviruses (Kasza and Griesemer 1962; Cheville 1966a,b; Conroy and Meyer 1971; Meyer and Conroy 1972; De Boer 1975). The virus replicates in the stratum spinosum causing hydropic degeneration. Sections stained with hematoxylin and eosin reveal one to three eosinophilic-staining intracytoplasmic inclusion bodies (ICIBs) in some cells during all stages of the infection. Characteristic central nuclear clearing, which is also observed with capipoxvirus infection, occurs in infected epithelial cells containing ICIBs. There may be intercellular edema, which could account for the transient vesicular stage. Acantholysis, the separation of individual cells of the stratum spinosum with loss of desmosomes and detachment into the vesicular fluid, was not found with SwPV infection (Meyer and Conroy 1972). Necrosis of epithelial cells and the presence of neutrophils and macrophages in the dermis and epidermis is common in later stages of the pox lesion (Fig. 28.2). Predominately granulomatous infiltrates with necrosis, as seen with capripoxvirus infection, are not seen. The pustules involve the full thickness of epithelium and may heal, leaving a light scar. Poxvirus particles may be observed in the cytoplasma of infected cells by electron microscopy. Margination of chromatin with nuclear filamentous matrix formation accounts for the central nuclear clearing observed histologically (Fig. 28.3).

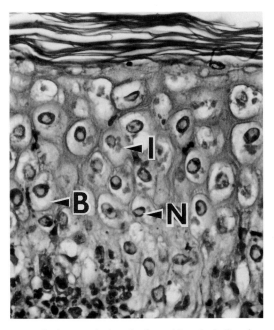

28.2. Swine pox lesions in the epidermis; ballooning degeneration of cytoplasm (*B*), intracytoplasmic inclusion bodies (*I*), and central nuclear clearing (*N*).

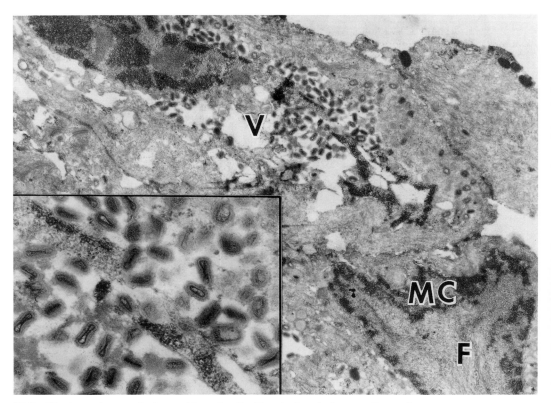

28.3. Electron micrograph of an epidermal cell with cytoplasmic degeneration and numerous poxvirus particles (*V*); a second cell has marginated chromatin (*MC*) and a filamentous matrix (*F*) in the nucleus, which corresponds to the central nuclear clearing seen histologically. Insert shows typical poxvirus particles. (Courtesy of D. A. Gregg.)

DIAGNOSIS. Swine pox is typified by the presence of pox lesions on the skin of the belly, ears, snout, vulva, and back. Secondary bacterial infections may cause more extensive lesions and local abscess formation. Diseases to consider in the differential diagnosis of SwP include VV infection, vesicular diseases, bites from needle teeth, pityriasis rosea, parakeratosis, parasitic skin disorders, allergic skin reactions, early stages of ringworm, and staphylococcal or streptococcal epidermitis.

The SwPV infection may be confirmed by detection of viral antigens using immunofluorescence and electron microscopy. The presence of ICIBs along with central nuclear clearing in affected epithelial cells is pathognomonic for SwP. VV infection does not cause the central nuclear clearing (Teppema and De Boer 1975). SwPV may be isolated by multiple passages in swine cell cultures and definitively identified by neutralization with specific-reference antiserum.

Serological diagnosis may be done using the agar gel immunodiffusion test or a more sensitive counterelectrophoresis test (De Boer 1975). Swine do not develop high levels of neutralizing antibody (Shope 1940; Kasza et al. 1960), and negative results on the virus neutralization test should not be interpreted as the absence of SwPV infection.

TREATMENT. There is no known treatment for swine pox, although antibiotics may diminish the complications caused by infection with secondary bacteria. Affected animals should be isolated. Ectoparasites should be controlled by the use of licensed insecticides, and the premises should be cleaned and disinfected.

PREVENTION. Vaccines for SwP have not been developed due to the relatively low economic importance of this disease. Recovered animals are specifically immune to SwP (Shope 1940) even in the absence of demonstrable neutralizing antibody, implying the importance of cell-mediated immunity.

Animals introduced into herds should be carefully inspected for skin lesions and ectoparasites. Good hygienic practices are essential for the prevention and control of SwP.

REFERENCES
Borst, G. H. A.; Kimman, T. G.; Gielkens, A. L. J.; and Van der Kamp, J. S. 1990. Four sporadic cases of congenital swinepox. Vet Rec 127:61–63.
Cheville, N. F. 1966a. The cytopathology of swinepox in the skin of swine. Am J Pathol 49:339–352.
———. 1966b. Immunofluorescent and morphologic studies on swinepox. Pathol Vet 3:556–564.
Conroy, J. D., and Meyer, R. C. 1971. Electron microscopy of swinepox virus in germfree pigs and in cell culture. Am J Vet Res 32:2021–2032.
Datt, N. S. 1964. Comparative studies of pigpox and vaccinia viruses. I. Host range pathogenicity. J Comp Pathol 74:62–80.
De Boer, G. F. 1975. Swinepox. Virus isolation, experimental infections and the differentiation from vaccinia virus infections. Arch Virol 49:141–150.
Kasza, L., and Griesemer, R. A. 1962. Experimental swine pox. Am J Vet Res 23:443–450.
Kasza, L.; Bohl, E. H.; and Jones, D. O. 1960. Isolation and cultivation of swinepox virus in primary cell cultures of swine origin. Am J Vet Res 21:269–273.
McNutt, S. H.; Murray, C.; and Purwin, P. 1929. Swinepox. J Am Vet Med Assoc 74:752.
Manninger, R.; Csontos, J.; and Salyi, J. 1940. Uber die Atiologie des pockenartigen Ausschlags der Ferkel. Arch Tierheilkd 75:159.
Matthews, R. E. F. 1979. Classification and nomenclature of viruses. Intervirology 12:160–164.
Meyer, R. C., and Conroy, J. D. 1972. Experimental swine pox in gnotobiotic piglets. Res Vet Sci 13:334–338.
Miller, R. B., and Olson, L. D. 1978. Epizootic of concurrent cutaneous streptococcal abscesses and swinepox in a herd of swine. Am J Vet Med Assoc 172:676–680.
———. 1980. Experimental induction of cutaneous Streptococcal abscesses as a sequela to swinepox. Am J Vet Res 41:341–347.
Schwarte, L. H., and Biester, H. E. 1941. Pox in swine. Am J Vet Res 2:136–140.
Shope, R. E. 1940. Swine pox. Arch Gesamte Virusforsch 1:457–467.
Spinola, M. 1842. Krankheiten der Schweine. Berlin: A. Hieschwald, p. 204.
Teppema, J. S., and De Boer, G. F. 1975. Ultrastructural aspects of experimental swinepox with special reference to inclusion bodies. Arch Virol 49:151–163.

29 Transmissible Gastroenteritis

L. J. SAIF
R. D. WESLEY

TRANSMISSIBLE GASTROENTERITIS (TGE) is a highly contagious, enteric viral disease of swine characterized by vomiting, severe diarrhea, and a high mortality (often 100%) in piglets under 2 weeks of age. Although swine of all ages are susceptible to this viral infection, the mortality in swine over 5 weeks of age is very low.

The disease was first reported by Doyle and Hutchings (1946) as occurring in the United States in 1945, although it undoubtedly had existed prior to this time. Subsequent to its recognition in the United States, TGE was reported in Japan in 1956 (Sasahara et al. 1958) and England in 1957 (Goodwin and Jennings 1958). Since then it has been reported in many European countries, Central and South America, Canada, Taiwan, Korea, the Philippines, and China.

The disease is most frequently diagnosed and causes the most loss when occurring in herds at farrowing time. In contrast, TGE often goes undiagnosed when occurring in growing, finishing, or adult swine because of the mild clinical signs, which usually consist only of inappetence and diarrhea of a few days duration. Because of these undiagnosed infections, serologic surveys are a more accurate indication of the prevalence of TGE virus (TGEV). Such surveys indicated 19–54% of sampled swine herds in Europe and North America were seropositive for TGEV antibodies (Gagnon et al. 1974; Witte 1974; Toma et al. 1978; Egan et al. 1982). Currently in many European countries, nearly 100% of swine herds are seropositive for TGEV antibodies. This situation is due to a TGEV respiratory variant termed porcine respiratory coronavirus (PRCV) that has rapidly spread in pigs since 1986 (Brown and Cartwright 1986; Pensaert et al. 1986; Pensaert 1989; Pensaert and Cox 1989). Economic losses from TGE can be severe, as reviewed in several studies (Toma et al. 1978; Miller et al. 1982; Pritchard 1982, 1987; Arendonk and Renkema 1983; Mousing et al. 1988).

In the densely swine-populated areas of the midwestern United States, TGE is recognized as one of the major causes of sickness and death in piglets. Swine producers are especially apprehensive about this disease because (1) mortality is high in newborn pigs; (2) there is no effective, practical treatment; (3) entrance of the virus into a herd in winter months is difficult to prevent because of the probable role of birds, especially starlings; and (4) the commercial vaccines available are of limited effectiveness (Bohl et al. 1975; Moxley and Olson 1989a; Saif and Theil 1990).

ETIOLOGY. The viral etiology of TGE was suggested by the initial report of Doyle and Hutchings (1946) when they described the filterable nature of the infectious agent. TGEV belongs to the genus *Coronavirus* of the family Coronaviridae (Siddell et al. 1983a).

Size, Morphology, and Morphogenesis. TGEV is enveloped and pleomorphic, with an overall diameter of 60–160 nm as viewed by negative-staining electron microscopy (Fig. 29.1) (Okaniwa et al. 1968; Phillip et al. 1971; Granzow et al. 1981). It has a single layer of club-shaped surface projections that are 12–25 nm in length and widely spaced.

The morphogenesis of coronaviruses has been reviewed (Siddell et al. 1983a,b). TGEV antigen

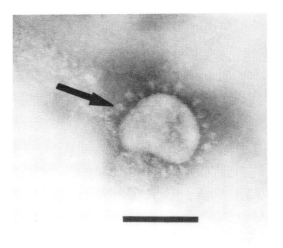

29.1. Electron micrograph of a TGEV particle showing typical coronavirus morphology. Arrow points to the virus peplomers or spikes. Bar = 100 nm.

The authors thank Dr. E. H. Bohl for his previous contributions to this chapter.

can be demonstrated in the cytoplasm by immunofluorescence (IF) as early as 4–5 hours postinfection (Pensaert et al. 1970a). Maturation of virus occurs in the cytoplasm by budding through endoplasmic reticulum, and viral particles (65–90

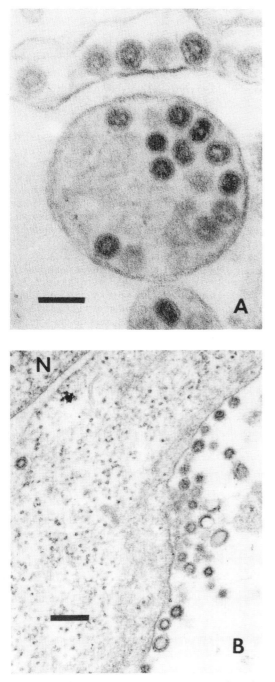

29.2. (A) TGEV in vesicles of the endoplasmic reticulum of a pig kidney cell (36 hours postinfection). Bar = 100 nm. (B) TGEV lining the cell membrane of a pig kidney cell (36 hours postinfection). N = nucleus; bar = 200 nm.

nm in diameter) are often observed within cytoplasmic vacuoles (Fig. 29.2A) (Thake 1968; Pensaert et al. 1970b; Wagner et al. 1973). Virus is frequently seen lining the host cell membranes after exit from infected cells (Fig. 29.2B). Recently, TGEV glycoproteins have been identified on the surface of infected swine testicular (ST) cells (Laviada et al. 1990).

Molecular Properties. TGEV is a pleomorphic, enveloped virus containing one large, polyadenylated, single-stranded, genomic RNA (>23 kb) of positive-sense polarity (Siddell et al. 1983a; Laude et al. 1990). RNA extracted from virions is infectious (Brian et al. 1980). During virus replication, 6–7 subgenomic mRNAs with common 3′ ends are synthesized for the production of viral proteins (Jacobs et al. 1986; Britton et al. 1989; Laude et al 1990; Wesley et al. 1990a). The nucleotide sequence at the 3′ end of the genome corresponding to the subgenomic mRNAs has been determined (Kapke and Brian 1986; Rasschaert and Laude 1987; Rasschaert et al. 1987). Intact virions have a buoyant density of 1.18–1.20 g/ml in sucrose (Brian et al. 1980; Jimenez et al. 1986). The phospholipids and glycolipids incorporated into the virus envelope are derived from the host cell, and thus, the envelope composition is host-cell dependent (Pike and Garwes 1977). TGEV contains three major structural proteins: a nucleocapsid protein (N); a small, integral-membrane glycoprotein (M); and a large spike or peplomer glycoprotein (S) (Garwes and Pocock 1975; Spaan et al. 1988). In the mature virus, the N protein binds viral RNA to form a helical ribonucleoprotein complex. The 29–31 kD M glycoprotein is firmly embedded in the viral envelope by three membrane-spanning domains. The hydrophilic N terminus of the M protein protrudes out from the virion, has a single accessible glycosylation site, and is presumed to be responsible for mediating complement-dependent neutralization and interferon induction (Charley and Laude 1988; Woods et al. 1988). The S glycoprotein or peplomer, (molecular weight 195–220 kD), is visualized in electron micrographs as the virus corona (Fig 29.1). Functions attributed to the S glycoprotein include cell attachment, membrane fusion, and complement-independent virus neutralization. Garwes et al. (1978/79) has shown that the purified S glycoprotein elicited the production of TGEV-neutralizing antibodies, which neutralize at multiple steps in the virus replication cycle (Nguyen et al. 1986; Sune et al. 1990). Convalescent serum from TGEV-recovered pigs contains precipitating TGEV antibodies to the S and M proteins, and frequently, antibodies are present that precipitate a 14-kD virus-coded intracellular protein (Wesley et al. 1987).

Monoclonal antibodies (MAbs) have been produced against attenuated (Jimenez et al. 1986; Laude et al. 1986; Correa et al. 1990; Delmas et al. 1990) and virulent (Welch and Saif 1988; Zhu et al. 1990) strains of TGEV and used to characterize TGEV proteins and map epitopes which elicit antibodies. The major neutralization determinants were associated with the viral S glycoprotein; these epitopes were highly conserved on most TGEV strains (Jimenez et al. 1986; Laude et al. 1986; Garwes et al. 1987; Welch and Saif 1988; Sanchez et al. 1989). Anti-M MAbs had little or no neutralizing activity (Jimenez et al. 1986; Laude et al. 1986; Welch and Saif 1988), but the neutralizing activity was enhanced by complement (Woods et al. 1988; Laude et al. 1990). Use of neutralizing MAbs to map epitopes on the S glycoprotein revealed four to six different antigenic sites, with sites A and B containing the highly conserved epitopes recognized by strongly neutralizing MAbs (Garwes et al. 1987; Correa et al. 1990; Delmas et al. 1990; Sanchez et al. 1990). In the latter two studies, the locations of each of the four major antigenic sites (A–D) were mapped on the primary structure of the S glycoprotein.

Biologic Properties. The virus is very stable when stored frozen, but somewhat labile at room temperature or above. Young et al. (1955) reported no detectable drop in titer when virus of pig intestine origin was stored at −20°C for 6 months, while Haelterman and Hutchings (1956) reported a drop in titer from 10⁶ to 10⁵ after storage at −18°C for 18 months. In contrast, virus of pig intestine origin, when allowed to dry and putrefy at 21°C, was rather labile; after 3 days only two of four inoculated pigs became sick; and after 10 days no viable virus was detected by pig inoculation (Bay et al. 1952). When held at 37°C, there was a log 10 reduction in infectivity titer every 24 hours (Young et al. 1955). Storage of cell-cultured virus at −20, −40, or −80°C for 365 days did not result in any significant drop in titer, while storage at 37°C for 4 days resulted in total loss of infectivity (Harada et al. 1968).

The virus is highly photosensitive. Haelterman (1963) reported that fecal material containing 10⁵ pig-infectious doses (PID) was inactivated within 6 hours when exposed in a petri dish to sunlight. Cartwright et al. (1965) reported the photosensitivity of a cytopathic strain when it was exposed to ultraviolet light on a laboratory bench.

In terms of chemical stability, TGEV is inactivated by exposure to 0.03% formalin, 1% Lysovet (phenol and aldehyde), 0.01% beta propiolactone, sodium hypochlorite, NaOH, iodines, quaternary ammonium compounds, ether, and chloroform (Harada et al. 1968; Nakao et al. 1978; Brown 1981).

As reported for other enteric viruses, TGEV field strains are trypsin resistant, relatively stable in pig bile, and stable at pH 3 (Harada et al. 1968; Moscari 1980a; Laude et al. 1981). These properties allow the virus to survive in the stomach and small intestine. However, attenuated strains as well as field strains of TGEV vary in these properties, and most studies failed to show a correlation between susceptibility to these various treatments and cell culture passage level or degree of virulence (Furuuchi et al. 1975; Hess and Bachmann 1976; Moscari 1980a; Laude et al. 1981).

Antigenic Relationships. Only one serotype of TGEV is known (Kemeny 1976) and this encompasses the PRCV strains that are antigenically indistinguishable (in neutralization tests) from enteropathogenic strains of TGEV (Pensaert 1989; Pensaert and Cox 1989). TGEV is not antigenically related to two other porcine coronaviruses, hemagglutinating encephalomyelitis virus and porcine epidemic diarrhea virus (PEDV or CV777) (Chasey and Cartwright 1978; Pensaert and DeBouck 1978; Pensaert et al. 1981). Although PEDV causes a disease syndrome similar to TGEV, this disease has only been documented in swine in Europe and Taiwan. Antibodies to PEDV have not been detected in a limited survey of adult swine sera from the United States (DeBouck et al. 1982; Saif and Pensaert 1990, unpublished).

TGEV, canine coronavirus (CCV), and a coronavirus of cats (feline infectious peritonitis virus—FIPV) are all antigenically related (Pedersen et al. 1978; Reynolds et al. 1980; Woods 1982), and it has been suggested that these three viruses may actually represent host range mutants of an ancestral virus strain (Horzinek et al. 1982). The following antigenic relationships have been reported from in vitro studies using virus-neutralization (VN) and IF tests: (1) antisera to CCV and TGEV reacted in IF and two-way cross-neutralization tests, but titers were consistently higher in homologous than heterologous reactions (Pedersen et al. 1978; Reynolds et al. 1980; Woods 1982); and (2) a two-way relationship between TGEV and FIPV was demonstrated by IF and cross-neutralization studies, but only a one-way relationship between FIPV and CCV was evident by cross-neutralization (Pedersen et al. 1978; Woods 1982). The observation that VN titers were consistently greater with homologous compared to heterologous virus suggests that these three viruses can be distinguished serologically (in sera from naturally infected animals) by employing two-way cross-neutralization tests (Reynolds et al. 1980).

Cross-reactivity also exists among these antigenically related coronaviruses at the level of the structural proteins. Horzinek et al. (1982) showed cross-reactivity between the homologous S, M, and N proteins of TGEV, FIPV, and CCV, using radioimmunoprecipitation, immunoblotting, and enzyme-linked immunosorbent assay (ELISA). Similar cross-reactivity was observed for the structural proteins of TGEV and PRCV using polyclonal antisera in immunoblotting assays (Callebaut et al. 1988).

Additional in vitro biologic differences also have been detected; whereas both TGEV and CCV will grow in either canine kidney cells (Welter 1965; Reynolds et al. 1980) or an established feline cell line (Woods 1982), neither CCV nor FIPV will grow in ST or porcine thyroid cells, both of which support the growth of TGEV isolates (Reynolds et al. 1980).

More recently, cDNA probes developed from the 5′ end of the S glycoprotein gene of TGEV were shown to react with TGEV but failed to recognize CCV or FIPV under conditions of high stringency, suggesting their possible application for differential diagnosis of these viruses. These same probes also differentiated U.S. strains of PRCV from prototype strains of TGEV (Bae et al. 1990). Similar differentiation of these viruses was possible using MAbs to nonneutralizing epitopes of the S glycoprotein of TGEV, which recognized TGEV strains but failed to react with PRCV, FIPV, or CCV (Laude et al. 1988; Callebaut et al. 1989; Sanchez et al. 1990).

In vivo biologic differences also exist among these three coronaviruses in their pathogenicity for neonatal pigs (Binn et al. 1974; Woods and Pedersen 1979). While virulent FIPV caused diarrhea and intestinal lesions similar to those of virulent TGEV, CCV caused no clinical signs and only slight villous atrophy. IF, detected using a porcine anti-TGEV serum conjugate, occurred in villous enterocytes of TGEV- and FIPV-infected pigs but predominated in crypt enterocytes of CCV-infected pigs. Although there are no reports of pigs being naturally infected with FIPV or CCV, this possibility cannot be excluded in light of the above findings. However, it is especially noteworthy that pigs infected with FIPV (Woods and Pedersen 1979) or CCV (Binn et al. 1974; Woods and Pedersen 1979) did not develop TGEV-neutralizing antibodies.

Besides the question of infection of swine with canine and feline coronaviruses, dogs and cats have also been suggested as possible carriers of TGEV. Dogs and cats fed TGEV showed no clinical signs (except after repeated passages in dogs, Klemm and Ristic 1976), but some shed infectious fecal virus for 2–3 weeks and became serologically positive for TGEV-neutralizing antibodies (Haelterman 1962; McClurkin et al. 1970; Witte et al. 1977; Reynolds and Garwes 1979). Cats infected with TGEV did not develop FIPV antibodies and were not protected when challenged with FIPV (Witte et al. 1977; Reynolds and Garwes 1979). It is presently unclear whether TGE VN and IF antibodies, which have been frequently detected in dogs (Norman et al. 1970; Reynolds et al. 1980) and cats (Osterhaus et al. 1977; Reynolds et al. 1977), are due to infection with TGEV or with the antigenically related CCV or FIPV respectively. However, the widespread occurrence of these antibodies in cats and dogs, especially in those with no previous contact with swine, favor the latter possibility (Reynolds et al. 1980).

Genomic Relationships. The nucleotide sequence of the 3′-most 8300 nucleotides of the genomic RNA of the TGEV Purdue cell-adapted strain has been determined (Laude et al. 1990). This region of the genome contains the three major TGEV structural genes with the consensus coronavirus orientation 5′ S-M-N 3′ and four large open reading frames (ORF) that encode potential viral proteins. The remaining 5′ portion of the TGEV genome is thought to encode the viral replicase/transcriptase as has been shown for infectious bronchitis virus (IBV) (Boursnell et al. 1987). Significant amino acid homologies among the structural proteins of TGEV and of antigenically unrelated coronaviruses suggest that these coronaviruses have a common evolutionary ancestry. However, nucleic acid cross-hybridization among antigenically unrelated coronaviruses is not observed because of low base sequence homologies (Shockley et al. 1987; Benfield et al. 1991).

Recently, the 3′ end of the PRCV genomic RNA has been sequenced (Rasschaert et al. 1990). Alignment of PRCV nucleotide and amino acid sequences with TGEV sequences revealed a 96% overall homology. The PRCV genome contained two distinctive features: (1) the S gene lacked 672 nucleotides in the 5′ region and encoded a smaller peplomer protein, and (2) the first ORF downstream from the S gene contained a double deletion. These genetic changes are thought to account for the altered tissue tropism of PRCV. Similarly an altered phenotype was reported for a small plaque (SP) variant of TGEV (Woods 1978; Woods et al. 1981). Although the S gene of the SP variant and wild-type TGEV are similar, a large deletion (462 nucleotides) is present in the SP viral genome just downstream from the S gene (Wesley et al. 1990a). This deletion eliminated the ORF of one potential viral encoded protein and eliminated the N-terminal portion of a second potential viral protein. Apparently, the pathogenicity of both PRCV and SP virus is reduced as a result of these genetic deletions.

The nucleotide sequence of the FIPV S gene has been determined and compared with the TGEV S gene sequence (Jacobs et al. 1987). Two distinct domains were identified based on nucleotide and amino acid homologies. One domain (amino acids 1–274) had a nucleotide homology of 39%, whereas the homology in the second domain (amino acids 275–1447) was 93%. A possible explanation for this high sequence divergence at the 3′ end could be that FIPV arose by RNA-RNA recombination of TGEV with a related virus. A high frequency of RNA-RNA recombination has been described for murine coronaviruses (Makino et al. 1986).

EPIDEMIOLOGY. The epizootiology of TGE has been reviewed (Haelterman 1962; Ferris 1973; Toma et al. 1978; Wood 1979; Pritchard 1982, 1987). On a herd basis, two epizootiologic forms of TGE can be described: epizootic and enzootic. In addition, infections with the TGEV variant PRCV present a different disease pattern and greatly complicate seroprevalence studies of the epizootiology of TGEV (Pensaert 1989; Pensaert and Cox 1989).

Epizootic TGE. Epizootic TGE refers to the occurrence of TGE in a herd where most if not all the animals are susceptible. When TGEV is introduced in such a herd, the disease usually spreads rapidly to swine of all ages, especially during the winter. Some degree of inappetence, vomition, or diarrhea will occur in most animals.

Suckling pigs become very sick, dehydrating rapidly; mortality in pigs under 2–3 weeks of age is very high but gradually decreases in older pigs. Lactating sows often become sick, developing anorexia and agalactia that further contribute to piglet mortality. The history and severe clinical signs aid in diagnosis of epizootic TGE in the United States, since other similar diseases have not been reported. However, in Europe, PED has similar clinical signs (Pensaert and DeBouck 1978).

Enzootic TGE. Enzootic TGE refers to a persistence of the virus and disease in a herd, occurring as a result of a continual or frequent influx of susceptible swine that, when infected, tend to perpetuate the disease. Enzootic TGE is limited to herds that have frequent farrowings (Stepanek et al. 1979) or have frequent additions of susceptible swine such as feeder pigs and represents a common sequel to a primary outbreak in large breeding herds. In these situations, TGEV spreads slowly among adult swine, particularly herd replacements. (Morin et al. 1978, 1983; Pritchard 1987). Females saved for breeding will be immune and will transfer via their colostrum and milk a variable degree of passive immunity to their progeny during the suckling period. In these herds, TGE viral diarrhea will be seen primarily in pigs from the age of about 6 days until about 2 weeks after weaning. The pig is clinically affected when viral exposure exceeds the pig's passive immunity, and the age when this occurs is related to, or reflects, the management system used in the herd and the degree of immunity of the sow. In some herds the disease "break" occurs primarily during the postweaning period. Affected pigs show rather mild but typical signs of TGE. Mortality is usually less than 10–20%, being determined by the age when infected and by the variable degree of immunity obtained from immune sows. Sows usually are not sick. Enzootic TGE in suckling or recently weaned pigs can be difficult to diagnose and must be differentiated from other types of enzootic diarrheal problems commonly occurring in young pigs, such as rotaviral diarrhea and colibacillosis. Enzootic TGE will persist in the herd as long as susceptible or partially immune swine are exposed to TGEV.

The recrudescence or reintroduction of TGEV may occur in herds that contain immune sows, resulting in discrete episodes of disease (Pritchard 1987). This situation commonly occurs in herds in the concentrated swine-rearing areas of the United States or other countries. Each winter, herds often become reinfected, and the disease is especially seen in growing and finishing swine. Such animals are susceptible, since the herd infection from the previous winter has usually terminated during the intervening summer and autumn. If the disease enters the farrowing house, the disease in suckling or weaned pigs will resemble that described above since the sows will usually be immune. It is unclear whether the source of virus in these circumstances comes from reactivation of virus shedding in carrier swine or reintroduction of virus into the herd.

Porcine Respiratory Coronavirus. In 1984, a serologic survey in Belgium showed a sudden increase in the prevalence of TGEV antibodies in culled sows. This situation occurred in the absence of vaccination and without any increase in clinical TGE the previous winter and spring. Subsequently a nonenteropathogenic virus, antigenically related to TGEV, was shown to be the etiologic agent and was isolated in cell culture (Pensaert et al. 1986). This TGEV variant infects epithelial cells of the respiratory tract and alveolar macrophages, and therefore, was designated PRCV (Pensaert 1989; Pensaert and Cox 1989). After experimental challenge, PRCV infects only a few unidentified cells in the small intestine, and thus, virus shedding in feces is limited or not detected (O'Toole et al. 1989; Cox et al. 1990a,b). PRCV-infected pigs produce antibodies that cross-neutralize TGEV.

PRCV infects pigs of all ages by the aerogenic route, and virus can spread to swine on neighboring farms that are several miles distant. The virus has spread extensively in Europe and has been reported in Belgium, England, France, the Netherlands, and Germany (Brown and Cartwright 1986; Jestin et al. 1987; Lange et al. 1988; Henningsen et al. 1989; Pensaert 1989; Van Nieuwstadt and Pol 1989). In addition it has spread into countries such as Denmark, which previously was free of TGEV (Pensaert 1989). Most recently PRCV was also identified in the United States, with isolates recovered from swine in Indiana and North Carolina (Hill et al. 1990; Wesley et al. 1990b).

PRCV has become enzootic in many European swine herds with the seroprevalence approaching 100% (Pensaert 1989). PRCV infections persist on closed breeding farms with cyclic episodes common during winter and spring. PRCV infections generally occur in the presence of passive serum antibodies after weaning in pigs 5–10 weeks of age. Generally, the infection is subclinical or accompanied by mild respiratory disease, with a mild interstitial pneumonia observed following histological examination of lung tissue. Diarrhea and fecal shedding of PRCV are not apparent.

Transmission and Reservoirs. One of the significant epizootiologic features of TGE is its seasonal appearance, i.e., during the winter months, usually from the middle of November to about the middle of April. Several explanations have been given for this seasonal occurrence. Haelterman (1962) has suggested that this is probably due to the characteristics of the virus, since the virus is very stable when frozen but rather labile when exposed to warm temperature or to sunlight. This would allow a greater opportunity for the virus to be transmitted in a viable state between herds in winter, particularly on inanimate objects, such as during transport of feed or animals. The observation has been made that reduced or fluctuating ambient temperatures markedly predispose feeder pigs to clinical manifestations of TGE (Shimizu et al. 1978; Shimizu and Shimizu 1979a), thus contributing to transmission in winter because of the diarrheic state.

What constitutes the reservoir of TGEV between seasonal epizootics? Haelterman (1962) proposed at least three reservoirs: associated pig farms in which the virus spreads subclinically, hosts other than swine, and carrier pigs. The most probable explanation for maintenance of the disease is that it exists in the enzootic form in feeder pig operations (Morin et al. 1978) or in herds that are on a continuous farrowing program. These situations could constitute foci for maintenance of the disease during the warmer months and for dissemination during the winter months. This concept becomes even more likely by the finding that TGEV infection can spread rather slowly through a group of growing swine under certain conditions such as during the summer months (Maes and Haelterman 1979).

There is also evidence for existence of TGEV in nonporcine hosts. Cats, dogs, and foxes have been suggested as possible carriers of TGEV from one herd to another since they can shed virus in their feces for variable periods (Haelterman 1962; McClurkin et al. 1970). Virus excreted by dogs was shown to be infectious for pigs (Haelterman 1962). Massive concentrations of starlings (*Sturnus vulgaris*) in winter in feeding areas of swine may provide a method by which TGEV can be mechanically carried from one farm to another. Pilchard (1965) reported that TGEV was detected in the droppings of starlings for as long as 32 hours after they were fed TGEV. House flies (*Musca domestica*) have also been proposed as possible vectors for TGEV. TGEV antigen was detected in flies within a swine herd in which TGE was enzootic, and experimentally inoculated flies excreted TGEV for 3 days (Gough and Jorgenson 1983).

A third possibility relating to the transmission of TGE is the length of time infected swine eliminate viable TGEV and the role of the carrier pig. Only one report (Lee et al. 1954) has indicated fecal shedding under natural conditions to be more than the commonly reported 2-week period (Pensaert et al. 1970a). However, TGEV has been isolated from intestinal contents or homogenates for postexposure periods up to 104 days (Underdahl et al. 1975). As for respiratory shedding of TGEV, virus has been detected in nasal swabs for postexposure periods up to 11 days (Kemeny et al. 1975). However, from lung homogenates, virus was detected for postexposure periods up to 104 days (Underdahl et al. 1975). The last authors suggested that TGE may also be a respiratory tract disease and that infection of the lungs may result in the chronic carrier animal. TGEV has also been recovered from milk of infected sows during the acute phase of the disease (Kemeny et al. 1975; Kemeny and Woods 1977) and following intramammary infusion or injection of lactating sows with TGEV (Saif and Bohl 1983). In the latter study, demonstration of TGEV antigen in mammary gland tissue indicates the virus may replicate in the mammary glands of lactating sows. Transmission of the virus via milk to nursing piglets, as suggested in the same study, may account, in part, for the rapid spread of the infection among a litter of piglets.

Although TGEV has been detected in the intestinal and respiratory tracts for periods of up to 104 days postinfection, it is unknown whether such virus can be eliminated from the body in a viable state that will result in new infections. Addition of sentinel pigs to a herd at 3, 4, and 5 months after a previous TGE outbreak resulted in no infections in the introduced pigs, as determined by serologic tests (Derbyshire et al. 1969). Nasal shedding of PRCV in experimentally infected pigs has been shown to occur through day 10 postexposure (Onno et al. 1989; Wesley et al. 1990b). It is unknown for how long pigs recovered from PRCV infections remain infectious. The possible role of the long-term carrier hog in transmitting TGE or PRCV is difficult to assess.

CLINICAL SIGNS. The typical clinical signs in piglets are transient vomiting, accompanied or rapidly followed by a watery and usually yellowish diarrhea, rapid loss of weight, dehydration, and high morbidity and mortality in pigs under 2 weeks of age. Diarrhea in young pigs is usually profuse, and feces will often contain small curds of undigested milk. The odor of the feces is very offensive. Severity of the clinical signs, duration of the disease, and mortality are inversely related to the age of the pig. Most pigs under 7 days of age will die in 2–7 days after first showing clinical signs. Most suckling pigs over 3 weeks of age will survive but are likely to remain unthrifty for a time.

Clinical signs in growing and finishing swine and in sows are usually limited to inappetence and diarrhea for 1 or a few days, with vomiting observed in an occasional animal. The very few deaths observed are probably due to complicating factors such as stress or concurrent infections, which frequently occur after weaning. However, Bachmann et al. (1972) reported a mortality between 25 and 30% in a group of 2- to 6-month-old swine in Germany. Some lactating sows become very sick, with an elevated temperature, agalactia, vomiting, inappetence, and diarrhea. These severe signs may be due to a high degree of exposure to the virus from close contact with their affected piglets or to hormonal factors that may influence susceptibility. In contrast, sows in the field having no contact with young infected pigs usually have rather mild clinical signs or none.

The incubation period is short, usually 18 hours to 3 days. Infection generally spreads rapidly through the entire group of swine so that in 2–3 days most animals are affected, but this is more likely to occur in winter than summer (Maes and Haelterman 1979).

Enzootic TGE. Enzootic TGE is most likely to occur in large herds that have frequent farrowings, as discussed under **EPIDEMIOLOGY.** The clinical signs shown by infected pigs will usually be similar but less severe than those seen in susceptible pigs of the same age. Death loss is usually low, especially if pigs can be kept warm. The clinical signs in suckling pigs can resemble those of "white scours," which is most commonly caused by a rotavirus (Bohl et al. 1978). In some herds, depending on management, enzootic TGE is manifested mainly in weaned pigs and may be confused with *Escherichia coli,* coccidia, or rotavirus infections (Morin et al. 1983; Pritchard 1987).

Porcine Respiratory Coronavirus. In swine of all ages, PRCV generally causes a subclinical respiratory infection. Fever and dyspnea were reported by Duret et al. (1988) following intratracheal inoculation with PRCV, while Van Nieuwstadt and Pol (1989) reported a fatal pneumonia after intranasal inoculation of 5-week-old pigs. However, the health status of the pigs in the former study has been questioned (Vannier 1990), and in the latter study, repeated lung lavages probably exacerbated the PRCV-induced respiratory infection. A transient weight loss was demonstrated after intratracheal inoculation of 90-day-old pigs (Vannier 1990) but was not observed following PRCV inoculation of 15-week-old pigs (Onno et al. 1989).

PATHOGENESIS. The pathogenesis of TGE has been reviewed (Hooper and Haelterman 1966; Moon 1978; Shepherd et al. 1979). The early events have been described as follows: TGEV is ingested, infects the mucosa of the small intestine, and causes a rapid and extensive loss of functional epithelial cells.

Intestinal Replication. Whether by the oral or nasal route, the virus is swallowed and, being able to resist the effects of a low pH and proteolytic enzymes, remains viable until it comes in contact with the highly susceptible villous epithelial cells of the small intestine. Infection and rapid destruction or alteration in function of a high proportion of these cells result in a marked reduction in enzymatic activity in the small intestine, which disrupts digestion and cellular transport of nutrients and electrolytes, causing an acute malabsorption syndrome (Moon 1978). Hooper and Haelterman (1966) suggested that the inability of infected pigs to hydrolyze lactose, and possibly other nutrients, results in the marked deprivation of nutrients that can be so critical to the young pig. Furthermore, they suggested that the presence of undigested lactose exerts an osmotic force in the lumen of the intestine, which causes a retention of fluid and even a withdrawal of fluid from the tissues of the body and thus contributes to diarrhea and dehydration.

Additional mechanisms contributing to diarrhea in TGEV-infected pigs include altered sodium transport in the jejunum, resulting in accumulation of electrolytes and water in the intestinal lumen (Butler et al. 1974), and loss of extravascular protein (Prochazka et al. 1975). The ultimate cause of death, as suggested by Cornelius et al. (1968), is probably dehydration and metabolic acidosis coupled with abnormal cardiac function resulting from hyperkalemia.

A marked shortening or atrophy of the villi occurs in the jejunum (Fig. 29.3) and to a lesser extent in the ileum, but it is often absent in the proximal portion of the duodenum (Hooper and Haelterman 1966). Both virus production and villous atrophy were greater in newborn pigs than in 3-week-old pigs (Moon et al. 1973; Norman et al. 1973), suggesting higher susceptibility of neonates to TGEV infection. Several mechanisms have been proposed to account for this age-dependent resistance to clinical disease. First, the rapidity with which infected villous epithelial cells can be replaced by migration of epithelial cells from crypts of Lieberkühn may partially account for the lower fatality rate in older than in newborn pigs. Moon (1978) reported that 3-week-old pigs normally replace villous enterocytes in the small intestine about three times more rapidly than newborn pigs. These newly replaced villous enterocytes are reportedly resistant to TGEV infection (Pensaert et al. 1970b; Shepherd et al. 1979), possibly due to onset of the immune response, presence of intestinal interferon (LaBonnardiere and Laude 1981), or inability of these regenerating cells to support virus growth. Second, TGEV accumulates and replicates in the apical tubulovascular system of villous absorptive cells in newborn pigs; this system is lacking in pigs older than 3 weeks (Wagner et al. 1973). Third, virus dose may play a major role in infections. Witte and Walther (1976) demonstrated that the infectious dose of TGEV needed to infect a market hog (about 6 months old) was 10^4 times greater than that needed to infect a 2-day-old piglet.

However, the severity of clinical signs due to TGE is also increased when pigs are (1) fed a zinc-deficient ration (Whitenack et al. 1978); (2) anemic (Ackerman et al. 1972); (3) exposed to a low temperature or a fluctuation in temperature (Shimizu et al. 1978); or (4) injected with a synthetic corticosteroid, dexamethazone (Shimizu and Shimizu 1979a). In regard to the last two items, the mechanism is thought to be due to an interference with the early initiation of a local cell-mediated immune response (Shimizu and Shimizu 1979a).

The failure of cell-cultured attenuated strains of TGEV to infect the epithelial cells located in the cranial portion of the small intestines of pigs probably explains why such strains do not cause diarrhea as severe as that observed with virulent strains (Frederick et al. 1976; Hess et al. 1977; Furuuchi et al. 1979; Pensaert 1979). Furthermore, there was a reverse correlation between the level of cell culture attenuation of TGEV and the extent of intestinal infection (Hess et al. 1977).

Cell-cultured strains of TGEV of reduced virulence in combination with a mildly virulent *E. coli* have been shown to cause a more severe disease in germfree pigs than when either organism was given alone (Underdahl et al. 1972). Concurrent infections with TGEV and *E. coli* or porcine rotavirus have been reported (Hornich et al. 1977; Theil et al. 1979).

Extraintestinal Replication Sites: TGEV. Although ingestion is undoubtedly the most common portal of entry for the virus, the nasal route or airborne infection may be important. Macroscopic lung lesions were observed in gnotobiotic pigs inoculated intranasally (IN)/orally with TGEV, but no clinical pneumonia resulted (Underdahl et al. 1975). A preliminary report also indicated that TGEV was present in alveolar macrophages of infected neonatal pigs, suggesting a possible role for these cells in lung infection. However, only cell culture–adapted but not virulent TGEV replicated in cultures of alveolar macrophages in vitro (Laude et al. 1984). Highly attenuated strains of TGEV have also been reported that replicate in the upper respiratory tract and lung but not in the intestine of newborn pigs (Furuuchi et al. 1979). Moreover, nasal shedding of TGEV was detected in lactating sows exposed to infected piglets (Kemeny et al. 1975).

In addition, studies have shown that TGEV is capable of replicating in mammary tissue of lactating sows (Saif and Bohl 1983) and that infected sows shed virus in milk (Kemeny and Woods 1977). The significance of possible mammary gland infection with TGEV under field conditions is unclear. Whether it plays a role in the agalactia, often seen in TGEV-infected sows, or rapid spread of infection among piglets warrants investigation.

Although natural infection of the porcine fetus with TGEV has not been reported, intrafetal inoculation results in the production of villous atrophy and seroconversion to TGEV (Redman et al. 1978).

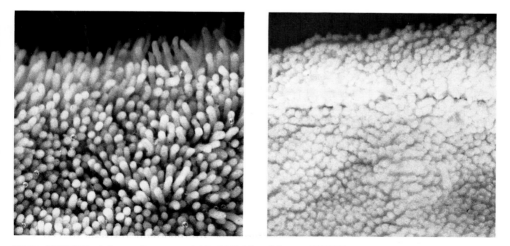

29.3. Villi of the jejunum from a normal pig (left) and from a TGEV-infected pig (right), as viewed through a dissecting microscope. Approximately × 10.

Extraintestinal Replication Sites: PRCV. The TGEV variant PRCV has an altered cell tropism. PRCV replicates to high titer in porcine lungs, infecting epithelial cells of the nares, trachea, bronchi, bronchioles and alveoli, and alveolar macrophages (Pensaert et al. 1986; O'Toole et al. 1989). Viremia occurs following primary infection and virus spreads to parenchymal organs and lymph nodes.

Only a few scattered cells containing PRCV antigen are found in the small intestine even when virus is directly inoculated into the intestinal lumen. These infected cells are located in or underneath the epithelial layer of the intestinal villi and crypts, and the virus does not spread to adjacent cells (Cox et al. 1990a,b). This limited intestinal replication of PRCV explains why infectious virus is seldom recovered in feces of PRCV-infected swine.

LESIONS

Gross Lesions. Gross lesions are usually confined to the gastrointestinal tract, with the exception of dehydration. The stomach is often distended with curdled milk. Congestion of the mucosa is a variable sign. Hooper and Haelterman (1969) reported that about 50% of the pigs killed during the first 3 days of infection had a small area of hemorrhage on the diaphragmatic side of the stomach at the border of the diverticulum ventriculus.

The small intestine is distended with yellow and frequently foamy fluid and usually contains flecks of curdled undigested milk. The wall is thin and almost transparent, probably due to atrophy of the villi. Although lung lesions have been observed in experimentally infected gnotobiotic pigs (Underdahl et al. 1975), they have not been reported in pigs naturally infected with TGEV.

Subgross Lesions. A highly significant lesion of TGE is the markedly shortened villi of the jejunum and ileum that Hooper and Haelterman (1969) referred to as villous atrophy (Fig. 29.3). However, this is also seen in rotavirus diarrhea but is not usually as severe or extensive as in TGE (Bohl et al. 1978). Some strains of *E. coli* (Hornich et al. 1977) and coccidia infections have also been reported to produce this lesion. However, the pathologic findings and extent of villous atrophy were highly variable in pigs from enzootically infected herds (Pritchard 1987).

Microscopic Lesions. The degree of villous atrophy can be judged in histologic sections by comparing the length of the jejunal villi with the depth of the crypts of Lieberkühn. In normal piglets these figures average about 795 μ and 110 μ respectively, giving a villi-crypt ratio of about 7:1; in infected piglets the corresponding figures are about 180 μ and 157 μ, giving a ratio of

about 1:1 (Hooper and Haelterman 1969). Other lesions reported in experimentally challenged 8-week-old pigs include microulceration of the dome epithelium over Peyer's patches, especially in the cranial portion of the small intestine (Chu et al. 1982a).

Scanning electron microscopy (EM) has been used to reveal the development of intestinal lesions of TGE and correlates well with lesions observed by light microscopy (Waxler 1972; Moxley and Olson 1989b).

Using scanning EM, Moxley and Olson (1989b) showed that the level of passive immunity in TGEV-infected pigs influenced not only the degree of villous atrophy, but also its segmental distribution. Villous atrophy was minimal in pigs nursing sows previously infected with virulent TGEV, compared to pigs nursing seronegative sows or sows given live-attenuated vaccines. In partially protected pigs, villous atrophy was seen primarily in the ileum instead of the jejunum. Similar observations were noted in pigs from herds with enzootic TGE.

Transmission EM of TGEV-infected epithelial cells of the small intestine has revealed alterations in the microvilli, mitochondria, endoplasmic reticulum, and other cytoplasmic components. Virus particles, primarily in cytoplasmic vacuoles, were observed in villous enterocytes and in M cells, lymphocytes, and macrophages in the dome regions of Peyer's patches (Thake 1968; Wagner et al. 1973; Chu et al. 1982a).

In the case of PRCV, as noted earlier, villous atrophy is not observed. However, microscopic examination of lungs from asymptomatic pigs reveals that PRCV causes a diffuse interstitial pneumonia in a high percentage of inoculated animals (O'Toole et al. 1989; Van Nieuwstadt and Pol 1989; Cox et al. 1990a).

DIAGNOSIS

Laboratory Diagnosis. This subject has been reviewed by Bohl (1981). Collection and preservation of appropriate clinical specimens is necessary for reliable diagnosis. Although villous atrophy is a consistent lesion in severely affected pigs, it frequently occurs in other enteric infections as well (rotavirus, PED, coccidia, and sometimes, *E. coli*). Laboratory diagnosis of TGE may be accomplished by one or more of the following procedures: detection of viral antigen, detection of viral nucleic acids, microscopic detection of virus, isolation and identification of virus, or detection of a significant antibody response.

Unfortunately, the serologic assays are complicated by the failure of polyclonal antibodies to differentiate between PRCV and TGEV (discussed under each subsequent heading). However, evaluation of clinical signs, histologic lesions, and tissue distribution of viral antigen may provide a presumptive diagnosis, since PRCV does not cause diarrhea or villous atrophy and replicates almost exclusively in respiratory tissues (Pensaert 1989; Pensaert and Cox 1989).

DETECTION OF VIRAL ANTIGEN. The detection of TGE viral antigen in epithelial cells of the small intestine is probably the simplest and most common method for diagnosing TGE in young pigs. Either the IF (Pensaert et al. 1970a) or the immunoperoxidase (Becker et al. 1974; Chu et al. 1982b) techniques may be used, but the former is more common. For best results, pigs in the early stages of diarrhea are killed. Mucosal scrapings (Black 1971) or frozen sections from the jejunum and ileum are prepared and stained by either the direct (Fig. 29.4) or indirect IF method. Mucosal scrapings generally yield a greater sampling of the intestinal mucosa. Problems that may be encountered in IF tests include (1) lack of sensitivity or specificity of reagents (primary or secondary reagents used must be free of antibodies to other enteric organisms, particularly rotavirus), (2) failure to obtain specimens early after onset of diarrhea before the loss of infected cells (piglets must be euthanized to obtain specimens), and (3) cross-reactions with FIPV, CCV, and PRCV. However, replication of PRCV in villous enterocytes is unreported, and IF staining of villous enterocytes in conjunction with diarrhea is almost certainly TGEV. Although polyclonal antibodies will not differentiate between TGEV and PRCV, certain MAbs have been produced that react with TGEV but fail to recognize PRCV. These differentiating MAbs have been used in IF and immunoperoxidase tests (Garwes et al. 1988; Van Nieuwstadt and Pol 1989). PRCV has been detected in respiratory tissues and nasal epithelial cells by IF, but use of differentiating MAbs is necessary for confirmation, since enteric strains of TGEV may also replicate in these tissues.

TGE viral antigens have also been detected in alkaline intestinal extracts by immunodiffusion (Bohac et al. 1975; Stone et al. 1976) and by immunoelectrophoresis and counterimmunoelectrophoresis (Bohac and Derbyshire 1975), but these methods have not been commonly used for routine diagnosis.

DETECTION OF VIRAL NUCLEIC ACIDS. Recently, nucleic acid hybridization probes have been developed to detect TGEV genome sequences in fecal samples or infected tissues (Shockley et al. 1987; Benfield et al. 1991). Moreover, nucleic acid probes derived from the 5' end of the TGEV peplomer gene can distinguish between PRCV and TGEV. In a hybridization assay, these probes selectively differentiated enteric TGEV isolates from the United States, Japan, and England, including live-attenuated TGEV vaccine strains from U.S. isolates of PRCV, FIPV, and CCV (Bae et al. 1990; Wesley et al. 1991).

ELECTRON MICROSCOPY (EM). TGEV has been demonstrated in the intestinal contents and feces of infected pigs by negative-contrast transmission EM (Fig. 29.5) (Saif et al. 1977). For laboratories having access to an electron microscope and personnel trained in virus recognition by EM, this procedure has had increasing use. Furthermore, immune EM (IEM) has advantages over conventional EM techniques in that it is more sensitive for detecting TGEV and can provide serologic

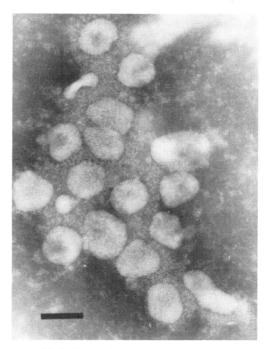

29.5. Typical virus-antibody aggregates observed by IEM of TGEV and gnotobiotic pig anti-TGEV serum. Bar = 100 nm.

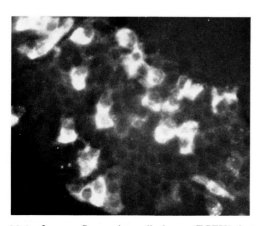

29.4. Immunofluorescing cells from a TGEV-infected pig. A compression smear was made from a mucosal scraping of the jejunum and stained by the direct fluorescent antibody test. ×350.

identification of the virus from either clinical specimens or cell culture harvests. In addition, use of IEM enables one to more readily differentiate TGEV from common enveloped membranous debris and to concurrently detect the presence of other enteric viruses (Saif et al. 1977). IEM is at least as sensitive as IF for detection of TGEV. IEM is also applicable for detection of PRCV-shedding in nasal secretions (Saif 1990, unpublished). However, this method cannot distinguish between TGEV and PRCV unless MAb are used for IEM, although shedding of large numbers of PRCV in feces would not be expected. (Saif 1977, unpublished).

ISOLATION AND IDENTIFICATION OF VIRUS. Oral exposure of young pigs is probably the most sensitive method for isolating or detecting TGEV (Dulac et al. 1977). However, this procedure is very expensive; consequently, cell cultures are more frequently used.

Primary and secondary pig kidney cells (Harada et al. 1963) or pig kidney cell lines (Laude et al. 1981), primary porcine salivary gland cells (Stepanek et al. 1971), porcine thyroid cells (Witte 1971b), and the McClurkin swine testicle (ST) cell line (McClurkin and Norman 1966) have been successfully used for detecting TGEV. The virus also replicates in organ cultures from pig esophagus, ileum, cecum, and colon (Rubenstein et al. 1970). However, parvovirus contamination of some batches of cells prepared from porcine thyroid glands may be a disadvantage to the use of these cells (Dulac et al. 1977). Distinct cytopathogenic effect (CPE) may be negligible upon primary isolation of field strains; additional passages may be required before CPE is evident. A characteristic type of CPE usually seen in ST or porcine thyroid cells consists of greatly enlarged, rounded, or elongated cells that have a balloonlike appearance (Kemeny 1978).

The ST cell line has been used for detecting field strains of TGEV by CPE, plaques, or IF (Kemeny 1978; Bohl 1979). For detecting viral CPE or plaques, the sensitivity of ST cells can be further enhanced by adding pancreatin or trypsin to cell culture media (Bohl 1979; Woods 1982) and using older cells (Stark et al. 1975). Pocock and Garwes (1975) reported that TGEV replicated at highest titer in a slightly acidic media in secondary pig thyroid cells. Primary pig kidney and particularly ST cells have been the cells of choice for isolation of PRCV. The CPE resembles that produced by TGEV strains, with syncytia formation frequently observed for PRCV (Pensaert 1989; Pensaert and Cox 1989). Identification of cell culture virus can be done by VN, IF, or IEM using specific TGEV antiserum. Monoclonal antibodies specific for TGEV are required to identify TGEV and exclude PRCV (Garwes et al. 1988; Laude et al. 1988). Confusion with cross-reacting CCV and FIPV should not occur, since these viruses do not replicate in ST or secondary pig thyroid cells (Reynolds et al. 1980).

SEROLOGIC DIAGNOSIS. The detection of TGEV antibodies can assist in diagnosis and control in several different ways. However, the serologic diagnosis of TGEV is complicated by the finding that both TGEV and PRCV induce neutralizing antibodies that are qualitatively and quantitatively similar (Pensaert 1989; Pensaert and Cox 1989). A blocking ELISA test (described later) is necessary to differentiate these antibodies. A rise in antibody titer between acute and convalescent serum samples provides retrospective evidence for epizootic TGE or PRCV infections. However, the history of the herd in respect to disease and serologic status is needed to help interpret serologic findings. To determine if enzootic TGE or PRCV is a problem in a herd, serum samples from 2- to 6-month-old swine can be tested for antibodies. At this age, passively acquired antibodies should be absent (Derbyshire et al. 1969); thus positive results suggest an enzootic TGEV or PRCV. Serologic tests can also be used to monitor the TGE or PRCV infection status of a herd. The entrance of only serologically negative swine will also help maintain a herd free of TGEV and PRCV. Neutralizing antibodies to TGEV can be detected in serum as early as 7–8 days after infection and may persist for at least 18 months: little is known about the persistence of neutralizing antibodies to PRCV within a herd (Cartwright 1968; Vannier et al. 1982).

TGEV antibodies have been detected by several different serologic tests. The VN test has been most common, using cell culture–adapted viruses in cell culture systems by a variety of procedures: inhibition of CPE in tubes (Harada et al. 1963) or in microtiter plates (Toma and Benet 1976), stained monolayer test (Witte and Easterday 1968), microcolor test (Witte 1971a), and plaque reduction (Bohl and Kumagai 1965; Thomas and Dulac 1976). An indirect fluorescent antibody test was developed (Benfield et al. 1978) but was less sensitive and reliable than the VN test (Hortig et al. 1980). An immunodiffusion test can detect antibodies, but it is rather insensitive (Bohac and Derbyshire 1976; Stone et al. 1976). Very sensitive passive hemagglutination tests (Labadie et al. 1977; Shimizu and Shimizu 1977) and ELISA tests (Nelson and Kelling 1984; Paul et al. 1986; Hohdatsu et al. 1987; Garwes et al. 1988; Bernard et al. 1989; Callebaut et al. 1989; Van Nieuwstadt 1989; Berthon et al. 1990) have been described, but both require concentrated purified virus for sensitizing red blood cells or coating ELISA plates. Other recently developed serologic tests include: an indirect immunoperoxidase test adapted to detect immunoglobulin (Ig) class-specific antibodies (Kodama et al. 1981); radioimmunoprecipitation (Kodama et al. 1980); and a modified autoradiographic test (Stepanek et al.

1982). Complement-fixing antibodies could not be demonstrated in convalescing swine (Stone et al. 1976; Dulac et al. 1977).

BLOCKING ELISA TEST FOR SEROLOGIC DIFFERENTIATION OF PRCV AND TGEV. MAb studies have shown that certain antigenic sites on TGEV are not present on the spike protein of PRCV (Laude et al. 1988; Callebaut et al. 1989; Sanchez et al. 1990). Thus some antigenic determinants on the spike protein of TGEV are modified or absent in PRCV. This and perhaps similar antigenic differences in the capacity of monoclonal antibodies to bind either virus serve as the basis of serological tests to determine if a swine herd is infected with TGEV or PRCV (Garwes et al. 1988; Bernard et al. 1989; Callebaut et al. 1989; Van Nieuwstadt et al. 1989). In the blocking ELISA, TGEV antigen is reacted with either TGEV or PRCV antiserum followed by the distinguishing MAb. TGEV antiserum contains competing antibody that blocks the binding of the MAb, whereas the PRCV antiserum allows the MAb to bind. The test should only be evaluated on a herd basis because some pigs with low TGEV titers may go undiagnosed (Callebaut et al. 1989). Presently, to export TGE-free swine, only this test provides the differential information required for animals testing seropositive to TGEV in countries where PRCV infections occur.

TREATMENT

Antiviral Agents and Interferon. Antiviral agents have not yet been developed for the specific treatment of TGE. Some inhibition of TGEV replication in cell culture has been reported for the antiviral compounds amantadine and isathiazone (Dimitrov 1982; Potopalsky et al. 1983 respectively). Although high levels of type 1 interferon were detected in the intestine in pigs in the early phase of TGEV infection, the role of interferon in the recovery or pathogenesis of TGE was undetermined (LaBonnardiere and Laude 1981). Recent studies suggest that interferon may activate natural killer cells in newborn pigs, thereby contributing a degree of resistance to challenge with TGEV (Lesnick and Derbyshire 1988; Loewen and Derbyshire 1988).

The only treatment presently available is to alleviate starvation, dehydration, and acidosis. Appropriate injections of fluids, electrolytes, and nutrients would be effective in treating young pigs, but this treatment was not practical under farm conditions. The following measures are suggested: provide a warm (preferably above 32°C), draft-free, and dry environment and provide water or an electrolyte or nutrient solution freely accessible to the thirsty TGEV-infected pigs. Such measures will tend to reduce mortality in pigs that are infected at more than 3–4 days of age. Antibacterial therapy might be beneficial in 2- to 5-week-old pigs, especially if there is a concurrent infection with pathogenic strains of *E. coli.* Cross-suckling or putting infected or susceptible litters onto TGE-immune sows was found useful in various field outbreaks (Stepanek et al. 1979; Pritchard 1982).

PREVENTION

Management

PREVENTING ENTRANCE OF TGEV INTO A HERD. Swine in the incubative stage of the disease or those in the viral shedding or carrier state can provide a source of entrance of TGEV into a herd. Some precautions to help avoid these possibilities are to introduce swine that originate from herds known to be free of TGE, are serologically negative, and/or are placed in isolation on the farm for 2–4 weeks before adding them to the herd proper. A frequent question, especially from feeder pig producers or buyers, is, How soon after a TGE outbreak can feeder pigs be moved to another herd without spreading the disease? It seems that a practical answer to this question is that a period of 4 weeks should elapse from the last sign of disease before introducing such animals into a "clean" herd.

Starlings have been incriminated as a means by which the disease is spread between herds in winter months, owing largely to their tendencies to gather in large flocks and feed around swine. Attempts have been made to control the starling population on some farms by the use of poison bait, but it is difficult to know if this approach is useful in preventing the spread of TGE. Cats, dogs, or foxes might play a role in spreading TGE between herds under certain situations (see **EPIDEMIOLOGY**).

Feces from TGEV-infected swine can be carried on boots, shoes, clothing, truck beds, feeds, etc., and can be a source of infection to other herds. Especially in winter these are probably important means by which TGEV is transmitted, as they are present coincidentally with transport of livestock and feed. Consequently, precautions should be taken to minimize such occurrences. If visitors, especially animal and feed truckers, have direct contact with swine during the winter months, it is well to provide them with clean footwear.

AFTER ONSET OF TGE. When TGE has occurred on a farm and pregnant animals have not yet been exposed, two possible procedures to minimize losses of the forthcoming newborn pigs are: (1) If the animals are due to farrow more than 2 weeks hence, purposely expose them to virulent virus—such as the guts of infected pigs—so they will be immune at farrowing time. (2) If the animals will farrow in less than 2 weeks, attempt to provide facilities and management procedures so they will not be exposed to TGEV until at least 3 weeks postfarrowing. To minimize death losses, provide young pigs with a warm, dry, draft-free environment and access to water, electrolyte solution, or milk replacer (see **TREATMENT**).

Some success has been achieved in elimination of TGEV from epizootically infected closed breeder herds without depopulation by the following procedures (Harris et al. 1987): (1) In the face of an outbreak, feed back TGEV-infected minced intestines simultaneously to all pigs in the herd (including replacement stock) to eliminate susceptible hosts, thereby shortening the time the disease progresses through the herd and assuring more uniform exposure levels in all pigs. (2) Maintain strict all-in/all-out production in farrowing and nursery units. (3) Add sentinel seronegative pigs about 2 months after clinical signs of TGE disappear and monitor these pigs for seroconversion to TGEV. Potential hazards associated with feed-back control of TGE include possible spread of other pathogens to pregnant sows and throughout the herd.

ENZOOTIC TGE. Two approaches can be considered in attempting to control or terminate an enzootic TGE herd problem. First, pregnant seropositive sows can be vaccinated intramuscularly (IM) or intramammarily late in gestation or shortly after farrowing with live attenuated TGEV to boost immunity. Although only limited information is available, this procedure should boost milk antibody levels (Saif and Bohl 1983), providing longer passive immunity to suckling pigs (Leopoldt and Meyer 1978; Stepanek et al. 1979; Lutter et al. 1982). Although this procedure may only delay the onset of TGE in exposed pigs, it can be beneficial in reducing mortality.

Second, an alteration in management can be made to break the cycle of infection by eliminating reservoirs of susceptible pigs in a unit. Some considerations are: prevent the continual influx of susceptible animals into the herd, e.g., by temporarily altering the farrowing schedule; temporarily utilize other facilities; and have smaller farrowing and nursing units to better approach the "all-in/all-out" management system.

Immunoprophylaxis

ACTIVE IMMUNITY. The mechanism and duration of active immunity in swine after oral infection with virulent TGEV has not been well characterized. Intestinal infection of breeding age swine results in detectable serum antibodies that persist for at least 6 months to possibly several years, but precise information is not available (Stepanek et al. 1979). It is well documented that these circulating antibodies (actively or passively acquired) provide little protection against a subsequent TGEV infection (Haelterman 1965; Harada et al. 1969). The serum antibody titer, therefore, al-though providing means for a serologic diagnosis of TGE, provides little indication of the degree of active immunity. Conversely, swine that have recovered from TGE are usually immune to subsequent challenge, presumably due to local immunity within the intestinal mucosa. The age and immune status of the animal at initial infection and the severity of the challenge may greatly influence the completeness and duration of this active immunity.

The mechanism of active immunity in the gut, although not specifically demonstrated with TGE, probably relates to stimulation of the secretory IgA (SIgA) immune system with production of intestinal SIgA antibodies by lymphoid cells within the lamina propria (Porter and Allen 1972; Husband and Watson 1978). SIgA TGEV antibodies have been detected in intestinal fluids and serum of pigs after oral, but not parenteral, inoculation with TGEV (Kodama et al. 1980; Sprino and Ristic 1982). Kodama et al. (1980) proposed that detection of IgA antibody in the serum, presumably intestinally derived, might serve as an indicator of active immunity to TGE. In another study, oral inoculation of gnotobiotic pigs with TGEV resulted in development of both serum and intestinal TGEV-neutralizing antibodies detectable from 5 to at least 35 days postexposure (DPE). Initially, only IgM (5–15 DPE), but later IgA, immunocytes (which remained predominant 7–35 DPE) were detected in the intestinal lamina propria of the TGEV-infected gnotobiotic pigs. Few IgM or IgA intestinal immunocytes and no TGEV antibodies were evident in control gnotobiotic pigs (Saif 1976). More recently, an enzyme-linked immunospot (ELISPOT) technique have been used to investigate the kinetics of IgA and IgG TGEV antibody production by pig mesenteric lymph node cells (Van Cott and Saif 1989; Berthon et al. 1990). These and other studies (Stone et al. 1982) indicate the pig is fully immunocompetent at birth in regard to humoral and mucosal antibody production, but in the intestine, additional maturational time may be required for antibody responses to reach adult levels.

Besides local antibody-mediated immunity, cell-mediated immune (CMI) responses may also be important in active immunity against TGEV infections. A number of tests have been used to demonstrate CMI to TGEV, including macrophage migration inhibition (Frederick and Bohl 1976), leukocyte migration-inhibition (Woods 1977; Liou 1982), direct lymphocyte cytotoxicity (Shimizu and Shimizu 1979b), lymphocyte proliferative response (Shimizu and Shimizu 1979c; Welch et al. 1988), spontaneous cell-mediated cytotoxicity (SCMC) and antibody-dependent cell-mediated cytotoxicity (ADCMC) (Cepica and Derbyshire 1983). Only indirect evidence exists concerning the role of CMI in resistance to TGE infection. CMI was demonstrated with lymphocytes obtained from gut-associated lymphoid tissue of swine orally infected with virulent TGEV (Frederick and Bohl 1976; Shimizu and Shimizu 1979c; Welch et al. 1988); swine parenterally or orally inoculated with attenuated virus developed CMI only in systemic sites (spleen or periphenal blood lymphocytes). CMI persisted with gut-associated lymphoid tissue but not systemic lymphocytes for at least 110 days after oral infection of 6-month-old swine (Shimizu and Shimizu 1979c) but only about 14 days after infection of younger (7-day-old) pigs (Welch et al. 1988). A recent study reported the absence of lymphocyte cytotoxicity in newborn piglets and its decrease in parturient sows. It was proposed that such a lack of K and NK cell activity against TGEV-infected cells may correlate with the increased susceptibility of newborn piglets and parturient sows to TGEV infection (Cepica and Derbyshire 1984). Thus CMI may play a role in either recovery from TGEV infection or resistance to reinfection via the rapid elimination of TGEV-infected epithelial cells by any one or all of a combination of SCMC, ADCMC, or sensitized T lymphocyte–mediated cytotoxicity.

VACCINATION OF NEONATAL OR WEANED PIGS. Neonatal pigs have been orally vaccinated with attenuated TGEV in an attempt to induce rapid protection via either interference or local immunity. No early interference has been demonstrated, and generally ≥5 days were required before protection due to active immunity could be induced (Pensaert 1979). One study reported a slightly earlier onset of protection by 3–4 days postvaccination after maintaining vaccinated pigs at a lowered temperature (18–20°C) to enhance replication of the attenuated virus (Furuuchi et al. 1976). Failure to induce an early interference phenomenon and the delay required for development of active immunity make neonatal vaccination an unlikely method of providing immediate protection against TGEV within the critical first few days of life.

Active immunization of suckling or feeder pigs could be important for control of enzootic infections, especially in newly weaned pigs in which TGEV infections may result in increased mortality. Live-attenuated and inactivated TGEV vaccines have been federally licensed for oral or intraperitoneal administration respectively shortly after birth. One limited preliminary study reported greater protection in vaccinated compared to control seropositive suckling pigs even though serum antibody levels were not enhanced but were comparable in the two groups (Graham 1980). However, challenge in older piglets usually is much more difficult to standardize, due to age resistance to infection. Two further studies reported that presence of maternal antibodies in vaccinates decreased (Hess et al. 1982) or completely suppressed (Furuuchi et al. 1978) active antibody production following oral administration of live-attenuated TGEV. The latter study was conducted in suckling piglets nursing naturally infected sows, whereas the former study was done in weaned piglets of vaccinated sows; higher levels of both passive circulating and intestinal antibodies in the suckling piglets probably accounted for the complete interference with active immunization.

Two further approaches have been used in attempts to actively immunize young pigs against TGEV. Woods and Pedersen (1979) noted 33% mortality in challenged pigs (3 of 9) vaccinated IN and intraperitoneally with two doses of the antigenically related live virulent FIPV. In comparison, 100% of the challenged pigs (3 of 3) died that were orally vaccinated once with an attenuated SP variant of TGEV. Gough et al. (1983a) reported that 10 young weaned pigs inoculated IM with two or three doses of an adjuvanted TGEV subunit vaccine were protected against virus challenge.

PASSIVE IMMUNITY. Passive immunity is of primary importance in providing newborn piglets with immediate protection against TGEV infection. Swine are born devoid of Igs, which they acquire after birth via colostrum. Colostral Igs, which consist primarily of IgG, represent a serum transudate that is transferred from the dam across the piglet's intestinal epithelium to its circulation, thus providing the neonate with the same complement of serum antibodies as in the dam (Porter and Allen 1972; Bourne 1973). These humoral antibodies function mainly in protection against systemic infection but do not protect against intestinal infection (Hooper and Haelterman 1966). The concentration of IgG decreases about 30-fold during the first week of lactation, while SIgA concentrations decline only about 3-fold, becoming the predominant Ig in milk (Porter and Allen 1972). SIgA is produced locally in the mammary tissue by cells seeded from the intestine (Roux et al. 1977). SIgA milk antibodies are not absorbed by the piglet, but they play an important role in passive intestinal immunity.

Mechanisms of passive immunity to TGEV infections have been reviewed (Pensaert 1979; Saif and Bohl 1979a, 1981a; Saif 1985; Saif and Theil 1990). Swine that have recovered from TGE can transmit passive immunity to their suckling pigs (Bay et al. 1953). Suckling pigs are protected as a result of the frequent ingestion of colostrum or milk that contains TGEV-neutralizing antibodies. Such antibodies in the lumen of the intestine will tend to neutralize any ingested TGEV and thus protect the susceptible epithelial cells of the small intestine. Haelterman (1963, 1965) referred to this immunogenic mechanism as lactogenic immunity. This is accomplished naturally when immune sows allow their pigs to suckle about every 2 hours. Passive protection can also be accomplished artificially by continuous feeding of antiserum to piglets (Haelterman 1963; Noble 1964). Although presently impractical because of the expense of the antiserum and problem of frequent administration, these problems might eventually be overcome by use of monoclonal antibodies in some type of slow-release delivery system. A question of major importance in possible application of monoclonal antibodies is whether they could be used in the face of an outbreak to reduce morbidity and mortality.

TGEV antibodies in colostrum and milk of sows are primarily associated with IgA or IgG (Abou-Youssef and Ristic 1972; Bohl et al. 1972; Saif et al. 1972). TGEV milk antibodies of the IgA class provide the most effective protection, but IgG antibodies were also protective if high titers could be maintained in milk (Bohl and Saif 1975) or by artificial feeding of colostral IgG (Stone et al. 1977). Probable reasons for the greater efficacy of IgA TGEV antibodies include: (1) they occur in higher levels in milk (Porter and Allen 1972); (2) they are more resistant to proteolytic enzymes (Underdown and Dorrington 1974); and (3) they selectively bind to gut enterocytes (Nagura et al. 1978). Antibodies in milk of the IgA class are produced by the lactating sow as a consequence of an intestinal infection, while those of the IgG class are produced as a result of a parenteral or systemic antigenic stimulation. To explain the occurrence of IgA TGEV antibodies in the milk following an intestinal infection, it was proposed that after antigenic sensitization in the gut, IgA immunocytes migrate to the mammary gland where they localize and secrete IgA antibodies into the colostrum and milk (Saif and Bohl 1979a, 1981a; Saif 1985; Saif and Theil 1990). This "gut-mammary" immunologic axis is an important concept in designing optimal vaccination procedures to provide effective lactogenic immunity.

VACCINATION OF THE PREGNANT DAM. Vaccination of pregnant swine has been attempted using a variety of viral preparations (virulent, attenuated, inactivated, and subunit viruses) and routes of administration (oral, intranasal (IN), intramuscular (IM), and intramammary) (Kaji and Shimizu 1978; Pensaert 1979; Saif and Bohl 1979a; Voets et al. 1980; Moxley and Olson 1989a; Saif and Theil 1990). Oral administration of live virulent virus generally results in the highest level of immunity, consistently producing high titers of persisting IgA TGEV antibodies in milk.

There are presently several federally licensed TGEV vaccines. All contain inactivated or live-attenuated TGEV and are approved for use in pregnant or neonatal swine. These vaccines and their efficacy will be considered in the following sections according to their respective routes of administration. Many variables complicate the evaluation of both experimental and commercial TGEV vaccines, often resulting in conflicting data. These include the challenge dose and strain of TGEV; the age of the pig at challenge; environmental conditions, especially temperature; the milking efficiency of the vaccinated sow; and the immune status of the dam at the time of vaccination.

ORAL AND/OR INTRANASAL VACCINATION. Based on the observation that sows infected with TGEV during gestation could transmit immunity to their piglets, "planned" infection of pregnant swine with virulent TGEV has been used to mimic this natural immunity. This procedure, which should provide a more uniform level of virus exposure, is usually accomplished by feeding virulent autogenous virus to pregnant swine at least 2 weeks before farrowing. The virus may consist of minced guts from young pigs acutely infected with TGEV and is administered to sows with food or in frozen gelatin capsules given orally by means of a balling gun.

Oral vaccination of pregnant swine with attenuated TGEV would appear to be the logical route of vaccination for stimulating milk IgA TGEV antibodies so as to duplicate the natural route of infection and induction of immunity. The IN route has been used alone or together with the oral route, since attenuated strains of TGEV are known to replicate in the respiratory tract (Furuuchi et al. 1979) and upon being swallowed might seed additional virus to the gut. However, results using attenuated strains orally and/or IN have generally been disappointing (Saif and Bohl 1979a, 1981a; Voets et al. 1980; Henning and Thomas 1981; Moxley and Olson 1989a). In previous studies using the high-passaged Purdue strain of TGEV orally, or orally and IM, few IgA TGEV antibodies were evident, and mortality rates among challenged pigs from vaccinated dams ranged from 25 to 100% (Saif and Bohl 1979a,b; Voets et al. 1980; Moxley and Olson 1989a; Saif and Theil 1990).

Concerns that attenuated strains of TGEV might not survive passage through the acidic environment of the stomach prompted studies using lyophilized-attenuated virus in enteric-coated gelatin capsules (Hess et al. 1978; Voets et al. 1980). Hess et al. (1978), using high-titered B1 strain of TGEV (300 cell culture passages), reported high levels of IgA TGEV antibodies in milk and only 10% piglet mortality. Voets et al. (1980) used the high-passaged Purdue strain and found six of nine sows failed to seroconvert after oral vaccination; even the three sows that seroconverted had a 44% piglet mortality rate. Fichtner et al. (1982) noted 30% mortality in challenged piglets after feeding attenuated Riems virus to their dams for 10 days during gestation. In further efforts to assure that vaccinal virus reached the small intestine, two studies used direct inoculation of attenuated viruses into the intestinal lumen. Again, protection was poor (62% mortality) (Voets et al. 1980) in challenged piglets from dams given a single intralumenal inoculation of attenuated Purdue TGEV during gestation, while greater protection (10% mortality) was noted in challenged piglets after their dams received intralumenal inoculation of attenuated Riems TGEV for several days during gestation (Fichtner et al. 1982).

Other researchers selected variants of high- and low-passaged TGEV strains resistant to low pH and proteolytic enzymes in vitro and used these strains as vaccines for passive protection studies (Aynaud et al. 1985; Chen 1985; Shirai et al. 1988; Bernard et al. 1989). They reported inconsistent results with mortality varying from 0 to 73% among litters challenged with virulent TGEV. In the latter two studies, data interpretation was confounded somewhat by variations in the ages of the pigs at challenge, a factor shown in other studies to dramatically influence piglet survivability (Moxley and Olson 1989a).

Moscari (1980b) reported induction of IgA TGEV antibodies in milk after oral administration of the Ckp-attenuated strain of TGEV; however, protection studies were not described. Inconsistent results were noted in vaccination studies using a commercial vaccine (Ambico, Inc.) administered twice orally (in feed) and once IM. Whereas Welter (1980) reported 8% mortality among challenged pigs, others reported higher mortality, similar to that in piglets suckling unvaccinated sows (Saif and Bohl 1981b; Bohl et al. 1982; Moxley and Olson 1989a).

The generally poor results obtained with oral or IN vaccination of sows using attenuated TGEV strains may be attributed to the superficial or limited replication of most attenuated strains in the sow's intestine (Frederick et al. 1976; Hess et al. 1977). Consequently, this results in little antigenic stimulation of underlying intestinal IgA plasma cells and correspondingly little IgA antibody secretion in milk. Attempts to use a low cell culture–passaged TGEV to induce passive immunity led to erratic results both in terms of seroconversion in orally/IN exposed sows and protection in piglets (Saif and Bohl 1979b). The dilemma remains of how to commercially develop vaccine strains of TGEV capable of stimulating an IgA response in the gut of sows but being sufficiently attenuated so as not to produce disease in newborn pigs.

PARENTERAL VACCINATION. Various experimental and two commercial vaccines have also used live-attenuated virus administered IM about 6 and 2 weeks prefarrowing. Experimental evaluations of this vaccination regime have generally indicated reduced piglet mortality (38–56% in vaccinates compared with 71–92% in controls) but not morbidity (Bohl et al. 1975; Voets et al. 1980; Moxley and Olson 1989a). However, vaccination results were poor when compared with almost complete protection (0–9% mortality) in litters of naturally

infected sows. Henning and Thomas (1981) and Matisheck et al. (1982) reported more favorable vaccination results with mortality of 10 and 18% using two commercial vaccines.

The IM vaccination procedure has two major disadvantages: (1) Vaccinated swine develop little or no gut immunity; they usually get sick when exposed to TGEV. If this occurs during lactation, their suckling pigs will be deprived of adequate milk. (2) The TGEV antibodies found in the milk of these vaccinated sows are of low level and of the IgG class that does not provide optimal protection to the gut.

Intramammary injection of seronegative pregnant swine with TGEV resulted in high titers of primarily IgG TGEV antibodies in milk, while similar injections in lactating sows resulted in IgA and IgM TGEV antibodies. Specific antibody activity was found not only in milk from injected glands but also in milk from noninjected glands (Bohl and Saif 1975; Saif and Bohl 1983). Protection was good (14–26% mortality) in litters of intramammarily vaccinated pregnant swine, presumably because exceptionally high levels of IgG antibodies persisted in the milk at the time of challenge, 3 days postfarrowing (DPF) (Shibley et al. 1973; Bohl and Saif 1975). A similar, greatly enhanced, predominantly IgG milk antibody titer was noted in two sows vaccinated IM/IN with high-titered (10^8–$10^{9.3}$ TCID50) attenuated TO163 strain of TGEV. No mortality occurred in either of these litters, suggesting the protective ability of IgG TGEV antibodies when present in high levels in milk (Kaji and Shimizu 1978).

NEW TYPES OF EXPERIMENTAL VACCINES

Heterologous Vaccine. The antigenic relationship between TGEV and FIPV was the basis for studies of the possible efficacy of FIPV as a heterologous coronavirus vaccine in swine. Preliminary studies indicated that some immunity (25% mortality) against TGE was conferred in pigs nursing two sows vaccinated during gestation orally/IN and intramammarily with live virulent FIPV. However, this FIPV was also pathogenic in newborn pigs (Woods and Pedersen 1979). Subsequent studies using cell culture–adapted attenuated FIPV in sows by the same routes of inoculation resulted in higher litter mortality (52%) and low TGEV antibody titers in the IgG class in milk (Woods 1984).

SP Variant Vaccine. A live-attenuated SP variant TGEV grown in a persistently infected porcine leukocyte cell line, has been used to vaccinate pregnant swine by the oral/IN and/or intramammary routes (Woods 1978, 1984). Challenge of the suckling pigs resulted in mortality of 14–34%. In the latter study the author reported generally high TGEV antibody titers in both IgA and IgG fractions of 3–4 DPF milk. However, three of eight sows vaccinated with SP TGEV became mildly sick after challenge exposure of their nursing pigs. Although diarrhea was observed in pigs nursing SP-TGEV vaccinates (48% morbidity), it was reportedly mild and delayed in onset (3 DPE). The SP TGEV has been reported to be avirulent for newborn pigs, replicating within the intestinal lamina propria but not epithelial cells (Woods et al. 1981). Recently, the SP virus has been shown to be a deletion mutant of the parent Miller virulent strain of TGEV (Wesley et al. 1990a). Further investigation of the site and mechanism of replication and antibody induction by this virus strain is warranted.

Native and rDNA Subunit Vaccines. In two studies, virus subunits purified from virulent TGEV and administered with adjuvants by parenteral routes were evaluated as vaccines (Garwes et al. 1978/79; Gough et al. 1983b). Garwes et al. (1978/79) injected pregnant sows intramammarily with virus surface projections (S glycoprotein) or subunit particles; neutralizing antibodies were present only in serum and colostrum of sows injected with S glycoproteins. Colostral antibodies were associated with IgG, except one sow that had both IgG and IgA antibodies. However, protection of challenged piglets was poor (100% mortality in four of six litters).

Gough et al. (1983b) used a low molecular weight undefined subunit (about 23,000) purified from TGEV to IM inject pregnant gilts. These investigators detected neutralizing antibodies in serum and milk and observed only 4% mortality among challenged piglets. The Ig class of TGEV antibodies in the milk of vaccinates was not determined. Although it would currently be very expensive commercially to produce TGEV subunits using the procedures described in the above studies, recombinant DNA technology might eventually provide the means to produce large quantities of the virus subunits at a moderate price. However, in view of the conflicting protection data generated in these two studies (Garwes et al. 1978/79; Gough et al. 1983b), further work is needed to characterize the virus subunits and the immune responses they elicit in swine.

Only preliminary data exists concerning the immunogenicity of rDNA-produced viral subunits or peptides of TGEV. The S protein fragments expressed in *E. coli* were not glycosylated, were difficult to isolate due to aggregation and insolubility, and did not induce neutralizing antibodies to TGEV in mice. However, these authors reported that the S glycoproteins expressed in vaccinia induced low neutralizing-antibody titers to TGEV in mice (Hu et al. 1985). Recently, Posthumus et al. (1990) noted that a peptide from the S region (amino acids 377–391) raised antibodies in rabbits with neutralizing activity to TGEV. No analysis of the immune responses to these proteins or peptides in swine has been reported.

Partial Natural Immunity with PRCV. Since PRCV became widespread in the European swine population, the incidence of epizootic TGE in countries with PRCV has declined (Pensaert and Cox 1989), which suggests that previous exposure of swine to PRCV imparts a degree of immunity to a subsequent TGEV infection but does not entirely prevent diarrhea (Pensaert 1989; Pensaert and Cox 1989). Bernard et al. (1989) reported partial lactogenic immunity in litters of sows naturally infected with PRCV. The mortality rate following a TGEV challenge of 6- to 10-day-old piglets nursing these sows was reduced to 44% (compared to 91% in seronegative control litters). Additional field observations of clinical TGE diarrhea in PRCV-infected swine herds also suggested only an incomplete lactogenic immunity to TGEV (Pensaert 1989; Pensaert and Cox 1989). Sows primed by a PRCV infection developed rapid secondary immune responses upon exposure to TGEV, with increased antibody levels in milk. This enhanced level of passive immunity apparently moderates the severity of TGE epizootics such that piglet mortality is decreased and the disease course is shortened. However, experimental studies by Paton and Brown (1990) showed no evidence for protective lactogenic immunity against TGEV induced by prior infection with PRCV.

Van Nieuwstadt et al. (1989) reported that active intestinal immunity was also incomplete when 9-week-old, PRCV-infected pigs were challenged with TGEV. Clearly, additional studies are necessary to clarify the levels and mechanisms of active and passive immunity to TGEV established in swine by previous exposure to PRCV. In particular, it is important to elucidate the mechanism by which IgA antibodies are induced after infection with PRCV, why they occur only in some sows, and the effectiveness of these IgA antibodies in protecting suckling pigs against intestinal TGEV infections.

VACCINATION OF PREVIOUSLY INFECTED SWINE. Vaccines have been used on two populations of pregnant swine: those that have and those that have not previously been naturally infected with TGEV. There are significant differences in the immune responses and consequently piglet protection in these two groups of animals following vaccination. These differences may account for some of the discrepant results seen in vaccine challenge studies if previously infected swine were unknowingly used. This possibility can only be eliminated by using a very sensitive test (such as plaque-reduction VN) to measure TGEV antibodies and by knowing the herd history of test animals in terms of previous TGE outbreaks. Occurrence of PRCV in herds may further complicate future TGEV vaccine studies.

Limited laboratory research indicated that parenteral inoculation during gestation of previously infected swine using attenuated TGEV resulted in a boost in TGEV milk antibodies in both the IgA and IgG classes (Saif and Bohl 1981a,b, 1983; Saif 1985). Others have also reported greatly increased milk TGEV antibody titers after intramammary inoculation of previously infected swine with inactivated TGEV (Thorsen and Djurickovic 1971). These titers were about 4- to 7-fold greater than in seronegative intramammarily vaccinated gilts or nonvaccinated infected sows. Currently available parenterally administered TGEV vaccines may be more effective in boosting immunity in previously infected pregnant swine than in initiating immunity in previously uninfected seronegative pregnant swine. These vaccines may be especially useful in herds in which enzootic TGE is a problem (Leopoldt and Meyer 1978; Stepanek et al. 1979; Lutter et al. 1982).

REFERENCES

ABOU-YOUSSEF, M. F., AND RISTIC, M. 1972. Distribution of antibodies to transmissible gastroenteritis virus in serum and milk of sows: Isolation and identification of the immunoglobulin classes of swine serum and milk. Am J Vet Res 33:975–979.

ACKERMAN, L. J.; MOREHOUSE, L. G.; AND OLSON, L. D. 1972. Transmissible gastroenteritis in three-week-old pigs: Study of anemia and iron absorption. Am J Vet Res 33:115–120.

ARENDONK, J. A. M., VAN, AND RENKEMA, J. A. 1983. Stimulatie als hulpmiddel bij het bestuderen van het verloop en de effecten van een besmettelijke dierziekte. Tijdschr Diergeneeskd 108:608–614.

AYNAUD, J. M.; NGUYEN, T. D.; BOTTREAU, E.; BRUN, A.; AND VANNIER, P. 1985. Transmissible gastroenteritis (TGE) of swine: Survivor selection of TGE virus mutants in stomach juice of adult pigs. J Gen Virol 66:1911–1917.

BACHMANN, P. A.; HANICHE, T.; DANNER, K.; AND BIBRACK, B. 1972. Epidemiology of TGE in the pig. Zentralbl Veterinaermed [B] 19:166–174.

BAE, I.; JACKWOOD, D. J.; BENFIELD, D. A.; SAIF, L. J.; WESLEY, R. D.; AND HILL, H. 1990. Differentiation of transmissible gastroenteritis virus from porcine respiratory coronavirus and other antigenically related coronaviruses by using cDNA probes specific for the 5′ region of the S glycoprotein gene. J Clin Microbiol 29:215–218.

BAY, W. W.; DOYLE, L. P.; AND HUTCHINGS, L. M. 1952. Some properties of the causative agent of transmissible gastroenteritis in swine. Am J Vet Res 13:318–321.

———. 1953. Transmissible gastroenteritis in swine. A study of immunity. J Am Vet Med Assoc 122:200–202.

BECKER, W.; TEUFEL, P.; AND MIELDS, W. 1974. The immunoperoxidase method for detection of viral and chlamydial antigens. III. Demonstration of TGE antigen in pig thyroid cell cultures. Zentralbl Veterinaermed [B] 21:59–65.

BENFIELD, D. A.; HAELTERMAN, E. O.; AND BURNSTEIN, T. 1978. An indirect fluorescent antibody test for antibodies to transmissible gastroenteritis of swine. Can J Comp Med 42:478–482.

BENFIELD, D. A.; JACKWOOD, D. J.; BAE, I.; SAIF, L. J.; AND WESLEY, R. D. 1991. Detection of transmissible gastroenteritis virus using cDNA probes. Arch Virol 116:91–106.

BERNARD, S.; BOTTREAU, E.; AYNAUD, J. M.; HAVE, P.; AND SZYMANSKY, J. 1989. Natural infection with the porcine respiratory coronavirus induces protective lactogenic immunity against transmissible gastroenteritis. Vet Microbiol 21:1–8.

BERTHON, P.; BERNARD, S.; SALMON, H.; AND BINNS, R. 1990. Kinetics of the in vitro antibody response to transmissible gastroenteritis virus from pig mesenteric lymph node cells using ELISASPOT and ELISA tests. J Immunol Methods 131:173–182.

BINN, L. N.; LAZAR, E. C.; KEENAN, K. P.; HUXSOLL, D. L.; MARCHWICKI, R. H.; AND STRANO, A. J. 1974. Recovery and characterization of a coronavirus from military dogs with diarrhea. Proc US Anim Health Assoc 78:359–366.

BLACK, J. W. 1971. Diagnosis of TGE by FA: Evaluation of accuracy on field specimens. Proc US Anim Health Assoc 75:492–498.

BOHAC, J., AND DERBYSHIRE, J. B. 1975. The demonstration of transmissible gastroenteritis viral antigens by immunoelectrophoresis and counterimmunoelectrophoresis. Can J Microbiol 21:750–753.

———. 1976. The detection of transmissible gastroenteritis viral antibodies by immunodiffusion. Can J Comp Med 40:161–165.

BOHAC, J.; DERBYSHIRE, J. B.; AND THORSEN, J. 1975. The detection of transmissible gastroenteritis viral antigens by immunodiffusion. Can J Comp Med 39:67–75.

BOHL, E. H. 1979. Diagnosis of diarrhea in pigs due to transmissible gastroenteritis virus or rotavirus. In Viral Enteritis in Humans and Animals. Ed. F. Bricout and R. Scherrer. INSERM (Paris) 90:341–343.

———. 1981. Coronaviruses: Diagnosis of infections. In Comparative Diagnosis of Viral Diseases, vol. 4. Ed. E. Kurstak and C. Kurstak. New York: Academic Press, pp. 301–328.

BOHL, E. H., AND KUMAGAI, T. 1965. The use of cell cultures for the study of swine. Proc US Livest Sanit Assoc 69:343–350.

BOHL, E. H., AND SAIF, L. J. 1975. Passive immunity in transmissible gastroenteritis of swine: Immunoglobulin characteristics of antibodies in milk after inoculating virus by different routes. Infect Immun 11:23–32.

BOHL, E. H.; GUPTA, R. K. P.; OLQUIN, M. V. F.; AND SAIF, L. J. 1972. Antibody responses in serum, colostrum and milk of swine after infection or vaccination with transmissible gastroenteritis virus. Infect Immun 6:289–301.

BOHL, E. H.; FREDERICK, G. T.; AND SAIF, L. J. 1975. Passive immunity in transmissible gastroenteritis of swine: Intramuscular injection of pregnant swine with a modified live-virus vaccine. Am J Vet Res 36:267–271.

BOHL, E. H.; KOHLER, E. M.; SAIF, L. J.; CROSS, R. F.; AGNES, A. G.; AND THEIL, K. W. 1978. Rotavirus as a cause of diarrhea in pigs. J Am Vet Med Assoc 172:458–463.

BOHL, E. H.; SAIF, L. J.; AND JONES, J. E. 1982. Observations on the occurrence of transmissible gastroenteritis (TGE) in a vaccinated herd. Ohio Swine Res Ind Rep, Anim Sci Ser 82-1, Ohio State Univ, pp. 66–69.

BOURNE, F. J. 1973. Symposium on nutrition of the young farm animal: The immunoglobulin system of the suckling pig. Proc Nutr Soc 32:205–214.

BOURSNELL, M. E. G.; BROWN, T. D. K.; FOULDS, I. J.; GREEN, P. F.; TOMLEY, F. M.; AND BINNS, M. M. 1987. Completion of the sequence of the genome of the coronavirus avian infectious bronchitis virus. J Gen Virol 68:57–77.

BRIAN, A. B.; DENNIS, D. E.; AND GREY, J. S. 1980. Genome of porcine transmissible gastroenteritis virus. J Virol 34:410–415.

BRITTON, P.; LOPEZ OTIN, C.; MARTIN ALONSO, J. M.; AND PARRA, F. 1989. Sequence of the coding regions from the 3.0 kb and 3.9 kb mRNA. Subgenomic species from a virulent isolate of transmissible gastroenteritis virus. Arch Virol 105:165–178.

BROWN, I., AND CARTWRIGHT, S. 1986. New porcine coronavirus? Vet Rec 119:282–283.

BROWN, T. T. 1981. Laboratory evaluation of selected disinfectants as viricidal agents against porcine parvovirus, pseudorabies virus, and transmissible gastroenteritis virus. Am J Vet Res 42:1033–1036.

BUTLER, D. G.; GALL, D. G.; KELLY, M. H.; AND HAMILTON, J. R. 1974. Transmissible gastroenteritis: Mechanisms responsible for diarrhea in an acute enteritis in piglets. J Clin Invest 53:1335–1342.

CALLEBAUT, P.; CORREA, I.; PENSAERT, M.; JIMENEZ, G.; AND ENJUANES, L. 1988. Antigenic differentiation between transmissible gastroenteritis virus of swine and a related porcine respiratory coronavirus. J Gen Virol 69:1725–1730.

CALLEBAUT, P.; PENSAERT, M. B.; AND HOOYBERGHS, J. 1989. A competitive inhibition ELISA for the differentiation of serum antibodies from pigs infected with transmissible gastroenteritis virus (TGEV) or with the TGEV-related porcine respiratory coronavirus. Vet Microbiol 20:9–19.

CARTWRIGHT, S. F. 1968. Transmissible gastroenteritis of swine (TGE). Br Vet J 124:410–413.

CARTWRIGHT, S. F.; HARRIS, H. M.; BLANDFORD, T. B.; FINGHAM, I.; AND GITTER, M. 1965. A cytopathic virus causing a transmissible gastroenteritis in swine. I. Isolation and properties. J Comp Pathol 75:386–395.

CEPICA, A., AND DERBYSHIRE, J. B. 1983. Antibody-dependent cell-mediated cytotoxicity and spontaneous cell-mediated cytotoxicity against cells infected with porcine transmissible gastroenteritis virus. Can J Comp Med 47:298–303.

————. 1984. Antibody-dependent and spontaneous cell-mediated cytotoxicity against transmissible gastroenteritis virus-infected cells by lymphocytes from sows, fetuses and neonatal piglets. Can J Comp Med 48:258–261.

CHARLEY, B., AND LAUDE, H. 1988. Induction of alpha interferon by transmissible gastroenteritis coronavirus: Role of transmembrane glycoprotein E1. J Virol 62:8–11.

CHASEY, D., AND CARTWRIGHT, S. F. 1978. Virus-like particles associated with porcine epidemic diarrhoea. Res Vet Sci 25:255–256.

CHEN, K. S. 1985. Enzymatic and acidic sensitivity profiles of selected virulent and attenuated transmissible gastroenteritis viruses of swine. Am J Vet Res 46:632–636.

CHU, R. M.; GLOCK, R. D.; AND ROSS, R. F. 1982a. Changes in gut-associated lymphoid tissues of the small intestine of eight-week-old pigs infected with transmissible gastroenteritis virus. Am J Vet Res 43:67–76.

CHU, R. M.; LI, N. J.; GLOCK, R. D.; AND ROSS, R. F. 1982b. Application of peroxidase staining technique for detection of transmissible gastroenteritis virus in pigs. Am J Vet Res 43:77–81.

CORNELIUS, L. M.; HOOPER, B. E.; AND HAELTERMAN, E. O. 1968. Changes in fluid and electrolyte balance in baby pigs with transmissible gastroenteritis. Am J Clin Pathol 2:105–113.

CORREA, I.; GEBAUER, F.; BULLIDO, M. J.; SUNE, C.; BAAY, M. F. D.; ZWAAGSTRA, K. A.; POSTHUMUS, W. P. A.; LENSTRA, J. A.; AND ENJUANES, L. 1990. Localization of antigenic sites of the E2 glycoprotein of transmissible gastroenteritis virus. J Gen Virol 71:271–279.

COX, E.; HOOYBERGHS, J.; AND PENSAERT, M. B. 1990a. Sites of replication of a porcine respiratory coronavirus related to transmissible gastroenteritis virus. Res Vet Sci 48:165–169.

COX, E.; PENSAERT, M. B.; CALLEBAUT, P.; AND VAN DEUN, K. 1990b. Intestinal replication of a porcine coronavirus closely related antigenically to the enteric transmissible gastroenteritis virus. Vet Microbiol 23:237–243.

DEBOUCK, P.; CALLEBAUT, P.; AND PENSAERT, M. 1982. Prevalence of the porcine epidemic diarrhea (PED) virus in the pig population of different countries. Proc 7th Int Congr Pig Vet Soc, Mexico City, p. 45.

DELMAS, B.; RASSCHAERT, D.; GODET, M.; GELFI, J.; AND LAUDE, H. 1990. Four major antigenic sites of the coronavirus transmissible gastroenteritis virus are located on the amino-terminal half of spike glycoprotein S. J Gen Virol 71:1313–1324.

DERBYSHIRE, J. B.; JESSETT, D. M.; AND NEWMAN, G. 1969. An experimental epidemiological study of porcine transmissible gastroenteritis. J Comp Pathol 79:445–452.

DIMITROV, P. 1982. Effect of amantadine on different stages of replication of porcine transmissible gastroenteritis virus. Vet Med Nauki 19:90–96. In Bulgarian with English abstract.

DOYLE, L. P., AND HUTCHINGS, L. M. 1946. A transmissible gastroenteritis in pigs. J Am Vet Med Assoc 108:257–259.

DULAC, G. C.; RUCKERBAUER, G. M.; AND BOULANGER, P. 1977. Transmissible gastroenteritis: Demonstration of the virus from field specimens by means of cell culture and pig inoculation. Can J Comp Med 41:357–363.

DURET, C.; BRUN, A.; GUILMOTO, H.; AND D'AUVERGNE, M. 1988. Isolement, identification et pouvoir pathogene chez le porc d'un coronavirus apparente au virus de la gastro-enterite transmissible. Rec Med Vet 164:221–226.

EGAN, I. T.; HARRIS, D. L.; AND HILL, H. T. 1982. Prevalence of swine dysentery, transmissible gastroenteritis, and pseudorabies in Iowa, Illinois and Missouri swine. Proc 86th Annu Meet US Anim Health Assoc, pp. 497–502.

FERRIS, D. H. 1973. Epizootiology of porcine transmissible gastroenteritis (TGE). In Advances in Veterinary Science and Comparative Medicine, vol. 17. New York, London: Academic Press, pp. 57–86.

FICHTNER, D.; LEOPOLDT, D.; AND MEYER, U. 1982. Untersuchungen zur Ermittlung der minimalen Antigenmenge bei der oralen Muttertierimmunisierung gegen die Transmissible Gastroenteritis der Schweine mit Riemser TGE-Vakzine. Arch Exp Veterinaermed 36:577–585.

FREDERICK, G. T., AND BOHL, E. H. 1976. Local and systemic cell-mediated immunity against transmissible gastroenteritis, an intestinal viral infection of swine. J Immunol 116:1000–1004.

FREDERICK, G. T.; BOHL, E. H.; AND CROSS, R. F. 1976. Pathogenicity of an attenuated strain of transmissible gastroenteritis virus for newborn pigs. Am J Vet Res 37:165–169.

FURUUCHI, S.; SHIMIZU, Y.; AND KUMAGAI, T. 1975. Comparison of properties between virulent and attenuated strains of TGE. Natl Inst Anim Health Q 15:159–164.

————. 1976. Vaccination of newborn pigs with an attenuated strain of transmissible gastroenteritis virus. Am J Vet Res 37:1401–1404.

FURUUCHI, S.; SHIMIZU, M.; AND SHIMIZU, Y. 1978.

Field trials on transmissible gastroenteritis live virus vaccine in newborn piglets. Natl Inst Anim Health Q (Tokyo) 18:135–142.

FURUUCHI, S.; SHIMIZU, Y.; AND KUMAGAI, T. 1979. Multiplication of low and high cell culture passaged strains of transmissible gastroenteritis virus in organs of newborn piglets. Vet Microbiol 3:169–178.

GAGNON, A. N.; DULACK, G. C.; MARSOLAIS, G.; LUSSIER, G.; AND MAROIS, P. 1974. Maladies porcines a etiologie virale dans la Province de Quebec. II. Gastro-enterite transmissible. Can Vet J 15:316–318.

GARWES, D. J., AND POCOCK, D. H. 1975. The polypeptide structure of transmissible gastroenteritis virus. J Gen Virol 29:25–34.

GARWES, D. J.; LUCAS, M. H.; HIGGINS, D. A.; PIKE, B. V.; AND CARTWRIGHT, S. F. 1978/79. Antigenicity of structural components from porcine transmissible gastroenteritis virus. Vet Microbiol 3:179–190.

GARWES, D. J.; STEWART, F.; AND ELLEMAN, C. J. 1987. Identification of epitopes of immunological importance on the peplomer protein of porcine transmissible gastroenteritis virus. Adv Exp Med Biol 218:509–515.

GARWES, D. J.; STEWART, F.; CARTWRIGHT, S. F.; AND BROWN, I. 1988. Differentiation of porcine coronavirus from transmissible gastroenteritis virus. Vet Rec 122:86–87.

GOODWIN, R. F. W., AND JENNINGS, A. R. 1958. A highly infectious gastroenteritis of pigs. Vet Rec 70:271–272.

GOUGH, P. M.; AND JORGENSON, R. D. 1983. Identification of porcine transmissible gastroenteritis virus in house flies (*Musca domestica* Linneaus). Am J Vet Res 44:2078–2082.

GOUGH, P. M.; ELLIS, C. H.; FRANK, C. J.; AND JOHNSON, C. J. 1983a. A viral subunit immunogen for porcine transmissible gastroenteritis. Antiviral Res 3:211–221.

GOUGH, P. M.; FRANK, C. J.; MOORE, D. G.; SAGONA, M. A.; AND JOHNSON, C. J. 1983b. Lactogenic immunity to transmissible gastroenteritis virus induced by a subunit immunogen. Vaccine 1:37–41.

GRAHAM, J. A. 1980. Induction of active immunity to TGE in neonatal pigs nursing seropositive dams. Vet Med Small Anim Clin 75:1618–1619.

GRANZOW, H.; MEYER, U.; SOLISCH, P.; LANGE, E.; AND FICHTNER, D. 1981. Die Morphologie der Koronaviren-Elektronmikroskopische Darstellung des Virus der Transmissible Gastroenteritis des Schweines im Negativekontrastverfahren. Arch Exp Veterinaermed 35:177–186.

HAELTERMAN, E. O. 1962. Epidemiological studies of transmissible gastroenteritis of swine. Proc US Livest Sanit Assoc 66:305–315.

———. 1963. Transmissible gastroenteritis of swine. Proc 17th World Vet Congr, Hannover, 1:615–618.

———. 1965. Lactogenic immunity to transmissible gastroenteritis of swine. J Am Vet Med Assoc 147:1661.

HAELTERMAN, E. O., AND HUTCHINGS, L. M. 1956. Epidemic diarrheal diseases of viral origin in newborn swine. Ann NY Acad Sci 66:186–190.

HARADA, K.; KUMAGAI, T.; AND SASAHARA, J. 1963. Cytopathogenicity of transmissible gastroenteritis virus in pigs. Natl Inst Anim Health Q (Tokyo) 3:166–167.

HARADA, K.; KAJI, T.; KUMAGAI, T.; AND SASAHARA, J. 1968. Studies on transmissible gastroenteritis in pigs. IV. Physicochemical and biological properties of TGE virus. Natl Inst Anim Health Q (Tokyo) 8:140–147.

HARADA, K.; FURUUCHI, S.; KUMAGAI, T.; AND SASAHARA, J. 1969. Pathogenicity, immunogenicity and distribution of transmissible gastroenteritis virus in pigs. Natl Inst Anim Health Q (Tokyo) 9:185–192.

HARRIS, D. L.; BEVIER, G. W.; AND WISEMAN, B. S. 1987. Eradication of transmissible gastroenteritis virus without depopulation. Proc Am Assoc Swine Pract, Des Moines, Iowa, p. 555.

HENNING, E. R., AND THOMAS, P. C. 1981. Comparison of intramuscular and oral modified live virus TGE vaccines. Vet Med Small Anim Clin 76:1789–1792.

HENNINGSEN, D.; MOUSING, J.; AND AALUND, O. 1989. Porcint corona virus (PCV) i Danmark. En epidemiologisk traersnitsanalyse baseret pa screeningomrade sporgeskema data. Dansk Vet Tidsskr 71:1168–1177.

HESS, R. G., AND BACHMANN, P. A. 1976. In vitro differentiation and pH sensitivity of field and cell culture attenuated strains of transmissible gastroenteritis. Infect Immun 13:1642–1646.

HESS, R. G.; BACHMANN, P. A.; AND HANICHEN, T. 1977. Attempts to establish an immunoprophylaxis for transmissible gastroenteritis virus infection of pigs. I. Pathogenicity of the B1 strain after serial passages. Zentralbl Veterinaermed [B] 24:753–763.

HESS, R. G.; BACHMANN, P. A.; AND MAYR, A. 1978. Attempts to develop an immunoprophylaxis against transmissible gastroenteritis (TGE) in pigs. III. Passive immune transfer after oral vaccination with attenuated TGE virus strain B1. Zentralbl Veterinaermed [B] 25:308–318.

HESS, R. G.; CHEN, Y. S.; AND BACHMANN, P. A. 1982. Active immunization of feeder pigs against transmissible gastroenteritis (TGE): Influence of maternal antibodies. Proc 7th Int Congr Pig Vet Soc, Mexico City, p. 1.

HILL, H.; BIWER, J.; WOOD, R.; AND WESLEY, R. 1990. Porcine respiratory coronavirus isolated from two U.S. swine herds. Proc Am Assoc Swine Pract, Des Moines, Iowa, p. 333.

HOHDATSU, T.; EIGUCHI, Y.; IDE, S.; BABA, K.; YAMAGISHI, H.; KUME, T.; MATUMOTO, M. 1987. Evaluation of an enzyme-linked immunosorbent assay for the detection of transmissible gastroenteritis virus antibodies. Vet Microbiol 13:93–97.

HOOPER, B. E., AND HAELTERMAN, E. O. 1966. Concepts of pathogenesis and passive immunity in transmissible gastroenteritis of swine. J Am Vet Med Assoc 149:1580–1586.

———. 1969. Lesions of the gastrointestinal tract of pigs infected with transmissible gastroenteritis. Can J Comp Med 33:29–36.

HORNICH, M.; SALAJKA, E.; AND STEPANEK, J. 1977. Malabsorption in newborn piglets with diarrhoeic *Escherichia coli* infection and transmissible gastroenteritis. Zentralbl Veterinaermed [B] 24:75–86.

HORTIG, H.; RODER, B; AND BRUSKE, R. 1980. Vergleichende Untersuchungen zur Verwendbarkeit des Microneutralisationstests, des indirekten Immunofluoreszenztests und des Virus-Inhibitionstests zum Nachweis von Antikorpen gegen das Virus der Transmissible Gastroenteritis (TGE) des Schweines. DTW 87:192–196.

HORZINEK, M. C.; LUTZ, H.; AND PEDERSEN, N. C. 1982. Antigenic relationships among homologous structural polypeptides of porcine, feline, and canine coronaviruses. Infect Immun 37:1148–1155.

HU, S.; BRUSZEWSKI, J.; SMALLING, R.; AND BROWNE, J. K. 1985. Studies of TGEV spike protein gp 195 expressed in E. coli and by a TGE-vaccinia virus recombinant. In Immunobiology of Proteins and Peptides–III. Ed. M. Zauhair-Atassi and H. L. Cachrach. New York: Plenum Press, p. 63.

HUSBAND, A. J., AND WATSON, D. L. 1978. Immunity in

the intestine. Vet Bull 48:911–920.

JACOBS, L.; VAN DER ZEIJST, B. A. M.; AND HORZINEK, M. C. 1986. Characterization and translation of transmissible gastroenteritis virus mRNAs. J Virol 57:1010–1015.

JACOBS, L.; DE GROOT, R.; VAN DER ZEIJST, B. A.; HORZINEK, M. C.; AND SPAAN, W. 1987. The nucleotide sequence of the peplomer gene of porcine transmissible gastroenteritis (TGEV): Comparison with the sequence of the peplomer protein of feline infectious peritonitis virus (FIPV). Virus Res 8:363–371.

JESTIN, A.; LE FORBAN, Y.; VANNIER, P.; MADEC, F.; AND GOURREAU, J. M. 1987. Un nouveau coronavirus porcin. Etudes sero-epidemiologiques retrospectives dans les elevages de Bretagne. Rec Med Vet 163:567–571.

JIMENEZ, G.; CORREA, I.; MELGOSA, M. P.; BUILLIDO, M. J.; AND ENJUANES, L. 1986. Critical epitopes in transmissible gastroenteritis virus neutralization. J Virol 60:131–139.

KAJI, T., AND SHIMIZU, Y. 1978. Passive immunization against transmissible gastroenteritis virus in piglets of ingestion of milk of sows inoculated with attenuated virus. Natl Inst Anim Health Q (Tokyo) 18:43–52.

KAPKE, P. A., AND BRIAN, D. A. 1986. Sequence analysis of the porcine transmissible gastroenteritis coronavirus nucleocapsid protein gene. Virology 151:41–49.

KEMENY, L. J. 1976. Antibody response in pigs inoculated with transmissible gastroenteritis virus and cross reactions among ten isolates. Can J Comp Med 40:209–214.

———. 1978. Isolation of transmissible gastroenteritis virus from pharyngeal swabs obtained from sows at slaughter. Am J Vet Res 39:703–705.

KEMENY, L. J., AND WOODS, R. D. 1977. Quantitative transmissible gastroenteritis virus shedding patterns in lactating sows. Am J Vet Res 38:307–310.

KEMENY, L. J.; WILTSEY, V. L.; AND RILEY, J. L. 1975. Upper respiratory infection of lactating sows with transmissible gastroenteritis virus following contact exposure to infected piglets. Cornell Vet 65:352–362.

KLEMM, R. C., AND RISTIC, M. 1976. The effect of propagation of transmissible gastroenteritis (TGE) virus in pups and the lungs of baby pigs on the immunologic properties of the virus. Proc 4th Int Congr Pig Vet Soc, Iowa State Univ, p. K11.

KODAMA, Y.; OGATA, M.; AND SHIMIZU, Y. 1980. Characteristics of immunoglobulin A antibody in serum of swine inoculated with transmissible gastroenteritis virus. Am J Vet Res 40:740–745.

———. 1981. Serum immunoglobulin A antibody response in swine infected with transmissible gastroenteritis virus, as determined by indirect immunoperoxidase antibody test. Am J Vet Res 42:437–442.

LABADIE, J. P.; AYNAUD, J. M.; VAISSAIRE, J.; AND RENAULT, L. 1977. Porcine transmissible gastroenteritis. Antibody detection by passive haemagglutination test: Applications to diagnosis and epidemiology. Rec Med Vet 153:931–936.

LABONNARDIERE, C., AND LAUDE, H. 1981. High interferon titer in newborn pig intestine during experimentally induced viral enteritis. Infect Immun 32:28–31.

LANGE, E.; SCHIRRMEIER, H.; GRANZOW, H.; FICHTNER, D. P.; AND LEOPOLDT, D. 1988. Isolierung und erste charakterisierung eines coronavirus aus lungen und tonsillen klinisch gesunder schweine. Monatsh Veterinaermed 43:273–274.

LAUDE, H.; GELFI, J.; AND AYNAUD, J. M. 1981. In vitro properties of low- and high-passaged strains of trans-

missible gastroenteritis coronavirus of swine. Am J Vet Res 42:447–449.

LAUDE, H.; CHARLEY, B.; AND GELFI, J. 1984. Replication of transmissible gastroenteritis coronavirus (TGE) in swine alveolar macrophages. J Gen Virol 65:327–332.

LAUDE, H.; CHAPSAL, J. M.; GELFI, J.; LABIAU, S.; AND GROSCLAUDE, J. 1986. Antigenic structure of transmissible gastroenteritis virus. I. Properties of monoclonal antibodies directed against virion proteins. J Gen Virol 67:119–130.

LAUDE, H.; GELFI, J.; RASSCHAERT, D.; AND DELMAS, B. 1988. Caracterisation antigenique du coronavirus respiratoire porcin a l'aide d'anticorps monoclonaux diriges contre le virus de la gastro-enterite transmissible. J Rech Porcine Fr 20:89–94.

LAUDE, H.; RASSCHAERT, D.; DELAMS, B.; GODET, M.; GELFI, J.; AND CHARLEY, B. 1990. Molecular biology of transmissible gastroenteritis. Vet Microbiol 23:147–154.

LAVIADA, M. D.; VIDEGAIN, S. P.; MORENO, L.; ALONSO, F.; ENJUANES, L.; AND ESCRIBANO, J. M. 1990. Expression of swine transmissible gastroenteritis virus envelope antigens on the surface of infected cells: Epitopes externally exposed. Virus Res 16:247–254.

LEE, K. M.; MORO, M.; AND BAKER, J. A. 1954. Transmissible gastroenteritis in pigs. Am J Vet Res 15:364–372.

LEOPOLDT, D., AND MEYER, U. 1978. Transmissible gastro-enteritis of swine-A model of infectious diarrhoea. Arch Exp Veterinaermed 32:417–425.

LESNICK, C. E., AND DERBYSHIRE, J. B. 1988. Activation of natural killer cells in newborn piglets by interferon induction. Vet Immunol Immunopathol 18:109–117.

LIOU, P. P. 1982. Cellular immunity in transmissible gastroenteritis virus-infected pigs: Influence of viral antigens in leukocyte migration. J Chin Soc Vet Sci 8:135–141.

LOEWEN, K. G., AND DERBYSHIRE, J. B. 1988. The effect of interferon induction in parturient sows and newborn piglets on resistance to transmissible gastroenteritis. Can J Vet Res 52:149–153.

LUTTER, K.; KLAHN, J.; AND KOKLES, R. 1982. Erfahrungen bei der Sanierung der Transmissible Gasroenteritis nach dem Selektionsverfahren in einer Schweinezuchtanlage mit 1200 produktiven Sauen. Monatsh Veterinaermed 37:121–126.

MCCLURKIN, A. W., AND NORMAN, J. O. 1966. Studies on transmissible gastroenteritis of swine. II. Selected characteristics of a cytopathogenic virus common to five isolates from transmissible gastroenteritis. Can J Comp Med 30:190–198.

MCCLURKIN, A. W.; STARK, S. L.; AND NORMAN, J. O. 1970. Transmissible gastroenteritis (TGE) of swine: The possible role of dogs in the epizootiology of TGE. Can J Comp Med 34:347–349.

MAES, R. K., AND HAELTERMAN, E. O. 1979. A seroepizootiological study of five viruses in a swine-evaluation station. Am J Vet Res 40:1642–1645.

MAKINO, S.; KECK, J. G.; STOHLMAN, S. A.; AND LAI, M. M. C. 1986. High frequency RNA recombination of murine coronaviruses. J Virol 57:729–737.

MATISHECK, P.; EMERSON, W.; AND SEARL, R. C. 1982. Results of laboratory and field tests of TGE vaccine. Vet Med Small Anim Clin 77:262–264.

MILLER, G. Y.; KLIEBENSTIN, J.; AND KIRTLEY, C. 1982. Some micro and macroeconomic impacts of swine disease: The case of transmissible gastroenteritis. Proc 3d Int Symp Vet Epidemiol Econ, pp. 527–534.

MOON, H. W. 1978. Mechanisms in the pathogenesis of

diarrhea: A review. J Am Vet Med Assoc 172:443–448.

MOON, H. W.; NORMAN, J. O.; AND LAMBERT, G. 1973. Age dependent resistance to TGE of swine. I. Clinical signs and some mucosal dimensions in the small intestine. Can J Comp Med 37:157–166.

MORIN, M.; SOLORZANO, R. F.; MOREHOUSE, L. G.; AND OLSON, L. D. 1978. The postulated role of feeder swine in the perpetuation of the transmissible gastroenteritis virus. Can J Comp Med 42:379–384.

MORIN, M.; TURGEON, D.; JOLETTE, J.; ROBINSON, Y.; PHANEUF, J. B.; SAUVAGEAU, R.; BEAUREGARD, M.; TEUSCHER, E.; HIGGINS, R.; AND LARIVERE, S. 1983. Neonatal diarrhea of pigs in Quebec: Infectious causes of significant outbreaks. Can J Comp Med 47:11–17.

MOSCARI, E. 1980a. Physicochemical properties of field and cell culture attenuated strains of swine transmissible gastroenteritis (TGE) coronavirus. Acta Vet Acad Sci Hung 28:341–350.

_____. 1980b. Vaccination experiments against transmissible gastroenteritis (TGE) of swine. VII. Immunoglobulin characteristics of antibodies in milk of sows vaccinated with the "CKp" strain of TGE virus. Acta Vet Acad Sci Hung 28:131–145.

MOUSING, J.; VAGSHOLM, I.; CARPENTER, T. E.; GARDNER, I. A.; AND HERD, D. W. 1988. Financial impact of transmissible gastroenteritis in pigs. J Am Vet Med Assoc 192:756–759.

MOXLEY, R. A., AND OLSON, L. D. 1989a. Clinical evaluation of transmissible gastroenteritis virus vaccination procedures for inducing lactogenic immunity in sows. Am J Vet Res 50:111–118.

_____. 1989b. Lesions of transmissible gastroenteritis virus infection in experimentally inoculated pigs suckling immunized sows. Am J Vet Res 50:708–716.

NAGURA, H.; NAKANE, D. K.; AND BROWN, W. R. 1978. Breast milk IgA binds to jejunal epithelia in suckling rats. J Immunol 120:1330–1339.

NAKAO, J.; HESS, R. G.; BACHMANN, P. A.; AND MAHNEL, H. 1978. Tenacity and inactivation of transmissible gastroenteritis (TGE) virus of pigs. Berl Munch Tieraerztl Wochenschr 91:353–357.

NELSON, L. D., AND KELLING, C. L. 1984. Enzyme-linked immunosorbent assay for detection of transmissible gastroenteritis virus antibody in swine sera. Am J Vet Res 45:1654–1657.

NGUYEN, T. D.; BOTTREAU, E.; BERNARD, S.; LANTIER, I.; AND AYNAUD, J. M. 1986. Neutralizing secretory IgA and IgG do not inhibit attachment of transmissible gastroenteritis virus. J Gen Virol 67:939–943.

NOBLE, W. A. 1964. Methods used to combat transmissible gastroenteritis. Vet Rec 76:51.

NORMAN, J. O.; MCCLURKIN, A. W.; AND STARK, S. L. 1970. Transmissible gastroenteritis (TGE) of swine: Canine serum antibodies against an associated virus. Can J Comp Med 34:115–117.

NORMAN, J. O.; LAMBERT, G.; MOON, H. W.; AND STARK, S. L. 1973. Age dependent resistance to transmissible gastroenteritis (TGE). II. Coronavirus titer in tissues of pigs after exposure. Can J Comp Med 37:167–170.

OKANIWA, A.; HARADA, K.; AND PARK, D. K. 1968. Structure of swine transmissible gastroenteritis virus examined by negative staining. Natl Inst Anim Health Q (Tokyo) 8:175–181.

ONNO, M.; JESTIN, A.; CARIOLET, R.; AND VANNIER, P. 1989. Rapid diagnosis of TGEV-like coronavirus in fattened pigs by indirect immunofluorescence labelling in nasal cells. J Vet Med [B] 36:629–634.

OSTERHAUS, A. D. M. E.; HORZINEK, M. C.; AND

REYNOLDS, D. J. 1977. Seroepidemiology of feline infectious peritonitis virus infections using transmissible gastroenteritis virus as antigen. Zentralbl Veterinaermed [B] 24:835–841.

O'TOOLE, D.; BROWN, I.; BRIDGES, A.; AND CARTWRIGHT, S. F. 1989. Pathogenicity of experimental infection with 'pneumotropic' porcine coronavirus. Res Vet Sci 47:23–29.

PATON, D. J., AND BROWN, I. H. 1990. Sows infected in pregnancy with porcine respiratory coronavirus show no evidence of protecting their suckling piglets against transmissible gastroenteritis. Vet Res Commun 14:329–337.

PAUL, P. S.; MENGELING, W. L.; SAIF, L. J.; AND VAN DERESEN, R. A. 1986. Detection of classes of antibodies to TGE and rotavirus of swine using monoclonal antibodies to porcine immunoglobulins. Proc Int Pig Vet Congr, Barcelona, p. 190.

PEDERSEN, N. C.; WARD, J.; AND MENGELING, W. L. 1978. Antigenic relationship of the feline infectious peritonitis virus to coronaviruses of other species. Arch Virol 58:45–53.

PENSAERT, M. B. 1979. Immunity in TGE of swine after infection and vaccination. In Viral Enteritis in Humans and Animals. Ed. F. Bricout and R. Scherrer. INSERM (Paris) 90:281–293.

_____. 1989. Transmissible gastroenteritis virus (respiratory variant). In Virus Infections of Porcines. Ed. M. B. Pensaert. Amsterdam: Elsevier Science, pp. 154–165.

PENSAERT, M. B., AND COX, E. 1989. Porcine respiratory coronavirus related to transmissible gastroenteritis virus. Agri-Pract 10:17–21.

PENSAERT, M. B., AND DEBOUCK, P. 1978. A new coronavirus-like particle associated with diarrhea in swine. Arch Virol 58:243–247.

PENSAERT, M. B.; HAELTERMAN, E. O.; AND BURNSTEIN, T. 1970a. Transmissible gastroenteritis of swine: Virus-intestinal cell interactions. I. Immunofluorescence, histopathology and virus production in the small intestine through the course of infection. Arch Gesamte Virusforsch 31:321–334.

PENSAERT, M. B.; HAELTERMAN, E. O.; AND HINSMAN, E. J. 1970b. Transmissible gastroenteritis of swine: Virus-intestinal cell interactions. II. Electron microscopy of the epithelium in isolated jejunal loops. Arch Gesamte Virusforsch 31:335–351.

PENSAERT, M. B.; DEBOUCK, P.; AND REYNOLDS, D. J. 1981. An immunoelectron microscopic and immunofluorescent study on the antigenic relationship between the coronavirus-like agent, CV 777, and several coronaviruses. Arch Virol 68:45–52.

PENSAERT, M.; CALLEBAUT, P.; AND VERGOTE, J. 1986. Isolation of a porcine respiratory, non-enteric coronavirus related to transmissible gastroenteritis. Vet Q 8:257–261.

PHILLIP, J. I. H.; CARTWRIGHT, S. F.; AND SCOTT, A. C. 1971. The size and morphology of T. G. E. and vomiting and wasting disease of pigs. Vet Rec 88:311–312.

PIKE, B. V., AND GARWES, D. J. 1977. Lipids of transmissible gastroenteritis virus and their relation to those of two different host cells. J Gen Virol 34:531–535.

PILCHARD, E. I. 1965. Experimental transmission of transmissible gastroenteritis virus by starlings. Am J Vet Res 26:1177–1179.

POCOCK, D. H., AND GARWES, D. J. 1975. The influence of pH on the growth and stability of transmissible gastroenteritis virus in vitro. Arch Virol 49:239–247.

PORTER, P., AND ALLEN, W. D. 1972. Classes of immunoglobulins related to immunity in the pig: A review. J Am Vet Med Assoc 160:511–518.

POSTHUMUS, W. P.; LENSTRA, J. A.; SCHAAPER, W. M.; VAN NIEUWSTADT, A. P.; ENJUANES, L.; AND MELOEN, R. H. 1990. Analysis and simulation of a neutralizing epitope of transmissible gastroenteritis virus. J Virol 64:3304–3309.

POTOPALSKY, A. I.; SPIVAK, N. Y.; SHVED, A. D.; MELNICHENKO, V. S.; AND KRASNOVA, E. F. 1983. Activity of certain chemopreparations with respect to the transmissible gastroenteritis virus and pig enterovirus. Mikrobiol Zh 45:75–78. In Russian with English abstract.

PRITCHARD, G. C. 1982. Observations on clinical aspects of transmissible gastroenteritis of pigs in Norfolk and Suffolk, 1980–81. Vet Rec 110:465–469.

_____. 1987. Transmissible gastroenteritis in endemically infected breeding herds of pigs in East Anglia, 1981–1985. Vet Rec 120:226–230.

PROCHAZKA, Z.; HAMPL, J.; SEDLACEK, M.; MAASEK, J.; AND STEPANEK, J. 1975. Protein loss in piglets infected with transmissible gastroenteritis virus. Zentralbl Veterinaermed [B] 22:138–146.

RASSCHAERT, D., AND LAUDE, H. 1987. The predicted primary structure of the peplomer protein E2 of the porcine coronavirus transmissible gastroenteritis virus. J Gen Virol 68:1883–1890.

Rasschaert, D.; Gelfi, J.; and Laude, H. 1987. Enteric coronavirus TGEV: Partial sequence of the genomic RNA, its organization and expression. Biochim 69:591–600.

RASSCHAERT, D.; DUARTE, M.; AND LAUDE, H. 1990. Porcine respiratory coronavirus differs from transmissible gastroenteritis virus by a few genomic deletions. J Gen Virol 71:2599–2607.

REDMAN, D. R.; BOHL, E. H.; AND CROSS, R. F. 1978. Intrafetal inoculation of swine with transmissible gastroenteritis virus. Am J Vet Res 39:907–911.

REYNOLDS, D. J., AND GARWES, D. J. 1979. Virus isolation and serum antibody responses after infection of cats with transmissible gastroenteritis virus. Arch Virol 60:161–166.

REYNOLDS, D. J.; GARWES, D. J.; AND GASKELL, C. J. 1977. Detection of transmissible gastroenteritis virus neutralizing antibody in cats. Arch Virol 55:77–86.

REYNOLDS, D. J.; GARWES, D. J.; AND LUCEY, S. 1980. Differentiation of canine coronavirus and porcine transmissible gastroenteritis virus by neutralization with canine, porcine and feline sera. Vet Microbiol 5:283–290.

ROUX, M. E.; MCWILLIAMS, M.; PHILLIPS-QUAGLIATA, J. M.; WEISZ-CARRINGTON, P.; AND LAMM, M. E. 1977. Origin of IgA-secreting cells in the mammary gland. J Exp Med 146:1311.

RUBINSTEIN, D.; TYRRELL, A. J.; DERBYSHIRE, J. B.; AND COLLINS, A. P. 1970. Growth of porcine transmissible gastroenteritis virus in organ cultures of pig tissue. Nature 227:1348–1349.

SAIF, L. J. 1976. The immune response of swine to transmissible gastroenteritis virus. Ph.D. thesis, Ohio State Univ.

_____. 1985. Passive immunity to coronavirus and rotavirus infections in swine and cattle: Enhancement by maternal vaccination. In Infectious Diarrhoea in the Young. Ed. S. Tzipori. Amsterdam: Elsevier Science, p. 456.

SAIF, L. J., AND BOHL, E. H. 1979a. Role of SIgA in passive immunity of swine to enteric viral infections. In Immunology of Breast Milk. Ed. P. L. Ogra and D. H. Dayton. New York: Raven.

_____. 1979b. Passive immunity in transmissible gastroenteritis of swine: Immunoglobulin classes of milk antibodies after oral-intranasal inoculations of sows with a live low cell culture-passaged virus. Am J Vet Res 40:115–117.

_____. 1981a. Keynote address: Passive immunity against enteric viral infections. Proc 3d Int Symp Neonatal Diarrhea. VIDO, Saskatoon, Canada.

_____. 1981b. Experimental studies using TGE vaccines. Ohio Swine Res Ind Rep, Anim Sci Ser 81-2, Ohio State Univ, pp. 58–59.

_____. 1983. Passive immunity to transmissible gastroenteritis virus: Intramammary viral inoculation of sows. Ann NY Acad Sci 409:708–723.

SAIF, L. J.; AND THEIL, K. W., eds. 1990. Viral Diarrheas of Man and Animals. Boca Raton, Fla: CRC Press.

SAIF, L. J.; BOHL, E. H.; AND GUPTA, R. K. P. 1972. Isolation of porcine immunoglobulins and determination of the immunoglobulin classes of transmissible gastroenteritis viral antibodies. Infect Immun 6:600–609.

SAIF, L. J.; BOHL, E. H.; KOHLER, E. M.; AND HUGHES, J. H. 1977. Immune electron microscopy of transmissible gastroenteritis virus and rotavirus (reovirus-like agent) of swine. Am J Vet Res 38:13–20.

SANCHEZ, C. M.; JIMENEZ, G.; LAVIADA, M. D.; CORREA, I.; SUNE, C.; BULLIDO, M. J.; GEBAUER, F.; SMERDOU, C.; CALLEBAUT, P.; ESCRIBANO, J. M.; AND ENJUANES, L. 1990. Antigenic homology among coronaviruses related to transmissible gastroenteritis virus. Virology 174:410–417.

SASHARA, J.; HARADA, K.; HAYASHI, S.; AND WATANABE, M. 1958. Studies on transmissible gastroenteritis in pigs in Japan. Jpn J Vet Sci 20:1–6.

SHEPHERD, R. W.; GALL, D. G.; BUTLER, D. G.; AND HAMILTON, J. R. 1979. Determinates of diarrhea in viral enteritis: The role of ion transport and epithelial changes in the ileum in transmissible gastroenteritis in piglets. Gastroenterology 76:20–24.

SHIBLEY, G. P.; SALSBURY, D. L.; DJURICKOVIC, S. M.; AND JOHNSON, G. 1973. Application of an intramammary route of vaccination against transmissible gastroenteritis in swine. Vet Med Small Anim Clin 68:59–61.

SHIMIZU, M., AND SHIMIZU, Y. 1977. Micro-indirect hemagglutination test for detection of antibodies against transmissible gastroenteritis virus of pigs. J Clin Microbiol 6:91–95.

_____. 1979a. Effects of ambient temperatures on clinical and immune responses of pigs infected with transmissible gastroenteritis virus. Vet Microbiol 4:109–116.

_____. 1979b. Demonstration of cytotoxic lymphocytes of virus-infected target cells in pigs inoculated with transmissible gastroenteritis virus. Am J Vet Res 40:208–213.

_____. 1979c. Lymphocyte proliferative response to viral antigen in feeder pigs infected with transmissible gastroenteritis. Infect Immun 23:239–243.

SHIMIZU, M.; SHIMIZU, Y.; AND KODAMA, Y. 1978. Effects of ambient temperatures on induction of transmissible gastroenteritis in feeder pigs. Infect Immun 21:747–752.

SHIRAI, J.; LANTIER, I.; BOTTREAU, E.; AYNAUD, J. M.; AND BERNARD, S. 1988. Lactogenic immunity to transmissible gastroenteritis of swine induced by attenuated Nouzilly strain of TGE virus: Neutralizing antibody classes and protection. Ann Rech Vet 19:267–272.

SHOCKLEY, L. J.; KAPKE, P. A.; LAPPS, W.; BRIAN, D. A.; POTGIETER, L. D.; AND WOODS, R. 1987. Diagnosis of porcine and bovine enteric coronavirus infections using cloned cDNA probes. J Clin Microbiol 25:1591–1596.

SIDDELL, S. G.; ANDERSON, R.; CAVANAGH, D.; FUJIWARA, K.; KLENK, H. D.; MACNAUGHTON, M. R.; PENSAERT, M.; STOHLMAN, S. A.;

STURMAN, L.; AND VAN DER ZEIJST, B. A. M. 1983a. Coronaviridae. Intervirology 20:181–189.

SIDDELL, S.; WEGE, H.; AND TER MEULEN, V. 1983b. The biology of coronaviruses. J Gen Virol 64:761–776.

SPAAN, W.; CAVANAGH, D.; AND HORZINEK, M. C. 1988. Coronaviruses: Structure and genomic expression. J Gen Virol 69:2939–2952.

SPRINO, P. J., AND RISTIC, M. 1982. Intestinal, pulmonary, and serum antibody responses of feeder pigs exposed to transmissible gastroenteritis virus by oral and oral-intranasal routes of inoculation. Am J Vet Res 43:255–261.

STARK, S. L.; FERNELIUS, A. L.; BOOTH, G. D.; AND LAMBERT, G. 1975. Transmissible gastroenteritis (TGE) of swine: Effect of age of swine testes cell culture monolayers on plaque assays of TGE virus. Can J Comp Med 39:466–468.

STEPANEK, J.; POSPISIL, Z.; AND MESAROS, E. 1971. Growth activity of transmissible gastroenteritis (TGE) virus in primary cultures of pig kidney cells and pig salivary gland cells. Acta Vet Brno 40:235–240.

STEPANEK, J.; MENSIK, J.; FRANZ, J.; AND HORNICH, M. 1979. Epizootiology, diagnosis and prevention of viral diarrhoea in piglets under intensive husbandry conditions. Proc 21st World Vet Congr, Moscow, 6:43.

STEPANEK, J.; HAMPL, J.; FRANZ, J.; MENSIK, P.; AND SKROBAK, F. 1982. Prukax protilatek proti viru virove gastroenteritidy prasat modifikvanym autoradiografickym testem. Vet Med (Praha) 27:473–482.

STONE, S. S.; KEMENY, L. J.; AND JENSEN, M. T. 1976. Partial characterization of the principal soluble antigens associated with the coronavirus of transmissible gastroenteritis by complement fixation and immunodiffusion. Infect Immun 13:521–525.

STONE, S. S.; KEMENY, L. J.; WOODS, R. D.; AND JENSEN, M. T. 1977. Efficacy of isolated colostral IgG, IgA and IgM(A) to protect neonatal pigs against the coronavirus of transmissible gastroenteritis. Am J Vet Res 38:1285–1288.

STONE, S. S.; KEMENY, L. J.; AND JENSEN, M. T. 1982. Serum antibody responses of neonatal and young adult pigs to transmissible gastroenteritis coronavirus. Vet Immunol Immunopathol 3:529–533.

SUNE, C.; JIMENEZ, G.; CORREA, I.; BULLIDO, M. J.; GEBAUER, F.; SMERDOU, C.; AND ENJUANES, L. 1990. Mechanisms of transmissible gastroenteritis coronavirus neutralization. Virology 177:559–569.

THAKE, D. C. 1968. Jejunal epithelium in transmissible gastroenteritis of swine (an electron microscopic and histochemical study). Am J Pathol 53:149–168.

THEIL, K. W.; SAIF, L. J.; BOHL, E. H.; AGNES, A. G.; AND KOHLER, E. M. 1979. Concurrent porcine rotaviral and transmissible gastroenteritis viral infections in a three-day-old conventional pig. Am J Vet Res 40:719–721.

THOMAS, F. C., AND DULAC, G. C. 1976. Transmissible gastroenteritis virus: Plaques and a plaque neutralization test. Can J Comp Med 40:171–174.

THORSEN, J., AND DJURICKOVIC, S. 1971. Experimental immunization of sows with inactivated TGE virus. Can J Comp Med 35:99–102.

TOMA, B., AND BENET, J. J. 1976. A technique of research on microplates of the antibodies neutralizing transmissible gastroenteritis virus of swine. Rec Med Vet 152:565–568.

TOMA, B.; VANNIER, P.; AND AYNAUD, J. M. 1978. Epidemiological studies on porcine transmissible gastroenteritis in France. Rec Med Vet 154:853–858.

UNDERDAHL, N. R.; MEBUS, C. A.; STAIR, E. L.; AND TWIEHAUS, M. J. 1972. The effect of cytopathogenic transmissible gastroenteritis-like viruses and/or *Escherichia coli* on germfree pigs. Can Vet J 13:9–16.

UNDERDAHL, N. R.; MEBUS, C. A.; AND TORRES-MEDINA, A. 1975. Recovery of transmissible gastroenteritis virus from chronically infected experimental pigs. Am J Vet Res 36:1473–1476.

UNDERDOWN, B. J., AND DORRINGTON, K. J. 1974. Studies on the structural and conformational basis for the relative resistance of serum and secretory immunoglobulin A to proteolysis. J Immunol 112:949–959.

VAN COTT, J. L., AND SAIF, L. J. 1989. An ELISPOT assay for the detection of antibody-secreting cells to transmissible gastroenteritis virus (TGEV). Proc Conf Res Workers Anim Dis CRWAD, Chicago, Abst 145, p. 27.

VANNIER, P. 1990. Disorders induced by the experimental infection of pigs with the porcine respiratory coronavirus (P.R.C.V.). J Vet Med [B] 37:177–180.

VANNIER, P.; TOMA, B.; MADEC, F.; AND AYNAUD, J. M. 1982. Valuation of duration of TGE virus spread among sows of 2 infected herds by means of a serological survey of antibodies persistence. Proc 7th Int Congr Pig Vet Soc, Mexico City, p. 3.

VAN NIEUWSTADT, A. P., AND POL, J. M. A. 1989. Isolation of a TGE virus-related respiratory coronavirus causing fatal pneumonia in pigs. Vet Rec 124:43–44.

VAN NIEUWSTADT, A. P.; ZETSTRA, T.; AND BOONSTRA, J. 1989. Infection with porcine respiratory coronavirus does not fully protect pigs against intestinal transmissible gastroenteritis virus. Vet Rec 125:58–60.

VOETS, M. TH.; PENSAERT, M.; AND RONDHUIS, P. R. 1980. Vaccination of pregnant sows against transmissible gastroenteritis with two attenuated virus strains and different inoculation routes. Vet Q 2:211–219.

WAGNER, J. E.; BEAMER, P. D.; AND RISTIC, M. 1973. Electron microscopy of intestinal epithelial cells of piglets infected with a transmissible gastroenteritis virus. Can J Comp Med 37:177–188.

WAXLER, G. L. 1972. Lesions of transmissible gastroenteritis in the pig as determined by scanning electron microscopy. Am J Vet Res 33:1323–1328.

WELCH, S.-K. W.; AND SAIF, L. J. 1988. Monoclonal antibodies to a virulent strain of transmissible gastroenteritis virus: Comparison of reactivity against the attenuated and virulent virus strain. Arch Virol 101:221–235.

WELCH, S.-K. W.; SAIF, L. J.; AND RAM, S. 1988. Cell-mediated immune responses of nursing pigs inoculated with attenuated or virulent transmissible gastroenteritis virus. Am J Vet Res 49:1228–1234.

WELTER, C. J. 1965. TGE of swine. I. Propagation of virus in cell cultures and development of a vaccine. Vet Med Small Anim Clin 60:1054–1058.

————. 1980. Experimental and field evaluation of a new oral vaccine for TGE. Vet Med Small Anim Clin 75:1757–1759.

WESLEY, R.; WOODS, R.; AND KAPKE, P. 1987. Antibody response in swine to individual transmissible gastroenteritis virus (TGEV) proteins. Adv Exp Med Biol 218:475–481.

WESLEY, R. D.; WOODS, R. D.; AND CHEUNG, A. K. 1990a. Genetic basis for the pathogenesis of transmissible gastroenteritis virus. J Virol 64:4761–4766.

WESLEY, R. D.; WOODS, R. D.; HILL, H. T.; AND BIWER, J. D. 1990b. Evidence for a porcine respiratory coronavirus, antigenically similar to transmissible gastroenteritis virus, in the United States. J Vet Diagn Invest 2:312–317.

WESLEY, R. D.; WESLEY, I. V.; AND WOODS, R. D. 1991. Differentiation between transmissible gastroenteritis virus and porcine respiratory coronavirus using a cDNA probe. J Vet Diagn Invest 3:29–32.

WHITENACK, D. L.; WHITEHAIR, C. K.; AND MILLER,

E. R. 1978. Influence of enteric infection on zinc utilization and clinical signs and lesions of zinc deficiency in young swine. Am J Vet Res 39:1447–1454.

WITTE, K. H. 1971a. Micro-color test for assay of transmissible gastroenteritis virus-neutralizing antibodies. Arch Gesamte Virusforsch 33:171–176.

_____. 1971b. Isolation of the virus of transmissible gastroenteritis (TGE) from naturally infected piglets in cell cultures. Zentralbl Veterinaermed [B] 18:770–778.

_____. 1974. Haufigkeit und Verbreitung Transmissible Gastroenteritis (TGE) Virus-neutralisierender Antikorper bei Mastschweinen in acht Kreisen Nordwestdeutschlands. Zentralbl Veterinaermed [B] 21:376–384.

WITTE, K. H., AND EASTERDAY, B. C. 1968. Stained monolayer test: A color test in disposable plastic trays for titrating transmissible gastroenteritis virus and neutralizing antibodies. Am J Vet Res 29:1409–1417.

WITTE, K. H., AND WALTHER, C. 1976. Age-dependent susceptibility of pigs to infection with the virus of transmissible gastroenteritis. Proc 4th Int Congr Pig Vet Soc, Iowa State Univ, p. K3.

WITTE, K. H.; TUCH, K.; DUBENKROPP, H.; AND WALTHER, C. 1977. Untersuchungen uber die Antigenverwandtschaft der Viren der Felinen Infektiosen Peritonitis (IFP) und der Transmissible Gastroenteritis (TGE) des Schweines. Berl Munch Tieraerztl Wochenschr 90:396–401.

WOOD, E. N. 1979. Transmissible gastroenteritis epidemic diarrhoea of pigs. Br Vet J 135:305–314.

WOODS, R. D. 1977. Leukocyte migration-inhibition procedure for transmissible gastroenteritis viral antigens. Am J Vet Res 38:1267–1269.

_____. 1978. Small plaque variant transmissible gastroenteritis virus. J Am Vet Med Assoc 173:643–647.

_____. 1982. Studies of enteric coronaviruses in a feline cell line. Vet Microbiol 7:427–435.

_____. 1984. Efficacy of vaccination of sows with serologically related coronaviruses for control of transmissible gastroenteritis in nursing pigs. Am J Vet Res 45:1726–1729.

WOODS, R. D., AND PEDERSEN, N. C. 1979. Cross-protection studies between feline infectious peritonitis and porcine transmissible gastroenteritis viruses. Vet Microbiol 4:11–16.

WOODS, R. D.; CHEVILLE, N. F.; AND GALLAGHER, J. E. 1981. Lesions in the small intestine of newborn pigs inoculated with porcine, feline, and canine coronaviruses. Am J Vet Res 42:1163–1169.

WOODS, R. D.; WESLEY, R. D.; AND KAPKE, P. A. 1988. Neutralization of transmissible gastroenteritis virus by complement dependent monoclonal antibodies. Am J Vet Res 49:300–304.

YOUNG, G. A.; HINZ, R. W.; AND UNDERDAHL, N. R. 1955. Some characteristics of transmissible gastroenteritis in disease-free antibody-devoid pigs. Am J Vet Res 16:529–535.

ZHU, X. L.; PAUL, P. S.; VAUGHN, E.; MORALES, A. 1990. Characterization and reactivity of monoclonal antibodies to the Miller strain of transmissible gastroenteritis virus of swine. Am J Vet Res 51:232–238.

30 Vesicular Diseases

J. A. House
C. A. House

VESICULAR DISEASES of swine can be caused by infection with foot-and-mouth disease (FMD), swine vesicular disease (SVD), vesicular stomatitis (VS), vesicular exanthema of swine (VES), and San Miguel sea lion (SMS) viruses (Table 30.1). A vesicular disease was first described in Italy by Fracastorius in 1546; it is likely that FMD virus (FMDV) was the cause. While VS was historically recognized in horses in the United States during the Civil War, infection in swine was not reported until 1943 (Schoening 1943). The first appearance of VES was in 1932 in California; it was recognized as a new disease by Traum (1934). Smith et al. (1973) identified a new viral isolate from marine mammals that was able to cause a vesicular disease in swine, and SMS viruses (SMSV) were identified as serotypes of caliciviruses, closely related to VES viruses (VESV). As diagnostic techniques for FMD became more sophisticated, another new disease, SVD, was shown to be present in Italy in 1966 (Nardelli et al. 1968). It is possible that additional new viral agents, able to cause infections clinically similar to FMD, may be identified as disease surveillance increases.

ETIOLOGY. Vesicular diseases are caused by infection of swine with a wide spectrum of viruses (Table 30.2).

Foot-and-Mouth Disease. Foot-and-mouth disease virus is a picornavirus (family Picornaviridae, genus *Aphthovirus*). The international name for FMDV is aphthovirus, from the Greek aphtha, "vesicles in the mouth." These viruses are acid labile and have a single-stranded, positive-sense RNA, which serves as messenger RNA and is directly translated into viral proteins. There are four viral proteins, of which viral protein 1 (VP1) has been shown to produce protective immunity in cattle. Variants of FMDV may become evident in immune or partially immune cattle during persistent infection; this may account for the appearance of new subtypes (Gebauer et al. 1988). The viral RNA polymerase, termed virus infection–associated (VIA) antigen, is group reactive among the seven serotypes of FMDV. Antibody to the VIA antigen was historically used to differentiate active infection from vaccination, although it is now recognized that repeated vaccination with killed FMD vaccine may elicit a transient antibody to VIA antigen (Pinto and Garland 1979).

Swine Vesicular Disease. Swine vesicular disease virus is also a picornavirus (family Picornaviridae, genus *Enterovirus*). The virions are acid stable and have a single-stranded, positive-sense RNA, and four viral proteins in the viral capsid.

Table 30.1. Chronologic and geographic distribution of vesicular diseases

Virus	Disease First Reported	Agent Identified	Distribution	Areas Free
Foot-and-mouth disease	1514	1897	Sporadic: Europe Endemic: South America, Asia, Africa	North and Central America, Australia, New Zealand, Panama, Scandinavia, Japan, Caribbean Basin
San Miguel sea lion	None	1973	Pacific Coast of North America	Remainder of world
Swine vesicular disease	1966	1968	Europe, Japan, Hong Kong, Taiwan	North, Central, and South America; Africa, United Kingdom
Vesicular exanthema of swine	1932	1933	Last North American case in 1956	World
Vesicular stomatitis	Civil War	1927	North, Central, and South America	Remainder of world

Table 30.2.   Characteristics of the etiologic agents of vesicular diseases

Disease Agent	Classification	Nucleic Acid	Size/ Stability	Serotypes	Features
Foot-and-mouth disease virus	Picornaviridae *Apthovirus*	SS RNA[a]	22 nm; labile below pH 6.5; ether resistant	7; numerous subtypes show varied degrees of cross-protection	4 viral proteins, plus a group reactive virus infection− associated (VIA) antigen
Swine vesicular disease virus	Picornaviridae *Enterovirus*	SS RNA	28 nm; acid stable; ether resistant	1	Related to Coxsackie B-5 virus
Vesicular exanthema of swine/San Miguel sea lion viruses	Caliciviridae *Calicivirus*	SS RNA	35 to 40 nm; labile below pH 3; ether resistant	25 or more	1 polypeptide in coat; have group reactive antigens
Vesicular stomatitis virus	Rhabdoviridae *Vesiculovirus*	SS RNA	70 × 170 nm; bullet-shaped; ether labile; acid labile	2 of importance to swine	1 immunogenic glycoprotein

[a]Single-stranded RNA.

Vesicular Exanthema of Swine and San Miguel Sea Lion Viruses.

The VESVs and SMSVs are caliciviruses, named from the Latin calices for the cup-shaped depressions on the virion. There are 13 known serotypes of VESVs designated (except for strains 1934B and 101) by a letter and the year of isolation (e.g., VESV A$_{48}$). The SMSV serotypes are numbered consecutively in order of discovery except for SMSV 3. Twelve serotypes of SMSV have been described in the literature, as well as five other serotypes of caliciviruses associated with marine animals (Barlough et al. 1986). Caliciviruses contain single-stranded, positive-sense RNA. The capsomers of the caliciviruses are composed of one major polypeptide. Group-reactive antigens of caliciviruses are useful for serodiagnosis.

Vesicular Stomatitis.

The bullet-shaped viruses of the family Rhabdoviridae, genus *Vesic-ulovirus*, contain single-stranded, negative-sense RNA and have a surface glycoprotein (G) that induces neutralizing and hemagglutinating antibodies, which are serotype specific. The viral nucleoprotein (N) and, to a lesser degree, the matrix (M) proteins account for serological group cross-reactions. The vesiculoviruses are ether labile and unstable at pH 3 or lower (Patterson et al. 1958).

EPIDEMIOLOGY. The epidemiological features of the vesicular diseases are compared in Table 30.3.

Foot-and-Mouth Disease. Foot-and-mouth disease is highly contagious and produces acute clinical signs in susceptible animals; aerosol exposure is the major means of spread. The disease is also spread by exposure to infected animals, contaminated semen, meat and milk products, fom-

Table 30.3.   Epidemiologic features of vesicular disease agents

Disease Agent	Main Species Affected	Transmission	Morbidity	Carrier State	Contamination of Meat and By-Products
Foot-and-mouth disease virus	Swine, cattle, sheep, goats	Aerosol, contact, fomites	High	Cattle, sheep, goats, African buffalo	Fast frozen meat, lymph nodes, bone marrow, milk products
Swine vesicular disease virus	Swine, humans	Contact, aerosal, fomites, oral	Moderate	Swine	Glands, gland extracts, low level of virus in bled-out meat
Vesicular exanthema of swine/San Miguel sea lion virus	Swine, various marine animals	Oral, contact, fomites	Moderate	No	Meat
Vesicular stomatitis virus	Swine, horses, cattle, humans	Likely insect bites, contact (biting) fomites	Moderate to low, summer	No	Not documented

ites, and viral aerosols carried by air currents over long distances. High humidity, cloud cover, and moderate temperatures favor long-distance airborne spread. Even with rigorous enforcement of regulations, the introduction of FMD into a disease-free country remains a possibility; therefore, FMD should be a part of the differential diagnosis in any vesicular disease of swine, cattle, or other cloven-footed animals. Almost all cloven-footed species are susceptible to FMD, with infected animals shedding large quantities of virus into their surroundings for at least 10 days; human infections are extremely rare and may occur with or without clinical symptoms (Hyslop 1973). Swine produce aerosols up to 1000 times greater in viral concentration than cattle (Donaldson and Ferris 1980) and may produce up to 10^8 infectious aerosolized particles per day (Sellers et al. 1971).

FMD has long been considered a major influence in international agriculture, producing economic loss directly through the loss of meat, milk, and draft power, and indirectly through embargoes and loss of trade. On the North American continent, FMD last occurred in Mexico in 1946–54 and in Canada in 1952. It has occurred nine times in the United States; the last outbreak was in 1929. Serotypes A, O, and C are prevalent in South America and are sporadically found in Western Europe. Six serotypes (A, O, and C, South African Territories 1 [SAT 1], South African Territories 2 [SAT 2], and South African Territories 3 [SAT 3]) occur in Africa. On the Asian continent, A, O, C, and Asia 1 occur. Japan, Australia, New Zealand, and certain Pacific islands are free of the disease. Stringent importation regulations (Section 306A of the Tariff Act of 1930 and Acts of 1890 and 1903) on animals and animal products have effectively protected the FMD-free status of the United States. Only the Agricultural Research Service (ARS) and the Animal and Plant Health Inspection Service (APHIS), U.S. Department of Agriculture (USDA) high-containment facilities (greater than biosafety level 3) at the Plum Island Animal Disease Center (PIADC) are permitted to perform research on FMDV in the United States. The Foreign Animal Disease Diagnostic Laboratory (FADDL) at the PIADC is a division of the National Veterinary Services Laboratories (NVSL), APHIS, and receives vesicular disease diagnostic samples from cloven-footed animals. If an outbreak of FMD ever does occur in the United States, prompt measures will be taken to eradicate the disease.

A carrier state for FMDV has not been described for swine. Carrier states in cattle, sheep, and goats for FMDV are readily demonstrated, but transmission to susceptible animals has not been demonstrated. The cape buffalo (*Syncerus caffer*) remains a carrier of FMDV for many months after infection and may, on rare occasion, be responsible for transmission of virus to livestock (Gainoru 1986; Bengis et al. 1987).

Cattle semen from infected cattle contained and transmitted FMDV by artificial insemination (AI) (Cottral et al. 1968); in contrast, semen from infected swine contained FMDV but did not transmit FMD by AI (McVicar et al. 1978).

Swine Vesicular Disease. In contrast to FMD, SVDV affects only swine, humans, and, experimentally, mice. SVD is moderately infectious and is spread primarily by contact with infected swine, their excretions, or by garbage feeding of SVDV-contaminated meat products. Swine shed SVDV in their feces for up to 23 days after experimental infection (Burrows et al. 1973). Byproducts from infected animals (glands, gland extracts) represent another source of infection. Because the virus is very stable and acid resistant, disinfection procedures must be rigorous. Earthworms from soil above pits used to bury infected pigs yielded SVDV when their gut tract and surfaces were sampled, thus emphasizing the ability of SVDV to persist in the environment (Coombs 1973). Persons working with or around infected pigs had SVDV in their nasal passages (Sellers and Herniman 1974).

SWD is important because of its clinical similarity to FMD and the costs associated with eradication, loss of meat, and embargoes. A 1966 outbreak in Lombardy, Italy, was determined to be due to a new enterovirus different from FMDV, now called SVDV. The closest relative of SVD is the human enterovirus Coxsackie B-5 (Graves 1973). Cell culture–passaged Coxsackie B-5 virus does not cause clinical disease in swine; however, SVDV causes human illness. Outbreaks of SVD in Hong Kong (1970) and in England (1972) once defined the eastern and western limits of SVDV; Great Britain was declared free of SVD in 1980. The prevention of SVD has been facilitated by controlling importation of swine, meat, and animal products.

Vesicular Exanthema of Swine. Vesicular exanthema of swine clinically affects only swine. It was confined to California swine from its first description in 1932 until 1951, when pork trimmings were removed from an interstate California passenger train and fed to swine in Wyoming. The ensuing epidemic involved 42 states plus the District of Columbia. It was controlled in 1956, costing $33 million in direct costs and indemnities (Mulhern 1953). After enactment of laws prohibiting feeding of raw garbage to swine and requiring the slaughter of infected animals, VES was eradicated from three large garbage-feeding operations in Secaucus, N.J.; the United States has since remained free of the disease. VES was declared an exotic disease in 1959.

The only cases outside the United States were in butcher hogs aboard ships enroute to Hawaii in 1946 and 1947, which were intercepted at Honolulu, and pigs fed uncooked garbage from a U.S.

military base in Iceland in 1955. These episodes were promptly controlled (Bankowski 1965).

VESV is a moderately contagious disease, spread by contact and fomites. Aerosol spread has not been clearly defined. The VESV was shown to be present in the meat of infected swine (Mott et al. 1953). Long-term carriers have not been shown for VES.

The epidemiologic relationship of caliciviruses capable of causing vesicular diseases in swine to related marine caliciviruses began with the isolation of SMSV 1 (Smith et al. 1973). Marine animals (fish, sea lions, fur seals, elephant seals, etc.) are apparently the natural hosts of at least 12 SMSV serotypes and at least 5 other caliciviruses.

Serotypes of the closely related SMSVs infect a variety of marine mammals along the Pacific coast; antibodies have been found in terrestrial mammals (swine, fox, buffalo, donkeys, and cattle) on the West Coast and on Santa Barbara Channel Islands (Smith and Latham 1978), but their relationship to natural disease is not clear.

When SMSV was passaged serially in swine, it increased in virulence (Bankowski et al. 1955). A SMSV was isolated from frozen meat of fur seals that was fed to mink (Sawyer et al. 1978). Since swine are sometimes on the premises of mink-raising operations, the possibility exists that seal meat or other marine-origin feed supplements could serve as a source of infection for swine. The potential threat of SMSVs and other caliciviruses to produce disease in swine warrants attention, but the role of these viruses as swine pathogens under current management conditions has not been documented.

Bovine calicivirus (BCV, Tillamook virus), a calicivirus serotype, isolated from three dairy calves in Oregon did not produce notable disease in experimentally inoculated cattle but caused vesicular lesions in experimentally inoculated swine (Smith et al. 1983). Antibodies to the BCV were found in various marine mammals, inferring that the virus was of marine origin (Barlough et al. 1987).

Vesicular Stomatitis. Vesicular stomatitis infects a wide range of animals including swine, cattle, horses, humans, and many species of wildlife including rodents. The disease outbreaks in 1925 and 1926 were shown to be due to infection with two distinct serotypes, later called Indiana and New Jersey (Cotton 1927). In the Americas, VS results in economic losses of meat, milk, and draft power; it also causes major consternation, as it must be decisively and rapidly differentiated from FMD when it affects swine and cattle. It first appeared in U.S. swine used for the production of hog cholera antiserum in Missouri in 1943. The disease occurred in pigs being hyperimmunized; contact transmission was also observed (Schoening 1943).

VS is not a highly contagious disease, and the origin of outbreaks and means of dissemination are not thoroughly understood. VS is endemic in the coastal regions of the Carolinas and Georgia (Stallknecht et al. 1985), and in Central and South America, infecting cattle, horses, feral swine, raccoon, and deer. Some infections are inapparent. The reasons for the specific geographical distribution (river basins, wooded areas) and methods of transmission remain unknown. Major seasonal epizootics in cattle and horses with occasional spillover to swine occur about every 10 years or more, starting in early summer and ending with the first frost. These epizootics sometimes extend into the northern United States, primarily affecting horses and cattle. The 1982–83 epizootic persisted into winter, causing speculation that VS may be altering its patterns. Movement of infected animals has sometimes extended outbreaks. Insects may play a role in transmission, particularly in horses and cattle on pasture. Studies on Ossabaw Island, Georgia, have shown that feral swine become seropositive to VSV NJ during late spring months when insect activity resumes (Stallknecht et al. 1985).

Serotypes New Jersey (NJ) and Indiana 1 have been associated with vesicular disease in swine under natural conditions. Both serotypes have been associated with vesicular disease in cattle, horses, and swine on an annual basis in Mexico and Central and South America. Indiana 2 and Indiana 3 (Federer et al. 1967), which occur respectively in Central and South America, cause vesicular disease in cattle and horses, but apparently do not produce clinical disease in swine under field conditions. There are numerous other serotypes of vesiculoviruses but none has been related to vesicular or other diseases of swine. The reservoirs of VS have not been fully defined.

VSV serotypes Indiana 1 and NJ have been isolated from sandflies (*Lutzomyia shannoni*), and transovarial transmission was demonstrated (Tesh et al. 1971; Comer et al. 1990). Comer et al. (1990) also have shown that sandflies infected with VSV NJ transmitted the virus to suckling mice. It was suggested that the VSV was a plant virus (Johnson et al. 1969), which could account for its reservoir and recurrence. Fomites play a significant role in the spread of VS in swine and milking cattle. Contact transmission in swine apparently requires abrasions in the epithelium (Patterson et al. 1955). A carrier state for VSV was not detected by virus isolation or nucleic acid hybridization studies (Redelman et al. 1989).

CLINICAL SIGNS. The clinical signs of FMD, VS, VES, SVD, and SMSV are essentially identical. Generally, within 1–5 days postexposure, the body temperature rises sharply to 40.5°C or higher. Areas of epithelium become blanched, followed by the formation of vesicles and, after the loss of epithelium, erosions. Vesicles up to 3 cm in diameter may be found on the snout (Figs. 30.1A,B,C), with vesicular lesions extending into the nares; on the lips, tongue (Fig. 30.1D), hard and soft palate, coronary band (Fig. 30.1E); on the soft tissues of the feet (interdigital clefts and bulbs) (Fig. 30.1F), and soft tissues around the dewclaws (Figs. 30.2A,B). Lesions may occur in other areas of the skin, especially where abrasion of tissues occurs. Vesicles are most apparent and deepest where there is mechanical pressure or abrasion. Nursing sows may have vesicles on the teats. Slobbering and chomping are common. The vulva and scrotum are less frequently involved. Pregnant sows may abort due to fever. The viruses of FMD, SVD, VES, and VS are not reported to infect the fetus.

The vesicles yield a serous fluid as they rupture (usually 6–24 hours after formation), and the epithelial layers above the stratum germinativum may detach. Eroded, hyperemic, hemorrhagic surfaces are seen. The hoof may become detached (Fig. 30.2C) if the vesicles have coalesced around the coronary band, and severe laminitis may be followed by a chronically deformed foot (Figs. 30.2D,E). After the initial stage of infection, the animal's temperature may drop to 40°C. The lesions heal within 7–14 days if no secondary bacterial infection occurs; however, there have been occasional reports of specific FMD isolates causing high mortality in mature animals.

Foot-and-mouth disease is highly contagious, infecting virtually 100% of the animals with no immunity. In partially immune populations, morbidity is decreased. VES is moderately contagious, with certain highly pathogenic strains infecting greater numbers. With SVD the entire herd may not be affected, and subclinical cases may occur. Patterns of VS infection are variable due to unknown features of transmission but, in general, VS is not considered to be a highly contagious disease in swine.

Low mortality (<5%) is usually seen with vesicular diseases. In young animals infected with FMDV or SVDV, myocardial necrosis may occur and mortality may reach 50% or higher.

PATHOGENESIS

Foot-and-Mouth Disease. The major route of transmission for FMDV is by aerosol (Sellers and Parker 1969; Donaldson et al. 1970). Particles of various sizes adhere to the upper respiratory tract (3–6 μ or greater) or reach the lower respiratory tract (3 μ or less). Tremendous aerosols are generated by swine, which are often referred to as an "amplifier host" (Sellers and Parker 1969; Donaldson and Ferris 1980; Donaldson et al. 1987). The main means of dissemination of virus from the initial site of entry is likely to be macrophages of either the pharyngeal lymph nodes or alveoli. Following seeding of secondary targets (epithelium, mucosa, and myocardium), the virus replicates

and high levels of viremia generally persist for 3–5 days (Sutmoller and McVicar 1976). Recent studies employing in situ nucleic acid–hybridization techniques on guinea pigs inoculated with FMDV indicate that FMDV infects a wide range of epithelial sites shortly after experimental inoculation (Brown et al. 1989; Olander et al. 1990). Within 2–3 days, vesicles develop where stress and mechanical abrasions occur, which in swine includes the snout, feet, and mouth. In addition, FMDV replication is well documented in the epithelial cells of the mammary gland. The FMDV is generally shed in the milk of cattle for up to about 10 days postexposure, corresponding to the development of virus-neutralization antibody. In some cattle, however, virus may be shed in the milk up to 7 weeks, even in the presence of neutralizing antibody in the serum (Burrows et al. 1971). Similar patterns of virus shedding in milk likely occur in swine. Virus is found in large quantities in pharyngeal fluids 2–7 days postexposure. A carrier state for FMDV lasted for at least 26 weeks in 5 of 10 cattle infected with FMDV (Burrows 1966); the carrier state is not documented for swine. High mortality rates may occur in young animals due to the FMDV causing severe myocardial necrosis, which results in a grossly mottled appearance, or "tiger heart."

Swine Vesicular Disease. SVD is spread by contact, particularly with feces from infected pigs. Lesions are evident 3–11 days after eating contaminated food (McKercher and Graves 1981) and as early as 2–4 days after experimental inoculation (Burrows et al. 1973; Lai et al. 1979). The first lesions generally appear on the coronary band. A fever, which persists for up to 5 days, essentially coincides with the development of a cell-free viremia and vesicular lesions. The peak viremia occurs 2–4 days postexposure to SVDV and persists for 6 days. Virus persists for at least 10 days in the tissues of the snout, tongue, coronary band, tonsil, cardiac muscle, and central nervous system. The stratum spinosum is the primary site of viral replication in the epithelium. A nonsuppurative meningoencephalitis most frequently occurs in the cerebrum, thalamus, brain stem, and olfactory lobes. Necrosis and an inflammatory reaction occur in the endocardium and myocardium (Lai et al. 1979).

Vesicular Exanthema of Swine. Vesicular exanthema of swine is primarily introduced by the feeding of contaminated raw garbage, even though oral infection with VESV is estimated to require 100–1000 times the amount of virus needed to produce a lesion by intradermal inoculation into the snout (Mott et al. 1953). Following entry of the virus into the epithelium via an abrasion, it multiplies in the stratum germinativum of the epidermis. Hydropic degeneration occurs, followed by necrosis of infected cells. Intracellular

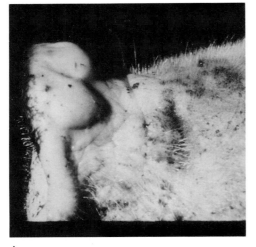

A

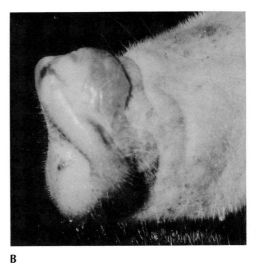

B

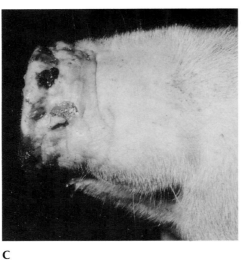

C

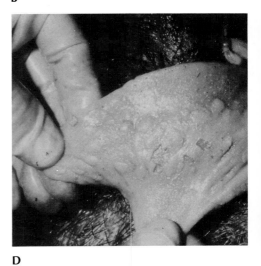

D

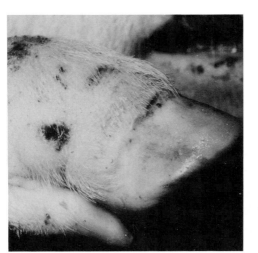

E

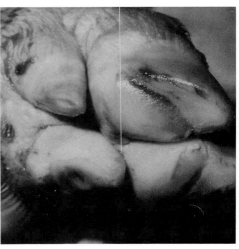

F

30.1. Signs of vesicular disease on swine. (A) VS vesicles on the snout; (B) VES vesicles on the snout; (C) ruptured VES vesicle; (D) tongue vesicles of FMD; (E) early foot lesions of VES showing coronary band blanching; (F) blanching and VES vesicles on the bulbs of the foot. (Courtesy of D. A. Gregg.)

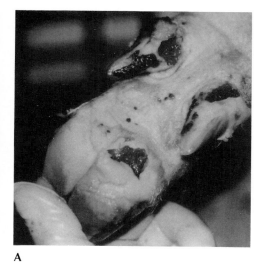

A

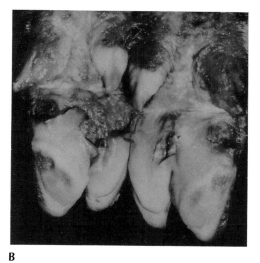

B

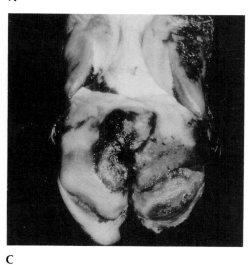

C

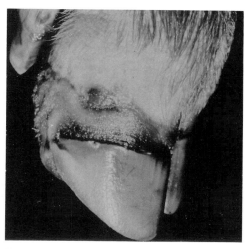

D

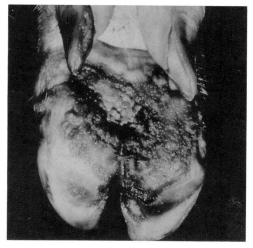

E

30.2. Lesions of vesicular disease on the feet of swine. (A) Ruptured SVD vesicles on the foot and dewclaw area; (B) ruptured FMD vesicles; (C) a sloughed hoof from FMD; (D) cellulitis with a chronic coronary band VES lesion; (E) granulation from a resolving VES foot lesion. (Courtesy of D. A. Gregg.)

edema accounts for vesicle formation (Madin and Traum 1955). Virus spreads from cell to cell as the infection progresses. Local lymph nodes may become involved, with extensive lymphocyte destruction and congestion; a low-level viremia occurs, likely accounting for secondary lesions.

Vesicular Stomatitis. Vesicular stomatitis virus apparently requires introduction into the epithelium through insect bites or via fomites into minor abrasions (Patterson et al. 1955) of the oral or nasal mucosa, teats, or feet. Swine inoculated intravenously develop a viremia (Shahan et al. 1946). Using intradermal inoculation in the snout approximating the natural route of infection, virus was isolated from local lymph nodes but not blood (Redelman et al. 1989). Virus replicates in the stratum spinosum. A vesicle and a transudate form, usually 2–3 days postinoculation. Without secondary infection, which may involve the subcutaneous tissue, the lesion heals in 1–2 weeks.

LESIONS. The principal lesion, the vesicle, of FMD, SVD, VES, and VS, is identical by gross pathology. Vesicles occur in the epithelium of the oral and nasal mucosa, feet, teats, interdigital space, and around the coronary band (Jubb et al. 1985).

Grossly, vesicular lesions begin as small blanched areas and progress to blanched, slightly raised areas that expand with the vesiculation process. The epithelium may separate from the stratum basale, leaving a red lesion with shreds of torn epithelium, or the vesicular fluid may desiccate through the stratum corneum without the formation of a true vesicle (Seibold and Sharp 1960). In either case, the stratum basale remains intact and, if secondary bacterial infection does

not occur, the epithelium is regenerated in 1–2 weeks. Since vesicles are most often seen at the site of mechanical stress, they usually rupture quickly, leaving a red erosion. Foot lesions of VES may be associated with a cellulitis with persistent swelling and lameness.

Histopathology. The histopathology for FMD, SVD, and VES is considered quite similar. The lesions begin in the stratum spinosum where vesicles form as a result of intercellular edema and necrosis of keratinocytes, which become spherical and float as single or clustered cells in the vesicular fluid (spongiosa) (Fig. 30.3A). The stratum basale essentially remains intact but has a tendency to be somewhat disrupted by VESV infection.

The histopathology of VSV in cattle, as carefully studied by Seibold and Sharp (1960) and described by Jubb et al. (1985), is considered equivalent for swine. The lesions develop in the stratum germinativum with intercellular edema that stretches the intercellular bridges (desmosomes). The cells remain attached at the ends parallel to the stratum germinativum but are separated lengthwise by intercellular edema, giving a "Japanese lantern" appearance (Fig. 30.3B). The cells become necrotic late in the progression of the lesion. The epithelial layers above the stratum basale separate in about 30% of the cases, but loss of vesicular fluid through the stratum corneum results in inspissation in the majority of lesions.

DIAGNOSIS. The diagnosis of FMD, SVD, VES, and VS must be conducted in the laboratory, for the diseases are clinically indistinguishable from each other. In countries where vesicular

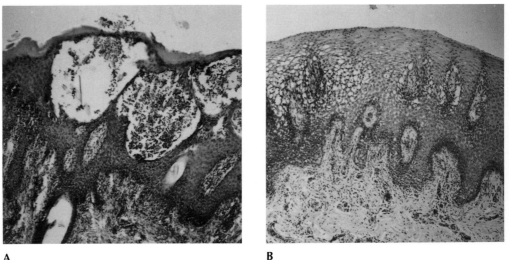

A   B

30.3. (A) A multilocular microvesicle of FMD with necrosis of the stratum spinosum. (B) Severe intercellular edema of the stratum germinativum and the "Japense lantern" appearance of the VS lesion. (Courtesy of D. A. Gregg.)

diseases are endemic, national animal disease diagnostic laboratories are generally available. Samples may be shipped to the World Reference Laboratory for Foot-and-Mouth Disease at Pirbright, Great Britain, or to regional vesicular disease diagnostic laboratories including the FADDL, Plum Island, N.Y., United States, or the Pan American Foot-and-Mouth Disease Laboratory in Rio de Janeiro, Brazil. The director of the respective laboratory should be contacted prior to shipment, proper permits must be obtained, and international shipping regulations for diagnostic samples must be followed. Samples from acutely ill swine should include vesicular tissue from gently washed, active lesions on the tongue, lips, gums, nares, feet, or teats, and if possible, vesicular fluid; heparinized and clotted blood should be collected for virus isolation and serology. If cattle on the same premises are affected, esophageal-pharyngeal fluid, vesicular tissue, and appropriate blood samples should be taken. Necropsy samples of tissues from any acutely ill, moribund, or recently dead animals, particularly newborn or young animals, should include skeletal muscle and myocardium. For histopathology, a complete set of tissues representative of all organ systems, but with emphasis on organs showing lesions, should be collected and preserved in buffered 10% formalin.

The differential diagnosis of FMD, SVD, VES, and VS should include parsnip or celery contact dermatitis (Montgomery et al. 1987), swine pox, chemical burns, trauma, and mycotic stomatitis.

Epithelial and vesicular fluid samples are tested immediately upon receipt by complement-fixation (CF) or ELISA for the presence of viral antigens of FMD, SVD, VES, and VS. A antigen-capture ELISA test employing serotype-specific rabbit antisera as the capture antibody, and a purified serotype-specific guinea pig indicator antibody, detected and identified serotypes of FMD viral antigens at lower levels than the CF test under experimental (Roeder and LeBlanc Smith 1987) and field (Westbury et al. 1988) conditions. Virus isolation in cell cultures (Snowdon 1966; House and House 1989) of suckling mice, electron microscopy (EM), and animal inoculation studies may be performed. The results of CF and ELISA studies for detection of vesicular disease agents are generally completed within 6 hours of receipt of the sample. A positive FMDV isolation with serotype identification may be completed as early as 24–72 hours of receipt of the sample. A negative virus isolation study may take up to 2 weeks, as multiple passages are required. Sequential serological testing of experimentally inoculated animals for up to 3 weeks postinoculation may be required for confirmation of a negative result.

Serum samples from unaffected, acutely ill, and recovering animals may be tested for immunoprecipitating antibody to the FMD VIA antigen, virus neutralizing antibody (VN) to FMDV,

SVDV, VESV/SMSV, and VSV, and CF antibody to VSV. Preliminary results of tests for antibody to the FMD VIA antigen are available at 24 hours, with a final reading at 48 hours. Serological tests can be completed within 3 days.

RNA fingerprinting, which uses ribonuclease T1 to specifically cleave the RNA at unique sites and produce a spectrum of different oligonucleotides, has been used to study the relationship of FMDVs (DeMello et al. 1986). However, nucleotide sequence determination, which provides the order of the nucleotides in the native RNA, is a more specific tool to study the variable areas of the genome of FMDV and other agents (Beck and Strohmaier 1987; Marquardt and Adam 1990). Experimental techniques, such as the polymerase chain reaction (PCR) combined with nucleotide sequencing and in situ hybridization, are being employed at the research level.

TREATMENT. No specific treatments are known for the vesicular diseases. Palliative measures such as feeding soft feeds, removing from hard-surfaced or concrete floors, and providing access to clean water at all times are advised.

Good hygienic conditions, the use of antiseptic solutions on affected epithelium, and administration of antibiotics may help prevent and control secondary infections.

PREVENTION

Exotic Vesicular Diseases. Prevention of FMD and SVD is accomplished primarily by the strict regulation of importation of animals and animal products. The ultimate international control and possible eradication of vesicular diseases depend on the ability to regulate movements of animals and animal products. Testing and quarantine of disease-free animals have been effectively used to import cattle from FMD-endemic areas to the United States (House et al. 1983); similarly, swine and swine semen were imported into the United States from China in 1989. An alternative approach to acquiring valuable genetic improvements is the international shipment of certified semen and embryos. Bovine embryos from infected donors have been shown to be free of FMD using prescribed methods for collection, washing, and preservation (Mebus and Singh 1988). The use of similar technology for swine may be complicated by the depth of sperm tracts causing physical entrapment of viral agents. Researchers continue to explore techniques to diminish this risk.

The data developed by research on the inactivation of disease agents in animal products forms the basis for regulations for the international movement of animal products. Regulations for cooking of garbage fed to swine account for the control and eradication of VES (Madin and Traum 1953). Studies to define times and temperatures to inactivate FMDV and SVDV in meat products have been reviewed (Blackwell 1984). Also, prolonged curing of hams from swine infected with FMDV and SVDV has resulted in a virus-free product (McKercher et al. 1985; McKercher et al. 1987). Virus in the milk of FMD-infected cattle was inactivated by pasteurization at ultrahigh temperatures for a short time (148°C for 2 seconds) (Cunliffe et al. 1979).

In cases of an outbreak of exotic vesicular disease in swine, the emergency disease guidelines of the USDA call for immediate quarantine of the premises, restriction of animal movement, public alert statements, and identification of the causative agent followed with eradication by slaughter. A bank of inactivated, safety- and potency-tested FMD vaccine antigens is maintained by USDA in cooperation with Canada and Mexico in the event that vaccination may be required to assist in the control and eradication of an FMD outbreak. Vaccinated animals would be permanently identified, and their movement would be restricted for life.

Vaccines for FMD, used throughout the world in FMD-endemic areas, are inactivated adjuvanted vaccines available as monovalent or polyvalent vaccines. The majority of vaccine is produced in suspension cell cultures and inactivated with ethylenimine derivatives, although the Frenkel method, employing thinly sliced bovine tongue epithelium in suspension cultures and formalin as an inactivant, is used in some production facilities. Vaccination with the prevalent serotypes is recommended 2–4 times a year. The traditional aluminum hydroxide–saponin adjuvanted FMD vaccines used for cattle are, in general, less efficacious for swine than oil-adjuvanted FMD vaccines (McKercher and Giordano 1967).

The gene for the key immunogenic FMD viral protein 1 (VP1) was cloned into *Escherichia coli* and successfully expressed for FMDV type A_{12} (Kleid et al. 1981). The cloned protein protected inoculated cattle and swine against challenge inoculation with virulent FMDV A_{12}. The system was successful with some other subtypes of A and C serotypes; but for type 0, the most prevalent serotype, the cloned proteins have not provided consistent protection.

The amino acid sequence of critical polypeptides, which could induce neutralizing antibody to serotype 0, was deduced from the nucleotide sequence. Synthetic polypeptides protected guinea pigs (Bittle et al. 1982) and cattle (DiMarchi et al. 1986) against challenge inoculation with virulent homologous virus. To achieve maximum immunogenicity, peptide antigens may be produced with repeated sequences and areas that react with sites on helper T cells or may even be combined with hepatitis B core protein (Brown 1989). Roosien et al. (1990) have synthesized what appear to be empty capsids of FMDV in insect cells using baculovirus-expression vectors; these particles may possess all the epitopes necessary for eliciting a brood-protective response in vaccinated animals.

There is no vaccine available for SVD or VES, since eradication is the preferred method of control. No country is currently considered to have VES. If a calicivirus vesicular disease became a problem, a vaccine could not be prepared until the outbreak occurred, for caliciviruses exhibit a wide antigenic spectrum.

Domestic Vesicular Diseases. Vaccination cannot be used to prevent VS in swine in the United States. While killed VS vaccines were produced and provisionally licensed for use in cattle during the 1982–83 epizootic, they were not approved for use in swine (Buisch 1983). Because as the epidemiology and transmission of VS remains unclear, preventative measures are recommended but not proven. The segregation of swine from infected cattle, horses, and wildlife, including feral swine, in endemic regions during epizootics is a practical suggestion. The role of insects in the spread of VS justifies an insect control program during a VS epizootic. Good sanitation may decrease the incidence of secondary infections, and many disinfectants (Patterson et al. 1958) used at the manufacturer's most-concentrated recommended dose inactivate VSV. Trauma and abrasions to the snout and feet should be avoided, as broken skin may be a route for the entry of the virus.

REFERENCES

BANKOWSKI, R. A. 1965. Vesicular exanthema. Adv Vet Sci 10:23–64.

BANKOWSKI, R. A.; PERKINS, A. G.; STUART, E. E.; AND KUMMER, M. 1955. Epizootiology of vesicular exanthema in California. Proc 59th Annu Meet US Livest Sanit Assoc, pp. 356–367.

BARLOUGH, J. E.; BERRY, E. S.; SKILLING, D. E.; AND SMITH, A. W. 1986. The marine calicivirus story, part II. Compend Cont Ed Proc Vet 8:F75–F82.

BARLOUGH, J. E.; BERRY, E. S.; SMITH, A. W.; AND SKILLING, D. E. 1987. Prevalence and distribution of serum neutralizing antibodies to Tillamook (bovine) calicivirus in selected populations of marine mammals. J Wildl Dis 23:45–51.

BECK, E., AND STROHMAIER, K. 1987. Subtyping of European foot-and-mouth disease virus strains by nucleotide sequence determination. J Virol 61:1621–1629.

BENGIS, R. J.; THOMSON, G. R.; AND DE VOS, V. 1987. Foot-and-mouth disease and the African buffalo: A review. J S Afr Vet Assoc 58:160–162.

BITTLE, J. L.; HOUGHTEN, R. A.; ALEXANDER, H.; SHINNICK, T. M.; SUTCLIFFE, J. G.; LERNER, R. A.; ROWLANDS, D. J.; AND BROWN, F. 1982. Protection against foot-and-mouth disease by immunization with a chemically synthesized peptide produced from viral nucleotide sequence. Nature 298:30.

BLACKWELL, J. H. 1984. Foreign animal disease agent survival in animal products: Recent developments. J Am Vet Med Assoc 184:674–679.

BROWN, C. C.; OLANDER, H. J.; AND MEYER, R. F. 1989. Pathogenesis of foot-and-mouth disease in guinea pigs using *in situ* hybridization. Proc 93rd Annu Meet US Anim Health Assoc, pp. 321–323.

BROWN, F. 1989. The next generation of foot-and-mouth disease vaccine. In Synthetic Peptides: Approaches to Biological Problems. Philadelphia: Alan R. Liss Inc, pp. 127–142.

BUISCH, W. W. 1983. Fiscal year 1982–1983 vesicular stomatitis outbreak. Proc 87th Annu Meet US Anim Health Assoc, pp. 78–84.

BURROWS, R. 1966. Studies on the carrier state of cattle exposed to foot-and-mouth disease virus. J Hyg (Camb) 64:81–90.

BURROWS, R.; MANN, J. A.; GREIG, A.; CHAPMAN, W. G.; and GOODRIDGE, D. 1971. The growth and persistence of foot-and-mouth disease virus in the bovine mammary gland. J Hyg (Camb) 69:307–321.

BURROWS, R.; GREIG, A.; and GOODRIDGE, D. 1973. Swine vesicular disease. Res Vet Sci 15:141–144.

COMER, J. A.; TESH, R. B.; MODI, G. B.; COIN, J. T.; and NETTLES, V. F. 1990. Vesicular stomatitis virus New Jersey serotype: Replication in and transmission by *Lutzomyia shannoni* (Diptera: Psychodidae). Am J Trop Med Hyg 42:483–490.

COOMBS, G. P. 1973. A study of swine vesicular disease in England. Proc 77th Annu Meet US Anim Health Assoc, pp. 332–335.

COTTON, W. E. 1927. Vesicular stomatitis. Vet Med 22:169–175.

COTTRAL, G. E.; GAILIUNAS, P.; and COX, B. F. 1968. Foot-and-mouth disease virus in semen of bulls and its transmission by artificial insemination. Arch Gesamte Virusforsch 23:362–377.

CUNLIFFE, H. R.; BLACKWELL, J. H.; DORS, R.; and WALKER, J. S. 1979. Inactivation of milk-borne foot-and-mouth disease virus at ultrahigh temperatures. J Food Prot 42(2):135–137.

DeMELLO, P. A.; OLASCOAGA, R. C.; GIOMI, M. P. C.; FERNANDEZ, A. A.; SCODELLER, E. A.; LaTORRE, J. L.; and BERGMANN, I. E. 1986. RNA fingerprinting of South American prototype aphthovirus strains. Vaccine 4:105–110.

DiMARCHI, R.; BROOKE, G.; GALE, C.; CRACKNELL, V.; DALE, T.; and MOWAT, N. 1986. Protection of cattle against foot-and-mouth disease by a synthetic peptide. Science 232:639–641.

DONALDSON, A. I., AND FERRIS, N. P. 1980. Sites of release of airborne foot-and-mouth disease virus from infected pigs. Res Vet Sci 29(3):315–319.

DONALDSON, A. I.; HERNIMAN, K. A. J.; PARKER, J.; and SELLERS, R. F. 1970. Further investigations on the airborne excretion of foot-and-mouth disease virus. J Hyg (Camb) 68:557–564.

DONALDSON, A. I.; GIBSON, C. F.; OLIVER, R.; HAMBLIN, C.; and KITCHING, R. P. 1987. Infection of cattle by airborne foot-and-mouth disease virus: Minimal doses with O₁ and SAT 2 strains. Res Vet Sci 43:339–346.

FEDERER, K. E.; BURROWS, R.; and BROOKSBY, J. B. 1967. Vesicular stomatitis virus: The relationship between some strains of the Indiana serotype. Res Vet Sci 8:103–117.

FRACASTORIUS, H. 1546. De contagione et contagiosis morbis et curatione. Libri iii. Cited by W. Bulloch. 1927. J Comp Pathol 40:75–76.

GAINORU, M. D.; THOMSON, G. R.; BENGIS, R. G.; ESTERHUYSEN, J. J.; BRUCE, W.; and PINI, A. 1986. Foot-and-mouth disease and the African buffalo (*Syncersus caffer*). II. Virus excretion and transmission during acute infection. Onderstepoort J Vet Res 53:75–85.

GEBAUER, F.; DE LA TORRO, J. C.; GOMES, I.; MATEU, M. G.; BARAHONA, H.; TIRABOSCHI, B.; BERGMANN, I.; DeMELLO, P. A.; and DOMINGO, E. 1988. Rapid

selection of genetic and antigenic variants of foot-and-mouth disease virus during persistence in cattle. J Virol 62:2041–2049.

GRAVES, J. H. 1973. Serological relationship of swine vesicular disease virus and Coxsackie B-5 virus. Nature (Lond) 245:314.

HOUSE, C., AND HOUSE, J. A. 1989. Evaluation of techniques to demonstrate foot-and-mouth disease virus in bovine tongue epithelium: Comparison of the sensitivity of cattle, mice, primary cell cultures, cryopreserved cell cultures, and established cell lines. Vet Microbiol 20:99–109.

HOUSE, J. A.; YEDLOUTSCHNIG, R. J.; DARDIRI, A. H.; HERRICK, D. E.; and ACREE, J. A. 1983. Procedures used for the importation of Brazilian Zebu cattle into the United States. Proc 26th Annu Meet Am Assoc Vet Lab Diagn, pp. 13–24.

HYSLOP, N. St. G. 1973. Transmission of the virus of foot-and-mouth disease between animals and man. Bull World Health Organ 49: 577–585.

JOHNSON, K. M.; TESH, R. B.; and PERALTA, P. H. 1969. Epidemiology of vesicular stomatitis virus: Some new data and a hypothesis for transmission of the Indiana serotype. J Am Vet Med Assoc 155:2133–2140.

JUBB, K. V. F.; KENNEDY, P. C.; and PALMER, N. 1985. Pathology of Domestic Animals, vol 2. New York: Academic Press, pp. 90–110.

KLEID, D. G.; YANSURA, D.; SMALL, B.; DOWBENKO, D.; MOORE, D. M.; GRUBMAN, M. J.; McKERCHER, P. D.; MORGAN, D. O.; ROBERTSON, B. H.; and BACHRACH, H. L. 1981. Cloned viral protein vaccine for foot-and-mouth disease: Responses in cattle and swine. Science 214:1125–1129.

LAI, S. S.; McKERCHER, P. D.; MOORE, D. M.; and GILLESPIE, J. H. 1979. Pathogenesis of swine vesicular disease in pigs. Am J Vet Res 40:463–468.

McKERCHER, P. D., AND GIORDANO, A. R. 1967. Foot-and-mouth disease in swine. I. The immune response of swine to chemically treated and nontreated foot-and-mouth disease virus. Arch Gesamte Virusforsch 20:39–53.

McKERCHER, P. D., AND GRAVES, H. J. 1981. Swine vesicular disease. In CRC Handbook Series in Zoonoses, Sec B. Viral Zoonoses, vol 2. Ed. J. H. Steele. Boca Raton, Fla.: CRC, pp. 161–167.

McKERCHER, P. D.; BLACKWELL, J. H.; MURPHY, R.; CALLIS, J. J.; PANINA, G. F.; CIVARDI, A.; BUGNETTI, M.; DeSIMONE, F.; and SCATOZZA, F. 1985. Survival of swine vesicular disease virus in "Prosciutto di Parma" (Parma Ham). Can Inst Food Sci Technol J 18:163–167.

McKERCHER, P. D.; YEDLOUTSCHNIG, R. J.; CALLIS, J. J.; MURPHY, R.; PANINA, G. F.; CIVARDI, A.; BUGNETTI, M.; FONI, E.; LADDAMADA, A.; SCARANO, C.; and SCATOZZA, F. 1987. Survival of viruses in "Prosciutto di Parma" (Parma Ham). Can Inst Food Sci Technol J 20:267–272.

McVICAR, J. W.; EISNER, R. J.; JOHNSON, L. A.; and PURSEL, V. G. 1978. Foot-and-mouth disease and swine vesicular disease viruses in boar semen. Proc 81st Annu Meet US Anim Health Assoc, pp. 221–230.

MADIN, S. H., AND TRAUM, J. 1953. Experimental studies with vesicular exanthema of swine. II. Studies on stability. Vet Med 48:443–450.

MADIN, S. H., AND TRAUM, J. 1955. Vesicular exanthema of swine. Bacteriol Rev 19:6–19.

MARQUARDT, O., AND ADAM, K. 1990. Foot-and-mouth disease virus subtyping by sequencing VP1 genes. Vet Microbiol 23:175–183.

MEBUS, C. A., AND SINGH, E. L. 1988. Failure to transmit foot-and-mouth disease via bovine embryo transfer. Proc 92nd Annu Meet US Anim Health Assoc, pp. 183–185.

MONTGOMERY, J. F.; OLIVER, R. E.; POOLE, W. S. H. 1987. A vesiculo-bullous disease in pigs resembling foot-and-mouth disease. I. Field cases. NZ Vet J 35:21–26.

MOTT, L. O.; PATTERSON, W. C.; SONGER, J. R.; AND HOPKINS, S. R. 1953. Experimental infections with vesicular exanthema. II. Feeding of viral suspensions and infected tissues. Proc 57th Annu Meet US Livest Sanit Assoc, pp. 349–360.

MULHERN, F. J. 1953. Present status of vesicular exanthema eradication program. Proc 57th Annu Meet US Livest Sanit Assoc, pp. 326–333.

NARDELLI, L.; LODETTI, E.; GUALANDI, G. L.; BURROWS, R.; GOODRIDGE, D.; BROWN, F.; AND CARTWRIGHT, B. 1968. A foot-and-mouth disease syndrome in pigs caused by an enterovirus. Nature 219:1275–1276.

OLANDER, H. J.; BROWN, C. C.; AND MEYER, R. F. 1990. The pathogenesis of foot-and-mouth disease infection in swine. Meet Int Pig Vet Soc, Lausanne.

PATTERSON, W. C.; JENNEY, E. W.; AND HOLBROOK, A. A. 1955. Experimental infections with vesicular stomatitis in swine. I. Transmission by direct contact and feeding infected meat scraps. Proc 59th Ann Meet US Livest Sanit Assoc, pp. 368–378.

PATTERSON, W. C.; HOLBROOK, A. A.; HOPKINS, S. R.; AND SONGER, J. R. 1958. The effect of chemical and physical agents on the viruses of vesicular stomatitis and vesicular exanthema. Proc 62nd Annu Meet US Livest Sanit Assoc, pp. 294–307.

PINTO, A. A., AND GARLAND, A. J. M. 1979. Immune response to virus-infection-associated (VIA) antigen in cattle repeatedly vaccinated with foot-and-mouth disease virus inactivated by formalin or acetylethyleneimine. J Hyg (Camb) 82:41–50.

REDELMAN, D.; NICHOL, S.; KLEEFORTH, R.; VAN DER MATTEN, M.; AND WHETSTONE, C. 1989. Experimental vesicular stomatitis virus infection of swine: Extent of infection and immunological response. Vet Immunol Immunopathol 20:345–361.

ROEDER, P. L., AND LEBLANC SMITH, P. M. 1987. Detection and typing of foot-and-mouth disease virus by enzyme-linked immunosorbent assay: A sensitive, rapid, and reliable technique for primary diagnosis. Res Vet Sci 43:225–232.

ROOSIEN, J.; BELSHAM, G. J.; RYAN, M. D.; KING, A. M. Q.; AND VLAK, J. M. 1990. Synthesis of foot-and-mouth disease virus capsid proteins in insect cells using baculovirus expression vectors. J Gen Virol 71:1703–1711.

SAWYER, J. C.; MADIN, S. H.; AND SKILLING, D. E. 1978. Isolation of San Miguel sea lion virus from samples of an animal food product produced from Northern fur seal (*Callorhinus ursinus*) carcasses. Am J Vet Res 39:137–139.

SCHOENING, H. W. 1943. Vesicular stomatitis in swine. Proc 47th Ann Meet US Livest Sanit Assoc, pp. 85–86.

SEIBOLD, H. R., AND SHARP, J. B. 1960. A revised concept of the pathological changes of the tongue in cattle with vesicular stomatitis. Am J Vet Res 21:35–51.

SELLERS, R. F., AND HERNIMAN, K. A. J. 1974. The airborne excretion by pigs of swine vesicular disease virus. J Hyg (Camb) 72:61–65.

SELLERS, R. F., AND PARKER, J. 1969. Airborne excretion of foot-and-mouth disease virus. J Hyg (Camb) 67:671–677.

SELLERS, R. F.; HERNIMAN, K. A. J.; AND DONALDSON, A. I. 1971. The effects of killing or removal of animals affected with foot-and-mouth disease on the amounts of airborne virus present in loose boxes. Brit Vet J 127:358–365.

SHAHAN, M. S.; FRANK, A. H.; AND MOTT, L. O. 1946. Studies on vesicular stomatitis with special reference to a virus of swine origin. J Am Vet Med Assoc 108:5–19.

SMITH, A. W., AND LATHAM, A. B. 1978. Prevalence of vesicular exanthema of swine antibodies among feral mammals associated with the southern California coastal zones. Am J Vet Res 39:291–296.

SMITH, A. W.; AKERS, T. G.; MADIN, S. H.; AND VEDROS, N. A. 1973. San Miguel sea lion virus isolation, preliminary characterization, and relationships to vesicular exanthema of swine virus. Nature 244:108–109.

SMITH, A. W.; MATTSON, D. E.; SHILLING, D. E.; AND SCHMITZ, J. A. 1983. Isolation and partial characterization of a calicivirus from calves. Am J Vet Res 44:851–855.

SNOWDON, W. A. 1966. Growth of foot-and-mouth disease virus in monolayer cultures of calf thyroid cells. Nature 210:1079–1080.

STALLKNECHT, D. E.; NETTLES, V. F.; FLETCHER, W. D.; AND ERICKSON, G. A. 1985. Enzootic vesicular stomatitis New Jersey type in an insular feral swine population. Am J Epidemiol 122:876–883.

SUTMOLLER, P., AND MCVICAR, J. W. 1976. Pathogenesis of foot-and-mouth disease: The lung as an additional portal of entry of the virus. J Hyg (Camb) 77:235–243.

TESH, R. B.; CHANIOTIS, B. H.; AND JOHNSON, K. M. 1971. Vesicular stomatitis virus (Indiana serotype) transovarial transmission by phlebotomine sandflies. Science 175:1477–1499.

TRAUM, J. 1934. Vesicular exanthema of swine, vol 2. Proc 12th Int Vet Congr, New York, pp. 5–9.

WESTBURY, H. A.; DOUGHTY, W. J.; FORMAN, A. J.; SUCHINTA TANGCHAITRONG; AND KONGTHAN, AB. 1988. A comparison of enzyme-linked immunosorbent assay, complement fixation, and virus isolation for foot-and-mouth disease diagnosis. Vet Microbiol 17:21–28.

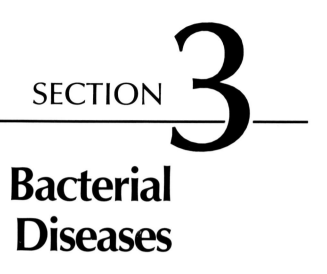

SECTION 3

Bacterial Diseases

D. J. Taylor, EDITOR

31 _Actinobacillus pleuropneumoniae_

J. Nicolet

Actinobacillus pleuropneumoniae is established as the etiologic agent of pleuropneumonia in pigs. The first observations of this disease were made by Pattison et al. (1957), Matthews and Pattison (1961), and Olander (1963). Shope (1964) later described an acute outbreak of a similar infection on a farm in Argentina. At that time the name _Haemophilus pleuropneumoniae_ was proposed for the well-characterized infectious agent (Shope et al. 1964; White et al. 1964). Kilian et al. (1978) confirmed this designation; thus, California strains (Olander 1963; Biberstein et al. 1963) and Swiss isolates (Nicolet and König 1966; Nicolet 1968) labelled as _H. parahaemolyticus_ are considered synonyms.

Since DNA homology studies showed the close relationship of _H. pleuropneumoniae_ to _A. ligniere-sii,_ it was proposed to transfer _H. pleuropneumoniae_ to the genus _Actinobacillus,_ using the new designation _A. pleuropneumoniae_ (Pohl et al. 1983). Furthermore, the _Pasteurella haemolytica_-like organism, described by Bertschinger and Seifert (1978) as a causative agent of necrotizing pleuropneumonia, is considered a nicotinamide-adenine dinucleotide (NAD)-independent biovar of _A. pleuropneumoniae_ (Pohl et al. 1983).

ETIOLOGY. The etiologic agent _A. pleuropneumoniae_ (syn. _H. pleuropneumoniae, H. para-haemolyticus_), neotype strains Shope 4074 and ATCC 27088, is a small, gram-negative capsulated rod with typical coccobacillary morphology. Hemolytic activity (complete hemolysis) on blood agar media (sheep red cells give more constant results) is a distinguishing characteristic. Biovar 1 is NAD-dependent, and biovar 2 is NAD-independent but requires the presence of specific pyridine nucleotides or pyridine nucleotide precursors for its NAD biosynthesis (Niven and Levesque 1988). Furthermore, _A. pleuropneumoniae_ produces an increased zone of hemolysis within the zone of partial lysis surrounding a beta-toxinogenic _Staphylococcus aureus_ (CAMP phenomenon) (Nicolet 1970; Kilian 1976). Additional detailed morphologic and biochemical characteristics may be found in original reports (Shope 1964; Nicolet 1968; Kilian et al. 1978).

For diagnostic purposes, _A. pleuropneumoniae_ must be distinguished from other haemophili occurring in pigs; e.g., _H. parasuis, Haemophilus_ sp. "minor group," _Haemophilus_ sp. "Taxon C," and _Haemophilus_ sp. "urease-negative" in the case of biovar 1, and from actinobacilli commonly isolated from pigs in the case of biovar 2 (Rapp et al. 1985).

Presently, 12 serovars have been described. Serovars 1–5 were well recognized by Kilian et al. (1978); however, serotype 5 was subdivided into subtypes 5A and 5B (Nielsen 1986a). Subsequently, serovars 6, 7 (Rosendal and Boyd 1982), 8 (Nielsen and O'Connor 1984), 9 (Nielsen 1985a), 10 (Nielsen 1985b), 11 (Kamp et al. 1987), and 12 (Nielsen 1986b) have been proposed. It must be noted that serovar 10, erroneously proposed by Kamp et al. (1987), is now referred to as serovar 11 (Nielsen 1986b).

The serologic specificity is given by the capsular polysaccharides and cellular lipopolysaccharides (LPS). However, some serovars show either structural similarities or identity of the LPS 0-chains, thus explaining the cross-reactions observed between the serovars 1–9 and 11; serovars 3, 6, and 8; and serovars 4 and 7 (Perry et al. 1990).

EPIDEMIOLOGY. Pleuropneumonia of the pig is widely distributed. Its epidemiologic significance is correlated with industrialization of pig production. Outbreaks have been reported from practically all European countries, including a few in East Europe, and from different parts of the United States and Canada, Mexico, South America, Japan, Taiwan, and Australia. Although some serovars are prevalent in certain countries (e.g., serovar 2 in Switzerland, Denmark, and Sweden or serovars 1 and 5 in the United States and Canada), various serovars may occur in the same country. Some serovars (e.g., serovar 3), considered to be of low virulence and of no epidemiologic importance in certain countries, may be epidemic in others (Desrosiers et al. 1984; Brandreth and Smith 1985). The international relationship of the different serovars is of special interest, for it points to a transmission through international exchange of animals. For further information of the geographic distribution see the reviews of Sebunya and Saunders (1983).

The economic importance of the disease is principally due to the mortality and medical costs in acute outbreaks. In chronically infected herds the rate of daily weight gain does not seem to be affected (Hunneman 1986).

401

Actinobacillus pleuropneumoniae is a parasite of the respiratory tract with a high host specificity for pigs. In peracute and acute infections it can be found not only in pneumonic lesions or in septicemia but also in large numbers in the nasal discharges. Survivors of acute infections become carriers, and the infectious agent is located mainly in necrotic lung lesions and/or in the tonsils, less frequently in the nasal cavity (Kume et al. 1984).

The incubation period can be quite variable. Experimental infections show that a high exposure leads to death within a few hours to a few days. Low exposures, however, may lead to subclinical disease.

All age categories are susceptible. In the acute phase of the disease the morbidity is generally high. Depending on the virulence of the strain and on the particular environment, the mortality may vary but is generally high. Extensive reviews of epidemiologic features are given by Nielsen (1982), Nielsen and Mandrup (1977), and Rosendal and Mitchell (1983).

The main route of spread is airborne and the disease is transmitted mainly by direct contact from pig to pig or by droplets within short distances. In acute outbreaks the infection may "jump" from one pen to another, suggesting the possible role of aerosols in connection with long distances or the indirect transmission of contaminated exudate from acutely infected pigs by farm personnel. Possible transmission by small rodents or birds is doubtful, and humans are not common hosts of *A. pleuropneumoniae.* Survival of the organism in the environment is considered to be of short duration. When protected with mucus or other organic matter, it can, however, survive for a few days.

Transmission between herds occurs through the introduction of carriers to populations without previous experience of the disease. Airborne transmission from farm to farm must be taken into consideration but has not yet been demonstrated. Moving and mixing pigs increases the risk of pleuropneumonia. Stress factors such as crowding and particularly adverse climatic conditions such as rapid changes of temperature, high relative humidity, and insufficient ventilation greatly support the onset and spread of the disease and, consequently, also affect the rates of morbidity and mortality. It is, therefore, not surprising that the highest incidence of outbreaks is observed in feeder pigs, mainly in seasons with adverse weather conditions. As a rule, large herds with frequent mixing of pigs are more at risk than small herds or herds with separate units.

Introduction of the disease by artificial insemination is improbable, since the genital tract is not a common site of infection, and penicillin contained in the diluent would prevent survival of the contaminating organism.

PATHOGENESIS. The pathogenesis of pleuropneumonia is not fully understood. However, the peracute and acute forms of the disease resemble the septic shock of humans (Kiorpes et al. 1990). Coagulation and inflammatory pathways have been shown to be central in the early development of lesions. The pathogenicity of *A. pleuropneumoniae* is considered to be multifactorial. Besides endogeneous host factors, different virulence attributes of the infectious agent, including capsule, endotoxin, exotoxins (e.g., hemolysins and cytotoxins), and others, play important roles in the pathogenesis (Bertram 1990; Fenwick 1990; Inzana 1990; Nicolet 1990). Differences in the virulence between the serovars or even within the same serovar have often been observed (Desrosiers et al. 1984; Rosendal et al. 1985; Brandreth and Smith 1987). It is suggested that such differences are due to capsular structure (Jacques et al. 1988), LPS composition (Jensen and Bertram 1986), or type of hemolysin (Frey and Nicolet 1990). In general, strains of serovars 1, 5, 9, 10, and 11 are found to be more virulent than those from other serovars. Concomitant infections with other pathogens of the respiratory tract may also aid the development of pleuropneumonia (Caruso and Ross 1990).

Experimental or natural infections stimulate the immune response. Circulating antibodies can be detected approximately 10–14 days postinfection, also in subclinically affected animals, thus conferring a herd immunity. These antibodies reach a maximum level within 4–6 weeks postinfection and may persist at low levels for many months or even disappear after a bacteriologic cure (Nicolet 1970; Nicolet et al. 1971; Bachmann 1972; Nielsen 1982; Nielsen 1988). Immune sows confer passive immunity on their offspring. Such colostral antibodies may persist about 5–9 weeks (Bachmann 1972), but the protection does not last for more than 3 weeks (Nielsen 1975).

CLINICAL SIGNS. These vary with the state of immunity of the animals, the stress of adverse environmental conditions, and the degree of exposure to the infectious agent. The clinical course can be peracute, acute, or chronic (Nicolet et al. 1969; Nielsen 1982; Shope 1964).

In the peracute form, one or more pigs in the same or different pens suddenly become very ill with fever to 106.7°F (41.5°C), apathy, and anorexia. There is a short period of slight diarrhea and vomiting. The affected animals lie on the floor without distinct respiratory signs, the pulse rate increases very early, and a cardiac and circulatory failure develops. The skin on the nose, ears, legs, and later the whole body becomes cyanotic. In the terminal phase, there is a severe dyspnea with mouth breathing in a sitting posture. Shortly before death, there is usually a copious foamy, blood-tinged discharge through the mouth and nostrils. Death occurs within 24–36 hours. Occasionally an animal may die suddenly without premonitory symptoms. In neonatal pigs the disease occurs as a septicemia with fatal results.

In the acute form, many pigs in the same or different pens are affected. Body temperature rises to 105–106°F (40.5–41°C); the animals are depressed and refuse food. Severe respiratory symptoms with dyspnea, cough, and sometimes mouth breathing are evident. Cardiac and circulatory failure are usually present. The course of the disease differs from animal to animal, depending on the extent of the lung lesions and the time of initiation of therapy. All stages of disease, from intermediate to fatal, subacute, or chronic, are possible.

The subacute and chronic forms develop after disappearance of acute signs. There is little or no fever, and a spontaneous or intermittent cough of varying intensity develops. The animals show loss of appetite and, consequently, a decreased rate of gain in body weight. In chronically infected herds there are often many subclinically diseased animals. The clinical signs may be exacerbated by other respiratory infections (mycoplasmal, bacterial, or viral). In primary outbreaks abortions may be observed (Wilson and Kierstead 1976), especially in specific-pathogen-free (SPF) herds. Complications such as arthritis, endocarditis, and abscesses in different sites may ocur in individual animals and are due principally to serotype 3 of *A. pleuropneumoniae* (Nicolet 1970).

LESIONS. The gross pathologic lesions are located mainly in the respiratory tract. The pneumonia is mostly bilateral, with involvement of the cardiac and apical lobes, as well as at least part of the diaphragmatic lobes where pneumonic lesions are often focal and well demarcated (Fig. 31.1). The pneumonic areas are dark and solid; the cut surface is friable (peracute course). The fibrinous pleurisy is very obvious, and the thoracic cavity contains a blood-tinged fluid. In rapidly fatal cases the trachea and bronchi are filled with a foamy, blood-tinged, mucous exudate. In more chronic cases nodules of different sizes develop, mostly in the diaphragmatic lobes. These abscesslike nodules are delimited by a thick capsule of connective tissue (Fig. 31.2). There are some areas of adhesive pleurisy. In many cases the lung lesion resolves and only a residual focal adhesive pleurisy is present. A high prevalence of chronic pleuritis at slaughter is very suggestive of pleuropneumonia. In the early stages of the disease, the histopathologic changes are characterized by necrosis, hemorrhage, neutrophil infiltration, macrophage and platelet activation, vascular thrombosis, widespread edema, and fibrinous exudate (Bertram 1985, 1986, 1988; Liggett and Harrison 1987). Following the acute response,

macrophage infiltration, marked fibrosis around areas of necrosis, and fibrous pleuritis are characteristic (Häni et al. 1973). Further descriptions are given in early works by Pattison et al. (1957), Olander (1963), and Shope (1964).

DIAGNOSIS. Pleuropneumonia may be suspected clinically in acute outbreaks. In such cases the presence of characteristic lung lesions with pleurisy at postmortem examination enhances suspicion. In chronic infections the necropsy findings are very suggestive. In view of the epidemiologic significance and the therapeutic approach to this disease, bacteriologic confirmation of the diagnosis is needed in each case.

It is easy to demonstrate and isolate the etiologic agent from bronchial or nasal exudate and pneumonic lesions. However, isolation may fail in very old chronic lesions. In peracute cases it is possible to isolate the agent from other organs (septicemia). Gram-stained smears show numerous gram-negative coccobacilli; a rapid specific diagnosis is afforded by a fluorescent antibody test (Nicolet 1970) or by detection of serotype-specific antigens in lung extracts with a coagglutination test (Mittal et al. 1983).

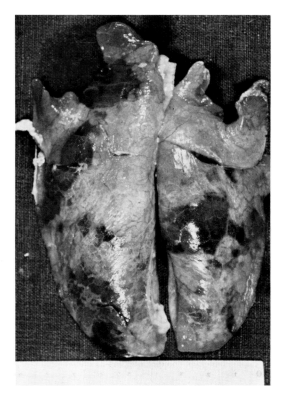

31.1. Gross lesions of a peracute case of pleuropneumonia showing a well-circumscribed pneumonic area in different lobes with fibrinous pleurisy. (Courtesy Prof. H. König, Institute of Animal Pathology, University of Berne.)

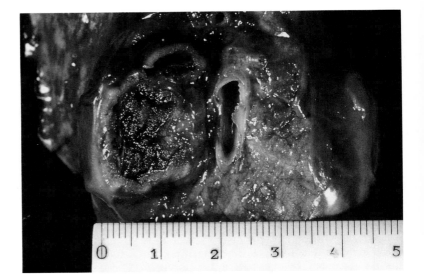

31.2. Chronic pleuropneumonia. Cross section of a well-capsulated nodule in the diaphragmatic lobe. (Courtesy Prof. H. König, Institute of Animal Pathology, University of Berne.)

Primary isolation on 5% sheep blood agar with a cross streak of *Staphylococcus epidermidis* has a great advantage over chocolate agar after overnight incubation, showing small colonies in the neighborhood of the streak (NAD requirement) surrounded by a clear zone of complete hemolysis. This allows a rapid presumptive bacteriologic diagnosis. Routine identification can be made by demonstrating the CAMP phenomenon, urease activity, and the fermentation of mannitol. In the case of mixed infections, particularly with *P. multocida,* or contamination with other bacteria, the use of selective media is recommended (Little and Harding 1971; Gilbride and Rosendal 1983).

Serotyping can be routinely achieved by slide agglutination from a subculture on a pleuropneumonialike organism medium enriched with serum (Nicolet 1971) or by the coagglutination test (Mittal et al. 1987). In many cases the final identification can only be achieved by agar gel diffusion and by indirect hemagglutination. A critical evaluation of available serotyping methods is given by Nicolet (1988). The serotyping of isolates is recommended for rapid confirmation of the bacteriologic diagnosis; it further demonstrates the local distribution of serovars and allows the epidemiologic situation to be estimated and the performance of specific serologic tests to be monitored. The detection of antibodies is of little diagnostic value in recent outbreaks but provides an important tool in epidemiologic investigations (Nielsen 1988).

Hog cholera, erysipelas, and streptococcal infections must be considered in the possible differential diagnosis of peracute and acute cases. In subacute and chronic infections the involvement of pyogenic bacterial agents such as *A. pyogenes, S. aureus,* diphtheroid rods, and *Fusobacterium necrophorum* must be excluded.

TREATMENT. *A. pleuropneumoniae* is particularly susceptible in vitro to penicillin, ampicillin, cephalosporin, chloramphenicol, tetracyclines, colistin, sulfonamide, cotrimoxazole (trimethoprim + sulfamethoxazole), and gentamicin to which it has low minimal inhibitory concentrations (MIC). High MIC values are found for streptomycin, kanamycin, spectinomycin, spiramycin, and lincomycin (Nicolet and Schifferli 1982; Gilbride and Rosendal 1984; Nadeau et al. 1988; Inoue et al. 1984).

The emergence of resistance to ampicillin, streptomycin, sulfonamides, tetracyclines, and chloramphenicol is of serious concern. It seems to be frequent in serovars 1, 3, 5, and 7 (Gilbride and Rosendal 1984; Vaillancourt et al. 1988) but rare in other serovars, particularly serovar 2 (Nicolet and Schifferli 1982; Inoue et al. 1984). The antibiotic resistance is plasmid mediated (Hirsh et al. 1982; Huether et al. 1987; Wilson et al. 1989).

According to a general rule, the antimicrobial of first choice would be the one with the lowest MIC and with the most satisfactory pharmacokinetic properties. Consequently, the betalactams, principally penicillin and cephalosporin; chloramphenicol; cotrimoxazole; and, to some extent, tetracyclines are considered to be most active. Recently available substances such as the quinolone derivatives (enrofloxacin) (Kobisch et al. 1990) or the semisynthetic cephalosporin ceftiofur sodium (Stephano et al. 1990) have been shown to be particularly effective after experimental challenge. Satisfactory results in the field have been reported with tiamulin (Anderson and Williams 1990) and a combination of lincomycin and spectinomycin (Hsu 1990). The determination of an antibiogram is recommended where problems are being experienced with treatment.

Antibiotic therapy is efficient only in the initial

phase of the disease, when it can reduce mortality. Antibiotics should be applied parenterally (subcutaneously or intramuscularly) and in high dosage. To ensure effective and durable blood concentrations, repeated injections according to the pharmacokinetic properties of the antibiotic used are recommended. The final success of therapy depends mainly on early detection of clinical signs and on rapid therapeutic intervention. Feed medicated with cotrimoxazole or chloramphenicol may be used successfully if all pigs have a normal food and water intake. Feed medication should be reserved for the prophylactic treatment of animals at risk during the acute phase of an outbreak (1–2 weeks). A combination of parenteral and peroral medication in a recent outbreak often yields the best results. In spite of apparent clinical success, it must be remembered that antibiotic therapy does not eliminate infection in a herd. Chronic infections in lung abscesses or on the tonsils of carriers persist to form an important source of infection for other animals.

PREVENTION. Prevention and control of pleuropneumonia may be accomplished in different ways. Once the infection has been established on a farm, it is difficult to eliminate the infectious agent in spite of the healthy appearance of the herd. Whatever strategy is chosen, it is essential to consider the epidemiologic features of pleuropneumonia. Control of environmental factors, purchase of healthy stock from monitored herds, a system of production with separate units in breeding farms, or all-in/all-out in fattening units would considerably reduce the risk of infection. For pleuropneumonia-free herds it is further recommended to organize, prior to the introduction of new animals, quarantine accommodation with serologic testing. Serologic blood testing has proved to be an effective means of detecting carriers and infected herds. Several methods such as the complement-fixation (CF) test, enzyme-linked immunosorbent assay (ELISA) (Nicolet et al. 1981; Morrison et al. 1984), or a 2-mercaptoethanol (2-ME) tube agglutination (Mittal et al. 1984) are suitable for this purpose.

In chronically infected herds, purchased seronegative animals should be vaccinated before introduction into the herd. Vaccination is serovar specific (Nielsen 1984) with possible cross-immunity with cross-reacting serovars (Nielsen 1985). The quality of the vaccines in terms of antigenic properties often determines the protection given. The type of adjuvant may enhance efficacy, whereas certain adjuvants can produce undesirable granulomatous lesions at the site of infection (Straw et al. 1985).

Vaccines provide high levels of protection in experiments, but field observations are less conclusive (Hunneman 1986). However, some commercially available vaccines may afford beneficial effects, mostly in reducing mortality, but do not prevent the carrier state. Consequently, long-term vaccination programs should be established, and the economic consequences must be carefully evaluated. Presently there is active research into the development of more efficient vaccines, however, these have to be evaluated in field situations (various reports in Proceedings International Congress Pig Veterinary Society, Rio de Janeiro 1988, pp. 81–88, and Lausanne 1990, pp. 6–13).

In an ideal situation all attempts to control pleuropneumonia have to proceed with health schemes aiming at pleuropneumonia-free breeding and multiplying herds, serologic monitoring, control of management, and controlled pig traffic (serologic testing, quarantine).

For herds infected with *A. pleuropneumoniae*, an eradication program can be considered after careful evaluation of the economic consequences. First, the prevalence of infected animals has to be assessed. In herds with a high rate of seropositive animals, depopulation and restocking with pigs originating from certified pleuropneumonia-free herds is the method of choice. This method is very expensive and may lead to the loss of important bloodlines. As an alternative, eradication has been achieved by providing an eradication program in the existing herd area but weaning at another farm, at the same time supported by a program of vaccination, medication, and culling and repopulation with disease-free gilts (Larsen et al. 1990).

In breeding herds with a relatively low percentage of seropositive animals (up to 30%), the "test-and-removal" of seropositive animals under medication has proved to be successful (Nicolet 1970; Nielsen et al. 1976). The principle is based on the serologic testing of sows shortly before farrowing and by weaning the piglets at 2 weeks of age under strict separation from the potentially infected stock. These piglets, which are seronegative up to the age of 12 weeks, would serve to restock the herd. Seropositive sows are systematically eliminated until the entire breeding stock is seronegative. This program can take 6–12 months. During the elimination procedure the whole herd is protected from reinfection by medicated feed, e.g., cotrimoxazole (trimethoprim + sulfamethoxazole 1:20, 250 mg/kg feed). Certain reports suggest that only partial success (Larivière et al. 1990) or even failure (Hunneman 1986) resulted from the application of such eradication programs. Some factors, e.g., virulence of the strain, the particular epidemiologic situation, management conditions, efficacy of medication, and fallibility of the diagnostic procedures, may influence the success of the program.

REFERENCES

ANDERSON, M. D., AND WILLIAMS, J. A. 1990. Effects of tiamulin base administered intramuscularly to pigs for treatment of pneumonia associated with *Actinoba-*

cillus pleuropneumoniae. Proc 11th Int Congr Pig Vet Soc, Lausanne, p. 15.

BACHMANN, Ph. 1972. Beitrag zur Epidemiologie der kontagiösen Pleuropneumonie beim Schwein. Schweiz Arch Tierheilkd 114:362–382.

BERTRAM, T. A. 1985. Quantitative morphology of peracute pulmonary lesions in swine induced by *Haemophilus pleuropneumoniae*. Vet Pathol 22:598–609.

———. 1986. Intravascular macrophages in lungs of pigs infected with *Haemophilus pleuropneumoniae*. Vet Pathol 23:681–691.

———. 1988. Pathobiology of acute pulmonary lesions in swine infected with *Haemophilus (Actinobacillus) pleuropneumoniae*. Can Vet J 29:574–577.

———. 1990. *Actinobacillus pleuropneumoniae*: Molecular aspects of virulence and pulmonary injury. Can J Vet Res 54:S53–S56.

BERTSCHINGER, H. U., AND SEIFERT, P. 1978. Isolation of a *Pasteurella haemolytica*-like organism from porcine necrotic pleuropneumonia. Proc 5th Int Cong Pig Vet Soc, Zagreb, Abstr M19.

BIBERSTEIN, E. L.; MINI, P. D.; AND GILLS, M. G. 1963. Action of *Haemophilus* cultures on α-aminolevulinic acid. J Bacteriol 86:814–819.

BRANDRETH, S.R., AND SMITH, I. M. 1985. Prevalence of pig herds affected by pleuropneumonia associated with *Haemophilus pleuropneumoniae* in eastern England. Vet Rec 117:143–147.

———. 1987. Comparative virulence of some English strains of *Haemophilus pleuropneumoniae* serotypes 2 and 3 in the pig. Res Vet Sci 42:187–193.

CARUSO, J. P., AND ROSS, R. F. 1990. Effects of *Mycoplasma hyopneumoniae* and *Actinobacillus (Haemophilus) pleuropneumoniae* infections on alveolar macrophage functions in swine. Am J Vet Res 51:227–231.

DESROSIERS, R.; MITTAL, K. R.; AND MALO, R. 1984. Porcine pleuropneumonia associated with *Haemophilus pleuropneumoniae* serotype 3 in Quebec. Vet Rec 115:628–629.

FENWICK, B. W. 1990. Virulence attributes of the lipopolysaccharides of the HAP group of organisms. Can J Vet Res 54:S28–S32.

FREY, J., AND NICOLET, J. 1990. Hemolysin patterns of *Actinobacillus pleuropneumoniae*. J Clin Microbiol 28:232–236.

GILBRIDE, K. A., AND ROSENDAL, S. 1983. Evaluation of a selective medium for isolation of *Haemophilus pleuropneumoniae*. Can J Comp Med 47:445–450.

———. 1984. Antimicrobial susceptibility of 51 strains of *Haemophilus pleuropneumoniae*. Can J Comp Med 48:47–50.

HÄNI, H.; KÖNIG, H.; NICOLET, J.; AND SCHOLL, E. 1973. Zur *Haemophilus*-Pleuropneumonie beim Schwein. V. Pathomorphologie. Schweiz Arch Tierheilkd 115:191–203.

HIRSH, D. C.; MARTIN, L. D.; AND LIBAL, M. C. 1982. Plasmid-mediated antimicrobial resistance in *Haemophilus pleuropneumoniae*. Am J Vet Res 43:269–272.

HSU, F. S. 1990. Evaluation of lincospectin sterile solution and Linco-Spectin 44 Premix in the treatment of pleuropneumonia. Proc 11th Int Congr Pig Vet Soc, Lausanne, p. 15.

HUETHER, M. J.; FEDORKA-CRAY, P. J.; PFANNENSTIEL, M. A.; AND ANDERSON, G. A. 1987. Plasmid profiles and antibiotic susceptibility of *Haemophilus pleuropneumoniae* serotype 1, 3, 5 and 7. FEMS Microbiol Lett 48:179–182.

HUNNEMAN, W. A. 1986. Incidence, economic effects, and control of *Haemophilus pleuropneumoniae* infections in pigs. Vet Q 8:83–87.

INOUE, A.; YAMAMOTO, K.; HIRANO, N.; AND MURA-

KAMI, T. 1984. Drug susceptibility of *Haemophilus pleuropneumoniae* strains isolated from pigs. Jpn J Vet Sci 46:175–180.

INZANA, T. J. 1990. Capsules and virulence in the HAP group of bacteria. Can J Vet Res 54:S22–S27.

JACQUES, M.; FOIRY, B.; HIGGINS, R.; AND MITTAL, K.R. 1988. Electron microscopic examination of capsular material from various serotypes of *Actinobacillus pleuropneumoniae*. J Bacteriol 170:3314–3318.

JENSEN, A. E., AND BERTRAM, T. A. 1986. Morphological and biochemical comparison of virulent and avirulent isolates of *Haemophilus pleuropneumoniae* serotype 5. Infect Immun 51:419–424.

KAMP, E. M.; POPMA, J. K.; AND VAN LEENGOED, L. A. M. G. 1987. Serotyping of *Haemophilus pleuropneumoniae* in the Netherlands: With emphasis on heterogeneity within serotype 2 and (proposed) serotype 9. Vet Microbiol 13:249–257.

KILIAN, M. 1976. The haemolytic activity of *Haemophilus* species. Acta Pathol Microbiol Scand [B] 84:339–341.

KILIAN, M.; NICOLET, J.; AND BIBERSTEIN, E. L. 1978. Biochemical and serological characterization of *Haemophilus pleuropneumoniae* (Matthews and Pattison 1961) Shope 1964 and proposal of a neotype strain. Int J Syst Bacteriol 28:20–26.

KIORPES, A. L.; MACWILLIAMS, P. S.; SCHENKMAN, D. I.; AND BÄCKSTRÖM, L. R. 1990. Blood gas and hematological changes in experimental peracute porcine pleuropneumonia. Can J Vet Res 54:164–169.

KOBISCH, M.; VANNIER, P.; DELAPORTE, S.; AND DELLAC, B. 1990. The use of experimental models to study in-vivo the antibacterial activity of Enrofloxacin against *Actinobacillus (Haemophilus) pleuropneumoniae* and *Mycoplasma hyopneumoniae* in combination with *Pasteurella multocida*. Proc 11th Int Congr Pig Vet Soc, Lausanne, p. 16.

KUME, K.; NAKAI, T.; AND SAWATA, A. 1984. Isolation of *Haemophilus pleuropneumoniae* from the nasal cavities of healthy pigs. Jpn J Vet Sci 46:641–647.

LARIVIÈRE, S.; D'ALLAIRE, S.; DE LASALLE, F.; NADEAU, M.; MOORE, C.; AND ETHIER, R. 1990. Eradication of *Actinobacillus pleuropneumoniae* serotype 1 and 5 infections in four herds. Proc 11th Int Congr Pig Vet Soc, Lausanne, p. 17.

LARSEN, H.; HOGEDAHL JORGENSEN, P.; AND SZANCER, J. 1990. Eradication of *Actinobacillus pleuropneumoniae* from a breeding herd. Proc 11th Int Congr Pig Vet Soc, Lausanne, p.18.

LIGGETT, A. D., AND HARRISON, L. R. 1987. Sequential study of lesion development in experimental haemophilus pleuropneumonia. Res Vet Sci 42:204–221.

LITTLE, T. W. A., AND HARDING, J. D. J. 1971. The comparative pathogenicity of two porcine *Haemophilus* species. Vet Rec 88:540–545.

MATTHEWS, P. R. J., AND PATTISON, I. H. 1961. The identification of a *Haemophilus*-like organism associated with pneumonia and pleurisy in the pig. J Comp Pathol 71:44–52.

MITTAL, K. R.; HIGGINS, R.; AND LARIVIÈRE, S. 1983. Detection of type-specific antigens in the lungs of *Haemophilus pleuropneumoniae*-infected pigs by coagglutination test. J Clin Microbiol 18:1355–1357.

———. 1987. An evaluation of agglutination and coagglutination techniques for serotyping of *Haemophilus pleuropneumoniae* isolates. Am J Vet Res 48:219–226.

MITTAL, K. R.; HIGGINS, R.; LARIVIÈRE, S.; AND LEBLANC, D. 1984. A 2-mercaptoethanol tube agglutination test for diagnosis of *Haemophilus pleuropneumoniae* infection in pigs. Am J Vet Res 45:715–719.

MORRISON, R. B.; BAHDAT, F.; HILLEY, H. D.; PIJOAN,

C.; AND HILL, H. T. 1984. An enzyme-linked immunosorbent assay using heat-treated antigen for the detection of *Haemophilus pleuropneumoniae* antibodies. Proc 8th Int Congr Pig Vet Soc, Ghent, p. 102.

NADEAU, M.; LARIVIÈRE, S.; HIGGINS, R.; AND MARTINEAU, G. P. 1988. Minimal inhibitory concentrations of antimicrobial agents against *Actinobacillus pleuropneumoniae*. Can J Vet Res 52:315-318.

NICOLET, J. 1968. Sur l'hémophilose du porc. I. Identification d'un agent fréquent: *Haemophilus parahaemolyticus*. Pathol Microbiol 31:215-225.

_____. 1970. Aspects microbiologiques de la pleuropneumonie contagieuse du porc. Thèse d'habilitation, Berne.

_____. 1971. Sur l'hémophilose du porc. III. Différenciation sérologique de *Haemophilus parahaemolyticus*. Zentralbl Bakteriol Hyg [Orig A] 216:487-495.

_____. 1988. Taxonomy and serological identification of *Actinobacillus pleuropneumoniae*. Can Vet J 29:578-580.

_____. 1990. Overview of the virulence attributes of the HAP group of bacteria. Can J Vet Res 54:S12-S15.

NICOLET, J., AND KÖNIG, H. 1966. Zur *Haemophilus*-Pleuropneumonie beim Schwein. Bakteriologische, pathologisch-anatomische und histologische Befunde. Pathol Microbiol 29:301-306.

NICOLET, J., AND SCHIFFERLI, D. 1982. In vitro susceptibility of *Haemophilus pleuropneumoniae* to antimicrobial substances. Proc 7th Int Congr Pig Vet Soc, Mexico City, p. 71.

NICOLET, J.; KÖNIG, H.; AND SCHOLL, E. 1969. Zur *Haemophilus*-Pleuropneumonie beim Schwein. II. Eine kontagiöse Krankheit von wirtschaftlicher Bedeutung. Schweiz Arch Tierheilkd 111:166-174.

NICOLET, J.; DE MEURON, P. A.; AND BACHMANN, PH. 1971. IV. L'Epreuve de fixation du complément, un test de dépistage des infections à *Haemophilus parahaemolyticus*. Schweiz Arch Tierheilkd 113:191-200.

NICOLET, J.; PAROZ, PH.; KRAWINKLER, M.; AND BAUMGARTNER, A. 1981. An enzyme-linked immunosorbent assay, using an EDTA-extracted antigen for the serology of *Haemophilus pleuropneumoniae*. Am J Vet Res 42:2139-2142.

NIELSEN, R. 1975. Colostral transfer of immunity to *Haemophilus parahaemolyticus* in pigs. Nord Vet Med 27:319-328.

_____. 1982. *Haemophilus pleuropneumoniae* infection in pigs. Thesis. Copenhagen.

_____. 1984. *Haemophilus pleuropneumoniae* serotypes—cross protection experiments. Nord Vet Med 36:221-234.

_____. 1985. *Haemophilus pleuropneumoniae* (*Actinobacillus pleuropneumoniae*) serotypes 8, 3 and 6—serological response and cross immunity in pigs. Nord Vet Med 37:217-227.

_____. 1985a. Serological characterization of *Haemophilus pleuropneumoniae* (*Actinobacillus pleuropneumoniae*) strains and proposal of a new serotype: Serotype 9. Acta Vet Scand 26:501-512.

_____. 1985b. Serological characterization of *Haemophilus pleuropneumoniae* (*Actinobacillus pleuropneumoniae*) strains and proposal of a new serotype: Serotype 10. Acta Vet Scand 26:581-585.

_____. 1986a. Serology of *Haemophilus* (*Actinobacillus*) *pleuropneumoniae* serotype 5 strains. Establishment of subtypes A and B. Acta Vet Scand 27:49-58.

_____. 1986b. Serological characterization of *Actinobacillus pleuropneumoniae* strains and proposal of a new serotype: serotype 12. Acta Vet Scand 27:453-455.

_____. 1988. Seroepidemiology of *Actinobacillus pleuropneumoniae*. Can Vet J 29:580-582.

NIELSEN, R., AND MANDRUP, M. 1977. Pleuropneumonia in swine caused by *Haemophilus parahaemolyticus*. A study of the epidemiology of the infection. Nord Vet Med 29:465-473.

NIELSEN, R., AND O'CONNOR, P. J. 1984. Serological characterization 8 *Haemophilus pleuropneumoniae* strains and proposal of a new serotype: Serotype 8. Acta Vet Scand 25:96-106.

NIELSEN, R.; THOMSEN, A. D.; AND VESTERLUND, S. D. 1976. Pleuropneumonia caused by *Haemophilus parahaemolyticus*. An attempt to control the disease at two progeny testing stations by serological blood testing followed by removal of the seropositive animals and their litter mates. Nord Vet Med 28:349-352.

NIVEN, D. F., AND LEVESQUE, M. 1988. V-factor-dependent growth of *Actinobacillus pleuropneumoniae* biotype 2 (Bertschinger 2008/76). Int J Syst Bacteriol 38:319-320.

OLANDER, H. J. 1963. A septicaemic disease of swine and its causative agent *Haemophilus parahaemolyticus*. Ph.D. diss., Univ. California.

PATTISON, I. H.; HOWELL, D. G.; AND ELLIOT, J. 1957. A *Haemophilus*-like organism isolated from pig lung and the associated pneumonic lesions. J Comp Pathol 67:320-329.

PERRY, M. B.; ALTMAN, E.; BRISSON, J. R.; BEYNON, L. M.; AND RICHARDS, J. C. 1990. Structural characteristics of the antigenic capsular polysaccharides and lipopolysaccharides involved in the serological classification of *Actinobacillus pleuropneumoniae* strains. Div Biol Sci. Natl Res Council Can, Ottawa.

POHL, S.; BERTSCHINGER, H. U.; FREDERIKSEN, W.; AND MANNHEIM, W. 1983. Transfer of *Haemophilus pleuropneumoniae* and the *Pasteurella haemolytica*-like organism causing porcine necrotic pleuropneumonia to the genus *Actinobacillus* (*Actinobacillus pleuropneumoniae* comb. nov.) on the basis of phenotypic and deoxyribonucleic acid relatedness. Int J Syst Bacteriol 33:510-514.

RAPP, V. J.; ROSS, R. F.; AND YOUNG, T. F. 1985. Characterization of *Haemophilus* spp. isolated from healthy swine and evaluation of cross-reactivity of complement-fixing antibiotics to *Haemophilus pleuropneumoniae* and *Haemophilus* Taxon "Minor group". J Clin Microbiol 22:945-950.

ROSENDAL, S., AND BOYD, D. A. 1982. Serotyping of *Haemophilus pleuropneumoniae*. J Clin Microbiol 16:840-843.

ROSENDAL, S., AND MITCHELL, W. R. 1983. Epidemiology of *Haemophilus pleuropneumoniae* infection in pigs: A survey of Ontario pork producers, 1981. Can J Comp Med 47:1-5.

ROSENDAL, S.; BOYD, D. A.; AND GILBRIDE, K. A. 1985. Comparative virulence of porcine *Haemophilus* bacteria. Can J Comp Med 49:68-74.

SEBUNYA, T. N. K., AND SAUNDERS, J. R. 1983. *Haemophilus pleuropneumoniae* infection in swine: A review. J Am Vet Med Assoc 182:1331-1336.

SHOPE, R. E. 1964. Porcine contagious pleuropneumonia. I. Experiment transmission, etiology and pathology. J Exp Med 119:357-368.

SHOPE, R. E.; WHITE, D. C.; AND LEIDY, G. 1964. Porcine contagious pleuropneumonia. II. Studies of the pathogenicity of the etiological agent *Haemophilus pleuropneumoniae*. J Exp Med 119:369-375.

STEPHANO, A.; NAVARRO, R.; RAYO, C. D.; AND OSORIO, M. 1990. Effect of the use of ceftiofur sodium injectable (Excenel sterile powder) for the treatment of induced *Actinobacillus pleuropneumonia*: Multiple dose titration study. Proc 11th Int Congr Pig Vet Soc, Lausanne, p. 41.

STRAW, B. E.; MACLACHLAN, N. J.; CORBETT, W. T.; CARTER, P. B.; AND SCHEY, H. M. 1985. Comparison of tissue reactions produced by *Haemophilus pleuro-*

pneumoniae vaccines made with six different adjuvants in swine. Can J Comp Med 49:149–151.

VAILLANCOURT, J. P.; HIGGINS, R.; MARTINEAU, G. P.; MITTAL, K. R.; AND LARIVIÈRE, S. 1988. Changes in the susceptibility of *Actinobacillus pleuropneumoniae* to antimicrobial agents in Quebec (1981–1986). J Am Vet Med Assoc 193:470–473.

WHITE, D. C.; LEIDY, G.; JAMIESON, J. D.; AND SHOPE, R. E. 1964. Porcine contagious pleuropneumonia. III. Interrelationship of Haemophilus pleuropneumoniae to other species of Haemophilus: Nutritional, metabol-ic, transformation and electron microscopy studies. J Exp Med. 120:1–12.

WILSON, R. W., AND KIERSTEAD, M. 1976. *Haemophilus parahaemolyticus* associated with abortion in swine. Can Vet J 17:222.

WILSON, P. J.; DENEER, H. G.; POTTER, A.; AND ALBRITTON, W. 1989. Characterization of a streptomycin-sulfonamide resistance plasmid from *Actinobacillus pleuropneumoniae*. Antimicrob Agents Chemother 33:235–238.

32 Anthrax

J. R. Walton

THE HISTORY of anthrax is intimately associated with the history of bacteriology and infectious diseases, since it was with anthrax that Robert Koch in 1877 first conclusively demonstrated the role of microorganisms in the cause of disease.

Swine are generally considered rather resistant to anthrax as compared to sheep and cattle, which are highly susceptible. Swine may become infected, however, along with other species of farm animals and may become important as a reservoir of infection.

Since anthrax is a zoonosis, infections in swine represent a threat to human health. Infected swine represent a hazard to the farmworker and veterinarian, to the abattoir worker, and to those preparing and eating contaminated pig products. The importance of this relatively rare disease in swine is increased by the public health requirement for abattoir disinfection and the disposal of carcasses after the discovery of an infected animal at meat inspection. Meat processors are becoming unwilling to slaughter pigs from infected farms, and the safe disposal of manures can be a major problem. These factors add a wider importance to the disease.

Anthrax is present throughout the world, and the FAO-WHO report (1973) indicates that the disease occurred in swine in every continent during 1972. The incidence remains low and sporadic but presents a local problem in some areas.

ETIOLOGY. Anthrax is caused by *Bacillus anthracis,* a large gram-positive, aerobic, spore-forming, nonmotile rod. The individual bacilli are 1–1.5 μm in diameter and 3–8 μm long. When observed in tissue from an infected animal, the organisms are commonly seen in short chains surrounded by a well-developed capsule. Under suitable aerobic conditions, spores highly resistant to disinfectants, heat, and desiccation may be produced.

B. anthracis grows very luxuriantly on most common laboratory media. On blood agar plates, colonies can usually be detected within 12 hours. After 24 hours at 37°C the colonies have a "ground glass" appearance, with irregular, wavy borders that give them the "medusa head" characteristic. No hemolysis is produced on blood agar; this is useful in distinguishing the colonies from those of certain nonpathogenic species of the

genus (Nordberg 1953). The colony of *B. anthracis* growing on blood agar on primary isolation possesses a stickiness that can be readily detected by touching with the bacteriologic loop. The colonial growth tends to adhere to the loop and forms tenacious threads.

Bacteria in these colonies do not produce capsules unless grown on special media or in 5% carbon dioxide but do produce spores. *B. anthracis* may be distinguished from other members of the genus by biochemical tests. Those used to differentiate the organism from related bacilli are listed under diagnosis below. *B. anthracis* is pathogenic to laboratory animals and humans. Culture should not be attempted unless appropriate safety precautions such as safety cabinets and adequate disposal facilities are available. Personnel handling the organism should be vaccinated.

EPIDEMIOLOGY. Anthrax is generally considered a soilborne infection in cattle, sheep, and horses. Animal-to-animal spread does not commonly occur, but rather, *B. anthracis* is deposited in the soil by the infected animal at the time of or following death. Spores are formed by some of the organisms, and these highly resistant bodies may remain viable for years, even under adverse conditions. Subsequently, the spores may be ingested by susceptible animals and anthrax may develop.

Swine can presumably become infected in this manner; however, because of the small number of spores likely to be picked up and the higher degree of resistance in swine, it probably occurs only rarely. Rather, anthrax in swine generally occurs following ingestion of feed that contains a large number of *B. anthracis* or viable spores. Swine that are permitted to eat the carcass of an animal dead of anthrax may consume large numbers of organisms and may therefore become infected. The use of bone meal or other animal products containing spores of *B. anthracis* in feed is the most common source of infection in swine. Davies and Harvey (1955) isolated *B. anthracis* from 5 of 41 cargoes of bone meal shipped to England from the Near and Middle East. Direct cultural methods were unsuccessful, but the authors isolated the organism from guinea pigs that were first protected from the various anaerobic species common in bone meal by means of clostridial antisera and antitoxins, followed by injection of the concentrated infusion from the bone meal specimen.

The role of feed contaminated with spores of *B. anthracis* in the transmission of anthrax can be illustrated by a brief account of the 1952 outbreak that occurred in the midwestern states (Ferguson 1986). Anthrax was confirmed on a farm in southern Ohio in February 1952 and further outbreaks occurred in rapid succession in widely separated areas. Within a week of the recognition of the first case, feed was incriminated as the source of infection. A number of feed companies were involved, but all had incorporated bone meal obtained from a company in Columbus, Ohio, which had processed part of a shipment of 100 tons of raw bone meal obtained from Belgium into a meat scrap concentrate. The companies purchased the concentrate and included it in many hundreds of tons of swine feed sold throughout Ohio and adjoining states. The organism was isolated from the raw bone meal and from the meat scrap concentrate but not from any of the finished feeds.

The organism appears to be spread in wet feed systems but rarely affects more than 1–2 animals in an infected herd. This was the classic picture, but accounts of continuing outbreaks exist (Jackson 1967; Jackson and Taylor 1989; Edgington 1990). The outbreak referred to by Jackson and Taylor (1989) and Edgington (1990) occurred in a 500-sow unit and persisted for 14 weeks, resulting in at least 18 cases in sows, sucking pigs, and weaned pigs. The development of disease in weaners may have been delayed by maternal immunity in this continuing outbreak. The origin of the outbreak was considered to be feed, but the disease persisted within the herd in spite of antimicrobial treatment. Persistence may have been in carrier pigs or as spores in slurry and housing. The role of flies in persistence and transmission was not clear although recent studies in the United States indicate that biting flies (*Stomoxys calcitrans*) and mosquitoes (*Aedes aegypti* and *A. taeniorhynchus*) transmit the disease experimentally 4 hours after feeding (Turell and Knudson 1987). Ticks (*Dermacentor marginatus*) were shown to harbor the organism for 76 days at 4°C and for 35 days at 22–25°C in the Soviet Union (Akhmerov et al. 1982).

PATHOGENESIS. There are two major groups of antigens in *B. anthracis:* somatic antigens and components of the complex exotoxin. The somatic antigens include a cell wall polysaccharide of a single antigenic type and a capsular polypeptide composed of a polypeptide of D-glutamic acid. Antibodies specific for the cell wall polysaccharide have no protective effect, while antibodies to the capsular antigen may inhibit establishment of infection by way of effect on phagocytosis.

The exotoxin (Smith et al. 1955b; Harris-Smith et al. 1958; Davis et al. 1973) is composed of three fractions that are either protein or lipoprotein: factor I, the *edema factor,* which causes edema; factor II, *protective antigen,* which induces protective antibodies; and factor III, the *lethal factor,* which is responsible for death of experimental animals. All three fractions of the exotoxin are required to produce the typical naturally occurring disease.

Molecular biology studies have shown that toxin production results from the possession of a 110-megadalton (MD) plasmid and that capsulation is related to the possession of a smaller 60-MD plasmid (Uchida et al. 1985; Mikesell et al. 1983).

The organism appears to enter the pig through the gut or tonsil. Septicemic disease is rare and the organism multiplies locally, resisting phagocytosis by means of the polyglutamic acid capsule. Edema is commonly produced locally. Neutrophils and other phagocytes are killed by factor II and organisms multiply until factor III is produced, resulting in the death of the animal as a result of its effect on the mitochondria. Immunity against anthrax is associated with antibodies against the exotoxin or certain fractions of the exotoxins (Sargeant et al. 1960; Thorne et al. 1960).

CLINICAL SIGNS. The first indications of an outbreak of the disease may be an increase in mortality. Investigation of these extra deaths may indicate the presence of anthrax and the clinical signs described below may be identified. Three forms of anthrax have been observed in swine: pharyngeal, intestinal, and septicemic. The usual portal of entry is the oral cavity, and invasion occurs in the tonsils or mucosa of the pharynx. In some cases the infection may remain localized in the lymph nodes of this region, and the disease is classified as pharyngeal. In other cases the organisms may pass into the intestinal tract, where primary invasion may also occur. When *B. anthracis* is not localized but gains access to the general circulation, the septicemic form of the disease develops.

The clinical signs commonly observed in pharyngeal anthrax are cervical edema and dyspnea. General depression, inappetence, and vomiting are commonly seen. Fever with temperatures to 41.7°C may occur, but it is not consistent, and in some affected swine the temperature may be subnormal. Death follows in many of the swine within 24 hours after the cervical edema is noticed. It is not uncommon for swine to recover even in the absence of treatment. The swelling may disappear gradually, and complete recovery appears to occur; however, such animals may continue to remain carriers of *B. anthracis*.

Clinical signs of intestinal anthrax are not obvious as are those in the pharyngeal form. In severe cases an acute digestive disturbance may be evident, with vomiting, complete loss of appetite, and diarrhea with bloody feces. Death may follow in the most severely affected swine; however, recovery occurs in many affected with the milder forms (Brennan 1953).

Intestinal anthrax has been reported only rarely in the United States. Many cases may be unrecognized because of the usual practice of avoiding a complete necropsy of animals suspected of anthrax. It is possible that some of the animals dying of pharyngeal anthrax may also have had lesions in the intestinal tract. Brennan (1953) reported that intestinal anthrax was the most common form of the disease seen in a 1952 outbreak of anthrax in swine in England.

Septicemic anthrax is the highly acute form that results from the entrance of *B. anthracis* into the bloodstream, followed by rapid reproduction of the organisms throughout the body. Death frequently occurs in animals so affected, without any period of illness being noticed by the owner. In swine it is the uncommon form of the disease. Walker et al. (1967) reported the presence of viable spores of *B. anthracis* in the lungs of dwarf swine for as long as 7 days following respiratory exposure. These authors suggested that resistance of swine may be related to some mechanism that inhibits germination of the spores. Goldstein (1957) reported that of 30 swine examined at necropsy during the anthrax outbreak of 1952 in Ohio, only 3 had the enlarged, dark spleen so characteristically seen in cattle. It is possible that young pigs develop septicemia more frequently than older swine.

LESIONS

Pathologic Changes. In the interest of controlling anthrax, complete necropsy of animals is strongly discouraged. Pigs with anthrax may not be identified before necropsy for the disease is relatively rare. Large pigs that have died from the disease may have a bloody nasal discharge (Edgington 1990), and small ones may appear very pale and dehydrated. The cervical region is edematous, but otherwise no superficial lesions are evident. Incision of the region reveals an extensive infiltration of the subcutaneous tissues with fluid, which is usually straw colored but may appear pink or hemorrhagic. The tissue, containing large amounts of fluid, may appear to possess a gelatinous consistency. The tonsils are usually covered with a fibrinous exudate or extensive necrotic changes may be evident. The pharyngeal mucosa is frequently inflamed and swollen.

The mandibular and suprapharyngeal lymph nodes are enlarged to several times their normal size. The cut surface of the affected node may vary in color from deep brick red to strawberry red. In more chronic cases the color may be grayish yellow, indicative of necrotic changes in the node. In cases of the septicemic and intestinal forms, the carcass may be opened before anthrax

is suspected. The intestinal form is most common and there is usually copious pinkish peritoneal fluid, which may clot on exposure to air. The small intestine is usually inflamed with fibrinous adhesions on the serous surface. The mesenteric lymph nodes may be swollen, hemorrhagic, or necrotic, and edema of the mesentery is common. The intestinal mucosa is covered with a diphtheritic membrane and may be hemorrhagic. The intestinal wall may be grossly thickened. In the septicemic form, little may be seen other than the presence of blood-stained fluid in the peritoneal cavity and local petechiation. In some cases the spleen is enlarged and there may be marked petechiation of the kidney.

Microscopic lesions in the lymph nodes usually consist of hemorrhage and necrosis with encapsulated bacilli. These may also be seen in the necrotic diphtheritic lesions of the intestinal mucosa and in the capillaries of any organ in septicemia.

DIAGNOSIS. Anthrax should be suspected when swine show cervical edema and dyspnea. However, erysipelas or malignant edema from *Clostridium septicum* may also provoke similar clinical signs. In malignant edema, which in swine has also been called para-anthrax, the edema will often be more prominent in the shoulders or axillary spaces. The edematous fluid and enlarged cervical or mesenteric lymph nodes, as seen on necropsy, are also very suggestive of anthrax. When the carcass has been opened, the presence of blood-stained fluid in the peritoneum, petechiation of the kidney or serosal surfaces, enlargement of the spleen, and thickening and inflammation of the small intestine should lead to suspicion of anthrax. A history of the type of feed products eaten by the affected swine is always of value.

The accurate diagnosis of anthrax is very important and in most cases is dependent upon the isolation and identification of *B. anthracis*.

Microscopic Examination. Impression smears and cultures should be made from cut surfaces of the cervical lymph nodes, spleen, mesenteric lymph nodes, intestinal mucosa, or kidney, for appropriate and peritoneal fluid should also be sampled when present. Smears should be fixed in Zenker's fluid, which kills spores, or by gentle heat, which does not, and then stained by polychrome methylene blue for 2 minutes and washed with water. The anthrax bacilli appear as squared-ended blue rods in a pinkish capsule. In smears made from decayed carcasses, other bacilli may be present, and where antimicrobial treatment has been given, the bacilli may only be present as capsules or in aberrant forms. The failure to find anthrax bacilli immediately should not rule out the disease as up to a 30-minute examination may be required. Peritoneal fluid is more often positive than splenic smears in septicemia. Slides and reagents used for diagnosis should be disposed of by incineration or formaldehyde fixation.

Spores are not observed in slides prepared from fresh tissue or from freshly cut surfaces. Spore-forming anaerobes are frequently encountered in tissues of animals that have been dead several hours prior to necropsy. Differentiation is important in such cases, and the following points are helpful. Spores are rarely seen in *B. anthracis* in fresh tissue preparations, while spores are regularly seen in clostridia. In the latter organism the rod is usually enlarged somewhat by the spore. Capsules are not observed on the clostridia.

Cultural Studies. *B. anthracis* grows readily on many common culture media and is characterized by very rapid colonial development. Typical colonies can be observed after 12–18 hours of incubation. This rapid growth is useful in differentiating *B. anthracis* from other pathogens.

B. anthracis is readily cultivated from the enlarged lymph glands, and it may also be demonstrated from the surrounding connective tissue in some cases. In the occasional septicemic case the organisms can be isolated from the blood, spleen, or liver—in fact, from essentially any tissue of the body. Since *B. anthracis* grows more rapidly than most of the saprophytic bacteria likely to be encountered, except other species of *Bacillus,* one should always examine the cultures after incubation of 12–18 hours.

Suspect colonies can be identified as *B. anthracis* by their biochemical characters using API systems or by the absence of hemolysis, lack of motility, growth on chloral hydrate agar, and susceptibility to anthrax phage. Final confirmation of pathogenic *B. anthracis* depends on the inoculation of culture into scratches on the foot pad of a guinea pig or mouse under strict containment. All cultures and experimental animals should be fixed in formaldehyde and incinerated.

CONTROL. Control of the spread of anthrax differs significantly from control of most of the other important animal diseases. The highly resistant spore formed by *B. anthracis* accounts for this difference. Some swine may become inapparent carriers, but there is little evidence to indicate that this forms an important source of infection to susceptible animals. Otherwise, animals that become infected do show clinical signs and generally develop an acute disease that terminates in death within a few days. Transmission from animal to animal rarely occurs, but soil contaminated by the organisms serves as a source from which susceptible animals subsequently ingest the spores. Because of this common form of transmission, anthrax can be controlled by preventing susceptible animals from contacting viable spores of *B. anthracis.*

Van Ness and Stein (1956) pointed out the importance of soil types in the survival of anthrax spores. The principal areas of enzootic anthrax are in regions characterized by soils high in nitrogen and with adequate calcium. Where such soil types are lacking (central and eastern states) anthrax does not appear to persist.

The spores can survive for years under a variety of environmental conditions. In the unopened carcasses of animals dead of anthrax, few spores are formed except at the body openings. When the animal is opened for a complete necropsy or when carnivorous animals are permitted to eat the carcass, there is usually extensive spore formation as the heavily infected blood and viscera are exposed to the oxygen of the air. The orifices and any cuts in a carcass should be covered with disinfectant-soaked cotton wool to prevent sporulation and spread of infection. The most productive control measures include the complete destruction of the carcasses of animals dead of anthrax by incineration or deep burial.

When an animal dies in the open, it is generally recommended that it be burned on the spot. If the animal must be moved, the carcass should be placed on a sled or other vehicle that can be thoroughly disinfected and then hauled, not dragged, to an area for disposal. When this is not possible, deep burial can be used. The carcass should be covered with lime and at least 4 feet of dirt. When carefully completed, either of these methods will minimize the chances of transmission of the infection.

Disinfection can be achieved with 5% freshly prepared sodium hydroxide or, more controllably, with 10% formaldehyde and the use of appropriate respirators. Only disinfectants capable of inactivating anthrax spores, such as those containing glutaraldehyde and formaldehyde, should be used. Disinfectants should be used prior to cleaning up infected premises and contaminated articles should be burned. Exposed surfaces should be scrubbed or pressure washed with the disinfectant.

Edgington (1990) gives an account of the procedure adopted in depopulating and disinfecting a chronically infected 500-sow unit from which purchasers would no longer take pigs. All 5000 pigs were slaughtered and burned, all 300,000 gallons of slurry were disinfected with 10% formaldehyde and disposed of in an approved toxic waste site, and the buildings were formaldehyde-fumigated and cleaned at a cost of £1,000,000 (US $1,700,000). Similar precautions may have to be adopted in contaminated meat plants to safeguard public health.

Following the outbreaks of anthrax in the Midwest in 1952, which were conclusively traced to imported bone meal, regulations were established that prohibit the importation of raw bone meal into the United States (Stein 1953). Comparable preventive legislation was adopted in Canada (Moynihan 1963). Bone meal processed by an acceptable steam treatment may be imported under these regulations. In addition to this federal regulation, some states have laws pertaining to the operation of rendering plants and the use of animal products in feed. These regulations have proved effective. Similar regulations apply in most developed countries.

TREATMENT. Treatment of animals infected with *B. anthracis* is possible. Since swine may develop a chronic form of the disease, treatment can be successfully administered in some cases. In the outbreak in Ohio in 1952, penicillin in oil was used at a dosage level of 10,000 units/lb body weight. According to Goldstein (1957), pigs that were showing clinical signs of anthrax recovered completely after this treatment, and the losses were reduced considerably when the disease was recognized early in its course. Anthrax antiserum in doses of 20–75 ml was also used in treatment of a limited number of animals. The results were comparable to those following treatment with penicillin in that the pigs in the early stages of anthrax recovered promptly. Oxytetracycline is effective against *B. anthracis* and may be used parenterally in daily doses of 4.4–11.0 mg/kg body weight. Edgington (1990) reported the successful use of penicillin, oxytetracycline, and chlortetracycline:sulphonamide:penicillin combinations to treat or suppress infection but had to withdraw treatment from animals intended for slaughter.

PREVENTION. Kaufmann et al. (1973) evaluated the Sterne strain anthrax vaccine, an avirulent spore vaccine, in an outbreak of the disease in Louisiana. The results supported the efficacy of the vaccine in swine, but the number involved was too small to provide significant data for this species. Similar findings were obtained by Jackson (1967) in a continuing outbreak in the United Kingdom. Immunization of swine would probably reduce the incidence of infection when they are exposed to massive doses of *B. anthracis*. Immunization on a large scale has not been recommended, however, since swine possess a level of natural resistance adequate to prevent the disease, except following heavy exposure to *B. anthracis*.

Human infection can be prevented by the safe disposal of all contaminated carcasses, articles, and fluids on farms by the methods outlined above. Persons exposed to the infection can be given prophylactic antimicrobials such as penicillin and tetracyclines, and any cases can be treated with them. Where longer-term exposure is likely, vaccination should be carried out.

REFERENCES

AKHMEROV, D. SH.; KUSOV, V. N.; AND CHERNOVA, A. A. 1982. Survival of *Bacillus anthracis* in the tick *Dermacentor marginalis*. Rep Kaganskii Vet Inst, pp. 101–103.

BRENNAN, A. D. J. 1953. Anthrax, with special reference to the recent outbreak in pigs. Vet Rec 65:255.

DAVIES, D. G., AND HARVEY, R. W. S. 1955. The isolation of *Bacillus anthracis* from bones. Lancet 2:86.

DAVIS, B. D.; DULBECCO, R.; EISEN, N. H.; GINSBERG, H. S.; WOOD, W. B.; AND MCCARTY, M. 1973. Microbiology, 2d ed. New York: Harper & Row.

EDGINGTON, A. B. 1990. An outbreak of anthrax in pigs: A practitioner's account. Vet Rec 127:321–324.

FAO/WHO. 1973. Animal Health Yearbook for 1972. Rome: FAO.

FERGUSON, L. C. 1986. Anthrax. In Diseases of Swine, 6th ed. Ed. A. D. Leman, B. Straw, R. D. Glock, W. L. Mengeling, R. H. C. Penny, and E. Scholl. Ames: Iowa State Univ Press, pp. 622–627.

GOLDSTEIN, H. 1957. Personal communication.

HARRIS-SMITH, P. W.; SMITH, H.; AND KEPPIE, J. 1958. Production in vitro of the toxin of *Bacillus anthracis* previously recognized in vivo. J Gen Microbiol 19:91.

JACKSON W. T. 1967. Anthrax in pigs—a series of deaths. State Vet J 22:67–71.

JACKSON, W. T., AND TAYLOR, K. C. 1989. Anthrax in pigs—a series of deaths. State Vet J 43:119–125.

KAUFMANN, A. F.; FOX, M. D.; AND KOLB, R. C. 1973. Anthrax in Louisiana, 1971: An evaluation of the Sterne strain anthrax vaccine. J Am Vet Med Assoc 163:442.

MIKESELL, P.; IVINS, B. E.; RISTROPH, J. D.; AND DREIER, T. M. 1983. Evidence for plasmid mediated toxin production in *Bacillus anthracis*. Infect Immun 39:371–376.

MOYNIHAN, W. A. 1963. Anthrax in Canada. Can Vet J 4:283.

NORBERG, B. K. 1953. Continued investigations of some important characteristics in anthrax-like microorganisms as viewed from a point of view of differential diagnosis. Nord Vet Med 5:915.

SARGEANT, K.; STANLEY, J. L.; AND SMITH, H. 1960. The serological relationship between purified preparations of factors I and II of the anthrax toxin produced in vivo and in vitro. J Gen Microbiol 22:219.

SMITH, H.; KEPPIE, J.; AND STANLEY, J. L. 1955. The chemical basis of the virulence of *Bacillus anthracis*. V. The specific toxin produced by *B. anthracis* in vivo. Br J Exp Pathol 36:460.

STEIN, C. D. 1953. A review of anthrax in livestock during 1952 with reference to outbreaks in the first eight months of 1953. Proc US Livest Sanit Assoc, p. 101.

THORNE, C. B.; MOLNAR, D. M.; AND STRANGE, R. E. 1960. Production of toxin in vitro by *Bacillus anthracis* and its separation into two components. J Bacteriol 79:450.

TURELL, M. J., AND KNUDSON, G. B. 1987. Mechanical transmission of *Bacillus anthracis* by stable flies (*Stomoxys calcitrans*) and mosquitoes (*Aedes aegypti* and *Aedes taeniorhynchus*). Infect and Immun 55:1859–1861.

UCHIDO, I.; SEKIZAKI, T.; HASHIMOTO, K.; AND TERAKADO, N. 1985. Association of the encapsulation of *Bacillus anthracis* with a 60 Megadalton plasmid. J Gen Microbiol 131:363–367.

VAN NESS, G., AND STEIN, C. D. 1956. Soils of the United States favorable for anthrax. J Am Vet Med Assoc 128:7.

WALKER, J. S.; KLEIN, F.; LINCOLN, R. E.; AND FERNELIUS, A. L. 1967. A unique defense mechanism against anthrax demonstrated in dwarf swine. J Bacteriol 93:2031.

33 (Progressive) Atrophic Rhinitis

M. F. De Jong

ATROPHIC RHINITIS (AR) (synonyms: infectious atrophic rhinitis, chronic atrophic rhinitis, progressive atrophic rhinitis (PAR) is a serious, widely prevalent, contagious disease of swine. The disease is now divided into a nonprogressive form, caused by toxigenic *Bordetella bronchiseptica* and a progressive form, caused by toxigenic *Pasteurella multocida,* alone or in combination with other agents (e.g., *Bordetella bronchiseptica*). The characteristic lesion is a hypoplasia of the nasal turbinate bones (conchal atrophy); in moderate to severe outbreaks this is accompanied by degrees of facial distortion (including brachygnathia superior, lateral deviation of the snout and septum deviation) and nasal hemorrhage as a result of frequent sneezing.

The disease is of global economic significance to swine production, since in PAR, these signs are accompanied by poor growth among fattening pigs. Toxigenic *B. bronchiseptica* is widespread in swine production. The toxigenic *P. multocida* is still spreading in the pig population, especially where disease control measurements are carried out ineffectively. The PAR toxigenic *P. multocida* can also be dangerous for other species, such as rabbits, goats, sheep, and cattle. Even humans can become infected, and lesions comparable to those in swine can be the result. Other animals such as rats, cats, dogs, and poultry are described as potential carriers.

A disease of the pig characterized by a shrinkage in development or total disappearance of the nasal turbinates (so called "turbinate atrophy") has been recognized for over 160 years and was first described as "Schnüffelkrankheit" in Germany (Franque 1830), where it came to be prevalent in several areas. Later it was reported from the United States (Doyle et al. 1944) and from the United Kingdom (Anon. 1954); it has subsequently been recognized in most areas of the world with major swine-producing industries and has become widely prevalent in some.

The precise etiology of this "condition" has been actively debated, with intermittent attempts at definition for well over a century. Since the 1930s, observations (Ratke 1938; Thunberg and Carlstrom 1940; Philips 1946) implied that the disease was contagious. Shortly thereafter it was demonstrated experimentally that turbinate atrophy was transmissible between pigs; when young pigs were inoculated intranasally with crude material from atrophic turbinates, they themselves frequently developed turbinate atrophy (Jones 1947; MacNabb 1948; Philips et al. 1948; Gwatkin et al. 1949, 1951; Terpstra and Akkermans 1960). Much research has since been directed toward defining the precise microbiological agent(s) responsible. While several management and husbandry factors can influence the severity and clinical expression of this disease, PAR is now established primarily as an infectious disease despite attempts at one time to redefine it as a disorder fundamentally of nutritional origin (Brown et al. 1966).

In 1956 Switzer suggested that turbinate atrophy may be caused by several agents, including trichomonads (Switzer 1951), filter-passing agents (Switzer 1953), viruses (Switzer and L'Ecuyer 1960; Edington et al. 1976) and mycoplasmas (Switzer 1955; Edington et al. 1976; Gois et al. 1977). Only special (AR-toxigenic) strains of *B. bronchiseptica* and *P. multocida* have consistently produced turbinate atrophy when sufficient quantities of pure (broth) cultures have been inoculated intranasally into young susceptible (e.g., colostrum-deprived specific-pathogen-free [SPF]) pigs. Despite these observations, however, clinical (and pathological) disease cannot be attributed solely to infection with either one or both agents, since these infections can occur in the field in the (temporary) absence of clinical disease (the so-called subclinical stage of PAR). Interruptions between periods of clinical disease that can vary in duration from approximately 2 months to about 2 years can occur in infected herds. Herd monitoring based on clinical (and or pathological) features, therefore, cannot guarantee the absence of infectious PAR in a pig herd. Complementary monitoring of a herd or connected breeding herds for at least 2 years, based on bacteriologic and/or serologic detection of the PAR-toxigenic *P. multocida,* may be necessary to obtain sufficient information concerning the PAR-infected or PAR-free status of the herd.

Definition: All diseases that cause turbinate atrophy in swine are called infectious atrophic rhinitis. It may be desirable to reserve the term "infectious progressive atrophic rhinitis" for the disease produced by one etiologic agent. Pedersen and Nielsen (1983) published the first recommendations as the result of a European Economic Community Commission of specialists on PAR. To obtain a consensus in a worldwide forum, the proposal was repeated by Pedersen and co-workers in 1988. The first agreement among specialists in swine diseases from Europe, North and South America, and Asia was achieved in 1988 (De Jong and Nielsen 1990). It was agreed to define PAR as a disease caused by infection with toxigenic *P. multocida*. In herds where suspicious manifestations such as sneezing; nose bleeding; and snout deformation, growth retardation, turbinate atrophy, and septum deviation are observed, and toxigenic *P. multocida* is detected (bacteriologically or serologically), the diagnosis of PAR can be confirmed. However, the disease may also develop in or be transmitted by pigs from herds harboring toxigenic *P. multocida* even though only slight or subclinical disease is present. The advantage of an etiologic definition of PAR rests in the possibility of identifying those herds that are able to transmit or develop the severe clinical disease independent of actual clinical status (Bollwahn 1988).

Estimates of the economic impact of this disease in swine have varied, but in moderate to severe outbreaks it can be of considerable economic importance (Pedersen and Nielsen 1983). From clinical and pathological points of view it is probably useful to continue regarding atrophic rhinitis as a single disease complex (Giles 1986), even though separate chapters on bordetellosis (Chap. 34) and pasteurellosis (Chap. 45) are found in this edition.

ETIOLOGY.   Research suggests that toxigenic strains of both *B. bronchiseptica* and *P. multocida* are the primary infectious etiologic factors. The severity of the disease that develops in a pig is related to the amount of toxin absorbed by the animal. The susceptibility of pigs to a certain amount of toxin that causes turbinate bone reduction has been shown to be age related. Toxigenic strains of *P. multocida* have been shown to produce severe PAR, including extreme growth retardation, even in pigs older than 3 months of age; toxigenic strains of *B. bronchiseptica* produce turbinate hypoplasia only in pigs until about the age of 6 weeks. The conditions for the growth and/or colonization of *P. multocida* or *B. bronchiseptica* necessary to produce a sufficient amount of toxin are influenced by bacteriologic and virologic damage to the mucosa and by certain environmental, management, and husbandry factors that create the (multifactorial) disease complex. When these factors are present, clinical PAR results. Since growth retardation and clinical PAR also occur after parenteral dosing with the toxin of *P. multocida*, colonization of toxigenic *P. multocida* in the nose may not be necessary for the development of the disease. Tonsils and lungs also have to be considered as locations for toxin production.

Infectious Agents

BORDETELLA BRONCHISEPTICA.   In the United States during the 1960s, *B. bronchiseptica* was said to be the principal cause of atrophic rhinitis (Switzer and Farrington 1975). After intranasal instillation of pure cultures of *B. bronchiseptica* in colostrum-deprived pigs a few days old, Cross and Claflin (1962) were able to produce typical experimental turbinate atrophy. This work was repeated by Ross et al. (1967), who were able to reproduce turbinate atrophy with pure cultures of AR pathogenic *B. bronchiseptica* in 95% of pigs inoculated at 1–3 days of age but in only 66% of 4-week-old pigs. Brassinne et al. (1976) reported that only high numbers of AR toxigenic *B. bronchiseptica* caused turbinate lesions. A toxigenic strain that caused 100% turbinate atrophy in 3-week-old colostrum-deprived SPF pigs did not cause typical atrophy when intranasally instilled during 4 successive days in 6-week-old pigs (De Jong and Akkermans 1986). This indicated that between 3 and 6 weeks of age the sensitivity to a heavy infection with an AR-producing *B. bronchiseptica* strain dropped drastically. Duncan et al. (1966) had already stated that experimental infections with *B. bronchiseptica* did not cause severe progressive lesions. Pearce and Roe (1966) were unsuccessful in producing turbinate atrophy with cultures of *B. bronchiseptica* in naturally farrowed pigs, but were able to produce the lesions when the culture was inoculated into colostrum-deprived pigs. This indicated protection against AR lesions by colostrum. Bacteriologic data from nose swabbings of pigs at different ages suggested that *B. bronchiseptica* infection starts to build up in conventional herds with and without clinical signs of PAR in the third week of age, when the sensitivity for toxigenic *B. bronchiseptica* has already started to decrease (Pedersen and Nielsen 1983; De Jong 1985). This meant that, under natural (conventional) conditions, the influence of *B. bronchiseptica* as a primary cause of PAR has been overestimated by different authors. In exceptional situations, such as after a primary *B. bronchiseptica* infection in SPF herds (Schöss 1982) and after experimental infections in piglets free of antibodies, turbinate atrophy can occur in 2- to 3-month-old piglets. Partial or total regeneration of such atrophy has been described and such infections seem to result in only a limited and low percentage of transient clinical snout deviations; animals with lesions caused by *B. bronchiseptica* did not develop significant growth depression (Pedersen and Barfod 1982). Nearly all *B. bronchiseptica* strains from pigs produced the thermolabile AR toxin. *B. bronchiseptica* can also affect the lower respiratory system (Chap. 34), and toxin production from such regions may have some influence on clinical AR.

Discrepancies in the results obtained in different countries could arise from variation in virulence or the amount of toxin produced by the organism concerned. This has been reported for isolates of *B. bronchiseptica* in the United States (Ross et al. 1967; Skelly et al. 1980), Canada (Miniats and Johnson 1980), the United Kingdom (Collings 1983), and in Hungary (Elias et al. 1982). However, even the most virulent of 10 United Kingdom isolates did not cause progressive turbinate atrophy or significant snout deformation in experimental infections (Rutter and Rojas 1982). More importantly in the United Kingdom, strains isolated from herds with or without progressive disease all caused nonprogressive lesions of similar severity (Rutter and Rojas 1982; Giles and Smith 1983). From observations in this laboratory, it appeared that strains isolated in AR-diseased herds and in herds not suspected of AR produced roughly the same amount of toxin. Only a few strains differed from this pattern (De Jong and Akkermans 1986). Thus, there is strong evidence, contrary to the opinions of Kielstein (1983) and Nakai et al. (1986), that although there are differences in the virulence of isolates of *B. bronchiseptica,* the severe lesions of clinical PAR cannot be attributed to this organism.

PASTEURELLA MULTOCIDA. Early studies (reviewed by Gwatkin 1959) established that *P. multocida* could experimentally produce turbinate atrophy in pigs and rabbits and that it was frequently but not always isolated from field outbreaks.

Several workers subsequently examined the ability of this organism to produce turbinate atrophy under controlled experimental conditions. Some strains studied produced a mild rhinitis but were unable to induce marked turbinate hypoplasia (Harris and Switzer 1968; Smith 1971; Koshimizu et al. 1973; Nakagawa et al. 1974; Edington et al. 1976), whereas in other studies, particularly from Europe, cultures of *P. multocida* produced nasal deformity and turbinate atrophy (Dirks et al. 1973) and even severe AR (Nielsen et al. 1976). In Germany and in the Netherlands particularly, *P. multocida* was considered to be an important primary pathogen in PAR (Dirks et al. 1973). Medication and vaccination with *Bordetella* vaccines in PAR herds reduced *B. bronchiseptica* successfully but failed to affect PAR. In these herds *P. multocida* was found to be the major pathogen. Reducing *P. multocida* in these herds decreased PAR (De Jong 1976–1979, 1980).

A major step in resolving these conflicting opinions began in the Netherlands when De Jong (1976–1979) and De Jong et al. (1980) began to test different *P. multocida* strains isolated from herds with and without PAR in colostrum-deprived SPF piglets, as described earlier by Ross et al. (1967) for *B. bronchiseptica.*

Because *P. multocida* does not grow on a solid medium under natural conditions and is not washed off and resuspended, but grows in a semifluid condition on the mucous membrane in the nose, a change to broth cultures was made. These broth cultures also contained substances excreted by the bacteria. It was then easy to reproduce AR lesions with the same strain in 3-week-old pigs instead of in 3-day-old pigs.

Martineau et al. (1982) showed the importance of using broth cultures instead of cultures washed from solid media, and explained that this could be a possible reason for the differences between investigators (Nakai et al. 1986). Pure cultures of both dermonecrotic and nondermonecrotic type D and type A isolates of *P. multocida* establish themselves poorly in the nasal cavity in conventional (Voets 1990), SPF (De Jong 1985), or gnotobiotic piglets (Rutter and Rojas 1982; Rutter 1983). Nasal instillations of pure broth cultures needed to be repeated for approximately 4 days to produce a severe *P. multocida* nasal infection that resulted in PAR. Uninoculated pigs that were kept in contact with inoculated pigs became infected, but only mild lesions were noticed 4 weeks later. Sneezing was sporadic in these experiments with gnotobiotic and SPF pigs. In contrast, *P. multocida* experiments with conventional pigs pretreated with chemical irritants or with *B. bronchiseptica,* resulted in sneezing, and PAR lesions occurred in the contact pigs. The strains that caused PAR lesions were called AR pathogenic. This characteristic correlated with the ability to produce a thermolabile toxin. PAR could be reproduced completely with bacteria-free filtrates of these unheated toxins. The severity depended on the amount of toxin administered to the pig.

The first publication explaining the role of toxigenic *P. multocida* in AR was by Ilina and Zasukhin (1975) in Russia. This publication encouraged the development of tests for selecting the toxigenic *P. multocida* isolates. Instead of using a rabbit test, the guinea pig skin test was chosen, because it also selected AR pathogenic *B. bronchiseptica* strains (De Jong 1980; Blobel and Schliesser 1981; De Jong and Akkermans 1986). Differences between infections with toxigenic *B. bronchiseptica* and toxigenic *P. multocida* strains were revealed when pure broth cultures were instilled intranasally in groups of colostrum-deprived SPF pigs aged 3, 6, 9, 12, and 16 weeks. In pigs infected with *B. bronchiseptica,* turbinate lesions were only noticed in 3- and 6-week-old pigs, not in pigs 9 weeks and older. The toxigenic *P. multocida* still induced typical snout and turbinate alterations, including septum deviation in pigs infected at 12 and at 16 weeks of age. The severity of nose lesions decreased with increasing age.

Other Factors. Most experienced clinicians have concluded that the severity of the disease is markedly influenced by extrinsic factors (Penny 1977; Goodwin 1980). A useful review of these noninfectious determinants has been given by

Smith (1983). Despite the major role of infectious agents, other factors contribute to the cause or at least the clinical expression of AR, but they have proved difficult to evaluate and have been inadequately defined quantitatively.

NUTRITION. Although the role of the dietary calcium:phosphorus imbalance is now discounted as a primary cause (Brown et al. 1966), a nutritional deficiency of any kind may enhance the severity of infectious disease. Feed consumption may be influenced by AR, since piglets with an acute rhinitis may accept feed less readily and become stunted and weak. Growing pigs with conchal damage may also have reduced feed intake, thus contributing to the reduced daily gain associated with the condition.

GENETIC INFLUENCES. In the past it has been suggested that heredity played a major role, but heritability estimates have varied greatly and attempts to control the disease solely by genetic selection have failed. There is probably a measure of genetically linked predisposition to AR, since breeds and strains that vary in liability to the disease and are susceptible to genetic pressure do occur. In the United Kingdom for example, Large White pigs are now generally considered more vulnerable than Landrace pigs, although 30 years ago the reverse could have been the case. The subject has been reviewed by Smith (1983), Voets et al. (1986a), and Martineau et al. (1988).

MANAGEMENT, HOUSING, AND ENVIRONMENT. Severe growth-retarding AR is a disease closely associated with intensive methods of production; it is undoubtedly severest when successive batches of pigs are housed in densely stocked, continuously occupied, poorly ventilated buildings (Smith and Giles 1980). Penny (1977) has identified several management factors that tend to predispose to an increased severity of AR (Table 33.1).

Most authorities agree that poor ventilation is the most important determinant, although overcrowding, continuous throughput of pigs, and substandard housing and hygiene are also major factors.

Instances have been observed where the disease was controlled, or at least reduced to economically acceptable levels, solely by the manipulation of housing and environment and improved management. It is also a common belief that the disease may be more severe in a dusty atmosphere, particularly where dry and dusty feed is delivered by automatic equipment. The influences of housing and the feed and delivery system on respiratory diseases of the pig have been reviewed by Owen (1982) and Strang (1982) respectively.

EPIDEMIOLOGY

Prevalence. Ways in which a disease is introduced and spread within a population depend on numerous factors, including the nature of the etiologic agent, the host, and the structure of the population. In intensive pig rearing, many animals are in close contact and there is often widespread movement of breeding and replacement stock between herds. The main risks of introducing infection are associated with purchased pigs, and disease may then spread rapidly within a seronegative herd. Early reports clearly recognized that AR was introduced by carrier pigs. The disease appeared in many Norwegian herds that had imported pigs, several of which eventually developed severe clinical signs. This led Braend and Flatla (1954) to conclude that "atrophic rhinitis was practically unknown in Norway prior to [World War II] after which it has been rather common, most certainly because of importation of pigs from Sweden where the disease is common." It was, therefore, assumed that a new infectious organism had been imported. The disease was declared notifiable and a slaughter policy was carried out. This strategy was also fol-

Table 33.1.   Management factors influencing the severity of atrophic rhinitis

Increase	Decrease
Large herds, open herds	Small herds, closed herds
Expanding herds	Static herd size
High proportion of gilts	Mainly old sows
Large farrowing unit	Small or single farrowing unit (all-in/all-out)
Multiple suckling	Single suckling
Large weaner pools	More isolation, modular systems (all-in/all-out)
Large number in one airspace	Small number in one airspace
Frequent movement and mixing	Little movement and mixing
Intensive systems indoors	Outdoor rearing
High stocking density	Low stocking density
Poor ventilation and no temperature control	Good ventilation and temperature control
Poor hygiene, little disinfection	Good hygiene and disinfection
Continual pig throughput	Buildings rested
Dry feeding, dusty atmosphere	Wet feeding, clean atmosphere
Mechanical food handling	

Source: After Penny 1977.

lowed in other European countries, such as in the United Kingdom until 1959 and in the Netherlands until 1980. Similarly, the introduction of AR into the United Kingdom was attributed to the importation of Swedish stock (Anon. 1954). There are at least two possible explanations for these observations: either that *B. bronchiseptica* was introduced in infected animals and exacerbated existing infections with toxigenic *P. multocida* or, more likely, that toxigenic *P. multocida* was introduced in the imported stock.

Estimates of the prevalence of PAR, whether from an individual farm or larger population, are usually conducted by an examination of the heads of pigs after slaughter. Such surveys have indicated that macroscopic nasal turbinate atrophy is widespread in pig populations. It occurred in about 40% of Danish and British herds (Nielsen 1983) in the late 1970s, although a later estimate from England showed a decline to 25% (Cameron et al. 1980). Such a high level of turbinate atrophy, however, does not reflect an equivalent level of clinical disease, since mild lesions are common in commercial fattening pigs and mild or even moderate atrophy in individuals may occur in herds without obvious clinical disease or adverse economic effects. The degree of growth retardation associated with more severe outbreaks has proved difficult to quantify, and some observers (Straw et al. 1983) have found no correlation between the degree of turbinate atrophy and production parameters. Nevertheless, where clinically apparent disease occurs there is frequently a reduction in average daily gain; this has been conservatively estimated as 5–8% for pigs with severe atrophy (Nielsen 1983).

Transmission of Infectious Agents. *B. bronchiseptica* colonizes the ciliated mucosa of the porcine respiratory tract very effectively; it is frequently isolated from the tonsils and large numbers (10^6/g) have been found in the intestinal contents of infected gnotobiotic pigs (Rutter 1985). Thus, direct contact, droplet infection, and perhaps ingestion of fecal material are likely to be the main routes of transmission. The cycle of infection appears to be maintained by a small proportion of breeding females. Litters within the farrowing house become infected at an early age, but in the United Kingdom as well as in the Netherlands, the major spread seems to occur after 2–3 weeks of age or after weaning, especially in large groups on flat decks, when 70–80% of a group can become infected. Infection persists for several months, with a gradual reduction in the intensity and rate of infection. The age at which animals first become infected with *B. bronchiseptica* has an important effect on the development of lesions. The most severe lesions occur in nonimmune animals infected during the first week of life (Duncan et al. 1966). Animals infected at 4 weeks show less-severe lesions, while those infected at 9 weeks show virtually no lesions (De Jong and Akkermans 1986).

The amount and type of immunity also influence the epidemiology of *Bordetella* infection. The presence of passive antibody in the sera of piglets born to naturally infected dams (with toxigenic *Bordetella*) appeared to provide protection against the development of turbinate lesions (Rutter 1981), but not against infection (Kobisch and Pennings 1989; Voets 1990). However, vaccination of sows appeared to delay infection in their piglets until 12–16 weeks of age as compared to nonvaccinated herds in which litters became infected by 2 weeks of age (Rutter et al. 1984).

B. bronchiseptica has been isolated from most domestic and wild animal species (Goodnow 1980) and, because it is a ubiquitous pathogen, there is always the risk that infection could be introduced by nonporcine vectors. Most isolates from other species appear to be poorly virulent in pigs, but it is possible that rodents might become infected with pig strains and transmit them. Virtually every pig herd is infected with *B. bronchiseptica,* and variable amounts of brachygnathia superior (BS) and moderately severe turbinate atrophy might be expected in all herds. For this to occur, pigs from nonimmune dams must become infected within the first 4 weeks of life and develop lesions that persist to slaughter, but mostly, regeneration of turbinates starts approximately 4 weeks after the start of infection, when the scrolls are not totally damaged. Lesions such as septal deviation, turbinate bone hyperplasia, and brachygnathia may be apparent at slaughter.

In the field, however, the picture is likely to be more complicated, e.g., there are reports that *Haemophilus parasuis* in combined infections with type A strains of *P. multocida* can produce mild turbinate lesions (Gois et al. 1983a). Others could not repeat these results.

The epidemiology of *P. multocida* infection in pigs is less well understood. The organism colonizes the tonsils, but some factor(s), the mechanism of which is not understood, are needed to assist colonization of the nasal mucosa. Nontoxigenic and toxigenic type A strains can be isolated from the lungs of pigs with pneumonia (Baekbo 1988), but *P. multocida* is much less effective than *B. bronchiseptica* in colonizing the trachea. In contrast to type A strains, toxigenic and nontoxigenic type D strains are isolated less frequently in the lungs but more frequently in the nose. *P. multocida* has also been isolated from most animal species and is well recognized as an important pathogen in cattle, poultry, and turkeys (Carter 1967). In some studies its distribution in pig herds was limited; only 9% were infected in one report (Harris and Switzer 1969), but such results may be attributable to the presence of the commensal flora in the nasal cavity (Chanter and Rutter 1989). Today in most laboratories, selective media and the technique of mouse passage can be used for isolation of the organism. Material from herds examined in this way (Rutter 1985) has yielded toxigenic and nontoxigenic isolates of types A or D, and mixed infections can occur with these two types in the same pig.

In contrast, the distribution of toxigenic isolates of *P. multocida* appears to be limited to those herds with PAR, or a history of the disease (Rutter 1985). In Germany, the Netherlands, and Denmark (Pedersen 1983), the picture is similar, indicating that the majority of herds infected with toxigenic *P. multocida* exhibit clinical signs of progressive disease. In the Netherlands, however, toxigenic *P. multocida* has been isolated from 15% of those herds with no history or clinical signs of progressive disease at the moment of the first detection of the toxigenic *P. multocida*. Most of these herds became clinically diseased within 2 years after this detection. Only 5% of pigs 4–12 weeks of age were infected in these herds. A few herds remain clinically unsuspected for some years (De Jong 1983a; Goodwin et al. 1990) which indicates that toxigenic strains may be present in some clinically unaffected herds, and these could transmit progressive disease if infected stock were purchased from them.

The main source of *P. multocida* infection for young pigs appears to be pharyngeal carriage of the organism among breeding stock; 10–15% of sows in farrowing houses were infected with toxigenic isolates (De Jong 1983b), and piglets became infected with these strains within a week after birth. Toxigenic *P. multocida* was isolated from the vaginas of a few sows. The age at which piglets first become infected with *P. multocida* affects the severity of the lesions produced, but unlike *B. bronchiseptica* infection, older pigs may still develop lesions. Significant turbinate atrophy occurred in pigs infected with toxigenic *P. multocida* up to 16 weeks of age, while Rutter et al. (1984) found that pigs that became naturally infected between 12 and 16 weeks of age had turbinate lesions. Injection of *P. multocida* toxin (125 μg/kg) produced significant atrophy in conventional pigs 10 weeks of age (Rutter 1985).

The prevalence of toxigenic *P. multocida* may be related to the extent of clinical disease. The organism was isolated from 50 to 60% of young pigs sampled in a herd in which almost 30% of fattening pigs had twisted snouts. In less severely affected herds, larger numbers of young pigs had to be sampled before toxigenic strains were isolated (Rutter 1985, De Jong et al. 1988). The distribution of toxigenic *P. multocida* in other species has still to be determined; Pedersen (1983), De Jong (1985), Rutter (1985), Baalsrud (1987), Ohkubo et al. (1987), and Kamp et al. (1990) reported that dermonecrotic strains occurred in cattle, rabbits, dogs, cats, rats, poultry, goats, and sheep. A toxigenic strain from pasteurellosis in turkeys produced severe turbinate atrophy in gnotobiotic pigs, but a toxigenic strain thought to

have been isolated from ovine pneumonia colonized the nasal cavity of pigs poorly, and did not produce significant lesions in combined infection with *B. bronchiseptica* (Rutter 1983, 1985). Toxigenic strains were isolated from humans suffering from tonsilitis, rhinitis, sinusitis, pleuritis, appendicitis, and septicemia, and were pathogenic for pigs (Nielsen and Frederiksen 1990). This implies special risks for all persons who have contact with herds or animals infected with toxigenic *P. multocida*: farmers and their families, farmhands, drivers, merchants, vets, consultants, butchers, and employees of slaughterhouses. Limitation of the risk of getting infected or spreading the infection, protection, and prevention can be effected by wearing masks that filter the air.

Problems of Diagnosis. Should pigs from a herd with no clinically apparent disease that have no obvious growth retardation but with mild turbinate atrophy at slaughter be considered as suffering from AR? It is suggested that where BS, lateral deviation, and poor growth are obvious within the herd and atrophy at slaughter is marked, the herd should be described as having clinical PAR. Conversely, where no turbinate atrophy is seen in slaughtered pigs, the herd must be regarded as clinically free from PAR. However, defining the status of herds where mild atrophy occurs in the absence of clinical disease presents problems, since there is no satisfactory single cutoff point between affected and unaffected herds (Goodwin 1988). These low levels of atrophy have been regarded as representing degrees of subclinical PAR but are probably better viewed as representing a potential risk of clinical PAR developing. It is often a matter of reasoned clinical judgment as to what level of atrophy is satisfactory or acceptable for a given enterprise. With the help of bacteriologic and serologic investigations this problem can be avoided.

Sources of Infection

SOWS AND GILTS. The dam has been considered a possible source of the important nasal infections for her sucking piglets, and she has been reliably incriminated as a source of *B. bronchiseptica* and *P. multocida*. However, her precise role in the transmission of *P. multocida* infection remains incomplete; the transmission does not always result in AR-diseased litters. Transmission also occurs between sows and boars. Although traditionally viewed as important, some observers have concluded that the sow's role might be minor, since clinically AR-free progeny have resulted when sows from an affected herd were reared under improved conditions (Bercovich 1978).

PIGS. Whether or not the sow is important in transmission, the recognized infectious agents pass readily between populations of young weaned pigs. Infection of pigs at an early age may be vital, even when the clinical disease seems to manifest itself late in the fattening period. But it has been shown that apparently healthy 3-month-old pigs can develop PAR when introduced into a commercial production unit where severe disease was occurring (Nielsen et al. 1976).

PRIMARY OUTBREAKS. The infectious agents are usually introduced into a previously unaffected herd by carrier pigs. Recently purchased breeding stock is commonly held responsible, although the evidence for their involvement is often circumstantial. The introduction of toxigenic strains of *P. multocida* is the principal event preceding an outbreak. Poorly colonizing strains with a low toxin production may represent an exception. Outbreaks by infections from other sources are rare, but seem to become more important if the spread of toxigenic *P. multocida* in pigs is not stopped.

PATHOGENESIS. The mechanism by which *B. bronchiseptica* colonizes the nasal epithelium and induces hypoplastic changes in the developing turbinate bones has been studied in detail; a description is given in Chapter 34. Much less is known about the mechanisms of colonization by *P. multocida* and the subsequent processes affecting the turbinate bone cells and leading to progressive atrophy and clinical PAR. Furthermore, the mechanisms by which these chronic nasal changes and their associated malfunctions cause growth retardation could be clarified to a large extent (Becker et al. 1986; Williams et al. 1986; Doster et al. 1990; Dugal and Jacques 1990).

P. multocida apparently colonizes the nasal cavity poorly unless there is preexisting mucosal damage (Elling and Pedersen 1983). Given this preconditioning, the organism will set up a nasal infection and, if toxigenic, the toxin will be elaborated. The nasal cavity, however, may not necessarily be the only possible site of toxin production. The toxin appears to be of crucial significance in the pathogenesis of AR, since only toxigenic strains of *P. multocida* produce progressive atrophic lesions; furthermore, the toxin will produce progressive snout shortening and turbinate atrophy when given to pigs intranasally (Ilina and Zasukhin 1975) and by a variety of parenteral routes (Rutter and Mackenzie 1984).

The precise mechanism of action of the *P. multocida* toxin has not been clearly defined; but it will produce a variety of changes in the ventral turbinates, consisting of epithelial hyperplasia, atrophy of mucosal glands, osteolysis, and a proliferation of mesenchymal cells. These eventually will replace the bone trabeculae and osteogenic and osteoclastic tissues (Rutter and Mackenzie 1984). PAR, therefore, seems to result from a combination of early osteoblastic damage followed by a series of toxin-induced chronic changes that result in osteolysis and subsequent replacement fibrosis (Martineau-Doize et al. 1990).

CLINICAL SIGNS. Clinical signs of PAR are not usually seen in pigs until about 4–12 weeks of age or later, depending on the severity of the outbreak, but sneezing and snuffling in baby pigs are commonly recorded as the first signs. They are not, however, specific or diagnostic of the condition, since they frequently occur in the absence of subsequent clinical PAR. Sneezing and snuffling in baby pigs is merely a reflection of an acute catarrhal rhinitis, which may be due to bordetellosis and/or infection with porcine cytomegalovirus; but other agents may possibly be involved, e.g., *Mycoplasma* sp., *Actinobacillus* sp., and Aujeszky's disease and influenza viruses. In herds where subsequent infectious and other factors combine to cause progression to clinical AR, affected pigs will continue to sneeze, snuffle, and snort throughout the growing period; this is accompanied by a variable amount of a serous to mucopurulent nasal discharge. In severely affected animals, sneezing may be pronounced and occasionally nasal bleeding may occur. Hemorrhage is usually unilateral and varies in severity. It may be seen on the walls of the pen or backs of the pigs; mucopurulent material and even pieces of turbinate debris may be expelled from the nose following episodes of forceful violent sneezing. In gilts and sows the hemorrhage in late gestation and farrowing can be life threatening to the dam and her piglets. The most characteristic clinical signs of PAR are due to disturbances of normal bone development of the nose; conspicuous deformities of the face may occur. The most common is BS in which the upper jaw is shortened in relation to the lower, as a result of growth depression of the ossa nasales and maxillares, giving the face a "pushed-up" appearance. The skin and subcutis over the dorsum of the shortened snout are thrown into folds; where the disturbance of bone growth affects one side of the face more than the other, lateral deviation of the snout occurs (Figs. 33.1, 33.2). This may vary in severity from a barely perceptible misalignment to severe twisting (possibly by as much as 50°). These facial deformities reflect an underlying turbinate atrophy; in the case of lateral deviation the atrophy is more pronounced on the side of the deviation. The prevalence of facial distortion varies among outbreaks, and not all pigs with significant turbinate atrophy develop marked facial distortion.

Dirty streaks on the face radiating from the medial canthus of the eye, caused by tearstaining and the entrapment of dust following occlusion of the nasolachrymal duct, are common in PAR outbreaks (Fig. 33.1). However, they are not diagnostic and may occur in the absence of PAR.

In moderate to severe herd outbreaks of PAR,

Some clinical parameters have been used in an attempt to monitor and quantify disease levels. The prevalence of gross distortion among growing pigs is a crude measure of disease level but is not a sensitive index of turbinate atrophy. The prevalence and degree of BS in weaned pigs can provide useful information (Bercovich and De Jong 1976), but is not always diagnostic (Schöss 1983), and confusion can arise with breeds that are naturally brachygnathic (e.g., Large White) (Van Groenland 1984). Sneeze counts have been used in an attempt to assess the effects of treatment (Douglas and Ripley 1984; Kobisch and Pennings 1989).

LESIONS. The gross lesions of PAR are restricted to the nasal cavity and adjacent structures of the skull, although in severe cases the pig may also be stunted. At necropsy both BS and facial distortion are observed in the intact head. The dominant lesion is an atrophy of the ventral and dorsal turbinates, and this can vary greatly in severity. The atrophy is assessed by a cross section of the snout at the level of the first/second upper premolar, at which point the conchae, dorsal and ventral, are symetrically and maximally developed in the normal pig (Fig. 33.3). In mild to moderate cases the ventral scroll of the ventral turbinate is by far the most consistently and severely affected area; it varies in appearance from a slightly shrunken scroll to complete atrophy (Figs. 33.4, 33.5).

In more severe cases, atrophy of the dorsal scrolls of the ventral turbinate and the dorsal and ethmoidal turbinates may occur (Figs. 33.6, 33.7); in the severest form there is a complete absence of all turbinate structures (Fig. 33.8). In between these mild and severe forms, a whole spectrum of atrophic changes may be observed; occasionally the turbinates may appear in bizarre shapes (Fig. 33.6), which have been considered to represent some degree of regrowth of the conchae (Done 1985). Another gross change that may be observed is bowing or buckling of the nasal septum (Fig. 33.8); this is not uncommon and is often associated with BS, facial distortion, and/or asymmetrical atrophy. Irregular formation of the ossa nasales and maxillares also occurs in PAR (De Jong 1985) and should not be neglected (Figs. 33.7, 33.8).

Exudate may be found in the nasal cavity but is not a constant finding. The amount and character depend on the age of the lesion and the type of infection; it consists of variable amounts of mucopurulent to purulent material, possibly flecked with blood. The mucosa lining the frontal sinus is sometimes inflamed, and the sinus itself may contain mucopurulent material. The bones surrounding the nasal cavity may have undergone thinning or may be irregularly shaped to some extent. Hyperplasia/hyperostosis can be observed in older pigs (De Jong 1985).

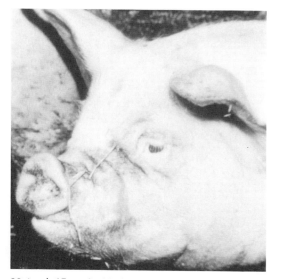

33.1. A 17-week-old pig with clinical PAR showing marked brachygnathia superior, wrinkling of the skin on the dorsum of the nose, and tearstaining.

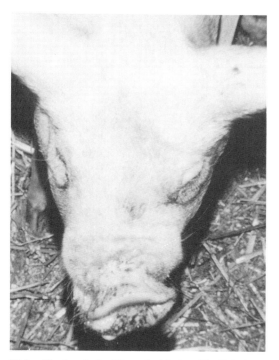

33.2. The head of a 15-week-old pig with clinical PAR showing severe lateral deviation of the snout. The anatomy of the skull is distinctly abnormal due to a failure of normal bone development.

the clinical signs are frequently accompanied by growth retardation and reduction in the efficiency of feed utilization. Feed utilization is particularly reduced in severely diseased pigs. The amount of *P. multocida* toxin may be of influence on growth performance (Doster et al. 1990).

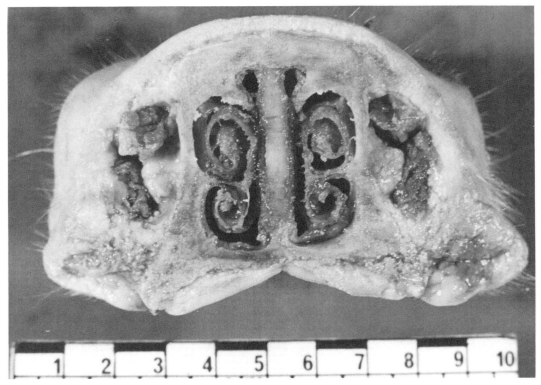

33.3. Cross section of the snout of an 18-week-old pig showing normal anatomy of the turbinates.

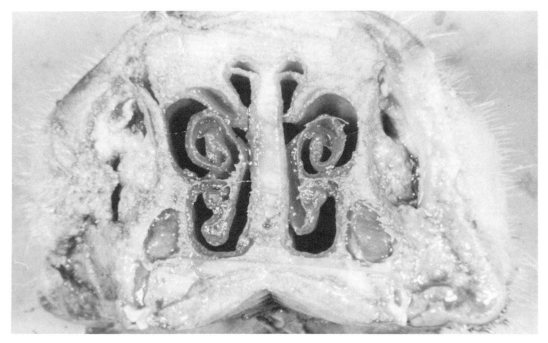

33.4. Cross section of the snout of an 18-week-old pig. Slight distortion of the ventral scrolls of the ventral turbinate is present, a common finding.

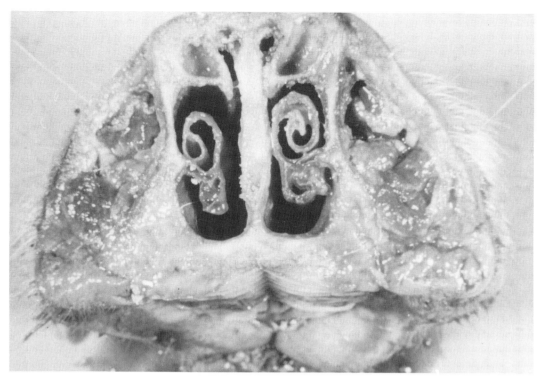

33.5. Cross section of the snout of an 18-week-old pig showing modest but definite turbinate atrophy.

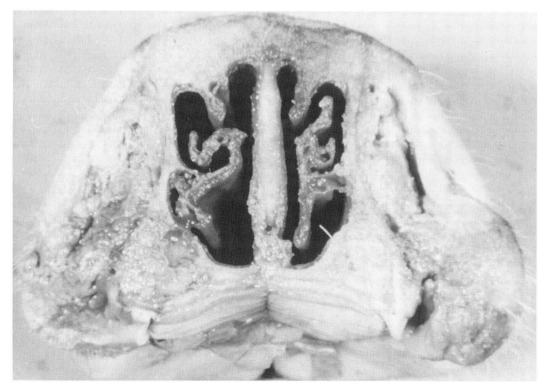

33.6. Cross section of the snout of an 18-week-old pig showing severe bilateral turbinate atrophy.

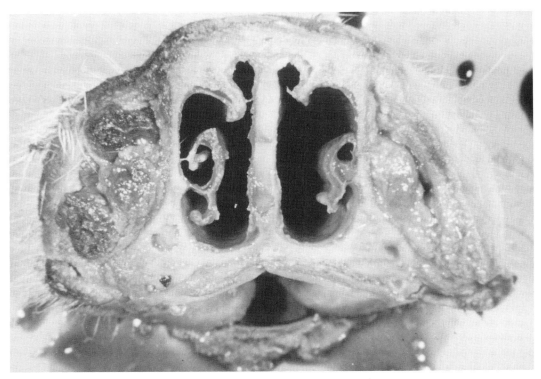

33.7. Cross section of the snout of an 18-week-old pig; the atrophic turbinates have developed into a bizarre shape.

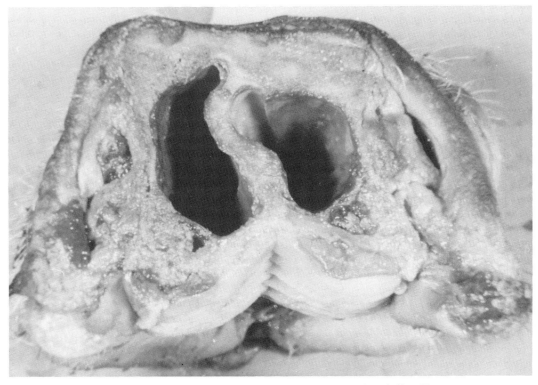

33.8. Cross section of the snout of a 22-week-old pig. There is total atrophy of all turbinate structures, with severe bending of the nasal septum.

Assessment of Turbinate Atrophy. The varying severity of the atrophic changes has led to the development of methods of quantitative assessment, but unfortunately, no one system has gained universal acceptance. Subjective scoring of snouts, e.g., on a 0–5 scale as in the British system (Anon. 1978), has proved very useful in evaluating treatment and monitoring schemes. As well as wide variation between systems, there is also considerable interobserver variation within a system (D'Allaire et al. 1988). At least one reason for this is probably the clinician's unwillingness to score a herd as having PAR, despite a degree of mild atrophy, when there has never been any clinical evidence of disease. Today, bacteriologic or serologic tests can be helpful in confirming the downgrading of a herd, e.g., when toxigenic *P. multocida* is present. The cutoff point between normality and being affected is imprecise, and the condition should not be regarded as a simple all-or-nothing phenomenon (Done 1985). The situation in many herds with only mild atrophy probably represents only the effects of a normally transient and often-resolving hypoplastic rhinitis without the tendency to progression characteristic of clinical PAR (see Definition).

Objective measures of assessing atrophy on a continuous scale have also been developed, including a morphometric index (area of free space as a percentage of total cross-sectional area of snout section) (Done et al. 1984). Such systems provide parametric data suitable for analysis, but as diagnostic tools they offer few advantages over subjective snout scoring (Collins et al. 1988, 1989).

Histologic Changes. Depending on the type of process active at the time of necropsy, acute, subacute, or chronic histologic changes may be observed. These changes in *B. bronchiseptica*–induced rhinitis are described in Chapter 34. The pathognomonic lesion of PAR by toxigenic *P. multocida* is a fibrous replacement of the bony plates of the ventral conchae (Done 1983a; Elling and Pedersen 1983; Martineau-Doize et al. 1990). Additionally, there may be a variable metaplasia of the respiratory epithelium and inflammation of the mucosal lamina propria; subacute cases of rhinitis in conventional pigs will show various mixtures of degenerative, inflammatory, dystrophic, and reparative processes. In SPF pigs an infection with toxigenic *P. multocida* did not induce a typical inflammatory reaction but did induce toxic alterations. The histologic changes in pigs with PAR that show retarded growth have been described by Yoshikawa and Hanada (1981).

Lesions in parenchymatous organs may also be present in cases of severe infection with toxigenic *P. multocida* (De Jong 1983a; Rutter 1983). Parenteral injections with *P. multocida* toxin induced liver cirrhosis, renal failure, marked decrease of peripheral blood lymphocytes without lysis, and growth retardation (Becker et al. 1986; Williams et al. 1986; Cheville et al. 1988).

DIAGNOSIS

Clinical Diagnosis. When the full range of clinical signs is present, a diagnosis of PAR on clinical signs alone is possible, but none of the snout deformations by itself is pathognomonic of PAR. Animals showing lateral deviation of the snout and/or marked BS, especially at an age of 10–12 weeks, almost always have pronounced turbinate atrophy (Bercovich and De Jong 1976; De Jong 1985; Kobisch and Pennings 1989). However, when these signs are not apparent or are of decreasing prevalence (e.g., following treatment), it is not possible for even experienced observers to assess the extent of turbinate atrophy in the live animal. The presence of a few twisted snouts or sneezing alone is not sufficient evidence to justify a diagnosis of PAR (see Definition).

Radiographic Diagnosis. Radiographic examination of the snout has been developed to facilitate improved diagnosis of turbinate atrophy in the live animal; a suitable procedure is described by Done (1976). In some countries this method has enjoyed widespread popularity, but it is beset with technical difficulties and problems in interpretation of the radiographs. The method may not detect mild lesions reliably, and its value has been questioned (Eikelenboom et al. 1978; Webbon et al. 1978); furthermore, pigs must be sedated, anaesthetized, or physically immobilized, and the procedure is costly and time consuming. With experience, however, some observers consider radiographic examination a useful aid (Schöss 1983). The same disadvantages are related to rhinoscopy (Plonait et al. 1980). Modern methods such as computerized tomography, used as a diagnostic tool for PAR, facilitate the macroscopic grading of the nasal structures in live pigs of any age (Jolie et al. 1990).

Postmortem Diagnosis. The prevalence and severity of turbinate atrophy is best estimated by examination of snouts after slaughter. Snouts should be transversely sectioned at the level of the first/second upper premolar; sectioning cranial to this should be avoided, since this will reveal a different pattern of turbinate development. Pigs 4 weeks old or older that died during weaning or prefattening can present turbinate atrophy at an early stage, and cross-sectioning can be carried out with a simple iron saw by qualified local veterinarians during regular herd inspections. Material from tonsils, lungs, and the nose can be sent to laboratories to assure a proper diagnosis. To determine a herd diagnosis, examine pigs at slaughter at regular intervals. As many pigs as practical should be examined; between 20 and 30 per time is often a suitable number (Goodwin

1988). Atrophy is scored on subjective grading systems (Bendixen 1971; Anon. 1978; Done 1983a, b; De Jong 1985). With low levels it is not possible to define a single cutoff point as representing freedom from PAR. An acceptable level for an individual (toxigenic *P. multocida*–infected) herd is a matter of reasoned clinical judgment but must be one in which the economic effects of the disease are minimal (Goodwin 1988). A monitoring scheme that could serve as a useful model with a diagrammatic representation of snout grading is described by Goodwin (1980). Computerized versions have been developed by Collins et al. (1988), Barfod et al. (1990), and Jolie and Thacker (1990).

Cultural and Serologic Diagnosis. Today, a definite diagnosis of PAR cannot be based solely on clinical and pathomorphologic observations, but requires laboratory tests (Pedersen 1983). Detection of the two most significant bacterial pathogens is possible by the culture of nasal and tonsillar swabs or tonsillar biopsies. The live pig should be adequately restrained and the external nares cleaned; slender cotton-tipped swabs with plastic or metal shafts should be inserted with slight rotation deep into both sides of the nasal cavity. Swabbing the tonsillar surface or tonsillar biopsies can aid the isolation and differention of *P. multocida* and toxigenic *P. multocida* (Van Leengoed 1986; De Jong et al. 1988). Swabs should be transported to the laboratory within 24 hours, preferably in a transport medium under cooled conditions (8°C). Nutrient transport media that support the growth of fast-growing contaminants are best avoided, but sterile phosphate-buffered saline is suitable (Pedersen 1983).

DETECTION OF *B. BRONCHISEPTICA*. Methods for the cultural diagnosis of bordetellosis are given in Chapter 34. Special selective media are described on which both *B. bronchiseptica* and *P. multocida* can grow (De Jong and Borst 1985).

DETECTION OF *P. MULTOCIDA*. The cultural isolation of *P. multocida* from nasal swabs and the testing of their toxigenicity is detailed by Pedersen (1983). When the nasal cavity is heavily infected with *P. multocida*, the organism can be recovered on simple blood agars (Smith and Baskerville 1983). However, field specimens frequently contain low numbers of organisms, and the other nasal flora may well mask the presence of *P. multocida* on nonselective media. Mouse inoculation greatly improves the recovery rate from field specimens, but a good in vitro method would be preferable. Some selective media are described by Smith and Baskerville (1983), Rutter and Luther (1984), De Jong and Borst (1985), Leblanc et al. (1986a, b), Chanter and Rutter (1989), and Avril et al. (1990). Evidence suggests that the tonsil is the preferred habitat for *P. multocida* in the

pig, and improved detection rates may be achieved by the collection of tonsillar swabs or biopsies in combination with nasal swabs (De Jong et al. 1988). Tonsils and lungs can also be collected in the slaughterhouse and examined in the laboratory. Swabs from noses of pigs sampled after immersion in the hot water tank are unsatisfactory for the detection of toxigenic *P. multocida* (Chanter and Rutter 1989).

DETECTION OF *P. MULTOCIDA* TOXIN. The central etiologic importance for toxigenic strains of *P. multocida* means that classification of field isolates into PAR toxin-positive or toxin-negative strains is necessary in understanding the epidemiology of the disease. The toxin is thermolabile, dermonecrotic in the guinea pig, and lethal for the mouse when administered intraperitoneally. Both tests give broadly comparable results; the methods are described by De Jong (1980, 1985), Pedersen (1983) and Rutter (1983) respectively. An in vitro system of detection by assessing the cytopathogenic effect in monolayers of Vero cells or embryonic bovine lung cells has been developed (Pennings and Storm 1984; Rutter and Luther 1984). Today, enyzme-linked immunosorbent assays are replacing the earlier tests (Foged et al. 1988). DNA probes have been developed to detect the gene responsible for toxin production in the toxigenic *P. multocida* (Andresen et al. 1990; Kamps et al. 1990; Lax and Chanter 1990).

***P. MULTOCIDA* SEROTYPES.** Determination of the capsular serotype of *P. multocida* is also often useful; most toxin-positive strains are type D, although toxin-positive type A strains also occur. In some regions the toxigenic type D is prevalent; in others it seems to be type A (Cowart and Bäckström 1984; Iwamatsu and Sawada 1988; Pijoan et al. 1988). The usual method of capsular serotyping is the indirect hemagglutination test with rabbit antisera (Carter 1955). The hyaluronidase test (Carter and Rundell 1975) and acriflavine test (Carter and Subronto 1973) are simpler methods for the detection of type A and D strains respectively, but not all porcine isolates are typable by these methods (Pedersen 1983). Piliation, hemagglutination, and capsular serotypes did not show a correlation with toxin production (Trigo and Pijoan 1988). An atypical *P. multocida* strain producing a toxin similar to the dermonecrotic toxin of *P. multocida* ssp. *multocida* is described in cattle (Kamp et al. 1990). Not only are the capsule and somatic structure of epidemiologic interest, the phage types and plasmid types also are indicated as interesting tools to follow the distribution pattern of the different toxigenic strains (Lugtenberg 1984; Nielsen and Rosdahl 1988, 1990; Hoje et al. 1990).

SEROLOGIC TESTS. Although agglutinating antibodies to *B. bronchiseptica* can be detected in pig serum (Giles and Smith 1983), this is of little diagnostic value. Serologic tests to detect antibodies against toxigenic *P. multocida* resulting from vaccination or infection have been described (De Jong and Akkermans 1986; Bechmann and Schöss 1990; Foged et al. 1990; Schimmelpfennig 1990). The toxin in natural infection is a weak immunogen, and antibodies to it takes 3 months or longer to detect and only then in some pigs (Bording et al. 1990). This means that serology may only be of importance in detecting antibodies in the sow population. A skin test is described to detect antibodies in sow herds that have been infected (Schimmelpfennig and Jahn 1988; Breuer and Schimmelpfennig 1990).

Differential Diagnosis. Sneezing in young pigs occurs in herds with active PAR, but it is not diagnostic itself, since it regularly occurs due to uncomplicated bordetellosis or porcine cytomegalovirus infection (Rondhuis et al. 1980). Both agents are widely spread in the pig industry and can cause severe mucous membrane damage, which is necessary for colonization with a toxigenic *P. multocida*. The frequency of severe sneezing can be used in clinical monitoring of PAR (Kobisch and Pennings 1989).

A variety of other conditions (reviewed by Done 1977) may cause facial deformity in pigs; these are likely to cause confusion in clinical and postmortem diagnosis, since malformations of the turbinates can be observed. A localized bacterial infection entering via wounds may produce a paranasal abscess (bullnose) in young pigs.

BS can occur as a breed-associated characteristic in certain lines of the Large White/Yorkshire breed. Breed-associated BS increases with age and cannot be influenced by a medication program intended to combat the influence of a *Bordetella* and/or a *Pasteurella* infection in these pigs. The breed-associated level of BS can easily be assessed by such a medication method. All BS grading higher than this lower genetic level may be a result of PAR. A warning limit can be chosen, e.g., at an age of 8–12 weeks, to select early clinically diseased animals and to take action to limit further damage in growing-out or fattening pigs. Breed-associated BS is easily distinguished from AR by the absence of turbinate atrophy, except where regeneration of the turbinates has occurred.

Sows and gilts kept in stalls often bite, chew, or play with bars or drinkers, and this can give rise to asymmetric bone development causing protrusion of the lower jaw or mandibular misalignment. These conditions can be confused with the facial deformity of AR, especially in the older pig, but careful inspection should reveal that the lower jaw is abnormally placed rather than the snout being shortened or laterally deviated. A useful technique is to draw an imaginary line between the center of the ears and eyes and project it

forward onto the snout. Some sows keep their snouts more to one side. This can induce misinterpretation. By pressing the molar teeth on top of each other and comparing the diastema between the incisor teeth in the upper and lower jaw, distortion can be noticed clinically at an early stage. This method can be carried out in combination with the BS-grading method. With thin nasal swabs an increase in internasal space can be observed clinically, but some experience is necessary for the interpretation.

TREATMENT. The effective treatment of an outbreak of AR requires a selected combination of management, environmental, chemotherapeutic, and vaccination procedures. No one combination is equally applicable to all affected herds. The overall aims of treatment are (1) to reduce the prevalence and load of the important specific bacterial infections (bordetellosis and pasteurellosis) in young pigs by sow vaccination, medication of feed, and antibiotic treatment of piglets; (2) to treat growing pigs with an acute rhinitis to reduce the weight of bacterial infection and severity of the hypoplastic changes and maintain efficient growth and feed utilization; and (3) to manipulate housing, ventilation, and management to improve the overall environment for the pigs (De Jong and Bartelse 1980; Smith 1983).

Sow Vaccination. Vaccination of the sow with a potent *B. bronchiseptica* vaccine is an effective way to reduce the prevalence and severity of nasal bordetellosis in sucking and weaned piglets (De Jong 1985), but this exerts only a limited effect on clinical PAR (Giles and Smith 1983). Pathogenic determinants important in vaccines include the toxigenic characters, the pilus-producing factor, and outer-membrane proteins. Lack of antibody to some of these properties seems to influence the reduction of *B. bronchiseptica* in sows and piglets. *B. bronchiseptica/P. multocida* vaccines have been evaluated experimentally and in the field, and in some countries these combined vaccines are available commercially. Such vaccines have reduced the prevalence of clinical PAR (Schuller et al. 1980; Baars et al. 1982; De Jong et al. 1984) but do not eliminate the condition. As might be expected, the thermolabile toxin from *P. multocida* appears to be an important determinant in eliciting protection, since experimental vaccination of sows with crude toxin significantly protected their offspring against PAR (Baars et al. 1982, 1986; Pedersen and Barfod 1982). Since then the specific importance of the toxoid fraction has been elucidated (Nagy et al. 1986; Foged et al. 1989; Frymus et al. 1989; Chanter and Rutter 1990). The antigens and mechanisms of protection against toxigenic *P. multocida* infection and associated disease have yet to be fully defined; reports show that toxoid preparations of *P. multocida* produce an antitoxin response, with an effect on colonization (Chanter and Rutter 1990). Claims made for *B. bronchiseptica* vaccines in the control of AR were not fully substantiated in field use (Giles and Smith 1983); thus, a rush to develop further combined vaccines without full appraisal of the required antigens is undesirable.

Some of the currently available combined *B. bronchiseptica/P. multocida* vaccines may be of benefit in controlling bordetellosis and toxigenic pasteurellosis and of value in reducing the prevalence and severity of PAR when combined with housing and management changes (De Jong et al. 1984). The marked reduction in toxigenic *P. multocida* in the nose following vaccination with a potent toxoid vaccine requires further evaluation to determine whether the expression of high antibody levels can eradicate toxigenic *P. multocida*. Vaccination of sows with combined vaccines can be as effective as piglet medication. However, neither procedure constitutes a means of protection against the condition nor necessarily obviates the need for medication. Such a vaccination program, once started in an infected herd, has to be continued constantly.

Medication of Sows and Piglets. To reduce the prevalence and severity of nasal infections acquired from their dams, the feed of the sow can be medicated during the final month of gestation. Sulfadimidine (sulfamethazine) (400–2000 g/ton) or oxytetracycline (400–1000 g/ton) are the products most widely used.

Sucking piglets are best medicated by strategic injections of antibacterial agents in therapeutic dosages four to eight times during the first 3–4 weeks of life. The most useful are potentiated sulfonamides, oxytetracycline, and penicillin/streptomycin. If bordetellosis is the major infection in sucking piglets, potentiated sulfonamides are the drugs of choice (12.5 mg/kg sulfadiazine or sulfadoxine + 2.5 mg/kg trimethoprim). Injections of oxytetracycline (20–80 mg/kg) once or twice a week are also clinically effective in PAR (De Jong and Oosterwoud 1977; Mefford et al. 1983). The long-acting formulation (20–80 mg/kg) may be the preferred product and is best given once or twice during each of the first 3 or 4 weeks of life. If not resistant, the drug is effective against pasteurellosis, since experimentally, long-acting oxytetracycline has reduced the prevalence of nasal infection and the severity of turbinate atrophy induced by *P. multocida* (Gois et al. 1983b); others prefer doxycycline (Pijpers et al. 1988). In the Netherlands, intranasal spraying of oxytetracycline in a 5% solution is used in piglets two times a week, when starting the treatment. If effective after 2–3 months, a reduction from twice to once a week can be recommended (De Jong 1983). This withdrawal of medication also depends on the average antibody titer against the toxin of *P. multocida* in the dams obtained by the vaccination program. Other antibiotics to which *P. multocida*

may be sensitive and that are frequently used in therapeutic concentrations against pneumonia caused by pasteurellosis include penicillin/streptomycin (20,000 IU/10–25 mg/kg), tylosin (10–25 mg/kg), lincomycin/spectinomycin (50/100 mg/kg), ampicillin (10–20 mg/kg), amoxycillin (10–20 mg/kg), spiramycin (25 mg/kg), quinolone derivatives (0.5–5 mg/kg), cephalosporins (1–5 mg/kg), or tiamulin (10–20 mg/kg) (Plonait and Bickhardt 1988). The benefits of these treatments have not been critically evaluated as far as nasal and pulmonary protection and/or elimination of the toxigenic *P. multocida* are concerned.

Vaccination of Piglets. *B. bronchiseptica* vaccine has been widely employed. Although some observers have concluded that it has little benefit against clinical PAR and is generally less effective than sow vaccination (Giles and Smith 1982, 1983), in some countries (notably the United States) the procedure nevertheless still enjoys fairly widespread use. *B. bronchiseptica/P. multocida* bacterin vaccines are also widely employed, but considering the composition, few may be of benefit in the field. In a study in which both sows and piglets were inoculated with a combined vaccine, Mefford et al. (1983) demonstrated that vaccination alone did not influence turbinate atrophy and only marginally improved profitability.

Only vaccination of the piglets born of inadequately vaccinated or unvaccinated dams is of value in the case of *P. multocida* toxoid vaccines. When sows are properly vaccinated and produce good levels of antitoxin antibodies, piglets may not respond to vaccination. If the dams show good titers, the colostral protection in pigs can last for 3–4 months. Vaccinations of the young breeding stock can be started after this age. A high antitoxin titer seems to reduce the colonization by toxigenic *P. multocida*.

The additional use of therapeutics (e.g., long-acting oxytetracycline) in piglets significantly reduced turbinate atrophy at slaughter and markedly improved profitability (Pejsak et al. 1990). Furthermore, some commercially available vaccines contain neither toxigenic strains nor *P. multocida* toxoid, the manufacturers only claiming efficacy against pneumonic pasteurellosis.

Medication of Weaners and Growers. The PAR in weaned pigs that leads eventually to marked turbinate atrophy at slaughter can be controlled to some extent by medication of creep in weaner and/or grower rations or by the addition of antibiotics to the drinking water. Such medication also assists in the maintenance of growth and efficiency of feed utilization in the face of active PAR, but as might be expected, medication is always much more effective when the environment of the pigs is improved. Various antibacterial agents alone or in combination are effective. The sulfonamides are frequently included in rations because of their known efficacy against bordetellosis. Their use in this respect and the problems of the development of drug resistance are discussed in Chapter 34. Well-established drugs or combinations suitable for the control of PAR are (1) sulfadimidine (sulfamethazine) (400–2000 g/ton) in feed or sulfathiazole (0.08–0.13 g/L) in the drinking water, (2) chlortetracycline (165 g/ton)/sulfadimidine (sulfamethazine) (165 g/ton)/penicillin G (83 g/ton) in feed, (3) tylosin (100 g/ton)/sulfadimidine (sulfamethazine) (100 g/ton) in feed, (4) carbadox (50 g/ton)/sulfadimidine (sulfamethazine) (100 g/ton) in feed, (5) oxytetracycline in feed (400 g/ton) or in drinking water (0.18 g/L)(Giles 1986). Various other antibacterial agents, alone or in combination, also have broadly similar beneficial effects on PAR lesions and help to maintain growth; e.g., lincomycin (220 g/ton), lincomycin (220 g/ton)/sulfamethazine (550 g/ton), lincomycin/spectinomycin and amoxicillin trihydrate (10–20 g/ton) in combination in feed have been demonstrated as clinically effective. When a number of drugs are used in feed, a decrease of bioavailability can occur, which may result from the amount of calcium, the feed processing, and the water ration given to the treated pigs (Counotte 1984; Froe 1990; Sutter and Wanner 1990). The availability of some of these drugs and the regulations regarding their use in food-producing animals vary between countries.

Selection of an appropriate antibiotic or combination depends partly on cost, legislation, and clinical experience but should also be related to the antibiotic sensitivity patterns of *B. bronchiseptica* and *P. multocida* isolates and the established minimum inhibitory concentrations (MIC) (Pijpers et al. 1988; Fales et al. 1990). Differences in MIC between *P. multocida* type D and A strains may occur in the same herd (Schimmelpfennig 1990). In a severe outbreak, treatment should be directed at pigs of all age groups other than those immediately destined for slaughter; as the severity declines, reducing antibiotic use for the older fatteners should be the first priority. The appropriate withdrawal times before slaughter must always be adhered to. It is usually necessary for pigs to receive medicated feed for a minimum period of 4–5 weeks and frequently for longer periods, depending on the results of the vaccination program and the improvement of housing, ventilation, and management.

Housing and Husbandry. Medication and vaccination procedures should never be introduced without concurrent attempts to improve swine management and husbandry. Although the noninfectious factors that contribute to the severity of PAR are inadequately defined quantitatively, steps should always be taken to reduce their influence. All-in/all-out systems are favored for farrowing, weaner, and preferably fattener management; allowing the age of the sow herd to rise and

avoiding the introduction of large numbers of infected new gilts; reducing the stocking density; implementing strict hygiene measures; and maintaining correct ventilation rates to reduce the airborne concentration of bacterial pathogens, noxious gases, and dust. Steps should also be taken to reduce factors that stress young pigs, including large temperature variations, chilling, and drafts. Replacement breeding stock should not only be free from clinical signs of disease but also be raised in herds free from infections with toxigenic *P. multocida;* introduced weaners should be free from active rhinitis and the associated sneezing and typical BS. Newly purchased stock should originate from toxigenic *P. multocida*–free herds, be isolated (quarantined), tested bacteriologically or serologically for freedom from toxigenic *P. multocida,* and then integrated slowly. Severely affected pigs with obvious and severe growth retardation should be culled. Vaccination programs should be started if breeding stock free from toxigenic *P. multocida* infection are brought into infected herds. Vaccination can reduce colonization with toxigenic *P. multocida* when infection cannot be avoided. Such an AR vaccination program needs to be carried out continuously in the whole sow population of the infected herd. Effective vaccination with potent vaccines in sows alone can also limit the economic damage in weaners. The risk to breeders, multipliers, and fatteners of becoming infected by the toxigenic *P. multocida* can be limited by asking or giving guarantees that the pigs bought or sold originate directly from herds certified free from the organism. This certification can be carried out under governmental legislation. Only by means of such a system of enforced restrictions can the spread of toxigenic *P. multocida* via sales or auctions be prevented.

Depopulation. Depopulation and restocking with swine from a source known to be free from the toxigenic *P. multocida* is often the only viable solution. Buildings should be thoroughly cleaned and disinfected, then fumigated and left empty for about 1–2 months, depending on the effectivity and quality of the hygiene program. Eradication of rats and mice must be carried out properly and continually. Replacement pigs should be from sources known to be free from PAR and toxigenic *P. multocida* infection, based on clinical, abattoir, bacteriologic, and or serologic monitoring.

PREVENTION. PAR can be prevented effectively only by rearing swine free from the specific infections required for disease to develop. The adoption of an SPF system of production and the maintenance of an effective microbiologic barrier is the only sure way of achieving this. Medicated early weaning (Alexander et al. 1980) may well be a viable alternative to the established methods of producing SPF stock free from toxigenic *P. multocida* (James 1989; Blaha et al. 1990; Larsen et al.

1990). Traditional vaccination or medication regimes applied to infected herds are not likely to create herds free from the infections; thus, the infected herds pose a serious threat for free herds in their neighborhood and also pose risks to other branches of animal production, such as poultry, rabbits, goats, sheep, and cattle (Nielsen et al. 1986). In a preventive disease control program, eradication schemes have to be carried out in all types of herds and in all kinds of animals infected with toxigenic *P. multocida*. *B. bronchiseptica* appears to be very widespread in the pig population, but the prevalence of infection with toxigenic strains of *P. multocida* is less well defined. A positive correlation exists between the prevalence of toxigenic strains of *P. multocida* in the herd and the known occurrence of PAR (De Jong 1983; Nielsen 1983; Pedersen 1983; Cowart and Bäckström 1984; Leblanc et al. 1986b; Bechmann and Schöss 1988; Cowart et al. 1989), although the mere presence of this infection does not always mean clinical disease. The potential risk of clinical PAR developing in a herd could be eliminated simply by ensuring that pigs are free from toxigenic *P. multocida* infection. Therefore, it is desirable to monitor breeding stock for this pathogen and to take steps to reduce its dissemination and introduction into unaffected herds. It is definitely beneficial to maintain herds with no history of PAR and low scores of atrophy at slaughter behind effective barriers or to bring in pigs only from sources known to be free from the condition. Breeding companies that sell and export pigs from infected herds, inadequately monitored for infectious diseases like PAR, are involved more and more in financial claims by new owners who will not accept the cost of medication and vaccination and the degradation of the health status of their own breeding herds. Because aerogenic spread has been described (Baekbo and Nielsen 1988; Stehmann et al. 1989) and spread of infection may be possible from surrounding herds, special attention to air filtration and decontamination systems (Rutter et al. 1986; Voets et al. 1986b) could be necessary if distances become too small (probably within 200–1000 m, depending on the size of the surrounding herds). PAR has also been found in outdoor systems. Prevention against toxigenic *P. multocida* infection in outdoor systems can be difficult. Prevention by artificial insemination seems possible, but some risks exist when the antibiotics used in the semen diluter do not eliminate the toxigenic *Pasteurella* (Overby 1990).

Monitoring. Commercial producers should be aware of the current disease status of their herds. This applies to herds that have past or present evidence for the clinical condition, as well as to producers who need to monitor the effects of control measures or whose herds have remained free from the condition and who appreciate early warning of any change in herd status. Hence, ideally, herds need monitoring systems that can quantify not only the presence but also the effects of PAR (Done 1983b), especially in the case of an infected herd. Since this disease is not a simple all-or-nothing condition, merely relying on the presence of clinical disease disguises moderate-to-low levels of infection and recognizes it too late for the introduction of prophylactic measures.

Parameters that can be usefully measured are indirect production or economic data, such as liveweight gain or efficiency of feed utilization, and clinical/pathologic data related to PAR, including the amount of sneezing, the incidence of facial distortion, and the two most useful criteria, the prevalence and extent of BS in weaned pigs and the prevalence and severity of turbinate atrophy at slaughter. The latter is the most popular in some countries. In large, modern slaughterhouses the gathering of snouts and cross sections is difficult; in such situations a scoring system on longitudinally opened snouts can be useful (Visser et al. 1988). Sophisticated methods of monitoring have been developed, one of which is the plotting of cumulative-sum charts with decision boundaries, since it gives early signals of deterioration or improvement. Done (1983b) has reviewed the methods of monitoring PAR. Use of computer technology in slaughterhouses and on pig farms means that important disease-monitoring systems may be effectively employed without laborious clerical work (Collins et al. 1988). Because the antibody titer against the toxin of *P. multocida* correlates with increased protection against turbinate atrophy (Sorensen et al. 1990), serological monitoring becomes of interest in determining a possible increase of PAR risk when a decrease in the titers occurs in herds with a sow vaccination program. A program in which only sows are vaccinated can also protect the pigs during the fattening period. Recent investigations have shown a relationship between antitoxin titers and some protection against colonization with the toxigenic pasteurellas (Chanter and Rutter 1990). Modernized methods for the detection of toxigenic *P. multocida* by DNA probes from samples of noses, tonsils, or lungs may soon become useful in monitoring systems (Kamps et al. 1990). Positive results have already been achieved by bacteriologic (Schöss 1982; Schöss and Thiel 1984; De Jong et al. 1988) or serologic monitoring (De Jong et al. 1988; Bechmann and Schöss 1990; Foged et al. 1990; Schimmelpfennig 1990).

REFERENCES

ALEXANDER, T. J. L.; THORNTON, K.; BOON, G.; LYSONS, R. J.; AND GUSH, A. F. 1980. Medicated early weaning to obtain pigs free from pathogens endemic in the herd of origin. Vet Rec 106:114.

ANDRESEN, L. O.; PETERSEN, S. K.; CHRISTIANSEN, C.; AND NIELSEN, J. P. 1990. Studies on the location of the *Pasteurella multocida* toxin gene, tox A. Proc Int Congr Pig Vet Soc, Lausanne, p. 60.

Anon. 1954. New pig disease in Britain. Vet Rec 66: 316.

Anon. 1978. Atrophic rhinitis: A system of snout grading. Ministry of Agriculture, Fisheries and Food Booklet LPD 51. Pinner, United Kingdom.

AVRIL, J. L.; DONNIO, P. Y.; AND POUEDRAS, P. 1990. Selective medium for *Pasteurella multocida* and its use to detect oropharyngeal carriage in pig-breeders. J Clin Microbiol 28:1438–1440.

BAALSRUD, K. J. 1987. Atrophic rhinitis in goats in Norway. Vet Rec 121:350–353.

BAARS, J. C.; DE JONG, M. F.; STORM, P. K.; WILLEMS, H.; AND PENNINGS, A. 1982. Atrophic rhinitis and its control with an adjuvant vaccine consisting of B. *bronchiseptica* and P. *multocida* strains. Proc Int Congr Pig Vet Soc, Mexico City, p. 121.

BAARS, J. C.; PENNINGS, A.; AND STORM, P. K. 1986. Challenge and field experiments with an experimental atrophic rhinitis vaccine, containing *Pasteurella multocida* DNT-toxoid and *Bordetella bronchiseptica*. Proc Int Congr Pig Vet Soc, Barcelona, p. 247.

BAEKBO, P. 1988. Pathogenic properties of *Pasteurella multocida* in the lung of pigs. Proc Int Congr Pig Vet Soc, Rio de Janeiro, p. 58.

BAEKBO, P., AND NIELSEN, J. P. 1988. Airborne *Pasteurella multocida* in pig fattening units. Proc Int Congr Pig Vet Soc, Rio de Janeiro, p. 51.

BARFOD, K.; SORENSEN, V.; AND NIELSEN, J. P. 1990. Methods of evaluation of the degree of atrophic rhinitis. Proc Int Congr Pig Vet Soc, Lausanne, p. 70.

BECHMANN, G., AND SCHÖSS, P. 1988. Untersuchungen über das Vorkommen toxinbildener Pasteurella-multocida-Stämme in Tonsillen und Nasen von Ferkeln aus Rhinitis-atrophicans-unverdächtigen Zuchtbeständen. Dtsch Tieraerztl Wochenschr 95:257–312.

———. 1990. Neutralizing activity against *Pasteurella multocida* toxin in sera of pigs with atrophic rhinitis. Proc Int Congr Pig Vet Soc, Lausanne, p. 50.

BECKER, H. N.; REED, P.; WOODARD, J. C.; AND WHITE, E. C. 1986. The effects of P. *multocida* type D toxin on turbinates, body weight gains, and liver weight in piglets when injected intramuscularly. Proc Int Congr Pig Vet Soc, Barcelona, p. 249.

BENDIXEN, H. C. 1971. Om nysesyge hos svinet. Chronic dystrophic s. atrophic s. infectious rhinitis in pigs. Vet Med [Suppl 1] 23:177.

BERCOVICH, Z. 1978. Contamination and age as factors in the pathogenesis of atrophic rhinitis. Tijdschr Diergeneeskd 103:833.

BERCOVICH, Z., AND DE JONG, M. F. 1976. Shortening of the upper jaw (Brachygnathia superior) as a clinical feature of atrophic rhinitis in approximately 8-week-old piglets. Tijdschr Diergeneeskd 101:1011–1022.

BLAHA, Th.; SCHIMMEL, D.; ERLER, W.; AND BURCH, D. G. S. 1990. Use of tiamulin for the production of pigs with healthy lungs, suitable for research into respiratory diseases. Proc Int Congr Pig Vet Soc, Lausanne, p. 110.

BLOBEL, H., AND SCHLIESSER, T. 1981. Handbuch der bakteriellen Infektionen bei Tieren. Band III V.E.B. Jena: Gustav Fischer Verlag.

BOLLWAHN, W. 1988. Forensische Aspekte der Rhinitis atrophicans der Schweine. Tieraerztl Prax [Suppl] 3:59–61.

BORDING, A.; PETERSEN, S.; AND FOGED, N. T. 1990. Immunological and pathological characterization of the *Pasteurella multocida* toxin and its derivates. Proc Int Congr Pig Vet Soc, Lausanne, p. 62.

BRAEND, M., AND FLATLA, J. L. 1954. Rhinitis infectiosa atroficans hos gris. Nord Vet Med 6:81–122.

BRASSINNE, M.; DEWAELE, A.; AND GOUFFAUX, M. 1976. Intranasal infection with *Bordetella bronchisepti-ca* in gnotobiotic piglets. Res Vet Sci 20:162–166.

BREUER, J., AND SCHIMMELPFENNIG, H. 1990. Skin-testing for P. *multocida* antitoxic antibodies in breeding herds. Proc Int Congr Pig Vet Soc, Lausanne, p. 51.

BROWN, W. R.; KROOK, L.; AND POND, W. G. 1966. Atrophic rhinitis in swine. Etiology, pathogenesis and prophylaxis. Cornell Vet [Suppl 1] 56:1–107.

CAMERON, R. D. A.; GILES, C. J.; AND SMITH, I. M. 1980. The prevalence of *Bordetella bronchiseptica* and turbinate (conchal) atrophy in English pig herds in 1978–1979. Vet Rec 107:146.

CARTER, G. R. 1955. Studies on *Pasteurella multocida*. I. A haemagglutination test for the identification of serological types. Am J Vet Res 16:481–484.

———. 1967. Adv Vet Sci Comp Med 11:321–379.

CARTER, G. R., AND RUNDELL, S. W. 1975. Identification of type A strains of P. *multocida* using staphylococcal hyaluronidase. Vet Rec 96:343.

CARTER, G. R., AND SUBRONTO, P. 1973. Identification of type D strains of *Pasteurella multocida* with acriflavine. Am J Vet Res 34:293.

CHANTER, N., AND RUTTER, J. M. 1989. Comparison of methods for the sampling and isolation of toxigenic *Pasteurella multocida* from the nasal cavity of pigs. Res Vet Sci 47:355–358.

———. 1990. The role of osteolytic toxin in colonisation by toxigenic P. *multocida*. Proc Int Congr Pig Vet Soc, Lausanne, p. 67.

CHEVILLE, N. F.; RIMLER, R. B.; AND THURSTON, J. R. 1988. A toxin from *Pasteurella multocida* type D causes acute hepatic necrosis in pigs. Vet Pathol 25:518–520.

COLLINGS, L. A. 1983. The pathogenicity of *Bordetella bronchiseptica* in porcine atrophic rhinitis. Ph.D. diss., Univ of Reading, United Kingdom.

COLLINS, M. T.; BÄCKSTRÖM, L. R.; AND CONRAD, T. A. 1988. Evaluation of a semi-automatic digitizer-tablet snout morphometry technique. Proc Int Congr Vet Soc, Rio de Janeiro, p. 37.

COLLINS, M. T.; BÄCKSTRÖM, L.; AND BRIM, A. 1989. Turbinate perimeter ratio as an indicator of conchal atrophy for diagnosis of atrophic rhinitis in pigs. Am J Vet Res 50:421–424.

COUNOTTE, G. H. M.; EEFTING, T.; AND BOSCH, A. 1984. Stability and distribution of oxytetracycline hydrochloride during the manufacture and storage of pig-rearing pellets under field conditions. Tijdschr Diergeneeskd 109(9):339–344.

COWART, R. P., AND BÄCKSTRÖM, L. 1984. Prevalence of dermonecrotic, toxin-producing *Pasteurella multocida* strains in Illinois swine herds with varying levels of atrophic rhinitis and pneumonia. Proc Int Congr Pig Vet Soc, Ghent, p. 159.

COWART, R. P.; BÄCKSTRÖM, L.; AND BRIM, T. A. 1989. *Pasteurella multocida* and *Bordetella bronchiseptica* in atrophic rhinitis and pneumonia in swine. Can J Vet Res 53(3):295–300.

CROSS, R. F., AND CLAFLIN, R. M. 1962. *Bordetella bronchiseptica* induced porcine atrophic rhinitis. J Am Vet Med Assoc 141:1467–1468.

D'ALLAIRE, S.; BIGRAS-POULIN, M.; PARADIS, M. A.; AND MARTINEAU, G. P. 1988. Evaluation of AR: Are the results repeatable? Proc Int Congr Pig Vet Soc, Rio de Janeiro, p. 38.

DE JONG, M. F. 1976–1979. Atrofische Rhinitis onderzoek. Annual Central Veterinary Institute, C.D.I. Postbus 65, Lelystad, Netherlands.

DE JONG, M. F. 1980. Some aspects of the study of atrophic rhinitis in pigs. Tijdschr Diergeneesk 105:711–714.

DE JONG, M. F. 1983a. Atrophic rhinitis caused by intranasal or intramuscular administration of broth-culture and broth-culture filtrates containing AR toxin of *Pasteurella multocida*. In Atrophic Rhinitis of Pigs. Ed. K. B. Pedersen and N. C. Nielsen. Comm Eur Communities Rep EUR 8643 EN, Luxembourg, p. 136.

DE JONG, M. F. 1983b. Atrophic Rhinitis of Pigs. Ed. K. B. Pedersen and N. C. Nielsen. Comm Eur Communities Rep EUR 8643 EN, Luxembourg.

DE JONG, M. F. 1985. Atrophic rhinitis in pigs. Thesis, Univ of Utrecht. Elinkwijk B. V. Utrecht.

DE JONG, M. F., AND AKKERMANS, J. P. W. M. 1986. I. Atrophic rhinitis caused by *Bordetella bronchiseptica* and *Pasteurella multocida* and the meaning of a thermolabile toxin of *P. multocida*. Vet Q 8(3): 204–214.

DE JONG, M. F., AND BARTELSE, A. 1980. The influence of management and housing on the isolation frequency of *Bordetella bronchiseptica* in piglet populations. Proc Int Congr Pig Vet Soc, Copenhagen, p. 212.

DE JONG, M. F., AND BORST, G. H. A. 1985. Selective medium for the isolation of *P. multocida* and *B. bronchiseptica*. Vet Rec 9:167.

DE JONG, M. F., AND NIELSEN, J. P. 1990. Definition of progressive atrophic rhinitis. Vet Rec 27:93.

DE JONG. M. F., AND OOSTERWOUD, R. A. 1977. Treatment with oxytetracycline hydrochloride in the prevention of atrophic rhinitis in baby pigs. Tijdschr Diergeneeskd 102:266.

DE JONG, M. F.; OEI, H. L.; AND TETENBURG, G. J. 1980. AR pathogenicity tests for *Pasteurella multocida* isolates. Proc Int Congr Pig Vet Soc, Copenhagen, p. 211.

DE JONG, M. F.; OOSTERWOUD, R. A.; AND BOUWKAMP, F. T. 1984. A field evaluation of the Nobi-Vac AR vaccine. Proc Int Congr Pig Vet Soc, Ghent, p. 174.

DE JONG, M. F.; WELLENBERG, G.; SCHAAKE, J.; AND FRIK, K. 1988. Selection of pig breeding herds free from atrophic rhinitis by means of a bacteriological screening of pigs on DNT producing *Pasteurella multocida;* a field evaluation from 1981 until 1987. Proc Int Congr Pig Vet Soc, Rio de Janeiro, p. 49.

DIRKS, C.; SCHÖSS, P.; AND SCHIMMELPFENNIG, H. 1973. Aetiology of atrophic rhinitis of swine. DTW 80:342.

DONE, J. T. 1976. Porcine atrophic rhinitis: Snout radiography as an aid to the diagnosis and detection of the disease. Vet Rec 98:23.

_____. 1977. Facial deformity in pigs. Vet Annu 17:96.

_____. 1983a. Atrophic rhinitis: Pathomorphological diagnosis. In Atrophic Rhinitis of Pigs. Ed. K. B. Pedersen and N. C. Nielsen. Comm Eur Communities Rep EUR 8643 EN, Luxembourg, p. 3.

_____. 1983b. Monitoring of atrophic rhinitis. In Atrophic Rhinitis of Pigs. Ed. K. B. Pedersen and N. C. Nielsen. Comm Eur Communities Rep EUR 8643 EN, Luxembourg, p. 193.

_____. 1985. Porcine atrophic rhinitis–an update. Vet Annu 25:180–191.

DONE, J. T.; UPCOTT, D. H.; FREWIN, D. C.; AND HEBERT, C. N. 1984. Atrophic rhinitis: Snout morphometry for quantitative assessment of conchal atrophy. Vet Rec 113:33.

DOSTER, A. R.; FRANTZ, J. C.; BROWN, A. L.; HUSEMAN, B. R.; AND HOGG, A. 1990. Effects of *Pasteurella multocida* serotype D dermonecrotic toxin in swine. Proc Int Congr Pig Vet Soc, Lausanne, p. 72.

DOUGLAS, R. G. A., AND RIPLEY, P. H. 1984. Sneeze counts as a diagnostic aid in pig production. Vet Rec 114:321.

DOYLE, L. P.; DONHAM, C. R.; AND HUTCHINGS, L. M. 1944. Report of a type of rhinitis in swine. J Am Vet Med Assoc 105:132.

DUGAL, F., AND JACQUES, M. 1990. Enchanced adherence of *Pasteurella multocida* to porcine tracheal rings pre-infected with *Bordetella bronchiseptica*. Proc Int

Congr Pig Vet Soc, Lausanne, p. 73.

DUNCAN, J. R.; ROSS, R. F.; SWITZER, W. P.; AND RAMSEY, F. K. 1966. Pathology of experimental *Bordetella bronchiseptica* infection in swine atrophic rhinitis. Am J Vet Res 27:457–466.

EDINGTON, N.; SMITH, I. M.; PLOWRIGHT, W.; AND WATT, R. G. 1976. Relationship of porcine cytomegalovirus and *B. bronchiseptica* to atrophic rhinitis in gnotobiotic piglets. Vet Rec 98:42.

EIKELENBOOM, G.; DIK, K. J.; AND DE JONG, M. F. 1978. De waarde van het rontgenologisch onderzoek voor de diagnostiek van Atrofische Rhinitis. Tijdschr Diergeneeskd 103:1002–1008.

ELIAS, B.; KRUGER, M.; AND RATZ, F. 1982. Epizootiologische Untersuchung der Rhinitis Atrophicans des Schweines. II. Biologische Eigenschaften der von Schweinen isolierten *Bordetella bronchiseptica* Stamme. Zentralbl Veterinaermed [B] 29:619–635.

ELLING, E., AND PEDERSEN, K. B. 1983. Atrophic rhinitis in pigs induced by a dermonecrotic type A strain of *Pasteurella multocida*. In Atrophic Rhinitis of Pigs. Ed. K. B. Pedersen and N. C. Nielsen. Comm Eur Communities Rep EUR 8643 EN, Luxembourg, p. 123.

FALES, W. H.; TURK, J. R.; MILLER, M. A.; BEANKNUDSEN, C.; NELSON, S. L.; MOREHOUSE, G. L.; AND GOSSEN, H. S. 1990. Antimicrobial susceptibility of *P. multocida* type D from Missouri swine. J Vet Diagn Invest 2:80–81.

FOGED, N. T.; NIELSEN, J. P.; AND SCHRIMER, A. L. 1988. Use of monoclonal antibodies in the diagnosis of atrophic rhinitis. Proc Int Congr Pig Vet Soc, Rio de Janeiro, p. 33.

FOGED, N. T.; NIELSEN, J. P.; AND JORSAL, S. E. 1989. Protection against progressive atrophic rhinitis by vaccination with *Pasteurella multocida* toxin purified by monoclonal antibodies. Vet Rec 125(1):7–11.

FOGED, N. T.; NIELSEN J. P.; AND BARFOD, K. 1990. The use of ELISA determination of *Pasteurella multocida* toxin antibodies in the control of progressive atrophic rhinitis. Proc Int Congr Pig Vet Soc, Lausanne, p. 49.

FRANQUE. 1830. Was ist die Schnuffelkrankheit der Schweine? Dtsch Z Gesammte Tierheilkd 1:75.

FROE, D. L., II. 1990. Oral tetracyclines: Factors affecting serum levels and efficacy. Proc Int Congr Pig Vet Soc, Lausanne, p. 353.

FRYMUS, T.; MULLER, E.; FRANZ, B.; AND PETZOLD, K. 1989. Protection by toxoid-induced antibody of gnotobiotic piglets challenged with dermonecrotic toxin of *P. multocida*. J Vet Med [B] 36:674–680.

GILES, C. J. 1986. Atrophic rhinitis. In Diseases of Swine, 6th ed. Ed. A. D. Leman, B. Straw, R. D. Glock, W. L. Mengeling, R. H. C. Penny, and E. Scholl. Ames: Iowa State Univ Press, pp. 455–469.

GILES, C. J., AND SMITH, I. M. 1982. The value of vaccinating pigs with *Bordetella bronchiseptica*. Pig Vet Soc Proc 9:61.

_____. 1983. Vaccination of pigs with *Bordetella bronchiseptica*. Vet Bull 53:327.

GOIS, M.; KUKSA, F.; AND SISAK, F. 1977. Experimental infection of gnotobiotic piglets with *Mycoplasma hyorhinis* and *Bordetella bronchiseptica*. Zentralbl Veterinaermed 24:89.

GOIS, M.; BARNES, H. J.; AND ROSS, R. F. 1983a. Potentiation of turbinate atrophy in pigs by long-term nasal colonization with *Pasteurella multocida*. Am J Vet Res 44:372.

GOIS, M.; FARRINGTON, D. O.; BARNES, H. J.; AND ROSS, R. F. 1983b. Long-acting oxytetracycline for control of induced *Pasteurella multocida* rhinitis in swine. J Am Vet Med Assoc 183:445.

GOODNOW, R. A. 1980. Biology of *Bordetella bronchisepti-*

ca. Microbiol Rev 44:722–738.

GOODWIN, R. F. W. 1980. Atrophic rhinitis of pigs. Vet Rec [Pract Suppl] 2:5.

_____. 1988. Monitoring for atrophic rhinitis; the problem of higher snout scores. Vet Rec 123: 566–568.

GOODWIN, R. F. W.; CHANTER, N.; AND RUTTER, J. M. 1990. Detection and distribution of toxigenic *Pasteurella multocida* in pig herds with different degrees of atrophic rhinitis. Vet Rec 126:452–456.

GWATKIN, R. 1959. Rhinitis of swine. XII. Some practical aspects of the rhinitis complex. Can J Comp Med Vet Sci 23:338.

GWATKIN, R.; PLUMMER, P. J. G.; BYRNE, J. L.; AND WALKER, R. V. L. 1949. Rhinitis of swine. III. Transmission to baby pigs. Can J Comp Med Vet Sci 13:15.

_____. 1951. Rhinitis of swine. V. Further studies on the aetiology of infectious atrophic rhinitis. Can J Comp Med Vet Sci 15:32.

HARRIS, D. L., AND SWITZER, W. P. 1968. Turbinate atrophy in young pigs exposed to *Bordetella bronchiseptica, Pasteurella multocida* and combined inoculum. Am J Vet Res 29:777.

_____. 1969. Nasal and tracheal resistance of swine against reinfection by *Bordetella bronchiseptica*. Am J Vet Res 30:1161–1166.

HOJE, S.; NORBY, K.; AND FALK, K. 1990. Plasmid profiles of selected strains of *P. multocida* from pneumonic lesions of slaughterweight swine. Proc Int Congr Pig Vet Soc, Lausanne, p. 104.

ILINA, Z. M., AND ZASUKHIN, M. I. 1975. Sb Nauch Rab, Sib Zonal' Nauchno-Issled Vet Inst, Omsk 25:76.

IWAMATSU, S., AND SAWADA, T. 1988. Relationship between serotypes, dermonecrotic toxin production of *Pasteurella multocida* isolates and pneumonic lesions of porcine lung. Jpn J Vet Sci 50(6):1200–1206.

JAMES, A. 1989. The manifestation and attempted eradication of atrophic rhinitis in a newly established Duroc herd. Pig Vet J 23:113–121.

JOLIE, R.; AND THACKER, B. 1990. Comparison of atrophic rhinitis morphometric measurements and macroscopic grades of nasal cross sections on computerized tomography scans in pigs. Proc Int Congr Pig Vet Soc, Lausanne, p. 53.

JOLIE, R.; DE ROOSE, P.; AND TUYTTENS, N. 1990. Diagnosis of atrophic rhinitis by computerized tomography: A preliminary report. Vet Rec 126:591–594.

JONES, T. L. 1947. Rhinitis in swine. Agric Inst Rev 2:274.

KAMP, E. M.; TER LAAK, E. A.; AND DE JONG, M. F. 1990. Atypical pasteurella strains producing a toxin similar to the dermonecrotic toxin of *P. multocida*. subsp. *multiocida*. Vet Rec 126:434–437.

KAMPS, A. M. I. E.; BUYS, W. E. C. M.; KAMP, E. M.; AND SMITS, M. A. 1990. Specificity of DNA probes for the detection of toxigenic *Pasteurella multocida* subsp. *multocida* strains. J Clin Microbiol 28:1858–1861.

KIELSTEIN, P. 1983. Zur Bordetelleninfektion des Schweines und die Bedeutung von Tiermodellen zum Nachweis protektiver Eigenschaften von *Bordetella bronchiseptica*. Monatsh Vet Med 38:504–509.

KOBISCH, M., AND PENNINGS, A. 1989. An evaluation in pigs of Nobi-Vac AR and an experimental atrophic rhinitis vaccine containing *P. multocida* DNT-toxoid and *B. bronchiseptica*. Vet Rec 124:57–61.

KOSHIMIZU, K.; KODAMA, Y.; OGATA, M.; SANBYAKU-DA, S.; OTAKE, J.; AND MIMURA, M. 1973. Studies on the etiology of infectious atrophic rhinitis of swine. V. Experimental *Bordetella bronchiseptica* infection in conventional piglets. Jpn J Vet Sci 35:223.

LARSEN, S.; HOGEDAL JORGENSEN, P.; AND NIELSEN, P. A. 1990. Elimination of specific pathogens in 3 to 4

week old piglets by use of strategic medication. Proc Int Congr Pig Vet Soc, Lausanne, p. 387.

LAX, A. J., AND CHANTER, N. 1990. Cloning of the toxin gene from *Pasteurella multocida* and its role in atrophic rhinitis. Proc Int Congr Pig Vet Soc, Lausanne, p. 61.

LEBLANC, R.; DENICOURT, M.; LARIVIÈRA, S.; AND MARTINEAU, G. P. 1986a. Comparison of isolation methods for the recovery of *Bordetella bronchiseptica* and *Pasteurella multocida* from the nasal cavities of piglets. Proc Int Congr Pig Vet Soc, Barcelona, p. 226.

LEBLANC, R.; LARIVIÈRA, S.; MARTINEAU, G. P.; AND MITTAL, K. R. 1986b. Characterization of *P. multocida* isolated from the nasal cavities of piglets from farms with or without atrophic rhinitis. Proc Int Congr Pig Vet Soc, Barcelona, p. 225.

LUGTENBERG, B.; BOXTEL, R. V.; AND DE JONG, M. F. 1984. Atrophic rhinitis in swine, correlation of *Pasteurella multocida* pathogenicity with membrane protein and lipopolysaccharide patterns. Infect Immun 46:48–54.

MACNABB, A. L. 1948. Rhinitis. Ont Vet Col Rep.

MARTINEAU, G. P.; BROES, A.; DE JONG, M. F.; AND MARTINEAU-DOIZE, B. 1982. Experimental reproduction of atrophic rhinitis with *P. multocida* in gnotobiotic and conventional piglets. Proc Int Congr Pig Vet Soc, Mexico City, p. 88.

MARTINEAU, G. P.; DENICOURT, M.; CHARETTE, P.; LAMBERT, J.; DESILETS, A.; SAUVAGEAU, R.; AND COUSINEAU, G. 1988. Retrospective study on atrophic rhinitis and enzootic pneumonia found in pigs at Quebec central testing station. Pt 2. Breed effect. Med Vet Quebec 18(4):175–179.

MARTINEAU-DOIZE, B.; FRANTZ, J. C.; AND MARTINEAU, G. P. 1990. Cartilage and bone lesions: An explanation of the severity of conchal atrophy induced by *Pasteurella multocida* type D dermonecrotic toxin. Proc Int Congr Vet Soc, Lausanne, p. 68.

MEFFORD, D. E.; VINSON, R. A.; SWAFFORD, W. S.; AND PINKSTON, M. L. 1983. The efficacy of long-acting oxytetracycline and/or *Bordetella/Pasteurella* bacterin in a swine herd with enzootic atrophic rhinitis. Vet Med Small Anim Clin 78:1911.

MINIATS, O. P., AND JOHNSON, J. A. 1980. Experimental atrophic rhinitis in gnotobiotic pigs. Can J Comp Med 44:358.

NAGY, L. K.; MACKENZIE, T.; AND SCARNELL, J. 1986. Serum antibody values to *Pasteurella multocida* type D toxin and susceptibility of piglets to experimental challenge with toxigenic type D of *P. multocida*. Proc Int Congr Pig Vet Soc, Barcelona, p. 224.

NAKAGAWA, M.; SHIMIZU, T.; AND MOTOI, Y. 1974. Pathology of experimental atrophic rhinitis in swine infected with *Alcaligenes bronchisepticus* or *Pasteurella multocida*. Natl Inst Anim Health Q (Tokyo) 14:61.

NAKAI, T.; KUME, K.; YOSHIKAWA, H.; OYAMADA, T.; AND YOSHIKAW, T. 1986. Changes in the nasal mucosa of specific-pathogen-free neonatal pigs infected with *Pasteurella multocida* or *Bordetella bronchiseptica*. Jpn J Vet Sci 48(4):693–701.

NIELSEN, N. C. 1983. Prevalence and economic significance of atrophic rhinitis. In Atrophic Rhinitis of Pigs. Ed. K. B. Pedersen and N. C. Nielsen. Comm Eur Communities Rep EUR 8643 EN, Luxembourg, p. 35.

NIELSEN, J. P.; AND FREDERIKSEN, W. 1990. Atrophic rhinitis in pigs caused by a human isolate of toxigenic *Pasteurella multocida*. Proc Int Congr Pig Vet Soc, Lausanne, p. 75.

NIELSEN, J. P., AND ROSDAHL, V. T. 1988. Phage-typing of toxigenic *Pasteurella multocida*. Proc Int Congr Pig Vet Soc, Rio de Janeiro, p. 34.

_____. 1990. Development and epidemiological applications of a bacteriophage typing system for typing *P. multocida.* J Clin Microbiol 28:103–107.

NIELSEN, N. C.; RIISING, H. J.; AND BILLE, N. 1976. Experimental reproduction of atrophic rhinitis in pigs reared to slaughter weight. Proc 4th Int Congr Pig Vet Soc, Iowa State Univ, p. 202.

NIELSEN, J. P.; BISGAARD, M.; AND PEDERSEN, K. B. 1986. Occurrence of toxin-producing strains of *P. multocida* in different mammalian and avian species. Proc Int Congr Pig Vet Soc, Barcelona, p. 232.

OHKUBO, Y.; HIRAMUNE, T.; AND KIKUCHI, N. 1987. Sero-types and dermonecrotic activity of *Pasteurella multocida* isolates from nares of rabbits. J of the College of Dairying, Japan. Nat Sci 12(1):279–285.

OVERBY, E. 1990. Determination of a possible survival rate of *Actinobacillus pleuropneumoniae* bacteria in an EDTA semen dilution experimentally infected. Proc Int Congr Pig Vet Soc, Lausanne, p. 45.

OWEN, J. E. 1982. The influence of buildings on respiratory disease. Pig Vet Soc Proc 9:24.

PEARCE, H. G., AND ROE, C. K. 1966. Infectious atrophic rhinitis: A review. Can Vet J 7:243.

PEDERSEN, K. B. 1983. Cultural and serological diagnosis of atrophic rhinitis in pigs. In Atrophic Rhinitis of Pigs. Ed. K. B. Pedersen and N. C. Nielsen. Comm Eur Communities Rep EUR 8643 EN, Luxembourg, p. 22.

PEDERSEN, K. B., AND BARFOD, K. 1982. Effect on the incidence of atrophic rhinitis of vaccination of sows with a vaccine containing *Pasteurella multocida* toxin. Nord Vet Med 34:293.

PEDERSEN, K. B., AND NIELSEN, N. C., eds. 1983. Atrophic Rhinitis of Pigs. Comm Eur Communities Rep EUR 8643 EN, Luxembourg, p. 205.

PEDERSEN, K. B.; NIELSEN, J. P.; FOGED, N. T.; ELLING, F.; NIELSEN, N. C.; AND WILLEBERG, P. 1988. Atrophic rhinitis in pigs: Proposal for a revised definition. Vet Rec 20:190.

PEJSAK, Z.; HOGG, A.; FOREMAN, K.; AND WASINSKA, B. 1990. The effect of terramycin LA in combination with a *Bordetella/Pasteurella* vaccine in controlling atrophic rhinitis in swine. Proc Int Congr Pig Vet Soc, Lausanne, p. 76.

PENNINGS, A. M. M. A., AND STORM, P. K. 1984. A test in Vero-cell monolayers for toxin production by strains of *Pasteurella multocida* isolated from pigs suspected of having atrophic rhinitis. Vet Microbiol 9:503–508.

PENNY, R. H. C. 1977. The influence of management changes on the disease picture in pigs. Vet Annu 17:111.

PHILIPS, C. E. 1946. Infectious rhinitis in swine (bull nose). Can J Comp Med Vet Sci 10:33.

PHILIPS, C. E.; LONFIELD, H. F.; AND MILTIMORE, J. E. 1948. Porcine infectious atrophic rhinitis experiments. Can J Comp Med Vet Sci 12:268.

PIJOAN, C.; TRIGO, E.; AND HOGG, A. 1988. Atrophic rhinitis in pigs associated with a toxigenic strain of *Pasteurella multocida* serotype A. Proc Int Congr Pig Vet Soc, Rio de Janeiro, p. 32.

PIJPERS, A.; VAN KLINGEREN, B.; SCHOEVERS, E. J.; VERHEYDEN, J. H. M.; AND VAN MIERT, A. S. P. 1988. The in vitro activity of some antimicrobial agents against 4 porcine respiratory tract pathogens. Proc Int Congr Pig Vet Soc, Rio de Janeiro, p. 98.

PLONAIT, H., AND BICKHARDT, K. 1988. Lehrbuch der Schweinekrankheiten. Berlin: Verlag Paul Parey.

PLONAIT, H.; HEINEL, K. G.; AND BOLLWAHN, W. 1980. Vergleich von Endoskopie und Rontgenaufnahmen als Hilfsmittel zur Diagnose der Rhinitis atrophicans am lebenden Schwein. Prakt Tieraerztl 61:1056–1064.

RATKE, G. 1938. Untersuchungen uber die Ursache und das Wesen der Schuffelkrankheit des Schweines. Ar-

chiv Wiss Prakt Tierheilkd 72:371.

RONDHUIS, P. R.; DE JONG, M. F.; AND SCHEP, J. 1980. Indirect fluorescence antibody studies of porcine cytomegalovirus infections in the Netherlands. Vet Q 2:65–68.

ROSS, R. F.; SWITZER, W. P.; AND DUNCAN, J. R. 1967. Comparison of pathogenicity of various isolates of *Bordetella bronchiseptica* in young pigs. Can J Comp Med Vet Sci 31:53–57.

RUTTER, J. M. 1981. Quantitative observations on *Bordetella bronchiseptica* infection in atrophic rhinitis of pigs. Vet Rec 108:451–454.

_____. 1983. Virulence of *Pasteurella multocida* in atrophic rhinitis of gnotobiotic pigs infected with *Bordetella bronchiseptica.* Res Vet Sci 34:287.

_____. 1985. Atrophic rhinitis in swine. Adv Vet Sci Comp Med 29:239–279.

RUTTER, J. M., AND LUTHER, P. D. 1984. Cell culture assay for toxigenic *Pasteurella multocida* from atrophic rhinitis of pigs. Vet Rec 114:393–396.

RUTTER, J. M., AND MACKENZIE, A. 1984. Pathogenesis of atrophic rhinitis in pigs. A new perspective. Vet Rec 114:89.

RUTTER, J. M., AND ROJAS, X. 1982. Atrophic rhinitis in gnotobiotic piglets: Differences in the pathogenicity of *Pasteurella multocida* in combined infection with *Bordetella bronchiseptica.* Vet Rec 110:531.

RUTTER, J. M.; TAYLOR, R. J.; CRIGHTON, W. G.; ROBERTSON, I. B.; AND BENTSON, A. J. 1984. Epidemiological study of *Pasteurella multocida* and *Bordetella bronchiseptica* in atrophic rhinitis. Vet Rec 115:615–619.

RUTTER, J. M.; BEARD, M.; CARPENTER, G. A.; AND FRYER, J. T. 1986. The effect of air filtration on the performance and health of pigs. Proc Int Congr Pig Vet Soc, Barcelona, p. 400.

SCHIMMELPFENNIG, H. 1990. Rhinitis atrophicans (Ra) des Schweines: Zur Neutralisation des Toxins von *Pasteurella multocida.* Dtsch Tieraerztl Wochenschr 97:195–196.

SCHIMMELPFENNIG, H., AND JAHN, B. 1988. Rhinitis atrophicans (R.a.) des Schweines: Ein Hauttest zum Nachweis antitoxischer *Pasteurella multocida* Antikorper. Dtsch Tieraerztl Wochenschr 95:285–286.

SCHÖSS, P. 1982. *Bordetella bronchiseptica* Infektionen in einem SPF Schweinebestand. Ein Beitrag zur Atiologie der Rhinitis atrophicans. Dtsch Tieraerztl Wochenschr 89:177–181.

_____. 1983. Clinical diagnosis of atrophic rhinitis. In Atrophic Rhinitis of Pigs. Ed. K. B. Pedersen and N. C. Nielsen. Comm Eur Communities Rep EUR 8643 EN, Luxembourg, p. 13.

SCHÖSS, P., AND THIEL, C. P. 1984. Occurrence of toxin-producing strains of *Pasteurella multocida* and *Bordetella bronchiseptica* in pig herds with atrophic rhinitis and in unaffected herds. Proc 8th Int Congr Pig Vet Soc, Ghent, p. 94.

SCHULLER, W.; TRUBRICH, H.; KOSZTOLICH, O.; FLATSCHER, J.; AND JAHN, J. 1980. Vaccination against atrophic rhinitis in swine with a combined *Bordetella bronchiseptica, Pasteurella multocida* vaccine. Zentralbl Veterinaermed 27:125.

SKELLY, B. J.; PRUSS, M.; PELLEGRINO, R.; ANDERSEN, D.; AND ABRUZZO, G. 1980. Variation in degree of atrophic rhinitis with field isolants of *Bordetella bronchiseptica.* Proc Int Congr Pig Vet Soc, Copenhagen, p. 210.

SMITH, I. M. 1971. Studies on the role of some microorganisms in respiratory infections of the pig with special reference to the involvement of *Pasteurella septica.* Ph.D. diss., Univ. of London.

SMITH, I. M., AND BASKERVILLE, A. J. 1983. A selective medium for the isolation of *P. multocida* in nasal specimens from pigs. Br Vet J 139:476.

SMITH, I. M., AND GILES, C. J. 1980. Vaccines for atrophic rhinitis. Pig Farming Suppl (Oct.):83.

SMITH, W. J. 1983. Infectious atrophic rhinitis: Noninfectious determinants. In Atrophic Rhinitis of Pigs. Ed. K. B. Pedersen and N. C. Nielsen. Comm Eur Communities Rep EUR 8643 EN, Luxembourg, p. 151.

SORENSEN, V.; BARFOD, K.; NIELSEN, J. P.; AND FOGED, N. T. 1990. Effect of degree of atrophy and serum antitoxin titer on the daily weight gain and feed conversion. Proc Int Congr Pig Vet Soc, Lausanne, p. 57.

STEHMANN, R.; MEHLHORN, G.; AND NEUPARTH, V. 1989. Detection of *Bordetella bronchiseptica* in the air of farrowing and weaned piglet pens. Monatsh Vet Med 44:307–311.

STRANG, M. M. 1982. The influence of feed and feed delivery systems on respiratory disease. Pig Vet Soc Proc 9:36.

STRAW, B. E.; BURGI, E. J.; HILLEY, H. D.; AND LEMAN, A. D. 1983. Pneumonia and atrophic rhinitis in pigs from a test station. J Am Vet Med Assoc 182:607.

SUTTER, M. TH., AND WANNER, M. 1990. Higher bioavailability of tetracyclines given with liquid feed in weaned pigs. Proc Int Congr Pig Vet Soc, Lausanne, p. 353.

SWITZER, W. P. 1951. Atrophic rhinitis and trichomonads. Vet Med 46:478.

_____. 1953. Studies on infectious atrophic rhinitis of swine. I. Isolation of a filterable agent from the nasal cavity of swine with infectious atrophic rhinitis. J Am Vet Med Assoc 123:45.

_____. 1955. Studies on infectious atrophic rhinitis. IV. Characterization of a pleuropneumonia-like organism isolated from the nasal cavities of swine. Am J Vet Res 16:540.

_____. 1956. Studies on infectious atrophic rhinitis. V. Concept that several agents may cause turbinate atrophy. Am J Vet Res 17:478.

SWITZER, W. P., AND FARRINGTON. D. O. 1975. Infectious atrophic rhinitis. In Diseases of Swine, 4th ed. Ed. H. W. Dunne and A. D. Leman. Ames: Iowa State Univ Press, p. 687.

SWITZER, W. P., AND L'ECUYER, C. 1960. Detection of swine nasal viruses in cell culture. Am J Vet Res 21:967.

TERPSTRA, J. I., AND AKKERMANS, J. P. W. M. 1960. Enkele aantekeningen over Atrofische Rhinitis. Tijdschr Diergeneeskd 85:1222–1233.

THUNBERG, E., AND CARLSTROM, B. 1940. Om nyssjuka hos svin fran epizootisynpunkt. Skand Vet 30:711. Can J Comp Med Vet Sci 10:169.

TRIGO, E., AND PIJOAN, C. 1988. Effect of piliation, hemagglutination and capsular serotype of *Pasteurella multocida* on the production of atrophic rhinitis in swine. Proc Int Congr Pig Vet Soc, Rio de Janeiro, p. 31.

VAN GEENGOED, L. A.; KAMP, E. M.; AND VECHT, U. 1986. Tonsil biopsy: A tool in epidemiological studies of atrophic rhinitis and streptococcal meningitis in pigs. Proc Int Congr Pig Vet Soc, Barcelona, p. 227.

VAN GROENLAND, G. J. 1984. Measuring the distance between tooth edges in piglets as a way to monitor breeding farms for atrophic rhinitis. Proc Int Congr Vet Soc, Ghent.

VISSER, I. J. R; VAN DEN INGH, T. S. G. A. M.; DE KRUIJF, J. M.; TIELEN, M. J. M.; URLINGS, H. A. P.; AND GRUYS, E. 1988. Atrofische rhinitis: The use of longitudinal sections of pigs' heads in the diagnosis of atrophy of the turbinate bones at the slaughter line. Tijdschr Diergeneeskd 113(24):1345–1355.

VOETS, M. TH. 1990. Evaluation of the challenge model to test AR vaccines. Proc Int Congr Pig Vet Soc, Lausanne, p. 56.

VOETS, M. TH.; TIELEN, M. J. M.; AND HUNNEMAN, W. 1986a. The heritability of conchal atrophy in a slight AR-infection. Proc Int Congr Pig Vet Soc, Barcelona, p. 391.

_____. 1986b. UV-ray treatment of air to prevent atrophic rhinitis. Proc Int Congr Pig Vet Soc, Barcelona, p. 404.

WEBBON, P. M.; PENNY, R. H. C.; AND GRAY, J. 1978. Atrophic rhinitis. The value of radiography for diagnosis in piglets. Br Vet J 134:193.

WILLIAMS, P. R.; HALL, R. M.; AND RIMLER, R. B. 1986. Effect of purified *Pasteurella multocida* turbinate atrophy toxin on porcine peripheral blood lymphocytes in vivo and in vitro. Proc Int Congr Pig Vet Soc, Barcelona, p. 234.

YOSHIKAWA, T., AND HANADA, T. 1981. Histological studies on pigs with atrophic rhinitis showing retarded growth. Jpn J Vet Sci 43:221.

34 Bordetellosis

C. J. Giles

IN PIGS, *Bordetella bronchiseptica* was first isolated from pneumonic lungs (Thorp and Tanner 1940; Phillips 1943), and although this organism may, on occasion, be responsible for a primary bronchopneumonia in young pigs, and may also occur as a secondary pathogen of the lower respiratory tract in older animals, its chief importance results from its ability to colonize the nasal cavity and induce inflammatory lesions in the nasal mucosa and hypoplastic changes in the developing turbinate bones (conchae) of young pigs.

B. bronchiseptica was first isolated from the nasal cavity by Switzer (1956), who subsequently demonstrated the unaided ability of this organism to induce hypoplastic (atrophic) changes in the turbinates and consequently laid the foundation for its implication as a primary pathogen in atrophic rhinitis (AR), in which turbinate atrophy is the dominant lesion. Following this discovery, nasal bordetellosis and AR have been inextricably linked and were even, for a period, regarded as virtually synonymous by some authorities (Ogata et al. 1970; Switzer and Farrington 1975; Switzer 1981). This view failed, however, to gain worldwide acceptance and a substantial body of opinion, especially from Western Europe, persisted with the opinion that the precise extent or manner of the involvement of *B. bronchiseptica* in AR was much less clear-cut (Done 1975; De Jong et al. 1976; Tornøe et al. 1976; Giles et al. 1980; Goodwin 1980; Pedersen and Barfod 1981; Rutter 1981; Whittlestone 1982), and this view has now gained wide acceptance.

Over the last decade many experimental and field studies have now clearly established that bordetellosis and AR should no longer be regarded as equivalent and have more clearly defined both the etiology of AR and the pathogenic significance of *B. bronchiseptica* in pigs. The key information is summarized below.

1. In commercial pig herds the prevalence of infection with *B. bronchiseptica* greatly exceeds that of clinical AR, the organism being found in herds both with and without the clinical disease (Tornøe et al. 1976; Giles et al. 1980). Furthermore, there may be no differences in the prevalence or relative intensity of nasal infection with this organism among young pigs in herds from either category (Rutter 1981).

2. Turbinate hypoplasia induced experimentally by *B. bronchiseptica* can be quite marked in pigs up to 8 weeks old, but these lesions neither progress, intensify, nor develop into clinical AR despite persistent nasal infection when the pigs are reared to slaughter weight in an environment free from spontaneous cases of the disease (Pedersen and Barfod 1981; Smith et al. 1982).

3. There is good evidence that such hypoplastic turbinates may regenerate by the time the pigs have reached conventional slaughter weight (Duncan et al. 1966a; Tornøe and Nielsen 1976; Rutter 1981; Smith et al. 1982).

4. Major advances have now been made by our understanding of the bacterial pathogens involved in AR following definition of the primary etiological role played by infection with toxigenic strains of *Pasteurella multocida* in this condition (De Jong et al. 1980). Most aspects of clinical AR have now been reproduced experimentally by a combined infection of the two bacteria (Pedersen and Barfod 1981; Rutter and Rojas 1982).

5. The pathogenesis of *B. bronchiseptica* infection has been more clearly elucidated. Differences are known to exist among porcine strains and the ability of the organism to induce turbinate hypoplasia in young pigs is dependent on its capacity to produce a cytotoxin (Magyar et al. 1988). Such toxigenic strains are, however, widely distributed in pig herds (Rutter 1989).

6. Prior infection of the nasal cavity of the young pig by toxigenic strains of *B. bronchiseptica* is able to increase the ability of toxigenic *P. multocida* to colonize the nasal mucosa (Chanter et al. 1989).

The importance of *B. bronchiseptica* as a pathogen of the pig is now able to be more clearly defined. *B. bronchiseptica* can be a significant nasal pathogen of the young pig in which, acting alone, it is capable of inducing a mild to moderately severe degree of turbinate hypoplasia. In uncomplicated field infections this hypoplasia is often of little clinical significance, but when the required infectious and other factors necessary for the development of AR are also present within the herd, such lesions may progress to clinical AR. The major significance of *B. bronchiseptica* infection in pig herds is its ability to initiate turbinate damage and assist the colonization of the nasal cavity by toxigenic strains of *P. multocida,* and as such, is therefore a significant predisposing or contributory factor in the pathogenesis of AR.

Atrophic rhinitis is considered in greater detail in Chapter 33. A large volume of knowledge has accumulated specifically about bordetellosis, and the present chapter is concerned mainly with the effects of this uncomplicated infection and those of Chapter 33 deal more widely with clinical AR; however, when considering the complex problem of AR, readers are recommended to study both chapters.

ETIOLOGY. *Bordetella bronchiseptica* is a motile, gram-negative rod or coccobacillus (approx. size 1.0×0.3 μm). The bacterium is aerobic, does not ferment carbohydrates, utilizes citrate, and splits urea.

Switzer (1956) first reported that a bacterium, described originally as an *Alcaligenes* sp. but subsequently identified as *B. bronchiseptica,* was capable of inducing turbinate atrophy when pure cultures were inoculated intranasally into young pigs free from respiratory disease. This experimental effect has been widely examined and the unaided ability of the prevailing porcine strains of the organism to induce a hypoplastic rhinitis in young conventional or gnotobiotic pigs has been consistently verified (Duncan et al. 1966a; Harris and Switzer 1968; Shimizu et al. 1971; Nakagawa et al. 1974; Edington et al. 1976; Tornøe and Nielsen 1976; Rutter et al. 1982; Magyar et al. 1988). At times a variable degree of bronchopneumonia may also occur (Duncan et al. 1966b; Meyer and Beamer 1973).

Observations on the experimental disease are thus numerous and the clinical and pathological effects of the infection well documented. *B. bronchiseptica* has been isolated widely from young pigs with rhinitis, from outbreaks of infectious atrophic rhinitis, from pigs with pneumonia, and also from animals in herds showing no clinical signs of respiratory disease. It is also a pathogen or potential pathogen of many other mammals, including dogs, cats, and rats.

EPIDEMIOLOGY

Prevalence. *B. bronchiseptica* is widely prevalent in the pig population in countries with major swine-producing industries. In the United States estimates based on the culture of nasal swabs from young pigs have shown that 25–54% of pig herds (Ross et al. 1963; Harris et al. 1969) and about 11% of pigs (Farrington and Switzer 1977; Jenkins et al. 1977) were infected with the organism. Prevalence estimates from Western Europe have been broadly similar or higher. In general, estimates of prevalence based on serological testing have been greater than those from culture (Kang et al. 1971; Jenkins et al. 1977).

The prevalence of *B. bronchiseptica* infection greatly exceeds that of clinical AR or marked turbinate atrophy at slaughter (Cameron et al. 1980),

and although *B. bronchiseptica* is frequently isolated from young pigs in outbreaks of AR, the infection also occurs widely in herds without the condition (Tornøe et al. 1976; Giles et al. 1980; Rutter 1981; Whittlestone 1982).

Transmission of Infection. The chief mode of transmission of *B. bronchiseptica* from pig to pig is by aerosol droplet infection. The high prevalence of infection among growing pigs suggests that transmission may occur at any age, but it is probably more common and more readily accomplished in susceptible young pigs in which an active rhinitis with sneezing develops. The infection can certainly spread rapidly among populations of susceptible (nonimmune) piglets (Smith et al. 1982).

Factors Influencing Infection

AGE. The ability of the sucking piglet to resist infection depends not only on the weight of challenge but also on the degree of immunity conferred by the passive transfer of colostral antibody. In the field the degree of passive protection afforded by different sows varies both within and between infected herds (Giles 1981), and at least while it operates, bordetellosis often tends to be a litter infection. The infection becomes more widely disseminated, however, following the mixing of piglets after weaning. The peak prevalence occurs in pigs of about 12 weeks (Switzer and Farrington 1972; Jenkins et al. 1977) or later in some herds (Giles 1981); a high proportion remain infected until 18–20 weeks (Cameron et al. 1980). Thereafter, an age-related decline in infection rate ensues (Switzer and Farrington 1972; Tornøe et al. 1976). The age when the pig initially acquires the infection is of key importance, since the damage the infection can produce declines with age (Duncan et al. 1966a) and infections acquired initially in the late-weaning or fattening stages of production are of little clinical significance (Giles et al. 1980).

Source of Infection

PIGS. The sow can act as a major source of infection to her sucking piglets (Switzer and Farrington 1972, 1975). Repeated nasal swabbing of sows in infected herds (Farrington 1974) indicated that a proportion do carry the organism, which in turn can be transmitted to the susceptible piglets of the litter. Once established, the infection in sucking pigs acts as a source for aerosol transmission to adjacent litters. The degree of resistance to natural *B. bronchiseptica* infection among sows does not appear to be marked, but younger sows are more likely to be active shedders of the organism. While infection from the dam is probably the chief method of at least initiating the infection among populations of sucking piglets, infection in weaner houses may often be endemic, infection passing laterally between different batches, particularly in systems where an "all-in/all-out" approach is not practiced.

B. bronchiseptica is primarily introduced into a previously uninfected herd by the introduction of carrier pigs; recently purchased breeding stock are often held responsible, although the evidence for their involvement is often merely circumstantial.

OTHER SOURCES. Sources of infection other than pigs have also been considered important (Switzer 1981), since the organism has been recovered from cats, rats, rabbits, and other wildlife (Ross et al. 1967; Farrington and Jorgensen 1976) that may gain access to pig farms, but their significance remains doubtful. Although some of these isolates will produce a degree of turbinate hypoplasia in young pigs (Ross et al. 1967), there are undoubtedly differences in virulence for pigs between porcine strains and those isolated from other species. Rutter and Collings (1983) concluded that infection of pigs with strains from other species is not likely to be hazardous, since in their experiments, significant turbinate lesions were only induced in gnotobiotic pigs infected with strains of porcine origin and this was associated with better colonization of the nasal cavity and greater toxin production.

Virulence. Variations in virulence among porcine strains are known to exist, but the significance of any differences in the field remains uncertain. Collings and Rutter (1985) determined that only those strains in phase 1 and isolated from pigs caused turbinate atrophy, and they established that the ability to both colonize the nasal cavity in large numbers and produce a cytotoxin were important virulence determinants. The role of the cytotoxin was clearly established by Magyar et al. (1988), who also examined the role of several other putative virulence determinants, including a hemolysin, adenylate cyclase, and an adhesin. By comparing the pathogenic effects of a porcine cytotoxic phase 1 strain with a noncytotoxic phase 1 strain also of porcine origin, they established that it is the cytotoxin (which is probably the same as the mouse lethal factor and dermonecrotic toxin) that is the key virulence determinant in the production of turbinate atrophy.

PATHOGENESIS. In an attempt to explain the mechanism of development of the turbinate atrophy in atrophic rhinitis, the pathogenesis of *B. bronchiseptica* infection of the nasal cavity has been studied in detail, particularly with regard to the nature and effects of putative toxic factors from the organism and the osteoblastic damage produced in the developing cancellous bone. However, the precise mechanism by which the organism produces the lesions of the turbinate

scrolls still remains uncertain. It is considered that colonization of the nasal cavity by *B. bronchiseptica* is by adherence of the organism to the nasal mucosa, where it probably preferentially attaches to the ciliated epithelial cells (Yokomizu and Shimizu 1979). This is followed by multiplication at the mucosal surface and toxin production leading to inflammatory, proliferative, and degenerative changes in the nasal epithelium, including the loss of cilia (Duncan et al. 1966a; Edington et al. 1976). The organism is not considered to invade the deeper tissues.

It is assumed that the organism at the mucosal surface elaborates a toxin that diffuses into the osseous core of the nasal turbinate and is responsibile for the osteopathy. The nature of this toxic factor has received much attention. Cell-free sonicated extracts from phase 1 *B. bronchiseptica* were originally shown to contain a heat-labile and dermonecrotic toxin, and it was assumed that this was probably an important factor in pathogenesis, since when such bacteria-free extracts containing high levels of this toxin were repeatedly inoculated intranasally into piglets, they produced nasal lesions similar to those seen in naturally occurring AR (Hanada et al. 1979; Nakase et al. 1980). The studies of Roop et al. (1987) confirmed that a dermonecrotic toxin is required for turbinate atrophy to develop. It is probable that this dermonecrotic toxin and the cytotoxin (Magyar et al. 1988) are the same factor. There is some variation in the toxigenicity of different strains of *B. bronchiseptica;* porcine phase 1 strains are more toxigenic than phase 3 or nonporcine isolates (Collings and Rutter 1985).

It has long been considered (Schofield and Jones 1950) that a defective osteogenesis rather than osteolysis is the basic mechanism underlying the development of turbinate hypoplasia in the young pig. Ultrastructural observations tend to confirm this, since they have revealed that it is the osteoblasts (on the inner aspect of the periosteum) that are the bone cells where (ultrastructural) abnormalities occur in bordetella-induced hypoplastic rhinitis (Fetter et al. 1975; Silveira et al. 1982).

Turbinate Regeneration. There is considerable field and experimental evidence that the hypoplasia of the turbinates produced by the uncomplicated infection of young pigs (up to about 8 weeks old) is capable of (sometimes even complete) regeneration (Duncan et al. 1966a; Tornøe and Nielsen 1976; Rutter 1981; Smith et al. 1982).

A degree of turbinate hypoplasia in young pigs, with a variable amount of subsequent regeneration as the pig grows to slaughter weight, may thus occur in most herds infected with *B. bronchiseptica*. This probably accounts for the high prevalence of mild lesions of turbinate atrophy seen at slaughter in the many bordetella-infected herds free from obvious clinical AR, especially in cases where the nasal cavity remains infected with other species, particularly with nontoxigenic *P. multocida* or *Haemophilus* sp. However, in herds where further infections (particularly with toxigenic *P. multocida*) and other factors operate, the initial bordetella-induced hypoplasia becomes progressive and intensifies, and clinical AR with severe turbinate atrophy and snout deformations becomes manifest as detailed in Chapter 33.

CLINICAL SIGNS. The principal signs seen in bordetellosis are sneezing and snuffling in young pigs. This can occur in piglets as young as 1 week but is frequently seen at or about the time of weaning, which may be related both to the waning of maternal colostral protection and the mixing of pigs at this stage. As an example, where pigs are weaned at 3 weeks, the sneezing frequently starts about a week after weaning.

Affected piglets sneeze, snuffle, and snort with a variable degree of catarrhal rhinitis producing a variable amount of serous or frequently mucopurulent nasal discharge, which may be observed by swabbing the nasal cavity. Generally, the younger the piglet when initially affected, the more severe the clinical signs. The appetite is usually only moderately to slightly impaired. The clinical signs increase in severity for a time, then tend to abate after a few weeks except in herds with clinical AR, where continued progressive turbinate damage causes frequent sneezing to continue. Uncomplicated *B. bronchiseptica* infections in older pigs produce only mild signs or remain clinically inapparent.

Not all sneezing in young pigs is attributable solely to *B. bronchiseptica,* since infection with porcine cytomegalovirus or other agents may also produce or exacerbate these signs.

Bronchopneumonia. A more severe manifestation of infection is bronchopneumonia, which is usually seen as a primary condition in very young piglets (3–4 days). Although this type of disease is relatively uncommon compared with the wide prevalence of nasal infection, *B. bronchiseptica* is an important pathogen in those cases of pneumonia with bronchitis that occur in young pigs. The condition only affects young pigs and is most common in winter (Whittlestone 1982). The major clinical sign is coughing, perhaps with whooping and dyspnea. Pyrexia is not usually marked (Switzer and Farrington 1975). Morbidity is high within litters, and mortality may be so in untreated cases.

B. bronchiseptica is not infrequently isolated from pneumonic lesions in older fattening pigs, but it is considered to be a secondary opportunist pathogen and the clinical significance of its presence remains largely unknown.

LESIONS. The lesions in bordetellosis are restricted to the respiratory tract. The principal lesion is a catarrhal rhinitis accompanied by a variable amount of turbinate hypoplasia in young pigs up to about 8 weeks of age. On occasion and usually restricted to animals a few days to weeks of age, a degree of bronchopneumonia may also occur. The degree of severity of the hypoplastic lesions seen in young pigs varies, and only rarely does severe hypoplasia result (Figs. 34.1, 34.2, 34.3).

The ventral scroll of the ventral turbinate is the area most commonly and consistently affected; grossly it varies in appearance from a slightly shrunken and distorted scroll to virtual complete absence. In the more severe cases the dorsal scrolls of the ventral turbinate and the dorsal turbinate are also usually additionally affected. The important factors that affect the severity of the hypoplasia are the degree of resistance of the pig to the infection (Smith et al. 1982) and the age when it was first acquired, since as the pig gets older its susceptibility to the damage the infection can produce declines.

The histologic changes in bordetella-induced hypoplastic rhinitis have been reported by Duncan et al. (1966a) and are detailed in Switzer and Farrington (1975). Briefly, there is a hyperplasia of the epithelium and, in places, a metaplasia, the epithelium becoming more stratified in structure with polyhedral cells devoid of cilia. There is a degree of cellular infiltration (principally with neutrophils and mononuclear cells), a fibroblastic proliferation in the lamina propria, and a reduction in size and replacement fibrosis of the osseous core. There are increased numbers of osteoblasts around the trabeculae, but osteoclasts are rarely found.

Bronchopneumonia. Pneumonic lesions occur principally in young pigs and have a characteristic scattered monolobular or bilobular distribution, mainly in the apical and cardiac lobes. Affected areas are initially dark red, become brown, then yellowish brown after a time and develop a contracted appearance.

Histologically, the pneumonic lesions in bordetellosis are characteristic. Detailed descriptions of the histopathology of experimental *B. bronchiseptica* bronchopneumonia are given by Duncan et al. (1966b) and Meyer and Beamer (1973) in conventional and germ-free swine respectively. The lesions from these experimental cases are similar to those of field cases. Briefly, the most severe cases affect the pneumonic vasculature, and there are areas of extensive alveolar hemorrhage with necrosis and interlobular edema. In areas where hemorrhagic changes are less extensive, there is an acute inflammatory reaction with cellular infiltration, principally with neutrophils. There is an accompanying bronchiolitis with neutrophilic exudate. As the lesions age, vascular changes become less prominent and epithelialization of the alveoli, fibroblastic activity, and deposition of col-

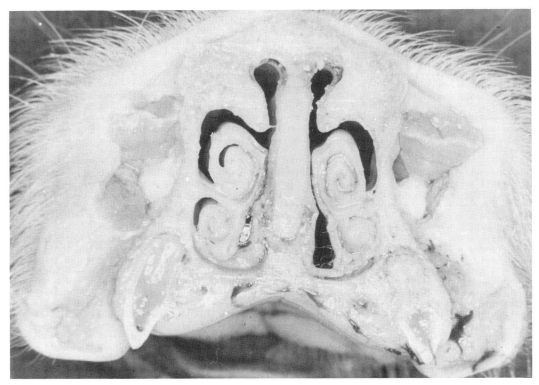

34.1. Cross section of the snout of an uninfected 8-week-old pig showing normal anatomy of the turbinate scrolls (conchae).

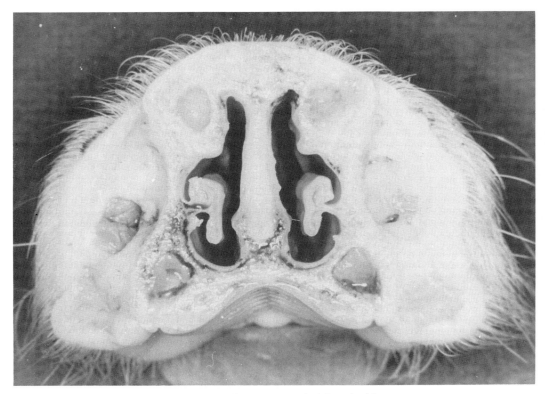

34.2. Turbinate hypoplasia in an 8-week-old pig spontaneously infected with *B. bronchiseptica* when 4 days old (littermate to pig in Fig. 34.1).

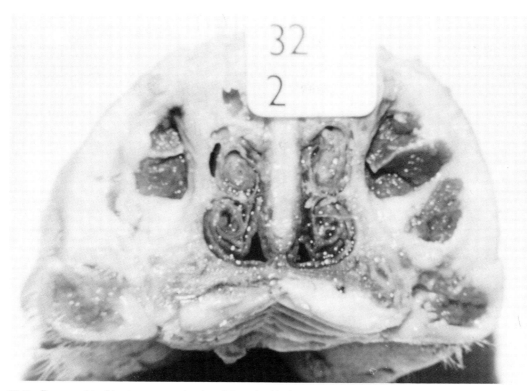

34.3. Presumed turbinate regeneration in a 22-week-old pig spontaneously infected with *B. bronchiseptica* when 4 days old (littermate to pigs in Figs. 34.1 and 34.2) and reared to slaughter weight in a good environment.

lagen occur. Large alveolar macrophages are present in some alveoli.

DIAGNOSIS.   Although the clinical signs are suggestive of infection, a definitive diagnosis of bordetellosis in pigs is only possible by the bacteriologic examination of nasal secretions. These are best collected on cotton-tipped swabs with either metal or plastic stems. Wooden-stemmed swabs should be avoided, since sudden movement of the pig may break the shaft. The live pig should be adequately restrained, preferably in dorsal recumbency, and the external nares cleaned. Swabs are carefully inserted in a naris with a gentle rotating motion and pushed carefully along the ventral meatus so as to avoid trauma to the delicate turbinates. The swabs are then submitted for laboratory examination, preferably in a bacteriologic transport medium.

The organism grows well on blood agar or MacConkey agar plus 1% glucose, but its isolation from field specimens is often complicated by the overgrowth of other organisms (Smith and Baskerville 1979); hence, culture on more selective media is recommended. Procedures for isolating and indentifying the organism from field specimens from pigs are given by Farrington and Switzer (1977), Smith and Baskerville (1979), and Rutter (1981).

The serologic diagnosis of bordetella infection by the detection of agglutinating antibodies in the serum has been described. The various methods of antigen preparation, details of some of the tests employed, and their interpretation have been reviewed by Giles and Smith (1983). Agglutinating antibodies to *B. bronchiseptica* are widespread in the pig population, but although their detection by serologic tests can be useful in making a herd diagnosis of bordetellosis, these are not commonly employed for routine diagnostic purposes, since, practically, serologic tests offer few advantages over the culture of nasal swabs.

TREATMENT.   The control of bordetellosis in commercial pig herds can be attempted by a combination of management and therapeutic measures. These are required or usually deemed necessary by experienced clinicians only in herds where this infection is associated with clinically significant disease, whether rhinitis, bronchopneumonia, or infectious AR, since the mere presence of the infection within an ordinary commercial herd is not, on its own, usually sufficient grounds for initiating therapeutic measures against it. This may not apply, however, in the case of high-health-status or specific-pathogen-free (SPF) herds, which may wish to remain free from the infection. Therapeutic measures to control bordetellosis are thus chiefly required as part of the clinician's armament against clinical infectious AR, especially in those cases where early infection of the young pig with *B. bronchiseptica* is a major predisposing or initiating factor. The overall treatment of AR is discussed in Chapter 33. Where such therapy is required, the management of the sow, her litter, and the newly weaned pigs should first be examined. Bordetellosis is likely to be of more significance where stress, principally from chilling, overcrowding, poor ventilation, or inadequate nutrition are evident. Modular accommodation is advisable and an all-in/all-out approach to weaner production is beneficial.

To reduce the pressure of infection among populations of young pigs, parenteral or in-feed medication of the sow during the latter part of gestation, parenteral medication of the sucking piglet, and medication of the creep, weaner, and grower rations or drinking water of the pigs have all been variously practiced. The sulphonamides were the first drugs to be used successfully in this respect (Switzer 1963) and are still widely employed, either alone, in combination with antibiotics, or potentiated with trimethoprim.

Specific therapeutic measures include (1) infeed sulphadimidine (sulphamezathine) (100 g/ton) to the sow for 1 month before farrowing; (2) three injections of potentiated sulphonamides (e.g., sulphadoxine or sulphadiazine at 12.5 mg/kg, plus trimethoprim at 2.5 mg/kg) or long-acting oxytetracycline (20 mg/kg) by parenteral injection to sucking piglets at approximately weekly intervals from 2 days of age; (3) sulphadimidine (sulphamezathine) (100–200 g/ton) alone or with tylosin (100 g/ton), or chlortetracycline (165 g/ton) with penicillin (83 g/ton) added to the ration; (4) sulphathiazole (0.08–0.13 g/L) in the drinking water.

Sulphonamides potentiated with trimethoprim are the drugs of choice in treating the infection in young pigs, although in some countries their use is not permitted in food-producing animals. Bronchopneumonia in piglets should be treated with parenteral injections of sulphadoxine or sulphadiazine at 12.5 mg/kg with trimethoprim at 2.5 mg/kg daily for 3–5 days. For infectious AR associated with bordetellosis, it is usual to give injections at approximately 2, 7, and 14 days. Although these strategic injections do not entirely rid the nasal mucosa of the infection, continuous medication of the drinking water at 13.3 and 66.7 µg/ml of trimethoprim and sulphadiazine respectively will do so in about 3 weeks, even in the face of continuous nasal challenge from untreated piglets (Giles et al. 1981). Such treatment also significantly reduces the amount of turbinate hypoplasia induced by the infection.

For economic reasons, the use of potentiated sulphonamides is mainly restricted to suckers and weaners. In older animals reliance must be placed on the sulphonamides alone, or in combination with antibiotics as detailed above. Pigs should generally be medicated for 3–6 weeks for the control of *B. bronchiseptica* infections, although often longer periods are required in infectious AR.

Antibiotic Resistance. A major problem in the widespread use of sulphonamides and potentiated sulphonamides has been the development of drug resistance. Following extensive use of sulphonamides in the United States, for example, in vitro resistance has been recorded in 71–81% of isolates (Harris and Switzer 1969; Farrington 1974). Similarly in Europe, of 138 strains of *B. bronchiseptica* examined by Smith et al. (1980) in England, 43% showed resistance to potentiated sulphonamides and a further 11% to sulphonamides alone. In this study there was a clear association between the long-term use of potentiated sulphonamides in the herd and the development of resistance. Although many of the herds in these various studies were examined specifically because of problems with infectious AR, the overall prevalence of sulphonamide resistance among porcine bordetellae is nevertheless high, since in England, 25% of the isolates from 86 randomly selected herds showed resistance (Cameron et al. 1980). The in vitro activity of 12 sulphonamide drugs against *B. bronchiseptica* was compared by Mengelers et al. (1989), who showed that the minimal inhibitory concentration (MIC)50 ranged from 0.5 to 8 µg/ml. Against a selection of the pathogenic respiratory bacteria of swine, sulphamethoxazole had the highest antimicrobial activity and sulphamezathine had an overall low activity. Isolates of *B. bronchiseptica* from pigs have been shown to have transmissible R factors that carry antibiotic resistance (Terakado et al. 1974).

Alternatives to the sulphonamide drugs have been examined. Most porcine isolates of *B. bronchiseptica* appear to be sensitive to the tetracyclines (Sisak et al. 1978; Smith et al. 1980; Pijpers et al. 1989), and these drugs, particularly a long-acting formulation of oxytetracyline given by parenteral injection to young pigs, would seem to be suitable for the control of bordetellosis. However, although they have been reported as clinically effective in infectious AR (De Jong and Oosterwoud 1977), their ability to reduce the weight of nasal infection with *B. bronchiseptica* is limited, since when given in feed or water, they are unable to eliminate an established infection (Switzer 1963; Woods et al. 1972) or even reduce its prevalence or relative intensity (Giles 1981). This is presumably because the drug fails to reach sufficiently high levels in the nasal mucus (Striz 1973). Given prophylactically to young pigs, however, a long-acting formulation of oxytetracycline will significantly reduce both the tendency of the organism to establish itself among the group and the intensity of the nasal infection that arises

(Giles 1981). The new flouroquinolones are also active against porcine bordetellae (Hannan et al. 1989).

PREVENTION. Since *B. bronchiseptica* is widely prevalent in the pig population, its total exclusion from a herd is only possible by the development of an SPF system and the strict maintenance of an effective barrier.

Vaccination. *B. bronchiseptica* vaccines have been developed and used in several countries in an attempt to control both the infection and clinical AR by immunologic methods. Killed whole-culture vaccines with aluminium salt adjuvants were the first to be available commercially and have been licensed for use in several countries since the 1970s. Other types of vaccine have also been investigated, including live avirulent strains and subunit vaccines, but generally have not been greatly successful. Killed whole-culture adjuvanted vaccines were at one time widely employed in pig herds, since several reports, mainly from the United States and Japan (e.g., Nakase et al. 1976; Goodnow 1977; Goodnow et al. 1979) indicated that such products were highly effective in the control of field outbreaks of clinical AR. In Europe, however, these benefits were much less obvious (Bercovich and Oosterwoud 1977; Pedersen and Barfod 1977; Giles and Smith 1982); later, further studies from the United States have also concluded that such bordetella vaccines are of limited efficacy in the overall control of AR. A critical review of bordetella vaccines (Giles and Smith 1983) concluded that, as single antigens, their beneficial effects in the control of AR are indeed limited and the previous claims for their usefulness overstated. In the light of new knowledge, combined vaccines have been developed consisting of *B. bronchiseptica/P. multocida* bacterins or *B. bronchiseptica* bacterin combined with *P. multocida* toxoid. Such vaccines are of use in the field, provided their limitations are fully realized by the clinician.

SOW VACCINATION. Vaccination of the sow induces a significant degree of passive colostral protection against *B. bronchiseptica* in the serum of her sucking piglets (Koshimizu et al. 1973; Smith et al. 1982); in the field, this protection will often persist until about the time of weaning. The colostral protection afforded by sow vaccination is thus an effective aid in controlling *B. bronchiseptica* infections among populations of young sucking piglets, and in herds where early piglet infection occurs and rhinitis and/or bronchopneumonia develops in young pigs, sow vaccination should be recommended. Initially two doses should be given 6 and 2 weeks before farrowing, followed by revaccination at 2 weeks before each subsequent farrowing.

As might be expected, however, in herds with clinical AR the immunologic control of bordetellosis per se can exert positive benefits, but it often has only a limited effect on the subsequent development of clinical disease among fatteners or the prevalence or severity of turbinate atrophy at slaughter.

PIGLET VACCINATION. Vaccination of the piglets (usually at 7 and 28 days of age) farrowed from vaccinated sows was at one time widely recommended and extensively used in the belief that the passively acquired antibody does not usually interfere with the development of an active response (Switzer 1981). The value of this procedure, however, remains equivocal.

Undoubtedly, under experimental conditions, vaccination (at 7 and 28 days) of SPF piglets (from *B. bronchiseptica*–free herds) produces a marked active agglutinin response, but detailed and critical study has demonstrated that only piglets farrowed from sows with no previous exposure to *B. bronchiseptica* respond in this manner (Smith et al. 1982) and that vaccination of the sows prior to farrowing prevents this active humoral response from developing in the sucking piglets (Pedersen and Jensen 1980; Smith et al. 1982).

Giles and Smith (1982) concluded that, in the field, there was likewise no serologic response among vaccinated piglets from vaccinated sows; even when a weak response was recorded (among the progeny of unvaccinated sows), this was of no clinical or bacteriologic benefit. These workers concluded that vaccination of piglets from vaccinated sows, or indeed vaccination of piglets alone, therefore appeared to be of little benefit. Vaccination of older pigs undoubtedly produces an active humoral response but its value is debatable, since the main effects of the infection occur in younger animals.

A variety of other methods of control have been described, including the culling of infected breeding stock (Farrington and Switzer 1977), but such procedures are expensive and not recommended.

Unless a herd is to remain free from *B. bronchiseptica* by adopting an SPF system and maintaining strict isolation, the mere presence of the organism in the herd may be of little significance and does not justify measures to exclude it. Where the infection is prevalent in sucking pigs or young weaners and bronchopneumonia and rhinitis occur and where infection with toxigenic *B. bronchiseptica* in young pigs is associated with infectious AR in growers, control measures should be adopted as part of a planned strategy to control AR. Specific measures against *B. bronchiseptica* infection should be directed toward preventing the infection from arising in sucking pigs (by management, sow vaccination, or chemotherapy) or mitigating its effects in young pigs (by management and/or chemotherapy).

REFERENCES

BERCOVICH, Z., AND OOSTERWOUD, R. A. 1977. Vaccination with *Bordetella bronchiseptica* vaccine on a farm with atrophic rhinitis: An evaluation of a field experiment. Tijdschr Diergeneeskd 102:485.

CAMERON, R. D. A.; GILES, C. J.; AND SMITH, I. M. 1980. The prevalence of *Bordetella bronchiseptica* and turbinate (conchal) atrophy in English pig herds in 1978–1979. Vet Rec 107:146.

CHANTER, N.; MAGYAR, T.; AND RUTTER, J. M. 1989. Interactions between *Bordetella bronchiseptica* and toxigenic *Pasteurella multocida* in atrophic rhinitis of pigs. Res Vet Sci 47:48.

COLLINS, L. A., AND RUTTER, J. M. 1985. Virulence of *Bordetella bronchiseptia* in the porcine respiratory tract. J Med Microbiol 19:247.

DE JONG, M. F., AND OOSTERWOUD, R. A. 1977. Treatment with oxytetracycline hydrochloride in the prevention of atrophic rhinitis in baby pigs. Tijdschr Diergeneeskd 102:266.

DE JONG, M. F.; BERCOVICH, Z.; AND AKKERMANS, J. P. W. M. 1976. Atrophic rhinitis control in the Netherlands. Proc 4th Int Congr Pig Vet Soc, Ames, p. 5.

DE JONG, M. F.; OEI, H. L.; AND TETENBURG, G. J. 1980. AR-Pathogenicity-tests for *Pasteurella multocida* isolates. Proc 6th Int Congr Pig Vet Soc, Copenhagen, p. 211.

DONE, J. T. 1975. Infectious atrophic rhinitis of pigs: Rational control at the herd level. Vet A 15:105.

DUNCAN, J. R.; ROSS, R. K.; SWITZER, W. P.; AND RAMSEY, R. K. 1966a. Pathology of experimental *Bordetella bronchiseptica* infection in swine: Atrophic rhinitis. Am J Vet Res 27:457.

DUNCAN, J. R.; RAMSEY, R. K.; AND SWITZER, W. P. 1966b. Pathology of experimental *Bordetella bronchiseptica* infection in swine: Pneumonia. Am J Vet Res 27:467.

EDINGTON, N.; SMITH, I. M.; PLOWRIGHT, W.; AND WATT, R. G. 1976. Relationship of porcine cytomegalovirus and *Bordetella bronchiseptica* to atrophic rhinitis in gnotobiotic piglets. Vet Rec 98:42.

FARRINGTON, D. O. 1974. Evaluation of nasal culturing procedures and immunization as applied to the control of *Bordetella bronchiseptica* rhinitis in swine. Ph.D. diss., Iowa State Univ, Ames.

FARRINGTON, D. O., AND JORGENSEN, R. D. 1976. Prevalence of *Bordetella bronchiseptica* in certain wild mammals and birds in central Iowa. J Wildl Dis 12:523.

FARRINGTON, D. O., AND SWITZER, W. P. 1977. Evaluation of nasal culturing procedures for the control of atrophic rhinitis caused by *Bordetella bronchiseptica* in swine. J Am Vet Med Assoc 170:34.

FETTER, A. W.; SWITZER, W. P.; AND CAPEN, C. C. 1975. Electron microscopic evaluation of bone cells in pigs with experimentally induced *Bordetella* rhinitis. Am J Vet Res 36:15.

GILES, C. J. 1981. Atrophic rhinitis of pigs: Studies on the naturally occurring and experimental disease in England with particular reference to *Bordetella bronchiseptica* infection. Ph.D. diss., Univ of London.

GILES, C. J., AND SMITH, I. M. 1982. The value of vaccinating pigs with *Bordetella bronchiseptica*. Pig Vet Soc Proc 9:61.

———. 1983. Vaccination of pigs with *Bordetella bronchiseptica*. Vet Bull 53:327.

GILES, C. J.; SMITH, I. M.; BASKERVILLE, A. J.; AND BROTHWELL, E. 1980. Clinical, bacteriological and epidemiological observations on infectious atrophic rhinitis of pigs in southern England. Vet Rec 106:25.

GILES, C. J.; SMITH, I. M.; BASKERVILLE, A. J.; AND

OLIPHANT, J. 1981. Treatment of experimental *Bordetella bronchiseptica* infection in young pigs with potentiated sulphonamide in the drinking water. Vet Rec 108:136.

GOODNOW, R. A. 1977. Control of atrophic rhinitis with a *Bordetella bronchiseptica* bacterin. Vet Med Small Anim Clin 72:1210.

GOODNOW, R. A.; SHADE, F. J.; AND SWITZER, W. P. 1979. Efficacy of *Bordetella bronchiseptica* bacterin in controlling enzootic atrophic rhinitis in swine. Am J Vet Res 40:58.

GOODWIN, R. F. W. 1980. Atrophic rhinitis of pigs. Vet Rec [Pract Suppl] 2:5.

HANADA, M.; SHIMODA, K.; TOMITA, S.; NAKASE, Y.; AND NISHIYAMA, Y. 1979. Production of lesions similar to naturally occurring atrophic rhinitis by cell-free sonicated extract of *Bordetella bronchiseptica*. Jpn J Vet Sci 41:1.

HANNAN, P. C. T.; O'HANLON, P. J.; AND ROGERS, N. H. 1989. In vitro evaluation of various quinolone antibacterial agents against veterinary mycoplasmas and porcine respiratory bacterial pathogens. Res Vet Sci 46:202.

HARRIS, D. L., AND SWITZER, W. P. 1968. Turbinate atrophy in young pigs exposed to *Bordetella bronchiseptica*, *Pasteurella multocida* and combined inoculum. Am J Vet Res 29:777.

———. 1969. Nasal and tracheal resistance of swine against reinfection by *Bordetella bronchiseptica*. Am J Vet Res 30:1161.

HARRIS, D. L.; ROSS, R. F.; AND SWITZER, W. P. 1969. Incidence of certain micro-organisms in nasal cavities of swine in Iowa. Am J Vet Res 30:1621.

JENKINS, E.M.; ANTHONY, V.; VANCE, R. T.; CLEVELAND, J.; AND GBADAMOSI, S. G. 1977. Prevalence of *Bordetella bronchiseptica* infection in swine of southeastern Alabama. Am J Vet Res 38:2071.

KANG, B. K.; KOSHIMIZU, K.; AND OGATA, M. 1971. Studies on the etiology of infectious atrophic rhinitis of swine. III. Field survey by agglutination test in relation to incidence of *Bordetella bronchiseptica* and turbinate atrophy. Jpn J Vet Sci 33:17.

KOSHIMUZU, K.; KODAMA, Y.; OGATA, M.; KINO, T.; SANBYAKUDA, S.; AND MIMURA, T. 1973. Studies on the etiology of infectious atrophic rhinitis of swine. VI. Effect of vaccination against nasal establishment of *Bordetella bronchiseptica*. Jpn J Vet Sci 35:411.

MAGYAR, T.; CHANTER, N.; LAX, A. J.; RUTTER, J. M.; AND HALL, G. A. 1988. The pathogenesis of turbinate atrophy in pigs caused by *Bordetella bronchiseptica*. Vet Microbiol 18:135.

MENGELERS, M. J. B.; VAN KLINGEREN, B.; AND VAN MIERT, A. S. J. P. A. M. 1989. In vitro antimicrobial activity of sulfonamides against some porcine pathogens. Am J Vet Res 50:1022.

MEYER, R. C., AND BEAMER, P. D. 1973. *Bordetella bronchiseptica* infections in germ-free swine: An experimental pneumonia. Vet Pathol 10:550.

NAKAGAWA, M.; SHIMIZU, T.; AND MOTOI, Y. 1974. Pathology of experimental atrophic rhinitis in swine infected with *Alcaligenes bronchisepticus* or *Pasteurella multocida*. Natl Inst Anim Health Q (Tokyo) 14:61.

NAKASE, Y.; KUME, K.; SHIMODA, K.; AND SAWATA, A. 1980. Experimental atrophic rhinitis produced by cell-free extract of *Bordetella bronchiseptica*. Proc 6th Congr Int Pig Vet Soc, Copenhagen, p. 202.

OGATA, M.; KOSHIMIZU, K.; KANG, B. K.; ATOBE, H.; YAMAMOTO, K.; KINO, T.; AND IKEDA, A. 1970. Studies on the etiology of infectious atrophic rhinitis of swine. I. Relationship between the disease and bacterial flora of nasal cavity of pigs. Jpn J Vet Sci 32:185.

PEDERSEN, K. B., AND BARFOD, K. 1977. Effect of vaccination of sows with *Bordetella bronchiseptica* on the incidence of atrophic rhinitis in swine. Nord Vet Med 29:369.

———. 1981. The aetiological significance of *Bordetella bronchiseptica* and *Pasteurella multocida* in atrophic rhinitis of swine. Nord Vet Med 33:513.

PEDERSEN, K. B., AND JENSEN, P. T. 1980. The influence of passively acquired antibodies on the immune response of piglets immunised with a *Bordetella bronchiseptica* vaccine. Proc 6th Congr Int Pig Vet Soc, Copenhagen, p. 176.

PHILLIPS, C. E. 1943. *Alcaligenes (Brucella) bronchisepticus* as a factor in porcine pneumonias. Can J Comp Med 7:58.

PIJPERS, A.; VAN KLINGEREN, B.; SCHOEVERS, E. J.; VERHEIJDEN, J.; AND VAN MIERT, A. S. J. P. A. M. 1989. In vitro activity of five tetracyclines and some other antimicrobial agents against four porcine respiratory tract pathogens. J Vet Pharmacol Therap 12:267.

ROOP, R. M.; VEIT H. P.; SINSKY, R. J.; VEIT, S. P.; HEWLETT, E. L.; AND KORNEGAY, E. T. 1987. Virulence factors of *Bordetella bronchiseptica* associated with the production of infectious atrophic rhinitis and pneumonia in experimentally infected neonatal swine. Infect Immun 55:217.

ROSS, R. F.; SWITZER, W. P.; AND MARE, C. J. 1963. Incidence of certain micro-organisms in Iowa swine. Vet Med 58:563.

ROSS R. F.; SWITZER, W. P.; AND DUNCAN, J. R. 1967. Comparison of pathogenicity of various isolates of *Bordetella bronchiseptica* in young pigs. Can J Comp Med 31:53.

RUTTER, J. M. 1981. Quantitative observations on *Bordetella bronchiseptica* infection in atrophic rhinitis of pigs. Vet Rec 108:451.

———. 1989. Atrophic rhinitis. Vet Rec [Pract Suppl] 11:74.

RUTTER, J. M., AND COLLINGS, L. A. 1983. The virulence of *Bordetella bronchiseptica* in atrophic rhinitis of pigs. In Atrophic Rhinitis of Pigs. Ed. K. B. Pedersen and N. C. Nielsen. Comm Eur Communities Rep EUR 8643 EN, Luxembourg, p. 77.

RUTTER, J. M., AND ROJAS, X. 1982. Atrophic rhinitis in gnotobiotic piglets: Differences in the pathogenicity of *Pasteurella multocida* in combined infection with *Bordetella bronchiseptica*. Vet Rec 110:531.

RUTTER, J. M.; FRANCIS, L. M. A.; AND SANSOM, B. F. 1982. Virulence of *Bordetella bronchiseptica* from pigs with or without atrophic rhinitis. J Med Microbiol 15:105.

SCHOFIELD, F. W., AND JONES, T. L. 1950. The pathology and bacteriology of infectious atrophic rhinitis in swine. J Am Vet Med Assoc 116:120.

SHIMIZU, T.; NAKAGAWA, M.; SHIBATA, S.; AND SUZUKI, K. 1971. Atrophic rhinitis produced by intranasal inoculation of *Bordetella bronchiseptica* in hysterectomy-produced colostrum-deprived pigs. Cornell Vet 61:696.

SILVEIRA, D.; EDINGTON, N.; AND SMITH, I. M. 1982. Ultrastructural changes in the nasal turbinate bone of pigs in early infection with *Bordetella bronchiseptica*. Res Vet Sci 33:37.

SISAK, F.; GOIS, M.; AND KUKSA, F. 1978. The sensitivity of the strains of *Bordetella bronchiseptica, Pasteurella multocida* and *Mycoplasma hyorhinis,* isolated from pigs, to antibiotics and chemotherapeutics. Vet Med (Praha) 23:531.

SMITH, I. M., AND BASKERVILLE, A. J. 1979. A selective medium facilitating the isolation and recognition of *Bordetella bronchiseptica* in pigs. Res Vet Sci 27:187.

SMITH, I. M.; OLIPHANT, J.; BASKERVILLE, A. J.; AND GILES, C. J. 1980. High prevalence of strains of *Bordetella bronchiseptica* resistant to potentiated sulphonamide in English pig herds in 1978–1979. Vet Rec 106:462.

SMITH, I. M.; GILES, C. J.; AND BASKERVILLE, A. J. 1982. The immunisation of pigs against experimental infection with *Bordetella bronchiseptica*. Vet Rec 110:488.

STRIZ, J. 1973. The persistence of oxytetracycline in the nasal cavity of piglets with atrophic rhinitis. Acta Vet Brno 42:423.

SWITZER, W. P. 1956. Studies on infectious atrophic rhinitis. V. Concept that several agents may cause turbinate atrophy. Am J Vet Res 17:478.

———. 1963. Elimination of *Bordetella bronchiseptica* from the nasal cavity of swine by sulphonamide therapy. Vet Med 58:571.

———. 1981. Bordetellosis. In Diseases of Swine, 5th ed. Ed. A. D. Leman, R. D. Glock, W. L. Mengeling, R. H. C. Penny, E. Scholl, and B. Straw. Ames: Iowa State Univ Press, p. 497.

SWITZER, W. P., AND FARRINGTON, D. O. 1972. Progress in the control of atrophic rhinitis caused by *Bordetella bronchiseptica* in swine. J Am Vet Med Assoc 161:1325.

———. 1975. Infectious atrophic rhinitis. In Diseases of Swine, 4th ed. Ed. H. W. Dunne and A. D. Leman. Ames: Iowa State Univ Press, p. 687.

TERAKADO, N.; AZECHI, H.; NINOMIYA, K.; FUKUYASU, T.; AND SHIMIZU, T. 1974. Incidence of R factors in *Bordetella bronchiseptica* isolated from pigs. Jpn J Microbiol 18:45.

THORP, F., JR., AND TANNER, F. W. 1940. A bacteriological study of the aerobic flora occurring in pneumonic lungs of swine. J Am Vet Med Assoc 96:149.

TORNØE, N., AND NIELSEN, N. C. 1976. Inoculation experiments with *Bordetella bronchiseptica* strains in SPF pigs. Nord Vet Med 28:233.

TORNØE, N.; NIELSEN, N. C.; AND SVENDSEN, J. 1976. *Bordetella bronchiseptica* isolations from the nasal cavity of pigs in relation to atrophic rhinitis. Nord Vet Med 28:1.

WHITTLESTONE, P. 1982. Infectious agents associated with porcine respiratory diseases. Pig Vet Soc Proc 9:71.

WOODS, G. T.; JENSEN, A. J.; GOSSLING, J.; RHOADES, H. E.; AND NICKELSON, W. F. 1972. The effect of medicated feed on the nasal microflora and weight gain of pigs. Can J Comp Med 36:49.

YOKOMIZO, Y., AND SHIMIZU, T. 1979. Adherence of *Bordetella bronchiseptica* to swine nasal epithelial cells and its possible role in virulence. Res Vet Sci 27:15.

35 Brucellosis

A. P. MacMillan

BRUCELLOSIS of swine is an infectious disease that has been recognized as a specific entity since 1914 when Traum (1914) isolated the organism from aborted swine fetuses in Indiana. For many years it was thought to be a specially pathogenic form of *Brucella abortus,* until Huddleston (1929) named it as a separate species. Brucellosis occurs in most countries throughout the world where swine exist in the wild or domesticated state.

In the United States swine brucellosis was recognized as a major swine disease, causing considerable economic loss from reduced reproduction during the 1920s–50s. Since that time, changes in swine management combined with regulatory programs to eradicate the disease have gradually eliminated brucellosis in swine as a major disease problem from large areas of the country. By 1989, all states were participating in the federal eradication program; regions where the majority of swine are raised appear to be now virtually free of brucellosis. Swine in the southeastern United States seem to have the highest incidence of brucellosis, although these are classified as Class B states with a herd infection rate of less than 1.5%. According to USDA statistical information (Huber et al. 1989), 0.04% or 691 of 1.9 million sows and boars tested on farms, at livestock markets, and at slaughter establishments during fiscal year 1989 were serologic reactors. This information indicates a higher incidence than actually exists, since single serologic reactors in noninfected herds are a frequent occurrence. The actual number of herds classified as infected in 1989 was 59, and these were for the most part small herds in endemic areas.

According to international data in the FAO-WHO-OIE Yearbook of 1989, the disease is reported in 12 out of 29 South American countries making a return. In Europe apart from Britain and Scandinavia, which are free, there is a general low prevalence of porcine brucellosis reported by 9 countries. In Africa, the disease is reported by 5 states, but there are not a large number of pigs on the continent, and the true position is not entirely clear. Asia, particularly Southeast Asia, seems to have a generally high prevalence of the disease. In Australia, the disease is confined to feral swine in Queensland (Alton 1990).

Swine brucellosis also has noteworthy public health implications. Until recently the source of the majority of human brucellosis has been *Brucella suis*–infected swine (Fox and Kaufmann 1977). The public health hazard caused by swine brucellosis is out of proportion to the incidence of brucellosis in other livestock, primarily because *B. suis* (biotypes 1 and 3) appears to have a much higher degree of pathogenicity for humans than other *Brucella* species found in the United States, and infected swine tend to have much higher numbers of *B. suis* organisms in their tissues than cattle infected with *B. abortus,* thus proving a greater exposure to persons who come in contact with infected swine. Since pigs do not produce dairy products, the incidence of *B. suis* in humans is almost entirely occupational – in farmers, veterinarians, and abattoir workers. Interestingly, although the infection of cattle with *B. suis* is rare, Cook and Noble (1984), working in Australia, reported several cases probably contracted following contact with feral swine. Persistent excretion in the milk may give rise to human epidemics (Borts et al. 1943).

ETIOLOGY. The genus *Brucella* is divided into six species: *B. melitensis, B. abortus, B. suis, B. neotomae, B. ovis,* and *B. canis* (Brinley-Morgan and McCullough 1974; Alton et al. 1975). The genus appears to be genetically very homogeneous (Verger et al. 1985) but does not appear to be closely related to any other animal pathogens (De Ley et al. 1987). The first three species are further divided into 3, 9, and 5 biotypes, respectively. The principal hosts for *B. melitensis* are goats and sheep; for *B. abortus,* cattle; for *B. neotomae,* desert wood rats; for *B. ovis,* sheep; and for *B. canis,* dogs. The most common host for *B. suis* types 1 and 3 is swine, and these biotypes are worldwide in distribution. *B. suis* type 2 occurs in Europe where the hosts are swine and the European hare (*Lepus capinensis*), which can form a reservoir for both wild and domestic pigs. The disease in pigs caused by this biovar differs slightly from that caused by biovars 1 and 3 in that miliary brucellosis of the uterus is a feature, and unlike them, it does not appear to be pathogenic for humans. *B. suis* type 4 is enzootic in reindeer and caribou (*Rangifer* spp.) in Siberia, Alaska, and Canada, and although it causes many cases of human brucellosis it is apparently not pathogenic for swine. *B. suis* biovar 5 causes murine brucellosis.

B. suis is the only recognized *Brucella* species

that causes systemic or generalized infection leading to reproductive failure in swine. Swine can be infected naturally or experimentally with other *Brucella* species, but a characteristic of the infection is almost invariably a symptomless, self-limiting localized infection of lymph nodes, regional to the point of entry. It should be noted, however, that the differentiation of *B. suis* biovar 3 and *B. melitensis* biovar 2 can be accomplished by using methods available only in large reference centers; this probably accounts for the frequent reports before the early 1960s of the isolation of *B. melitensis* from pigs (Alton 1990).

Primary isolations of *B. suis,* like the other species in the genus, appear as small, convex, translucent colonies on the surface of agar media after incubation at 37°C for 3–7 days. All *Brucella* species and biotypes, except *B. ovis* and *B. canis,* are of smooth colonial morphology in their most pathogenic form. *B. ovis* and *B. canis* are rough and mucoid respectively. All smooth forms of brucellae may dissociate into intermediate, rough, or mucoid forms under certain artificially induced environmental conditions. This frequently occurs if cultures are left for long periods without being subcultured, and it renders them unable to be assigned to species or biovar. Microscopically, brucellae are small, gram-negative bacilli or coccobacilli and are nonmotile and arranged singly. *B. suis* organisms from different sources may vary considerably in size but are generally 0.4–0.8 × 0.6 to 3.0μm.

Several commercially available agar media are suitable for isolation and propagation of *B. suis*; those more commonly used include tryptose, trypticase-soy, Albimi, serum dextrose, Farrell's, and potato infusion. The addition of serum to the media to a final concentration of 5% frequently enhances the growth of brucellae, particularly on primary isolation. Increased carbon dioxide (CO_2) tension does not enhance the growth of *B. suis*. A more complete discussion of biotyping procedures, types, and formulation of growth media, as well as descriptive characteristics of the entire genus, can be obtained from Alton et al. (1988).

In general, all biotypes of *B. suis* have a noticeably greater urease and catalase activity than other species of *Brucella*. Classification of *B. suis* into biotypes is based on the combined findings of a variety of conventional and specialized tests. Briefly, *B. suis* type 1 produces large amounts of hydrogen sulfide, whereas types 2, 3, and 4 produce little or none; growth of types 1 and 2 is inhibited to a greater degree by basic fuchsin than growth of types 3 and 4; all types of *B. suis* are inhibited less by thionin than by basic fuchsin; *B. suis* is not affected by routine test dilutions (RTD) of Tbilisi *Brucella* phage but may be partially lysed by 10,000 × RTD. Of the four recognized serotypes (A, M, AM, and R) among *Brucella, B. suis* types 1, 2, and 3 are serotype A, while type 4 is AM (the only distinguishing feature separating

types 3 and 4). *B. suis* type 2 is inhibited to a greater extent by all aniline dyes than other *B. suis* types, and although there are finite differences in oxidative metabolic characteristics between types 1 and 2 and 3 and 4, all *B. suis* tend to oxidatively metabolize carbohydrate substrates and urea cycle amino acids to a greater extent than other amino acid substrates.

Among the *B. suis,* only types 1 and 3 are known to occur in swine-raising areas of the United States. Until 1946 the only recognized cause of swine brucellosis in the United States was the organism now known as *B. suis* type 1. At that time, *B. suis* type 3 (originally classified as American *B. melitensis*) was first isolated from tissues of infected swine by S. H. McNutt (Borts et al. 1946). Since the 1950s, reported isolations of *B. suis* type 1 have become comparatively less frequent, while isolations of *B. suis* type 3 have become more frequent. There is little doubt that type 3 is now the predominant biotype in swine brucellosis in the United States. It seems likely that type 3 evolved from type 1 and is somehow better adapted to persist in nature. There is bacteriologic evidence for this evolutionary proposal (Meyer 1990).

EPIDEMIOLOGY. Most evidence indicates that most *B. suis* infection is transmitted to susceptible swine through direct association with infected swine. The most important routes of infection are through the alimentary and genital tracts. The habits of swine and usual character of the disease strongly suggest that the alimentary tract is the most common entry. Swine of all ages will eat food or drink fluid contaminated with discharges from infected swine. Suckling pigs are frequently infected by nursing infected dams. When breeding swine are confined in common pens or lots, aborted fetuses and fetal membranes are readily consumed.

Brucellosis is a venereal disease in swine. Sows and gilts are readily infected when bred to boars with genital infection or when artificially inseminated with semen containing *B. suis*. Experimentally, swine can easily be infected by conjunctival or intranasal exposure with suspensions of *B. suis*. It is possible that organisms could also enter through scarified or, possibly, intact skin.

The survival of brucellae under environmental conditions is a relatively important factor in transmission of the disease. Experimentally, brucellae in a dried state are more resistant to environmental changes, and the survival rate decreases as the temperature increases. Brucellae are resistant to freezing; therefore, the most suitable methods for preserving *Brucella* organisms for long periods are lyophilization and/or storage at subfreezing temperatures. Experimental evidence indicates that *B. suis* is readily killed by pasteurization, 2–4 hours of direct sunlight, and the most commonly used disinfectants. Brucellae can survive in organic matter at freezing or near-freezing temperatures in excess of 2 years. Consequently, efforts to eliminate brucellosis from swine-raising premises must include an effective sanitation program (Luchsinger et al. 1965).

There are few known reservoirs of *B. suis* infection other than infected domestic swine. Only the European hare and feral swine have been established as significant potential reservoirs. The European hare was incriminated as a natural host for *B. suis* type 2 as early as 1954 (Bendsten et al. 1954) and was apparently responsible for periodic outbreaks of brucellosis of swine in Europe. Feral swine in the southeastern United States have been discovered to have a high rate of serologic reactors, with isolation of *B. suis* type 1 from selected specimens (Wood et al. 1976; Becker et al. 1978). The epizootiologic importance of feral hogs in maintenance of swine brucellosis depends largely on the degree of contact between wild and domestic swine. If swine management systems in regions where feral swine exist prevent cohabitation, *B. suis* infection in feral swine may be of greater public health importance than a threat to the swine industry. There have been numerous instances of *B. suis* infection or seropositivity in rodents or carnivorous species trapped near areas where brucellosis in domesticated swine has occurred. However, general indications are that these species acquired infection from the swine and are terminal hosts of the infection. With few or no exceptions, epidemiologic investigation of newly infected swine herds has revealed the source as another herd of domesticated swine.

Experimental studies have shown that swine can be infected with *B. suis* type 4, *B. abortus, B. melitensis, B. canis,* and *B. neotomae.* However, there has been no evidence that these organisms invade the genital tract, are transmissible between swine, or localize in any tissues other than cephalic lymph nodes. All available evidence indicates that these biotypes or species are not highly pathogenic for swine, swine are not likely to show clinical evidence of disease, and the infection is self-limiting and usually persists less than 60 days. Nevertheless, these infections do have importance in public health, if not in swine disease. In particular, swine are associated with *B. abortus* infection in packinghouse workers.

Swine infected with *B. suis* types 1, 2, or 3 can serve as a source of infection for other domesticated animal species. *B. suis* infection can occur naturally in horses, cattle, dogs, and fowl. Although the most common *Brucella* infection in horses is *B. abortus,* fistulous withers and other similar ailments have been recorded as caused by *B. suis* when horses were associated with infected swine. Cattle are rarely infected with *B. suis;* when it does occur, the characteristic infection is mastitis, with *B. suis* organisms excreted in the milk. There are no recorded cases of abortion in cattle caused by *B. suis,* but it can cause an acute

infection in dogs, with pregnant bitches frequently aborting. There is a possibility that *B. canis,* a significant pathogen in dogs, evolved from *B. suis* type 3. Brucellosis in fowl, regardless of the *Brucella* species involved, appears to be self-limiting and is only an incidental finding in birds intimately associated with infected swine herds where abortions have occurred.

PATHOGENESIS. Available literature and comparative studies indicate that the pathogenesis of *B. suis* types 1, 2, and 3 infection is very similar (Thomsen 1934; Hutchings 1950; Hoerlein et al. 1954; Deyoe 1967). Differences are generally related to factors such as method of exposure, environmental conditions, age and breed of swine, and possibly minor differences between strains of the same biotype. However, the characteristics of the disease produced are usually indistinguishable.

Regardless of the route of infection, the organism must be able to attach to and penetrate the mucosal epithelium, although the mechanism allowing this crucial event has never been documented. Following the initial penetration, submucosal aggregations of lymphocytes and plasma cells form in response. Invading organisms are carried to local lymph nodes, although it is not known whether they travel as free organisms or within phagocytes, or infected nodes become enlarged due to lymphoid and reticuloendothelial hyperplasia and infiltration. Brucellae surviving regional node colonization enter a phase of bacteremia, now protected from humoral immune mechanisms by their intracellular location within neutrophils and macrophages.

In *B. suis* infection of swine, bacteremia is an invariable finding in acute stages of the disease if frequent blood samples are collected and examined bacteriologically. In general, the onset of bacteremia ranges from 1 to 7 weeks postexposure, with a mean of about 2 weeks postexposure. Bacteremia persists an average of about 5 weeks and is generally continuous during that time. Intermittent bacteremia in individual swine has been observed to be as brief as 1 week to as long as 34 months. It is this bacteremia that is probably responsible for the wide range of tissues secondarily infected during the course of the disease.

Within a short time after the bacteremia stage, *B. suis* can be isolated from a large number of sites in the body (Deyoe and Manthei 1967). The entire lymphatic system is often affected for a period of time. With increasing time after exposure, there are fewer sites of localization of the organism. Among lymph nodes, the most frequent sources of *B. suis* are mandibular, gastrohepatic, internal iliac, and suprapharyngeal, in that order, depending essentially on the route of infection. Organs of the genital system, containing high levels of erythritol, become involved in many swine and may remain persistently infected. The placenta is a privileged site, and brucellae localize in the rough endoplasmic reticulum of the chorionic trophoblasts. Despite severe placental infection, only mild inflammation of the endometrium is observed. The spleen, liver, kidney, bladder, mammary gland, and brain may be involved (Jubb et al. 1985), although not as regularly as lymph nodes. Other significant sources of *B. suis,* particularly in chronically infected swine, are joint fluids and bone marrow.

The response of defense mechanisms to invasion by *B. suis* becomes evident with the appearance of humoral antibody, activation of the cell-mediated immune system, and development of microscopic lesions. These manifestations may occur simultaneously but usually are subsequent to the appearance of detectable bacteremia, which may precede detectable antibody levels by as much as 6–8 weeks. As swine recover from *B. suis* infection (i.e., when viable organisms are no longer present in their tissues), other manifestations such as antibody levels, cellular hypersensitivity, and microscopic lesions recede and disappear also. Unfortunately, many swine remain permanently infected.

In a series of experiments, infection was established in 248 sexually mature swine (Deyoe 1972a). They were killed at various intervals after exposure to *B. suis* and their tissues were subjected to thorough bacteriologic examination. Three-fourths of the swine in each group of females had recovered from infection by 4–6 months or longer after exposure, whereas the recovery rate in males never exceeded 50%. In contrast, Goode et al. (1952) and Manthei et al. (1952) isolated *B. suis* from only 12 of 474 adult swine exposed as suckling pigs. This information demonstrates beyond doubt that the majority of swine infected with *B. suis* would eventually recover spontaneously. Nevertheless, sufficient numbers of permanently infected animals would remain to serve as a continual source of infection.

CLINICAL SIGNS. Clinical evidence of *B. suis* infection varies considerably in different herds. The majority of affected herds may have no signs of brucellosis recognizable by the herd owner. The classic manifestations of swine brucellosis are abortion, infertility, orchitis, posterior paralysis, and lameness. Infected swine fail to show any persisting or undulating pyrexia. Clinical signs may be transient and death is a rare occurrence.

Abortions may occur at any time during gestation and are influenced more by the time of exposure than by the time of gestation. The rate of abortion is highest in sows or gilts exposed via the genital tract at the time of breeding (Deyoe and Manthei 1969). Abortions have been observed as early as 17 days following natural insemination by boars disseminating *B. suis* in the semen. Early abortions are usually overlooked under field conditions, and the first indication is a large percentage of sows or gilts showing signs of estrus 30–45 days after the service that resulted in conception. Little or no vaginal discharge is observed with early abortions. Abortions that occur during the middle or late stages of gestation are usually associated with females that acquire infection after pregnancy has advanced past 35 or 40 days. The persistence of genital infection in females varies considerably.

A small percentage of sows has been shown to shed *B. suis* in vaginal discharges for as long as 30 months. However, the majority have ceased shedding organisms within 30 days. A clinically apparent abnormal vaginal exudate is seldom observed in sows that have uterine infection except just prior to and for a short time after abortions. The majority of female swine eventually recover from genital infection.

When genital infection in sows persists only a short time after abortion, parturition, or breeding to an infected boar and the sows are permitted two or three estrous cycles of sexual rest, subsequent conception rates and reproductive capacity are usually very good.

Genital infection tends to be more persistent in boars than in sows. Some infected boars do not develop a localized genital infection. However, boars that do develop genital infection seldom recover from it. Pathologic changes in the male accessory glands or testes are generally more extensive and irreversible than in the uterus. Infertility and lack of sexual drive may occur in infected boars and are frequently associated with testicular involvement. More commonly, however, boars have infection in accessory genital glands and as a result disseminate large numbers of *B. suis* in their semen. These boars do not necessarily have reduced fertility (Vandeplassche et al. 1967). In most circumstances, clinically apparent lesions of *B. suis* type 1, 2, or 3 infection in boars are seldom encountered.

Brucellosis in suckling and weaning pigs usually appears as spondylitis associated with posterior paralysis. These clinical signs are also occasionally observed in swine of any age.

LESIONS. Macroscopic pathologic changes produced by *B. suis* in swine are quite variable.

Abscess formation in affected organs may occur enough to result in necrosis and desquamation of a significant proportion of the mucous membrane. Generally, the histopathologic changes consist of uterine glands filled with leukocytes, cellular infiltration of the endometrial stroma, and hyperplasia of periglandular connective tissue. Diffuse suppurative inflammation is usually present in affected placentas. There also may be considerable necrosis of epithelium and diffuse hyperplasia of fibrous connective tissue.

Focal microscopic granulomatous lesions frequently can be observed in livers of swine with brucellosis, particularly during bacteremic phases of the disease. These foci frequently are necrotic areas infiltrated with lymphocytes, macrophages, neutrophilis, and giant cells, with sheets of histocytic and epithelioid cells with a central zone of caseous or coagulative necrosis. The lesions are usually partially or completely enclosed by a fibrous capsule. The necrotic portions of the granulomas are heavily infiltrated with neutrophils and liquefaction and mineralization may occur (Enright 1990). These lesions are not specific for brucellosis, since similar hepatic lesions are associated with other bacterial infections.

Microscopic lesions of bones are sometimes caused by *B. suis* infection. These occur both in vertebrae and long bones. The lesions are most frequently located adjacent to the epiphyseal cartilage and usually consist of caseous centers surrounded by a zone of macrophages and leukocytes and often by an outer zone of fibrous connective tissue.

Focal areas of chronic lymphocytic and macrocytic inflammation or focal abscesses are found infrequently in kidneys, spleen, brain, ovaries, adrenal glands, lungs, and other tissues of infected swine.

DIAGNOSIS. The most accurate and possibly the most sensitive method of diagnosis of swine brucellosis is isolation of *Brucella* organisms by direct culture methods. It has been shown that routine culture of a small sample of lymph nodes from carcasses will reveal as many positives as serologic diagnosis (Alton 1990). This is a very practical survey strategy, as virtually all the produce of the industry passes through abattoirs and the material can be removed without damage to the carcasses. Culture of other material that becomes available is often fruitful, such as vaginal swabs or products of abortion, semen samples or castrated testicles, or the contents of swollen joints and blood samples. However, this is often not feasible because of inadequate or unavailable laboratory facilities and trained personnel (Deyoe 1969). *B.suis* can readily be grown on all the normal *Brucella* media in the absence of added CO_2, the techniques being fully described by Alton et al. (1988).

Attempts at detection of *B. suis* antigen in tissues of infected swine have been investigated, primarily using fluorescent antibody (FA) techniques. The general conclusion has been that *Brucella* are seldom detectable in lymph node impression smears with FA procedures because of the relatively low numbers of organisms typically present (Deyoe 1972b). Nevertheless, FA tests could probably be useful for examining aborted materials, since large numbers of *B. suis* are typical in such specimens.

Serologic procedures to detect antibodies against *Brucella* in infected swine are generally the most practical and most common means of diagnosis, but the results obtained are far from perfect. Market swine surveys have shown that as many as 18% of normal swine may react at a level of 1:25 when plate agglutination tests are used (Deyoe 1969). On the contrary, some swine produce little or no antibody against *Brucella*. Because of variable stages of disease, an infected herd of swine will nearly always contain some infected individuals that have no detectable *Brucella* antibody. Some strains of *B. suis* apparently do not stimulate antibody production as well as others (Deyoe 1967). Swine exposed to a minimal infective dose of *B. suis* generally have a prolonged incubation period before the appearance of significant quantities of antibody.

Because of the foregoing factors, serologic tests often achieve disappointing results in diagnosis of individual swine. However, most serologic tests are entirely adequate for herd tests. Characteristically, infected herds include a majority or large numbers of infected individuals. Because of close contact between animals and the tendency of brucellosis to spread rapidly through a herd, 50–80% is a common morbidity range (Spencer and Mattison 1975). When large herds have only a single serologic reactor disclosed during a herd test, it can generally be concluded that *B. suis* infection is not present.

Numerous serologic tests are available or have been investigated for use in diagnosing swine brucellosis (Alton et al. 1988). Many of these were developed for diagnosing bovine brucellosis and have been adapted for testing swine serums. Most tests utilize *B. abortus* whole cell antigens. Since the commonly used antigen strains of *B. abortus* 1119-3 and S99 have the same or very similar surface lipopolysaccharide complex as smooth *B. suis,* the standardized antigens produced and distributed by the Animal and Plant Health Inspection Service (APHIS) of the USDA, or the Central Veterinary Laboratory, Weybridge, United Kingdom, are equally useful for diagnosing both bovine and porcine brucellosis. This has been confirmed by extensive laboratory testing of swine sera with both *B. abortus* and *B. suis* antigens.

The original test methods for swine brucellosis diagnosis were tube and plate agglutination procedures. Interpretation of results were based on the finding that most infected swine herds contained one or more animals with >100 international units (IU) of agglutination. Therefore, all animals in such herds with >25 IU of *Brucella* agglutination were considered to be infected. It is now known that standard agglutination tests, although highly sensitive, are not sufficiently specific to be reliable diagnostic tools when used alone. Some of the inaccuracies can be overcome in situations where frequent and repeated testing is practicable and the trend of antibody titers can be determined.

Efforts to develop more specific serologic tests made use of early findings that incubation of the tube agglutination tests for a shorter time at higher temperatures tended to suppress the reaction of nonspecific IgM. However, the 56°C, 18-hour test developed by Hoerlein (1953) never gained widespread use because it had few clear-cut advantages over other tests in use or under development at that time.

Reducing the pH of antigen-serum mixtures to 3–4 was also found to suppress the agglutination of *Brucella* antigens by nonspecific agglutinations. Consequently, methods such as acidified plate antigen tests were developed. Such procedures were further refined by buffering the antigen at pH 3.65 to overcome the instability found with acidified plate antigens. The buffered *Brucella* antigen became the basis of the brucellosis card test and similar procedures, such as buffered plate antigen and Rose-Bengal tests. These tests are the most practical methods of diagnosis for swine brucellosis at present and are possibly still the preferred method for large-scale surveillance testing. It has a distinct advantage over standard agglutination tests because it is relatively unaffected by nonspecific agglutinins and it is generally as sensitive as any other serologic test for diagnosis of swine brucellosis.

Other tests such as Rivanol precipitation–serum agglutination, 2-mercaptoethanol, and complement-fixation are frequently used for diagnosis of brucellosis in swine and are very useful in confirming results of card tests. The above tests very seldom or never detect IgM *Brucella* antibodies in swine serum, therefore, they are highly specific. However, the relative sensitivity of these methods is usually low in early stages of brucellosis. By the time the antibody response peaks and thereafter in chronic stages, the Rivanol, mercaptoethanol, or complement-fixation methods are generally as sensitive as the card test. Regardless of the serologic test used for diagnosis, detection of 80–90% of individual, infected swine must be regarded as the best that can be achieved at present because of factors previously discussed.

Limited investigation of the enzyme-linked immunosorbent assay (ELISA) has been conducted, and it appears that this method may be equal or slightly superior to other serologic procedures for diagnosis of swine brucellosis in the future. Further investigation of this test for use in eradication campaigns is warranted.

Experimental studies reviewed by Corbel (1985) have shown that infection with organisms of several other genera can produce antibodies reactive in brucellosis diagnostic tests. These organisms include *Escherischia coli* serogroup O:157, *Salmonella* serotypes of Kaufman-White group N, and most importantly *Yersinia enterocolitica* serogroup O:9. Infection of pigs with this latter organism has often been confirmed, and the cross-reaction that results is highly significant due to the dominant O polysaccharide antigen being chemically identical to the A antigen present on the surface of all smooth brucellae. In some situations, yersiniosis poses a greater threat to the agricultural industry than does brucellosis itself, due to the confusion of brucellosis diagnosis. Great Britain has always been free of *B. suis* infection, and enjoys a thriving export trade as a result of the generally high health status of its stock. During the 7 years prior to 1988, the number of pigs tested for export certification giving a complement-fixation test (CFT) reaction of greater than 20 international complement-fixation test units (ICFTU) has never exceeded 0.004%, while the figures for 1988, 1989, and 1990 were 0.42%, 0.70%, and 1.5% respectively. During 1988 and 1989 at least 5% of exporting herds gave more than 5% CFT-positive reactions, with some herds reaching levels of more than 50% of animals tested failing at this level. *Y. enterocolitica* O:9 has been isolated from most herds involved and despite extensive investigation, *B. suis* could not be recovered (Wrathall et al. 1991).

Lymphocyte transformation tests have been used to measure cell-mediated immune responses in infected swine on a limited scale (Kaneene et al. 1978). There was high correlation between recovery of *B. suis* from tissues and detectable lymphocyte stimulation responses. However, the complexity of the method probably eliminates it from consideration as a diagnostic tool except in specialized instances.

Tests for delayed hypersensitivity, using intradermal injection of *Brucella* allergens, have been studied, but results have not stimulated much enthusiasm in the United States. However, they are of similar accuracy to serologic tests, and would be more appropriate for farm testing in some circumstances, although they are more difficult to apply and read, and would not be applicable in market swine–testing programs. Nevertheless, skin tests are used frequently for diagnosis of brucellosis of swine in many countries, particularly in eastern Europe.

One of the most important aids to diagnosis is an adequate herd history. Good records of clinical manifestations, movement of animals, additions to the herd, breeding records, and illnesses in persons working with the swine provide invaluable information necessary to arrive at a diagnosis of brucellosis. Accurate epidemiologic information is an essential supplement to laboratory tests.

TREATMENT. No treatments, such as antibiotic therapy, dietary supplements, or other chemotherapy, have proven effective and economically feasible in curing swine of brucellosis. Large doses of tetracylines, streptomycin, or sulfonamides given over relatively long periods have been investigated. In some trials these antibiotics alone or in combination appeared promising. In general, however, antibiotic therapy was effective in limiting the bacteremic stage of the disease;

but after therapy was discontinued, viable *B. suis* was still present in tissues. Although treatments have not been effective in eliminating all organisms from the host, chemotherapy in carefully selected circumstances could probably suppress multiplication of *B. suis* in vivo sufficiently to alleviate clinical manifestations and shedding of organisms. Even though such an approach may have limited practicability, it could have beneficial effects in an infected herd and should not be dismissed as impossible.

PREVENTION

Immunity. Safe and reliable vaccines that produce serviceable immunity against brucellosis in swine have not been developed. Significant resistance can be stimulated, but persistence of immunity has been a limiting factor (Deyoe 1972a). Interest in vaccination of swine in the United States has declined along with the decline in incidence of the disease. With the present incidence of swine brucellosis in this country, the cost of developing and applying vaccination cannot be justified.

There have been no basic studies specifically directed toward the mechanism of immunity against *B. suis* infection in swine. Nevertheless, one must assume from the overwhelming evidence accumulated in research on brucellosis in other species that the fundamental mechanism is a cell-mediated immunity, with humoral immunity having only a minor or nonexistent role.

A compilation of investigations on anti-*Brucella* immunity in swine can be summarized as follows: (1) some swine are naturally resistant to *Brucella* infection and this resistance could be enhanced markedly by selective breeding programs (Cameron et al. 1941) if all other genetic factors could be ignored; (2) the majority of swine infected with virulent *B. suis* will recover from the disease but subsequent resistance induced by the virulent infection may be transient, as most will be susceptible to reexposure, probably within 6–12 months after the initial infection; (3) trials with attenuated *B. suis* or *B. abortus* strain 19 have been unsuccessful in producing a persistent immunity with products considered to be safe for use; and (4) bacterins or extracts of killed *B. suis* have generally been ineffective in stimulating immunity or else there has been no conclusive evidence that the persistence of immunity is adequate.

CONTROL. Experiences in control of swine brucellosis indicate that eradication of the disease from swine in the United States is desirable and feasible. Marked reduction in the incidence of the disease has occurred since 1950. One significant factor in this reduction has been the tendency for swine production to become more specialized and less a part of diversified farming operations. Consequently, the occurrence of reproductive disease

in swine has become proportionally more important, confinement systems and closed herds have eliminated many opportunities for interfarm spread of disease, and larger units have eliminated the "community boar" in most instances. Another important instrument in control of swine brucellosis has been the establishment and maintenance of validated brucellosis-free herds, particularly purebred herds or those selling breeding stock. Implementation of effective surveillance programs such as market swine (sows and boars) identification and testing have been instrumental in locating and eliminating large numbers of infected herds. Finally, it has been found that whenever recommended procedures to eradicate brucellosis from an individual herd or an enzootic area are conscientiously followed, there is very seldom any recurrence of the disease in that locality (Spencer and Mattison 1975).

The current brucellosis eradication program in the United States is a joint state-federal and livestock industry program. The program is administered, supervised, and funded by cooperative efforts between state and federal animal health regulatory agencies. The livestock industries have input into procedures to be used through representation on advisory committees that ultimately determine the Uniform Methods and Rules for Brucellosis Eradication, the principal guideline for conducting the program. These rules and guidelines are revised frequently; therefore, current information regarding the program as it applies in each state is always available from each state veterinarian.

There are three acceptable alternative plans recommended for use when swine herds are found to be, or suspected of being, infected with *B. suis*. Plan 1 consists of depopulation of the entire herd, which is by far the most successful and the most economical in the long run. Plan 2 is a procedure designed to salvage irreplaceable bloodlines and basically consists of marketing the adult swine for slaughter and retaining weanling pigs for breeding stock, a plan that is not always successful and necessitates considerable isolation and retesting requirements. Plan 3 consists of removing only serologic reactors and retesting the herd as many times as necessary. This latter procedure is rarely successful if the herd is actually infected but is the plan of choice if it contains only a single reactor or if a very low proportion of animals are reactors and there is reasonable doubt that brucellosis exists.

REFERENCES

ALTON, G. G. 1990. *Brucella suis.* In Animal Brucellosis. Boca Raton: CRC Press Inc.

ALTON, G. G.; JONES, L. M.; AND PIETZ, D. E. 1975. Laboratory Techniques in Brucellosis, 2d ed. Geneva: World Health Organization.

ALTON, G. G.; JONES, L. M.; ANGUS, R. D.; AND VERGER, J. M. 1988. Techniques for the Brucellosis Laboratory. Paris: INRA.

BECKER, H. N.; BELDEN, R. C.; BREAULT, T.; BUR-RIDGE, M. J.; FRANKENBERGER, W. B.; AND NICOLET-TI, P. 1978. Brucellosis in feral swine in Florida. J Am Vet Med Assoc 173:1181–1182.

BENDTSEN, H.; CHRISTIANSEN, M.; AND THOMSEN, A. 1954. Brucella enzootics in swine herds in Denmark – presumably with hare as a source of infection. Nord Vet Med 6:11–21.

BORTS, I. H.; HARRIS, D. M.; JOYNT, M. F.; JENNINGS, J. R.; AND JORDAN, C. F. 1943. A milk-borne epidemic of brucellosis caused by the porcine type of Brucella (Brucella suis) in a raw milk supply. J Am Vet Med Assoc 121:319.

BORTS, I. H.; McNUTT, S. H.; AND JORDAN, C. F. 1946. Brucella melitensis isolated from swine tissues in Iowa. J Am Med Assoc 130:966.

BRINLEY-MORGAN, W. J., AND McCULLOUGH, N. B. 1974. Genus Brucella. In Bergey's Manual of Deter-minative Bacteriology, 8th ed. Baltimore: Williams and Wilkins, pp. 278–282.

CAMERON, H. S.; GREGORY, P. W.; AND HUGHES, E. H. 1941. Studies on genetic resistance in swine to Brucel-la infection. II. A bacteriological examination of re-sistant stock. Cornell Vet 31:21–24.

COOK, D. R., AND NOBLE, J. W. 1984. Isolation of B. suis from cattle. Aust Vet J 61:263–264.

CORBEL, M. J. 1985. Effect of atrophic rhinitis vaccines on the reaction of pigs to serological tests for brucello-sis. Vet Rec 117:150.

DE LEY, J.; MANNHEIM, W.; SEGERS, P.; LIEVENS, A.; DENIJIN, M.; VANHOUKE, M.; AND GILLIS, M. 1987. Ribonucleic acid cistron similarities and taxonomic neighborhood of Brucella and CDC group Vd. Int J Syst Bacteriol 37:35–42.

DEYOE, B. L. 1967. Pathogenesis of three strains of Bru-cella suis in swine. Am J Vet Res 28:951–957.

_____. 1969. Diagnostic tests for swine brucellosis. Proc 53d Annu Meet Livest Conserv, pp. 20–22.

_____. 1972a. Immunology and public health signifi-cance of swine brucellosis. J Am Vet Med Assoc 160:640–643.

_____. 1972b. Research findings applicable to eradica-tion of swine brucellosis. Proc 76th Annu Meet US Anim Health Assoc, pp. 108–114.

DEYOE, B. L., AND MANTHEI, C. A. 1967. Sites of locali-zation of Brucella suis in swine. Proc 71st Annu Meet US Livest Sanit Assoc, pp. 102–108.

_____. 1969. Swine brucellosis Proceedings of the 1967 Symposium on Factors Producing Embryonic and Fe-tal Abnormalities, Death, and Abortion in Swine. ARS 91-73, pp. 54–60.

ENRIGHT, F. M. 1990. The pathogenesis and pathobiolo-gy of Brucella infection in domestic animals. In Ani-mal Brucellosis. Boca Raton: CRC Press Inc.

FOX, M. D., AND KAUFMANN, A. F. 1977. Brucellosis in the United States, 1965–1974. J Infect Dis 136:312–316.

GOODE, E. R., JR.; MANTHEI, C. A.; BLAKE, G. E.; AND

AMERAULT, T. E. 1952. Brucella suis infection in suckling and weanling pigs. J Am Vet Med Assoc 121:456–464.

HOERLEIN, A. B. 1953. Studies of swine brucellosis. III. The differentiation of specific and nonspecific ag-glutination titers. Cornell Vet 43:28–37.

HOERLEIN, A. B.; HUBBARD, E. D.; LEITH, T. S.; AND BIESTER, H. E. 1954. Swine brucellosis. Vet Med Res Inst, Iowa State Coll.

HUBER, J. D.; KOPEK, J. D.; AND STEWART, W. C. 1989. Status report – 1989 cooperative state/federal brucel-losis eradication program. Proc 93rd Annu Meet US Anim Health Assoc, pp. 157–180.

HUDDLESTON, I. F. 1929. The differentiation of the spe-cies of the genus Brucella. 1929 Bull Mich Agric Exp Stn No. 100.

HUTCHINGS, L. M. 1950. Swine brucellosis. In Brucello-sis: American Association for the Advancement of Science Symposium. Washington, D.C.: Waverly Press, pp. 188–198.

JUBB, K. V. F.; KENNEDY, P. C.; AND PALMER, N. 1985. Pathology of Domestic Animals, vol 3. Orlando: Aca-demic Press, pp. 349.

KANEENE, J. M.; ANDERSON, R. K.; JOHNSON, D. W.; ANGUS, R. D.; MUSCOPLATE, C. C.; PIETZ, D. E.; VANDERWAGON, L. C.; AND SLOANE, E. E. 1978. Cell-mediated immune responses in swine from a herd in-fected with Brucella suis. Am J Vet Res 39:1607–1611.

LUCHSINGER, D. W.; ANDERSON, R. K.; AND WERRING, D. F. 1965. A swine brucellosis epizootic. J Am Vet Med Assoc 147:632–636.

MANTHEI, C. A.; MINGLE, C. K.; AND CARTER, R. W. 1952. Brucella suis infection in suckling and weaning pigs. J Am Vet Med Assoc 121:373–382.

MEYER, M. E. 1990. Current Concepts in the Taxonomy of the Genus Brucella. Boca Raton: CRC Press Inc.

SPENCER, P. L., AND MATTISON, J. R. 1975. Pike Coun-ty, Illinois, swine brucellosis project. Proc 79th Annu Meet US Anim Health Assoc, pp. 86–91.

THOMSEN, A. 1934. Brucella infection in swine. Acta Pathol Microbiol Scand [Suppl] 21.

TRAUM, J. 1914. Report to the chief. Bureau of Animal Industry, USDA, p. 30.

VANDEPLASSCHE, M.; HERMAN, J.; SPINCEMAILLE, J.; BOUTERS, R.; DEKEYSER, P.; AND BRONE, E. 1967. Brucella suis infection and infertility in swine. Meded Veeartsenijsch Rijksuniv (Ghent) 11:1–40.

VERGER, J. M.; GREYMONT, F.; GREMONT, P. A. D.; AND GRAYON, M. 1985. Brucella, a monospecific genus as shown by deoxyribonucleic acid hybridisation. Int J Syst Bacteriol 35:292–295.

WOOD, G. W.; HENDRICKS, J. B.; AND GOODMAN, D. E. 1976. Brucellosis in feral swine. J Wildl Dis 12:579–582.

WRATHALL, A. E.; BROUGHTON, E. S.; GILL, K. P. W.; AND GOLDSMITH, G. P. 1991. Serological reactions to Brucella in British pigs. Vet Rec. In press.

36 Clostridial Infections

D. J. Taylor
M. E. Bergeland

A NUMBER OF species of clostridia are involved in disease in swine. *Clostridium perfringens* (*welchii*) types A and C, *C. tetani, C. novyi, C. botulinum* and, to a lesser extent, *C. chauvoei* and *C. septicum* are the causes of recognizable clinical syndromes. These include *C. perfringens* type C enteritis, *C. perfringens* type A enteritis, tetanus, botulism, sudden death in sows associated with *C. novyi,* and blackleg (*C. chauvoei* and *C. septicum*). Some species are also involved as contaminants of wounds and lesions and may affect the clinical signs and the pathologic and bacteriologic findings. Species that may invade existing lesions include *C. perfringens* types A and C, *C. novyi, C. septicum,* and *C. chauvoei.* Other species may be recorded in swine from time to time and carcasses that are not chilled immediately after death are frequently invaded by clostridia from the gut. This invasion can be so rapid that it may be difficult to identify the actual cause of death. The presence of clostridia in specific or nonspecific disease in swine affects the prognosis of the disease and requires specific treatment, supportive and preventive measures appropriate to the control of the organism(s) present.

Clostridia are all large, gram-positive spore-forming bacilli. All are anaerobic and can be grown in culture under appropriate conditions. Species can be identified by the size and shape of the bacterial cell, the presence or absence of spores and their shape and position, their colonial morphology, biochemical characters, the presence of specific antigens, and the production of toxins. These toxins can also be used to distinguish between different varieties or types of a species. In some cases the organisms can be identified in fixed smears by their morphology or antigenicity, or toxins can be identified in pathologic material, allowing confirmation of diagnosis without isolation.

All clostridial species mentioned above cause disease by the elaboration of specific toxins or enzymes; these are described in the appropriate section below. This fact is of vital importance when considering treatment and prevention—clostridia are sensitive to a wide range of antimicrobials, which can only be effective in treatment and prevention of disease when tissue destruction is not very far advanced. Once toxins have been produced and are fixed to tissues, antimicrobials can only eliminate the bacteria, not reverse the damage. They may be of value in treatment, particularly in the early stages of disease, but are of most use in short-term prevention. Antitoxin may affect the course of disease in some cases and protect in the short term, but most recognizable clostridial diseases can be prevented reliably by vaccinating the animal at risk or the sow to provide colostral protection.

Clostridium perfringens Type C Enteritis

FATAL NECROTIC enteritis in nonimmune pigs is caused by *C. perfringens* and is commonest in piglets less than 1 week of age. Affected animals may be found dead or develop hemorrhagic diarrhea, rapidly followed by death in acute cases. Subacute cases occur in which mortality is less common. All are associated with a necrotic enteritis caused by multiplication of the organism in the small intestine. The disease was first identified in 1955 in the United Kingdom (Field and Gibson 1955) and Hungary (Szent-Iványi and Szabo 1955) but was subsequently identified in the United States (Barnes and Moon 1964), Denmark (Høgh 1965), Germany (Matthias et al. 1968), the Netherlands (Plaisier 1971), Canada (Morin et al. 1983), and Japan (Azuma et al. 1983). It has now been identified in most swine-rearing areas of the world.

Etiology. *C. perfringens* is an encapsulated, gram-positive bacillus measuring 1–1.5 μm × 4.8 μm. Spores are rarely visible but are ovoid and eccentric. The colonies are clearly visible on horse or bovine blood agar after a 24-hour incubation in anaerobic conditions and are 3–5 mm in diameter, grayish, circular, and surrounded by a variable zone of beta hemolysis. Type C organisms produce alpha and beta toxins most consistently as well as smaller amounts of other toxins. *C. perfringens* type B has been recovered from a syndrome resembling that described below (Bakhtin 1956) and also produces beta toxin, but type D has also been isolated (Harbola and Khera 1990) from a slightly different syndrome. Most isolates from the disease are identified as belonging to type C, which is not only a primary cause of disease, but can colonize the lesions caused by diseases of piglets, such as transmissible gastroenteritis (TGE).

Epidemiology.   Outbreaks of *C. perfringens* type C enteritis have been recorded in large numbers of herds in an area over a short period of time, as in the epizootic reported from Minnesota and Iowa (Bergeland et al. 1966) when 41 herds were affected. Once the disease has been identified in a country or area, it occurs more commonly in individual herds as outbreaks that may last up to 2 months. In a few units, the acute disease may occur over longer periods, and in these cases nonimmune gilts or sows may be introduced to an infected area or unit or piglets may not receive adequate levels of specific antibody in the colostrum. The age incidence of the disease is marked, for it normally occurs in pigs aged from 12 hours to 7 days, usually at around 3 days, although the disease has been recorded in pigs aged 2–4 weeks (Bergeland et al. 1966; Høgh 1974) and in weaned pigs (Meszaros and Pesti 1965; Matthias et al. 1968). Clinically affected pigs usually die, and mortality rates within affected litters may reach 100% in the progeny of nonimmune sows. When protective immunity develops in the sow as a consequence of disease in her litter, subsequent litters are usually unaffected. Morbidity rates vary from herd to herd according to the immune status of the sows in the herd and the time period over which morbidity is measured. In 20 herds from Minnesota and Iowa, the incidence of affected litters ranged from 9 to 100%, and the total herd mortality ranged from 5 to 59%, with a mean herd mortality of 26% (Bergeland et al. 1966). An average mortality rate of 54% was observed in 24 herds in Denmark (Høgh 1967b).

The organism may be transmitted as a vegetative organism from piglet to piglet in an infected farrowing house or may be acquired from maternal feces. It may persist in the environment as a vegetative organism or in the spore form, and the disease may affect litters over long periods of time if vaccination is not practiced. Spores are resistant to boiling for up to 1 hour and can persist in contaminated buildings for periods of at least 1 year. The purchase of carrier sows is the most likely source of the disease for farms, but it could be introduced by fecal contamination of boots and clothing.

Pathogenesis.   Infection is oral and newborn piglets become infected within minutes or hours of birth. The organisms multiply in the gut and become attached to the jejunal epithelial cells at the apexes of the villi (Arbuckle 1972; Walker et al. 1980). Desquamation of these epithelial cells is accompanied by proliferation of the organisms along the basement membrane and complete necrosis of the lamina propria of the villi (Fig. 36.1). In peracute cases hemorrhage accompanies the necrosis. The necrotic zone later advances to involve the crypts, the muscularis mucosae and submucosa, and occasionally the muscular layers. Some organisms penetrate the intestinal wall to cause emphysema in the muscle layers; some occasionally penetrate beneath the peritoneum and in the draining mesenteric lymph nodes. Thrombosis may develop in emphysematous areas. Most bacteria remain adherent to the necrotic villi or are shed into the intestinal lumen along with cell debris and blood and may sporulate there (Kubo and Watase 1985).

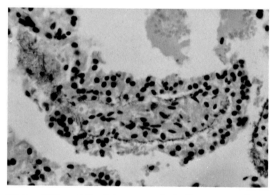

36.1.   Villus of the jejunum early in the course of *C. perfringens* type C infection in a 12-hour-old piglet. Numerous bacilli are present beneath the desquamated epithelium in the area of the epithelial basement membrane. H & E.

The lethal, necrotizing beta toxin is the most important factor in the pathogenesis of the disease. Strains isolated from piglets consistently produce alpha toxin (lecithinase), beta toxin (Warrack 1963, Høgh 1967a), and a variety of minor toxins, including the delta toxin. Evidence for the importance of the toxin comes from the widespread use of the toxoid alone in the prevention of the disease. Experimental evidence is more equivocal. The disease was reproduced by the oral administration of the toxin to pigs subsequently found to be carrying the organism (Field and Goodwin 1959; Bergeland 1965) and by the inoculation of gut loops with whole-broth cultures (Bergeland 1972), but no necrosis was produced by the inoculation of beta toxin alone. The sensitivity of the toxin to trypsin may account for these results and for the occurrence of the disease in pigs of less than 4 days of age in which trypsin secretion is absent.

Death results primarily from the effects of the intestinal damage and to a lesser extent from the extraintestinal effects of the toxin. The toxin can cause sudden death following intravenous infusion in high doses; at lower doses it causes polioencephalomalacia, adrenal cortical necrosis, nephrosis, and pulmonary edema (Bergeland 1965). Toxin has been demonstrated both in the intestinal contents of affected pigs and in the peritoneal fluid. Hypoglycemia occurs in field cases (Field and Goodwin 1959; Høgh 1967b) and may be a factor in mortality, along with secondary bacteremia due to *C. perfringens* or *E. coli.*

Clinical Signs. These vary according to the immune status and age of the piglets affected within a herd and from herd to herd. Peracute, acute, subacute, and chronic disease can be distinguished. The onset of clinical signs normally occurs within the first 2–3 days of life in all forms of the disease.

PERACUTE FORM. Affected piglets remain normal for the first 10 hours of life, but may be found dead within 12–36 hours of birth. They develop hemorrhagic diarrhea in most cases, and this may stain the perineum but can be overlooked. Piglets become weak, move with reluctance, rapidly become moribund, and may be crushed by the sow. The rectal temperature falls to 35°C and the abdominal skin may blacken before death. Death may occur in some animals without diarrhea being seen.

ACUTE FORM. Acute cases survive 2 days after the onset of clinical signs and commonly die when 3 days old. Throughout the course of the disease they have reddish brown liquid feces that contain shreds of gray necrotic debris. They lose condition and become gaunt and weak, making only feeble attempts to suck on the last day of life.

SUBACUTE FORM. These pigs have a persistent nonhemorrhagic diarrhea and usually die when about 5–7 days of age. They remain active and alert and have a fair appetite but become progressively more emaciated and may be extremely thin and dehydrated at the time of death. The feces tend to be yellow at first and then change to a clear liquid containing flecks of necrotic debris.

CHRONIC FORM. Chronic cases may have an intermittent or persistent diarrhea for 1 or more weeks. The feces are yellow-gray and mucoid, and the tail may be coated with dried feces. Affected pigs may remain alert and vigorous for 10 days or more, but their rate of growth is depressed. These pigs may eventually die after several weeks or be killed because of their failure to gain weight.

Lesions. Piglets that die from the peracute form are often in good condition and do not appear dehydrated. There may be blackish discoloration of the abdominal skin, even in animals killed in extremis. The umbilical cord is usually still present. Reddish feces may be present on the perineum. The abdominal wall is often edematous when cut. The most immediate and striking findings are the presence of intensely hemorrhagic small intestines (Fig. 36.2) and the presence of blood-stained fluid in the abdominal cavity.

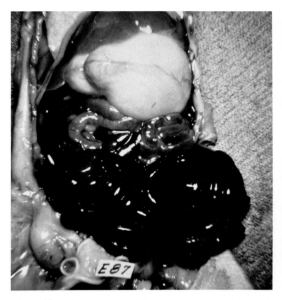

36.2. Necrohemorrhagic jejunitis in a 1-day-old piglet with peracute *C. perfringens* type C enteritis.

The lesions vary in extent, occurring in the jejunum but extending into the ileum. They may extend from 14 cm posterior to the pylorus to the cecum or affect only 2–3 cm of bowel. Lesions are reddish or black, and there may be gas bubbles in the intestinal wall. The mesenteric lymph nodes may be reddened. The contents of the affected area are hemorrhagic and hemorrhagic contents may be found in the intestine distal to the lesion, often as far as the rectum. The mucosa is intensely hemorrhagic and no villi can be distinguished. Microscopically, the villi in the affected portion of the jejunum are necrotic and covered by large gram-positive bacilli. The epithelium of the crypts may or may not be necrotic and there is profuse hemorrhage throughout the mucosa and submucosa (Figs. 36.3, 36.4). Large numbers of gram-positive bacilli are present in smears of the lesions.

Acute cases may be dehydrated or show loss of body condition, and there may be scalding of the perineum and adherent reddish feces. The intestines are less frequently reddened and any reddish lesions may be localized. Emphysema of a

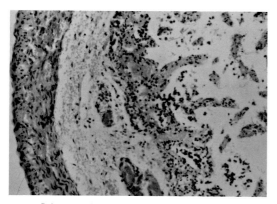

36.3. Jejunum of a piglet with peracute *C. perfringens* type C enteritis. There is acute necrosis of the mucosa and massive hemorrhage in the submucosa. H & E.

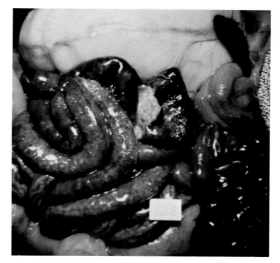

36.5. Acute *C. perfringens* type C enteritis in a 3-day-old piglet. There is an emphysematous segment of upper jejunum (left) that is held together by acute peritonitis. Mucosal necrosis of the lower jejunum (right) is seen from the serosal surface.

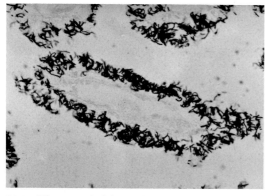

36.4. The necrotic jejunal villi from a piglet with peracute *C. perfringens* type C infection are covered by numerous gram-positive bacilli. Gram.

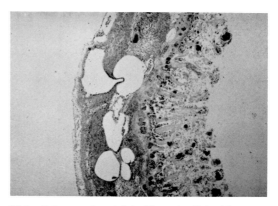

36.6. Jejunum of a piglet with acute *C. perfringens* type C enteritis. The mucosa is completely necrotic and there is emphysema of the submucosa and tunica muscularis. H & E.

sharply demarcated portion of up to 40 cm of the jejunum may be present from 30 cm posterior to the pylorus; this portion of the intestine may be loosely adherent to adjacent segments by acute fibrinous peritonitis (Fig. 36.5).

The wall of the intestine is usually thickened and the contents are sometimes bloodstained and often contain some necrotic debris. The mucosa is yellow or grayish and covered with loosely adherent necrotic debris. Microscopic lesions include the absence of most villi and those that survive are necrotic and covered with bacteria. The luminal surface is covered with a necrotic membrane comprised of bacteria, shed epithelial cells, fibrin, and degenerating inflammatory cells lying directly over the submucosa. The submucosal vessels are necrotic and many contain thrombi. Emphysema may be evident in the submucosa, tunica muscularis, and under the serosa (Fig. 36.6). Large gram-positive bacteria may be present in deeper layers of the intestinal wall.

Subacute cases are usually in poor condition and there may be adhesions between affected areas of the small intestine. The intestinal wall is thickened and friable, and the mucosal surface is covered by a tightly adherent necrotic membrane, which may be seen from the serosal surface as longitudinal grayish yellow bands (Fig. 36.7).

Chronically affected pigs may have lesions resembling those described above, but they may not be obvious from the serosal surface of the intestine. There may be local thickening of the intestinal wall and local, well-defined areas to which necrotic membrane is adherent. These areas may be only 1–2 cm in length and consist of areas in which the mucosa has been replaced by a necrotic membrane with a variety of bacteria along the deep edge. Deeper layers of the intestinal wall show evidence of chronic inflammation (Fig. 36.8).

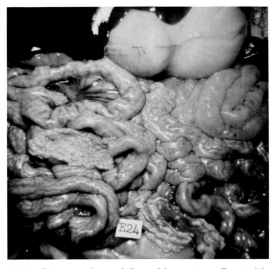

36.7. Subacute form of *C. perfringens* type C enteritis in a 6-day-old piglet. The entire jejunum is lined by a necrotic membrane.

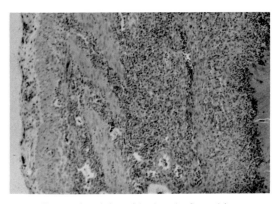

36.8. Ileum of a piglet with chronic *C. perfringens* type C enteritis. The mucosa is replaced by a necrotic membrane containing a variety of bacterial species. The submucosa, tunica muscularis, and serosa are infiltrated by chronic inflammatory cells. H & E.

Diagnosis. The clinical signs and gross postmortem findings are sufficient for a presumptive diagnosis of *C. perfringens* type C enteritis to be made. Hemorrhagic diarrhea in young piglets, the pattern of mortality, and the presence of the hemorrhagic, necrotic lesions in the small intestine are the most important features on which to base this diagnosis. The presence of emphysematous sections of the small intestine in freshly dead piglets is also significant. Diagnosis of the chronic disease is more difficult and may depend upon a history of previous infection in the herd, the elimination of other causes of necrotic enteritis, and laboratory confirmation of the presence of the agent in the lesions. Coccidiosis (*Isospora suis*) and other causes of villous atrophy, such as rotavirus, transmissible gastroenteritis, and porcine

epidemic diarrhea, may all cause lesions that are colonized by bacteria including *C. perfringens* type C (Bergeland 1977). *C. perfringens* type A (see below) may also cause clinical signs and lesions resembling those of the subacute and chronic forms and may only be distinguished from them by laboratory means.

Diagnosis can be supported in the laboratory by examination of smears of intestinal contents and mucosal lesions and histologic sections of the intestinal wall for the presence of large, gram-positive rods. The microscopic appearance of the hemorrhagic lesions is characteristic and is almost pathognomonic. Diagnosis can be confirmed beyond doubt by the demonstration of the beta toxin of *C. perfringens* type C in supernates of hemorrhagic intestinal contents and sometimes in peritoneal fluid. Mouse inoculation and protection tests using type-specific antisera may be used to detect the toxin itself, as may enzyme-linked immunosorbent assay tests.

In more chronic cases and in some acute ones the toxin cannot be identified; less satisfactory confirmation can be obtained by directly inoculating blood agar plates with *C. perfringens* type C from scrapings of the intestinal mucosa and identifying and toxin-typing the isolated colonies. This method of confirmation is less satisfactory because the organism has been found as a secondary agent colonizing the lesions of piglets with TGE and other viral diseases. When the disease is chronic the organism may be impossible to isolate, and in those instances, earlier cases of the disease must be sought in the herd to confirm a diagnosis.

Treatment and Prevention. Once clinical signs are present little can be done, for the intestinal damage is already extensive (Szabo and Szent Iványi 1957; Høgh 1967b). Even where the organism is eliminated, the animal still dies or remains stunted. Prophylaxis is of more value than therapy.

In an outbreak, the disease can be prevented in a herd by passive immunization with antitoxin to *C. perfringens* type C in litters of nonimmune sows. Parenteral injection of antitoxin should be carried out as soon after birth as possible, for the disease may already be occurring in piglets only a few hours old. Oral antimicrobials such as ampicillin may also be given as soon after birth as possible and should prevent the development of the disease. Treatment should be repeated daily for the first 3 days of life. Recent studies suggest that *C. perfringens* may develop resistance to antimicrobials commonly used on a farm; tetracycline-resistant plasmids have been identified in this species (Rood et al. 1985).

Prevention of the disease on a more permanent basis relies on vaccination of sows with *C. perfringens* type C toxoid on two occasions: first, at service or midgestation and the second, 2–3 weeks before farrowing. Piglets will be protected, provided they suck colostrum (Ripley and Gush 1983). The level of passive antibody in the piglet is related to that in the sow at farrowing. These can vary markedly from 4.5 IU to 123 IU/ml (Matishek and McGrinley 1986). Booster injections should be given about 3 weeks before subsequent farrowings. Toxoid may also be of value in protecting weaned pigs (Meszaros and Pesti 1965).

Clostridium perfringens Type A Enteritis

C. PERFRINGENS type A has been isolated from the intestines of pigs for many years and has been considered to form part of the normal flora (Mansson and Smith 1962). Evidence has gradually accumulated that this organism is involved in enteric disease, both in neonatal piglets and in older pigs in the postweaning period (Jestin et al. 1985). The organism is present in every pig and is distributed worldwide. In recent years reports of its involvement in clinical disease or the reproduction of disease have come from Germany (Amtsberg et al. 1976), France (Ramisse et al. 1979), the United Kingdom (Olubunmi 1982), the Netherlands (Nabuurs et al. 1983), and Romania (Secasiu 1984).

Etiology. *C. perfringens* type A resembles *C. perfringens* type C, but colonies are often surrounded by a double zone of hemolysis, the outer of which is caused by the alpha toxin and the inner by theta toxin. The organism does not produce beta toxin or the other major toxins used in typing, but some strains produce a powerful enterotoxin upon sporulation. An ability to sporulate is generally considered a prerequisite for enterotoxin production. Spores may require heat shocking to germinate. Enterotoxin-producing strains rarely produce large amounts of alpha toxin and there appear to be two separate syndromes associated with the two types of *C. perfringens* type A. Both sporulating and enterotoxin-producing strains of *C. perfringens* type A have been demonstrated in pigs (Estrada and Taylor 1989), although Damme-Jongsten et al. (1990) failed to demonstrate the gene concerned.

Epidemiology. The organism is ubiquitous in gut contents and in soil. Spores can survive freezing and boiling for up to 10 minutes, but the vegetative cells are fully susceptible to heat. The epidemiology of *C. perfringens* type A is not completely known. The organism can be isolated on all farms and antibody is widespread in finishing pigs and sows (Estrada Correa and Taylor 1989). Outbreaks of disease in litters and on farms appear to be associated with organisms with similar cultural characteristics, but no detailed studies have yet determined whether these are individual strains. It must be assumed that the major source of the organism for intensively housed pigs is pig feces, but the organism can be demonstrated in some diets and in the environment.

Enterotoxigenic strains are capable of causing human food poisoning, usually following growth in slowly cooling joints of meat following cooking. It is not known whether strains causing food poisoning found in cooked pork are the same as those causing disease in the live animal.

Pathogenesis. Infection with *C. perfringens* type A occurs in most piglets within a few hours of birth and the organism can be demonstrated in the first feces following the clearance of meconium. In nonimmune piglets infected with pathogenic strains, numbers build up in the ileum and jejunum to levels of 10^8–10^9/g of contents. Similar levels may be found in large intestinal contents and feces. Vegetative forms produce alpha toxin and possibly other toxins that cause necrosis of the intestinal epithelium in experimental infections in vivo. No consistent changes have been produced by the inoculation of gut loops with purified alpha toxin (Estrada Correa 1986). Sporulating forms produce enterotoxin that causes dramatic villous necrosis and outpourings of fluid into the intestinal lumen. The toxin fixes to the colonic epithelial cells and may be responsible for failure to resorb water. Antibody to both toxins is present in colostrum, and disease associated with enterotoxin is commonly seen after maternal antibody disappears in weaned pigs 5–7 weeks of age (Estrada Correa 1986).

C. perfringens type A also colonizes existing lesions.

Clinical Signs. Piglets develop a creamy or pasty diarrhea within 48 hours of birth and lose condition when infected with vegetative forms of *C. perfringens* type A. Affected piglets appear hairy and have fecal staining of the perineum. There is no fever and animals rarely die. If they do, there is often discoloration of the abdominal skin, similar to that seen in *C. perfringens* type C infections. Diarrhea lasts for up to 5 days and feces on the pen floor appears mucoid and may be pink. Recovered piglets remain in poor condition for some time. Infections caused by the sporulating form cause a transient watery diarrhea, which may only last for 24–48 hours.

Weaned pigs 5–7 weeks of age develop diarrhea or soft feces lasting 4–7 days. This diarrhea does not result in death but affected animals lose condition and become covered with feces. The rate of daily liveweight gain is depressed. Onset of the diarrhea can be delayed by the use of antimicrobial feed additives that affect clostridia. The clinical signs may form part of the "colitis" complex (see Swine Dysentery, Chapter 49, and Spirochetal Diarrhea, Chapter 47).

Lesions

GROSS LESIONS. Piglets are usually dehydrated with fecal staining of the perineum. The small intestine is flaccid and thick walled, with pasty contents and no blood. The mucosa is mildly inflamed and necrotic material may be adherent to it. The absence of villi is obvious under a hand lens. The large intestine is distended with whitish pasty contents. The mucosa is often normal or may be coated with necrotic debris. In weaned pigs there are few if any gross lesions in the mucosa, but there may be frothy, mucoid contents in both ileum and the cecum.

MICROSCOPIC LESIONS. In piglets there is villous atrophy with superficial necrosis and accumulations of fibrin. Although there is capillary dilatation, the hemorrhage seen in *C. perfringens* type C infections is absent. There may also be an inflammatory colitis. Gram-positive rods may be seen adjacent to the mucosa in Gram-stained sections. In the weaned pig, there may be some villous atrophy in the ileum and superficial colitis, but in some cases the mucosa appears normal.

BACTERIOLOGY. Clostridia are obvious in fecal smears or gut contents, and large numbers of spores are present when enterotoxin-producing strains are involved. *C. perfringens* type A can be isolated from the small intestine in profuse culture in affected piglets and from the large intestinal contents in weaned pigs. Sporulating bacteria can be isolated by heating samples to 80°C for 10 minutes before culture.

Diagnosis. The clinical signs of disease in piglets resemble those of mild *C. perfringens* type C infection. There is little or no blood in the feces and there is little or no mortality. The condition can be confirmed by isolation of the organism and by failure to demonstrate the presence of other agents. In weaned pigs the organism rarely occurs alone; a diagnosis of uncomplicated *C. perfringens* type A infection requires the failure to demonstrate other enteropathogens, coupled with the presence of high numbers of sporulating organisms and the demonstration of preformed enterotoxin in fecal filtrates by reverse passive agglutination tests or counter immunoelectrophoresis (CIE). Toxin levels of 1:32 were considered significant by Jestin and Popoff (1987) and maximum levels of 1:160 were recorded.

Treatment. The disease in piglets can be treated by using antimicrobials in the same way as with *C. perfringens* type C infection, but with more likelihood of success. Vaccination is not possible as no commercial clostridial vaccine currently includes alpha toxin or enterotoxin. Experimental vaccination of the sow has shown that vaccination is possible, but the ubiquitous nature of the organism means that it is usually sufficient to ensure that piglets ingest sufficient colostrum. In weaned pigs it is usually sufficient to include a growth promoter, such as avoparcin, in the ration at a level capable of inhibiting the organism (Taylor and Estrada Correa 1988).

Cellulitis and Gas Gangrene

INFECTED WOUNDS in swine often contain several types of bacteria. When the histotoxic clostridia become established in a wound, however, they rapidly become the most predominant and significant pathogen. These clostridial wound infections are highly fatal and are characterized by intense acute inflammation with abundant edema and varying amounts of gas and local tissue necrosis. The inflammation spreads rapidly from the primary infection site, and there usually is terminal generalized sepsis.

C. septicum, C. perfringens type A, *C. novyi,* and *C. chauvoei* are the common causes of clostridial cellulitis and gas gangrene in swine.

CLOSTRIDIUM SEPTICUM INFECTION (MALIGNANT EDEMA)

Etiology. *C. septicum* appears to be the most common etiologic agent of clostridial cellulitis and gas gangrene of swine.

The organism is an anaerobic gram-positive rod, approximately 0.6–0.8μ wide and 3–8μ long, which forms oval subterminal spores. It is known to produce four toxins of which the alpha toxin is hemolytic, necrotizing, and lethal. In addition, hyaluronidase, deoxyribonuclease, and an oxygen-labile hemolysin are produced (Moussa 1958).

Epidemiology. *C. septicum* is a common potential wound contaminant, since it is a widespread inhabitant of the soil (MacLennan 1962). The incidence of malignant edema is particularly high on certain premises. These often are lots that have had high populations of livestock for many years, which suggests that there is a buildup of spore numbers in the environment of these farms.

Pathogenesis. Since *C. septicum* infection nearly always involves the skin and subcutis, it appears that most cases result from perforated wounds, even though evidence of a wound may sometimes not be found. Tissue damage at the site of inoculation favors the initial establishment of the infection. It is probable that the local lesion is largely the result of the necrotizing effect of the alpha toxin. It has been proposed that the hyaluronidase produced by *C. septicum* causes disappearance of the endomysium (Aikat and Dible 1960), which may aid the spread of the infection through muscle.

Toxemia undoubtedly is a major factor in causing death of the animal. Experimental intravenous infusion of *C. septicum* toxins in the cat causes a specific constriction in the coronary and pulmonary circulations, with the development of pulmonary edema (Kellaway et al. 1941). On the basis of this evidence, it could be speculated that the pulmonary edema and the serofibrinous exudates found in the pericardial and pleural cavities of some cases of malignant edema in swine are the result of bacterial toxemia.

Clinical Signs. *C. septicum* infection has an acute course and is often fatal in less than 24 hours. Gross swelling may be located in any area of the body. Common sites include the inguinal and ventral abdominal region, the head and ventral cervical area, and the shoulder. The swelling spreads rapidly from the primary site, but it usually remains confined to one general region of the body. If the limbs are involved, there is reluctance to bear weight on the affected leg. The skin overlying the swollen area has a blotchy reddish purple discoloration. Palpation of the swollen area reveals a pitting edema, and crepitation may also be evident late in the course of the disease. In the terminal stage, affected swine lie in lateral recumbency and commonly make a groaning noise during forced expiration.

Lesions. There is conspicuous swelling in the general region of the primary infection site (Fig. 36.9). Incision of the erythematous skin overlying the infection reveals subcutaneous edema that may be colorless with focal hemorrhages or may be uniformly sanguinous. Gas is present in varying quantities. The adjacent skeletal muscle may be edematous with essentially normal color or may have the features of typical gas gangrene in

which there are black, dry, and crepitant areas (Fig. 36.10). Affected muscle may have a butyric odor indistinguishable from the characteristic odor of *C. chauvoei* infection in the ruminant. The regional lymph nodes are enlarged, hemorrhagic, and may be emphysematous. There is commonly an acute fibrinohemorrhagic peritonitis. The spleen is only slightly enlarged. There is moderate pulmonary edema and congestion. Varying amounts of amber fluid and fibrin may be found in the pleural cavity and pericardial sac.

Postmortem decomposition occurs rapidly, and subcutaneous gas accumulates progressively until the subcutis of the entire carcass is emphysema-

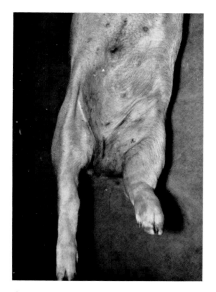

36.9. *C. septicum* infection. The grossly swollen area involves the entire left rear leg and extends cranially to the umbilicus. The overlying skin has a blotchy reddish purple discoloration.

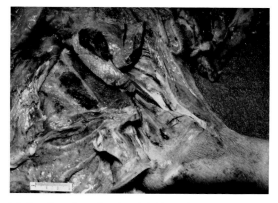

36.10. Rear leg of a pig with *C. septicum* infection. There is prominent subcutaneous edema. The infection extends into the ham, which has foci of black, dry necrotic muscle.

tous. Focal postmortem lysis of the liver is commonly seen, with resulting grayish tan foci being evident within several hours after death. As postmortem decomposition progresses, the foci become confluent, giving the liver a uniform tan color with numerous gas bubbles.

Microscopically, there is edema of the subcutis that contains large numbers of degenerating acute inflammatory cells and bacteria. Septic thrombi in subcutaneous veins and lymphatics are commonly found (Fig. 36.11). Affected skeletal muscle fibers undergo coagulation necrosis with fragmentation and lysis, and bacteria are readily found between the degenerating muscle fibers (Fig. 36.12).

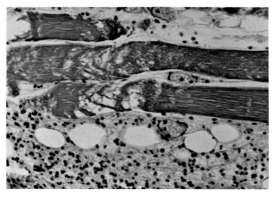

36.11. Acute septic thrombophlebitis involving the subcutaneous vein of a pig with *C. septicum* infection. The thrombus contains many long, slender rods and degenerating leukocytes. H & E.

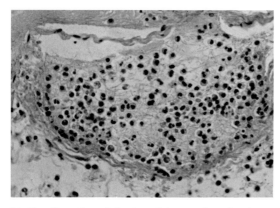

36.12. *C. septicum* infection of the rear leg of a pig. Skeletal muscle fibers are undergoing fragmentation and lysis. The adjacent connective tissues are edematous and contain bacteria, degenerating inflammatory cells, and emphysema. H & E.

Diagnosis. A presumptive diagnosis is made by observation of typical gross lesions in the freshly dead animal. Laboratory confirmation is based on pathologic findings, together with exclusion of other diseases, and identification of the organism.

Many bacteria are seen on direct smears of the affected subcutis or muscle. Fluorescent-labelled antibody staining (Batty and Walker 1963) of direct impression smears of the local lesion is a rapid and accurate method of positively identifying *C. septicum*. An alternate method is isolation of the organism by anaerobic culture and identification by biochemical tests; however, this is more time consuming and less reliable than the use of immunofluorescence (Martig 1966).

Treatment and Prevention. Treatment with antibiotics may be successful if given early in the course of the disease. There is little specific information available on the therapy of malignant edema in swine. Zeller (1956) mentions the recovery of two pigs after treatment with oxytetracycline. Experimentally, the prophylactic use of tetracyclines, penicillin, or chloramphenicol would prevent the disease in mice; however, their effectiveness was greater when administered locally at the inoculation site than when given systemically (Taylor and Novak 1952).

Prevention of the disease involves good sanitation and prevention of injuries. Sharp objects that may cause perforating wounds should be removed from the environment. In many instances *C. septicum* infection is a sequel of hypodermic injections in swine; therefore, adequate sanitary procedures should be followed when making injections or performing surgery. On premises where there are recurrences of the disease, immunization with *C. septicum* bacterin could be considered; however, this is seldom done in swine.

CLOSTRIDIUM PERFRINGENS TYPE A INFECTION (GAS GANGRENE). *C. perfringens* is occasionally involved in wound infections in swine. The infection is acute and highly fatal and usually of only sporadic incidence.

A high herd incidence of *C. perfringens* gas gangrene is occasionally seen in young piglets as a complication of injection of iron-containing preparations used for the prevention of nutritional anemia. Circumstantial evidence suggests that injection of iron preparations creates a microenvironment in tissue that favors the growth of *C. perfringens*. Jaartsveld et al. (1962) reported the occurrence of *C. perfringens* infection in two herds following intramuscular injection of an iron preparation. Twelve of 25 piglets in one herd died the morning following injection. It was assumed that contaminated hypodermic needles were the source of the infection. The author has seen a similar problem in several herds in which *C. perfringens* occurred as a pure infection in some cases and as a mixed infection with *E. coli* and staphylococci in others. When the problem occurs, the herd incidence is usually high, with mortality approaching 50%. The affected piglets have marked swelling of the entire rear limb that was injected, and the swelling extends cranially to the umbilical area. The skin overlying the swollen area has a dark reddish brown discoloration. Incision of the affected area reveals extensive edema, and there may be a copious quantity of gas in the muscle and subcutis. The inflammatory exudate is brownish red, due largely to staining by the injected iron preparation. The lesion usually has a putrid odor. Postmortem decomposition occurs rapidly, and the liver of pigs dead more than a few hours may have conspicuous gray foci of lysis that surround minute gas bubbles. Microscopically, acute thrombophlebitis may be evident, and affected muscle fibers undergo fragmentation and liquefaction necrosis.

The alpha toxin (lecithinase) of *C. perfringens* has been shown to be almost solely responsible for the production of the local lesion (Aikat and Dible 1956). It is proposed that the lecithinase causes cellular necrosis by action on lipoprotein complexes of cell membranes. In addition there is evidence that the mu toxin (hyaluronidase) causes separation of the muscle sarcolemma from the endomysium.

The diagnosis is based on clinical and pathologic findings, together with the isolation and identification of *C. perfringens*. In mixed infections, direct Gram-stained smears of the lesion are helpful in estimating the relative numbers of different bacteria present. *C. perfringens* is evident as a robust gram-positive bacillus that seldom contains spores. Isolation of the organism is easily accomplished by anaerobic incubation for 18–24 hours of blood agar and egg yolk agar plates streaked directly from the lesion.

Treatment of *C. perfringens* infections with antibiotics may be successful if instituted early in the course of the disease. Experimentally, penicillin injections given at the same time as inoculation of *C. perfringens* in mice gave almost complete protection; however, a delay in penicillin injection of over 3 hours appreciably lowered the survival rate (Hac and Habert 1943). Jaartsveld et al. (1962) mention the recovery of some clinically sick pigs following penicillin injection.

Prevention of *C. perfringens* gas gangrene in swine involves preventing the occurrence of deep, contaminated wounds.

CLOSTRIDIUM CHAUVOEI INFECTION (BLACKLEG).

The pig is generally considered to be quite resistant to *C. chauvoei* infection, and historically there have been very few substantiated reports of this disease in swine. Sterne and Edwards (1955) reported the occurrence of blackleg in swine kept under very poor hygiene in a lot where there previously had been high losses of cattle from blackleg. Four pigs were examined, 2 of which were found to be infected with *C. chauvoei* and 2 with *C. septicum*. Gualandi (1955) reported an outbreak of *C. chauvoei* infection in which 15 of 34 pigs died in 2 days. Edema of the

pharynx was a constant finding. Eggleston (1950) described the losses of 3 pigs, weighing 100–140 pounds, which had been fed a blackleg calf carcass. There was swelling of the face and throat region, including the ears, and the odor of the lesions resembled rancid butter.

C. chauvoei is a pleomorphic, anaerobic, gram-positive rod, measuring 0.5–1 μ by 3–8 μ, which readily forms central to subterminal spores. It produces several exotoxins, of which the alpha toxin is lethal, necrotizing, and possibly hemolytic. In addition, deoxyribonuclease, hyaluronidase, and an oxygen-labile hemolysin are produced (Moussa 1958).

The pathogenesis of *C. chauvoei* infection is not completely understood. It is assumed that the organism usually has an oral portal rather than being a wound infection. It is postulated that the bacteria sometimes may lie dormant in various tissues until there is a favorable microenvironment for their growth. Tissue damage such as bruising may then be the factor that triggers the disease. Once bacterial growth occurs, the disease appears to be a manifestation of the effects of bacterial toxins and pathologically may closely resemble *C. septicum* infection.

Because of the pathologic similarity between *C. septicum* and *C. chauvoei* infections and the apparent higher incidence of *C. septicum* infection in swine, a diagnosis of blackleg can be made only by bacterial identification. The fluorescent antibody test (Batty and Walker 1963) applied to direct impression smears of infected tissue is a rapid and practical method of identification. Isolation by anaerobic culture may be difficult in decomposing specimens, since *C. chauvoei* is relatively fastidious and easily overgrown by other bacteria, such as *C. septicum*.

The prevention of *C. chauvoei* infection involves minimizing exposure to the organism. Even though *C. chauvoei* has not been demonstrated to be a common soil organism, circumstantial evidence from the few reports of the disease in pigs suggests that keeping swine on known contaminated premises or allowing them to eat carcasses of ruminants dead of blackleg are factors in its incidence.

CLOSTRIDIUM NOVYI INFECTION (SUDDEN DEATH).

C. novyi may cause sudden death in swine. Batty et al. (1964) reported the sudden death of 12 pigs over a 3-week period. Postmortem decomposition progressed unusually rapidly. The lungs were congested, the trachea contained blood-stained froth, and there was some hemorrhage on the surface of the kidney. They reported the loss 4 days after farrowing of an adult sow that showed marked decomposition, and the internal organs contained massive numbers of *C. novyi*.

Four cases of sudden death in sows on grass were described by Bourne and Kerry (1965). Necropsy findings included rapid postmortem tympany; submandibular swellings; bloodstained fluid in the pleural, pericardial, and peritoneal cavities; serosal hemorrhages; splenic enlargement; and marked degeneration and emphysema of the liver. *C. novyi* was demonstrated in various tissues, including heart blood. An obvious feature of pigs that have died from this disease is the bronze color of the liver and the presence of large numbers of small gas bubbles in the substance of the organ when it is cut. These are particularly significant when the remainder of the carcass is fresh.

C. novyi is an anaerobic, spore-forming, gram-positive rod that varies in size but generally is the largest of the clostridia encountered in swine. The organism produces highly potent exotoxins, and the species is subdivided into four types (A–D) based on toxin production. The lethal, necrotizing alpha toxin is considered to be the principal toxin of types A and B strains. Death in infected ruminants is attributed to bacterial toxemia. The type involved in swine infections has been identified as type B by Itoh et al. (1987).

A positive diagnosis of *C. novyi* infection in swine is made with difficulty, since suspect cases are usually found dead and some interval of time elapses between death and necropsy. The organism is a common and early postmortem invader, especially of adult swine in warm weather. Therefore, a detailed examination to exclude other possible causes of death must always be made. The disease should be suspected when there is a history of sudden death, together with necropsy findings that may include submandibular swelling, pulmonary edema and tracheal froth, serofibrinous or serosanguinous exudates in pericardial and pleural cavities, and unusually rapid decomposition with accumulation of gas in the liver. The presence of gas bubbles in an otherwise fresh carcass is particularly significant.

The organism is rapidly identified by fluorescent antibody staining of direct smears of infected tissue. Isolation and typing of the organism are difficult since it has the most fastidious growth requirements of the clostridia commonly encountered in swine but isolation has been described by Itoh et al. (1987).

Information on pathogenesis and epidemiology in swine awaits further study of the disease. The disease can be controlled by reducing the incidence of pneumonias and enteritis in affected groups of pigs, coupled with vaccination of finishing pigs and sows against the disease using alum-adjuvanted vaccines such as those readily available for sheep.

Tetanus

TETANUS is a disease characterized by uncontrollable spasms of voluntary muscles, which is caused by the toxin of *C. tetani* elaborated at the site of a deep infection. Swine of all ages may be affected; however, the majority of cases involve young pigs, usually as a complication of either castration wound infection or umbilical infection.

C. tetani is a slender, anaerobic, gram-positive rod, measuring $0.3–0.6$ μ by $2–8$ μ, which characteristically forms terminal spherical spores. Its major lethal toxin, tetanospasmin, is a highly potent neurotoxic protein. An oxygen-labile hemolysin, tetanolysin, is also produced.

Epidemiology. *C. tetani* is a common inhabitant of the soil. Sergeeva and Matveev (1966) conducted a survey of 5338 soil samples collected from various regions of the USSR and found that the highest level of soil contamination was in the southern regions having fertile black soil, long periods of vegetation for plants and soil organisms, and highly developed agriculture and cattle breeding. In some regions the rate of isolation was as high as 40–62% of the samples examined. In areas where the soil was not fertile, regions with concentrated cattle raising and fields fertilized with animal manure had a significantly higher incidence of soil contamination than regions without livestock. Tetanus morbidity in various areas of the USSR correlated directly with the prevalence of the organism in the soil. Sakurai (1966) also reported a high incidence of tetanus in areas of Japan where stock farms and pastures had been located since early times.

Pathogenesis. The development of tetanus is dependent upon the presence of *C. tetani* in tissue in an environment that will permit its growth and toxin production, and the toxin formed must subsequently reach the central nervous system (CNS) tissue in sufficient quantity to produce overt disease. The organism gains entrance to the tissue via a defect in the normal barriers to infection, usually via a deep skin wound. Since spores are commonly present in soil, any contaminated wound should be regarded as a possible site of *C. tetani* infection. Tetanus bacilli have little or no invasive ability and tend to remain localized at the primary site of infection.

C. tetani is a strict anaerobe; thus its growth requires a microenvironment with lowered oxidation-reduction potential. Deep foci of devitalized tissue provide a suitable environment for growth of the organism. Such foci may be formed by traumatic tissue injury, the presence of foreign bodies, or infection by histotoxic bacteria introduced during or subsequent to wounding. In swine the most commonly reported location of tetanus infection is castration wounds. Sakurai (1966) reported that 202 of 220 cases in Japan, in which the infection site was known, were postcastration infections. Kaplan (1943) reported the loss of 60 of 250 young pigs from tetanus; 40 cases were postcastration and 20 probably were umbilical infections. Wounds inflicted by unclipped canine teeth as well as infected dental alveoli during eruption of teeth have also been suggested as possible sources of infection (Morrill 1964).

The incubation period (interval between establishment of the infection focus and onset of clinical signs) ranges from several days to several weeks. In general, cases with a short incubation period run a more acute and fulminating course with a higher fatality rate than cases with a long incubation period.

The precise mechanism by which toxin passes from the infection site to the CNS and the exact mode of action of the toxin on the nervous tissues are not yet fully understood despite extensive investigation throughout this century. Evidence has been accumulated supporting pathways of toxin spread from the peripheral infection site to the CNS via peripheral nerves (including axons of peripheral nerves, endoneural tissue spaces, perineural tissue spaces, epineural lymphatics, and cerebrospinal fluid).

Many factors may contribute to the cause of death. The consequences of prolonged recumbency and deprivation of nutrients may be factors in animals with a relatively long survival time. In acute cases, respiratory failure resulting from severe skeletal muscle spasms is likely to be the single most important factor. Whether or not the toxin produces a specific metabolic lesion that is directly involved in causing death in the pig is not known.

Clinical Signs and Lesions.

The clinical features of tetanus relate to spasms of skeletal muscle, which occur in the generalized form in swine. The earliest sign is a stiffened gait. The disease progresses rapidly and usually is fully developed in 1–2 days. As the disease progresses, the pig has difficulty walking, the ears are erect, the tail tends to be extended straight posteriorly, the head is slightly elevated, and there may be some protrusion of the nictitating membrane. Further progression of the disease renders the pig incapable of walking, and the skeletal muscles are very firm on palpation. Ultimately the pig lies in lateral recumbency in opisthotonus, with both thoracic and pelvic limbs rigidly extended and directed posteriorly (Fig. 36.13). The tetanic spasms are noticeably heightened by sudden sensory stimuli such as noise, touch, or motion of a visible object. Terminally, there are tachycardia and increased

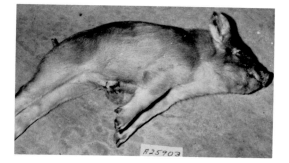

36.13. Generalized tetanus in a 10-day-old pig, which apparently resulted from umbilical infection. The ears are erect and the limbs are rigidly extended.

respiration rate, and white froth may be present around the mouth and external nares.

No lesions specific for tetanus are found at necropsy. Conspicuous abrasions of the skin over pressure points may be seen, and there may be pulmonary congestion and edema.

Diagnosis.

The diagnosis of tetanus in swine is based on observation of typical clinical signs. An obvious area of infection such as a castration wound or umbilical abscess is apparent in many cases. Direct Gram-stained smears of exudate from the lesion may reveal bacteria with typical *C. tetani* morphology, i.e., slender gram-positive bacilli with terminal spherical spores ("drumstick" forms) among the bacterial flora. The organism may be isolated by anaerobic culture or can be identified by immunofluorescence (Batty and Walker 1964); however, this usually is not necessary if there is adequate antemortem clinical observation of the affected animals.

Treatment and Prevention.

The prognosis in affected swine is poor, and there is little evidence that treatment by currently practical methods is of real benefit. Mihaljevic (1966) reported that all 6 tetanus cases submitted to the clinic at Zagreb during 1948 through 1965 succumbed to the disease. Kaplan (1943) described 4 recoveries of 60 affected pigs; however, the recovered cases may have been mild and were not necessarily associated with therapy. Only 11 of 240 cases described in a report from Japan survived the disease (Sakurai 1966). Various suggested treatments include reopening castration wounds and flushing them with hydrogen peroxide, administration of antitoxin in an attempt to neutralize toxin not already fixed by nervous tissue, administration of antibiotics, and use of tranquilizers or barbiturates as muscle relaxants.

Since there is no practical way to eliminate the spores of *C. tetani* from the soil, control is directed toward the prevention of wound contamination by soil or feces. Good sanitation in the farrowing house, treatment of the umbilical cord with antiseptics soon after birth, and prompt clipping of the canine incisors are recommended preventive measures against neonatal tetanus. Sharp objects that may cause skin wounds should be removed from the environment. Because most tetanus in swine follows castration, particular emphasis should be placed on proper surgical technique, with the establishment of good wound drainage and provision of clean quarters for the pigs after castration to prevent undue contamination of the castration wound by soil or feces.

If reasonable preventive measures cannot be followed or if valuable animals are wounded, passive immunization with tetanus antitoxin, the pro-phylactic use of antibiotics, and/or active immunization with tetanus toxoid may be indicated. Veronesi (1966) concluded that the prophylactic use of large doses of long-acting penicillin or tetracyclines (or repeated injections of short-acting preparations of these drugs for 5 days) may be superior to antitoxin in preventing experimental tetanus in mice if treatment is instituted within a few hours after infection. An appreciable amount of active immunity may be obtained from a single injection of alum-precipitated tetanus toxoid, and excellent protection for a year or more can be expected if three doses are given several weeks apart (Morrill 1964).

Botulism

BOTULISM is a toxicosis characterized by rapidly progressive flaccid paralysis and caused by the toxins of *C. botulinum*. The toxin is produced by the organism as it grows in decomposing organic matter of animal or vegetable origin, and poisoning follows oral consumption of toxin-containing material by a susceptible animal.

Swine are considered to be quite highly resistant to botulism, and there are few authentic reports of naturally occurring botulism in this species.

Etiology. The organism is an anaerobic, gram-positive bacillus, usually having a size range of 0.6–1.2 μ by 4–6 μ; however, much longer forms may be found in some cultures (Smith and Holdeman 1968). It forms oval, usually subterminal, spores. Growth requires rather strictly anaerobic conditions and occurs within a wide range of temperatures up to body temperature but is perhaps optimal at about 30°C.

The lethal toxin, a protein, is an extremely potent poison. There is variation among different strains of the organism with respect to neurotoxin production. These differences involve the antigenic properties of the toxin as well as the spectrum of animal species susceptible to the toxin. *C. botulinum* is currently divided into six types (A–F) on the basis of major toxin antigenic structure. Type C strains are further subdivided into types C_a and C_b, whose toxins are antigenically related but not identical. Regardless of the type of toxin involved or the species of animal affected, however, all animals with botulism exhibit similar clinical signs.

Epidemiology. *C. botulinum* is commonly present in soil throughout the world. There are geographic variations in the incidence of the different types. The prevalence appears to be associated with the quantity of organic matter in the soil, and factors such as fertilization with manure may increase bacterial numbers.

The occurrence of botulism is dependent upon the consumption of a sufficient quantity of toxin by a susceptible pig to produce disease, which implies that a potential foodstuff must provide an environment suitable for growth and toxin elaboration by *C. botulinum*. The tissues of dead animals, including crustaceans, fish, birds, and mammals, that decompose during warm or hot weather are the most common source of toxin for animals. Since botulism rarely occurs in swine, there are few recorded sources of toxin for this species. The death of five adult swine after eating dead fish from the edge of a partially dried-up lagoon was reported by Beiers and Simmons (1967). The loss of pigs being fed swill and decomposing brewer's waste has also been reported (Doiurtre 1967). Type C strains were incriminated in these cases.

The eating habits of nonconfined pigs should make them likely candidates for botulism. The very low incidence of the disease in swine is explained on the basis of innate resistance. In 1919 Thom et al. reported that toxin produced by a strain isolated from spoiled canned asparagus failed to affect a pig when administered orally. The pig succumbed, however, when the toxin was injected subcutaneously. Dack and Gibbard (1926a) reported similar findings. Two pigs fed 10 million and 7.5 million mouse lethal doses (LD) of type A toxin failed to develop signs. One of these pigs was later injected intraperitoneally with a large dose of toxin and died 4 days later. They indicated (1926b) that the hog's intestine has a low permeability for the toxin. More recently, Scheibner (1955) found young swine resistant to 1 million mouse LD of types B, C, D, and E toxins given orally. A similar dose of type A toxin produced typical signs and death; however, 60,000 mouse LD of type A toxin had no effect.

Smith et al. (1971) found weanling pigs to be moderately susceptible to type B toxin when it was infused intravenously, but they were highly resistant to the toxin when given orally (oral:intravenous ratio = 16,700:1). The intravenous LD of type B toxin was approximately 180 mouse LD/kg body weight. This group of experimental pigs was moderately resistant to intravenous infusion of types A, C_b, E, and F toxins (LD = 4000–20,000 mouse LD/kg), at least moderately resistant to C_a toxin (LD = 18,000 mouse LD/kg), and highly resistant to type D toxin (LD = 67,000 mouse LD/kg). They were highly resistant to all types given orally.

Pathogenesis. Botulism is generally considered to be strictly a food poisoning, i.e., any significant quantity of the toxin is elaborated in the foodstuff before it is eaten, and poisoning results from absorption of preformed toxin. The bacteria are, of course, consumed along with the toxin, and it has been proposed that there may be further toxin production in the intestine.

Absorption of type A toxin was found to occur much more readily in the upper small intestine than in the ileum of rats, rabbits, and mice, and absorption from the stomach was poor in these species (May and Whaler 1958). These workers also found that the toxin was absorbed by the lymphatics, with passage into the general circulation by way of thoracic lymph rather than portal blood.

The principal site of action of the toxin is at the myoneural junction, where the toxin produces its effect by preventing the release of acetylcholine from its binding sites, thereby preventing muscular contraction (Burgen et al. 1949).

Death is generally ascribed to asphyxia resulting from paralysis of the muscles of respiration.

Clinical Signs. The latent period between consumption of toxic material and onset of signs ranges from 8 hours to 3 days or more. The clinical features are a manifestation of progressive flaccid paralysis of voluntary muscles. The initial signs are weakness, incoordination, and staggering. Morrill and Bajwa (1964) stated that weakness often appears in the forelegs of swine first, followed by involvement of the hind legs. The paralysis may then progress to lateral recumbency with complete flaccidity. Smith et al. (1971) observed an initial weakness of the pelvic limbs and lumbar region, followed by general motor paralysis and dilation of the pupils of the eyes. Other clinical signs include anorexia; lordosis; reduced vision or complete blindness; aphonia; excessive salivation; involuntary urination and defecation; and deep, labored breathing (Smintzis and Durin 1950; Beiers and Simmons 1967).

The time interval between onset of signs and death or recovery is variable and probably is largely determined by the amount of toxin consumed. Five adult swine that consumed decomposing fish died between 19 and 52 hours after

eating the fish, and two that staggered recovered later (Beiers and Simmons 1967). Smintzis and Durin (1950) reported mortality on the sixth day of the disease.

No lesions specific for botulism are found at necropsy. Significant findings might include the presence in the stomach of the material suspected as the toxin source and occurrence of aspiration pneumonia consequent to paralysis of the muscles of deglutition (Beiers and Simmons 1967).

Diagnosis. Because the pig apparently is quite highly resistant to botulism, a diagnosis should be made only after thorough investigation and exclusion of other possible diagnoses. A presumptive diagnosis is based on observation of typical clinical signs, i.e., a progressive flaccid paralysis. Disclosure of a possible toxin source such as spoiled canned goods or a decomposing animal carcass is also helpful.

Methods of laboratory confirmation of the disease in swine are not clearly defined. Valuable confirmatory evidence can be obtained by demonstrating the presence of toxin in the suspected source material or in the poisoned animal's gastrointestinal content or serum. Toxin is readily detected in the serum of some species by mouse protection tests and employing type-specific diagnostic antitoxins, but this does not appear to be the case in swine. On the 4 days following intravenous inoculation of a pig with 21,400 mouse LD type A toxin/kg body weight, Smith et al. (1971) demonstrated 100, 100, 30, and 10 mouse LD toxin/ml serum. No toxin was found in the serum of pigs 1 day after giving large doses of types B, C_b, or D toxin, and no toxin was demonstrated in urine from pigs inoculated with any of the types. Identification of type C toxin in filtrates of small intestine content from a poisoned sow has been reported (Beiers and Simmons 1967).

The isolation and identification of *C. botulinum* may also be of some value in establishing the diagnosis. Narayan (1967) reported recovery of *C. botulinum* from swine that were silent carriers of the organism. Müller (1967), however, stated that type C_b organisms were isolated from only 3–4% of the livers from healthy slaughtered cattle and swine in Denmark, whereas this type was isolated from 90% of cattle and horses that had died from botulism.

Treatment and Prevention. If botulism is suspected, an effort should be made to find the toxin source and prevent further consumption of any remaining suspect material by the herd.

The only specific treatment for botulism is the use of antitoxin. Antitoxins have been effective in reducing mortality in humans when given after consumption of food suspected of containing toxin. It has been suggested that antitoxin may be beneficial not only when given parenterally but orally as well in an attempt to neutralize toxin in the alimentary tract (Lamanna and Carr 1967). As pointed out by Burgen et al. (1949), the toxin appears to produce an irreversible neuromuscular block; therefore, the principal benefit of antitoxin probably is to prevent additional fixation of toxin at myoneural junctions, thereby impeding the progressive severity of the disease. If antitoxins are to be of value, they must contain antibodies to the specific type of toxin involved. Therapy therefore indicates the use of polyvalent antitoxins that incorporate the types most commonly present in a geographic area.

Therapy aimed at reducing continued absorption of toxin from the intestine was suggested by Beiers and Simmons (1967). They fed affected sows 1 gallon of skim milk containing 4 ounces of magnesium sulfate, repeating this treatment three times at 12-hour intervals. Only 2 of 4 sows that were weak and staggering consumed the preparation and both subsequently recovered, whereas the other 2 died. The use of sedatives also has been recommended.

Prevention of botulism involves preventing the consumption of potentially toxic material such as spoiled garbage and decomposing animal tissue. Prophylactic immunization with toxoids is not practical in swine because of the infrequent occurrence of the disease.

REFERENCES

Clostridium perfringens Type C Enteritis

ARBUCKLE, J. B. R. 1972. The attachment of *Clostridium welchii* (*Cl. perfringens*) type C to intestinal villi of pigs. J Pathol 106:65.

AZUMA, R.; HAMAOKA, T.; SHIOI, H.; TANJI, T.; YAMAGUCHI, H.; AND SHIGA, K. 1983. Case report of necrotic enteritis in neonatal pigs caused by *Clostridium perfringens* type C. Nippon Juigaku Zasshi 45:135.

BAKHTIN, A. G. 1956. Dysentery of newborn piglets. Veterinariia (Moscow) 33:30. Abstr Vet Bull 26:562.

BARNES, D. M., AND MOON, H. W. 1964. Enterotoxemia in pigs due to *Clostridium perfringens* type C. J Am Vet Med Assoc 144:1391.

BERGELAND, M. E. 1965. Studies of a porcine enterotoxemia caused by *Clostridium perfringens* type C. Ph.D. diss., Univ of Minnesota.

———. 1972. Pathogenesis and immunity of *Clostridium perfringens* type C enteritis in swine. J Am Vet Med Assoc 160:658.

———. 1977. Necrotic enteritis in nursing piglets. Proc Am Assoc Vet Lab Diagn 20:151.

BERGELAND, M. E.; DERMODY, T. A.; AND SORENSEN, D. K. 1966. Porcine enteritis due to *Clostridium perfringens* type C. I. Epizootiology and diagnosis. Proc US Livest Sanit Assoc 70:601.

FIELD, H. I., AND GIBSON, E. A. 1955. Studies on piglet mortality. II. *Cl. welchii* infection. Vet Rec 67:31.

FIELD, H. I., AND GOODWIN, R. F. W. 1959. The experimental reproduction of enterotoxemia in piglets. J Hyg (Camb) 57:81.

HARBOLA, P. C., AND KHERA, S. S. 1990. Porcine enteritis due to *Clostridium perfringens* and its immunoprophylaxis. Proc Int Pig Vet Soc 11:164.

HØGH, P. 1965. Enterotoksaemi hos pattegrise forårsa-

get of *Clostridium perfringens* type C. Nord Vet Med 17:1.

———. 1967a. Necrotizing infectious enteritis in piglets, caused by *Clostridium perfringens* type C. I. Biochemical and toxigenic properties of the *Clostridium*. Acta Vet Scand 8:26.

———. 1967b. Necrotizing infectious enteritis in piglets, caused by *Clostridium perfringens* type C. II. Incidence and clinical features. Acta Vet Scand 8:301.

———. 1974. Porcine infectious necrotizing enteritis caused by *Clostridium perfringens*. Ph.D. diss., Royal Veterinary Agriculture Univ., Copenhagen.

KUBO, M., AND WATASE, H. 1985. Electron microscopy of *Clostridium perfringens* in the intestine of pigs with necrotic enteritis. Jpn J Vet Sci 47:497–501.

MATISHEK, P. H. AND McGRINLEY, M. 1986. Colostral transfer of *Clostridium perfringens* type C beta antitoxin in swine. Am J Vet Res 46:2147–2148.

MATTHIAS, D.; ILLNER, F.; AND BAUMAN, G. 1968. Untersuchungen zur Pathogenese der Magen-Darm-Veranderungen bei der infektiosen Gastroenteritis der Schweine. Arch Exp Veterinaermed 22:417.

MESZAROS, J., AND PESTI, L. 1965. Studies on the pathogenesis of gastroenteritis in swine. Acta Vet Acad Sci Hung 15:465.

MORIN, M.; TURGEON, D.; JOLETTE, J.; ROBINSON, Y.; PHANEUF, J. B.; SAUVAGEAU, R.; BEAUREGARD, M.; TEUSCHER, E.; HIGGINS, R.; AND LARIVIERE, S. 1983. Neonatal diarrhea of pigs in Quebec: Infectious causes of significant outbreaks. Can J Comp Med 47:11.

PLAISIER, A. J. 1971. Enterotoxemia in piglets caused by *Clostridium perfringens* type C. Tijdschr Diergeneeskd 96:324.

RIPLEY, P. H., AND GUSH, A. F. 1983. Immunization schedule for the prevention of infectious necrotic enteritis caused by *Clostridium perfringens* type C in piglets. Vet Rec 112:201.

ROOD, J. I.; BUDDLE, J. R.; WALES, A. J.; AND SIDHU, R. 1985. The occurrence of antibiotic resistance in *Clostridium perfringens* from pigs. Aust Vet J 62:276–279.

SZABO, ST., AND SZENT-IVÁNYI, TH. 1957. Infectious necrotic enteritis in sucking pigs. II. Incidence and control of the disease in Hungary. Acta Vet Acad Sci Hung 7:413.

SZENT-IVÁNYI, TH., AND SZABO, ST. 1955. I. *Clostridium welchii* type C causing infectious necrotic enteritis in newborn piglets. Magy Allatorv Lapja 10:403. Abstr Vet Bull 26:259.

WALKER, P. D.; MURRELL, T. G. C.; AND NAGY, L. K. 1980. Scanning electronmicroscopy of the jejunum in enteritis necroticans. J Med Microbiol 13:445.

WARRACK, G. H. 1963. Some observations on the typing of *Clostridium perfringens*. Bull Off Int Epizoot 59:1393.

Clostridium perfringens Type A Enteritis

AMTSBERG, G. W.; BISPING, W.; EL-SULKHON, S. N.; MATTHIESEN, I.; AND KROBISCHI, P. 1976. *Clostridium perfringens* type A infectie. Berl Munch Tieraerztl Wochenschr 21:409–414.

DAMME-JONGSTEN, M. VAN; HAAGSMA, J.; AND NOTERMANS, S. 1990. Enterotoxin gene not found in *Clostridium perfringens* isolates from pigs. Vet Rec 126:191–192.

ESTRADA CORREA, A. E. 1986. Studies of *Clostridium perfringens* type A enteritis in the pig. Ph.D. diss., Univ of Glasgow.

ESTRADA CORREA, A. E., AND TAYLOR, D. J. 1989. *Clostridium perfringens* type A spores, enterotoxin and antibody to enterotoxin. Vet Rec 124:606–611.

JESTIN, A., AND POPOFF, M. R. 1987. L'enterotoxine de *Clostridium perfringens* de type A. Interet de son etude dans la pathologie digestive du porc a l'engrais. Rec Med Vet 163:33–38.

JESTIN, A.; POPOFF, M. R.; AND MAHE, S. 1985. Epizootiologic investigations of a diarrheic syndrome in fattening pigs. Am J Vet Res 46:2149–2151.

MANSSON, I., AND SMITH, L. D. S. 1962. Atypical strains of *Clostridium perfringens* from swine. Acta Pathol Microbiol Scand 55:342–348.

NABUURS, M.; HAAGSMA, J.; MOLEN, E.; AND HEIJDEN, J. 1983. Diarrhoea in one to three week-old piglets associated with *Clostridium perfringens* type A. Ann Rech Vet 14:408–411.

OLUBUNMI, P. A. 1982. Bacteria associated with inflammatory enteric lesions in pigs. Ph.D. diss., Univ of Glasgow.

POPOFF, M. R., AND JESTIN, A. 1985. Enteropathogenicity of purified *Clostridium perfringens* enterotoxin in the pig. Am J Vet Res 47:1132–1133.

RAMISSE, J.; BREMENT, A.; POIRIER, J.; RABREAUD, C.; AND SIMONNET, P. 1979. Flore microbienne isolee au cours de diarrhees neonatales mortelles chez le veau, l'agneau et le porcelet. Rev Vet Med 130:111–122.

SECASIU, V. 1984. Diagnosticul bacteriologic welchiozei porcine (enterotoxiema anaeroba). Rev Cresterea Anim 2:38–45.

TAYLOR, D. J., AND ESTRADA CORREA, A. E. 1988. Avoparcin in the prevention of enterotoxigenic *C. perfringens* type A infections and diarrhoea in pigs. Proc Int Pig Vet Soc 10:140.

Cellulitis and Gas Gangrene

AIKAT, B. K., AND DIBLE, J. H. 1956. The pathology of *Clostridium welchii* infection. J Pathol 71:461.

————. 1960. The local and general effects of cultures and culture-filtrates of *Clostridium oedematiens, Cl. septicum, Cl. sporogenes,* and *Cl. histolyticum.* J Pathol 79:227.

BATTY, I., AND WALKER, P. D. 1963. Differentiation of *Clostridium septicum* and *Clostridium chauvoei* by the use of fluorescent-labeled antibodies. J Pathol 85:517.

BATTY, I.; BUNTAIN, D.; AND WALKER, P. D. 1964. *Clostridium oedematiens:* A cause of sudden death in sheep, cattle, and pigs. Vet Rec 76:1115.

BOURNE, F. J., AND KERRY, J. B. 1965. *Clostridium oedematiens* associated with sudden death in the pig. Vet Rec 77:1463.

EGGLESTON, E. L. 1950. Blackleg in swine. Vet Med 45:253.

GUALANDI, G. L. 1955. L'infezione da *"Clost. chauvoei"* nel. suino. Arch Vet Ital 6:57.

HAC, L. R., AND HABERT, A. C. 1943. Penicillin in treatment of experimental *Clostridium welchii* infection. Proc Soc Exp Biol Med 53:61.

ITOH, H.; UCHIDA, M.; SUGIURA, H.; OGUSO, S.; AND YAMAKAWA, K. 1987. Outbreak of *Clostridium novyi* infection in swine and its rapid diagnosis. J Jpn Vet Med Assoc 40:365–369.

JAARTSVELD, F. H. J.; JANSSENS, F. T. M.; AND JOBSE, C. J. 1962. *Clostridium* infectie bij biggen. Tijdschr Diergeneeskd 87:768.

KELLAWAY, C. H.; REID, G.; AND TRETHEWIE, E. R. 1941. Circulatory and other effects of the toxin of *Cl. septique.* Aust J Exp Biol Med Sci 19:277.

MACLENNAN, J. D. 1962. Histotoxic clostridial infections of man. Bacteriol Rev 26:177.

MARTIG, J. 1966. Zur Differentialdiagnose zwischen Rauschbrand und Pararauschbrand mit Hilfe der Immunofluoreszenz. Schweiz Arch Tierheilkd 108:303.

MOUSSA, R. S. 1958. Complexity of toxins from *Clostridium septicum* and *Clostridium chauvoei.* J Bacteriol 76:538.

STERNE, M., AND EDWARDS, J. B. 1955. Blackleg in pigs caused by *Clostridium chauvoei.* Vet Rec 67:314.

TAYLOR, W. I., AND NOVAK, M. 1952. Antibiotic prophylaxis of experimental clostridial infections. Antibiot Chemother 2:639.

ZELLER, M. 1956. Enzootischer Pararauschbrand in einer Schweinemastanstalt. Tieraerztl Umsch 11:406.

Tetanus

BATTY, I., AND WALKER, P. D. 1964. The identification of *Clostridium novyi* (*Clostridium oedematiens*) and *Clostridium tetani* by the use of fluorescent labelled antibodies. J Pathol 88:327.

KAPLAN, M. M. 1943. An unusual epizootic of tetanus in young pigs. Middx Vet 3:8.

MIHALJEVIC, K. 1966. A contribution to the study of lockjaw in animals. Vet Arh 36:152.

MORRILL, C. C. 1964. Clostridial infections. In Diseases of Swine, 2d ed. Ed. H. W. Dunne. Ames: Iowa State Univ Press, p. 378.

SAKURAI, N. 1966. The relation between human and veterinary tetanus in a Japanese prefecture. Principles on Tetanus. Proc 2d Int Conf Tetanus, p. 91.

SERGEEVA, T. I., AND MATVEEV, K. I. 1966. Geographical distribution of *Clostridium tetani* in the soil of the U.S.S.R. Principles on Tetanus. Proc 2d Int Conf Tetanus, p. 77.

VERONESI, R. 1966. Antibiotics versus antitetanic serum in the prevention of human tetanus. Principles on Tetanus. Proc 2d Int Conf Tetanus, p. 417.

Botulism

BEIERS, P. R., AND SIMMONS, G. C. 1967. Botulism in pigs. Aust Vet J 43:270.

BURGEN, A. S. V.; DICKENS, F.; AND ZATMAN, L. J. 1949. The action of botulinum toxin on the neuromuscular junction. J Physiol 109:10.

DACK, G. M., AND GIBBARD, J. 1926a. Studies on botulinum toxin in the alimentary tract of hogs, rabbits, guinea-pigs and mice. J Infect Dis 39:173.

————. 1926b. Permeability of the small intestine of rabbits and hogs to botulinum toxin. J Infect Dis 39:181.

DOIURTRE, M. P. 1967. Botulism in animals in Senegal. Bull Off Int Epizoot 67:1497.

LAMANNA, C., AND CARR, C. J. 1967. The botulinal, tetanal, and enterostaphyloccoccal toxins: A review. Clin Pharmacol Ther 8:286.

MAY, A. J., AND WHALER, B. C. 1958. The absorption of *Clostridium botulinum* type A toxin from the alimentary canal. Br J Exp Pathol 39:307.

MORRILL, C. C., AND BAJWA, G. S. 1964. Botulism. In Diseases of Swine, 2d ed. Ed. H. W. Dunne. Ames: Iowa State Univ. Press, p. 605.

MÜLLER, J. 1967. On the occurrence of *Clostridium botulinum* type C beta in the livers of slaughter animals in Denmark. Bull Off Int Epizoot 67:1473.

NARAYAN, K. G. 1967. Incidence of clostridia in pigs. Acta Vet Acad Sci Hung 17:179.

SCHEIBNER, VON G. 1955. Die Emfanglichkeit des Schweines fur Botulinustoxin der Typen A–E. DTW 62:355.

SMINTZIS, G., AND DURIN, D. 1950. Epizootie de botulisme chez le porc. Bull Soc Sci Vet (Lyon), p. 71.

SMITH, L. DS.; AND HOLDEMAN, L. V. 1968. The Pathogenic Anaerobic Bacteria. Springfield, Ill.: Charles C Thomas.

SMITH, L. DS.; DAVIS, J. W.; AND LIBKE, K. G. 1971. Experimentally induced botulism in weanling pigs. Am J Vet Res 32:1327.

THOM, C.; EDMONDSON, R. B.; AND GILTNER, L. T. 1919. Botulism from canned asparagus. J Am Med Assoc 73:907.

37 Eperythrozoonosis

A. R. Smith

EPERYTHROZOONOSIS in swine is caused by the rickettsial organism, *Eperythrozoon suis* (Ristic and Kreier 1974). Historically, eperythrozoonosis has been a disease of feeder pigs under stress, expressed as a febrile condition with development of an acute icteroanemia (Splitter 1950 a,b). More recently, eperythrozoonosis has been observed in a wide age range, from piglets to pregnant sows (Berrier and Gouge 1954; Henry 1979). The organism has been hard to demonstrate in blood films except when obtained from febrile pigs early in the disease.

Anemia observed following acute eperythrozoonosis is similar to that induced by anaplasmosis in cattle and *Haemobartonella* (feline infectious anemia) in cats. Sheep infected with *E. ovis* gain at less than a normal rate (Daddow 1979). Subclinical infections and the carrier state persist for extended periods with these agents. Protective antibodies do not develop following infections, since carriers relapse following introduction of sufficient stress (Kreier and Ristic 1968).

ETIOLOGY. *E. suis* organisms are obligate intracellular parasites of porcine erythrocytes. Organisms are coccoid, with an average diameter of $0.8-1\mu m$ and multiple organisms (up to five erythrocytes) may be observed. Free organisms in the plasma are also sometimes seen.

EPIDEMIOLOGY. Eperythrozoonosis caused by *E. suis* organisms has been observed only in domestic pigs. Serologic tests on serum from wild pigs have been uniformly negative for *E. suis* in the indirect hemagglutination (IHA) test.

Early reports of swine eperythrozoonosis noted that the majority of clinical cases occurred in the summer, and it was believed that arthropod vectors were implicated in transmission (Splitter 1950a). Presence of the hog louse, *Hematopinus suis,* has been suspected. Others have suggested mosquitoes and biting flies. Experiments proving arthropod transmissions in swine have not been reported, however.

The percent of swine positive in the IHA test does not vary with season. With the popularity of rearing swine in confinement units, the higher density of animals and possibly additional stress may be factors. Also, ample opportunities for mechanical transmission through blood-contaminated needles and surgical instruments exist in many units. In utero and oral transmission have been accomplished at the University of Illinois.

CLINICAL SIGNS

Field Cases. Pigs under 5 days of age are most likely to show clinical signs of skin pallor and icterus in a herd (Henry 1979). The pigs appeared to recover when approximately 1 week old, since anemia and icterus would resolve. Henry reported that recovered pigs showed effects of infection by wide variation in size and vigor. By weaning time, an anemic group of pigs was the principal clinical sign. However, icterus and anemia were also occasionally observed at weaning. Preston and Greve (1965) also reported eperythrozoonosis in 4-week-old pigs. The anemia appeared to persist in herds with concurrent bacterial or parasitic diseases. A general unthriftiness would develop and control of chronic bacterial pneumonia and enteritis were more difficult.

Feeder Pigs. The classic icteroanemia (Robb 1943) is not now commonly observed. No explanation has been given for this, except that the widespread use of feed additives and more balanced rations may possibly minimize this form of the disease. Henry (1979) reported observing icteroanemia in feedlots where pigs of different origins were grouped.

Sows. Henry (1979) reported sows had acute and chronic infections. Acutely affected sows typically were anorectic for 1–3 days, had temperatures ranging from 104 to 107°F (40–41.7°C), and were most commonly limited to those under stress immediately prepartum. Fever often persisted following farrowing. Occasionally, sows developed mammary and vulval edema. In such sows, milk flow was depressed and maternal behavior was subnormal or lacking. Predictably, the most severely affected pigs were from such sows. Recovery without treatment occurred by the third day after farrowing. A similar condition of acute infection was observed in sows at weaning, with a marked decrease in first-breeding conception rate. Immunity apparently was weak, inasmuch as some individuals developed the same signs at subsequent farrowings.

Chronic infection in sows had much the same clinical appearance as seen in chronically affected pigs; i.e., a portion of the herd would become debilitated, pale, and icteric. Many of these sows would not conceive on repeated mating, and sows did not show estrus, causing a decrease in conception rates. Concurrent infectious disease, especially sarcoptic mange, along with poor environmental and nutritional conditions may have contributed to development of debility and anemia. Death from secondary infections was common, and affected sows did not gain weight even when segregated and fed ad libitum.

Laboratory Infection. Splenectomized pigs, 10–17 weeks of age, have been injected with eperythrozoon-infected blood. A febrile response occurred 7–8 days following subcutaneous injection of 1 ml blood containing detectable organisms. Pigs were inappetent, temperatures varied from 105.9 to 107°F (41.1–41.7°C), eperythrozoon organisms were numerous in the erythrocytes, and the pigs were hypoglycemic at patency. If animals were untreated, fever persisted until shortly before death. When blood glucose dropped to less than 10 mg/dl, pigs would commonly go into convulsions and coma followed by death. Glucose values returned to near normal within 24 hours in animals surviving the initial hypoglycemic crisis. Anemia developed gradually, often requiring 1 week after onset of clinical disease to be obvious. At this time, respiration was increased (anemia and possibly icterus were visible). Blood appeared thin and watery, and the erythrocyte sedimentation rate was increased. Thrombocytes decreased rapidly and preceded the drop in packed-cell volume (PCV) and hemoglobin values.

Affected pigs were listless, depressed, weak, and constipated. Hemoglobinuria was not observed nevertheless. Weight loss often exceeded 10% of body weight during the 24-hour period preceding death (Barnett 1963).

Postmortem lesions observed in swine diagnosed as having eperythrozoonosis have been fairly well characterized for the classical icteroanemia form of the disease. In field cases of naturally infected swine, lesions are similar to those described in experimental cases produced by infection of splenectomized pigs with *E. suis* or those produced by reactivation of the clinical disease following splenectomy of latent carriers (Splitter 1950a). The appearance of specific postmortem lesions from pig to pig or herd to herd can be variable and inconsistent.

Macroscopic and microscopic lesions usually appear directly or indirectly related to the severity of the hemolytic and/or immune-mediated anemia produced following infection. The severity of the anemia appears related to the degree of erythroparasitemia, the virulence of the organism, and the physical and nutritional status of the host. Anemia and icterus are the major macroscopic lesions. Mucous membranes and skin are pale;

blood is thin and watery but will clot after exposure to the atmosphere. A generalized icterus is frequently but inconsistently observed and usually appears in the most severe cases. The liver is yellowish brown, swollen, and firm. The gallbladder contains a thick gelatinous bile. A frequent finding is an enlarged, soft spleen; less-frequent findings are pale flabby heart and kidney. Lymph nodes may be swollen and edematous. Ascites, hydrothorax, and hydropericardium are frequently reported. These serous effusions may contain bile. Petechial hemorrhages may be observed in the bladder mucosa of some cases. The bone marrow is reddened, cellular, and not fatty, but this finding appears related to the duration of the clinical disease. Microscopic changes observed are variable hepatic hemosiderosis, hepatic fatty change, centrolobular degeneration and necrosis (the latter is probably due to tissue hypoxia secondary to hypoxemia), lymphocytic infiltrates within the liver, and hyperplastic bone marrow. Organisms are difficult to demonstrate in tissue sections stained with hematoxylin, eosin, and Giemsa.

DIAGNOSIS

Acute Cases. Diagnosis of acute cases is made by detection of organisms in a stained blood film obtained from a febrile pig with a history compatible with that described under Clinical Signs. To demonstrate organisms, blood films should be prepared from suspect febrile pigs. Organisms are generally easier to detect in young pigs that are febrile. They may or may not be anemic. Blood films should be stained with Wright-Giemsa or Diff-Quik stain. The Diff-Quik stain requires 5 seconds to fix with the fixative triarylmethane, 10 seconds to stain with solution 1 (xanthine), and 20 seconds to stain with solution 2 (thiazine). Veterinarians submitting blood to clinical pathology or diagnostic laboratories equipped with fluorescent microscopes should collect blood in anticoagulant (heparin or acid citrate dextrose) and transfer 1 ml blood to a blood tube. One ml 10% formalin (10 cm³ formaldehyde added to 90 ml physiologic saline) should be added and the contents mixed. The formalin fixes and preserves the blood. The submitter should request acridine orange staining for detection of eperythrozoon organisms. A history including age, temperature, and serologic status of the herd should be sent with the fixed blood. Organisms are difficult to detect in blood obtained from pigs that are not febrile.

Subclinical Infection. The difficulty in finding organisms in recovered swine that were proven carriers led to the development of the IHA test for eperythrozoonosis (Smith and Rahn 1975). The test consists of attaching eperythrozoon antigen to sheep erythrocytes with the fixative glutaraldehyde. Swine serums to be tested, including known positive and negative controls, are inactivated and absorbed. Serial twofold dilutions (1:10–1:1280) of the serums, are made in U-shaped microtitration trays following inactivation and absorption. The titer is reported as a reciprocal of the highest dilution in which agglutination occurs. Experimental, infected, splenectomized pigs develop titers of 40 or greater following experimental infection.

Development of the IHA test led to the observation that eperythrozoon antibodies are common in swine in the United States. Serum samples from 15,000 swine were tested for eperythrozoon antibodies in 1979 with the following results: 85% were negative, 7% were suspect at a titer of 40, and 8% were positive at a titer of 80 or above. The test has also shown that the gestating or lactating sow is most likely to possess eperythrozoon antibodies. Sows at term, during lactation, or at rebreeding reacted at a higher percentage and with a higher geometric mean titer than all other groups in the herd. The following, listed in descending order of serologic reactivity, are sows at term, during lactation, or at rebreeding; gestating sows; gilts at term, during lactation, or at rebreeding; gestating gilts; boars; pigs over 3 months of age; and pigs less than 3 months of age. It is rare for pigs under 3 months of age to react serologically. In a limited number of infected herds, the incidence of eperythrozoon antibodies is correlated with age; the oldest sows have the highest titers. At this time it is premature to consider this as universally true.

The IHA test for eperythrozoonosis is controversial since sows are sometimes found to be serologically positive, but clinical disease of eperythrozoonosis is not observed. Historically, eperythrozoonosis has been a disease associated with stress. Clinical signs may be observed only at certain times of the year. This stress requirement still appears to exist at the present time. However, the carrier state of eperythrozoonosis has been verified in serologically positive animals. In addition, pure infection of eperythrozoonosis alone probably exists only in experimentally inoculated germ-free pigs. Other agents, in combination with eperythrozoonosis, probably occur in the field and are involved in the eperythrozoonosis complex disease.

Veterinarians have associated reproductive problems with eperythrozoon titers. These include reproductive problems in sows with either anestrus or delayed estrus, embryonic death with absorption of fetuses, and abortions (Holter and Andrews 1979). However, a variety of other infectious disease agents and management conditions can contribute to the same symptomology. Control studies in the laboratory have not been conducted to prove that the reproductive problems are due to eperythrozoonosis. Circumstantial evidence implicates eperythrozoonosis, since serum samples collected shortly after abortion have been negative or low titer and have converted to high titers 2 weeks later. Improvement has occurred following addition of either arsenicals or tetracyclines to the rations.

The diagnosis of eperythrozoonosis can be verified by splenectomizing swine that have eperythrozoon titers and demonstrating organisms after the animals become febrile. A simpler approach is to inject normal splenectomized pigs with fresh blood containing anticoagulants obtained from sows that are serologically positive.

The IHA test measures immunoglobulin (Ig) M antibody rather than IgG. Therefore, this may be why titer and the carrier state are correlated. The test is used as a herd test rather than to identify individually infected animals. Serologically positive animals are felt to be carriers; however, animals serologically negative may be also. Intact animals injected with blood containing eperythrozoon organisms have remained negative, but following splenectomy they have become febrile and subsequently developed eperythrozoon antibodies. Therefore, 10 serum samples obtained from sows from the farrowing house should be submitted to ascertain the eperythrozoonosis status of the herd. Also, eperythrozoonosis should not be eliminated from consideration on the basis of a negative serologic test from pigs, gilts, or boars.

PREVENTION AND CONTROL. The Food and Drug Administration has not approved any product for the treatment of eperythrozoonosis in swine. However, laboratory and field studies have shown beneficial effects following treatment with tetracyclines and/or organic arsenicals. Experimentally infected splenectomized swine have not been cleared to the carrier state by oxytetracycline injected at 11 mg/kg once daily for 14 consecutive days (Splitter and Castro 1957). Also, serologic titers have not decreased following tetracycline in gestating rations at 200 g/ton.

The mechanism of action of organic arsenicals is not well understood. They have frequently been used to improve feed efficiency and weight gains in swine and poultry. Organic arsenicals have also been used for treatment of swine dysentery and trypanosome infections in humans.

Since Splitter (1950c) had stated that neoarsphenamine suppressed parasitemia, arsanilic acid was fed to splenectomized swine that were eperythrozoon carriers. Arsanilic acid was commercially available and cleared as a feed additive for swine, whereas neoarsphenamine was not available. In the absence of arthropod vectors, mange mites, and mechanical transmission, animals serologically positive to eperythrozoons became negative. In addition, anemic sows have shown increased PCV and hemoglobin values following the addition of arsanilic acid to the ration. Herds that are serologically negative and receiving therapy with arsenicals should be retested after the arsenical has been removed from the ration for 1 month.

Manufacturers of arsanilic acid and sodium arsanilate in the United States are Fleming Laboratories, Charlotte, N.C., and Whitmoyer Laboratories, Myerstown, Pa. The 3-nitro-4-hydroxyphenylarsonic acid (3-Nitro) and its water-soluble derivative (3-Nitro-W) are available from Salsbury Laboratories, Charles City, Iowa.

Anemic Pigs. Litters of pigs that are anemic and from eperythrozoonosis-positive herds (diagnosed either by demonstration of the organism or by serologic test on sows) are treated with iron dextran and oxytetracycline (Hottell 1980). Injections with 200 mg iron dextran and 25 mg oxytetracycline are made at 1–2 days of age. A follow-up injection of iron dextran is given at 2 weeks of age. The rationale for the additional iron is replacement of iron eliminated by destroyed erythrocytes.

Pigs that relapse or stall out following weaning are harder to treat successfully. Affected pigs usually do not consume adequate feed to respond to oxytetracycline or arsenicals incorporated into the ration. Injected oxytetracycline is probably most effective but often is not practical because of the labor input required. Water medication with sodium arsanilate, 3-Nitro-W, or water-soluble tetracyclines can be used for 10 days postweaning in problem herds. Herds with anemic piglets may also incorporate 150 g tetracycline and 45 g arsanilic acid in the farrowing ration. Tetracycline at 200 g/ton may also be helpful in the nursery ration, or arsenicals could be substituted for the tetracycline (arsanilic acid at 90 g/ton or 3-Nitro at 45 g/ton).

Breeding Herd. Various arsenical treatment regimens are being used in attempts to control eperythrozoonosis in breeding herds. The products manufactured in the United States appear to be of higher quality than some of the imported arsenicals. It is often difficult to ascertain the origin of the arsenicals when purchased through feed dealers and distributors.

Arsenicals are being used in the following ways: (1) The gestation ration may contain 90 g/ton arsanilic acid (each animal to receive approximately 250 mg daily) from day 21 to day 105 of gestation. With this regimen, arsanilic acid may or may not be continued in the lactation ration. If continued, a 45 g/ton level appears to be safe. If 3-Nitro is used, reduce to 50% of the arsanilic acid dosage. (2) Arsanilic acid alone may be incorporated in the lactation ration. A dosage maintained at 90 g/ton is fed for the entire period the females are in the farrowing house (typically, a daily dose of 450–500 mg/sow for a 4- to 6-week period). (3) Following a positive diagnosis, the whole herd can be placed on a 180 g/ton level of

arsanilic acid for 1 week. The dosage should then be dropped to 90 g/ton level for 1 month. The dosage in the farrowing house should never be above the 90 g/ton level. (4) When replacement gilts are selected from eperythrozoon-affected herds, arsanilic acid at the 90 g/ton level should be administered for 1 month.

Acute clinical signs of organic arsenical poisoning include incoordination, inability to control body limb movements, and ataxia. After a few days pigs may become quadriplegic but will continue to eat and drink. Arsanilic acid and the sodium salt may produce blindness, but the effect rarely is seen with 3-Nitro. When the arsenicals are given, adequate supplies of drinking water should be provided. The organic arsenicals are excreted via the kidneys. Toxicity is increased when given to animals with diarrhea.

There are no feed additives listed in the *Feed Additive Compendium* for treatment of eperythrozoonosis; therefore, feed mills are unable to add arsanilic acid or tetracycline at medication levels for this purpose. Veterinarians recommending on-farm mixing of these drugs assume legal responsibility for any problems that occur.

A number of herds with eperythrozoonosis have moderate to severe sarcoptic mange and lice infestations. Field experience has shown that eperythrozoonosis cannot be controlled in the absence of mange and lice control. Transmission with needles and surgical instruments contaminated with blood can be limited in sows by changing needles between injections and bleeding and in pigs between litters. At least two sets of surgical instruments should be used; the contaminated set should be placed in properly diluted disinfectant and alternated between litters. A major effort must be directed to control sarcoptic mange, pediculosis, and helminth infections.

No vaccines are available to prevent eperythrozoonosis. If a herd is free, new additions should be from eperythrozoon-free herds. Negative serologic tests of serum of 10 sows in the farrowing house on an arsenic-free ration should be adequate to minimize the introduction of eperythrozoonosis. If the herd is already positive, the need to obtain serologically negative animals is not apparent.

REFERENCES

Barnett, S. F. 1963. *Eperythrozoon parvum* in pigs in Kenya. Bull Epizoot Dis Afr 11:185.

Berrier, H. H., and Gouge, R. E. 1954. Eperythrozoonosis transmitted in utero from carrier sows to their pigs. J Am Vet Med Assoc 124:98.

Daddow, K. N. 1979. *Eperythrozoon ovis* – A cause of anemia, reduced production, and decreased exercise tolerance in sheep. Aust Vet J 55(9):433–434.

Henry, S. C. 1979. Clinical observations on eperythrozoonosis. J Am Vet Med Assoc 174(6):601–603.

Holter, J. A., and Andrews, J. J. 1979. Evaluation of current diagnostic methods for causes of abortions. Annu Proc Am Assoc Vet Lab Diagn 22:85.

Hottel, J. D. 1980. Personal communication.

KREIER, J. P., AND RISTIC, M. 1968. Haemobartonellosis, eperythrozoonosis, grahamellosis, and erlichosis. In Infectious Blood Diseases in Man and Animal, vol. 2. Ed. D. Weinman and M. Ristic. New York: Academic Press, pp. 387–472.

PRESTON, K. S., AND GREVE, J. H. 1965. Eperythrozoonosis in 4-week-old pigs. Iowa State Univ Vet 3:119.

RISTIC, M., AND KREIER, J. P. 1974. Family III Anaplasmataceae. In Bergey's Manual of Determinative Bacteriology, 8th ed. Ed. R. E. Buchanan and N. E. Gibbons. Baltimore: Williams & Wilkins, pp. 906–914.

ROBB, A. D. 1943. Ictero-anemia in growing swine. Vet Med 38:271.

SMITH, A. R., AND RAHN, T. 1975. An indirect hemagglutination test for the diagnosis of *Eperythrozoon suis* infection in swine. Am J Vet Res 36:1319.

SPLITTER, E. J. 1950a. *Eperythrozoon suis,* the etiologic agent of ictero-anemia or an anaplasmosis-like disease in swine. Am J Vet Res 11:324.

_____. 1950b. *Eperythrozoon suis* n. sp., and *E. parvum* n. sp., two new blood parasites in swine. Science 111:513.

_____. 1950c. Neoarsphenamine in acute eperythrozoonosis of swine. J Am Vet Med Assoc 117:371.

SPLITTER, E. J., AND CASTRO, E. R. 1957. Antibiotic therapy in acute eperythrozoonosis of swine. J Am Vet Med Assoc 131:293.

38 Erysipelas

R. L. Wood

SWINE ERYSIPELAS, (SE) or its equivalent in other languages – *Schweinerotlauf, vlekziekte, rouget du porc, mal rossino, entrace eresipelatoso, rozyca,* and *erisipela del cerdo* – is a disease caused by the bacterium *Erysipelothrix rhusiopathiae* (Sneath et al. 1986) and manifested by acute or subacute septicemia and chronic proliferative lesions. The disease is worldwide in distribution and is of economic importance throughout Europe, Asia, and the Australian and American continents.

The identification of SE as a disease entity began in 1878 when Koch isolated from an experimental mouse an organism that he called "the bacillus of mouse septicemia." In 1882–83 Pasteur and Thuillier briefly described the organism isolated from pigs with *rouget.* In 1886 Löffler published the first accurate description of the causative agent of *Schweinerotlauf* and described the infection in swine.

In the United States the history of SE began in 1885 when Theobald Smith isolated the causative organism from the kidney of a pig and noted that it resembled the one Pasteur had isolated from pigs with *rouget.* Over the next 40 years reports of cases of acute and chronic SE in the United States appeared occasionally, but the disease was not considered important. In 1928 serious outbreaks were reported in South Dakota; by 1937 acute SE was present in 28 states. Since 1959 when the disease was reported in 44 states, prevalence of SE apparently has decreased overall (Wood 1984). However, the disease is still considered to be of economic importance, especially in the chronic form, and outbreaks of acute SE continue to occur sporadically in endemic areas.

E. rhusiopathiae occurs in most parts of the world, and SE occurs in most areas where domestic swine are produced. The organism also causes polyarthritis of sheep and lambs and serious death losses in turkeys. It has been isolated from body organs of many species of wild and domestic mammals and birds as well as reptiles, amphibians, and the surface slime of fish.

In humans *E. rhusiopathiae* causes erysipeloid, a local skin lesion that occurs chiefly as an occupational disease of persons engaged in handling and processing meat, poultry, and fish as well as of rendering-plant workers, veterinarians, game handlers, leather workers, laboratory workers, and the like. The organism occasionally is isolated from cases of endocarditis in humans and rarely causes acute septicemic disease.

ETIOLOGY. *E. rhusiopathiae* (formerly *E. insidiosa*), the causative agent of SE, is a gram-positive bacillus with a marked tendency to form elongated filaments.

Physicochemical Characteristics

MORPHOLOGY AND STAINING. The morphology of *E. rhusiopathiae* is variable. In smears or cultures made directly from tissues in cases of acute infection, the organism appears as slender, straight, or slightly curved rods, 0.2–0.4 by 0.8–2.5 μm, occurring singly or in short chains (Fig. 38.1). An occasional coccoid or clubbed form may be seen. Palisades and angular formations ("snapping division") are common. The organism is nonmotile, noncapsulated, nonsporeforming, and nonacid-fast. It stains readily with ordinary dyes and is gram-positive but is easily decolorized. After several subcultures on artificial medium, filamentous forms of the organism begin to appear. These forms may predominate in old cultures, in media containing specific antiserum, or in chronic lesions. Filamentous forms are somewhat thickened, greatly elongated (4–60 μm), and may form a mass resembling mycelia, especially in liquid medium (Fig. 38.1). Branching is not known to occur. The filamentous forms sometimes have a beaded appearance when Gram's stain is used.

GROWTH CHARACTERISTICS. The appearance of growth of *E. rhusiopathiae* in a tryptose or meat infusion broth culture at 24 hours was best described by Smith (1885) as "a faint opalescence . . . , which on shaking was resolved for the moment into delicate rolling clouds." Slight sedimentation will be seen after 36–48 hours of incubation. Growth is much heavier in broth enriched with serum, usually forming a powdery sediment by 24 hours. There is no pellicle. In gelatin stabs incubated at 22°C for 4–8 days, growth of the organism radiates out from the stab in all directions, resembling a test-tube brush.

The short, slender, curved rods of *E. rhusiopathiae* isolated from acutely affected animals typically form smooth colonies, which at 48 hours of incubation are usually round, convex, colorless to bluish gray, nearly transparent, and 0.5–0.8

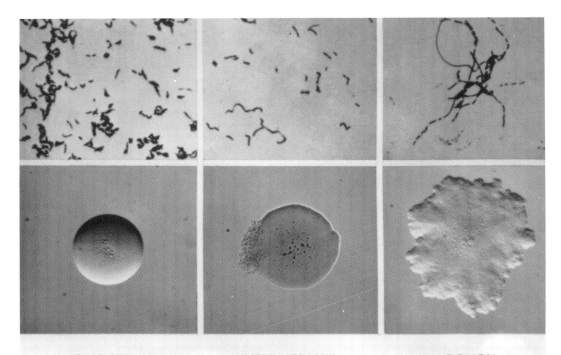

SMOOTH INTERMEDIATE ROUGH

38.1. Cellular and colonial morphology of *E. rhusiopathiae.* Upper row ×1200, crystal violet; lower row ×32. (Courtesy National Animal Disease Center, Ames, Iowa.)

mm in diameter (Fig. 38.1). Colonies of most strains have entire edges, but some strains form colonies that are slightly larger and have somewhat undulate edges. Granulelike structures usually appear under a colony just below the surface of the agar. The filamentous form produces rough colonies that are larger than smooth colonies (1–2 mm); are flattened, opaque, and irregular in shape; and have rough, uneven surfaces and edges (Fig. 38.1). Dissociation from smooth to rough form may occur during the development of a colony, producing a sector (Fig. 38.1). Such colonies are sometimes called intermediate forms; morphology of cells from these will include a variety of shapes from short, curved rods to short filaments.

Most strains of *E. rhusiopathiae* produce a narrow zone of partial hemolysis on blood agar, usually with a greenish color. Rough colonies do not induce hemolysis.

BIOCHEMICAL PROPERTIES. *E. rhusiopathiae* is relatively inactive in commonly used tests of biochemical activity (Cottral 1978). The organism produces acid but no gas from certain fermentable carbon compounds and produces hydrogen sulfide in triple-sugar iron agar (Vickers and Bierer 1958; White and Shuman 1961).

ANTIGENIC STRUCTURE. Most if not all strains of *E. rhusiopathiae* have one or more common heat-labile antigens, which are proteins or protein-saccharide-lipid complexes. The presence of common antigens is indicated by cross-agglutination and cross-immunity studies. The organism does not possess capsular or flagellar antigens, since neither a capsule nor flagella are present.

Heat-stable antigens consisting of peptidoglycan fragments from the cell wall form the basis for division of the species into serotypes, which are identified by precipitin reactions with specific hyperimmune rabbit sera, usually in a gel double-diffusion system. Most isolates of the organism (75–80%) from swine fall into two major serotypes originally designated A and B by Dedié (1949). About 20% of isolates make up a group of less-common serotypes. Under a numerical system introduced by Kucsera (1973), a total of 25 serotypes have been described so far (Wood et al. 1978; Nørrung 1979; Xu et al. 1984, 1986; Nørrung et al. 1987). In this system, now generally preferred, the former types A and B are designated 1 and 2 respectively. Strains that do not possess type-specific antigen are referred to as type N.

Immunizing antigen is discussed in the section on Prevention.

Biologic Characteristics

GROWTH REQUIREMENTS. *E. rhusiopathiae* is facultatively anaerobic; some strains grow better in an atmosphere of reduced oxygen containing 5–10% carbon dioxide. The organism will grow at temperatures of 5–42°C. Optimum growth occurs at 30–37°C and at a pH range of 7.4–7.8. Growth is enhanced by serum, glucose, protein hydrolysates, or surfactants such as Tween-80. Specific nutrient requirements are not known, but one or more peptides are required as well as small amounts of riboflavin and oleic acid.

RESISTANCE. *E. rhusiopathiae* is relatively resistant to adverse conditions for a nonsporeforming organism (see also **EPIDEMIOLOGY**). The organism is somewhat resistant to drying and can remain viable for several months in animal tissues under a variety of conditions. Thus it can persist in frozen or chilled meat, decaying carcasses, dried blood, or fish meal. It is remarkably resistant to salting, pickling, and smoking and can survive several months in cured and smoked hams. The organism can survive in swine feces or fish slime for 1–6 months if temperatures remain below 12°C. It is resistant to 0.2% phenol, 0.5% potassium tellurite, and 0.001% crystal violet; it is very tolerant to sodium azide, growing in the presence of a 0.1% concentration. The organism is sensitive to penicillin and usually to the tetracyclines; it is quite resistant to polymyxin B, neomycin, and kanamycin and is relatively resistant to streptomycin and the sulfonamides (see **TREATMENT**). It is killed readily by common disinfectants, heat (15 minutes at 60°C), and gamma irradiation.

EPIDEMIOLOGY

Sources of Infection.   The most important reservoir of *E. rhusiopathiae* is probably the domestic pig. It is estimated that 30–50% of healthy swine harbor the organism in their tonsils and other lymphoid tissues. These carriers can discharge the organism in their feces or oronasal secretions, creating an important source of infection. Swine affected with acute erysipelas shed *E. rhusiopathiae* profusely in feces, urine, saliva, and nasal secretions. Soil, bedding, feed, and drinking water therefore are contaminated by infected pigs and can serve as media for indirect transmission. The movement of surface water may transport the organism from one farm to another, particularly water from an area in which manure from infected swine or turkeys has accumulated. In addition, contamination of surface water and soil by infected rodents and sewage from meat-packing plants has been reported. The presence of the organism in the surface slime of fish creates a source of infection for swine through contaminated fish meal used in feed.

Although probably secondary to swine in importance as an immediate source of infection, the large variety of mammals and birds known to harbor *E. rhusiopathiae* provides an extensive reservoir. The organism has been isolated from at least 50 species of wild mammals, nearly half of which were rodents (Wood and Shuman 1981), and from over 30 species of wild birds (Shuman 1971). Obviously, the potential of certain wild animals, particularly rodents commonly found on the farm, as sources of indirect transmission of *E. rhusiopathiae* to susceptible swine is significant. Various species of domestic animals from which the organism has been isolated (cattle, horses, sheep, poultry, dogs, cats) provide an additional potential reservoir on swine-producing farms; however, with the possible exception of turkeys and sheep, their importance is doubtful.

The role of the soil in the epidemiology of SE has not been clearly defined. The belief that *E. rhusiopathiae* can lead a saprophytic existence in the soil, living on dead and decaying organic material, has persisted for many years. However, available research data have consistently indicated that the organism, like most other nonsporeforming pathogenic bacteria, finds an unfavorable environment in the soil and dies out in a relatively short time, most likely because of the action of protozoa. *E. rhusiopathiae* can be found in the soil of swine pens and in feces of apparently healthy swine inhabiting the pens. However, Wood (1973) found no evidence of growth or maintenance of the organism in test soils under various conditions of temperature, pH, moisture content, and organic matter content or in samples of swine-pen soils from which *E. rhusiopathiae* had been isolated previously. Survival time did not exceed 35 days under any conditions, was longest at low temperature, and was shortest at high temperature and low moisture content. This failure to establish a stable population of the organism in soil is similar to results reported by other investigators since 1955. It is perhaps possible that lysogenic cells, L-forms, or mutants of the organism can live for an extended time in the soil, but no information on this subject is available. Present information indicates that swine-pen soil, more or less continually inoculated by infected animals, probably provides a temporary but significant medium for transmission of *E. rhusiopathiae*.

According to some reports, SE tends to occur more frequently in geographic areas having alkaline soils than in areas having acid soils. However, such observations fail to account for numerous other factors that can influence the incidence of disease in the field.

The possibility of transmission of SE by insects cannot be overlooked. Transmission by various species of biting flies and ticks has been demonstrated; however, their significance has not been established.

Factors of Susceptibility

AGE.   Swine less than 3 months or more than 3 years of age are generally least predisposed to

SE. Age related to susceptibility may be explained by naturally acquired passive immunity in the young and active immunity following subclinical infection in older animals. Suckling pigs of immune sows are immune to infection for several weeks after birth. The degree and duration of passive immunity is related to the immune status of the sow.

GENETICS. Around the beginning of the twentieth century, the observation was sometimes made that the common country pig appeared to be less susceptible than the so-called refined or improved breeds. Efforts to confirm such observations have not given conclusive results, however, and it is probable that the apparent resistance (or susceptibility) of certain breeds or families is mainly from the presence of varying degrees of naturally acquired passive or active immunity.

NATURAL ACTIVE IMMUNITY. For many years after SE research was begun in the 1880s, a major problem existed in the inability to consistently induce acute SE in swine by experimental infection with *E. rhusiopathiae*. The problem eventually was eliminated by use of specific-pathogen-free (SPF) pigs delivered aseptically by surgery, deprived of colostrum, and raised in isolation. This development revealed the importance of naturally acquired immunity as a factor of susceptibility to erysipelas.

Naturally acquired active immunity is induced by previous infection with *E. rhusiopathiae*. It is well known that immunity to acute SE follows clinical disease. Less well recognized is the immunity that can be induced by organisms of low virulence, which are capable of causing mild unnoticed subacute disease or subclinical infection.

PREDISPOSING FACTORS. SE can occur with other swine diseases, but the significance of preexisting infectious disease as a predisposing factor is uncertain. Parasitic infestations have been reported to increase the severity of clinical SE. In addition, Cysewski et al. (1978) showed that the susceptibility of swine to acute SE can be enhanced by subclinical toxicity from aflatoxin in the feed. This treatment also interfered with the induction of immunity to SE by vaccination.

Environmental and stress factors such as nutrition, ambient temperature, and fatigue, particularly sudden changes in these conditions, have long been linked to the appearance of SE. For example, acute disease has occurred following sudden changes in diet such as accidental access to tankage or to a field of corn, feeding new corn, or placing pigs on new pasture. Experimentally, sudden exposure to either excessive heat or cold or exposure to a sustained high temperature (30°C) has been reported to enhance susceptibility. Under natural conditions, sudden changes in weather involving extreme temperature changes may have the same effect. Variations in prevalence of SE believed to be related to cyclic years or to season of the year have been reported, but consistent patterns of prevalence corresponding to these factors have not emerged. Except for a possible relationship to temperature changes, the variations remain unexplained.

When attempting to evaluate factors that may be related to the occurrence of SE on the farm, it should be kept in mind that a variety of stimuli in the animal's total environment can affect the level of susceptibility existing at any given time. Sudden outbreaks of acute SE may be the result of a combination of susceptibility of the animals and virulence of the causative organism, both of which are variable.

PATHOGENESIS. Investigations using germ-free pigs have demonstrated that *E. rhusiopathiae* is the sole causative agent of SE and does not require the presence of any other infectious agent for its disease-producing ability.

Mode of Entrance. SE organisms can gain entry to the body by a variety of routes. Infection through ingestion of contaminated feed and water is considered a common mode. There is no information on specific areas within the digestive system where entry may occur, nor is it known whether the organism can invade normal mucosa. Early investigators postulated it gained entrance through lesions produced by intestinal parasites; however, their presence is unnecessary. It seems likely that the organism can readily gain access to the body through the palatine tonsils or other lymphoid tissue in the wall of the digestive tract, but entrance is probably not limited to these areas.

Natural infection no doubt can result from infected skin wounds, which may be concealed or too small to be readily noticeable. Experimental infection can be accomplished easily by inoculation of scarified skin (Shuman 1951); therefore, it seems likely that infection in this manner from a contaminated environment would not be uncommon.

Acute SE. Acute or subacute systemic SE begins with bacteremia, which quickly results in clinical signs of generalized infection (septicemia). A nonsystemic infection consisting only of a local skin lesion may occur upon cutaneous exposure to a strain of low virulence or when the pig is partly immune. In such cases the organism is eliminated without inducing septicemia and the lesion disappears. In the more typical systemic infection caused by virulent organisms, bacteremia usually develops within 24 hours after exposure. The organism usually can no longer be cultured from blood or most body organs after a few days but may persist, often for months, in the joints and in lymphoid tissue such as tonsils, Peyer's patches, and spleen.

According to Schulz et al. (1975b, 1977), pathogenesis of the early septicemic phase consists of changes involving capillaries and venules of most body organs, including synovial tissues. As early as 36 hours after subcutaneous exposure of swine to virulent *E. rhusiopathiae,* they observed swelling of endothelium, with adherence of monocytes to vascular walls and evidence of widespread hyaline thrombosis. This process was referred to as a shocklike generalized coagulopathy leading within 4 days to fibrinous thrombosis, diapedesis, invasion of vascular endothelium by bacteria, and deposition of fibrin in perivascular tissues. They stated that this process leads eventually to connective tissue activation in predisposed sites such as joints, heart valves, and blood vessels.

In severe acute SE, hemolysis is commonly observed. Ischemic necrosis of perivascular tissues may occur, caused by interference with microcirculation. Drommer et al. (1970) observed a high incidence of encephalomalacia in acute experimental SE and theorized that certain strains of the organism are endotheliotropic and damage the endothelial cell barrier in the central nervous system (CNS).

Mild, delayed hypersensitivity responses to *E. rhusiopathiae* can be elicited and transferred by lymphoid cells. It is doubtful, however, that delayed hypersensitivity has a significant part in the pathogenesis of acute SE.

Chronic SE. Information on the pathogenesis of chronic SE is derived primarily from studies on development of the arthritic lesion, which has stimulated interest because of its apparent similarity to the lesion of rheumatoid arthritis of humans.

According to observations by Schulz et al. (1975a, 1977), the joint lesion in chronic SE begins with acute synovitis that may occur as early as 4–10 days after exposure to *E. rhusiopathiae.* Within 3 months fibrinous exudation, proliferation, and pannus formation occur, developing further into severe fibrosis and destruction of articular cartilage in 5–8 months. These investigators describe the earliest changes in the synovial tissue as consisting of coagulopathy and fibrinous exudate into perivascular tissues. Fibrin deposited during the vascular phase, not bacterial colonization, is believed to act as mediator of the subsequent connective tissue proliferation.

Affected joints appear to become culture-negative after 3–6 months, yet the arthritic lesions usually continue a progressive development that can continue at least 2 years. The development of such lesions in the apparent absence of the infectious agent has stimulated investigation of the role of immunopathologic processes in chronic arthritis. Hypersensitivity may be a significant factor in the chronic proliferative and destructive

changes but probably not in initiation of the lesion.

There is evidence that the bacteria do not entirely disappear from chronically affected joints, and the long-term progressive lesion may occur in response to the continued presence of either whole bacterial cells or their antigens. Schulz et al. (1977) reported that living *E. rhusiopathiae* was occasionally isolated from such joints for up to 2 years. Furthermore, they stated that *E. rhusiopathiae* antigen could be detected by immunofluorescence and whole or fragmented bacteria could be seen with the electron microscope in culturally negative joints. Denecke and Trautwein (1986) reported detection of *E. rhusiopathiae* in arthritic joints microbiologically and immunohistologically for up to 3 years. Specific antibodies to the SE organism have been detected in synovial fluid of chronically arthritic joints and apparently are produced locally by plasma cells in the synovial tissue, which can assume a lymphoid function. It is not known whether the chronicity of the joint lesion is maintained entirely by specific immune reactions against *E. rhusiopathiae* antigen or whether superimposed autoimmune reactions are involved.

A preponderance of evidence exists to indicate that erysipelatous arthritis is initiated by active infection of the joint. Mild synovitis and arthritis have been induced in rabbits and rats by massive intravenous or intraarticular injections with nonliving whole cells or fractions of the organism (White et al. 1975; Hermanns et al. 1982), but the lesions were not as severe as those typically caused by infection. White et al. (1975) suggested that the mild response induced by such antigens may predispose the joint to infection during a subsequent transient septicemia.

Studies on the pathogenesis of endocarditis indicate that the valvular lesions begin with vascular inflammation and myocardial infarcts, possibly resulting from bacterial emboli. These processes, together with exudation of fibrin, lead to destruction of valvular endocardium.

Mechanism of Pathogenicity. The mechanism by which *E. rhusiopathiae* incites disease processes is not clearly understood. The organism is not known to produce toxins. For a time hyaluronidase was thought to play a part in pathogenicity, but its production by individual strains was eventually found to be inconsistent with pathogenic properties. Considerable evidence has accumulated indicating that neuraminidase, an enzyme produced by a number of species of pathogenic bacteria, is a factor in pathogenicity of *E. rhusiopathiae.* This enzyme specifically cleaves alpha-glycosidic linkages in neuraminic acid (sialic acid), a reactive mucopolysaccharide on surfaces of body cells. The enzyme is produced by *E. rhusiopathiae* during logarithmic growth, and the amount of activity is reported to be less in avirulent strains or strains of low virulence than in fully virulent strains (Nikolov 1978; Müller 1981). Specific antibody activity against *E. rhusiopathiae* neuraminidase has been demonstrated in serum of swine with chronic SE, in commercial equine antierysipelas serum, and in serum of rabbits hyperimmunized with a preparation of neuraminidase from the organism. This latter preparation also induced a low level of protection in mice to *E. rhusiopathiae* infection. There is no evidence of a relationship between serotype and amount of neuraminidase activity.

The specific role of *E. rhusiopathiae* neuraminidase in pathogenesis of the disease is speculative. The enzyme is not a toxin; it must be produced in large amounts to be pathogenically active. It can act on substrates in cell walls throughout the body, and no doubt its activity reaches high levels in an acute septicemia.

Neuraminidase may not be the only factor responsible for pathogenicity of the organism. For example, Krasemann and Müller (1975) reported a lower growth rate in strains of low virulence than in those of high virulence; this factor and neuraminidase production were not interdependent. The ability to adhere to cell surfaces may play a role in pathogenicity of *E. rhusiopathiae.* Takahashi et al. (1987) reported that virulent strains of the organism adhered better to porcine kidney cells in vitro than did avirulent strains. Therefore, neuraminidase activity could be a major factor in what may be a multiple mechanism mediating the widespread vascular damage, thrombosis, and hemolysis described.

It has been known for many years that strains of *E. rhusiopathiae* vary in virulence, but the factors responsible for this variation are not known. There has been no evidence of a relationship between virulence and chemical structure, antigenic structure, or morphology. Attempts to relate virulence with various biochemical activities also have been negative, with the single exception of neuraminidase activity.

Serotype and Clinical Form. Most surveys of field cases have described serotype 1 (usually subtype 1a) as the predominant isolate from acute septicemic disease and serotype 2 as the most common isolate from subacute and chronic cases of erysipelas, but some surveys have provided contradictory information. Experimentally, all clinical forms can be induced readily in susceptible swine by strains of serotypes 1 or 2 as well as other serotypes (Wood and Harrington 1978).

CLINICAL SIGNS. The clinical signs of SE can be divided into three general headings: acute, subacute, and chronic. In addition, subclinical infection can occur in which no visible signs of acute disease are evident but which can lead to chronic SE.

Acute SE. Acute SE is characterized by sudden onset, sometimes with sudden death of one or more animals. Other animals in the herd may be noticeably sick, and some of these may subsequently die. Those visibly sick will have temperatures of 104–108°F (40–42°C) and over, and those with the higher temperatures may show signs of chilling. Some pigs may appear normal and yet have temperatures of around 106°F (41°C). In surviving pigs, temperatures usually return to normal within 5–7 days.

Affected animals withdraw from the herd and will be found lying down. When approached, they resent being disturbed but usually will get up and move away. This usually is accompanied by squealing; when walking, they manifest a stiff, stilted gait. Upon stopping, they may be seen to shift their weight in an apparent effort to ease the pain in their legs. If left alone, they will soon lie down carefully. Pigs showing severe depression are nevertheless usually aware of activities around them. They may evidence some resentment at being disturbed but will make little or no effort to rise. Upon being forced to get up, they may stand for only a few moments before lying down again. While standing, the feet are carried well under them and the head is hung dejectedly, giving the back line a marked arched appearance. Others will not be able to stand even when assisted.

Most affected animals will show partial or complete inappetence. Bowel movements are usually retarded and the feces firm and dry in pigs of market age and older, although as the disease progresses, a diarrhea may appear in younger animals. Abortion may occur in sows that contract acute or subacute SE during pregnancy.

Cutaneous lesions (urticarial, or "diamond-skin" lesions) appear as early as the second and usually by the third day after exposure to *E. rhusiopathiae* (Fig. 38.2). On the light-skinned pig they can be seen as small, light pink to dark purple areas that usually become raised, are firm to the touch, and in most instances are easily palpated. In animals with dark-pigmented skin, one must rely mainly on palpation, although when observed from a proper perspective, the weltlike lesions can be seen. The lesions may be few in number and thus easily overlooked or so numerous it would be difficult to count them all. An animal also may die before recognizable urticarial lesions can be felt or seen. Individual lesions, by extension of the borders, assume a characteristic square or rhomboid shape. In acute nonfatal erysipelas, these lesions may spread considerably but will gradually disappear within 4–7 days after their first appearance, with no subsequent effect other than a superficial desquamation to mark the site. The intensity of skin lesions has a direct relationship to the outcome of the disease. Light pink to light purplish red lesions are characteristic of acute

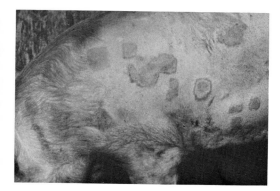

38.2. Typical rhomboid urticarial lesions ("diamond skin lesions") of SE. (Courtesy National Animal Disease Center, Ames, Iowa.)

nonfatal SE, whereas angry dark purplish red lesions usually precede death of the animal. In acute fatal disease, extensive dark purplish discoloration often occurs over the belly, ears, tail, posterior aspect of the thighs, and jowls. Infrequently, severely affected pigs do not die, and skin necrosis may follow the severe cutaneous lesions. The areas of necrotic skin are dark, dry, and firm and eventually become separated from the healing underlying tissue. Affected areas, particularly the ears and tail, will eventually slough. Healing may require many weeks as a result of secondary infection.

Subacute SE. Subacute SE includes signs that are less severe in their manifestations than the acute form. The animals do not appear as sick; temperatures may not be as high or may not persist as long; appetite may be unaffected; a few skin lesions may appear that may be easily overlooked; and, if visibly sick, the animals will not remain so for as long as those acutely ill. Some cases of subacute SE are so mild as to remain unnoticed.

Chronic SE. Chronic SE may follow acute or subacute disease or subclinical infection and is characterized most commonly by signs of arthritis. Signs of cardiac insufficiency may be seen occasionally and will be most noticeable following exertion, sometimes causing sudden death. Chronic arthritis results in joints that show various degrees of stiffness and enlargement, sometimes as early as 3 weeks after infection. Interference with locomotion ranges from a slight limp to complete refusal to put weight on the limb, depending upon the extent of damage. Arthritis is the most important clinical manifestation of SE from an economic standpoint. The condition not only affects growth rate but is responsible for significant losses of prime cuts at the packing plant.

LESIONS. Rhomboid urticarial lesions ("diamond-skin" lesions) are characteristic of acute SE, and when generalized (Fig. 38.2) they are a reliable indicator of septicemia. This observation is important in meat inspection as well as in field diagnosis (see also **Clinical Diagnosis**).

Acute SE. Most lesions of acute SE are similar to those of septicemia caused by a variety of organisms.

MACROSCOPIC LESIONS. In swine dead from acute SE, evidence of diffuse cutaneous hemostasis is often prominent, particularly in skin of the snout, ears, jowls, throat, abdomen, and thighs. The lungs may be congested and edematous. Petechial and ecchymotic hemorrhages may be seen on the epicardium and in the musculature of the atria, particularly the left atrium. Catarrhal to hemorrhagic gastritis is common, and hemorrhage of the serosa of the stomach may be present. The liver usually is congested. The appearance of the spleen is of particular note, for it may be congested and markedly enlarged, particularly in animals affected for several days. Petechial hemorrhages may be present in the cortex of the kidneys. The appearance of the lymph nodes will depend upon the degree of involvement in the area they drain. There is some degree of enlargement with moderate to marked congestion; subcapsular hemorrhage of peripheral nodes may be seen after several days of illness. The mucosa of the urinary bladder usually appears normal but may present areas of congestion.

MICROSCOPIC LESIONS. A histologic examination of skin lesions reveals damage to the capillaries and venules, with perivascular infiltration by lymphoid cells and fibroblasts. The pathologic changes occur in the papillae and upper layers of the derma. Blood vessels of the papillae are congested and may contain microthrombi and bacteria. The papillae may also present focal necrotic areas as a result of circulatory stasis. Vascular lesions can be seen in the heart, kidney, lung, liver, nervous system, skeletal muscle, and synovial membranes. Cellular response to infection by *E. rhusiopathiae* consists predominantly of mononuclear leukocytes and macrophages. Neutrophils may appear but do not predominate. Purulent lesions are not characteristic of *E. rhusiopathiae* infection.

Affected lymph nodes usually show acute hyperplastic lymphadenitis, with hyperemia and hemorrhage. In some nodes there may be evidence of thrombosis and necrosis of small blood vessels and capillaries. Hemorrhagic nephritis with inflammatory changes in glomeruli may be seen occasionally. In addition, necrosis of renal tubules with hyaline and granular casts has been reported. Focal accumulations of mononuclear cells may be seen in subcapsular sinuses of the adrenal cortex. Lesions of skeletal muscle may occur, associated with vascular lesions. These consist of a segmented hyaline and granular necrosis of muscle fibers, which may be followed by fibrosis, calcification, and regeneration. Lesions of the CNS have been described, consisting of angiopathies with disturbances in permeability, degeneration of neurons, swelling of endothelial cells, and malacic foci in the cerebrum, brain stem, and spinal cord.

Chronic SE. The predominant lesion of chronic SE in swine is a proliferative, nonsuppurative arthritis, occurring most commonly in hock, stifle, elbow, and carpal joints. Spondylitis is occasionally seen. Vegetative proliferation on the heart valves is less common.

MACROSCOPIC LESIONS. Animals affected with chronic arthritis have an enlargement of one or more joints, most readily visible in hock and carpal joints. The joint capsule is thickened with fibrous connective tissue. The joint cavity contains an excessive amount of serosanguinous synovial fluid, which may be slightly cloudy, indicating a small amount of purulent material. The presence of frank pus, however, is not characteristic of the lesion. The synovial membrane presents varying degrees of hyperemia and proliferation (Fig. 38.3), which gives the tissue a swollen, somewhat granular appearance, and often takes irregular forms, producing fringes ("tags") that project into the joint cavity. These fringes may be caught between the articulating surfaces and produce severe pain. The proliferating tissue also may extend across the surface of articular cartilage, forming a pannus that leads to destruction of the articular surface and eventually to fibrosis and ankylosis of the joint. Lymph nodes associated with arthritic joints are usually enlarged and edematous.

Vegetative endocarditis consists of proliferative granular growths on the heart valves and may be accompanied by lesions resulting from cardiac insufficiency. Other internal organs may show chronic inflammatory changes such as infarcts of kidneys and spleen. Enlargement of the adrenal gland has been reported.

MICROSCOPIC LESIONS. Lesions of the synovial tissue may vary in severity, from slight perivascular accumulation of mononuclear cells to an extensive proliferative process. The typical synovial lesion in chronic SE is characterized by pronounced hyperplasia of the synovial intima and subintimal connective tissue, with vascularization and accumulation of lymphoid cells and macrophages, forming a villous pad of inflammatory tissue. Deposition and organization of fibrin may be seen. As the lesion progresses, proliferation of fibrous connective tissue becomes more prominent, and long fronds of hyperplastic synovium may be seen. The surface lining may become necrotic, with deposition of a fibrinous to fibrinopurulent exudate. Some tendency to follicle formation may be evident in the heavy accumulations of lymphoid cells. There may be erosion of the articular cartilages along with periostitis and osteitis. In old lesions ankylosis of the involved joint by fibrous adhesion may be accompanied by calcification.

Vegetative growths on the heart valves are composed of granulation tissue and superimposed masses of fibrin. Connective tissue proliferation occurs with additional fibrin formation, which can be the source of emboli.

CLINICAL PATHOLOGY. Leukocytosis may occur in field cases of erysipelas after several days duration, or possibly from mixed bacterial infection, but in uncomplicated acute SE a leukopenia accompanied by a relative lymphocytosis is characteristic during the first 3–5 days. There may be

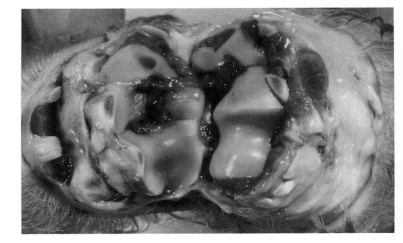

38.3. Synovitis and arthritis of chronic SE in a hock joint 8 weeks after exposure. Note hyperemia and proliferation of synovial tissue. (Courtesy National Animal Disease Center, Ames, Iowa.)

a relative increase in the number of eosinophils.

Hemoglobin and hematocrit values decrease during acute disease, followed later by appearance of nucleated erythrocytes. Sedimentation rate increases. Changes in plasma components during acute SE include a decrease in glucose and increases in glutamic oxaloacetic transaminase activity, blood creatinine, and blood urea nitrogen.

DIAGNOSIS. Clinical and bacteriologic examinations are the most reliable means of diagnosis of acute SE.

Clinical Diagnosis. Acute SE often cannot readily be differentiated clinically from other septicemic diseases, such as *Actinobacillus suis* septicemia (Miniats et al. 1989). Nevertheless, certain clinical features of an outbreak in a herd are more characteristic of SE than of other diseases if viewed in combination. For example, the following are presumptive of SE: a history of a few sudden deaths with no prior evidence of illness; several others sick with high temperatures and apparent stiffness in legs; reluctance of sick pigs to move but unexpected vitality when aroused; and clear, alert eyes. Other characteristic signs include a fair appetite in some visibly sick animals; normal to dry feces; death or recovery of sick animals within a few days; and, when present, the characteristic rhomboid skin lesions. Marked improvement within 24 hours after treatment with penicillin supports the diagnosis. At necropsy the presence of an enlarged spleen is suggestive.

Bacteriologic Diagnosis. Isolation of *E. rhusiopathiae* from the acutely affected animal provides a definite laboratory diagnosis of SE. Hemoculture is a useful diagnostic aid in living animals, but specimens should be taken from several affected animals in the herd, as the presence of the organism in the blood of an individual may be inconstant. At necropsy of a pig that has died in the acute phase, the organism is easily cultured from a variety of body organs (heart, lungs, liver, spleen, kidneys, joints). If the illness has persisted for several days, however, the organism often can no longer be cultured from internal organs but may still be found in the joints. Under these conditions it is important to take several specimens of fluid and synovial tissue from as many synovial sacs of a joint as possible, because the organisms may be present in small numbers and limited to certain areas.

Culture of *E. rhusiopathiae* from tissue specimens is relatively simple and requires only basic laboratory equipment and culture media such as tryptose or meat infusion media with or without blood or serum added. Care should be taken to avoid accidental skin infection, as the organism is pathogenic for humans. Selective culture methods for isolation of the organism from contaminated specimens are described elsewhere (Cottral 1978).

The use of immunofluorescence for rapid identification of *E. rhusiopathiae* has been reported; however, the method may not be sufficiently specific and sensitive for routine diagnostic purposes (Harrington et al. 1974).

Serologic Diagnosis. A variety of serologic tests have been used in attempts to diagnose SE. These include plate, tube, and microtitration agglutination; passive hemagglutination; hemagglutination-inhibition; complement-fixation; enzyme-linked immunosorbent assay (ELISA); and indirect immunofluorescence. An agglutination test involving the use of growing culture as antigen was developed by Wellmann (1955). In this test, called the *Wachstumsprobe* or growth-agglutination test, a culture of *E. rhusiopathiae* growing in liquid medium in the presence of sterile test serum agglutinates if sufficient specific antibody is present.

No serologic test has proved useful for routine diagnosis of acute infection or for differentiation between immune and susceptible pigs. Serologic diagnosis may have some value in detection of chronic infection, primarily on a herd basis. Microtitration agglutination, growth agglutination, and ELISA are probably the most reliable for this purpose but may be difficult to interpret. It can be concluded that serologic testing has limited practical application in clinical diagnosis of SE in the field. The chief value of serologic procedures resides in research.

TREATMENT. The treatment of SE with hyperimmune serum, usually obtained from horses, was introduced in 1899, several years after it had been developed for use in conjunction with live-culture vaccination. Until the introduction of antibiotics nearly 50 years later, the administration of antiserum was the only worthwhile available form of treatment. Although now considered obsolete by some veterinarians, antiserum can still be useful. For maximum effectiveness the serum must be given early in the course of the disease. The recommended therapeutic dose, given subcutaneously, varies from 5 to 10 ml for pigs weighing less than 50 pounds to 20–40 ml for pigs weighing more than 100 pounds.

It is generally accepted that the treatment of choice for acute erysipelas is administration of penicillin. The SE organism is highly sensitive to this antibiotic, and treatment early in an acute outbreak usually results in dramatic response within 24–36 hours. Specific treatment regimens generally involve giving penicillin alone or in combination with other antibiotics or antiserum (occasionally both) to provide a longer action. For example, long-acting penicillin (available under various proprietary names), consisting of a combination of 150,000 units procaine penicillin G and 150,000 units benzathine penicillin G/cm³, may be given intramuscularly at a single dose of 5000–10,000 units/pound to visibly sick pigs, and the entire herd may be treated with tetracycline in the drinking water (500 mg/gallon) until 5 days after no sick pigs are observed. The entire herd may also be given antiserum if the outbreak is very severe. As an alternative, long-acting penicillin may be given in severe outbreaks and procaine penicillin G in less severe cases. The use of antiserum for treatment of suckling pigs is a fairly common practice. Initiation of a vaccination program in previously unvaccinated herds where outbreaks occur is strongly recommended.

Although penicillin has been consistently found to be the most effective antibiotic for treatment of acute SE, satisfactory results have been reported also with tetracyclines (including chlortetracycline and oxytetracycline), lincomycin, and tylosin. The organism is sensitive in vitro to erythromycin, but this antibiotic has been reported to be relatively ineffective in vivo. Streptomycin, dihydrostreptomycin, chloramphenicol, bacitracin, polymyxin B, neomycin, and sulfonamides are not effective against erysipelas. There have been no published reports of development of resistance by *E. rhusiopathiae* to penicillin in the field since use of the antibiotic for treatment of SE was first reported in 1949. However, some isolates of the organism from swine have been found to be resistant to tetracyclines.

There is no practical treatment for chronic SE. Experimentally, the administration of antiinflammatory agents has provided some alleviation of the effects of chronic arthritis, and they may be used in treatment of especially valuable individual animals.

PREVENTION. Prevention of SE is best accomplished by sound practices of herd health management, including a program of immunization.

General Management Practices. Swine should be raised according to sound husbandry practice relative to nutrition, housing, and condition of lots and pastures, and they should be observed regularly for deviations from their usual attitude. Replacements should be obtained from clean sources. The recent introduction of a new boar is a relatively common history preceding acute outbreaks in a herd. Newly purchased animals should be isolated for at least 30 days.

Good sanitation is important in general herd management and is essential following the cessation of an outbreak. Walls and floors should be cleaned and disinfected. Phenolic, alkali, hypochlorite, or quaternary ammonium disinfectants are effective against the organism but must be applied to clean surfaces.

It is advisable to eliminate chronically affected swine from the herd, as they can remain carriers of the organism indefinitely. Lots or pastures in which the disease appeared can be vacated for several months, preferably including a summer season.

Although there is at present no evidence that *E. rhusiopathiae* can exist in soil for periods longer than a few weeks, certain empirical practices seem to be beneficial. For example, the risk of SE outbreaks is apparently less if the swine are kept on concrete and away from contact with the soil, probably because soil is a more effective medium of transmission of the organism.

Immunization. A variety of biologic products have been produced for the purpose of conferring immunity to SE in swine. The simultaneous or serum-culture method of immunization was introduced in 1893 and consists of concomitant injections of virulent culture and antiserum. This method was first used in the United States in 1938, and its use continued for about 20 years until safer products became available. The method is no longer used. Active immunization against SE is now carried out by the use of either attenuated (so-called avirulent) vaccines or nonliving products (bacterins).

ATTENUATED VACCINES. Vaccines made from *E. rhusiopathiae* of reduced virulence were first licensed in the United States in 1955. Attenuation of virulence has been accomplished by passage through rabbits or chicken embryos, by air-drying, or by growth in media containing acridine dyes. Although these vaccines are commonly referred to as avirulent, they are in fact strains of extremely low virulence for swine, often retaining some virulence for mice. They stimulate immunity in swine by limited multiplication in the body; therefore, the response to vaccination is subject to such variables as status of passive or active immunity already existing in the animal. In addition, there is some evidence that antiserum given concomitantly may interfere with development of immunity in response to attenuated vaccines. Manufacturers generally do not recommend use of serum with their attenuated products except when immediate protection is necessary, as in the case of suckling pigs being given both vaccine and serum during a herd outbreak. In this case, repeated vaccination at weaning is recommended.

Attenuated vaccines should not be given to swine being treated with antibiotics to which *E. rhusiopathiae* is sensitive. Antibiotic treatment should be discontinued at least 8–10 days before vaccination.

Attenuated vaccines are usually given by injection or administered orally in drinking water. Some manufacturers provide a product that can be given either way. In some parts of Europe and the U.S.S.R., vaccination by aerosol is gaining popularity. Elaborate equipment for generating and distributing the aerosol is necessary.

Use of living vaccines leaves open the possibility, however remote, of vaccinated animals becoming carriers and disseminators of the organism, which conceivably could undergo increased virulence through serial passage. There is no experimental evidence, however, that attenuated SE vaccines can regain their virulence and pose a hazard to susceptible swine.

BACTERINS. Use of a bacterin consisting of a formalin-killed whole culture adsorbed on aluminum hydroxide gel was first reported in East Germany in 1947. This type of product has been used in the United States since 1953. It is made from selected strains of serotype 2 that form a soluble immunizing product when grown in a complex medium containing serum. This product, which is released into the medium, has been described as a glyco-lipoprotein (White and Verwey 1970). Its formation is enhanced specifically by serum, and it is considered by most investigators to be a necessary component for stimulation of immunity by the bacterin. The combination of the soluble antigenic product and whole killed bacteria, adsorbed and concentrated on aluminum hydroxide gel or other suitable adjuvant, constitutes the basic features of an SE bacterin. Lysate bacterin, developed in France in 1953, has been used in the United States since 1955.

Bacterins are given by subcutaneous or intramuscular injection; a second injection in 3–5 weeks and annually thereafter is generally recommended for breeding animals. An effective level of protection is reached in 2–3 weeks.

PASSIVE IMMUNITY. Temporary passive immunity can be induced by administration of commercially available antiserum. Pigs given antiserum subcutaneously receive immediate passive protection, which persists for about 2 weeks. The preventive dose is half the therapeutic dose (see **TREATMENT**). Antiserum may be useful during a herd outbreak for temporary protection of suckling pigs until they are old enough to be vaccinated.

EFFICACY OF BIOLOGICS. No presently available immunizing product adequately fills the need for effective long-term protection against SE. Some veterinarians consider living vaccines to be superior to bacterins, but Shuman (1959) found no significant difference in their efficacy under experimental conditions. According to most reports, vaccination generally can be expected to induce immunity lasting 3–5 months. A second injection (double treatment) may increase this duration to 6 months and is recommended, especially for bacterins. Development of immunity in vaccinated swine may be adversely affected by such environmental factors as overheating or poor nutrition.

A serious deficiency of SE vaccination is its inability to prevent the chronic form. Most investigators agree that there is little effect of vaccination on the incidence of arthritis caused by *E. rhusiopathiae,* although this observation is difficult to evaluate in the field, since SE vaccination is not universally practiced in the United States. It is possible that vaccination reduces the overall prevalence of arthritis by reducing the prevalence of acute erysipelas. On the other hand, some believe vaccination actually causes an increase in arthritic lesions by initiating a state of hypersensitivity to subsequent contact with the organism. An alternative explanation for the failure of vaccination to prevent arthritis may exist, however. The organism may be carried to synovial tissues by loaded macrophages soon after exposure, thereby escaping the opsonic effects of humoral immunity (Drommer et al. 1970).

There is some evidence of serotype specificity in immunity to *E. rhusiopathiae* induced in swine by vaccination. A slight degree of specificity between the common serotypes 1 and 2 was reported by White (1962). Other studies have demonstrated that certain isolates of unusual serotypes may be refractory to the immunity induced in mice and swine by standard erysipelas vaccines. However, such serotypes are usually isolated from healthy carrier pigs or nonporcine sources, and none have been directly associated with cases of acute SE in the field.

A possible relationship of serotype to immunizing potential of specific strains of *E. rhusiopathiae* has been recognized for many years. Effective living vaccines have been produced from strains of both serotypes 1 and 2, but only certain strains of serotype 2 are known to produce good SE bacterins. This characteristic, first pointed out by Dedié (1949), has never been explained.

Although vaccination against SE is not entirely effective in preventing the disease, it provides a worthwhile means of control when used with other good management practices. A regular vaccination program for both breeding and market animals is recommended. Because of the ubiquity of *E. rhusiopathiae,* together with its poorly understood ability to exist in nature, the possibility of eradication of SE seems remote.

REFERENCES

COTTRAL, G. E. 1978. Manual of Standardized Methods for Veterinary Microbiology. Ithaca, N. Y.: Cornell Univ Press, pp. 429–436, 671, 672, 679, 687.

CYSEWSKI, S. J.; WOOD, R. L.; PIER, A. C.; AND BAETZ, A. L. 1978. Effects of aflatoxin on the development of acquired immunity to swine erysipelas. Am J Vet Res 39:445–448.

DEDIÉ, K. 1949. Die saureloslichen Antigene von *Erysipelothrix rhusiopathiae.* Monatsh Veterinaermed 4:7–10.

DENECKE, R., AND TRAUTWEIN, G. 1986. Lokale Antigenpersistenz und Chronizität der experimentellen Rotlauf-Polyarthritis. Berl Münch Tieraerztl Wochenschr 99:200–208.

DROMMER, W.; SCHULZ, L. C.; AND POHLENZ, J. 1970.

Experimenteller Rotlauf beim Schwein. Permeabilitatsstorungen und Malazien im zentralen Nervensystem. Pathol Vet 7:455–473.

HARRINGTON, R., JR.; WOOD, R. L.; AND HULSE, D. C. 1974. Comparison of a fluorescent antibody technique and cultural method for the detection of *Erysipelothrix rhusiopathiae* in primary broth cultures. Am J Vet Res 35:461–462.

HERMANNS, W.; JESSEN, H.; SCHULZ, L. C.; KERLEN, G.; AND BÖHM, K. H. 1982. Ueber die Induktion einer chronischen Polyarthritis mit Bestandteilen von Rotlaufbakterien (*Erysipelothrix rhusiopathiae*). II. Mitteilung: Versuche zur Arthritis-Induktion bei Ratten. Zentralbl Veterinaermed [B] 29:85–98.

KRASEMANN, C., AND MÜLLER, H. E. 1975. Die Virulenz von *Erysipelothrix rhusiopathiae* – Stammen und ihre Neuraminidase – produktion. Zentralbl Bakteriol [Orig A] 231:206–213.

KUCSERA, G. 1973. Proposal for standardization of the designations used for serotypes of *Erysipelothrix rhusiopathiae* (Migula) Buchanan. Int J Syst Bacteriol 23:184–188.

MINIATS, O. P.; SPINATO, M. T.; AND SANFORD, S. E. 1989. *Actinobacillus suis* septicemia in mature swine: Two outbreaks resembling erysipelas. Can Vet J 30:943–947.

MÜLLER, H. E. 1981. Neuraminidase and other enzymes of *Erysipelothrix rhusiopathiae* as possible pathogenic factors. In Arthritis: Models and Mechanisms. Ed. H. Deicher. Berlin: Springer-Verlag, p. 58.

NIKOLOV, P. 1978. Virulence and neuraminidase activity in *Erysipelothrix rhusiopathiae*. Acta Microbiol Bulg (2):62–65.

NØRRUNG, V. 1979. Two new serotypes of *Erysipelothrix rhusiopathiae*. Nord Vet Med 31:462–465.

NØRRUNG, V.; MUNCH, B.; AND LARSEN, H. E. 1987. Occurrence, isolation and serotyping of *Erysipelothrix rhusiopathiae* in cattle and pig slurry. Acta Vet Scand 28:9–14.

SCHULZ, L. C.; DROMMER, W.; SEIDLER, D.; EHARD, H.; LEIMBECK, R.; AND WEISS, R. 1975a. Experimenteller Rotlauf bei verschiedenen Spezies als Modell einer systemischen Bindegewebskrankheit. II. Chronische Phase mit besonderer Berucksichtigung der Polyarthritis. Beitr Pathol 154:27–51.

SCHULZ, L. C.; DROMMER, W.; SEIDLER, D.; EHARD, H.; VON MICKWITZ, G.; HERTRAMPF, B.; AND BÖHM, K. H. 1975b. Experimenteller Rotlauf bei verschiedenen Spezies als Modell einer systemischen Bindegewebskrankheit. I. Systemische vaskulare Prozesse bei der Organmanifestation. Beitr Pathol 154:1–26.

SHULZ, L. C.; DROMMER, W.; EHARD, H.; HERTRAMPF, B.; LEIBOLD, W.; MESSOW, C.; MUMME, J.; TRAUTWEIN, G.; UEBERSCHÄR, S.; WEISS, R.; AND WINKLEMANN, J. 1977. Pathogenetische Bedeutung von *Erysipelothrix rhusiopathiae* in der akuten und chronischen Verlaufsform der Rotlaufarthritis. DTW 84:107–111.

SHUMAN, R. D. 1951. Swine erysipelas induced by skin scarification. Proc Am Vet Med Assoc, p. 153.

_____. 1959. Comparative experimental evaluation of swine erysipelas bacterins and vaccines in weanling pigs, with particular reference to the status of their dams. Am J Vet Res 20:1002–1009.

_____. 1971. *Erysipelothrix*. In Infectious and Parasitic Diseases of Wild Birds. Ed. J. W. Davis, R. C. Anderson, L. H. Karstad, and D. O. Trainer. Ames: Iowa State Univ Press, p. 141.

SMITH, T. 1885. Second Annual Report of the Bureau of Animal Industry. Washington, D.C.: USDA, p. 187.

SNEATH, P. H. A.; MAIR, N. S.; SHARPE, M. E.; AND HOLT, J. G. 1986. Bergey's Manual of Systematic Bacteriology, vol. 2. Baltimore: Williams & Wilkins, pp. 1245–1249.

TAKAHASHI, T.; HIRAYAMA, N.; SAWADA, T.; TAMURA, Y.; AND MURAMATSU, M. 1987. Correlation between adherence of *Erysipelothrix rhusiopathiae* strains of serovar 1a to tissue culture cells originated from porcine kidney and their pathogenicity in mice and swine. Vet Microbiol 13:57–64.

VICKERS, C. L., AND BIERER, B. W. 1958. Triple sugar iron agar as an aid in the diagnosis of erysipelas. J Am Vet Med Assoc 133:543–544.

WELLMANN, G. 1955. Die subklinische Rotlaufinfektion und ihre Bedeutung fuer die Epidemiologie des Schweinerotlaufs. Zentralbl Bakteriol [Orig A] 162:265–274.

WHITE, R. R., AND VERWEY, W. F. 1970. Solubilization and characterization of a protective antigen of *Erysipelothrix rhusiopathiae*. Infect Immun 1:387–393.

WHITE, T. G. 1962. Type specificity in the vaccination of pigs with killed *Erysipelothrix rhusiopathiae*. Am J Vet Res 23:752–755.

WHITE, T. G., AND SHUMAN, R. D. 1961. Fermentation reactions of *Erysipelothrix rhusiopathiae*. J Bacteriol 82:595–599.

WHITE, T. G.; PULS, J. L.; AND HARGRAVE, P. 1975. Production of synovitis in rabbits by fractions of a cell-free extract of *Erysipelothrix rhusiopathiae*. Clin Immunol Immunopathol 3:531–540.

WOOD, R. L. 1973. Survival of *Erysipelothrix rhusiopathiae* in soil under various environmental conditions. Cornell Vet 63:390–410.

_____. 1984. Swine erysipelas: A review of prevalence and research. J Am Vet Med Assoc 184:944–949.

WOOD, R. L.; AND HARRINGTON, R., JR. 1978. Serotypes of *Erysipelothrix rhusiopathiae* isolated from swine and from soil and manure of swine pens in the United States. Am J Vet Res 39:1833–1840.

WOOD, R. L., AND SHUMAN, R. D. 1981. *Erysipelothrix* infection. In Infectious Diseases of Wild Mammals, 2d ed. Ed. J. W. Davis, L. H. Karstad, and D. O. Trainer. Ames: Iowa State Univ Press.

WOOD, R. L.; HAUBRICH, D. R.; AND HARRINGTON, R., JR. 1978. Isolation of previously unreported serotypes of *Erysipelothrix rhusiopathiae* from swine. Am J Vet Res 39:1958–1961.

XU, K.; HU, X.; GAO, C.; AND LU, Q. 1984. A new serotype of *Erysipelothrix rhusiopathiae*. Anim Infect Dis 4(1984):11–14.

XU, K.; GAO, C.; AND HU, X. 1986. Study on a new serotype of *Erysipelothrix rhusiopathiae* isolated from marine fishes. Anim Infect Dis 3(1986):6–7, 48.

39 *Escherichia coli* Infections

H. U. Bertschinger

J. M. Fairbrother

N. O. Nielsen

J. F. Pohlenz

Introduction

H. U. Bertschinger

THE GENUS *Escherichia* is named after the German pediatrician Theodor Escherich (1857–1911). It is classified with the family Enterobacteriaceae, which belongs to the gram-negative, facultatively anaerobic rods. The species *Escherichia (E.) coli* brings together normal inhabitants of the gastrointestinal tract and organisms causing a broad variety of intestinal and extraintestinal diseases in the porcine species.

BACTERIOLOGY. *E. coli* are gram-negative, peritrichous flagellated rods of variable length, with a diameter of about 1 μm. Colonies on solid media reach their full size within 1 day of incubation. Colonial diameters range from 2 to several millimeters, and the appearance of the growth may vary from smooth to rough or mucoid. There is a broad range of selective media available. Some strains produce hemolysins. Species identification relies mainly on biochemical characters. It should be borne in mind that there are exceptions with every single biochemical character. Commercially available identification kits therefore make use of up to 50 characters to achieve a high level of accuracy. The interpretation may be facilitated by computer-assisted processing of the data. The determination of DNA relatedness, the theoretical base of discrimination between species, is restricted to research laboratories.

SEROTYPING. There are several ways to subdivide the species into types. So far serotypes have shown the best association with certain virulence traits. Complete serotyping includes determination of O (somatic), K (capsular or microcapsular), H (flagellar), and F (fimbrial) antigens. Unlike salmonellae, only a small percentage of *E. coli* isolates are typable with available antisera, since serotyping has been limited to isolates of proven or suspected pathogenicity. Currently, at least 170 O, 70 K, 56 H, and a fast-growing number of F antigens are officially recognized.

In diagnostic laboratories serotyping is often reduced to one or two classes of antigens and to a limited spectrum of antisera. This may be quite suitable, since in a given region, animal species and organ pathogenic serotypes maintain their characteristic antigenic makeup. Thus, one may deduce the complete serotype from a simple slide agglutination with a living culture. Serotyping is diagnostically helpful in communicable types of disease caused by a limited number of serotypes, such as postweaning enteric infections.

VIRULENCE FACTORS. Bacterial traits involved in pathogenesis are called virulence factors. Much has been learned in this fast-progressing field (Sussman 1985; Roth 1988), but we are far from understanding every step in the development of the different kinds of disease caused by *E. coli*. Potent exotoxins trigger the secretion of fluid into the gut lumen in enterotoxigenic *E. coli* (ETEC) infections and are responsible for systemic pathology caused by enterotoxemic *E. coli* (ETEEC) strains. Endotoxin is present in the outer membrane of most *E. coli* strains. Its significance is well documented only in extraintestinal infections, such as septicemia, mastitis, and urinary tract infections.

Many *E. coli* infections require the colonization of mucous membranes. With ETEC and ETEEC, adhesion to the small intestine is mediated by extracellular proteinaceous appendages, which are called fimbriae or pili and are highly specific. In some strains capsular polysaccharide has been shown to enhance the ability to colonize. Enteropathogenic *E. coli* (EPEC) colonizing the lower gastrointestinal tract adhere by an attaching and effacing mechanism, which is not yet well elucidated. In the pig, colonization of the urinary tract has received little attention so far.

Some *E. coli* utilize high-affinity iron-uptake systems to compete with the host for available iron. In extraintestinal sites *E. coli* have to resist the natural bactericidal activity of serum, a characteristic called serum resistance. A given pathogenic strain may harbor a whole set of virulence factors, i.e., more than one toxin and up to three adhesion factors. Detection of more virulence factors can be expected.

GENETICS OF VIRULENCE. Very specific sets of virulence factors are needed to cause a particular disease. Thus, strains causing enteric diseases are not associated with extraintestinal infections and vice versa. Most virulence factors examined so far are plasmid determined. This applies in particular to hemolysins, toxins, and adhesins of ETEC. In strains from human urinary tract infections, however, the genes encoding for some fimbriae are chromosomally located. In the laboratory, plasmids can easily be transmitted from donor to recipient strains. However, such exchanges of genetic material do not appear to play a major role in the field. The genetic makeup of pathogenic *E. coli* strains is remarkably stable. This may be because a whole set of virulence factors is involved in the virulence of a particular strain, and certain recipient strains may not express transmitted plasmid-determined functions.

The time-consuming and sometimes cumbersome assays for virulence factors are increasingly being replaced by gene probes hybridizing with corresponding gene sequences of test strains. However, these techniques have not yet gained access to diagnostic laboratories. The molecular biology of bacterial virulence genes has a great potential for the prevention of *E. coli* diseases in the future.

ECOLOGY. The particular ecology of pathogenic *E. coli* strains has been somewhat neglected. Intestinal infections caused by ETEC and ETEEC are often contagious in character. The same strain is usually found in many sick pigs and often repeatedly in consecutive batches of pigs. These strains may sometimes appear in healthy pigs without overt disease (Hinton et al. 1985). They are usually shed in high numbers for a period of a few days only. The ensuing dramatic decrease seems to be due to the development of local immunity.

Extraintestinal infections, however, do not behave like communicable diseases. Individual pigs in a given herd are affected most often by different strains. Mixed infections by more than one strain are frequent. In humans the fecal flora is obviously the reservoir of such pathogenic strains. In 18 out of 67 sows with mastitis, *E. coli* of the same O types present in samples of mammary secretion were isolated from the feces (Awad-Masalmeh et al. 1990). This underlines the endogenous character of most extraintestinal infections in the pig as well.

The primary habitat of porcine *E. coli* is the gastrointestinal tract. The *E. coli* flora of individual pigs is extremely complex. When strains were distinguished by the combined application of O serogrouping, biotyping, and resistogram typing, up to 25 strains were identified in the gastrointestinal tract of one individual (Hinton et al. 1985). Numerically dominant strains change at intervals from one day to several weeks leading to successive waves of dominant strains (Craven and Barnum 1971). Proliferation of *E. coli* takes place mainly in the course of the passage through the small intestine. Increase from the ileum to the rectum is minimal or absent (McAllister et al. 1979). Numbers in the large intestine fluctuate around 10^7 colony-forming units/g. However, *E. coli* contributes less than 1% to the total bacterial count. When found elsewhere (feed, water, soil, etc.), *E. coli* is derived from this habitat, usually by fecal contamination. Long survival times in the environment are promoted among other factors by low temperature and sufficient available water. In an experiment with five slurry samples, a porcine *E. coli* O139:K82(B) retained viability for between 5 and over 11 weeks (Burrows and Rankin 1977).

REFERENCES

Awad-Masalmeh, M.; Baumgartner, W.; Passernig, A.; Silber, R.; and Hinterdorfer, F. 1990. Bakteriologische Untersuchungen bei an puerperaler Mastitis (MMA-Syndrom) erkrankten Sauen verschiedener Tierbestände Österreichs. Tieraerztl Umsch 45:526–535.

Burrows, M. R., and Rankin, J. D. 1970. A further examination of the survival of pathogenic bacteria in cattle slurry. Br Vet J 126:xxxii–xxxiv.

Craven, J. A., and Barnum, D. A. 1971. Ecology of intestinal *Escherichia coli* in pigs. Can J Comp Med 35:324–331.

Hinton, M.; Hampson, D. J.; Hampson, E.; and Linton, A. H. 1985. A comparison of the ecology of *Escherichia coli* in the intestine of healthy unweaned pigs and pigs after weaning. J Appl Bacteriol 58:471–478.

McAllister, J. S.; Kurtz, H. J.; and Short, E. C., Jr. 1979. Changes in the intestinal flora of young pigs with postweaning diarrhea or edema disease. J Anim Sci 49:868–879.

Roth, J. A. 1988. *Virulence Mechanisms of Bacterial Pathogens.* Washington, D.C.: American Society for Microbiology.

Sussman, M. 1985. The Virulence of *Escherichia coli:* Reviews and Methods. London: Academic Press.

Enteric Colibacillosis

J. M. Fairbrother

DIARRHEA HAS become an economically important disease in pigs as a result of increasing intensification of farrowing management. It may be classified into three main entities: neonatal diarrhea (within the first few days of birth), young piglet diarrhea (from the first week of birth to weaning), and postweaning diarrhea. *Escherichia coli* is the most important etiologic agent of neonatal and postweaning diarrhea. Etiologic agents of diarrhea in young piglets are more numerous and include transmissible gastroenteritis (TGE) virus, rotavirus, coccidia, and *E. coli* (Biehl and Hoefling 1986). *E. coli* is a normal inhabitant of the intestinal tract of animals but may also cause disease. Pathogenic enteric *E. coli* belong to a restricted number of serogroups and produce one or more virulence factors, which are not usually found in nonpathogenic *E. coli*. Over the last several years, our knowledge of enteric *E. coli* virulence factors and their role in the pathogenesis of enteric disease has rapidly expanded. The terminology used to describe pathogenic *E. coli* has greatly changed; thus, *E. coli* may now be categorized by pathotype, based on their production of virulence factors. Specific *E. coli* pathotypes are associated with each of the main disease entities. A less frequently encountered manifestation of enteric *E. coli* infection is hemorrhagic gastroenteritis. Another more frequent manifestation, edema disease, is discussed below.

ETIOLOGY. Neonatal diarrhea associated with *E. coli* is observed most commonly in pigs from 0 to 4 days old. Causative strains produce one or more enterotoxins and have been designated enterotoxigenic *E. coli* (ETEC). ETEC adhere to the small intestinal mucosa by means of one or more of the fimbrial adhesins F4 (K88), F5 (K99), F6 (987P), or F41 (Table 39.1). They colonize the small intestine and produce one or more of the enterotoxins STa (STI), STb (STII), or LT. Until recently, the most commonly observed ETEC in cases of neonatal diarrhea belonged to the classical serogroups O149, O8, O147, and O157, were F4-positive, and produced the enterotoxins LT and STb (Wilson and Francis 1986; Soderlind et al. 1988; Harel et al. 1990). An increasing number of ETEC of serogroups such as O8, O9, O64, and O101, which are F5-, F6-, and/or F41-positive and mainly produce the enterotoxin STa, or less often

Table 39.1. Serogroups and virulence factors of pathogenic *E. coli* in pigs

Serogroup	Clinical Disease	Category	STa	STb	LT	VT	F4	F5	F6	F41
08:K"S16"	Diarrhea in neonates, young pigs	ETEC	+					+	+	
09:K35			+					+		
09/0101:K30			+					+		
09/0101:K103			+							+
09:(group)			+						+	
020:K101			+					+	+	+
064:K"V142"			+	(+)				+	+	(+)
08:K"4627"	Diarrhea in neonates, young pigs, weanlings; hemorrhagic gastroenteritis	ETEC		+	+		+			
08:(group)				+	+		+			
0157:K"V17"			+	+	+	(+)	+			
0147:K89			(+)	+	+		+	(+)		
0149:K91			(+)	+	+	(+)	+			
08:(group)	Diarrhea in young pigs, weanlings	ETEC		+	+					
0147:K"1285"				+	(+)					
0115:K"V165"				+						
0138:K81	Diarrhea in weanlings	ETEC and VTEC	+	+	+	+				
0139:K82				+	+	+				
0141:K85			(+)	+		+				
045:K"E65"	Diarrhea in weanlings	AEEC		(+)	(+)		(+)			

Note: + virulence determinant often found in this serogroup; (+) virulence determinant occasionally found in this serogroup.

STb, are now being isolated. These ETEC cause diarrhea mainly in pigs aged from 0 to 6 days, and to a lesser extent in pigs aged from 7 to 21 days, whereas F4-positive ETEC are now more often isolated in diarrheic pigs aged from 7 to 21 days. Fewer F4-positive ETEC within the classical serogroups, especially O157, are now being isolated. ETEC isolated from cases of diarrhea in young pigs aged from 1 to 6 weeks often belong to serogroups O8, O115, or O147 and are negative for the known fimbrial adhesins (Broes et al. 1988; Fairbrother et al. 1988).

Diarrhea is often observed in pigs following the stress and dietary changes of weaning and in many cases may be attributed to ETEC. The most commonly encountered serogroups are O8, O138, O139, O141, O147, O149, and O157 (Nagy et al. 1990). Whereas ETEC of the classical serogroups mostly produce LT and STb and are F4-positive, those of serogroups O138, O139, and O141, and sometimes O147 and O157, produce STb or STa, and more often one of the verocytotoxins (VT) (Gannon et al. 1988). However, known fimbrial adhesins are rarely found on these strains. Other as yet uncharacterized fimbrial antigens may mediate the adherence of these strains to the small intestine. *E. coli* of serogroup O45 are also isolated from pigs with postweaning diarrhea and may be F4-positive and produce LT and STb (Woodward et al. 1990), but have also been associated with lesions of attaching and effacing *E. coli* (AEEC) (Hélie et al. 1990). The frequency of AEEC among isolates of other serogroups has not yet been determined.

Hemorrhagic gastroenteritis also occurs in young pigs before and after weaning. *E. coli* associated with this disease commonly belong to serogroups O149:K91, O157:KV17, and O8:K4627, are F4-positive, produce STb and LT, but only occasionally produce VT (Faubert and Drolet 1991).

EPIDEMIOLOGY.   The occurrence of *E. coli* diarrhea depends on an interaction between the causative bacteria, environmental conditions, and certain host factors. Only *E. coli* that carry virulence factors as described in the previous section, ingested in large numbers, are able to cause diarrhea. The newborn pig, on leaving the uterus and before reaching the teats of the sow, encounters the heavily contaminated environment of the farrowing crate and the skin of the dam, resulting in ingestion of microbes from the intestinal flora of the sow. Thus, in conditions of poor hygiene or in a continuous farrowing system, a buildup of pathogenic *E. coli* in the environment could lead to an outbreak of neonatal *E. coli* diarrhea. The colostrum contains nonspecific bactericidal factors and specific antibody (IgA), which inhibit the proliferation of pathogenic *E. coli* in the intestine. If the dam has not been exposed to the pathogenic *E. coli* present in the environment of the

piglets, specific antibodies are not present in the colostrum and the piglets are susceptible to infection. Similarly, when individual piglets do not have access to colostrum, due to injury or inability to compete or due to agalactia or insufficient teats of the sow, they are more susceptible to infection. Ambient temperature in the farrowing house is also very important. In pigs kept at temperatures of less than 25°C, intestinal peristaltic activity is greatly reduced and passage of bacteria and protective antibodies through the intestine is delayed (Sarmiento 1983). Increased numbers of pathogenic *E. coli* in the intestinal tract of these pigs results in a more severe diarrhea than in pigs kept at 30°C.

Following the neonatal period, a concurrent decrease in the maternal antibody level in the piglet and increased exposure to pathogenic *E. coli* or other etiologic agents in the environment may lead to a greater incidence of diarrhea. It is probable that pathogenic *E. coli* are present in the intestinal flora of pigs at the time of weaning. Several factors could be responsible for the increased occurrence of diarrhea at this time (Fahy et al. 1987). Piglets are deprived of lactogenic antibodies that may have helped to control the numbers of pathogenic *E. coli* present in the intestine. The diet is changed from being highly digestible to one that is new to the digestive enzymes of the pig, resulting in a buildup of undigested material in the intestine, which would be available as a substrate for pathogenic *E. coli*. Variations in environmental temperature seem to play an important role in the development of postweaning diarrhea, possibly by similar mechanisms to those described for neonatal diarrhea. The stress associated with dietary change and handling at weaning would also be an important factor in the development of diarrhea.

PATHOGENESIS.   In the presence of the appropriate predisposing environmental conditions and host factors, pathogenic *E. coli* proliferate in the intestine and cause diarrhea by means of specific virulence factors. Pathogenesis will be discussed with respect to the *E. coli* categories defined by the production of these virulence factors.

Enterotoxigenic E. coli.   Most pathogenic *E. coli* produce one or more fimbrial adhesins, which mediate their attachment to specific receptors on mucosal epithelial cells and in the adjacent mucous layer. These fimbriae (or pili) are hairlike appendages extending from the bacterial cell and consist of structural protein subunits, which in many cases act as a support for a separate adhesive protein found at the tip of the fimbriae. Fimbriae are classified by serologic reactivity or by receptor specificity, the latter being manifested by agglutination of red blood cells from different animal species. The nomenclature for fimbriae has been very diverse. For example, the first fimbrial adhesins demonstrated on porcine ETEC were thought to be capsular antigens and were named K88 and K99. A more standardized nomenclature based on serologic activity in crossed immunoelectrophoresis and using an F designation has been proposed (Orskov and Orskov 1983) and is slowly being accepted. The latter nomenclature will be used in this chapter. Although an increasing number of fimbrial adhesins have been described (more than 30), most fimbrial adhesins, with the exception of F1 (type 1) common fimbriae, are associated with *E. coli* of particular serogroups isolated from specific animal species. F1 fimbriae are found on most *E. coli* isolates and cause an agglutination of guinea pig red cells, which is inhibited by D-mannose. Their role in attachment of porcine ETEC to the intestinal mucosa is still unclear (To et al. 1984; Jayappa et al. 1985). We have found only F1 and no other known fimbrial adhesins on certain diarrheagenic ETEC strains (Broes et al. 1988). The four important fimbrial adhesins of porcine ETEC are F4 (K88), F5 (K99), F6 (987P), and F41. F4 or K88 fimbriae have been divided into three variants, K88ab, K88ac, and K88ad, based on serologic cross-reactions (Guinee and Jansen 1979). Many ETEC isolates produce more than one fimbrial adhesin, and common combinations are F5 and F6, F5 and F41, and F4 and F6. Production of fimbriae is controlled by genes on the bacterial chromosome (F1, F41) or on plasmids (F4, F5, F6). Many fimbriae, such as F1 and F6, undergo phase variation and may be very poorly expressed after several passages in culture conditions. Other fimbriae (F5 and F41) undergo quantitative variation and are only well expressed in culture media low in glucose or alanine in culture, such as Minca medium (Guinee et al. 1977). Other fimbrial antigens have been more recently associated with porcine ETEC. The fimbria F165 has occasionally been found on O8 ETEC isolates, but is more commonly isolated from non-ETEC isolates able to cause septicemia in piglets (Fairbrother et al. 1989). Fimbriae CS1541 and F42 have also been found on porcine ETEC, but their role in the development of enterotoxigenic diarrhea has not been definitively demonstrated (Yano et al. 1986; Broes et al. 1988).

Fimbriae adhere to specific receptors on the cell wall of intestinal epithelial cells and to specific receptors or nonspecifically in the mucus coating the epithelium. ETEC producing fimbriae F5, F6, or F41 mostly colonize the posterior jejunum and ileum, whereas F4-positive ETEC tend to colonize the length of the jejunum and the ileum. Certain pigs do not have receptors for the F4 adhesin on intestinal epithelial cells and are thus resistant to infection by F4-positive ETEC (Sellwood et al. 1975). This genetic resistance to infection is inherited in a simple Mendelian way and the allele for the receptor is dominant. Subsequent studies have demonstrated at least five pig phenotypes, based on susceptibility of brush borders of different pigs to adherence of isolates that produce the different variants K88ab, K88ac, and K88ad (Bijlsma et al. 1982). A similar genetic resistance has not been observed for the other fimbriae of porcine ETEC. On the other hand, there appears to be an age resistance to infection by F5-positive isolates, which is not observed for F4-positive isolates. Piglets are most susceptible to infection with F5-positive ETEC during the first several days of life and subsequently become more resistant. This susceptibility could be related to a reduction of the number of receptors present on intestinal epithelial cells with age (Runnels et al. 1980).

ETEC that adhere to the intestinal mucosa produce enterotoxins, which change the water and electrolyte flux of the small intestine and may lead to diarrhea if the excess fluid from the small intestine is not absorbed in the large intestine. Two major classes of enterotoxin are produced by porcine ETEC: heat-stable toxin (ST), which is resistant to heat treatment at 100°C for 15 minutes, and heat-labile toxin (LT), which is inactivated at 60°C for 15 minutes (Guerrant et al. 1985). ST has been further divided into STa and STb, based on solubility in methanol and biologic activity (Robichaud et al. 1978).

LT is a high molecular weight toxin complex, which consists of five B subunits able to bind to ganglioside receptors on the intestinal epithelial cell surface and a biologically active A subunit (Gill et al. 1981). After binding, the latter activates adenylate cyclase, which stimulates the production of cyclic adenosine monophosphate (cAMP). High levels of cAMP in the cell result in increased secretion of Cl, Na, HCO3, and water into the intestinal lumen. Excessive secretion leads to dehydration, metabolic acidosis, and eventually death. Two subgroups of LT, LTI, and LTII, have been described (Holmes et al. 1986). Only LTI is neutralized by anticholera toxin. LT produced by porcine isolates belongs to the LTI subgroup. The LTs produced by human and porcine ETEC have been designated LTh and LTp, based on slight differences in the genes coding for the toxin.

STa (STI, ST1, and ST mouse) is a small, nonimmunogenic protein with a molecular weight of 2000 (Lallier et al. 1982). STa activates guanylate cyclase, which stimulates production of cyclic guanosine monophosphate (cGMP). High levels of cGMP in the cell inhibits the Na/Cl cotransport system and reduces the absorption of electrolytes and water from the intestine (Dreyfus et al. 1984). STa is active in infant mice and young piglets of less than 2 weeks of age, but is less active in older pigs. As with LT, STa produced by human and porcine ETEC has been designated STaH and STaP, based on differences in the genes coding for the toxin.

STb (STII, ST2, ST pig) is a small 5000-MW

protein, which is antigenically and genetically un-related to STa and is poorly immunogenic (Dubreuil et al. 1991). STb stimulates cyclic nucleotide–independent fluid secretion in the gut, but its mode of action has not been further characterized (Kennedy et al. 1984). STb is active in the pig intestine but not in infant mice. It is inactivated by trypsin and, in the presence of trypsin-inactivator, is active in intestines of mice, rats, and calves (Whipp 1990). STb is found in over 75% porcine *E. coli* isolates. Only 33% of ETEC from older pigs with enteric colibacillosis are positive for STb (Moon et al. 1986). The role of STb in the development of diarrhea is not yet known, although ETEC producing only STb can induce diarrhea in experimentally infected newborn pigs (Fairbrother et al. 1989); STb induces some villous atrophy in pig intestinal gut loops (Rose et al. 1987).

Verocytotoxigenic *E. coli*. Many *E. coli* of serogroups O138, O139, and O141 isolated from pigs with postweaning diarrhea produce VT. Although the role of VT in the pathogenesis of edema disease (see below) has been determined, the role of VT in development of postweaning diarrhea is not known.

Attaching and Effacing *E. coli*. Porcine AEEC attach to the intestinal mucosa and cause lesions similar to those observed for enteropathogenic *E. coli* (EPEC) isolated from human infantile diarrhea (Hélie et al. 1990). The latter attach initially to microvilli by means of a plasmid-coded EPEC-attachment factor, then attach more intimately to the epithelial cell membrane, efface the microvilli, and invade the epithelial cells. These steps are coded by genes on the chromosome and on plasmids. The mechanisms by which porcine AEEC cause diarrhea are not yet known.

CLINICAL SIGNS. Enteric *E. coli* infection is usually manifested by diarrhea, the severity of which depends on the virulence factors of the *E. coli* and the age and immune status of the piglets. In severe cases, dehydration, metabolic acidosis, and death are observed. In certain cases, particularly in young animals, the infection may be so rapid that death occurs before the development of diarrhea.

Neonatal diarrhea may first be observed 2–3 hours after birth and may affect single pigs or whole litters. Gilt litters are more often affected than sow litters. A large number of piglets in a farrowing house may be affected and mortality may be very high in the first few days of life. Diarrhea may be very mild with no evidence of dehydration or may be clear and watery. The feces vary from clear to whitish or various shades of brown. The fecal material may just dribble from the anus down the perineum and only be detected by close examination of the perineal area. In very severe outbreaks, a small proportion of affected animals may vomit. In severe cases, 30–40% of total body weight may be lost as fluid into the intestinal lumen and result in signs of dehydration. The abdominal musculature is flaccid and atonic, the pigs are depressed and sluggish, the eyes may be sunken, and the skin may be bluish gray and resemble parchment in texture. The loss of fluid and weight results in the exaggerated appearance of the bony prominences. These animals usually die. In more chronic or less severely affected cases, the anus and perineum may be inflamed from contact with the alkaline fecal material. Pigs with less severe dehydration may continue to drink and, if treated appropriately, may recover with only minimal long-term effects.

Diarrhea in pigs from the neonatal to the postweaning period is similar to that observed in neonatal piglets but tends to be less severe. Morbidity may be the same as in the neonatal period but mortality is invariably lower. The feces vary from grayish to whitish in unweaned piglets to brownish in recently weaned piglets. Postweaning *E. coli* infection usually occurs within the first week after weaning and is usually mild. Nevertheless, a dramatic reduction in weight gain may be observed, not only in affected animals, but in the entire group.

Hemorrhagic gastroenteritis occurs both in unweaned pigs from 8 days of age and in recently weaned pigs (Faubert and Drolet 1991), in contrast to earlier reports. Apparently healthy pigs die suddenly, or decline rapidly with cyanosis of the extremities. A yellowish to brownish diarrhea is sometimes observed.

LESIONS. Few specific pathologic changes may be attributed to enteric *E. coli* infection. Gross lesions that may be observed include dehydration; dilation of the stomach, which may contain undigested milk curd or feed in the case of postweaning diarrhea; venous infarcts on the greater curvature of the stomach; and dilation of the small intestine, with some congestion of the small intestinal wall. In cases of hemorrhagic gastroenteritis, characteristic lesions include marked congestion of the small intestinal and stomach wall and blood-tinged intestinal contents.

Histologic lesions depend on the category of *E. coli* involved. In ETEC infections, layers of *E. coli* are observed adhering to the mucosal epithelial cells of most of the jejunum and ileum in the case of F4-positive ETEC isolates, and of the posterior jejunum and/or the ileum in the case of other ETEC isolates. Adhering bacteria may be found only in the crypts of Lieberkühn, or more often covering the crypts and the tips of the villi. On transmission electron microscopy, bacteria are usually located approximately half a bacterium width away from the microvilli; fimbriae may sometimes be visualized between the bacteria and the microvilli (Fig. 39.1). Histologic lesions, if observed, may include vascular congestion in the lamina propria with some hemorrhages into the intestinal lumen, increased numbers of neutrophils and macrophages in the lamina propria and migrating into the lumen, and some villous atrophy.

In pigs infected with AEEC isolates, a multifocal colonization of the brush border of mature enterocytes by *E. coli* arranged in palisades with enterocyte degeneration and light to moderate inflammation of the lamina propria is observed, mostly in the ileum (Hélie et al. 1990). In newborn pigs experimentally infected with an AEEC isolate, colonization was most intense in the duodenum and cecum, bacteria were sometimes observed in intracytoplasmic vacuoles in enterocytes, and there was a light to moderate villous atrophy in the small intestine. On transmission electron microscopy, bacteria are intimately attached to the cytoplasmic membrane of mature enterocytes and arranged in regular palisades, parallel to the microvilli, with effacement of adjacent villi (Fig. 39.2). The bacterial cell wall and the apical cell membrane of the enterocyte are separated by a narrow regular gap of 10 nm at the cupping pedestal, and apical dense regions are seen at attachment sites. In cases of hemorrhagic gastroenteritis, *E. coli* are found adhering to the mucosal epithelial cells of the small intestine. Congestion, some hemorrhages, and in severe cases, villous necrosis and microvascular fibrinous thrombi are observed in the lamina propria of the stomach, small intestine, and colon.

DIAGNOSIS. Enteric *E. coli* infection in young, unweaned pigs must be differentiated from other common infectious causes of diarrhea in pigs of this age group. These include TGE virus, rotavirus, and coccidia. More than one etiologic agent may be associated with a particular animal or outbreak. A presumptive diagnosis may be made by determinating the fecal pH. Secretory diarrheic fluid, as a result of enteric ETEC infection, has an alkaline pH, whereas that from diarrheas associated with malabsorption, as a result of TGE virus or rotavirus infection, are acid. Diagnosis of enteric *E. coli* infection is based on clinical signs, histopathologic lesions, and the presence of gram-negative organisms usually closely adhering to the small intestinal mucosa (Wilson and Francis 1986). This diagnosis is strengthened by the isolation of *E. coli* of the appropriate serogroup, or more importantly, possessing one or more of the above-mentioned virulence factors. Detection of production of en-

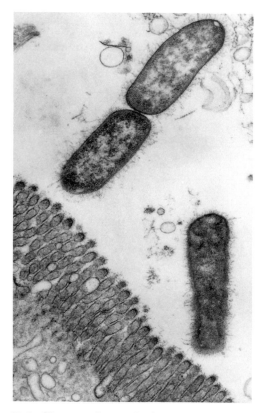

39.1. Electron micrograph of attachment of 987P positive strain in the intestine.

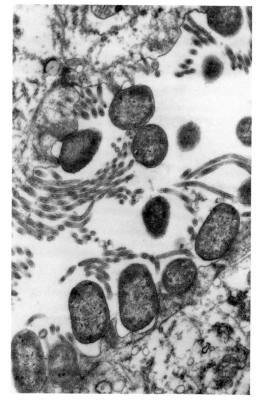

39.2. Electron micrograph of attaching effacing lesions.

terotoxins and cytotoxins has been arduous. Until recently, it has been based on detection of toxin biologic activity. STa activity is determined using the infant-mouse test; STb activity is determined using ligated pig and, more recently, rat gut loops; and LT and VT are determined using cell culture assays. Fimbrial adhesins are detected by serologic assays, such as agglutination, immunofluorescence, and enzyme-linked immunosorbent assay (ELISA), using rabbit polyclonal antisera. However, F5 and F41 are only produced when *E. coli* are grown on special minimal media and F6 is often poorly produced in vitro. Alternatively, *E. coli* adhering to the intestinal mucosa may be demonstrated directly in infected pigs by examination of frozen sections using indirect immunofluorescence or by examination of formalin-fixed, paraffin-embedded tissues using the immunoperoxidase technique.

Recent technologic advances have greatly improved the detection of *E. coli* virulence factors. Use of monoclonal antibodies has led to more specific, sensitive, and reproducible assays for the detection of STa, F4, F5, F6, and F41. Such antibodies could be used in diagnostic kits for the rapid detection and identification of pathogenic *E. coli* directly in the feces or intestinal contents of affected piglets. Probes have now been developed for the detection of the genes coding for the fimbrial adhesins and enterotoxins of swine ETEC (Moon et al. 1986; Nagy et al. 1990). There is a high correlation between the results of the standard serologic and biologic assays and those of gene probes for the detection of fimbrial adhesins and enterotoxins of swine ETEC (Harel et al. 1990). Probes are currently used in many diagnostic laboratories for the identification of

ETEC isolates and for the detection of ETEC directly in the feces of pigs with diarrhea (Monckton and Hasse 1988). At present, gene probe techniques involve the use of radioactivity and thus must be performed in controlled laboratory conditions. Nonradioactive gene probes are being developed and could feasibly be used in kits by the veterinary practitioner for the detection of pathogenic *E. coli* directly in the fecal or intestinal contents of diarrheic pigs. In the future, use of the polymerase chain reaction (PCR) technique will greatly enhance the sensitivity of current gene probe techniques.

However, the traditional approach for identification of pathogenic *E. coli* by serotyping will still be necessary, at least in reference laboratories, to monitor changing trends and to identify new, emerging *E. coli* virulence determinants, which could gain importance due to the pressure of vaccination of sows against the currently predominant determinants.

TREATMENT. Treatment of enteric *E. coli* infection should be aimed at removing the pathogenic *E. coli*, correcting their harmful effects, and providing optimal environmental conditions. Therapy should be rapidly instituted to be as effective as possible. It is important to confirm the diagnosis of *E. coli* infection by culture and to perform antibiotic sensitivity tests, since antibiotic sensitivity varies greatly between *E. coli* isolates. A broad-spectrum antibiotic treatment could be used initially until the results of antibiotic sensitivity are known. In vitro sensitivity of *E. coli* isolates to a wide range of antimicrobial agents has greatly increased over the last several years (Table 39.2). Whereas over a decade ago most *E.*

Table 39.2. Antibiotic sensitivity patterns of *E. coli* isolates from swine with diarrhea in Quebec, 1987–90

Year	Ampicillin	Cephalothin	Gentamicin	Neomycin	Spectinomycin	Tetracycline	Sulfisoxazole	Trimethoprim/Sulfamethoxazole	Kanamycin	Amikacin	Apromycin
						(%)					
1987											
R	47	4	4	36	68	86	85	16	39		
S	52	80	92	61	32	12	15	84	59		
I	1	16	4	3	0	2	0	0	2		
1988											
R	50	15	7	24	59	86	79	22	34		
S	47	60	89	67	38	12	20	78	65		
I	3	25	4	9	3	2	1	0	1		
1989											
R	45	15	7	27	65	88	84	8	38	1	2
S	54	61	89	59	32	11	15	81	59	97	96
I	1	24	4	14	3	1	1	1	3	2	2
1990											
R	49	19	10	31	72	93	89	22	37	0	3
S	49	57	88	64	24	6	11	75	62	99	93
I	2	24	2	5	4	1	0	3	1	1	4

Note: R = resistant; S = sensitive; I = intermediate.

coli isolates were sensitive to gentamycin and the trimethoprim/sulfamethoxazole combination, a recent study of isolates from diarrheic piglets in Quebec showed a substantial level of resistance. Resistance to cephalothin and gentamycin has steadily increased over the last 4 years. Most isolates are sensitive to two newer antibiotics, amikacin and apramycin. An alternative approach to the treatment of enteric *E. coli* infection is the use of bacteriophages, an approach that has been successful experimentally but has not been extensively applied in the field.

Fluid therapy, consisting of electrolyte-replacement solutions containing glucose given orally, is useful for the treatment of dehydration and acidosis. Drugs that inhibit the secretory effects of enterotoxin, such as chlorpromazine and berberine sulfate, may be useful for the treatment of diarrhea, although many of these drugs have undesirable side effects. It is important to ensure that younger piglets are maintained at a constant temperature of 30–34°C and that recently weaned pigs are held in a draft-free environment at a constant temperature of about 29.5°C.

PREVENTION. A program for prevention of enteric *E. coli* infection should be aimed at reducing the numbers of pathogenic *E. coli* in the environment by good hygiene, maintaining suitable environmental conditions, and providing a high level of immunity. Because most pathogenic *E. coli* belong to a limited number of serogroups, enteric *E. coli* infection could be eliminated from some herds.

HUSBANDRY. One of the most important factors in preventing enteric *E. coli* infection is maintaining the piglets at an adequate environmental temperature (32–34°C for unweaned and 28–30°C for newly weaned pigs), free of draughts and on a low-heat-conducting floor. This is particularly true for piglets of below average weight that lose heat more rapidly because they have a greater skin surface area per unit body weight.

Good hygiene in the farrowing area leads to a reduction in the numbers of *E. coli* being presented to the piglet to a level that the piglet is able to control through its own defense mechanisms.

Farrowing-crate design is important because it affects the position at which feces are deposited by the sow. In crates that are too long, the feces are deposited over a large area of the available floor space, thereby increasing the heavily contaminated area. Ideally, the crate should be adjustible, allowing for a shorter crate for gilts than for sows. Crates on raised, perforated floors allow fecal material to drop through and away from the piglets, and litters farrowed onto such floors have a noticeably lower incidence of diarrhea than those on solid concrete floors.

A dry, warm environment reduces the moisture

available to enhance the survival of *E. coli*. This is largely affected by ventilation rates, although if room temperature is too high, sows tend to spread water over their lying area to cool themselves, thereby defeating other hygienic procedures. The sow should be at a temperature of approximately 22°C, necessitating a warmer creep area for the piglets.

Quarantine should be used to control the introduction of different *E. coli* pathotypes or other infectious agents into the herd. Animals in the herd will have little immunity to *E. coli* fimbrial antigens with which they have not had contact. Farrowing crates should be thoroughly cleaned and disinfected between litters. An all-in/all-out farrowing system with thorough disinfection of the farrowing room between batches would reduce the *E. coli* population in the environment.

Diet may be modified in order to reduce colonization of the intestine by *E. coli*. Addition of lactic acid to the drinking water may decrease gastric pH and inhibit the multiplication of *E. coli* (Thomlinson and Lawrence 1981). Feeding cultures of *Streptococcus faecium* to young pigs may reduce the incidence of diarrhea (Morkoc et al. 1984).

Careful attention to diet after weaning can reduce the incidence of postweaning diarrhea (Hampson 1987). If the diet is of low digestibility, restricting access is the most effective way to control postweaning diarrhea. A highly digestible, milk-based diet, fed in liquid form at regular intervals, reduces proliferation and adherence of ETEC in the small intestine and results in improved growth rates. High levels of nonmilk sugars and low-quality protein should be avoided. Highly antigenic dietary material should be avoided immediately after weaning if hypersensitivity to diet, manifested as increased crypt cell production rates, occurs.

IMMUNITY. Immunity to enteric *E. coli* infections is humoral and is provided initially through the maternal colostrum and subsequently by a local intestinal immune response. Specific antibodies inhibit bacterial adherence to receptors on the intestinal epithelial cells and neutralize the activity of the enterotoxins or cytotoxins produced by *E. coli*.

Colostrum from the sow contains high levels of immunoglobulin (Ig) G, which rapidly decrease during lactation and IgA becomes the main Ig class (Bourne 1976). The latter protects the gut against *E. coli* infection. It appears that most IgA, IgM, and IgG in the milk of the sow is produced within the mammary gland. During pregnancy, a proportion of the lymphocytes stimulated by antigens in the intestine migrate to the mammary gland and produce specific antibody against enteric pathogens. These antibodies are actively transported to the colostrum and then to the milk during lactation.

The newborn piglet begins to synthesize specific Ig and develop intestinal immunity during the first week of life (Butler 1973). At first IgM predominates but after 2–3 weeks is replaced by IgA as the most important Ig class in the intestine. Thus, during the first weeks of life, colostrum is the main source of immunologic protection for the piglet.

Breakdown in the protection provided by colostrum may occur for several reasons. If the dam has not been exposed to ETEC present in the environment of the piglets, her colostrum will not contain the specific antibodies necessary for protection against adherence and proliferation of ETEC. Any disease process causing agalactia in the sow will diminish transfer of colostrum. Generalized systemic infection may cause a total reduction in colostrum production, whereas mastitis or injured teats may affect production in one or several glands. Piglets failing to receive colostrum due to deformities, infection, small size, or damage at birth will also be more susceptible to ETEC infection.

Maternal vaccination has been one of the most effective ways of controlling neonatal ETEC diarrhea in piglets. Identification of virulence factors important in the pathogenesis of ETEC diarrhea and application of recombinant DNA technology has resulted in the production of more efficient vaccines over the last several years. One of the earliest vaccination techniques consisted of culturing in milk the small intestinal contents from a piglet with diarrhea and feeding the culture to pregnant sows, usually about a month before parturition (Kohler 1974). This technique is effective and is still used, particularly in the United States. Commonly used commercially available vaccines are given parenterally and may consist of killed whole cell bacterins or purified fimbrial vaccines. Both types of vaccines appear to work equally well (Fahy 1987). Bacterins usually contain strains representing the most important serogroups and producing the fimbrial antigens F4, F5, F6, and F41 (Nagy 1986). They are usually given parenterally at about 6 weeks and 2 weeks prior to parturition. Addition of the common fimbrial antigen F1 to a fimbrial bacterin appears to be protective in one study (Jayappa et al. 1985) but not protective in another study (To et al. 1984). Recombinant DNA technology has enabled the production of large quantities of purified fimbrial antigens for use in parenteral vaccines for immunization of the dam (Clarke et al. 1985). However, more widespread vaccination has lead to a change in the bacterial population. Fewer F4-positive ETEC are being isolated from neonatal piglets (Soderlind et al. 1988), and F4-negative isolates from classical F4-positive serogroups are emerging (Harel et al. 1990). In cases where vaccination is ineffective, it is important to identify the serotypes involved for possible inclusion into an autogenous bacterin. Further characterization

of these isolates may identify new or variant fimbrial adhesins important in the pathogenesis of ETEC diarrhea. An alternative approach to the problem of emerging ETEC negative for the known fimbriae has been the use of vaccines containing the nontoxic form of the enterotoxin LT-B conjugated to the nonimmunogenic STa (Klipstein 1986). Following conjugation, STa becomes immunogenic, and this vaccine has given protection in experimental animals. Addition of these components to fimbrial vaccines will provide protection in neonates against emerging ETEC with new fimbrial antigens and against ETEC negative for the known fimbrial antigens commonly found in older pigs. Oral or parenteral immunization of young piglets with live or killed ETEC vaccines may reduce the incidence of postweaning diarrhea and improve the growth rate of early weaned pigs (Fahy et al. 1987).

REFERENCES

BIEHL, L. G., AND HOEFLING, D. C. 1986. Diagnosis and treatment of diarrhea in 7- to 14-day-old pigs. J Am Vet Assoc 188:1144–1146.

BIJLSMA, I. G. W.; DE NIJS, A.; VAN DER MEER, C.; AND FRIK, J. F. 1982. Different pig phenotypes affect adherence of *Escherichia coli* to jejunal brush borders by K88ab, K88ac, or K88ad antigen. Infect Immun 37:891–894.

BOURNE, F. J. 1976. Humoral immunity in the pig. Vet Rec 98:499–501.

BROES, A.; FAIRBROTHER, J. M.; LARIVIÈRE, S.; JACQUES, M.; AND JOHNSON, W. M. 1988. Virulence properties of enterotoxigenic *Escherichia coli* O8:KX105 strains isolated from diarrheic piglets. Infect Immun 56:241–246.

BUTLER, J. E. 1973. Synthesis and distribution of immunoglobulins. J Am Vet Med Assoc 163:795–800.

CLARKE, S.; CAHILL, A.; STIRZAKER, C.; GREENWOOD, P.; AND GREGSON, R. 1985. Prevention by vaccination-animal bacteria. In Infectious Diarrhea in the Young. Amsterdam: Elsevier Science Publishers B. V., p. 481.

DREYFUS, L. A.; JASO-FRIEDMANN, L.; AND ROBERTSON, D. C. 1984. Characterization of the mechanism of action of *Escherichia coli* heat stable enterotoxin. Infect Immun 44:493–501.

DUBREUIL, J. D.; FAIRBROTHER, J. M.; LALLIER, R.; AND LARIVIÈRE, S. 1991. Production and purification of heat-stable enterotoxin b from a porcine *Escherichia coli* strain. Infect Immun. 59:198–203.

FAIRBROTHER, J. M.; LARIVIÈRE, S.; AND JOHNSON, W. M. 1988. Prevalence of fimbrial antigens and enterotoxins in nonclassical serogroups of *Escherichia coli* isolated from newborn piglets with diarrhea. Am J Vet Res 44:1325–1328.

FAIRBROTHER, J. M.; BROES, A.; JACQUES, M.; AND LARIVIÈRE, S. 1989. Pathogenicity of *Escherichia coli* O115:K"V165" strains isolated from pigs with diarrhea. Am J Vet Res 50:1029–1036.

FAHY, V. A. 1987. Preweaning colibacillosis. Proc Conf Australasian Pig Sci Assoc, Albury, p. 177.

FAHY, V. A.; CONNAUGHTON, I. D.; DRYDEN, S. J.; AND SPICER, E. M. 1987. Postweaning colibacillosis. Proc Conf Australasian Pig Sci Assoc, Albury, p. 189.

FAUBERT, C., AND DROLET, R. 1991. *Escherichia coli* hemorrhagic gastroenteritis in the piglet: Clinical, pathological, and microbiological findings. Can Vet J. Submitted.

GANNON, P. J.; GYLES, C. L.; AND FRIENDSHIP, R. W. 1988. Characteristics of verotoxigenic *Escherichia coli* from pigs. Can J Vet Res 52:331–337.

GILL, D. M.; CLEMENTS, J. D.; ROBERTSON, D. C.; AND FINKLESTEIN, R. A. 1981. Subunit number and arrangement in *Escherichia coli* heat-labile enterotoxin. Infect Immun 33:677–682.

GUERRANT, R. L.; HOLMES, R. K.; ROBERTSON, C. C.; AND GREENBERG, R. N. 1985. Roles of enterotoxins in the pathogenesis of *Escherichia coli* diarrhea. In Microbiology–1985. Ed. L. Leive, P. F. Bonventre, J. A. Morello, S. Schlesinger, S. D. Silver, and H. C. Wu. Washington, D.C.: Am Soc Microbiol, pp. 68–73.

GUINEE, P. A. M., AND JANSEN, W. H. 1979. Behavior of *Escherichia coli* K antigens K88ab, K88ac, and K88ad in immuno-electrophoresis, double diffusion, and hemagglutination. Infect Immun 23:700–705.

GUINEE, P. A. M.; VELDKAMP, J.; AND JANSEN, J. 1977. Improved Minca medium for the detection of K99 antigen in calf enterotoxigenic strains of *Escherichia coli*. Infect Immun 15:676–678.

HAMPSON, D. J. 1987. Dietary influences on porcine post-weaning diarrhea. Proc Conf Australasian Pig Sci Assoc, Albury, p. 222.

HAREL, J.; LAPOINTE, H.; FALLARA, A.; LORTIE, L. A.; BIGRAS-POULIN, M.; LARIVIÈRE, S.; AND FAIRBROTHER, J. M. 1990. Detection of genes for fimbrial antigens and enterotoxins associated with *Escherichia coli* serogroups isolated from pigs with diarrhea. J Clin Microbiol. 29:745–752.

HÉLIE, P.; MORIN, M.; JACQUES, M.; AND FAIRBROTHER, J. M. 1990. Experimental infection of newborn pigs with an attaching and effacing *Escherichia coli* O45:K"E65" strain. Proc Int Congr Pig Vet Soc, Lausanne.

HOLMES, R. K.; TWIDDY, E. M.; AND PICKETT, C. L. 1986. Purification and characterization of type II heat-labile enterotoxin of *Escherichia coli*. Infect Immun 53:464–473.

JAYAPPA, H. G; GOODNOW, R. A.; AND GEARY, S. J. 1985. Role of *Escherichia coli* Type 1 pilus in colonization of porcine ileum and its protective nature as a vaccine antigen in controlling colibacillosis. Infect Immun 48:350–354.

KENNEDY, D. J.; GREENBERG, R. N.; DUNN, J. A.; ABERNATHY, R.; RYERSE, J. S.; AND GUERRANT, R. L. 1984. Effects of *Escherichia coli* heat-stable enterotoxin STb on intestines of mice, rats, rabbits, and piglets. Infect Immun 46:639–643.

KLIPSTEIN, F. A. 1986. Development of *Escherichia coli* vaccines against diarrheal disease in humans. Development of Drugs and Vaccines against Diarrhea. 11th Nobel Conf Stockholm 1985. Stdentlitteratur, Lund, p. 53.

KOHLER, E. M. 1974. Protection of pigs against neonatal enteric colibacillosis with colostrum and milk from orally infected sows. Am Vet J 35:331–338.

LALLIER, R.; BERNARD, F.; GENDREAU, M.; LAZURE, C.; SEIDAH, N. G.; CHRETIEN, M.; AND ST-PIERRE, S. 1982. Isolation, purification, and structure of *Escherichia coli* heat-stable enterotoxin of porcine origin. Anal Biochem 127:267–275.

MONCKTON, R. P., AND HASSE, D. 1988. Detection of enterotoxigenic *Escherichia coli* in piggeries in Victoria by DNA hybridization using K88, K99, ST1, and ST2 probes. Vet Microbiol 16:273–281.

MOON, H. W; SCHNEIDER, R. A.; AND MOSELY, S. L.

1986. Comparative prevalence of four enterotoxin genes among *Escherichia coli* isolated from swine. Am J Vet Res 47:210–212.

MORKOC, A.; BACKSTROM, L.; AND SAVAGE, D. 1984. *Streptococcus faecium* in prevention of neonatal colibacillosis in piglets. Proc 8th Int Congr Pig Vet Soc, Ghent, p. 76.

NAGY, B. 1986. Vaccines against toxigenic *Escherichia coli* disease in animals. Development of Drugs and Vaccines against Diarrhea. 11th Nobel Conf Stockholm 1985. Stdentlitteratur, Lund, p. 53.

NAGY, B.; CASEY, T. A.; AND MOON, H. W. 1990. Phenotype and genotype of *Escherichia coli* isolated from pigs with post-weaning diarrhea in Hungary. J Clin Microbiol 28:651–653.

ORSKOV, I., AND ORSKOV, F. 1983. Serology of *Escherichia coli* fimbriae. Prog Allergy 33:80–105.

ROBICHAUD, N.; LALLIER, R.; AND LARIVIÈRE, S. 1978. Comparison of the various test systems for the detection of *Escherichia coli* enterotoxin. In Proceedings of the 2nd International Symposium on Neonatal Diarrhea. Ed. S. D. Acres. Saskatoon, Canada, pp. 149–150.

ROSE, R.; WHIPP, S. C.; AND MOON, H. W. 1987. Effects of *Escherichia coli* heat-stable enterotoxin b on small intestinal villi in pigs, rabbits, and lambs. Vet Pathol 24:71–79.

RUNNELS, P. L.; MOON, H. W.; AND SCHNEIDER, R. A. 1980. Development of resistance with host age to adhesion of K99+ *Escherichia coli* to isolated intestinal epithelial cells. Infect Immun 28:298–300.

SARMIENTO, J. I. 1983. Environmental temperature: A predisposing factor in the enterotoxigenic *Escherichia coli*-induced diarrhea of the newborn pig. M.S. thesis, Univ of Guelph, Ontario.

SELLWOOD, R.; GIBBONS, R. A.; JONE, G. W.; AND RUTTER, J. M. 1975. Adhesion of enteropathogenic *Escherichia coli* to pig intestinal brush borders: The existence of two pig phenotypes. J Med Microbiol 8:405–411.

SODERLIND, O.; THAFVELIN, B.; AND MOLLBY, R. 1988. Virulence factors in *Escherichia coli* strains isolated from Swedish pigs with diarrhea. J Clin Microbiol 26:879–884.

THOMLINSON, J. R., AND LAWRENCE, T. J. L. 1981. Dietary manipulation of gastric pH in the prophylaxis of enteric disease in weaned pigs: Some field observations. Vet Rec 109:120–122.

TO, S. C. M.; MOON, H. W.; AND RUNNELS, P. L. 1984. Type 1 pili (F1) of porcine enterotoxigenic *Escherichia coli*: Vaccine trial and tests for production in the small intestine during disease. Infect Immun 43:1–5.

WHIPP, S. C. 1990. Assay of enterotoxigenic *Escherichia coli* heat-stable toxin b in rats and mice. Infect Immun 58:930–934.

WILSON, R. A., AND FRANCIS, D. H. 1986. Fimbriae and enterotoxins associated with *Escherichia coli* serogroups isolated from pigs with colibacillosis. Am J Vet Res 47:213–217.

WOODWARD, M. J.; KEARSLEY, R.; WRAY, C.; AND ROEDER, P. L. 1990. DNA probes for detection of toxin genes in *Escherichia coli* isolated from diarrhoeal disease in cattle and pigs. Vet Microbiol 22:277–290.

YANO, T.; LEITE, D. S.; DE CARMARGO, I. J. B.; AND DE CASTRO, A. F. P. 1986. A probable new adhesive factor (F42) produced by enterotoxigenic *Escherichia coli* isolated from pigs. Microbiol Immunol 30:495–508.

Edema Disease

H. U. Bertschinger
N. O. Nielsen

EDEMA DISEASE (ED) is a communicable tox-emia caused by absorption from the intestine of a toxin that is produced by a few serotypes of *E coli.* The names "edema disease," "bowel edema," or "gut edema" were coined because edema of the submucosa of the stomach and the mesocolon is often a prominent feature of the disease. The syndrome was first reproduced by inoculation of pigs with fluid from the intestinal contents of pigs that had died from the disease (Timoney 1949). Therefore, the name "enterotoxemia" was suggested as being more appropriate (Schofield 1953). This term has found some currency in literature, and it is consistent with present views about the pathogenesis of ED. ED and *E. coli* enterotoxemia will be handled as synonyms in this chapter.

ED was first described in the scientific literature in 1938 by Shanks, based on observations of the disease over several years in Ireland. Subsequently, edema disease was identified in many countries where such a syndrome had also been observed sporadically for some time. ED became particularly prevalent in the years just after World War II, when the pig industry was not restrained by shortage of feedstuffs (Timoney 1950). Schofield and Schroder (1954) speculated that ED had been recognized in earlier times as the disease "pig staggers" or "stomach staggers," and they considered that the introduction of more complete rations had roughly paralleled the increased incidence of ED.

Schofield and Davis (1955) and Gregory (1955) first reported the occurrence of large numbers of hemolytic *E. coli* in the intestine of pigs dying with ED. Relatively few specific serotypes were involved. More direct evidence for the etiologic role of these *E. coli* strains was provided when cell-free extracts from cultures of these organisms were found to reproduce the disease following intravascular inoculation (Erskine et al. 1957; Timoney 1957). The early research on ED has been reviewed in detail by Sojka (1965).

ED continues to occur widely throughout the world where more modern pig husbandry is practiced, although incidence changes with time and geographic location. Since ED is caused by strains of *E. coli* that are endemic in most pig herds, it is reasonable to assume that its occurrence will continue to be widespread and that eradication is impractical.

It would appear that there has been a remarkable drop in the incidence of ED in North America. On the other hand, in the United Kingdom and some parts of continental Europe, the disease remains an important cause of death in weaned pigs. In Switzerland, ED was diagnosed in 7.3% of a total of 6628 pigs examined postmortem. In the age group between 4 and 12 weeks, the prevalence amounted to about 22% (Häni et al. 1976). In what was then East Germany, with 750,000 productive sows, Jahn and Uecker (1987) reported a mortality rate in weaned pigs of 1.8%; postweaning *E. coli* diarrhea may be included in this figure. Direct and indirect annual losses were estimated at about 50 million East German marks. The explanation for the variation in incidence is not readily apparent.

ED bears substantial similarities to the human diseases caused by enterohemorrhagic strains of *E. coli* (EHEC), which produce closely related, but not identical, shiga-like toxins. However, the human EHEC strains colonize the porcine digestive tract by a mechanism distinct from enterotoxemic *E. coli* (ETEEC) (Tzipori et al. 1986). Gnotobiotic piglets experimentally infected with EHEC strains develop lesions distinct from those in humans (Francis et al. 1989).

ETIOLOGY. ED is caused by infection of the small intestine with certain pathogenic strains of *E. coli.* It was recognized early that the majority of cases of ED are caused by not more than four serotypes reported from all over the world (Sojka 1965). The official serotype designations are O138:K81:NM, O139:K12 (formerly K82):H1, O141:K85a,b:H4, and O141:K85a,c:H4 (Ørskov and Ørskov 1984). Other serotypes were sporadically associated with the disease. However, their etiologic role is not beyond doubt.

Only a bacterium furnished with a set of virulence factors is able to cause edema disease. First of all, colonization of the small intestine is essential and requires some mechanism to resist the flushing action of peristalsis. Early attempts to demonstrate adhesive structures on *E. coli* causing ED were unsuccessful (Bertschinger and Pohlenz 1983). Adhesive fimbriae were recently detected on bacteria colonizing the small intestine of pigs inoculated with an ETEEC strain serogroup O139:K12. The fimbriae are not found in cultures of these bacteria. However, a mutant (strain 107) expresses antigenically related fimbriae in vitro. The fimbriae were designated 107. They are antigenically distinct from other fimbriae of porcine *E. coli,* have no hemagglutinating activity, and adhere to intestinal brush borders in vitro (Bertschinger et al. 1990). A study of field cases of ED and postweaning diarrhea revealed a high prevalence of fluorescing bacteria in mucosal smears stained with antiserum against fimbriae 107 in an indirect immunofluorescence test. High numbers of *E. coli* of serogroups O139:K12 or O141:K85a,b, which were not agglutinated by antifimbrial antiserum when grown on usual media (Stamm et al. 1990), were isolated from these pigs. The existence of additional adhesins cannot be excluded at this time.

The term "edema disease principle" (EDP) was coined to describe the substance responsible for causing ED before it became clear that this substance was in fact a true toxin (Nielsen and Clugston 1971). Its presence has been demonstrated in intestinal contents and some bacterial extracts (Erskine et al. 1957; Timoney 1957). Experimentation with EDP was hampered by contamination of EDP with endotoxin (Schimmelpfennig 1970; Nielsen and Clugston 1971). The terms neurotoxin (Schimmelpfennig 1970) and vasotoxin (Clugston and Nielsen 1974) were proposed in view of the functional and morphologic effects of EDP. A useful toxin assay became available when Konowalchuk et al. (1977) described toxic effects of culture filtrates prepared from certain strains of *E. coli*, including a strain from ED on cultured Vero cells. The toxic principle was called verotoxin (VT) and was detected in a high proportion of isolates of the serotypes mentioned above as well as in some other types from diarrheic pigs (Dobrescu 1983; Smith et al. 1983; Gonzales and Blanco 1985; Baloda et al. 1987; Linggood and Thompson 1987; Gannon et al. 1988). Further study of the VTs produced by a variety of *E. coli* strains revealed the existence of a family of toxins differing slightly in antigenicity, heat resistance, and biologic activities. Due to the close similarity to the toxin produced by *Shigella dysenteriae*, the VTs of *E. coli* were renamed shiga-like toxins (SLT). The toxin of the ED strains is neutralized by antiserum to SLT type II but has different activity on certain cell lines and experimental animals. Therefore, Marques et al. (1987) proposed the designation shiga-like toxin type-II variant (SLT-IIv). Differences in cytotoxicity of SLT-II and SLT-IIv are due to differences in the glycolipid structures to which the B subunits bind (Weinstein et al. 1988; Samuel et al. 1990). Assay of the toxin may be performed by animal inoculation, tests in tissue cultures, immunologic tests (Schimmelpfennig 1970; Timoney 1986), or DNA hybridization (Pohl et al. 1989).

A single SLT-IIv is produced by the above mentioned serotypes of *E. coli* isolated from ED and postweaning diarrhea (PWD) in many countries, but not by *E. coli* from other sources. The toxin is a protein with a molecular weight of about 70,000 (Clugston and Nielsen 1974; Timoney 1986; MacLeod and Gyles 1990). Analysis of the nucleotide sequence of the genes encoding SLT-IIv revealed very close relationship with SLT-II and a structure similar to other exotoxins comprising one subunit A and five smaller B subunits (Gyles et al. 1988). SLT-IIv inhibits protein synthesis by enzymatic cleavage of a single base from ribosomal RNA (Saxena et al. 1989). MacLeod and Gyles (1990) developed a purification scheme resulting in a homogeneous preparation of SLT-IIv free of endotoxin. As little as 3 ng of pure SLT-IIv per kg of body weight administered intravenously to young pigs induces disease. Clinical signs, gross and microscopic lesions, are characteristic of ED thus confirming that SLT-IIv and EDP are identical. SLT-IIv has less enterotoxic activity than SLT-I in the ligated intestinal loop of rabbits and no such activity in the pig (Gannon and Gyles 1990). Incubation time and severity of disease are directly related to the toxin dose.

Location of the genes encoding SLT-IIv seems to vary in different bacterial strains. Smith et al. (1983) and Timoney (1986) concluded from transfer experiments that SLT-IIv was plasmid rather than phage mediated, whereas others have evidence for their chromosomal location (Weinstein et al. 1988).

ED and *E. coli* PWD have a different pathogenesis but may be caused by the same bacterial strain. Canadian VT-positive isolates were examined by Gannon et al. (1988) for enterotoxin production. Heat-stable enterotoxins STa and/or STb were detected in a high proportion of strains from serogroups O138:K81, O141:K85, and more rarely O139:K82, and heat-labile enterotoxin was determined in about half of the isolates O141:K85. Prevalence of these toxins varies in different regions.

It was observed very early that *E. coli* associated with ED have alpha-hemolytic activity (Smith 1963). At least in the ETEC strain examined by Smith and Linggood (1971a), this attribute is not related to virulence.

EPIDEMIOLOGY. The epidemiology of ED has many features in common with PWD. Factors that allow infection and colonization of the intestine by pathogenic *E. coli* appear similar in these diseases.

ED usually occurs 1–2 weeks after weaning; therefore, the usual age of affected animals ranges from 4 to 12 weeks, but there may be exceptions. ED has been diagnosed in 4-day-old nursing piglets and in sows (Shanks 1938; Austvoll 1957). Typically, ED is seen in rapidly growing, apparently healthy animals, and often the best animals in the litter are affected (Shanks 1938; Timoney 1950; Schofield and Schroder 1954). The morbidity in an affected herd is extremely variable. The morbidity within a particular litter may be up to 80% or more, but the average is 30–40% (Timoney 1950; Kernkamp et al. 1965; Sweeney 1976). The case fatality rate ranges from 50% to over 90%, most cases tending toward the higher value. The course of the disease in the herd varies from 4 to 14 days, the average being slightly under a week. The disease disappears as abruptly as it appears. Recurrence on premises is common (Timoney 1950; Schofield and Davis 1955; Kurtz et al. 1969).

The environment of the weaner unit appears to be the most likely source of pathogenic *E. coli* strains. Unweaned pigs may acquire infection in the farrowing house, presumably from the same source, and carry it into the weaning unit. Routine cleaning and disinfection are usually insufficient to break the cycle of infection (Hampson et al. 1987). Under experimental conditions, however, transmission can be prevented by rigid hygienic measures (Smith and Halls 1968; Kausche 1989); the minimal infectious dose is not known. In transmission experiments with a K88-positive ETEC strain, airborne transmission between pigs in wire cages 1.5 m apart was repeatedly observed (Wathes et al. 1989).

Outbreaks of ED tend to involve only one strain of *E. coli* at any one time. Occasionally, two potential pathogens are isolated, but one usually predominates (Sweeney 1972). Multiple infections of herds involving more than one serogroup were detected in 47% out of 84 herds (Awad-Masalmeh et al. 1988).

The spread of pathogenic *E. coli* is presumed to occur via aerosols; feed; and other vehicles, pigs, and possibly other animals. Introduction of new pathogenic strains of *E. coli* into closed primary SPF herds with a high isolation standard was observed at intervals of 1–2 years. Once a site is contaminated with a particular strain, it can remain so for an extended period. The serotypes associated with ED tend to be similar in broad geographic areas (Sweeney 1976).

PATHOGENESIS. For the sake of clarity, intestinal colonization and toxemia will be presented separately. However, there may be mutual interactions.

Colonization of the Small Intestine. An *E. coli* strain O group 141 causing PWD and ED (Smith and Halls 1968) as well as two strains of O group 139 devoid of enterotoxins (Bertschinger and Pohlenz 1983; Bertschinger et al. 1990) reach high population densities throughout the intestinal tract, including the upper small intestine. Such colonization requires both mucosal adhesion and proliferation. The degree of colonization determines whether or not disease will result from infection. Adhering microcolonies or layers of bacteria were observed on the small intestinal mucosae of pigs experimentally infected with two strains of O group 139 (Fig. 39.3) (Bertschinger and Pohlenz 1983; Methiyapun et al. 1984; Bertschinger et al. 1990). ETEEC adhere to the brush border in a similar manner as do ETEC, whereas other producers of SLTs show the "attaching and effacing" phenomenon. Since colonization depends on a multiplicity of factors, it is not reliably reproducible. Some of the known factors are discussed here.

A hereditary susceptibility to colonization was suggested by Smith and Halls (1968). In a series of trials involving standardized exposure of more than 5000 pigs in a closed herd, Bertschinger et al. (1986) observed a highly significant influence of the sire on the incidence of ED in his progeny. The colonization, i.e., the numbers of organisms shed with the feces, was correlated with mortality. The authors discussed a genetic mechanism comparable to that observed with F4 (K88) fimbriae.

The newly weaned pig is particularly susceptible to intestinal colonization with ETEEC and ETEC strains. Salajka et al. (1975) and Svendsen

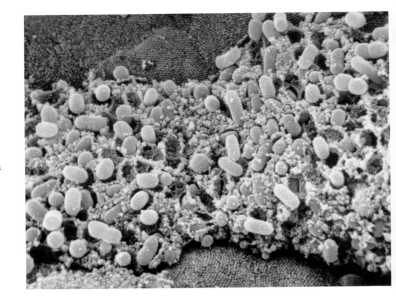

39.3. Bacteria adhering patchwise to microvilli of small intestinal epithelium of a weaner 6 days after oral inoculation with a culture of *E. coli* O139:K12:H1.

and Larsen (1977) detected specific antibodies in milk and suggested that milk antibody would protect the piglets as long as they were nursing. A daily dose of 525 ml, but not of 270 ml, milk obtained from sows in late lactation fed to weaned pigs completely inhibits colonization, whereas pigs fed 525 ml of cow's milk shed high numbers of the ETEEC bacteria (Deprez et al. 1986). Spray-dried blood plasma fed at a dose equivalent to 1 L of fresh plasma/pig/day has a similar inhibitory effect that lasts only as long as the plasma is fed (Deprez et al. 1990).

Actively acquired immunity against colonization has received little attention. In the experiments with oral inoculation of weaned pigs (Smith and Halls 1968), eight pigs that recovered from clinical disease resisted colonization by the same *E. coli* strain again given by mouth 15–18 days after initial inoculation. Bertschinger et al. (1984) reported an experiment in which weaned pigs were first inoculated with an ETEEC of serogroup 139 of low virulence and later challenged with a virulent strain of the same serogroup. Fewer pigs became colonized by the challenge strain as compared to litter mates without preinoculation. Protection was dose-dependent and considered to demonstrate active immunization. In another experiment the period needed for active immunization was assessed to be between 5 and 11 days (Bertschinger et al. 1981).

Some authors consider ED to be a consequence of a disequilibrium of the gastrointestinal flora. However, comparison of the main bacterial categories at different sites along the gastrointestinal tract of nursing pigs and weaned, affected pigs revealed no consistent differences except an enormous proliferation of ETEEC in the small intestine (Schulze 1977). Interference by specific species or types of bacteria may nevertheless be a factor. Nielsen et al. (1988) reported partial inhibition of intestinal colonization and disease by repeated administration of a mixture of five strains of lactobacilli. Reuterin, an inhibitory substance with a broad antimicrobial spectrum, is produced by *Lactobacillus reuteri,* a species occurring in the digestive organs of pigs (Axelsson et al. 1989).

A variety of viruses infect the porcine intestine and may thereby change the bacterial environment. In an experimental PWD model, an F4-positive ETEC strain colonizes weaned pigs in the absence of rotaviral infection (Sarmiento et al. 1988). Dual infection of pigs with rotavirus and with an ETEC strain without F4 results in a more severe diarrhea than inoculation with either agent alone (Lecce et al. 1982). The investigators concluded that viral damage of the epithelium favors colonization by *E. coli.* In a different experimental system, Cox et al. (1988) found an opposite effect of viral infection. Adhesion to intestinal villi of an ETEC strain with F4 adhesin was examined in vivo and in vitro. Pigs with and without an experimental transmissible gastroenteritis (TGE) infec-

tion were compared. Numbers of adherent bacteria on shortened villi of TGE-infected pigs were significantly lower when compared to villi of non-TGE-infected pigs.

An acid environment has an inhibitory effect on *E. coli.* In the gastrointestinal tract, an increase in the pH of the stomach contents of weaned in comparison to unweaned pigs was described by Bolduan et al. (1988), who assumed the high pH to be the essential factor allowing colonization of the small intestine by ETEEC. However, other investigators reported nearly identical pH values in the stomachs of weaned and unweaned pigs (Schulze 1977; Rohrmann and Uecker 1987). This inconsistency may be explained by divergent experimental protocols. Addition of 5% citric acid to two types of compounded rations lowers the feed pH from 5.9 to 4.1, but does not reduce numbers of fecal ETEEC or mortality due to ED in experimentally infected weaners (Bertschinger et al., unpublished observation).

Veterinary practitioners and farmers were convinced years ago that nutritious feed would play an important role. Thus ED was named "protein intoxication." Smith and Halls (1968) inoculated pigs on various feed regimens with an ETEEC strain serogroup O141:K85a,c. They found that severe feed restriction resulted in much lower fecal numbers of the bacteria and absence of disease. A similar effect was achieved by feeding pigs ad libitum a diet extremely rich in fiber and low in nutrients. The authors concluded that the physiologic state of the intestinal epithelium might influence bacterial adhesion. These experiments were extended by Bertschinger et al. (1978), using an ETEEC strain serogroup O139:K12 for inoculation. The findings of Smith and Halls (1968) were confirmed. However, the poor diets inhibited growth of the pigs. When these diets were replaced by a conventional type of feed, colonization and clinical disease developed. The inhibitory effect of the poor diet was abolished by supplementation with fish meal but not with starch or fat. The precise mechanism behind these phenomena remains to be elucidated. When protein-deficient diets are fed to growing rats, significant shortening of the intestinal villi is observed. The shortening is not due to a different turnover but to a reduced mitotic rate of small intestinal epithelial cells as compared to control rats (Syme and Smith 1982).

Other environmental factors potentially involved were studied with respect to PWD due to ETEC with F4 adhesin (Sarmiento et al. 1988; Wathes et al. 1989). No experimental data pertaining to ED are available.

Enterotoxemia. EDP (now called SLT-IIv) has been detected on numerous occasions in the small intestinal contents of pigs affected with ED (Sojka 1965). The highly purified toxin induces a disease indistinguishable from ED when administered intravenously (IV) to pigs (MacLeod and Gyles 1990). However, details such as amounts of toxin present in the gut, transport mechanisms into circulation, distribution, and target cells remain to be elucidated.

The most consistent injury detected in natural cases, after injection of partially purified toxin (Clugston et al. 1974b; Gannon et al. 1989), and in pigs inoculated orally with live cultures, is a degenerative angiopathy of small arteries and arterioles (Methiyapun et al. 1984; Kausche 1989). The edema fluid found in various tissues is low in protein and could be the result of a mild increase of vascular permeability. Information on pathophysiology of ED is scarce. Clugston et al. (1974a) observed an increase of blood pressure after IV administration of EDP. Hypertension developed later than clinical edema and was therefore thought to be the result of vascular injury rather than its cause. Hypertension might exacerbate the lesions in the already damaged vessels. The development of injuries in the nervous system may be due to hypoxia resulting from impaired blood flow (Clugston et al. 1974b).

A distinct type of ED is characterized by terminal bloody diarrhea and hemorrhagic lesions in the cardiac region of the stomach, the ileum, and the large intestine (Fig. 39.4) (Bertschinger and Pohlenz 1983). According to Gannon et al. (1989) and MacLeod and Gyles (1990), acute hemorrhagic gastroenteritis occurs in some of the pigs to which a high dose of SLT-IIv is administered. Epithelial necrosis secondary to necrosis of small ar-

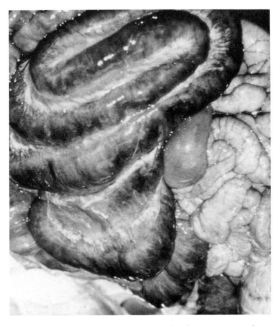

39.4. Extended hemorrhages and minor mesenteric edema in the colon of a pig developing bloody diarrhea 5 days after inoculation with a culture of *E. coli* O139:K12:H1.

teries and arterioles may be responsible for luminal hemorrhage.

Smith and Linggood (1971b) observed passive protection by parenteral administration of a large volume of antiserum against the live homologous bacteria of pigs orally inoculated with ETEEC serogroup O141:K85a,c. The authors suspected that protection was directed against the product of the bacteria causing ED. Active immunity against IV challenge with EDP was induced in young pigs by a toxoid vaccine prepared from EDP by treatment with glutaraldehyde (Dobrescu 1982). A similar toxoid was used for vaccination of pigs 1 week before weaning (Awad-Masalmeh et al. 1989). The vaccine conferred highly significant protection against ED after the pigs were orally challenged with ETEEC serogroup O139:K12. Vaccinated principals shed lower numbers of the inoculated bacteria and had better weight gains than placebo-vaccinated littermates. Sera from neonatal and from weaned pigs from herds with and without clinical ED do not contain neutralizing antibody against SLT-IIv (Gannon et al. 1988).

A variable proportion of ETEEC isolates produce one or more enterotoxins in addition to SLT-IIv (Smith and Halls 1968; Smith et al. 1983; Gannon et al. 1988; Nagy et al. 1990). Enterotoxic effects may change the course of ED. If they induce significant dehydration, edematous lesions may be minimal or absent. Clinicians as well as pathologists should be aware of this complication. The role of endotoxin in the pathogenesis of ED is not clear. Based on limited similarities between endotoxin shock and ED, it was speculated that endotoxin effects could be a significant component of some forms of ED and PWD (Schulz et al. 1961). The effective protection against ED conferred by a vaccine prepared from EDP seems to exclude at least a primary role of endotoxin. On the other hand, endotoxin administered at the appropriate time has been shown to enhance the toxic effects of SLT-II in rabbits and mice (Barrett et al. 1989).

CLINICAL SIGNS. Clinical signs characteristic of the late stages dominate descriptions of field cases (Sojka 1965). Often, pigs are found dead without preceding clinical illness. Others are ataxic or recumbent and show running or paddling movements. Affected pigs may display an altered, hoarse squeal, which is ascribed to laryngeal edema. Early signs and the course of the disease can be followed most easily when the disease is reproduced experimentally.

Reproduction of ED by the oral administration of *E. coli* was first reported by Smith and Halls (1968). The pigs were inoculated with 10^{10} colony-forming units (CFU) of a strain of serogroup O141:K85a,c, obviously a producer of SLT-IIv and of enterotoxin(s). The first sign was anorexia, which started at the onset of shedding bacterial numbers above 10^9 CFU/g of feces, 3 (2–5) days postinoculation (PI), and was observed in 20 out of 21 experimental pigs. Anorexia lasted for several days in the 2 pigs that recovered and until euthanasia in the 19 pigs killed when death was imminent. Diarrhea appeared on day 4 (1–8) PI. Usually it was severe, but of short duration. It was fatal in only 1 out of 17 diarrheic pigs. In most pigs diarrhea was no longer present, when signs of nervous involvement became apparent, i.e., on day 6 (5–13) PI. Swollen eyelids were seen at about the same time. Ataxia was accompanied with varying degrees of mental confusion and was usually progressive. Affected pigs soon became completely recumbent. Severe dyspnea was usually present at this final stage. Nine out of 13 pigs with ataxia had to be killed on the day the nervous signs appeared. Three others survived for 2–4 days. Pigs were moribund 7 (5–13) days PI. The rectal temperature always remained within the normal range.

A very similar disease was seen in pigs inoculated with a nonenterotoxigenic ED strain of serotype O139:K12:H1 (Bertschinger et al. 1978, 1986). Exceptions were that diarrhea was not regularly associated with colonization, and that more pronounced edema developed in some cases. In such cases ears, subcutaneous tissue over the frontal bones, nose, and lips were swollen (Fig. 39.5). In mild cases, subcutaneous edema was accompanied by pruritus, which disappeared after recovery. In some pigs with or without dyspnea, respiration was coupled with a snoring sound. Watery diarrhea with clots of fresh blood became apparent in a few pigs at the terminal stage (Bertschinger and Pohlenz 1983).

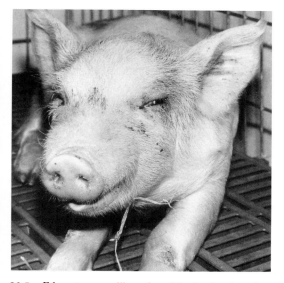

39.5. Edematous swelling of eyelids, forehead, and lips, breathing through open mouth, and inability to rise in a weaner 4 days after oral inoculation with a culture of *E. coli* O139:K12:H1.

Clinical signs may occur as early as 7 hours after intravenous injection of a high dose of purified SLT-IIv toxin (MacLeod and Gyles 1990). Early symptoms are edema of the eyelids and inappetence. Neurologic signs comprising incoordination, confusion, and ataxia develop with severe illness. Paralysis, tremors, paddling of the limbs, convulsions, dyspnea, altered squeal, and coma are observed in advanced stages. Hemorrhagic colitis develops in pigs to which high doses of toxin were administered. Gannon et al. (1989) described a similar hemorrhagic colitis in some pigs inoculated with a less-purified preparation. Pigs with colitis suffered from bloody diarrhea 18–24 hours PI.

Chronic ED develops in a variable, but mostly low, proportion of pigs recovering from acute attacks of ED or PWD (Bertschinger and Pohlenz 1974; Nakamura et al. 1982). The condition was called cerebrospinal angiopathy before its association with ED became apparent. At times varying from days to several weeks after intestinal infection, growth stops, and sick pigs often show unilateral nervous disturbances such as circling movements, twisting of the head, or atrophy of limb muscles with progressive weakness. Subcutaneous edema is rare. Affected pigs have to be destroyed.

LESIONS

Gross Lesions. The external appearance of a pig dead of ED is not especially remarkable. Irregular reddening of the skin in the ventral parts of the body trunk may be present.

ED is a disease of vasculature, and while edema at specific sites appears to be a manifestation of this lesion, its presence is variable and may be absent in some animals. Subcutaneous edema may be present as noted above. Edema in the submucosa of the stomach is characteristic when present and is located in the region of the glandular cardia (Fig. 39.6). It may vary from being barely detectable to 2 cm or more in thickness. This edema fluid is usually serogelatinous in nature and occasionally may be sanguine adjacent to the mucosa. If severe, the edema may extend into the fundic submucosa, but it would appear to originate from the cardiac region. Edema of the gastric submucosa can be evaluated best by incising the serosa and muscularis over the greater curvature beginning at the cardia. Palpation of the glandular cardia can also be helpful in locating edematous lesions. Inflammatory edema associated with acute ulceration of the esophageal cardia must not be confused with that of ED. Such acute ulcers occur at the margin of the esophageal cardia on either side of the cardial orifice, and the associated inflammatory edema is in the submucosa of the adjacent glandular cardia. Chronic ulceration of the esophageal cardia is not associated with edema.

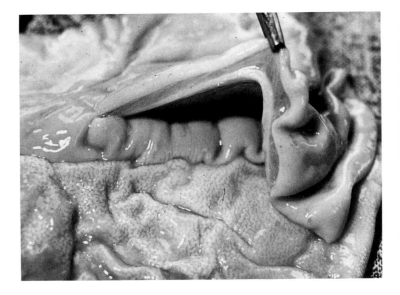

39.6. Edematous swelling of glandular mucosa of the cardiac region and gelatinous submucosal edema of the cut stomach wall with a field case from which *E. coli* O139:K12:H1 was isolated.

Edema of the gallbladder is sometimes seen. The mesocolon is a common site for edema. Occasionally, a segment of small intestine or rectum may display submucosal edema (Shanks 1938). In experimental cases the submucosa of the cecum is frequently involved (Nielsen and Clugston 1971). Careful inspection of the peritoneal cavity may reveal occasional fibrin strands and a slight increase in serous fluid. The mesenteric and colic nodes vary in appearance from normal to being swollen, edematous, and congested. A few *E. coli* may be isolated from this tissue. Typically, the stomach is full of dry, fresh-looking feed, and the small intestine is relatively empty. Colonic contents may be diminished in amount. It may be inferred that this is a manifestation of delayed gastric emptying, since some animals have a period of anorexia before death. Also, it has been shown experimentally that pigs with ED may eat very little for 48 hours before death and at necropsy have full stomachs (Smith and Halls 1968). The suggestion that some pigs with ED are affected by constipation is also in accord with these observations.

The pleural cavity may contain excess serous fluid, and the lungs may display varying degrees of edema (Timoney 1950). In some cases this has been the only observable lesion (Schofield and Schroder 1954). Cases with laryngeal edema have also been observed. The pericardial cavity may contain excess serous fluid in which fibrin may be present, and a few epicardial and endocardial petechiae may occur (Timoney 1950). This lesion must not be confused with mulberry heart disease.

If the offending strain of *E. coli* is also capable of producing enterotoxin, usually O138:K81 or O141:K85, lesions of PWD may be added, and edema may be mild or absent.

Microscopic Lesions. The microscopic appearance of edema lesions suggests that they are not associated with inflammation of the affected interstitial tissue, since leukocytes are not prominent. The most important microscopic lesions are those of a degenerative angiopathy affecting small arteries and arterioles (Kurtz et al. 1969; Clugston et al. 1974b). The lesions may occur in many organs and tissues. The dense arterial network in the mesocolon adjacent to the colic lymph nodes is frequently affected. The early acute lesion is one of necrosis of smooth muscle cells in the tunica media characterized by pyknosis and karyorrhexis of nuclei and hyaline change in cytoplasmic elements. In some affected vessels infiltration with fibrinoid material occurs (Fig. 39.7). Swelling of endothelial cells has also been observed. In older lesions there may be proliferation of adventitial and medial cells (Fig. 39.8). Vascular lesions may be difficult to detect in acute cases, but in surviving pigs or those affected subclinically, they are more readily apparent (Kausche 1989). Thrombosis is not usually a feature of uncomplicated naturally occurring ED. In pigs with experimental ED induced by feeding pathogenic *E. coli,* transmission electron microscopic studies of intestinal microcirculation have demonstrated endothelial swelling, vacuolation and proliferation, microthrombus formation, subendothelial fibrin, medial necrosis, and perivascular edema (Methiyapun et al. 1984).

In pigs that have recovered from natural outbreaks or survived for several days following acute signs, there are lesions of focal encephalomalacia in the brain stem together with lesions in the small arteries and arterioles (Fig. 39.9) (Kurtz et al. 1969). These are thought to be the result of vascular injury leading to edema and ischemia. In acute experimental cases, edema of the lepto-

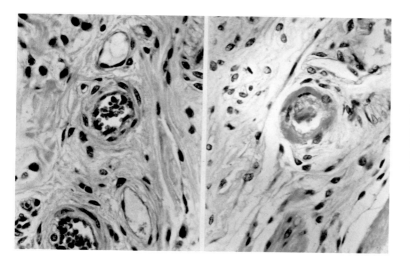

39.7. Arterioles in submucosa of the urinary bladder: (left) normal; (right) fibrinoid or hyaline change, acute experimental ED. (Clugston et al. 1974b.)

meninges and perivascular spaces has been demonstrated. A cerebrospinal angiopathy of pigs has been recognized as a clinicopathologic entity for some years (Harding 1966). Its microscopic features are those described above plus the occurrence of eosinophilic, periodic acid–Schiff (PAS)-positive droplets around affected vessels (Nakamura et al. 1982). This angiopathy is considered most likely to be a manifestation of edema disease (Bertschinger and Pohlenz 1974).

DIAGNOSIS. The diagnosis of acute ED is based on typical epidemiology—principally, sudden appearance and clinical signs of neurologic disease in thriving pigs 1–2 weeks after weaning. In the live pig the most important and constant diagnostic sign is partial ataxia or a staggering gait. Subcutaneous edema in the orbit and over the frontal bones is also a cardinal sign when present. At necropsy the characteristic lesions of edema, when present, are helpful in confirming

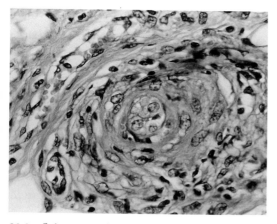

39.8. Submucosa of cardial gland region of the stomach 17 days after inoculation with EDP; arteriole with proliferative arteriopathy. (Clugston et al. 1974b.)

the diagnosis but may be absent in a significant number of cases.

Bacteriologic examination of the small intestine and colon should yield nearly pure cultures of hemolytic *E. coli*. However, bacterial numbers may already be dropping in more protracted cases (Bertschinger and Pohlenz 1983). After death the small numbers of organisms may be overgrown by other enterobacteriaceae. In contrast to ETEC infections, a negative bacteriologic result does not, therefore, exclude the diagnosis of ED. Serologic identification of the common types associated with ED is additional evidence. Serotyping is essential, because hemolytic *E. coli* not associated with ED are frequently encountered in the intestinal flora, and may be present in high numbers (Smith 1963).

Subacute or chronic ED is diagnosed by the demonstration of arteriopathy and eventually lesions of focal encephalomalacia. ED may be more difficult to diagnose if associated with severe forms of PWD.

In cases of sudden death, differential diagnosis will have to include microangiopathia dietetica and circulatory failure as seen after severe fighting. When pigs show nervous signs, viral encephalitis (enteroviral polioencephalomyelitis, pseudorabies) and bacterial meningoencephalitis (*Streptococcus suis*, *Haemophilus parasuis*) as well as water deprivation should be considered.

TREATMENT. While an understanding of the pathogenesis of ED is not yet complete, it does allow for some degree of rational therapy. A primary therapeutic objective is to reduce the number of pathogenic *E. coli* in the intestinal tract. For animals with clinical signs of the disease, this approach is probably too late. For those incubating disease and harboring pathogenic *E. coli*, it may be possible to reduce the intestinal *E. coli* populations with antimicrobials before lethal amounts of EDP have been produced and ab-

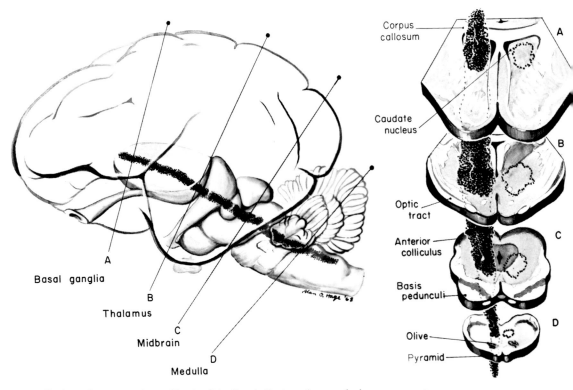

39.9. Brain and cross sections of brain. Stippling indicates where malacia occurs most commonly in pigs with ED. (Kurtz et al. 1969.)

sorbed from the intestine.

For animals showing ED, therapy should be directed at ameliorating the vascular lesions and their consequences, especially brain edema. If hypertension proves to be an important feature of the clinical disease, therapy directed at reducing blood pressure may offer some benefit. Whether this is so remains to be determined. Melperone at a dose of 4–6 mg/kg body weight has been advocated as a useful treatment if given early in the course of the disease (Olsson and Olsson 1982).

PREVENTION. In view of the unpredictable, erratic occurrence of ED in sequential batches of weaners and even in contemporaneously weaned litters, efficiency of prophylactic measures is hard to assess. Most prophylactic measures are intended to reduce intestinal colonization.

Once ED is diagnosed, management must be directed at deterring the development of clinically significant infections of the intestine with pathogenic strains of *E. coli* in the animals at risk. There may be a direct approach through use of antibacterial drugs in the feed and, ideally, the sensitivity of the organism should be known. Development of multiple antibiotic resistance is very common and may occur within days or weeks after introduction of a new drug into a herd. At present, colistin and the fluoroquinolones are the only known antimicrobial agents that in general do not induce multiple resistance. Chemoprophylaxis requires a therapeutic dose. Drug loss due to adsorption to or inactivation by the feed has to be taken into account with in-feed medication. Chemoprophylaxis may postpone outbreaks until medication is stopped 2–3 weeks after weaning (Böhringer 1986).

Management in the first instance should attempt to minimize the risk of introduction of pathogenic strains of *E. coli* into the herd. Where such strains are already present, weanling pigs should be managed to minimize the opportunity for pathogenic *E. coli* to establish a clinically significant level of infection in the intestine. Creep feeding should be initiated well before weaning to allow maximal opportunity for physiologic adaptation to solid feed.

Restriction of feed intake, high-fiber diets, or ad libitum feeding of fiber have been reported as effective deterrents to the development of ED and weanling diarrhea (Smith and Halls 1968; Bertschinger et al. 1978). Total feed intake may be restricted to 300 g/day at weaning and then gradually increased to normal levels over a 2- to 3-week period. Alternatively, the nutritive value of the feed may be reduced by increasing fiber content to 15–20% and reducing crude protein and digestible energy to one-half normal values (Bertschinger et al. 1978). The addition of fiber to normal diets may be beneficial. Dunne (1975) advocated feeding high-quality alfalfa coupled with restriction of daily feed intake to 450 g. To be effective, nutrient intake has to be low enough to maintain daily gain in the 2 weeks after weaning below 1% of body weight. Such diets prevent colonization and impair the development of immunity in the same way as antimicrobials. Later outbreaks are frequently seen. A lower mortality due to *E. coli* enterotoxemia and improved weight gains were reported by Bolduan et al. (1988) after introduction of compounded rations with a reduced acid-binding capacity. A similar effect is ascribed to organic acids, and a pH of the feed of about 5.0 is recommended. Crude fiber contents of about 5% reduce transit times of ingesta. Results obtained with lactic acid–producing bacteria are conflicting (Nielsen 1988; Deprez et al. 1989). They may depend on strains used.

Management of the weanling pig should minimize environmental and other forms of stress such as unnecessary mixing of litters, chilling, transportation, assignment to new pens, etc.

Resistance of the herd to ED may be increased through genetic selection, which involves culling breeding stock that has produced susceptible animals. Clinical reports have clearly established that certain breeding stock may produce successive affected litters and that some are markedly predisposed to this disease while others are resistant (Bertschinger et al. 1986).

Immunoprophylaxis of ED will have to be directed at either prevention of small intestinal colonization to clinically significant levels or at neutralizing the effects of EDP. Bertschinger et al. (1981) have had partial success in developing clinical immunity to edema disease by inoculating pigs orally with a live pathogenic strain of *E. coli* after weaning and during restricted feeding. More normal diets are introduced after 2–3 weeks. In herds where ED is a severe problem, it may occur following the period of feed restriction. The prevention of weanling diarrhea by oral immunization or parenteral inoculation with formalized autogenous vaccine has met with some success and may imply promise for a similar vaccine in ED (Husband and Seaman 1979; Svendsen 1979). Toxoid vaccines (Awad-Masalmeh et al. 1989) are not yet on the market. Passive protection by incorporation of dried blood plasma into the feed holds some promise (Deprez et al. 1990).

In summary, no universally effective prevention has been developed so far.

REFERENCES

Austvoll, J. 1957. Gut oedema in a litter of four day old pigs. Vet Rec 69:104.

Awad-Masalmeh, M.; Reitinger, H.; Quakyi, E.; Hinterdorfer, H.; Silber, R.; and Willinger, H. 1988. Observations on the isolation and characterization of *E. coli* derived from edema disease cases. Proc 10th Int Congr Pig Vet Soc, Rio de Janeiro, p. 114.

Awad-Masalmeh, M.; Schuh, M.; Köfer, J.; and Quakyi, E. 1989. Überprüfung der Schutzwirkung eines Toxoidimpfstoffes gegen die Ödemkrankheit des Absetzferkels im Infektionsmodell. Dtsch Tieraerztl Wochenschr 96:397–432.

Axelsson, L. T.; Chung, T. C.; Dobrogosz, W. J.; and Lindgren, S. E. 1989. Production of a broad-spectrum antimicrobial substance by *Lactobacillus reuteri*. Microbiol Ecol Health Dis 2:131–136.

Baloda, S. B.; Yuk, Y. R.; Krovacek, K.; Sethi, S. K.; and Wadström, T. 1987. Detection of *Shiga*-like (SL) toxins of enteropathogenic *Escherichia coli* (EPEC) of human, porcine, calf, and lamb origin on Vero and HeLa S3 cells: A comparative study. Zentralbl Bakt Hyg [A] 264:33–40.

Barrett, T. J.; Potter, M. E.; and Wachsmuth, I. K. 1989. Bacterial endotoxin both enhances and inhibits the toxicity of *Shiga*-like toxin II in rabbits and mice. Infect Immun 57:3434–3437.

Bertschinger, H. U., and Pohlenz, J. 1974. Cerebrospinale Angiopathie bei Ferkeln mit experimenteller Coli-Enterotoxämie. Schweiz Arch Tierheilk 116:543–554.

———. 1983. Bacterial colonization and morphology of the intestine in porcine *Escherichia coli* enterotoxemia (edema disease). Vet Pathol 20:99–110.

Bertschinger, H. U.; Eggenberger, U.; Jucker, H.; and Pfirter, H. P. 1978. Evaluation of low nutrient, high fibre diets for the prevention of porcine *Escherichia coli* enterotoxemia. Vet Microbiol 3:281–290.

Bertschinger, H. U.; Jucker, H.; Halter, H. M.; and Pfirter, H. P. 1981. Zur Prophylaxe der Colienterotoxämie des Schweines: Dauer der oralen Immunisierung mit virulenten Erregern unter dem Schutz eines Diätfutters. Schweiz Arch Tierheilk 123:61–68.

Bertschinger, H. U.; Jucker, H.; and Pfirter, H. P. 1984. Orale Vakzination von Ferkeln gegen Colienterotoxämie mit einer Streptomycin-Dependenz-Revertante von *Escherichia coli*. Schweiz Arch Tierheilk 126: 497–509.

Bertschinger, H. U.; Munz-Müller, M.; Pfirter, H. P.; and Schneider, A. 1986. Vererbte Resistenz gegen Colienterotoxämie beim Schwein. Zschr Tierzüchtung Züchtungsbiol 103:255–264.

Bertschinger, H. U.; Bachmann, M.; Mettler, C.; Pospischil, A.; Schraner, E. M.; Stamm, M.; Sydler, T.; and Wild, P. 1990. Adhesive fimbriae produced in vivo by *Escherichia coli* O139:K12(B):H1 associated with enterotoxaemia in pigs. Vet Microbiol 25:267–281.

Böhringer, U. 1986. Behandlung von experimentellen enteralen Coliin-fektionen bei Absetzferkeln mit dem Aminoglykosid-Antibiotikum BAY V1 4718. Thesis (printed), Zurich.

Bolduan, G.; Jung, H.; Schnabel, E.; and Schneider, R. 1988. Recent advances in the nutrition of weaner piglets. Pig News Inform 9:381–385.

Clugston, R. E., and Nielsen, N. O. 1974. Experimental edema disease of swine (*E. coli* enterotoxemia). I. Detection and preparation of an active principle. Can J Comp Med 38:22–28.

Clugston, R. E.; Nielsen, N. O.; and Roe, W. E. 1974a. Experimental edema disease of swine (*E. coli* enterotoxemia). II. The development of hypertension after the intravenous administration of edema disease principle. Can J Comp Med 38:29–33.

Clugston, R. E.; Nielsen, N. O.; and Smith, D. L. T. 1974b. Experimental edema disease of swine (*E. coli* enterotoxemia). III. Pathology and pathogenesis. Can J Comp Med 38:34–43.

Cox, E.; Cools, V.; Thoonen, H.; Hoorens, J.; and Houvenaghel, A. 1988. Effect of experimentally-induced villus atrophy on adhesion of K88ac-positive *Escherichia coli* in just-weaned piglets. Vet Microbiol 17:159–169.

DEPREZ, P.; VAN DEN HENDE, C.; MUYLLE, E.; AND OYAERT, W. 1986. The influence of the administration of sow's milk on the post-weaning excretion of hemolytic *E. coli* in the pig. Vet Res Commun 10:469–478.

DEPREZ, P.; VAN DEN BRANDEN, J.; DE GEEST, J.; DE-MEULENAERE, D.; AND MUYLLE, E. 1989. The influence of *Streptococcus faecium* feeding to weaned piglets on the excretion of *Escherichia coli* and the occurrence of edema disease. Vlaams Diergeneeskd Tijdschr 58:113–117.

DEPREZ, P.; DE CUPERE, F.; AND MUYLLE, E. 1990. The effect of feeding dried plasma on experimental *Escherichia coli* enterotoxemia in piglets. Proc 11th Int Congr Pig Vet Soc, Lausanne, p. 149.

DOBRESCU, L. 1982. Immunological studies in pigs using edema disease principle (*E. coli* neurotoxin). Proc 7th Int Congr Pig Vet Soc, Mexico City, p. 19.

———. 1983. New biological effect of edema disease principle (*Escherichia coli* neurotoxin) and its use as an in vitro assay for this toxin. Am J Vet Res 44:31–34.

DUNNE, H. W. 1975. Colibacillosis and edema disease. In Diseases of Swine, 4th ed. Ed. H. W. Dunne and A. D. Leman. Ames: Iowa State Univ Press, p. 674.

ERSKINE, R. G.; SOJKA, W. J.; AND LLOYD, M. K. 1957. The experimental reproduction of a syndrome indistinguishable from oedema disease. Vet Rec 69:301–303.

FRANCIS, D. H.; MOXLEY, R. A.; AND ANDRAOS, C. Y. 1989. Edema disease-like brain lesions in gnotobiotic piglets infected with *Escherichia coli* serotype O157:H7. Infect Immun 57:1339–1342.

GANNON, V. P. J., AND GYLES, C. L. 1990. Characteristics of the *Shiga*-like toxin produced by *Escherichia coli* associated with porcine edema disease. Vet Microbiol 24:89–100.

GANNON, V. P. J.; GYLES, C. L.; AND FRIENDSHIP, W. 1988. Characteristics of verotoxigenic *Escherichia coli* from pigs. Can J Vet Res 52:331–337.

GANNON, V. P. J.; GYLES, C. L.; AND WILCOCK, B. P. 1989. Effects of *Escherichia coli* *Shiga*-like toxins (verotoxins) in pigs. Can J Vet Res 53:306–312.

GONZALEZ, E. A., AND BLANCO, J. 1985. Production of cytotoxin VT in enteropathogenic and non-enteropathogenic *Escherichia coli* strains of porcine origin. FEMS Microbiol Lett 26:127–130.

GREGORY, D. W. 1955. Role of beta hemolytic coliform organisms in edema disease of swine. Vet Med 1:609–610.

GYLES, C. L.; DE GRANDIS, S. A.; MACKENZIE, C.; AND BRUNTON, J. L. 1988. Cloning and nucleotide sequence analysis of the genes determining verocytotoxin production in a porcine edema disease isolate of *Escherichia coli*. Microbiol Pathog 5:419–426.

HAMPSON, D. J.; FU, Z. F.; AND ROBERTSON, I. D. 1987. Investigation of the source of haemolytic *Escherichia coli* infecting weaned pigs. Epidemiol Inf 99:149–153.

HÄNI, H.; BRÄNDLI, A.; NICOLET, J.; VON ROLL, P.; LUGINBÜHL, H.; AND HÖRNING, B. 1976. Vorkommen und Bedeutung von Schweinekrankheiten: Analyse eines Sektionsguts (1971–1973). III. Pathologie des Digestionstraktes. Schweiz Arch Tierheilk 118:13–29.

HARDING, J. D. J. 1966. A cerebrospinal angiopathy in pigs. Pathol Vet 3:83–88.

HUSBAND, A. J., AND SEAMAN, J. T. 1979. Vaccination of piglets against *Escherichia coli* enteritis. Aust Vet J 55:435–436.

JAHN, S., AND UECKER, E. 1987. Ökonomische Untersuchungen zur Kolienterotoxämie des Schweines. Monatsh Vet Med 42:769–771.

KAUSCHE, F. M. 1989. An experimental model for edema disease (*Escherichia coli* enterotoxemia) in swine. Thesis, Iowa State Univ, Ames.

KERNKAMP, H. C. H.; SORENSEN, D. K.; HANSON, L. J.; AND NIELSEN, N. O. 1965. Epizootiology of edema disease in swine. J Am Vet Med Assoc 146:353–357.

KONOWALCHUK, J.; SPEIRS, J. I.; AND STAVRIC, S. 1977. Vero response to a cytotoxin of *Escherichia coli*. Infect Immun 18:775–779.

KURTZ, H. J.; BERGELAND, M. E.; AND BARNES, D. M. 1969. Pathologic changes in edema disease of swine. Am J Vet Res 30:791–806.

LECCE, J. G.; BALSBAUGH, R. K.; CLARE, D. A.; AND KING, M. W. 1982. Rotavirus and hemolytic enteropathogenic *Escherichia coli* in weanling diarrhea of pigs. J Clin Microbiol 16:715–723.

LINGGOOD, M. A., AND THOMPSON, J. M. 1987. Verotoxin production among porcine strains of *Escherichia coli* and its association with oedema disease. Med Microbiol 25:359–362.

MACLEOD, D. L., AND GYLES, C. L. 1990. Purification and characterization of an *Escherichia coli* *Shiga*-like toxin II variant. Infect Immun 58:1232–1239.

MARQUES, L. R. M.; PEIRIS, J. S. M.; CRYZ, S. J.; AND O'BRIEN, A. D. 1987. *Escherichia coli* strains isolated from pigs with edema disease produce a variant of *Shiga*-like toxin II. FEMS Microbiol Lett 44:33–38.

METHIYAPUN, S.; POHLENZ, J. F. L.; AND BERTSCHINGER, H. U. 1984. Ultra-structure of the intestinal mucosa in pigs experimentally inoculated with an edema disease-producing strain of *Escherichia coli* (O139:K12:H1). Vet Pathol 21:516–520.

NAGY, B.; CASEY, T. A.; AND MOON, H. W. 1990. Phenotype and genotype of *Escherichia coli* isolated from pigs with postweaning diarrhea in Hungary. J Clin Microbiol 28:651–653.

NAKAMURA, K.; KUBO, M.; SHOYA, S.; KASHIWAZAKI, M.; KOIZUMI, S.; AND ONAI, M. 1982. Swine cerebrospinal angiopathy with demyelination and malacia. Vet Pathol 19:140–149.

NIELSEN, N. C.; SUHR-JESSEN, T.; AND JENSEN, M. M. 1988. Inhibitive effect of 5 probiotic porcine lactobacillus strains on the incidence and severity of experimentally induced post weaning *E. coli* syndrome in pigs. Proc 10th Int Congr Pig Vet Soc, Rio de Janeiro, p. 111.

NIELSEN, N. O., AND CLUGSTON, R. E. 1971. Comparison of *E. coli* endotoxin shock and acute experimental edema disease in young pigs. Ann NY Acad Sci 176:176–189.

OLSSON, T., AND OLSSON, S. O. 1982. Melperone treatment of edema disease of pigs. Proc 7th Int Congr Pig Vet Soc, Mexico City, p. 26.

ØRSKOV, I., AND ØRSKOV, F. 1984. Serotyping of *Escherichia coli*. In Methods in Microbiology, vol. 14. Ed. T. Bergan. New York: Academic Press, pp. 43–112.

POHL, P.; LINTERMANS, P.; MAINIL, J.; AND DEPREZ, P. 1989. Production de vérocytotoxine par les *Escherichia coli* du porc. Ann Méd Vét 133:31–38.

ROHRMANN, H., AND UECKER, E. 1987. Experimentelle Untersuchungen zur Bedeutung des Ingesta-pH-Wertes in der Pathogenese der Kolienterotoxämie des Schweines. Monatsh Vet Med 42:422–425.

SALAJKA, E.; CERNOHOUS, J.; AND SARMANOVA, Z. 1975. Association of the colonization of the intestine by pathogenic strains of haemolytic *E. coli* in weaned piglets with withdrawal of antibody contained in the dams' milk. Docum Vet Brno 8:43–55.

SAMUEL, J. E.; PERERA, L. P.; WARD, S.; O'BRIEN, A. D.; GINSBURG, V.; AND KRIVAN, H. C. 1990. Comparison of the glycolipid receptor specificities of *Shiga*-like toxin type II and *Shiga*-like toxin type II variants. Infect Immun 58:611–618.

SARMIENTO, J. I.; CASEY, T. A.; AND MOON, H. W. 1988. Postweaning diarrhea in swine: Experimental model of enterotoxigenic *Escherichia coli* infection. Am J Vet Res 49:1154–1159.

SAXENA, S. K.; O'BRIEN, A. D.; AND ACKERMAN, E. J. 1989. *Shiga* toxin, *Shiga*-like toxin II variant, and ricin are all single-site RNA N-glycosidases of 28 S RNA when microinjected into *Xenopus* oocytes. J Biol Chem 264:596–601.

SCHIMMELPFENNIG, H. H. 1970. Untersuchungen zur Aetiologie der Oedemkrankheit des Schweines. In Beiheft 13 zum Zentralblatt fur Veterinarmedizin. Berlin: Paul Parey, pp. 1–80.

SCHOFIELD, F. W. 1953. Should the name "oedema disease" be changed to "entero-toxaemia" of swine? Vet Rec 65(28):443.

SCHOFIELD, F. W., AND DAVIS, D. 1955. Oedema disease (enterotoxaemia) in swine. II. Experiments conducted in a susceptible herd. Can J Comp Med 19:242–245.

SCHOFIELD, F. W., AND SCHRODER, J. D. 1954. Some important aspects of oedema disease in swine (enterotoxaemia). Can J Comp Med 18:24–28.

SCHULZ, L. C.; BRASS, W.; AND NÜSSEL, M. 1961. Experimentelle Untersuchungen zur Pathogenese schockartiger und rheumatoider Krankheiten des Schweines. I. Schockartige Erkrankungen und die Beteiligung des zentralen Nervensystems. Dtsch Tieraerztl Wochenschr 68:289–296.

SCHULZE, F. 1977. Quantitative Magen-Darm-Flora-Analysen beim Ferkel vor und nach dem Absetzen unter Berücksichtigung der Pathogenese der Kolienterotoxämie. Arch Exper Vet Med 31:299–316.

SHANKS, P. L. 1938. An unusual condition affecting the digestive organs of the pig. Vet Rec 50:356–358.

SMITH, H. W. 1963. The haemolysins of *Escherichia coli.* J Pathol Bacteriol 85:197–211.

SMITH, H. W., AND HALLS, S. 1968. The production of oedema disease and diarrhoea in weaned pigs by the oral administration of *Escherichia coli:* Factors that influence the course of the experimental disease. J Med Microbiol 1:45–59.

SMITH, H. W., AND LINGGOOD, M. A. 1971a. Observations on the pathogenic properties of the K88, HLY and ENT plasmids of *Escherichia coli* with particular reference to porcine diarrhoea. J Med Microbiol 4:467–485.

———. 1971b. The effect of antisera in protecting pigs against experimental *Escherichia coli* diarrhoea and oedema disease. J Med Microbiol 4:487–493.

SMITH, W. H.; GREEN, P.; AND PARSELL, Z. 1983. Vero cell toxins in *Escherichia coli* and related bacteria:

Transfer by phage, conjugation and toxic action in laboratory animals, chickens and pigs. J Gen Microbiol 129:3121–3137.

SOJKA, W. J. 1965. *Escherichia coli* in domestic animals and poultry. Commonw Agric Bur, Farnham Royal, Bucks, England, pp. 104–156.

STAMM, M.; BERTSCHINGER, H. U.; AND SYDLER, T. 1990. Prevalence of fimbriae 107 in the intestine of pigs with oedema disease or postweaning *E. coli* diarrhoea. Proc 11th Int Congr Pig Vet Soc, Lausanne, p. 142.

SVENDSEN, J. 1979. Enteric *Escherichia coli* infections in suckling pigs and in pigs at weaning. Aspects of pathogenesis, prevention and control. Thesis (printed), Swedish Univ of Agricultural Sciences.

SVENDSEN, J., AND LARSEN, J. L. 1977. Studies of the pathogenesis of enteric *E. coli* infections in weaned pigs. The significance of the milk of the dam in preventing the disease. Nord Vet Med 29:533–538.

SWEENEY, E. J. 1972. *Escherichia coli* enterotoxaemia of swine: A bacteriological study of Irish outbreaks during 1971. Ir Vet J 26:69–73.

———. 1976. Enterotoxaemia *Escherichia coli* in swine: Some aspects of current interest. Vet Serv Bull 6:15–25.

SYME, G., AND SMITH, M. W. 1982. Intestinal adaptation to protein deficiency. Cell Biol Intern Rep 6:573–578.

TIMONEY, J. F. 1949. Experimental production of oedema disease of swine. Vet Rec 61:710.

———. 1950. Oedema disease of swine. Vet Rec 62:748–756.

———. 1957. Oedema disease in swine. Vet Rec 69:1160–1175.

TIMONEY, J. F., JR. 1986. Genetic and characterization studies on edema disease toxin. Proc 9th Int Congr Pig Vet Soc, Barcelona, p. 199.

TZIPORI, S.; WACHSMUTH, I. K.; CHAPMAN, C.; BIRNER, R.; BRITTINGHAM, J.; JACKSON, C.; AND HOGG, J. 1986. The pathogenesis of hemorrhagic colitis caused by *Escherichia coli* O157:H7 in gnotobiotic piglets. J Infect Dis 154:712–716.

WATHES, C. M.; MILLER, B. G.; AND BOURNE, F. J. 1989. Cold stress and postweaning diarrhoea in piglets inoculated orally or by aerosol. Anim Prod 49:483–496.

WEINSTEIN, D. L.; JACKSON, M. P.; SAMUEL, J. E.; HOLMES, R. K.; AND O'BRIEN, A. D. 1988. Cloning and sequencing of a *Shiga*-like toxin type II variant from an *Escherichia coli* strain responsible for edema disease of swine. J Bacteriol 170: 4223–4230.

Systemic Infection

H. U. Bertschinger

SYSTEMIC *E. coli* infection comprises both septicemia and local extraintestinal infection resulting from bacteremia. Systemic infection is a relatively common finding in suckling piglets. In a prospective 2-year study of the losses in 17 Danish herds covering 28,002 live born pigs, systemic *E. coli* infection was diagnosed postmortem in 115 piglets, i.e., 0.4% (Nielsen et al. 1975b). At least three types of systemic infections can be distinguished: primary systemic infection, septicemia complicating an enteric ETEC infection, terminal bacteremia secondary to a variety of debilitating diseases.

ETIOLOGY. In the material of Nielsen et al. (1975b) already mentioned, about one-third of the 115 cases yielded *E. coli* with hemolytic activity. From additional 9 cases *Klebsiella* were isolated and from 1 case *Pseudomonas* (Nielsen et al. 1975b). Thirty isolates from primary systemic infections represented at least 12 different O groups (Nielsen et al. 1975a). Not every *E. coli* strain is able to induce septicemia when fed to gnotobiotic pigs. The disease was reproduced with isolates from pigs, from a cat, and from a chicken (Meyer et al. 1971; Murata et al. 1979).

EPIDEMIOLOGY. Primary systemic infection is most often seen as sporadic cases (Nielsen et al. 1975a). Very rarely, small outbreaks are recorded. Piglets are most often affected during the first and second week of life. However, the disease may occur throughout the suckling period, with exceptional cases in pigs up to 80 days old. Epidemiology of the secondary systemic infection is determined by the underlying disease.

PATHOGENESIS. Primary systemic *E. coli* infection does not develop in pigs without some defect of the immune system. Colostrum deprivation is a requisite for the reproduction of this disease entity (Waxler and Britt 1972). Even colostrum-deprived pigs develop resistance against systemic infection, if they are fed a diet containing macromolecules (Murata et al. 1979). Bacteria may invade the host by endocytotic uptake into intestinal epithelial cells. Observation of a high incidence of *E. coli* septicemia in the progeny of two half-sib boars led to the assumption that increased susceptibility to this condition might be inherited (Wijeratne et al. 1970).

Secondary systemic invasion by enterotoxigenic *E. coli* (ETEC) has been observed in conventional as well as in gnotobiotic pigs. In many cases postmortem signs are indicative of a septicemia that is assumed to be of pathogenic significance (Svendsen et al. 1975). Orally applied colostrum from nonvaccinated sows did much to enhance the clearing of ETEC bacteria from the blood of colostrum-deprived pigs, whereas purified colostral IgG from vaccinated sows was almost ineffective (Brandenburg and Wilson 1974).

In most cases without underlying ETEC infection, development of septicemia is assumed to be favored by undersupply of colostrum, low birth weight, and sublethal malformations. Death following perforating lesions of the gastrointestinal tract is often due to *E. coli* septicemia.

CLINICAL SIGNS. Piglets with a primary systemic infection characteristically show marked depression, rough hair coat, anorexia, distention of the abdomen, and labored respiration (Nielsen et al. 1975a). In experimentally inoculated gnotobiotic pigs the incubation period varied from 1 to 5 days and the time of survival from 1 to 8 days, depending on the bacterial strain (Meyer et al. 1971; Waxler and Britt 1972; Murata et al. 1979). Experimental pigs exhibited fever, depression, loss of appetite, and occasional mild diarrhea without dehydration. Terminal respiratory distress was seen in some pigs with prolonged survival time (Meyer et al. 1971). Articular pain and nervous signs may develop.

LESIONS. Primary *E. coli* septicemia often leads to severe fibrinous polyserositis (Waxler and Britt 1972; Nielsen et al. 1975a). Liver, spleen, and subcutaneous and mesenteric lymph nodes are enlarged and hyperemic. There may be fibrinopurulent arthritis and meningitis. More severe polyserositis and some pneumonia are observed in slowly developing cases (Meyer et al. 1971). Histologic examination of the lung reveals interalveolar interstitial pneumonia with edema and neutrophilic infiltration, but alveoli are free of exudates (Waxler and Britt 1972).

Less prominent lesions, such as icterus, petechial hemorrhages in the serosal membranes, and splenomegaly, were reported in pigs with underlying ETEC infections (Svendsen et al. 1975). They were accompanied by severe diarrhea and dehydration. In many cases of secondary systemic *E. coli* infection, presumably occurring at a very late stage of the underlying disease, the changes are slight or no lesions at all are recorded.

DIAGNOSIS. Systemic *E. coli* infection may be suspected on a clinical basis, if cases are sporadic, and if underlying primary diseases are evident. In many cases, however, postmortem examination and bacteriology may be indispensable. Polyserositis caused by *Hemophilus parasuis* is seen mostly in pigs 2–3 months old, after introduction into other herds. *Mycoplasma hyorhinis* should be considered as well.

PREVENTION AND TREATMENT. Prevention should concentrate on underlying primary causes as well as on early and plentiful supply of colostrum. Treatment may be attempted with the antimicrobials used for the treatment of other extraintestinal *E. coli* diseases but is usually ineffective once the clinical signs are apparent in neonates.

REFERENCES

BRANDENBURG, A. C., AND WILSON, M. R. 1974. Immunity to *Escherichia coli* in pigs: IgG and blood clearance. Res Vet Sci 16:171–175.

MEYER, R. C.; SAXENA, S. P.; AND RHOADES, H. E. 1971. Polyserositis induced by *Escherichia coli* in gnotobiotic swine. Infect Immun 3:41–44.

MURATA, H.; YAGUCHI, H.; AND NAMIOKA, S. 1979. Relationship between the intestinal permeability to macromolecules and invasion of septicemia-inducing *Escherichia coli* in neonatal piglets. Infect Immun 26:339–347.

NIELSEN, N. C.; BILLE, N.; RIISING, H.-J.; AND DAM, A. 1975a. Polyserositis in pigs due to generalized *Escherichia coli* infection. Can J Comp Med 39:421–426.

NIELSEN, N. C.; RIISING, H.-J.; LARSEN, J. L.; BILLE, N.; AND SVENDSEN, J. 1975b. Preweaning mortality in pigs. 5. Acute septicaemias. Nord Vet Med 27:129–139.

SVENDSEN, J.; BILLE, N.; NIELSEN, N. C.; LARSEN, J. L.; AND RIISING, H.-J. 1975. Preweaning mortality in pigs. 4. Diseases of the gastrointestinal tract in pigs. Nord Vet Med 27:85–101.
WAXLER, G. L., AND BRITT, A. L. 1972. Polyserositis and arthritis due to *Escherichia coli* in gnotobiotic pigs. Can J Comp Med 36:226–233.
WIJERATNE, W. V. S.; CROSSMAN, P. J.; AND GOULD, C. M. 1970. Evidence of a sire effect on piglet mortality. Br Vet J 126:94–99.

Coliform Mastitis

H. U. Bertschinger
J. Pohlenz

THE TERM coliform mastitis (CM) has been introduced to denominate puerperal mastitis in the pig. The term should end the confusing terminology in this field. In addition, this expression points out the parallels to CM in the cow. A cumulative tabulation of necropsies performed on agalactic sows revealed that 59 of 72 sows (82%) had gross lesions of mastitis (Ross et al. 1981). Because of the hidden character of the disease, the practicing veterinarian will perhaps continue to use less precisely defined expressions describing the more prominent symptoms of CM, i.e., milk fever, farrowing fever, lactational failure, hypogalactia, and agalactia. Other expressions such as mastitis-metritis-agalactia (MMA), agalactia toxemia, puerperal mastitis, and puerperal toxemia reflect views of different authors on pathogenesis.

Early publications on postparturient disorders associated with agalactia have been reviewed in detail by Ringarp (1960). Most dealt predominantly with clinical aspects of the syndrome. However, there are some early reports on the isolation of coliform bacteria from the milk of sows with mastitis. In the past, authors attributed to mastitis only those cases of lactational failure that displayed symptoms of mastitis on clinical examination. The remaining cases were thought to result from either a septicemia or a toxemia. The former concept was supported by bacteriologic findings in exceptional fatal cases of puerperal fever. It was speculated that a toxemia resulted from either puerperal metritis or gastrointestinal disorders. However, metritis only rarely contributes to lactational failure. Excessive vulval discharge was observed in a similar proportion of sows with and without agalactia (Nachreiner and Ginther 1972; Jones 1976). Measurements and gross and microscopic appearance of the genital tract did not differ in healthy and agalactic sows (Nachreiner and Ginther 1972). Following experimental inoculation, the bacteria colonized the uterus without signs of systemic disease or agalactia (Jones 1976). Significant evidence of the existence of a toxemia originating in the digestive system is still lacking (Elmore et al. 1982). Careful investigations did not reveal morphologic or functional changes in the gastrointestinal tract (Nachreiner and Ginther 1972).

CM has a worldwide distribution. Hermansson et al. (1978) disclosed an average incidence of agalactia postpartum of 12.8%, with a variation for individual herds from 0.5 to 50%. In a Danish study covering more than 72,000 farrowings in farms with a high management level, the incidence amounted to 9.5% of the farrowings (Jorsal 1986).

Economic loss results from a number of factors and therefore is difficult to estimate. The death rate of affected sows is low. The cost of extra care and of treatment is hard to assess. The piglets suffer more than the affected dam. Bäckström et al. (1984) reported mortality of piglets nursing pluriparous sows with MMA was 55.8%, whereas that of piglets nursing healthy sows was 17.2%. Mortality of piglets may result from elongated farrowing time, crushing by the sow, starvation, and impaired immunity to infectious agents because of insufficient uptake of colostral immunoglobulins. The average milk yield of three sows affected with CM on the first 2 days after farrowing was about half the yield of healthy sows, and the piglets of the sick sows lost some weight (Ross et al. 1975). Piglets sucking glands with mastitis of sows with subclinical CM had smaller weight gains only for days 1–4 postpartum (Bertschinger et al. 1990).

ETIOLOGY. The term "coliform," when used in the context of mastitis, covers the bacterial genera *Escherichia*, *Klebsiella*, *Enterobacter*, and *Citrobacter*. However, the methods used for identification in several studies were not adequate to determine the genera and even less the species of the bacterial isolates. *E. coli* was the organism most often identified in either milk samples or affected mammary tissue (Ringarp 1960; Glawischnig 1964; Armstrong et al. 1968; Bertschinger et al. 1977a; Ross et al. 1981; Wegmann et al. 1986). *Klebsiella*, mostly *K. pneumoniae*, was prevalent in the cases investigated by Ross et al. (1975) and Jones (1976). *Enterobacter aerogenes* (Ringarp 1960; Glawischnig 1964; Armstrong et al. 1968) was isolated repeatedly, whereas *E.*

cloacae (Bertschinger et al. 1977a) and *C. freundii* (Armstrong et al. 1968) were detected in not more than one sow each. *Staphylococcus epidermidis* and a variety of streptococci were also found in the mammary glands of sows with signs of mastitis, either mixed with coliforms or as pure cultures. The noncoliform organisms were occasionally associated with microscopic lesions of mastitis (Bertschinger et al. 1977a; Ross et al. 1981).

EPIDEMIOLOGY. CM of the sow appears to be noncontagious. Serologic typing of isolates from mastitis revealed an extreme multiplicity of serologic types not only within a herd but also within distinct glands of one sow. A significant proportion of subcomplexes harbor more than one type (Bertschinger et al. 1977a; Awad-Masalmeh et al. 1990). The great variety of coliform bacteria associated with CM indicates an abundant reservoir of potentially pathogenic bacteria. The coliforms causing mastitis may originate from the flora of the sow as well as from the environment. In about one-third of the sows with mastitis, identical isolates were found in mastitic glands, the uterine contents, and the urinary bladder (Bertschinger et al. 1977a). The intestinal flora of the sow, the oral flora of the neonatal piglet, and environmental bacteria may significantly contribute to contamination of the nipples. Awad-Masalmeh et al. (1990) found identical O serotypes of *E. coli* in mammary secretion and in feces of about one-fourth of 67 sows with CM. Muirhead (1976) considered the bedding of the sow of paramount importance. Dung and urine contaminate the udder. *Klebsiella* sp. may also originate from wood shavings used for bedding. Bertschinger et al. (1990) compared 12 farrowings, each in conventional farrowing crates and in an experimental pen where the sows were to lie down in a clean resting area. Sows in the experimental pen had much lower counts of coliform bacteria on their teat ends and an incidence of intramammary *E. coli* infections 10 times lower than in the crate.

PATHOGENESIS

Invasion of Mammary Gland. Mastitis was reproduced in the sow by intramammary instillation of not more than 120 organisms of a strain of *K. pneumoniae*. Following massive external contamination of the nipples with the same strain, the bacteria were recovered from 60 out of 142 subcomplexes examined. External contamination of the nipples was as successful on gestation day 111 as 2 hours after completion of farrowing (Bertschinger et al. 1977b). It is largely unknown at what time spontaneous invasion of the cistern takes place. McDonald and McDonald (1975) found significant numbers of coliform bacteria in about one-fourth of mammary glands cultured just before parturition. In a sequential examination of the mammary secretions *E. coli* was iso-

lated from 17 out of 30 totally infected glands, before the first piglet was born (Bertschinger et al. 1990). New infections appeared not later than day 2 postpartum.

The bacteria are located in the ductular and alveolar lumina, either free or within phagocytic cells. Adhesion to surfaces is not observed. At postmortem examination the causative bacteria are frequently isolated from regional lymph nodes, whereas isolations from liver, spleen, or kidney are rare (Armstrong et al. 1968; Bertschinger et al. 1977a, b; Ross et al. 1981).

Multiplication of bacteria in the mammary secretion is controlled by antimicrobial mechanisms, which so far have been studied in the pig with respect to piglet enteritis only. The antimicrobial activity of cow's milk is due to a variety of inhibitors acting in concert and conferring to the dry udder a nearly total resistance to coliform proliferation (Bramley 1976). Growth in vitro of a given strain of *E. coli* in secretions of individual sows varies enormously. The secretion of atrophic glands exerts a bactericidal effect (Wegmann 1985). CM is a self-curing disease. The bacteria disappear between 1 and 6 days after parturition (Wegmann and Bertschinger 1984; Bertschinger et al. 1990).

Mammary Inflammation. CM in the sow is associated with massive accumulation of neutrophils in the lumina of affected glands. Simultaneous induction of CM in several mammary subcomplexes of sows, from which the piglets had been removed, resulted in severe leukopenia within 24 hours (Bertschinger et al. 1977b). Intracisternal instillation of identical bacterial inocula following a standardized protocol leads to a spectrum of reactions, reaching from very severe local and general signs to subclinical mastitis (Bertschinger, unpublished observations). In the experiments of Löfstedt et al. (1983) susceptibility to experimental infection was associated with impaired function of circulating neutrophils. Cytological findings must be interpreted with caution. Mammary glands not chosen by a piglet undergo atrophy soon after parturition. Atrophy is accompanied by an increase in the total somatic cell count as well as of the proportion of polymorphonuclear (PMN) cells (Wegmann and Bertschinger 1984). In some sows many glands show mild to severe increases of total somatic and PMN cells in the absence of cultivable bacteria (Bertschinger et al. 1990). Wegmann and Bertschinger (1984) proposed classifying glands as mastitic, if the total cell count surpasses 10^6 cells/ml and the rate of PMN cells is higher than 70%. However, even the combined use of the two parameters does not always permit accurate distinction between atrophic and inflamed glands.

Systemic Reaction. The clinical symptoms as well as the endocrinologic, hematologic, and blood chemical changes after intramammary infusion of endotoxin are much the same as in spontaneous cases of agalactia (Nachreiner and Ginther 1974; Elmore et al. 1978). Small amounts of endotoxin cause a decrease in prolactin plasma levels and a significant depression of piglet growth (Smith and Wagner 1984). Endotoxin was more often detected in the blood of 25 affected sows than of 13 contemporary healthy control sows (Morkoc et al. 1983). De Ruijter et al. (1988) observed in sows rendered refractory to intravenous injection of endotoxin a marked increase of rectal temperature after intramammary infusion of a small toxin dose. The authors concluded that local release of acute-phase mediators in the mammary gland is the predominant cause of systemic signs. These mediators are known to act on thermoregulatory centers.

Immunity. CM apparently does not result in protective immunity (Bertschinger and Bühlmann 1990). Ringarp (1960) reported a higher incidence in sows than in gilts as well as the repeated occurrence in individual sows up to 10 times. Vaccination is not a promising method for control of mastitis. Even when an autogenous vaccine was used, protection was unsatisfactory (Ross 1983, unpublished data).

CLINICAL SIGNS. Most clinical work on CM was done before lactational failure was traced to mastitis. Ross et al. (1975) described the clinical findings in sows with proven CM and demonstrated changes quite similar to those described earlier in sows with lactational failure. Interpretation of clinical parameters is rendered difficult by the presence of subclinical CM in apparently healthy sows (Nachreiner and Ginther 1972; Middleton-Williams et al. 1977).

The initial signs are most often detected on the first or second day and more rarely on the third day after farrowing. However, they may be observed as early as during parturition (Martin et al. 1967). The first symptoms are temperature response, listlessness, weakness, and loss of interest in the piglets. Affected sows prefer sternal recumbency. In severe cases they become stiff and dizzy, do not stand up, and may even become comatose. Feed and water consumption are either reduced or absent. Body temperature is moderately elevated and only rarely exceeds 42°C. A febrile cases have been reported; however, the temperature was not taken continuously. On the other hand many normal sows will have rectal temperatures that exceed the 39.7°C limit on the day of parturition and for 2 days thereafter (King et al. 1972). In affected sows respiratory and heart rates are increased. In general the symptoms described do not last for more than 2–3 days.

On hematologic examination a more or less pronounced leukopenia with a left shift is common early in sows with mastitis (Ross et al. 1975;

Bertschinger et al. 1977b). Subsequently, leukocytosis is observed (Nachreiner and Ginther 1972). The ratio of plasma protein to fibrinogen was lowered (Ross et al. 1975). The plasma cortisol level is increased in sows with agalactia (Nachreiner and Ginther 1972).

The behavior of the piglets is very helpful in the early detection of lactational failure. Undernourished piglets look gaunt. They frequently try to suck, move from nipple to nipple, nibble at litter, and lick urine from the floor. If access to the nipples is given by the sow, the periods of suckling are shortened. After suckling, the piglets stray about instead of resting in close contact with their littermates.

Precise localization of mammary lesions is often not possible because reddening and heat of the skin extend over several subcomplexes. The reliable clinical assessment of the state of the actual mammary tissue is rendered difficult by subcutaneous fat and considerable subcutaneous edema. If palpable, the mastitic tissue is firmer and palpation may cause pain (Glawischnig 1964). The red color of the skin is blanched by finger pressure, which causes a depression of the tissue lasting for some time. Mere clinical examination will at best detect some of the affected subcomplexes. The inguinal lymph nodes may be swollen.

The fluid expressed from a nipple originates from more than one subcomplex, because two or, rarely, three teat canals end in each nipple. Therefore, in samples taken from a nipple, secretion from the unaffected, productive subcomplex dominates. The exudate from inflamed subcomplexes looks serous to creamy, like pus. It may contain clots of fibrin or blood. Whereas the pH is of limited diagnostic value (Glawischnig 1964; Ross et al. 1981), the cytologic examination allows differentiation between healthy and mastitic complexes at least during the first 48 hours after parturition (Wegmann and Bertschinger 1984).

LESIONS. Despite the high incidence of CM, there are not many reports on necropsy findings (Martin et al. 1967; Jones 1976; Middleton-Williams et al. 1977; Ross et al. 1981). In general, lesions are confined to the mammary glands and regional lymph nodes. The subcutaneous tissue may be edematous over affected parts of the udder. For reliable demonstration of mastitis, Middleton-Williams et al. (1977) recommended a longitudinal section on the level of the nipples through each row of glands. Using this technique, irregularly scattered foci of mastitis were detected in 1–23 subcomplexes (Fig. 39.10). The appearance of affected mammary tissue varied from slightly increased firmness and grayish discoloration to sharply demarcated, red-mottled, hard, and dry areas (Fig. 39.11). The secretion was sparse and sometimes mixed with clots.

By histologic examination additional lesions

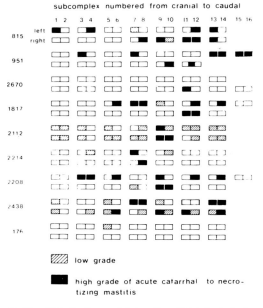

39.10. Distribution and intensity of histologic lesions in nine field cases of CM. (Modified from Middleton-Williams et al. 1977.)

were detected that had not been recognized at gross examination. In every case there was an acute purulent exudative mastitis with congestion. An extreme variability of severity ranging from a small number of neutrophils in the alveolar lumina to severe purulent infiltration with necrosis was obvious (Fig. 39.12). The severity of the lesions varied not only between but also within subcomplexes where unaffected tissue was found adjacent to severely inflamed areas. Acute purulent lymphadenitis was present in the inguinal and iliac lymph nodes (Middleton-Williams et al. 1977).

DIAGNOSIS. Any hypogalactia at the beginning of lactation arouses suspicion of CM. The diagnosis may be supported by fever, anorexia, reluctance to stand up, lying on the gland, and disinterest in the piglets. In severe cases some affected glands may be reddened, swollen, and firm, and the secretion may look abnormal. A reliable rapid test for use in the barn is not available. Due to the higher cell content of sow milk, tests developed for use with the cow cannot be recommended. Bacteriologic and cytologic examinations of the secretion make sense only if all glands are sampled or if affected glands are known. The differential diagnosis of CM is reviewed in Chapter 4.

TREATMENT. Therapeutic measures are usually not taken before the sow shows signs of dysgalactia. Thus treatment may at best shorten the period of underfeeding of the piglets.

Chemotherapy is complicated by the heterogeneous pattern of antimicrobial susceptibility of individual isolates, not only within a herd but also within a sow. Therefore, sensitivity testing is of little value in individual cases. The data in Table 39.3 indicate that the percentage of sensitive isolates is still decreasing.

The pharmacokinetics of antimicrobials has received but limited attention. One injection of 20 mg/kg body weight of a slow-release formulation of oxytetracycline results in milk levels not surpassing 2 μg/ml, i.e., just above the minimal inhibitory concentration (MIC) of susceptible *E. coli* (Schoneweis et al. 1982). Enrofloxacin, a quinolone antibiotic, given at 2.5 mg/kg body weight orally every half day, is concentrated in colostrum and milk to mean levels of 1.2 μg/ml, which is 20 times higher than the MIC (Oliel and Bertschinger 1990). Awad-Masalmeh et al. (1990) tested 107 strains of *E. coli* isolated from sows

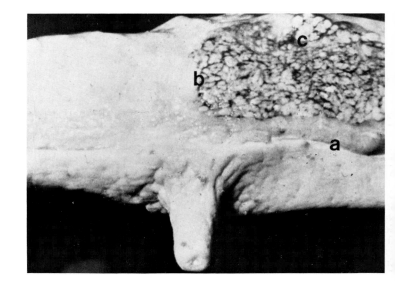

39.11. Acute CM of one subcomplex adjacent to unaltered glandular tissue in longitudinal cut surface: (*a*) subcutaneous edema, (*b*) demarcation from adjacent subcomplex, (*c*) mottled appearance of affected tissue.

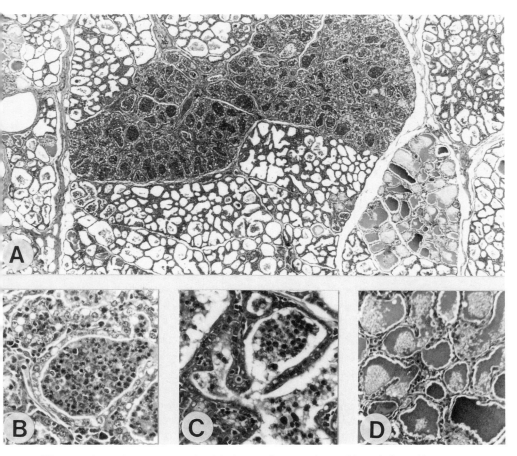

39.12. Histopathology of a mammary gland 24 hours after experimental inoculation with a culture of *Klebsiella pneumoniae*. (A) Low-power magnification within a single subcomplex different types of mastitis next to secreting alveoli. (B) Dark area filled with densely packed polymorphonuclear leukocytes and local destruction of epithelium. (C) Nearly empty-looking alveoli containing low numbers of polymorphonuclear leukocytes. (D) Alveoli with normal-looking secretion (Institute of Veterinary Pathology, Univ of Zurich).

with CM from 43 herds and found no resistance to enrofloxacin. Therapeutic trials are generally difficult to evaluate, because the curing effect is not quantified and often hardly distinguishable from spontaneous improvement.

The additional injection of a glucocorticosteroid (50–100 mg prednisolone) results in a signifi-cant reduction of piglet mortality (Ringarp 1960). In sows with endotoxin-induced hypogalactia, the repeated intravenous application of oxytocin (30 IU) raises the milk intake of the piglets signifi-cantly (Garcia et al. 1980).

Much attention should be given to the piglets. They may either be fostered by other sows or

Table 39.3. Sensitivity to antimicrobials of coliform isolates from mammary glands in Switzerland and Austria

	Sensitive Isolates (%)		
Substance	Bertschinger et al. 1977a n = 80	Wegmann et al. 1986 n = 107	Awad-Masalmeh et al. 1990 n = 107
Ampicillin	90	86	74
Tetracycline	19	42	16
Chloramphenicol	95	81	64
Streptomycin	21	21	21
Neomycin	96	92	86
Gentamicin	100	100	100
Trimethoprim plus sulfamethoxazole	100	84	51
Enrofloxacin	not tested	not tested	100

remain with their mother and receive a milk substitute. Sweetened condensed milk diluted with water 1:1 can be used instead of commercial products. Sterile 5% glucose solution in a dose of approximately 15 ml can be repeatedly injected intraperitoneally several hours apart, or a more concentrated solution may be applied intragastrically. When the pig obtains insufficient amounts of milk, protection against chilling is particularly important.

PREVENTION

Hygiene Measures. Muirhead (1976) and Jones (1979) suggested that protection of the teats from bacterial contamination might be an effective prophylaxis of CM. Bertschinger et al. (1990) performed a prospective study of farrowing in two types of pens. They concluded that the density of the coliform flora on the teat apex reflects the degree of contamination of the lying area. Optimal prophylaxis is achieved by designing farrowing accommodation in such a manner that the sow is prevented from lying down in her own excreta. On the other hand, washing and disinfection of the pen and of the newly housed sow contribute much less to efficient prophylaxis. If cases of CM accumulate, the bedding materials should be checked.

Nutrition of the Sow. Drastic reduction of the sow's ration shortly before parturition is a widespread practice. In a carefully designed long-term study using pairs of full sibs, the reduction of the daily feed allowance from 3.2 to 1.0 kg of a commercial-type feed lowered the incidence of agalactia from 26.6% to 14.4% (Persson et al. 1989). Udder changes were registered in a high percentage of the agalactic sows and significant numbers of bacteria were found in more than 80% of the agalactic sows. Plonait et al. (1986) reported a corresponding observation. Experimentally induced CM takes a similar course with sows on high and low rations (Bertschinger and Bühlmann, unpublished data). This finding led to the suggestion that feed reduction might act through reduced exposure of the teats due to the much smaller amounts of feces and urine contaminating the laying area.

Immunoprophylaxis. Induction of specific immunity is hampered by the wide range of antigenic types of coliforms isolated from sows with CM. Use of an *E. coli* bacterin induced poor protection in sows against intramammary challenge with the same strain used to prepare the bacterin (Ross 1982, 1983, unpublished data).

Hormones. Some investigators found an extended period of gestation in sows developing lactational failure. The length of gestation can be controlled by use of prostaglandins. However, the prophylactic application led to conflicting results. Studies focussing on CM are not known.

Chemoprophylaxis. For the time being, chemoprophylaxis appears to be the most promising method of control, where accommodation cannot be improved. The prevalence of drug resistance and the wide variety of bacteria associated with the disease in a given herd must be considered when the drug is selected. Feed medication should be replaced by individual application of the drug in a small amount of feed because the feed consumption of the sow in the periparturient period is quite variable. Keeping the period of treatment as short as possible helps to postpone the emergence of drug resistance. In field trials the morbidity from MMA was reduced from 30 to 12% by giving 0.4 g trimethoprim, 1 g sulfadimidine, and 1 g sulfathiazole/150 kg body weight twice a day. The treatment began on gestation day 112 and lasted for 4 days regardless of the day of farrowing (Bollwahn 1978). Six intramuscular injections of apramycin (6.25 mg/kg) at 12-hour intervals reduced the severity of experimentally induced mastitis (Ross and Zimmermann 1982).

Oliel and Bertschinger (1990) tested oral chemoprophylaxis with enrofloxacin of experimentally induced CM. Three glands of each sow were inoculated with *E. coli* and three glands with *K. pneumoniae*. Eight sows were not treated (group I), eight sows received 2.5 mg (group II), and eight sows 5.0 mg/kg body weight twice a day (group III). The inoculated bacteria were reisolated in group I from 100%, in group II from 10%, and in group III from 2% of the inoculated glands. A beneficial effect on milk productivity would be expected but could not be demonstrated because the control sows did not develop systemic signs.

REFERENCES

ARMSTRONG, C. H.; HOOPER, B. E.; AND MARTIN, C. E. 1968. Microflora associated with agalactia syndrome of sows. Am J Vet Res 29:1401–1407.

AWAD-MASALMEH, M.; BAUMGARTNER, W.; PASSERNIG, A.; SILBER, R.; AND HINTERDORFER, F. 1990. Bakteriologische Untersuchungen bei an puerperaler Mastitis (MMA-Syndrom) erkrankten Sauen verschiedener Tierbestände Oesterreichs. Tieraerztl Umsch 45:526–535.

BÄCKSTRÖM, L.; MORKOC, A. C.; CONNOR, J.; LARSON, R.; AND PRICE, W. 1984. Clinical study of mastitis-metritis-agalactia in sows in Illinois. J Am Vet Med Assoc 185:70–73.

BERTSCHINGER, H. U., AND BÜHLMANN, A. 1990. Absence of protective immunity in mammary glands after experimentally induced coliform mastitis. Proc 11th Int Congr Pig Vet Soc, Lausanne, p. 175.

BERTSCHINGER, H. U.; POHLENZ, J.; AND HEMLEP, I. 1977a. Untersuchungen ueber das Mastitis-Metritis-Agalaktie-Syndrom (Milchfieber) der Sau. II. Bakteriologische Befunde bei Spontanfallen. Schweiz Arch Tierheilkd 119:223–233.

BERTSCHINGER, H. U.; POHLENZ, J.; AND MIDDLETON-WILLIAMS, D. M. 1977b. Untersuchungen ueber das Mastitis-Metritis-Agalaktie-Syndrom (Milchfieber) der Sau. III. Galaktogene Erzeugung von Klebsiellen-Mastitis. Schweiz Arch Tierheilkd 119:265–275.

BERTSCHINGER, H. U.; BÜRGI, E.; ENG, V.; AND WEGMANN, P. 1990. Senkung der Inzidenz von puerperaler Mastitis bei der Sau durch Schutz des Gesäuges vor Verschmutzung. Schweiz Arch Tierheilkd 132:557–566.

BOLLWAHN, W. 1978. Effect of strategic TMP/S treatment on puerperium and conception in sows. Proc 5th Int Congr Pig Vet Soc, Zagreb, p. KA16.

BRAMLEY, A. J. 1976. Variations in the susceptibility of lactating and non-lactating bovine udders to infection when infused with *Escherichia coli.* J Dairy Res 43:205–211.

DE RUIJTER, K.; VERHEIJDEN, J. H. M.; PIJPERS, A.; AND BERENDS, J. 1988. The role of endotoxin in the pathogenesis of coliform mastitis in sows. Vet Q 10:186–190.

ELMORE, R. G.; MARTIN, C. E.; AND BERG, J. N. 1978. Absorption of *Escherichia coli* endotoxin from the mammary glands and uteri of early postpartum sows and gilts. Theriogenology 10:439–445.

ELMORE, R. G.; VOGELWEID, C. M.; AND BERG, J. N. 1982. Fate of *Escherichia coli* endotoxin infused into jejunums of pigs. Proc 7th Int Congr Pig Vet Soc, Mexico City, p. 24.

GARCIA, M. C.; FIRST, N. L.; GINTHER, O. J.; AND RUTLEDGE, J. J. 1980. Effect of gram-negative bacterial endotoxin, oxytocin and dexamethasone on lactation in sows. Proc 6th Int Congr Pig Vet Soc, Copenhagen, p. 67.

GLAWISCHNIG, E. 1964. Das puerperale Schweineeuter und seine klinischen Veranderungen wahrend der Laktation. Wien Tieraerztl Monatsschr 51:576–596, 675–702.

HERMANSSON, I.; EINARSSON, S.; LARSSON, K.; AND BÄCKSTRÖM, L. 1978. On the agalactia postpartum in the sow: A clinical study. Nord Vet Med 30:465–473.

JONES, J. E. T. 1976. Bacterial mastitis and endometritis in sows. Proc 4th Int Congr Pig Vet Soc, Ames, p. E6.

———. 1979. Acute coliform mastitis in the sow. Vet Annu 19:97–101.

JORSAL, S. E. 1986. Epidemiology of the MMA-syndrome, a field survey in Danish sow herds. Proc 9th Int Congr Pig Vet Soc, Barcelona, p. 93.

KING, G. J.; WILLOUGHBY, R. A.; AND HACKER, R. R. 1972. Fluctuations in rectal temperature of swine at parturition. Can Vet J 13:72–74.

LÖFSTEDT, J.; ROTH, J. A.; ROSS, R. F.; AND WAGNER, W. C. 1983. Depression of polymorphonuclear leukocyte function associated with experimentally induced *Escherichia coli* mastitis in sows. Am J Vet Res 44:1224–1228.

MCDONALD, T. J., AND MCDONALD, J. S. 1975. Intramammary infections in the sow during the peripartum period. Cornell Vet 65:73–83.

MARTIN, C. E.; HOOPER, B. E.; ARMSTRONG, C. H.; AND AMSTUTZ, H. E. 1967. A clinical and pathologic study of the mastitis-metritis-agalactia syndrome of sows. J Am Vet Med Assoc 151:1629–1634.

MIDDLETON-WILLIAMS, D. M.; POHLENZ, J.; LOTT-STOLZ, G.; AND BERTSCHINGER, H. U. 1977. Untersuchungen ueber das Mastitis-Metritis-Agalaktie-Syndrom (Milchfieber) der Sau. I. Pathologische Befunde

bei Spontanfallen. Schweiz Arch Tierheilkd 119:213–222.

MORKOC, A.; BÄCKSTRÖM, L.; LUND, L.; AND SMITH, A. R. 1983. Bacterial endotoxin in blood of dysgalactic sows in relation to microbial status of uterus, milk, and intestine. J Am Vet Med Assoc 183:786–789.

MUIRHEAD, M. R. 1976. Veterinary problems of intensive pig husbandry. Vet Rec 99:288–292.

NACHREINER, R. F., AND GINTHER, O. J. 1972. Porcine agalactia: Hematologic, serum chemical, and clinical changes during the preceding gestation. Am J Vet Res 33:799–809.

———. 1974. Induction of agalactia by administration of endotoxin (*Escherichia coli*) in swine. Am J Vet Res 35:619–622.

OLIEL, N., AND BERTSCHINGER, H. U. 1990. Prophylaxis of experimentally induced coliform mastitis in the sow with enrofloxacin (BAYTRIL®). Proc 11th Int Congr Pig Vet Soc, Lausanne, p. 186.

PERSSON, A.; PEDERSEN, A. E.; GÖRANSSON, L.; AND KUHL, W. 1989. A long-term study on the health status and performance of sows on different feed allowances during late pregnancy. I. Clinical observations, with special reference to agalactia post partum. Acta Vet Scand 30:9–17.

PLONAIT, H.; KUMP, A. W.-S.; AND SCHÖNING, G. 1986. Prophylaxis of the MMA-syndrome by antibacterial medication and restricted feeding. Proc 9th Int Congr Pig Vet Soc, Barcelona, p. 96.

RINGARP, N. 1960. Clinical and experimental investigation into a post-parturient syndrome with agalactia in sows. Acta Agric Scand [Suppl] 7.

ROSS, R. F., AND ZIMMERMANN, B. J. 1982. Control of *Escherichia coli*–induced mastitis in sows with apramycin. Proc 7th Int Congr Pig Vet Soc, Mexico City, p. 14.

ROSS, R. F.; ZIMMERMANN, B. J.; WAGNER, W. C.; AND COX, D. F. 1975. A field study of coliform mastitis in sows. J Am Vet Med Assoc 167:231–235.

ROSS, R. F.; ORNING, A. P.; WOODS, R. D.; ZIMMERMANN, B. J.; COX, D. F.; AND HARRIS, D. L. 1981. Bacteriologic study of sow agalactia. Am J Vet Res 42:949–955.

SCHONEWEIS, D. A.; HUMMELS, S.; AND SCHULTEIS, L. 1982. Levels of oxytetracycline in plasma and milk in pig. Proc 7th Int Congr Pig Vet Soc, Mexico City, p. 291.

SMITH, B. B., AND WAGNER, W. C. 1984. Suppression of prolactin in pigs by *Escherichia coli* endotoxin. Science 224:605–607.

WEGMANN, P. 1985. Zur Pathogenese der Colimastitis beim Mutterschwein. DVM thesis, Zurich.

WEGMANN, P., AND BERTSCHINGER, H. U. 1984. Sequential cytological and bacteriological examination of the secretions from sucked and unsucked mammary glands with and without mastitis. Proc 8th Int Congr Pig Vet Soc, Ghent, p. 287.

WEGMANN, P.; BERTSCHINGER, H. U.; AND JECKLIN, H. 1986. A field study on the prevalence of coliform mastitis (MMA) in Switzerland and the antimicrobial susceptibility of the coliform bacteria isolated from the milk. Proc 9th Int Congr Pig Vet Soc, Barcelona, p. 92.

Urinary Tract Infection

H. U. Bertschinger

URINARY TRACT infection (UTI) is present whenever any of the typically sterile sections of the urinary tract is colonized by microbes. UTI may or may not be accompanied by clinically manifest or subclinical disease. In the pig, specific UTI caused by *Eubacterium* (*E.*) *suis* (Chapter 51) is distinguished from nonspecific UTI caused by a variety of microbes and dealt with in this chapter.

Severe acute UTI is important to the veterinarian caring for breeding stock (Stirnimann 1984), and UTI is the predominant cause of death in pigs over 1 year of age (Häni et al. 1976). In a survey of culled sows, significant bladder colonization was detected in 17% of the sows (Colman et al. 1988); 80% of the colonized bladders exhibited histologic lesions of cystitis.

Many authors suggested a relationship between bacteriuria and reproductive disorders, including mastitis-metritis-agalactia (MMA). Sows developing MMA have a much higher prevalence of UTI in the preceding gestation period than sows with a normal puerperium (Miquet et al. 1990). According to Petersen (1983), examination of urine in late pregnancy allows recognition of sows at risk to develop MMA at subsequent farrowing. However, this view is not beyond controversy. Similar prevalences of UTI in herds with and without MMA were reported by Becker et al. (1985). Potential pathogenetic relations between UTI and MMA were discussed in detail by Berner (1988).

ETIOLOGY. Stirnimann and Tschudi (1985) gave a description of postmortem bacteriologic findings in 12 sows with acute urinary tract disease. *E. suis* was diagnosed in 9 sows, 3 of them monoinfected, by means of an immunofluorescence technique. Two or three bacterial species were isolated from the 9 sows not monoinfected: *E. coli* (7 sows), *Streptococcus* sp. (5 sows), *Staphylococcus epidermidis* (2 sows), *Klebsiella* sp. (1 sow), *Pseudomonas* sp. (1 sow), *Aeromonas* sp. and *Bacteroides* sp. (1 sow).

Urine was obtained from 90 sows with severe acute urinary tract disease by means of a catheter (Stirnimann 1984). *E. suis* was again looked for by immunofluorescence, but was detected in only 10 sows. Thirty-seven sows were monoinfected. The bacterial spectrum was comparable to that described above.

In aspirates taken at a slaughterhouse from 114 sow bladders with significant colonization, Colman et al. (1988) identified *E. coli* (81 sows), diverse gram-negative rods (4 sows), *S. aureus* (11

sows), *S. hyicus* (3 sows), *Enterococcus faecalis* (6 sows), *Enterococcus faecium* (3 sows), *S. dysgalactiae* (5 sows) and diverse gram-positive bacteria (7 sows). *E. suis* was not detected by anaerobic culture. These figures suggest a higher prevalence of *E. suis* in sows with severe urinary tract disease. Furthermore, nonspecific UTI cannot be regarded as a disease exclusively caused by *E. coli*.

The urinary tract is a dynamic microbiologic ecosystem (Berner 1981a,b). Components of the flora may increase and decrease in numbers and eventually disappear. Dominant bacterial species change spontaneously in a significant proportion of sows surveyed over prolonged periods (Berner 1990). These changes become more frequent when sows are treated with antimicrobials.

EPIDEMIOLOGY. Nonspecific UTI behaves like a noncontagious infectious disease of endogenous origin. In the canine species, *E. coli* isolates from urine and from rectal samples of the same dog show identity in extended phenotypic and genotypic tests (Low et al. 1988). Corresponding studies with the pig are lacking. The fecal flora may achieve access to the urinary tract more efficiently in females than in males. Under intensive confinement conditions the vulva of sows is often placed in direct contact with feces (Smith 1983). The dog-sitting position helps to force fecal material into the vagina. Sows resting for long periods void urine at longer intervals. However, housing conditions have not yet been studied with respect to UTI.

The age distribution of UTI favors the concept of continuous exposure to fecal contamination. The prevalence of UTI increases from 18% in young sows with 1–3 litters to 38% in old sows with 7 and more litters (Becker et al. 1985). In another study the prevalence of cystitis rises from about 16% in gilts and young sows with 1–4 litters to 42% in old sows with 8 and more litters (Akkermans 1984).

PATHOGENESIS. In humans colonization of the lower genital tract and of the urinary tract by *E. coli* is greatly facilitated by adhesive fimbriae. Such fimbriae are also present in canine *E. coli* isolates from the urinary tract (Low et al. 1988), whereas porcine isolates have not yet been checked for adhesins. It is assumed that most agents ascend through the urethra (Smith 1983). Invasion is favored by the short, wide urethra of the female pig; the relaxation of the sphincter muscle in late pregnancy and puerperium; trauma to urethra and bladder at coitus and parturition;

abnormal bacterial colonization of the sinus urogenitalis and the genital organs; incomplete closure of the vulva; and catheterization of the bladder (Berner 1988). Repeated examination of individual sows led to the conclusion that asymptomatic bacteriuria may temporarily deteriorate to cystitis with spontaneous remission (Berner 1988). Carr et al. (1990) postulate that bacterial colonization leads to shortening and deformation of the ureteric valve and thereby promotes vesicoureteric reflux. The latter could be easily demonstrated postmortem in cases of acute pyelonephritis.

Serum antibody against the infecting *E. coli* strain can regularly be detected in sows with pyelonephritis, less often in sows with cystitis, and rather rarely in sows with asymptomatic bacteriuria (Wagner 1990). *E. coli* strains may persist in the urinary tract despite high antibody concentrations in the urine.

UTI predisposes to MMA in one or several ways (Berner 1988). Ascending invasion of the uterus at parturition and of the mammary glands from contamination of the lying area appear most likely. However, other routes cannot be ruled out. Identical OK serotypes of *E. coli* were found in the urinary bladder and in the uterus of three sows and in the bladder and in the mammary gland of one out of nine sows with MMA, killed for postmortem examination (Bertschinger et al. 1977).

CLINICAL SIGNS.

In the vast majority of nonspecific UTI cases there are no clinical signs (Berner 1988). Akkermans and Pomper (1980) concluded from an extended field study that sows with a significant bacteriuria tend to wean small litters, have increased intervals between litters, show a lower fertility rate, and exhibit an inferior body condition. In many sows with cystitis, careful observation reveals abnormal urination (Becker et al. 1988). The sows stand in one place before they void urine in small quantities with straining. They are more often seen in a dog-sitting position.

Vulval discharge may appear as dried deposits around the vulva or more often as a pool on the floor underneath the sows (Dial and MacLachlan 1988a). The discharge may be mucoid, mucohemorrhagic, or purulent and is observed most often during the final phase of urination. However, discharge may result from inflammation of any part of the urogenital tract. Significant discharge is more often the consequence of endometritis than of UTI.

Severe pyelonephritis becomes clinically manifest during the first 2 weeks postpartum in 40% of the cases (Stirnimann 1984). Typical cases exhibit a rectal temperature below 38.0°C, a heart rate over 120, polypnea, cyanosis, ataxia, and more rarely generalized tremor (Stimimann and Tschudi 1985). The blood concentrations of urea and creatinine are higher than normal.

LESIONS.

Berner (1981) examined 118 culled sows for bacteria and lesions. Twenty-six out of 29 sows with a UTI presented a cystitis, and 12 sows presented an additional pyelonephritis.

The gross lesions of cystitis begin as focal or diffuse mucosal hyperemia (Dial and MacLachlan 1988b). Subsequently, there may be mucosal ulceration with fibrinopurulent exudate over affected areas. The bladder wall becomes thickened. Similar lesions occur in the ureters and the renal pelvis if infection ascends the urinary tract. In pyelonephritis the inflammatory process extends into the renal parenchyma. Wedge-shaped foci extend from the distorted pelvis to the cortex. Fibrosis of the kidneys may occur with time.

DIAGNOSIS.

Mere clinical examination of the animal is of little value in the diagnosis of UTI (Stirnimann 1984); urine must be examined in most cases. Bacteriology of the urinary tract is complicated by the normal flora colonizing the vagina and the distal part of the urethra and by comprising species associated with UTI as well. Therefore, distinction between contamination and infection is based on the number of bacteria in the urine. In human medicine, a viable count of 10^5 CFU/ml is interpreted as indicative of infection and 10^4 CFU/ml as suspicious. These limits are used in porcine medicine as well (Berner 1971; Stirnimann 1984; Colman et al. 1988). High bacterial density results in cloudiness of the urine and can be recognized if counts exceed 10^7 CFU/ml (Berner 1971). Dip slides, i.e., commercially available slides covered by bacterial culture media give satisfactory quantitative results when used with porcine urine (Berner 1971; Akkermans and Pomper 1980). Dip slides have the shortcoming that anaerobes such as *E. suis* and slow growers will be missed. Urine samples can be obtained from sows either by means of a catheter or by spontaneous voiding. Catheterization of the sow is possible (Stirnimann 1984) but does not circumvent contamination and involves the risk of setting up a new UTI. Voiding can be induced by rousing the sows in the morning before feeding time (Becker et al. 1985). When collecting midstream urine, the attendant should avoid contact with the urine, which may contain zoonotic agents such as leptospires.

Diagnostic test strips are applicable to the urine of pigs except for nitrite. The latter test has a too-low sensitivity due to the low nitrate concentration in porcine urine (Becker et al. 1985). The most useful parameters are protein, hemoglobin, and pH. Cytologic examination may allow discrimination between mere bacteriuria, cystitis, and pyelonephritis. The presence and concentrations of antibodies in the urine are not well correlated with the severity of the condition (Wagner 1990). Test strips permit the rapid determination of blood urea (Stirnimann 1984). Concentrations greater than 10 mmol/L indicate uremia. In the case of vaginal discharge, differential diagnosis may be based on infertility in sows with endometritis (Dial and MacLachlan 1988a).

TREATMENT. Nearly all the treatments recommended in the literature are aimed at elimination of the bacteria by antimicrobials. The variable susceptibilities of the diverse bacteria involved and the frequent acquisition of R factors pose considerable problems (Table 39.4). With regard to the observed changes of infecting bacterial species or types in the course of antimicrobial treatments, Berner (1990) recommended the use of either broad-spectrum or combined antimicrobials and suggested intensifying the search for alternative strategies.

Becker et al. (1988) treated 9 sows twice daily for 2 weeks via feed with sulfadimidine, 1.0 g; sulfathiazole, 1.0 g; and trimethoprim, 0.4 g/sow. Significant bacteriuria was present in 2 sows 1 week after the treatment and in 3 sows 7 weeks later. The same substances applied over 4 days gave much inferior results. Gentamicin, 2.5 mg/kg body weight, was injected intramuscularly to 15 sows on the first day, followed by 2.0 mg on the next 3 days. One week after this treatment, 10 sows were free of significant bacteriuria. The authors concluded that prolonged treatment should be preferred. Antimicrobial resistance was not checked.

Treatment of severely affected sows was reported by Stirnimann (1988). With 34 sows each, injection of ampicillin, 3 g/sow daily, for 4 days was compared with the same antibiotic combined with novaminsulfon 10 g/sow. The combined treatment led to a smaller number of emergency slaughters. Subclinical UTI persisted in about half of the successfully treated sows.

Dial and MacLachlan (1988b) concluded that treatment of urogenital infections of swine generally is frustrating.

PREVENTION. Results of long-term prospective studies are not available. Berner (1988) recommended that all pregnant sows be checked repeatedly for UTI and that positive sows be treated with antimicrobials shortly before parturition. Smith (1983) suggested medicating all dry sows on problem farms for 7–10 days at 6-week intervals. The interval between treatments can be increased gradually as experience dictates. Antibiotics such as tetracyclines or a suitable form of penicillin have been successfully used in the diet. In view of the disappointing results reported by Berner (1990), these recommendations should be viewed with caution.

According to Wagner (1990), immunoprophylaxis holds little promise. Thus, Smith (1983) recommended to reduce environmental exposure by improving fecal drainage and housing conditions. These factors as well as the role of water intake should be further investigated. Frequency of urination was increased by giving access to an exercise yard and by increasing water intake, which was achieved by a salt content of 1% in the diet (Smith 1983).

REFERENCES

AKKERMANS, J. P. W. M. 1984. Analysis of pathological observations in 1445 sows. Proc 8th Int Congr Pig Vet Soc, Ghent, p. 366.

AKKERMANS, J. P. W. M., AND POMPER, W. 1980. The significance of a bacteriuria with reference to disturbances in fertility. Proc 6th Int Congr Pig Vet Soc, Copenhagen, p. 44.

Table 39.4. Antimicrobial sensitivity of significant isolates from porcine UTI in Belgium and Switzerland

| | Rate of Sensitive Isolates (%) | | |
| | Colman et al. 1988 | | Stirnimann 1988 |
Substance	Gram-negative (n = 62)	Gram-positive (n = 18)	E. coli (n = 21)
Penicillin G	NT	44	NT
Penicillinase-stable penicillins	NT	72	NT
Ampicillin	68	44	71
Amoxicillin and clavulanic acid	100	72	NT
Streptomycin	40	44	NT
Neomycin	98	61	86
Spectinomycin	85	72	NT
Gentamicin	100	61	100
Tetracycline	47	61	33
Chloramphenicol	82	83	67
Nitrofuran	95	94	14
Sulfonamide	37	50	52
Trimethoprim	76	61	NT
Trimethoprim and sulfonamide	NT	NT	76
Macrolide	NT	61	NT
Lincomycin	NT	72	NT

Note: NT = not tested.

Becker, H.-A.; Kurtz, R.; and Von Mickwitz, G. 1985. Chronische Harnwegsinfektionen beim Schwein, Diagnose und Therapie (I). Prakt Tieraerztl 66:1006–1011.

———. 1988. Chronische Harnwegsinfektionen beim Schwein, Diagnose und Therapie (III). Prakt Tieraerztl 69:41–45.

Berner, H. 1971. Die Bedeutung chronischer Erkrankungen der Harnwege bei der Entstehung von Puerperalstörungen und Mastitiden der Muttersau. Dtsch Tieraerztl Wochenschr 78:233–256.

———. 1981a. Untersuchungen zum Vorkommen von Harnwegsinfektionen beim Schwein. 1. Mitteilung: Harnwegsinfektionen bei Muttersauen in Ferkelerzeugerbetrieben. Tieraerztl Umsch 36:162–171.

———. 1981b. Untersuchungen zum Vorkommen von Harnwegsinfektionen bei Muttersauen. 2. Mitteilung: Harnwegsinfektionen bei Schlachtschweinen. Tieraerztl Umsch 36:250–255.

———. 1988. Cystitis in der MMA–Diagnostik. Prakt Tieraerztl 69: 124–131.

———. 1990. Erregerwechsel als Ursache von Misserfolgen bei der Therapie bakteriell bedingter Krankheiten der Urogenitalorgane des Schweines. Dtsch Tieraerztl Wochenschr 97:20–24.

Bertschinger, H. U.; Pohlenz, J.; and Hemlep, I. 1977. Untersuchungen über das Mastitis-Metritis-Agalaktie-Syndrom (Milchfieber) der Sau. Schweiz Arch Tierheilkd 119:223–233.

Carr, J.; Walton, J. R.; and Done, S. H. 1990. Observations on the intravesicular portion of the ureter from healthy pigs and those with urinary tract disease. Proc 11th Int Congr Pig Vet Soc, Lausanne, p. 286.

Colman, J.; Devriese, L.; and Verdonck, M. 1988. Bacteriuria and urinary tract infection in sows. Vlaams Diergeneesk Tijdschr 57:192–198.

Dial, G., and MacLachlan, N. J. 1988a. Urogenital infections of swine. I. Clinical manifestations and pathogenesis. Compend Contin Educ 10:63–71.

———. 1988b. Urogenital infections of swine. II. Pathology and medical management. Compend Contin Educ 10:529–540.

Häni, H.; Brändli, A.; Luginbühl, H.; and König, H. 1976. Vorkommen und Bedeutung von Schweinekrankheiten: Analyse eines Sektionsgutes (1971–1973). Schweiz Arch Tierheilkd 118:1–11.

Low, D. A.; Braaten, B. A.; Ling, G. V.; Johnson, D. L.; and Ruby, A. L. 1988. Isolation and comparison of *Escherichia coli* strains from canine and human patients with urinary tract infections. Infect Immun 56:2601–2609.

Miquet, J. M.; Madec, F.; and Paboeuf, F. 1990. Epidemiology of farrowing disorders in the sow. Preliminary results of a prospective inquiry in 2 farms. Proc 11th Int Congr Pig Vet Soc, Lausanne, p. 472.

Petersen, B. 1983. Methods of early recognition of puerperal and fertility disorders in the sow. Livest Prod Sci 10:253–264.

Smith, W. J. 1983. Cystitis in sows. Pig News Inf 4:279–281.

Stirnimann, J. 1984. Akute Harnwegsentzündung bei der Muttersau. Schweiz Arch Tierheilkd 126:597–605.

———. 1988. Zur Behandlung der akuten Harnwegsentzündung bei der Muttersau. Schweiz Arch Tierheilkd 130:605–611.

Stirnimann, J., and Tschudi, P. R. 1985. Beurteilung der Nierenfunktion bei Muttersauen mit akuter Harnwegsentzündung. Schweiz Arch Tierheilkd 127:575–582.

Wagner, S. 1990. Die Immunreaktion bei der durch *Escherichia coli* bedingten chronischen Harnwegsinfektion des weiblichen Schweines. DVM thesis, Univ of München, Germany.

40 Exudative Epidermitis

D. J. Taylor

EXUDATIVE EPIDERMITIS has been known by its clinical signs for nearly 150 years (Spinola 1842). The classic disease occurs in piglets in which a generalized dermatitis leads to dehydration and death; weaners and even adults may also be affected. Early occurrence and distribution have been comprehensively reviewed by Jones (1956), who provided a good description of the disease and its effects on production. It has been recorded in most pig-rearing countries both in piglets and weaners. Major studies have been carried out by Sompolinsky (1953), Jones (1956), Underdahl et al. (1963; 1965), L'Ecuyer (1966), L'Ecuyer and Jericho (1966), and Hunter et al. (1970). The condition is of sporadic occurrence in all countries but may be of importance in individual herds (Pepper and Taylor 1977).

ETIOLOGY. *Staphylococcus hyicus* ssp. *hyicus* is the causal agent of the generalized form of the disease seen in piglets, but although it is present in profuse culture in the lesions of adult pigs, the disease has not been reproduced in that age group. It has been shown to colonize skin lesions produced by swine pox and can be isolated from superficial wound infections in pigs on infected farms. *S. hyicus* was first described by Sompolinsky (1953) as *Micrococcus hyicus* and then defined as a staphylococcus by Baird-Parker (1965). *S. hyicus* ssp. *hyicus* was first separated from *S. hyicus* ssp. *chromogenes,* a nonpathogen, by Devriese et al. (1978). The organism is a grampositive coccus, which forms 3- to 4-mm white nonhemolytic colonies on sheep blood agar after 24-hours incubation. It is generally coagulase negative, and is DNAase positive, phosphatase positive, mannitol and acetoin negative, and hyaluronidase positive. These biochemical characteristics are of value in distinguishing the organism by conventional means from other staphylococci found in pigs (Devriese 1977). At least six serologic types have been identified (Hunter et al. 1970; Park and Kang 1987) and at least five of these may be isolated from clinically affected animals. There are antigenic and other differences between pig strains of *S. hyicus* ssp. *hyicus* and those isolated from cattle and other animals.

EPIDEMIOLOGY. The disease occurs most commonly following the introduction of carrier animals to a nonimmune herd and affects successive litters of piglets, usually those born to nonimmune sows. All litters in an affected herd may be affected and up to 70% of affected piglets may die. Outbreaks are usually self-limiting and last 2–3 months but may persist if fresh nonimmune sows are brought into infected buildings or exposed to infected animals. Disease may persist where husbandry conditions such as coarse sawdust bedding, fighting in piglets, and poorly finished or worn caging are present. High humidity may also increase the incidence of the disease. Reasons for the spread of the acute localized disease in adults are not clear and it may be associated with mange, other mite infections, or causes of local abrasions. It is not clear whether cases occur only in nonimmune sows. *S. hyicus* ssp. *hyicus* can be recovered from nasal mucosa of healthy pigs (7%), from conjunctiva (12%), skin of the snout or ear (16%) (Hajsig et al. 1985), and from the vagina in sows (17%) (Elliott 1986). The organism can persist for some weeks on fittings and has been recovered from a number of other species such as horses, dogs, cattle, goats, and chickens, but these hosts may be of little importance as sources of infection for pigs. Phage-typing studies indicate that diseased pigs, healthy pigs, cattle, and poultry share phage types of *S. hyicus* ssp. *hyicus* (Shimizu et al. 1987); however, recent work on isolates from pigs suggests that only they carry plasmids (Schwarz and Blobel 1989) and that protein A is absent from cattle and chicken isolates (Takeuchi et al. 1988), suggesting that they represent separate populations.

PATHOGENESIS. Application of pure cultures of *S. hyicus* ssp. *hyicus* to the skin of a nonimmune pig is sufficient to reproduce the disease (Underdahl et al. 1965; L'Ecuyer and Jericho 1966), but it can also be produced by subcutaneous injection in specific-pathogen-free (SPF) piglets (Underdahl et al. 1965; Wegener 1990). Conventional animals may be resistant to such applications. Immunity may be an important protective factor, but recent studies suggest that other elements of the skin flora, especially other staphylococci, may contribute to this resistance to colonization (Jones 1985). Trauma from fighting, unclipped teeth, rough bedding, or pen walls may allow the organism to cause disease. The earliest changes are seen as skin reddening accompanying the multiplication of the organism on the skin surface and its growth between the corneocytes of the epidermis where microcolonies develop. Inflammation occurs and there is a marked hyperplasia of the stratum corneum, invasion by neutrophils, with an increase in thickness of the epidermis, followed by its erosion. The stratum germinativum becomes disorganized and penetrates deeply into the dermis. Clinical signs develop in gnotobiotic piglets when the number of organisms on the skin exceeds $10^5/cm^2$ (Allaker et al. 1988). Attachment of the organism may be associated with the production of protein A, for strains producing the protein have been shown to adhere to tissue culture cells (Teranishi et al. 1988), resistance to phagocytosis may result from the production of a capsule, and the epidermal erosion may be associated with the production of exfoliative factors demonstrable in culture supernates of the organism (Wegener 1990). These changes are accompanied by an excess in sebaceous secretion and serous exudate. The organism is present in large numbers in the skin and may be isolated from the draining lymph nodes, but it does not cause septicemia consistently. The mortality associated with this disease results from dehydration.

CLINICAL SIGNS.   Piglets develop the disease between 4–6 days and 5 weeks of age. Clinical signs begin with dejection and a reddish or coppery skin color. Thin, pale brown scales of exudate develop in the axillae and groin and within 3–5 days spread to all parts of the body and rapidly become dark in color and greasy in texture (Fig. 40.1).

The skin of affected piglets is often hot to the touch, the hair coat is matted, and exudate may extend to the eyelashes. Ulcers may occur in the mouth and separation of horn may occur at the bulbs of the heels. Anorexia and dehydration are

features of this disease. Severely affected piglets lose weight rapidly and may die within 24 hours; death usually occurs within 3–10 days. There is no pruritis and fever is not common. Not all piglets in a litter are affected to the same extent and some individuals will suffer from chronic disease in which smaller areas of the body are involved. Mildly affected piglets may have a yellowish skin, appear hairy, and have only a few flakes of exudate in the axillae or groin or near facial scratches, damage on the knees, or adjacent to badly clipped teeth. Growth depression is marked in survivors and productivity of the herd may be depressed by up to 35% during an outbreak and up to 9% in the year following infection (Pepper and Taylor 1977). Disease may occur in weaned pigs, but in this age group presents as an acute disease resulting in growth depression rather than death.

Disease in adults varies in severity but occurs as localized lesions on the back or flanks. Mild forms may appear as brownish areas of exudative epidermitis, but in some cases, there may be ulceration (Smith et al. 1990).

LESIONS

Gross Lesions.   The carcasses of pigs that have died from exudative epidermitis are dehydrated and emaciated. The skin is thickened and sometimes edematous. The superficial lymph nodes are usually edematous and swollen. Few other gross lesions are present. Most animals have empty stomachs, and urate crystals may be seen in the medulla of the kidney on section. There is often an accumulation of mucoid or crystalline material in the pelvis of the kidney and pyelonephritis may be present.

Microscopic Lesions.   Inflammatory changes are seen in histologic sections of the skin with

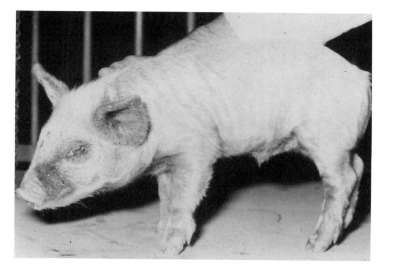

40.1. 10-day-old piglet with exudative epidermitis.

bacterial microcolonies in the keratinized layer of the epidermis accompanied by neutrophil infiltration and capillary dilatation in the dermis. The stratum germinativum often extends into the dermis in the form of rete pegs.

Bacteriology. *S. hyicus* ssp. *hyicus* can usually be isolated from the lesions and from the superficial lymph nodes in early untreated cases, but may be difficult to demonstrate if treatment has been given or if secondary infection by *Proteus* sp. and *Pseudomonas aeruginosa* has occurred. *Dermatophilus* sp. has been recovered from some cases.

DIAGNOSIS. The clinical signs are generally sufficient to reach a diagnosis in young piglets. The lack of fever or of pruritis and the generalized nature of the lesions, their appearance, and the variation in severity within an affected litter are all features suggestive of the disease. Confirmation may be obtained by histologic and bacteriologic means. It may be necessary to confirm the identity of the staphylococci isolated as *S. hyicus* ssp. *hyicus* by conventional bacteriologic means (Devriese 1977) or by use of strip tests such as the Staph-Zym test (Lammler 1989). These have the advantage of revealing the identity of non–*S. hyicus* staphylococci. Diagnosis is less easy when the lesions are mild, localized around predisposing lesions such as fight wounds, or have been treated. The demonstration of *S. hyicus* and response to antimicrobials may help confirm uncomplicated disease of this type, but the organism may be present in lesions caused by a number of initiating agents. Other skin conditions that may be confused with exudative epidermitis include swine pox (localized lesions, rarely fatal), mange (pruritis, demonstration of mites), ringworm (expanding superficial lesions, isolation of fungus), pityriasis rosea (expanding circles, nonfatal, lesions not greasy), zinc deficiency (weaners, symmetrical, dry lesions), dermatosis vegetans (inherited in Landrace, fatal pneumonitis), and local wounds such as facial fight wounds and abraded knees in piglets and crate injuries in adults.

The organism may be isolated from other pathologic conditions such as arthritis in piglets (Noda and Fukui 1986) and cystitis in sows as well as from the skins of healthy pigs.

TREATMENT. Treatment is most successful if carried out early in the disease; severely affected animals may not respond. *S. hyicus* is sensitive to many antibiotics but resistance to one or more antimicrobials may occur as in other staphylococcal infections (Teranishi et al. 1987). Antimicrobial treatment with a suitable antimicrobial such as penicillin, ampicillin, tylosin, lincomycin, trimethoprim sulphonamide, or cephalosporins should be accompanied by the provision of a fluid replacer or at least clean water for affected

piglets and by local treatment with skin disinfectants such as cetrimide or hexocil. Treatment may have to be continued for up to 5 days, and clinically affected piglets may make a slow recovery or remain stunted.

There are suggestions that vaccination of sows with autogenous bacterins made from strains isolated on the affected farm may be of value in protecting the litters of newly purchased sows when given before farrowing. Recovery of single serologic types from related outbreaks and from all piglets in affected litters (Park and Kang 1987) suggests that this approach may be effective.

The incidence of the disease may be reduced by clipping the teeth of litters at risk, by ensuring that pen surfaces are not abrasive, and by providing soft bedding, such as softwood sawdusts or chaffed straw. Sows entering farrowing accommodations should be washed and disinfected and placed in clean, disinfected, or fumigated pens. Prompt treatment of local lesions on both sows and piglets may also help. The prevention of disease by early colonization of the skin using nonpathogenic strains has been demonstrated experimentally in gnotobiotic piglets (Allaker et al. 1988) but has not yet been shown to work in the field.

REFERENCES

ALLAKER, R. P.; LLOYD, D. H.; AND SMITH, I. M. 1988. Prevention of exudative epidermitis in gnotobiotic piglets by bacterial interference. Vet Rec 123:287–288.

BAIRD-PARKER, A. C. 1965. The classification of staphylococci and micrococci from world-wide sources. J Gen Microbiol 38:363–387.

DEVRIESE, L. A. 1977. Isolation and identification of *Staphylococcus hyicus*. Am J Vet Res 38:787–792.

DEVRIESE, L. A.; HAJEK, V.; OEDING, P.; MEYER, S. A.; AND SCHLIEFER, K. H. 1978. *Staphylococcus hyicus* (Sompolinsky 1953) comb. nov. and *Staphylococcus hyicus* subsp. *chromogenes* subsp. nov. Int J Syst Bacteriol 28:482–490.

ELLIOTT, G. 1986. Porcine bacterial flora. Vet Rec 118:251.

HAJSIG, D.; BABIC, T.; AND MADIC, J. 1985. Exudative epidermitis in piglets. II. Distribution of *Staphylococcus hyicus* subsp. *hyicus*. Findings in healthy piglets. Vet Arh 55:45–51.

HUNTER, D.; TODD, J. N.; AND LARKIN, M. 1970. Exudative epidermitis of pigs. Br Vet J 126:225–229.

JONES, L. D. 1956. Exudative epidermitis of pigs. Am J Vet Res 17:179–193.

JONES, M. A. 1985. Studies on the bacterial flora of the skin of the pig with particular reference to *Staphylococcus hyicus*. M.S. thesis, Royal Veterinary College, Univ of London.

LAMMLER, C. 1989. Evaluation of the Staph-Zym system for identification of *Staphylococcus hyicus* and *Staphylococcus intermedius*. J Vet Med [B] 36:180–184.

L'ECUYER, C. 1966. Exudative epidermitis in pigs. Clinical studies and preliminary transmission trials. Can J Comp Med 30:9–16.

L'ECUYER, C., AND JERICHO, K. 1966. Exudative epidermitis in pigs. Etiological studies and pathology. Can J Comp Med 30:94–101.

NODA, K., AND FUKUI, T. 1986. Outbreaks of pyogenic arthritis in newborn piglets and stillbirth caused by *S.*

hyicus subsp. *hyicus.* Jpn J Vet Med Assoc 39:305–310.

PARK, C. K., AND KANG, B. K. 1987. Studies on exudative epidermitis in pigs. II. Serological typing of *Staphylococcus hyicus* subsp. *hyicus* isolated from pigs. Korean J Vet Res 27:47–52.

PEPPER, T. A., AND TAYLOR, D. J. 1977. The effect of exudative epidermitis on weaner production in a small pig herd. Vet Rec 101:204–205.

SCHWARZ, S., AND BLOBEL, H. 1989. Plasmids and resistance to antimicrobials and heavy metals in *Staphylococcus hyicus* from pigs and cattle. J Vet Med [B] 36:669–677.

SHIMIZU, A.; TERANISHI, H.; KOWANO, J.; AND KIMURA, S. 1987. Phage patterns of *Staphylococcus hyicus* subsp. *hyicus* isolated from chickens, cattle and pigs. Zentralbl Bakteriol Microbiol Hyg 265:57–61.

SMITH, W. J.; TAYLOR, D. J.; AND PENNY, R. H. C. 1990. A Colour Atlas of Diseases and Disorders of the Pig. London: Wolfe Publishing Ltd, pp. 113–114.

SOMPOLINSKY, D. 1953. De l'impetigo contagiosa suis. Schweiz Arch Tierheilkd 95:302–309.

SPINOLA, J. 1842. Die Krankheiten der Schweine. Berlin: Verlag Hirschwald, pp. 146–148.

TAKEUCHI, S.; KOBAYASHI, Y.; MOROSUMI, T.; AND MORI, Y. 1988. Protein A in *Staphylococcus hyicus* subsp. *hyicus* isolated from pigs, chickens and cows. Jpn J Vet Sci 50:153–157.

TERANISHI, H.; SHIMIZU, A.; KOWANO, J.; AND KIMURA, S. 1987. Antibiotic resistance of *Staphylococcus hyicus* subsp. *hyicus* strains isolated from pigs, cattle and chickens. Jpn J Vet Sci 49:427–432.

_____. 1988. Comparative adhesion of Protein A positive and Protein A negative strains of *Staphylococcus hyicus* subsp. *hyicus* to Vero cells. Jpn J Vet Sci 50:825–827.

UNDERDAHL, N. R.; GRACE, P. D.; AND YOUNG, G. A. 1963. Experimental transmission of exudative epidermitis of pigs. J Am Vet Med Assoc 142:754–762.

UNDERDAHL, N. R.; GRACE, P. D.; AND TWIEHAUS, M. J. 1965. Porcine exudative epidermitis: Characterisation of bacterial agent. Am J Vet Res 26:617–624.

WEGENER, H. C. 1990. Studies on *Staphylococcus hyicus* virulence in relation to exudative epidermitis in piglets. Proc Int Pig Vet Soc 11:197.

41 *Haemophilus parasuis*

J. Nicolet

SINCE THE observation of a small gram-negative organism (Glässer 1910) associated with a fibrinous serositis and polyarthritis and the isolation of *H. influenzae suis* from the respiratory tract of swine affected with the virus of swine influenza (Lewis and Shope 1931), many observations have been made on this subject. The entity of the serositis-arthritis syndrome was settled by Hjärre and Wramby (1943), and the name of the etiologic agent was shortened to *H. suis.* Although its identity with *H. influenzae suis* was assumed, the exact role of *H. suis* in the respiratory tract was not clearly defined, since this bacterium was not only found associated with pathologic lesions but also in the bacterial flora of normal pigs. This rather unclear situation existed because *Haemophilus* bacteria are fastidious organisms, the characterization of which has been neglected for a long time.

Extensive taxonomic studies by Kilian (1976) showed that collected strains designated as *H. suis* are in reality *H. parasuis.* This generic name is accepted for the designation of the infectious agent of porcine polyserositis and arthritis and of strains found opportunistically in the respiratory tract of swine.

ETIOLOGY. The etiologic agent of porcine polyserositis and arthritis (or Glässer's disease) is *H. parasuis.* It is a small pleomorphic gram-negative rod, varying from a coccobacillary form to slender filaments. Growth is supported only on media containing nicotinamide-adenine dinucleotide (NAD) (heated blood agar, Levinthal agar) or on blood agar in the vicinity of a streak of a staphylococcus strain (satellitism). Visible growth occurs generally after 36–48 hours incubation.

A serologic investigation by Bakos (1955) showed that strains isolated from Glässer's disease belong mostly to groups B and C; a few others belong to groups A, D, and N. However, serologic group B contains only strains from Glässer's disease; other groups also have strains from the respiratory tract. Morozumi and Nicolet (1986a) pointed out the heterogeneity of *H. parasuis* strains isolated from different pathologic conditions. Using extracts from autoclaved cells, seven distinct serovars have so far been identified with an agar-gel-precipitation test (Bloch 1985; Morozumi and Nicolet 1986b), including strains of Bakos's groups A and B. It has further been

demonstrated by DNA-hybridization assays that serovar 5 (corresponding to Bakos's group B), with a 40% rate of homology with other strains, may even represent a subspecies of *H. parasuis* (Morozumi et al. 1986). Serovar 5 is commonly isolated from cases of septicemia or polyserositis-arthritis.

EPIDEMIOLOGY. Porcine polyserositis-arthritis is found worldwide. It is sporadic in occurrence and is generally limited to one farm with a variable rate of morbidity. The disease usually affects young pigs (2 weeks to 4 months), principally after the weaning period (5–8 weeks old). Mortality may reach 50%. However, the epidemiologic picture in specific-pathogen-free (SPF) swine may be different, since when older pigs contract the disease, they may have a much higher morbidity (Baehler et al. 1974; Nielsen and Danielsen 1975).

Haemophilus parasuis is also commonly found in the nasal cavities of swine (Harris et al. 1969; Bertschinger and Nicod 1970) but not (or rarely) in normal lungs (Little 1970). On the other hand, *H. parasuis* is commonly involved (45.5%) in pneumonia lesions resembling enzootic pneumonia (Little 1970). This suggests that *H. parasuis* is a common opportunistic invader causing pulmonary infection only in association with viral, mycoplasmal, or other bacterial agents as in swine influenza (Lewis and Shope 1931).

It is obvious that the virulence properties of the *H. parasuis* strains differ remarkably. Although many attempts have been made to associate virulence with phenotypic features by polyacrylamide gel electrophoresis (PAGE) with whole cell proteins (Nicolet et al. 1980), PAGE with outer membrane proteins (OMPs) (Rapp et al. 1986), and serovars (Morozumi and Nicolet 1986a, b; Kielstein et al. 1990), the situation remains unclear. However, it seems that, in addition to serovar, OMP may be an important indicator of pathogenic potential of an isolate (Rapp-Gabrielson and Gabrielson 1990).

CLINICAL SIGNS. The onset of clinical signs is usually sudden; symptoms can also occur over a period of several days in a single pig or in several animals. Even an enzootic outbreak is possible (Nielsen and Danielsen 1975). The course of the disease is peracute or acute, and often the

526

heaviest pigs are affected.

The clinical signs are described as various syndromes, depending on the localization of the inflammatory lesions. Initially, the body temperature increases, ranging from 104.9°F (40.5°C) to 107.6°F (42°C). Apathy, inappetence, and finally anorexia follow. The peripheral circulation fails, and cyanosis is visible on the skin of the peripheral parts of the body. Subcutaneous edema of the eyelids and the ears is occasionally observed. The conjunctivae are often reddened. The respiration can be normal but can also be altered in the form of dyspnea. Diseased animals get up often and indicate pain by squealing. They walk slowly with lameness and often sit like dogs. One or more joints are swollen, warm, and painful. The carpal and tarsal joints seem to be more often affected than others.

In many cases pigs show symptoms of a meningoencephalitis. The affected pigs show muscular tremor. They walk slowly, with incoordination of the hind legs. Often, pigs are in lateral recumbency and make struggling attempts to rise. The septicemic form of the disease in 1- to 2-week-old piglets has been reported by Thomson and Ruhnke (1963).

LESIONS. The necropsy findings are principally of a fibrinous or serofibrinous meningitis, pleuritis, pericarditis, peritonitis, and arthritis that occur in various combinations and occasionally singly. The involvement of the central nervous system is predominant. This was confirmed in an outbreak in SPF pigs, where 62.2% of the animals showed a leptomeningitis (Nielsen and Danielsen 1975).

The histopathologic features are those of a fibrinopurulent inflammation with infiltration of many neutrophils and some mononuclear cells (Hjärre and Wramby 1943).

DIAGNOSIS. The diagnosis of porcine polyserositis-arthritis is based on the history (mixing of animals of different origin), clinical signs, and necropsy findings. A bacteriologic confirmation is required. However, the isolation of the etiologic agent is not in every case successful (Nielsen and Danielsen 1975). The most reliable medium for isolation seems to be sheep, horse, or ox blood agar streaked with a staphylococcus. Some improvement of the isolation rate may be reached by using a selective medium containing bacitracin or crystal violet (Little 1970) or by culturing pathologic specimens in broth with added NAD. After 48 hours incubation, the presence of *Haemophilus* is detected by subculturing on suitable plates (Neil et al. 1969). Final identification, particularly of respiratory isolates, must include differentiation between microaerophilic *Haemophilus* sp. of taxon C (Kilian 1976), urease-negative and indolpositive *Haemophilus* sp. (Rapp et al. 1985), and hemolytic urease-positive *Haemophilus* sp. of the

"minor group" taxon (Kilian et al. 1978).

Other septicemic bacterial infections (*Streptococcus suis, Erysipelothrix rhusiopathiae*) must be considered in the differential diagnosis. Infections caused by *Mycoplasma hyorhinis* also should be taken into account. However, the symptoms of mycoplasmosis are generally milder and more chronic, with a low morbidity and are rarely accompanied by meningitis. When nervous symptoms are observed, the suspicion of *Escherichia coli* enterotoxemia and a viral infection (Teschen or Aujeszky's disease) must be eliminated on the basis of epidemiologic, microbiologic, and histopathologic investigations.

TREATMENT. It is important to start therapeutic measures as early as possible after the manifestation of clinical signs. The initial treatment must be given parenterally. Treatment should be repeated after an interval of 24 hours. All pigs in an affected group must be treated in addition to those showing clinical symptoms. High therapeutic doses are usually required for penetration of cerebrospinal and other tissue fluids and for diffusion into the affected joints.

H. parasuis is particularly sensitive to penicillin, ampicillin, chloramphenicol, cotrimoxazole (trimethoprim + sulfonamide), and tetracyclines, which are considered as the drugs of choice. Aminoglycosides (streptomycin, neomycin, and gentamicin) and sulfonamides seem, at least in vitro, to be less effective.

PREVENTION. In the prevention of the disease, great care is to be taken to mix nonimmune animals, e.g., from SPF-primary herds, with others. Furthermore, the reduction of stress situations decreases the risk of infection. In risk situations vaccination is an effective way to prevent outbreaks of the Glässer's disease (Riising 1981; Miniats and Smart 1988).

REFERENCES

BAEHLER, J. F.; BURGISSER, H.; DE MEURON, P. A.; AND NICOLET, J. 1974. Infection à *Haemophilus parasuis* chez le porc. Schweiz Arch Tierheilkd 116:183–188.

BAKOS, K. 1955. Studien über *Haemophilus suis,* mit besonderer Berücksichtigung der serologischen Differenzierung seiner Stämme. Diss., Stockholm.

BERTSCHINGER, H. U., AND NICOD, B. 1970. Untersuchungen über die Nasenflora bei Schweinen. Vergleich zwischen SPF-Herden und schwedisch sanierten Herden. Schweiz Arch Tierheilkd 112:493–499.

BLOCH, I. 1985. Beitrag zur Epidemiologie, Serologie und Polyacrylamidgel-Elektrophorese von *Haemophilus parasuis.* DVM thesis, Univ of Berne.

GLÄSSER, K. 1910. Die fibrinöse Serosen- und Gelenkentzündung der Ferkel. In Die Krankheiten des Schweines. Hannover: M. & H. Schaper, pp. 122–125.

HARRIS, D. L.; ROSS, R. F.; AND SWITZER, W. P. 1969. Incidence of certain microorganisms in nasal cavities of swine in Iowa. Am J Vet Res 30:1621–1624.

HJÄRRE, A., AND WRAMBY, G. 1943. Ueber die fibrinöse Serosa-Gelenkentzündung (Glässer) beim Schwein. Z Infektionskr Parasitenkd Krankheit Hyg Haustiere 60:37–64.

KIELSTEIN, P.; ROSNER, H.; AND MÜLLER, W. 1990. Relationship between serology, virulence and protein pattern of *Haemophilus parasuis*. Proc 11th Int Congr Pig Vet Soc, Lausanne, p. 180.

KILIAN, M. 1976. A taxonomic study of the genus *Haemophilus*, with the proposal of a new species. J Gen Microbiol 93:9–62.

KILIAN, M.; NICOLET, J.; AND BIBERSTEIN, E. L. 1978. Biochemical and serological characterization of *Haemophilus pleuropneumoniae* (Matthews and Pattison 1961) Shope 1964 and proposal of a neotype strain. Int J Syst Bacteriol 28:20–26.

LEWIS, A., AND SHOPE, R. E. 1931. Swine influenza. II. A haemophilic bacillus from the respiratory tract of infected swine. J Exp Med 54:361–371.

LITTLE, T. W. A. 1970. *Haemophilus* infection in pigs. Vet Rec 87:399–402.

MINIATS, O. P., AND SMART, N. L. 1988. Immunization of primary SPF pigs against Glässer's disease. Proc 10th Int Congr Pig Vet Soc, Rio de Janeiro, p. 157.

MOROZUMI, T., AND NICOLET, J. 1986a. Morphological variations of *Haemophilus parasuis* strains. J Clin Microbiol 23:138–142.

———. 1986b. Some antigenic properties of *Haemophilus parasuis* and a proposal for serological classification. J Clin Microbiol 23:1022–1025.

MOROZUMI, T.; PAULI, U.; BRAUN, R.; AND NICOLET, J. 1986. Deoxyribonucleic acid relatedness among strains of *Haemophilus parasuis* and other *Haemophilus* spp. of swine origin. Int J Syst Bacteriol 36:17–19.

NEIL, D. H.; McKAY, K. A.; L'ECUYER, C.; AND CORNER, A. H. 1969. GLÄSSER'S disease of swine produced by intratracheal inoculation of *Haemophilus suis*. Can J Comp Med 33:187–193.

NICOLET, J.; PAROZ, P.; AND KRAWINKLER, M. 1980. Polyacrylamide gel electrophoresis of whole cell proteins of porcine strains of *Haemophilus*. Int J Syst Bacteriol 30:69–76.

NIELSEN, R., AND DANIELSEN, V. 1975. An outbreak of Glässer's disease. Studies on etiology, serology and the effect of vaccination. Nord Vet Med 27:20–25.

RAPP, V. J.; ROSS, R. F.; AND YOUNG, T. F. 1985. Characterization of *Haemophilus* spp. isolated from healthy swine and evaluation of cross-reactivity of complement-fixing antibodies to *Haemophilus pleuropneumoniae* and *Haemophilus* Taxon "minor group." J Clin Microbiol 22:945–950.

RAPP, V. J.; ROSS, R. F.; AND NICOLET, J. 1986. Characterization of the outer membrane proteins of *Haemophilus parasuis*. Proc 9th Int Congr Pig Vet Soc, Barcelona, p. 262.

RAPP-GABRIELSON, V. J., AND GABRIELSON, D. A. 1990. Serotyping of *Haemophilus parasuis* by agar-gel-precipitation test (AGPT). Proc 11th Int Congr Pig Vet Soc, Lausanne, p. 181.

RIISING, H. J. 1981. Prevention of Glässer's disease through immunity to *Haemophilus parasuis*. Zentralbl Veterinaermed [B] 28:630–638.

THOMSON, R. G., AND RUHNKE, L. 1963. *Haemophilus* septicaemia in piglets. Can Vet J 4:271–275.

42 Leptospirosis

W. A. Ellis

LEPTOSPIROSIS is a cause of reproductive loss in breeding herds and has been reported in swine from all parts of the world; however, knowledge of the incidence and economic impact of the disease is largely confined to the intensive pig industries of the northern hemisphere, Australia, Argentina, and Brazil.

Endemic infection in a herd of swine may produce little evidence of clinical disease, but when it is first introduced into a susceptible breeding herd, or during periods of waning herd immunity, it can cause very appreciable losses through abortion, or the full-term birth of dead pigs, or weak pigs of reduced viability.

ETIOLOGY. Leptospirosis of swine is a disease caused by a variety of morphologically similar, but antigenically distinct, small, motile, aerobic spirochaetes belonging to the genus *Leptospira*. They are flexible helicoidal gram-negative rods, 0.1 μm in diameter and 6–12 μm in length, and usually hooked at each end. They stain poorly with aniline dyes. Unstained cells are visible only by dark-field microscopy. Motility is accomplished by rotating along the long axis in liquid medium, but this changes to an undulating action in semisolid media. They require special media containing mammalian serum or albumin for cultivation.

The taxonomy of this genus is in a period of change. Until recently those strains found in animals (the parasitic strains) and those found in water (the saprophytic strains) were given the species names of *interrogans* and *biflexa* respectively, and differentiation was by growth requirements and biochemical reactions. However, as a result of DNA-relatedness studies and guanine (G) and cytosine (C) content of DNA, the *interrogans* species has been divided into the *interrogans, weilii, borgpetersenii, noguchi,* and *santarosai* species (Yasuda et al. 1987). While leptospires infecting swine are known to be members of these species, the exact species allocation of all the important swine pathogens has not been determined yet.

As a further taxonomic tool and as an aid to epidemologic studies, the parasitic leptospires are subdivided into serogroups on the basis of antigenic relationships, as determined by cross-agglutination reactions and further subdivided into serovars by agglutination-absorption patterns. There are now some 23 serogroups recognized containing 212 serovars. Strains belonging to at least 10 serogroups have been isolated from pigs. Genotyping by the use of restriction endonuclease analysis is widely used as a supplementary typing system and as an epidemiologic tool.

EPIDEMIOLOGY. The epidemiology of swine leptospirosis is potentially very complicated, since swine can be infected by any of the pathogenic serovars. Fortunately, only a small number of serovars will be endemic in any particular region or country. Furthermore, leptospirosis is a disease that shows a natural nidality and each serovar tends to be maintained in specific-maintenance hosts. Therefore, in any region pigs will be infected by serovars maintained by pigs or by serovars maintained by other animal species present in the area. The relative importance of these incidental infections is determined by the opportunity that prevailing social, management, and environmental factors provide for contact and transmission of leptospires from other species to pigs.

Pigs act as maintenance hosts for serovars belonging to the Pomona, Australis, and Tarassovi serogroups, while strains belonging to the Canicola, Icterohaemorrhagiae, and Grippotyphosa serogroups are among the more commonly identified incidental infections in swine.

Pomona Infection. Serovar *pomona* has been the most common serovar isolated from pigs worldwide. Infection with this serovar has been extensively studied and it provides a suitable model with which to illustrate general concepts of swine leptospirosis. Many strains of serovar *pomona*, especially those of the kennewicki genotype found in the United States and Canada, are adapted to swine. Serovar *pomona* has been the cause of widespread clinical disease in swine in North and South America, Australia, New Zealand, parts of Asia, and eastern and central Europe and is endemic in many of these regions. Such strains are apparently absent from the more westerly parts of Europe. Furthermore, not all strains of serovar *pomona* are adapted to pigs as are the other serovars of the Pomona serogroup, but they have rodent hosts (Sebek et al. 1983).

In parts of North America, the prevalence of *pomona* infection in pigs has fallen from the high levels observed in the 1950s and early 1960s: no

529

carriers were detected in a 1989 meat-plant survey carried out in Iowa (Bolin 1990). In contrast, Baker et al. (1989) recovered *pomona* (genotype kennewicki) from almost 10% of pigs in a small survey in Canada.

Leptospires have a particular affinity for the kidneys of infected pigs, where they persist, multiply, and are voided in urine. This characteristic is very important in the transmission of infection.

Infection is introduced into a susceptible herd by three possible routes: the introduction of infected stock, exposure to a contaminated environment, or contact with an alternative infected animal vector (Hathaway 1983). Carrier pigs are probably the most common route of introduction. Replacement gilts (Edwards and Daines 1979) or infected boars (Kemenes and Suveges 1976) have been identified as important means of introducing infection.

The importance of free-living species as possible sources of *pomona* infection of pigs depends on geographical location. In North America, the skunk has been incriminated as a source of *pomona* outbreaks in pigs (Mitchell et al. 1966).

Once *pomona* has been introduced into a pig population, a high prevalence of infection is established. Only low infective doses are required to transmit infection (Chaudhary et al. 1966a,b). If direct contact is prevented, indirect contact through contaminated effluent, water, or soil ensures transmission (Michna 1970; Buddle and Hodges 1977; Kingscote 1986). The presence of moisture is critical for indirect transmission; the organisms cannot withstand dessication, but when infected urine is deposited in damp soil or water with a pH around or slightly on the alkaline side, the organisms may survive for extended periods (Mitscherlich and Marth 1984).

During the initial herd infection, clinical disease may occur in all ages of sows.

Following the initial establishment of infection, an endemic cycle typical of that in a maintenance host population is set up (Hathaway 1981). Piglets are passively protected in the first weeks of life by colostrum-derived immunoglobulins from infected dams (Fish et al. 1963). The duration of this passive protection depends primarily on the quantity of immunoglobulins received in colostrum (Chaudhary et al. 1966b). Infection between groups of fattening pigs is often by urine-contaminated effluent from a common drainage system (Buddle and Hodges 1977).

In herds with endemic infection, clinical disease is usually restricted to gilts that have either been reared in isolation since weaning and reintroduced into the herd, or more commonly brought in from an uninfected herd.

Tarassovi Infection. There is much less information available on the epidemiology of *tarassovi* infection in pigs. The pig acts as a maintenance host for some strains of *tarassovi* found in Eastern Europe and Australia. In these regions, it does not spread as rapidly in a pig population as does *pomona* (Kemenes and Suveges 1976), but endemic infection is readily maintained (Ryley and Simmons 1954b; Kemenes and Suveges 1976).

Many strains of *tarassovi* have been recovered from free-living animals (Anon. 1966, 1975) and these may give rise to incidental pig infections; e.g., *tarassovi* has not been recovered from swine in the United States, but there is serologic evidence of infection in pigs (Cole et al. 1983) in the southeastern states where it has been isolated from racoons, skunks, and opossums (McKeever et al. 1958; Roth 1964).

Australis Infection. Serovar *bratislava* and to a lesser extent the closely related serovar *muenchen* have emerged as major swine-maintained leptospiral infections in the last few years. Serologic data has indicated widespread *bratislava* infection in Germany (Weber and Fenske 1978), the United Kingdom (Hathaway and Little 1981; Hathaway et al. 1981), Czechoslovakia (Propopcakova et al. 1981), the Netherlands (Bercovich et al. 1983), Sweden (Sandstedt and Engvall 1985), Denmark (Jensen and Binder 1989; Nissen 1989), the United States (Hanson 1985, 1987), and Canada (Kingscote 1988).

Serovar *bratislava* was first recovered from a pig in the Netherlands by Hartmann et al. (1975); initially this strain was wrongly identified as *lora,* but it has since been shown to be *bratislava.* This serovar has now been recovered from pigs in the United Kingdom (Ellis et al. 1986a,b,c), the United States (Ellis and Thiermann 1986; Bolin and Cassells 1990), and Germany (Schonberg 1989).

The epidemiology of these strains is complicated and poorly understood. There are specific pig-adapted strains, strains that are maintained by pigs, dogs, horses, and hedgehogs, and strains that are found only in wildlife.

While the renal-carrier state does become established, urinary excretion is poor compared with *pomona* excretion, and transmission within the fattening house is inefficient. Important additional carrier sites have been identified, namely, the upper genital tracts of sows and boars (Ellis et al. 1986b,c). Venereal transmission is thought to play an important role in the spread of *bratislava* infection.

Canicola Infection. Although organisms belonging to this serogroup have been recovered from swine in at least 11 countries (Hanson and Tripathy 1986), little is known of the epidemiology of *canicola* infection in pigs. The dog is the recognized maintenance host for this serovar and is the probable vector whereby this serovar enters a piggery. The long period of leptospiruria observed in infected pigs (at least 90 days) (Michna 1962) and the ability of *canicola* to survive for up to 6 days in undiluted pig urine (Michna 1962) suggest that there would be an opportunity for intraspecies transmission, but no studies have been done on this subject (Hathaway 1983).

Icterohaemorrhagiae Infection. Serologic evidence of Icterohaemorrhagiae serogroup infection has been reported in many countries but few isolations have been made from pigs (Hathaway 1985). It appears that both serovars *copenhageni* and *icterohaemorrhagiae* may be involved. The maintenance host for these serovars is the brown rat (*Rattus norvegicus*), and it is probable that *copenhageni* and *icterohaemorrhagiae* are introduced to susceptible stock via an environment contaminated with infected rat urine. Field investigation suggests that intraswine transmission is inefficient (Hathaway 1985). Schnurrenberger et al. (1970) found that urinary excretion lasted less than 35 days in naturally infected pigs, while Fennestad and Borg-Petersen (1966) failed to demonstrate leptospiruria in experimentally infected pigs. Low prevalences of renal infection have been found in those microbiologic surveys in which Icterohaemorrhagiae strains have been recovered; Hathaway et al. (1981) reported a 0.7% prevalence in England while McErlean (1973) found a 0.4% prevalence in Ireland.

Grippotyphosa Infection. Serovar *grippotyphosa* infection is maintained by wildlife hosts, and incidental infection of pigs gives rise to low prevalences of antibodies in swine in various regions, particularly eastern and central Europe and the United States. It has been recovered from pigs in the U.S.S.R. (Gorshanova 1964) and the United States (Hanson et al. 1965; 1971).

Sejroe Infection. Serovar *hardjo* infection is maintained by cattle worldwide, and where cattle and pigs come in close contact, the opportunity arises for infection in pigs to occur. There are now reports of the isolation of *hardjo* from pigs in the United Kingdom (Hathaway et al. 1983; Ellis et al. 1986a) and the United States (Bolin 1990). Persistence in renal tissue was not a feature of experimental infection (Hathaway et al. 1983); therefore, intraspecies transmission is unlikely.

Serovar *sejroe,* which is maintained by small rodents, has also been isolated from swine in Europe (Brandis 1956; Fuzi et al. 1957; Combiesco et al. 1958), while another serovar in this group (serovar *balcanica*) has been recovered from swine in the U.S.S.R (Matveeva et al. 1977).

PATHOGENESIS. The most important route of natural infection has not been determined; however, it is thought to be via the mucous membranes of the eye, mouth, or nose (Alston and Broom 1958; Alexander et al. 1964; Michna and Campbell 1969). Infection via the vaginal route is also possible (Ferguson and Powers 1956; Chaudhary et al. 1966a). Transmission of lepto-

spires through milk from an infected dam has been demonstrated experimentally (Tripathy et al. 1981). One or 2 days after infection there is a period of bacteremia, which may last for a week. During this period leptospires can be isolated from most organs of the body and also from cerebrospinal fluid. This primary bacteremic phase ends with the appearance of circulating antibodies, which are detectable usually after 5–10 days (Hanson and Tripathy 1986). A secondary bacteremic period (after 15–26 days) has been reported in experimental *hardjo* infection (Hathaway et al. 1983).

Antileptospiral agglutinins appear at detectable levels in the blood at approximately 5–10 days after infection and reach maximum levels at around 3 weeks (Ryley and Simmons 1954b; Ferguson and Powers 1956; Morse et al. 1958). Peak titers vary considerably (1:1000 to 1:100,000 in the microscopic agglutination test) and these may be maintained for up to 3 weeks, after which a subsequent gradual decline occurs. Low titers may be detectable for several years in many animals.

Following the period of leptospiremia, the leptospires localize in the proximal renal tubules where they multiply and are voided in the urine. The duration and intensity of urinary shedding varies from pig to pig and with the infecting serovar. In the case of *pomona* infection, the intensity of excretion is highest during the first month of shedding, when more than a million leptospires may be present in each milliliter of urine (Morse et al. 1958); leptospiruria is very constant during this period (Hodges et al. 1979). A variable period of intermittent, low-intensity leptospiruria then ensues, and this may last for up to 2 years in some cases (Ryley and Simmons 1954a; Morse et al. 1958; Mitchell et al. 1966). Low levels of antibody may be detected in the urine of pigs (Morse et al. 1958), but the immunologic mechanism whereby infection is ultimately eliminated from the kidneys is not known.

Leptospires also localize in the uterus of pregnant sows and abortion, production of stillborn pigs, and neonatal disease frequently result from intrauterine infections occurring in the last half of the gestation period. Abortions and stillbirths usually occur 1–4 weeks following infection of the gilt or sow (Hanson and Tripathy 1986), by which time most sows have developed detectable antibody titers. Since pig fetuses are capable of producing antibodies during the latter stages of gestation, some stillborn piglets will have detectable titers.

The pathogenesis of reproductive disease is poorly understood, but it is generally believed that transplacental infection, which only occurs during the very limited period of maternal leptospiremia, is the sole cause (Fennestad and Borg-Petersen 1966). The possibility of transplacental infection during leptospiremia appears to increase with the stage of pregnancy (Wrathall 1975). From midpregnancy onward, it is likely that the majority of fetuses in a litter at risk will become infected. Fennestad and Borg-Petersen (1966) have suggested that horizontal transmission to littermates not infected during the period of maternal leptospiremia may also occur. Once the placental barrier is breached, septicemia results in large numbers of leptospires in all fetal tissues (Preston and Morter 1960). It is unlikely that placental insufficiency plays a role in fetal death (Wrathall 1975); abortion is probably initiated by toxic products released from dead and autolysing fetuses.

An additional feature seen in *bratislava* infection but not reported for the other swine leptospiral infections is the persistence of leptospires in the oviduct and uterus of nonpregnant sows (Ellis et al. 1986c) and in the genital tracts of boars (Ellis et al. 1986b).

CLINICAL SIGNS

Acute Leptospirosis. This phase usually coincides with the period of bacteremia (Morse et al. 1958; Sleight and Lundberg 1961; Chaudhary et al. 1966a,b). In experimental infections, many pigs exhibit transient anorexia, pyrexia, and listlessness at this time (Hanson and Tripathy 1986). However, the mild nature of these signs means that in natural infections, especially in endemically infected herds where perhaps only one or two animals may be affected, this phase of infection usually goes unrecognized.

There have been a few reports of jaundice and hemoglobinuria in naturally occurring outbreaks (Ferguson et al. 1956), particularly in cases of infection in piglets under 3 months of age by strains belonging to the Icterohaemorrhagiae serogroup (Klarenbeek and Winsser 1932; Field and Sellers 1951; Urban and Androsov 1976). A high proportion of these undergo spontaneous recovery within a week of when symptoms develop. The small number of such reports suggests that this more severe form of disease is rare.

Chronic Leptospirosis. Abortions, stillbirths, and the birth of weak piglets of reduced viability are primary signs of chronic leptospirosis, particularly *pomona* infection, in pigs (Bohl et al. 1954; Fennestad and Borg-Petersen 1966) and it is this aspect of leptospirosis that can cause considerable economic loss.

Information as to the importance of leptospirosis as a cause of abortion in national swine herds is not available, and if it were it must vary from country to country depending on prevalence, epidemiologic and management factors, including the implementation of control measures. From the limited information available it would appear that even in countries were vaccination has been widely practiced, leptospirosis is a common cause of swine abortion. In Ontario for example, 6% of swine abortions were attributed to *pomona* infection (Anon. 1986). Endemic *tarassovi* infection was considered to be the cause of a 3% abortion rate in herds in Poland investigated by Wandurski (1982). Acute outbreaks can still give rise to severe losses; Saravi et al. (1989) described an outbreak in a herd in which 19% of pregnant sows aborted, while the number of dead piglets/sow rose from 8% prior to the outbreak to 28% during the outbreak.

A very high prevalence of serovars belonging to the Australis serogroup in aborted pig litters has been observed in part of the United Kingdom; Ellis et al. (1986a) isolated either serovar *bratislava* or *muenchen* from 71% of litters they examined. Similar strains have also been recovered from aborted piglets in the United States (Bolin and Cassells 1990), where a high prevalence in aborted fetuses has also been noted (Bolin 1990). Published experimental evaluations of the significance of such isolations are not available. There has, however, been an absence of significant isolations of other abortifacient agents from these cases, and the farrowing rate and the number of live piglets born/sow improves significantly following either *bratislava* vaccination (Frantz et al. 1989) or the use of an antibiotic medication program (Ellis 1989).

Following abortions due to *pomona*, there does not appear to be any subsequent limitation on reproductive performance, even in pigs that remain infected for long periods (Ferguson and Powers 1956; Mitchell et al. 1966; Kemenes and Suveges 1976).

Infertility is a feature of *bratislava* infection. An analysis of serologic and clinical data by Hathaway and Little (1981) has shown a statistically significant relationship between Australis serogroup titers and infertility in sows. Split-herd trials, carried out using a *bratislava* bacterin, have demonstrated significant improvements in sow fertility (Frantz et al. 1989).

LESIONS. Pathologic changes in acute *pomona* infection are very limited, reflecting the mild nature of acute clinical disease. Hanson and Tripathy (1986) reported little gross or histopathologic change in swine killed during the acute phase of leptospirosis. Burnstein and Baker (1954) reported that petechial and echymotic hemorrhages could be seen in the lungs of some pigs and histologic examinations have revealed minor renal tubular damage, focal liver necrosis, lymphocytic infiltration of the adrenal glands, and meningoencephalitis with perivascular lymphocytic infiltration (Burnstein and Baker 1954; Sleight et al. 1960; Chaudhary et al. 1966a).

In chronic leptospirosis, lesions are confined to the kidneys and consist of scattered small gray foci, often surrounded by a ring of hyperemia. Microscopic examination shows these lesions to be a progressive focal interstitial nephritis (Burnstein and Baker 1954; Langham et al. 1958; Cheville et al. 1980). The interstitial leukocytic infiltrations, which consist mainly of lymphocytes, macrophages, and plasma cells, may be extensive in some areas. Focal damage may also involve glomeruli and renal tubules. Some affected glomeruli are swollen, some atrophic, and others are replaced by fibrosis. The Bowman's capsule may be thickened, containing eosinophilic granular material (Langham et al. 1958). Tubular changes involve atrophy, hyperplasia, and the presence of necrotic debris in the lumen in some areas. Occasionally, petechial hemorrhages may be present in interstitial spaces.

Older lesions mainly consist of fibrosis and interstitial infiltration. Chronic lesions with accompanying acute inflammatory changes are still noticeable as long as 14 months postinfection (Morter et al. 1960).

Experimental studies indicate leptospires can invade the mammary gland of pigs and produce a mild, focal nonsuppurative mastitis (Tripathy et al. 1981).

The gross pathology of fetuses aborted as a sequela of *pomona* infection is nonspecific and includes edema of various tissues, serous or blood-stained fluid in body cavities, and sometimes petechial hemorrhages in the renal cortex (Ryley and Simmons 1954b; Fennestad and Borg-Petersen 1966; Wrathall 1975). These changes are probably the result of intrauterine autolysis. Jaundice may be seen in some aborted piglets (Hathaway et al. 1983). Focal necrosis, presenting as small grayish-white spots, is a frequent finding in liver (Ryley and Simmons 1954b; Fish et al. 1963; Fennestad and Borg-Petersen 1966). Histologic examination may reveal small foci of interstitial nephritis.

Placentas from aborted fetuses are grossly normal (Fish et al. 1963; Fennestad and Borg-Petersen 1966).

DIAGNOSIS. A diagnosis of leptospirosis in swine may be required not only for the clinician to confirm leptospirosis as a cause of clinical disease but also for other reasons, such as (1) the assessment of the infection and/or the immune status of a herd for the purposes of a control or eradication program on either a herd or national basis; (2) epidemiologic studies; and (3) an assessment of the infectivity status of an individual animal to assess its suitability for international trade or for introduction into an uninfected herd.

The mild, often inapparent, clinical signs of acute leptospirosis make clinical diagnosis difficult, therefore, diagnosis is usually based on the results of laboratory procedures.

Laboratory diagnostic procedures for leptospirosis fall into two groups. The first group consists of tests for antibody detection; the second contains the tests for the demonstration of leptospires in pig tissues. The selection of tests to be carried out depends on the purpose for which a diagnosis is to be made and the resources available.

Serologic Tests. Serologic testing is the most widely used method for diagnosing leptospirosis, and the microscopic agglutination (MA) test (Cole et al. 1980; Faine 1982) is the standard serologic test. The minimum antigen requirements are that the test should employ representative strains of all the serogroups known to exist in the particular country, plus those known to be maintained by pigs elsewhere.

The MA test is used primarily as a herd test. To obtain useful information, at least 10 animals or 10% of the herd, whichever is the greater (Cole et al. 1980), should be tested. A retrospective diagnosis of both acute leptospirosis and *pomona* abortion may be made when the majority of affected animals have titers of 1:1000 or greater. Increasing the sample size and sampling a number of different cohorts markedly improves epidemiologic information, investigations of clinical disease, assessments of vaccination needs, and public health tracebacks.

As an individual animal test, the MA test is very useful in diagnosing acute infection; rising antibody titers in paired acute and convalescent serum samples are diagnostic. The presence of antibody in fetal serum is diagnostic of leptospiral abortion.

The MA test has severe limitations in the diagnosis of chronic infection in individual pigs, both in the diagnosis of abortion and in the identification of renal or genital carriers. Infected animals may have MA titers below the widely accepted minimum significant titer of 1:100 (Ellis et al. 1986b, c).

Demonstration of Leptospires in Pig Tissues. The isolation of leptospires from, or their demonstration in, the internal organs (such as liver, lung, brain) and body fluids (blood, cerebrospinal, thoracic, and peritoneal) of clinically affected animals gives a definitive diagnosis of acute clinical disease, or in the case of a fetus, a diagnosis of leptospiral abortion and probable chronic infection of its mother.

Their presence in the male or female genital tract, the kidney, or urine, in the absence of evidence of generalized infection, is diagnostic of chronic infection. Failure to demonstrate leptospires in the urine of a pig does not rule out the possibility of the animal being a chronic renal carrier; it merely indicates that the pig was not excreting detectable numbers of leptospires at the time of testing.

ISOLATION. Isolation, especially from clinical material, is difficult and time consuming and is a job for laboratories specializing in the identification of isolates. Isolation from renal carriers is very useful in epidemiologic studies to determine which serovars are present in an animal species, or in a particular group of animals or geographic location.

The isolation of leptospires is the most sensitive method of demonstrating their presence, provided that antibiotic residues are absent, that tissue autolysis is not advanced, and that tissues for culture have been stored at a suitable temperature (4°C) and, in the case of urine, at a suitable pH since collection.

Culture should be carried out in a semisolid (0.1–0.2% agar) bovine serum–albumin medium containing either Tween 80 (Johnson and Harris 1967) or a combination of Tween 80 and Tween 40 (Ellis 1986), and preferably a small amount of fresh rabbit serum (0.4–2%). A dilution culture method should be used (Ellis 1986). Contamination may be controlled by a variety of selective agents, e.g., 5-fluorouracil, nalidixic acid, fosfomycin, and a cocktail of rifamycin, polymyxin, neomycin, 5-fluorouracil, bacitracin, and actidione. The use of selective agents will reduce the chance of isolation where there are only small numbers of viable leptospires. Culture media containing 5-fluorouracil at levels between 200 and 500 μg/ml should be used as transport media for the submission of samples (Ellis 1990).

Cultures should be incubated at 29–30°C for at least 12 weeks, preferably for 26 weeks (Ellis 1986). They should be examined by dark-ground microscopy every 1–2 weeks.

OTHER METHODS OF DEMONSTRATING LEPTO-SPIRES. Leptospires do not stain satisfactorily with the aniline dyes, and silver-staining techniques lack sensitivity and specificity (Baskerville 1986). Dark-ground microscopy of fetal fluids or urine has been widely used in the diagnosis of leptospirosis and can be a useful tool in the hands of an experienced diagnostician, but many tissue artifacts can be mistakenly identified as leptospires.

The demonstration of leptospires by immunochemical tests (immunofluorescence, immunoperoxidase, and immunogold) is more suited to most laboratory situations; however, these tests are "number-of-organisms" dependant and lack the sensitivity of culture. They provide no information as to the infecting serovar (Ellis 1990) and require high IgG titer antileptospire sera, which are not available commercially. Immunofluorescence is the method of choice for the diagnosis of fetal leptospirosis. The use of specific DNA probes, polymerase chain reaction, and time-resolved fluoroimmunoassays is being investigated, but there are no published evaluations of their use as diagnostic reagents for leptospirosis in swine.

CONTROL. Control of leptospirosis is dependant on the combined use of three strategies: anti-

biotic therapy, vaccination, and management. Unfortunately, not all these options are available in every country; e.g., vaccines are not available in many western European countries including the United Kingdom, while problems of antibiotic residues may make the use of antibiotic therapy difficult in other situations. Control programs must therefore be modified to meet local conditions.

Vaccination induces immunity of relatively short duration. Immunity to infection is probably never 100% and, at best, lasts little more than 3 months (Kemenes and Suveges 1976; Ellis et al. 1989); immunity to clinical disease is believed to last somewhat longer, although exact duration is not known. Vaccination will markedly reduce the prevalence of infection in a herd (Wrathall 1975; Kemenes and Suveges 1976) but will not eliminate infection (Hodges et al. 1976; Edwards and Daines 1979; Cargill and Davos 1981).

Antibiotics alone will not eliminate pig-maintained leptospiral infections from the individual carrier animal or control infection in herds. Despite claims by some authors that either systemic streptomycin at 25 mg/kg body weight (Dobson 1974) or oral tetracyclines at levels of 800 g/ton of feed (Stalheim 1967) will eliminate carriers, others have reported that these regimes do not work (Doherty and Baynes 1967; Hodges et al. 1979).

The main management factor in the control of leptospirosis is the prevention of direct or indirect contact with free-living vectors or other domestic stock. When faced with an outbreak of clinical disease, the best option is to treat both affected and at-risk stock with streptomycin at 25 mg/kg body weight, to immediately vaccinate the at-risk stock, and then to introduce a regular vaccination program. If vaccination is not an available option, then a feed medication program, using either chlor- or oxytetracycline at 600 gm/ton of feed, should be introduced. This ration is fed either continuously or on a 1-month-on/ 1-month-off basis. Alternatively, it may be fed for two periods of 4 weeks in the year, preferably, one in the spring and the other in the autumn.

REFERENCES

ALEXANDER, A. D.; YAGER, R. H.; AND KEEFE, T. J. 1964. Leptospirosis in swine. Bull Off Epizoot 61:273–304.
ALSTON, J. M., AND BROOM, J. C. 1958. Leptospirosis in Man and Animals. Edinburgh: E. and S. Livingstone Ltd., pp. 65–75.
ANON. 1966. Zoonoses surveillance. Leptospiral serotype distribution lists. U.S.D.H.E.W. Altanta, Ga.
ANON. 1975. Zoonoses surveillance. Leptospiral serotype distribution lists according to host and geographic area. July 1966–July 1973. U.S.D.H.E.W. Atlanta, Ga.
ANON. 1986. Diagnosis of abortions, V. L. S., Guelph. Can Vet J 27:A20.
BAKER, I. F.; McEWAN, S. A.; PRESCOTT, J. F.; AND MEEK, A. H. 1989. The prevalence of leptospirosis and its association with multifocal interstitial

nephritis in swine at slaughter. Can J Vet Res 53:290–294.

BASKERVILLE, A. 1986. Histological aspects of diagnosis of leptospirosis. The Present State of Leptospirosis Diagnosis and Control. Dordrecht, Nether.: Martinus Nijhoff, pp. 33–43.

BERCOVICH, Z.; SPEK, C. W.; AND COMVALIUS-ADRIAAN, I. 1983. Occurrence of antibodies to various serotypes of *Leptospira interrogans* among swine in the Netherlands between 1975 and 1980. Tidjschr Diergeneeskd 108:133–138.

BOHL, E. H.; POWERS, T. E.; AND FERGUSON, L. C. 1954. Abortions in swine associated with leptospirosis. J Am Vet Med Assoc 124:262.

BOLIN, C. A. 1990. Personal communication.

BOLIN, C., AND CASSELLS, J. A. 1990. Isolation of *Leptospira interrogans* serovar *bratislava* from stillborn and weak pigs in Iowa. J Am Vet Med Assoc 196:1601–1604.

BRANDIS, H. 1956. Ueber Leptospirosen durch den typ. L. saxkoebing. Klin Wochenschr 34:521.

BUDDLE, J. R., AND HODGES, R. T. 1977. Observations on some aspects of the epidemiology of leptospirosis in a herd of pigs. NZ Vet J 25:56, 65–66.

BURNSTEIN, T., AND BAKER, J. A. 1954. Leptospirosis in swine caused by *Leptospira pomona*. J Infect Dis 94:53–54.

CARGILL, C. F., AND DAVOS, D. E. 1981. Renal leptospirosis in vaccinated pigs. Aust Vet J 57:236–238.

CHAUDHARY, R. K.; FISH, N. A.; AND BARNUM, D. A. 1966a. Experimental infection with *Leptospira pomona* in normal and immune piglets. Can Vet J 7:106–112.

_____. 1966b. Protection of piglets from immunised sows via colostrum against experimental *Leptospira pomona* infection. Can Vet J 7:121–127.

CHEVILLE, N. F.; HUHN, R.; AND CUTLIP, R. C. 1980. Ultrastructure of renal lesions in pigs with acute leptospirosis caused by *Leptospira pomona*. Vet Pathol 17:338–351.

COLE, J. R.; ELLINGHAUSEN, H. C.; AND RUBIN, H. L. 1980. Laboratory diagnosis of leptospirosis of domestic animals. Proc US Anim Health Assoc 83:189–199.

COLE, J. R.; HALL, R. F.; ELLINGHAUSEN, H. C.; AND PURSELL, A. R. 1983. Prevalence of leptospiral antibodies in Georgia cattle and swine, with emphasis on *Leptospira interrogans* serovar *tarassovi*. Proc US Anim Health Assoc 87:199–210.

COMBIESCO, D.; STURDZA, N.; SEFER, M.; AND RADU, I. 1958. Recherches sur les leptospirosis. Arch Roum Pathol Exp Microbiol 17:245.

DOBSON, K. J. 1974. Eradication of leptospirosis in commercial pig herds. Aust Vet J 50:471.

DOHERTY, P. C., AND BAYNES, I. D. 1967. The effects of feeding oxytetracycline on leptospira in pigs infected with *L. pomona*. Aust Vet J 43:135–137.

EDWARDS, J. D., AND DAINES, D. 1979. A leptospirosis outbreak in a piggery. NZ Vet J 27:247–248.

ELLIS, W. A. 1986. The diagnosis of leptospirosis in farm animals. In The Present State of Leptospirosis Diagnosis and Control. Dordrecht, Nether.: Martinus Nijhoff, pp. 13–31.

_____. 1989. Leptrospira Australis infection in pigs. Pig Vet J 22:83–92.

_____. 1990. Leptospirosis. OIE manual of recommended diagnostic techniques and requirements for biological products for List A and B diseases, vol 2, Sect 7, pp. 1–11. Paris.

ELLIS, W. A., AND THIERMANN, A. B. 1986. Isolation of *Leptospira interrogans* serovar *bratislava* from sows in Iowa. Am J Vet Res 47:1458–1460.

ELLIS, W. A.; McPARLAND, P. J.; BRYSON, D. G.; AND CASSELLS, J. A. 1986a. Prevalence of leptospira infec-tion in aborted pigs in Northern Ireland. Vet Rec 118:63–65.

_____. 1986b. Boars as carriers of leptospires of the Australis serogroup on farms with an abortion problem. Vet Rec 118:563.

ELLIS, W. A.; McPARLAND, P. J.; BRYSON, D. G.; THIERMANN, A. B.; AND MONTGOMERY, J. 1986c. Isolation of leptospires from genital tract and kidneys of aborted sows. Vet Rec 118:294–295.

ELLIS, W. A.; MONTGOMERY, J. M.; AND McPARLAND, P. J. 1989. An experimental study with a *Leptospira interrogans* serovar *bratislava* vaccine. Vet Rec 125:319–321.

FAINE, S. 1982. Guidelines for the control of leptospirosis. WHO. Geneva.

FENNESTAD, K. L., AND BORG-PETERSEN, C. 1966. Experimental leptospirosis in pregnant sows. J Infect Dis 116:57–66.

FERGUSON, L. C., AND POWERS, T. E. 1956. Experimental leptospirosis in pregnant swine. Am J Vet Res 17:471–477.

FERGUSON, L. C.; LOCOCO, S.; SMITH, H. R.; AND HANDY, A. H. 1956. The control and treatment of swine leptospirosis during a naturally occurring outbreak. J Am Vet Med Assoc 129:263–265.

FIELD, H. I., AND SELLERS, K. C. 1951. *Leptospira icterohaemorrhagiae* infection in piglets. Vet Rec 63:78–81.

FISH, N. A.; RYU, E.; AND HULLAND, T. J. 1963. Bacteriological and pathological studies of natural and experimental swine abortion due to *Leptospira pomona*. Can Vet J 4:317–327.

FRANTZ, J. C.; HANSON, L. E.; AND BROWN, A. L. 1989. Effect of vaccination with a bacterin containing *Leptospira interrogans* serovar *bratislava* on the breeding performance of swine herds. Am J Vet Res 50:1044–1047.

FUZI, M.; ALFOLDY, Z.; KISZEL, J.; AND RADITZ, I. 1957. Die Leptospiren-Infection der Feldnagetiere in einem Gebiet von Westungarn. Acta Microbiol Acad Sci Hung 4:155–156.

GORSHANOVA, E. N. 1964. Domestic animals as a source of leptospirosis in Dagestan. J Microbiol (Moscow) 41:120.

HANSON, L. E. 1985. Report of the committee on leptospirosis. Proc 90th Meet US Anim Health Assoc, p. 217.

_____. 1987. *Bratislava* – a newly recognised leptospiral serovar in swine. Swine Consultant (Spring):1–8.

HANSON, L. E., AND TRIPATHY, D. N. 1986. Leptospirosis. In Diseases of Swine, 6th ed. Ed. A. D. Leman, B. Straw, R. D. Glock, W. L. Mengeling, R. H. C. Penny, and E. Scholl. Ames: Iowa State Univ Press, pp. 591–599.

HANSON, L. E.; SCHNURRENBERGER, P. R.; MARSHALL, R. B.; AND SCHERRICK, G. W. 1965. Leptospiral serotypes in Illinois cattle and swine. Proc US Livest Sanit Assoc 69:164.

HANSON, L. E.; REYNOLDS, H. A.; AND EVANS, L. B. 1971. Leptospirosis in swine caused by serovar *grippotyphosa*. Am J Vet Res 32:855.

HARTMANN, E. G.; BRUMMELMAN, B.; AND DIKKEN, H. 1975. Leptospirae of serotype *lora* of the serogroup Australis isolated for the first time from swine in the Netherlands. Tidjschr Diergeneeskd 100:421–425.

HATHAWAY, S. C. 1981. Leptospirosis in New Zealand: An ecological view. NZ Vet J 29:109–112.

_____. 1983. Leptospirosis in pigs in England. FRCVS thesis. Royal College of Veterinary Surgeons, London.

_____. 1985. Porcine leptospirosis. Pig News Inf 6:31–34.

HATHAWAY, S. C., AND LITTLE, T. W. A. 1981. Prevalence and clinical significance of leptospiral antibodies in pigs in England. Vet Rec 108:224–228.

HATHAWAY, S. C.; LITTLE, T. W. A.; AND STEVENS, A. E. 1981. Serological and bacteriological survey of leptospiral infection in pigs in southern England. Res Vet Sci 31:169–173.

HATHAWAY, S. C.; ELLIS, W. A.; LITTLE, T. W. A.; STEVENS, A. E.; AND FERGUSON, H. W. 1983. *Leptospira interrogans* serovar *hardjo* in pigs: A new host-parasite relationship in the United Kingdom. Vet Rec 113:153–154.

HODGES, R. T.; STOCKER, R. P.; AND BUDDLE, J. R. 1976. *Leptospira interrogans* serotype *pomona* infection and leptospiruria in vaccinated pigs. NZ Vet J 24:37–39.

HODGES, R. T.; THOMPSON, J.; AND TOWNSEND, K. G. 1979. Leptospirosis in pigs: The effectiveness of streptomycin in stopping leptospiruria. NZ Vet J 27:124–126.

JENSEN, A. M., AND BINDER, M. 1989. Serological reactions for leptospires in reproductive failure in Danish pigs. Is there a connection? A preliminary investigation. Dansk Vet 72:1181–1187.

JOHNSON, R. C., AND HARRIS, V. G. 1967. Differentiation of pathogenic and saprophytic leptospires. 1. Growth at low temperatures. J Bacteriol 94:27–31.

KEMENES, F., AND SUVEGES, T. 1976. *Leptospira*-induced repeated abortion in sows. Acta Vet Hung 26:395–403.

KINGSCOTE, B. F. 1986. Leptospirosis outbreak in a piggery in southern Alberta. Can Vet J 27:188–190.

———. 1988. Leptospiral serovars in Canada. Can Vet J 29:70–71.

KLARENBEEK, A., AND WINSSER, J. 1937. Ein Fall von spontaner Weilscher Krankheit bei Ferkeln. Dtsch Tieraerztl Wochenschr 45:434–435.

LANGHAM, R. F.; MORSE, E. V.; AND MORTER, R. L. 1958. Experimental leptospirosis. V. Pathology of *Leptospira pomona* infection in swine. Am J Vet Res 19:395–400.

McERLEAN, B. A. 1973. The isolation of leptospirae from the kidneys of bacon pigs. Irish Vet J 27:185–186.

McKEEVER, S.; GORMAN, G. W.; CHAPMAN, J. F.; GALTON, M. M.; AND POWERS, D. K. 1958. Incidence of leptospirosis in wild mammals from southwestern Georgia with a report of new hosts of six serotypes of leptospires. Am J Trop Med Hyg 7:646.

MATVEEVA, A. A.; SAKHAROVA, P. V.; SHARBAN, E. K.; AND DRAGOMIR, A. V. 1977. [Etiology of leptospires in animals in the Moldavian Republic USSR]. Veterinariya (Moscow) 1:61–63.

MICHNA, S. W. 1962. Abortion in the sow due to infection by *Leptospira canicola*. A prelimary report. Vet Rec 74:917–919.

———. 1970. Leptospirosis. Vet Rec 86:484–496.

MICHNA, S. W., AND CAMPBELL, R. S. F. 1969. Leptospirosis in pigs: Epidemiology, microbiology and pathology. Vet Rec 84:135–138.

MITCHELL, D.; ROBERTSON, A.; CORNER, A. H.; AND BOULANGER, P. 1966. Some observations on the diagnosis and epidemiology of leptospirosis in swine. Can J Comp Med 30:211–217.

MITSCHERLICH, E., AND MARTH, E. H. 1984. Microbial Survival in the Environment. Berlin: Springer-Verlag, pp. 202–243.

MORSE, E. V.; BAUER, D. C.; LANGHAM, R. F.; LANG, R. W.; AND ULLREY, D. E. 1958. Experimental leptospirosis. IV. Pathogenesis of porcine *Leptospira pomona* infections. Am J Vet Res 19:388–394.

MORTER, E. V.; MORSE, E. V.; AND LANGHAM, R. F. 1960. Experimental leptospirosis. VII. Re-exposure of

pregnant sows with *Leptospira pomona*. Am J Vet Res 21:95.

NISSEN, O. D. 1989. Leptospirosis in pigs. A review of the literature and a study of the development of titres against *L. bratislava* in two herds. Dansk Vet 72:619–635.

PRESTON, K. S., AND MORTER, R. L. 1960. Rapid laboratory confirmation of clinical diagnosis of *Leptospira pomona* infection in pregnant sows. Allied Vet 31:104–107.

PROPOPCAKOVA, H.; POSPISIL, R.; CISLAKOVA, L.; AND KOZAK, M. 1981. Determination of antibodies to leptospirosis in animals and man in eastern Slovakia in the past ten years. Veterinarstvi 31:275–277.

ROTH, E. E. 1964. Leptospirosis in wildlife in the United States. Proc Am Vet Med Assoc 101:211.

RYLEY, J. W., AND SIMMONS, G. C. 1954a. *Leptospira pomona* as a cause of abortion and neonatal mortality in swine. Queensl J Agric Sci 11:61–74.

———. 1954b. Leptospirosis of pigs with special reference to birth of dead pigs and neonatal mortality. Aust Vet J 30:203–208.

SANDSTEDT, K., AND ENGVALL, A. 1985. Serum antibodies to *Leptospira bratislava* in Swedish pigs and horses. Nord Vet Med 37:312–313.

SARAVI, M. A.; MOLINAR, R.; SORIA; E. H.; AND BARRIOLA, J. L. 1989. Serological and bacteriological diagnosis, and reproductive consequences of an outbreak of porcine leptospirosis caused by a member of the *Pomona* serogroup. Res Sci Tech Off Int Epix 8:709–718.

SCHNURRENBERGER, P. R.; HANSON, L. E.; AND MARTIN, R. J. 1970. Long term surveillance of leptospirosis on an Illinois farm. Am J Epidemiol 92:223–239.

SCHONBERG, A. 1989. Personal communication.

SEBEK, Z.; TREML, F.; AND VALOVA, M. 1983. Experimental infection with the virulent central European murine *Leptospira pomona* strain in the pig. Folia Parasitol 30:269–275.

SLEIGHT, S. D., AND LUNDBERG, A. M. 1961. Persistence of *Leptospira pomona* in porcine tissues. J Am Vet Med Assoc 139:455–456.

SLEIGHT, S. D.; LANGHAM, R. F.; AND MORTER, R. L. 1960. Experimental leptospirosis: The early pathogenesis of *Leptospira pomona* infection in young swine. J Infect Dis 106:262–269.

STALHEIM, O. H. V. 1967. Chemotherapy of renal leptospirosis in swine. Am J Vet Res 28:161–166.

TRIPATHY, D. N.; HANSON, L. E.; MANSFIELD, M. E.; AND THILSTED, J. P. 1981. Pathogenesis of *Leptospira pomona* in lactating sows and transmission to piglets. Proc US Anim Health Assoc 85:188.

URBAN V. P., AND ANDROSOV, V. A. 1976. [Titer of leptospiral antibodies as a function of time and course of infectious process]. Dokl Vses Acad Sci-Khoz Nauk 2:39–42.

WANDURSKI, A. 1982. Effect of infections with various serotypes of *Leptospira interrogans* on the fertility of swine. Med Weter 38:218–220.

WEBER, B., AND FENSKE, G. 1978. Unterschungen zur *Leptospira bratislava* Infection beim Schwein. Monatsh Vet Med 33:652–656.

WRATHALL, A. E. 1975. Reproductive disorders in pigs. Commonwealth Agricultural Bureaux. Anim Health Rev Ser No. 11.

YASUDA, P. H.; STEIGERVALT, A. G.; SULZER, K. R.; KAUFMANN, A. F.; ROGERS, F.; AND BRENNER, D. J. 1987. Deoxyribonucleic acid relatedness between serogroups and serovars in the family Leptospiraceae with proposals for seven new *Leptospira* species. Int J Syst Bacteriol 37:407–415.

43 Mycoplasmal Diseases

R. F. Ross

MYCOPLASMAL PNEUMONIA of swine (MPS) or enzootic pneumonia, caused by *Mycoplasma hyopneumoniae,* is one of the most important causes of disease-associated loss in swine production. Economic loss associated with MPS is often the result of a complex interaction between mycoplasmal and bacterial infections, poor management, and poor environmental conditions. *M. hyorhinis,* another common inhabitant of the respiratory tract of swine, is not a primary cause of pneumonia, but occasionally causes polyserositis and arthritis in young pigs; *M. hyosynoviae* causes arthritis in growing and finishing swine. Other swine isolates, not known to be pathogenic or not common, include *M. flocculare, M. sualvi, M. hyopharyngis,* and several species of acholeplasmas.

Mycoplasmal Pneumonia of Swine

CHRONIC PNEUMONIA of swine has been recognized as a serious impediment to swine production for almost 100 years. Definitive characterization of enzootic pneumonia, particularly its distinction from swine influenza, resulted from the work of Pullar (1948) and Gulrajani and Beveridge (1951). Because the agent was filterable, the term virus pneumonia of pigs was used widely. In 1965, a mycoplasma was isolated from pneumonic lung and demonstrated to reproduce the disease in the United States (Maré and Switzer 1965) and England (Goodwin et al. 1965). The American and British isolates, named *M. hyopneumoniae* and *M. suipneumoniae* respectively, were shown to be identical, and the former name was found to have priority. Enzootic pneumonia has been reported from many countries and is one of the most common and economically important diseases occurring in swine. Information on the distribution and significance of the disease, reviewed by Whittlestone (1973, 1979) and Switzer and Ross (1975), represents the current situation.

ETIOLOGY. Isolation of the organism is complicated by its extremely fastidious growth requirements and the frequent presence of *M. hyorhinis* in swine pneumonias. The most widely used medium is that described by Friis (1975). Media and methods for isolation of *M. hyopneumoniae* were reviewed by Ross and Whittlestone (1983).

In primary broth cultures, *M. hyopneumoniae* grows slowly, producing a faint turbidity and an acid color shift after 3–30 days incubation. Generally, cultures are passaged several times in broth, then inoculated on agar medium and incubated in a 5–10% carbon dioxide atmosphere. Colonies of the organism become barely visible after 2–3 days incubation, and they increase in size to about 0.25–1 mm diameter in about 10 days. Information concerning the biologic and biochemical properties of *M. hyopneumoniae* and methods for specific identification were reviewed by Ross and Whittlestone (1983). *M. flocculare,* a nonpathogen common in swine lungs, has many morphologic, growth, and antigenic similarities to *M. hyopneumoniae.*

EPIDEMIOLOGY. Field observations have strongly implicated carrier swine as a major source of infection with *M. hyopneumoniae.* In an early report, Pullar (1948) summarized data on outbreaks of pneumonia in 190 Australian swine herds; 80% of outbreaks were associated with introduction and commingling of store (feeder) pigs with swine already present on the farm, and 20% were associated with introduction of adult breeding stock.

Current evidence indicates that transmission of *M. hyopneumoniae* is effected by direct contact with respiratory tract secretions from infected swine. Goodwin (1972a) demonstrated that the organism could be isolated from nasal samples from affected pigs. Farrington (1976) and Etheridge et al. (1979a) demonstrated that transmission of the organism occurs among penmate swine; however, transmission does not always take place even among commingled penmates (Goodwin 1972b). Because of the fastidious nature of the organism and the large inoculum required for experimental

537

transmission of the disease, dogma has held that it could not be easily transmitted between herds unless carrier swine were involved. However, many breakdowns have occurred in pneumonia-free herds that were thought to be rather strictly isolated (Whittlestone 1973, 1979). In Britain, Goodwin (1985) found that breakdowns occurred most frequently when herds were less than 3.2 km apart. Jorsal and Thomsen (1988) found that reinfections occurred most frequently in Danish herds during the autumn and winter and when specific-pathogen-free (SPF) herds were close to non-SPF herds. Transmission was especially likely when the latter contained more than 500 swine.

MPS is maintained in many herds by sow-to-pig transmission of *M. hyopneumoniae*. Once infection is established in a few pigs, transmission among penmates occurs, especially after animals are pooled together at weaning time. In continuous-production systems *M. hyopneumoniae* and a number of other important respiratory pathogens may be transmitted in large numbers from older to younger pigs. Overt signs of MPS usually are not seen until piglets are 6 weeks of age or older. Although *M. hyopneumoniae* infections are commonly thought to begin in the nursing pig, microbiologic evidence that it is common in such lesions has not been presented. Kott (1983) found no evidence of *M. hyopneumoniae* in lungs of 55 baby pigs with pneumonia. Predominant organisms isolated were *Haemophilus parasuis, M. hyorhinis,* and *Bordetella bronchiseptica*. Pigs of various ages seem to be equally susceptible to the disease (Piffer and Ross 1984). Undoubtedly, the long incubation period, slow spread of the organism in litters, increased animal density, spread of other infectious agents, and environmental factors that develop following weaning contribute to the peak prevalence of *M. hyopneumoniae* disease in growing and finishing swine.

Chronic pneumonia of swine is extremely common and causes considerable economic loss in all areas where swine are raised. Surveys conducted in a variety of countries have indicated that lesions typical of those seen with MPS occur in 30–80% of slaughter-weight swine (Whittlestone 1973, 1979; Switzer and Ross 1975). In the United States, a study of slaughter hogs from 337 herds from 13 states indicated that 99% of the herds had hogs with lesions of pneumonia (Muller and Abbott 1986). The frequency of isolation of *M. hyopneumoniae* from chronic swine pneumonia has been reported to range from 25% (Goiš et al. 1980) to 93% (Yamamoto and Ogata 1982). In a survey of Iowa breeding swine of various ages, Young et al. (1983) found that animals in 60% of 597 herds had complement-fixing antibodies to *M. hyopneumoniae*. In another survey of Iowa swine, primarily slaughter-weight swine, Owen (1990) found complement-fixing antibodies to the organism in sera from 80% of 88 herds and 32%

of 2077 animals in these herds.

Economic loss attributable to MPS has long been associated with reduced rate of gain and feed efficiency (Switzer and Ross 1975). Braude and Plonka (1975) found that an outbreak of MPS in a British herd resulted in an estimated increased cost of production of £0.75 ($1.50) per pig. Pointon et al. (1985) reported that growth rate of pigs held in contact with MPS-affected pigs was reduced by 12.7% between 50- and 85-kg body weight. In another trial, they found that growth rate of pigs exposed to infected dams was reduced by 15.9% (between 8- and 85-kg body weight), and feed conversion was decreased by 13.8% (between 10- and 25-kg body weight). Losses were estimated to be approximately $2.80 (Australian) for each pig produced.

Much information about prevalence of MPS and the related economic loss has been based on evaluation of lungs at slaughter weight. Recent reports indicate that caution must be exercised in using data collected in slaughter examinations (Morrison et al. 1986). Scheidt et al. (1990a) found no correlation between average daily gain and severity of pneumonia at slaughter, and Noyes et al. (1988) found little correlation between extent of lesions detected at slaughter and those detected radiologically earlier in life.

PATHOGENESIS. The incubation period of MPS was reported to be 10–16 days under natural conditions (Betts 1952); however, other reports have indicated considerable variability in duration. Onset of disease is probably dependent on the intensity of infection with the organism on the tracheal and bronchial mucosal surfaces. Disease has been reported in pigs 2 weeks of age (Holmgren 1974), but it generally spreads slowly and many pigs do not evidence disease until they are 3–6 months old.

In the early stages of infection, large numbers of mycoplasmas have been detected by electron microscopy as well as by immunofluorescence (IF) tests, primarily on the surface of the trachea, bronchi, and bronchioles. Very few organisms have been found in the small bronchioles and alveoli. Scanning (Mebus and Underdahl 1977) and transmission (Blanchard et al. 1990) electron microscopy of MPS-affected lungs revealed a close association of mycoplasmas with the cilia as well as extensive loss of cilia. No evidence of a specialized attachment or orientation of the organism to the epithelial cells has been demonstrated. Consolidation patterns in MPS reflect a bronchogenic distribution of the infection, compromised mucociliary clearance, and gravitational settling of byproducts of the primary mucosal infection into the terminal airways and alveoli. The microscopic changes in mycoplasmal pneumonias of other animals, especially peribronchial and perivascular lymphoreticular hyperplasia, are widely thought to reflect significant involvement of the immune response in lesion development.

Recent efforts have been directed toward elucidation of the pathogenetic mechanisms utilized by *M. hyopneumoniae* in induction of pneumonia. Adherence of the organism to ciliated cells of the respiratory epithelia appears to be an important event (Mebus and Underdahl 1977). Efforts to study adhesion in vitro revealed that the organism adhered to red blood cells (Young et al. 1989) and to tissue culture monolayers (Zielinski et al. 1990). However, convincing evidence that these in vitro models are good correlates of the *M. hyopneumoniae*/respiratory epithelial cell interaction in infected pigs was not obtained. Infected airways evidence ciliary and epithelial cell damage. DeBey and Ross (1990) produced similar damage in vitro with tracheal ring cultures inoculated with pneumonic lung homogenate containing *M. hyopneumoniae*. In addition, membranes from the organism have been shown to cause cytotoxic damage to monolayers of tissue cultures (Geary and Walczak 1985). Another potentially important event in the pathogenesis of the disease is the interaction of the mycoplasma with lymphoid cells. Membranes of the organism were mitogenic for porcine lymphocytes in vitro (Messier and Ross 1990), and swine infected with the organism have altered alveolar macrophage function (Caruso and Ross 1990) and are immunosuppressed (Wannemuehler et al. 1988; Weng and Lin 1988).

Virtually all naturally occurring cases of MPS are mixed infections involving mycoplasmas, bacteria, viruses, or nematodes. L'Ecuyer et al. (1961) and Goiš et al. (1975) present ample evidence of the role of *M. hyorhinis* and *P. multocida* (Chap. 45) in the disease. Experimentally induced *M. hyopneumoniae* pneumonia has been shown to predispose swine to pneumonia caused by *P. multocida* (Ciprian et al. 1988) and *Actinobacillus*

pleuropneumoniae (Yagihashi et al. 1984). The importance of environmental factors in respiratory disease losses is discussed by Curtis and Backstrom in Chapter 71.

Lloyd and Etheridge (1981) found that intravenous administration of some strains of *M. hyopneumoniae* resulted in a severe chronic arthritis. Evidence that arthritis or any other extrapulmonary disease occurs in naturally occurring infections with *M. hyopneumoniae* has not been presented.

CLINICAL SIGNS. Betts (1952) described MPS as a chronic disease with a high morbidity and a low mortality. The principal clinical sign is a chronic, nonproductive cough. Onset of the disease is gradual, with coughing continuing for a few weeks or even months, although some affected pigs evidence little or no coughing. Intensity of coughing is often greatest in growing and finishing swine. Respiratory movements are normal unless extensive lung involvement, especially secondary bacterial infection, develops. Death loss associated with secondary bacterial infection and stress may occur at 4–6 months of age. Animals with this "secondary breakdown" may evidence inappetence, labored breathing or "thumping," increased coughing, elevated temperatures, and prostration. Most pigs with MPS evidence no malaise but appear unthrifty, their hair coat lacking a normal "bloom." Growth may be retarded and stunting may occur, although appetites are usually normal.

LESIONS. Gross lesions in lungs of swine with MPS consist of purple to gray areas of consolidation. The lesions are virtually always in the ventral portions of the cranial and middle lobes, the accessory lobe, and the cranial portion of the caudal lobes of the lungs (Fig. 43.1). The gross

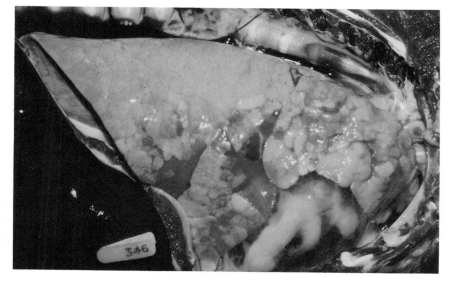

43.1. The lung of a pig with *M. hyopneumoniae* pneumonia.

appearance of the involved lung resembles that of atelectatic lung, particularly during the chronic stages of disease. When the affected lung is incised, the consistency is "meaty" but not excessively firm. In early and middle stages of disease, there is usually a catarrhal exudate in the airways. Bronchial and mediastinal lymph nodes are often enlarged.

Microscopic changes in the lungs of pigs with experimentally induced MPS have been described by Whittlestone (1972). The lesions are very similar to those described in reports on the naturally occurring disease. Early lesions consist of small accumulations of neutrophils in the lumina and around airways as well as in the alveoli. Infiltrating lymphocytes are seen in adventitia of arterioles and venules and around airways. As the disease progresses, there are increased numbers of lymphocytes in perivascular, peribronchial, and peribronchiolar tissues as well as in the lamina propria of the airways. Alveoli may contain eosinophilic edema fluid and increased numbers of mononuclear, septal, and polymorphonuclear cells (Fig. 43.2). By about 15–20 days there is appreciable cuffing or lymphoid hyperplasia around the airways, more extensive accumulations of edema fluid, and large mononuclear and other inflammatory cells in alveoli, and thickening of interalveolar septa. More advanced lesions, 17–40 days postinfection as described by Whittlestone (1972), consist of extensively proliferated lymphoreticular tissue in perivascular and peribronchiolar areas (Fig. 43.3). In recovering lesions described by Whittlestone, there were collapsed alveoli, alveolar emphysema, and rather extensive hyperplastic lymphoid nodules (Fig. 43.4), especially in association with the airways.

MPS lesions are markedly influenced by secondary bacterial infections, stress, poor air quality, and bad management (Chaps. 7 and 71).

DIAGNOSIS. Clinical signs that are helpful and lead one to suspect MPS include a chronic nonproductive cough, retarded growth and stunt-

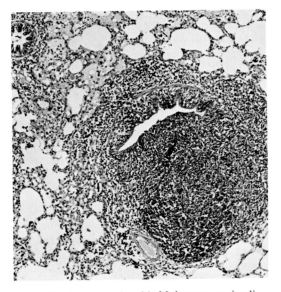

43.3. The lung of a pig with *M. hyopneumoniae* disease. More advanced lesion with resolving alveolar inflammation and peribronchiolar lymphocytic hyperplasia. H & E. ×287.

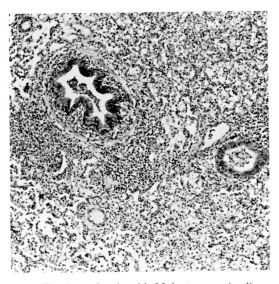

43.2. The lung of a pig with *M. hyopneumoniae* disease. Early stage with mixed alveolar exudate and some peribronchiolar lymphocytic infiltration. H & E.

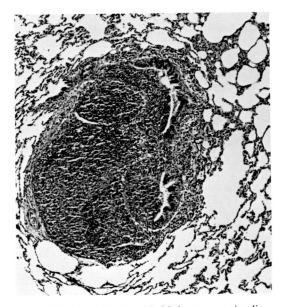

43.4. The lung of a pig with *M. hyopneumoniae* disease. Advanced lymphocytic hyperplasia, including obliteration of bronchioles. H & E. ×287.

ing, low mortality, slow onset and spread, and repeated occurrence of the disease. Lesions of MPS, described in the previous section, are characteristic for MPS but are not specific in that similar lesions may be seen in pneumonias caused by other agents.

Serologic methods found useful for diagnosis of MPS include indirect hemagglutination (IHA), complement-fixation (CF), and enzyme-linked immunosorbent assay (ELISA) (Ross and Whittlestone 1983). Other tests that have been evaluated include agglutination, latex agglutination, and indirect IF tests.

The CF test is relatively sensitive and specific for MPS, although cross-reactions with *M. flocculare* and *M. hyorhinis* have been detected. Pigs develop CF antibodies by 1–5 weeks postexposure and become seronegative by 13–15 weeks postexposure (Slavik and Switzer 1972). Some infected pigs do not develop CF antibodies.

The IHA test appears to be specific and sensitive; however, it has not been used extensively because it is difficult to perform. Freeman et al. (1984b) found that results obtained with IHA correlated poorly with other indicators of MPS, such as CF and ELISA titers and IF results.

Bruggmann et al. (1977b) described use of the ELISA with sodium dodecyl sulfate extract as antigen in diagnosis of *M. hyopneumoniae* disease in swine. The test was found to be highly sensitive and relatively specific, although in later work it was reported that cross-reactions were detected between *M. hyopneumoniae* and *M. hyorhinis* (Bruggmann 1978) and *M. flocculare* (Freeman et al. 1984a). ELISA antibodies develop in susceptible pigs as early as 2 weeks postexposure to infected pigs (Piffer et al. 1984) and persist for as long as 52 weeks postexposure (Armstrong et al. 1983; Bereiter et al. 1990). Use of Tween 20 extract instead of sodium dodecyl sulphate (SDS) extract resulted in improved specificity of the ELISA for detection of antibodies to *M. hyopneumoniae* (Nicolet et al. 1980; Bommeli and Nicolet 1983). Cross-reactions resulting from *M. flocculare* infections were minimized using a slight modification of the Tween 20 ELISA (Bereiter et al. 1990).

L'Ecuyer and Boulanger (1970), Meyling (1971), and others have found the IF test to be a highly reliable diagnostic method for detection of *M. hyopneumoniae* in infected lung. Direct as well as indirect modifications have been used, and positive results obtained have correlated well with positive findings obtained by other methods. IF seems particularly suited for acute-stage disease when larger amounts of mycoplasmal cells are present. The organism can be found principally on the bronchial and bronchiolar lining of affected lung. *M. hyopneumoniae* has been detected in pneumonic lungs also by use of an enzyme-linked immunoperoxidase technique (Bruggmann et al. 1977a), a radiolabelled DNA probe (Chan and

Ross 1984), the polymerase chain reaction (PCR) (Harasawa et al. 1990), and a capture ELISA (Pedersen et al. 1990).

M. hyopneumoniae is one of the most difficult mycoplasmas to isolate and identify. It grows slowly and is often overgrown by *M. hyorhinis,* a common secondary invader in swine pneumonia. Although methods for isolation have been improved and more laboratories have developed the capability to isolate the organism, diagnosis by culture is not feasible in most situations.

TREATMENT. Early evidence that *M. hyopneumoniae* disease could be controlled at least in part by medication with tetracycline antibiotics has been reviewed by Whittlestone (1973) and Switzer and Ross (1975). Huhn (1971a) demonstrated that chlortetracycline given at 50–200 g/ton feed prevented development of pneumonia. The drug does not prevent establishment of infection, and lesions apparently develop after cessation of medication. Repeated administration of long-acting oxytetracycline during the suckling and early nursery periods may have potential for reducing pneumonias occurring at later stages (Scheidt et al. 1990b). In vitro studies have confirmed the sensitivity of *M. hyopneumoniae* to tetracyclines, although Williams (1978) and Yamamoto and Koshimizu (1984) found chlortetracycline to be less active than oxytetracycline and doxycycline. Etheridge et al. (1979b) found a wide variation in the minimal inhibitory concentration (1.6–25 μg/ml) of chlortetracycline for the organism.

Feed medication with 1000 g/ton tylosin phosphate (Maré and Switzer 1966) and water medication with 2 g/gallon tylosin tartrate (Huhn 1971b) did not prevent MPS. Goodwin (1972a) presented evidence that intramuscular injection of 10 mg/kg tylosin daily, starting the day before exposure and continuing for 3 additional days, reduced the severity of the disease. However, intramuscular inoculation with tylosin at 8.8 mg/kg for 5 days beginning 14 days after intratracheal challenge had no effect on incidence or severity of experimentally induced MPS (Ross 1981). In another study Ross and Skelly (1982) found that tylosin phosphate at 100 g/ton feed for 8 weeks had no effect on severity of lung lesions in pigs with naturally acquired MPS.

Evidence has been presented that lincomycin fed at 200 g/ton for 3 weeks reduces the incidence and severity of MPS and results in improved performance (Van Buren 1983; Graham et al. 1984). However, we found that medication with lincomycin at 500 g/ton of feed continuously did not prevent transmission of *M. hyopneumoniae* from pigs with clinically overt MPS to in-contact susceptible pigs, nor did it reduce the severity of pneumonia in pigs with early-stage established disease (Ross 1985). Administration of several doses of lincomycin intramuscularly to baby pigs was reported to improve gains and efficiency in herds with MPS (Kunesh 1981; Lukert and Mulkey 1982).

Tiamulin at 200 ppm in feed for 10 days reduced severity of experimentally induced (Schuller et al. 1977a) and naturally occurring (Stipkovits et al. 1978a; Martineau et al. 1980) MPS. Tiamulin at 200 ppm in the feed for 10 days (Martineau et al. 1980) improved growth rates; given at 30 ppm continuously (Burch 1984b), it improved weight gains and feed efficiency in the presence of MPS. Administration of 0.006% tiamulin in the drinking water (Johnson et al. 1978) or parenterally at 12.5 mg/kg for 5 days (Hsu et al. 1982) or 15 mg/kg for 3 days (Burch 1984a) was reported to result in clinical improvement and improved growth in the presence of naturally occurring MPS. Yamamoto and Koshimizu (1984) reported that tiamulin had high in vitro activity against *M. hyopneumoniae*. However, in spite of the many published reports on efficacy of tiamulin, we were unable to detect a beneficial effect when the drug was administered in the drinking water at 60, 120, or 180 ppm for 10 days to pigs with experimentally induced MPS (Ross and Cox 1988).

Newer quinolone antibiotics have good in vitro activity against *M. hyopneumoniae* (Hannan et al. 1989). At least three quinolones, enrofloxacin (Simon et al. 1990), danofloxacin (Ross et al. 1990), and norfloxacin (Hannan and Goodwin 1990), have been reported to be effective in treating the disease.

Sulfonamides have long been known to have little influence on *M. hyopneumoniae,* although they are widely used for control of bacterial infections responsible for a great part of the economic loss associated with MPS. Penicillin, streptomycin, and erythromycin are of no value in treatment of MPS.

PREVENTION. Early methods for prevention of MPS were reviewed by Whittlestone (1973) and Switzer and Ross (1975). Effective control of the disease depends on providing an optimal environment including air quality, ventilation, and temperature, and proper stocking density. Use of a strict all-in/all-out production scheme is possibly the most effective way to control the disease in infected herds (Clark et al. 1990; Scheidt et al. 1990c). Clark et al. (1989) have recommended no more than 3 weeks variation in age in stocking a room. The strategy of using repopulation to gain improved performance may be in part related to reduction in the severity of, or complete elimination of, the retarding effects of MPS. Leman (1990) has advocated consideration of repopulation when a pork producer is not competitive; indicators may include poor gains, poor feed efficiency, or excessive mortality.

Various health control schemes have been developed that place emphasis on certification of herds free of MPS and other diseases. Methods used included on-farm inspection, rigid isolation, and periodic examination of lungs from slaughter pigs reared in close confinement (Goodwin and Whittlestone 1967). Whittlestone (1973, 1979) has reviewed problems attendant to breakdowns in various systems for maintenance of MPS-free herds.

It has been known for many years that older sows that have recovered from MPS are less likely to carry *M. hyopneumoniae*. A number of systems have been devised to take advantage of this natural adjunct to disease control. Serotesting of older sows to detect those that are seropositive with the objective of culling them to establish a MPS-free herd has been investigated with variable success (Preston 1976; Schuller et al. 1977b). Renewed efforts to utilize a serotest and cull strategy for controlling MPS should be tried utilizing the Tween 20 ELISA discussed earlier. In work with the Tween 20 ELISA, Zimmermann et al. (1986) found substantially more positive animals when colostrum was tested rather than serum.

The SPF pig program has found wide application in the control of MPS (Twiehaus and Underdahl 1975). Pigs are procured by hysterectomy or cesarean section; reared on colostrum-free diets; and used to repopulate vacated, cleaned swine facilities. Producers that have repopulated according to this system or with second-generation stock derived from primary herds have benefited greatly, although breakdowns have posed a problem. Monitoring for continued freedom from MPS should encompass use of the most sensitive and specific tests such as IF and Tween 20 ELISA for detection of subclinical *M. hyopneumoniae* infections.

Alexander et al. (1980) developed the medicated early weaning (MEW) system, wherein intensive medication of the sow during late gestation and immediately following parturition and of the newborn piglet is used to derive pigs free of *M. hyopneumoniae*. Pigs derived were free of MPS, and monitoring revealed no evidence of *M. hyopneumoniae* or *Bordetella bronchiseptica* in representative pigs examined from 5 weeks of age to slaughter. Harris (1990) has devised a similar strategy (Isowean) utilizing early weaning and rearing in three isolated sites to prevent transmission of a variety of diseases, including *M. hyopneumoniae*, from the sow to the piglet. Pigs reared utilizing the Isowean strategy gained substantially better than those reared in the traditional manner (Harris et al. 1990). Zimmermann et al. (1989) reported that a control program based on removal of all young swine and gilts, coupled with feeding tiamulin or chlortetracycline/tylosin/sulfadimidine to remaining older sows, resulted in elimination of *M. hyopneumoniae* from 16 of 17 Swiss herds. Continued surveillance to assure that the organism had not reentered the herd was accomplished with a four-prong program of clinical observation, commingling of progeny with known susceptible swine during growing and finishing, slaughter examination of lungs, and milk and blood serology with the Tween 20 ELISA.

Protective immunity develops in swine recovered from MPS. *M. hyopneumoniae* vaccines consisting of adjuvanted whole cell preparations have been shown to induce at least partial protection against development of gross lesions of experimentally induced MPS (Goodwin and Whittlestone 1973). Commercial development of adjuvanted whole cell vaccines has been reported recently (Dayalu and Ross 1990; Peterson et al. 1990). Data indicated that these products provided significant reduction in severity of induced MPS. French workers (Kobisch et al. 1987) have shown that a *M. hyopneumoniae* membrane preparation administered to sows enabled passive protection in piglets or, when administered to piglets (Kobisch et al. 1990), rendered them actively immune. Several groups have partially characterized the protective activity of *M. hyopneumoniae* extract or subunit antigens (Lam and Switzer 1971; Ross et al. 1984; Ose et al. 1990). Certain extract vaccines have provided variable protective activity and, in some instances, have enhanced development of lesions (Ross et al. 1984). Widespread adoption of mycoplasma vaccines in the field will depend on clear evidence of significant reduction in overall losses caused by pneumonia in swine.

M. hyorhinis Polyserositis and Arthritis

RESPIRATORY TRACT infection with *M. hyorhinis* has been reported in swine from many different countries. It is the first mycoplasma isolated when an investigator begins searching for these organisms in swine tissue. The organism is an extremely common contaminant in cell culture lines, even in laboratories far removed from contact with swine or swine specimens. The origin of these contaminants has not been determined.

ETIOLOGY. Media and methods for isolation and growth of *M. hyorhinis* have been summarized by Ross and Whittlestone (1983). For isolation, 3–5 days incubation are required; whereas established cultures grow within 1–2 days. The organism requires sterols for growth, ferments glucose, but does not utilize arginine or hydrolyze urea. Colonies produced by *M. hyorhinis* develop with 2–5 days incubation and measure 0.5–1 mm in diameter.

EPIDEMIOLOGY. *M. hyorhinis* infections are transmitted to young pigs from infected sows or from older pigs in a nursery or grower unit. The organism can be isolated from nasal or sinus secretions of about 10% of sows (Ross and Spear 1973) and from the nasal secretions of about 30–40% of weanling swine. The organism is also common (51–64%) in pneumonic lungs of slaughter swine (L'Ecuyer et al. 1961; Goiš et al. 1975). Nasal and tracheobronchial infections with *M. hyorhinis* appear to spread rapidly once one pig in a group becomes infected. Many infected pigs evidence no clinical disease, although experimental work with gnotobiotic pigs and a field study by Kott (1983) suggest that it may play an important role in pneumonias of baby pigs.

PATHOGENESIS. *M. hyorhinis* is very common in nasal and tracheobronchial secretions of young swine. It seems likely that other diseases such as pneumonia or stress facilitate septicemic infection of pigs already colonized with the organism. When this occurs, the organism may localize in the joints and the serous membrane–lined body cavities, where it then elicits acute serofibrinous inflammation. As the disease progresses, pigs develop marked increases in serum proteins, especially gamma globulin, and low levels of antiglobulin may develop.

M. hyorhinis can be isolated from acute-stage lesions. During the subacute disease (i.e., 2 weeks to 3 months after onset) it can still be isolated but is present in a decreasing number of sites. The organism persists for as long as 6 months in some affected joints.

Some strains of the organism produce pneumonia in gnotobiotic pigs (Goiš and Kuksa 1974). Less clear is its capability of acting as a primary cause of pneumonia in naturally born pigs. It is possible that the pulmonary pathogenicity of *M. hyorhinis* is strain variable. Although *M. hyorhinis* is a frequent isolate from pneumonia with lymphoreticular hyperplasia characteristic of that produced by *M. hyopneumoniae,* it is also frequent in lesions of other bronchopneumonias (Schulman et al. 1970). No difference has been detected in severity between pneumonias with or without *M. hyorhinis.*

CLINICAL SIGNS. Outbreaks of polyserositis generally occur in swine 3–10 weeks of age, although occasionally the disease occurs in young adult swine. The first clinical evidence of illness occurs 3–10 days postexposure or after a precipitating stress. Acute-phase signs consist of a roughened hair coat, moderate temperature elevations, listlessness, moderate inappetence, reluctance to move, abdominal tenderness, lameness, and swollen joints. Evidence of abdominal and thoracic involvement is manifested by a tucked-up appearance, labored breathing, stretching movements, and lying in a sternal recumbency. The duration and degree of clinical change during the acute phase varies, depending on the severity of the lesions.

Ten to 14 days after onset, acute-phase signs begin to abate, and the main clinical signs thereafter consist of lameness and swollen joints. Joint involvement is most severe during the subacute stage of the disease. Two to 3 months after onset, lameness and joint swelling may become less severe, although some pigs are still lame 6 months later.

LESIONS. Acute-stage lesions consist of acute serofibrinous and fibrinopurulent pericarditis, pleuritis, and to a lesser extent peritonitis (Fig. 43.5). Acute joint lesions consist of swelling and hyperemia of the synovial membranes and increased amounts of serosanguineous synovial fluid.

Microscopic changes in acute lesions consist of thickening of serosal membrane; infiltration of subserosal tissue with lymphocytes, plasma cells, and some neutrophils; and fibrinopurulent exudate on the serosal surface. Acute-stage joint lesions consist of mild villous hypertrophy; thickening of the synovial cell layer; infiltration of the subsynovial tissue with lymphocytes, plasma cells, and macrophages; and some fibrinopurulent surface exudate.

Subacute-phase serosal membrane lesions consist of organized fibrous adhesions and thickened, cloudy serosal membranes. Microscopically, there are fibrous connective tissue and scattered foci of lymphocytes (Fig. 43.6). Synovial membranes may be quite thickened, and villous hypertrophy is evident (Fig. 43.7). Synovial fluid is serosanguineous and increased markedly in amount. Microscopically, diffuse and perivascular accumulations of lymphocytes, and in some cases nodules of lymphocytes, are seen in the synovium. Villous hypertrophy and a thickened lining cell layer are seen.

In later stages, 3–6 months, lesions appear less active, although cartilage erosion and pannus formation may be seen. Lymphocytic nodules are common in the synovium. Serosal lesions consist of organized fibrous adhesions.

DIAGNOSIS. Gross lesions of serofibrinous to fibrinopurulent polyserositis and arthritis in 3- to 10-week-old swine are suggestive of *M. hyorhinis* disease, although similar lesions are also caused by *Haemophilus parasuis* and other agents. The organism generally can be isolated from acute- and early subacute-phase lesions. Animals examined for diagnosis should be killed in the acute stage of the disease. Autolytic changes in dead animals may reduce the chances of isolating *M. hyorhinis.*

Swine with *M. hyorhinis* polyserositis and arthritis evidence strong complement-fixing antibody responses. However, serodiagnosis has been little used in this disease, and it is possible that many normal swine have titers developed from subclinical or respiratory infection with *M. hyorhinis.*

TREATMENT. Although *M. hyorhinis* is generally quite sensitive to tylosin or lincomycin in vitro, antibiotic therapy of swine clinically ill with

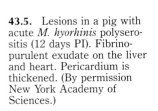

43.5. Lesions in a pig with acute *M. hyorhinis* polyserositis (12 days PI). Fibrinopurulent exudate on the liver and heart. Pericardium is thickened. (By permission New York Academy of Sciences.)

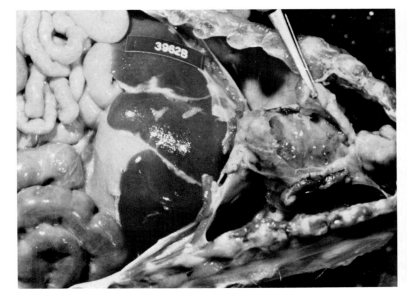

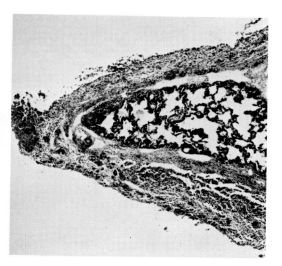

43.6. Lung and pleura of a pig with *M. hyorhinis* pleuritis (45 days PI). H & E. ×160.

43.7. Synovial membrane from a pig joint with *M. hyorhinis* arthritis (14 days PI). Villi are hypertrophied and contain lymphocytic cellular infiltrate. H & E. ×176. (By permission New York Academy of Sciences.)

M. hyorhinis disease is not very satisfactory. The inflammatory response seems to either prevent antibiotic penetration or to be self-perpetuating. Treatment with tylosin or lincomycin on a herd basis may be beneficial.

PREVENTION. Control programs should emphasize control of other conditions such as respiratory or enteric disease or stress that might predispose to *M. hyorhinis* disease. No data is available on the efficacy of prophylactic feed medication with tylosin, lincomycin, or other antibiotics.

M. hyosynoviae Arthritis

ARTHRITIS associated with *M. hyosynoviae* infection has been reported principally in the United States, although the disease also has been reported in England (Roberts et al. 1972) and Germany (Ross et al. 1977). Nielsen (1988) reported severe outbreaks of bursitis associated with *M. hyosynoviae* infection in Danish slaughter pigs.

ETIOLOGY. *M. hyosynoviae* can be isolated best in mycoplasma medium containing mucin (Ross and Karmon 1970). The organism requires sterols for growth and utilizes arginine but does not ferment glucose or hydrolyze urea. Colonies of *M. hyosynoviae* develop on agar medium within 2- to 4-days incubation and measure 0.5–1 mm in diameter. A selective procedure for isolation of *M. hyopneumoniae* in the presence of *M. hyorhinis* has been reported (Friis et al. 1990).

EPIDEMIOLOGY. The organism is common in nasal and pharyngeal secretions of sows (Ross and Spear 1973), apparently persisting in such carrier swine indefinitely. Transmission from adult carrier swine to young piglets generally does not occur until the pigs are 4–8 weeks of age. Shedding of large numbers of the organism in mucosal secretions occurs during the acute stage of the disease.

Nasal and pharyngeal infection with *M. hyosynoviae* occurs first in a few pigs at 4–8 weeks of age (Ross and Spear 1973). The spread among penmates has not been studied thoroughly; however, it seems that in some herds most pigs have experienced nasal and/or pharyngeal infection by 12 weeks of age. Rate of spread might be related to population density and environment.

PATHOGENESIS. Two to 4 days following intranasal exposure, *M. hyosynoviae* can be isolated from the blood. The septicemia persists for 8–10 days, and during this time joint infection may occur. The duration and severity of joint infection is variable. Many infected joints do not have lesions of arthritis and are infected for only a few days. Other joints evidence acute arthritis; the organism probably grows to higher titers and persists longer in these joints. *M. hyosynoviae* has been isolated as long as 24 days postinoculation.

Factors that contribute to development of lesions in joints have not been determined. The arthritis is especially severe in heavily muscled swine that have poor leg action and conformation, i.e., stilted gait with especially straight legs. Osteochondrosis, a degenerative disease of the epiphyseal and subchondral osteoid tissue, is also extremely common in the same type of pig. It seems likely that joint lesions developing as a result of osteochondrosis or trauma-induced bursal lesions (Nielsen 1988) might predispose to infection with *M. hyosynoviae.*

CLINICAL SIGNS. Clinical evidence of *M. hyosynoviae* disease occurs principally in pigs 12–24 weeks of age. Lameness appears suddenly and may occur in one or more limbs. Temperature elevations generally are not detected. Severely affected pigs may have slight to moderate inappetence and loss of weight.

Rear leg involvement is evidenced as limping, frequent flexion of the affected leg, shifting of weight from one leg to another, or one or both legs positioned abnormally forward. Front leg involvement appears as limping, stiffness, kneeling on the fetlock, or uneven leg stance. Animals with the disease usually have difficulty rising or in some instances are not able to rise. Joint swelling is usually not observed because joints covered with muscle are most often involved. Pseudocysts or calluses on the cranial surface of the carpal joint or the plantar and lateral surface of the tarsal joint may become swollen (Nielsen 1988).

Acute-phase signs persist for 3–10 days, and following that, severity of lameness generally decreases. Many animals recover and evidence no further lameness, or only stiffness. Some pigs may be lame for several weeks or months; however, clinical signs in such animals are often a reflection of osteochondrosis as well. Morbidity

of *M. hyosynoviae* arthritis varies from 1 to 50% in affected herds. Mortality is very low, occurring only when affected animals cannot eat or are killed by penmates.

LESIONS. Synovial membranes in acute *M. hyosynoviae* arthritis are swollen, edematous, and hyperemic (Fig. 43.8). Synovial fluid is increased markedly in volume and is serofibrinous to serosanguineous. Periarticular tissues may be edematous. Pigs with subacute disease have yellow to brown, thickened hyperemic membranes. Mild villous hypertrophy may be seen. In chronic stages the membranes are more thickened, and pannus formation may be seen. Articular cartilage changes may be seen, but these are usually focal and are very likely the result of osteochondrosis. The periarticular fibrosis seen in erysipelas is not observed.

Microscopic changes have not been well characterized; however, the lesions in acute disease are very similar to those seen in *M. hyorhinis* arthritis. There is mild villous hypertrophy; thickening of the synovial cell layer; and infiltration of subsynovial tissues with lymphocytes, plasma cells, and macrophages (Fig. 43.9).

DIAGNOSIS. An outbreak of acute lameness in 10- to 20-week-old swine that is not responsive to penicillin is suggestive of *M. hyosynoviae* arthritis. Definitive diagnosis of the disease should be based on isolation of the organism from typical lesions. Animals examined should be representative of the herd problem, be in the acute stage of the disease, and be unmedicated. Fluids may be aspirated from joints of live animals or from slaughtered or necropsied animals. It is best to examine several representative fluids, since some will be culture-negative.

Antibodies detectable by means of the CF test develop quickly during *M. hyosynoviae* disease

43.8. Femorotibial joint of a pig with *M. hyosynoviae* arthritis (14 days PI). Synovial membrane is darkened and hypertrophied. Articular cartilage is normal. (By permission New York Academy of Sciences.)

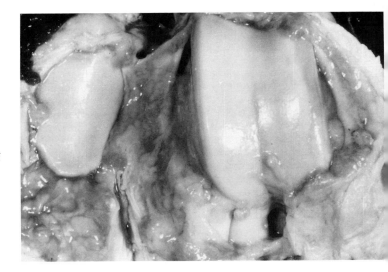

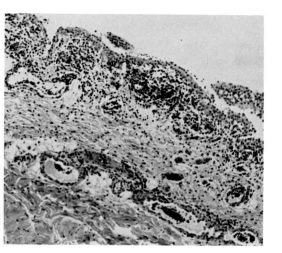

43.9. Synovial membrane from a pig joint with *M. hyosynoviae* arthritis (14 days PI). There are hyperplasia of lining cells and infiltration with mononuclear cells, primarily lymphocytes. H & E. × 184. (By permission New York Academy of Sciences.)

(Zimmermann and Ross 1982). Many pigs have subclinical disease and develop antibodies to the organism; therefore, such tests should be used with paired serums collected during the acute and early convalescent stages of the disease to ascertain that an antibody rise coincides with the clinical problem. Serologic testing for *M. hyosynoviae* is not generally available.

TREATMENT. Treatment of *M. hyosynoviae* disease is best achieved by use of injectable tylosin, lincomycin, or tiamulin, possibly in combination with a corticosteroid. Burch (1984a) reported that intramuscular treatment with 10 mg/kg tiamulin or lincomycin for 3 days resulted in reduced lameness and improved gains in swine with naturally occurring mycoplasmal arthritis. Roberts et al. (1972) reported that complete recovery resulted if affected swine were given 8 mg of betamethasone within 24 hours of onset of lameness. Pigs with bone and joint damage caused by osteochondrosis will not respond well to any treatment.

PREVENTION. Preventive measures should include selecting breeding stock with good leg action and conformation, preventing stress during the susceptible age, and allowing new young breeding stock time to adjust to a new location. Protective immunity results from infection with *M. hyosynoviae*. It is likely that pigs experiencing the infection prior to 12 weeks of age are protected against the clinical disease at an older age. Vaccines have been shown to be efficacious (Ross 1978) but have not been made available commercially.

Other Mycoplasmas from Swine

INFORMATION on mycoplasmas other than *M. hyorhinus, M. hyopneumoniae,* and *M. hyosynoviae* isolated from swine has been reviewed by Switzer and Ross (1975) and Whittlestone (1979). Isolates reported include mycoplasmas that normally are isolated from some other animal species; previously unreported strains that represent new species but are not yet associated with disease in swine; and acholeplasmas, saprophytic organisms that are common in a wide variety of animal and plant sources.

M. flocculare is a species that has been isolated from lungs and nasal cavities of swine in Denmark (Meyling and Friis 1972), England, and the United States (Armstrong and Friis 1981). Friis (1978) indicated that it is widespread in the upper respiratory tracts of Danish swine, including SPF swine. Friis (1973) presented evidence that *M. flocculare* produced lymphocytic infiltration in the nasal mucosa and peribronchial areas of gnotobiotic pigs inoculated with the organism. Evidence that it is of significance in naturally occurring respiratory disease has not been presented. Freeman et al. (1984b) reported that serums from swine frequently have antibodies detectable with ELISA that react with both *M. hyopneumoniae* and *M. flocculare;* however, Bereiter et al. (1990) found that the Tween 20 antigen allowed good discrimination between the two organisms.

The genitourinary tract is a common site of infection with mycoplasmas in several animal species. Evidence for a consistent mycoplasma flora in the genitourinary tracts of swine has not been presented. Mycoplasmas have been incriminated in the mastitis-metritis-agalactia (MMA) syndrome of sows; however, as reviewed by Switzer and Ross (1975), comprehensive efforts to confirm that mycoplasmas play a role in MMA have been unsuccessful.

Stipkovits et al. (1978b) reported isolation of ureaplasmas from 15 of 47 boar semen samples. The animals had antibodies against the organisms isolated. Kuksa and Goiš (1982) isolated ureaplasmas from vaginal swabs, genital tracts of sows collected at slaughter, and aborted fetuses. Attempts by a number of other workers to isolate ureaplasmas from porcine reproductive tract disease have been nonproductive (Porcine Team 1980, 1982).

Gourlay et al. (1978) reported a mycoplasma

from rectal, intestinal, and vaginal samples from swine, which they named *M. sualvi.* The organism has not been shown to cause disease in swine. Mycoplasmas have also been isolated from, or detected by electron microscopy in, specimens from pigs with conjunctivitis (Friis 1976; Rogers et al. 1990). Other mycoplasmas reported as occasional or incidental isolates from swine include *M. hyopharyngis, M. arginini, M. bovigenitalium, M. buccale, M. gallinarum, M. iners, M. mycoides,* and *M. salivarium.*

Acholeplasmas have many characteristics in common with members of the genus *Mycoplasma.* They differ in having a larger genome and being capable of growth in medium not containing sterols. These organisms are occasionally isolated from respiratory disease in swine. Evidence was presented that *Acholeplasma axanthum* caused pneumonia in disease-free pigs following inoculation with the organism (Stipkovits et al. 1974); however, convincing evidence that these organisms are important in naturally occurring swine respiratory disease has not appeared.

Acholeplasmas, nonpathogenic relatives of the mycoplasmas, may be isolated from nasal and pharyngeal secretions of swine or from environmental sources such as fecal material or recycled effluent used to remove manure from swine facilities. Goiš et al. (1969) demonstrated that acholeplasmas may be the only mycoplasmas isolated from respiratory tracts of swine in respiratory disease-free herds. The source of such strains is not known, but it is likely that they can be carried into closed herds by humans or inanimate materials such as feed. Species of acholeplasmas isolated from swine include *A. laidlawii, A. granularum, A. axanthum,* and *A. oculi.*

REFERENCES

ALEXANDER, T. J. L.; THORNTON, K.; BOON, G.; LYSONS, R. J.; AND GUSH, A. F. 1980. Medicated early weaning to produce pigs free from pathogens endemic in the herd of origin. Vet Rec 106:114–119.

ARMSTRONG, C. H., AND FRIIS, N. F. 1981. Isolation of *Mycoplasma flocculare* from swine in the United States. Am J Vet Res 42:1030–1032.

ARMSTRONG, C. H.; FREEMAN, M. J.; SANDS-FREEMAN, L.; LOPEZ-OSUNA, M.; YOUNG, T.; AND RUNNELS, L. J. 1983. Comparison of the enzyme-linked immunosorbent assay and the indirect hemagglutination and complement fixation tests for detecting antibodies to *Mycoplasma hyopneumoniae*. Can J Comp Med 47:464–470.

BEREITER, M.; YOUNG, T. F.; JOO, H. S.; AND ROSS, R. F. 1990. Evaluation of the ELISA, and comparison to the complement fixation test and radial imunodiffusion enzyme assay for detection of antibodies against *Mycoplasma hyopneumoniae* in swine serum. Vet Microbiol 25:177–192.

BETTS, A. O. 1952. Respiratory diseases of pigs. V. Some clinical and epidemiological aspects of virus pneumonia of pigs. Vet Rec 64:283–288.

BLANCHARD, B.; CAVALIER, A.; LELANNIC, J.; AND KOBISCH, M. 1990. Electron microscopic observation of respiratory tract from gnotobiotic piglets inoculated with *Mycoplasma hyopneumoniae*. IOM Lett 1 (8):480–481.

BOMMELI, W. R., AND NICOLET, J. 1983. A method for the evaluation of enzyme-linked immunoassay results for diagnosing enzootic pneumonia in pig herds. Proc Int Symp World Assoc Vet Lab Diag 3(2):439–442.

BRAUDE, R., AND PLONKA, S. 1975. Effect of enzootic pneumonia on the performance of growing pigs. Vet Rec 96:359–360.

BRUGGMANN, S. 1978. Immunochemical characterization of *Mycoplasma suipneumoniae* by the enzyme linked immunosorbent assay (ELISA). Proc 5th Int Congr Pig Vet Soc, Zagreb, p. KA8.

BRUGGMANN, S.; ENGBERG, B.; AND EHRENSPERGER, F. 1977a. Demonstration of *M. suipneumoniae* in pig lungs by the enzyme-linked immunoperoxidase technique. Vet Rec 101:137.

BRUGGMANN, S.; KELLER, H.; BERTSCHINGER, H. U.; AND ENGBERG, B. 1977b. Quantitative detection of antibodies to *Mycoplasma suipneumoniae* in pigs' sera by an enzyme-linked immunosorbent assay. Vet Rec 101:109–111.

BURCH, D. G. S. 1984a. The evaluation of tiamulin by injection for the treatment of enzootic pneumonia and mycoplasmal arthritis of pigs. Proc 8th Int Congr Pig Vet Soc, Ghent, p. 117.

_____. 1984b. Tiamulin feed premix in the improvement of growth performance of pigs in herds severely affected with enzootic pneumonia. Vet Rec 114:209–211.

CARUSO, J., AND ROSS, R. F. 1990. Effects of *Mycoplasma hyopneumoniae* and *Actinobacillus (Haemophilus) pleuropneumoniae* infections on alveolar macrophage functions in swine. Am J Vet Res 51:227–231.

CHAN, H. W., AND ROSS, R. F. 1984. Restriction endonuclease analyses of two porcine mycoplasma deoxyribonucleic acids; sequence-specific methylation in the *Mycoplasma hyopneumoniae* genome. Int J Syst Bacteriol 34:16–20.

CIPRIAN, A.; PIJOAN, C.; CRUZ, T.; CAMACHO, J.; TORTORA, J.; COLMENARES, G.; LOPEZ-REVILLA, R.; AND DE LA GARZA, M. 1988. *Mycoplasma hyopneumoniae* increases the susceptibility of pigs to experimental *Pasteurella multocida* pneumonia. Can J Vet Res 52:434–438.

CLARK, L. K.; SCHEIDT, A. B.; MAYROSE, V. B.; ARMSTRONG, C. H.; CLINE, T. R.; AND KNOX, K. 1989. Methodology to reduce days to market in swine herds with enzootic pneumonia. Proc Iowa Vet Med Assoc 107:129–135.

CLARK, L. K.; SCHEIDT, A. B.; MAYROSE, V. B.; ARMSTRONG, C. H.; AND KNOX, K. 1990. Prevention of the development of enzootic pneumonia within an infected swine herd. Proc 11th Int Congr Pig Vet Soc, Lausanne, p. 91.

DAYALU, K. I., AND ROSS, R. F. 1990. Evaluation of experimental vaccines for control of porcine pneumonia induced by *Mycoplasma hyopneumoniae*. Proc 11th Int Congr Pig Vet Soc, Lausanne, p. 83.

DEBEY, M. C., AND ROSS, R. F. 1990. Ciliostatic and cytotoxic effects of *Mycoplasma hyopneumoniae* in vitro. IOM Lett 1 (8):315–316.

ETHERIDGE, J. R.; COTTEW, G. S.; AND LLOYD, L. C. 1979a. Isolation of *Mycoplasma hyopneumoniae* from lesions in experimentally infected pigs. Aust Vet J 55:356–359.

ETHERIDGE, J. R.; LLOYD, L. C.; AND COTTEW, G. S. 1979b. Resistance of *Mycoplasma hyopneumoniae* to chlortetracycline. Aust Vet J 55:40.

FARRINGTON, D. O. 1976. Immunization of swine against mycoplasmal pneumonia. Proc 4th Int Congr Pig Vet Soc, Ames, p. 4.

FREEMAN, M. J.; ARMSTRONG, C. H.; SANDS-FREEMAN, L. L.; AND LOPEZ-OSUNA, M. 1984a. Serological cross-reactivity of porcine reference antisera to *Mycoplasma hyopneumoniae, M. flocculare, M. hyorhinis* and *M. hyosynoviae* indicated by the enzyme-linked immunosorbent assay, complement fixation and indirect hemagglutination test. Can J Comp Med 48:202–207.

FREEMAN, M. J.; LOPEZ-OSUNA, M.; ARMSTRONG, C. H.; AND SANDS-FREEMAN, L. 1984b. Evaluation of the indirect hemagglutination assay as a practical serodiagnostic test for mycoplasmal pneumonia of swine. Vet Microbiol 9:259–270.

FRIIS, N. F. 1973. The pathogenicity of *Mycoplasma flocculare.* Acta Vet Scand 14:344–346.

――――. 1975. Some recommendations concerning primary isolation of *Mycoplasma suipneumoniae* and *Mycoplasma flocculare.* Nord Vet Med 27:337–339.

――――. 1976. A serologic variant of *Mycoplasma hyorhinis* recovered from the conjunctiva of swine. Acta Vet Scand 17:343–353.

――――. 1978. Personal communication.

FRIIS, N. F.; LARSEN, H.; AND AHRENS, P. 1990. Propagation of *Mycoplasma hyosynoviae* in the presence of specific suppressing factors against *Mycoplasma hyorhinis.* IOM Lett 1 (8):377–378.

GEARY, S. J., AND WALCZAK, E. M. 1985. Isolation of a cytopathic factor from *Mycoplasma hyopneumoniae.* Infect Immun 48:576–578.

GOIŠ, M., AND KUKSA, F. 1974. Intranasal infection of gnotobiotic piglets with *Mycoplasma hyorhinis:* Differences in virulence of the strains and influence of age on the development of infection. Zentralbl Veterinaermed [B] 21:352–361.

GOIŠ, M.; CERNY, M.; ROZKOSNY, V.; AND SOVADINA, J. 1969. Studies on the epizootiological significance of some species of mycoplasma isolated from nasal swabs and lungs of pigs. Zentralbl Veterinaermed [B] 16:253–265.

GOIŠ, M.; SISAK, F.; KUKSA, F; AND SOVADINA, M. 1975. Incidence and evaluation of the microbial flora in the lungs of pigs with enzootic pneumonia. Zentralbl Veterinaermed [B] 22:205–219.

GOIŠ, M.; KUKSA, F.; AND SISAK, F. 1980. Microbiological findings in the lungs of slaughter pigs. Proc 6th Int Congr Pig Vet Soc, Copenhagen, p. 214.

GOODWIN, R. F. W. 1972a. Isolation of *Mycoplasma suipneumoniae* from the nasal cavities and lungs of pigs affected with enzootic pneumonia or exposed to this infection. Res Vet Sci 13:262–267.

――――. 1972b. Experiments on the transmissibility of enzootic pneumonia of pigs. Res Vet Sci 13:257–261.

――――. 1985. Apparent reinfection of enzootic pneumonia-free pig herds: Search for possible causes. Vet Rec 116:690–694.

GOODWIN, R. F. W., AND WHITTLESTONE, P. 1967. The detection of enzootic pneumonia in pig herds. I. Eight years general experience with a pilot control scheme. Vet Rec 181:643–647.

――――. 1973. Enzootic pneumonia of pigs: Immunization attempts inoculating *Mycoplasma suipneumoniae* antigen by various routes and with different adjuvants. Br Vet J 129:456–464.

GOODWIN, R. F. W.; POMEROY, A. P.; AND WHITTLESTONE, P. 1965. Production of enzootic pneumonia in pigs with a mycoplasma. Vet Rec 77:1247–1249.

GOURLAY, R. N.; WYLD, S. G.; AND LEACH, R. H. 1978. *Mycoplasma sualvi,* a new species from the intestinal and urogenital tracts of pigs. Int J Syst Bacteriol 28:289–292.

GRAHAM, R.; LENS, S.; AND JANSEGERS, L. 1984. The effect of lincomycin as medicated feed on reduction of incidence and severity of mycoplasmal pneumonia in growing swine. Proc 8th Int Congr Pig Vet Soc, Ghent, p. 119.

GULRAJANI, T. S., AND BEVERIDGE, W. I. B. 1951. Studies on respiratory diseases of pigs. IV. Transmission of infectious pneumonia and its differentiation from swine influenza. J Comp Pathol 61:118–139.

HANNAN, P. C. T., AND GOODWIN, R. F. W. 1990. Efficacies of norfloxacin and its 6-chloro analogue in experimentally-induced *M. hyopneumoniae* pneumonia in pigs. IOM Lett 1 (8):351–352.

HANNAN, P. C. T.; O'HANLON, P. J.; AND ROGERS, N. H. 1989. In vitro evaluation of various quinolone antibacterial agents against veterinary mycoplasmas and porcine respiratory bacterial pathogens. Res Vet Sci 46:202–211.

HARASAWA, R.; KOSHIMIZU, K.; AND ASADA, K. 1990. Species-specific detection of *Mycoplasma hyopneumoniae* by using polymerase chain reaction (PCR). IOM Lett 1 (8):383.

HARRIS, D. L. 1990. The use of Isowean 3 site production to upgrade health status. Proc 11th Int Congr Pig Vet Soc, Lausanne, p. 374.

HARRIS, D. L.; EDGERTON, S. L.; AND WILSON, E. R. 1990. Large thymus glands in Isowean pigs. Proc 11th Int Congr Pig Vet Soc, Lausanne, p. 291.

HOLMGREN, N. 1974. Swine enzootic pneumonia: Immunologic studies in infected sow-herds. Res Vet Sci 17:145–153.

HSU, F. S.; YANG, P. C.; AND WUNG, S. C. 1982. Tiamulin injectable for the treatment of swine bacterial pneumonia. Proc 7th Int Congr Pig Vet Soc, Mexico City, p.104.

HUHN, R. G. 1971a. Swine enzootic pneumonia: Age susceptibility and treatment schemata. Can J Comp Med 35:77–81.

――――. 1971b. The action of certain antibiotics and ether on swine enzootic pneumonia. Can J Comp Med 35:1–4.

JOHNSON, R. J.; MAPLESDEN, D. C.; AND SZANTO, J. 1978. Efficacy of tiamulin in the treatment of mycoplasmal pneumonia of swine. Proc 5th Int Congr Pig Vet Soc, Zagreb, p. M25.

JORSAL, S. E., AND THOMSEN, B. L. 1988. A Cox regression analysis of risk factors related to *Mycoplasma suipneumoniae* reinfection in Danish SPF-herds. Acta Vet Scand [Suppl] 29:436–438.

KOBISCH, M.; QUILLIEN, L.; TILLON, J. P.; AND WROBLEWSKI, H. 1987. The *Mycoplasma hyopneumoniae* plasma membrane as a vaccine against porcine enzootic pneumonia. Ann Inst Past/Immunol 138:693–705.

KOBISCH, M.; MILWARD, F.; DESMETTRE, PH.; AND MORVAN, P. 1990. Prevention of *Mycoplasma hyopneumoniae* experimental infection by vaccination: Active and passive protection. IOM Lett 1 (8):125–126.

KOTT, B. E. 1983. Chronological studies of respiratory disease in baby pigs. M.S. thesis, Iowa State Univ.

KUKSA, F., AND GOIŠ, M. 1982. Personal communication.

KUNESH, J. P. 1981. A comparison of two antibiotics in treating mycoplasma pneumonia in swine. Vet Med Small Anim Clin 76:871–872.

LAM, K. M., AND SWITZER, W. P. 1971. Mycoplasmal pneumonia of swine: Active and passive immunizations. Am J Vet Res 32:1737–1741.

L'ECUYER, C., AND BOULANGER, P. 1970. Enzootic pneumonia of pigs: Identification of a causative mycoplasma in infected pigs and in cultures by immunofluorescent staining. Can J Comp Med 34:38–46.

L'ECUYER, C.; SWITZER, W. P.; AND ROBERTS, E. D.

1961. Microbiological survey of pneumonic and normal swine lungs. Am J Vet Res 22:1020–1025.

LEMAN, A. 1990. Repopulation technology. Proc Iowa Vet Med Assoc 108:199–200.

LLOYD, L. C., AND ETHERIDGE, J. R. 1981. Production of arthritis by intravenous inoculation of *Mycoplasma hyopneumoniae:* Tests on five strains. Res Vet Sci 30:124–126.

LUKERT, P. D., AND MULKEY, G. 1982. Treatment of mycoplasmosis in young swine. Mod Vet Pract 63:107–110.

MARÉ, C. J., AND SWITZER, W. P. 1965. New species: *Mycoplasma hyopneumoniae,* a causative agent of virus pig pneumonia. Vet Med 60:841–846.

———. 1966. Virus pneumonia of pigs: Drug and ether sensitivity of a causative agent. Am J Vet Res 27:1671–1675.

MARTINEAU, G.; MARTINEAU-DOIZE, B.; COIGNOUL, F.; AND DEWAELE, A. 1980. Bilan econmique apres traitment de la broncho-pneumonie enzootique par la tiamuline. Ann Med Vet 124:369–377.

MEBUS, C. A., AND UNDERDAHL, N. R. 1977. Scanning electron microscopy of trachea and bronchi from gnotobiotic pigs inoculated with *Mycoplasma hyopneumoniae.* Am J Vet Res 38:1249–1254.

MESSIER, S., AND ROSS, R. F. 1990. Interactions of *Mycoplasma hyopneumoniae* membranes with porcine lymphocytes. Am J Vet Res. In press.

MEYLING, A. 1971. *Mycoplasma suipneumoniae* and *Mycoplasma hyorhinis* demonstrated in pneumonic pig lungs by the fluorescent antibody technique. Acta Vet Scand 12:137–141.

MEYLING, A., AND FRIIS, N. F. 1972. Serological identification of a new porcine mycoplasma species, *M. flocculare.* Acta Vet Scand 13:287–289.

MORRISON, R. B.; PIJOAN, C; AND LEMAN, A. D. 1986. Association between enzootic pneumonia and performance. Pig News and Inf 7:23–31.

MULLER, R. D., AND ABBOTT, P. B. 1986. Estimating the cost of respiratory disease in hogs. Anim Health Nutr (Feb):30–35.

NICOLET, J.; PAROZ, P.; AND BRUGGMANN, S. 1980. Tween 20 soluble proteins of *Mycoplasma hyopneumoniae* as antigen for an enzyme-linked immunosorbent assay. Res Vet Sci 29:305–309.

NIELSEN, N. C. 1988. Mycoplasma-associated enzootic bursitis in growing pigs. Proc 10th Int Congr Pig Vet Soc, Rio de Janeiro, p. 240.

NOYES, E.; PIJOAN, C.; AND FEENEY, D. 1988. Radiographic study of the evolution of the pneumonic process in slaughter pigs. Proc Am Assoc Swine Pract, p. 277.

OSE, E. E.; TONKINSON, L. V.; KO, C.; AND KUNER, J. M. 1990. Effectiveness of experimental *Mycoplasma hyopneumoniae* (Mhp) vaccines. I. Synergen proteins. IOM Lett 1 (8):371–372.

OWEN, W. J. 1990. Food animal disease monitoring. Ames, Iowa.

PEDERSEN, M. W.; FRIIS, N. F.; AND AHRENS, P. 1990. Detection of *Mycoplasma hyopneumoniae* in pneumonic pig lungs by an ELISA using monoclonal antibodies. IOM Lett 1 (8):399–400.

PETERSON, G.; WEISS, D.; EGAN, J.; KORSHUS, J.; PETERS, R.; AND MIRON, M. 1990. Response to *Mycoplasma hyopneumoniae* vaccination in nursing piglets. Proc 11th Int Congr Pig Vet Soc, Lausanne, p. 84.

PIFFER, I. A., AND ROSS, R. F. 1984. Effect of age on susceptibility of pigs to *Mycoplasma hyopneumoniae* pneumonia. Am J Vet Res 45:478–481.

PIFFER, I. A.; YOUNG, T. A.; PETENATE, A.; AND ROSS, R. F. 1984. Comparison of complement fixation test and enzyme-linked immunosorbent assay for detec-

tion of early infection with *Mycoplasma hyopneumoniae.* Am J Vet Res 45:1122–1126.

POINTON, A. M.; BYRT, D.; AND HEAP, P. 1985. Effect of enzootic pneumonia of pigs on growth performance. Aust Vet J 62:13–18.

PORCINE TEAM. 1980. Report of Consultations. Blue Bell Lodge, Custer, S. D. IOM Int Res Prog Comp Mycoplasmol.

———. 1982. Report of Consultations. Tokyo. IOM Int Res Prog Comp Mycoplasmol.

PRESTON, K. S. 1976. The uses of the microtitration complement fixation test as an aid in controlling mycoplasmal pneumonia of swine. Proc 4th Int Congr Pig Vet Soc, Ames, p. 7.

PULLAR, E. M. 1948. Infectious pneumonia of pigs. I. General description, differential diagnosis and epidemiology. Aust Vet J 24:320–330.

ROBERTS, D. H.; JOHNSON, C. T.; AND TEW, N. C. 1972. The isolation of *Mycoplasma hyosynoviae* from an outbreak of porcine arthritis. Vet Rec 90:307–309.

ROGERS, D. G.; Frey, M. L.; and Hogg, A. 1990. Conjunctivitis associated with a mycoplasma-like organism in swine. Proc 11th Int Congr Pig Vet Soc, Lausanne, p. 184.

ROSS, R. F. 1978. Immunization of swine against *Mycoplasma hyosynoviae.* Zentralbl Bakteriol [Orig A] 241:246.

———. 1981. Unpublished data.

———. 1985. Unpublished data.

ROSS, R. F., AND COX, D. F. 1988. Evaluation of tiamulin for treatment of mycoplasmal pneumonia in swine. J Am Vet Med Assoc 193:441–446.

ROSS, R. F., AND KARMON, J. A. 1970. Heterogeneity among strains of *Mycoplasma granularum* and identification of *Mycoplasma hyosynoviae,* sp. nov. J Bacteriol 103:707–713.

ROSS, R. F., AND SKELLY, B. J. 1982. Unpublished data.

ROSS, R. F., AND SPEAR, M. L. 1973. Role of the sow as a reservoir of infection for *Mycoplasma hyosynoviae.* Am J Vet Res 34:373–378.

ROSS, R. F., AND WHITTLESTONE, P. 1983. Recovery of, identification of and serological response to porcine mycoplasmas. In Methods in Mycoplasmology, vol. 2. Ed. J. G. Tully and S. Razin. New York: Academic Press.

ROSS, R. F.; WEISS, R.; AND KIRCHHOFF, H. 1977. Nachweis von *M. hyorhinis* und *M. hyosynoviae* in arthritischen Gelenken von Schweinen. Zentralbl Veterinaermed [B] 24:741–745.

ROSS, R. F.; ZIMMERMANN-ERICKSON, B. J.; AND YOUNG, T. F. 1984. Characteristics of protective activity of *Mycoplasma hyopneumoniae* vaccine. Am J Vet Res 45:1899–1905.

ROSS, R. F.; JACKSON, J. A.; TANNER, A. C.; ANDREWS, J. J.; AND MAGONIGLE, R. A. 1990. In vitro and in vivo efficacy of danofloxacin against *Mycoplasma hyopneumoniae.* Proc 11th Int Congr Pig Vet Soc, Lausanne, p. 85.

SCHEIDT, A. B.; MAYROSE, V. B.; HILL, M. A.; CLARK, L. K.; CLINE, T. R.; KNOX, K. E.; RUNNELS, L. J.; FRANTZ, S.; AND EINSTEIN, M. E. 1990a. Relationship of growth performance to pneumonia and atrophic rhinitis detected in pigs at slaughter. J Am Vet Med Assoc 196:881–884.

SCHEIDT, A.; FROE, D.; CLINE, T.; MAYROSE, V.; AND EINSTEIN, M. 1990b. The use of long-acting oxytetracycline (LA200$_{tm}$) in two swine herds for control of enzootic pneumonia. Proc 11th Int Congr Pig Vet Soc, Lausanne, p. 87.

SCHEIDT, A.; CLARK, K.; MAYROSE, V.; CLINE, T.; JONES, D.; AND FRANTZ, S. 1990c. All-in, all-out as a means for improving growth in a swine herd affected by enzootic pneumonia. Proc 11th Int Congr Pig Vet Soc, Lausanne, p. 92.

SCHULLER, W.; LABER, G.; AND WALZL, H. 1977a. Chemotherapeutische Untersuchungen mit 81723 hfu (Tiamulin), einem neuen Pleuromutilin-Derivat, an der experimentellen Mykoplasma-Pneumonie des Schweines. DTW 84:333–372.

SCHULLER, W.; NEUMEISTER, E.; AND VOGL, D. 1977b. Zur Sanierung von mit Enzootischer Pneumonie versuchten Schweinebestanden. Wien Tieraerztl Monatsschr 64:156–160.

SCHULMAN, A.; ESTOLA, T.; AND GARRY-ANDERSSON, A.-S. 1970. On the occurrence of *Mycoplasma hyorhinis* in the respiratory organs of pigs, with special reference to enzootic pneumonia. Zentralbl Veterinaermed [B] 17:549–553.

SIMON, F.; SEMJEN, G.; DOBOS-KOVACS, M.; LACZAY, P.; AND CSEREP, T. 1990. Efficacy of enrofloxacin against enzootic pneumonia in swine. Proc 11th Int Congr Pig Vet Soc, Lausanne, p. 96.

SLAVIK, M. F., AND SWITZER, W. P. 1972. Development of a microtitration complement-fixation test for diagnosis of mycoplasmal swine pneumonia. Iowa State J Res 47:117–128.

STIPKOVITS, L.; ROMARY, J.; NAGY, Z.; BODON, L.; AND VARGA, L. 1974. Studies on the pathogenicity of *Acholeplasma axanthum* in swine. J Hyg (Camb) 72:289–296.

STIPKOVITS, L.; LABER, G.; AND SCHUTZE, E. 1978a. Tiamulin, ein neues Antibiotikum zur Behandlung der enzootischen Pneumonie (EP) beim Schwein. DTW 85:475–496.

STIPKOVITS, L.; RASHWAN, A.; TAKACS, J.; AND LAPIS, K. 1978b. Occurrence of ureaplasmas in swine semen. Zentralbl Veterinaermed [B] 25:605–608.

SWITZER, W. P., AND ROSS, R. F. 1975. Mycoplasmal diseases. In Diseases of Swine, 4th ed. Ed. H. W. Dunne and A. D. Leman. Ames: Iowa State Univ Press, pp. 741–764.

TWIEHAUS, M. J., AND UNDERDAHL, N. R. 1975. Control and elimination of swine diseases through repopulation with specific-pathogen-free stock. In Diseases of Swine, 4th ed. Ed. H. W. Dunne and A. D. Leman. Ames: Iowa State Univ Press, pp. 1163–1179.

VAN BUREN, J. W. 1983. Lincomycin and swine mycoplasmal pneumonia indications and efficacy. Proc Am Assoc Swine Pract, Cincinnati, pp. 29–40.

WANNEMUEHLER, M. W.; MINION, F. C.; AND ROSS, R. F. 1988. Immune suppression of *Mycoplasma hyopneumoniae* infected swine. Proc Int Org Mycoplasmol 7:72.

WENG, C. N., AND LIN, W. H. 1988. Cell-mediated immune response in pig after *Mycoplasma hyopneumoniae* infection: Effect of immunosuppression on pneumonia in pig induced by *M. hyopneumoniae.* J Chin Soc Vet Sci 14:267–273.

WHITTLESTONE, P. 1972. The role of mycoplasmas in the production of pneumonia in the pig. In Pathogenic Mycoplasmas. Amsterdam: Associated Scientific Publishers, pp. 263–283.

———. 1973. Enzootic pneumonia of pigs (EPP). Adv Vet Sci Comp Med 17:1–55.

———. 1979. Porcine mycoplasmas. In The Mycoplasmas. Vol. 2: Human and Animal Mycoplasmas. Ed. J. G. Tully and R. F. Whitcomb. New York: Academic Press, pp. 133–176.

WILLIAMS, P. P. 1978. In vitro susceptibility of *Mycoplasma hyopneumoniae* and *Mycoplasma hyorhinis* to fifty-one antimicrobial agents. Antimicrob Agents Chemother 14:210–213.

YAGIHASHI, T.; NUNOYA, T.; MITUI, T.; AND TAJIMA, M. 1984. Effect of *Mycoplasma hyopneumoniae* infection on the development of *Haemophilus pleuropneumoniae* pneumonia in pigs. Jpn J Vet Sci 46:705–713.

YAMAMOTO, K., AND KOSHIMIZU, K. 1984. In vitro susceptibility of *Mycoplasma hyopneumoniae* to antibiotics. Proc 8th Int Congr Pig Vet Soc, Ghent, p. 116.

YAMAMOTO, K., AND OGATA, M. 1982. Mycoplasmal and bacterial flora in the lungs of pigs. Proc 7th Int Congr Pig Vet Soc, Mexico City, p. 94.

YOUNG, T. F.; ROSS, R. F.; AND DRISKO, J. 1983. Prevalence of antibodies to *Mycoplasma hyopneumoniae* in Iowa swine. Am J Vet Res 44:1946–1948.

YOUNG, T. F.; ERICKSON, B. Z.; ROSS, R. F.; AND WANNEMUEHLER, Y. 1989. Hemagglutination and hemagglutination inhibition of turkey red blood cells with *Mycoplasma hyopneumoniae.* Am J Vet Res 50:1052–1055.

ZIELINSKI, G. C.; YOUNG, T.; ROSS, R. F.; AND ROSENBUSCH, R. F. 1990. Adherence of *Mycoplasma hyopneumoniae* to cell monolayers. Am J Vet Res 51:339–343.

ZIMMERMANN, B. J., AND ROSS, R. F. 1982. Antibody response of swine experimentally infected with *Mycoplasma hyosynoviae.* Vet Microbiol 7:135–146.

ZIMMERMANN, W.; TSCHUDI, P.; AND NICOLET, J. 1986. Elisa-serologie in Blut und Kolostralmilch: Eine Moglichkeit zur Uberwachung der enzootischen Pneumonie (EP) in Schweine-Bestanden. Schweiz Arch Tierheilkd 128:299–306.

ZIMMERMANN, W.; ODERMATT, W.; AND TSCHUDI, P. 1989. Enzootische Pneumonie (EP): Die Teilsanierung EP-Reinfizierter Schweinezuchtbetriebe als alternative zur Totalsenierung. Schweiz Arch Tierheilkd B1:179–191.

44 Pneumonic Pasteurellosis

C. Pijoan

PNEUMONIC PASTEURELLOSIS, the result of *Pasteurella multocida* infection of the lung, represents the common final stage of the enzootic pneumonia or mycoplasma-induced respiratory disease syndrome. This syndrome is one of the most common and costly diseases of pigs, especially when they are raised under confinement. Recent data suggests that pneumonic lesions at slaughter are very common, even in well-managed herds. Pointon (personal communication) recently found that all 125 herds from the Midwest had pneumonic lesions at slaughter, with 74.9% of pigs affected on average. In these same herds, 71.8% had pleurisy, with 14.5% of pigs affected.

Pneumonia in pigs appears to be a very costly disease. In the same study, Pointon found that 41.7% of pigs were affected in the best 20% of herds, while 97.4% were affected in the worst 20%. Regarding pleurisy, the best 20% of herds also had no detectable lesions, while the worst 20% had an average of 30.6% animals with lesions. Noyes et al. (1990) performed a radiographic study of pigs' lungs in a commercial herd, to evaluate lifetime pneumonia and found a significant correlation between the extent of lifetime pneumonic lesions and the weight of the animals at 180 days.

Pneumonic pasteurellosis is found worldwide and can be demonstrated in all climates and husbandry conditions. Specific-pathogen-free (SPF) schemes, especially at the national level, do achieve a degree of control, presumably through the eradication of *Mycoplasma hyopneumoniae.* However, *P. multocida,* which is a common inhabitant of the pig's nasal flora, is extremely difficult to eradicate and can be found in most high-health herds, such as SPF, or minimal-disease herds.

ETIOLOGY. *P. multocida* is a gram-negative coccobacillus, 0.5–1 μ × 1–2 μ in size. The organism is a facultative anaerobe, growing well in most enriched media. It is oxidase positive, nonmotile, indole positive, and urease negative. It does not grow well in MacConkey and is nonhemolytic and does not require X and V factors. These reactions are helpful in differentiating *P. multocida* from a group of closely related bacteria that are also involved in pulmonary diseases of pigs, namely *P. haemolytica, Actinobacillus suis,* and *A. pleuropneumoniae* (Table 44.1).

P. multocida has 5 capsular serotypes, A, B, D, E, and F of which A, B, and D have been reported in swine. Serotype B, however, is atypical in that it produces a much more severe disease. It is also rare, confined to regions of Southeast Asia, China, and India (Verma 1988). It has not been reported from natural outbreaks in pigs in North America or Europe. The most common serotype isolated from pneumonic lungs is A, although a small proportion of serotype D strains are also found (Pijoan et al. 1983a; 1984; Kielstein 1986; Cowart et al. 1989). *P. multocida* also has 16 somatic serotypes. Strains of serotypes 3 and 5 are commonly detected in pigs with strains A:3, A:5, D:5, and D:3 being the most prevalent in that order.

Virulence Factors. The virulence factors of *P. multocida* are not well defined. In particular, the importance of the dermonecrotic toxin (DNT) is unresolved. This toxin is central to the production of atrophic rhinitis (see Chapter 33), where only toxigenic strains of *P. multocida* are involved in the disease. Toxigenic strains of *P. multocida* from lungs were first reported by Pijoan et al. (1984). Since then, a number of authors have found increasing numbers of toxigenic strains (both types A and D) in pneumonic lungs. Recent reports (Kielstein 1986; Iwamatsu and Sawada 1988) show that between 25–45% of strains isolated from lungs are toxigenic. Kielstein (1986) found

Table 44.1. Differential biochemical reactions of common pasteurellae and actinobacilli from pigs

	P. multocida	*P. haemolytica*	*A. suis*	*A. pleuropneumoniae*
Oxidase	+	+	+	+
Motility	–	–	–	–
Growth in MacConkey	–	+	+	–
Hemolysis	–	+	+	+
V factor required	–	–	–	+
Indole	+	–	–	±
Urease	–	–	+	+

that toxigenic strains were frequently isolated from acute cases but not from slaughterhouse lungs suggesting enhanced virulence. However, Baekbo (1988) recently reported that toxigenicity was not important in determining the virulence of *P. multocida* in experimentally infected animals.

The capsule is an important virulence factor, especially of serotype A, for it helps the organism avoid phagocytosis by alveolar macrophages. Maheswaran and Thies (1979) reported that *P. multocida* uptake by swine alveolar macrophages was very low, even in the presence of opsonins. Similar results were found by Fuentes and Pijoan (1986).

Some strains of *P. multocida* are able to produce pleuritis and abscessation in experimentally infected pigs (Pijoan and Fuentes 1987). The virulence factors that distinguish these strains from less virulent pneumonic strains are not defined. However, Iwamatso and Sawada (1988) found that strains of serotype D or toxigenic strains (of both serotypes) were associated with abscesses but not with pleuritis.

Cytoadhesion. The colonization of mucous surfaces by *P. multocida* has received some attention lately, as it is of paramount importance in understanding the pathogenesis of this organism. Jacques (1987) found that both serotypes A and D adhered poorly to isolated tracheal epithelial cells, although serotype A strains were more adherent. He later showed that serotype A strains adhered mostly to ciliated epithelial cells. Pijoan and Trigo (1989) also found sparse colonization by both serotype A and D strains, but found that serotype D strains adhered mostly to nonciliated cells. It appears, therefore, that serotype A and D strains have different receptors for cell attachment. In contrast to their poor attachment to epithelial surfaces, *P. multocida* strains have been shown to attach readily to nasal mucus, raising questions as to where normal attachment and colonization take place.

EPIDEMIOLOGY. The epidemiology of *P. multocida* is not well understood. The organism is present in practically all herds, and can be readily isolated from the nose of normal, healthy individuals. Transmission of the disease by aerosols has been postulated, but is unlikely to be of importance. Baekbo and Nielsen (1988) measured airborne *P. multocida* in herds suffering from atrophic rhinitis. They were able to isolate the organism in 29 of 44 herds studied. However, the low number of organisms isolated (144 cfu/m³) led them to conclude that there was no relationship between the number of organisms recovered and the severity of the clinical problem.

Although aerosol transmission may occasionally occur within the herd, it is probable that nose-to-nose contact is the common route of infection. Both vertical and horizontal transmission probably occur, although this has not been proven. External sources of the organism include mice and other rodents, although chickens and chicken manure have also been postulated. These are commonly infected with *P. multocida* and may explain why it is nearly impossible to keep a herd free of the organism.

PATHOGENESIS. Experimental infections with *P. multocida* are very difficult to establish. Healthy pigs will readily tolerate large doses of organisms instilled intranasally or even intratracheally. Pulmonary clearance is very effective, and the bacteria cannot be reisolated 30 minutes after challenge. Experimental models of the disease have relied on using serotype B organisms (Farrington 1986), previous infections with immunosuppressive virus or mycoplasmas (Fuentes and Pijoan 1986; Ciprian et al. 1988), or by massive instillation of infected fluids into the lung (Hall et al. 1988). This has led to the conclusion that *P. multocida* is not a primary agent of pneumonia but rather that it follows infections with other agents. Vaccination against hog cholera virus (Pijoan and Ochoa 1978) as well as infection with pseudorabies virus (Fuentes and Pijoan 1987) or *Mycoplasma hyopneumoniae* (Ciprian et al. 1988) have all been shown to predispose the pig to superinfections with *P. multocida*. Death appears to be the result of endotoxic shock and respiratory failure.

CLINICAL SIGNS. The clinical signs vary in severity depending on the strain of *P. multocida* involved, together with the immune status of the animals.

Acute Form. This form is most commonly associated with serotype B strains. The animals show dyspnea, labored breathing with abdominal "thumps" (sudden contractions of the abdomen), prostration, and high fever (up to 42.2°C, 108°F). Mortality may be high (5–40%) in these cases. Dead and moribund animals may show purplish discoloration of the abdominal region, suggesting endotoxic shock.

Subacute Form. This is associated with *P. multocida* strains that produce pleuritis. In these cases, cough and abdominal breathing can be detected in grower or finishing pigs up to market weight. Cough in this age pig is usually the hallmark of severe disease. Clinically, this form of the disease is very similar to pleuropneumonia due to *Actinobacillus pleuropneumoniae* (see Chapter 31). The main distinguishing feature is that pleuritic pasteurellosis rarely results in sudden deaths. Rather, pigs become extremely emaciated but may survive for a long time.

Chronic Form. This is the most common form of the disease, characterized by occasional cough, thumping, and low or nonexistent fever. Animals affected are usually in the later stages of the nursery or are growers (10–16 weeks of age). The signs are indistinguishable from those following *Mycoplasma hyopneumoniae* infections, for *P. multocida* represents a continuation and exacerbation of primary mycoplasmosis.

LESIONS. Lesions of *P. multocida* are confined to the thoracic cavity and are superimposed on those of *M. hyopneumoniae*. Typically, anteroventral consolidation of the lung is seen, together with froth in the trachea. There is a clear line of demarcation between affected and healthy lung tissue. The affected portion of the lung will have discoloration ranging from red to grayish-green, depending on the course of the infection (Fig. 44.1).

Severe cases may present varying degrees of pleuritis and abscessation. Pleural adhesions to the thoracic wall are common in these cases and the pleura has a translucent, dry appearance (Fig. 44.2, 44.3). This is useful in differentiating pneumonic pasteurellosis from actinobacillus pleuropneumonia, where moist, yellowish pleural adhesions with massive fibrin infiltration are more common (Pijoan 1989).

Histologically, a lobular, exudative bronchopneumonia is found. Severe bronchopneumonia, alveolar epithelial hyperplasia, and the presence of abundant neutrophils are seen with mucopurulent exudate in the bronchial lumen and in alveolar spaces. These lesions are not specific to *P. multocida* infections and are similar for most bacterial pneumonias.

DIAGNOSIS. Since the lesions of *P. multocida* infections are not pathognomonic, they cannot be used as the only criteria to establish a definite diagnosis. History of the outbreak, together with histopathology and isolation of the organism, should be used to confirm the original presumptive diagnosis. Serology has not proven effective for diagnosis, and no serologic test is routinely available for *P. multocida* infections. However, some experimental techniques, such as Western blot analysis of membrane protein, show promise that serologic diagnosis will be available in the future.

P. multocida is a relatively easy organism to culture, provided proper specimens are submitted to the laboratory. Specimens yielding the best isolations include swabs of tracheobronchial exudate, or affected lung tissue obtained from the border area between affected and normal tissue. Swabs should be immersed in an appropriate transport medium, such as Stuart's. Lung samples should be obtained as aseptically as possible. All samples should be refrigerated (but preferably not frozen) until cultured.

Culture of *P. multocida* can be successfully achieved in laboratories with minimal facilities.

Good-quality specimens will yield the organism on direct culture onto blood agar or glucose agar plates. If the samples are more contaminated, they can be serially diluted tenfold in brain-heart infusion (BHI) broth, grown overnight and then plated (Pijoan et al. 1983b). Alternatively, selective media can be used; Baekbo and Nielsen (1988) used blood agar containing neomycin sulphate (2 μg/ml) and bacitracin (3.5 μg/ml) to culture *P. multocida* successfully from the air. Isolation can also be enhanced by injecting the specimen intraperitoneally into mice and then recovering the pasteurella 24 hours later from liver and ascitic fluid.

Differential diagnosis must include influenza virus, *A. pleuropneumoniae*, *Bordetella bronchiseptica*, *Salmonella choleraesuis*, and pure *M. hyopneumoniae* infections. Accurate clinical differentiation based on the epidemiology and lesions can be readily achieved for most of these conditions, but may be difficult in cases of influenza, *B. bronchiseptica*, or *M. hyopneumoniae*. In this case, histology and bacterial culture will be needed. Ramirez and Pijoan (1982) and Straw (1986a) have published tables for the differential diagnosis of these conditions.

TREATMENT. Treatment of *P. multocida* field infections with antibiotics is usually difficult or unsuccessful. This is partly due to widespread antibiotic resistance in *P. multocida* isolates in the United States and also to difficulties in achieving adequate antibiotic concentrations in consolidated, pneumonic lung.

A variety of antibiotics and antibiotic combinations are commonly used (Farrington 1986). These include parenteral antibiotics such as oxytetracycline, 11 mg/kg; long-acting oxytetracycline, 20 mg/kg; procaine penicillin, 66,000 units/kg; benzathine penicillin, 32,000 units/kg; tiamulin, 10–12.5 mg/kg; and ampicillin, 6.6 mg/kg. Treatment via feed antibiotics has also been suggested, although, as in the case of other pneumonias, it is probably not very effective. Recommended oral antimicrobials include tetracyclines, 400 ppm, and sulphonamide, 500–1000 ppm.

The effectiveness of all these antimicrobials will vary considerably depending on strain susceptibility. Since *P. multocida* readily exhibits resistance to various antimicrobials, antibiograms should be performed before instituting treatment. The importance of strain susceptibility can be seen in the case of oxytetracycline. Several authors have found good results with this antibiotic while others have not. Pijpers et al. (1989) clarified this issue when they reported the existence of both susceptible strains with minimal inhibitory concentrations (MIC) of 0.25–0.5 μg/ml and resistant strains (MIC = 64 μg/ml).

As in other respiratory infections, antibiotics are more effective when used as prophylactic

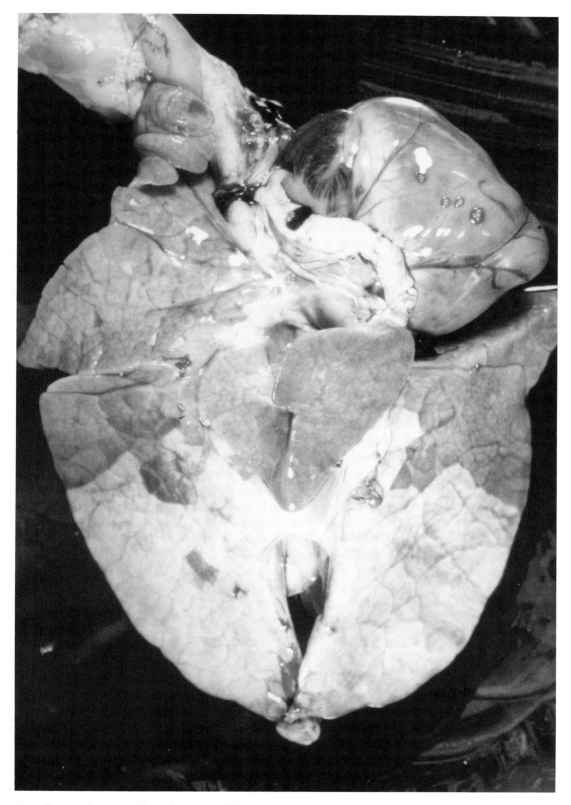

44.1. Pneumonic pasteurellosis. Lung consolidation is anteroventral with a clear demarcation line between affected and healthy tissue.

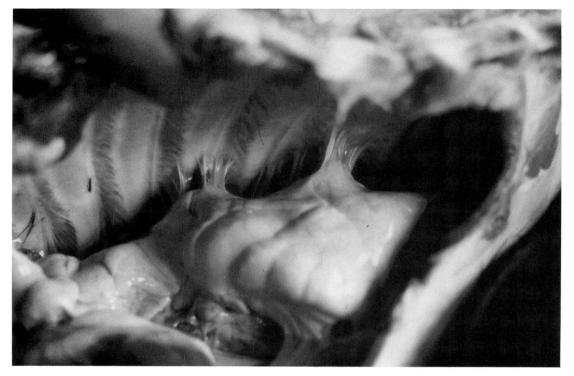

44.2. Pleural adhesions of lung to the thoracic wall in a case of pleuritic pasteurellosis. Note that the pleura has a translucent, dry aspect.

rather than therapeutic agents. Tetracyclines alone, combined with sulphamethazine or sulphathiazole and penicillin, and tylosin combined with sulphamethazine have been recommended for this purpose. It is probable that the most effective compound in these mixtures is sulphamethazine. This antimicrobial has recently been the focus of controversy over residues. Because of this, its use has been severely limited and monitored. Tiamulin (40 ppm in feed) has been shown, in a number of trials, to improve average daily gain. However, since pneumonic lesions are not significantly reduced by this antibiotic (Pott and Edwards 1990), the mode of action by which these improvements are obtained is unclear.

Some new antibiotics with claims for *P. multocida* treatment are not available in the United States, but are used extensively in other countries. These include injectable lincomycin-spectinomycin, cephalosporins (ceftiofur and cefquinome), and various quinolones including enroflaxin and danofloxacin.

PREVENTION. Since antibiotic therapy is often unsuccessful and even when successful may not prove cost effective, prevention of pneumonia has received much attention. Prevention is usually obtained through changes in management. The management techniques that result in decreased pneumonia have been reviewed by several authors (Pijoan 1986; Straw 1986b). Caution must be taken when implementing these recommendations, since they derive mostly from retrospective epidemiologic studies and not from experimental data. Also, they are intended to reduce pneumonia as a whole (and other respiratory problems) and do not differentiate between conditions of different etiology.

Management changes can be either directed at modifying the pig's environment, or at reducing the possibilities of spreading the organism.

Environmental changes such as increasing ventilation flow rate, decreasing ammonia, and minimizing temperature fluctuations and dust are usually recommended. Some of these recommendations are antagonistic; increasing air flow, especially in winter, results in a decrease of both temperature and humidity, with an increase in dust. Most of these changes have not proven valuable in controlled, experimental conditions. Noyes et al. (1986) found that decreasing ventilation below minimal recommended levels (0.5 cfm/pig) had no effect on weaned pigs inoculated with both *B. bronchiseptica* and *P. multocida*. Similarly, Rafai et al. (1987) found that cold stress, even while it reduced immune function in suckling pigs, had no effect on the course of an experimental *P. multocida* infection.

Environmental changes frequently entail extensive remodeling. They are, therefore, expensive

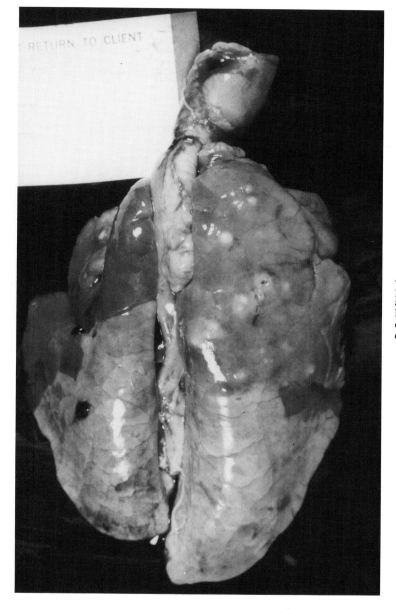

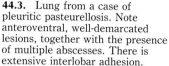

44.3. Lung from a case of pleuritic pasteurellosis. Note anteroventral, well-demarcated lesions, together with the presence of multiple abscesses. There is extensive interlobar adhesion.

to institute and maintain. It is not clear that these changes are cost effective in terms of reducing respiratory disease.

On the other hand, a considerable improvement may be obtained by instituting management changes that reduce the spread of the organism. These include

1. All-in/all-out production. Backstrom and Bremer (1978) showed that all herds in their study with lowest levels of pneumonia were all-in/all-out, while herds with highest levels had continuous flow and purchased pigs.

2. Closed herds. Minimizing purchase of outside pigs, especially fatteners, results in a de-crease of pneumonia and other respiratory conditions.

3. Minimal mixing and sorting. This is a source of stress to the pigs, while also intensifying the probabilities of disease transmission. Pigs should be mixed as few times as possible during their productive life.

4. Reduction in building and pen size. Smaller rooms and smaller pens both have been shown to reduce levels of pneumonia. Rooms should have a maximum of 250 pigs, and pens a maximum of 20–25 pigs each.

5. Decrease animal density. Decreasing animal density has been shown by many authors to reduce levels of pneumonia. Lindqvist (1974) found

that stocking densities of less than 0.7 m²/pig resulted in increased respiratory disease.

VACCINATION. Although several killed vaccines for the prevention of pneumonic pasteurellosis are available, their effectiveness is questionable. Since no reliable model of experimental disease exists, potency testing is usually performed in mice. It is doubtful, therefore, that this model truly replicates the disease in the pig.

Under field conditions, clinicians frequently find disappointing results with these vaccines, and they do not appear to be cost effective.

On the other hand, Awad-Masalmeh et al. (1990) reported the disappearance of *P. multocida* from the nasal flora of pigs receiving autogenous vaccines, thereby suggesting that the problems associated with vaccination may be due to improper strain selection or to loss of protective antigens through culture.

OTHER PASTEURELLA INFECTIONS IN PIGS. Several authors have sporadically isolated of *P. haemolytica*-like organisms from cases of severe necrotizing pleuropneumonia. The lesions seen are similar to those found in *A. pleuropneumoniae* infections, but tend to be less severe. In this regard, they are also similar to lesions reported from *A. suis*.

All these organisms are very similar, and differ in minor biochemical reactions such as indole formation or V-factor requirement. Bisgaard (1984) did a comprehensive study of these strains and concluded that they were different from *P. haemolytica* sensu stricto and classified them as "taxon 15." Since the lesions produced (and the serologic reactions) are indistinguishable from *A. pleuropneumoniae,* it is possible that some field outbreaks have been misdiagnosed. At present, it is very difficult to assess the true prevalence and economic impact of these strains.

REFERENCES

Awad-Masalmeh, J.; Kofer, J.; and Schuh, M. 1990. On the occurrence of chronic respiratory disease at swine herds in Austria. Bacteriological findings on efficacy of autogenous vaccines. Proc Int Congr Pig Vet Soc, Lausanne, p. 107.

Backstrom, L., and Bremer, H. 1978. The relationship between disease environmental factors in herds. Nord Vet Med 30:526–533.

Baekbo, P. 1988. Pathogenic properties of *Pasteurella multocida* in the lungs of pigs. Proc Int Congr Pig Vet Soc, Rio de Janeiro, p. 58.

Baekbo, P., and Nielsen, J. P. 1988. Airborne *Pasteurella multocida* in pig fattening units. Proc Int Congr Pig Vet Soc, Rio de Janeiro, p. 51.

Bisgaard, M. 1984. Comparative investigations of *Pasteurella haemolytica sensu stricto* and so-called *P. haemolytica* isolated from different pathological lesions in pigs. Acta Pathol Microbiol Immunol Scand [B]92:203–207.

Ciprian, A.; Pijoan, C.; Cruz, T.; Camacho, J.; Tortora, J.; Colmenares, G.; Lopez-Revilla, R.; and Garza, M. De la. 1988. *Mycoplasma hyopneumoniae*

increases the susceptibility of pigs to experimental *Pasteurella multocida* pneumonia. Can J Vet Res 52:434–438.

Cowart, R. P.; Backstrom, L.; and Brim, T. 1989. *Pasteurella multocida* and *Bordetella bronchiseptica* in atrophic rhinitis and pneumonia in swine. Can J Vet Res 53:295–300.

Farrington, D. O. 1986. Pneumonic Pasteurellosis. In Diseases of Swine, 6th ed. Ed. A. D. Leman, B. Straw, R. D. Glock, W. L. Mengeling, R. H. C. Penny, and E. Scholl. Ames: Iowa State Univ Press, p. 436.

Fuentes, M., and Pijoan, C. 1986. Phagocytosis and killing of *Pasteurella multocida* by pig alveolar macrophages after infection with pseudorabies virus. Vet Immunol Immunopathol 13:165–172.

———. 1987. Pneumonia in pigs induced by intranasal challenge exposure with pseudorabies virus and *Pasteurella multocida.* Am J Vet Res 48:1446–1448.

Hall, W.; Bane, D.; Kilroy, C.; and Essex-Sorlie, D. 1988. A model for the induction of pneumonia caused by *Pasteurella multocida* type A. Proc Int Congr Pig Vet Soc, Rio de Janeiro, p. 59.

Iwamatsu, S., and Sawada, T. 1988. Relationship between serotypes, dermonecrotic toxin production of *Pasteurella multocida* isolates and pneumonic lesions of porcine lungs. Jpn J Vet Sci 50:1200–1206.

Jacques, M. 1987. Adherence of *Pasteurella multocida* to porcine upper respiratory tract cells. Current Microbiol 15:115–119.

Kielstein, P. 1986. On the occurrence of toxin-producing *Pasteurella multocida* strains in atrophic rhinitis and in pneumonias of swine and cattle. J Vet Med [B] 33:418–424.

Lindqvist, J. 1974. Animal health and environment in the production of fattening pigs. Acta Vet Scand 515:1–78.

Maheswaran, S., and Thies, E. 1979. Influence of encapsulation on phagocytosis of *Pasteurella multocida* by bovine neutrophils. Infect Immun 26:76–81.

Noyes, E.; Pijoan, C.; and Jacobson, L. 1986. Ventilating environment for the weaned pig. Proc Int Congr Pig Vet Soc, Barcelona, p. 401.

Noyes, E.; Feeney, D.; and Pijoan, C. 1990. Comparison of the effect of pneumonia detected during a lifetime with pneumonia detected at slaughter on growth in swine. J Am Vet Med Assoc 197:1025–1029.

Pijoan, C. 1986. Respiratory system. In Diseases of swine, 6th ed. Ed A. D. Leman, B. Straw, R. D. Glock, W. L. Mengeling, R. H. C. Penny, and E. Scholl. Ames: Iowa State Univ Press, p. 152.

———. 1989. Pleuritis effect on growth underestimated. Int Piglett 9:17–19.

Pijoan, C., and Fuentes, M. 1987. Severe pleuritis associated with certain strains of *Pasteurella multocida* in swine. J Am Vet Med Assoc 191:823–826.

Pijoan, C., and Ochoa, G. 1978. Interaction between a hog cholera vaccine strain and *Pasteurella multocida* in production of porcine pneumonia. J Comp Pathol 88:167–170.

Pijoan, C., and Trigo, E. 1989. Bacterial adhesion to mucosal surfaces with special reference to *Pasteurella multocida* isolates from atrophic rhinitis. Can J Vet Sci 54:516–521.

Pijoan, C.; Morrison, R. B.; and Hilley, H. D. 1983a. Serotyping of *Pasteurella multocida* isolated from swine lungs collected at slaughter. J Clin Microbiol 17:1074–1076.

———. 1983b. Dilution technique for isolation of *Haemophilus* from swine lungs collected at slaughter. J Clin Microbiol 18:143–145.

Pijoan, C.; Lastra, A.; Ramirez, C.; and Leman, A. 1984. Isolation of toxigenic strains of *Pasteurella multocida* from lungs of pneumonic swine. J Am Vet Med Assoc 185:522–523.

PIJPERS, A.; KLINGEREN, B. VAN; SCHOEVERS, E. J.; VERJEIJDEN, J.; AND MIERT, A. S. VAN. 1989. *In vitro* activity of five tetracyclines and some other antimicrobial agents against four porcine respiratory tract pathogens. J Vet Pharmacol Ther 12:267–276.

POTT, J., AND EDWARDS, J. 1990. Beneficial effects of tiamutin administered in feed at 40 ppm to pigs with enzootic pneumonia. Proc Int Congr Pig Vet Soc, Lausanne, p. 86.

RAFAI, P.; NEUMANN, R.; LEONHARDT, W.; FRENYO, L.; RUDAS, P.; FODOR, L.; AND BOROS, G. 1987. Effect of environmental temperature on pigs infected with *Pasteurella multocida* type A. Acta Vet Hung 35:211–223.

RAMIREZ, N., AND PIJOAN, C. 1982. Diagnostico de las Enfermedades del Cerdo. Ed. R. R. Necoechea and C. A. Pijoan. Mexico City: Necoechea and Pijoan, p. 227.

STRAW, B. E. 1986a. Differential diagnosis of swine diseases. In Diseases of Swine, 6th ed. Ed. A. D. Leman, B. Straw, R. D. Glock, W. L. Mengeling, R. H. C. Penny, and E. Scholl. Ames: Iowa State Univ Press, p. 214.

_____. 1986b. A look at factors that contribute to the development of swine pneumonia. Vet Med (Aug): 747–755.

VERMA, N. D. 1988. *Pasteurella multocida* B:2 in haemorrhagic septicaemia outbreak in pigs in India. Vet Rec 123:63.

45 Porcine Proliferative Enteropathies

A. C. Rowland
G. H. K. Lawson

PROLIFERATIVE ENTEROPATHIES (PE) are a group of conditions of widely differing gross appearance but which have a common underlying pathologic change; namely, a thickening of the mucous membrane of the small, and sometimes the large, intestine. Histologically, the affected tissues show proliferation and immaturity of the intestinal epithelium (Biester and Schwarte 1931; Biester et al. 1939), and this primary pathologic lesion may be manifested by a variety of clinical symptoms, depending on the age of the animal affected and whether or not destructive changes occur within the altered mucosa.

The name given to the condition resulting from uncomplicated proliferation is porcine intestinal adenomatosis (PIA); the other members of the complex, in which additional changes are superimposed on the basic abnormality, are necrotic enteritis (NE), regional ileitis (RI), and proliferative hemorrhagic enteropathy (PHE) (Field et al. 1953; Hoorens 1962; O'Hara 1972; Rowland and Rowntree 1972; Martinsson et al. 1974; Rowland and Lawson 1975).

Whenever these proliferative changes in pigs have been studied at either an ultrastructural level or using silver stains, bacterial profiles have been found within the abnormal proliferating cells (Rowland and Lawson 1974). These intracellular bacteria are curved to straight rods with either tapered or rounded ends measuring 1.25–1.75 μm in length by 0.25–0.43 μm in width. The outer wall is a wavy trilaminar membrane separated from the cytoplasmic membrane by an electron-lucent zone. The bacteria lie free in the apical cytoplasm of the enterocyte, not within phagosomes during the important stages of infection.

The disease is worldwide in distribution and has been described in Australia, Belgium, Brazil, Canada, Denmark, Finland, France, Greece, Holland, India, Japan, South Africa, Sweden, Taiwan, the United Kingdom, the United States, and Yugoslavia.

PE has also been described in a number of other mammalian species, notably the hamster (Frisk and Wagner 1977), but also in the fox (Eriksen and Landsverk 1985), ferret (Fox and Lawson 1988), horse (Duhamel and Wheeldon 1982), rat (Vandenberghe and Marsboom 1982), and rabbit (Fox and Lawson 1989). In all these species intracellular bacteria have been observed in proliferating epithelium, and there is some evidence that the agent may be common to all species affected.

In this chapter PIA describes a thickening of the intestinal mucosa relatively free from or with only minor inflammatory surface lesions; NE is a deep, coagulative necrosis of an adenomatous mucosa; and RI is a progressive proliferation of granulation tissue in the lamina propria and submucosa of a case of PIA, with consequential hypertrophy of both outer muscle coats. Intermediate forms may occur. PHE is a massive hemorrhage into the lumen in the absence of visible bleeding points in the thickened proliferated mucosa of PIA.

Other terms in the literature used to describe similar conditions include terminal or regional ileitis, regional enteritis, intestinal adenoma, porcine proliferative ileitis, and muscular hypertrophy with stenosis of the ileum.

Necrosis of the mucosa is a feature of many enteric infections and the term "necrotic enteritis" accurately describes the end stage of a number of specific diseases. We believe that, rather than attempting to introduce yet another specific name, the simple definition should be retained and qualified where appropriate by cause, e.g., NE associated with PIA.

Particular care must be taken to avoid confusion between the condition described in this chapter as PHE, wherein the intestinal wall is thickened and the lumen contains free blood, and a form of intestinal catastrophe showing a major vascular component variously named colonic bloat, torsion of the mesentery, and intestinal hemorrhage syndrome, in all of which the intestine remains thin-walled and intensely congested.

ETIOLOGY. A variety of campylobacters, but particularly *Campylobacter mucosalis* (Lawson and Rowland 1974) and *C. hyointestinalis* (Gebhart et al. 1983), are morphologically similar to the intracellular bacteria and can be recovered in large numbers from proliferative lesions. This association has focused attention on these or other campylobacters as candidate etiologic agents. Most workers have found that gnotobiotic piglets are easy to infect with campylobacters and despite prolonged colonization of the intestine, neither lesions, disease, nor substantial intracellular colonization occurs (Roberts et al. 1980; McCartney et al. 1984; Boosinger et al. 1985). This host/parasite relationship is not altered by the presence of other viral pathogens or bacteria commensals (McCartney et al. 1984); the only reported successful transmission of the disease involving cultivated bacteria (Lomax et al. 1982c) does not appear to have been repeated.

In contrast to exposure to cultivated bacteria, exposure of pigs to diseased mucosa frequently results in intestinal lesions and clinical disease (Roberts et al. 1977; Mapother et al. 1987; McOrist and Lawson 1989a). Intestinal lesions that develop as a result of artificial exposure have all the characteristics of the field disease including the presence of intracellular bacteria.

Attempts to identify the intracellular agent in the tissues by immunologic techniques have provided conflicting results (Rowland and Lawson 1974; Chang et al. 1984), probably due to the presence of a "natural" rabbit antibody reactive with the intracellular organism (Lawson et al. 1985). Elimination of this source of confusion allows specific hyperimmune sera and monoclonal antibodies to be prepared. These react with the intracellular bacteria and do not react with cells of any cultivated *Campylobacter* sp. in immunofluorescent antibody (IFA) techniques (Lawson et al. 1985; McOrist et al. 1987). Specific reactivity of monoclonal and polyclonal antibody raised to the intracellular organism mainly lies in a 25–27 kD fragment on the outer aspect of the envelope (McOrist et al. 1989a,b).

Both the outer membrane proteins (McOrist et al. 1989a) and the fragment pattern of DNA endonuclease digests (McOrist et al. 1990) of the intracellular bacteria differ from those of known *Campylobacter* spp. These results confirm that the intracellular campylobacterlike organisms (CLO) are distinct from known *Campylobacter* spp. It is also possible that this new agent cannot be cultivated using conventional bacteriologic techniques. The part played by these other *Campylobacter* spp., if any, in the disease process has yet to be resolved.

EPIDEMIOLOGY. Documented information on the occurrence of the disease complex in the pig herds of the world is still scarce. The main reason for this deficiency is that in many instances clinical signs are not dramatic, and that until recently specific tools for the diagnosis of the disease in the live animal have not been available.

Abattoir monitoring has been used to assess the presence and possible impact of the disease; the extent to which the incidence at slaughter may reflect the occurrence of disease in life or production loss is largely unknown. The presence of lesions in animals at slaughter is a consequence of the management system on the farm. Other farms may suffer equivalent effects without showing animals with lesions, for in most instances, the disease is believed to resolve naturally.

Various authors have demonstrated lesions in pigs at normal slaughter; the incidence of animals with lesions has often been low, 0.7–1.63% (Emsbo 1951; Rowland and Hutchings 1978; Kubo et al. 1984). However, some more recent reports have indicated much higher levels of lesions. In one report 35% of herds had pigs with lesions at slaughter and the incidence of lesions in particular herds reached 40% (Pointon 1989). Estimates of clinical occurrence of the nonhemorrhagic or wasting disease suggest that between 0.89 and 2.5% of pigs may be affected (Roberts et al. 1979; Jackson and Baker 1980) with 1.0% mortality of throughput (Lawson et al. 1980).

PHE generally is much more dramatic in its appearance, has all the characteristics of an infectious disease, and may clinically affect a high proportion (12%, Love et al. [1977] to 50%, Lomax et al. [1982b]) of animals in a susceptible herd. Boar and gilt testing stations in the United Kingdom have shown an incidence of the condition in 0.25% of the throughput, with a distinct predominance of the Large White breed among those affected, although no breed susceptibility has been noted elsewhere.

Excretion of the intracellular organisms in the feces of pigs, at levels that can at present be detected by IFA techniques, is rare. Where clinical disease occurs the organism is present in the feces and asymptomatic adjacent animals can be found to be excreting at this time (McOrist and Lawson 1989b). Excretion of other campylobacters, particularly *C. coli*, is common in all ages of pigs and unrelated to disease.

Pathologically similar diseases are present in a number of other species and the majority, but not all, of these conditions show intracellular bacteria in the cytoplasm of the enterocytes. Reports of these conditions have mainly been sporadic. However, in some animals, namely the hamster, ferret, and rabbit, the disease may have clinical significance and the CLO is antigenically closely related to the pig organism (Lawson et al. 1985; Fox and Lawson 1988). Hamsters are susceptible to the pig disease (Gebhart 1987; McOrist and Lawson 1987). These findings taken together suggest that sources of infection other than pigs may on occasion have importance in the introduction of infection into high–health status herds.

PATHOGENESIS. PE can be reproduced by exposing susceptible pigs to diseased mucosa containing CLO (Lomax et al. 1982a; Mapother et al. 1987; McOrist and Lawson 1989a). Many attempts at transmission have failed for reasons that are poorly understood. Young piglets have frequently shown diarrhea 5–6 days postexposure, the significance of which remains unclear, since animals that fail to develop the disease often show similar signs. Histologic changes, CLO-cell parasitism, and on occasion, gross lesions are evident 8–10 days after exposure to infection; in experimental studies, lesions reach their maximum around 21 days postexposure or shortly thereafter. Organisms associated with one pathologic type of lesion appear capable of producing the range of pathologic sequelae, and specific strains are not associated with a specific type of disease. Thus, pigs exposed to diseased mucosa may develop either the necrotic or hemorrhagic form of the disease (Mapother et al. 1987).

PE develops as a progressive proliferation of the immature epithelial cells populated by CLO. To persist and multiply within the epithelium, CLO must penetrate the dividing crypt cells. Both CLO and campylobacters migrate to the crypt lumen where the CLO become closely associated with the cell membrane (McOrist et al. 1989b). Bacteria then enter the enterocyte and multiply; the infected cells fail to mature, continue to undergo mitosis, and, possibly as a consequence of this immaturity, are not shed. Glands therefore become enormously elongated and often branched.

Degrees of degenerative and reparative changes may be superimposed on the essential enterocyte proliferation. These changes range from a superficial fibrinous reaction to extensive, deep, coagulative necrosis, which is the lesion of NE, and from a mainly mononuclear leukocyte infiltration of the lamina propria to a substantial granulation tissue proliferation leading to the muscular hypertrophy of RI. Heavy, mixed bacterial contamination of such lesions is the rule.

PHE is marked by severe bleeding into the lumen of the intestine from established lesions of PIA. The hemorrhage occurs possibly concurrently with the widespread destruction of intracellular campylobacters, degeneration and desquamation of many epithelial cells, and leakage from the capillary bed.

CLINICAL SIGNS. Clinical cases of PIA, NE, or RI are observed most commonly in the postweaned fattening pig between 6 and 20 weeks of age.

In many cases of PIA, the clinical signs are very slight, and little more is seen than failure to sustain growth and a degree of anorexia, characterized by curiosity about food but refusal to eat. Thus, affected animals vary from the clinically unremarkable to those showing marked dullness and apathy. Diarrhea is not always a feature of this form of the disease, and when PIA is endemic in a herd, these milder cases can be relatively common but difficult to detect. However, in fattening herds during the postweaning period, wasting of a well-grown animal with anorexia and irregular diarrhea is frequently seen. Such cases are often associated with varying degrees of inflammatory or necrotic change in the affected mu-

cosa, and those that develop NE or the "hose pipe" ileum of RI show severe loss of condition and often persistent scours. Death is not uncommon and in RI is frequently associated with perforations of the hypertrophied ileal wall, leading to a generalized terminal peritonitis. In uncomplicated PIA, careful monitoring of weight gain may be the only guide to the presence of the disease, and in these circumstances the use of cumulative summation techniqes to identify nonthriving animals may be of value (Roberts et al. 1979).

Cases of PHE occur more commonly in young adults than in younger growing animals and present a clinical picture of acute hemorrhagic anemia. If the disease is prolonged, black tarry feces will be passed and these may become loose. However, some animals die without fecal abnormality and show only marked pallor. Up to half the animals clinically affected will succumb, the remainder recovering over a short period of time. Marked loss of condition is not a feature of the hemorrhagic disease. Pregnant animals that are clinically affected may abort, the majority within 6 days of the onset of clinical signs (Beers 1984).

Recovery from uncomplicated PIA is the rule and occurs abruptly 4–6 weeks after the onset of clinical signs with a return of appetite and growth rate to normal levels. Indeed, as judged by abattoir surveys, progress to slaughter weight can take place despite extensive residual lesions (Emsbo 1951; Rowland and Hutchings 1978).

LESIONS

Porcine Intestinal Adenomatosis. PIA occurs most commonly in, but is not restricted to, the terminal 50 cm of the small intestine and the upper third of the spiral colon, including the cecum. The magnitude of the proliferation varies widely, but in the developed case the wall is visibly thickened and the overall diameter increased. Some subserosal and mesenteric edema is common, and the normal reticulated pattern of the serosal surface is emphasized. The mucosal surface is moist but not mucoid, sometimes with loosely adherent flecks of inflammatory exudate. The mucosa itself is thrown into deep longitudinal or transverse folds, (Fig. 45.1); similar changes in the large intestine may result in sharply defined plaques or marked multiple-polyp formation (Fig. 45.2).

Histologically, the mucosa is composed of large, branching glands (Fig. 45.3) lined by immature columnar epithelium showing nuclei varying from vesicular structures to densely staining elongate spindles. Mitotic figures occur at all levels. Goblet cells are absent, and their reappearance in the deep glands is an indication of impending resolution. In uncomplicated disease the lamina propria is normal. Electron microscopy reveals CLOs, often in considerable numbers and dividing, lying in the apical cytoplasm of the affected epithelium (Fig. 45.4). In recovered cases

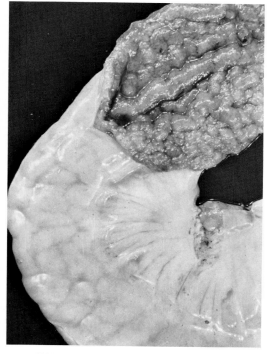

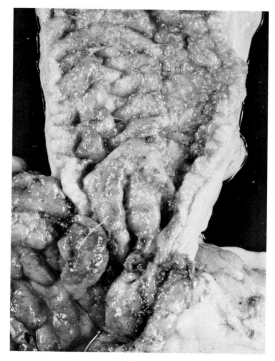

45.1. PIA. Lower ileum showing thickened ridged mucosa with marked reticulation of the serosal surface.

45.2. PIA. Ileocecal junction showing thickening of mucosa in the ileum and cecum, with some superficial inflammation.

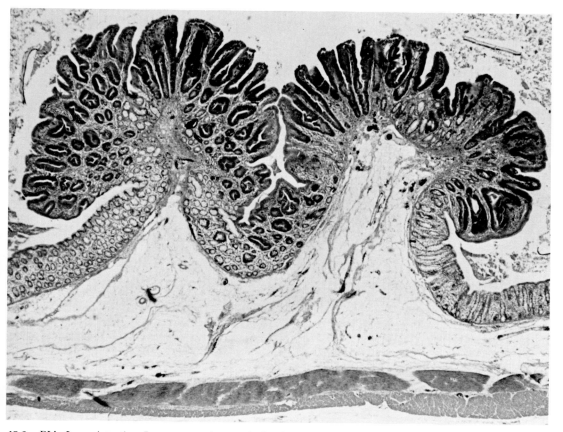

45.3. PIA. Large intestine. Low-power micrograph showing two polyps composed of proliferating glands lined by immature epithelium. H & E. ×20.

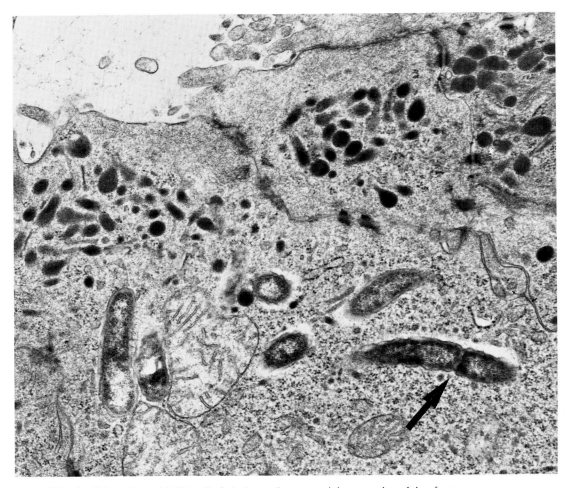

45.4. PIA. Small intestine epithelial cell. Apical cytoplasm containing organisms lying free and undergoing division (arrow). Uranyl acetate and lead citrate. × 10,000.

the organisms become shrunken, aggregated, and occasionally envesicled and may be extruded from the cell into the lamina propria or lumen. Many cases show little evidence of inflammatory reaction. When it occurs, recovery is notable for the development of a population of mature epithelial cells, with goblet cells in the deep crypts and a rapid disappearance of the adenomatous cells from the surface.

Necrotic Enteritis. Coagulative necrosis with some degree of inflammatory exudation of an established PIA lesion results in yellow-gray cheesy masses that adhere tightly to the wall and closely follow the original architecture. Histologically, the coagulative necrosis is clearly defined, together with varying degrees of fibrin, and remnants of the adenomatous epithelium can often be observed in the deep layers. In more chronic cases, granulation tissue may become prominent.

Regional Ileitis. RI is easily recognized as a smoothly contracted, almost rigid length of lower small intestine, and here the traditional name of "hose pipe gut" is appropriate (Fig. 45.5). When the lumen is opened, usually linear ulceration can be seen with adjacent islands or strips of surviving mucosa. Granulation tissue may be prominent, but the most striking feature is hypertrophy of the outer muscle coats.

Proliferative Hemorrhagic Enteropathy. PHE shows a distribution similar to PIA, although lesions of the large intestine are rare. The ileum is thickened and somewhat turgid with peripheral edema. The lumen of the ileum may contain a formed blood clot, and the colon may contain black, tarry feces of mixed blood and digesta (Fig. 45.6). The contents are seldom fluid. The mucosal surface of the affected small intestine shows little gross damage except for the adenomatous thickening; bleeding points, ulcers, or erosions are not observed. Histologic examination is necessary to demonstrate the extensive degeneration of the adenomatous epithelium, with the accumulation of cellular debris in the crypt lumina

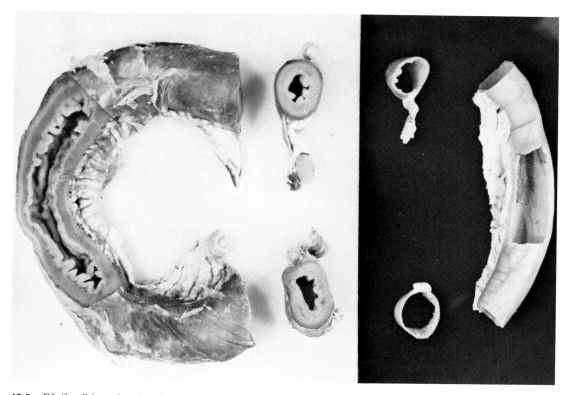

45.5. RI. Small intestine showing marked muscular hypertrophy. Normal intestine adjacent.

and the formation of goblet cells in the deep crypts that are characteristic of this condition (Fig. 45.7).

DIAGNOSIS. Confirmation of a clinical diagnosis may be obtained either by demonstration of CLO in feces using hyperimmune or preferably monoclonal antibody and IFA techniques, or by serologic techniques. When using the IFA test, clinical cases are usually found to be excreting the agent (McOrist et al. 1987; McOrist and Lawson 1989b), but the test is unlikely to prove sufficiently sensitive for the diagnosis of all infections. Serologic diagnosis employs CLO extracted from the tissues as antigen and an indirect IFA test (Lawson et al. 1988); the antibody response is

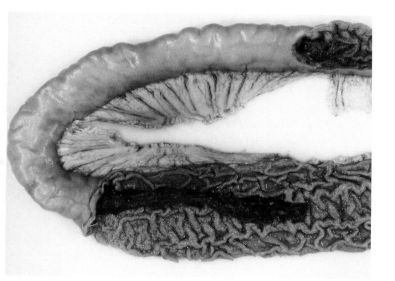

45.6. PHE. Small intestine showing thickened mucosa and blood clot in lumen.

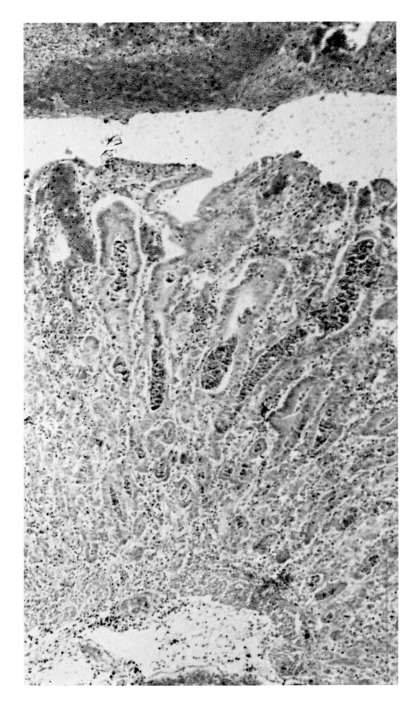

45.7. PHE. Small intestine showing widespread degeneration and early necrosis of proliferating mucosal epithelium with hemorrhage on the surface. H & E. ×100.

short-lived, involves predominantly IgM, and its specificity relates well to the presence of lesions. Exposure to infection itself does not induce seroconversion and as with the demonstration of CLO in feces, the serotest indicates that many more animals have lesions than can be detected clinically.

At necropsy the use of modified Ziehl-Neelsen stain on mucosal smears to demonstrate the intracellular organisms is a simple confirmatory tech-

nique, especially in cases where lesions are minimal. Histologic examination of affected tissues will reveal the morphology of the lesions, and specific diagnosis can be achieved by IFA or immunoperoxidase staining of fixed embedded tissues (Lawson et al. 1985; McOrist et al. 1987). In the absence of specific reagents silver-staining techniques will show the presence of intracellular bacteria (Fig. 45.8), the authors have found Young's modification of the Warthin-Starry silver-

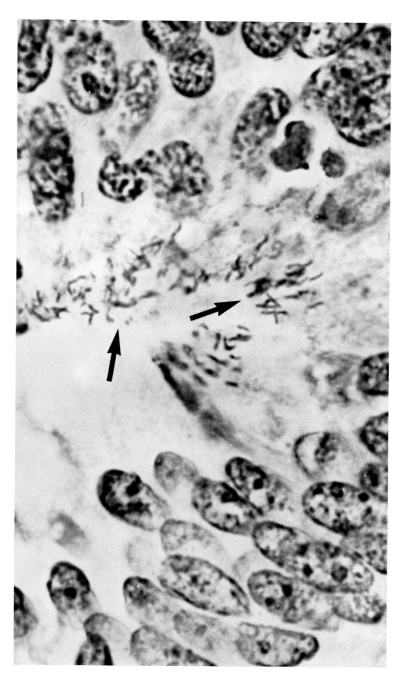

45.8. PIA. Small intestine stained by silver impregnation technique to show bacteria (arrows) in the apical cytoplasm of affected epithelium. Warthin-Starry. × 2000.

impregnation technique (Young 1969) satisfactory for routine use, and the method of Levaditi is sometimes of value.

Where electron microscopic facilities are available, identification of the intracellular location of the organism can be undertaken and may be necessary where other techniques give equivocal results.

TREATMENT AND PREVENTION. There is little or no authenticated evidence that treatment of clinical PIA or PHE is of value; there is, however, the widespread clinical impression supported by limited controlled field studies that disease may be prevented by antibacterial treatment. Three different approaches to medication are possible. First, animals introduced into infected premises are allowed a period of exposure followed by therapeutic levels of antimicrobials to obviate the occurrence of clinical disease. The preferred treatment is tetracycline, with or without the addition of other drugs, at 300–400 ppm for 14 days; the period of exposure should not exceed 3 weeks before the introduction of antibiotics (Love and Love 1977). Such an approach is most suited to the management of PHE in mature animals.

Second, clinical disease manifested as necrotic enteritis will often appear to be moderated either by tylosin/sulphonamide combinations or dimetridazole (100–500 ppm). If sufficient numbers of clinical cases are occurring in growers, removal of affected animals to separate accommodation with supportive therapy may limit losses.

The final approach to treatment is continuous medication to slaughter, to minimize production loss caused by the disease. Certain drugs appear ineffective (olaquindox, 50; furazolidine, 100; dimetridazole, 200; and nitrovin, 100 ppm) (Pointon 1989), and despite their usage at the levels indicted, intestinal pathology still develops. It is easier to obtain information on lack of efficacy of drugs than to demonstrate positive effects. The performance of drugs believed not to work may be influenced by a variety of other on-farm factors; more data is therefore required before reliable drugs therapies can be promoted. There is evidence that resistance to the tetracycline groups of drugs, used alone, takes place following prolonged usage.

Throughout the world the PIA complex appears to be endemic in many pigs herds, with clinical disease at a low level and largely unrecognized. Until the extent of the economic loss is evaluated, there is possibly little justification for attempting to control this form of the disease.

It remains a matter of concern that PHE continues to be a serious problem in minimally diseased herds, and it would appear possible that the entry of infection is not necessarily connected with the introduction of pigs. Presently, sustained isolation of the herd with rigorous control of access appears the most appropriate precaution. This means that purchased stock must be derived either by hysterectomy or medicated early weaning (MEW) or from herds produced in this way and in which it can be certain PE has not been observed. Doubt must exist as to the status of animals derived from any other environment.

It cannot be overemphasized that in the conventional herd the absence of clinical PIA, even over a period of years, is no guarantee of freedom from the disease and infection. Apparently clean animals from such herds may be responsible for the introduction of PE into a hitherto uncontaminated environment, followed by the explosive development of PHE and later by a low level of endemic PIA.

REFERENCES

BEERS, P. T. 1984. Studies on porcine adenomatosis with particular reference to proliferative haemorrhagic enteropathy. Ph.D. diss., Sidney Univ, Australia.

BIESTER, H. E., AND SCHWARTE, L. H. 1931. Intestinal adenoma in swine. Am J pathol 7:175–185.

BIESTER, H. E.; SCHWARTE, L. H.; AND EVELETH, D. F. 1939. Studies on a rapidly developing intestinal adenoma in a pig. Am J Pathol 15:385–389.

BOOSINGER, T. R.; THACKER, H. L.; AND ARMSTRONG, C. H. 1985. *Campylobacter sputorum* subsp. *mucosalis* and *Campylobacter hyointestinalis* infections in the intestine of gnotobiotic pigs. Am J Vet Res 46:2152–2156.

CHANG, K.; KURTZ, H. J.; WARD, G. E.; AND GEBHART, C. J. 1984. Immunofluorescent demonstration of *Campylobacter hyointestinalis* and *Campylobacter sputorum* subspecies *mucosalis* in swine intestine with lesions of proliferative enteritis. Am J Vet Res 45:703–710.

DUHAMEL, G. E., AND WHEELDON, E. B. 1982. Intestinal adenomatosis in a foal. Vet Pathol 19:447–450.

EMSBO, P. 1951. Terminal or regional ileitis in swine. Nord Vet Med 3:1–28.

ERIKSEN, K., AND LANDSVERK, T. 1985. Intestinal adenomatosis in the Blue Fox. Nord Vet Med 37:254–255.

FIELD, H. I.; BUNTAIN, D.; AND JENNINGS, A. R. 1953. Terminal or regional ileitis in pigs. J Comp Pathol 63:153–158.

FOX, J. G., AND LAWSON, G. H. K. 1988. Campylobacter-like omega intracellular antigen in proliferative colitis of ferrets. Lab Anim Sci 38:34–36.

———. 1989. Unpublished observations.

FRISK, C. S., AND WAGNER, J. E. 1977. Experimental hamster enteritis: An electron microscopic study. Am J Vet Res 38:1861–1868.

GEBHART, C. J. 1987. Role of various *Campylobacter* species in swine proliferative enteritis. Ph.D. diss., Minnesota Univ, St. Paul.

GEBHART, C. J.; WARD, G. E.; CHANG, K.; AND KURTZ, H. J. 1983. *Campylobacter hyointestinalis* (new species) isolated from swine with proliferative ileitis. Am J Vet Res 45:361–367.

HOORENS, J. 1962. Regional enteritis in the pig. Thesis, Univ of Ghent, Belgium.

JACKSON, G. H., AND BAKER, J. R. 1980. The occurrence of unthriftiness in piglets post-weaning. Proc 6th Int Congr Pig Vet Soc, Copenhagen, 7:63.

KUBO, M.; OHYA, T; AND WATASE, H. 1984. Proliferative hemorrhagic enteropathy detected at an abattoir in Kagoshima. Jpn J Vet Sci 46:413–417.

LAWSON, G. H. K., AND ROWLAND, A. C. 1974. Intestinal adenomatosis in the pig: A bacteriological study. Res Vet Sci 17:331–336.

LAWSON, G. H. K.; ROWLAND, A. C.; SMITH, W. J.; ROBERTS, L.; AND LUNNE, D. 1980. Immunisation of pigs with *Campylobacter sputorum* subspecies *mucosalis* vaccine. Vet Rec 107:424–425.

LAWSON, G. H. K.; ROWLAND, A. C.; AND McINTYRE, N. 1985. Demonstration of a new intracellular antigen in porcine intestinal adenomatosis and hamster proliferative ileitis. Vet Microbiol 10:303–313.

LAWSON, G. H. K.; McORIST, S.; ROWLAND, A. C.; McCARTNEY, E.; AND ROBERTS, L. 1988. Serological diagnosis of the porcine proliferative enteropathies: Implications for etiology and epidemiology. Vet Rec 122:554–557.

LOMAX, I. G.; GLOCK, R. D.; AND HOGAN, J. E. 1982a. Experimentally induced porcine proliferative enteritis in specific-pathogen free pigs. Am J Vet Res 43:1615–1621.

———. 1982b. Porcine proliferative enteritis (intestinal adenomatosis): Field studies. Vet Med 77:1777–1786.

LOMAX, L. G.; GLOCK, R. D.; HARRIS, D. L.; AND HOGAN, J. E. 1982c. Porcine proliferative enteritis: Experimentally induced disease in cesarean-derived pigs. Am J Vet Res 43:1622–1630.

Love, R. J., and Love, D. N. 1977. Control of proliferative haemorrhagic enteropathy in pigs. Vet Rec 100:473.

Love, R. J.; Love, D. N.; and Edwards, M. J. 1977. Proliferative haemorrhagic enteropathy in pigs. Vet Rec 100:65–68.

McCartney, E.; Lawson, G. H. K.; and Rowland, A. C. 1984. Behaviour of *Campylobacter sputorum* subspecies *mucosalis* in gnotobiotic pigs. Res Vet Sci 36:290–297.

McOrist, S., and Lawson, G. H. K. 1987. Possible relationship of proliferative enteritis in pigs and hamsters. Vet Microbiol 15:293–302.

_____. 1989a. Reproduction of proliferative enteritis in gnotobiotic pigs. Res Vet Sci 46:27–33.

_____. 1989b. Failure to demonstrate *Campylobacter*-like organisms of the proliferative enteropathies in pigs excreting *Campylobacter* sp. Vet Rec 124:41.

McOrist, S.; Boid, R.; Lawson, G. H. K.; and McConnell, I. 1987. Monoclonal antibodies to intracellular *Campylobacter*-like organisms of the porcine proliferative enteropathies. Vet Rec 121:421–422.

McOrist, S.; Boid, R.; and Lawson, G. H. K. 1989a. Antigenic analysis of *Campylobacter* species and an intracellular *Campylobacter*-like organisms associated with porcine proliferative enteropathies. Infect Immun 57:957–962.

McOrist, S.; Lawson, G. H. K.; Rowland, A. C.; and McIntyre, N. 1989b. Early lesions of proliferative enteritis in pigs and hamsters. Vet Pathol 26:260–264.

McOrist, S.; Lawson, G. H. K.; Roy, D. J.; and Boid, R. 1990. DNA analysis of intracellular *Campylobacter*-like organisms associated with the porcine proliferative enteropathies: Novel organism proposed. FEMS Microbiol Lett 69:189–194.

Mapother, M. E.; Joens, L. A.; and Glock, R. D. 1987. Experimental reproduction of porcine proliferative enteritis. Vet Rec 121:553–556.

Martinsson, K.; Holmgren, N.; Jonsson, L.; and Nordstrom, G. 1974. Studies in terminal ileitis in piglets. Sven Veterinaertidn 26:347–354.

O'Hara, P. J. 1972. Intestinal haemorrhage syndrome in the pig. Vet Rec 91:517–518.

Pointon, A. M. 1989. *Campylobacter* associated intestinal pathology in pigs. AustVet J 66:90–91.

Roberts, L.; Rowland, A. C.; and Lawson, G. H. K. 1977. Experimental reproduction of porcine intestinal adenomatosis and necrotic enteritis. Vet Rec 100:12–13.

Roberts, L.; Lawson, G. H. K.; Rowland, A. C.; and Laing, A. H. 1979. Porcine intestinal adenomatosis and its detection in a closed pig herd. Vet Rec 104:366–368.

Roberts, L.; Lawson, G. H. K.; and Rowland, A. C. 1980. The experimental infection of neonatal pigs with *Campylobacter sputorum* subspecies *mucosalis.* Res Vet Sci 28:145–147.

Rowland, A. C., and Hutchings, D. A. 1978. Necrotic enteritis and regional ileitis in pigs at slaughter. Vet Rec 103:338–339.

Rowland, A. C., and Lawson, G. H. K. 1974. Intestinal adenomatosis in the pig: Immunofluorescent and electron microscopic studies. Res Vet Sci 17:323–330.

_____. 1975. Porcine intestinal adenomatosis: A possible relationship with necrotic enteritis, regional ileitis and proliferative haemorrhagic enteropathy. Vet Rec 97:178–180.

Rowland, A. C., and Rowntree, P. G. M. 1972. A haemorrhagic bowel syndrome associated with intestinal adenomatosis in the pig. Vet Rec 91:235–241.

Vandenberghe, J., and Marsboom, R. 1982. *Campylobacter*-like bacteria in adenocarcinomas of the colon in two Wistar rats. Vet Rec 111:416–417.

Young, B. J. 1969. A reliable method for demonstrating spirochaetes in tissue sections. J Med Lab Technol 26:248–252.

46 Salmonellosis

B. P. Wilcock

K. J. Schwartz

INFECTION BY members of the genus *Salmonella* is of concern to veterinarians and swine producers as a cause of septicemia and diarrhea in weaned pigs and as a source of human foodborne salmonellosis. The first association of the bacteria with disease was made by Salmon and Smith (1886) when they described *S. choleraesuis* as the cause of hog cholera (HC). When the viral etiology of HC was established some 20 years later, salmonella was demoted to the ignoble role of an opportunistic pathogen in swine debilitated by HC. In North America it was only with the demise of HC that salmonellae gained appropriate recognition as a primary swine pathogen capable of inducing almost all the clinical and pathologic features previously attributed to that disease.

Infection with salmonellae may be clinically inapparent or may cause clinical disease referable to septicemia, to enterocolitis, or to bacteremic localization as pneumonia (Baskerville and Dow 1973), or occasionally as meningitis (Reynolds et al. 1967; McErlean 1968), encephalitis (Wilcock and Olander 1977c), caseous lymphadenitis (Barnes and Bergeland 1968), or abortion (Schwartz and Daniels 1987).

ETIOLOGY. Members of the genus *Salmonella* are a morphologically and biochemically homogeneous group of gram-negative, motile, facultatively anaerobic bacilli with peritrichous flagellae. The list of serologically distinct serotypes has grown to about 2000, usually named by the geographic site of first isolation.

Salmonellae are hardy and ubiquitous pathogens. They multiply at 7–45°C; survive freezing and desiccation well; and persist for weeks, months, or even years in suitable organic substrates. Salmonellae were reported to survive in meat-meal fertilizer for 8 months (Mittermeyer and Foltz 1969) and in manure oxidation ditches for 47 days (Will et al. 1973). Survival is greatly shortened below pH 5.0 (Henry et al. 1983). Numerous reports of prolonged survival in water have been cited (Williams 1975; Wray and Sojka 1977; Pokorny 1988). The cells are readily inactivated by heat and sunlight; do not form spores; and are destroyed by common phenolic, chlorine, and iodine-based disinfectants (Rubin and Weinstein 1977).

A major factor in the success of salmonellae as virtually universal pathogens is their ability to adapt to a seemingly endless list of hosts. The amusing parade of papers entitled, "*Salmonella* isolated from a . . . ," should be laid to rest by the observation by Taylor and McCoy (1969) that salmonellae have been isolated from all vertebrate hosts from which they have been sought, with the possible exception of fish in unpolluted waters. Techniques for isolation of salmonellae vary widely with the nature of the suspect material and sometimes with the specific serotypes sought. From materials like sewage, feed, and polluted water in which salmonella numbers are likely to be low compared to other organisms, there is a ritual of preenrichment, selective enrichment, and selective plating (Groves et al. 1971; Edwards and Ewing 1972; Skovgaard et al. 1985; Vassiliadis et al. 1987). Occasionally these methods are necessary for the isolation of salmonella from tissues or feces of carrier animals in which numbers are often low, but in clinically affected animals the numbers should be such that direct plating of internal organs and simple selective enrichment of intestinal samples are usually adequate (Committee on Salmonella 1969). In fact, if elaborate techniques are required for salmonella isolation from a sick pig, salmonella is unlikely to be the causal agent. The various isolation techniques are detailed in any standard text on clinical microbiology. Serotype identification is based on identification of specific somatic and flagellar antigens by agglutination serology. Epidemiologic investigations of zoonotic outbreaks occasionally demand more sophisticated techniques of phage-typing, plasmid characterization, or mapping of outer membrane proteins to trace the footprints of a specific isolant.

In marked contrast to the seemingly endless list of serotypes isolated from carcasses and pork products, the disease in swine is almost always caused by either *S. choleraesuis* var. *kunzendorf* or by *S. typhimurium;* localized epizootics of disease caused by the biochemically atypical *S. typhisuis* have been reported in the American Midwest (Barnes and Bergeland 1968; Andrews 1976) and at least historically in Europe (Barnes and Sorensen 1975). This organism grows poorly in standard selective mediums for salmonella isolation, thus infection may be more widespread than commonly thought. The disease produced by *S. typhisuis* is so characteristic, however, that outbreaks are not likely to remain unnoticed (Barnes and Bergeland 1968). Other serotypes probably are occasional causes of disease in swine, but convincing reports of naturally occurring disease are found only for *S. dublin* (Lawson and Dow 1966; McErlean 1968) and *S. enteritidis* (Reynolds et al. 1967) in which isolation was supported by clinical or pathologic evidence of salmonellosis. In the case of both *S. dublin* and *S. enteritidis,* the reports were of meningitis in suckling pigs.

S. choleraesuis, usually as the hydrogen sulfide–producing variant *kunzendorf,* has traditionally been considered the most frequent serotype causing disease in swine (Levine et al. 1945; Lawson and Dow 1966; Morehouse 1972; Wilcock et al. 1976; Mills and Kelly 1986; Schwartz and Daniels 1987). *S. typhimurium* is the second most frequent isolant, and usually causes enterocolitis. Disease caused by *S. typhimurium* occurs with greater than expected frequency in what could be considered unusually clean herds: university research herds, testing stations, closed specific-pathogen-free (SPF) herds, and purebred breeding herds (Heard et al. 1965; Gooch and Haddock 1969; Lynn et al. 1972).

EPIDEMIOLOGY. The epidemiology of salmonellosis in swine must be viewed as two relatively separate problems: salmonella infection of pork carcasses and retail products and salmonellosis as a disease of pigs. Failure by authors of prevalence surveys to distinguish the two conditions (and failure by later reviewers to recognize the presence or absence of such a distinction) has led to considerable confusion about the etiology and epidemiology of clinical salmonellosis in swine. Infection of swine by a wide variety of

serotypes is common, but clinical disease caused by serotypes other than *S. choleraesuis* or *S. typhimurium* is distinctly uncommon.

Salmonella in Pork. Data collected from various countries indicates wide variation in contamination of carcasses and retail pork products with salmonella. Variation is probably due in part to real variation in contamination and in part to differences in methods. Some of the largest surveys are summarized in Tables 46.1 and 46.2. The high level of infection demonstrated in these studies is mainly the result of abattoir cross-contamination in crowded holding pens prior to slaughter and mechanical transfer of contamination among carcasses by dehairing machines, scalding tanks, and polishers (Galton et al. 1954; Hansen et al. 1964; Kampelmacher et al. 1965; Williams and Newell 1970; Michaud 1978; Morgan et al. 1987). Nevertheless, it is the infected pig leaving the farm that must be considered the original source of abattoir infections. The stress of transport activates latent carriers, which then massively contaminate the environment of the truck and abattoir (Williams and Newell 1970). The prevalence of infection within the group continues to increase with increasing length of stay in the pens prior to slaughter, rising by about 50% for each 24-hour period (Craven and Hurst 1982; Morgan et al. 1987). It should be noted that *S. choleraesuis* is rarely associated with contamination of carcasses and pork products. Unusual as a cause of human disease, *S. choleraesuis* infection is severe when it does occur (Cherubin 1980). For further details concerning the epidemiology of porcine salmonellosis as a public health hazard, readers may consult Newell and Williams (1971), Morse and Duncan (1974), Wiener (1974), or Williams (1975).

Table 46.1. Salmonella isolations from pork carcasses

Year	Location	Sample	Samples	% Positive	Reference
1970	Australia	Mesenteric nodes Intestine	200	27	Riley (1970)
1972	England	Feces Tissues	976	9.9	Nottingham et al. (1972)
1973	England	Cecal content Mesenteric nodes	300	7.3	McCaughey et al. (1973)
1976	United States	Cecal content	658	44.8	Gustafson et al. (1976)
1978	United States	Feces	263	14.8	Tacal and Lawrence (1980)
1984	California	Mesenteric nodes	280	4.3	Morse and Hird (1984)
1989	Hungary	Feces	200	48.0	Jayarao et al. (1989)

Table 46.2. Salmonella isolations from pork products

Year	Location	Sample	Samples	% Positive	Reference
1970	Hawaii	Pork	885	4.15	Gooch and Goo (1971)
1972	United States	Sausage	560	28.0	Surkiewicz et al. (1972)
1975	England	Sausage	1467	29.7	Roberts et al. (1975)
1983	England	Sausage	115	35.9	Banks and Board (1983)
1984	United States	Sausage	175		Silas et al. (1984)
1987	Japan	Ground pork	120	30.0	Fukushima et al. (1987)

Salmonellosis as a Disease. In contrast to the abundant epidemiologic information on carcass infection, there is embarrassingly little information on the clinical disease of swine. Most outbreaks occur in intensively reared weaned pigs, and although disease in adults is not infrequent, disease in suckling pigs is distinctly uncommon but infection is not (Gooch and Haddock 1969; Wilcock et al. 1976). The rarity of salmonellosis in suckling pigs presumably results from lactogenic immunity, since neonatal swine are susceptible to oral challenge with salmonellae and develop a disease comparable to that in weaned pigs (Wilcock 1978).

Disease is worldwide but varies markedly in estimated prevalence and mortality. Much of the confusion arises from incautious extrapolation of data gathered in microbiologic surveys to actual disease incidence. All too often reviews containing estimates of the prevalence of "outbreaks" of salmonellosis are in fact reporting epidemiologic data from slaughterhouse or federal surveillance studies unsupported by clinical or pathologic criteria of salmonellosis. In one correlative study in Indiana in 1974–75, salmonellosis accounted for 19% of 327 consecutive porcine necropsies (Wilcock et al. 1976). In contrast, Hooper and Troutt (1971) reported that salmonella infection was considered the major disease process in only 2% of samples submitted in Missouri between 1967 and 1969. During a 4-year period in Ireland, salmonellosis was the diagnosis in 4.4% of 2180 swine necropsies (Lawson and Dow 1966). In Taiwan, *Salmonella* spp. were isolated from about 10% of scouring pigs and 48% of fatal diarrheas or septicemias in weaned pigs (Hsu et al. 1983).

S. choleraesuis has been the second most frequently isolated salmonella from all animal sources in the United States since 1979, isolated almost exclusively (>99%) from diseased swine (Ferris and Frerichs 1990).

Midwestern diagnostic laboratories and veterinarians report increasing frequency of salmonellosis due to *S. choleraesuis*. One laboratory in Iowa reported 256 isolations in 1981 with gradual increase to 788 in 1989. *S. choleraesuis* was isolated in >95% of swine salmonellosis with *S. typhimurium* present in 4% and others in less than 1% of salmonellosis outbreaks in Iowa in 1989 (Schwartz 1990). Salmonellosis as a disease in swine ranks second only to swine dysentery in total cost to Iowa swine producers (Owen 1990). We believe that the regional variation is loosely correlated to pig density, husbandry practices, and in particular, commingling of pigs of different ages and/or origins.

Sources of Infection. A poll of "salmonella experts" conducted as part of a task force study in the United States failed to reach a consensus as to the most important source of salmonella for pigs (Bixler 1978). If one recognizes that *S. chol-eraesuis* is the most frequent porcine isolate but is a very infrequent isolate from pig feeds or nonporcine salmonella reservoirs, the conclusion seems clear that the infected, shedding pig is the major source of new infections. During acute disease pigs will shed up to 10^6 *S. choleraesuis*/g feces (Smith and Jones 1967) or 10^7 *S. typhimurium* (Gutzmann et al. 1976). The minimum disease-producing dose of either serotype has not been established, and disease is frequently difficult to reproduce. There is one report of moderate disease following oral inoculation of 10^6 cells (Dawe and Troutt 1976), but most authors report successful disease production with doses of 10^8–10^{11} cells. High animal density, stress of transport, and intercurrent nutritional or infectious disease are assumed to increase the shedding by carriers and the susceptibility of exposed pigs (Committee on Salmonella 1969).

For serotypes other than *S. choleraesuis*, pigs should be thought of as biological filters for the low numbers of various salmonellae present in feed or water contaminated by birds, rodents, or other livestock. Feeds containing animal-origin protein may also be sources of infection (Allred et al. 1967; Williams et al. 1969; Nape and Murphy 1971), although evidence linking feed contamination to clinical outbreaks is generally lacking. In most instances the salmonellae establish clinically inapparent infection of unknown duration, which is of significance as a potential zoonosis, but not to the pig. Under conditions of concurrent disease or stress the usually nonpathogenic serotypes may cause disease, but ordinarily disease results only from infection with *S. choleraesuis* or *S. typhimurium.*

Shedding and Carrier States. The pattern of shedding and the duration of the carrier state after clinically apparent disease has been studied only in group-housed pigs with no barrier to repeated reinfection (Wilcock and Olander 1978; Wood et al. 1989). After experimentally induced infection with *S. typhimurium,* salmonella was isolated from feces daily during the first 10 days postinfection and frequently during the next 4–5 months. At slaughter 4–7 months after initial infection, over 90% of pigs were positive for *S. typhimurium* in the mesenteric lymph node, tonsil, cecum, or feces (Wilcock and Olander 1978; Wood et al. 1989). In naturally occurring infections with the same organism, prolonged but sporadic shedding necessitated repeated fecal cultures of each pig before the organism was finally isolated (Heard et al. 1968; Gooch and Haddock 1969).

The duration of shedding of *S. choleraesuis* and location(s) of organisms in carrier swine appears not to have been studied.

The influence of antibiotics on the frequency and duration of shedding of salmonellae in pigs has received little attention. In human enteric salmonellosis the use of antibiotics has long been recognized to prolong the carrier state (Dixon 1965; Aserkoff and Bennett 1969). In pigs with enterocolitis, antibiotics do not reduce the duration or magnitude of fecal shedding, but neither are they reported to prolong or intensify shedding (Finlayson and Barnum 1973; DeGeeter et al. 1976; Gutzmann et al. 1976; Wilcock and Olander 1978; Jones et al. 1983; Jacks et al. 1988). In contrast, vigorous antibacterial therapy early in the course of septicemia caused by *S. choleraesuis* may significantly reduce the magnitude and duration of fecal shedding (Jacks et al. 1981).

PATHOGENESIS. The clinical and pathologic features of salmonellosis reflect a host:parasite interaction that can be influenced by serotype virulence, natural and acquired host resistance, and route and size of infective dose. There is tremendously wide variation in serotype virulence and genetically conditioned host resistance to disease.

The sequence of events following ingestion of salmonellae was first described by Takeuchi (1967) and by Takeuchi and Sprinz (1967) in a classic experiment with *S. typhimurium* in guinea pigs. Following a brief period of intraluminal replication, salmonellae invaded the intestinal mucosa, particularly of the ileum. Passage through the epithelium resulted in mild and transient enterocyte damage. The organisms were phagocytized but not destroyed by macrophages in the lamina propria, and within 24 hours of challenge the bacilli were numerous within macrophages of gut-associated lymphoid tissue. Concurrent with bacillary spread was the appearance of an acute, predominantly macrophage, inflammatory reaction and prominent microvascular damage with thrombosis within the lamina propria and submucosa. In similar experiments in weaned pigs, the bacilli were seen free or within phagosomes within apparently healthy enterocytes within a few hours of ingestion. Spread to mesenteric lymph nodes is almost equally rapid, occurring within 2 hours of inoculation of ligated intestinal loops or 24 hours after oral challenge (Reed et al. 1985; 1986). Since *S. typhimurium* is frequently isolated from tonsil and mandibular lymph nodes, it is likely that this and other "gut-associated" serotypes are capable of limited invasion throughout the gastrointestinal tract (Pospischil et al. 1990). Mucosal invasion is probably an absolute prerequisite for disease (Giannella et al. 1973). Intraluminal salmonella replication is probably not necessary for disease production with large inocula but may be important with small inocula from contaminated feed or water.

Replication to about 10^7 organisms/g intestinal content is required for lesion production in pigs infected with *S. typhimurium* and probably applies to other serotypes causing enterocolitis. Alterations in normal intestinal defenses by antibiotic-induced changes in normal flora or cold-induced alteration in intestinal motility may reduce the amount of replication required for disease or increase the ease of salmonella replication (Bohnhoff et al. 1954). Infection with *S. choleraesuis* may not require such massive lumenal proliferation as prerequisite for disease inasmuch as it is inherently more invasive than other serotypes and regularly causes signs of septicemia 24–72 hours before the onset of diarrhea (Smith and Jones 1967; Cherubin et al. 1974; Wilcock 1979; Reed et al. 1986).

The pathogenesis of the diarrhea typical of enteric salmonellosis and of later stages of salmonella septicemia has traditionally been attributed to malabsorption and net fluid leakage by a necrotic, inflamed bowel. Several studies using rabbits, monkeys, calves, or pigs have demonstrated fluid secretion independent of mucosal necrosis or inflammation (Giannella et al. 1973; Rout et al. 1974; Kinsey et al. 1976; Clarke and Gyles 1987).

These studies present evidence that, at least early in the disease, the diarrhea is the result of decreased sodium resorption and increased chloride secretion, somewhat analogous to the secretory diarrheas of porcine colibacillosis or human cholera. Salmonellae are known to produce choleralike and shigalike enterotoxins, and these toxins may induce diarrhea independent of mucosal damage. Secretion stimulated by prostaglandins elaborated by endotoxin-stimulated neutrophils may also be important (Stephen et al. 1985). Most of the experimental work has been done using small intestine of rabbits or monkeys, species in which the lesions of salmonelloses are quite different from those in pigs. At the moment, the relative importance of the various toxins, of prostaglandins or other mediators, and of mucosal necrosis in the diarrhea seen in naturally occurring disease remains unknown.

Mucosal inflammation and necrosis occurs in concert with the diarrhea but perhaps independently of it. Microvascular thrombosis and endothelial necrosis in the submucosa and lamina propria are consistent early lesions in porcine salmonellosis (Lawson and Dow 1966; Wilcock et al. 1976; Jubb et al. 1985; Reed et al. 1986), probably in response to locally produced endotoxin. The salmonellae are not directly associated with the damaged vessels but direct the events from the protected intracellular niche of macrophages in the surrounding submucosa or lamina propria (Takeuchi and Sprinz 1967). Mucosal ischemia as a result of the microvascular thrombosis is probably a major contributor to the mucosal necrosis so typical of salmonellosis in all species. The second major contribution to mucosal necrosis is probably from the chemical products of mucosal inflammation, which for reasons still obscure is characteristically histiocytic rather than neutrophilic.

The systemic signs and lesions of septicemic salmonellosis, in swine almost exclusively *S. choleraesuis* infection, are most commonly attributed to endotoxemia from bacterial dissemination. The complex biology of endotoxin is beyond the scope of this chapter, and readers should consult Wolff (1973), Elin and Wolff (1976), or Cybulsky et al. (1988). Briefly, endotoxin interacts with plasma and with leukocytes to activate complement and intrinsic coagulation, initiate inflammation, and induce fever. Most of these effects are mediated by interleukin 1, a lymphokine produced by macrophages stimulated by the endotoxin (Rubin and Weinstein 1977). Information on the pathogenesis of the various systemic lesions (pneumonitis, hepatic microgranulomas, splenomegaly, fundic infarction) is as yet too incomplete to allow identification of each lesion as specifically endotoxic, immunologic, or ischemic in origin.

CLINICAL SIGNS AND DIAGNOSIS. The clinical signs of porcine salmonellosis may be the result of septicemia or enterocolitis. Pigs surviving the acute septicemia may develop clinical signs referable to bacteremic localization: pneumonia, hepatitis, enterocolitis, and, occasionally, meningoencephalitis. Pigs initially suffering from enterocolitis may later develop chronic wasting disease or rectal stricture.

Septicemic Salmonellosis. This form of disease, usually caused by *S. choleraesuis,* occurs mainly in weaned pigs less than 5 months old but may be seen occasionally in market swine or adult breeding stock as a cause of sudden death or abortion either in a single animal or as an epizootic. It is rare in conventionally reared sucking pigs.

CLINICAL SIGNS. Affected pigs are inappetent, reluctant to move, febrile with temperatures of 105–107°F (40.5–41.6°C), and often have a shallow, moist cough. A few individuals may be seen huddled in a corner of the pen. The first evidence of disease is frequently the finding of several dead pigs with purple extremities and abdomens. Diarrhea is not a feature of septicemic salmonellosis until the third or fourth day of disease, when watery yellow feces may be seen. In most outbreaks, mortality is high and morbidity is variable but usually less than 10%. The duration of the disease in individual surviving pigs and the duration and severity of each epizootic is unpredictable. This makes evaluation of therapeutic regimens in naturally occurring outbreaks very difficult. Disease spread is fecal-oral with an incubation period of at least 24–48 hours. The disease has been experimentally reproduced by intranasal inoculation, and aerosol transmission might explain those epizootics in which pneumonia is an unusually prominent clinical sign or in which barn design makes fecal transmission unlikely. Recovered pigs are carriers and fecal shedders, but the duration is unknown.

GROSS LESIONS. Lesions at necropsy include cyanosis of ears, feet, tail, and ventral abdominal skin; congestion progressing to infarction of gastric fundic mucosa; splenomegaly and less severe hepatomegaly; and moist, swollen mesenteric lymph nodes. Lungs are firm and diffusely congested, often with interlobular edema and hemorrhage. Icterus is not uncommon (Fig. 46.1). A le-

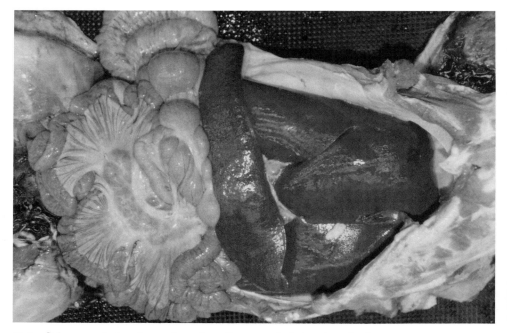

46.1. Splenomegaly, hepatomegaly, and swollen mesenteric lymph nodes from *S. choleraesuis* infection.

sion that is equally frequent but more subtle is miliary, random white foci of necrosis in the liver. In pigs surviving the first few days of disease there is serous to necrotic enterocolitis. The features of the intestinal lesion are described more fully in the section on salmonella enterocolitis. Petechial hemorrhage is not a common feature of salmonellosis but, when present, is usually best seen in the renal cortex and on the epicardium.

MICROSCOPIC LESIONS. Probably the best candidate for the diagnostic lesion of salmonellosis is the paratyphoid nodule. Throughout the liver are clusters of histiocytes amid foci of acute coagulative hepatocellular necrosis, corresponding to the white foci seen grossly. The lesions are consistently present (Lawson and Dow 1966) and, to the authors' knowledge, are not mimicked by any other lesion in pigs. Other lesions typical of salmonellosis include fibrinoid thrombi in venules of gastric mucosa, in cyanotic skin, in glomerular capillaries, and less regularly in pulmonary vessels. There is hyperplasia of reticular cells of spleen and lymph nodes as well as generalized swelling of endothelial cells and histiocytes typical of gram-negative sepsis. A similar proliferative reaction in lung is usually seen and may be interpreted as diffuse interstitial pneumonia. A complete discussion of the pathology of septicemic salmonellosis can be found in Lawson and Dow (1966) or Jubb et al. (1985).

DIAGNOSIS. The diagnosis of septicemic salmonellosis cannot be made on the basis of clinical signs alone, which are similar to those of other causes of septicemia in pigs, particularly erysipelas, streptococcal septicemia, or sudden death due to *Actinobacillus pleuropneumonia*. Gross lesions of splenomegaly, hepatomegaly, lymphadenopathy, or focal hepatic necrosis are very suggestive of septicemic salmonellosis, but are not seen in every case. In most situations, definitive diagnosis requires the isolation of large numbers of salmonellae from affected pigs, almost invariably *S. choleraesuis* var. *kunzendorf*. Samples of lung, liver, or spleen will yield pure cultures of the organism on brilliant green, bismuth sulfite, or even MacConkey's agar. Enrichment techniques are seldom required unless the organs have been contaminated by feces or careless handling, in which case tetrathionate-brilliant green broth at 42–43°C is the enrichment medium of choice. Selenite broth is inhibitory for *S. choleraesuis* and should be avoided (Edwards and Ewing 1972). Attempts to isolate salmonellae from animals that have received antimicrobial therapy are often unrewarding. Intestine or feces is not a reliable site for isolation of the organism in pigs with acute septicemia.

Differential diagnosis must include agents associated with the particular systems affected, including those that may cause septicemia, pneumonia, hepatitis, encephalitis, or enterocolitis (Schwartz 1991).

Salmonella Enterocolitis. Outbreaks of salmonellosis as enterocolitis are most frequent in pigs from weaning to about 4 months of age. Disease may be acute or chronic, and can usually be ascribed to *S. typhimurium* or, less frequently, to *S. choleraesuis*. Outbreaks due to *S. typhimurium* are not uncommon in breeding herds and testing stations, and these very susceptible herds may have unusually high mortality.

CLINICAL SIGNS. The initial sign is watery yellow diarrhea, initially without blood or mucus. The disease may spread rapidly to involve most pigs in a pen within a few days. The initial diarrhea in an individual pig usually lasts 3–7 days, but it typically may recur for second and third bouts, giving the impression of a waxing and waning diarrheal disease of several weeks duration. Blood may appear sporadically in the feces but rarely with the profuseness typical of swine dysentery. Affected pigs are febrile, have decreased food intake, and show dehydration paralleling the severity and duration of the diarrhea. Mortality usually is low and occurs only after several days of diarrhea, presumably the result of hypokalemia and dehydration. Most pigs make complete clinical recovery but remain as carriers and intermittent shedders for at least 5 months. There is no correlation between the severity of disease and the duration or magnitude of shedding. A few pigs may remain unthrifty, and some may develop rectal strictures.

GROSS LESIONS. In pigs that have died of diarrhea the major lesion is focal or diffuse necrotic colitis and typhlitis, which may also involve small intestine. The lesion is seen as adherent gray-yellow debris on the red, roughened mucosal surface of an edematous spiral colon and cecum (Fig. 46.2). Colon and cecal contents are bile stained and scant, often with black or sandlike gritty material. Mesenteric lymph nodes, especially ileocecal nodes, are greatly enlarged and moist. The gross lesion extends to involve the descending colon and rectum. The necrosis may be seen as sharply delineated button ulcers, particularly in resolving lesions. Necrotic ileitis has historically been attributed to numerous agents, including salmonella, but in confirmed cases of salmonellosis, ileal involvement usually is seen as reddening and slight roughening of the mucosa, suggesting mild superficial necrosis. Lesions of septicemia may be present in those cases involving *S. choleraesuis*. In cases of *S. typhimurium* enterocolitis, the liver and spleen are not enlarged except by terminal congestion.

MICROSCOPIC LESIONS. The typical enteric lesion is necrosis of cryptal and surface enterocytes

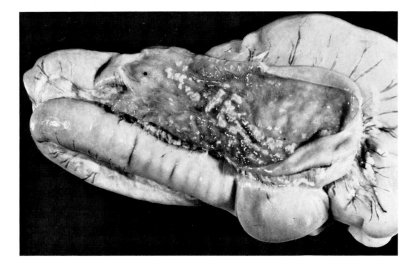

46.2. Coalescing colonic ulcers from *S. typhimurium* infection.

that varies from focal to diffuse. The lamina propria and submucosa contain numerous macrophages and moderate numbers of lymphocytes; neutrophils are numerous only in the very early lesions. Thrombi containing one or more of fibrin, platelets, and leukocytes are numerous (Fig. 46.3). The necrosis frequently extends to involve muscularis mucosa, submucosa, and lymphoid follicles. *Balantidium coli* is not uncommonly present in necrotic debris of chronic cases. In the ileum, necrosis is usually quite superficial and is often seen as villous atrophy. The Peyer's patches may be necrotic in acute disease, but in pigs dying of the naturally occurring disease, lymphoid atrophy or even regenerative hyperplasia is more common. The liver may contain typical paratyphoid nodules but not the necrosis usually seen in the septicemic disease. A more complete discussion of the pathology can be found in Wilcock et al. (1976), Jubb et al. (1985), or Reed et al. (1986).

DIAGNOSIS. The differential diagnosis of diarrhea in weaned pigs must include salmonellosis, swine dysentery, and porcine proliferative enteritis (*Campylobacter*). Other viral, bacterial, or parasitic diseases capable of causing diarrhea include rotaviral and coronaviral enteritis, postweaning colibacillosis, trichuriasis, and coccidiosis; but none of these mimics the clinical features of salmonellosis in weaned swine. Typical acute swine dysentery is distinguished from salmonellosis on the basis of the mucoid and bloody diarrhea in otherwise alert swine with dysentery, contrasted to the marked depression and less profuse yellow diarrhea of salmonellosis. However, in outbreaks of dysentery modified by therapy or immunity, the clinical signs may resemble salmonellosis and require differentiation by necropsy. Porcine proliferative enteritis may be seen as acute intestinal hemorrhage or acute to chronic diarrhea. In the latter manifestation, ne-

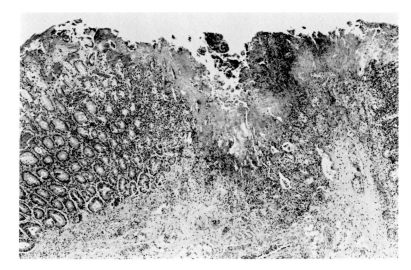

46.3. Histologic section, deep colonic ulceration, and inflammation from *S. typhimurium* infection.

cropsy is required to distinguish it from salmonellosis.

Differentiation among the three diseases at necropsy is primarily by recognition of differences in lesion distribution rather than by differences in character. Salmonellosis is primarily but not exclusively colonic, may be focal, and always involves marked mesenteric lymphadenopathy. The lesion of swine dysentery is diffuse, shallow, and restricted to large intestine; lymph node enlargement is absent or mild. In proliferative enteritis ileal involvement usually overshadows the milder colonic lesions, and the mucosa underlying the necrotic membrane is markedly hyperplastic (Table 46.3). Whipworms (*Trichuris suis*) may also cause diffuse mucohemorrhagic colitis.

The diagnosis of salmonellosis is confirmed by microbiologic and histologic examination. The wide distribution of environmental salmonellae makes isolation alone unreliable for disease diagnosis, and a positive isolation should always be supported by appropriate lesions before a diagnosis of salmonellosis is made. A pool of ileum and ileocecal lymph node should enable detection of virtually all active or recently recovered cases, although tissues such as tonsil or cecal wall will usually yield positive cultures as well (Wilcock et al. 1976; Wood et al. 1989). *S. choleraesuis* is readily isolated from spleen, liver, lung, and kidney in pigs that have died from septicemic salmonellosis. From live animals, large (10 g) aliquots of feces are preferable to rectal swabs for isolation, and tetrathionate enrichment is the method of choice.

Other Syndromes. Salmonella is occasionally involved in disease outbreaks in which the clinical signs may not suggest salmonella as the etiologic diagnosis. Outbreaks of neurologic disease resembling HC or pseudorabies have been reported (Wilcock and Olander 1978), and brain lesions are not uncommonly present with septicemic salmonellosis. The lesion in the brain is necrotic vasculitis and perivascular granulomatous lesions resembling typical paratyphoid nodules (Fig. 46.4). Rectal strictures in growing pigs have been ascribed to defective healing of ulcerative proctitis caused by *S. typhimurium* (Wilcock and Olander 1977a,b). The stricture reportedly represents fibrosis in an area of persistent ischemia, with the rectum predisposed because of a normally precarious blood supply (Fig. 46.5).

Infection with the fastidious, swine-adapted serovar *S. typhisuis* causes a relatively specific chronic syndrome of diarrhea and wasting in which caseous lymphadenitis, histiocytic interstitial pneumonia, or suppurative bronchopneumonia are added to the typical necrotic colitis (Barnes and Bergeland 1968; Andrews 1976; Fenwick and Olander 1987). In some pigs the intestinal lesions may have healed, leaving the lymphoid and pulmonary lesions to be distinguished from tuberculosis and infection with *Actinomyces* spp. (Barnes and Sorensen 1975).

TREATMENT. Whether septicemic or enteric salmonellosis occurs, the primary goals in an outbreak of salmonellosis are to minimize the severity of clinical disease, prevent spread of infection and disease, and prevent recurrence of the disease in the herd. With salmonellosis the attainment of these goals is particularly difficult. Both *S. choleraesuis* and *S. typhimurium* usually show in vitro resistance to many antibacterial agents used in swine (Barnes and Sorensen 1975; Wilcock et al. 1976; Blackburn et al. 1984; Schultz 1989; Fales et al. 1990; Schwartz 1991). During clinical disease, the organisms inhabit a protected intracellular niche inaccessible to many common antibacterial drugs. To date there is no procedure, including the use of antibiotics, that will measurably reduce the prevalence, magnitude, or duration of salmonella shedding by sick or recovered pigs (DeGeeter et al. 1976; Gutzmann et al. 1976; Wilcock and Olander 1978; Jones et al. 1983; Jacks et al. 1988).

Nonetheless, the use of various antibiotics to treat enteric salmonellosis is widely advocated

Table 46.3. Differential diagnosis of enterocolitis in swine at necropsy

Condition	Ileal lesion	Colonic lesion	Ileocecal nodes	Extraintestinal lesions
Salmonellosis	Mild, usually no pseudomembrane	Focal to diffuse, deep necrotic lesions	Always enlarged two to five times normal	Variable, gastric infarction, interstitial pneumonitis, miliary hepatic necrosis
Swine dysentery	Absent	Superficial and usually diffuse necrosis, blood and/or mucus	Often normal, slight enlargement	None except gastric fundic infarction in natural deaths
Porcine proliferative enteritis	Varies from hemorrhagic to necrotic or proliferative	Milder than in the ileum, usually only the proximal spiral colon	Variable with stage of disease	None

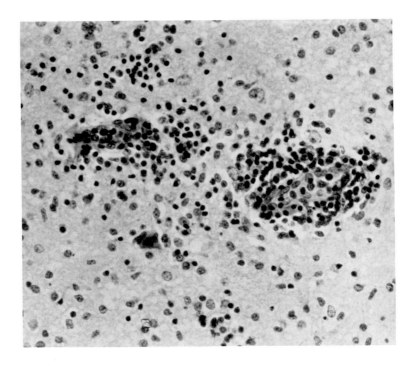

46.4. Histologic section showing vasculitis and perivascular granulomatous inflammation in the brain stem from *S. choleraesuis* encephalitis.

(Morehouse 1972; Barnes and Sorensen 1975; Blood et al. 1979), but much of the data to support this recommendation has inappropriately been taken from trials designed to test the prophylactic efficacy of drugs, not their therapeutic efficacy. Thus pigs on medicated feed, when inoculated orally with the salmonellae, have the antibiotic already in the stomach and intestine to interact with the salmonellae, resulting in milder disease because of what amounts to a decreased inoculum. In the few trials designed specifically to test antibacterial drug efficacy against clinical enteric salmonellosis, such therapy was considered to be of equivocal or no merit (Heard et al. 1968; Gutz-

mann et al. 1976; Olson et al. 1977; Wilcock and Olander 1978).

In contrast, vigorous therapy early in the course of septicemia caused by *S. choleraesuis* has been reported to significantly reduce the duration and severity of disease (Jacks et al. 1981). In that report, therapy was initiated after inoculation but prior to the onset of clinical signs. Critical studies of antimicrobial therapy for treatment of septicemic salmonellosis are generally lacking. Evaluation of efficacy under field conditions is difficult because of the unpredictability of the disease and because husbandry changes often accompany the use of antibacterials in an outbreak. Reports and

46.5. Rectal stricture at necropsy.

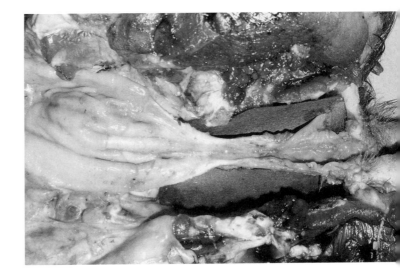

practitioner communications from the American Midwest, however, suggest visibly affected animals respond to aggressive therapy with parenteral antimicrobials (Schwartz 1991). Mass medication to decrease severity and transmission of *Salmonella* is also widely practiced. The choice of an appropriate antimicrobial is by antibiograms and previous herd experience. In the absence of either, amikacin, gentamicin, apramycin, and trimethoprim-sulfa are effective in vitro against most isolates (Barnes and Sorensen 1975; Wilcock et al. 1976; Mills and Kelly 1986; Schultz 1989; Evelsizer 1990; Fales et al. 1990). Antiinflammatory agents are sometimes administered to critically ill animals to combat the effects of endotoxin (Schwartz and Daniels 1987; Schultz 1989; Evelsizer 1990).

In addition to antimicrobial therapy, the control of salmonellosis involves routine husbandry procedures recommended for control of infectious disease. The diarrheic pig massively contaminates its environment and is the single most important source of infection for other pigs. In addition to removal and isolation of sick animals, minimizing exposure to infective material by scrupulous pen sanitation, frequent cleaning of water bowls, and restriction of animal or staff movement from potentially contaminated to clean areas is necessary. Efforts to modify management and environment to decrease stress and increase pig comfort are essential adjustments to specific therapy.

PREVENTION. Prevention of infection of swine with *Salmonella* spp. is not currently possible. The control of disease caused by serotypes other than *S. choleraesuis* rests on the recognition that the carrier pig and contaminated feed or environment are the significant sources of infection and that pigs are most likely to develop disease when exposed during periods of stress or when exposed to massive numbers of salmonellae. The commingling and transport of weanling pigs from different sources to finishing farms enhances activation of latent carriers and assures exposure of stressed pigs to salmonellae (Allred 1972).

The source of host-adapted *S. choleraesuis,* which is rarely, if ever, isolated from feed or feed ingredients, including animal by-products, would seem to be limited to carrier pigs and facilities previously contaminated with this serotype. The fact that many outbreaks occur in facilities with good sanitation suggests that other stresses likely contribute to occurrence of the disease.

Management practices that allow filling of grower and finishing rooms with single-source and -age pigs is of benefit. Minimizing the variety of stress often involved in acute outbreaks requires constant attention to details of management and husbandry, including proper animal density; maintaining dry, comfortable pens and temperatures; and adequate ventilation. On farms with enzootic disease, modifications to the facility and environment and implementation of management practices that emphasize all-in/all-out production should precede a prophylactic drug program. Antibiotics are probably useful as aids in preventing occurrence of disease when used prophylactically, but their use will not prevent infection. Drugs are ordinarily administered at maximum permissible levels in feed or water; ideally, the choice of antibacterial agent should be based on in vitro susceptibility testing of isolates from each outbreak. Since medication often must be initiated before such results are available, choices must be based on previous experience and results of controlled trials. Anecdotal reports suggest acidification of rations or water to be of benefit.

Vaccination against salmonellosis is controversial because of conflicting claims for safety and efficacy. Killed vaccines for *S. typhimurium* are safe but the bulk of the evidence is that they have little efficacy in preventing disease following strong challenge because resistance to disease rests primarily with cell-mediated immunity (Collins 1974; Davies and Kotlarski 1976). Extrapolation of information from experience in humans (Hornick et al. 1970; Welliver and Ogra 1978) and calves (Bairey 1978) suggests, however, that use of a potent killed vaccine may increase the dose necessary to cause disease and may offer some protection from septicemic salmonellosis, in which humoral immunity may probably play a significant role. Reports from midwestern practitioners suggest better efficacy from univalent or autogenous bacterins than from mixed bacterins.

The development and use of modified live salmonella vaccines holds much greater promise by virtue of their ability to stimulate both cell-mediated and humoral immunity. Most recent studies have concentrated on mutant strains that lack one or more enzymes essential to bacterial metabolism or cell wall integrity. The principle underlying their potential usefulness as live vaccines is that they should persist long enough to stimulate protective humoral and cellular immunity but not so long as to cause disease, and should present no risk of reversion to virulence. None of the mutant-strain live vaccines tested to date is completely free of side effects (fever, diarrhea) or protects completely against disease following challenge with virulent *S. typhimurium.* Almost no work has involved pigs. The only reports subsequent to that of Smith (1965) are on the use of attenuated live *S. choleraesuis* vaccines. In one study, the intramuscular vaccination of sows resulted in piglets with high titers of circulating maternally derived antibodies and these piglets resisted subsequent intranasal challenge (Hanna et al. 1979). The relevance of this work to the more usual oral challenge, and in weaned pigs, is dubious. In a second study, conjunctival or intramuscular vaccination protected weaned pigs from subsequent intratracheal challenge with virulent *S. choleraesuis.* However, even nonvaccinated pigs developed only mild disease with minimal colonization of parenchymal organs (Kramer et al. 1987). The efficacy of such attenuated or mutant strain vaccines under field conditions remains unproven. An attenuated live *S. choleraesuis* vaccine was used widely in the United Kingdom for many years but was withdrawn when *S. cholerasuis* infection decreased in that country to negligible proportions.

The detection of carrier animals is difficult because of the unpredictability of fecal shedding. Even repeated negative fecal or tonsilar cultures do not assure that a herd or individual is not a salmonella carrier and thus a potential shedder. The use of salmonella serology will determine if the animal has had previous exposure to salmonella, but this has no relevance to the carrier status or to the probability of shedding. Refusal to introduce any animal with a positive titer will surely eliminate the introduction of carriers, but at the same time it may eliminate genetically useful animals who are not, in fact, carriers.

Monitoring herds for salmonellae is not commonly practiced. Expectations are that detection of salmonellae by bacterial culture of feces and tonsils of diarrheic pigs in the nursery would be the most rewarding to identify infected herds. Isolation attempts from circulating neutrophils (buffy coat) has also offered some promise in detecting carrier swine (Roof 1991). Biotechnology offers the possibility of sensitive and specific methods to identify carriers but tests suitable for routine use have yet to be developed.

REFERENCES

ALLRED, J. N. 1972. Comments on salmonellosis in swine. J Am Vet Med Assoc 160:601–602.
ALLRED, J. N.; WALKER, J. W.; BEAL, V. C.; AND GERMAINE, F. W. 1967. A survey to determine the salmonella contamination rate in livestock and poultry feeds. J Am Vet Med Assoc 151:1857–1860.
ANDREWS, J. J. 1976. *Salmonella typhisuis* infection in swine. Proc North Cent Conf Vet Lab Diagn, p. 7.
ASERKOFF, B., AND BENNETT, J. V. 1969. Effect of antibiotic therapy in acute salmonellosis on the fecal excretion of salmonellae. N Engl J Med 281:636–640.
BAIREY, M. H. 1978. Immunization of calves against salmonellosis. J Am Vet Med Assoc 173:610–613.
BANKS, J. G., AND BOARD, R. G. 1983. The incidence and level of contamination of British fresh sausages and ingredients with salmonellas. J Hyg (Lond) 90:213–223.
BARNES, D. M., AND BERGELAND, M. E. 1968. *Salmonella typhisuis* infection in Minnesota swine. J Am Vet Med Assoc 152:1766–1769.
BARNES, D. M., AND SORENSEN, D. K. 1975. Salmonellosis. In Diseases of Swine, 4th ed. Ed. H. W. Dunne and A. D. Leman. Ames: Iowa State Univ Press, pp. 554–564.
BASKERVILLE, A., AND DOW, C. 1973. Pathology of experimental pneumonia in pigs produced by *Salmonella choleraesuis.* J Comp Pathol 83:207–215.
BIXLER, W. B. 1978. FDA salmonella control activities for animal feeds and feed ingredients. Proc Natl Salmonellosis Semin, Washington, D.C.

BLACKBURN, B. O.; SCHLATER, L. K.; AND SWANSON, M. R. 1984. Antibiotic resistance of members of the genus *Salmonella* isolated from chickens, turkeys, cattle, and swine in the United States during October 1981 through September 1982. Am J Vet Res 45:1245–1249.
BLOOD, D. C.; HENDERSON, J. A.; AND RADOSTITS, O. M. 1979. Veterinary Medicine, 4th ed. London: Baillière Tindall, pp. 476–486.
BOHNHOFF, M.; DRAKE, B. L.; AND MILLER, C. P. 1954. Effect of streptomycin on susceptibility of intestinal tract to salmonella infection. Proc Soc Exp Biol Med 86:133–137.
CHERUBIN, C. E. 1980. Epidemiologic assessment of antibiotic resistance in salmonella. In CRC Handbook Series in Zoonosis, I Sect D. Ed. J. H. Steele. pp. 173–200.
CHERUBIN, C. E.; NEU, H. C.; IMPERATO, P. J.; HARVEY, R. P.; AND BELLEN, N. 1974. Septicemia with nontyphoid salmonella. Medicine 53:365–376.
CLARKE, R. C., AND GYLES, C. L. 1987. Virulence of wild and mutant strains of *Salmonella typhimurium* in ligated intestinal segments of calves, pigs, and rabbits. Am J Vet Res 48:504–510.
COLLINS, F. M. 1974. Vaccines and cell-mediated immunity. Bacteriol Rev 38:371–402.
COMMITTEE ON SALMONELLA. 1969. An evaluation of the salmonella problem. Natl Acad Sci, Washington, D.C.
CRAVEN, J. A., AND HURST, D. B. 1982. The effect of time in lairage on the frequency of salmonella infection in slaughtered pigs. J Hyg (Camb) 88:107–111.
CYBULSKY, M. I.; CHAN, M. K. W.; AND MOVAT, H. Z. 1988. Biology of disease. Acute inflammation and microthrombosis induced by endotoxin, interleukin-1, and tumor necrosis factor and their implication in gram-negative infection. Lab Invest 58:365–378.
DAVIES, R., AND KOTLARSKI, I. 1976. The role for antibody in the expression of cellular immunity to *Salmonella typhimurium* C5. Aust J Exp Biol Med Sci 54:207–219.
DAWE, D. L., AND TROUTT, H. F. 1976. Treatment of experimentally induced salmonellosis in weanling pigs with trimethoprim and sulfadiazine. Proc 4th Int Congr Pig Vet Soc, Ames, Iowa. p. M4.
DEGEETER, M. H.; STAHL, G. L.; AND GENG, S. 1976. Effect of lincomycin on prevalence, duration and quantity of *Salmonella typhimurium* excreted by swine. Am J Vet Res 37:525–529.
DIXON, J. M. S. 1965. Effect of antibiotic treatment on duration of excretion of *Salmonella typhimurium* by children. Br Med J 2:1343–1345.
EDWARDS, P. R., AND EWING, W. H. 1962. Identification of Enterobacteriaceae, 2d ed. Minneapolis: Burgess.
———. 1972. Identification of Enterobacteriaceae, 3d ed. Minneapolis: Burgess, pp. 146–207.
ELIN, R. J., AND WOLFF, S. M. 1976. Biology of endotoxin. Ann Rev Med 27:127–141.
EVELSIZER, R. 1990. Salmonellosis in grow-finish pigs. Minnesota Swine Conf Vet, St. Paul.
FALES, W. H.; MADDOX, C. W.; OAKMAN, J. K. 1990. Antimicrobial susceptibility of *Salmonella choleraesuis* from Missouri swine. 33d Annu Meet AAVLD, Denver, Colo.
FENWICK, B. W., AND OLANDER, H. J. 1987. Experimental infection of weanling pigs with *Salmonella typhisuis:* Effect of feeding low concentrations of chlortetracycline, penicillin, and sulfamethazine. Am J Vet Res 48:1568–1573.
FERRIS, K., AND FRERICHS, W. 1990. Salmonella serotypes from animals and related sources. Proc 94th Annu Meet US Anim Health Assoc, Denver, Colo.

FINLAYSON, M., AND BARNUM, D. A. 1973. The effect of chlortetracycline feed additive on experimental salmonella infection of swine and antibiotic resistance transfer. Can J Comp Med 37:139–146.

FUKUSHIMA, H.; HOSHINA, K.; NAKAMURA, R.; AND ITO, Y. 1987. Raw beef, pork and chicken in Japan contaminated with *Salmonella* sp., *Campylobacter* sp., *Yersinia enterocolitica* and *Clostridium perfringens* – a comparative study. Zentralbl Bakteriol Mikrobiol Hyg 184:60–70.

GALTON, M. M.; SMITH, W. V.; McELRATH, H. B.; AND HARDY, A. B. 1954. *Salmonella* in swine, cattle, and the environment of abattoirs. J Infect Dis 95:236–245.

GIANNELLA, R. A.; FORMAL, S. B.; DAMMIN, G. J.; AND COLLINS, H. 1973. Pathogenesis of salmonellosis. Studies of fluid secretion, mucosal invasion, and morphologic reaction of the rabbit ileum. J Clin Invest 52:441–453.

GOOCH, J. M., AND GOO, V. 1971. Frequency of *Salmonella* isolation in selected foods of animal origin, Hawaii. (Cited by Tompkin, R. B. 1978.) The red meat processor's role in salmonella prevention. Proc Natl Salmonellosis Semin, Washington, D.C.

GOOCH, J. M., AND HADDOCK, R. L. 1969. Swine salmonellosis in a Hawaiian piggery. J Am Vet Med Assoc 154:1051–1054.

GROVES, B. I.; FISH, N. A.; AND MITCHELL, W. R. 1971. The occurrence of salmonella infection in market swine in Ontario. Can Vet J 12:11–15.

GUSTAFSON, R. H.; KOBLAND, J. D.; AND LANGNER, P. H. 1976. Incidence and antibiotic resistance of salmonella in market swine. Proc 4th Int Congr Pig Vet Soc, Ames, p. M2.

GUTZMANN, F.; LAYTON, H.; SIMKINS, K.; AND JAROLMEN, H. 1976. Influence of antibiotic-supplemented feed on the occurrence and persistence of *Salmonella typhimurium* in experimentally infected swine. Am J Vet Res 37:649–655.

HANNA, J.; ELLIS, W. A.; AND O'BRIEN, J. J. 1979. Immunization of pregnant sows with a live *Salmonella choleraesuis* vaccine. Vet Microbiol 3:303–309.

HANSEN, R.; ROGERS, R.; EMGE, S.; AND JACOBS, N. J. 1964. Incidence of *Salmonella* in the hog colon as affected by handling practices prior to slaughter. J Am Vet Med Assoc 145:139–140.

HEARD, T. W.; LINTON, A. H.; PENNY, R. H. C.; AND WILSON, M. R. 1965. *Salmonella typhimurium* infection in a hysterectomy-produced herd of pigs. Vet Rec 77:1276–1279.

HEARD, T. W.; JENNETT, N. E.; AND LINTON, A. H. 1968. The control and eradication of salmonellosis in a closed pig herd. Vet Rec 82:92–99.

HENRY, D. P.; FROST, A. J.; SAMUEL, J. L.; O'BOYLE, D. A.; AND THOMSON, R. H. 1983. Factors affecting the survival of *Salmonella* and *Escherichia coli* in anaerobically fermented pig waste. J Appl Bacteriol 55:89–95.

HOOPER, B. E., AND TROUTT, H. F. 1971. Swine salmonellosis. Proc Carbadox: Synthetic Antibacterial Agent, Kansas City, pp. 83–101.

HORNICK, R. B.; GRIESMAN, S. E.; AND WOODWARD, T. E. 1970. Typhoid fever: Pathogenesis and immunologic control. N Engl J Med 283:735–746.

HSU, F. S.; CHUECK, L. L.; AND SHEN, Y. M. 1983. Isolation, serotyping and drug resistance of salmonellae in scouring pigs in Taiwan. Chung Hua Min Kuo Wei Sheng Wu Chi Mien I Hsueh Tsa Chih 16:283–290.

JACKS, T. M.; WELTER, C. J.; FITZGERALD, G. R.; AND MILLER, B. M. 1981. Cephamycin C treatment of induced swine salmonellosis. Antimicrob Agents Chemother 19:562–566.

JACKS, T. M.; FRAZIER, E.; JUDITH, F. R.; AND OLSON, G. 1988. Effect of efrotomycin in feed on the quantity, duration, and prevalence of shedding and antibacterial susceptibility of *Salmonella typhimurium* in experimentally infected swine. Am J Vet Res 49:1832–1835.

JAYARAO, B. M.; BIRO, G.; KOVACS, S.; DOMJAN, H.; AND FABIAN, A. 1989. Prevalence of Salmonella serotypes in pigs and evaluation of a rapid, presumptive test for detection of Salmonella in pig faeces. Acta Vet Hung 37:39–44.

JONES, F. T.; LANGLOIS, B. E.; CROMWELL, G. L.; AND HAYS, V. W. 1983. Effect of feeding chlortetracycline or virginiamycin on shedding of salmonellae from experimentally infected swine. J Anim Sci 57:279–285.

JUBB, K. V.; KENNEDY, P. C.; AND PALMER, N. C. 1985. Pathology of Domestic Animals, 3d ed., vol. 2. New York: Academic Press, pp. 120–127.

KAMPELMACHER, E. H.; GUINEE, P. A. M.; AND VAN KEULEN, A. 1965. Prevalence of salmonellosis in pigs fed decontaminated and normal feeds. Zentralbl Veterinaermed [B] 12:258–267.

KINSEY, M. D.; DAMMIN, G. J.; FORMAL, S. B.; AND GIANNELLA, R. A. 1976. The role of altered intestinal permeability in the pathogenesis of salmonella-diarrhea in the rhesus monkey. Gastroenterology 71:429–434.

KRAMER, T. T.; PARDON, P.; MARLY, J.; AND BERNARD, S. 1987. Conjunctival and intramuscular vaccination of pigs with a live avirulent strain of *Salmonella choleraesuis*. Am J Vet Res 48:1072–1076.

LAWSON, G. H. K., AND DOW, C. 1966. Porcine salmonellosis. J Comp Pathol 76:363–371.

LEVINE, N. D.; PETERSON, E. H.; AND GRAHAM, R. 1945. Studies on swine enteritis. II. *Salmonella* and other enteric organisms isolated from diseased and normal swine. Am J Vet Res 6:241–246.

LYNN, M.; DOBSON, A. W.; McCLUNE, E. L.; AND DORN, C. R. 1972. A study of *Salmonella typhimurium* infection in a swine-testing station. Vet Med Small Anim Clin 67:1022–1027.

McCAUGHEY, W. G.; McCLELLAND, T. G.; AND RODDY, R. M. 1973. *Salmonella* isolations in pigs. Vet Rec 92:191–194.

McERLEAN, B. A. 1968. *Salmonella dublin* meningitis in piglets. Vet Rec 82:257–258.

MICHAUD, R. P. 1978. Contributory sources of salmonella in the environment of swine slaughterhouses. M.S. thesis, Univ of Guelph.

MILLS, K. W., AND KELLY, B. L. 1986. Antibiotic susceptibilities of swine *Salmonella* isolants from 1979 to 1983. Am J Vet Res 47:2349–2350.

MITTERMEYER, F. C., AND FOLTZ, V. D. 1969. Salmonella survey of plant foods used in and around the home. Appl Microbiol 18:682–683.

MOREHOUSE, L. G. 1972. Salmonellosis in swine and its control. J Am Vet Med Assoc 160:594–601.

MORGAN, I. R.; KRAUTIL, F. L.; AND CRAVEN, J. A. 1987. Effect of time in lairage on caecal and carcass salmonella contamination of slaughter pigs. Epidemiol Infect 98:323–330.

MORSE, E. V., AND DUNCAN, M. A. 1974. Salmonellosis – an environmental health problem. J Am Vet Med Assoc 167:1015–1019.

MORSE, J. W., AND HIRD, D. W. 1984. Bacteria isolated from lymph nodes of California slaughter swine. Am J Vet Res 45:1648–1649.

NAPE, W. F., AND MURPHY, C. 1971. Recovery of salmonellae in feed mills, using terminally heated and regularly processed animal protein. J Am Vet Med Assoc 159:1569–1572.

NEWELL, K. W., AND WILLIAMS, L. P., JR. 1971. The

control of salmonellae affecting swine and man. J Am Vet Med Assoc 158:89–98.

NOTTINGHAM, P. M.; PENNEY, N.; AND WYBORN, R. 1972. Salmonella infection in calves and other animals. III. Further studies with pigs and calves. NZ J Agric Res 15:279–283.

OLSON, L. D.; RODEBAUGH, D. E.; AND MOREHOUSE, L. G. 1977. Comparison of furazolidone and carbadox in the feed for treatment of *Salmonella choleraesuis* in swine. Am J Vet Res 38:1471–1477.

OWEN, W. 1990. Food Animal Disease Monitoring in Iowa (NAHMS), p. 23.

POKORNY, J. 1988. Survival and virulence of salmonellae in water. J Hyg Epidemiol Microbiol Immunol 32:361–366.

POSPISCHIL, A.; WOOD, R. L.; AND ANDERSON, T. D. 1990. Peroxidase-antiperoxidase and immunogold labeling of *Salmonella typhimurium* and *Salmonella choleraesuis* var. *kunzendorf* in tissues of experimentally infected swine. Am J Vet Res 51:619–624.

REED, W. M.; OLANDER, H. J.; AND THACKER, H. L. 1985. Studies on the pathogenesis of *Salmonella heidelberg* infection in weanling pigs. Am J Vet Res 46:2300–2310.

————. 1986. Studies on the pathogenesis of *Salmonella typhimurium* and *Salmonella choleraesuis* var. *kunzendorf* infection in weanling pigs. Am J Vet Res 47:75–83.

REYNOLDS, I. M.; MINER, P. W.; AND SMITH, R. E. 1967. *Salmonella enteritidis* from porcine meningitis: A case report. Cornell Vet 58:180–185.

RILEY, M. G. I. 1970. The incidence of salmonellosis in normal slaughtered pigs in Australia. Aust Vet J 46:40–43.

ROBERTS, D.; BOAG, K.; HALL, M. L. M.; AND SHIPP, C. R. 1975. The isolation of salmonella from British pork sausage and sausage meat. J Hyg (Camb) 75:173–184.

ROOF, M. 1991. Personal communication.

ROUT, W. R.; FORMAL, S. B.; GIANNELLA, R. A.; AND DAMMIN, G. J. 1974. Pathophysiology of Salmonella diarrhea in the rhesus monkey: Intestinal transport, morphologic and bacteriological studies. Gastroenterology 67:59–70.

RUBIN, R. H., AND WEINSTEIN, L. 1977. Salmonellosis. New York: Stratton Intercontinental Medical Book Corp., p. 25.

SALMON, D. E., AND SMITH, T. 1886. The bacterium of swine plague. Am Mon Microbiol J 7:204.

SCHULTZ, R. A. 1989. Salmonellosis–The Problem–How do we handle it? Proc Am Assoc Swine Prod, Des Moines, Iowa.

SCHWARTZ, K. 1990. Salmonellosis in Midwestern Swine. Proc 94th Annu Meet US Anim Health Assoc, Denver, Colo.

————. 1991. Salmonellosis in Swine. Compend Contin Educ 13(1):139–148.

SCHWARTZ, K., AND DANIELS, G. 1987. Salmonellosis. Proc Minnesota Swine Herd Health Prog Conf Univ of Minnesota.

SILAS, J. C.; CARPENTER, J. A.; AND REAGAN, J. O. 1984. Update: Prevalence of *Salmonella* in pork sausage. J Anim Sci 59:122–124.

SKOVGAARD, N.; CHRISTENSEN, S. G.; AND CULISTANI, A. W. 1985. Salmonellas in Danish pigs: A comparison of three isolation methods. J Hyg (Lond) 95:69–75.

SMITH, H. W. 1965. The immunization of mice, calves and pigs against *Salmonella dublin* and *Salmonella choleraesuis* infections. J Hyg (Camb) 63:117–135.

SMITH, H. W., AND JONES, J. E. T. 1967. Observations on experimental oral infection with *Salmonella dublin* in calves and *Salmonella choleraesuis* in pigs. J Pathol 93:141–156.

STEPHEN, J.; WALLIS, T. S.; STARKEY, W. G.; CANDY, D. C. A.; OSBORNE, M. P.; AND HUDDON, S. 1985. Salmonellosis: In retrospect and prospect. In Microbial Toxins and Diarrhoeal Diseases. Ciba Foundation Symposium. London: Pitman.

SURKIEWICZ, B. F.; JOHNSTON, R. W.; ELLIOTT, E. P.; AND SIMMONS, E. R. 1972. Bacteriologic survey of fresh pork sausage produced at establishments under federal inspection. Appl Microbiol 23:515–520.

TACAL, J. V., AND LAWRENCE, W. 1980. A survey for salmonella among market swine in southern California 1980. Calif Vet 11:15–18.

TAKEUCHI, A. 1967. Electron-microscopic studies of experimental salmonella infection. I. Penetration into the intestinal epithelium by *Salmonella typhimurium*. Am J Pathol 50:109–136.

TAKEUCHI, A., AND SPRINZ, H. 1967. Electron microscopic studies of experimental salmonella infection in the preconditioned guinea pig. II. Response of the intestinal mucosa to the invasion by *Salmonella typhimurium*. Am J Pathol 51:137–161.

TAYLOR, J., AND McCOY, J. H. 1969. Salmonella and Arizona infections and intoxications. In Foodborne Infections and Intoxications. New York: Academic Press, pp. 3–71.

VASSILIADIS, P.; MAVROMATI, C.; TRICHOPOULUS, D.; KALAPOTHAKI, V.; AND PAPADAKIS, J. 1987. Comparison of procedures based upon Rappaport-Vassiliadis medium with those using Muller-Kauffmann medium containing Teepol for the isolation of *Salmonella* sp. Epidemiol Infect 99:143–147.

WELLIVER, R. C., AND OGRA, P. L. 1978. Importance of local immunity in enteric infection. J Am Vet Med Assoc 173:560–564.

WIENER, H. 1974. The origins of salmonellosis. Am Anim Health Inst, Washington, D.C., pp. 22–31.

WILCOCK, B. P. 1978. Experimental *Klebsiella* and *Salmonella* infection in neonatal swine. Can J Comp Med 43:100–106.

————. 1979. Serotype-associated virulence factors in porcine salmonellosis. Conf Res Workers, Anim Dis Res Inst, Ottawa.

WILCOCK, B. P., AND OLANDER, H. J. 1977a. The pathogenesis of porcine rectal stricture. I. Observations on the naturally occurring disease and its association with salmonellosis. Vet Pathol 14:36–42.

————. 1977b. The pathogenesis of porcine rectal stricture. II. Experimental salmonellosis and rectal stricture. Vet Pathol 14:43–55.

————. 1977c. Neurologic disease in naturally occurring *Salmonella choleraesuis* infection in pigs. Vet Pathol 14:113–120.

————. 1978. Influence of oral antibiotic feeding on the duration and severity of clinical disease, growth performance and pattern of shedding in swine inoculated with *Salmonella typhimurium*. J Am Vet Med Assoc 172:472–477.

WILCOCK, B. P.; ARMSTRONG, C. H.; AND OLANDER, H. J. 1976. The significance of the serotype in the clinical and pathologic features of naturally occurring porcine salmonellosis. Can J Comp Med 40:80–88.

WILL, L. A.; DIESCH, S. L.; AND POMEROY, B. X. 1973. Survival of *Salmonella typhimurium* in animal manure disposed in a model oxidation ditch. Am J Public Health 63:322–336.

WILLIAMS, C. B. 1975. Environmental considerations in salmonellosis. Vet Rec 93:317–321.

WILLIAMS, L. P., AND NEWELL, K. W. 1970. Salmonella excretion in joy-riding pigs. Am J Public Health 50:926–929.

WILLIAMS, L. P.; VAUGHN, J. P.; SCOTT, A.; AND BLAN-
TON, V. 1969. A ten-month study on salmonella con-
tamination in animal protein meals. J Am Vet Med
Assoc 155:167–174.

WOLFF, S. M. 1973. Biologic effects of bacterial endotoxins in man. J Infect Dis 128 [Suppl]:159–164.

WOOD, R. L.; POSPISCHIL, A.; AND ROSE, R. 1989. Distribution of persistent *Salmonella typhimurium* infection in internal organs of swine. Am J Vet Res
50:1015–1021.

WRAY, C., AND SOJKA, W. J. 1977. Reviews of progress
in dairy science: Bovine salmonellosis. J Dairy Res
44:383–425.

47 Spirochetal Diarrhea

D. J. Taylor

SPIROCHETAL DIARRHEA is a syndrome in which weaned pigs develop soft feces or diarrhea containing some mucus and little or no blood. The diarrhea lasts for several days and is associated with loss of condition and reduced growth rate. It is caused by spirochetes distinct from *Serpulina hyodysenteriae,* which infect the large intestine and cause a colitis less severe than that seen in swine dysentery. The disease was first reproduced by Taylor et al. (1980) but spirochetes were noted in ulcers of the colon by Smith (1894), Gilruth (1910), and King and Hoffman (1913). The latter considered them to be the cause of swine fever, for they were such a consistent finding in the colonic lesions of the disease, but this view was disproved by Bekensky (1916) who found that they only occurred in 58% of the pigs dying from the disease. Some of these accounts may have referred to *Serpulina (Treponema) hyodysenteriae,* but many antedate the description of swine dysentery by Whiting et al. (1921) and do not mention dysentery. Stanton et al. (1991) proposed the new genus name *Serpula.* This genus has subsequently been renamed *Serpulina* and includes the species *S. hyodysenteriae* and *S. innocens* (Stanton 1992). Classic disease was seen by Taylor (1970, unpublished observations) in a high-health herd in the United Kingdom where a mucoid diarrhea, loss of condition, and weight depression were associated with a patchy colitis in which spirochetes were present. Since the description of the disease by Taylor et al. (1980), the disease has been recognized in the United States, Canada (Spearman et al. 1988; Girard et al. 1989; Jacques et al. 1989), Poland, the Netherlands, France, and Denmark. It is commonly noticed in well-managed herds.

ETIOLOGY. The causal agent is a spirochete that is 6–10 μm in length, 0.25 μm in diameter, and possesses 5–7 fibrils in the axial filament. It forms weakly beta-hemolytic colonies on horse-blood agar after 3–5 days and can be cultured under the same conditions as *S. hyodysenteriae.* Biochemical testing by the API Zym test shows it to be distinct from that species and antigenically distinct both on immunofluorescence and disk inhibition tests (Taylor et al. 1980) and by immunoblots, where it is seen to lack the 16-kD band typical of *S. hyodysenteriae.* It is also distinct from *Treponema succinifaciens* (Cwyk and Canale-

Parola 1979). The relationship of the agent described by Taylor et al. (1980) to *S. innocens* (Kinyon and Harris 1979) is not clear, since much of the early pathogenicity testing carried out by Taylor (1972) and Hudson et al. (1976), on spirochetes of the type later assigned to this species simply showed that they did not cause swine dysentery. Joens and Marquez (1986) showed that *S. innocens* lacked the 12-kD protein of *S. hyodysenteriae,* and the causal spirochete of spirochetal diarrhea resembles it in this respect. Subsequent authors have identified the weakly hemolytic spirochetes from cases of spirochetal diarrhea as *S. innocens* on morphologic and biochemical grounds. Studies of *S. innocens* strains by Chatfield et al. (1988) suggest that *S. innocens* is not a homogeneous group; Lymbery et al. (1990) suggest that at least three different groups of weakly beta-hemolytic spirochetes exist within *S. innocens.* One of the strains of that species was found to possess a lipooligosaccharide antigen found in *S. hyodysenteriae* but not in other isolates assigned to the species (Halter and Joens 1988). Their work reinforces that of Binek and Szynkiewicz (1984), who found weakly beta-hemolytic spirochetes that they identified as intermediates between *S. hyodysenteriae* and *S. innocens.* Weakly hemolytic spirochetes fall into six biochemical groupings (Hunter and Wood 1979).

Pathogenicity testing of three weakly hemolytic spirochetes in the United Kingdom showed that the isolate described by Taylor et al. (1980) is not unique in terms of its ability to induce disease in pigs (Table 47.1).

EPIDEMIOLOGY. The detailed epidemiology of the disease is not known. Transmission is oral from infected feces. It occurs in weaned pigs from shortly after weaning to adulthood and the spirochete can be isolated from newly weaned pigs and from older animals within herds where the disease is occurring. Its ability to survive in the environment is not known but it appears to be introduced to herds in carrier pigs. Similar spirochetes have been isolated from rodents; circumstantial evidence exists for the infection of spirochete-free herds following rodent infestations.

PATHOGENESIS. Oral infection is followed by colonization of the colonic mucosa within 3–7 days. The crypts and luminal epithelium are col-

Table 47.1. Results of the infection of spirochete-free pigs with three poorly hemolytic porcine enteric spirochetes

Spirochetal Isolate	Clinical Signs	Spirochetes Reisolated	Gross Lesions	FCR	DLWG (g)
None	0/5	0/5	0/5	2.7	500
P70/4	0/5	4/5	0/5	2.7	500
IW2	2/5	5/5	0/5	3.0	495
PW1	5/5	5/5	3/5	2.7	300

Note: FCR = feed conversion ratio; DLWG = daily live-weight gain.

onized with the spirochetes arranged like a false brush border on the epithelial surface. Inflammation of the mucosa is preceded by edema of the bowel wall and is accompanied by an increase in the water content of the cecal and colonic contents; the inflammation is followed by necrosis, which leaves peaks of adherent necrotic material scattered over the colonic surface. The inflamed surface is rapidly colonized by *Balantidium coli.* Serum antibody to the causal spirochete can be demonstrated in recovered cases (Taylor et al. 1980).

CLINICAL SIGNS. The disease is most frequently seen in animals that have been weaned or mixed at least 1 week before and are not receiving feed medication with antimicrobials, which prevent swine dysentery. It can also occur in growing or finishing pigs. It is rare in adults but may be seen in recently introduced breeding stock. The incubation period is 6–14 days but may be longer. The first clinical signs are hollowing of the flanks and the passage of pasty feces. Affected animals stand with a humped back with tail hanging, and there is fecal staining of the perineum. The animal then loses condition but may not lose its appetite. Fever is not a feature of this disease. Diarrhea that is the texture of wet cement is then passed; it is shiny with clear mucus early in the course of the disease but later is flecked with blood, or small tags of thicker mucus may be seen. This diarrhea may persist for 3–14 days and is associated with a marked loss of condition and a decrease in the rate of daily live-weight gain. Animals rarely die from the uncomplicated disease. Spirochetal diarrhea may affect groups of pigs at the same age on a unit or be present in pigs of all ages within a house.

LESIONS

Gross Lesions. These are confined to the large intestine, which is flaccid in early cases; the serosal surface and mesocolon may be edematous. The contents are fluid, but there are few if any changes to be seen on the mucosa. Later, some inflammation may occur and in severe cases the mucosa may be thickened and inflamed with localized hemorrhages 2–5 mm in diameter. The severe inflammation seen in swine dysentery is absent and there is rarely any blood in the intestinal lumen. In older and resolving lesions, the hemorrhages are covered by 2- to 5-mm tags of fibrin and necrotic material, which appear as conical scales adherent to the surface of the large intestinal mucosa (Fig. 47.1). This material may be dislodged by rinsing and can be found as a deposit after decanting the washings. Since death rarely results from the uncomplicated condition, the lesions described here are those found in animals

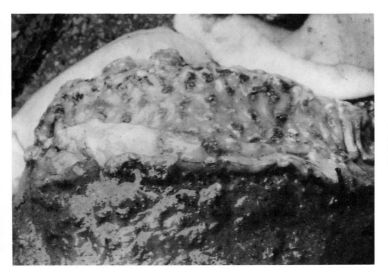

47.1. Colonic mucosa of a chronic case of spirochetal diarrhea. Note the isolated areas of necrotic material.

that have been killed. In those that have died from other causes, the lesions will not be so distinctive.

Microscopic Lesions.   The large intestinal mucosa is thickened and edematous, with dilated crypts and capillary dilatation beneath the mucosal epithelium. The luminal epithelium is usually intact and covered with a false brush border of spirochetes (Taylor et al. 1980, Jacques et al. 1989) (Fig 47.2). Spirochetes may also be seen within the dilated mucosal crypts and can be demonstrated by means of silver stains or immunoperoxidase staining. *Balantidium coli* is often seen in large numbers on the surface of the mucosa.

Bacteriology.   Large numbers of spirochetes can be seen in wet smears viewed by phase-contrast microscopy or in fixed Gram-stained smears. They appear subjectively to be thinner than *S. hyodysenteriae* and are weakly hemolytic when cultured on spectinomycin blood agar.

DIAGNOSIS.   A tentative diagnosis of spirochetal diarrhea can be made when mucoid diarrhea containing no blood and causing no mortality is found in weaned pigs receiving no antidysentery feed medication. Depression of growth rate is common. Confirmation is by demonstrating the spirochete in smears and by culture. The organism should be confirmed as belonging to this group by electron microscopy, slide agglutination tests, growth inhibition tests, and the API ZYM test (Hunter and Wood 1979). The lesions of a number of conditions may be colonized by the spirochetes of spirochetal diarrhea. These include swine dysentery, proliferative intestinal adenopathy, trichuriasis (Beer and Rutter 1972), salmo-

nellosis, and the possible presence of these conditions should be eliminated before a diagnosis of uncomplicated spirochetal diarrhea is reached. The organism must be distinguished from *S. hyodysenteriae* by immunofluorescence, reverse passive latex-agglutination tests, culture, and biochemical or serologic means.

TREATMENT AND CONTROL.   Affected pigs should be treated by water medicated with antimicrobials effective against swine dysentery. Tylosin may be used, for resistance is less common in non–*S. hyodysenteriae* spirochetes. Feed medicated with similar antimicrobials may be equally effective, since this disease is less severe than swine dysentery. Parenteral medication may not be necessary. The disease responds to treatment with antimicrobials but may recur in a herd once medication is removed. The causal organism is usually sensitive in vitro to all antimicrobials used for swine dysentery and is eliminated from the feces by treatment with them.

Control methods similar to those described above for swine dysentery (see Chapter 49) may be effective but few if any attempts to eliminate spirochaetal diarrhea have been recorded. The only study in which the elimination of this type of spirochaete is recorded was the original description of Medicated Early Weaning (Alexander et al. 1980). Some spirochetes survived the treatment or reinfection occurred subsequently.

REFERENCES
ALEXANDER, T. J. L.; THORNTON, K.; BOON, G.; LYSONS, R. J.; AND GUSH, A. F. 1980. Medicated Early Weaning to obtain pigs free from pathogens endemic in the herd of origin. Vet Rec 106:114–119.
BEER, R. J., AND RUTTER, J. M. 1972. Spirochaetal in-

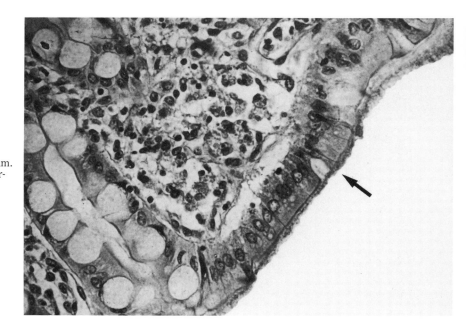

47.2.
Photomicrograph of the colonic epithelium. Note false brush border of spirochetes (arrow). ×400.

vasion of the colonic mucosa in a syndrome resembling swine dysentery following experimental *Trichuris suis* infection in weaned pigs. Res Vet Sci 29:593–595.

BEKENSKY, P. 1916. Contribution a l'etude des spirochetes des voies digestives des porcs dans leurs rapports avec la peste porcine. Rev Gen Med Vet 26:607–608.

BINEK, M., AND SZYNKIEWICZ, Z. M. 1984. Physiological properties and classification of strains of *Treponema* spp. isolated from pigs in Poland. Comp Immunol Microbiol Infect Dis 7:141–148.

CHATFIELD, S. N.; FERNIE, D. S.; BEESLEY, J.; PENN, C.; AND DOUGAN, G. 1988. Characterisation of the cell envelope of *Treponema hyodysenteriae*. FEMS Microbiol Lett 55:303–308.

CWYK, W. M., AND CANALE-PAROLA, E. 1979. *Treponema succinifaciens* sp. nov., an anaerobic spirochete from the swine intestine. Arch Microbiol 122:231–239.

GILRUTH, J. A. 1910. Spirochaeta in lesions affecting the pig. Vet J 17:528–532.

GIRARD, C.; JACQUES, M.; AND HIGGINS, R. 1989. Colonic spirochetosis in piglets. Can Vet J 30:68.

HALTER, M. R., AND JOENS, L. A. 1988. Lipooligosaccharides from *T. hyodysenteriae* and *T. innocens*. Infect Immun 56:3152–3156.

HUDSON, M. J.; ALEXANDER, T. J. L.; AND LYSONS, R. J. 1976. Diagnosis of swine dysentery: Spirochaetes which may be confused with *Treponema hyodysenteriae*. Vet Rec 99:498–500.

HUNTER, D., AND WOOD, T. 1979. An evaluation of the API ZYM system as a means of classifying spirochaetes associated with swine dysentery. Vet Rec 104:383–384.

JACQUES, M.; GIRARD, C.; HIGGINS, R.; AND GOYETTE, G. 1989. Extensive colonisation of the porcine colonic epithelium by a spirochete similar to *Treponema innocens*. J Clin Microbiol 27:1139–1141.

JOENS, L. A., AND MARQUEZ, R. B. 1986. Molecular characterisation of proteins from porcine spirochetes. Infect Immun 54:893–896.

KING, W. E., AND HOFFMAN, G. L. 1913. *Spirochaeta suis,* its significance as a pathogenic organism. Studies on Hog Cholera. J Infect Dis 13:463–498.

KINYON, J. M., AND HARRIS, D. L. 1979. *Treponema innocens,* a new species of intestinal bacteria and emended description of the type strain of *Treponema hyodysenteriae* Harris et al. Int J Syst Bacteriol 29:102–109.

LYMBERY, A. J.; HAMPSON, D. J.; HOPKINS, R. M.; COMBS, B.; AND MHOMA, J. R. L. 1990. Multilocus enzyme electrophoresis for identification and typing of *Treponema hyodysenteriae* and related spirochaetes. Vet Microbiol 22:89–99.

SMITH, T. 1894. Grosse und feine Spirillen in Darme eines Schweines. Zentralbl Bakt Parasitenkd 16:324.

SPEARMAN, J. G.; NAYAR, G.; AND SHERIDAN, M. 1988. Colitis associated with *Treponema innocens* in pigs. Can Vet J 29:747.

STANTON, T. B. 1992. Proposal to change the genus designation *Serpula* to *Serpulina* gen. nov. containing the species *Serpulina hyodysenteriae* comb. nov. and *Serpulina innocens* comb. nov. Int J Syst Bacteriol (January). In press.

STANTON, T. B.; JENSEN, N. S.; CASEY, T. A.; DEWHIRST, F. E.; AND PASTER, B. J. 1991. Reclassification of *Treponema hyodysenteriae* and *Treponema innocens* in a new genus, *Serpula,* gen. nov., as *Serpula hyodysenteriae* comb. nov. and *Serpula innocens* comb. nov. Int J Syst Bacteriol 41(1):50–58.

TAYLOR, D. J. 1972. Studies of bacteria associated with swine dysentery. Ph.D. diss., Univ of Cambridge.

TAYLOR, D. J.; SIMMONS, J. R.; AND LAIRD, H. M. 1980. Production of diarrhoea and dysentery in pigs by feeding pure cultures of a spirochaete differing from *Treponema hyodysenteriae*. Vet Rec 106:324–332.

WHITING, R. A.; DOYLE, L. P.; AND SPRAY, R. S. 1921. Swine Dysentery. Purdue Univ Agric Exp St Bull 257:1–15.

48 Streptococcal Diseases

S. E. Sanford

R. Higgins

SEVERAL SPECIES of streptococci can be found in pigs, some of which are commensals, others are pathogens. In addition to members of the genus *Enterococcus,* two species have been characterized as an important part of the intestinal flora in swine. They are *Streptococcus intestinalis* (Robinson et al. 1988), which appears to be the predominant bacterium isolated from the colons of healthy pigs, and *S. hyointestinalis* (Devriese et al. 1988), another inhabitant of the small and large intestines of pigs.

Among streptococci considered pathogenic for pigs are *S. suis,* responsible for epidemic outbreaks of meningitis, septicemia, and arthritis; *S. porcinus* (Collins et al. 1984), a species that includes Lancefield group E, associated with cervical lymphadenitis, pneumonia, and septicemia, and Lancefield groups P, U, and V, also isolated from different clinical conditions in pigs; "*S. equisimilis,*" responsible for sporadic cases of septicemia and arthritis in young pigs and endocarditis in feeder pigs; Lancefield group L streptococci; and occasionally other groups. The different conditions associated with these streptococci are discussed in this chapter, along with brief discussions on reproductive tract, mammary gland, and cutaneous and respiratory tract streptococcal infections in swine.

Infections Caused by *S. suis*

EPIDEMIC OUTBREAKS of disease associated with alpha-hemolytic streptococci in swine 1–6 months old and 2–6 weeks old, respectively, were initially reported by Jansen and Van Dorssen (1951) in the Netherlands and Field et al. (1954) in England. Elliott (1966) and Windsor and Elliott (1975) isolated streptococci from cases of septicemia, meningitis, and arthritis in young pigs, which were apparently identical to the organism from the earlier outbreaks that subsequently had been characterized by DeMoor (1963) as new Lancefield groups R, S, RS, and T. They demonstrated that these strains possessed the Lancefield group D antigen, and designated them *S. suis* types 1, 2, and 1/2 (DeMoor's groups S, R, and RS respectively) based on the capsular material. Group T was later designated as *S. suis* capsular type 15 (Gottschalk et al. 1989). *S. suis* was officially described as a new species in 1987 by Kilpper-Balz and Schleifer, who have shown that *S. suis* is a genetically homogeneous species different from other members of Lancefield group D.

There are now 29 known capsular types of *S. suis* and their number will increase, since there are many isolates that are untypable (Higgins and Gottschalk 1990; Gottschalk et al. 1991). Most capsular types have been associated with various infections in pigs, but some of them (capsular types 17, 18, 19, and 21) have been recovered almost exclusively from clinically healthy pigs.

Disease caused by *S. suis* has frequently been recognized across Europe (Windsor 1977; Clifton-Hadley et al. 1986; Arends and Zanen 1988; Hommez et al. 1988), in the Far East (Chau et al. 1983), and in Australia and New Zealand (Robertson and Blackmore 1989). In the Americas, reports have been published from Brazil (Coelho 1977), Canada (Sanford and Tilker 1982; Touil et al. 1988; Higgins et al. 1990a), and the United States (Erickson et al. 1984; Hoffman and Henderson 1985; Wilkins 1989). Capsular type 2 appears to be the most prevalent serotype in North America, followed by capsular types 1/2, 3, and 8 (Touil et al. 1988; Higgins et al. 1990a), whereas in Scandinavian countries capsular type 7 is most commonly found (Perch et al. 1983; Boetner et al. 1987; Sihvonen et al. 1988). Capsular type 2 is associated with outbreaks of meningitis, arthritis, polyserositis, valvular endocarditis, and pneumonia (Sanford and Tilker 1982; Sanford 1987). However, the majority of other capsular types have also been associated with similar lesions (Touil et al. 1988; Higgins et al. 1990). *S. suis* is also associated with rhinitis, vaginitis, and abortions (Hoffman and Henderson 1985; Sihvonen et al. 1988; Higgins et al. 1990a).

S. suis is a zoonotic agent, causing septicemia, meningitis, and endocarditis in humans (Chau et al. 1983; Arends and Zanen 1988; Peetermans et al. 1989). Disease in humans appears to be an occupational hazard, as most of more than 60 reported cases have occurred in butchers, pig farmers, veterinarians, and other pig handlers. Capsular types 2, 4, and 14 have been isolated from humans (Gottschalk et al. 1989).

Formerly reported from pigs and humans only, *S. suis* has now been cultured from a racoon dog (Keymer et al. 1983), sheep, goats, horses, and cattle. In ruminants, capsular types 2, 5, 8, 9, 16, and 20 of *S. suis* have been associated with extramammary infections (Hommez et al. 1988; Higgins et al. 1990b).

ETIOLOGY. On bovine blood agar, colonies of *S. suis* are 1–2 mm in diameter and are generally alpha-hemolytic. Microscopically, the cocci are small, gram-positive, ovoid or elongated, and arranged singly, in pairs, or rarely in short chains. Identification is based on biochemical tests and on capsular typing. If an isolate does not grow in broth with 6.5% NaCl, but produces acid from trehalose and salicin, and is negative for acetoin, it can be presumptively identified as *S. suis* and must then be confirmed by capsular typing (Higgins and Gottschalk 1990). If one of the reactions with carbohydrates is different, additional tests are required. Those proposed are production of acid from inulin, lactose, and sucrose and absence of production of acid from glycerol, mannitol, and sorbitol.

Capsular typing can be carried out on capsulated strains only. Capsulated strains exhibit a homogeneous growth in Todd-Hewitt broth. Because of the large number of capsular types, capsular typing is not accessible to every diagnostic laboratory. Moreover, nonspecific cross-reactions among several capsular types necessitate the use of the capillary precipitation or the capsular reaction tests to assist the coagulation test (Higgins and Gottschalk 1990).

EPIDEMIOLOGY. Infection is usually introduced into a herd by healthy carrier pigs (Clifton-Hadley et al. 1986). Organisms are present in tonsils and nasal cavities (Clifton-Hadley et al. 1986; Moreau et al. 1989; Brisebois et al. 1990). *S. suis* can persist in the tonsils of healthy carrier pigs in the presence of circulating and binding antibodies and in pigs receiving penicillin-medicated feed for up to 512 days. The introduction of healthy carrier pigs (breeding gilts and boars, weaners) into a noninfected herd usually results in the subsequent appearance of disease in weaners and/or growing pigs in recipient herds (Clifton-Hadley et al. 1986). Gilts presumably infect their own piglets via the respiratory route, and these piglets

infect others when they are mixed together after weaning.

Disease caused by *S. suis* is more prevalent in modern, intensive, totally confined systems with high population density. Although outbreaks might occur more frequently in the fall-to-spring period (Sanford and Tilker 1982; Erickson et al. 1984), or after sudden changes to colder weather (Clifton-Hadley et al. 1986), *S. suis* causes disease year round under modern management conditions (Windsor 1977; Hoffman and Henderson 1985; Higgins et al. 1990).

S. suis type 2 can survive in feces and dust at 0°C for up to 104 and 54 days respectively and for 10 and 25 days at 9°C, but could not be isolated from dust kept at room temperature for 24 hours. Because of its zoonotic capabilities, it is encouraging to note that *S. suis* is rapidly inactivated by commonly used disinfectants and cleansers at concentrations far below those recommended by the manufacturers (Clifton-Hadley et al. 1986).

PATHOGENESIS. The pathogenesis of *S. suis* infections is still unclear. Williams et al. (1973) reported that *S. suis* capsular type 1 is transmitted via the respiratory route and invades via the palatine tonsils. From that site it moves via the lymphatics to the mandibular lymph nodes. The organism may remain localized in these tissues with no evidence of clinical disease, or it may become septicemic and invade the meninges, joints, and other tissues. Death may occur within hours. Williams et al. (1988) postulated that *S. suis* capsular type 2 can survive and multiply intracellularly, allowing monocytes, via normal migratory pathways, to transport the bacterial cells into the cerebrospinal fluid compartment, thereby causing meningitis. Vecht et al. (1989) postulated that when *Bordetella bronchiseptica* adheres to ciliated nasal epithelial cells and causes cellular injury, this predisposes pigs to *S. suis* infections.

A polysaccharidic capsule protects the organism from phagocytosis in nonimmune animals, and opsonizing antibody against this antigen develops in pigs vaccinated with the capsular antigen (Clifton-Hadley et al. 1986). Nevertheless, Williams et al. (1988) demonstrated that monocytes are able to phagocytose *S. suis* capsular type 2 microorganisms in the absence of specific opsonins. The role of capsular antigens in protective immunity against *S. suis* disease has not been clarified. Finally, it seems that antigens other than capsular material are also implicated in virulence (Holt et al. 1989; Vecht et al. 1989). High molecular weight, muramidase-released proteins (MRPs) from the cell wall have been reported in virulent strains of *S. suis* type 2, and absent from avirulent strains (Vecht et al. 1989). These MRPs may be similar, but apparently not identical, to the M protein (Mogollon et al. 1990), which is an important virulence factor that enables virulent group A (and other) streptococci to resist phago-cytosis and adhere to human epithelial cells.

CLINICAL SIGNS AND LESIONS. In pera-cute cases, pigs may be found dead with no pre-monitory signs. Usually, however, signs of meningitis predominate. In most cases a progres-sion of anorexia, depression, reddening of the skin, fever, incoordination, paralysis, paddling, opisthotonus, tremors, and convulsions develops. Blindness, deafness, and lameness are also seen. Septicemia and arthritis in the absence of meningitis are less striking and may go unrec-ognized (Clifton-Hadley 1983).

Reddening of the carcass, enlargement and congestion of lymph nodes, congestion of par-enchymatous organs, and polyserositis may be seen at necropsy. Gross changes in the brain are not always seen. Sometimes edema and conges-tion of the brain and meninges, suppurative meningitis, and excess turbid cerebrospinal fluid are apparent (Fig. 48.1). Suppurative polyarthritis may be noted in affected pigs. Occasionally seen also are vegetative valvular endocarditis and hemorrhagic, necrotizing myocarditis. A cra-nioventral fibrinous bronchopneumonia has been reported (Sanford and Tilker 1982). Marked in-flammatory cell infiltration into the meninges (predominantly neutrophils), typical of a bacterial leptomeningitis, is seen histologically (Fig. 48.2). In chronic cases or treated pigs, mononuclear cells may predominate.

DIAGNOSIS. A tentative diagnosis may be made based on clinical signs, age of affected pigs, necropsy findings, and demonstration of gram-positive cocci in the lesions. Confirmation is based on isolation of *S. suis*. Determination of the capsular type is recommended for final identifica-tion and is very useful when vaccination is consid-ered (Higgins and Gottschalk 1990).

TREATMENT AND CONTROL. Early individ-ual therapy with penicillin and supportive nursing care prevent death and may result in complete recovery. Resistance of *S. suis* to penicillin has been observed (Hoffman and Henderson 1986; Sanford and Tilker 1989).

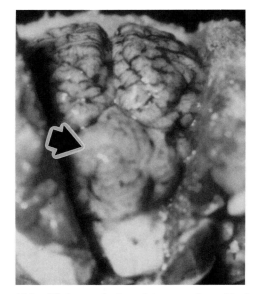

48.1. Fibrinopurulent exudate on surface of brain of weaned pig. Exudate is most obvious over cerebellum (arrow).

Management practices that minimize stress from overcrowding, poor ventilation, and mixing and moving of pigs are key factors in effecting some control. Strategic feed medication prior to known periods of heightened risk is beneficial but frequently results in shifting the expression of clinical cases to a later period in the production system. If the economic effects of the disease warrant it, eradication can be achieved by de-population and restocking with clean stock, or via medicated early weaning (MEW) or modified MEW techniques. Encouraging results with autogenous bacterins have been reported (Wilkins 1989). Commercial antisera and vaccines are now available in North America. Because of the large number of capsular types, however, overall success with commercial vaccines may be elusive until the specific virulence factors contrib-uting to the pathogenicity of the organism are better understood.

Streptococcic Lymphadenitis of Swine (Jowl Abscess) Caused by *S. porcinus* (Group E Streptococcus)

STREPTOCOCCIC LYMPHADENITIS of swine (SLS), also known as jowl abscess, cervical lymphadenitis, feeder boils, and swine strangles, has been of great importance to the swine in-

dustry in the United States because of the losses from trimming and condemnation of infected car-casses. Newsom (1937) first isolated streptococci from cervical abscesses. Collier (1956) experi-

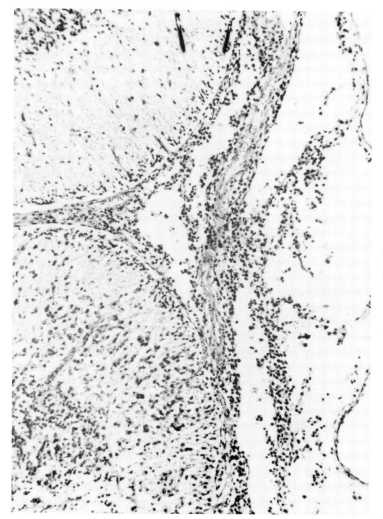

48.2. Acute fibrinopurulent meningitis caused by *S. suis* type 2. H & E. ×240.

mentally reproduced cervical abscesses by feeding cultures of beta-hemolytic streptococci to susceptible swine. The beta-hemolytic streptococcus was placed in Lancefield group E, and in 1985 it, along with streptococci of groups P, U, and V, was officially named *Streptococcus porcinus* (Anon. 1985).

ETIOLOGY. Colonies of group E streptococci are gray, 0.8 mm in diameter, and surrounded by zones of beta hemolysis 1–2 mm in diameter on blood agar after 48 hours incubation. Chains of 3–16 gram-positive cocci may be seen microscopically in preparations from broth cultures. Capsules as well as streptokinase and streptodornase are produced. The organism ferments glucose, sucrose, trehalose, salicin, glycerol, and mannitol. Lactose, xylose, and raffinose are not fermented. Definitive identification is accomplished by use of Lancefield typing sera.

Strains of the group E streptococcus belong to at least six serotypes, and some are untypable. Those from swine abscesses are predominantly serotype IV. Representatives of serotype II, serotype IV, untypable isolates, and isolates of uncertain type status (originally identified as types 1 or 3) have been demonstrated experimentally to be pathogenic for swine. The pathogenic potential of serotypes VI, VII, and VIII is not known. Isolates of bovine milk origin also have been shown to be pathogenic for swine.

EPIDEMIOLOGY. Carrier animals harbor the group E streptococci in their tonsils and possibly Peyer's patches (Collier 1956; Miller and Olson 1983a). They transmit the organisms by shedding them into and contaminating food, drinking water, soil, and feces or by direct contact exposure with susceptible swine (Collier 1956; Collier and Noel 1971; Ellis and Armstrong 1972; Miller and Olson 1983a). SLS develops most commonly in pigs from weaning to market age, although it occurs occasionally in suckling pigs and adult breeding stock (Miller and Olson 1983b). The disease is enzootic on certain farms where it occurs year after year in young swine.

PATHOGENESIS. Infection occurs via the pharyngeal mucosa after susceptible pigs ingest the group E streptococci with contaminated food or water (Collier 1956). Streptococci are detected in mandibular lymph nodes from 2 hours to 13 days postinfection (PI) (Gosser and Olson 1973). Two hours after pharyngeal exposure, leukocytes infiltrate the mandibular lymph nodes. Foci of neutrophils aggregate in the nodes by 48 hours PI, and necrosis occurs within 96 hours. Enlarged areas of liquefaction necrosis develop by 5 days. The abscesses are encapsulated as early as 7 days PI, and by 13 days small abscesses enlarge and coalesce to form larger ones.

Hematogenous spread by group E streptococci sometimes occurs and abscesses may occasionally develop at atypical sites other than in the cervicocephalic region (Miller and Olson 1983a). Few abscesses develop in swine inoculated by footpad scarification, suggesting that biting by carrier swine or the invasion of traumatized surface epithelium by bacteria from abscess exudates are not significant in the spread of SLS (Miller and Olson 1983a).

Daynes and Armstrong (1973) demonstrated that the group E streptococcus produced an antiphagocytic factor (APF) and suggested that it may have been associated with protective immunity rather than with the group- or type-specific polysaccharide antigens. Wessman and Wood (1979) demonstrated that swine vaccinated with extracts of the organism produced antibodies to the APF and were partially protected against the disease.

CLINICAL SIGNS AND LESIONS. Visible and palpable abscesses in the lymph nodes of the cervicocephalic region are evidence of SLS (Fig. 48.3). A febrile response of 2–8 days duration often ensues following exposure to the organism. Collier (1956) detected swelling of mandibular lymph nodes as early as 15 days PI. Concurrent with the febrile response, a rise in total white blood cell count of several days duration is usually detected. Schmitz and Olson (1971) found that anorexia, moderate depression, and a transient mild diarrhea occurred in some animals, especially those given large doses of the organism.

DIAGNOSIS. Enlargement of cervicocephalic lymph nodes is highly suggestive of SLS. Necropsy or slaughter inspection may be required for detection of small abscesses or abscesses located in deeper lymph nodes. The organism is usually easy to isolate by culture of abscess material on blood agar. Conclusive identification of a streptococcus as a group E is accomplished with Lancefield typing sera. A direct immunofluorescence technique has been used for identification of the

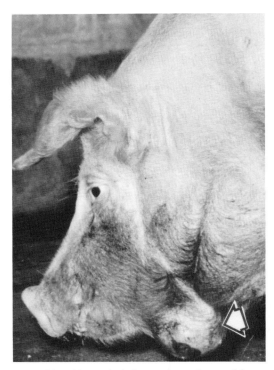

48.3. Pig with cervical abscess (arrow) caused by group E streptococcus. (Courtesy of National Animal Disease Center, Ames, Iowa.)

organism in cultures and lymph nodes (Schueler et al. 1973). Humoral antibodies to numerous soluble and whole cell antigens of group E streptococcus have been detected in sera of infected swine, but cross-reactions with antibodies to other groups of streptococci have been a major obstacle to development of a useful serologic test for diagnosis and detection of carrier swine (Wessman et al. 1971). A microtitration agglutination test, although not highly sensitive, is free of these cross-reactions and can detect active infection before abscesses are noticeable clinically and for long periods after they have healed (Armstrong et al. 1982; Miller and Olson 1983a).

TREATMENT AND PREVENTION. Superficial abscesses may be treated surgically. Antibacterial drugs are ineffective in swine with established abscesses.

A modified live-culture vaccine prepared from a type 4 group E streptococcus has been shown to be effective in preventing SLS (Engelbrecht and Dolan 1968; Collier et al. 1976). Generally, killed bacterins prepared from whole cells of virulent strains have not been found to be efficacious; however, Wessman and Wood (1979) indicated that autoclave extracts of the organism induced a degree of protection against the disease.

Schmitz and Olson (1973a) reported that feeding 138 g chlortetracycline/metric ton (125 g/ton) to pigs for 4–6 weeks after weaning and isolation, reduced the number of abscesses. In addition, they found that simultaneous treatment of breeding stock with 400 g/ton, and of all market swine with 200 g/ton of the same drug for 1 month resulted in a reduction in abscesses. In another study Schmitz and Olson (1973b) found that chlortetracycline or oxytetracycline given at 50 g/ton for 3 days prior to and 4½ weeks after exposure to the group E streptococcus prevented lymphadenitis.

The widespread use of broad-spectrum antibiotics in swine rations is generally credited with apparent reduction in occurrence of epizootic SLS; however, Miller and Olson (1983b) demonstrated that combining weaning and isolation of piglets with other current routine management procedures would prevent epizootic SLS. Hence the swine industry may have decreased SLS partially through changes in management methods— e.g., change from outdoor finishing lots (with mixing of ages) to confinement rearing and the all-in/all-out concept—and inadvertently attributed the decrease solely to antibiotic feeding.

Septicemia, Arthritis, and Endocarditis Caused by Group C ("*S. equisimilis*") and Group L Streptococci

COLLIER (1951) identified 39 of 67 beta-hemolytic streptococci isolated from various tissues in swine in the United States as "*S. equisimilis.*" In Sweden, Thal and Moberg (1953) found that 65 of 161 lesion-associated, beta-hemolytic streptococci from pigs were group C and 39 of the isolates were group L. Surveys in England (Anon. 1959, 1960) indicated that streptococci caused 30% of bacterial disease in the first week of life of piglets; thereafter the losses fell to 15% for 1–8 weeks of age and 4% at 1–2 months. Jones (1976a) reported that of 125 disease-associated streptococci from British pigs, 40% were group C and 16% were group L. In Denmark, Riising (1976) reported that 43.9% of 2275 beta-hemolytic streptococci isolated from suckling pigs were group C and 16% were group L. Most group C strains examined biochemically were "*S. equisimilis*" ("human" C). In his study of bacterial valvular endocarditis in pigs, Jones (1980) identified 23 of 30 cases associated with streptococci, principally groups C and L.

Some isolates from septicemia, arthritis, and endocarditis belong to Lancefield types other than group C and L or cannot be typed.

ETIOLOGY. "*S. equisimilis*" was well characterized by Frost and Engelbrecht (1940). It produces colonies that are 0.2–0.7 mm in diameter, flat to convex, and semitranslucent after 24 hours incubation on blood agar. Hemolytic zones average 4 mm in diameter at 24 hours. After 48 hours incubation, zones are 5 mm and colonies are 0.5–0.8 mm in diameter. Microscopically, cells are grampositive, ovoid to spherical in shape, and 0.6–1.0 μm in diameter. Pairs and short chains are seen in infected material, and longer chains are seen in preparations from broth cultures. The organism ferments dextrose, maltose, sucrose, and trehalose. Variable results are obtained with lactose and salicin. Raffinose, inulin, mannitol, and sorbitol are not fermented.

Group L streptococci produce colonies similar to group C. Using lactose, hippurate, salicin, and glycerol, Riising (1976) found 11 different biotypes among isolates of group L streptococci from swine.

EPIDEMIOLOGY. Group C streptococci, mainly "*S. equisimilis,*" are common in nasal and throat secretions, tonsils, vaginal secretions, and milk of normal swine (Hare et al. 1942; McDonald and McDonald 1975; Jones 1976b). In Denmark, Olsen (1964) isolated group L streptococci commonly from skin and from throat, vaginal, and preputial secretions of swine. Streptococcal infection is common in neonatal pigs, and the sow is the main source of infection.

In a detailed investigation of baby pig mortality in Danish herds Riising et al. (1976) reported that the incidence of streptococcal disease was higher after the introduction of new female breeding stock, in pigs born to gilts and in large litters, among male than female pigs, in winter than in summer, and in herds where tails were docked and needle teeth clipped. In Scotland, Smith and Mitchell (1976) showed that foot lesions caused by "new" concrete allowed streptococci to gain entry and produce disease.

Jones (1980) reported that pigs with valvular endocarditis were older than pigs with other streptococcal infections.

PATHOGENESIS. Streptococci gain entry to the bloodstream after invasion via skin wounds, the navel, and tonsils. A bacteremia or septicemia is produced and the organisms then settle in one or more tissues, giving rise to arthritis, endocarditis, or meningitis (Windsor 1978). Insufficient consumption of colostrum or milk or inadequate levels of antibodies, especially in gilts, may predispose to disease.

Roberts et al. (1968) demonstrated that disease could be produced experimentally by inoculating

"*S. equisimilis*" intravenously but not by intraarticular or intraperitoneal routes. Lameness and roughened hair coats are evident within 2–3 days after inoculation. Swelling of joints may be seen as early as 3 days PI. By 15 days PI, marked swelling with induration of the swollen tissue is evident. During the septicemic phase of infection, the organism localizes in the bone marrow. Pathologic changes occur in response to the infection in the growth plates, joint spaces, and periarticular tissues. "*S. equisimilis*" persists in joints for 3–6 months after onset of disease (Roberts 1965).

Jones (1981) produced endocarditis experimentally in pigs by a single intravenous inoculation of group L streptococci. Pigs developed endocarditis 3–14 days after inoculation. The endocardial lesions are probably initiated by the bacteremia immediately following inoculation, which allows some of the organisms the opportunity to adhere to the valves.

CLINICAL SIGNS AND LESIONS. Streptococcal disease is usually first seen in pigs at 1–3 weeks of age. Joint swelling and lameness are the most obvious and persistent clinical signs. Elevated temperatures, lassitude, roughened hair coats, and inappetence may also be apparent.

Early lesions of "*S. equisimilis*" disease consist of periarticular edema; swollen, hyperemic synovial membranes; and turbid synovial fluid. Necrosis of articular cartilage may be seen 15–30 days after onset and may become progressively more severe. Fibrosis and multiple focal abscessation of periarticular tissues and hypertrophy of synovial villi also occur (Fig. 48.4). Infections in bone may interfere with the formation of the metaphysis adjacent to the zone of hypertrophic cartilage. Young swine with suppurative arthritis often have a swollen urachus containing suppurative exudate.

Endocarditis is difficult to diagnose in the live animal. Experimentally, pigs with endocarditis are usually more severely ill than those with polyarthritis only; terminally they become depressed and prostrate and show signs of pain and discomfort in response to handling, reddening and cyanosis of the skin of the extremities, and a cold body surface (Jones 1981). Valves on the left side of the heart are affected 2–3 times as often as those on the right (Jones 1980, 1981). Lesions consist of yellow or white vegetations of differing sizes on and often covering the entire surface of the affected valve.

DIAGNOSIS. Diagnosis of streptococcal septicemia, arthritis, or endocarditis is best accomplished by necropsy and bacteriologic examination of representative affected pigs. Rather small numbers of organisms or no organisms may be isolated from affected joints, especially when the inflammatory process is advanced. Use of large

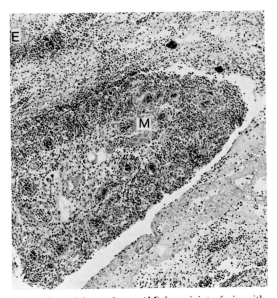

48.4. Synovial membrane (*M*) from joint of pig with "*S equisimilis*" arthritis (3 days PI). Extensive fibrinopurulent surface exudate (*E*) and destruction of synovial lining with mixed subsynovial infiltrate. H & E. ×287.

inoculums when making bacteriologic examinations enhances isolation of the organism. Organisms grow readily from portions of the vegetations in cases of endocarditis. The organism may be detected in smears of joint fluid or in the vegetations stained with Giemsa, methylene blue, or Gram stain.

TREATMENT AND CONTROL. Penicillin has long been recommended for treatment of streptococcus infections in baby pigs. Generally, strains of "*S. equisimilis*" have been sensitive in vitro to that drug as well as to the tetracycline antibiotics. However, unpublished reports indicate increasing resistance of the organisms to these commonly used antibiotics. Long-acting antibiotics may be more beneficial than conventional formulations, and treatment should be given before the inflammatory process is well advanced. Treatment for endocarditis is impractical.

Since baby pigs are virtually assured of being exposed to group C and/or group L streptococci, effective preventive measures should be followed. Adequate intake of colostrum may ensure that the piglet receives protective antibodies. Traumatic injuries to the feet and legs should be minimized by reducing the abrasiveness of the floor surface in the nursing area.

Navel dipping has long been advocated as a measure for control of "joint ill," although there is little controlled evidence of its efficacy in swine. Success is probably greatest when this measure is applied as early as possible following birth of the piglets.

Hare et al. (1942) reported favorable results using an autogenous bacterin in herds where the principal organisms were group C streptococci. Helms (1962) reported a reduction in incidence of navel infection when sows were vaccinated be-fore farrowing with either an autogenous bacterin or a commercially available product. Woods and Ross (1977) reported that pigs vaccinated with "*S. equisimilis*" bacterins were protected against the experimentally induced disease.

Other Infections

REPRODUCTIVE TRACT. Beta-hemolytic streptococci frequently are isolated from the reproductive tract of sows with infertility, abortion, or postparturient agalactia. Attempts to attach etiologic significance to these isolates are understandable, but conclusive evidence that any reproductive tract disorder in sows is caused by streptococci is lacking.

Ringarp (1960) isolated beta-hemolytic streptococci from 26 of 127 uterine tampon samples while studying the postpartum agalactia syndrome. Isolates were identified as group L (5), group D (2), group K (2), and group N (1), but 16 isolates were not grouped. Armstrong et al. (1968) examined 18 sows with agalactia at necropsy and isolated streptococci (*S. faecalis,* now *Enterococcus faecalis*) from the uterus of only 1. Ross et al. (1969) and Speer et al. (1971) found no correlation between poor pig growth and survival rates and isolation of beta-hemolytic streptococci from vaginal secretions of postpartum sows. Jones (1976b) concluded that beta-hemolytic streptococci were common in the genital tract of healthy adult sows and boars after isolating them from the vagina of 24 of 75 sows (32%) from one herd and the presperm fraction of semen from 8 of 40 boars (20%) from various sources. Swann and Kjar (1980), however, reported that streptococci were the etiologic agents responsible for a high percentage of infertility and abortions in breeding sows in one herd in Alabama after isolating hemolytic streptococci from the genitourinary tract of 46 of 75 (61%) sows examined. They further indicated a significant benefit in the reproductive performance of a random sample of 18 of these sows given penicillin therapy. The percentage distribution of streptococci isolated was 63.4% group C, 22% group D, and 7.3% each for groups A and G.

Streptococci also are isolated from aborted swine fetuses. Collier (1951) isolated "*S. equisimilis*" from two cases of abortion in his study. Saunders (1958) isolated beta- and alpha-hemolytic streptococci from several swine fetuses in a study of 67 outbreaks of abortion and stillbirth. These isolates were predominantly groups C and E. Two of 137 streptococci of swine origin examined by Krantz and Dunne (1965) were from cases of abortion. One isolate was classified as group A and the other was not grouped. Doty and Vorhies (1971) and Swann and Kjar (1980) also have reported isolation of streptococci from cases of abortion. Sanford and Tilker (1982) and Erickson et al. (1984) have reported isolating *S. suis* from aborted fetuses.

RESPIRATORY TRACT. Streptococci of many serologic groups are common in the nasal and pharyngeal secretions of swine; however, these infections are not known to be associated with disease of the upper respiratory tract. Beta- and alpha-hemolytic streptococci are also frequent in lungs of swine with pneumonia. Thal and Moberg (1953) found 33 group C, 7 group D, 27 group E, 19 group L, and 14 nongroupable streptococci among 100 isolates from pneumonic swine lungs. In a survey of 186 pneumonic swine lungs, L'Ecuyer et al. (1961) recovered 15 isolates of beta-hemolytic streptococci. The isolates were recovered in mixed culture with other bacteria and were not characterized biochemically. *S. suis* is commonly isolated from pneumonic lungs of suckling and weaned pigs (Sanford and Tilker 1982; Erickson et al. 1984) and although pneumonia has been experimentally reproduced in pigs (Vecht et al. 1989), the pathogenic mechanisms involved are not clear.

CUTANEOUS INFECTIONS. Localized cutaneous and subcutaneous abscesses of pigs may be caused by streptococci. Jones (1976a) noted that abscesses mainly were located in subcutaneous tissues, occasionally near joints. Lancefield groups C and L were most commonly isolated. Miller and Olson (1978) reported cutaneous streptococcal abscesses after a swine pox outbreak and experimentally reproduced the condition (Miller and Olson 1980).

Beta-hemolytic streptococci also have been implicated in the progression of ear necrosis lesions in pigs. Porcine ear necrosis is characterized by large erosions at the margin of the pinna (Richardson 1983). These lesions usually start after the ear has been traumatized from fighting, ear biting, cannibalism, or other effects of social dominance behavior among recently weaned and commingled pigs. The traumatized areas usually are invaded first by *Staphylococcus hyicus* and slowly heal. A few lesions, however, are invaded by more virulent organisms (especially beta-hemolytic streptococci) and develop cellulitis, vasculitis, thrombosis, ischemia, and necrosis in the dermis, progressing to deep necrotic ulcers at the margin of the pinna.

MISCELLANEOUS. Streptococci from many Lancefield groups are involved in septicemias in swine. It is therefore logical that these organisms are frequent isolates from a variety of diseased tissues and may be identified in cases of pleuritis, peritonitis, and dermatitis.

Enterococcus durans has been implicated in enteritis in piglets and has been shown to produce enteritis in gnotobiotic pigs (Duimstra et al. 1983).

MAMMARY GLANDS. Bacteria commonly isolated from mammary glands of sows with mastitis include *Escherichia coli, Klebsiella* spp., *Staphylococcus* spp., and *Streptococcus* spp. Mastitis has been produced experimentally in the sow with *Klebsiella* spp.; however, the pathogenicity of the other organisms has not been assessed.

Ringarp (1960) found a variety of bacteria in 167 samples of milk collected from sows with the agalactia syndrome. Although *E. coli* predominated, 37 samples were positive for streptococci. Twenty-two of the 37 isolates were identified as group L, while 6 were identified as group C. Ringarp found no specific infection in milk collected from 15 clinically healthy sows. In a study of 18 sows with the agalactia syndrome, Armstrong et al. (1968) found *Streptococcus* spp. in milk from 1 sow and *E. faecium* in milk from another. Streptococci were not recovered from mammary tissue of the 18 sows. In a clinical and microbiologic study of 18,403 sows on 43 farms, Chjerkasova and Ponomareva (1964) diagnosed 894 cases of mastitis. In that study, 56% of the milk samples collected from 77 cases of mastitis and 223 other sows with sick or dead piglets were positive for streptococci. Berner and Marx (1967) examined milk from 259 glands from 23 sows and found beta-hemolytic streptococci in 3 samples that were cytologically normal and 12 samples that had increased cell counts.

McDonald and McDonald (1975) examined the aerobic bacterial flora of mammary glands of 24 hysterectomized sows and of milk samples collected from 16 machine-milked sows. Slightly over 30% (178 of 590) of the samples collected from mammary tissue were positive for bacteria; 81% of the samples of milk were positive for bacteria. The most numerous organisms were *Staphylococcus epidermidis*, followed by beta-hemolytic streptococci, alpha-hemolytic streptococci, *E. coli,* and diphtheroids. Sixty-five of 86 isolates of beta-hemolytic streptococci were group C and were identified biochemically as "*S. equisimilis.*" Nine of the isolates were group E, while 12 did not react with typing sera against groups A through U.

Ross et al. (1981) concluded that although coliforms were the most significant bacteria in mastitis in sows, beta-hemolytic streptococci, when isolated in large numbers and pure culture from mastitic glands, may also be pathogenic.

REFERENCES

Anon. 1959. A survey of the incidence and cause of mortality in pigs. I. Sow survey. Vet Rec 71:777–786.

———. 1960. A survey of the incidence and causes of mortality in pigs. II. Findings at postmortem examination of pigs. Vet Rec 72:1240–1247.

———. 1985. Validation of the publication of new names and new combinations previously effectively published outside the IJSB. Int J Syst Bacteriol 35:224.

Arends, J. P., and Zanen, H. C. 1988. Meningitis caused by *Streptococcus suis* in humans. Rev Infect Dis 10:131–137.

Armstrong, C. H.; Hooper, B. E.; and Martin, C. E. 1968. Microflora associated with agalactia syndrome of sows. Am J Vet Res 29:1401–1407.

Armstrong, C. H; Wood, R. L.; and Wessman, G. E. 1982. A microtitration agglutination test for detecting group E streptococcus infection in swine. Can J Comp Med 46:201–205.

Berner, H., and Marx, D. 1967. Zur Entzundung der laktierenden Milchdruse beim Schwein unter besonderer Berucksichtigung der Coliinfektion. Berl Munch Tieraerztl Wochenschr 22:428–433.

Boetner, A. G.; Gindes, M.; and Bille-Hansen, V. 1987. *Streptococcus suis* infection in Danish pig and experimental infection with *Streptococcus suis* serotype 7. Acta Pathol Microbiol Immunol Scand [Sect B] 95:233–239.

Brisebois, L.; Charlebois, R; Higgins, R.; and Nadeau, M. 1990. Prevalence of *Streptococcus suis* in four to eight week-old clinically healthy piglets. Can J Vet Res 54:174–177.

Chau, P. Y.; Huang, C. Y.; and Kay, R. 1983. *Streptococcus suis* meningitis. An important underdiagnosed disease in Hong Kong. Med J Aust 1:414–417.

Chjerkasova, A. V., and Ponomareva, M. I. 1964. Laboratory diagnosis of mastitis in sows. Veterinariia 41:89. Abstr Vet Bull 35:112, 1965.

Clifton-Hadley, F. A. 1983. *Streptococcus suis* type 2 infections. Br Vet J 139:1–5.

Clifton-Hadley, F. A.; Alexander, T.; and Enright, M. R. 1986. The epidemiology, diagnosis, treatment and control of *Streptococcus suis* type 2 infection. Proc Am Assoc Swine Pract, pp. 473–491.

Coelho, A. M. B. 1977. Estudo das artrites bacterianas do suino. Arq Esc Vet Univ Fed Minas Gerais 29:358–359.

Collier, J. R. 1951. A survey of beta hemolytic streptococci from swine. Proc 88th Annu Meet Am Vet Med Assoc 88:169–172.

———. 1956. Streptococcic lymphadenitis of the pharyngeal region of swine. J Am Vet Med Assoc 129:543–548.

Collier, J. R., and Noel, J. 1971. Streptococcic lymphadenitis of swine. A contagious disease. Am J Vet Res 32:1501–1505.

Collier, J. R.; Schaffer, H. D.; and Shultz, M. 1976. Evaluation of a vaccine for control of streptococcic lymphadenitis of swine. J Am Vet Med Assoc 169:697–699.

Collins, M. D.; Farrow, J. A. E.; Katic, V.; and Kandler, O. 1984. Taxonomic studies on streptococci of serological groups E, P, U, and V; Description of *Streptococcus porcinus* sp. nov. Syst Appl Microbiol 5:402–413.

DAYNES, R. A., AND ARMSTRONG, C. H. 1973. An antiphagocytic factor associated with group E streptococcus. Infect Immun 7:298–304.

DeMoor, C. E. 1963. Septicaemic infections in pigs, caused by haemolytic streptococci of new Lancefield groups designated R, S and T. Antonie van Leeuwenhoek 29:272–280.

DEVRIESE, L. A.; KILPPER-BALZ, R.; AND SCHLEIFER, K. H. 1988. *Streptococcus hyointestinalis* sp. nov. from the gut of swine. Int J Syst Bacteriol 38:440–441.

DOTY, M. K., AND VORHIES, M. W. 1971. The role of *Streptococcus equisimilis* in swine infertility, fetal death, and abortion. Iowa State Univ Vet 33:89–91.

DUIMSTRA, J. R.; McADARAGH, J. P.; AND JOHNSON, D. D. 1983. Enteritis in gnotobiotic pigs infected with *Streptococcus durans.* Proc Am Conf Res Workers Anim Dis, p. 30.

ELLIOTT, S. D. 1966. Streptococcal infection in young pigs. I. An immunochemical study of the causative agent (PM streptococcus). J Hyg (Camb) 64:205–212.

ELLIS, R. P., AND ARMSTRONG, C. H. 1972. Humoral antibody responses of swine infected experimentally with group E streptococcus. II. Antistreptokinase and antistreptodornase responses. Can J Comp Med 36:210–220.

ENGELBRECHT, H., AND DOLAN, M. 1968. Vaccination of swine for jowl abscesses. Vet Med Small Anim Clin 63:872–875.

ERICKSON, E. D.; DOSTER, A. R.; AND, POKORNY, T. S. 1984. Isolation and identification of *Streptococcus suis.* J Am Vet Med Assoc 185:666–668.

FIELD, H. I.; BUNTAIN, D.; AND DONE, J. T. 1954. Studies on piglet mortality. I. Streptococcal meningitis and arthritis. Vet Rec 66:453–455.

FROST, W. D., AND ENGELBRECHT, M. A. 1940. The Streptococci. Madison, Wis.: Willdof Book Co.

GOSSER, H. S., AND OLSON, L. D. 1973. Chronologic development of streptococci lymphadenitis in swine. Am J Vet Res 34:77–82.

GOTTSCHALK, M.; HIGGINS, R.; JACQUES, M.; MITTAL, K.; AND HENRICHSEN, J. 1989. Description of 14 new capsular types of *Streptococcus suis.* J Clin Microbiol 27:2633–2635.

GOTTSCHALK, M.; HIGGINS, R.; JACQUES, M.; BEAUDOIN, M.; AND HENRICHSEN, J. 1991. Characterization of six new capsular types (23 through 28) of *Streptococcus suis.* J Clin Microbiol 29:2590–2594.

HARE, T.; FRY, R. M.; AND, ORR, A. B. 1942. First impressions of the beta haemolytic streptococcus infection of swine. Vet Rec 54:267–269.

HELMS, H. T. 1962. Uterine infections in sows and navel infections in pigs: Controlled field study. Fort Dodge Biochem Rev 31:8–27.

HIGGINS, R., AND GOTTSCHALK, M. 1990. An update in *Streptococcus suis* identification. J Vet Diagn Invest 2:249–252.

HIGGINS, R.; GOTTSCHALK, M.; MITTAL, K.; AND BEAUDOIN, M. 1990a. *Streptococcus suis* infection in swine: A sixteen month study. Can J Vet Res 54:170–173.

HIGGINS, R.; GOTTSCHALK, M.; FECTEAU, G.; SAUVAGEAU, R.; DeGUISE, S.; AND DuTREMBLAY, D. 1990b. Isolation of *Streptococcus suis* from cattle. Can Vet J 31:529.

HOFFMAN, L., AND HENDERSON, L. 1985. The significance of *Streptococcus suis* in swine diseases: Clinical, pathologic, and bacteriologic data from a two year study. Proc Annu Meet Am Assoc Vet Lab Diagn 28:201–210.

HOLT, M. E.; ENRIGHT, M. R.; AND ALEXANDER, T. J. L. 1989. Studies of the protective effect of different fractions of sera from pigs immune to *Streptococcus suis* type 2 infection. J Comp Pathol 100:435–442.

HOMMEZ, L.; WULLEPIT, J.; CASSIMON, P.; CASTRICK, F.; CEYSSENS, P.; AND DEVRIESE, L. A. 1988. *Streptococcus suis* and other streptococcal species as a cause of extramammary infection in ruminants. Vet Rec 123:626–627.

JANSEN, E. J., AND VAN DORSSEN, C. A. 1951. Meningoencephalitis bij varkens door streptococcen. Tijdschr Diergeneeskd 76:815–832.

JONES, J. E. T. 1976a. The serological classification of streptococci isolated from diseased pigs. Br Vet J 132:163–170.

————. 1976b. The carriage of beta-haemolytic streptococci by healthy pigs. Br Vet J 132:276–283.

————. 1980. Bacterial endocarditis in the pig with special reference to streptococcal endocarditis. J Comp Pathol 90:11–28.

————. 1981. Experimental streptococcal endocarditis in the pig: The development of lesions 3 to 14 days after inoculation. J Comp Pathol 91:51–62.

KEYMER, I. F.; HEATH, S. E.; AND WOOD, J. G. P. 1983. *Streptococcus suis* type II infection in a raccoon dog (*Nyctereutes procyonoide*), family Canidae. Vet Rec 113:624.

KILPPER-BALZ, R., AND SCHLEIFER, K. H. 1987. *Streptococcus suis* sp. nov.; nom. rev. Int J Syst Bacteriol 37:160–162.

KRANTZ, G. E., AND DUNNE, H. W. 1965. An attempt to classify streptococci isolates from domestic animals. Am J Vet Res 26:951–959.

L'ECUYER, C.; SWITZER, W. P.; AND ROBERTS, E. D. 1961. Microbiologic survey of pneumonic and normal swine lungs. Am J Vet Res 22:1020–1025.

McDONALD, T. J., AND McDONALD, J. S. 1975. Intramammary infections in the sow during the peripartum period. Cornell Vet 65:73–83.

MILLER, R. B., AND OLSON, L. D. 1978. Epizootic of concurrent cutaneous streptococcal abscesses and swinepox in a herd of swine. J Am Vet Med Assoc 172:676–680.

————. 1980. Experimental induction of cutaneous streptococcal abscesses in swine as a sequela to swinepox. Am J Vet Res 41:341–347.

————. 1983a. Distribution of abscesses and shedder state in swine inoculated with group E streptococci via routes other than oral. Am J Vet Res 44:937–944.

————. 1983b. Frequency of jowl abscesses in feeder and market swine exposed to group E streptococci as nursing pigs. Am J Vet Res 44:945–948.

MOGOLLON, J. D.; PIJOAN, C.; MURTAUGH, M.; AND COLLINS, J. E. 1990. Testing meningeal strains of *Streptococcus suis* for the presence of M-protein gene. Proc 11th Int Congr Pig Vet Soc, Lausanne, p. 171.

MOREAU, A.; HIGGINS, R.; BIGRAS-POULIN, M.; AND NADEAU, M. 1989. Rapid detection of *Streptococcus suis* serotype 2 in weaned pigs. Am J Vet Res 50:1667–1671.

NEWSOM, I. E. 1937. Strangles in hogs. Vet Med 32:137–138.

OLSEN, S. J. 1964. Undersogelser over gruppe L-Streptokokker. Forekomst og infektioner saerlig hos kvaeg og svin. Copenhagen: Carl Fr. Mortensen.

PEETERMANS, W. E. C.; MOFFIE, B. G.; AND THOMPSON, J. 1989. Bacterial endocarditis caused by *Streptococcus suis* type 2. J Inf Dis 159:595–596.

PERCH, B.; PEDERSEN, K. B.; AND HENRICHSEN, J. 1983. Serology of capsulated streptococci pathogenic for pigs: Six new serotypes of *Streptococcus suis.* J Clin Microbiol 17:993–996.

RICHARDSON, J. A. 1983. Ear necrosis in swine. Proc Annu Meet Am Assoc Swine Prac, pp. 75–81.

RIISING, H. J. 1976. Streptococcal infections in pigs. II. Serological and biochemical examinations. Nord Vet Med 28:80–87.

RIISING, H. J.; NIELSEN, N. C.; BILLE, N.; AND SVEND-SEN, J. 1976. Streptococcal infections in suckling pigs. I. Epidemiological investigations. Nord Vet Med 28:65–79.

RINGARP, N. 1960. Clinical and experimental investigations into a postparturient syndrome with agalactia in sows. Acta Agric Scand [Suppl] 7:1–166.

ROBERTS, E. D. 1965. Porcine suppurative arthritis and costochondral changes produced by *Streptococcus equisimilis.* Ph.D. diss., Iowa State Univ.

ROBERTS, E. D.; RAMSEY, F. K.; SWITZER, W. P.; AND LAYTON, J. M. 1968. Pathologic changes of porcine suppurative arthritis produced by *Streptococcus equisimilis.* Am J Vet Res 29: 253–262.

ROBERTSON, I. D., AND BLACKMORE, D. K. 1989. Prevalence of *Streptococcus suis* types I and II in domestic pigs in Australia and New Zealand. Vet Rec 124: 391–394.

ROBINSON, I. M.; STROMLEY, J. M.; VAREL, V. H.; AND CATO, E. P. 1988. *Streptococcus intestinalis:* A new species from the colons and feces of pigs. Int J Syst Bacteriol 38:245–248.

ROSS, R. F.; CHRISTIAN, L. L.; AND SPEAR, M. L. 1969. Role of certain bacteria in mastitis-metritis-agalactia of sows. J Am Vet Med Assoc 155:1844–1852.

ROSS, R. F.; ORNING, A. P.; WOODS, R. D.; ZIMMERMANN, B. J.; COX, D. F.; AND HARRIS, D. L. 1981. Bacteriologic study of sow agalactia. Am J Vet Res 42:949–955.

SANFORD, S. E. 1987. Gross and histopathological findings in unusual lesions caused by *Streptococcus suis* in pigs. I. Cardiac lesions. Can J Vet Res 51:481–485.

SANFORD, S. E., AND TILKER, A. M. E. 1982. *Streptococcus suis* type II-associated diseases in swine. Observation of a one-year study. J Am Vet Med Assoc 181:673–676.

_____. 1989. *Streptococcus suis* antimicrobial susceptibility. Can Vet J 30:679.

SAUNDERS, C. N. 1958. Abortion and stillbirths in pigs—an analysis of 67 outbreaks. Vet Rec 70:965–970.

SCHMITZ, J. A., AND OLSON, L. D. 1971. Streptococcic lymphadenitis. I. The febrile leucocytic and pathologic responses of swine fed varying quantities of group E streptococci. Proc US Anim Health Assoc 74:357–367.

_____. 1973a. Prevention of streptococcic lymphadenitis in swine: Effectiveness of medication with chlortetracycline and isolation from other swine in an infected herd. J Am Vet Med Assoc 162:55–57.

_____. 1973b. Prevention of streptococcic lymphadenitis in swine: Effectiveness of selected antibiotics and a modified live GES vaccine. J Am Vet Med Assoc 162:58–60.

SCHUELER, R. L.; MOREHOUSE, L. G.; AND OLSON, L. D. 1973. A direct fluorescent antibody test for iden-

tification of group E streptococci. Can J Comp Med 37:327–329.

SIHVONEN, L.; KURL, D. N.; AND HENRICHSEN, J. 1988. *Streptococcus suis* isolated from pigs in Finland. Acta Vet Scand 29:9–13.

SMITH, W. J., AND MITCHELL, C. D. 1976. Floor surface treatment to prevent lameness in suckling piglets. Farm Bldg Prog 43:17–19.

SPEER, V. C.; ROSS, R. F.; AND SPEAR, M. L. 1971. Relationship of an index to sow reproduction and vaginal bacteria. J Anim Sci 33:211.

SWANN, A. I., AND KJAR, H. A. 1980. Streptococcal infection as a source of reproductive tract problems of swine. Vet Microbiol 5:135–142.

THAL, V. E., AND MOBERG, K. 1953. Serologische Gruppenbestimmung der bei Tieren vorkommenden Beta-haemolytischen Streptokokken. Nord Vet Med 5:835–846.

TOUIL, F.; HIGGINS, R.; AND NADEAU, M. 1988. Isolation of *Streptococcus suis* from diseased pigs in Canada. Vet Microbiol 17:171–177.

VECHT, U.; ARENDS, M. D.; VAN DER MOLEN, E. J.; AND VAN LEENGOED, L. A. M. G. 1989. Difference in virulence between two strains of *Streptococcus suis* type II after experimentally induced infection of new germ-free pigs. Am J Vet Res 50:1037–1043.

WESSMAN, G. E., AND WOOD, R. L. 1979. Immune response in swine given soluble antigens from group E streptococcus. Am J Vet Res 40:1553–1557.

WESSMAN, G. E.; SHUMAN, R. D.; WOOD, R. L.; AND NORD, N. 1971. Swine abscesses caused by Lancefield's group E streptococci. IX. Comparison of the precipitin, hemagglutination and agglutination tests for their detection. Cornell Vet 61:400–415.

WILKINS, L. 1989. *Streptococcus suis* update. Proc The George A. Young Swine Conf and Annu Nebraska SPF Swine Conf, pp. 13–17.

WILLIAMS, A. E.; BLAKEMORE, W. F.; AND ALEXANDER, T. J. L. 1988. Observation on the pathogenesis of meningitis caused by *Streptococcus suis* type 2. Proc 10th Int Congr Pig Vet Soc, Rio de Janeiro, p. 151.

WILLIAMS, D. M.; LAWSON, G. H. K.; AND ROWLAND, A. C. 1973. Streptococcal infection in piglets: The palatine tonsils as portal of entry for *Streptococcus suis.* Res Vet Sci 15:352–362.

WINDSOR, R. S. 1977. Meningitis in pigs caused by *Streptococcus suis* type II. Vet Rec 101:378–379.

_____. 1978. Streptococcal infections in young pigs. Vet Annu 18:134–143.

WINDSOR, R. S., AND ELLIOTT, S. D. 1975. Streptococcal infection in young pigs. IV. An outbreak of streptococcal meningitis in weaned pigs. J Hyg (Camb) 75:69–78.

WOODS, R. D., AND ROSS, R. F. 1977. Immunogenicity of experimental *Streptococcus equisimilis* vaccines in swine. Am J Vet Res 38:33–36.

49 Swine Dysentery

D. L. Harris

R. J. Lysons

SWINE DYSENTERY (SD) is a severe muco-hemorrhagic diarrheal disease that primarily affects pigs during the growing-finishing period. This enteric disease is also referred to as vibrionic dysentery, bloody scours, bloody dysentery, black scours, or mucohemorrhagic diarrhea. SD was originally described in 1921 and since that time has been reported to occur in most swine-rearing areas of the world. An anaerobic spirochete, *Serpulina hyodysenteriae* is considered to be the primary etiologic agent of SD, and diagnostic tests are based on demonstrating the presence of this organism. However, other indigenous microbiota of the intestinal tract may also contribute to lesion production.

For veterinary practitioners familiar with SD and desiring specific directions concerning the formulation of advice to producers minimizing the detrimental economic effects of the disease, the authors suggest that **PRACTICAL VETERINARY ADVICE TO PRODUCERS** (later in chapter) be studied prior to referring to the other sections in the chapter.

ETIOLOGY. Although SD was first described in 1921 by Whiting et al., the etiology remained unknown for 50 years. In 1971 Taylor and Alexander at Cambridge University reported the successful propagation of a pathogenic anaerobic spirochete. Their work was simultaneously confirmed at Iowa State University and the organism was named *Treponema hyodysenteriae* (Glock and Harris 1972; Harris et al. 1972). The organism is now classified in the new genus *Serpulina*, which also includes the species *S. innocens* (Stanton 1992). The organism is a gram-negative, oxygen-tolerant, anaerobic spirochete. It is 6–8.5 μm in length, 320–380 nm in diameter, loosely coiled (Fig. 49.1), motile, and hemolytic. *S. hyodysenteriae* contains 7–13 endoflagella, which are inserted at each end of the cell and overlap at the middle of the protoplasmic cylinder. The whole cell, including the endoflagella, is covered by a loose outer membrane. (Fig. 49.2).

S. hyodysenteriae produces typical signs and lesions of SD when orally inoculated into conventional or specific-pathogen-free (SPF) pigs (Taylor and Alexander 1971; Glock and Harris 1972; Harris et al. 1972). Several animal models have

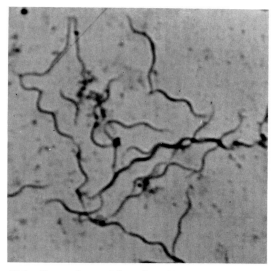

49.1. Pure culture of *Serpulina* (*Treponema*) *hyodysenteriae,* carbol fuchsin stain, as viewed by light microscopy. (Kinyon 1974.)

been developed for the study of SD. Lesions closely resembling SD can be produced with pure cultures of *S. hyodysenteriae* in a colonic segment of pigs prepared by surgical anastomosis (Hughes et al. 1975), in isolated ligated colonic loops of pigs (Whipp et al. 1978), and by oral inoculation of guinea pigs (Joens et al. 1978a) and mice (Joens and Glock, 1979); *S. hyodysenteriae* is also pathogenic for young chicks (Adachi et al. (1985).

Initial studies on the pathogenicity of *S. hyodysenteriae* in gnotobiotic pigs indicated that the organism could not establish itself in the gut when inoculated orally in the absence of other anaerobic bacteria (reviewed by Harris and Glock 1981). Studies in gnotobiotic mice (Joens et al. 1982) and pigs (Whipp et al. 1982) clearly showed that *S. hyodysenteriae* is not dependent upon other microorganisms for the production of lesions in the colon and cecum, although the disease produced in gnotobiotic pigs was less severe than in conventional pigs. Anaerobic indigenous bacteria of the colon and cecum are synergistic with *S. hyodysenteriae* by facilitating colonization and by augmenting lesion production. There is no doubt that *S. hyodysenteriae* is the only transmissible

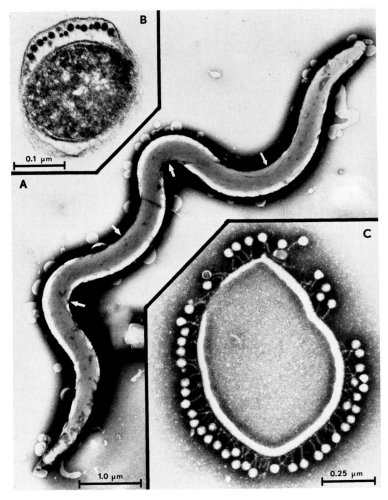

49.2. Electron micrographs of *S. hyodysenteriae:* (A) *S. hyodysenteriae* from the intestinal mucosa of a pig acutely affected with SD. The organism is negatively stained with potassium phosphotungstate. Arrows indicate areas of flagellar crossover (Ritchie and Brown 1974). (B) *S. hyodysenteriae,* isolate 3166 (Norway), in thin section. Transverse aspect illustrating flagellar diameters and apposition to the outer envelope. The differences in flagellar diameter are presumably due to different stages of morphogenetic assembly (Ritchie and Joens 1978). (C) Bacteriophages ubiquitously associated with *S. hyodysenteriae,* in potassium phosphotungstate–negative stain illustrating uniform morphology and close proximity of the receptor sites on a fragment of the outer envelope (Ritchie et al. 1978).

agent in natural outbreaks of SD.

In their original work, Taylor and Alexander (1971) demonstrated a second type of anaerobic spirochete in the feces of normal swine, which morphologically resembled pathogenic *S. hyodysenteriae.* This nonpathogenic type can be differentiated from pathogenic *S. hyodysenteriae* either by hemolytic pattern on blood agar plates (Fig. 49.3) or enteropathogenicity testing in pigs or mice. Nonpathogenic spirochetes probably exist in all pig herds (Hudson et al. 1976; Kinyon et al. 1976; Joens et al. 1979b). Kinyon and Harris (1979) proposed that nonpathogenic spirochetes isolated from the pig gut be named *Treponema (Serpulina) innocens.* Kinyon et al. (1977) and Kinyon and Harris (1979) showed that 25 of 25 beta-hemolytic isolates (*S. hyodysenteriae*) caused SD when orally inoculated into SPF pigs. Also, they showed that 13 weakly beta-hemolytic isolates (*S. innocens*) were not pathogenic for pigs.

There had been concern (Sellwood 1991) that these organisms were not typical of the genus *Treponema.* Analysis of 16S RNA sequence data

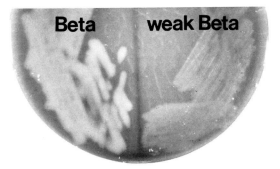

49.3. Zones of beta hemolysis (*S. hyodysenteriae*) and weak beta hemolysis (*S. innocens*) produced on bovine blood agar.

from strains of *T. hyodysenteriae* and *T. innocens* and data from other spirochetes and other bacteria enabled genetic relationships to be established. Taking this RNA homology, DNA-DNA reassociation, and SDS-Page profiles of whole cell proteins, Stanton et al. (1991) proposed the new genus *"Serpula"* (Latin, little serpent) for both *T. hyodysenteriae* and *T. innocens* strains. These were closely related to each other but only distantly related to treponemes and other bacteria. The genus name *Serpula* was found to be a duplicate of a fungal genus and has subsequently been changed to *Serpulina* (Stanton 1992).

In 1982, Lysons et al. described three isolates of *S. hyodysenteriae* that were cultured from three different pig herds without previous histories of SD. All three isolates were beta-hemolytic on blood agar and lacked pathogenicity for conventional experimental pigs by oral inoculation. These three isolates were indistinguishable from *S. hyodysenteriae* in biochemical, slide agglutination, and disk growth-inhibition tests. Agglutinin cross-absorption tests were used to differentiate the three isolates from a pathogenic isolate of *S. hyodysenteriae*. These three isolates appear to be avirulent strains of *S. hyodysenteriae*, distinct from *S. innocens*, which may confuse the laboratory diagnosis of SD based on routine cultural, biochemical, and antigenic analysis.

Initially, *S. hyodysenteriae* could not be grown in a liquid medium; both isolation and propagation were conducted on solid agar. In 1974, Kinyon and Harris reported the propagation of the organism in a liquid medium consisting of trypticase soy broth without dextrose but with 10% fetal calf serum under O_2-free H_2 and carbon dioxide (CO_2). Lemcke et al. (1979) described a procedure for growth of *S. hyodysenteriae* in trypticase soy broth with 10% rabbit serum under O_2-free N_2 and CO_2. Lemcke and Burrows (1980) propagated the organism in serum-free medium containing bovine serum albumin and cholesterol. Other media have been described by Kunkle et al. (1986) and also by Stanton and Lebo (1988), who used 1% O_2 in the culture atmosphere (*S. hyodysenteriae* can utilize oxygen with the aid of enzymes such as NADH oxidase; Stanton 1989). Kent et al. (1988) described a simple laboratory flask apparatus in which enhanced growth of the organism was demonstrated. Kinyon (1974), Kinyon and Harris (1979), and Lemcke and Burrows (1981) compared the cultural characteristics of *S. hyodysenteriae* and *S. innocens*. Both organisms produce acid from a limited number of carbohydrates, usually glucose and maltose; the end products of fermentation are acetate, small amounts of butyrate, H_2, and CO_2. The organisms degrade pyruvate but not lactate and are negative in tests for catalase, cytochrome oxidase, hydrogen sulfide, gelatin hydrolysis, meat hydrolysis, glycine tolerance, starch hydrolysis, and urease. They are positive in tests for bile tolerance, esculin hydrolysis, and iodoacetic acid tolerance. *S. hyodysenteriae* can be separated from some strains of *S. innocens* by differences in fructose fermentation and indole production; more reliable is the hemolytic pattern, with enteropathogenicity for pigs and mice being the ultimate test. Miao et al.

(1978) found that *S. hyodysenteriae* and *S. innocens* have an extremely low guanine-plus-cytosine content (25.8%). The two organisms have only 28% deoxyribonucleic acid (DNA) sequence homology. By contrast, different isolates of *S. hyodysenteriae* exhibit greater than 75% DNA sequence homology. Ritchie et al. (1978) demonstrated several different types of bacteriophages on the surfaces of pure cultures of *S. hyodysenteriae* and *S. innocens*.

The hemolysin of *S. hyodysenteriae* has been demonstrated in filtrates of cultures, the amount being enhanced if sodium (Na) RNA was added (Picard et al. 1978). Lemcke et al. (1982) used washed cells in a buffer with various "carriers"; yeast RNA core was more efficient than Na RNA, while bovine serum albumin fraction V and Tween 80 were worse. They also determined that the hemolysin of *S. hyodysenteriae* was oxygen-stable and resembled another carrier-dependent toxin, streptolysin S. It is a small peptide with a molecular weight of 19 kD (Kent et al. 1988), which has proved difficult to separate from the carrier. The hemolysin is cytotoxic for a number of tissue culture cells and also primary pig cells, lymphocytes being particularly sensitive (Kent and Lemcke 1984). It has also been shown to damage epithelial cells in pig ligated intestinal loops (Lysons et al. 1991).

Baum and Joens (1979a) serologically characterized phenol extracts of *S. hyodysenteriae* and *S. innocens*. Water-phase material (lipopolysaccharide, LPS) from phenol extracts of *S. hyodysenteriae* was utilized to classify isolates into four serotypes by agar gel diffusion tests. Mapother and Joens (1985) found three more LPS serotypes, designated 5, 6, and 7 (Table 49.1). Lemcke and Bew (1984), meanwhile, found three new serotypes, which have not been compared with those of Mapother and Joens. Having stud-

Table 49.1. Serotypes of *S. hyodysenteriae* based on water-soluble antigens as revised by Mapother and Joens (1985)

Serotype	Origin	Isolate
1	Iowa	Strain B78[a]
	Missouri	Dys 7, Den 191
	Missouri	B234[b]
	Denmark	Dys 7, Den 191
	Mexico	Strain G
	Iowa	T6
	Minnesota	T7
	Minnesota	B140
2	Iowa	B204[c]
	Iowa	T3, T4, T5
	Iowa	B9605
3	Canada	B169
4	England	A-1
5	Illinois	B6933
6	Missouri	B8044
7	Netherlands	Ack 300/8

[a]Type species: ATCC 27164; CCM 6063.
[b]ATCC 31287.
[c]ATCC 31212.

ied LPS antigens of North American, European, and Australian isolates, Hampson et al. (1989a,b; 1990) proposed that LPS serologic typing should be modified to serogroups (currently six), each of which contains several distinct serotypes. The situation in the United States appears relatively simple; most isolates belong to serotypes 1 and 2 of Baum and Joens (1979a), whereas European and Australian isolates are more diverse. There is no indication that virulence varies between serotypes of *S. hyodysenteriae*.

Other typing methods suggested have been agglutinin cross-absorption (Lemcke and Bew 1984), which was likely to be very complex, and multilocus enzyme electrophoresis (Lymbery et al. 1990). "Fingerprinting" of individual strains by restriction endonuclease analysis (Combs et al. 1989) may be a useful epidemiologic tool.

The LPS has been shown to resemble endotoxin by in vitro tests. Studies using LPS extracted by phenol/water (Nuessen et al. 1982) and endotoxin extracted by butanol/water (Greer and Wannemuehler 1989a) showed that it acts as a mitogen for murine splenocytes, generates a chemotoxin in fresh swine serum, causes an increase in uptake of red blood cells by murine peritoneal cells via Fc and C3 receptors, and is cytotoxic to murine peritoneal cells. The butanol/water preparation was also able to stimulate production of interleukin-1 and tumor necrosis factor from murine peritoneal exudate cells. However, the differences in virulence between *S. hyodysenteriae* and *S. innocens* could not be attributed to the biologic properties investigated. Oral inoculation of two types of conventional mice with *S. hyodysenteriae* has shown that the LPS may be involved in lesion production. Lesions were produced in the colons of endotoxin-sensitive mice but not in endotoxin-resistant mice (Nuessen et al. 1983).

Other morphologic types of spirochetes are present in colons of normal pigs and those affected with SD. These may be confused with *S. hyodysenteriae* when using dark-field or phase-contrast microscopy. A commonly recognized type is the small spirochete or pig feces spirochete. It has a corkscrew shape and is approximately 220 nm in diameter with 2–4 periplasmic fibrils. These should not be confused with the much larger and snakelike *S. hyodysenteriae* and *S. innocens*. Cwyk and Canale-Parola (1979) characterized the morphology and general physiologic characteristics of a small corkscrew-shaped anaerobic spirochete that had been isolated from the colon of a pig. They named this organism *T. succinifaciens*. This organism is nonpathogenic for pigs by oral inoculation.

EPIDEMIOLOGY. Egan et al. (1982) determined that 40% of all pig herds in Iowa, Illinois, and Missouri were affected with SD by testing sera collected at slaughter plants. In the United Kingdom, Taylor (1984) conducted a veterinary practitioner survey that indicated that 27% of the feeder pig–producing herds were affected with the disease. SD is the second most commonly diagnosed pig disease (after enteric colibacilosis) in UK Veterinary Investigation Centers, and the incidence has not dropped noticeably, despite some successful attempts at eradication by depopulation or cleaning/medication plus the availability of disease-free replacement breeding stock. Roncalli and Leaning (1976) reported that SD was present in most pig-producing countries of the world. It appears to continue to be prevalent in most countries.

Sweden has experienced an increase in SD in recent years and their experience will be of value to those in other countries where there is pressure for less frequent use of antibiotics in farm animals. First diagnosed in 1960, SD has been present in the southern counties of the country. From the beginning of 1986, all routine use of antibiotics was banned in pig feedstuffs. There was a rapid increase in enteric diseases, postweaning scours and swine dysentery in particular. The amount of specific SD drugs (dimetridazole, ronidazole, and tiamulin) for therapeutic use increased by 50% in 1987 (Wallgren 1988). Moreover, the disease spread into more northerly counties during 1988, probably aided by transport of animals from an area newly affected by the disease. SD was a serious problem as a region first became affected, decreasing as earlier treatment and appropriate husbandry measures were used.

SD is most commonly observed in 15- to 70-kg pigs, but the disease may also occur in adults, particularly in sows reared outdoors, and occasionally in suckling piglets. Transmission of the disease occurs primarily by ingestion of fecal material either from clinically affected pigs or from clinically normal pigs that carry the disease. Experimentally, transmission has been accomplished by exposure of susceptible pigs to previously affected animals that have had no clinical signs for 70 days. SD has also been transmitted by animal caretakers who did not change clothing or footwear between isolation units containing diseased and healthy pigs. Differences in susceptibility due to breed have not been reported.

SD causes a tremendous financial loss due to mortality, decreased rate of growth, poor feed conversions, and expenses for chemotherapy. Lysons (1983) calculated that in-feed medication for SD could cost £1.50–£5.00 ($2.60–$8.60)/pig. Wood and Lysons (1988) demonstrated that the feed-conversion efficiency (FCE) ratio in a herd deteriorated by 0.58 while it had SD, a cost increase of £7.31 ($12.60)/pig sold while the cost of medication was £1.38 ($2.40)/pig. Although there were pigs with clinical SD in the herd, the poor FCE ratio was attributed mainly to subclinical disease. In field cases, morbidity of SD in weanling pigs may approach 90% and mortality may be

30%, depending on the effectiveness of treatment. The severity in chronically affected herds may be mild and disease may not be clinically evident. This situation is due to protection afforded suckling pigs by the milk of chronically affected dams and the common use of drugs in creep and grower rations. Under experimental conditions in which pigs are not treated, mortality is often 50%. The severity of experimentally induced SD is related to the amount of stress on the pig, the quantity of infectious inocula administered, and the size of the pig.

Clinical signs of SD seem to occur in a cyclic manner. In large groups of pigs affected with the disease, symptoms may reappear at 3- to 4-week intervals. This reappearance of symptoms often occurs only after removal of therapeutic levels of drugs from the water or feed. Because *S. hyodysenteriae* survives in the rearing environment, some pigs may become reinfected and repeatedly show symptoms of the disease. By contrast, many pigs that survive the acute phase of the disease do recover from SD and are capable of resisting subsequent challenge. However, chemotherapy during the acute phase may not allow the pig to initiate an immune response.

Pigs that have recovered from SD may be asymptomatic but shed *S. hyodysenteriae* in their feces. Songer and Harris (1978) reported that pigs that had not had clinical signs of SD for 70 days would transmit the disease to susceptible sentinel pigs. *S. hyodysenteriae* shed in the feces of asymptomatic sows can cause infection of suckling pigs. Depending on the immune status of the sow, the suckling pigs may not show clinical symptoms until removal from the sow. Glock et al. (1975) showed that lagoon water containing effluent of a herd affected with SD would produce the disease when administered to susceptible pigs. The organism has been isolated from the pit of a slotted-floor building that housed pigs affected with the disease. *S. hyodysenteriae* was isolated from a dog that frequented pens containing pigs affected with SD (Songer et al. 1978). Similarly, the organism has been isolated by Joens and Kinyon (1982) from field mice captured on three farms on which there were pigs affected with the disease.

Experimentally, Glock et al. (1978) showed that oral inoculation of dogs and birds (starlings) resulted in fecal shedding of *S. hyodysenteriae* for 13 days and 8 hours respectively. Flies may carry the organism for at least 4 hours (Songer 1978). Experimentally inoculated mice shed *S. hyodysenteriae* in feces for over 180 days (Joens 1980), while rats shed it for only 2 days (Chia 1977). Conventional pigs exposed to the feces of infected mice developed clinical symptoms of SD within 11 days after the first contact with mouse feces (Joens 1980). Chia and Taylor (1978) demonstrated that *S. hyodysenteriae* will survive in dysenteric feces diluted in water for 61 days at 5°C. The organism survives in feces for 7 days at

25°C. Egan (1980) found that *S. hyodysenteriae* would survive in soil for 18 days at 4°C. However, her attempts to transmit the disease to susceptible pigs by placing them on contaminated dirt lots were unsuccessful. In pure culture, *S. hyodysenteriae* survives at −80°C for more than 10 years. The above observations indicate that although *S. hyodysenteriae* is an anaerobic bacterium, it may have the potential to survive under a wide range of environmental conditions.

The origin of most epizootics of SD can be explained by the fact that carrier pigs were introduced into a herd. However, outbreaks of the disease do occur in herds with no history of introduction of new animals. Other factors that play a role in the induction of symptoms of SD in infected pigs are stresses, including a change in feed, shipping, castration, overcrowding, and exposure to extreme changes in environmental temperatures. Where antibiotic medication is routine, any cause of loss of appetite, such as pneumonia, stops the intake of drug; the animal can then succumb to SD. The disease seems to occur frequently in the late summer and fall.

The incubation period of SD is variable. Specific reports range from 2 days to 3 months, but the disease usually occurs within 10–14 days in naturally exposed pigs. Olson (1974) showed that treatment with preventive levels of sodium arsanilate may be a factor in prolonging the incubation period.

Experimental oral inoculation of starvation-stressed pigs with colonic mucosa from acutely affected donors has resulted in lesion formation within 24 hours. Variation in incubation time occurs with varied doses of inoculum. Unfortunately, some animals may carry the infection for days with no clinical signs. Unknown circumstances usually described as "stress" may induce the active disease and spread of infection to other animals.

PATHOGENESIS. Swine dysentery is associated with the proliferation of *S. hyodysenteriae* and perhaps other synergistic supporting organisms within the large intestine. Although *S. hyodysenteriae* can be seen within epithelial cells and the lamina propria of tissues with typical lesions, invasion may not be essential for lesion production (Glock et al. 1974). The organism is efficient at moving through viscous material such as mucus and has been shown to be attracted to hog gastric mucin by chemotaxis (Kennedy et al. 1988). It is thus able to get close to epithelial cells in the colon (Wilcock and Olander 1979a,b). Knoop et al. (1979) and Bowden et al. (1989) demonstrated attachment of *S. hyodysenteriae* to animal cells in vitro. Bowden et al. (1989) concluded that binding adhesins on *S. hyodysenteriae* for cultured Henle intestinal epithelial (HIE 407) cells may contain sialic acid residues. Cellular damage and invasion did not occur. Whether attachment is an important feature in the disease has not been clearly demonstrated.

Although the mechanism of tissue destruction has not been fully elucidated, two toxins of *S. hyodysenteriae* have been described and characterized that may play a role in lesion production. The hemolysin produced by *S. hyodysenteriae* as extracted by Kent et al. (1988) is cytotoxic for several types of cell cultures. By contrast, hemolysin prepared from the avirulent strain of *S. hyodysenteriae* VS1 was less toxic for cell cultures (Kent and Lemcke 1984). Lysons et al. (1991) demonstrated damage to epithelial cells in germ-free pig ligated ileal and colonic loops injected with hemolysin. Damage occurred after 0.5–1 hours when cell organelles were disrupted; swelling and shedding of cells had occurred after 3 hours. The pattern of damage was similar to that observed by Kang and Olander (1990) when following early changes at intervals after injecting pig colonic loops with cultures of *S. hyodysenteriae*. The LPS described originally by Baum and Joens (1979) has endotoxic activity that may have a direct effect on the epithelial cells of the large intestine (Nuessen et al. 1983), and could elicit an inflammatory response via the stimulation of production of interleukin-1 (IL-1) and tumor necrosis factor (TNF) (Greer and Wannemuehler 1989b). However, treponemal endotoxin was less potent than *E. coli* endotoxin at stimulating IL-1 and TNF and causing death in galactosamine-sensitized BALB/cByJ mice (Greer and Wannemuehler 1989a,b).

Whipp et al. (1978) reported that sterile filtrates of broth cultures of *S. hyodysenteriae* caused no fluid accumulation in ligated colonic loops of pigs or in sucking mice. Furthermore, sterile filtrates did not produce changes in Y-1 adrenal cells. Inactivated whole cells and sonically disrupted suspensions of *S. hyodysenteriae* do not cause lesions or fluid accumulation in ligated colonic segments of pigs.

The causative organisms do not invade beyond the lamina propria of the large intestine, and the lack of *S. hyodysenteriae* and significant lesions in other organs implies that the entire pathogenesis of the disease can be directly attributed to the enteric lesions (Kinyon et al. 1980). The primary systemic effects of typical SD are the result of fluid and electrolyte imbalance induced by enteritis. The pathogenesis of peracute deaths is not known but could be attributable to endotoxin.

The pathophysiology of the disease has been studied by Argenzio et al. (1980), Argenzio (1981), and Schmall et al. (1983). In contrast to what would be expected from histologic interpretations, the diarrhea observed is not the result of increased mucosal permeability and leakage of protein and extracellular fluid from blood to lumen because of increased tissue hydrostatic pressures. Instead, the fluid loss appears to be the result of colonic malabsorption as a consequence of the failure of the epithelial transport mechanisms to actively transport sodium and chlorine from lumen to blood. Furthermore, cyclic adenosine monophosphate (cAMP) and cyclic guanosine monophosphate (cGMP) levels in colonic mucosa of infected pigs were normal, but their response to a stimulus (theophylline) was markedly attenuated. Thus, these studies strongly suggest that an enterotoxin and/or prostaglandins released from the inflamed mucosa are not involved in the production of diarrhea. Therefore, the pathogenesis of dysentery is unlike the diarrhea induced by enterotoxigenic *E. coli* or *Salmonella* spp.

Studies of small intestine function in infected pigs indicated that the glucose-stimulated fluid-absorptive mechanism was intact and that no additional small intestine secretory component was present. Therefore, the fluid losses are exclusively the result of failure of the colon to reabsorb the animals' own endogenous secretions. Because as much as 30–50% of the extracellular fluid volume of these animals, in the form of endogenous secretions, is presented daily to the colon for absorption, colonic absorptive failure alone is sufficient to explain the progressive dehydration and death associated with the disease. These studies also imply that oral glucose-electrolyte solutions would be useful as a therapeutic measure in restoring these extracellular fluid losses.

CLINICAL SIGNS. Diarrhea is the most consistent sign of SD, but the severity may be quite variable. The disease usually spreads gradually through an infected herd, with new animals being affected each day. The course varies not only between individual animals within a herd but also between herds.

Occasional animals are peracutely affected and die after a period of only a few hours with little or no evidence of diarrhea. This syndrome is, however, uncommon. The first evidence of the disease in most animals is soft, yellow to gray feces. Partial anorexia and increased rectal temperature of 104–105°F (40–40.5°C) may be evident in some animals, but not uniformly so. After a few hours to a few days following infection, there are large amounts of mucus and often flecks of blood in the feces. As the diarrhea progresses, watery stools containing blood, mucus, and shreds of white mucofibrinous exudate are seen with concurrent staining of the rear quarters. An arched back and occasional kicking at the abdomen suggests abdominal pain. Prolonged diarrhea leads to dehydration with increased thirst, and affected animals become gaunt, weak, incoordinated, and emaciated.

Most pigs follow the same general sequence of clinical signs, but the time involved may vary from hours to weeks, and arbitrary separation into acute, subacute, and chronic categories is often made. The feces in chronic forms often contain well-mixed dark blood leading to so-called black scours. A walk through the facilities housing an infected herd may permit the observation of soft, yellow or gray feces, some mucoid feces with partially mixed blood, and uniformly dark red or brown feces of variable consistency.

The ultimate cause of death in most animals is associated with dehydration, acidosis, and hyperkalemia, which are discussed in greater detail below. The cause of the occasional peracute deaths is not known.

Suckling pigs are not commonly affected and are an exception to the typical form of SD in that they may have catarrhal enteritis without hemorrhage.

LESIONS

Gross Lesions. The first obvious signs noted in pigs that have died from SD are emaciation and a hair coat that is often rough and stained with feces. Dehydration is usually evident. A consistent characteristic of the disease is the presence of lesions in the large intestine but not in the small intestine, often with a sharp line of demarcation at the ileocecal junction.

Typical changes in the acute stages of SD include hyperemia and edema of the walls and mesentery of the large intestine. Inflammation may also induce swelling of mesenteric lymph nodes and formation of small amounts of clear ascitic fluid. Colonic submucosal glands are often more prominent than normal and appear as white, slightly raised foci on the serosa. There is obvious swelling of the mucosa, with loss of the typical rugose appearance. The mucosa is usually covered by mucus and fibrin with flecks of blood, and the colonic contents are soft to watery and contain exudate.

As the condition progresses, the amount of edema within the wall of the large intestine may decrease. Mucosal lesions may become more severe with increased fibrin exudation and may form thick, mucofibrinous pseudomembranes containing blood. As lesions become more chronic, the mucosal surface is usually covered by a thin, dense, fibrinous exudate, often giving the appearance of marked necrosis, which is quite superficial. Lesions can be found in clinically healthy pigs and appear as discrete areas of reddening of the mucosa, usually covered with some mucus, but with colon contents of normal consistency.

Distribution of lesions within the large intestine varies. In some instances the entire organ may be involved, while at other times only certain segments may be affected. Lesions tend to become more diffuse in the later stages of the disease.

Other lesions may include hepatic congestion and hyperemia or hemorrhage of the gastric fundus. However, these lesions are also associated with other diseases and are not specific for SD. The fact that the stomach may be full is often interpreted as meaning the appetite was normal prior to death. It is probably more reasonable to associate the full stomach with gastric stasis. Pigs with enteritis also frequently ingest materials with a high fiber content.

Microscopic Lesions. The only significant microscopic lesions are found in the cecum, colon, and rectum. Typical acute lesions include obvious thickening of the mucosa and submucosa due to vascular congestion and extravasation of fluids and leukocytes. There is also hyperplasia of goblet cells, and the epithelial cells at the base of the crypts may be elongated and hyperchromic in appearance. Increased numbers of various types of leukocytes may be present in the lamina propria, but quantitative evaluation of this lesion is difficult because of the relatively numerous leukocytes present in normal animals. However, excessive accumulation of neutrophils in and around capillaries near the lumen is commonly observed.

Groups of epithelial cells on the luminal surface may separate from the lamina propria early in the course of the disease, resulting in exposure of capillaries. Focal areas of hemorrhage result and blood is trapped in the overlying mucus, producing the typical blood-flecked appearance of the colonic contents in the acute stages of the disease.

Later changes include accumulation of large amounts of fibrin, mucus, and cellular debris in mucosal crypts and on the luminal surface of the large intestine. Superficial necrosis of the mucosa may be extensive, but deep ulceration is not typical. Increased numbers of neutrophils may be seen throughout the lamina propria. Large spirochetes with the appearance of *S. hyodysenteriae* are found in the lumen and within crypts at all stages of the disease but are most numerous in the acute phase (Fig. 49.4).

Chronic changes are not very specific, with less hyperemia and edema. There is often more ad-

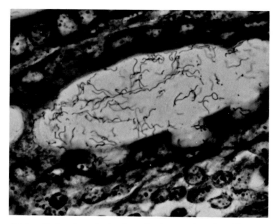

49.4. *S. hyodysenteriae* in colonic crypt and epithelium. Warthin-Starry. ×750.

vanced superficial necrosis of the mucosa, which usually has a thick, fibrinous pseudomembrane.

Ultrastructural changes of the intestine during the early stages of SD have been characterized. Large numbers of spirochetes with the appearance of *S. hyodysenteriae* are found at the luminal surface and within crypts (Fig. 49.5). Adjacent epithelial cells have lesions including destruction of microvilli, swelling of the mitochondria and endoplasmic reticulum, loss of other organelles, and decreased density. As damage becomes more pronounced, the epithelial cells often shrink and become dark. *S. hyodysenteriae* invade epithelial cells, goblet cells, and the lamina propria and may be found in large clusters within some epithelial cells, suggesting that intracellular multiplication may occur (Glock 1971; Taylor and Blakemore 1971; Taylor 1972; Glock et al. 1974).

Hematology. Hematologic changes in SD include marked alterations in many measurable factors. Total leukocyte counts may increase, but not consistently. However, a marked left shift usually occurs with high numbers of immature neutrophils in circulation.

Other changes include early transient increases in erythrocyte sedimentation rates and fibrinogen levels. Packed-cell volumes vary but do not indicate significant blood loss, and total plasma protein may be elevated as a result of dehydration. Serum glutamic-oxaloacetic transaminase levels remain normal.

The most significant changes occur in blood electrolytes. Serum sodium, chloride, and bicarbonate levels decrease and a marked metabolic acidosis develops, which may be fatal. Terminal hyperkalemia may be noted and may be a significant cause of death along with acidemia (Glock 1971).

DIAGNOSIS. The diagnosis of SD depends primarily on differentiation from other potential causes of diarrhea. Factors that should be considered include history, clinical signs, gross lesions, microscopic lesions, and isolation and identification of *S. hyodysenteriae*.

SD may occur as a persistent problem within a herd, with phases of increased or decreased severity. Diagnostic problems are most likely to occur in a herd in which the disease has not been previously diagnosed. History may be helpful, as it is not unusual to have an outbreak following the introduction of new animals, presumably carriers, into the herd. Other situations that disrupt the normal environment may also precipitate outbreaks in herds that have been exposed to *S. hyodysenteriae* but in which the overt disease has not been detected.

Clinical signs such as depression, dehydration, and diarrhea with mucus and/or blood in the feces are quite suggestive but offer only presumptive evidence. Temperature increases are too moderate and inconsistent to be of any diagnostic benefit. Hematologic changes as previously described are characteristic but not sufficiently unique to be of any great differential value.

Further evidence may be obtained by necropsy. Only acutely affected animals should be examined, since various secondary infectious agents may cause confusion in a chronically affected animal. The essential finding is a diffuse enteritis limited to the large intestine. Mucofibrinous exudate and free blood in the lumen are characteristic but do not eliminate some differential questions. Typical microscopic lesions of mucosal edema and microfibrinous enteritis with superficial erosion are helpful but not very definitive as diagnostic criteria.

Confirmation of a diagnosis of SD requires iso-

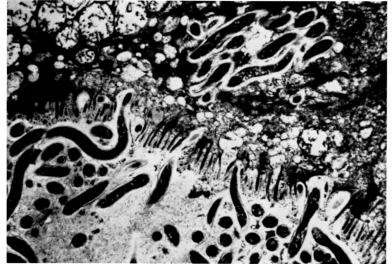

49.5. Electron photomicrograph of *S. hyodysenteriae* invading a colonic epithelial cell. (Glock and Harris 1972.)

lation and identification of *S. hyodysenteriae* from the colonic mucosa or feces. A selective isolation medium has been developed that utilizes 400 μg/ml spectinomycin hydrochloride incorporated in trypticase soy agar and 5% bovine or horse blood (Songer et al. 1976). Other antibiotics can be added to the medium (Jenkinson and Wingar 1981; Kunkle and Kinyon 1988). Lemcke and Williams (1984) showed that the addition of Na RNA (1%) to the selective medium containing spectinomycin increased the degree of hemolysis around colonies of *S. hyodysenteriae* and enhanced the viable counts of the organism. Fastidious Anaerobe Agar (Lab M) gives a more lush surface growth of *S. hyodysenteriae* (Burrows 1988). Swabs may be used to collect samples of colonic mucosa or feces. The samples should be stored at 4°C in phosphate-buffered saline or a transport medium until streaked onto the selective agar medium. The selective medium should be utilized within 3 days of preparation if stored at room temperature. Pure cultures are more readily obtained if the agar surface is kept free of moisture. After streaking, the plates should be placed in an anaerobic container with cold palladium catalyst and a mixture of H_2 and CO_2. The anaerobic container should contain an indicator (methylene blue) assuring that a reduced atmosphere has been obtained within 2–3 hours of closure. The plates should be incubated at 37°C or, preferably 42°C, for 24–48 hours prior to their initial observation. On primary isolation, *S. hyodysenteriae* produces zones of beta-hemolysis in which colonies are hard to distinguish, but a film of growth in the hemolytic zone is grossly visible. As a routine, plates without evidence of beta-hemolysis should be further incubated anaerobically and observed at 48-hour intervals for at least a total of 144 hours of incubation. Great care must be taken to distinguish the weakly beta-hemolytic zones of growth produced by *S. innocens* from those produced by *S. hyodysenteriae*. To adequately distinguish *S. hyodysenteriae* from *S. innocens*, serial passage on trypticase soy agar with 5% blood may be required. Serial passage is readily accomplished by removing plugs of agar from within the hemolytic zones (free of other colony-forming bacteria) and transferring the agar to fresh medium. The plugs of agar should be dispersed on fresh medium with a transfer loop to free the treponemes from the agar.

Kinyon (1974) has shown that 25 of 25 isolates of *S. hyodysenteriae* (beta-hemolytic), from various countries of the world, were enteropathogenic for pigs by oral inoculation. She also found that 13 of 13 isolates of *S. innocens* (weakly beta-hemolytic) were not enteropathogenic for pigs. Other models of in vivo testing for enteropathogenicity include isolated colonic loops in pigs (Whipp et al. 1978) and oral inoculation of mice (Joens et al. 1980). Other possible methods of distinguishing between *S. hyodysenteriae* and *S. innocens* include a fluores-cent antibody test with absorbed antisera, a growth-inhibition test (Lemcke and Burrows 1979), enzyme analysis (Hunter and Wood 1979), rapid slide agglutination (Burrows and Lemcke 1981), and biochemical differential tests. Improved identification methods depend on the use of a *S. hyodysenteriae*–specific antigen or monoclonal antibodies to such an antigen. Some candidate antigens have been identified. Baum and Joens (1979b) described a protein isolated and purified from phenol-phase material of a phenol/water extraction of isolate B169 of *S. hyodysenteriae* by starch-block electrophoresis. In agar gel diffusion tests this protein reacted against antisera prepared from all isolates of *S. hyodysenteriae* but not isolates of *S. innocens*. Sellwood et al. (1989) identified a 16-kD protein present on the outer membrane of *S. hyodysenteriae*, which may be species specific.

The direct culture of *S. hyodysenteriae* from colonic tissue or feces has aided greatly in confirming the diagnosis of the disease. But as with other enteric diseases, the sensitivity of this procedure is dependent upon the number of organisms present in the sample. Pigs acutely affected with SD possess large numbers (10^8–10^9/g) of *S. hyodysenteriae* in their colonic mucosa and feces. By contrast, pigs that are asymptomatic may only shed the organism periodically at detectable levels in their feces (Harris et al. 1978). Furthermore, medications commonly used to treat or prevent SD may reduce the number of organisms below culturally detectable levels. Therefore, great caution must be used in interpreting the results of negative attempts to culture the organism, particularly from fecal samples.

The isolation by Lysons et al. (1982) of avirulent treponemes that cannot be readily differentiated from *S. hyodysenteriae* in vitro may pose a problem for accurate diagnosis of SD by isolation and identification of the organism. To date, such organisms have only been isolated and identified in the United Kingdom, but diagnostic laboratories throughout the world should be aware of this and be prepared to conduct in vivo tests to determine if beta-hemolytic isolates from herds without typical signs and lesions of SD are truly pathogenic *S. hyodysenteriae*.

It is common practice to conduct direct examination of smears prepared on slides from colonic mucosa or feces of pigs suspected of being affected with SD. Workers in the United Kingdom have utilized an absorbed antiserum in an indirect fluorescent antibody test to detect *S. hyodysenteriae* (Hunter and Saunders 1977). Joens et al. (1978b) in the United States and Lysons and Lemcke (1983) in the United Kingdom have presented evidence that questions the specificity of this test regarding its cross-reactivity with *S. innocens*. However, improvements have been made to the test as used in the United Kingdom. The examination of smears for the presence of *S. hy-*

odysenteriae is less sensitive than isolation and identification of the organism (Lysons and Lemcke 1983). However, direct microscopic examination revealing large numbers of organisms resembling *S. hyodysenteriae* can be used as presumptive evidence of SD until completion of cultural examination. Mucosal or fecal smears may be examined as wet mounts by phase-contrast or dark-field microscopy or stained with crystal violet, dilute carbol fuchsin, or Victoria blue 4-R stains and viewed by light microscopy. *S. hyodysenteriae* and *S. innocens* are easily recognized by these techniques, but it is impossible to differentiate the two species. Electron microscopic examination of negative-stained preparations of intestinal or fecal fluids may detect the organisms but does not distinguish between the two species. The organisms can also be demonstrated but not differentiated by light microscopy in sections of the colonic mucosa by staining with Warthin-Starry, Victoria blue 4-R, or Goodpasture stains.

Campylobacter (synonym *Vibrio*) spp. may appear in increased numbers in some affected animals, but such organisms are often numerous in normal animals. Therefore, no diagnostic significance should be associated with the observation or isolation of *Campylobacter* spp.

Several serologic tests have been reported that detect antibodies to *S. hyodysenteriae* in serum of experimentally affected pigs. To date, these tests have not been based on species-specific antigens and have had low specificity and sensitivity. They include macroscopic agglutination (Joens et al. 1978c), indirect fluorescent antibody, passive hemolysis (Jenkins et al. 1976), enzyme-linked immunosorbent assay (ELISA) (Høgh 1979; Burrows et al. 1984), and agar gel diffusion (Joens 1979). Egan et al. (1983) designed a method for determining the accuracy of serologic testing for SD as a means of determining the prevalence of the disease and the usefulness of serology for diagnosis. They compared the accuracy and sensitivity of the microtitration agglutination test and ELISA (Joens et al. 1981) by evaluating the level of antibodies in the sera of three age groups of swine from 22 farms; 14 of the farms had a previous history of SD and 8 had no history that the disease had ever occurred. Egan et al. (1983) concluded that ELISA could be used for determination of the prevalence of SD but not for detection of pigs affected with the disease on an individual basis.

Further research must be done before national control schemes or import-export regulations are formulated based on serologic tests. The specificity of such tests could be improved by the identification of a *S. hyodysenteriae* antigen and/or monoclonal antibodies to it. A 16-kD molecular weight outer membrane protein may prove to be a useful species-specific antigen (Sellwood et al. 1989).

Porcine intestinal adenomatosis (synonym, proliferative enteritis) may clinically resemble the symptoms of SD. However, SD does not affect the small intestine, whereas proliferative enteritis usually occurs primarily in the small intestine. Necrotic debris and blood that originated in the anterior intestine will often be present in the large intestine and feces of pigs affected with proliferative enteritis. *S. innocens* is commonly isolated from cases of proliferative enteritis, although it is believed to play no role in the disease. A definitive diagnosis of proliferative enteritis depends on the lack of isolation of *S. hyodysenteriae*, lesions characteristic of proliferative enteritis, and the presence of organisms with the appearance of *Campylobacter* spp. in the intestinal epithelium.

Salmonellosis, in particular *Salmonella choleraesuis* infection, can be easily confused with SD because symptoms and lesions may be quite similar. It should be kept in mind that hemorrhage or necrosis in parenchymatous organs and lymph nodes may be expected with salmonellosis but not with SD. Mucosal lesions may be found in the small intestine with salmonellosis but not with uncomplicated SD. Deep ulcerative enteric lesions are also much more typical of salmonellosis. The definitive diagnosis depends on lack of *S. hyodysenteriae* in the mucosa of the large intestine and the isolation of *Salmonella* spp. from the intestine or other organs such as lymph nodes or spleen. The mere isolation of *Salmonella* spp. does not constitute a positive diagnosis, since both normal animals and animals with SD may harbor *Salmonella* spp.

Trichuriasis may be differentiated on the basis of the presence of numerous *Trichuris suis* in the large intestine and the lack of *S. hyodysenteriae*. It should be noted that concurrent infections can occur, and possible potentiation of swine dysentery by *T. suis* has been postulated. Here again, demonstration of the absence of *S. hyodysenteriae* is necessary to eliminate the possibility of both infections being present.

Gastric ulcers and other hemorrhagic conditions may cause the presence of blood in the feces and confusion with SD. These conditions are easily differentiated at necropsy since they generally involve the anterior digestive tract.

"Colitis" is a disease syndrome of growing pigs that can resemble SD both in clinical signs and postmortem appearance (Lysons et al. 1988). This may or may not be the same as spirochetal diarrhea (Taylor et al. 1980; Taylor, this volume). Typically, pigs aged 7 weeks or more are affected. They have a watery scour, or sometimes just soft feces, and lose body condition. Some pigs will have mucus and/or blood in feces. Lesions are confined to the colon. In the early stages of the disease, the entire large intestine is filled with liquid contents and there is a mild reddening of the colon. Pigs in which the disease persists can become thin, excrete mucus, and have a mucofibrinous exudate on the mucosal surface of the colon. To eliminate SD from the diagnosis, it is necessary to autopsy pigs in the early stages of the disease and to carry out extensive screening for the presence of *S. hyodysenteriae*.

TREATMENT. Pigs acutely affected with SD should be medicated via the water. Usually, animals in the early stages of the disease consume very low amounts of feed. This precludes placing therapeutic levels of drugs in the feed as a method of treatment. Occasionally, moribund animals may require systemic injection of drugs, but this is usually impractical in large herd situations. Medication is often added to the feed as a method of preventing SD.

Table 49.2 lists the dosage levels, duration of administration, and withdrawal times of various drugs used for the treatment and/or prevention of SD as approved by the United States Food and Drug Administration. Harris and Glock (1975, 1981, 1986) have reviewed other drugs that have been used to either treat and/or prevent SD.

Before the advent of chemotherapeutics and antibiotics, SD was routinely treated by administering oats that had been previously soaked in salt water or sodium hydroxide solution. The farmer was also advised to disperse the pigs into a larger area to decrease the reexposure of animals to infectious agents in the feces. This old remedy accomplished two purposes that may still be of benefit today: the diet was changed to a high-fiber content, and the chance of bacterial buildup in the environment was decreased. Treatment of SD is usually accomplished by administering either chemotherapeutics or antibiotics supplemented with electrolytes.

Various organic arsenical preparations were the first chemotherapeutic group of compounds to be reported as successful treatments for SD. The effectiveness of the organic arsenicals has diminished due to the development of resistance to the compound by *S. hyodysenteriae*. Extreme care should be taken in the administration of organic arsenicals to prevent toxicity and the occurrence of residues in the body organs of treated animals. This medication must be removed from the feed and water 5 days before slaughter.

Other chemicals that have been reported to be effective for the treatment and/or prevention of SD are sulfonamides, nitrofurans, quinoxalines, ionophores, mutilins, and the nitroimidazoles. The following antibiotics have been reported to be effective for the treatment and/or prevention of SD: streptomycin, bacitracin, neomycin, tylosin, gentamicin, chlortetracycline, virginiamycin, and lincomycin (Harris and Glock 1975).

Methods for in vitro sensitivity testing of antimicrobials have been developed utilizing either liquid or solid media (Kitai et al. 1979; Kinyon and Harris 1980). Resistant isolates of *S. hyodysenteriae* for sodium arsanilate, lincomycin, and tylosin have been reported (Kinyon and Harris 1980). In addition, such compounds as neomycin, streptomycin, chlortetracycline, and the nitrofurans have apparently decreased in effectiveness. Some of the other compounds are currently quite efficacious under field conditions, but not all have been cleared by regulatory authorities for administration to swine. As with the treatment of any infectious disease, successful therapy is dependent on an accurate differential diagnosis distinguishing SD from other enteric bacterial or parasitic diseases.

Elimination of SD by Medication and Cleaning. The use of drugs on all ages of pigs on the premises and careful cleanup and disinfection procedures have been successfully utilized to eradicate SD from affected herds without depopulation. Songer and Harris (1978) reported that *S. hyodysenteriae* could be completely eliminated

Table 49.2. Dosage level, duration of administration, and withdrawal time for various drugs used for the treatment and/or prevention of SD as approved by the US Food and Drug Administration

Drug	Dosage in Water	Duration (days)	Withdrawal (days)	Dosage in Feed	Duration (days)	Withdrawal (days)
Bacitracin MD	1 g/gal	7–14, up to 250 lb BW	None	250 g/t	Up to 250 lb BW	None
Carbadox	NA	NA	NA	50 g/t feed	Up to 75 lb BW	70
Gentamicin solution	50 mg/gal (1 ml)	3	3	NA	NA	NA
Lincomycin	250 mg/gal	5–10	6	40–100 g/t	Up to 250 lb BW	6
Tiamulin	227 mg/gal	5, up to 250 lb BW	3	35 g/t	Up to 250 lb BW	2
Tylosin	0.25 g/gal	3–10	2	100 g/t	3 wk, then 40 g/t thereafter	None
Tylosin injectable	4.0 ml/lb BW	3	14	NA	NA	NA
Virginiamycin	NA	NA	NA	25–100 g/t	[a]See below	None

Source: Harris et al. (1990).
Note: BW = body weight; NA = not applicable.
[a]For nonbreeding swine over 120 lb BW. For swine up to 120 lb BW, use 100 g/ton for 14 days, then 50 g/ton thereafter.

from pigs by treatment with dimetridazole or ronidazole when pigs were housed in conditions minimizing exposure to their feces. Rainier et al. (1980) showed that carbadox would also eliminate the organism from pigs under similar conditions. Veterinarians from several countries have reported the successful elimination of SD from affected herds by medication of all pigs on the premises (Glock 1979). During the medication period the facilities should be cleaned and disinfected frequently to minimize the environmental survival of *S. hyodysenteriae*. In addition, the rodent population on the farm should be reduced and eliminated from the pig buildings.

The regimes for eradication have varied greatly. The medication period has been as short as 5 days (Moller 1984), or as long as 6 months (Wood and Lysons 1988); the former approach depended on intensive, high-level medication to all pigs via drinking water or oral dosing, the latter concentrated on elimination of *S. hyodysenteriae* from sows as they came into the farrowing house.

General guidelines for eradicating swine dysentery from a herd without depopulation are given below (Harris 1984):

1. A warm season in which temperatures are higher than 15°C (59°F) is preferable.
2. The number of animals in the herd should be decreased to as few as possible.
3. If farrowings occur in batches, the recommended time to eradicate the disease is when no suckling pigs are on the farm.
4. An effective rodent control program, including renovation of buildings, should be instituted.
5. All liquids should be removed from pits within buildings in which pigs are housed.
6. Any buildings that do not contain pigs should be cleaned, disinfected, and fumigated.
7. All pigs on the farm should be medicated simultaneously with drugs known to eliminate *S. hyodysenteriae* from the pig intestinal tract. Care should be taken to ensure that inclusion rates of antibacterials in the diet of animals, such as adult stock, on restricted feeding is adjusted so that the animals receive the correct dose/kg of body weight.
8. After 1 week of medication, all equipment used for handling pigs, feed, and manure should be cleaned and disinfected.
9. During the medication period, an attempt should be made to clean and disinfect floors of buildings frequently. Animals should not be housed in overcrowded conditions.

This method of elimination of the disease without depopulation is not always successful. Muirhead (1984) reported 11 attempts to eliminate SD from six herds, i.e., the success rate for any one attempt was 54%. With careful selection of herds, including an assessment of the ability and commitment of the work force, the chances of success are likely to reach 80–90% (Wood and Lysons 1988). To determine if the disease has been eliminated, it is recommended that for 3–6 months following medication no antimicrobials be used that are efficacious for SD. Clinical evidence of the disease will usually reappear if the organism is still present. The increased feed-conversion efficiency of SD-free pigs means that the cost of the eradication program will usually be recovered in 6–12 months.

PREVENTION. The economically devastating effects of SD justify a serious effort to keep the disease from being introduced into a noninfected herd. Infectious materials may be carried into a herd by fomites such as workers' boots, farm implements, and trucks. Isolation of a herd and rigid sanitation are essential to reduce this potential hazard.

Introduction of new stock is an even greater hazard. A reliable history of the source herd is the only assurance of safety. Research efforts are being directed at various methods of identification of carrier animals, and it is hoped that serologic tests or other detection methods will soon be available for use in screening potential herd additions. Quarantine of all new animals is an excellent procedure, especially since clinical signs often appear in subclinically affected animals as a result of transportation. Furthermore, during quarantine, the newly purchased animals could be placed on one of the three drugs known to eliminate *S. hyodysenteriae* from the intestinal tract to preclude the introduction of the disease into the herd.

It is well accepted that, although SD is very prevalent, the disease may be readily eliminated by surgical procedures used for repopulation. Once a herd is established in the absence of the disease, such precautions as those taken by the specific-pathogen-free or minimal-disease associations, the Pig Health Control Association in the United Kingdom (Goodwin and Whittlestone 1984) and the Health Control Programs of certain breeding-stock companies (Alexander 1985) can prevent recurrence of *S. hyodysenteriae*. For example, newly established surgically derived herds in some locales may eventually become infected with such agents as *Bordetella bronchiseptica* and *Mycoplasma hyopneumoniae* but often can be maintained free of *S. hyodysenteriae*. The introduction of *S. hyodysenteriae* into a susceptible farm primarily occurs with the carrier pigs. Mice are considered only as reservoir hosts because mice do not usually migrate from farm to farm. Such mechanical vectors of infected feces as boots, coveralls, vehicles, migratory animals, and birds are also possible modes of introduction.

Losses in affected herds can also be reduced or prevented by various management procedures. Outbreaks of SD are often associated with conditions that produce stress such as handling, transportation, severe weather, or dietary changes. Minimizing stress or using preventive levels of various efficacious compounds may be useful aids. Sanitation is also extremely important, since the severity of the disease within an individual or a herd is directly related to the quantities of contaminated feces that are ingested. Reducing crowded conditions and providing a clean, dry environment can produce dramatic results. Conversely, poor sanitation will greatly enhance the distribution and severity of the disease within a herd. An example of this may be seen in occasional herds in northern latitudes where severe outbreaks have followed overfilling of waste pits under slatted-floor systems when outlets became frozen.

Depopulation is a rather drastic but frequently necessary measure to eliminate chronic SD. Because the causative agent is anaerobic and susceptible to heat, oxygen, drying, and disinfectants, it is recommended that depopulation be done during warm, dry weather if possible. Thorough cleaning and disinfection should be followed by enough time to reduce hazards of reinfection. *Serpulina hyodysenteriae* may survive in feces (pits and lagoons) for 60 days. The organism does not survive for long periods of time in feces-contaminated soil during seasonal temperatures of 15°C (59°F) or above (Egan 1981). Therefore, dirt lots that have held pigs affected with SD should remain free of pigs for at least 30 days during a warm period of the year. Any liquid feces such as pits and lagoons should be considered to contain *S. hyodysenteriae* for 90 days during periods of warm weather. Therefore, lagoon water used for recycling should not be utilized for several months after depopulation of the affected pigs.

Repopulation is extremely critical because any preventive procedures are for naught if carrier pigs are introduced into the herd. Only surgically derived pigs or animals from reliable sources should be considered as replacement stock.

Serious losses may be prevented even in exposed herds by use of preventive levels of various therapeutic compounds. Judicious use of these compounds as described in the section on therapy may be very beneficial, but they should not be relied upon as a substitute for good management.

Thus far no practical or reliable method of immunization is available for the prevention of SD. Among veterinarians and producers, there has been confusion regarding whether or not pigs that recover from SD are subsequently immune. Pigs with experimentally induced SD that recover without drug treatment can be immune to rechallenge (Joens et al. 1979a), or they may require more than one episode of disease before acquiring protective resistance (Rees et al. 1989).

Pigs that develop SD and recover without treatment usually continue to excrete *S. hyodysenteriae* in their feces (i.e., the immune status could be an infection immunity). This immunologic state can be maintained under conditions of good management. If some management stress is applied, clinical symptoms of the disease can reappear. If pigs that are acutely affected with the disease are given effective pharmaceuticals for treatment, the development of immunity may be impaired. Once the drug is withdrawn, the pig will be readily reinfected by *S. hyodysenteriae* present in the environment and exhibit clinical symptoms of SD.

Sows that have been exposed to *S. hyodysenteriae* protect their sucking piglets. The feces of these immune sows are the source of *S. hyodysenteriae* for the suckling pigs. Pigs that are not weaned until 8–10 weeks of age perhaps have a better chance to develop immunity, while pigs weaned at a younger age do not. Since a natural infected-immune state can exist for SD involving a secretory immune response (Joens et al. 1984; Rees et al. 1989), it is possible that a vaccine could be developed to prevent the disease. Several researchers have published information about experimental attempts to prevent SD by active immunization. Most use a parenteral administration of killed whole cells of *S. hyodysenteriae* (Fernie et al. 1983; Parizek et al. 1985; Coloe and Gerraty 1988), or subunits (Joens et al. 1990; Wannemuehler et al. 1990). Cloned endoflagella antigens were demonstrated to confer protection in the CF-1 mouse model (Boyden et al. 1989). A combination of killed whole cells given intramuscularly followed by an oral vaccination with live avirulent *S. hyodysenteriae* was a novel approach that gave better protection than intramuscular vaccination alone (Lysons et al. 1986). Only one vaccine is commercially available and reports suggest that partial protection is conferred.

PRACTICAL VETERINARY ADVICE TO PRODUCERS.

The most important mode of transmission of SD from farm to farm is the asymptomatic carrier pig. Reservoir hosts for *S. hyodysenteriae* are pigs and mice. The organism also survives readily in feces, particularly in waste pits (Table 49.3).

In herds known to be free of SD, the practitioner should determine that replacement breeding stock and purchased feeder pigs are free of the disease. In production facilities where the disease is endemic, reduction in production costs can be attained by eradication of the organism without depopulation; two-site production with partial depopulation; or total depopulation, cleanup, disinfection, and repopulation with SD-free stock.

Establishing a Diagnosis of SD.

A diagnosis of SD based on clinical signs and/or gross and histologic lesions should be confirmed by isolation and identification of *S. hyodysenteriae*. If no clinical signs of SD have been observed in the herd, the

Table 49.3. Survival time of *Serpulina hyodysenteriae* in animals and the environment

Location	Condition	Temp. °F	Temp. °C	Survival Time
Pigs	–	–	–	60 days
Mice	–	–	–	1 year
Rats	–	–	–	2 days
Dogs	–	–	–	13 days
Feces				
Pits	Moist	45	7	60 days
Hog lots	Dry	65	18	7 days
Hog lots	Cold or frozen	45	7	Until temp increases
Lagoons	–	–	–	60 days

Source: Harris et al. (1990).

veterinarian must be assured by the farmer that drugs and vaccines known to be effective for the treatment and prevention of SD are not being used and thus masking the disease. Clinical signs of SD should become apparent in 3–6 months, particularly in confinement facilities in the absence of drugs and vaccines.

Avoiding Introduction of *Serpulina hyodysenteriae* into Herds Free of SD. Herds that have been established as free of SD and are either closed or maintained in a closed pyramid will remain free of SD if situated in an isolated locale and precautions are taken to prevent contamination by feces from carrier pigs. If breeding stock or feeder pigs are introduced into the herd, care should be taken to limit the introductions to as few sources as possible and to procure the pigs from herds known to be free of SD. Pigs should be purchased from herds that do not use drugs or vaccines known to prevent the occurrence of SD. In addition, the source herd should not have made recent introductions of pigs from questionable or SD-positive herds. It is not recommended that tests be conducted to ascertain the SD status because cultural tests lack sensitivity (Harris et al. 1978) and serologic tests often have false-positive reactions (Egan et al. 1983). A fecal ELISA has been developed but it appears to be no more sensitive than culture, and false-positive reactions also occur (Taylor and Stevenson 1986).

If the SD status of the source herd(s) cannot be ascertained, then it is imperative that pigs be placed in quarantine prior to entry into the SD-free herd. In quarantine, the pigs should either be nonmedicated and observed for signs of SD or be medicated to eliminate carriers of *S. hyodysenteriae*. It is more practical to medicate, since it has been reported that unmedicated pigs may remain asymptomatic carriers of the disease for at least 60 days (Songer and Harris 1978).

Herd Elimination Programs. In some situations, pig producers must continually use medications and vaccines for control of SD. Quite often, however, the cost of such programs is prohibitive due to poor profitability. If the producer is capable of maintaining a herd free of SD then consid-

eration should be given to eliminating *S. hyodysenteriae* from the herd/facilities. The options are as follows:

1. Eradication of *S. hyodysenteriae* without depopulation. *S. hyodysenteriae* can be eliminated from endemic herds without depopulation but the procedure is not always successful. Several drugs used either alone or in combination have been reported to eliminate the infection from endemic herds when used in conjunction with sanitation and rodent control (Blaha et al. 1986; Coulson 1986; Larsen 1987; Wetzel 1987; Olson 1988). Drugs that are recommended for this procedure are as follows: lincomycin, carbadox, and tiamulin. The principle applied for elimination without depopulation is to medicate via feed, water, and/or injection to all pigs in the herd for a period of several days to months. During this medication period, a sanitation program is conducted, which eliminates the organism from the facility. In addition, the rodent population is exterminated. The reason for failure to eliminate the organism in this manner is believed to be caused by survival of *S. hyodysenteriae* either in slurry (Glock et al. 1975) or mice (Joens and Kinyon 1982). More research is needed to determine if vaccines could be of benefit in such programs.

2. Isowean 2- or 3-site production with partial depopulation. Endemic SD is often not difficult or costly to control in the adult population. Dams previously recovered from SD confer resistance to their young during the suckling period (Harris and Glock 1986). The cost of medication to control SD to 18–32 kg body weight is not prohibitive, since certain drugs at growth-promotion levels often control SD in this age of pig. Therefore, if pigs are removed from either the farrowing rooms after receiving colostrum as in Isowean (Alexander and Harris 1992) or the nursery accommodation up to 30 kg body weight, it is possible that the pigs will be free of *S. hyodysenteriae* at this time. The SD-free pigs should be isolated from the adult herd and moved to facilities not contaminated with *S. hyodysenteriae*. The use of a SD vaccine in the sow herd may also be helpful in this procedure.

3. Total depopulation, cleanup, disinfection,

and repopulation with SD-free stock. The decision to totally depopulate an ongoing pig operation should not be made without serious deliberation and accurate financial calculations (Wood and Lysons 1988). However, in some situations, this alternative is the only method available to eliminate *S. hyodysenteriae* from the herd/facilities. At warm temperatures, the organism does not survive well in soil (less than 7 days) (Egan 1981). Therefore, the most important reservoirs for the organism in a depopulated facility are the slurry and rodents. At temperatures above 60°F (16°C), facilities can be cleaned, disinfected, and repopulated very rapidly.

REFERENCES

ADACHI, Y.; SUEYOSHI, M.; MIYAGAWA, E.; MINATO, H.; AND SHOYA, S. 1985. Experimental infection of young broiler chicks with *Treponema hyodysenteriae*. Microbiol Immunol 29:683–688.

ALEXANDER, T. J. L. 1985. Methods of disease control. In Diseases of Swine, 6th ed. Ed. A. D. Leman, B. Straw, R. D. Glock, W. L. Mengeling, R. H. C. Penny, and E. Scholl. Ames: Iowa State Univ Press, pp. 778–800.

ALEXANDER, T. J. L., AND HARRIS, D. L. 1992. Methods of disease control. In Diseases of Swine, 7th ed. Ed. A. D. Leman, B. Straw, W. L. Mengeling, D. J. Taylor, and S. D'Allaire. Ames: Iowa State Univ Press, pp. 808–833.

ARGENZIO, R. A. 1981. Glucose-stimulated fluid absorption in the pig small intestine: An approach to oral fluid therapy in swine dysentery. Am J Vet Res 41:2000–2006.

ARGENZIO, R. A.; WHIPP, S. C.; AND GLOCK, R. D. 1980. Pathophysiology of swine dysentery: Colonic transport and permeability studies. J Infect Dis 142:676–684.

BAUM, D. H., AND JOENS, L. A. 1979a. Serotypes of beta-hemolytic *Treponema hyodysenteriae*. Infect Immun 25:792–796.

————. 1979b. Partial purification of a specific antigen of *Treponema hyodysenteriae*. Infect Immun 26:1211–1223.

BLAHA, TH.; ERLER, W.; AND BURCH, D. G. S. 1986. The evaluation of tiamulin injection for the elimination of the agent of swine dysentery under field conditions. Proc Int Congr Pig Vet Soc, Barcelona, p. 177.

BOWDEN, C. A.; JOENS, L. A.; AND KELLEY, L. M. 1989. Characterisation of the attachment of *Treponema hyodysenteriae* to Henle intestinal cells in vitro. Am J Vet Res 50:1481–1485.

BOYDEN, D. A; ALBERT, F. G.; AND ROBINSON, C. S. 1989. Cloning and characterization of *Treponema hyodysenteriae* antigens and protection in a CF-1 mouse model by immunization with a cloned endoflagellar antigen. Infect Immun 57:3808–3815.

BURROWS, M. R. 1988. Personal communication.

BURROWS, M. R., AND LEMCKE, R. M. 1981. Identification of *Treponema hyodysenteriae* by a rapid slide agglutination test. Vet Rec 108:187–189.

BURROWS, M. R.; LYSONS, R. J.; ROWLANDS, G. J.; AND LEMCKE, R. M. 1984. An enzyme-linked immunosorbent assay for detecting serum antibody to *Treponema hyodysenteriae*. Proc Int Congr Pig Vet Soc, Ghent, p. 186.

CHIA, S. P. 1977. Studies of the survival of *Treponema hyodysenteriae* and the epidemiology of swine dysentery. M.V.M. thesis, Univ of Glasgow, Scotland.

CHIA, S. P., AND TAYLOR, D. J. 1978. Factors affecting the survival of *Treponema hyodysenteriae* in dysenteric pig feces. Vet Rec 103:68–70.

COLOE, P. J., AND GERRATY, N. L. 1988. The use of vaccination against swine dysentery to improve health status and productivity in intensively housed pigs. Proc Int Congr Pig Vet Soc, Rio de Janeiro, p. 123.

COMBS, B.; HAMPSON, D. J.; MHOMA, J. R. L.; AND BUDDLE, J. R. 1989. Typing of *Treponema hyodysenteriae* by restriction endonuclease analysis. Vet Microbiol 19:351–359.

COULSON, A. 1986. An attempt to eliminate swine dysentery from a 400 sow herd by the use of lincomycin in their water and feed. Proc Int Congr Pig Vet Soc, Barcelona, p. 179.

CWYK, W. M., AND CANALE-PAROLA, E. 1979. *Treponema succinifaciens* sp. nov., an anaerobic spirochete from the swine intestine. Arch Microbiol 122:231–239.

EGAN, I. T. 1980. Personal communication.

————. 1981. The epidemiological aspects of swine dysentery in the midwestern United States. Ph.D. diss., Iowa State Univ.

EGAN, I. T.; HARRIS, D. L.; AND HILL, H. T. 1982. Prevalence of swine dysentery, transmissible gastroenteritis, and pseudorabies in Iowa, Illinois, and Missouri swine. Proc US Anim Health Assoc, pp. 497–502.

EGAN, I. T.; HARRIS, D. L.; AND JOENS, L. A. 1983. Comparison of the microtitration agglutination test and the enzyme-linked immunosorbent assay for the detection of herds affected with swine dysentery. Am J Vet Res 44:1323–1328.

FERNIE, D. S.; RIPLEY, P. H.; AND WALKER, P. D. 1983. Swine dysentery: Protection against experimental challenge following single dose parenteral immunisation with inactivated *Treponema hyodysenteriae*. Res Vet Sci 35:217–221.

GLOCK, R. D. 1971. Studies on the etiology, hematology and pathology of swine dysentery. Ph.D. diss., Iowa State Univ.

————. 1979. Swine dysentery: Is cleanup possible? Proc Livest Conserv Inst, p. 130.

GLOCK, R. D., AND HARRIS, D. L. 1972. Swine dysentery. II. Characterization of lesions in pigs inoculated with *Treponema hyodysenteriae* in pure and mixed culture. Vet Med Small Anim Clin 67:65–68.

GLOCK, R. D.; HARRIS, D. L.; AND KLUGE, J. P. 1974. Localization of spirochetes with the structural characteristics of *Treponema hyodysenteriae* in the lesions of swine dysentery. Infect Immun 9:167–178.

GLOCK, R. D.; VANDERLOO, K. J.; AND KINYON, J. M. 1975. Survival of certain pathogenic organisms in swine lagoon effluent. J Am Vet Med Assoc 166(3):277–278.

GLOCK, R. D.; KINYON, J. M.; AND HARRIS, D. L. 1978. Transmission of *Treponema hyodysenteriae* by canine and avian vectors. Proc Int Congr Pig Vet Soc, Zagreb, p. KB63.

GOODWIN, R. F. W., AND WHITTLESTONE, P. 1984. Monitoring for swine dysentery: Six years' experience with a control scheme. Vet Rec 115:240–241.

GREER, J. M., AND WANNEMUEHLER, M. J. 1989a. Comparison of the biological responses produced by lipopolysaccharide and endotoxin of *Treponema hyodysenteriae* and *Treponema innocens*. Infect Immun 57:717–723.

————. 1989b. Pathogenesis of *Treponema hyodysenteriae*: Induction of interleukin-1 and tumour necrosis factor by a treponema butanol/water extract (endotoxin). Microbiol Pathol 7:279–288.

HAMPSON, D. J.; MHOMA, J. R. L.; AND COMBS, B. 1989a. Analysis of lipopolysaccharide antigens of

Treponema hyodysenteriae. Epidemiol Infect 103:275–284.

HAMPSON, D. J.; MHOMA, J. R. L.; COMBS, B.; AND BUDDLE, J. R. 1989b. Proposed revisions to the serotyping system for *Treponema hyodysenteriae*. Epidemiol Infect 102:75–84.

HAMPSON, D. J.; MHOMA, J. R. L.; COMBS, B. G.; AND LEE, J. I. 1990. Serological grouping of *Treponema hyodysenteriae*. Epidemiol Infect 105:79–85.

HARRIS, D. L. 1984. The epidemiology of swine dysentery as it relates to the eradication of the disease. Comp Contin Educ 6:683–688.

HARRIS, D. L., AND GLOCK, R. D. 1975. Swine dysentery. In Diseases of Swine, 4th ed. Ed. H. W. Dunne and A. D. Leman. Ames: Iowa State Univ Press, p. 541.

———. 1981. Swine dysentery. In Diseases of Swine, 5th ed. Ed. A. D. Leman, R. D. Glock, W. L. Mengeling, R. H. C. Penny, E. Scholl, and B. Straw. Ames: Iowa State Univ Press, p. 432.

———. 1986. Swine dysentery and spirochetal diseases. In Diseases of Swine, 6th ed. Ed. A. D. Leman, B. Straw, R. D. Glock, W. L. Mengeling, R. H. C. Penny, and E. Scholl. Ames: Iowa State Univ Press, p. 494.

HARRIS, D. L.; GLOCK, R. D.; CHRISTENSEN, C. R.; AND KINYON, J. M. 1972. Swine dysentery. I. Inoculation of pigs with *Treponema hyodysenteriae* (new species) and reproduction of the disease. Vet Med Small Anim Clin 67:61–64.

HARRIS, D. L.; KINYON, J. M.; GLOCK, R. D.; SONGER, J. G.; AND EGAN, I. T. 1978. Cultural detection of swine infected with pathogenic *Treponema hyodysenteriae*. Proc Int Congr Pig Vet Soc, Zagreb, p. M3.

HARRIS, D. L.; McKEAN, J. D.; JOENS, L. A.; GLOCK, R. D.; AND SCHULTZ, R. 1990. Swine dysentery – practitioner planning guide for herd elimination programs. Livest Conserv Inst, Madison, Wis.

HØGH, P. 1979. Personal communication.

HUDSON, M. J.; ALEXANDER, T. J. L.; AND LYSONS, R. J. 1976. Diagnosis of swine dysentery: Spirochaetes which may be confused with *Treponema hyodysenteriae*. Vet Rec 99:498–500.

HUGHES, R.; OLANDER, H. J.; AND WILLIAMS, C. B. 1975. Swine dysentery: Pathogenicity of *Treponema hyodysenteriae*. Am J Vet Res 36:971–977.

HUNTER, D., AND SAUNDERS, C. N. 1977. Diagnosis of swine dysentery using an absorbed fluorescent antiserum. Vet Rec 101:303–304.

HUNTER, D. M., AND WOOD, T. 1979. An evaluation of the API ZYM system as a means of classifying spirochaetes associated with swine dysentery. Vet Rec 104:383–384.

JENKINS, E. M.; SINHI, P. P.; VANCE, R. T.; AND REESE, G. L. 1976. Passive hemolysis test for antibody to *Treponema hyodysenteriae*. Infect Immun 14:1106–1107.

JENKINSON, S. R., AND WINGAR, C. R. 1981. Selective medium for the isolation of *Treponema hyodysenteriae*. Vet Rec 109:384–385.

JOENS, L. A. 1979. Personal communication.

———. 1980. Experimental transmission of *Treponema hyodysenteriae* from mice to pigs. Am J Vet Res 41:1225–1226.

JOENS, L. A., AND GLOCK, R. D. 1979. Experimental infection in mice with *Treponema hyodysenteriae*. Infect Immun 25:757–760.

JOENS, L. A., AND KINYON, J. M. 1982. Isolation of *Treponema hyodysenteriae* from wild rodents. Infect Immun 15:994–997.

JOENS, L. A.; SONGER, J. G.; HARRIS, D. L.; AND GLOCK, R. D. 1978a. Experimental infection with *Treponema hyodysenteriae* in guinea pigs. Infect Immun 22:132–135.

JOENS, L. A.; KINYON, J. M.; BAUM, D. H.; AND HARRIS, D. L. 1978b. Immunofluorescent studies on *Treponema hyodysenteriae*. Proc Int Congr Pig Vet Soc, Zagreb, p. M2.

JOENS, L. A.; HARRIS, D. L.; KINYON, J. M.; AND KAEBERHLE, M. L. 1978c. Microtitration agglutination for detection of *Treponema hyodysenteriae* antibody. J Clin Microbiol 8:293–298.

JOENS, L. A.; HARRIS, D. L.; AND BAUM, D. H. 1979a. Immunity to swine dysentery in recovered pigs. Am J Vet Res 40:1352–1354.

JOENS, L. A.; SONGER, J. G.; AND HARRIS, D. L. 1979b. Comparison of selective culture and serologic agglutination of *Treponema hyodysenteriae* for diagnosis of swine dysentery. Vet Rec 105:463–465.

JOENS, L. A.; GLOCK, R. D.; AND KINYON, J. M. 1980. Differentiation of *Treponema hyodysenteriae* from *Treponema innocens* by enteropathogenicity testing in the CF1 mouse. Vet Rec 107:527–529.

JOENS, L. A.; ROBINSON, I. M.; GLOCK, R. D.; AND MATTHEWS, P. J. 1981. Production of lesions in gnotobiotic mice by inoculation with *Treponema hyodysenteriae*. Infect Immun 31:504–506.

JOENS, L. A.; NORD, N. A.; KINYON, J. M.; AND EGAN, I. T. 1982. Enzyme-linked immunosorbent assay for detection of antibody to *Treponema hyodysenteriae* antigens. J Clin Microbiol 15:249–252.

JOENS, L. A.; DEYOUNG, D. W.; CRAMER, J. C.; AND GLOCK, R. D. 1984. The immune response of the porcine colon to swine dysentery. Proc Int Congr Pig Vet Soc, Ghent, p. 187.

JOENS, L. A.; CRAMER, J. D.; AND MAPOTHER, M. E. 1990. Swine dysentery subunit vaccine and method. Patent Coop Treaty WO 90/02565.

KANG, B., AND OLANDER, H. J. 1990. Scanning electron microscopy of the colon inoculated with *Treponema hyodysenteriae* in colonic loops of swine. Proc Int Congr Pig Vet Soc, Lausanne, p. 117.

KENNEDY, M. J.; ROSNICK, D. K.; ULRICH, R. G.; AND YANCEY, R. J. 1988. Association of *Treponema hyodysenteriae* with porcine intestinal mucosa. J Gen Microbiol 134:1565–1567.

KENT, K. A.; AND LEMCKE, R. M. 1984. Purification and cytotoxic activity of a haemolysin produced by *Treponema hyodysenteriae*. Proc Int Congr Pig Vet Soc, Ghent, p. 185.

KENT, K. A.; LEMCKE, R. M.; AND LYSONS, R. J. 1988. Production, purification and molecular weight determination of the haemolysin of *Treponema hyodysenteriae*. J Med Microbiol 27:215–224.

KINYON, J. M. 1974. Characterization of *Treponema hyodysenteriae* isolated from outbreaks of swine dysentery. M.S. thesis, Iowa State Univ.

KINYON, J. M., AND HARRIS, D. L. 1974. Growth of *Treponema hyodysenteriae* in liquid medium. Vet Rec 95: 219–220.

———. 1979. *Treponema innocens*, a new species of intestinal bacteria and emended description of the type strain of *Treponema hyodysenteriae* Harris et al. Int J Syst Bacteriol 29:102–109.

———. 1980. In vitro susceptibility of *Treponema hyodysenteriae* and *Treponema innocens* by the agar dilution method. Proc Int Symp Vet Lab Diagn, Lucerne, Switzerland.

KINYON, J. M.; SONGER, J. G.; JANC, M.; AND HARRIS, D. L. 1976. Isolation and identification of *Treponema hyodysenteriae*: Aid to the diagnosis and treatment of swine dysentery. 19th Annu Proc Am Assoc Vet Lab Diagn, pp. 65–74.

KINYON, J. M.; HARRIS, D. L.; AND GLOCK, R. D. 1977. Enteropathogenicity of various isolates of *Treponema hyodysenteriae*. Infect Immun 15:638–646.

———. 1980. Isolation of *Treponema hyodysenteriae* from

experimentally infected pigs at various intervals post inoculation. Proc Int Congr Pig Vet Soc, Copenhagen.

KITAI, K.; KASHIWAZAKI, M.; ADACHI, Y.; KUME, T.; AND ARAKAWA, A. 1979. In vitro activity of 39 antimicrobial agents against *Treponema hyodysenteriae*. Antimicrob Agents Chemother 15:392–395.

KNOOP, F. C.; SCHRANK, G. D.; AND FERRARO, F. M. 1979. In vitro attachment of *Treponema hyodysenteriae* to mammalian epithelial cells. Can J Microbiol 25:399–405.

KUNKLE, R. A., AND KINYON, J. M. 1988. Improved selective medium for the isolation of *Treponema hyodysenteriae*. J Clin Microbiol 26:2357–2360.

KUNKLE, R. A.; HARRIS, D. L.; AND KINYON, J. M. 1986. Autoclaved liquid medium for propagation of *Treponema hyodysenteriae*. J Clin Microbiol 24:669–671.

LARSEN, L. P. 1987. Eradication of swine dysentery. Proc Am Assoc Swine Pract, Indianapolis, Ind., p. 565.

LEMCKE, R. M., AND BEW, J. 1984. Antigenic differences among isolates of *Treponema hyodysenteriae*. Proc Int Congr Pig Vet Soc, Ghent, p. 183.

LEMCKE, R. M., AND BURROWS, M. R. 1979. A disc growth-inhibition test for differentiating *Treponema hyodysenteriae* from other intestinal spirochetes. Vet Rec 104:548–551.

———. 1980. Sterol requirement for the growth of *Treponema hyodysenteriae*. J Gen Microbiol 116:539–543.

———. 1981. A comparative study of spirochaetes from the porcine alimentary tract. J Hyg Camb 86:173–182.

LEMCKE, R. M., AND WILLIAMS, L. A. 1984. Modification of the selective medium for *Treponema hyodysenteriae*. Proc Int Congr Pig Vet Soc, Ghent, p. 184.

LEMCKE, R. M.; BEW, J.; BURROWS, M. R.; AND LYSONS, R. J., 1979. The growth of *Treponema hyodysenteriae* and other porcine intestinal spirochaetes in a liquid medium. Res Vet Sci 26:315–319.

LEMCKE, R. M.; BURROWS, M. R.; KENT, K. A.; AND LYSONS, R. J. 1982. Studies on a haemolysin produced by *Treponema hyodysenteriae*. Proc Int Congr Pig Vet Soc, Mexico City, p. 39.

LYMBERY, A. J.; HAMPSON, D. J.; HOPKINS, R. M.; COMBS, B.; AND MHOMA, J. R. L. 1990. Multilocus enzyme electrophoresis for identifying and typing of *Treponema hyodysenteriae* and related spirochaetes. Vet Microbiol 22:89–99.

LYSONS, R. J. 1983. European perspectives on control of swine dysentery. Proc Am Assoc Swine Pract, Cincinnati, Ohio.

LYSONS, R. J., AND LEMCKE, R. M. 1983. Swine dysentery: To isolate or to fluoresce? Vet Rec 112:203.

LYSONS, R. J.; LEMCKE, R. M.; BEW, J.; BURROWS, M. R.; AND ALEXANDER, T. J. L. 1982. An avirulent strain of *Treponema hyodysenteriae* isolated from herds free of swine dysentery. Proc Int Congr Pig Vet Soc, Mexico City, p. 40.

LYSONS, R. J.; BURROWS, M. R.; DEBNEY, T. G.; AND BEW, J. 1986. Vaccination against swine dysentery—an effective novel method. Proc Int Congr Pig Vet Soc, Barcelona, p. 180.

LYSONS, R. J.; LEMCKE, R. M.; AND DUNCAN, A. L. 1988. "Colitis" of pigs—an emerging disease. Proc Int Congr Pig Vet Soc, Rio de Janeiro, p. 141.

LYSONS, R. J.; KENT, K. A.; BLAND, A. P.; SELLWOOD, R.; ROBINSON, W. P.; AND FROST, A. J. 1991. A cytotoxic haemolysin from *Treponema hyodysenteriae*: A probable virulence determinant in swine dysentery. J Med Microbiol 34(2):97–102.

MAPOTHER, M. E., AND JOENS, L. A. 1985. New sero-

types of *Treponema hyodysenteriae*. J Clin Microbiol 22:161–164.

MIAO, R. M.; FELDSTEEL, A. H.; AND HARRIS, D. L. 1978. Genetics of *Treponema*: Characterization of *Treponema hyodysenteriae* and its relationship to *Treponema pallidum*. Infect Immun 22:736–739.

MOLLER, A. F. N. 1984. Eradication of swine dysentery with a 5 day treatment of tiamulin. Dansk Vet Tidsskr 67:20. 15/10 1017–1022.

MUIRHEAD, M. R. 1984. With precise planning and implementation, swine dysentery can be eliminated from a herd. Int Piglett 4:1–3.

NUESSEN, M. E.; BIRMINGHAM, J. R.; AND JOENS, L. A. 1982. Biological activity of a lipopolysaccharide extracted from *Treponema hyodysenteriae*. Infect Immun 37:138–142.

NUESSEN, M. E.; JOENS, L. A.; AND GLOCK, R. D. 1983. Involvement of lipoplysaccharide in the pathogenicity of *Treponema hyodysenteriae*. J Immun 131:997–999.

OLSON, L. D. 1974. Clinical and pathological observations on the experimental passage of swine dysentery. Can J Comp Med 28:7–13.

OLSON, S. 1988. Eradication of swine dysentery from a farrow to finish herd using lincomycin. Proc Am Assoc Swine Pract, St. Louis, Mo, p. 301.

PARIZEK, R.; STEWART, R.; BROWN, K.; AND BLEVINS, D. 1985. Protection against swine dysentery with an inactivated *Treponema hyodysenteriae* bacterin. Vet Med 80:80–86.

PICARD, B.; MASSICOTTE, L.; AND SAHEB, S. A. 1978. Effect of sodium ribonucleate on the growth and the hemolytic activity of *Treponema hyodysenteriae*. Experientia 35:484–486.

RAINIER, R. H.; HARRIS, D. L.; GLOCK, R. D.; KINYON, J. M.; AND BRAUER, M. A. 1980. Effects of carbadox and lincomycin for treatment and carrier state control of swine dysentery. Am J Vet Res 41(9):1349–1356.

REES, A. S.; LYSONS, R. J.; STOKES, C. R.; AND BOURNE, F. J. 1989. Antibody production in the colon during infection with *Treponema hyodysenteriae*. Res Vet Sci 47:263–269.

RITCHIE, A. E.; ROBINSON, I. M.; JOENS, L. A.; AND KINYON, J. M. 1978. A bacteriophage for *Treponema hyodysenteriae*. Vet Rec 102:34–35.

RONCALLI, R. A., AND LEANING, W. H. D. 1976. Geographical distribution of swine dysentery. Proc Int Congr Pig Vet Soc, Ames, p. L17.

SCHMALL, M. S.; ARGENZIO, R. A.; AND WHIPP, S. C. 1983. Pathophysiologic features of swine dysentery: Cyclic nucleotide-independent production of diarrhea. Am J Vet Res 44:1309–1316.

SELLWOOD, R. 1991. Antigenic characterisation and genetics of *Treponema hyodysenteriae*. In Genetics and Molecular Biology of Anaerobes. Ed. M. Sebald. New York: Springer-Verlag.

SELLWOOD, R.; KENT, K. A.; BURROWS, M. R.; LYSONS, R. J.; AND BLAND, A. P. 1989. Antibodies to a common outer envelope antigen of *Treponema hyodysenteriae* with antibacterial properties. J Gen Microbiol 135:2249–2257.

SONGER, J. G. 1978. Personal communication.

SONGER, J. G., AND HARRIS, D. L. 1978. Transmission of swine dysentery by carrier pigs. Am J Vet Res 39:913–916.

SONGER, J. G.; KINYON, J. M.; AND HARRIS, D. L. 1976. Selective medium for isolation of *Treponema hyodysenteriae*. J Clin Microbiol 4:57–60.

SONGER, J. G.; GLOCK, R. D.; SCHWARTZ, K. J.; AND HARRIS, D. L. 1978. Isolation of *Treponema hyodysenteriae* from sources other than swine. J Am Vet Med Assoc 172:464–466.

STANTON, T. B. 1989. Glucose metabolism and NADH recycling by *Treponema hyodysenteriae*, the agent of swine dysentery. Appl Environ Microbiol 55:2365–2371.

———. 1992. Proposal to change the genus designation *Serpula* to *Serpulina* gen. nov. containing the species *Serpulina hyodysenteriae* comb. nov. and *Serpulina innocens* comb. nov. Int J Syst Bacteriol (January). In press.

STANTON, T. B., AND LEBO, D. F. 1988. *Treponema hyodysenteriae* growth under various culture conditions. Vet Microbiol 18:177–190.

STANTON, T. B.; JENSEN, N. S.; CASEY, T. A.; DEWHIRST, F. E.; AND PASTER, B. J. 1991. Reclassification of *Treponema hyodysenteriae* and *Treponema innocens* in a new genus, *Serpula,* gen. nov., as *Serpula hyodysenteriae* comb. nov. and *Serpula innocens* comb. nov. Int J Syst Bacteriol 41(1):50–58.

TAYLOR, D. J. 1972. Studies of bacteria associated with swine dysentery. Ph.D. diss., Univ of Cambridge, England.

———. 1984. Swine dysentery survey. Vet Rec 115:110–111.

TAYLOR, D. J., AND ALEXANDER, T. J. L. 1971. The production of dysentery in swine by feeding cultures containing a spirochaete. Br Vet J 127(11):58–61.

TAYLOR, D. J., AND BLAKEMORE, W. F. 1971. Spirochaetal invasion of the colonic epithelium in swine dysentery. Res Vet Sci 12:177–179.

TAYLOR, D. J., AND STEVENSON, R. 1986. A fecal ELISA test for *Treponema hyodysenteriae* in pig feces and slurry. Proc Int Congr Pig Vet Soc, Barcelona, p. 175.

TAYLOR, D. J.; SIMMONS, J. R.; AND LAIRD, H. M. 1980. Production of diarrhoea and dysentery in pigs by feeding pure cultures of a spirochaete differing from *Treponema hyodysenteriae.* Vet Rec 106:326–332.

WALLGREN, P. 1988. The relationship between swine dysentery and the ban of infeed prophylactic antibiotics. Proc Annu Gen Vet Meet [Suppl II]:305–315.

WANNEMUEHLER, M. J.; OSTLE, A. G.; NIBBLELINK, S. K.; COYLE, D. C.; AND WALTER, C. J. 1990. Pathogenesis of swine dysentery: Preparation of a protective vaccine. Proc Int Congr Pig Vet Soc, Lausanne, p. 124.

WETZEL, T. 1987. A case report: The use of Carbadox to eradicate swine dysentery. Proc Am Assoc Swine Pract, Indianapolis, p. 375.

WHIPP, S. C.; HARRIS, D. L.; KINYON, J. M.; SONGER, J. G.; AND GLOCK, R. D. 1978. Enteropathogenicity testing of *Treponema hyodysenteriae* in ligated colonic loops of swine. Am J Vet Res 39:1293–1396.

WHIPP, S. C.; POHLENZ, J.; HARRIS, D. L.; ROBINSON, I. M.; GLOCK, R. D.; AND KUNKLE, R. 1982. Pathogenicity of *Treponema hyodysenteriae* in uncontaminated gnotobiotic pigs. Proc Int Congr Pig Vet Soc, Mexico City, p. 31.

WHITING, R. A.; DOYLE, L. P.; AND SPRAY, R. S. 1921. Swine dysentery. Purdue Univ Agric Exp Stn Bull 257:3–15.

WILCOCK, B. D., AND OLANDER, H. J. 1979a. Studies on the pathogenesis of swine dysentery. I. Characterization of the lesions in colons and colonic segments inoculated with pure cultures or colonic content containing *Treponema hyodysenteriae.* Vet Pathol 16:450–465.

———. 1979b. Studies on the pathogenesis of swine dysentery. II. Search for a cytotoxin in spirochetal broth cultures and colon content. Vet Pathol 16:567–573.

WOOD, E. N., AND LYSONS, R. J. 1988. The financial benefit from the eradication of swine dysentery. Vet Rec 121:277–279.

50 Tuberculosis

C. O. Thoen

DURING 1989 in the United States, 33,517,563 cattle (exclusive of tuberculin reactors) were slaughtered under federal inspection; of these, 143 carcasses (0.0004%) were designated as being tuberculous. In contrast, of 82,110,688 swine slaughtered during the same period, 551,378 (0.67%) had lesions attributed to tuberculosis (USDA 1990). The percentage of swine carcasses with lesions attributed to tuberculosis is almost 1700 times greater than that for cattle, and this is cause for concern.

Increased interest in swine tuberculosis was aroused by changes in the regulations of the Meat and Poultry Inspection Program of the USDA. These regulations require that unaffected portions of swine carcasses with tuberculous lesions in more than one primary site, such as cervical and mesenteric lymph nodes, be cooked at 170°F (76.7°C) for 30 minutes before being approved for human food (Anon. 1973). The processing of tuberculous swine carcasses is costly and results in significant economic losses.

The public health significance of *Mycobacterium avium* complex infections has been recognized (Guthertz et al. 1989). Of special interest are reports on the isolation of certain serovars of *M. avium* complex from patients with acquired immune deficiency syndrome (Good 1985).

There has been no direct campaign to eradicate tuberculosis in swine. It was once believed that the campaign to eradicate bovine tuberculosis, which was started in 1917, would result in a reduction of the disease in swine in the United States. However, the percentage of swine with tuberculous lesions continued to increase for a number of years (Table 50.1).

ETIOLOGY. Swine are susceptible to infection with *Mycobacterium tuberculosis, M. avium,* and *M. bovis.* The investigations of Van Es and Martin (1925) showed that in the United States most of the tuberculosis in swine was caused by avian tubercle bacilli. *M. avium* serovars 1, 2, 4, and 8 are the most common isolates from tuberculous lesions in swine in the United States (Mitchell et al. 1975; Thoen et al. 1975b). At least 15 other *M. avium* serovars have been isolated from swine in the United States (Thoen et al. 1975b; Payeur et al. 1981) as well as in other countries: Australia (Tammemagi and Simmons 1971), Brazil (Pestana de Castro et al. 1978), Denmark (Jorgensen 1978), France and Germany (Meissner et al. 1978), Hungary (Szabo et al. 1975), Japan (Yugi et al. 1972), and South Africa (Kleeberg and Nel 1973).

Table 50.1. Incidence of tuberculosis in swine in the United States as determined by inspection in abattoirs under federal supervision

Year	Number Slaughtered	Percent Tuberculosis[a]	Percent Condemned[b]
1912	34,966,378	4.69	0.12
1917	40,210,847	9.89	0.19
1922	34,416,439	16.38	0.20
1927	42,650,443	13.54	0.14
1932	45,852,422	11.38	0.08
1937	36,226,309	9.48	0.08
1942	50,133,871	7.96	0.026
1947	47,073,370	8.50	0.023
1952	63,823,263	4.40	0.015
1956	66,781,940	4.76	0.010
1962	67,109,539	2.25	0.008
1968	72,325,507	1.35	0.005
1972	83,126,396	0.85	0.007
1978	71,805,911	0.75	0.006
1983	79,992,743	0.41	0.003
1989	82,110,688	0.67	0.002

Note: Data compiled from USDA 1922, 1973, 1979, 1984, 1990; Feldman 1963.
[a]Includes all carcasses with evidence of tuberculosis, varying in extent from only small foci in cervical lymph nodes to generalized involvement.
[b]Includes carcasses with evidence of generalized tuberculosis. Owing to a change in reporting in 1978, carcasses restricted and passed for cooking are included with the number condemned.

These reports indicate the worldwide distribution of tuberculosis in swine due to *M. avium.* The similarity of *M. avium* and so-called *M. intracellulare* has led to the proposal that the latter be considered serovars of *M. avium* (Wolinsky and Schaefer 1973; Meissner et al. 1974; Thoen et al. 1984); this has been done in this chapter.

A numbering scheme has been developed for reporting *M. avium* serovars (Wolinsky and Schaefer 1973). Serovars 1, 2, and 3 occur mainly in animals but also in humans, whereas serovars 4–8 are found in human patients and less commonly in animals. A micromethod has been developed for identifying serovars of *M. avium* allowing for savings in time and materials (Thoen et al. 1975a).

The decrease in prevalence of tuberculosis in swine in the United States is largely attributable to a lowering of the incidence of tuberculosis in poultry, which in turn is the result of the increasing practice of maintaining all-pullet flocks of chickens. The control of tuberculosis in swine is thus incidental to and a beneficial but secondary effect of a changing practice of poultry husbandry. Perhaps a more rapid decline in tuberculosis among swine will occur if a direct and effective attack is made on tuberculosis in poultry.

A new aspect of swine tuberculosis has been observed in large confined herds in which the infection is caused by *M. avium* serovars 4 and 8. Outbreaks usually result in large losses involving 30–60% of slaughter swine (Pritchard et al. 1977). The problem has been associated with the use of sawdust for litter (Dalchow and Nassal 1979; Songer et al. 1980).

EPIDEMIOLOGY. Because swine are not routinely tested with tuberculin, the only sources of information on the prevalence and geographic distribution of tuberculosis in this species are the data obtained from meat inspection records. On this basis an increase in the rate of infection occurred in the United States until 1922 (Table 50.1). During 1922, 16.38% of all swine slaughtered under federal supervision had tuberculous lesions; in 0.2% the disease was so extensive that the entire carcass was condemned. Since 1922, there has been a gradual decline; by 1983, the incidence had decreased to 0.41%, with only 0.003% having evidence of generalized tuberculous disease.

Since most of the tuberculosis in swine in the United States is of avian origin, the disease among swine is expected to be greater in the north central states where tuberculosis among chickens is greater (Thoen and Karlson 1991). However, data from meat inspection records may be misleading because in the United States swine may be shipped great distances from the state of origin for slaughter. Data on the prevalence of tuberculosis in swine from meat inspection records may also be misleading because the

diagnoses are made on the basis of the macroscopic appearance of lesions. A certain number of tuberculous infections will escape detection because the lesions are not grossly visible. Avian tubercle bacilli have been isolated from tonsils (Feldman and Karlson 1940) and lymph nodes (Pestana de Castro et al. 1978; Langenegger and Langenegger 1981) of apparently normal swine as well as from grossly normal lymph nodes of carcasses that were "passed for food" (Payeur et al. 1981).

In studies in the United States and Canada, where presumably tuberculous lymph nodes of swine were collected at abattoirs and examined bacteriologically, a varying percentage failed to yield tubercle bacilli (Table 50.2). Similar observations have been made by workers in Australia (Clapp 1956), Brazil (Pestana de Castro et al. 1978), Denmark (Plum 1946; Jorgensen et al. 1972), England (Cochin 1943), Finland (Vasenius 1965), France (LaFont and LaFont 1968), and Germany (Retzlaff 1966; Dalchow and Nassal 1979). The failure to demonstrate tubercle bacilli in lesions that appear grossly to be tuberculous may be due to inadequacy of present-day methods for isolating tubercle bacilli, occurrence of healed processes that contain no viable tubercle bacilli, or cause of the lesions by some microorganism other than tubercle bacilli, such as *Rhodococcus* (*Corynebacterium*) *equi* or *R. sputi* (to be discussed later).

SOURCES OF INFECTION AND CONTROL. Swine are susceptible to infection with *M. tuberculosis, M. bovis,* and *M. avium.* The occurrence of tuberculosis in swine, therefore, is related to the opportunity for direct or indirect contact with tuberculous cattle, humans, and fowl and to the prevalence of tuberculosis in all of these species.

The bovine tubercle bacillus is not a frequent cause of tuberculosis in swine in localities where the disease in cattle is controlled by a campaign of eradication. In the United States and Canada, for example, bovine tubercle bacilli are rarely found in lesions of swine (Table 50.2). In Great Britain during 1952–55, the bovine type of tuberculosis in swine gradually declined concurrently with the eradication of the disease in cattle. The percentage of avian-type infection increased from 44% during the first 5 years of the study to 92% for the last 5 years (Lesslie et al. 1968). However, the occasional finding of bovine tubercle bacilli in swine is a reminder that the disease in cattle is a constant threat. Efforts to eradicate bovine tuberculosis should not be diminished. Infection from *M. bovis* has been found among feral swine in Hawaii where it occurred among cattle and deer (Essey et al. 1981).

Where tuberculosis does occur in cattle, the infection may be transmitted to swine by the feeding of unpasteurized milk and dairy by-products.

Table 50.2. Summary of data compiled from reports in North America on the occurrence of tubercle bacilli in tuberculous lymph nodes of swine

Reference	Date[a]	Origin of Swine	Specimens	Avian only	Mammalian only	Mixed	None[b]
					Type of Tubercle Bacillus (%)		
Van Es	1925	Nebraska	248	74.6	4.4	5.6	15.4
Van Es and Martin	1925	Michigan	14	92.9	None	7.1	None
Mitchell et al.	1934	Canada	96	38.5	None	None	61.5
Feldman	1938b	Southeastern Minnesota	30[c]	80.0	6.6 (bovine)	None	13.3
Feldman	1939	Minnesota	75[d]	46.6	16.0 (human)	None	37.3
Feldman and Karlson	1940	Minnesota	89	61.8	None	None	38.2
Pullin	1946	Eastern Canada	232	44.8	0.9 (bovine)	None	54.3
Bankier	1946	Alberta, Canada	102	88.0	1.0 (bovine)	None	11.0
Karlson and Thoen	1971	Minnesota	36	72.0	None	None	28.0
Thoen et al.	1975b	USA	2036	76.0	<1.0	<1.0	22.0
Pritchard et al.	1977	Idaho	31	80.0	None	None	22.0
Cole et al.	1978	Georgia	112	53.6	None	None	46.4

Note: Specimens obtained from abattoirs under federal supervision.
[a]Several papers indicated that the work was done from 1 to 2 years before publication.
[b]Tubercle bacilli not demonstrated by cultural or animal inoculation tests.
[c]Selected cases of generalized tuberculosis; some of the specimens were portions of lung, liver, or spleen.
[d]Garbage-fed swine.

Feces of tuberculous cattle may contain viable tubercle bacilli; this provides an obvious hazard where swine and cattle are maintained in a common feedlot.

The practice of feeding swine the offal from abattoirs or feeding uncooked garbage is obviously unwise, because such material may contain tuberculous material from beef carcasses. Fichandler and Osborne (1966) described an epizootic of tuberculosis in a herd of swine in Connecticut that was fed improperly cooked offal from tuberculous cattle. A serious outbreak of avian tuberculosis in a swine-feeding establishment in Denmark was traced to the improper cooking of offal from poultry plants (Biering-Sorensen 1959). The human type of bacilli is occasionally isolated from tuberculous lesions in swine. No person known to have active tuberculosis should be permitted to have contact with swine or other animals.

Uncooked garbage is a potential means of transmitting tuberculosis to swine. Feldman (1939) recorded that of 264 garbage-fed swine, 75 (28.4%) were found to have tuberculous lesions at the time of slaughter. Of these, 47 contained tubercle bacilli, of which 35 were avian type and 12 were human type. It was concluded that garbage may contain the offal of tuberculous chickens and that material from tuberculous human patients is not properly disposed of. The frequent occurrence of avian tubercle bacilli in lesions limited to the cervical and mesenteric lymph nodes in naturally infected swine indicates that infection usually occurs by ingestion. Janetschke (1963) found that the primary complex involved the alimentary tract in 97.3% of 1000 carcasses with tuberculous lesions; a pulmonary route of infection was noted

in only 2.7%, as indicated by involvement of the bronchial lymph nodes.

Schalk et al. (1935) found that swine contracted tuberculosis when placed on ground that had not been occupied by tuberculous chickens for the previous 2 years. Viable and pathogenic avian tubercle bacilli were found in the soil and litter of a chicken cage after 4 years. Schalk and co-workers concluded that soil contaminated by feces of tuberculous fowl is the most important source of infection for swine. No success was obtained in controlling the disease merely by use of the tuberculin test and elimination of reactors, because the soil remained contaminated. They recommended that an ideal program to control avian tuberculosis is to rear young birds on clean ground and to dispose regularly of all fowl more than 1 year old.

Schliesser and Weber (1973) studied the survival of *M. avium* in sawdust. At 18–22°C, the survival time of two virulent strains was 153–160 days and of two avirulent strains, 169–214 days. The survival times were greatly reduced when the contaminated sawdust was maintained at 37°C.

Wild birds may be incriminated as a source of avian tuberculosis in swine. Tuberculosis was found in starlings on a farm with a high incidence of tuberculosis in the swine but where no poultry had been kept for 8 years (Bickford et al. 1966). Tuberculosis due to *M. avium* has been found in various wild birds, some of which frequent feedlots (Thoen and Karlson 1991).

The close contact of swine in yards and feeding pens provides opportunity for transmission of tuberculosis from animal to animal. The occurrence of intestinal lesions (Fig. 50.1) allows spread of

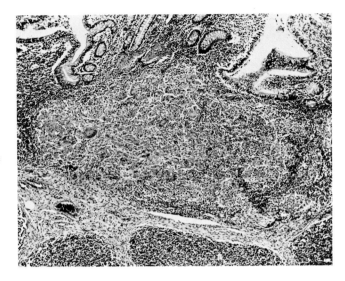

50.1. Submucosal tuberculous lesion due to avian tubercle bacilli in the intestinal tract of the pig. The lesion appears to be extending toward the surface, where it may ulcerate and discharge bacilli into the lumen. Diffuse cellular proliferation with little necrosis is typical of avian tubercle bacillus infection in swine. H & E. ×50.

tubercle bacilli in feces. Feldman and Karlson (1940) and Pullar and Rushford (1954) demonstrated avian tubercle bacilli in the tonsils of pigs. The latter workers suggested that this may be a source of infection for other animals. Smith (1958) found avian tubercle bacilli in apparently normal lymph nodes of 7% of swine, 5% of sheep, and 5% of cattle but was unable to find them in adult normal chickens; he suggested, therefore, that domestic mammals may contract avian tuberculosis from each other as well as from tuberculous fowl.

Pulmonary, uterine, and mammary tuberculous lesions in swine constitute sources of infection for other animals. Jorgensen et al. (1972) described an enzootic of pulmonary tuberculosis resulting from *M. avium* in pigs. Lesslie and Birn (1967) found *M. avium* in the udder or milk of 18 cows and concluded that such animals may be a source of avian tuberculosis in pigs. Bille and Larsen (1973) reported congenital infection in swine caused by avian tubercle bacilli, suggesting that infected pregnant sows may have a role in the transmission of this infection.

Where sawdust is used for bedding, various serovars of *M. avium* have been isolated from lesions in swine as well as from the sawdust. Reactions to avian and bovine tuberculin have been reported in boars exposed to sawdust from which *M. avium* or other nonphotochromogenic mycobacteria were isolated (Fodstad 1977). Schliesser and Weber (1973) found that *M. avium* would survive as long as 214 days in sawdust. In Hungary, Szabo et al. (1975) found that the incidence of tuberculous adenitis in swine was greater when sawdust was used as litter; when the use of sawdust was discontinued, the occurrence of such lesions decreased significantly. Dalchow and Nassal (1979) recorded that the same serovars of avian tubercle bacilli as found in swine could be isolated from sawdust. These workers also reported that

sawdust could contain infectious mycobacteria even after 4 years of storage. Songer et al. (1980) investigated herds of swine in Arizona and found in at least one herd that the source was sawdust and wood shavings.

PATHOGENESIS. The development of disease in swine depends on the ability of the tubercle bacillus to multiply within tissues of the host and to induce a host response. Although acid-fast bacilli initially encounter granulocytes and humoral components, activated mononuclear macrophages are considered to be more important in protection of the host against mycobacteria.

The capacity of tubercle bacilli (*M. tuberculosis*, *M. avium*, or *M. bovis*) to produce progressive disease in swine may be related to certain complex lipids present in the cell wall, such as trehalose-6, 6′dimycolate, sulfur-containing glycolipids (sulfatides), or strongly acidic lipids (Thoen and Himes 1986). However, it appears that the effect of these components alone or together on phagolysosome fusion cannot account for virulence. Available information suggests that a combination of toxic lipids and factors released by virulent tubercle bacilli may cause disruption of the phagosome, interfere with phagolysosome formation, alter the release of hydrolytic enzymes from the attached lysosomes, and/or inactivate the lysosomal enzymes released into the cytoplasmic vacuole (Thoen and Himes 1985). The role of cyclic nucleotides in altering mononuclear cell functions in naturally occurring swine tuberculosis needs investigation. Certain serovars of *M. avium* are susceptible to oxidative bactericidal mechanisms of macrophages (Bermudez and Young 1989). However, the importance of reactive oxygen radicals and hydrogen peroxide in macrophages of swine exposed to virulent tubercle bacilli remains to be elucidated.

Although the mechanisms by which mycobacteria produce disease in swine have not been clearly defined, experimental studies in piglets revealed that nonspecific esterase activity was elevated in mononuclear macrophages of lymph nodes 7 days following inoculation of *M. avium* complex (*M. intracellulare*) serovar 8 (Momotani et al. 1980). Granulomas of varying stages were observed in mesenteric and mandibular lymph nodes and intestinal mucosa at 14 days postinoculation. In other investigations, sensitized lymphocytes and detectable mycobacterial antibodies have been reported to occur at 14–28 days postexposure to *M. avium* or *M. bovis* (Muscoplat et al. 1975; Thoen et al. 1979a).

Evidence has been presented in humans suggesting that deficiencies in mononuclear function have been associated with certain mycobacterial diseases (Uchiyama et al. 1981; Mason et al. 1982). This abnormality may be mediated by an imbalance of the metabolic products of arachidonic acid, since in vitro responses to specific antigens were improved in cultures containing indomethacin. Studies are needed to determine the importance of these observations in swine tuberculosis.

LESIONS

Tubercle Bacilli. Detailed discussions of the pathologic anatomy of tuberculosis in swine may be found in Pallaske (1931), Feldman (1938a), Francis (1958), and Kramer (1962).

As seen in the abattoirs, tuberculous lesions in swine are usually limited to lymph nodes of the cervical and the mesentery regions. The lesions vary in appearance from small, yellowish white, caseous foci a few millimeters in diameter to diffuse enlargement of the entire node. The disease may be localized in one group of nodes or may involve a number of lymph nodes along the digestive tract.

Gross differentiation between tuberculous adenitis caused by avian tubercle bacilli and that by mammalian tubercle bacilli is difficult, but in general, some features are characteristic of each. In an infection of avian origin the lymph nodes may be enlarged and firm with no discrete purulent foci, or there may be one or more soft caseous areas with indistinct borders. Calcification is seldom demonstrable. The cut surface of the lesion has a neoplastic appearance with a few caseous foci. Although there may be diffuse fibrosis, there is little tendency to encapsulation. Relatively large areas of caseation may be present and occasionally will involve the entire lymph node. The lesions due to tubercle bacilli of the avian type are generally not easily enucleated. In contrast, when the infection is of mammalian origin (either bovine or human), the lesions tend to be well encapsulated and are relatively easy to separate from the surrounding tissue. In addition, calcification is usually prominent in lesions caused by infection with mammalian tubercle bacilli. The individual foci appear to be discrete and caseous. These distinctions are by no means absolute, and there are many variations in the gross appearance of tuberculous lesions in lymph nodes of swine.

Clapp (1956) examined, by bacteriologic procedures, 420 lymph nodes (mostly submaxillary) designated as tuberculous upon meat inspection. There was some association between the gross appearance and the cause. Localized lesions that were not easily enucleated and large, dry calcareous processes involving an entire lymph node were usually due to avian tubercle bacilli. Indistinctly mottled and streaked lesions, large encapsulated purulent abscesses, and lesions that could be easily enucleated were usually not caused by tubercle bacilli. Some of these yielded *Corynebacterium equi,* now reclassified as *Rhodococcus equi* (Goodfellow et al. 1982), which Clapp considered important in producing tuberculosislike lymphadenitis in swine. In the series of 420 specimens, only 5 were from swine with generalized tuberculosis, and all of these were associated with bovine tubercle bacilli. Microscopically, the changes induced in swine tissues by avian tubercle bacilli are characterized by diffuse proliferation of epithelioid cells and giant cells. There may be some necrosis and calcification, especially in older lesions, but calcification is not usually prominent. Similar changes are observed in sows and slaughter pigs (Thoen et al. 1976). Proliferation of connective-tissue elements accompanies the process. Lesions caused by mammalian tubercle bacilli have a tendency to become encapsulated by a well-developed zone of connective tissue. In addition, there is often early caseation and marked calcification (Fig. 50.2). However, consistent histopathologic differentiation between lesions caused by mammalian and avian tubercle bacilli is not possible (Himes et al. 1983).

Generalized tuberculosis in swine is not commonly seen. In most instances it is from infection with bovine tubercle bacilli, but it may also result from the avian type (Feldman 1938b; Jorgensen et al. 1972). The extent and character of generalized involvement vary from the occurrence of a few small foci in several organs to extensive nodular processes involving the liver, spleen, lungs, kidneys, and many lymph nodes. Generalized lesions from infection with avian tubercle bacilli tend to be diffuse. The cut surface is usually smooth, and there is no great tendency toward encapsulation by fibrosis. There may be foci of caseation, but calcification is not pronounced. Lesions resulting from infection with mammalian tubercle bacilli, however, are likely to be discrete, caseous, and well circumscribed by fibrosis. Calcification is prominent.

Bacteria Other than Tubercle Bacilli. Various species of mycobacteria other than tubercle bacil-

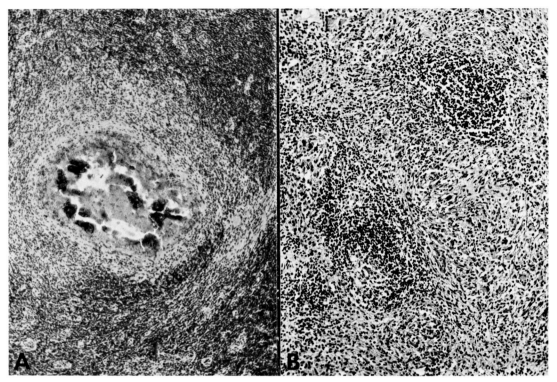

50.2. Tuberculous changes in cervical lymph nodes of swine. (A) Mammalian tubercle bacillus infection. Peripheral fibrosis, necrosis, and calcification are typical of lesions due to bovine or human types of tubercle bacilli. H & E. ×40. (B) *M. avium* infection. Diffuse cellular proliferation with little necrosis. H & E. ×95.

li have been isolated from swine and other animals in different countries, but reports of such are few and usually concern only sporadic cases (Schliesser 1976). The significance of finding *M. kansasii, M. xenopi,* or *M. fortuitum* is not clear. It may be important, however, to learn if animals and humans become infected from the same sources. Of potential importance is the recovery of *M. chelonei* from swine because this bacterium has been isolated from prosthetic heart valves that were prepared from swine (Thoen and Himes 1977).

In Norway, *M. paratuberculosis* was isolated by culture from lesions in the mesenteric lymph nodes of swine as well as from normal swine that were closely associated with a herd of cattle in which Johne's disease was present (Ringdal 1963). This microorganism was isolated in the United States from a slaughter pig (Thoen et al. 1975b). Jorgensen (1969) and Larsen et al. (1971) found that swine may be infected with *M. paratuberculosis* after oral administration of the organism. *M. xenopi* was isolated from tissues of slaughtered swine that originated in the southeastern region of the United States (Jarnagin et al. 1971). Another rare finding was the isolation of the vole bacillus, *M. microti,* from lymph nodes of three swine (Huitema and Jaartsveld 1967).

Mention must be made of the occurrence of *R. equi* in localized lesions that cannot be easily differentiated from tuberculous processes either macroscopically or histologically (Feldman et al. 1940). Holth and Amundsen (1936) in Norway reported that of 162 tuberculous lymph nodes from swine, only 103 yielded tubercle bacilli (97 were typed, with 80 avian and 16 human strains and 1 bovine strain). Of the other 59, 38 contained a variably acid-fast "coccobacillus." The acid-fastness, however, was not constant and was lost on subculture. The presence of this microorganism in localized tuberculosislike lesions in swine was soon confirmed by other Scandinavian workers. Plum (1946) in Denmark studied a large number of tuberculous lymph nodes from swine and concluded that it is difficult for inspectors in abattoirs to differentiate. Barton and Hughes (1980) recorded 32 reports of *R. equi* infection in swine. Ottosen (1945) has shown that *R. equi* occurs more frequently in the soil of hog pens than elsewhere. More recently, *R. sputi* was isolated from tuberculosislike lesions in the mesenteric lymph nodes of swine (Tsukamura et al. 1988).

DIAGNOSIS. A clinical diagnosis of tuberculosis in swine is presumptive at best. Generally, the tuberculous lesions are limited to small foci in a few lymph nodes of the digestive tract. It is difficult to conceive that such nonprogressive morbid changes may elicit signs detectable by physical examination. In extensive tuberculous infection, signs may be suggestive of an infectious disease, but the symptoms and changes are not sufficiently characteristic to establish a diagnosis of tuberculosis.

The necropsy and histopathologic appearance of tuberculosis in swine has been described. Although the morbid changes are sufficiently characteristic to permit a tentative diagnosis of tuberculosis, they are not specific. The great similarity between localized tuberculous lesions and those associated with *R. equi* and other bacteria has already been discussed. Also, chronic granulomatous lesions may be difficult to differentiate grossly because of parasitic nodules and neoplasms.

Enzyme-linked immunosorbent assay (ELISA) has been described for detecting antibodies in swine infected with *M. avium* (Thoen et al. 1979a,b). Positive ELISA reactions were observed in pigs experimentally infected and in those naturally infected. The ELISA reaction is a rapid test that can be automated. It may be of value in identifying herds from which slaughter swine originated and also in testing replacement breeding animals.

The mere demonstration of acid-fast bacilli in exudates or in lesions may be misleading. Some workers have recorded that *R. equi* is acid-fast in smears of necrotic material from lymph nodes of swine (Ottosen 1945). Acid-fast microorganisms other than tubercle bacilli have been isolated from swine (Karlson and Feldman 1940; Brandes 1961).

The characteristic pathologic feature of tuberculosis in swine and the presence of acid-fast microorganisms in such lesions provide important indications on which to base a diagnosis of tuberculosis. However, an unequivocal diagnosis can be made only on the basis of bacteriologic procedures designed for the isolation, identification, and typing of the tubercle bacillus.

TUBERCULIN TEST. The tuberculin test for the diagnosis of tuberculosis in swine appears to be a useful procedure on a herd basis. Of the various techniques described for this test in swine, the operator should select the method that proves by experience to be most suitable. Separate simultaneous tests with avian and mammalian types of tuberculin must be made (Thoen and Karlson 1970). A number of investigators have found that some tuberculous swine may fail to react to the intradermal tuberculin test. Therefore, tests should be repeated in a herd in which animals with positive reactions have been found and excluded.

The intradermal test, usually on the ear or vulva, may be employed. Because swine are susceptible to infection with avian and mammalian tubercle bacilli, avian and mammalian tuberculin should be used. The tuberculins may be diluted (1:100) to minimize nonspecific cross-reactions (Meyn et al. 1959). Fichandler and Osborne (1966) described an extensive outbreak of bovine tuberculosis in swine in which animals reacted to mammalian tuberculin by developing erythema and swelling of the ear, as compared with slight reactions to the avian tuberculin.

Feldman (1938a) recommended the use of 0.2 ml 25% Old Tuberculin applied into the dermis on the dorsal surface of the ear, slightly anterior to the base. A positive reaction is indicated in 24 hours by a flat, reddish swelling up to 3 cm in diameter, which in 48 hours reaches its maximal intensity. At this time the erythema and swelling are more pronounced; the central area becomes hemorrhagic, and ulceration may occur. McDiarmid (1956) described a means of testing swine in which restraint is not necessary. While the animals are feeding from a trough, 0.1 ml tuberculin is injected at a right angle into the skin at the junction of the ear and neck using a needle only 3.5 mm long. With this short needle, most of the tuberculin is deposited in the skin. By using a syringe in each hand, avian tuberculin can be injected on one side and mammalian tuberculin on the other. Reactions are recorded in 48 hours. A positive reaction varies from "puffy" edema to inflammation, with purple discoloration and necrosis. McDiarmid used Weybridge purified protein derivative (PPD), which, according to Paterson (1949), has 3 mg protein/ml for mammalian tuberculin and 0.8 mg protein/ml for avian.

Lanz (1955) recommended injecting the tuberculin in the skin of the back about 10–20 cm caudal to the shoulders and slightly to the right of the midline. This was easier and less time consuming than trying to use the ear. A dose of 0.1 ml PPD (as used for cattle in Switzerland) is injected intradermally. A positive reaction reaches its peak in 72 hours and consists of a painful erythematous swelling 22–35 mm in diameter. As determined by necropsy, no false-negative or atypical reactions were found among 316 animals.

Luke (1952) described observations on the tuberculin test in 100 sows, 3 years old or older, using avian and mammalian tuberculin intradermally in the ear and recording the results in 24 hours. A positive reaction was ascribed when there was an increase of 2 mm in thickness of the skin at the site of injection. Of 39 reactors only 22 had visible lesions, chiefly of lymph nodes of the digestive tract. Tubercle bacilli were demonstrable in only 3 of the 22 animals with lesions, and each was a mammalian strain. Lesions considered to be tuberculous were found in 8 animals that were nonreactors, but tubercle bacilli were apparently not demonstrable in these. In Luke's opinion, there is a large percentage of error in the tuberculin test in swine because of nonspecific sensitivity or residual sensitivity from healed tuberculous lesions. Negative reactions in animals with lesions may, according to Luke (1958), be ascribed to the ability of the pig to overcome and apparently sterilize existing lesions. Luke (1953) studied various aspects of the tuberculin test in swine, including the specific effect of tuberculin on the leukocyte count.

Lesslie et al. (1968), using Weybridge PPD, tested 84 White pigs from a herd known to have tuberculosis. The avian tuberculin was given in injections of 0.1 ml, each containing 2500 tuberculin units (TU); and the mammalian tuberculin was given in injections of 0.1 ml, each containing 10,000 TU. The injections were made simultaneously, each at the base on an ear; in 48–72 hours a positive reaction was recorded when the reaction consisted of edema and erythema. Guinea pigs experimentally sensitized with *M. avium* serovars 3, 4, 5, 6, 8, and 9 each reacted similarly to tuberculin prepared from serovars 2 and 7 (Anz et al. 1970). Swine experimentally infected with *M. avium* serovars 4 and 8 reacted well to the USDA avian Old Tuberculin and to PPD prepared from *M. avium* serovar 1 (Thoen et al. 1976; Thoen et al. 1979b). Further studies must be made in swine to determine whether the serovar of the infecting strain will influence the specificity of the tuberculin test.

At present, intradermal infection of PPD tuberculin in the dorsal surface of the ear is recommended procedure for applying the tuberculin test in swine. The injection site should be observed at 48 hours.

PREVENTION.   The eradication of tuberculosis in swine as well as other species is dependent on the availability of an economical and specific means of detecting infected animals. Studies should be extended to explore the efficacy of a blood test such as ELISA, which would require only one handling of the animal. Furthermore, a routine blood test for tuberculosis could be performed on blood specimens submitted for other tests such as those for brucellosis.

Additional information is needed to determine adequate measures for cleaning and disinfecting the premises where *M. avium* persists in the soil, in buildings, or on equipment. Also, we need to know how long these organisms will remain viable in the environment. Investigations also should be made to determine the sources and modes of transmission of all the different serovars of *M. avium.* Information is needed on the stability of the serovars and the genetic relationships of the *M. avium* isolated from tuberculous swine and those that cause disease in humans. This is of increased importance since serovars 1, 4, and 8, which are most commonly isolated from patients with acquired immune deficiency syndrome, are also isolated from tuberculous lesions in swine.

REFERENCES

Anon. 1973. Code of federal regulations, animal and animal byproducts. Title 9, Chap. 3, Subchap. A, Pt. 311. Gen Serv Adm, Washington, D.C.

Anz, W.; Lauterback, D.; Meissner, G; and Willers, I. 1970. Vergleich von Sensitin-Testen an Meerschweinchen mit Serotyp und Huhnervirulenz bei *M. avium*- and *M. intracellulare*-Stammen. Zentralbl Bakteriol [Orig A] 215:536–549.

Bankier, J. C. 1946. Tuberculous lesions of swine. II. Survey of lesions found in the prairie provinces, especially in Alberta. Can J Comp Med 10:250–253.

Barton, M. D., and Hughes, K. L. 1980. *Corynebacterium equi:* A review. Vet Bull 50:65–80.

Bermudez, L. E. M., and Young, L. S. 1989. Oxidative and nonoxidative killing of *Mycobacterium avium* complex. Microb Pathog 7:289–298.

Bickford, A. A.; Ellis, G. H.; and Moses, H. E. 1966. Epizootiology of tuberculosis in starlings. J Am Vet Med Assoc 149:312–318.

Biering-Sorensen, U. 1959. Ophobning af tilfaelde af aviaer tuberkulose i en svinebesaetning. Medd Dan Dyrlaegeforen 42:550–552.

Bille, N., and Larsen, J. L. 1973. Porcine congenital infection due to *Mycobacterium tuberculosis typus avium:* Report of a case. Nord Vet Med 25:139–143.

Brandes, T. 1961. Zur makroskopischen Unterscheidung zwischen tuberkulosen und tuberkuloseahnlichen Veranderungen in den Mesenteriallymphknoten des Schweines. Arch Lebensmittelhyg 12:53–56.

Clapp, K. H. 1956. Tuberculosis-like lesions in swine in South Australia. Aust Vet J 32:110–113.

Cochin, E. 1943. Tubercle bacilli in lesions of the submaxillary lymph nodes of swine. J Comp Pathol 53:310–314.

Cole, J. R.; Sangster, L. T.; Thoen, C. O.; Pursell, A. R.; Williams, D. J.; DuBois, P. R.; and McDaniel, H. T. 1978. Mycobacteriosis in a Georgia swine herd. Proc 21st Meet Am Assoc Vet Lab Diagn, pp.195–208.

Dalchow, W., and Nassal, J. 1979. Mykobakteriose beim Schwein durch Sagemehleinstreu. Tieraerztl Umsch 34:253–261.

Essey, M. A.; Payne, R. L.; Himes, E. M.; and Luchsinger, D. W. 1981. Bovine tuberculosis surveys of axis deer and feral swine on the Hawaiian island of Molokai. Proc 85th Annu Meet US Anim Health Assoc, pp.538–549.

Feldman, W. H. 1938a. Avian Tuberculosis Infections. Baltimore: Williams & Wilkins.

_____. 1938b. Generalized tuberculosis of swine due to avian tubercle bacilli. J Am Vet Med Assoc 92:681–685.

_____. 1939. Types of tubercle bacilli in lesions of garbage-fed swine. Am J Public Health 29:1231–1238.

_____. 1963. Tuberculosis. In Diseases Transmitted from Animals to Man, 5th ed. Ed. T. G. Hull. Springfield, Ill.: Charles C. Thomas, p. 5.

Feldman, W. H., and Karlson, A. G. 1940. Avian tubercle bacilli in tonsils of swine. J Am Vet Med Assoc 96:146–149.

Feldman, W. H.; Moses, H. E.; and Karlson, A. G. 1940. *Corynebacterium equi* as a possible cause of tuberculous-like lesions of swine. Cornell Vet 30:465–481.

Fichandler, P. D., and Osborne, A. D. 1966. Bovine tuberculosis in swine. J Am Vet Med Assoc 148:167–169.

Fodstad, F. H. 1977. Tuberculin reactions in bulls and boars sensitized with atypical mycobacteria from sawdust. Acta Vet Scand 18:374–383.

FRANCIS, J. 1958. Tuberculosis in Animals and Man: A Study in Comparative Pathology. London: Cassell, p.177.

GOOD, R. C. 1985. Opportunistic pathogens in the genus *Mycobacterium*. In Annual Review of Microbiology. Palo Alto, Calif.: Annual Reviews Inc., pp.347–369.

GOODFELLOW, M.; BECKHAM, A. R.; FELDMAN, W. H.; AND BARTON, M. D. 1982. Numerical classification of *Rhodococcus equi*. J Appl Bacteriol 53:199–207.

GUTHERTZ, L. S.; DAMSKER, B; BUTTONE, J.; FORD, E. G.; MIDURA, T. F.; AND JANDA, J. M. 1989. *Mycobacterium avium* and *Mycobacterium intracellulare* infections in patients. J Infect Dis 160:1037–1041.

HIMES, E. M.; MILLER, L. D.; AND THOEN, C. O. 1983. Swine tuberculosis: Histologic similarities of lesions from which *Mycobacterium tuberculosis, M. avium* complex or *M. bovis* was identified. Proc 26th Meet Am Assoc Vet Lab Diagn, pp.63–76.

HOLTH, H., AND AMUNDSEN, H. 1936. Fortsatte undersokelser over baciltypene ved tuberkulose hos svinet pa Ostlandet. Nor Vet Tidsskr 48:2–17.

HUITEMA, H., AND JAARTSVELD, F. H. J. 1967. *Mycobacterium microti* infection in a cat and some pigs. Antonie van Leeuwenhoek 33:209–212.

JANETSCHKE, P. 1963. Ueber die tuberkulose beim Schwein. Monatsschr Veterinaermed 18:860–864.

JARNAGIN, J. L.; RICHARDS, W. D.; MUHM, R. L.; AND ELLIS, E. M. 1971. The isolation of *Mycobacterium xenopi* from granulomatous lesions in swine. Am Rev Respir Dis 104:763–765.

JORGENSEN, J. B. 1969. Paratuberculosis in pigs: Experimental infection by oral administration of *Mycobacterium paratuberculosis*. Acta Vet Scand 10:275–287.

———. 1978. Serological investigation of strains of *Mycobacterium avium* and *Mycobacterium intracellulare* isolated in animal and non-animal sources. Nord Vet Med 30:155–162.

JORGENSEN, J. B.; HAARBO, K.; DAM, A.; AND ENGBAEK, H. C. 1972. An enzootic of pulmonary tuberculosis in pigs caused by *M. avium*. I. Epidemiological and pathological studies. Acta Vet Scand 13:56–57.

KARLSON, A. G., AND FELDMAN, W. H. 1940. Studies on an acid-fast bacterium frequently present in tonsillar tissue of swine. J Bacteriol 39:461–472.

KARLSON, A. G., AND THOEN, C. O. 1971. *Mycobacterium avium* in tuberculous adenitis of swine. Am J Vet Res 32:1257–1261.

KLEEBERG, H. H., AND NEL, E. E. 1973. Occurrence of environmental atypical mycobacteria in South Africa. Ann Soc Belg Med Trop 53:405–417.

KRAMER, H. 1962. Zur Beurteilung tuberkuloseahnalicher Veranderungen in den Gekroslymphknoten des Schweines unter besonderer Beruchsichigung der bakterioskopischer Prufung. Arch Lebensmittelhyg 13:264–271.

LAFONT, P., AND LAFONT, J. 1968. Etude microbiologique a des adenites cervicales du porc. II. Adenites a mycobacteries atypiques. Rec Med Vet 144:611–630.

LANGENEGGER, C. H., AND LANGENEGGER, J. 1981. Prevalence and distribution of serotypes of mycobacteria of the MAIS-complex isolated from pigs in Brazil. Pesqui Vet Bras 1:75–80.

LANZ, E. 1955. Uber die Tuberkulose und die intrakutane Tuberkulinisierung beim Schwein. Schweiz Arch Tierheilkd 97:229–245.

LARSEN, A. B.; MOON, H. W.; AND MERKAL, R. S. 1971. Susceptibility of swine to *Mycobacterium paratuberculosis*. Am J Vet Res 32:589–595.

LESSLIE, I. W., AND BIRN, K. J. 1967. Tuberculosis in cattle caused by the avian type tubercle bacillus. Vet Rec 80:559–564.

LESSLIE, I. W.; BIRN, K. J.; STUART, P.; O'NEILL, P. A. F.; AND SMITH, J. 1968. Tuberculosis in the pig and the tuberculin test. Vet Rec 83:647–651.

LUKE, D. 1952. Studies in tuberculous sensitivity in the pig. III. The tuberculin skin reaction in the sow. Vet Rec 64:344–345.

———. 1953. The intradermal tuberculin test in the pig. Vet Rec 65:533–535.

———. 1958. Tuberculosis in the horse, pig, sheep and goat. Vet Rec 70:529–536.

MCDIARMID, A. 1956. Tuberculin testing of pigs. Vet Rec 68:298–299.

MASON, U. G.; GREENBERG, L. E.; YEN, S. S.; AND KIRKPATRICK, C. H. 1982. Indomethacin-responsive mononuclear cell dysfunction in "atypical" mycobacteriosis. Cell Immunol 71:54–65.

MEISSNER, G.; SCHRODER, K. H.; AMADIO, G. E.; Anz, W.; CHAPARAS, S.; ENGLE, H. W. B.; JENKINS, P. A.; KAPPLER, W.; KLEEBERT, H. H.; KUBALA, E.; KUBIN, M.; LAUTERBACH, D.; LIND, A.; MAGNUSSON, M.; MIKOVA, Z. D.; PATTYN, S. R.; SCHAEFER, W. B.; STANFORD, J. L.; TSUKAMURA, M.; WAYNE, L. G.; WILLERS, I.; AND WOLINSKY, E. 1974. A co-operative numerical analysis of nonscoto- and nonphotochromogenic slowly growing mycobacteria. J Gen Microbiol 83:207–235.

MEISSNER, G.; VIALLIER, J.; AND COULLIOUD, D. 1978. Identification serologique de 1,590 souches de *Mycobacterium avium* isolees en France et en Allemagne Federale. Ann Microbiol (Paris) 129A:131–137.

MEYN, A.; SCHLIESSER, T.; AND BEDERKE, G. 1959. Zur Frage der Abklarung unspezifischer Tuberkulinreaktionen mit verdunntem Rinder-Einheitstuberkulin. Rindertuberk Brucell 8:179–185.

MITCHELL, C. A.; WALKER, R. V. L.; AND HUMPHREY, F. A. 1934. Types of tubercle bacilli found in swine of two accredited areas. Rep Vet Dir Gen Dep Agric Can, pp.43–44.

MITCHELL, M. D.; HUFF, I. H.; THOEN, C. O.; HIMES, E. M.; AND HOWDER, J. W. 1975. Swine tuberculosis in South Dakota. J Am Vet Med Assoc 167:152–153.

MOMOTANI, E.; YOKOMIZO, Y.; SHOYA, S.; NAKAMURA, K.; AND YUGI, H. 1980. Experimental granuloma formation with *Mycobacterium intracellulare* in HPCD piglets. J Tokyo Vet Zootec Sci 29:25–32.

MUSCOPLAT, C. C.; THOEN, C. O.; CHEN, A. W.; RAKICH, P. M.; AND JOHNSON, D. W. 1975. Development of specific lymphocyte immunostimulation and tuberculin skin reactivity in swine infected with *Mycobacterium bovis* and *Mycobacterium avium*. Am J Vet Res 36:1167–1171.

OTTOSEN, H. E. 1945. Undersogelser over Corynebacterium Magnusson-Holth, specielt med Henblik paa dens serologiske Forhold. A/S Carl Fr Mortensen, Copenhagen.

PALLASKE, G. 1931. Studien zum Ablauf, Zur Pathogenese und pathologischen Anatomie der Tuberkulose des Schweines. (Beitrag zum Vergleichenden Studium der Tiertuberkulose.) Z Infektionskr Parasitenkd Krankheit Haustiere 39:211–260.

PATERSON, A. B. 1949. Tuberculosis in animals other than cattle. III. Vet Rec 61:880–881.

PAYEUR, J. B.; BROWN, J.; AND HIGGINBOTHAM, A. A. 1981. Mycobacterial isolations from swine tissues. Proc 85th Annu Meet US Animal Health Assoc, pp. 475–484.

PESTANA DE CASTRO, A. F.; CAMPEDELLI FILHO, O; AND WAISBICH, E. 1978. Opportunistic mycobacteria isolated from the mesenteric lymph nodes of apparently healthy pigs in Sao Paulo, Brazil. Rev Microbiol (Brazil) 9:74–83.

PLUM, N. 1946. Om Vaerdien af den Makroskopiske Diagnose af de Holthske Processer. Maandsskr Dyrlaegeforen 58:27–37.

PRITCHARD, W. D.; THOEN, C. O.; HIMES, E. M.; MUSCOPLAT, C. C.; AND JOHNSON, D. W. 1977. Epidemiology of mycobacterial lymphadenitis in an Idaho swine herd. Am J Epidemiol 106:222–227.

PULLAR, E. M., AND RUSHFORD, B. H. 1954. The accuracy of the avian intradermal tuberculin test in pigs. Aust Vet J 30:221–231.

PULLIN, J. W. 1946. Tuberculous lesions of swine. I. Survey of lesions found in eastern Canada. Can J Comp Med 10:159–163.

RETZLAFF, N. 1966. Histologische Untersuchungen an Lymphknoten von mit Mykobakterien infizierten Schlachtschwein. Arch Lebensmittelhyg 17:56–62.

RINGDAL, G. 1963. Johne's disease in pigs. Nord Vet Med 15:217–238.

SCHALK, A. F.; RODERICK, L. M.; FOUST, H. L.; AND HARSHFIELD, G. S. 1935. Avian tuberculosis: Collected studies. ND Agric Exp Stn Tech Bull 279.

SCHLIESSER, T. 1976. Vorkommen und Bedeutung von Mykobakterien bei Tieren. Zentralbl Bakteriol [Orig A] 235:184–194.

SCHLIESSER, T., AND WEBER, A. 1973. Untersuchungen ueber die Tenazitat von Mykobakterien der Gruppe III nach Runyon in Sagemehleinstreu. Zentralbl Veterinaermed [B] 20:710–714.

SMITH, H. W. 1958. The source of avian tuberculosis in the pig (letter to the editor). Vet Rec 70:586.

SONGER, J. G.; BICKNELL, E. J.; AND THOEN, C. O. 1980. Epidemiological investigations of swine tuberculosis in Arizona. Can J Comp Med 44:115–120.

SZABO, I; TUBOLY, S.; SZEKY, A.; KEREKES, J.; AND UDVARDY, N. 1975. Swine lymphadenitis due to *Mycobacterium avium* and atypical mycobacteria. II. Studies on the role of littering in mycobacterial lymphadenitis incidence in large-scale pig units. Acta Vet Acad Sci Hung 25:77–83.

TAMMEMAGI, L., AND SIMMONS, G. C. 1971. Pathogenicity of *Mycobacterium intracellulare* to pigs. Aust Vet J 47:337–339.

THOEN, C. O., AND HIMES, E. M. 1977. Isolation of *Mycobacterium chelonei* from a granulomatous lesion in pig. J Clin Microbiol 6:81–83.

_____. 1985. Pathogenesis of *Mycobacterium bovis* infections. In Advances in Veterinary Microbiology and Immunology, vol. 2. Ed. R. Pandy. Basel: S. Karger.

_____. 1986. *Mycobacterium.* In: Pathogenesis of Bacterial Infections in Animals. Eds. C. L. Gyles and C. O. Thoen. Ames: Iowa State Univ Press, pp. 26–34.

THOEN, C. O., AND KARLSON, A. G. 1970. Epidemiologic studies on swine tuberculosis. Proc US Anim Health Assoc, pp. 459–464.

_____. 1991. Avian Tuberculosis. In: Diseases of Poultry, 9th ed. Eds. B. W. Calnek, H. J. Barnes, C. W. Beard, W. M. Reid, and H. W. Yoder, Jr. Ames: Iowa State Univ Press, pp. 172–183.

THOEN, C. O.; JARNAGIN, J. L.; AND CHAMPION, M. L. 1975a. Micromethod for serotyping strains of *Mycobacterium avium.* J Clin Microbiol 1:469–471.

THOEN, C. O.; JARNAGIN, J. L.; AND RICHARDS, W. D. 1975b. Isolation and identification of mycobacteria from procine tissues: A three-year summary. Am J Vet Res 36:1383–1386.

THOEN, C. O.; HIMES, E. M.; WEAVER, D. E.; AND SPANGLER, G. W. 1976a. Tuberculosis in brood sows and pigs slaughtered in Iowa. Am J Vet Res 37:775–778.

THOEN, C. O.; JOHNSON, D. W.; HIMES, E. M.; MENKE, S. B.; AND MUSCOPLAT, C. C. 1976b. Experimentally induced *Mycobacterium avium* serotype 8 infection in swine. Am J Vet Res 37:177–181.

THOEN, C. O.; ARMBRUST, A. L.; AND HOPKINS, M. P. 1979a. Enzyme-linked immunosorbent assay for detecting antibodies in swine infected with *Mycobacterium avium.* Am J Vet Res 40:1096–1099.

THOEN, C. O.; OWEN, W. J.; AND HIMES, E. M. 1979b. *Mycobacterium avium* serotype 4 infection in swine. Proc 83d Annu Meet US Anim Health Assoc, pp.468–479.

THOEN, C. O.; HIMES, E. M.; AND KARLSON, A. G. 1984. *Mycobacterium avium* complex. In The Mycobacteria: A Sourcebook. Ed. G. P. Kubica and L. G. Wayne. New York: Marcel Dekker.

TSUKAMURA, M.; KOMATSUZAKI, C.; SAKAI, R.; KANEDA, K.; KUDO, K.; AND SEINO, A. 1988. Mesenteric lymphadenitis of swine caused by *Rhodococcus sputi.* J Clin Microbiol 26:155–157.

UCHIYAMA, N.; GREEN, G. R.; WARREN, B. J.; MORGUMI, P. A.; SPEAR, G. S.; AND GALLANT, S. P. 1981. Possible monocyte killing defect in familial atypical mycobacteriosis. J Pediatr 98:785–788.

USDA. 1922. Yearbook of Agriculture, Washington, D. C.

_____. 1973. Statistical Summary. Federal Meat and Poultry Inspection for Calendar Year 1972. MPI-1.

_____. 1990. Statistical Summary. Federal Meat and Poultry Inspection for Calendar Year 1989. MPI-1.

VAN ES, L. 1925. Tuberculosis of swine. Univ of Nebr Agric Exp Stn Circ 25.

VAN ES, L., AND MARTIN, H. M. 1925. An inquiry into the cause of the increase of tuberculosis of swine. Univ of Nebr Agric Exp Stn Res Bull 30.

VASENIUS, H. 1965. Tuberculosis-like lesions in slaughter swine in Finland. Nord Vet Med 17:17–21.

WOLINSKY, E., AND SCHAEFER, W. B. 1973. Proposed numbering scheme for mycobacterial serotypes of agglutination. Int J Syst Bacteriol 23:182–183.

YUGI, H.; NEMOTO, H.; AND WATANABE, K. 1972. Serotypes of *Mycobacterium intracellulare* of porcine origin. Natl Inst Anim Health Q (Tokyo) 12:168–169.

51 Miscellaneous Bacterial Infections

D. J. Taylor

S. E. Sanford

J. E. T. Jones

J. A. Yager

Pseudomonas

D. J. Taylor

PSEUDOMONAS is a genus of gram-negative bacteria consisting of a large number of species. Most of these live freely in the environment and are of little or no importance to the pig. Three species are of relevance, however, all in different ways: *P. methylotropha* is used to produce microbial protein from methyl alcohol, and this protein is used in pig feed; *P. pseudomallei* produces melioidosis, a disease characterized by widespread granulomas in pigs in tropical and subtropical regions; *P. aeruginosa* has been isolated worldwide from a large number of different pathologic conditions. In most of these it is clearly not a cause of the lesions in which it is found, and no single distinctive clinical syndrome can be attributed to it. It may have to be considered, however, when designing control and treatment programs for a number of syndromes.

P. aeruginosa is the species most likely to be encountered in disease situations. Since it is antimicrobial resistant and easy to cultivate and identify presumptively, it is often reported by laboratories, particularly in samples submitted by mail in which it can grow at room temperature. Little experimental evidence exists for a causal role in any distinct syndrome. The organism is widely distributed in the environment.

ETIOLOGY. *P. aeruginosa* is a thin, gram-negative bacillus, 1.5 μm in length and 0.5 μm in diameter. It is aerobic and microaerophilic and grows readily on even the simplest of laboratory media to produce colonies 3–5 mm in diameter, grayish in color, and nonhemolytic in young cultures; it produces a distinctive green pigment (pyocyanin) that diffuses into the medium. This green color and its characteristic smell make it readily detectable in culture even in small numbers. On MacConkey and other media that detect nonlactose-fermenting organisms such as *Salmonella* spp., it appears as a nonlactose fermenter and may initially be confused with salmonellae. The organism is resistant to many antimicrobials and is sensitive in general to only a few (gentamicin, carbenicillin, polymyxin B), although some isolates may also be sensitive in vitro to neomycin, streptomycin, and occasionally to chloramphenicol and tetracyclines. It is also capable of growth on or in some disinfectants; can grow readily in products such as cetrimide, especially when diluted for use; and can survive treatment with low concentrations of phenols. It is, however, a nonsporing organism and can readily be destroyed by heat; it is not very resistant to drying or chlorine disinfectants.

EPIDEMIOLOGY. *P. aeruginosa* can be isolated from feeds and water and is probably present at low levels in almost any environment. In the normal pig it may be found in small numbers in the gut and feces. These reservoirs of the organism can lead to the infection of wounds by contact or inhalation. In superficial wound infections, high environmental humidity, serous discharge from the wound, or antimicrobial treatment can all increase the likelihood of infection with *P. aeruginosa*.

PATHOGENESIS. The pathogenesis of *P. aeruginosa* infections in the pig has rarely been studied in detail. It produces a number of toxins, can survive phagocytosis, and may be seen within neutrophils in abscesses. Experimental studies of its role in atrophic rhinitis suggested that it was unable alone to initiate disease in the nasal cavities of specific-pathogen-free pigs (Miniats and Johnson 1980). There is evidence that some strains may produce enterotoxin, and gut loop

627

studies have shown that strains of porcine origin produce fluid accumulation (Baljer and Barrett 1979; Choudhary et al. 1983). Baljer and Barrett attributed their results to enterotoxin production, but *P. aeruginosa* enterotoxin appears to act only in the anterior part of the jejunum and its elaboration is unlikely to account for all the changes seen in enteric infections with *P. aeruginosa*. In cystitis, vaginal infections, and mastitis, it appears to enter as an ascending infection and produce its effects by the elaboration of toxins and endotoxin release. In the urinary tract its ability to produce urease and split urea may increase the irritation produced.

Skin infections appear to result from surface contamination and the organism is rarely recovered from the body tissues, although it can be recovered from local lymph nodes in some cases. Septicemias in the newborn are usually the result of spread from umbilical infections. In older animals they are associated with some form of immunodepression.

CLINICAL SIGNS. There are no specific clinical signs associated with *P. aeruginosa* infection. The organism is associated with chronic disease and inflammation. In some tissues such as the lung or kidney it may give rise to abscesses, and discharges associated with it often contain pus. Conditions in which it is present rarely respond easily to antibiotic treatment.

P. aeruginosa is commonly isolated from the nasal conchae in chronic atrophic rhinitis, especially where some antimicrobial has been given. It can be recovered from chronic cases of pneumonia. Pigs with pneumonias complicated by *P. aeruginosa* often have a fever (to 40°C), may have bronchitis, and may be emaciated. Apart from a failure to respond to antimicrobials, there is no distinct clinical feature of *P. aeruginosa* pneumonia, and the involvement of the organism is usually sporadic and late.

In enteritis the organism may be associated with chronic watery, brownish diarrheas, but again these provide no obvious clue to the presence of the organism. Infection is commonly found after antimicrobial therapy. Septicemia with high fever may occur in neonates and resembles "colisepticemia" and may also occur in immunocompromised older animals. Mastitis and cystitis in the sow are also caused by the organism and clinically resemble those produced by *Escherichia coli* or *Klebsiella* strains. Perhaps the only site in which *P. aeruginosa* may be identified clinically is in skin lesions. When these are chronic, moist, and suppurating or with serum exudation, crusted, and chronically inflamed, the presence of *P. aeruginosa* may be suspected. Such lesions respond poorly to treatment and animals are often debilitated. It is commonly found in the late stages of exudative epidermitis and may prolong the condition.

LESIONS. Few specific lesions can be associated with *P. aeruginosa* infection. Its involvement in atrophic rhinitis cannot easily be identified on gross inspection. Varying degrees of bronchitis may be present in the lung; it can be isolated from pneumonias in which hemorrhagic areas, congestion, and edema are common. Gram-negative rods may be seen in neutrophils in clumps in microabscesses and capillaries or other sites that have undergone postmortem change. There are few distinctive features except perhaps for the dilation of capillaries in the lamina propria and the presence of large numbers of neutrophils crossing into the lumen in addition to changes associated with the underlying cause of the enteritis. Changes in the mammary gland, bladder, and vagina are similar to those associated with coliform infections. In skin lesions there is often evidence of edema or fibrosis in the thickness of the dermis; serous exudates are common. In histologic sections of *P. aeruginosa*–complicated exudative epidermitis, the presence of bacilli rather than the otherwise predominant clumps of cocci may be apparent.

DIAGNOSIS. Diagnosis is almost entirely bacteriologic and relies upon culture. The involvement of *P. aeruginosa* may be suspected if any chronic skin condition fails to heal in humid conditions or after routine antimicrobial therapy with compounds specifically active against gram-positive organisms.

The organism is not sufficiently distinctive to be identified in Gram-stained smears but is readily isolated in bacterial culture on a number of media. Presumptive identification by its colonial morphology, smell, appearance as a nonlactose-fermenting colony on MacConkey agar, and production of green pigment is usually sufficient.

TREATMENT. *P. aeruginosa* is resistant to many antimicrobials. Infections can be treated using aminoglycosides, especially gentamicin, and chloramphenicol or tetracyclines. Polymyxin B and carbenicillin are extremely useful, but because of toxicity or cost they would be unsuitable for most uses in pigs. In vitro sensitivity testing of isolates may be the easiest way to determine the most suitable antimicrobial. Antimicrobial treatment should be supplemented by hygiene and, in the case of skin wounds, by washing with cetrimide-based compounds. Affected animals should be allowed to recover in warm, dry environments and reinfection prevented by cleaning of water systems and chlorination of the water supply.

PREVENTION. Prevention is best carried out by prompt control of diseases likely to cause lesions that can be colonized by *P. aeruginosa* (e.g., atrophic rhinitis, swine dysentery, neonatal diarrhea, exudative epidermitis) and by attention to other predisposing causes such as teat damage (mastitis) and perineal soiling (cystitis and metritis). Maintenance of a dry, clean environment and clean water will also be of value. Use of chlorinated water prevents infection by this route.

MELIOIDOSIS.   In tropical and subtropical regions such as those of Asia and northern Australia, pigs may become infected by *P. pseudomallei,* which is a short, gram-negative rod, 0.8 by 1.5 μm that produces rough or mucoid colonies on a wide variety of laboratory media. It is present in water and soil in tropical and subtropical areas and may infect pigs when water supplies are contaminated. Infection is often clinically inapparent but has been associated with clinical signs (Olds and Lewis 1955; Omar et al. 1962; Laws and Hall 1964; Rogers and Andersen 1970). Clinical signs include a raised rectal temperature (40–42°C, 104–108°F) for up to 4 days, unsteady gait, lameness or weakness, slight nasal discharge, and subcutaneous swellings of the limbs. Deaths may occur but are rare in adults in which abortions and uterine discharges have been recorded.

Lesions are found in slaughter pigs in which clinical signs have not been seen and in those that have died from the disease. They consist of large abscesses in the lungs, liver, spleen, kidney, and mesenteric and subcutaneous lymph nodes. The organism can be isolated from them. Melioidosis may be suspected on clinical grounds especially when prolonged raised rectal temperatures and unsteady gait are associated with subcutaneous swellings of the limbs. More frequently, diagnosis is based on the creamy abscesses found at slaugh-

ter or on the bacteriologic results needed to confirm the presence of *P. pseudomallei* (Ketterer et al. 1986). A hypersensitivity test resembling a tuberculin test (the melioidin test) and serum-agglutination and complement-fixation tests have all been described and can be used to confirm a diagnosis in the live pig.

Treatment with tetracyclines has been described, and the disease can be prevented by use of clean or chlorinated water supplies and preventing access to contaminated soil. As the disease is of public health importance, infected carcasses should be disposed of safely.

REFERENCES
BALJER, G., AND BARRETT, J. T. 1979. Demonstration of enterotoxin-forming strains of *P. aeruginosa* by the ligated ileal loop test in piglets. Zentralbl Veterinaermed [B] 26:740–747.
CHOUDHARY, S. P.; SINGH, S. N.; AND NARAIJAN, K. G. 1983. *Pseudomonas aeruginosa* as an aetiological agent of piglet diarrhoea. Indian J Anim Sci 53:629–634.
KETTERER, P. J.; WEBSTER, W. R.; SHIELD, J.; ARTHUR, R. J.; BLACKALL, P. J.; AND THOMAS, A. D. 1986. Melioidosis in intensive piggeries in South Eastern Queensland. Aust Vet J 63:146–149.
LAWS, L., AND HALL, W. T. K. 1964. Melioidosis in animals in North Queensland. IV. Epidemiology. Aust Vet J 40:309–314.
MINIATS, O. P., AND JOHNSON, J. A. 1980. Experimental atrophic rhinitis in growing pigs. Can J Comp Med 44:358–365.
OLDS, R. J., AND LEWIS, F. A. 1955. Melioidosis in a pig. Aust Vet J 31:273–274.
OMAR, A. R.; CHEAH, K. K.; AND MAHENDRANATHAN, T. 1962. Observations on porcine melioidosis in Malaya. Br Vet J 118:421–429.
ROGERS, R. J., AND ANDERSEN, D. J. 1970. Intrauterine infection of a pig by *Pseudomonas pseudomallei.* Aust Vet J 46:292.

Chlamydia

D. J. Taylor

CHLAMYDIAS are small intracellular bacteria that cause disease in many mammalian species and are widespread in birds. The most widespread species is *Chlamydia psittaci,* which has been demonstrated in cases of pneumonia, pleurisy, pericarditis, arthritis, orchitis, and uterine infections. The last two are often associated with abortion. Most recent work on *C. psittaci* in pigs has been carried out in Germany, and a comprehensive review of the literature and experimental studies has been published (Stellmacher et al. 1983). Elsewhere, chlamydial infections in pigs have been reported relatively rarely, possibly because the organism may be difficult to identify in material from clinical cases unless the laboratory concerned is familiar with it.

ETIOLOGY.   *C. psittaci* is a gram-negative bacterium that can only multiply inside living cells. It is unusual among bacteria in that it exists outside the cell only as an inactive, trypsin-resistant, infectious particle 0.2–0.3 μm (200–300 nm) in diameter known as an elementary body (Fig. 51.1). This body has an electron-dense core packed with DNA and surrounded by a trilaminar cytoplasmic membrane, outside of which lies a further trilaminar envelope and then a cell wall with projections that may be associated with attachment to cells. Within 6–9 hours after the elementary body has entered a cell, it forms a reticulate body 1 μm (1000 nm) in diameter. This body divides by binary fission to form further reticulate bodies in an inclusion within the host cell. At this

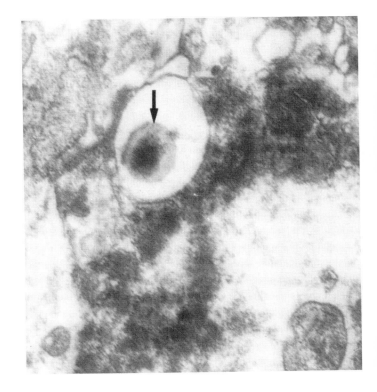

51.1. Electron micro-graph of elementary body (arrow) of *Chlamydia* sp. in an aborted placenta. × 52,500.

stage the infected host cell may divide to infected daughter cells, which may account for latent infections seen in animal hosts. Within 20 hours of the first division of the reticulate body, some begin to mature into elementary bodies. The chlamydial inclusions may occupy up to three-quarters of the cell volume and contain up to 10,000 elementary bodies. Infected cells may lyse to release the elementary bodies or these may be budded from persistently infected cells.

C. psittaci can be grown in the laboratory by inoculation of the yolk sac of 6- to 8-day-old embryonated hens eggs and in neonatal mice. Most laboratories now use cell cultures, usually McCoy or L929 cells in which the chlamydia grow readily. In some cases, isolation can be improved by treatment of the cells, using irradiation or cycloheximide (1 μg/ml), and by centrifugation of the chlamydia onto the cells.

Several biotypes of *C. psittaci* have been identified by their differential growth in cell cultures in the presence of tissue culture medium supplemented with amino acids such as arginine, isoleucine, and methionine (Johnson 1984), but there is no information about the biotypes present in pigs.

Antigenic differences between strains have also been described in *C. psittaci* isolates obtained from animal and bird species other than pigs, but once again the situation in the pig is not known.

EPIDEMIOLOGY. *C. psittaci* occurs in many avian species and is particularly common in pi-

geons and doves but may occur in almost any bird. Some mammals such as sheep, cattle, and rodents may be infected. All these species may form a reservoir of infection for the pig. The major routes of transmission are by inhalation of aerosols of *C. psittaci* elementary bodies, either fresh or in dust, from respiratory, genital tract, or enteric infections; by ingestion of contaminated feed; and by contact, particularly venereal, in the case of genital tract infections.

Infection in the pig has been poorly documented but has been reported from the United States (Willigan and Beamer 1955; Popischil and Wood 1987), Britain (Wilson and Plummer 1966; Harris 1976), Rumania (Sorodoc et al. 1961), Germany (Stellmacher et al. 1983), and in other countries.

Serologic surveys suggest that complement-fixing and microagglutinating antibodies may be present in up to 23% of slaughter pigs (Wilson and Plummer 1966). Most antibody titers are low (1:8–1:128), but titers as high as 1:1024 have been recorded (Wilson and Plummer 1966). It is clear, therefore, that the infection or exposure to it is widespread among pigs.

Studies of the distribution of infection within infected herds are less common, but *C. psittaci* was isolated from 73 of 309 samples from 13 infected herds. Samples from which the organism was isolated included semen samples from boars; fetuses, both live and aborted; sows; lungs, joints, and organs such as liver and spleen from piglets; store pigs; and pigs at slaughter. It is therefore clear that all ages of pig may be infected. The presence of low levels of antibody in piglets may suggest maternal antibody transfer.

PATHOGENESIS. Elementary bodies of *C. psittaci* enter by the respiratory, oral, or genital routes and enter epithelial cells in which they multiply or are taken up by macrophages and distributed to lymph nodes. Infection may be local at the portal of infection and remain inapparent or latent; may cause local disease such as pneumonia, enteritis, or disturbances of reproduction; or may become generalized. *C. psittaci* isolates of avian, bovine, ovine, and porcine origin have been used in experimental infections; but strains of porcine origin appear to be most virulent for the pig, provided they have not become yolk sac or tissue culture adapted. There appears to be some adaptation of strains to the method of transmission, in that strains of genital origin (Kielstein et al. 1983) do not appear to cause severe pneumonia and parenteral inoculation was found necessary to reproduce arthritis with an arthritis isolate. Pneumonia has been consistently produced by intranasal or intratracheal inoculation with porcine strains (Kielstein et al. 1983; Martin et al. 1983; Stellmacher et al. 1983), but spread of infection to other organs were found consistently. These studies suggest that an acute exudative or interstitial pneumonia with peribronchiolar cellular cuffing and a lobular distribution occurs within 4–8 days of infection. Lesions are fully developed by 8–12 days postinfection and are largely resolved by 4 weeks after infection, although infection may still be present in the lungs. Contact infections suggest that natural infection is normally less severe and that reinfection after 3–4 weeks results in little or no further disease. This development of immunity is accompanied by development of complement-fixing antibodies to *C. psittaci*, which appear within 2 weeks and remain detectable for a variable period.

In genital infections, infected semen given to sows has resulted in the birth of weak piglets and continued shedding of chlamydia for up to 20 months.

CLINICAL SIGNS. Many chlamydial infections are inapparent, but consistent features of respiratory tract and generalized infections include an incubation period of 3–11 days followed by inappetence and a rise in rectal temperature to 39–41°C. Pneumonia and conjunctivitis may occur. Evidence of pleurisy or pericarditis may be detected by auscultation, and articular involvement by lameness in one or more joints. In slaughter pigs, polyarthritis associated with synovitis has been reported. Other disturbances of gait include weakness in piglets and nervous signs in pigs of all age groups. Fatal infections are most commonly reported in younger animals.

Diarrhea has been reported to be associated with chlamydial infection (Popischil and Wood 1987), but many reports deal with genital tract infection and disturbances in reproduction. In the boar, infection is associated with orchitis, epididymitis, and urethritis; while infections in gilts and sows have resulted in late abortions and the birth of dead or weak piglets. Serologic and isolation studies suggest that many genital tract infections are clinically inapparent.

LESIONS. Lesions in which *C. psittaci* has been demonstrated often contain other agents, and many descriptions of the lesions found in field cases may not take into account the presence of agents such as mycoplasmas or viruses. The large body of work on respiratory disease suggests that lung lesions are distributed posteriorly in most cases, although occasional patches of pneumonia may occur in the anterior lobes (Harris et al. 1984).

Lesions are irregular and raised, of firm consistency, extending deep into the lung tissue, limited by lobular boundaries, and clearly demarcated from adjacent grossly normal tissue. Early lesions are pale red, becoming grayish as they age. Enlarged bronchial lymph nodes may be present. The microscopic findings include thickening of the alveolar septae by capillaries, septal edema, and neutrophils in peribronchial and subepithelial sites. Neutrophils and macrophages are common in the alveolar lumina, and in some areas this exudate occludes terminal bronchioles. Edema and massive epithelial cell shedding have been reported in severely affected lung lobules (Martin et al. 1983). Peribronchiolar accumulations of plasma cells, lymphocytes, and macrophages are also common. There appears to be no pleurisy in experimental infections, and no gross changes in other organs were reported beyond enlargement of the bronchial lymph nodes.

The other lesions reported to occur in field cases include pericarditis, pleurisy, hemorrhages of kidney and bladder, and enlargement of the spleen. There is little doubt that synovitis accompanies the arthritic changes and that orchitis in boars is accompanied by interstitial edema and tubular degeneration. Aborted piglets may be mummified; stillborn or weak piglets may have lung, liver, or enteric lesions. The organism has been isolated from pseudomembranous colitis in experimental *S. typhimurium* infections (Popischil and Wood 1987).

DIAGNOSIS. The clinical signs of *C. psittaci* infection are not distinctive, but it must be considered as a possible cause of pneumonia, polyarthritis, enteritis, late abortion, stillbirths, and mummified piglets and of orchitis in boars. The gross lesions in the lung may be more suggestive of *C. psittaci* infection, but any firm diagnosis involves laboratory tests. These are serologic (complement fixation, using heat-stable *C. psittaci* antigen), microscopic agglutination (Wilson and Plummer 1966), and indirect immunofluorescence. Complement-fixing antibodies should ideally be found to rise in paired serum samples, but the presence of high levels of antibody (1:256) may be sufficient. As only low levels of complement-fixing antibodies may arise from infections in sites such as the respiratory, enteric, and genital tracts, the absence of high levels of complement-fixing antibody does not rule out *C. psittaci* as a cause of disease.

C. psittaci itself may be detected in smears of discharges or postmortem specimens and in histologic specimens after staining by Giemsa's method. The organisms are tiny (0.2–1.0 mµ) and are present in large numbers in cells. A more satisfactory method is to use Koster's stain in which a fixed smear is stained for 5 minutes with carbol fuchsin, decolorized for 30 seconds with 0.25% acetic acid, and counterstained for 1 minute with 1% aqueous Loeffler's methylene blue. The chlamydia appear as clusters of intracellular red dots against a blue background (Fig. 51.2). Most specific of all is the immunofluorescence test using specific fluorescein-conjugated antibody to *C. psittaci* (e.g., Imagen) to demonstrate infected cells. Immunoperoxidase tests have been described (Chasey et al. 1981).

Isolation can also be carried out by the inoculation of young mice and of 6–8 day fertile hens eggs. More than one subculture may be necessary before infection can be detected. Cell cultures us-

ing L929 or McCoy cell lines treated with cycloheximide (1 µg/ml) may be inoculated by centrifugation (Farmer et al. 1982) in a tissue culture medium at pH 7.0. Inclusions are at a maximum after 48 hours of incubation at 35–37°C.

Transport media for chlamydia should contain streptomycin (50–100 mg/l) or gentamicin (10–20 mg/l) with vancomycin (100 µg/l) and nystatin (25 mg/l). Samples can be stored at 4°C or at −60°C. Handling *C. psittaci* is dangerous and severe human infections and death can result. Appropriate safety precautions should be observed.

TREATMENT. A number of antimicrobials have some effect on *C. psittaci* in vitro, but the most satisfactory compounds for treatment are the tetracyclines. Treatment for inadequate times may result in relapse; for complete elimination or suppression of infection to the latent state, 21-day treatment should be given at the therapeutic level. Tetracycline, oxytetracycline, and chlortetracycline can all be used in drinking water or feed. Long-acting oxytetracycline injections are useful for treating individual infected animals.

PREVENTION. Pigs should be prevented from coming into contact with infected birds or their droppings or with other infected mammalian species. Infected pigs should be maintained in separate air and drainage spaces from susceptible animals. Any infected breeding stock should be used only after tetracycline treatment or kept with

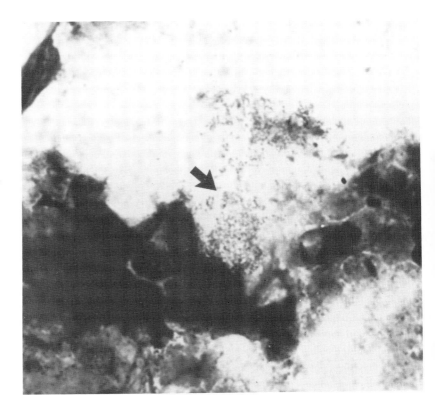

51.2. Photomicrograph of elementary bodies of *Chlamydia* sp. (arrow) in an aborted placenta. ×1200.

other infected stock in isolation until sufficient uninfected animals are available to replace them. Disinfection with phenols and formalin fumigation will eliminate elementary bodies from buildings.

REFERENCES

CHASEY, D.; DAVIS, P.; AND DAWSON, M. 1981. Immunoperoxidase detection of *Chlamydia ovis* in experimentally infected cell culture. Br Vet J 137:634–638.

FARMER, H.; CHALMERS, W. S. K.; AND WOOLCOCK, P. R. 1982. *Chlamydia psittaci* isolated from the eyes of domestic ducks (*Anas platyrhynchos*) with conjunctivitis and rhinitis. Vet Rec 110:59.

JOHNSON, F. W. A. 1984. Isolation of *C. psittaci* from nasal and conjunctival exudate of a cat. Vet Rec 114:342–344.

HARRIS, J. W. 1976. Chlamydial antibodies in pigs in Scotland. Vet Rec 98:505–506.

HARRIS, J. W.; HUNTER, A. R.; AND MARTIN, D. A. 1984. Experimental chlamydial pneumonia in pigs. Comp Immun Microbiol Infect Dis 7:19–26.

KIELSTEIN, P.; STELLMACHER, H.; HORSCH, F.; AND MARTIN, J. 1983. Zur Chlamydien Infektion des Schweines I. Mitteilung zur experimentellen Chlamydien-Pneumonie des Schweines. Arch Exp Veterinaermed 37:569–586.

MARTIN, J.; KIELSTEIN, P.; STELLMACHER, P.; AND HORSCH, F. 1983. Zur Chlamydien Infektion des Schweines. II. Mitteilung: Pathologische-histologische Besonderhecten der experimentellen Chlamydien Pneumonie des Schweines. Arch Exp Veterinaermed 37:939–949.

POSPISCHIL, A., AND WOOD, R. L. 1987. Intestinal *Chlamydia* in pigs. Vet Pathol 24:568–570.

SORODOC, G.; SURDAN, C.; AND SARATEANU, D. 1961. Cercetari asupra identificarii virusului pneumoniei enzootice a porcilor. Stud Cerc Inframicrobiol 12[Suppl]:355–364.

STELLMACHER, H.; KIELSTEIN, P.; HORSCH, F.; AND MARTIN, J. 1983. Zur Bedeutung der Chlamydien-Infektion des Schweines unter besonder Berucksichtigung der Pneumonien. Monatsh Veterinaermed 38:601–606.

WILLIGAN, D. A., AND BEAMER, P. D. 1955. Isolation of a transmissible agent from pericarditis of swine. J Am Vet Med Assoc 126:118–122.

WILSON, M. R., AND PLUMMER, P. A. 1966. A survey of pig sera for the presence of antibodies to the P.L.V. group of organisms. J Comp Pathol 76:427–433.

Actinobacillus suis

S. E. Sanford

SEPTICEMIA and death caused by *Actinobacillus suis* and occasionally by *A. equuli* in sucking and recently weaned pigs have been reported sporadically from several pig-rearing countries (Van Dorssen and Jaartsveld 1962; Cutlip et al. 1972; Windsor 1973; Mair et al. 1974; MacDonald et al. 1976). *A. suis* outbreaks resembling erysipelas have been reported in older pigs and sows in Canada (Miniats et al. 1989). Most outbreaks occur as sudden death of one or several piglets in one, two, or rarely, multiple litters in individual herds. Infection with *A. suis* is probably widespread but disease is seldom reported.

ETIOLOGY. *A. suis* is a gram-negative, nonmotile, noncapsulated, aerobic and facultative anaerobic coccobacillus, 0.5–3 μm long and about 0.8 μm wide. Filamentous forms occur. The organism grows on MacConkey agar. Grayish adherent, circular, translucent colonies measuring 1–2 mm form on blood agar within 24 hours. On horse blood agar, colonies are surrounded by a narrow but distinct zone of alpha hemolysis and a wide zone of beta (complete) hemolysis on calf and sheep blood agars. Biochemically, *A. suis* can be differentiated from other related bacteria isolated from pigs by its ability to produce catalase, oxidase, and urease; hydrolysis of esculin; and acid production without gas from arabinose, lactose, salicin, and trehalose, but not from mannitol or sorbitol. *A. equuli* differs from *A. suis* by being nonhemolytic; producing acid from mannitol but not from arabinose, cellulose, and salicin; and not splitting esculin. *A. suis* is pathogenic for mice; *A. equuli* is not. *A. suis* and *A. equuli* are killed within 15 minutes at 60°C and are sensitive to most disinfectants. They die out within a few days in culture and pathologic material.

EPIDEMIOLOGY. *A. suis* can be carried in the tonsils and nostrils of healthy pigs of any age, and the vaginas of apparently healthy sows (Ross et al. 1972). Clinical disease occurs in neonates and sucking pigs and up to just after weaning age, and less commonly in sows and mature swine (Miniats et al. 1989; Sanford et al. 1990). With the separation of pigs and horses in modern farming systems, infection in pigs by *A. equuli* seems to have diminished.

Outbreaks of *A. suis* infections occur more frequently in minimal disease and other high–health status herds (Miniats et al. 1989; Sanford et al. 1990), possibly because the lack of immunity in these pigs allows virulent *A. suis* organisms to express their pathogenic potential.

PATHOGENESIS. The pathogenesis of *A. suis* infection has not been defined. Infection probably occurs via the upper respiratory tract although invasion through abrasions in the skin and mucous membranes is also likely. In susceptible animals, septic emboli then spread rapidly to multiple organs and tissues throughout the body and are either trapped in vessels or adhere to vessel walls, forming microcolonies surrounded by areas of hemorrhage and necrosis. Virulence factors of *A. suis* have not been specifically determined but lipopolysaccharide, polysaccharides in the cell wall, outer-membrane proteins, and a 104-kD hemolysin are all potential virulence factors likely to be involved in pathogenesis. Pigs may die within 15 hours of infection.

CLINICAL SIGNS. Sudden death of sucking piglets, 2 days to 4 weeks old, in one or more litters is often the first indication of an outbreak of actinobacillosis. Deaths are sometimes mistakenly attributed to crushing. Cyanosis, petechial hemorrhages, fever (up to 40°C, 104°F), and panting, sometimes accompanied by shaking and/or paddling, may be seen prior to death in sucking pigs. Congestion of extremities (leading to necrosis of feet, tail, and ears) and swollen joints may occur. In weaned pigs, anorexia, fever, a persistent cough, and pneumonia are reported; recovered animals may remain unthrifty. In outbreaks in mature animals, fever, round and rhomboid erythematous skin lesions, inappetence, and sudden deaths are characteristic, but mortality is usually low. Metritis, meningitis, and abortion have been reported in sows. The disease may be confused with erysipelas, especially when skin lesions develop.

LESIONS. The most striking gross lesions are petechial to ecchymotic hemorrhages in any of the following organs: lung, kidney, heart, liver, spleen, skin, and intestines. The lesions are especially prominent and most frequently seen in the lung where lobular necrosis and serofibrinous exudates also occur (Fig. 51.3). Increased serous or serofibrinous exudates may occur in the thorax

and the pericardium. Pleurisy, pericarditis, and miliary abscesses in the lung, liver, skin, mesenteric lymph nodes, and kidney may be seen in older sucking or weaned pigs. Arthritis (Van Dorssen and Jaartsveld 1962) and valvular endocarditis (Jones and Simmons 1971) have been reported. In mature animals, numerous round, rhomboid, or irregular skin lesions are common (Fig. 51.4).

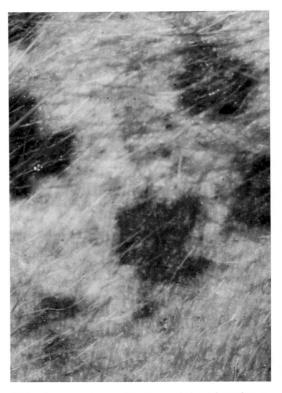

51.4. Irregular to roughly diamond-shaped erythematous skin lesions resembling erysipelas in a sow with *A. suis* septicemia.

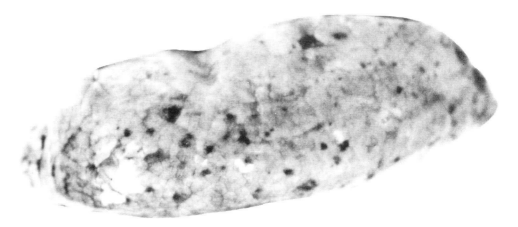

51.3. Lung of 3-day-old piglet with actinobacillosis. Note the hemorrhages.

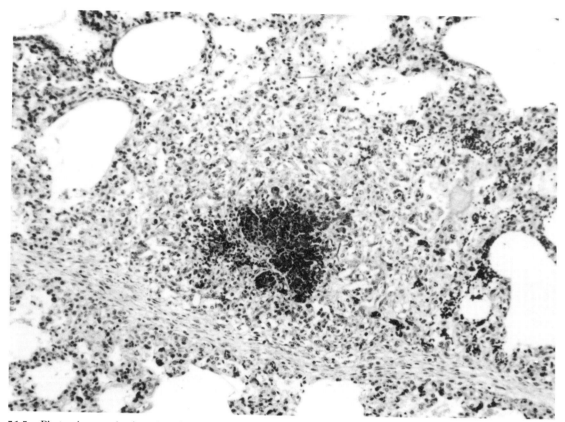

51.5. Photomicrograph of a microabscess in the lung as shown in Figure 51.3. Note the microcolonies of bacteria. H & E. × 110.

Histologically, bacterial thromboemboli with accompanying fibrinohemorrhagic necrosis in randomly scattered vessels in the lung, liver, kidney, skin, spleen, heart, pericardium, meninges, and brain are characteristic (Fig. 51.5). Bacterial emboli may be surrounded by radiating eosinophilic clublike colonies. Most frequently and usually most severely affected is the lung where there may be large coalescing areas of necrosis.

DIAGNOSIS. Sudden mortality in sucking pigs in individual litters in herds with previous *A. suis* outbreaks usually indicates a new outbreak. The gross lesions of hemorrhages and necrosis in the lung and/or skin and kidney, and splenic enlargement are suggestive of *A. suis* infection. In mature pigs, fever, inappetence, and skin lesions resembling erysipelas, especially in herds already vaccinated against erysipelas, should raise a suspicion of *A. suis*. Microscopic lesions consisting of bacterial emboli, necrosis, and inflammatory cells in the lung and other organs are also suggestive. Diagnosis, however, depends on isolation of *A. suis* or *A. equuli* from the lesions.

TREATMENT. *A. suis* is sensitive to most commonly used antibiotics. Since outbreaks in suck-

ing pigs are so acute and unpredictable, however, treatment is usually too late. In older pigs, response to treatment with ampicillin (5 mg/kg) orally or parenterally, injectable benzathine-procaine penicillin G (2.25–3.0 × 10⁶ IU) intramuscularly (IM), injectable procaine penicillin (1.8–2.4 × 10⁶ IU) IM, or in-feed medication with oxytetracycline hydrochloride (550 g/ton) and/or streptomycin for periods up to 1 week has all been excellent.

PREVENTION. Autogenous bacterins have not been critically evaluated but have been used in herds with repeated *A. suis* outbreaks with apparent success.

REFERENCES
CUTLIP, R. C.; AMTOWER, W. C.; AND ZINOBER, M. R. 1972. Septic embolic actinobacillosis of swine: A case report and laboratory reproduction of the disease. Am J Vet Res 33:1621–1626.
JONES, J. E. T., AND SIMMONS, J. R. 1971. Endocarditis in the pig caused by *Actinobacillus equuli*. A field and an experimental case. Br Vet J 127:25–29.
MACDONALD, D. W.; HEWITT, M. P.; WILTON, G. S.; RAWLUK, S.; AND CHILDS, L. 1976. *Actinobacillus suis* infections in Alberta swine, 1973–1975: Pathology and bacteriology. Can Vet J 17:251–254.
MAIR, N. S.; RANDALL, C. J.; THOMAS, G. W.; HAR-

BOURNE, J. F.; McCREA, C. T.; AND COWL, K. P. 1974. *Actinobacillus suis* infection in pigs: A report of four outbreaks and two sporadic cases. J Comp Pathol 84:113–119.

MINIATS, O. P.; SPINATO, M. T.; AND SANFORD, S. E. 1989. *Actinobacillus suis* septicemia in mature swine. Two outbreaks resembling erysipelas. Can Vet J 30:943–947.

ROSS, R. F.; HALL, J. E.; ORNING, A. P.; AND DALE, S. E. 1972. Characterization of an *Actinobacillus* isolated from the sow vagina. Int J Syst Bacteriol 22:39–46.

SANFORD, S. E.; JOSEPHSON, G. K. A.; REHMTULLA, A. J.; AND TILKER, A. M. E. 1990. *Actinobacillus suis* infection in pigs in southwestern Ontario. Can Vet J 31:443–447.

VANDORSSEN, C. A.; AND JAARTSVELD, F. H. J. 1962. *Actinobacillus suis* (novo species), a bacterium occurring in swine. Tijdschr Diergeneeskd 87:450–458.

WINDSOR, R. S. 1973. *Actinobacillus equuli* infection in a litter of pigs and a review of previous reports on similar infections. Vet Rec 92:178–180.

Yeasts

D. J. Taylor

YEASTS ARE FUNGI that are normally single celled but can form filaments or pseudohyphae. Some can sporulate to produce resistant spores. They occur in the food of the pig and in dusts. Some species are commonly found on the skin and mucous membranes. In certain situations, yeasts of a number of species (but principally *Candida albicans*) may be isolated from inflammatory lesions of the oral cavity, gastrointestinal tract, urogenital tract, and skin. Their isolation from such lesions is often associated with use of therapeutic antimicrobials, especially in piglets.

Yeasts may also form a major part of the diet of the pig, as either yeast wastes from brewing or distilling or yeast grown and treated specifically as a component of rations. These yeasts can provide high protein and, in particular, high lysine. Traces of paraffin waxes have been found in the fat of pigs fed on yeasts grown on that substrate, and there are some reports of diarrhea and increased kidney weights in yeast-fed pigs. Most reports indicate that inclusion of yeasts in the ration does not adversely affect the health of pigs.

ETIOLOGY. Yeasts identified in infections in pigs belong to a number of genera. Those of the genus *Candida* are most commonly isolated, although species of *Torulopsis, Trichosporon, Rhodotorula, Pichia, Pityrosporum,* and *Cryptococcus* have been recorded. *Cryptococcus neoformans* has been isolated from cryptococcosis in pigs, but the disease is rare in this species and occurs only where the organism is commonly found in other livestock.

Candida albicans is the species of *Candida* most frequently reported; but *C. tropicalis, C. pseudotropicalis, C. brumptii, C. sloofii, C. rugosa, C. lipolytica, C. krusei,* and *C. scottii* have been isolated from lesions or feces of apparently healthy pigs. Since *C. albicans* is associated most frequently with specific lesions, both it and its relationship to these lesions will be described here.

Candida spp. are spherical cells, 2.5–6 μm in diameter. They reproduce by budding (blastospores) and chlamydospores, which bud from filaments (or pseudohyphae) on chlamydospore agar, particularly under reduced oxygen tension at 25°C (Carter 1979). Pseudohyphae and oval yeast forms are found in lesions. *Candida* spp. grow readily on Sabouraud agar, malt agar, and often on blood agar incubated aerobically. They form 1–2 mm, creamy white, opaque circular colonies within 24–48 hours at 37°C and within 2–4 days at 25°C. *C. albicans* produces chlamydospores and germ tubes but no pellicle when grown in broth and ferments glucose, maltose, and galactose, but not sucrose or lactose. It is not known to produce toxins, although there have been suggestions that it can produce keratolytic enzymes in the presence of glucose.

EPIDEMIOLOGY. *C. albicans* has been identified in the bedding, feed, and water supplies of pigs. It occurs on the skin and in the oral cavity, stomach, and intestines of normal pigs in small numbers. It can be shed in the feces and exhaled in droplets by animals with oral infections. It may be isolated from the feces of birds, rodents, and other animal species and may cause disease in those species that may form a source of the organism for pigs. Organisms in the environment may multiply in moist conditions in the presence of suitable substrates such as spilled meal or garbage.

PATHOGENESIS. *C. albicans* appears to colonize debilitated skin surfaces and lesions on other mucous surfaces. The predisposing factors appear to include the effects of artificial rearing of piglets (Osborne et al. 1960) and chronic enteritis often associated with treatment with broad-spectrum antimicrobials. Gastric ulcers appear to be colonized by yeasts rather than initiated by them, and cutaneous candidiasis often results from exposure to continually warm moist conditions that are accompanied by poor hygiene and food residues (Reynolds et al. 1968).

Invasion of mucous surfaces appears to follow accumulation of yeast forms on the debilitated surface and develops with pseudohyphal invasion of the superficial layers of the epithelium. Systemic invasion is rare and the inflammatory response to infection is slight.

CLINICAL SIGNS. Yeasts have been implicated in chronic gastroenteritis in piglets, gastric ulceration, and cutaneous and oropharyngeal infections. Piglets are often 3–5 days old (more commonly, 7–14 days) before yeast infection complicates the underlying problem. The clinical signs of gastroenteritis complicated by yeasts are not specific, but there is often a history of dullness, inappetence, vomiting, and chronic diarrhea that may be grayish or blackish depending on the diet and has failed to respond to the use of broad-spectrum antibiotics such as tetracyclines. Piglets may die after 10–14 days of illness. In many cases there are characteristic yellowish white, circular, 2–5 mm lesions on the tongue and hard palate, which resemble colonies of *C. albicans* on artificial media. When scraped off, no macroscopic changes are seen beneath them. Cutaneous candidiasis often presents as a moist gray exudate on the surface of the skin of the abdomen with little or no effect on the hair in early lesions, but later resulting in hair loss and thickening of the skin. Affected animals are often kept in moist conditions and exposed to food residues.

LESIONS. Piglets with candidiasis are often in poor condition with chronic diarrhea. There may be lesions in the oral cavity and throughout the gastrointestinal tract. These consist of white specks and circular patches 2–5 mm in diameter on the dorsum of the tongue, less frequently on the pharynx, and sometimes on the soft or hard palate. These patches may coalesce to form larger areas of pseudomembranous material that may occlude the lumen of the esophagus. The lesions may extend down the esophagus and may be seen on the gastric mucosa. There may be small hemorrhages in the cardiac area and white pseudomembranous lesions in the esophageal area. Descriptions of the lesions distal to the stomach are rarely published, but in heavily infected animals they resemble those of chronic enteritis, with villous atrophy and thickening of the mucosa. When the white pseudomembranous material is removed, congestion of the mucosal surface may be seen, but ulceration is rare. In older pigs, *C. albicans* may be isolated from gastric ulcers, but these do not differ grossly from uninfected ones. Gross lesions may be seen in cutaneous candidiasis and include a grayish surface deposit, thickening of the skin, and hair loss.

Microscopic lesions include the presence of numerous yeasts on the epithelial surface, with pseudohyphal filaments visible as 1.5–2.0 μm deeply staining threads in the epithelium. In lesions on the tongue, yeast cells and pseudohyphae may be seen in cavities beneath the papillae. They may also be present in large numbers in the periphery of infected gastric ulcers. Degenerative changes are frequently present in the infected epithelium. They include desquamation of epithelial cells, capillary dilation, edema of the submucosa or dermis (depending on the epithelial surface attacked), and presence of inflammatory cells. These are neutrophils in the early lesions, later (in 4- to 5-day-old lesions) accompanied by eosinophils, macrophages, plasma cells, and lymphocytes.

DIAGNOSIS. In piglets the appearance of the white 2–5 mm lesions in the oral cavity may suggest that candidiasis is present, but diarrhea and association of infection with gastric ulceration may not be identified on clinical grounds. Skin changes may also suggest a diagnosis of candidiasis. A history of chronic enteritis and broad-spectrum antibiotic use or housing in moist conditions is often suggestive of candidiasis.

Confirmation of diagnosis is based on demonstration of the organism concerned in the lesions or, in life, isolation of large numbers from the feces. The presence of yeasts in lesions or the intestine may be established by their demonstration in Gram-stained smears in which oval or round gram-positive, often budding, 2.5–6 μm cells may be seen (Fig. 51.6). Similar bodies may be seen in histologic sections stained by hemalum and eosin or, more easily, when stained by periodic acid–Schiff or silver stains such as Grocott's (Fig. 51.7). None of these allow the complete identification of the organism.

Yeasts may be isolated using Sabouraud's agar with or without chloramphenicol (Carter 1979). Some, such as *C. albicans,* will grow readily on horse blood agar. Incubation at 25°C yields colonies 1–2 mm in diameter after 3–4 days, but incubation at 37°C can allow colonies to be identified within 24–48 hours. The genera can be separated using characters such as shape of the cells, presence or absence of pseudomycelium, presence or absence of capsule, production of chlamydospores, ability to split urea, and other characters (Carter 1979).

Isolation of large numbers of yeasts from lesions may confirm a diagnosis of candidiasis, but their isolation in small numbers from the skin, vagina, or feces and intestines of clinically normal pigs may not be significant.

TREATMENT. *Candida albicans* and other yeasts are sensitive in vitro to a number of compounds such as nystatin, miconazole, and amphotericin B, but only nystatin and amphotericin B have been used in treatment (Osborne et al.

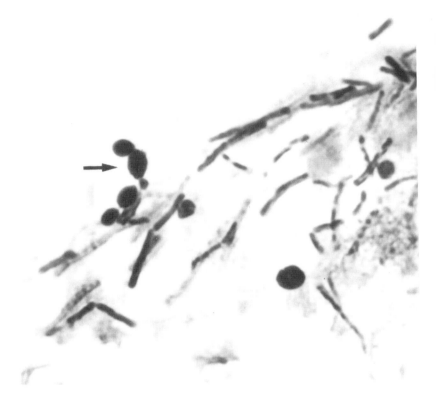

51.6. Photomicrograph of yeast cells (arrow) from the ileal mucosa in a 10-day-old piglet. Gram. ×1200.

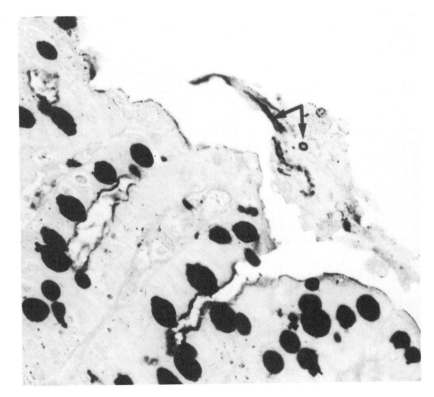

51.7. Photomicrograph of yeast cells and pseudo-hyphae adjacent to the ileal mucosa in a 10-day-old piglet. Grocott. ×400.

1960). Nystatin suppressed the clinical signs but did not eliminate infection. Amphotericin B may be effective in young piglets given at a rate of 0.5 mg/kg twice daily. In many instances, correction of underlying disease or husbandry factors is sufficient. Cleaning up waste food and providing a dry environment caused resolution of cutaneous candidiasis (Reynolds et al. 1968). Treatment should also include discontinuation of the use of broad-spectrum antibiotics and their replacement with narrow-spectrum ones if they are a factor in yeast colonization. Animals with cutaneous candidiasis may also be scrubbed with a suitable detergent or with hexetidine-based shampoos.

PREVENTION. Pigs should be maintained in warm, dry, clean conditions, and accumulations of moist fermenting food should be prevented. Enteric diseases in piglets should be treated with appropriate antimicrobials and lengthy treatment with broad-spectrum antibiotics should be avoided. Disinfection of pens and pen fittings can be carried out by using formaldehyde vapor or 2% formaldehyde; cleaning and drying of the pens will reduce levels of yeasts to normal background levels.

REFERENCES

CARTER, G. R. 1979. Diagnostic Procedures in Veterinary Bacteriology and Mycology, 3d ed. Springfield: Charles C Thomas, Chap. 30.
OSBORNE, A. D.; MCCREA, M. R.; AND MANNERS, M. J. 1960. Moniliasis in artificially reared pigs and its treatment with nystatin. Vet Rec 72:237–241.
REYNOLDS, I. M.; MINER, P.; AND SMITH, R. E. 1968. Cutaneous candidiasis on swine. J Am Vet Med Assoc 152:182–186.

Infection with *Yersinia*

D. J. Taylor

A NUMBER OF species of *Yersinia* have been isolated from pigs, and reports of association between infection and clinical disease are increasing. The organisms are, however, potential pathogens; one species (*Y. enterocolitica*) has increasingly become recognized as a cause of human food poisoning and enteritis since the late 1960s. The source of these infections varies, but the pig is considered to be important. There are reports in the literature of many surveys of pig carcasses, offal, and feces for the presence of *Y. enterocolitica* (Doyle et al. 1981; Schieman and Fleming 1981; Hunter et al. 1983). Results of these surveys suggest that infection is distributed worldwide in pigs, and serotypes considered pathogenic to man are commonly present. This relationship to human disease has stimulated a number of reports of pathogenic determinants (Mosimbale and Gyles 1982) that have been demonstrated in *Y. enterocolitica* in laboratory studies. Further reports deal with the antigenic relationships between *Yersinia* spp. and *Brucella* spp., since infections with certain strains of the former can cause interference with serologic tests for both *B. abortus* and *B. suis*. This interference is described in Chapter 35.

Infection in pigs is usually inapparent, but *Y. pseudotuberculosis* and *Y. enterocolitica* have been isolated from pigs with fever, enteritis, and diarrhea.

ETIOLOGY. Yersinias are aerobic or facultatively anaerobic, gram-negative coccobacilli or short rods, 1.2 μm in length and 0.5–1.0 μm in diameter. They are nonmotile at 37°C, but some are motile at lower temperatures. The genus was separated from *Pasteurella* in 1944 and now contains a number of species. These include *Y. pseudotuberculosis* ssp. *pseudotuberculosis*, *Y. pseudotuberculosis* ssp. *pestis* (the plague bacillus), *Y. enterocolitica*, *Y. intermedia*, *Y. fredrikensii*, and *Y. kristensenii*, all of which have been demonstrated in pigs. Only two species (*Y. pseudotuberculosis* ssp. *pseudotuberculosis* and *Y. enterocolitica*) have yet been associated with clinical disease in pigs.

They may be isolated in routine media upon which they appear as grayish 1–2 mm colonies within 24–48 hours and as similar-sized nonlactose-fermenting colonies on MacConkey agar. The species are distinguished by biochemical tests. *Y. pseudotuberculosis* ssp. *pseudotuberculosis* is motile at 22°C, grows on citrate media at 22°C, splits urea, and does not ferment sucrose or raffinose but does ferment mannose. *Y. pseudotuberculosis* ssp. *pestis* is negative for all these characters. *Y. enterocolitica* is also motile and splits urea but ferments sucrose and does not grow on citrate or ferment mannose. Individual species can be divided into biotypes and serotypes. Capsules, attachment antigens, and enterotoxins have been described in organisms of this genus.

Y. enterocolitica has been subdivided into at least 46 O groups and at least 5 biotypes. Of these, most human infections are associated with biotype 2, O9 and biotype 4, O3. Biotype 1, O8 is also associated with some human infections. *Y. enterocolitica* of a number of O groups have been recorded from pigs. The actual O groups isolated may vary from one part of a country to another (Schieman and Fleming 1981) but include O3, O5, O6, O7, O8, O9, O13, O18, and O46.

EPIDEMIOLOGY. *Y. enterocolitica* is found throughout the world and has been recorded from pigs in many countries (Bockemuhl et al. 1979; Cantoni et al. 1979; Barcellos and Castro 1981; Doyle et al. 1981; Schieman and Flemming 1981; Hunter et al. 1983). Infection may not be general, since not all herds are infected (Christensen 1980). It is shed in the feces of infected pigs for up to 30 weeks and has been shown to be transmitted to human food and elsewhere on farms by flies (Fukushima et al. 1979). Feed has been found to be infected, and studies of the dissemination of infection in pig facilities (Fukushima et al. 1983) indicate that infection is transmitted from contaminated pens in which infection can persist for 3 weeks. Other studies suggest that feces can remain infected for up to 12 weeks and that, in suitable substrates, the organism may multiply at 20–22°C. It appears that transmission from pig to pig is via fecal contamination of accommodation, water, and feed.

Y. pseudotuberculosis ssp. *pseudotuberculosis* is less commonly demonstrated in America than in Europe or Japan and is less commonly identified in pigs than *Y. enterocolitica*. It is commonly found in rodents, which probably represent the main source of infection for pigs.

Y. pseudotuberculosis ssp. *pestis* may infect wild pigs in California, presumably from infection present in rodents (Clark et al. 1983).

PATHOGENESIS. *Y. enterocolitica* has been shown to infect pigs orally, to multiply and be found in the feces within 2–3 weeks of infection, and to disappear from the feces within 30 weeks (Fukushima et al. 1984). No clinical signs or lesions were described and none were found following infection of 6 pigs with the isolate obtained from the clinical outbreak described above. Studies in sucking mice have indicated that 10 of the 12 pig isolates tested produced enterotoxin and that one isolate could produce fluid in piglet gut loops. The Sereny test for invasiveness was negative in typical pig strains (Mosimbale and Gyles 1982). Recent studies by Erwerth and Natterman (1987) suggest that oral infection is followed by establishment of infection in the tonsils and the development of enteritis in the ileum and large intestine. Similar colonization was reported by Schiemann (1988).

CLINICAL SIGNS. Clinical disease has been associated only with *Y. enterocolitica* and *Y. pseudotuberculosis* ssp. *pseudotuberculosis*. *Y. pseudotuberculosis* ssp. *pestis* is clearly capable of producing serologic reactions (Clark et al. 1983), but no clinical disease has been described.

Y. enterocolitica was isolated in profuse culture from outbreaks of diarrhea in weaned pigs from which no other infectious agents could be recovered. Mild fever (to 39.4°C, 103°F) was present and the diarrhea contained no blood or mucus and was blackish in color. Clinical signs resembling those described above have been seen in animals receiving tiamulin or lincomycin. Blood-stained mucus may also be found in some diarrheic feces and on solid feces passed by pen mates. The organism has been isolated from the rectal mucosa in cases of rectal stricture.

Y. pseudotuberculosis ssp. *pseudotuberculosis* has been associated with clinical signs by Morita et al. (1968), who described an outbreak in Japan. Affected pigs were dull and showed inappetence; blood-stained diarrhea; and edema of eyelids, lower face, and dependent parts of the abdomen. Diarrhea was also observed by Barcellos and Castro (1981). The organism has been isolated from pigs with the rectal stricture syndrome.

LESIONS. The lesions caused by *Y. enterocolitica* infection have been described in detail by Erwerth and Natterman (1987) and consist of catarrhal enteritis in the small and large intestines. Microcolonies of the organism can be seen in the disrupted intestinal epithelium and in pigs with rectal lesions, bacterial penetration and inflammation reach the muscularis mucosae.

Lesions of *Y. pseudotuberculosis* ssp. *pseudotuberculosis* have been described (Morita et al. 1968). They resembled those of pseudotuberculosis in other species, with miliary gray-white spots on the liver and spleen and swollen gray-white mesenteric lymph nodes. A catarrhal and diphtheritic change was described in the colon and rectum, as edema and ascites also occurred. Microscopic lesions included necrotic foci containing masses of bacteria surrounded by a thin layer of granulation tissue in the lung, liver, spleen, mesenteric lymph nodes, and lymphoid follicles of the large intestine. *Y. pseudotuberculosis* ssp. *pseudotuberculosis* was isolated from the liver, spleen, lungs, duodenum, rectum, and mesenteric lymph nodes. *Y. pseudotuberculosis* ssp. *pseudotuberculosis* can also be isolated from inflammatory lesions of the rectal mucosa similar to those described above.

DIAGNOSIS. The clinical signs are not distinctive, but the occurrence of mild fever and blood and mucus on solid feces can indicate *Yersinia* infection in the absence of swine dysentery. Where rectal stricture is common, the organism may be responsible for diarrhea in younger age groups. Diagnosis of infection with most *Yersinia* spp. in pigs depends upon isolation of the organism and its identification. Serology has been used to identify *Y. pseudotuberculosis* ssp. *pestis* (Clark et al. 1983), but most accounts of *Yersinia* infections suggest that, although agglutinating antibody may result from infection, isolation methods are adequate for diagnosis. *Y. pseudotuberculosis* ssp. *pseudotuberculosis* can readily be isolated at 37°C on blood and MacConkey agar from lesions of the type described by Morita et al. (1968) and so may *Y. enterocolitica*. Most isolation methods for all *Yersinia* involve use of a cold-enrichment technique in which tissues or samples under investigation are placed in phosphate-buffered saline M/15 at pH 7.6 at 4°C for 6 weeks, with subculture at 3 and 6 weeks onto a selective medium (Hunter et al. 1983). The selective medium may be MacConkey agar incubated at 30°C or a specific medium for *Y. enterocolitica*. These methods may be used for direct isolation. Media are described by Hunter et al. (1983) and six are reviewed by Catteau et al. (1983).

Criteria for separation of *Yersinia* isolates into species are given by Hunter et al. (1983) and Brewer and Corbel (1983).

TREATMENT. There is at present no general indication for the treatment of *Yersinia* infections, since clinical signs are so rare. In vitro studies suggest that isolates are often sensitive to oxytetracycline, furazolidone, neomycin, sulphonamides, and spectinomycin. Tetraclines have been used in feed to eliminate infection and clinical signs.

PREVENTION. Since spread of *Y. enterocolitica* from pig to pig appears to occur from contact with feces, hygiene coupled with housing groups of pigs in separate drainage areas will reduce infection. Control of flies and rodents and disinfection of pens before restocking will reduce transmission. Morita et al. (1968) found that pseudotuberculosis could be prevented by excluding birds and rodents.

REFERENCES
BARCELLOS, D. E. S. N. DE, AND CASTRO, A. F. P. DE. 1981. Isolation of *Yersinia pseudotuberculosis* from diarrhoeas in pigs. Br Vet J 137:95–96.
BOCKEMUHL, J.; SCHMITT, H.; ROTH, J.; AND SAUPE, E. 1979. Die jahreszeitliche Haufigkeit der Ausscheidung von *Yersinia enterocolitica* im Kot gesunder Schlachtschweine. Zentralbl Bakteriol [Orig A]244:494–505.
BREWER, R. A., AND CORBEL, M. J. 1983. Characterisation of *Yersinia enterocolitica* strains isolated from cattle, sheep and pigs in the U.K. J Hyg (Camb) 90:425–433.
CANTONI, C.; D'AUBERT, S.; BUOGO, A.; AND GUIZZARDI, F. 1979. *Yersinia enterocolitica* nelli feci di suino. Arch Vet Ital 30:134–136.
CATTEAU, M.; KREMBEL, C.; AND WAUTERS, G. 1983. Isolement de *Yersinia enterocolitica* de langues de porc. Rec Med Vet 159:89–94.
CHRISTENSEN, S. G. 1980. *Yersinia enterocolitica* in Danish pigs. J Appl Bacteriol 48:377–382.
CLARK, R. K.; JESSUP, D. A.; HIRD, D. W.; RUPANNER, R.; AND MEYER, M. E. 1983. Serologic survey of California wild hogs for antibody against selected zoonotic disease agents. J Am Vet Med Assoc 183:1248–1251.
DOYLE, M. P.; HUGDAHL, M. B.; AND TAYLOR, S. L. 1981. Isolation of *Yersinia enterocolitica* from porcine tongues. Appl Environ Microbiol 41:661–666.
ERWERTH, W., AND NATTERMAN, H. 1987. Histopathologische Untersuchengen bei der experimentellen oralen *Yersinia enterocolitica* Infektion des Jungschweines. Monatsh Vet 42:319–324.
FUKUSHIMA, H.; ITO, Y.; SAITO, K.; TSUBOKURA, M.; AND OTSUKI, K. 1979. Role of the fly in the transport of *Yersinia enterocolitica*. Appl Environ Microbiol 38:1009–1010.
FUKUSHIMA, H.; NAKAMURA, R.; ITO, Y.; SAITO, K.; TSUBOKURA, M.; AND OTSUKI, K. 1983. Ecological studies of *Y. enterocolitica* in pigs. I. Dissemination of *Y. enterocolitica* in pigs. Vet Microbiol 8:469–483.
FUKUSHIMA, H.; NAKAMURA, R.; ITO, Y.; AND SAITO, K. 1984. Ecological studies of *Yersinia enterocolitica*. II. Experimental infection with *Y. enterocolitica* in pigs. Vet Microbiol 9:375–389.
HUNTER, D.; HUGHES, S.; AND FOX, E. 1983. Isolation of *Yersinia enterocolitica* from pigs in the United Kingdom. Vet Rec 112:322–323.
MORITA, M.; NAKAMATSU, M.; AND GOTO, M. 1968. Pathological studies on pseudotuberculosis rodentium. III. Spontaneous swine cases. Jpn J Vet Sci 30:233–239.
MOSIMBALE, F., AND GYLES, C. L. 1982. The pathogenicity of *Yersinia enterocolitica* strains isolated from various sources for four test systems. Can J Comp Med 46:70–75.
SCHIEMANN, D. A., AND FLEMING, C. A. 1981. *Yersinia enterocolitica* isolated from throats of swine in eastern and western Canada. Can J Microbiol 27:1326–1333.
SCHIEMANN, D. A. 1988. The pathogenicity of *Yersinia enterocolitica* for piglets. Can J Vet Res 52:325–330.

Staphylococci

D. J. Taylor

STAPHYLOCCCOCI are ubiquitous. They are present on every pig farm and involved in a wide range of lesions in pigs of all ages. The most easily recognized are those of exudative epidermitis caused by *Staphylococcus hyicus* and described elsewhere. Few if any of the other lesions can be unequivocally identified as being staphylococcal on clinical grounds; in the majority, staphylococcal involvement must be confirmed by laboratory means. In addition to their association with pig disease, some of the staphylococci that infect the pig, notably *S. aureus,* may be involved in human food poisoning if carcasses are contaminated or abscesses are present.

ETIOLOGY. Staphylococci are gram-positive, 0.5–1.5 μm in diameter, forming grapelike clusters when grown in serum broth or seen in pus. They grow primarily in aerobic conditions but can also grow anaerobically, are oxidase-negative but produce catalase, and metabolize a wide variety of sugars. They produce a wide range of enzymes and some toxins. The species are distinguished by the presence of enzymes such as coagulase, DNAase, hemolysins, phosphatase, and ability to utilize a variety of sugars. Major species reported from the pig are *S. aureus, S. hyicus,* and *S. epidermidis,* although *S. saprophyticus* has also been described.

S. aureus is the only species apart from *S. hyicus* to be consistently isolated from lesions in pigs. It forms yellowish white, opaque, circular, domed colonies, 1–2 mm in diameter, on blood agar after 24 hours of incubation. These colonies may be surrounded by a zone of complete hemolysis, caused by alpha hemolysins, on horse blood agar. On sheep blood agar, the ring of complete hemolysis is surrounded by a wider area of incomplete hemolysis caused by beta hemolysins; this becomes complete on cooling of the plate. In addition to these hemolysins, the organism produces coagulase, DNAase, proteinases, hyaluronidase, and toxins that include the alpha toxin and the enterotoxins. Both have been demonstrated in strains of porcine origin (Engvall and Schwan 1983). Isolates of *S. aureus* can be identified by phage typing, and those of public health significance may readily be traced. *S. aureus* is fairly resistant to drying but is readily inactivated by heat. It is sensitive to a wide range of disinfectants such as phenols, hypochlorites, iodine, and iodophors.

EPIDEMIOLOGY. *S. aureus* is widely distributed in the environment and has been recovered from pig feces, food, water following contamination of drinkers, pen floors and walls, and the air in pig facilities. The organism can be isolated from a wide range of hosts including birds, rodents, dogs, cats, and humans. The extent to which isolates from lesions in pigs are of nonporcine origin is not yet known. Porcine strains capable of enterotoxin production have been identified on carcasses and represent a source of infection or possible food poisoning to humans (Engvall and Schwan 1983).

The pig is probably the major source of infection for other pigs; *S. aureus* can be isolated from the skin, oral cavity, upper respiratory tract, prepuce, vagina, and gut of healthy pigs on a very wide scale. Transmission of the organism may be by aerosol to the upper respiratory tract, directly by skin contact, or indirectly by contact with contaminated walls or fittings. Ingestion of *S. aureus* from food, contaminated water, or litter is common. Venereal contact may be responsible for some genital infections; local invasion of the mammary gland, navel, and skin lesions is common.

PATHOGENESIS. *S. aureus* appears to multiply on damaged mucosal surfaces or skin and can invade to cause bacteremia. In some cases such as neonatal septicemia, animals may become fevered and die, but bacteremia usually leads to formation of multiple abscesses. These may occur in bones to give osteomyelitis; in joints; on the heart valves to give vegetative endocarditis; and in the liver, kidney, or lymph nodes. Vegetative endocarditis may give rise to septic emboli that cause abscess formation and infarction in the kidney. Most of these systemic infections occur in neonates or piglets and take 7–10 days to develop. They are also present in apparently normal pigs at slaughter. Abscesses contain neutrophils and microcolonies of bacteria in all stages of multiplication and heal by fibrosis.

Mastitis, vaginitis, and metritis appear to result from ascending infection. Abortion has been associated with the demonstration of serum antibody to alpha hemolysin in the sow (Kohler and Wille 1980), but the importance of this and other toxins in abortion is not known.

In enteric infection, experimental studies have shown that staphylococcal enterotoxin A will cause emesis when given orally in doses of 40–50 μg within 90–180 minutes (Taylor et al. 1982). Larger doses can cause behavioral changes, including inappetence, restlessness, and staggering. The piglet is clearly susceptible, but the ability of enteric staphylococcal infections to produce enterotoxin in vivo is not known.

CLINICAL SIGNS. The presence of *S. aureus* infection cannot readily be suspected on clinical grounds. *S. aureus* has been isolated from a wide variety of syndromes. Most of these occur in individual animals, and disease rarely spreads from animal to animal. It can cause neonatal septicemia and is often identified in small, hairy stunted piglets of 7–10 days of age with umbilical abscesses, joint ill, and signs of cardiac enlargement due to vegetative endocarditis. It is a cause of subcutaneous abscesses associated with abrasions and foot lesions, especially in piglets. These often result in arthritis of the distal phalangeal joints, enlargement of the hoof, and sinus formation at the coronary band. Creamy pus is often seen to exude from these.

It has been isolated from enteritis in piglets and in older animals and from the rectal skin of animals with lesions of rectal stricture. No particular features of diarrhea are associated with staphylococci except that the enteritis is often chronic and antibiotic treatment may have been given. It is also present in a small percentage of cases of mastitis and has been isolated from metritis and agalactia. The only reason to suspect staphylococcal involvement may be the presence of a creamy white or bloodstained pus, but this often contains other organisms. It has also been isolated from aborted fetuses and placentas (Kohler and Wille 1980).

LESIONS. No gross lesions may be seen in piglet septicemia. In chronic infections, an inflamed mucosa may be associated with staphylococcal infection, but there is no specific feature that allows their identification with staphylococcal infection. Abscesses may occur in the umbilicus, liver, lungs, lymph nodes, spleen, kidney, joints, and bones in osteomyelitis; the latter may give rise to pathologic fractures, especially when in the vertebrae. Body cavities (peritoneal cavity, pericardial cavity, uterine lumen) may contain pus, especially in younger animals, following umbilical infection. S. aureus is only one cause of such lesions. Both gross and microscopic lesions of mastitis may be found in the mammary glands, and in some cases fibrosis may be considerable. Occasionally, a granulomatous mass with fibrosis may be found in the abdominal cavity of piglets that have died after castration. In all cases, confirmation that the lesions are staphylococcal depends on demonstration of the organisms.

DIAGNOSIS. The clinical signs resulting from multiple abscess formation in individual pigs may be suggestive, and similar suspicions may arise from the postmortem findings. Confirmation of involvement of staphylococci rather than *Actinomyces pyogenes* or streptococci in abscesses and arthritis is obtained from Gram-stained smears of the pus in which gram-positive cocci may be seen singly or in clusters. Only the isolation of staphylococci in culture confirms that they are involved. *S. aureus* can be isolated readily on blood and MacConkey agar and its identity confirmed by coagulase and DNAase tests and its ability to ferment mannitol. Isolates may be phage typed if this is considered relevant, and any toxins produced may be identified.

In most abscesses the absence of other bacteria must be excluded before *S. aureus* is considered to be the sole cause; exclusion of other agents is even more important in diseases at mucous surfaces.

TREATMENT. Individual abscesses may be opened surgically after skin cleaning and disinfection, but most treatments rely on antimicrobial treatment. Since *S. aureus* infection is an individual animal problem, there is usually no need to treat the whole group. Parenteral treatment with an appropriate formulation and prompt treatment at any age can prevent the development of large and potentially extensive and fatal abscesses. The use of feed medication as a prophylactic cannot be justified unless a severe problem has been identified, since the development of antimicrobial resistance in staphylococci is likely to favor them over other organisms after a brief period during which they are suppressed. The use of bacterins has been described, but they are not widely available or extensively used.

REFERENCES

ENGVALL, A., AND SCHWAN, O. 1983. Isolation and partial characterization of bacteria recovered from abscesses of normally slaughtered pigs. Acta Vet Scand 24:74–83.

KOHLER, B., AND WILLE, H. 1980. Bakteriologische Untersuchungen bei abortierten Schweinefeten unter Berucksichtigung der atiologischen Bedeutung von *Staphylococcus aureus.* Monatsch Veterinaermed 35:506–510.

TAYLOR, S. L.; SCHLUNZ, L. R.; BEEREY, J. T.; CLIVER, D. O.; AND BERGDOLL, M. S. 1982. Emetic action of staphylococcal enterotoxin A on weanling pigs. Infect Immunol 36:1263–1266.

Eubacterium (Corynebacterium) suis

J. E. T. Jones

IN 1957 SOLTYS and Spratling in the United Kingdom isolated, anaerobically, a diphtheroid bacterium from the urine and diseased tissue of adult pigs affected with cystitis and pyelonephritis. They named the bacterium *Corynebacterium suis*. Soltys (1961) described the characteristics of *C. suis* in more detail.

The taxonomic position of *C. suis,* however, is not established; it seems to have been assigned to the genus *Corynebacterium* largely on morphologic criteria. It has no antigenic relationship with *C. renale* and it does not have the cell wall composition of true corynebacteria. Wegienek and Reddy (1982) proposed that *C. suis* be assigned to the genus *Eubacterium* but this is a questionable proposal. The genus *Eubacterium* has served as a depository for a wide and varied collection of gram-positive, nonspore-forming, obligately anaerobic bacteria (Jones and Collins 1986). *E. (C.) suis* is not an obligate anaerobe. It has some of the features of organisms belonging to the genus *Actinomyces* but Weiss (personal communication) believes that it may need to be assigned to a new genus. In the meantime many bacteriologists and clinicians will continue to call it *C. suis* rather than compound an error in spite of its current official name. The authors will use the *E.(C.) suis* designation throughout this book.

E. (C.) suis infection associated with urinary tract disease in sows was reported from Canada (Percy et al. 1966), Norway (Aalvik 1968), Holland (Dijkstra 1969; Frijlink et al. 1969; Narucka and Westendorp 1972), Denmark (Larsen 1970, 1973), Hong Kong (Munro and Wong 1972), Australia (Glazebrook et al. 1973), Switzerland (Schällibaum et al. 1976), Finland (Kauko et al. 1977), Malaysia (Too et al. 1985), Germany (Muller et al. 1986; Waldmann 1987), Brazil (De Oliveira et al. 1988), and the United States (Walker and MacLachlan 1989).

Cystitis and pyelonephritis are discussed in Chapter 10. Here, the principal features of *E. (C.) suis* are described and some aspects of the associated disease are briefly outlined.

ETIOLOGY. *E. (C.) suis* is a gram-positive pleomorphic rod, 2–3 μm long, and 0.3–0.5 μm wide; the organism tends to be larger in tissues than in cultures. In tissues and cultures it occurs in the form of so-called Chinese letters and in a palisade fashion. It is nonmotile and does not form spores.

E. (C.) suis grows well on blood agar under anaerobic conditions. Colonies are evident at 2 days, having a diameter of 2–3 mm; they then begin to flatten and develop a characteristic dry, gray, opaque surface with a crenated edge; some colonies attain a size of 4–5 mm in 5–6 days. There is no hemolysis. Growth on nutrient agar, even after subculture, is poor. In liquid media such as cooked meat broth and brain-heart infusion, slight turbidity is produced in 2–4 days; growth is more luxuriant in trypticase soy broth and is further enhanced by the addition of urea to a final concentration of 1.2% (w/v). The addition of maltose to either solid or liquid media improves growth. Although *E. (C.) suis* has always been described as an anaerobic organism, prolonged aerobic incubation on blood agar results in the development of colonies within 5–10 days; on subculture, aerobically, colonies are evident in 2–3 days.

The organism is relatively inactive when subjected to conventional biochemical tests. Most strains ferment maltose and xylose and hydrolyze starch but do not attack other commonly used "sugars"; all produce urease. Catalase, methyl red, Voges-Proskauer, indole, and nitrate-reduction tests are negative. Coagulated serum and egg medium are not liquefied. A slight alkalinity is produced in litmus milk.

EPIDEMIOLOGY AND PATHOGENESIS. Most male pigs, aged 6 months or more, harbor *E. (C.) suis* in the preputial diverticulum, which may become colonized when pigs are only a few weeks old. Uninfected males are readily infected when they are housed with carrier males (Jones and Dagnall 1984). The organism may be found on the floors of pens occupied by male pigs. Carr and Walton (1990) have isolated *E. (C.) suis* from the footwear of handlers working with boars but not from those working in the farrowing area. Only rarely is it found in the vagina of healthy females, but it may be that existing cultural techniques are insufficiently sensitive to demonstrate its presence there. Hitherto, there are no reports of *E. (C.) suis* being isolated from any sites in the pig other than the urogenital tract.

Cystitis and pyelonephritis, caused by *E. (C.) suis*, mainly affect adult females. Infection of the bladder and kidneys is by the ascending route. Most cases occur within 1–3 weeks of mating, suggesting that there are predisposing factors operating at this time but such factors have not yet been elucidated. However, the disease may become clinically evident at any time in relation to the breeding cycle of the sow, e.g., after parturition; in such cases it is not always clear whether infection of the urinary tract is recent or whether there has been a recrudescence of previously existing disease.

Studies on the adhesive properties of *E. (C.) suis* have been reported by Larsen et al. (1986). They have demonstrated that some strains are heavily fimbriated and are able to adhere to the epithelial cells of the porcine bladder; their findings support the hypothesis that glycoconjugates are specific receptor sites for the attachment of *E. (C.) suis*.

CLINICAL SIGNS AND LESIONS. Hematuria is the main sign in the acute phase. As the disease progresses there is loss of weight. Some sows may die suddenly, apparently from acute renal failure.

Inflammatory reactions in the mucosa of the urethra, bladder, and ureters may be catarrhal, fibrinopurulent, hemorrhagic, or necrotic. Affected kidneys often have irregular yellow areas of degeneration in the parenchyma that are visible on the surface. The renal pelvis may be dilated and contain mucoid fluid in which flakes of necrotic debris and altered blood are present. The medullary pyramids often show yellow or dark green to black foci of necrosis. There are no related lesions elsewhere in the body.

DIAGNOSIS. Diagnosis is based on clinical signs and bacteriologic examination of urine. *E. (C.) suis* is easily seen in Gram-stained films, often with other bacteria, notably streptococci. For cultural examination it is essential to incubate the medium (e.g., blood agar), which has been inoculated with urine or other appropriate material, anaerobically for 4 days. Results of cultural procedures should not be reported as negative before this time. Rapid diagnosis can be achieved by the use of immunofluorescent techniques (Schällibaum et al. 1976; Kauko et al. 1977). A selective medium for the isolation of *E. (C.) suis* has been described by Dagnall and Jones (1982).

TREATMENT AND PREVENTION. *E. (C.) suis* is sensitive in vitro to several antibiotics, including penicillin and tetracyclines. Administration of antibiotics is frequently effective, at least in the short term. However, relapses commonly occur, and often it is best to advise early slaughter of affected animals.

There are no proved methods of prevention. *E. (C.) suis* may be transmitted from boars to sows at the time of mating. Culling of carrier boars has been suggested as a method of preventing infection of sows; this does not seem worthwhile because replacement boars will almost certainly be infected. Culling might be of value if there are "pathogenic" and "nonpathogenic" strains of *E. (C.) suis*, but there is no evidence that such different strains exist. Currently, the only means of attempting prevention of the disease is to administer antibiotics to sows immediately after service or, if outbreaks of the disease are economically serious, to use artificial insemination.

REFERENCES

AALVIK, B. 1968. *Corynebacterium suis* isolert fra et tilfelle av pyelonefritt hos purke. Nord Vet Med 20:319–320.
CARR, J., AND WALTON, J. R. 1990. Investigation of the pathogenic properties of *Eubacterium (Corynebacterium) suis*. Proc 11th Int Congr Pig Vet Soc, Lausanne.
DAGNALL, G. J. R., AND JONES, J. E. T. 1982. A selective medium for the isolation of *Corynebacterium suis*. Res Vet Sci 32:389–390.
DE OLIVEIRA, S. J.; BARCELLOS, D. E. S. N.; AND BOROWSKI, S. M. 1988. Urinary tract infections in two pig breeding herds, with emphasis on the presence of *Corynebacterium suis*. Proc 10th Int Congr Pig Vet Soc, Rio de Janeiro.
DIJKSTRA, R. G. 1969. Cysto-pyelonefritis bij varkens veroorzaakt door *Corynebacterium suis*. Tijdschr Diergeneeskd 94:393–394.
FRIJLINK, G. P. A.; VAN DIJK, J. E.; AND GOUDSWAARD, J. 1969. Een hemorragische-necrotiserende cystopyelonefritis bij een drachtige zeug, veroorzaakt door *Corynebacterium suis*. Tijdschr Diergeneeskd 94:389–393.
GLAZEBROOK, J. S.; DONALDSON-WOOD, C.; AND

LADDS, P. W. 1973. Pyelonephritis and cystitis in sows associated with *Corynebacterium suis*. Aust Vet J 49:546.
JONES, D., AND COLLINS, M. D. 1986. Irregular nonsporing Gram positive rods. In *Bergey's Manual of Systematic Bacteriology*, vol. 2, sect. 15. Ed. P. H. A. Sheath, N. S. Mair, and M. E. Sharpe. Baltimore, London: Williams & Wilkins, pp. 1265, 1370.
JONES, J. E. T., AND DAGNALL G. J. R. 1984. The carriage of *Corynebacterium suis* in male pigs. J Hyg (Camb) 93:381–388.
KAUKO, L.; SCHILDT, R.; AND SANDHOLM, M. 1977. *Corynebacterium suis* emakoiden pyelonefriitin aiheuttajana suomessa. Suom Elainl 83:489–492.
LARSEN, J. L. 1970. *Corynebacterium suis* infektioner hos svin. Nord Vet Med 22:422–431.
———. 1973. Et enzootisk udbrud af cystitis og pyelonephritis forarsaget af *Corynebacterium suis*. Medlemsbl Dan Dyrlaegeforen 56:509–515.
LARSEN, J. L.; HOGH, P.; AND HOVIND-HOUGEN, K. 1986. Haemagglutinating and hydrophobic properties of *Corynebacterium (Eubacterium) suis*. Acta Vet Scand 27:520–530.
MULLER, E.; POZVARI, M.; AND MERKT, M. 1986. Zum Vorkommen von blutig-eitrigen Harnblasen und Nierenentzundungen bei Zuchtsauen in Verbindung mit *Corynebacterium suis*. Prakt Tieraerztl 67:1081–1083.
MUNRO, R., AND WONG, F. 1972. First isolation of *Corynebacterium suis* in Hong Kong. Br Vet J 128:29–32.
NARUCKA, U., AND WESTENDORP, J. F. 1972. *Corynebacterium suis* in pigs. Neth J Vet Sci 4:86–92.
PERCY, D. H.; RUHNKE, H. L.; AND SOLTYS, M. A. 1966. A case of infectious cystitis and pyelonephritis of swine caused by *Corynebacterium suis*. Can Vet J 7:291–292.
SCHÄLLIBAUM, VON M.; HÄNI, H.; AND NICOLET, J. 1976. Infektion des Harntraktes beim Schwein mit *Corynebacterium suis:* Diagnosis met Immunofluoreszenz. Schweiz Arch Tierheilkd 118:329–334.
SOLTYS, M. A. 1961. *Corynebacterium suis* associated with specific cystitis and pyelonephritis in pigs. J Pathol 81:441–446.
SOLTYS, M. A., AND SPRATLING, F. R. 1957. Infectious cystitis and pyelonephritis of pigs: A preliminary communication. Vet Rec 69:500–504.
TOO, H. L.; CHOOI, K. F.; AND BAHAMAN, A. R. 1985. Cystitis in a sow due to *Corynebacterium suis*. Kajian Veterinar 17:155–156.
WALDMANN, K. H. 1987. Die Pyelozystitis der Zuchtsau. Tieraerztl Prax 15:263–267.
WALKER, R. L., AND MacLACHLAN, J. J. 1989. Isolation of *Eubacterium suis* from sows with cystitis. J Am Vet Med Assoc 195:1104–1107.
WEGIENEK, J., AND REDDY, C. A. 1982. Taxonomic study of *Eubacterium suis* (nom. rev.) comb. nov. Int J Syst Bacteriol 32:218–228.

Rhodococcus Equi

J. A. Yager

RHODOCOCCUS EQUI is a minor pathogen of swine. The disease ascribed to *R. equi*, granulomatous lymphadenitis affecting the lymph nodes of the head and neck, is of importance only in that it is readily confused at slaughter with tuberculosis. Furthermore, the primary pathogenicity of *R. equi* has been questioned, because the bacterium is frequently isolated from normal cervical and submaxillary lymph nodes.

ETIOLOGY. Magnusson (1923) first isolated the gram-positive coccobacillus from the pneumonic lungs of a foal and named it *Corynebacterium equi*. The taxonomic history of *R. equi* has been confused, resulting in its current listing in the Approved List of Bacterial Names as both *Corynebacterium* and *Rhodococcus*. It is now accepted as belonging to the latter genus, a member of the nocardioform actinomycete group (Goodfellow et al. 1982). In common with other members of this genus, *R. equi* produces pinkish colonies on solid media. The mycolic acids of *R. equi* have a chain length of 34–48 C and the DNA base composition is 66–72 mol% guanine plus cytosine. Chemical properties used in defining the species are summarized by Goodfellow (1987).

Isolation of *R. equi* from clinical samples is easily achieved by aerobic culture on routine media at 37°C, although the optimum temperature is 28–30°C. Selective media, such as that developed by Woolcock et al. (1979), are required for fecal isolation. Colonies are slow growing, requiring 48 hours to reach a size of 2–4 mm. The typical colony is irregularly round, buff-pink, smooth, and mucoid, although colonial variation is common within and between strains (Mutimer and Woolcock 1981). *R. equi* is biochemically unreactive. It is not proteolytic and does not ferment carbohydrates. *R. equi* is catalase positive, usually urease positive, and oxidase negative. The API ZYM system has been found helpful in bacterial identification (Mutimer and Woolcock 1982). *R. equi* is not hemolytic but, in conjunction with the phospholipase D of *Corynebacterium pseudotuberculosis* or the beta toxin of *Staphylococcus aureus,* produces complete hemolysis of sheep or cattle erythrocytes (Prescott et al. 1982). Semipurification of this factor, known as "equi factor," has indicated that cholesterol oxidase is the major constituent (Linder and Bernheimer 1982).

R. equi possesses an abundant acidic polysaccharide capsule, which is the basis for several serotyping schemes. Prescott (1981) has identified 7 serotypes of which 1 is the most frequently isolated in Canada, Australia, and India. Japanese workers have identified 27 serotypes, with the most common being equivalent to Prescott serotype 1 (Nakazawa et al. 1983). There is no relationship between capsular serotype and origin of the isolates. The capsular polysaccharides of 4 Prescott serotypes have been purified.

EPIDEMIOLOGY AND PATHOGENESIS. *R. equi* is primarily a soil resident. Environmental distribution favors soils enriched with herbivore manure, since fecal matter potentiates bacterial multiplication (Barton and Hughes 1984). *R. equi* is also a transient in the intestinal tract of many species, including pigs, cattle, deer, horses, sheep, goats, and wild birds (Woolcock et al. 1979; Carman and Hodges 1987). Being an obligate aerobe, *R. equi* is not likely to be a member of the normal flora. The bacterium is found in soil samples collected from arable land that has not pastured animals for many years, emphasizing its durability. *R. equi* is present in dust and even in cobwebs of farm buildings. *R. equi* is relatively resistant to chemical disinfectants, such as treatment with 2.5% oxalic acid and 0.5% sodium hydroxide over periods of 15–60 minutes (Karlson et al. 1940).

Little is known of the epidemiology or pathogenesis of the naturally occurring disease in swine. As in horses, *R. equi* infection is likely to be acquired from the environment (Woolcock et al. 1980). Ingestion is the normal mode of exposure in foals (Takai et al. 1986a), leading to the development of solid protective immunity in the majority of animals (Prescott et al. 1980; Chirino-Trejo et al. 1987). A similar situation likely occurs in swine housed on pasture or in yards contaminated with *R. equi,* as the bacterium is readily isolated from the feces of such pigs (Barton and Hughes 1984). Several slaughterhouse studies have also demonstrated recovery of *R. equi* from normal cervical and submaxillary lymph nodes at rates varying from 7% to 35% (Mutimer and Woolcock 1980; Takai et al. 1986b). However, no epidemiologic studies have been carried out to correlate infection rates, disease prevalence, and environmental contamination of *R. equi* on pig farms, as has been done in horses.

The question of the primary role of *R. equi* in the pathogenesis of granulomatous lymphadenitis of the head and neck is unresolved. Arguments used to deny a primary role include the recovery of *R. equi* from normal nodes, the co-isolation of *R. equi* with *Mycobacteria* spp. in a small percentage of cases, and a failure to reproduce the nodal lesions experimentally (Karlson et al. 1940; Cotchin 1943). However, *R. equi* typically produces a granulomatous tissue reaction in lymph nodes of other species, consistent with its action as a facultative intracellular pathogen (Yager 1987). With the probable exception of the foal, *R. equi* is an opportunistic pathogen, requiring a diminution of host defenses before virulence is expressed. It is likely that other, as yet undetermined, predisposing factors are required for the expression of lesions in particular infected pigs.

The isolated reports in which *R. equi* has been associated with serious clinical disease, including one outbreak of oral abscesses and one of pneumonia (Thal and Rutqvist 1959; Rao et al. 1982), suggest abnormal susceptibility, for pigs are extremely resistant to experimental infection by *R. equi*. Following aerosolization, *R. equi* is cleared from the lungs very slowly, but clinical signs and pathological lesions of pneumonia are minimal despite exposure to 10^7 organisms on 7 consecutive days (Zink and Yager 1987). Pneumonia has, however, been induced by intratracheal inoculation of fluid inocula (Thal and Rutqvist 1959).

LESIONS. Lymphadenitis causes no significant clinical signs; lesions are detected only at slaughter. Affected submandibular and cervical nodes are enlarged, containing multiple yellow-tan foci, often in a subcapsular location. Caseation and calcification of these foci sometimes occurs. Histologically the lesion is granulomatous or pyogranulomatous. A similar granulomatous lymphadenitis, but affecting the mesenteric lymph nodes, has recently been associated with another member of the rhodococci, *Rhodococcus sputi* (Tsukamura et al. 1988).

DIAGNOSIS. Diagnosis is at postmortem. Microbiologic identification of *R. equi* is necessary for it is not possible to differentiate the gross lesions of *R. equi*–induced lymphadenitis from those caused by *Mycobacterium* spp.

TREATMENT AND PREVENTION. *R. equi*–induced disease is not sufficiently important to necessitate antemortem diagnosis and treatment in swine. Therapy, which in foals requires long-term administration of rifampicin and erythromycin, is not feasible on economic grounds. While some economic loss may accrue from condemnation at slaughter, there are no studies that indicate the extent of this loss and there appears to be no incentive to institute control measures. These would in any case be difficult; an effective vaccine is presently unavailable.

REFERENCES

BARTON, M. D., AND HUGHES, K. L. 1984. Ecology of *Rhodococcus equi.* Vet Microbiol 9:65–76.
CARMAN, M. G., AND HODGES, R. T. 1987. Distribution of *Rhodococcus equi* in animals, birds and from the environment. NZ Vet J 35:114–115.
CHIRINO-TREJO, J. M.; PRESCOTT, J. F.; AND YAGER, J. A. 1987. Protection of foals against experimental *Rhodococcus equi* pneumonia by oral immunization. Can J Vet Res 51:444–447.
COTCHIN, E. 1943. *Corynebacterium equi* in the submaxillary lymph nodes of swine. J Comp Pathol 53:298–309.
GOODFELLOW, M. 1987. The taxonomic status of *Rhodococcus equi.* Vet Microbiol 14:205–209.
GOODFELLOW, M.; BECKHAM, A. R.; AND BARTON, M. D. 1982. Numerical classification of *Rhodococcus equi* and related actinomycetes. J Appl Bacteriol 53:199–207.
KARLSON, A. G.; MOSES, H. R.; AND FELDMAN, W. H. 1940. *Corynebacterium equi* (Magnusson, 1923) in the submaxillary lymph nodes of swine. J Infect Dis 67:243–251.
LINDER, R., AND BERNHEIMER, A. W. 1982. Enzymatic oxidation of membrane cholesterol exidase in relation to lysis of sheep erythrocytes by corynebacterial enzymes. Arch Biochem Biophys 213:395–404.
MAGNUSSON, H. 1923. Spezifische Infektiose Pneumonie beim Fohlen. Ein neuer Eitererreger beim Pferde. Arch Wiss Prakt Tierheilk 50:22–38.
MUTIMER, M. D., AND WOOLCOCK, J. B. 1980. *Corynebacterium equi* in cattle and pigs. Vet Q 2:25–27.
_____. 1981. Some problems associated with the identification of *Corynebacterium equi.* Vet Microbiol 6:331–338.
_____. 1982. API ZYM for identification of *Corynebacterium equi.* Zentralbl Bakteriol Hyg Abt [Orig C3]:410–415.
NAKAZAWA, M.; KUBO, M.; SUGIMOTO, C.; AND ISAYAMA, Y. 1983. Serogrouping of *Rhodococcus equi.* Microbiol Immunol 27:837–846.
PRESCOTT, J. F. 1981. Capsular serotypes of *Corynebacterium equi.* Can J Comp Med 45:130–134.
PRESCOTT, J. F.; OGILVIE, T. J. H.; AND MARKHAM, R. J. F. 1980. Lymphocyte immunostimulation in the diagnosis of *Corynebacterium equi* pneumonia of foals. Am J Vet Res 41:2073–2075.
PRESCOTT, J. F.; LASTRA, M.; AND BARKSDALE, L. 1982. *Equi* factors in the identification of *Corynebacterium equi* Magnusson. J Clin Microbiol 16:988–990.
RAO, M. S.; ZAKI, S.; KESHAVAMURTHY, B. S.; AND SINGH, K. C. 1982. An outbreak of an acute *Corynebacterium equi* infection in piglets. Indian Vet J 59:487–488.
TAKAI, S.; OHKURA, H.; WATANABE, Y.; AND TSUBAKI, S. 1986a. Quantitative aspects of fecal *Rhodococcus* (*Corynebacterium*) *equi* in foals. J Clin Microbiol 23:794–796.
TAKAI, S.; TAKEUCHI, T.; AND TSUBAKI, S. 1986b. Isolation of *Rhodococcus (Corynebacterium) equi* and atypical mycobacteria from the lymph nodes of healthy pigs. Jpn J Vet Sci 48:445–448.
THAL, E., AND RUTQVIST, L. 1959. The pathogenicity of *Corynebacterium equi* for pigs and small laboratory animals. Nord Vet Med 11:298–304.
TSUKAMURA, M.; KOMATSUZAKI, C.; SAKAI, R.; KANEDA, K.; KUDO, T.; AND SEINO, A. 1988. Mesenteric lymphadenitis of swine caused by *Rhodococcus sputi.* J Clin Microbiol 26:155–157.
WOOLCOCK, J. B.; FARMER, A.-M. T.; AND MUTIMER, M. D. 1979. Selective medium for *Corynebacterium equi* isolation. J Clin Microbiol 9:640–642.
WOOLCOCK, J. B.; MUTIMER, M. D.; AND FARMER, A. M. T. 1980. Epidemiology of *Corynebacterium equi* in horses. Res Vet Sci 28:87–90.
YAGER, J. A. 1987. The pathogenesis of *Rhodococcus equi* pneumonia in foals. Vet Microbiol 14:225–232.
ZINK, M. C., AND YAGER, J. A. 1987. Experimental infection of piglets by aerosols of *Rhodococcus equi.* Can J Vet Res 51:290–296.

Actinomyces Pyogenes

J. A. Yager

ACTINOMYCES PYOGENES, formerly known as *Corynebacterium pyogenes,* is a common cause of suppurative lesions in pigs throughout the world. Disease is opportunistic, resulting from the invasion of skin or mucous membranes by resident *A. pyogenes.* Clinical manifestations are protean, including vertebral osteomyelitis, arthritis, pneumonia, endocarditis, mastitis, and subcutaneous abscesses.

ETIOLOGY. *A. pyogenes* is a small gram-positive pleomorphic rod. There is marked morphologic variation between and within strains. Growth is poor on simple media and is enhanced by the addition of serum or blood. *A. pyogenes* is aerobic or facultatively anaerobic. The optimal temperature for growth is 37°C. Colonies are translucent and small, taking 48 hours to achieve a diameter of 1 mm. *A. pyogenes* forms narrow zones of complete hemolysis after 24 hours on blood agar. Strains isolated from pigs are more hemolytic than those isolated from cattle. *A. pyogenes* produces a hemolysin and an exotoxin which is dermonecrotic in rabbits and guinea pigs and lethal following intravenous injection in rabbits and mice (Lovell 1944). Glucose is fermented by all strains but other carbohydrate reactions are variable. In general, porcine strains are more biochemically active than bovine strains (Roberts 1968; Tainaka et al. 1983). *A. pyogenes* is proteolytic.

A. pyogenes has been reclassified into the genus *Actinomyces* by Collins and Jones (1982), chiefly on the basis of cell wall composition. The guanine-cytosine content of DNA is 58 mol%. Identification of *A. pyogenes* is rapid and reliable with the API 20 Strep system (Morrison and Tillotson 1988).

EPIDEMIOLOGY AND PATHOGENESIS. *A. pyogenes* is a common resident of the mucous membranes of the upper respiratory tract and genital tract of several animal species, including the pig. Disease is therefore the result of endogenous infection and is sporadic, requiring some predisposing event, such as trauma, to initiate the process. For *A. pyogenes* to cause subcutaneous lesions, devitalized or inflamed tissue is an apparent prerequisite, since the inoculation of *A. pyogenes* subcutaneously does not, per se, lead to abscesses. Predisposing events include tail biting leading to abscessation and suppurative osteomyelitis, retention of the fetal membranes leading to endometritis, lacerations of the mammary gland

litis and arthritis, umbilical cord contamination leading to omphalophlebitis, and iatrogenic abscesses resulting from faulty injection or castration techniques. Local extension may produce pelvic lymphadenitis and peritonitis. *A. pyogenes* may act as a secondary invader in preexisting pneumonia.

Bacteremic spread from infective foci results in a variety of lesions including embolic pneumonia, endocarditis, arthritis, and vertebral osteomyelitis. Experimental intravenous inoculation of *A. pyogenes* shows bacterial localization within the marrow of vertebral body epiphyses, initiating osteolysis, abscessation, and the formation of osteophytes (Vladutiu et al. 1982). Valvular endocarditis may result from bacteremia following tail-biting lesions (Van den Berg et al. 1981). *A. pyogenes* is occasionally recovered from fetuses and fetal membranes but its role in abortion has not been established.

A. pyogenes, as denoted by its name, causes suppurative lesions. Surprisingly little, however, is known of the virulence factors important in disease causation. Both the hemolytic protein exotoxin and protease have been proposed (Kume et al. 1983). *A. pyogenes* also binds alpha-2 macroglobulin (Lammler et al. 1985), a property that could interfere with local regulation of inflammation.

CLINICAL SIGNS AND LESIONS. The clinical signs are very variable, since *A. pyogenes* is responsible for a range of pathological lesions. Some, such as endocarditis and adhesive peritonitis, may be fatal. Others, such as vertebral osteomyelitis leading to posterior paralysis, may necessitate euthanasia. Suppurative osteomyelitis generally affects the vertebral bodies, leading to transverse pathological fractures, vertebral collapse, and compression of the spinal cord. Lameness results from polyarthritis or from cellulitis and periarthritis. However, many lesions, including subcutaneous or intramuscular abscesses, are clinically inapparent and are discovered only at postmortem or slaughter. Such abscesses vary from a few millimeters to several centimeters in size, usually have a thick fibrous capsule, and contain a yellow-green pus of variable consistency. Mastitis may be confined to one gland or may involve several.

DIAGNOSIS. Diagnosis in individual cases requires the demonstration of the organism in lesional material and confirmation by laboratory culture and identification. Carcass abscesses typically yield mixed cultures, including clostridia,

Bacteroides spp., *Proprionobacterium granulosum, Pasteurella multocida,* and unidentified anaerobes (Hara 1980; Jones 1980). Diagnosis of infection within a herd has been attempted serologically using an immunodiffusion test for antibody to *A. pyogenes* protease (Takeuchi et al. 1979). However, in a slaughterhouse survey, only 34.4% of pigs with abscesses had an antiprotease titer (Hara 1980).

TREATMENT. *A. pyogenes* is sensitive to a wide range of antimicrobial agents including penicillin, tetracycline, and erythromycin. Some strains have been shown to be resistant to sulphonamides and trimethoprim. In vivo sensitivity does not necessarily reflect in vitro sensitivity, for the physicochemical properties of chronic abscesses tend to protect the bacteria from the action of antimicrobial drugs. Abscesses may be removed surgically.

PREVENTION. Surveys of serum antibodies to *A. pyogenes* protease show approximately one-third of pigs are positive (Hara 1980). Antitoxin antibodies are also demonstrable and may increase with age. However, mice vaccinated with preparations of whole cells with or without toxoid or even given live organisms are not adequately protected against subsequent challenge (Derbyshire and Matthews 1963; Durner and Werner 1983). There is no effective vaccine available for swine. Prevention requires management of the environment to reduce or abolish the various conditions that predispose the development of *A. pyogenes* lesions.

REFERENCES

COLLINS, M. D., AND JONES, D. 1982. Reclassification of *Corynebacterium pyogenes* (Glage) in the genus *Actinomyces,* as *Actinomyces pyogenes* Comb. nov. J Gen Microbiol 128:901–902.

DERBYSHIRE, J. B., AND MATTHEWS, P. R. J. 1963. Immunological studies with *Corynebacterium pyogenes* in mice. Res Vet Sci 4:537–542.

DURNER, K., AND WERNER, B. 1983. Untersuchungen zur Immunogenitat und zu den Pathogenitatsfaktoren von *Corynebacterium pyogenes.* Arch Exp Vet Med Leipzig 37:541–547.

HARA, F. 1980. A study on pig pyogenic infections. Results of clinical, pathological, bacteriological and serological examinations of slaughtered pigs. Bull Azabu Uni Vet Med 1:187–202.

JONES, J. E. T. 1980. Observations on the bacterial flora of abscesses in pigs. Br Vet J 136:343–348.

KUME, T.; TAINAKA, M.; SAITO, M.; HIRUMA, M.; NISHIO, S.; KASHIWAZAKI, M.; MITANI, K.; AND NAKAJIMA, Y. 1983. Research on experimental *Corynebacterium pyogenes* infections in pigs. Kitasato Arch Exp Med 56:119–135.

LAMMLER, C.; CHHATWAL, G. S.; AND BLOBEL, H. 1985. Binding of α_2-macroglobulin and haptoglobin to *Actinomyces pyogenes.* Can J Microbiol 31: 657–659.

LOVELL, R. 1944. Further studies on the toxin of *Corynebacterium pyogenes.* J Pathol Bacteriol 56:525–529.

MORRISON, J. R. A., AND TILLOTSON, G. S. 1988. Identification of *Actinomyces* (*Corynebacterium*) *pyogenes* with the API 20 Strep system. J Clin Microbiol 26:1865–1866.

ROBERTS, R. J. 1968. Biochemical reactions of *Corynebacterium pyogenes.* J Pathol Bacteriol 95:127–130.

TAINAKA, M.; KUME, T.; TAKEUCHI, S.; NISHIO, S.; AND SAITO, M. 1983. Studies on the biological and serological properties of *Corynebacterium pyogenes.* Kitasato Arch Exp Med 56:105–117.

TAKEUCHI, S.; AZUMA, R.; NAKAJIMA, Y.; AND SUTO, T. 1979. Diagnosis of *Corynebacterium pyogenes* infection in pigs by immunodiffusion test with protease antigen. Natl Inst Anim Health Q (Tokyo) 19:77–82.

VAN DEN BERG, J.; NARUCKA, U.; NOUWS, J. F. M.; OKMA, B. D.; PEELEN, J. P. J.; AND SOETHOUT, A. E. E. 1981. Lesions in slaughtered animals. II. Inflammation of the tail and embolic pneumonia in pigs. Tijdschr Diergeneeskd 106:407–410.

VLADUTIU, O.; FLORESCU, S.; AND MURGU, I. 1982. Research in the pathogenetic mechanisms of osteophytosis in pyobacillary polyarthritis. Arch Vet 16:75–95.

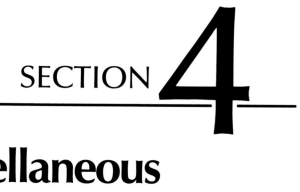

SECTION 4

Miscellaneous Conditions

S. D'Allaire, EDITOR

52 Behavioral Problems

P. H. Hemsworth

BEHAVIORAL PROBLEMS in farm animals can be defined as behavioral changes that compromise the production, health, or welfare of the animals. These changes include changes in the level of behavior or occurrence of a behavior that is inappropriate in the context of the performance of the behavior. This chapter will review the major behavioral changes that are observed in commercial pigs, with the objective of recommending possible solutions to improve the productivity, health, and welfare of these pigs.

LOW LEVELS OF SEXUAL BEHAVIOR IN THE BOAR.
While there is little documented evidence on poor sexual behavior in commercial boars, experience from artificial insemination centers and commercial piggeries indicate that up to 49% of culled boars are unable to copulate or copulate at sufficient frequency (Melrose 1966). Low levels of sexual behavior result from either low sexual motivation or poor mating competency. The latter, if not too serious, may be overcome in some situations where matings are supervised and assisted by stockpersons.

Poor Mating Competency.
Locomotor and penile injuries may not physically allow the achievement of copulation or may inhibit copulation because of pain (Christensen 1953), while injury sustained during copulation may produce a psychological effect for some time after physical recovery has occurred, again inhibiting copulation. Prevention of locomotor and penile injuries should include attention to the design and maintenance of the accommodation and mating areas, amount of supervision at mating, and selection for desirable conformational traits of the feet and legs. (See **Physical Environment at Mating** for a discussion on a suitable arena for mating.)

Poor orientation of the mounting response, such as head mounting, is often seen in the young boar. However, proper orientation is probably a learned response, and if the boar is of satisfactory sexual motivation, mating competency should improve with the positive reinforcement of copulation.

Social Environment.
The social environment during puberty can have serious long-term effects on the sexual behavior of the boar. Isolation of young postpubertal boars from 6 to 9 months of age from female pigs has been shown to depress the subsequent sexual behavior of the boars (Hemsworth et al. 1983). Therefore, housing procedures for selected pubertal and postpubertal boars and quarantine procedures applied to newly introduced young boars should include contact with female pigs. Housing these young postpubertal boars within several meters of females should provide them with sufficient female contact.

Isolation of mature boars from female pigs will also depress the sexual behavior of the boars (Hemsworth 1982), however, this effect is not permanent and housing these isolated boars near females will restore their sexual behavior within 4 weeks. The estrous status of the females does not influence the effectiveness of females in stimulating the sexual behavior of mature boars (Hemsworth 1982). It appears that olfactory and perhaps auditory stimuli from the female are most likely involved in stimulating the sexual behavior of mature boars (Hemsworth 1982).

As with the social environment at puberty, the social environment during rearing also appears to exert a long-term and perhaps even permanent effect on the sexual behavior of boars. Young boars up to 30 weeks of age require social contact, particularly tactile contact with other pigs, in order to develop high levels of sexual behavior (Hemsworth 1982). Failure to provide young boars with this contact will depress their subsequent sexual behavior. Therefore, it is recommended that prepubertal boars that may eventually be selected for breeding should be kept in groups for as long as practical, so that sexual behavior develops normally. Young boars kept in groups also display a fully coordinated mating response at an earlier age than boars reared individually (Thomas et al. 1979). If it is necessary to measure individual feed intake, separate feeding stalls could be provided in the group pens. Alternatively, since boars reared in individual pens with wire-mesh divisions can receive sufficient tactile contact with their neighbors to develop normal levels of sexual behavior (Hemsworth 1982), young boars can be reared in individual pens with wire-mesh or barred divisions.

Physical Environment at Mating.
The importance of the physical environment at mating on the reproductive performance of the pig is often

neglected. A common practice in intensive units is having pigs mate in the boar's accommodation pen, even though the physical conditions for mating may be far from ideal. For example, the pens are often small and the floors may be slippery. A recent study has demonstrated the importance of physical conditions at mating on the sexual behavior of the boar. Hemsworth et al. (1989a) found that the percentage of mating tests that resulted in copulations was lower for pigs mating in the boar's accommodation pen than for those mating in a specific mating pen that had a large, dry, nonslip floor. The sexual behavior of the gilts in the two treatments was similar, but there was a consistent trend toward a difference in the sexual behavior of the boars, suggesting that the low mating rate of pigs in the boar pen may have been mediated through an effect on the sexual behavior of the boar rather than that of the gilt. The male variables most affected were the time to first mount and the duration of ejaculation, indicating that the sexual motivation of the boar may have been adversely affected by the poor physical conditions at the time of mating. Therefore, it is recommended that matings should be conducted in separate, specially designed pens with a large floor area (minimum dimension of 2.5 m) to provide the boar with good access to the female's rear quarters; a nonslip floor surface, not abrasive to the animal's feet, that should be kept dry; and an area free of obstructions or other features, such as damaged or wire-mesh walls, that may trap the leg of an unbalanced boar.

To minimize moving the pigs, it is useful to have an area adjacent to the boar pens that can be used for both estrus detection and mating. A group of females can be briefly held in this area while the back-pressure test is conducted, and those in estrus can be separated and mated in this pen. Recent research indicates that gilts detected and mated in such an area have larger litters than those mated in the boar's accommodation pen (total litter size of 10.31 vs. 8.96, Hemsworth et al. 1991). If there is insufficient space available to build a mating pen, a number of these features can be incorporated into the boar pens.

Genetic and Climatic Factors.
Evidence from other species, together with breed comparisons of boars (Einarsson 1968), suggests that the sexual behavior of the boar may have a heritable basis. Elevated environmental temperatures may reduce the sexual behavior of the boar, but this effect is generally only temporary (Winfield et al. 1981). Insulation, adequate ventilation, and sprinkler cooling in the mating shed should minimize the adverse effects of high external temperatures.

LOW LEVELS OF SEXUAL BEHAVIOR IN THE FEMALE PIG.
Low levels of sexual behavior in female pigs will result in problems with estrus detection and sexual receptivity. It is generally recognized by pig producers that there is more difficulty in mating gilts than in mating sows (English et al. 1982) and thus this section will concentrate on gilts; however most of the principles considered apply to the sow. The literature indicates that in addition to delayed puberty, poor detection of estrus contributes to mating difficulties in commercial gilts (Hemsworth 1982). The incidence and consequences of poor sexual receptivity in those gilts detected in estrus are unknown, although this condition does occur (Cronin et al. 1982). Nevertheless, sexual receptivity and detection of estrus should be considered under the same behavioral category, since receptivity or the standing response is generally the criterion used in the main procedures for detecting estrus (e.g., use of boars or the back-pressure test).

Boar Contact. The most common procedure for detecting estrus other than the use of boars is the back-pressure test (BPT) or riding test (Signoret 1970). Females reacting to pressure on their back by displaying the "standing" or lordosis response for at least 10 seconds are generally classified as being sexually receptive (Hemsworth et al. 1988). The efficiency of this procedure depends on the female receiving intense boar contact at the time of testing. Signoret (1970) reported that the maximum percentage of gilts displaying the standing response to the BPT in the absence of boars was 59% between 24 and 36 hours after the start of estrus. This percentage increased to 90% by providing the gilts with auditory and olfactory contact with boars and further increased to 100% with the addition of visual and tactile contact with boars. Similarly, Hemsworth et al. (1984) demonstrated the importance of intense contact with the boar at the time of conducting the BPT. Testing the gilts at a distance of 1 m or more from the boar, which presumably reduced the amount of boar contact, reduced the efficiency of the test (52% of postpubertal gilts detected in estrus compared to 90% when gilts were tested adjacent to boars). Therefore, intense boar contact at the time of testing is vital in achieving a high efficiency with the BPT. Reducing boar contact will reduce sexual receptivity in estrous females.

While it appears that boar contact has an important role in stimulating the female's sexual behavior, there are situations where continuous stimulation from the boar may adversely affect sexual behavior. Research (Hemsworth et al. 1984, 1986a, 1988) has shown that housing postpubertal gilts adjacent to boars, with a wire-mesh divider separating them, results in a low estrus detection rate with the BPT (when gilts were tested adjacent to boars). It has been proposed that habituation by gilts to the important boar stimuli (e.g., auditory and olfactory stimuli), which facilitate the standing response of the estrous female to pressure on her back (Signoret

1970), is responsible for this detection problem (Hemsworth et al. 1988). This housing procedure, which is common in the industry, may also produce problems in detecting estrus when boars are used as determinants (Hemsworth et al. 1987). The results of these studies indicate that the common practice of housing postpubertal gilts adjacent to boars, with a wire-mesh or barred wall separating them, may adversely affect the sexual behavior of the gilts to the extent that there are difficulties in detecting estrus. Housing weaned sows adjacent to boars does not adversely affect the detection of estrus, perhaps because there is insufficient time for habituation to occur before the onset of estrus (Hemsworth and Hansen 1990).

There is substantial variability in the industry in procedures that use a boar to detect estrous females and yet these procedures have received little research attention. Hughes et al. (1985) indicate that 6- to 7-month-old boars may be less efficient at detecting estrous gilts than older boars because the young boars provide gilts with less olfactory and auditory stimulation. Clearly, further research is required to examine the effects of apparently important factors such as the sexual motivation and recent mating frequency of the boar, the testing time, and the group size of females on the efficiency of estrus detection using procedures that actively utilize boars. Until this research is conducted, these factors should be considered when assessing the efficiency of these procedures.

Space Allowance and Group Size. There is limited evidence that space allowance and, to a lesser extent, group size of group-housed gilts may influence the efficiency of detecting estrus. Hemsworth et al. (1986b) examined the effects of housing groups of adult postpubertal gilts (6 pigs/group) with a space allowance of 1, 2, or 3 m²/gilt on sexual behavior. A lower percentage of gilts were detected in estrus when housed with a space allowance of 1 m²/gilt than with a space allowance of 2 or 3 m²/gilt (detection rate of 79, 88, and 100%). A significant sustained increase in plasma-free-corticosteroid concentrations in gilts housed with a space allowance of 1 m²/gilt suggests that a chronic stress response may have reduced sexual receptivity. Clearly more comprehensive research is required, but in the meantime it is suggested that postpubertal gilts and weaned sows around the time of mating should be provided with at least 2 m²/animal.

In addition to this study on space allowance, several studies have examined the effects of group size. The literature on the effects of group size on the sexual behavior of female pigs is equivocal, perhaps because of suboptimal space allowances in these studies (Hemsworth and Barnett 1990), but there appear to be problems with detecting estrus in small groups (Christen-son 1984) and large groups (Christenson and Ford 1979; Cronin et al. 1983). The interaction between group size and space allowance must be examined to clarify the optimal social and spatial conditions for group-housed gilts.

Climatic Environment. Several studies have reported variation in the rate of detecting estrus in gilts between seasons. Christenson (1981) observed that a higher proportion of ovulating gilts were undetected in late summer than in the remainder of the year (16.7 and 8.4%, respectively). Cronin et al. (1983) reported that in the spring there was a lower percentage of unmated postpubertal gilts at 35 weeks of age that had not been detected in estrus than at other times of the year (3.2 and 6.5%, respectively). The effects of photoperiod and temperature are confounded in these two studies.

There is some limited evidence that indicates that increased environmental temperatures may affect sexual behavior of gilts. In two out of three trials, Warnick et al. (1965) reported that a total of 3 out of 13 gilts (23.1%) were not detected in estrus at an ambient temperature of 32°C although all had ovulated. In only one of a series of experiments reported by Godfrey et al. (1983), increased temperatures (38°C for 10 hours and 32°C for 14 hours) reduced the percentage of gilts detected in estrus (21 vs. 4% for control), however it was not determined whether ovulatory activity or detection of estrus was affected. Several studies reported that the duration of detected estrus was reduced by high temperatures (see review by Paterson and Pett 1987).

TAIL BITING. Although the incidence of tail biting appears to be highly variable, the problem appears widespread and the incidence may have increased with intensification of pig production (Smith and Penny 1986). The pathology of tail biting has been described by Smith and Penny (1986), and Van Putten (1969) lists the possible consequences of tail biting as restlessness, poor growth, possible paralysis and mortality due to infections, and condemnation of the carcass. There have been few experimental studies conducted on tail biting and consequently its cause(s) is poorly understood.

Outbreaks of tail biting have been attributed to numerous factors, including the physical and climatic environments and nutrition (see review by Smith and Penny 1986). However, the most likely explanation for outbreaks comes from the proposal originally made by Van Putten (1969) but which has been further developed by Fraser (1987). Van Putten (1969) argues that an outbreak of tail biting originates from the chewing and rooting of pen mates that generally occur with groups of pigs. These low-intensity behaviors are probably a result of the pig's natural tendency to root and chew on objects in its environment, but the behaviors are directed toward other pigs at least partly because of a lack of more suitable objects (Van Putten 1969). Since the tail is easy to chew and the chewing may not provoke an attack by the recipient, it is the tail that is most likely to receive a wound. According to Van Putten (1969), it is the vigorous tail waving, due to the irritation of a wound, that attracts further biting by other pen mates as well as by the original biter. Fraser (1987) has proposed that an attraction to blood from the wound may also lead to an escalation of tail biting. The large idiosyncratic differences between pigs in the degree of attraction to blood (Fraser 1987) could explain the variable incidence of tail biting.

Many farmers practice routine clipping of pigs' tails, and while this may reduce the incidence of tail biting, it may only mask the underlying problem (Fraser 1987). Attention to ventilation, temperature control, and space allowances may reduce the frequency of low-intensity chewing of pen mates (Fraser 1987), while the provision of distractions such as straw or other chewable objects may be beneficial (Van Putten 1969). Once an outbreak has occurred, the most useful approach may include the application of various preparations such as Stockholm tar to tails and rumps and restricting light.

EAR AND FLANK BITING. As with tail biting, the cause(s) of outbreaks of these behaviors is poorly understood. However, the origins of outbreaks of ear and flank biting may be similar to those of outbreaks of tail biting: chewing and rooting pen mates may lead to a wound on the ear or a lesion on the flank, which in turn stimulates an outbreak of more biting by pen mates. The pathology of ear and flank biting has been described by Smith and Penny (1986).

Treatment and control should be similar to that suggested for tail biting.

PEN FOULING. The excretory behavior of penned pigs indicates that they have highly localized excretory habits (Baxter 1984), and although many pens are designed with specific excreting areas such as partly slatted areas or dung passages, this does not guarantee the use of these areas by pigs for excretion (Baxter 1989). Only limited research has been conducted on the excretory behavior of pigs, however, Petherick (1983) and Baxter (1984, 1989) have suggested that the main factors affecting the excretory behavior of pigs are security and the thermal environment.

Although objective data are limited, Baxter (1989) proposed a set of rules that can be utilized when designing a pigpen; those rules relating to excretory behavior can be considered when addressing a problem of pen fouling:

1. Pigs will choose a dry, warm, draft-free area in which to rest.

2. Pigs will not choose to rest in areas subject to commotion and disturbance such as around ad libitum feeders, drinkers, and grooming points.

3. Pigs will rarely excrete in the area chosen for resting, but they will excrete in any space that is left after the resting area has been established.

4. Pigs may choose to lie in wet, excretory areas if environmental temperatures are high enough to raise their body temperatures to their upper critical level.

5. Pigs will tend to defecate next to walls or corners of the excretory space where they have some protection when they adopt the somewhat unstable posture during excretion. Subordinates may be displaced from an overcrowded excretory area and may then excrete anywhere; this may give rise to a new focus for excretion.

6. A minimum of two drinkers should be provided in every pen, since competition for the drinker (as with feeders) may cause commotion, which in turn may encourage pigs to excrete away from the disturbance.

FEAR OF HUMANS. In modern pig production there is frequent and often intense contact between humans and pigs, particularly young pigs and breeding pigs. In some circumstances commercial pigs may be highly fearful of humans (Hemsworth and Barnett 1987), and research on both experimental and commercial pigs has shown that high levels of fear of humans may markedly reduce the growth and reproductive performance of the pigs (Hemsworth and Barnett 1987, 1991). The mechanism involved appears to be a chronic-stress response, since in a number of experiments pigs that were highly fearful of humans had a sustained elevation of free-corticosteroid concentrations (Hemsworth and Barnett 1987). The results of these experiments have more implications for the breeding pig than for the grower pig, since the breeding pig is likely to receive more human contact. It should be emphasized that high levels of fear of humans may be a major limiting factor to the reproductive performance of commercial pigs: in one study, fear of humans by sows accounted for about 20% of the variation between commercial farms in reproductive performance (Hemsworth et al. 1989b).

In a study of the human factors that influence commercial pigs' fear of humans, it was found that the stockperson's behavior toward pigs was a good predictor of the level of fear of humans by pigs (Hemsworth et al. 1989b); a high proportion of physical interactions of a negative nature was consistently and strongly associated with a high level of fear of humans. Most of these negative interactions were hits, slaps, and kicks; however, many of these surprisingly were applied with only slight or moderate force. The positive interactions were mainly pats, strokes, and hands resting on the back of the pig. Thus, it appears that the frequent use of negative behaviors, irrespective of the amount of force used, and the infrequent use of positive behaviors by stockpersons will increase the fear of humans by pigs.

In situations where pigs are highly fearful of humans, there appears to be the opportunity to improve productivity through improving the behavior of stockpersons toward pigs; where breeding pigs appear to be highly fearful of humans, stockpersons should be encouraged to replace negative behaviors used on pigs with positive ones. While there are occasions when negative behaviors have to be used to move pigs, stockpersons should use these behaviors sparingly. When pigs baulk or are difficult to move, stockpersons should first examine the features of the environment that may be fear provoking, and if there are fear-provoking features, they should be improved before stockpersons resort to the use of negative behaviors. Environmental features that may cause pigs to baulk include unfamiliar objects and locations, changing or contrasting light patterns, and changing floor surfaces or levels.

A rough assessment of differences in the level of fear of humans by pigs between units or farms can be made by observing the approach and withdrawal behavior in the presence of humans. Techniques that can be used to reduce fear of humans include increasing the amount of human contact, replacing negative human behaviors with positive human behaviors toward pigs, avoiding situations where pigs may associate aversive events with humans, and using handling facilities such as corridors, gates, and races that promote ease of handling of pigs.

STEREOTYPIES. A useful definition of stereotypies is those behaviors that consist of morphological identical movements that are regularly repeated, have no obvious function, or are unusual in the context of their performance (Cronin et al. 1986). Examples of these behaviors are bar biting, sham chewing, and head weaving.

Numerous authors have proposed explanations for stereotypies in pigs, and these proposed causes range from frustration of feeding to lack of environmental stimulation (Barnett and Hemsworth 1990). While the cause(s) of the stereotypies is unclear, the function is even less clear. Some authors have proposed that the occurrence of stereotypies is indicative of poor welfare: it has been suggested that the welfare of the animal is at risk if the stereotypies occur for 10% of the animal's waking life (Broom 1983) and if they occur in more than 5% of all animals (Wiepkema 1983). However, these proposals are not substantiated, and in fact there is some limited evidence to indicate that the development of stereotypies may enable the animal to successfully adapt to a substantial environmental change. Dantzer et al. (1980) have shown that pigs able to chew a chain in a conflict situation have lower plasma corticosteroid concentrations; Cronin and Barnett (1987)

reported that the level of stereotypies by tethered sows was negatively correlated with plasma-free-corticosteroid concentrations.

Therefore, with the present knowledge of the cause and function of stereotypies, there are substantial difficulties in interpreting the implications of stereotypies for the welfare and productivity of pigs, except for those stereotypies that result in physical damage (e.g., the development of lesions in stall-housed sows that persistently rub their tail roots from side to side against stall fittings (Ewbank 1978).

MATERNAL BEHAVIOR. A significant proportion of live-born piglets do not survive the lactation period and a number of factors, such as the physical and climatic environments, health, and nutrition appear to be responsible (see Chapter 68). While savaging and overlaying of piglets by sows may account for up to a third of preweaning losses (Cutler et al. 1989), the contribution of changes in maternal behavior of sows to preweaning mortality has received surprisingly little research attention.

Savaging of piglets is more common in primiparous sows and the savaging attempt is often only directed to the first-born piglet (English et al. 1984; Spicer et al. 1985). Sows that savage their litters are more likely to be those mated at low body weights (Spicer et al. 1985). The cause(s) of savaging is unknown; however, in cases of observed savaging, an injection of a suitable tranquillizer (e.g., Azaperone; English et al. 1984) or separation of piglets from the sow until farrowing is complete is usually all that is needed to settle the sow.

While malnutrition or illness of piglets may be implicated in many cases of overlaying (English et al. 1984), many overlain piglets show no evidence of preexisting illness (Spicer et al. 1985). If a high incidence of overlaying is suspected, consideration should be given to the recommendations made by Cutler (Chapter 68) for the provision of a suitable thermal environment for the piglets and a suitable physical environment for the sow.

The possibility that piglet mortality may be affected by disturbances to the maternal behavior of sows is demonstrated by some recent research. Cronin and Van Amerongen (1991) found that the provision of straw to and a hessian cover over the farrowing crates of primiparous sows, in order to simulate a completed farrowing nest, reduced preweaning mortality. It is of interest that the sows in this treatment were more responsive to distress vocalizations of their piglets. Similarly, Cronin (unpublished data) found that the addition of small amounts of sawdust to the farrowing crates of young sows reduced the incidence of overlaying during and 6 hours after parturition. These limited results indicate that it may be possible to improve maternal behavior in order to reduce preweaning mortality by modifying the physical environment at parturition, and clearly further research is warranted on maternal behavior.

REFERENCES

BARNETT, J. L., AND HEMSWORTH, P. H. 1990. The validity of physiological and behavioural measures of animal welfare. Appl Anim Behav Sci 25:177–187.

BAXTER, S. H. 1984. Intensive Pig Production:Environmental Management and Design. London: Granada, pp. 210–254.

_____. 1989. Designing the pig pen. In Manipulating Pig Production. II. Werribee, Australia: Australasian Pig Science Association, pp. 191–206.

BROOM, D. M. 1983. Stereotypies as animal welfare indicators. In Indicators Relevant to Farm Animal Welfare. Ed. D. Smith. The Hague: Martinus Nijhoff, pp. 81–87.

CHRISTENSEN, N. O. 1953. Impotentia coeundi in boars due to arthrosis deformans. 15th Int Vet Congr, Part I, Vol. 2, pp. 742–745; Part II, pp. 332–333.

CHRISTENSON, R. K. 1981. Influence of confinement and season of the year on puberty and estrous activity of gilts. J Anim Sci 52:821–825.

_____. 1984. Influence of number of gilts per pen on oestrous traits in confinement reared gilts. Theriogenology 22:313–320.

CHRISTENSON, R. K., AND FORD, J. J. 1979. Puberty and estrus in confinement-reared gilts. J Anim Sci 49:743–751.

CRONIN, G. M., AND BARNETT, J. L. 1987. An association between plasma corticosteroids and performance of stereotypic behaviour in tethered sows. In Manipulating Pig Production. Werribee, Australia: Australasia Pig Science Association, p. 26.

CRONIN, G. M., AND VAN AMERONGEN, G. 1991. The effect of modifying the farrowing environment on sow behaviour and growth of piglets. Appl Anim Behav Sci 30:287–298.

CRONIN, G. M.; HEMSWORTH, P. H.; AND WINFIELD, C. G. 1982. Oestrous behaviour in relation to fertility and fecundity of gilts. Anim Reprod Sci 5:117–125.

CRONIN, G. M.; HEMSWORTH, P. H.; WINFIELD, C. G.; MULLER, B.; AND CHAMLEY, W. A. 1983. The incidence of, and factors associated with, failure to mate by 245 days of age in the gilt. Anim Reprod Sci 5:199–205.

CRONIN, G. M.; WIEPKEMA, P. R.; AND VAN REE, J. M. 1986. Endorphins implicated in stereotypies of tethered sows. Experientia 42:198–199.

CUTLER, R. S.; SPICER, E. M.; AND PRIME, R. W. 1989. Neonatal mortality: The influence of management. In Manipulating Pig Production. II. Werribee, Australia: Australasian Pig Science Association, pp. 122–126.

DANTZER, R.; ANNONE, M.; AND MORMEDE, P. 1980. Effects of frustration on behaviour and plasma corticosteroid levels in pigs. Physiol Behav 24:1–4.

EINARSSON, S. 1968. Fertility and serving ability of Swedish Landrace and Swedish Yorkshire boars. Nord Vet Med 20:616–621.

ENGLISH, P. R.; SMITH, W. J.; AND MacLEAN, A. 1984. The Sow–Improving Her Efficiency, 4th ed. Suffolk: Farming Press Limited, pp. 186–218.

EWBANK, R. 1978. Stereotypies in clinical veterinary practice. 1st World Congr Ethol Appl Zootech, Madrid, pp. 499–502.

FRASER, D. 1987. Attraction to blood as a factor in tail-biting by pigs. Appl Anim Behav Sci 17:61–68.

GODFREY, N. W.; MERCY, A. R.; AND EMMS, Y. 1983. The effect of high ambient temperature on reproductive performance in gilts. Proc Aust Pig Ind Res Comm Workshop Reprod, Tasmania, Australia.

HEMSWORTH, P. H. 1982. Social environment and reproduction. In Control of Pig Reproduction. Ed. D. J. A. Coles and G. R. Foxcroft. London: Butterworth, pp. 585–601.

HEMSWORTH, P. H., AND BARNETT, J. L. 1987. Human-animal interactions. Vet Clin North Am 3:339–356.

_____. 1990. Behavioural responses affecting gilt and sow reproduction. J Reprod Fert Suppl 40:343–354.

_____. 1991. The effects of aversively handling pigs, either individually or in groups, on their behaviour, growth and corticosteroids. Appl Anim Behav Sci 30:61–72.

HEMSWORTH, P. H., AND HANSEN, C. 1990. The effects of continuous boar contact on oestrus detection rate of weaned sows. Appl Anim Behav Sci 28:281–285.

HEMSWORTH, P. H.; WINFIELD, C. G.; HANSEN, C.; AND MAKIN, A. W. 1983. The influence of isolation from females and mating frequency on the sexual behaviour and semen quality of young post-pubertal boars. Anim Prod 37:49–52.

HEMSWORTH, P. H.; CRONIN, G. M.; HANSEN, C.; AND WINFIELD, C. G. 1984. The effects of two estrus detection procedures and intense boar stimulation near the time of estrus on mating efficiency of the female pig. Appl Anim Behav Sci 12:339–347.

HEMSWORTH, P. H.; WINFIELD, C. G.; BARNETT, J. L.; SCHIRMER, B.; AND HANSEN, C. 1986a. A comparison of the effects of two oestrus detection procedures and two housing systems on the oestrus detection rate of female pigs. Appl Anim Behav Sci 16:345–351.

HEMSWORTH, P. H.; BARNETT, J. L.; HANSEN, C.; AND WINFIELD, C. G. 1986b. Effects of social environment on welfare status and sexual behaviour of female pigs. II. Effects of space allowance. Appl Anim Behav Sci 16:259–267.

HEMSWORTH, P. H.; WINFIELD, C. G.; BARNETT, J. L.; HANSEN, C.; SCHIRMER, B.; AND FOOTE, M. 1987. The efficiency of boars to detect oestrous females housed adjacent to boars. Appl Anim Behav Sci 19:81–87.

HEMSWORTH, P. H.; WINFIELD, C. G.; TILBROOK, A. J.; HANSEN, C.; AND BARNETT, J. L. 1988. Habituation to boar stimuli: Possible mechanism responsible for the reduced detection rate of oestrous gilts housed adjacent to boars. Appl Anim Behav Sci 19:255–264.

HEMSWORTH, P. H.; HANSEN, C; AND WINFIELD, C. G. 1989a. The influence of mating conditions on the sexual behaviour of male and female pigs. Appl Anim Behav Sci 23:207–214.

HEMSWORTH, P. H.; BARNETT, J. L.; COLEMAN, C. J.; AND HANSEN, C. 1989b. A study of the relationships between the attitudinal and behavioural profiles of stockpersons and the level of fear of humans and reproductive performance of commercial pigs. Appl Anim Behav Sci 23:301–314.

HEMSWORTH, P. H.; HANSEN, C.; COLEMAN, G. J.; AND JONGMAN, E. 1991. The influence of conditions at the time of mating on reproduction of commercial pigs. Appl Anim Behav Sci 30:273–285.

HUGHES, P. E.; HEMSWORTH, P. H.; AND HANSEN, C. 1985. The effects of supplementary olfactory and auditory stimuli on the stimulus value and mating success of the young boar. Appl Anim Behav Sci 14:245–252.

MELROSE, D. R. 1966. A review of progress and of possible developments in artificial insemination of pigs. Vet Rec 78:159–168.

PATERSON, A. M., AND PETT, D. H. 1987. The role of high ambient temperature in seasonal infertility in the sow. In Manipulating Pig Production. Werribee, Australia: Australasian Pig Science Association, pp. 48–52.

PETHERICK, J. C. 1983. A biological basis for the design of space in livestock housing. In Farm Animal Housing and Welfare. Ed. S. H. Baxter, M. R. Baxter, and J. A. C. MacCormack. The Hague: Martinus Nijhoff, pp. 103–120.

SIGNORET, J. P. 1970. Swine behaviour in reproduction. In Effect of Disease and Stress on Reproductive Efficiency in Swine. Extension Service, Univ of Nebraska, pp. 28–45.

SMITH, W. J., AND PENNY, R. H. C. 1986. Behavioral problems, including vices and cannibalism. In Diseases of Swine. 6th ed. Ed. A. D. Leman, B. Straw, R. D. Glock, W. L. Mengeling, R. H. C. Penny, and E. Scholl. Ames: Iowa State Univ Press, pp. 761–772.

SPICER, E. M.; DRIESEN, S. J.; FAHY, V. A.; AND HORTON, B. J. 1985. Trauma, overlay and savaging. Aust Adv Vet Sci p. 122.

THOMAS, H. R.; KATTESH, H. G.; KNIGHT, J. W.; GWAZDAUSKAS, F. C.; MEACHAM, T. N.; AND KORNEGAY, E. T. 1979. Effects of housing and rearing on age of puberty and libido in boars. Anim Prod 28:231–234.

VAN PUTTEN, G. 1969. An investigation of tail-biting among fattening pigs. Br Vet J 125:511–517.

WARNICK, A. E.; WALLACE, H. D.; PALMER, A. Z.; SOSA, E.; DUERRE, D. J.; AND CALDWELL, V. E. 1965. Effect of temperature on early embryo survival in gilts. J Anim Sci 24:89–92.

WIEPKEMA, P. R. 1983. On the significance of ethological criteria for the assessment of animal welfare. In Indicators Relevant to Farm Animal Welfare. Ed. D. Smith. The Hague: Martinus Nijhoff, pp. 71–79.

WINFIELD, C. G.; HEMSWORTH, P. H.; GALLOWAY, D. B.; AND MAKIN, A. W. 1981. Sexual behaviour and semen characteristics of boars: Effects of high temperature. Aust J Exp Agric Anim Husb 21:39–45.

53 Coccidia and Other Protozoa

D. S. Lindsay

B. L. Blagburn

B. P. Stuart

Coccidiosis (*Isospora suis*)

COCCIDIA ARE obligatory intracellular protozoan parasites. *Eimeria, Isospora,* and *Cryptosporidium* are important coccidial parasites of mammals and birds. Domestic animals may be infected with several species of coccidia but usually only a few species are pathogenic for a given host.

Neonatal coccidiosis is the most important protozoal disease of swine. Although the causative agent, *Isospora suis,* was described from pigs in 1934 (Biester and Murray 1934), it was not until the middle 1970s that neonatal coccidiosis was recognized as a disease problem in nursing pigs (Sangster et al. 1976; Bergland 1977). In 1978, it was demonstrated that *I. suis* was the cause of neonatal piglet coccidiosis in natural cases and coccidiosis was experimentally reproduced in nursing pigs (Stuart et al. 1978). Neonatal piglet coccidiosis has a cosmopolitan distribution and is found anywhere pigs are raised in confinement (Stuart et al. 1978; Roberts et al. 1980; Coussement et al. 1981; Sanford and Josephson 1981; Vitovec and Koudela 1987).

ETIOLOGY

Life Cycle of *Isospora suis*. Coccidial life cycles are divided into three phases: sporogony, excystation, and endogenous development. Each phase is unique for each species and knowledge of life-cycle phases is important in diagnosis, treatment, prevention, and control of these parasites.

Sporogony is the process by which the oocysts (environmentally resistant cyst stages) develop from the unsporulated noninfectious stages passed in the feces to infective stages (Figs. 53.1–53.3). Proper temperature and moisture must be present for sporulation to take place. The oocysts of *I. suis* sporulate rapidly at temperatures between 20° and 37°C (Lindsay et al. 1982). Because supplemental heat of between 32° and 35°C are provided by producers for newborn piglets, these temperatures favor rapid development (within 12 hours) of *I. suis* oocysts in the farrowing crate. Oocysts are most sensitive to killing when in the unsporulated state and during

sporulation. Once the oocysts are sporulated they are resistant to most disinfectants. The sporulated oocysts of *I. suis* contain two sporocysts each with four sporozoites when fully sporulated.

Excystation is the phase of the life cycle that occurs immediately after the infectious oocysts are ingested. Passage through the stomach alters the oocyst wall and allows bile salts and digestive enzymes to activate the sporozoites. The activated sporozoites leave the sporocyst and oocyst and are freed into the intestinal lumen. The sporozoites then penetrate enterocytes and begin the endogenous phase of parasite multiplication.

The endogenous stages of the life cycle of *I. suis* occur in enterocytes throughout the small intestine with most stages being present in the jejunum and ileum. Occasionally, in heavy infections, parasites can be found in the cecum and colon. Stages are usually located on the distal por-

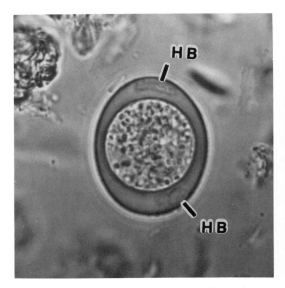

53.1. Unsporulated oocyst of *Isospora suis* in a fecal flotation demonstrating diagnostic hazy bodies (*HB).* (Lindsay et al. 1982, J Parasitol 68:861–865, with permission.)

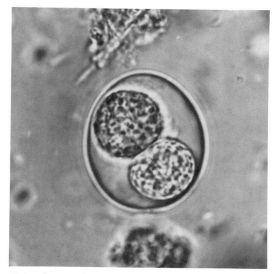

53.2. Oocyst of *Isospora suis* in the diagnostic two-celled stage in a fecal flotation.

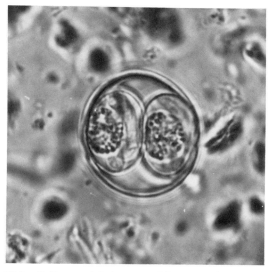

53.3. Fully sporulated oocyst of *Isospora suis* in a fecal flotation.

tions of the villi and are in a parasitophorous vacuole below the host-cell nucleus (Lindsay et al. 1980). In severe clinical or experimental cases, stages may also be located in crypt enterocytes.

There are two distinct types of asexual stages that occur in the endogenous life cycle of *I. suis*. Sporozoites enter enterocytes and become binucleated Type 1 meronts, which divide by endodyogeny in about 24 hours and produce two Type 1 daughter merozoites. The characteristic side-by-side appearance of these Type 1 merozoites is useful in diagnosis because none of the swine *Eimeria* species divide by endodyogeny (Lindsay et al. 1983). Several divisional cycles by endo-

dyogeny can occur and produce cells with many Type 1 merozoites. Type 2 meronts are multinucleated and form Type 2 merozoites, which may be seen as early as 4 days postinoculation (PI). Type 2 merozoites are smaller than Type 1 merozoites. Sexual stages consist of microgamonts that produce biflagellated microgametes and macrogamonts. The microgametes fertilize the macrogamonts and an oocyst is formed. These sexual stages also may be seen 4 days PI, while oocysts are first seen in the feces 5 days PI (rarely 4 days).

Immunity to *Isospora suis*. Pigs that have been infected with *I. suis* and recover are resistant to challenge infection (Stuart et al. 1982b). These challenged pigs excrete no or very few oocysts (in contrast to initial infection) and do not develop clinical signs. Administration of corticosteroids (methylprednisolone acetate) does not cause these previously exposed pigs to reexcrete oocysts, suggesting good immunity has developed. Little is known about the specific humoral or cell-mediated immune response of pigs to *I. suis* infection.

Pigs demonstrate age-related differences in susceptibility to experimental infection and disease (Stuart et al. 1982a). One to 2-day-old nursing pigs develop much more severe disease than do pigs inoculated with an identical number of oocysts at 2 or 4 weeks of age.

CLINICAL SIGNS. Signs of disease occur in formally healthy nursing pigs between 7 and 14 days of age (Stuart et al. 1978; Morin et al. 1983). Yellowish to grayish diarrhea is the major clinical sign. The feces are initially loose or pasty and become more fluid as the infection progresses. Piglets become covered with the liquid feces causing them to stay damp and have a rancid odor of sour milk. The piglets usually continue to nurse, develop a rough-hair coat, become dehydrated, and have depressed weight gains (Lindsay et al. 1985). Litters within the farrowing house vary in the degree to which they demonstrate clinical signs and not all piglets within a litter are equally affected. Morbidity is usually high but mortalities are usually moderate. Concurrent bacterial, viral, or other parasitic infections may lead to extreme mortalities and complicate diagnosis.

Occasionally *I. suis* oocysts are present in the feces of recently weaned pigs, some of which may have diarrhea. Although this indicates a patent infection, whether or not *I. suis* is the etiologic agent of the diarrhea is unknown because of complicating factors such as diet and other management changes that occur at weaning. *I. suis* infections do not cause disease in finishing pigs or in breeding stock.

PATHOLOGIC CHANGES. Experimental studies have shown that the degree of disease is dependent on the number of sporulated *I. suis* oocysts that a piglet ingests (Stuart et al. 1980, 1982a). Inoculation of 200,000 or more oocysts usually produces severe disease and moderate to extreme mortalities (Stuart et al. 1980; Lindsay et al. 1985). Inoculation of fewer oocysts generally produces clinical disease characterized principally by diarrhea, but few or no mortalities (Stuart et al. 1980; Robinson et al. 1983).

Necropsy examination may demonstrate gross lesions of neonatal coccidiosis characterized by a fibrinonecrotic membrane in the jejunum and ileum, but this is seen only in severely infected piglets (Fig. 53.4). Hemorrhage is not seen, even in extreme cases of natural infections or in experimental infections where large numbers of oocysts are given.

Microscopic lesions consist of villous atrophy, villous fusion, crypt hyperplasia, and necrotic enteritis (Stuart et al. 1980, 1982a; Eustis and Nelson 1981; Robinson et al. 1983). The columnar enterocytes at the tips of the villi may be destroyed, exposing the underlying lamina propria,

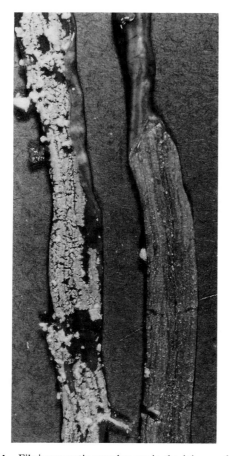

53.4. Fibrinonecrotic membranes in the jejunum from two piglets experimentally infected with *Isospora suis* oocysts, 4 days postinoculation. (Stuart et al. 1980, Vet Pathol 17:84–93, with permission.)

or they are replaced by flattened immature enterocytes. The functional ability for absorption is diminished in this altered epithelium, resulting in fluid loss and diarrhea. Lesions develop about 4 days PI and are associated with the presence of the asexual stages. In most natural cases few parasites are present in the sections and most of these parasites are asexual stages. In severe cases piglets may succumb to coccidiosis before the sexual stages are produced. The extent of microscopic lesions produced is dependent on the number of *I. suis* oocysts a pig ingests.

DIAGNOSIS. Diarrhea in nursing pigs 7–14 days of age that does not respond to antibiotic treatment is suggestive of neonatal *I. suis* infection. Other agents such as enteropathogenic *E. coli,* transmissible gastroenteritis virus, rotavirus, *Clostridium perfringens* type C, and *Strongyloides ransomi* should be considered in the differential diagnosis.

Diagnosis of *I. suis* is best achieved by finding *I. suis* oocysts in the feces of clinically affected piglets. This is the quickest method available for diagnosis. Fecal smears or fecal flotations should be made from several litters within the farrowing house that have been showing clinical signs for 2–3 days, because diarrhea starts about a day before oocysts are passed and peak oocyst production occurs about 2–3 days after clinical signs develop. The oocysts of *I. suis* have characteristic structures called "hazy bodies" between the oocyst wall and the sporont (Fig. 53.1). These are diagnostic for *I. suis* because none of the oocysts of the swine *Eimeria* species have this structure (Lindsay et al. 1982). Additionally, some of the oocysts may be in the 2-celled stage (Fig. 53.2), which is also diagnostic for *I. suis.*

Mucosal smears can be used in the diagnosis of *I. suis* infection (Stevenson and Andrews 1982; Lindsay 1989). The intestinal mucosa should be scraped with a scalpel using just enough pressure to dislodge villi and the scrapings prepared as a smear on a glass microscope slide. The smears are then stained with any of a number of routine blood stains. The presence of paired Type 1 merozoites (Fig. 53.5) is diagnostic. Other asexual stages such as binucleated Type 1 meronts, Type 2 meronts and merozoites, and sexual stages (microgamonts and macrogamonts) will probably be present also, but their identification is more difficult and not needed for the diagnosis.

Histologic diagnosis of *I. suis* in tissue sections is possible (Lindsay et al. 1983). As with mucosal smears, demonstration of paired Type 1 merozoites is diagnostic. The multinucleated Type 2 meronts of *I. suis* are elongated and are often found in the same host cell. This association of meronts is also characteristic for *I. suis.* Finally, the macrogamonts of *I. suis* lack the characteristic eosinophilic wall-forming bodies seen in *Eimeria* species.

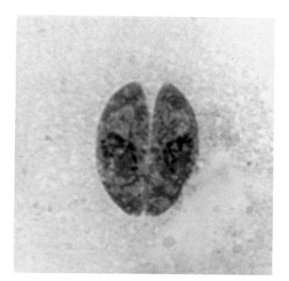

53.5. Paired Type 1 merozoites of *Isospora suis* in a mucosal scraping from an experimentally infected piglet, 3 days postinoculation. Note the side-by-side appearance of the merozoites. Wright's-Giemsa. (Lindsay et al. 1980, J Parasitol 66:771–779, with permission.)

EPIDEMIOLOGY

***Eimeria* Species.** There are eight species of *Eimeria* that occur in swine in the United States (Vetterling 1965; Greiner et al. 1982; Lindsay et al. 1984). Reports of coccidiosis in swine caused by *Eimeria* species are rare and are associated with animals on dirt lots (Hill et al. 1985). Experimental studies have demonstrated that inoculation of 3-day-old nursing pigs with up to 5 million oocysts of *Eimeria debliecki* does not cause clinical disease and that up to 10 million oocysts does not cause disease in 4-week-old weaned pigs (Lindsay et al. 1987). Similarly, *E. spinosa* is not pathogenic for pigs under experimental conditions (Ernst 1987). Coccidia vary in their inherent abilities to cause disease and it appears that the *Eimeria* species infecting swine are nonpathogenic.

Isospora suis. Once *I. suis* coccidiosis was recognized as a problem in nursing pigs, most veterinarians and researchers assumed that piglets were infected by ingesting *I. suis* oocysts from the sow's feces. However, studies have failed to confirm this assumption. Surveys of the swine population in the United States indicate that *Eimeria* infections are common (60–95%) in animals raised in lots or in the wild, but less than 3% of the animals sampled are excreting oocysts of *I. suis* (Vetterling 1966; Greiner et al. 1982; Lindsay et al. 1984). One study examined the species of oocysts excreted by sows on farms with and without a history of *I. suis* infections in nursing

pigs; sows on all the farms underwent gestation on dirt lots (Lindsay et al. 1984). The study reported that 82% of the sows on farms with a history of coccidiosis had *Eimeria* infections but no detectable *I. suis* infections. The sows from farms with no history of neonatal coccidiosis had an infection rate of 95% with *Eimeria* species and less than 1% with *I. suis*.

In the United States, Stuart and Lindsay (1986) examined the transmission of *I. suis* on two farms in Georgia. Daily fecal samples were collected rectally from sows typically 1 week prior to farrowing, the day of farrowing, and for about 1 week after farrowing. Colostrum and placentas from several sows were examined microscopically for parasites. A coccidiostat (amprolium HCl, Amprol 25% feed grade) was given to half of the sows on each farm. *Eimeria* species were the only coccidia seen in the feces of sows. None of the sows given amprolium HCl had oocysts in fecal samples at farrowing. No parasitic stages were seen in the colostrum or placentas examined. On Farm 1, 7 of 12 litters from nontreated sows and 9 of 12 litters from treated sows developed clinical coccidiosis. On Farm 2, all 11 litters from nontreated sows and 11 of 12 litters from treated sows developed clinical coccidiosis. *I. suis* was the only species of coccidia seen in these piglets.

The results of these studies indicate that sows are not the primary source of *I. suis* infection for nursing pigs. It is still not known how *I. suis* becomes established on a farm; once it is established, it is probably transmitted through contaminated farrowing crates. The temperature (32–35°C) and moisture in the farrowing crate favor rapid sporulation of *I. suis*. High temperatures (32–35°C) may inhibit sporulation of the *Eimeria* species and could explain the absence of these species in nursing pigs.

TREATMENT AND CONTROL

Anticoccidials. Sows do not appear to be a major source of infection for nursing pigs; therefore, using anticoccidial drugs in the sow's ration is of little value in controlling neonatal coccidiosis. Early studies that reported success with treating sows probably are due to improved sanitation once the producers were made aware that their pigs had a coccidia problem. Studies that demonstrate anticoccidial activity of drugs in weaned or finishing pigs are of no value in predicting the ability of these drugs to control disease in nursing pigs. Addition of anticoccidial drugs to the drinking water of piglets or mixing drugs in oral iron may be beneficial in treating coccidiosis, but there is no way to ensure that every piglet gets a therapeutic/preventive dose. There are no controlled studies that have documented the effectiveness of this type of treatment. Individual dosing is still the best way to ensure that each piglet gets a proper dose of anticoccidial drug.

The controlled studies conducted to date in nursing pigs have not identified an effective coccidiostat. In one study, neither amprolium HCl nor furazolidone were effective in preventing coccidiosis in 4-day-old pigs inoculated with *I. suis* (Girard and Morin 1987). Pigs were treated orally with 2 ml of 9.6% amprolium HCl (Amprol) daily for 5 days beginning on the day of infection, or with 1 ml of furazolidone (Furoxone) daily for 3 days beginning on the day of infection and then every other day thereafter until necropsy. Clinical disease was delayed 2–3 days in pigs treated with furazolidone, but no effect on oocyst production or weight gain was seen. Amprolium HCl did not delay clinical signs or prevent growth retardation, but did decrease oocyst production. Monensin did not prevent clinical disease, oocyst production, or microscopic intestinal lesions in pigs inoculated with *I. suis* at 3 days of age (Doré and Morin 1987). Piglets were treated orally with 15 mg/kg monensin (Rumensin) in 2 ml of milk beginning 1 day before infection and every other day thereafter until necropsy. A slight delay in the onset of clinical signs was seen in monensin-treated pigs.

Sanitation. Improved attention to sanitation has been the most successful method for reducing losses due to neonatal coccidiosis in pigs (Ernst et al. 1985; Stuart and Lindsay 1986). A good sanitation program entails thorough cleaning of the crates to remove organic debris, disinfection with bleach (at least 50%) or ammonia compounds for several hours or overnight, and steam cleaning. Buildings should be empty of animals when disinfecting is being done. Ventilation should be adequate to prevent excessive exposure of workers to fumes of bleach or ammonia, or a chemical mask must be worn by workers. Producers should limit access to farrowing crates by workers to avoid crate-to-crate contamination with oocysts carried on boots or clothing. Likewise, pets should be prevented from entering the farrowing house and spreading oocysts from crate to crate on their paws. Rodent populations should be controlled to prevent these animals from mechanically transmitting oocysts.

Facilities need to be sanitized after every farrowing. Producers should be made aware that even though clinical disease is under control, the potential for future outbreaks is still present. In some cases, outbreaks of moderate clinical disease have developed in the first farrowing after sanitation was not done (Ernst et al. 1985).

Cryptosporidiosis (*Cryptosporidium parvum*)

CRYPTOSPORIDIOSIS is caused by infection with *Cryptosporidium parvum,* a small coccidial parasite that can infect a wide variety of mammalian hosts including humans. Members of the genus *Cryptosporidium* differ from conventional coccidia that infect animals in that they develop in the microvillous border of enterocytes, rather than down deep in the host-cell cytoplasm. Additionally, oocysts of *Cryptosporidium* are completely sporulated when excreted in the feces and contain four sporozoites and no sporocysts (Upton and Current 1985).

CLINICAL SIGNS AND PATHOLOGIC CHANGES. Most cases of porcine cryptosporidiosis are asymptomatic and infection with this parasite does not appear to be a major production problem (Kennedy et al. 1977; Links 1982; Sanford 1987). If clinical signs are present they consist of nonhemorrhagic diarrhea. Most cases are seen in pigs from 6 to 12 weeks of age (Sanford 1987).

Microscopic lesions associated with cryptosporidial infection in pigs are minimal or not present (Links 1982; Sanford 1987). The parasites are found in the jejunum, ileum, cecum, and colon with most numbers of parasites being in the ileum. When lesions are present they consist of mild villous atrophy and invasion of the lamina propria by large numbers of mononuclear inflammatory cells and fewer eosinophils (Sanford 1987). Microvilli in the area of the parasites may be displaced or hypertrophic.

EPIDEMIOLOGY AND DIAGNOSIS. Pigs are infected with *Cryptosporidium* by ingesting oocysts in contaminated feed, from the environment, or in water. There is no seasonal pattern to the prevalence of infection (Sanford 1987).

Diagnosis can be achieved by finding the developmental stages of the parasite in histologic sections. The parasites are 2–6 μm, basophilic, and appear to be embedded in the microvillous border of the enterocytes. Diagnosis can also be made by finding the characteristic oocysts in fecal flotations. The oocysts are small, 5.0 by 4.5 μm, and have a pinkish color and residual body when observed with light microscopy. Sheather's sugar solution is the flotation media of choice; a microscope equipped with good objectives is needed to identify the oocysts in flotations. It is important to remember that in fecal flotations, the cryptosporidial oocysts will be in a slightly higher plane of focus than other coccidial oocysts. Several methods of staining fecal samples and examining for oocysts have been developed but these are not practical for use in pigs. Several serologic methods such as enzyme-linked immunosorbent assay and indirect fluorescent antibody have been developed for estimating the prevalence of cryptosporidial exposure, but these tests are not currently in widespread use.

TREATMENT AND CONTROL. There is no treatment for cryptosporidial infection. Sanitation methods used to control *I. suis* coccidiosis should also prove effective against cryptosporidial infections.

Toxoplasmosis (*Toxoplasma gondii*)

TOXOPLASMOSIS is caused by infection with *Toxoplasma gondii,* a protozoan parasite related to the coccidia. Infections are common in humans and animals. Adult animals become infected by ingesting sporulated *T. gondii* oocysts or by consuming meat containing tissue cysts. Cats (and other felines) are the only animals that can excrete oocysts in their feces and are important in the transmission of *T. gondii* to pigs and other animals. Tissue cysts are found mainly in the central nervous system and cardiac and skeletal muscles of infected animals, and contain bradyzoites that are slowly multiplying stages. Tissue cysts remain viable in the tissues for many years and probably the life of the animal. Bradyzoites can survive passage through the stomach. Once in the intestine of the host, the sporozoites or bradyzoites change into a fast-multiplying stage called tachyzoites, which cannot survive passage through the stomach; therefore, ingestion of meat that contains tachyzoites is not an effective mode of transmission. Tachyzoites multiply in the lamina propria of the intestine and eventually spread throughout the body. Transplacental infections may occur and are associated with tachyzoite dissemination. Tachyzoites cause tissue damage and eventually develop into the bradyzoite stage in tissue cysts. Toxoplasmosis is a zoonosis, and pork is considered a major source of human infection in the United States (Dubey 1990).

CLINICAL SIGNS. Most infections in swine are asymptomatic (Dubey 1986). Abortions due to *T. gondii,* although uncommon, may occur in sows. Transplacentally infected pigs may be born premature, dead, weak, or die soon after birth. Pigs that live may develop diarrhea, incoordination, tremors, or cough. Few reports exist on clinical disease in pigs that acquire infection postnatally. Young pigs (1–2 weeks old) that acquire infection by ingesting oocysts may exhibit diarrhea or even fatal infections (Dubey et al. 1979). On one farm, pigs that became infected with *T. gondii* by cannibalism did not develop clinical signs (Dubey et al. 1986). Experimental studies indicate that inoculation of pigs with *T. gondii* oocysts is more likely to produce disease than inoculation with tissue cysts (Dubey 1986). Severity of disease is dependent upon the number

of infective stages inoculated. Older animals are less likely to develop clinical disease. Experimental studies indicate that transplacental infections are difficult to produce in swine.

PATHOLOGIC CHANGES. Pathologic changes are associated with necrosis of host tissue caused by the rapidly multiplying tachyzoites. Ingestion of oocysts is more likely to give rise to intestinal lesions than does ingestion of tissue cysts. Lymphadenitis, splenitis, hepatitis, pneumonitis, and less frequently myositis and encephalitis are seen in naturally infected pigs (Dubey 1986).

DIAGNOSIS. Methods of diagnosis include bioassays of tissues in cats or mice, serology, and histology. Bioassays are the most sensitive but are costly and few laboratories perform these tests. Several serologic tests are available for determining antibodies to *T. gondii.* These include the Sabin-Feldman dye test (DT), indirect hemagglutination test, direct agglutination (DAG) test, latex agglutination test, indirect fluorescent antibody (IFA) test, and enzyme-linked immunosorbent assay (ELISA). The DT is best and considered the standard by which all other tests are judged. The DAG, IFA, and most ELISA tests compare favorably to the DT. Fetal fluids from aborted pigs should be examined for antibodies to *T. gondii* to confirm *T. gondii* abortion in sows. Histologic examination of tissues may be utilized for a presumptive diagnosis based on lesion characteristics and parasite structure following routine histologic staining (periodic acid–Schiff [PAS], silver, Giemsa) of tissue sections. For a definitive diagnosis, if parasites are found in tissue sections, then specific immunohistochemical tests (peroxidase-antiperoxidase test, avidin-biotin complex test) can be used.

EPIDEMIOLOGY. Serologic surveys indicate that from less than 1 to 69% of swine examined may have antibodies to *T. gondii.* A study conducted in Iowa indicated that farms with <100 sows and gilts were significantly more likely to be infected than farms with >100 sows and gilts (Zimmerman et al. 1990). The rate of infection was the same in total confinement farms and those farms that were under other management practices.

Pigs become infected by ingesting *T. gondii* oocysts in contaminated feed or water, by ingesting tissue cysts in infected meat, or by transplacental infection. Cats are the source of *T. gondii* oocysts for pigs, and pigs may ingest tissue cysts by killing and eating infected rodents, by cannibalism, by ear and tail biting, or by consumption of garbage.

TREATMENT AND CONTROL. Because most cases of porcine toxoplasmosis are asymptomatic, little is known about the treatment of the disease (Dubey 1986). In general, drugs used to treat toxoplasmosis in humans have been effective. These include pyrimethamine or trimethoprim in combination with a sulfonamide.

Control of *T. gondii* infection in pigs is important because of the public heath concerns over human infections. Following experimental infection, viable tissue cysts of *T. gondii* can be found in most commercial cuts of pork and studies have shown that the cysts will be viable for at least 2.5 years (Dubey 1988). Freezing ($-12°C$) for 3 days or heating pork to 58°C for 10 minutes will kill tissue cysts in pork (Dubey et al. 1990).

Prevention of *T. gondii* infection in pigs can be achieved by practicing good husbandry. To prevent oocyst-induced infections, cats should never be allowed in buildings where pigs are housed or where feed is stored. Rodenticides should be used to control rodents and eliminate this possible source of tissue cysts. Any pigs that die should be removed promptly to prevent cannibalism. Wild animal carcasses or uncooked garbage should never be fed to pigs.

Sarcocystis (*Sarcocystis miescheriana*)

SARCOCYSTIS spp. are coccidialike parasites that have a two-host life cycle. There are three species that use pigs as the intermediate host and form tissue cysts in the pig muscles. *Sarcocystis miescheriana* has a pig-dog life cycle and is the only species found in the United States. Dogs excrete infective stages (sporocysts) in their feces. The other species are *S. suihominis* that uses the human as the definitive host and *S. porcifelis* that uses cat as the definitive host (Dubey et al. 1989).

Surveys indicate that from 3 to 17% of the commercial breeding sows and 32% of wild swine examined in the United States have *Sarcocystis* infection. There are no reports of naturally occurring clinical disease due to *Sarcocystis* infection in swine (Dubey et al. 1989). Experimental infections indicate that *S. miescheriana* can cause abortion, death, dyspnea, weight loss, muscle tremors, and purpura of the skin. *Sarcocystis* infection in swine can be prevented by eliminating their exposure to canine feces. To prevent exposure in dogs, they should not be allowed to consume pig carcasses.

REFERENCES

BERGLAND, M. E. 1977. Necrotic enteritis in nursing piglets. Proc Am Assoc Vet Lab Diagn 20:151–156.
BIESTER, H. E., AND MURRAY, C. 1934. Studies in infectious enteritis of swine: VIII. *Isospora suis* N. sp. in swine. J Am Vet Med Assoc 85:207–219.
COUSSEMENT, W.; DUCATELLE, R.; GEERAERTS, G.; AND BERGHEN, P. 1981. Baby pig diarrhea caused by coccidia. Vet Q 3:57–60.
DORÉ, M., AND MORIN, M. 1987. Porcine neonatal coccidiosis: Evaluation of monensin as preventive therapy. Can Vet J 28:663–666.
DUBEY, J. P. 1986. A review of toxoplasmosis in pigs. Vet Parasitol 19:181–223.

————. 1988. Long-term persistence of *Toxoplasma gondii* in tissues of pigs inoculated with *T. gondii* oocysts and effect of freezing on viability of tissue cysts in pork. Am J Vet Res 49:910–913.
————. 1990. Status of toxoplasmosis in pigs in the United States. J Am Vet Med Assoc 196:270–274.
DUBEY, J. P.; WEISBRODE, S. E.; SHARMA, S. P.; AL-KHALIDI, N. W.; ZIMMERMAN, J. L.; AND GAAFAR, S. M. 1979. Porcine toxoplasmosis in Indiana. J Am Vet Med Assoc 174:604–609.
DUBEY, J. P.; MURRELL, K. D.; HANBURY, R. D.; ANDERSON, W. R.; DOBY, P. B.; AND MILLER, H. O. 1986. Epidemiologic findings on a swine farm with enzootic toxoplasmosis. J Am Vet Med Assoc 189:55–56.
DUBEY, J. P.; SPEER, C. A.; AND FAYER, R. 1989. Sarcocystis of Animals and Man. Boca Raton, Fla: CRC Press Inc.
DUBEY, J. P.; KOTULA, A. W.; SHARAR, A.; ANDREWS, C. D.; AND LINDSAY, D. S. 1990. Effect of high temperature on infectivity of *Toxoplasma gondii* tissue cysts in pork. J Parasitol 76:201–204.
ERNST, J. V. 1987. Pathogenicity in pigs experimentally infected with *Eimeria spinosa*. J Parasitol 73:1254–1256.
ERNST, J. V.; LINDSAY, D. S.; AND CURRENT, W. L. 1985. Control of *Isospora suis*-induced coccidiosis on a swine farm. Am J Vet Res 46:643–645.
EUSTIS, S. L., AND NELSON, D. T. 1981. Lesions associated with coccidiosis in nursing piglets. Vet Pathol 18:21–28.
GIRARD, C., AND MORIN, M. 1987. Amprolium and furazolidone as preventive treatment for intestinal coccidiosis of piglets. Can Vet J 28:667–669.
GREINER, E. C.; TAYLOR, C.; FRANKENBERGER, W. B.; AND BELDEN, R. C. 1982. Coccidia of feral swine from Florida. J Am Vet Med Assoc 181:1275–1277.
HILL, J. E.; LOMAX, L. G.; LINDSAY, D. S.; AND LYNN, B. S. 1985. Coccidiosis caused by *Eimeria scabra* in a finishing hog. J Am Vet Med Assoc 186:981–982.
KENNEDY, G. A.; KREITNER, G. L.; AND STRAFUSS, A. C. 1977. Cryptosporidiosis in three pigs. J Am Vet Med Assoc 170:348–350.

LINDSAY, D. S. 1989. Diagnosing and controlling *Isospora suis* in nursing pigs. Vet Med 83:443–448.

LINDSAY, D. S.; STUART, B. P.; WHEAT, B. E.; AND ERNST, J. V. 1980. Endogenous development of the swine coccidium *Isospora suis* Biester, 1934. J Parasitol 66:771–779.

LINDSAY, D. S.; CURRENT, W. L.; AND ERNST, J. V. 1982. Sporogony of *Isospora suis* Biester, 1934 of swine. J Parasitol 68:861–865.

LINDSAY, D. S.; CURRENT, W. L.; ERNST, J. V.; AND STUART, B. P. 1983. Diagnosis of neonatal porcine coccidiosis caused by *Isospora suis.* Vet Med Small Anim Clin 78:89–95.

LINDSAY, D. S.; ERNST, J. V.; CURRENT, W. L.; STUART, B. P.; AND STEWART, T. B. 1984. Prevalence of oocysts of *Isospora suis* and *Eimeria* spp. from sows on farms with and without a history of neonatal coccidiosis. J Am Vet Med Assoc 185:419–421.

LINDSAY, D. S.; CURRENT, W. L.; AND TAYLOR, J. R. 1985. Effects of experimental *Isospora suis* infection on morbidity, mortality and weight gains of nursing pigs. Am J Vet Res 46:1511–1512.

LINDSAY, D. S.; BLAGBURN, B. L.; AND BOOSINGER, T. R. 1987. Experimental *Eimeria debliecki* infections in nursing and weaned pigs. Vet Parasitol 25:39–45.

LINKS, I. J. 1982. Cryptosporidial infection of piglets. Aust Vet J 58:60–62.

MORIN, M.; TURGEON, D.; JOLETTE, J.; ROBINSON, Y.; PHANEUF, J. B.; SAUVAGEAU, R.; BEAUREGARD, M.; TEUSCHER, E.; HIGGINS, R.; AND LARIVIERE, S. 1983. Neonatal diarrhea of pigs in Quebec: Infectious causes of significant outbreaks. Can J Comp Med 47:11–17.

ROBERTS, L.; WALKER, E. J.; SNODGRASS, D. R.; AND ANGUS, K. W. 1980. Diarrhoea in unweaned pigs associated with rotavirus and coccidial infections. Vet Rec 107:156–157.

ROBINSON, Y.; MORIN, M.; GIRARD, C.; AND HIGGINS, R. 1983. Experimental transmission of intestinal coccidiosis to piglets: Clinical, parasitological, and pathological findings. Can J Comp Med 47:401–407.

SANFORD, S. E. 1987. Enteric cryptosporidial infection in pigs: 184 cases (1981–1985). J Am Vet Med Assoc 190:695–698.

SANFORD, S. E., AND JOSEPHSON, G. K. A. 1981. Porcine neonatal coccidiosis. Can Vet J 22:282–285.

SANGSTER, L. T.; SEIBOLD, H. R.; AND MITCHELL, F. E. 1976. Coccidial infections in suckling pigs. Proc Am Assoc Vet Lab Diagn 19:51–55.

STEVENSON, G. W., AND ANDREWS, J. J. 1982. Mucosal impression smears for diagnosis of piglet coccidiosis. Vet Med Small Anim Clin 77:111–115.

STUART, B. P., AND LINDSAY, D. S. 1986. Coccidiosis in swine. Vet Clin North Am Food Anim Pract 2:455–468.

STUART, B. P.; LINDSAY, D. S.; AND ERNST, J. V. 1978. Coccidiosis as a cause of scours in baby pigs. Proc Int Symp Neonatal Diarrhea 2:371–382.

STUART, B. P.; LINDSAY, D. S.; ERNST, J. V.; AND GOSSER, H. S. 1980. *Isospora suis* enteritis in piglets. Vet Pathol 17:84–93.

STUART, B. P.; GOSSER, H. S.; ALLEN, C. B.; AND BEDELL, D. M. 1982a. Coccidiosis in swine: Dose and age response to *Isospora suis.* Can J Comp Med 46:317–320.

STUART, B. P.; SISK, D. B.; BEDELL, D. M.; AND GOSSER, H. S. 1982b. Demonstration of immunity against *Isospora suis* in swine. Vet Parasitol 9:185–191.

UPTON, S. J., AND CURRENT, W. L. 1985. The species of *Cryptosporidium* infecting mammals. J Parasitol 71:625–629.

VETTERLING, J. M. 1965. Coccidia (Protozoa: Eimeriidae) of swine. J Parasitol 51:897–912.

————. 1966. Prevalence of coccidia in swine from six localities in the United States. Cornell Vet 56:155–166.

VITOVEC, J., AND KOUDELA, B. 1987. Pathology of natural isosporosis in nursing piglets. Folia Parasitol 34:199–204.

ZIMMERMAN, J. J.; DREESEN, D. W.; OWEN, W. J.; AND BERAN, G. W. 1990. Prevalence of toxoplasmosis in swine from Iowa. J Am Vet Med Assoc 196:266–270.

54 External Parasites

K. J. Dobson

P. R. Davies

THE EXTERNAL parasites of economic importance for swine are mites, lice, fleas, mosquitoes, flies, and ticks. Lice, fleas, flies, and mosquitoes belong to the class Insecta. Mites and ticks belong to the class Arachnida and are characterized by having four pairs of legs.

External parasites of pigs in general exert their deleterious effects by irritating the animal, interfering with growth, and sometimes transmitting disease-producing microorganisms. Loss at the slaughterhouse may occur because of skin damage. In addition, problems of insecticidal residues may result from treatment of these external parasites.

SARCOPTIC MANGE. The mite *Sarcoptes scabiei* var. *suis,* the cause of sarcoptic mange, is probably the most important ectoparasite of swine throughout the world. Its importance tends to be underrated because of the lack of recognition of its presence within many herds. It has significant economic importance because of its effect on growth rate and efficiency of food conversion.

The clinical manifestations of sarcoptic mange are seen within a herd either as a chronic skin condition affecting a few pigs or, more commonly, as an allergic response affecting great numbers of pigs.

Earlier descriptions of sarcoptic mange appear to have referred mainly to the condition now known as chronic or hyperkeratotic mange, in which skin lesions were present and from which mites were readily isolated (McPherson 1960; Seddon 1968; Sheahan 1970).

More recent studies have shown that a separate and distinct entity referred to as sarcoptic mite hypersensitivity exists (Sheahan 1974; Cargill and Dobson 1979a). This allergic pruritis occurs some 3–10 weeks after exposure to mites and causes a large proportion of pigs to exhibit rubbing.

Distribution. It is reasonable to assume that most if not all countries of the world have pig herds with sarcoptic mites. Because many pigs have inapparent infestations, trade would favor wide dissemination.

Reports include those from New Zealand (Brakenridge 1958), Britain (Brownlie and Harrison 1960), Scotland (McPherson 1960), Ireland (Sheahan 1970), the United States (Magee 1974; Wooten-Saadi et al. 1987), Czechoslovakia (Kamyszek 1975), Australia (Cargill and Dobson 1977), and the Netherlands (Smeets et al. 1989). Most of these indicate that a high proportion of herds are affected (70–90%) and many pigs within the herd (20–95%).

Etiology and Life Cycle. The sarcoptes mite is a small grayish white circular parasite about 0.5 mm in length and just visible to the naked eye when placed on a dark background. When viewed under a dissecting microscope, the mite readily moves away from bright light. It has four pairs of short stumpy legs, some of which are provided with long unjointed pedicles that terminate in suckerlike organs. These pedicles occur on the first two pairs of legs in the female and on the first, second, and fourth pairs in the male (Figs. 54.1 and 54.2).

The life cycle in the pig has been assumed to be similar to that in humans (Soulsby 1968), but no specific study has been carried out to prove this point. This classical description states that mites are permanent parasites of the epidermis, in which eggs, larvae, nymphs, and adults all develop below the surface of the skin. After the female mates, she lays eggs in tunnels carved into the upper two-thirds of the epidermis. A female can lay 40–50 eggs at a rate of 1–3 per day; she dies after about 1 month. Eggs hatch in about 5 days in the tunnels. Larvae molt to nymphs and nymphs molt to adults, all within the tunnels. Mating can occur in the molting pockets or near the skin surface, after which the ovigerous females initiate new burrows. The cycle from egg to ovigerous female requires 10–15 days.

Specific studies in the pig suggest that most of the mite activity is confined to the inner surface of the ear (Walton 1967; Sheahan 1975). In established infestations material from ear scrapings may contain very large numbers of mites, while in other parts of the body it is difficult to find any mites at all (Bogatko 1974; Dobson and Cargill 1979). Histologic studies of tissue dissected from mite-infested pigs have shown that mites burrow no deeper than the epidermis and make burrows parallel to the surface (Magee 1974).

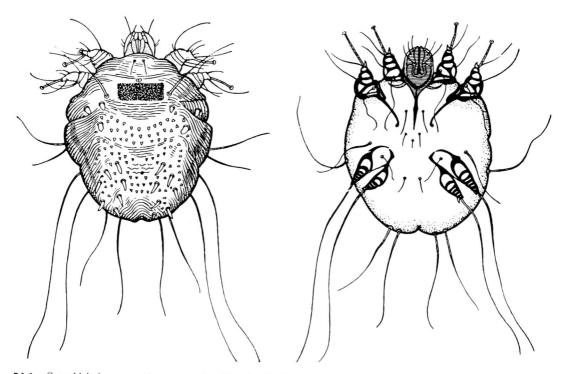

54.1. *S. scabiei,* the sarcoptic mange mite. Female. (Left) dorsal view; (right) ventral view. (From Belding 1952. Textbook of Clinical Parasitology. Courtesy Appleton-Century-Crofts.)

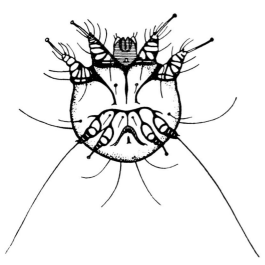

54.2. *S. scabiei,* the sarcoptic mange mite. Male, ventral view. (From Belding 1952. Textbook of Clinical Parasitology. Courtesy Appleton-Century-Crofts.)

Epidemiology. The main source of mites for spread within a herd is from animals with chronic lesions containing large numbers of mites. Such lesions are most common inside the ear of multiparous sows, but extensive hyperkeratotic lesions may occur on the body and hind legs in the absence of ear lesions (Martineau et al. 1984). The

authors have examined cases in which an estimated 18,000 mites/g of ear material have been recorded. Usually, high numbers occur in breeding animals, which are grouped together, thereby giving maximum opportunity to build up mite populations. The boar is often a source of infestation within the breeder herd because it is treated less often than sows. Chronic ear and body lesions are occasionally seen in grower pigs where control measures for mange are poor.

Spread from the affected breeder animal to the growing pig is by direct contact soon after the sow farrows. The newly fertilized adult female mite is thought to be the main means of spread. Maximum opportunity for spread exists because by nature pigs huddle together for warmth. Pig management practices of dry sow grouping and sorting of weaned litters according to size assist in the spread of mites, which ultimately gives rise to the mite hypersensitivity syndrome in a large number of pigs. Exposure for as little as 24 hours to pens that have been immediately vacated by previously infected pigs has resulted in infestation (Smith 1986).

Survival of the mite and eggs away from the host is limited to a short period only. Under optimum laboratory conditions the mites have been kept alive for 3 weeks (Soulsby 1968). In the colder climate of the Soviet Union, Mikhalochkina (1975) demonstrated that the mite would not survive for more than 12 days in the piggery at temperatures of 7–18°C and relative humidity of 65–75%. In the warmer climate of South Australia, clinical evidence of sarcoptic mite hypersensitivity could not be demonstrated when noninfected pigs were exposed on repeated occasions to contaminated bedding vacated 3 days previously in either autumn or spring (Cargill and Dobson 1977). This was supported by laboratory experiments in which it was found that mites did not survive longer than 96 hours at temperatures of less than 25°C or longer than 24 hours from 25 to 30°C; at temperatures above 30°C survival was for less than 1 hour.

Other hosts are unlikely sources of infestation for pigs. Magee (1974) was not able to develop reproducing populations of mites after transfer from pigs to calves, sheep, rabbits, or guinea pigs.

Transmission from one herd to another can readily occur from pigs with inapparent infestations. In a study of 187 clinically healthy pigs, Bogatko (1974) was not able to demonstrate mites in skin scrapings of the head and neck but did isolate mites from the ear scrapings of 18% of these animals.

Economic Importance.   Financial losses to the pig industry due to sarcoptic mange are considerable and may be associated with both the chronic and the allergic forms. Animals may also be condemned in part at the slaughterhouse, and there are considerable costs associated with control programs in many herds.

Chronic mange in growing pigs occurs mainly in poorly managed herds without a control program. The growth rate is severely affected, and pigs may become stunted and unthrifty (Seddon 1968). In better-managed herds, chronic ear mange may still occur and is economically important because it provides the source of mites for the more common allergic type of mange.

Mite hypersensitivity in pigs, characterized by frequent rubbing but sometimes without obvious skin lesions and unthriftiness, is the greatest source of economic loss because it affects large proportions of pigs in infested piggeries.

Studies attempting to quantify the production effects of sarcoptic mange have yielded varying results. In South Australia, experiments with Large White pigs housed under either intensive or semiintensive conditions on diets with either optimal or suboptimal protein levels have shown that growth rate and efficiency of feed conversion in pigs grown from 18 to 68 kg were reduced by approximately 10% (Cargill and Dobson 1979b). In Ireland, Sheahan (1974) was not able to demonstrate significant differences in pigs artificially infested under controlled conditions, but the hypersensitivity in these experiments differed from field conditions in being present for only 2–3 weeks. The same author in a subsequent examination of a field outbreak of mange in a prog-

eny testing station was able to demonstrate an improvement in the weekly body liveweight gain from 4.5 kg in the 3 weeks prior to treatment to 5.6 kg in the 4 weeks after treatment (Sheahan and Kelly 1974).

In the United Kingdom Hewett (1985) observed a 12% improvement in growth rate under commercial conditions from pigs treated with phosmet when compared to untreated controls. Dalton and Ryan (1988) demonstrated a 9% improvement in both growth rate and efficiency of feed conversion of grower pigs in a commercial herd in which the dams were treated with ivermectin prior to farrowing when compared to untreated controls.

In the United States Alva-Valdes et al. (1986) obtained only a 5.5% increase in growth rate but no significant increase in efficiency of feed conversion in pigs from weaning to 100 kg when a group was treated with ivermectin.

There is evidence that sarcoptic mites are more prevalent in the cooler months of the year (Wooten-Saadi et al. 1987; Smeets et al. 1989) and this could have a bearing on economic importance of mange treatment.

The cost of chemicals and labor for a control program may be considerable when mange is not properly controlled. A survey of 50 piggeries in South Australia showed that about half the producers interviewed sprayed all their pigs at 1-month intervals, and a further third sprayed at about 3-month intervals.

Clinical Signs, Pathogenesis, and Lesions.   The only constant clinical sign is pruritis. The newborn piglet of an infected dam may initially exhibit intermittent body scratching. True generalized pruritis does not occur until some weeks later. The reported length of this latent period from infestation to sensitization ranges from 2 to 3 weeks (Sheahan 1974) up to 7–11 weeks (Cargill and Dobson 1979a). This variation is in conformity with reported variations in human scabies in which the latent period given by five different researchers ranged from 9 to 10 days to 4–6 weeks (Sheahan 1974).

The intensity and duration of pruritis vary considerably. When control measures are inadequate, itching and rubbing are common in some pigs in most pens of growers up to the time of slaughter.

Lesions are first observed in natural infestations as early as 3 weeks after contact with mites. They begin as small encrustations in the ear and develop to plaquelike lesions about 5 mm in diameter, which may coalesce to cover up to 70% of the luminal surface of the ear (Fig. 54.3). Most regress and disappear in 12–18 weeks (Cargill and Dobson 1979a). The epidermal changes and sequence of events have been well documented using electron microscopy by Morsy et al. (1989).

Focal erythematous skin papules associated with hypersensitivity occur in most animals as the

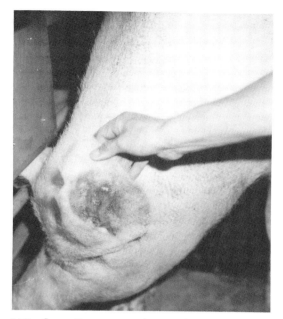

54.3. Sarcoptic mange on the ear of a sow.

ear lesions regress. They are seen particularly on the rump, flank, and abdomen. Histologically, they contain large numbers of eosinophils, mast cells, and lymphocytes, but no evidence of mites. Immunological studies have shown that immunoglobulin-secreting cells in the ears of pigs increase to a peak in the 2–5 weeks after infestation and then subside substantially after a few weeks (Morsy and Gaafar 1989). Repeated or multiple infestations give only a small increase in immunoglobulin-secreting cells. Without treatment the condition progresses, and rubbing results in the proliferation of connective tissue and keratinization, so that the skin becomes thickened and wrinkled. Hair loss and skin abrasion may occur over the flanks of animals that manifest frequent rubbing.

Lesions characteristic of chronic mange develop in only a few animals. In the ear they are seen as a thick asbestoslike scab, loosely attached to the skin and very rich in mites. Chronic scabs may progressively cover the head, neck, and other parts of the body, although this is uncommon.

The interrelationship between immunity, inadequate nutrition, poor management, and hyperkeratotic sarcoptic mange is worthy of note. Hyperkeratotic mange has often been described as a disease of poor management, and it is considered to be more common in poorly fed pigs. Studies have shown that low-protein diets and iron deficiency are associated with reduced hypersensitivity and a greater proportion of chronically affected animals (Sheahan 1974; Cargill and Dobson 1979a). However, some animals may fail to develop a hypersensitivity reaction. The overall clinical picture is substantially influenced by the effectiveness of treatment and herd management. Other disease conditions probably influence the severity of mange infestations.

Diagnosis. Sarcoptic mange is likely to be present in most herds unless these have been derived from specific-pathogen-free (SPF) sources or unless special measures have been taken to eradicate this parasite. Clinical signs of rubbing in grower pigs that have small red papules on the body are the most consistent and reliable indications of sarcoptic mange.

Diagnosis should be confirmed by demonstrating the presence of the mite within the herd. The surest method is to examine inside the ears of breeding animals with a flashlight until some are found with chronic ear scab. The presence of mites can be demonstrated on the farm by taking this material from the ear and breaking it onto a sheet of black paper. After a few minutes the scab residue can be tipped or gently blown off, leaving mites adhering to the paper by the suckers on their feet. Mites can be observed directly or with a magnifying glass (Brakenridge 1958).

The usual laboratory technique is to break down ear scab with 10% potassium hydroxide and observe it under a low-power microscope. In another method used particularly for harvesting large numbers of mites from encrusted ear lesions, vibration and low heat for 6–24 hours cause mites to emerge in great numbers and adhere to the bottom of a petri dish (Sheahan and Hatch 1975). Examination of carcasses of slaughter pigs for papular lesions may be a useful adjunct to diagnosis of mange and assessment of severity within the herd (see Chapter 79). Continued monitoring is useful to gauge control within the herd.

Differential diagnosis from other skin conditions is important, and the reader should seek information from other parts of the text. Conditions that can be confused with mange include parakeratosis, exudative epidermitis, niacin and biotin deficiencies, dermatomycosis, swine pox (SP), sunburn, and photosensitization.

Treatment, Control, and Eradication. Failure to control sarcoptic mange is due in part to poor understanding of the epidemiology and to apathy of the pig producer that results from lack of appreciation of the economic loss from mite hypersensitivity. In the past, producers have tended to regard signs of rubbing in pigs as a normal phenomenon, and treatment has been given too late and to the wrong animals.

Mange control in general involves identification of the badly affected animals, systematic and regular treatment of those that carry mite populations, and protection of the young—who are born free of mites—from exposure to older infected pigs.

A control program must begin with the breeding herd. Animals with chronic lesions should be identified by examination of individual sows in stalls or after restraint in the pen. These should be culled and the remainder treated thoroughly, either simultaneously for at least three times at weekly intervals or alternatively in segregated groups prior to farrowing. The boars should be treated as often as the sows, as they are likely to remain affected. Repeat treatments are most important because any eggs present in the skin tunnels would not be reached, although a single subcutaneous (SC) injection of ivermectin now seems likely to be at least as effective. If sows are free of mites and farrow in clean pens, litters of pigs can be reared that are also free of mites.

Agents for treating the sarcoptic mite have received considerable attention. The authors' experience in the field suggests that if mange is kept well under control, most registered acaracides will be effective. On the other hand, the best insecticides are useless when mange control programs are inadequate.

Older remedies to treat sarcoptic mange include used crankcase oil, diesel oil, and lime sulfur. Oil assists in softening the hard scab under which the mite can shelter, and it is still useful either as an alternating treatment or mixed with insecticides. Oil mixtures are more effective than water-soluble products.

Insecticides used in the 1970s were mainly confined to sprays of either the organochlorinated hydrocarbons—lindane and toxaphene—or the organophosphorus compounds—malathion, trichlorfon, and diazinon (Table 54.1). More recently developed insecticides include phosmet used as a pour-on, amitraz used as a spray, and ivermectin given as an injection. The precise products available are dependent on the legislation of the country in question. Instructions on dilutions, withholding periods, dangers, and any precautions are given by the manufacturer and should be followed carefully.

Lindane marketed as a wettable powder and applied as a 0.06% high-pressure spray is considered the most effective insecticide. It has the disadvantage of not being recommended for young pigs and sows near farrowing. A withholding period of 30 days is required, and the product is not permitted in some countries. The organophosphorus compounds are not as effective, but they have shorter withholding periods.

Phosmet formulated as a 20% oily pour-on and applied at the rate of 1 ml/10 kg body weight has been shown to be quite effective (Hewett and Heard 1982). It is recommended that a small amount of the product be placed in the inner aspect of each ear. Amitraz used as a 0.1% spray has also been shown to be efficient (Johansson et al. 1980).

The ivermectins are new wide-spectrum antiparasiticide compounds effective against most internal parasites as well as lice and sarcoptic mange. They can be given orally at 300–500 $\mu g/$kg (Lee et al. 1980; Alva-Valdes et al. 1984) or more conveniently by SC injection at 300 $\mu g/kg$ body weight (Courtney et al. 1983; Martineau et al. 1984; Dalton and Ryan 1988). They are more efficient because of their systemic action.

Eradication of sarcoptic mange is possible by using the techniques described under treatment and control. Keller et al. (1972) reported eradication of sarcoptic mange in Switzerland from six SPF herds into which mange was accidently introduced. They gave three to four treatments with diazinon and lindane at 9- to 15-day intervals to all animals and sprayed the surroundings. Frick et al. (1974) attempted eradication of lice and mange in a district of the German Democratic Republic by routine twice-yearly treatments of all herds with trichlorfon. The program included compulsory reporting of affected herds, which were treated twice at intervals of 8–10 days and checked at quarterly inspections. The program resulted in mange being eliminated from one-quarter of all herds in the district. Dobson and Cargill (1979) reported eradication from two commercial herds with longstanding mite hypersensitivity by treating the sows and boars for 3 consecutive weeks with oil and then trichlorfon prior to farrowing and segregating progeny from those of nontreated sows until the time of slaughter.

Work by Courtney et al. (1983) and more recently by Henriksen et al. (1987), White and Ryan (1987), and Dalton and Ryan (1988) would indicate that ivermectin given as a single SC injection could be used as the basis of eradication within a herd. However account should be taken of Alva-Valdes et al. (1984) using ivermectin orally at 300 and 500 $\mu g/kg$, which failed to eradicate mites with a single treatment. Similarly Thomas et al. (1986) using 300 $\mu g/kg$ SC on three occasions within a month failed to eradicate sarcoptic mange.

Eradication of mange requires a diligent approach, and equal care must be taken with pigs introduced from other herds. Eradication by the hysterectomy method used in obtaining SPF herds has proved very effective and is justified economically.

DEMODECTIC MANGE. In contrast to sarcoptic mange, demodectic mange is relatively unimportant in pigs. It is a condition identified occasionally at meat inspection and is seldom reported as a clinical entity in the field.

Distribution throughout the world and in pig populations is not well documented. It has been reported in many countries including Australia, the United States, Kenya, New Zealand, and several European countries.

The specific etiology of demodectic mange in the pig is the mite *Demodex phylloides* (Fig. 54.4). This spindle-shaped mite measures about 0.25 mm in length and has four pairs of short stumpy

Table 54.1. Guidelines for insecticidal treatments for external parasites of swine

Chemical	Concentration	Parasites Affected	Directions for Use
Amitraz	0.1% solution	Mites	Spray pigs, pens, and surroundings. Repeat in 7–10 days.
Ciodrin	0.25%	Lice	Spray with up to 4 gal/head. Respray 14 days later. No preslaughter interval.
Coumaphos (Co-Ral)	0.06% solution	Lice, horn flies	Spray. Repeat if necessary, but not more than once every 10 days. No preslaughter interval.
	0.12% solution	Ticks (*Amblyomma, Dermacentor, Ixodes*), mites	Spray.
	0.24% solution	Screwworms, blowflies	Treat all wounds thoroughly.
	1% dust	Lice	Apply to hogs; simultaneously apply 20 g/m² of fresh dry bedding.
	5% dust	Ear ticks (*Otobius*)	Apply to ears and adjacent areas of head.
Diazinon	0.05% emulsion	Lice and mites	Spray pigs 3 times at 10-day intervals.
Dioxathion (Delnav)	0.15% solution	Lice, ticks (*Amblyomma, Dermacentor, Ixodes*)	Spray or dip. Do not treat sows within 2 weeks of farrowing or while nursing. Do not repeat treatment within 2 weeks. No preslaughter interval.
Ivermectin	SC injection	Lice, mites	Give 300 µg/kg body weight.
	Oral dose		Give 300–500 µg/kg body weight.
Lindane	0.06% emulsion	Lice, sarcoptic mites	Dip or spray. Do not dip within 60 days or spray within 30 days of slaughter. Do not use benzene hexachloride.
	1% dust	Fleas	Dust heads, necks, and backs.
	3% formulated in smear, paste, or pressurized aerosol	Screwworms, blowflies	Treat all wounds thoroughly.
Malathion	0.5% emulsion	Lice, ticks, mites	Spray. No preslaughter interval.
	6% dust	Fleas, lice	Dust thoroughly.
	2.5% emulsion	Houseflies, stable flies, fleas	Spray houses and premises.
Phosmet	20% oily solution	Mites	Pour on 1 ml/10 kg body weight along back. Place some in inner ear.
Polysulfides	2%	Sarcoptic mange	Spray pigs.
Rabon	2% solution	Houseflies, stable flies	Spray 1 gal/12–24 m² of ceiling and wall space.
Ronnel (Korlan)	0.25% emulsion	Lice	Spray thoroughly.
	5% granules	Lice	Apply evenly over bedding at 25 g/m².
	5% pressurized aerosol	Screwworms, blowflies	Treat all wounds thoroughly.
Rotenone	1% powder	Fleas	Dust heads, necks, and backs.
Toxaphene	0.5% emulsion	Lice, ticks, mites	Spray. Do not apply within 28 days of slaughter.
Trichlorfon (Neguvon)	0.125% emulsion	Houseflies, stable flies, mites	Spray buildings. Do not contaminate feed or water.

Source: Based on compilation by Bennet (1975).

legs. It lives in the hair follicles, and for this reason the condition is often referred to as follicular mange. The life cycle of the mite is not well understood. The female lives in the hair follicle and lays spindle-shaped eggs from which larvae with three pairs of legs hatch. The larval stage progresses through three nymphal instars to an adult (Soulsby 1968). Approximately 2 weeks are required to complete the life cycle, and the life span

of the adult is 1–2 months.

Transmission of the mites is probably by direct contact of pigs, but it is difficult to produce artificial infestations. The parasites are fairly resistant, being able to survive for several days off the host in moist surroundings and up to 21 days under experimental conditions in pieces of skin kept moist and cool (Nutting 1976). However, the mites will live for only 1 or 2 days if removed

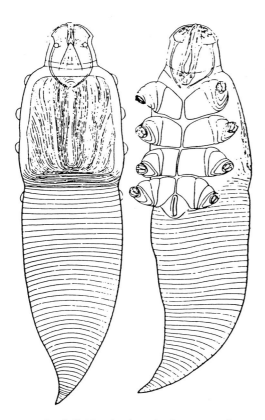

54.4. *D. phylloides,* the demodectic mange mite. Female. (Left) dorsal view; (right) ventral view. (From Hirst 1922. British Museum, Economic Series 13.)

from the host tissue and can be killed by desiccation in as little as 1 hour at 20°C on the skin surface.

Lesions observed are red pinpoint areas around the snout and eyelids, along the underside of the neck and abdomen, and inside the thighs (Walton 1967). Later, the lesions may take on a more scaly nodular appearance, particularly in the area of the mammary gland and flanks. These nodules resemble old pox lesions and when incised contain a thick, white cheeselike material with innumerable mites (Harland et al. 1971). Mites have been recovered in scrapings from the eyelids of swine that have shown no gross signs of infestation (Nutting et al. 1975). Diagnosis of the condition is confirmed by demonstration of *D. phylloides* in the lesions. Treatment with any form of medication, either topical or systemic, has not been successful. Severely affected animals should be culled from the herd.

LICE. Lice in pigs are readily observed and often blamed for damage due to mange because both conditions cause signs of rubbing. Herds treated routinely to effectively control mange seldom carry significant lice populations, and many are probably free of lice. Only one species

of lice affects pigs. The distribution of the pig louse is very widespread. A survey of market pigs in Indiana in 1980–81 indicated presence of lice in 22.5% of 821 herds surveyed (Wooten-Saadi et al. 1987).

The pig louse (*Haematopinus suis*) belongs to the suborder Anoplura, the members of which have piercing and sucking mouthparts. It is grayish brown in color and has black markings. The females are about 6 mm long and the males slightly smaller (Fig. 54.5).

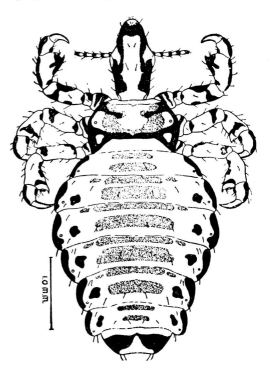

54.5. *H. suis,* the hog louse. (From Whitehead 1942. Macdonald College Farm Bull 7.)

In the life cycle as described by Florence (1921) the adult female lays 3–4 eggs (nits) each day, with a total of up to 90 over a period of about 25 days. Each egg is about 1–2 mm long and is attached by clear cement to the hair (Fig. 54.6). Eggs hatch in 12–20 days. The nymphs develop through three instars, all of which feed on blood that is generally from a tender part of the body such as the inner surface of the ear. The third instar nymphs develop into adults. The whole cycle requires 23–30 days (Walton 1967).

The epidemiology is uncomplicated in that the pig louse is host-specific and cannot live for more than 2–3 days away from the host. Lice are found on all parts of the body but particularly in the folds of the skin around the neck, jowl, and flanks and inside the legs. They often shelter inside the ears, where they are sometimes seen in "nests." The method of spread is by direct contact from

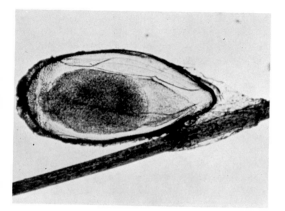

54.6. Egg (nit) of *H. suis* attached to a hair.

one pig to another during the period of huddling, although clean pigs placed in a yard just vacated by lousy pigs could become infested.

The economic importance of lice has not been critically evaluated to the same extent as sarcoptic mange. However, it is known that heavy infestations result in anemia in young pigs and may affect growth rate and efficiency of food conversion. One estimate of reduced growth was 50 g/day (Hiepe and Ribbeck 1975), though Davis and Williams (1986) failed to demonstrate any such effect. Lice have always been considered vectors of SP. It has also been reported that hides from pigs with lice are rendered unsuitable for manufacture into high-grade leather (Hiepe and Ribbeck 1975).

A diagnosis of lousiness should always be considered when pigs scratch and rub. Confirmation is readily made by identification of adult lice on the body and nits attached to the lower parts of hairs. Examination inside the ears of a number of breeding animals will assist in finding lice if they are present and will enable differential diagnosis from sarcoptic mange.

Treatment and Control. Treatment and control of lice are readily achieved because the parasites live on the skin surface and can survive for only a few days away from their host.

Therapeutic agents may be applied to the pig in the form of sprays, pour-ons, and dusting powders. Control can also be assisted by placing granules containing insecticides in the bedding. Pour-ons and powders have the advantage that pigs do not have to be sprayed in cold weather.

The older treatments of diesel oil and crankcase oil applied either directly to the pig or from rubbing posts are of limited value and have been largely superseded by insecticides of the organochloride and organophosphorus compounds, which are effective and easier to apply. Several of the organophosphorus compounds such as rabon, ciodrin, ronnel, coumaphos, and methoxychlor are suitable for lice control but are less commonly registered for treatment of sarcoptic mange (Table 54.1). In addition ivermectins have been shown to be effective in controlling lice (Barth and Brokken 1980).

All the points made in the treatment of sarcoptic mange apply equally to the treatment of lice. These include special attention to the ears, treatment of the boars, multiple treatment of sows prior to farrowing, segregation of clean and untreated animals if all the herd is not treated at one time, and treatment of all introduced animals. Eradication of lice by thorough treatment of the whole herd is an achievable goal.

FLEAS. Fleas are not host-specific and will generally choose any convenient mammal or bird for a blood meal. The two fleas most commonly associated with swine are *Pulex irritans,* the human flea, and *Echidnophaga gallinacea,* the stickfast flea. *Ctenocephalides felis,* the cat flea, is seen occasionally on young swine. *Tunga penetrans,* the chigger flea, has been associated with pigs in Africa.

The distribution of fleas in nature is wide, but they are seldom a serious problem in the well-managed piggery. These wingless insects are 2–4 mm in length, have a thick, brown chitinous exoskeleton, and have powerfully developed legs.

The life cycle is similar in all fleas. The female lays eggs about 0.5 mm long, which drop off the host into the animal bedding. Larvae hatch in 2–16 days and feed on dry blood, feces, and other organic material. With moderate temperature and high humidity the larvae mature in 1–2 weeks and pass through a pupal stage. The whole life cycle takes as little as 18 days but may take in excess of 1 year depending on environmental conditions (Soulsby 1968).

Only the adult flea is parasitic in that it requires periodic blood meals. The stickfast flea differs from the others, spending most of its adult life on a host animal.

Fleas can survive for many months in the absence of a host. Survival is dependent on whether they are fed and the degree of moisture in the environment. Under optimum conditions the human flea can live for over 2 years.

Fleas are relatively unimportant in pig production. However, instances have been reported where hundreds of fleas have been seen in sheds and have seriously disturbed the pigs (Hungerford 1975). Fleas are also capable of transmitting infectious diseases such as SP in pigs and bubonic plague in humans. An allergic dermatitis similar to that described in dogs (Nesbitt and Schmitz 1978) is likely to occur in pigs, and its signs would resemble those seen in the allergic form of sarcoptic mange.

T. penetrans infestation has been reported as being associated with agalactia in sows in the Republic of Zaire (Verhulst 1976). Clinical examination showed that the ovigerous females (chiggers) were localized in the teats and obstructed the ducts. This produced agalactia and death of piglets. An outbreak of *T. penetrans* was also reported in Tanzania in which adult pigs were affected around the feet, snout, and scrotum (Cooper 1967).

Diagnosis of flea infestation is not easy, as adult fleas may leave the host and larvae and eggs are difficult to find. The bites are not readily differentiated from those of mosquitoes, lice, and mites, so the presence of those other parasites should be carefully checked before a diagnosis is made.

Treatment and control are based on locating the flea-breeding area. Both the surroundings and animals should be sprayed with an insecticide (Table 54.1). Litter, bedding, dirt, and manure should be removed from the house and burned and the house thoroughly cleaned. Housing can then be sprayed with 2.5% malathion and the pigs dusted with a 1% rotenone powder, 1% lindane powder, or 6% malathion powder.

MOSQUITOES. Mosquitoes, although considered primarily as pests of humans, also attack livestock, causing discomfort and irritation. In some cases the affected carcasses of pigs must be skinned at slaughter.

Aedes spp. have been observed attacking swine in large numbers in Florida (Bennett 1975; Becker and Gross 1987). In South Australia the same species, which have been able to breed in brackish pools of seawater left by high tides, have caused troubles in nearby piggeries (Dobson 1973).

Lesions observed by the authors appeared on several or all the pigs within a pen in the form of raised edematous weals on the legs and abdomen. These tended to disappear spontaneously within 1–2 days but made pigs unacceptable for marketing at the time.

Control within the piggery was possible by using a diazinon aerosol spray in the late evening as a regular procedure. Mosquito screening and insect repellents are also helpful in minimizing the problem in the piggery. Where possible the breeding ground of the mosquitoes should be identified. The larvae can be destroyed by either draining water reservoirs or covering the surface with oil. A wide range of insecticides have been used successfully in breeding grounds.

FLIES. Flies are of importance in pig production for several reasons. In all piggeries they tend to be used as a measure of hygiene by local health authorities. Some flies annoy animals by their vicious bite, while others act only as a vehicle for transmission of infectious disease. Some species are a problem because they are associated with myiasis, i.e., invasion of the tissues of animals by fly larvae.

The common housefly (*Musca domestica*) is ubiquitous and most active in summer. The preferred breeding place is either in the feces of animals or in decaying organic matter. The housefly is well known for its ability to transfer pathogenic bacteria mechanically via its hairy feet and legs or by regurgitation of fluid from its crop. It can also act as the intermediate host of several worm parasites of domestic animals, and it may act as a disseminator of the eggs of many others (Soulsby 1968). It has been demonstrated experimentally that it is capable of spreading hog cholera (HC) virus from infected to susceptible pigs (Morgan and Miller 1976).

The stable fly (*Stomoxys calcitrans*) is also a common fly about the size of the housefly. Its preferred breeding ground is in decaying vegetable matter such as straw and hay, but moisture is necessary. The flies are most abundant in summer and prefer fairly strong light rather than dark stables or houses. Both male and female are blood suckers of humans and animals. When present in large numbers, the stable fly may become a source of annoyance, resulting in weight loss. However, Campbell et al. (1984) were not able to demonstrate reduced gain or feed conversion experimentally in Nebraska. In addition, it can be a carrier of infectious organisms including HC.

Horseflies of the Tabanidae family are large robust flies with clear powerful wings. The common breeding place is on the leaves of plants in the vicinity of water. Horseflies are active in summer, particularly on hot sultry days. They attack large animals, including pigs, by biting in a number of different places and then taking blood. They have been observed feeding on swine in the United States (Tidwell et al. 1972). They attack adult swine, feeding most frequently on the back, head, ears, ventral surface, and especially the udder of sows. They are capable of transmission of infectious diseases, including HC (Tidwell et al. 1972).

Blackflies of the family Simuliidae, also known as buffalo gnats, occur in all parts of the world and can be troublesome in warm countries. Their breeding place is below the surface of the water in running streams. Swarms of the flies will prevent stock from grazing. The fly attacks the legs, abdomen, head, and ears, causing vesicles and papules. In European countries considerable numbers of stock have been killed. Death of 3 sows and severe illness in another 27, together with interference with growth, have been recorded in East Germany (Gräfner et al. 1976).

Screwworm flies of the genus *Callitroga* cause myiasis in humans and animals. *C. hominovora* is present in North America and *C. bezziana*, the Old World screwworm fly, occurs in Africa and southern Asia. The adult fly is 10–15 mm long and has a metallic green sheen to its thorax and abdomen. It has three longitudinal stripes on the thorax. The life cycle differs from other flies in that breeding takes place in the wounds of the live animal and not in carcasses.

The female lays 150–500 eggs at the edge of a wound on the mammalian host. Larvae hatch in 10–12 hours and mature in 3–6 days, after which they leave the host to pupate in the ground. The pupal period lasts from 3 days to several weeks, depending on prevailing temperatures. Hibernation occurs most commonly in the pupal stage (Soulsby 1968).

Most cases of myiasis occur in rainy weather. Maggots penetrate the wound tissue, which they liquefy and thus extend the lesion. There is a foul-smelling exudate. Death from screwworm infection is not infrequent.

Loss can be prevented if surgical wounds are avoided during the fly season and prompt attention is given to lacerations and injuries. Close inspection is necessary so that treatment can be given to stricken animals before the larvae have caused irreversible damage.

Wounds can be protected from myiasis by the application of a prophylactic wound dressing. Smear 62 (containing diphenylamine, benzol, turkey red oil, and lampblack) or, alternatively, EQ335 (containing 3% lindane and 35% pine oil) will protect wounds for at least 3 days (Bennett 1975). After wounds are invaded by larvae they may be effectively treated with pressurized aerosols containing coumaphos, lindane, or ronnel (Table 54.1). These are quite effective in killing larvae in wounds if penetration is not too deep, but they will not protect wounds from invasion for as long as the prophylactic drugs.

Blowflies of the subfamily Calliphorinae differ from screwworm flies in that they deposit their eggs in necrotic wounds. Secondary blowflies deposit their eggs only on necrotic wounds that have been previously struck by either primary blowflies or screwworm flies. The damage caused by blowflies is similar to but less severe than that caused by screwworms. Treatment and prevention are similar.

Control of Flies. Fly control in all piggeries must be a continuing exercise in summer months because flies annoy pigs, staff, and neighboring people. Control is exercised by preventing flies from breeding and destroying adult flies within pig sheds.

Breeding of flies can be prevented if dung is removed regularly. At temperatures of 25°C or more the life cycle of the housefly takes only 15 days. This is shorter than the 3-week period between changeovers of sows, often the only time that complete cleaning of the shed is possible. In summer, manure should be removed at least weekly and spread thinly on soil so fly eggs and larvae are killed by desiccation. Dung should be disposed of in the center of effluent ponds rather than at the edge where flies can breed.

Destruction of flies within pig sheds can be carried out in a number of ways. Insecticides are effective in the form of sprays, baits, or vapona strips (Table 54.1). Some insecticides such as trichlorfon, given to pigs as a medication for internal parasites, are effective in destroying both the larvae and adult flies that settle on dung from treated pigs.

Sprays are applied to walls, ceilings, and pen partitions within sheds. With some insecticides, stock and feed may need to be removed first. Space or aerosol sprays (foggers) used twice daily with knockdown insecticides are also effective. Baits applied to clean concrete surfaces and pen divisions are effective and usually contain insecticides such as ronnel, diazinon, malathion, trichlorfon, and dichlorvos.

Fly electrocutors offer an automatic nonchemical method of controlling flies. Screen doors help limit the number of flies entering buildings. Electric-light traps can be used as an auxiliary in fly control but are considered more efficient for midges rather than flies (Schmidt 1987).

TICKS. Ticks are found on a wide variety of host animals and are not ordinarily very host specific. They are not considered to be common parasites of swine. The ticks of potential importance to pigs are of the suborder Ixodoidia, which includes two large families, the Ixodidae or hard tick and the Argasidae or soft tick.

In the United States the following ticks have been reported as occurring on swine:

Ixodidae
> *Dermacentor andersoni* (Rocky Mountain spotted fever tick)
> *D. variabilis* (American dog tick or wood tick)
> *D. nitens* (tropical horse tick)
> *Amblyomma maculatum* (Gulf Coast tick)
> *Ixodes scapularis* (black-legged tick or shoulder tick)

Argasidae
> *Ornithodoros turicata* (relapsing fever tick)
> *Otobius megnini* (spinose ear tick)

In Australia *I. holocyclus,* the dog paralysis tick, has been known to cause death in suckling pigs (Seddon 1968). In general, species of ticks are adapted to specific ranges of temperature and humidity, and the reader should seek local information to assist in identifying specific species.

The life cycle of the tick is characterized by the stages of egg, larva (seed tick), nymph, and adult. The six-legged seed tick, on hatching from the egg, climbs onto grass or shrubs and waits till a suitable host passes. It attaches itself to the host and engorges with lymph and blood. It then molts and an eight-legged nymph emerges. This feeds on the host and molts to become an adult tick. After mating, the female drops off the host, lays her eggs, and dies.

The economic importance of ticks for all species of animals is considerable because of the annoyance to the host and transmission of protozoan, rickettsial, and viral diseases. In pig production enterprises, ticks are seldom a problem because animals are raised in confinement. However, it has been shown that the African swine fever virus, when introduced experimentally to the tick *Ornithodoros moubata*, could be recovered 50 weeks after infection (Greig 1972). Therefore, ticks could be of significance in the spread of viral diseases from wild pigs to domestic animals.

The diagnosis of tick infestation is based on the known location of ticks and the access of pigs to these areas. Ticks are readily seen by gross visual examination. Although found on any part of the body, they are more often seen around the ears, neck, and flanks. The tick differs from other arthropod parasites in that it is attached to its host. The size and appearance varies according to the degree of blood engorgement. A careful check should be made in the ear for the *Otobius* ear tick.

The treatment and control of ticks in pigs is seldom a problem. If only a few ticks are present, these can be removed manually and the pigs confined away from infested pasture. Many insecticides are effective as a spray or dip. Toxaphene as a 0.5% spray is recommended because it will protect against reinfestation for 2 weeks or longer (McIntosh and McDuffie 1956). Other effective acaricides include coumaphos, dioxathion, and malathion (Table 54.1). A 5% coumaphos dust has been used effectively in the ears to control the spinose ear tick.

REFERENCES

ALVA-VALDES, R.; WALLACE, D. H.; BENZ, G. W.; FOSTER, A. G.; AND HOLSTE, J. E. 1984. Efficiency of ivermectin against the mange mite *Sarcoptes scabiei* var *suis* in pigs. Am J Vet Res 45:2113–2114.

ALVA-VALDES, R.; WALLACE, D. H.; FOSTER, A. G.; ERICSSON, G. F.; AND WOODEN, J. W. 1986. The effects of sarcoptic mange on the productivity of confined pigs. Vet Med 81:258–260.

BARTH, D., AND BROKKEN, E. S. 1980. The activity of 22, 23-dihydroavermecton B1 against the pig louse, *Haematopinus suis*. Vet Rec 106:388.

BECKER, H. N., AND GROSS, T. L. 1987. Porcine allergic dermatitis caused by insect bites. Agri-Practice 8:8–10.

BENNETT, D. G. 1975. External parasites. In Diseases of Swine, 4th ed. Ed. H. W. Dunne and A. D. Leman. Ames: Iowa State Univ Press.

BOGATKO, W. 1974. Studies in the occurrence of *Sarcoptes scabiei* in clinically healthy pigs. Med Weter 30:38.

BRAKENRIDGE, D. T. 1958. Mange in pigs. A survey. NZ Vet J 6:166–167.

BROWNLIE, W. M., AND HARRISON, J. R. 1960. Sarcoptic mange in pigs. Vet Rec 72:1022–1023.

CAMPBELL, J. B.; BOXLER, D. J.; DANIELSON, D. M.; AND CVENSHAW, M. A. 1984. Effects of house and stable flies on weight gain and feed efficiency by feeder pigs. S West Entomol 9:273–274.

CARGILL, C. F., AND DOBSON, K. J. 1977. Field and experimental studies of sarcoptic mange in pigs in South Australia. Proc 54th Annu Conf Aust Vet Assoc, p. 129.

_____. 1979a. Experimental *Sarcoptes scabiei* infestation in pigs. I. Pathogenesis. Vet Rec 104:11–14.

_____. 1979b. Experimental *Sarcoptes scabiei* infestation in pigs. II. Effects on production. Vet Rec 104:33–36.

COOPER, J. E. 1967. An outbreak of *Tunga penetrans* in a pig herd. Vet Rec 80:365–366.

COURTNEY, C. H.; INGALLS, W. L.; AND STITZLEIN, S. L. 1983. Ivermectin for the control of swine scabies: Relative values of prefarrowing treatment of sows and weaning treatment of pigs. Am J Vet Res 44:1220–1223.

DALTON, P. M., AND RYAN, W. G. 1988. Productivity effects of pig mange and control with ivermectin. Vet Rec 122:307–308.

DAVIS, D. P., AND WILLIAMS, R. E. 1986. Influence of hog lice, *Haematopinus suis*, on blood components, behaviour, weight gain and feed efficiency of pigs. Vet Parasitol 22:307–314.

DOBSON, K. J. 1973. External parasites of pigs. Mosquitoes. Univ Sydney Post Grad Comm Vet Sci Proc 19:349.

DOBSON, K. J., AND CARGILL, C. F. 1979. Epidemiology and economic consequence of sarcoptic mange in pigs. Proc 2d Int Symp Vet Epidemiol Econ. Aust Gov Pub Serv, Canberra, p. 401.

FLORENCE, I. 1921. The hoglouse *Haematopinus suis linne*, its biology, anatomy and histology. Cornell Univ Agric Exp Stn Mem 51.

FRICK, W.; KRAUS, H.; AND DANNEBERG, H. D. 1974. Results of ectoparasite control on pigs at district level. Monatsh Veterinaermed 29:612.

GRAFNER, G.; ZIMMERMANN, H.; KARGE, E.; MUNCH, J.; RIBBECK, R.; AND HIEPE, T. 1976. Occurrence and harmful effects of the black flies in the Schwerin district of East Germany. Angew Parasitol 17:2.

GREIG, A. 1972. The localisation of African swine fever virus in the tick *Ornithodoros moubata porcinus*. Arch Gesamte Virusforsch 39:24C.

HARLAND, E. C.; SIMPSON, C. F.; AND NEAL, F. C. 1971. Demodectic mange of swine. J Am Vet Med Assoc 159:1752–1754.

HENRIKSEN, S. A.; EBBESEN, T. J.; AND NIELSEN, K. V. 1987. Eradication of mange from a large sow and slaughter pig herd. Dansk Vet Tidsskr 70:575–579.

HEWETT, G. R. 1985. Phosmet for the systemic control of pig mange in growing pigs. Vet Parasitol 18:265–268.

HEWETT, G. R., AND HEARD, T. W. 1982. Phosmet for the systemic control of pig mange. Vet Rec 111:558.

HIEPE, T., AND RIBBECK, R. 1975. The pig louse (*Haematopinus suis*). Angew Parasitol 16 [Suppl].

HUNGERFORD, T. G. 1975. Fleas in pigs. In Diseases of Livestock, 8th ed. Sydney: McGraw-Hill.

JOHANSSON, L. E.; NILSSON, O.; AND OLEVALL, O. 1980. Amitraz (Taktik) for the control of pig mange. Nord Vet Med 32:161–164.

KAMYSZEK, F. 1975. Sarcoptic mange in pigs. A problem in large herds. Wiad Parazytol 21:281.

KELLER, H.; ECKERT, J.; AND TREPP, H. C. 1972. Eradication of sarcoptic mange in pigs. Schweiz Arch Tierheilkd 114:573–582.

LEE, R. P.; DOOGE, D. J. D.; AND PRESTON, J. M. 1980. Efficiency of ivermectin against *Sarcoptes scabiei* in pigs. Vet Rec 107:503–505.

MCINTOSH, A., AND MCDUFFIE, W. C. 1956. Ticks that affect domestic animals and poultry. In Animal Diseases. Yearbook of Agriculture. Washington, D.C.: USDA, p. 157.

MCPHERSON, E. A. 1960. Sarcoptic mange in pigs. Vet Rec 72:869–870.

MAGEE, J. C. 1974. Studies on *Sarcoptes scabiei* on swine

in Iowa. Proc North Cent Branch Entomol Soc Am 29:125.

MARTINEAU, G. P.; VAILLANCOURT, J.; AND FRÉ-CHETTE, J. L. 1984. Control of *Sarcoptes scabiei* infestation with ivermectin in a large intensive breeding piggery. Can Vet J 25:235–238.

MIKHALOCHKINA, E. I. 1975. Resistance of *Sarcoptes suis* to environmental factors. Uch Zap Vitebsk Vet Inst 28:179.

MORGAN, N. O., AND MILLER, L. D. 1976. Muscidae (Diptera). Experimental vectors of hog cholera virus. J Med Entomol 12:657.

MORSY, G. H., AND GAAFAR, S. M. 1989. Responses of immunoglobulin-secreting cells in the skin of pigs during *Sarcoptes scabiei* infestation. Vet Parasitol 33:165–175.

MORSY, G. H.; TUREK, J. J.; AND GAAFAR, S. M. 1989. Scanning electron microscopy of sarcoptic mange lesions in swine. Vet Parasitol 31:281–288.

NESBITT, G. H., AND SCHMITZ, J. A. 1978. Fleabite allergic dermatitis. A review and survey of 330 cases. J Am Vet Med Assoc 173:282–288.

NUTTING, W. B. 1976. Hair follicle mites (*Demodex* spp.) of medical and veterinary concern. Cornell Vet 66:214–231.

NUTTING, W. B.; KETTLE, P. R.; TENQUIST, J. D.; AND WHITTEN, L. 1975. Hair follicle mites (*Demodex* spp.) in New Zealand. NZ J Zool 2:219–222.

SCHMIDT, U. 1987. Use of electric light traps to control insects in a piggery. Fleischwirtschaft 68:1421–1425. Cited in Pig News Inf 9:1660. Abstr.

SEDDON, H. R. 1968. Sarcoptic mites: Sarcoptic mange. In Diseases of Domestic Animals in Australia. II. Arthropod Infestations, 2d ed. Rev. H. E. Albiston. Commonw Dep Health Serv Publ 7, p. 98.

SHEAHAN, B. J. 1970. Sarcoptic mange in Irish pigs: A survey. Ir Vet J 24:201–203.

———. 1974. Experimental *Sarcoptes scabiei* infection in pigs: Clinical signs and significance of infection. Vet Rec 94:202–209.

———. 1975. Pathology of *Sarcoptes scabiei* infection in

pigs. I. Naturally occurring and experimentally induced lesions. II. Histological, histochemical and ultrastructural changes at skin test sites. J Comp Pathol 85:87–110.

SHEAHAN, B. J., AND HATCH, C. 1975. A method for isolating large numbers of *Sarcoptes scabiei* from lesions in the ears of pigs. J Parasitol 61:350.

SHEAHAN, B. J., AND KELLY, E. P. 1974. Improved weight gains in pigs following treatment for sarcoptic mange. Vet Rec 95:169–170.

SMEETS, J. F. M.; SNIJDERS, J. M. A.; AND GRUYS, E. 1989. Dermatitis in slaughter pigs: Occurrence, pathology and economic significance. Tijdschr Diergeneeskd 114:603–610.

SMITH, H. J. 1986. Transmission of *Sarcoptes scabiei* in swine by fomites. Can Vet J 27:252–254.

SOULSBY, E. J. L. 1968. Helminths, arthropods and protozoa of domesticated animals. In Monnig's Veterinary Helminthology and Entomology, 6th ed. London: Baillière, Tindall and Cassell.

THOMAS, P.; BICKNELL, S. R.; HAMLET, E. J.; JANOWICZ, J.; GRIFFITHS, P.; WHERTON, C.; AND ROSS, D. B. 1986. Porcine sarcoptic mange, an eradication project. A preliminary report. Proc Pig Vet Soc 15:496.

TIDWELL, M. A.; DEAN, W. D.; COMBS, G. A.; ANDERSON, D. W.; COWART, W. D.; AND AXTELL, R. C. 1972. Transmission of hog cholera virus by horseflies (Tabanidae: Diptera). Am J Vet Res 33:615–622.

VERHULST, A. 1976. *Tunga penetrans* (*Sarcopsylla penetrans*) as a cause of agalactia in sows in the Republic of Zaire. Vet Rec 98:384.

WALTON, G. S. 1967. The young pig ectoparasitic infestations. Vet Rec 80 [Clin Suppl] 9:11–13.

WHITE, M. E. C., AND RYAN, W. G. 1987. Control of an outbreak of pig mange with ivermectin. Vet Rec 121:496.

WOOTEN-SAADI, E. L.; TOWELL-VAIL, C. A.; WILLIAMS, R. E.; AND GAAFAR, S. M. 1987. Incidence of *Sarcoptes scabiei* and *Haematopinus suis* on swine in Indiana. J Econ Entomol 80:1031–1034.

55 Gastric Ulcers

J. J. O'Brien

ULCERATION of the gastrointestinal tract in various animals has been described in the course of such diseases as foot-and-mouth disease, rinderpest, mucosal disease, malignant catarrhal fever, hog cholera, and purpura hemorrhagica (Kowalczyk et al. 1960). A more localized distribution of differing etiology that is restricted to the stomach and duodenum has been recognized in humans and animals (both domestic and wild captive) for many years (Halloran 1955; O'Brien 1969). In the pig some of the ulcers in the glandular areas of the stomach occur as a result of hog cholera, chronic erysipelas, and infestations by *Hyostrongylus rubidus.*

The literature relative to gastric ulceration in pigs indicates that authors differentiate between ulcers occurring in the glandular and the nonglandular areas of the stomach. Reviews by Kernkamp (1945) and Nutrition Reviews (Anon. 1963) failed to make the differentiation.

Curtin et al. (1963), Rothenbacher et al. (1963), Larenaudie (1964), Muggenburg et al. (1964), Huber and Wallin (1965), and O'Brien (1969) all make the distinction between the common peptic ulcer of the glandular mucosa, seen primarily in the fundic region and rarely in the cardiac and pyloric regions, and ulceration of the glandless esophageal area (pars oesophagea).

The syndrome described here is ulceration of the pars oesophagea. Descriptions of ulcers seen in the glandular areas may be found in standard pathology textbooks such as Jubb et al. (1985).

The term "ulceration of the pars oesophagea" is being used because other descriptions—e.g., "ulcerative gastric haemorrhage" (Hannan and Nyhan 1962), "stomach ulcer gastrorrhagia" (Rothenbacher et al. 1963), "esophagogastric ulcers" (Curtin et al. 1963), "proventricular ulcer" (Ito et al. 1974)—are either too vague or misleading. In addition, the pars oesophagea is usually the only area in the stomach affected by this ulceration; on rare occasions it is accompanied by ulceration of the fundic zone. Esophagogastric implies that the esophagus and any part of the stomach may be involved in the lesions. Very few authors have noted concomitant ulcers in the esophagus when ulcers of the pars oesophagea were present. The results of necropsies performed by the writer indicated that less than 0.5% of pigs affected with this condition showed lesions in the esophagus also.

INCIDENCE AND DISTRIBUTION. The original reference to pars oesophagea ulceration was by McIntosh (1897) in Illinois. Since then, published accounts of its occurrence have appeared from many countries, as indicated in Table 55.1. In addition to these citations, there is evidence to indicate its presence in New Zealand, Colombia, Germany, Holland, Puerto Rico, Portugal, India, and Russia.

Various accounts of the prevalence of the condition varying from 5 to 100% have been published (O'Brien 1969; Kowalczyk 1975). These results should only be accepted as a guide, as assessments of the ulcer condition may be quite subjective. The occurrence of ulcers has varied in time and distribution within geographic areas.

CLINICAL SIGNS. There is agreement among investigators that clinical manifestations of the disease usually follow definite patterns, depending on the duration of the condition. The forms seen are described as peracute, acute, subacute, and chronic (O'Connor 1958; McErlean 1962; Curtin et al. 1963; Kowalczyk and Muggenburg 1963; Rothenbacher et al. 1963; Larenaudie 1964).

In the peracute form apparently healthy animals of any age are found dead or collapsed after exercise or excitement. The whole carcass becomes extremely pale as a result of loss of blood. Necropsy examination reveals massive intragastric hemorrhage.

In the acute form affected animals become pale, anemic, and weak and show increased respiration rates. There may be grinding of teeth, presumably due to gastric pain. Periods of anorexia supervene. Vomiting may be noted. The passing of bloody, tarry feces is a fairly constant feature. Temperatures are usually normal or subnormal.

In the subacute and chronic forms the onset and duration of the symptoms are prolonged. There are signs of anemia, anorexia, and loss of weight. Some animals may pass dark feces continuously or intermittently. In certain mild cases of the chronic form few if any clinical signs may be seen; the only indication of the condition in such animals is the occasional passage of hard, pelleted feces and the finding of the lesion in the stomach at slaughter. The duration of the symptoms of the subacute or chronic forms has been given as 2–51 days (Curtin et al. 1963) and 8–50

Table 55.1. World distribution of pars oesophagea ulceration in swine

Country	Author and Year	Pigs Examined	Percent Affected	Comment
United States (Illinois)	Jensen and Frederick 1939	20,000	5.0	At abattoir
Sweden	Obel 1953	77	22.1	At necropsy
Czechoslovakia	Jelinek 1957			
Ireland	O'Connor 1958	70		At necropsy
Belgium	Thoonen and Hoorens 1961	600	4.8	At necropsy
England	Buntain 1961	92	29.3	At necropsy
France	Larenaudie 1964	65	12.8	At necropsy
Switzerland	Walzl 1964	2	10.0	At necropsy
Australia (Victoria)	Kinnard 1965	3800	4.7	At necropsy
Austria	Rembold 1965	17		At necropsy
Italy	Asdrubali and Mughetti 1965	4	10.0	At necropsy
Yugoslavia	Šenk and Šabec 1965	2345	2.5	At necropsy
Canada	Pocock 1966	198	69.0	At abattoir
Spain	Rico Lenza 1966		30.3	At abattoir
Norway	Nafstad 1967	72	65.2	On experiment
Rumania	Barzoi et al. 1968	2172	6.4	Majority at abattoir
Hungary	Kowács 1974	13,400	12.7	At abattoir
Brazil	Bivin et al. 1974	3113	77.6	At abattoir
Japan	Ito et al. 1974	73	100.0	At abattoir
Poland	Kaszubkiewicz and Bocianowski 1978	70		At necropsy
Cuba	Szemerédi and Solá 1979	2457	20.0	At abattoir

days (Larenaudie 1964). Pigs of either sex and any breed from 8 weeks of age are more usually affected. Seasonal incidence and sporadic outbreaks are noted. However, the early signs may be masked by other diseases such as enteric diseases and pneumonia. The condition terminates in death or the animal makes a slow, protracted recovery.

Hematologic findings will depend on the severity and duration of hemorrhage. The disease is mostly subclinical and may only be diagnosed in the live animal by endoscopic examination (Kowalczyk et al. 1968), although there is a suggestion from Russian literature that changes in serum leucine aminopeptidase activity and other blood proteins may be of diagnostic value (Shugam et al. 1979). It is usually detected at abattoirs by characteristic lesions in the pars oesophagea.

PATHOLOGY. There is general agreement among the many authors who have described this condition as to the gross and microscopic pathology of ulceration of the pars oesophagea (Kowalczyk et al. 1960; McErlean 1962; Curtin et al. 1963; O'Brien 1966; Nafstad 1967; Ito et al. 1974; Rivera and Gaafar 1976).

Macroscopic Description

NORMAL PARS OESOPHAGEA. The surface area of the pars oesophagea in the pig varies according to the size of the animal. It is about 50–80 mm long and 40–50 mm wide in the 70- to 90-kg pig. The pars oesophagea is covered by a stratified squamous epithelium continuous with that of the esophagus (Fig. 55.1). Normally this surface is white, smooth, and glistening; however, it may

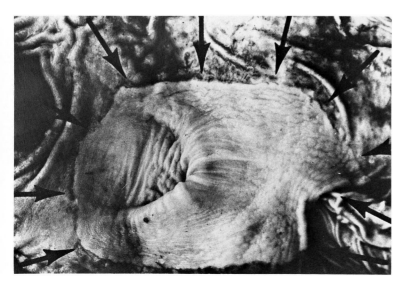

55.1. Normal pars oesophagea of the pig.

sometimes be bile stained. The layer of epithelium ends abruptly at the junction of the pars oesophagea and the cardiac zone. There are no glands in the pars oesophagea.

ULCERATION LESIONS. While several classifications have been used to describe the clinical and postmortem manifestations of ulceration (Curtin et al. 1963; Kowalczyk and Muggenburg 1963; Muggenburg et al. 1964; O'Brien 1966), it should be noted that these classifications are purely arbitrary to aid description; the degree, severity, or extent of the ulceration present will be in response to the insult offered to the tissue of the pars oesophagea. The lesion may be single or multiple, discrete and irregular in shape, and may vary in size from a few square millimeters to encompassing the whole area.

The first observed change is in the epithelial layers (Fig. 55.2). The surface becomes corrugated, elevated, irregular, and roughened. This roughened surface is at times very easily peeled off, removing most of the epithelial layer. The roughened surface and sloughing epithelial tissue appear to have a great affinity for staining with bile and the coloring matter from the stomach contents. Hence on inspection it frequently is yellow, yellow-brown, or yellow-green.

It appears that this change then leads to erosions and breaks in the continuity of the epithelial layer, resulting in active ulceration accompanied by hemorrhage (Fig. 55.3). At this stage the blood can be seen oozing from the underlying vessels of the lamina propria. There is very little fibrous tissue reaction at this stage, judging by visual inspection and palpation of the lesions. This active ulceration either continues to bleed and tends to enlarge, or it heals. If the repair process supervenes, either of two main types of chronic ulcer may arise. The first is characterized by the formation of fibrous tissue and contraction of the area of previously active ulceration. The pars oesophagea may be completely covered with fibrous tissue to give the characteristic deeply punched-out appearance of the chronic ulcer, or one or more discrete areas, even as small as 1 mm², may be affected. Hemorrhage from this ulcer is not apparent macroscopically but can be seen on microscopic examination.

The second type of chronic ulcer shows further activity (frank bleeding), presumably when it is subjected to further ulcerogenic influences (Fig. 55.4). Part of the pars oesophagea may be showing areas of chronic ulceration and areas of new or renewed activity at the same time. The renewed activity is quite apparent when the ulcer is lightly washed with water, as bleeding from surface blood vessels is readily seen. At other times small blood clots may be seen adhering to exposed blood vessels. Large blood clots may also be present in the lumen of the stomach (Fig. 55.5).

If the ulcerogenic influences cease, healing of ulcers may follow; on occasion it has been noted that the pars oesophagea has been severely contracted by cicatricial tissue, almost obliterating the opening of the esophagus into the stomach (Fig. 55.6). Reepithelialization of the area may take place from the surrounding glandular tissue.

STOMACH CONTENTS. Prior to the incision of the stomach along the greater curvature to carry out the macroscopic examination, it is frequently noted that the organ is flabby and lacks tone.

In the peracute form of this disease the stomach is often distended and filled with a mixture of blood clots, unclotted blood, and fibrinous exudate enclosing a variable amount of food. In the acute, subacute, and chronic forms the amount and especially the consistency and color of the

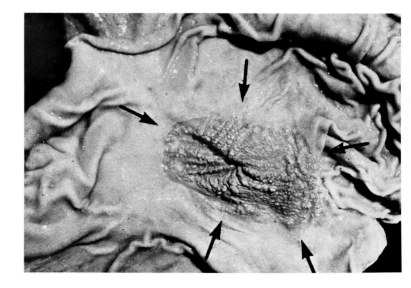

55.2. Initial epithelial changes: parakeratosis.

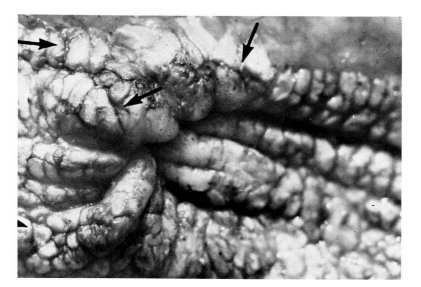

55.3. Close-up view of the fissuring and erosion of the surface epithelium.

ingesta of the stomach and intestines are related to the severity of the hemorrhage, its duration, and the interval of time between the bleeding and death of the animal. Almost all stomachs with chronic ulceration contain varying amounts of brownish yellow liquid ingesta that frequently is completely watery. Stomachs that show abnormality of the pars oesophagea almost invariably contain more fluid ingesta than normal ones. The stomach contents sometimes have a smell of fermentation.

Microscopic Description

NORMAL PARS OESOPHAGEA. The pars oesophagea of the pig is covered by stratified squamous epithelium, 8–20 cells in depth. The upper layers of this epithelium are keratinized, and pyknotic nuclei are visible at the outer border – the stratum corneum. At the deep limit of this is a pale line – the stratum lucidum. Immediately beneath this line is the granular layer – stratum granulosum – which is 2–4 cells deep. The deepest layer of the epithelial covering forms a stratum germinativum.

The lower limits of the covering form projections – rete pegs – into the lamina propria. These are seen to alternate with the upward projections of the lamina propria – the papillae of the lamina propria. The underlying lamina propria is thin and not many vessels are evident in it. It rests on a deep, broad muscularis mucosae. The pars oesophagea contains no secretory glands.

EPITHELIAL CHANGES. In the early stages of the ulceration process the chief change seen is one of

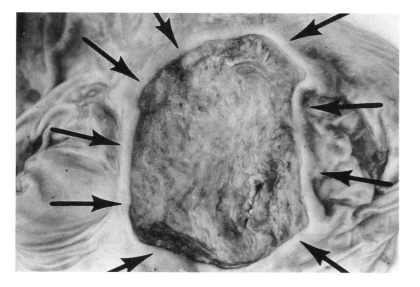

55.4. Chronic ulceration. Note deep crater formation.

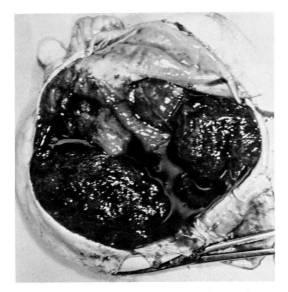

55.5. Large blood clots from pars oesophagea ulceration in the lumen of the stomach.

parakeratosis with or without focal surface erosion (Fig. 55.7). The surface epithelial cells, instead of undergoing cornification or hyalinization, show large, persistent, pale-staining nuclei surrounded by pale eosinophilic-staining cytoplasm. These cells extend right to the surface. The depth of the epithelium is also markedly increased. There are areas of gross vacuolation in the parakeratotic layer, and these spaces are filled with brightly eosinophilic-staining edemalike fluid. This is a change prior to sloughing. Gross irregularities of the surface of the whole epithelial layer can be seen.

The papillae of the lamina propria are very near the surface, and occasionally infiltrations of polymorphonuclear cells and degenerative changes of the basal epithelium cover them. Inflammatory cells are generally absent. The rete pegs show increased depth into the lamina propria and display great irregularity in shape (Fig. 55.8). There is no great increase in vascularity, dilatation, or change in the vessel walls of either the lamina propria or muscularis mucosae. The lymphoid tissue normally present in the submucosa in this area becomes hyperplastic, especially at the edges where the pars oesophagea adjoins the glandular mucosa. Lymphoid nodules form round vessels in the lamina propria as well. There are distinct germinal centers in this hyperplastic lymphoid tissue.

In the borders of the lymphoid tissue and in the surrounding tissue of the lamina propria, infiltration of eosinophils is often striking.

As a result of the parakeratosis, the epithelium of the pars oesophagea becomes weakened, and erosion eventually occurs (Fig. 55.9). This early erosion and cracking of the epithelium is most common where the papillae of the lamina propria are near the surface.

In the glandular area of the stomach immediately surrounding the pars oesophagea (about 2–3 cm) there is a marked mucoid metaplasia involving the loss of peptic and parietal cells and hypertrophy of the mucus-secreting cells of the neck of the glands. In some cases there is marked infiltration of plasma cells, macrophages, and lymphocytes into the interglandular connective tissue and the tissue just beneath the glands.

ACTIVE ULCERS. Once erosion of the epithelium takes place, the underlying tissue and the blood vessels of the lamina propria are exposed to the corrosive effect of the gastric contents, causing the diffuse necrosis and bleeding characteristic of an active ulcer.

The necrosis caused by exposure to the gastric

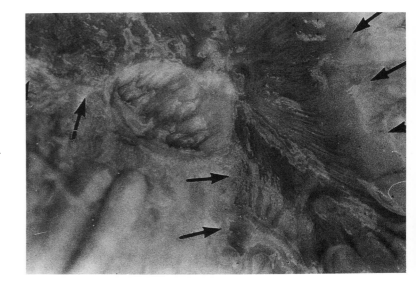

55.6. Cicatricial tissue formation causing occlusion of the entrance of the esophagus into the stomach.

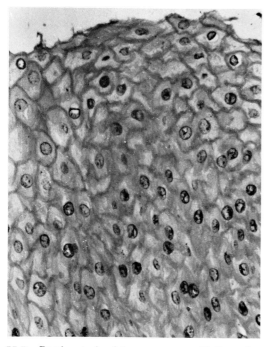

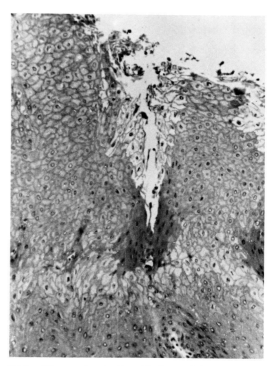

55.7. Parakeratosis of the squamous epithelium of the pars oesophagea. Note persistent pale-staining nuclei.

55.9. The parakeratotic epithelium of the pars oesophagea undergoing erosion. Note a papilla of the lamina propria just beneath this erosion (bottom right). Hemorrhage of the active ulcer appears to begin from such an area.

contents is characterized by a darkly basophilic-staining reaction zone on the surface (Fig. 55.10). This surface is composed of necrotic tissue containing large numbers of degenerating inflammatory cells, which appear to be a mixture of macrophages, neutrophils, and lymphocytes.

The underlying lamina propria is highly vascularized. In general, inflammatory cells are not particularly numerous, although in very active ulcers large numbers of eosinophils are frequently present. A varying amount of granulation tissue is seen. Vessels with large unorganized thrombi are sometimes present in the necrotic membrane and the underlying tissue.

In very acute, active ulceration there is considerable edema in the lamina propria, submucosa, and down into and involving the muscularis mucosae. Large quantities of eosinophilic-staining threads are seen throughout the lesion. Thrombosed blood vessels are very evident in the lamina propria, and deeper in the submucosa there is marked dilation of the lymphatic vessels, some of which are thrombosed. In some of the blood vessels margination by polymorphonuclear cells and subsequent contraction occur. In the serosa there is occasionally hypertrophy of the walls of the arterioles so that the muscle tissue of the walls becomes very thick in proportion to the lumen of the vessel.

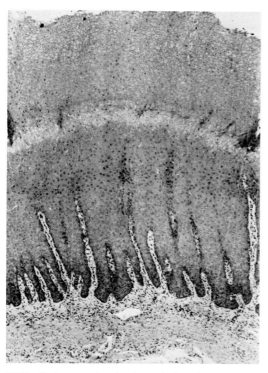

55.8. Rete pegs showing irregularity of shape and increased depth into the lamina propria. Note the marked parakeratotic changes of the surface layers of the epithelium.

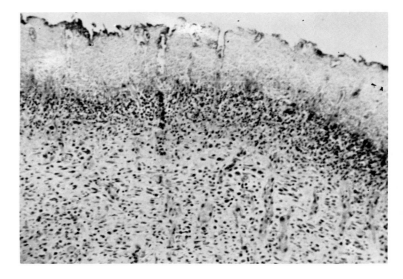

55.10. Active ulceration. Basophilic reaction zone on the surface. Note increased vascularity of the underlying lamina propria and varying amount of granulation tissue.

An interesting feature in many of these active ulcers is the persistence of a small pillar of epithelium between the ulcer itself in the pars oesophagea and the glandular tissue of the cardiac zone. This presumably should be a very weak spot where the ulcer would begin. As noted with the parakeratotic changes in the initial or precursor stages of the active ulceration, mucoid hyperplasia of the surrounding glandular tissue is also present.

CHRONIC ULCERS. The aging or development of the chronic state of ulceration is characterized by the laying down of a deep layer of fibrous connective tissue in the underlying lamina propria. As indicated earlier, two types of chronicity may be noted. In type A the reaction zone is of minimal thickness and the underlying fibrous tissue appears to be quiescent. The fibrous tissue forms a deep band, the depth of which appears to depend on the severity of the former active ulcer. There are, however, small focal hemorrhages from the surface blood vessels. In type B the reaction membrane is commonly increased in thickness and is composed of large numbers of inflammatory cells with pyknotic nuclei. These cells are apparently degenerating polymorphonuclear cells, fibroblasts, and numerous lymphocytes. Great fibroblast proliferation is evident where the ulcer is actively advancing. This tissue becomes very vascular. The following features are also common to both chronic types of ulceration.

Postulceration Parasites. A wide variety of organisms and branching fungal hyphae are usually present in the surface necrotic membrane.

Eosinophils. Eosinophils are present in abundance in the lamina propria, but they tend to congregate at the edge of the ulcer. They also tend to surround the lymphoid follicles of this region and accumulate at their edges. In certain cases eosinophils infiltrate the muscle bundles of the muscularis mucosae. However, in type B it is noticeable that small foci of eosinophils are sometimes scattered throughout the fibrous tissue in the depths of the ulcer.

Vascular Damage. In these chronic ulcers small thrombosed vessels usually are numerous in areas where the ulcer shows signs of recent activity. Deep in the submucosa there is at times slight endarteritis. Thrombi may also be present. Some vessels show deposition of fibrin in portions of the intima, i.e., fibrinoid necrosis.

Granulation Tissue. In areas of older ulcers where they show renewed activity, much granulation tissue is present.

Muscularis Mucosae: Hypertrophy. Depending on the severity and presumably the age of the ulcer, the muscular tissue of the muscularis mucosae undergoes focal hypertrophy. The muscle bundles are surrounded by collagen fibers and edema is present. There is a marked increase in blood supply to this muscle tissue.

Muscularis Mucosae: Degeneration. In some long-standing ulcers the necrotic zone actually involves the muscularis mucosae. When muscle degeneration takes place, it is replaced by heavily collagenized fibrous tissue. The nerve plexuses are also involved in this degeneration.

Serosa. The ulceration in certain cases actually shows the reaction membrane penetrating to the subserosal fat. There are thrombi in the lymphatics of the submucosa and deposits of fibrin in the serosal connective tissue. In such cases it is presumed that the progress of the lesion would lead to perforation of the ulcer into the abdominal cavity.

Lymphoid Hyperplasia. Lymphoid hyperplasia is present especially at the border of the pars oesophagea and the glandular area. In certain cases mucosal catarrh is visible above these lymphoid follicles.

Associated Lesions. Thoonen and Hoorens (1961), McErlean (1962), Curtin et al. (1963), Rothenbacher et al. (1963), and O'Brien (1966) noted concomitant tissue changes in the esophagus at the entrance to the stomach. The occurrence of ulceration of the pars oesophegea, hyaline degeneration, hepatosis dietetica, and mulberry heart disease (dietetic microangiopathy) have been seen either alone or in combination with each other by Obel (1953), Grant (1961), and O'Brien (1966).

ETIOLOGY. The etiology of this condition still needs clarification, although the circumstances under which it occurs are being understood more fully. The suggested causes of ulceration have been reviewed by O'Brien (1969) and Kowalczyk (1975). The condition occurs in all breeds regardless of age or sex, although strains bred for fast growth and lean backfat have shown a higher incidence of the condition (Berruecos and Robinson 1972; Grondalen and Vangen 1974).

Infectious Agents. Although many species of bacteria and fungi from typical ulcer lesions have been isolated (Thoonen and Hoorens 1961; Curtin et al. 1963; Griffing 1963; Rothenbacher et al. 1963), none of these is considered to be the causal agent of the condition. Qureshi et al. (1978) recorded the association of ulceration and infection with *Ascaris suum* infection. If infection was the main cause of ulceration, it is likely that more stomach ulcers would occur in connection with bacteremias or septicemias.

Copper Toxicity. Ulceration of the pars oesophagea has been noted where high levels of copper are fed as a growth-promoting factor to pigs (Buntain 1961; Allen and Harding 1962). Ulceration and subsequent deaths are eliminated by the inclusion of zinc carbonate at 110 ppm of diet.

Psychosomatic and Other Stress Factors. Various suggestions have been made, as an analogy from cases of human ulceration, that pigs develop ulceration as a result of present-day production methods that may involve fear, pain, fatigue, fasting, restraint, and other stress factors (Kowalczyk and Muggenburg 1963; Larenaudie 1964; Kowalczyk et al. 1966; Reese et al. 1966; Kaszubkiewicz and Bocianowski 1978; Driesen et al. 1987). Muggenburg et al. (1967) tested the effects of stress from transportation, deprivation of food, crowding, and mixing with unfamiliar pigs on the induction of ulcers. It was found that pigs mixed with an equal number of unfamiliar pigs

and starved (except for water) at the abattoir 18–26 hours before slaughter had significantly more ulcers than similar control pigs. It also appeared that the severity of the lesions increased with the length of time the pigs were so held.

Gastric Acidity. In human medicine the experience of many gastroenterologists that gastric and duodenal ulcers tend to heal under medical management devised to neutralize the hydrochloric acid (HCl) of gastric content around the clock must be regarded as evidence of ulcers being caused or exacerbated by gastric secretion of HCl and pepsin (Dragstedt and Woodward 1970). In pigs there is evidence that gastric hyperacidity may play an important role in causing ulceration of the pars oesophegea (Kowalczyk and Muggenburg 1963; Huber and Wallin 1965; Mahan et al. 1966; Muggenburg et al. 1966b; Reimann et al. 1967; Maxwell 1970; Arnot et al. 1979).

Feed Processing and Dietary Factors

FEED PROCESSING. Heat- and cold-pelleting and gelatinization processes in feed preparation have been shown to be associated with increased ulceration (Perry 1962; Chamberlain et al. 1967; Pocock et al. 1968).

FINENESS OF GRINDING. An increased incidence of ulceration was produced by the use of finely, as opposed to coarsely, ground diets (Reiman et al. 1967; Maxwell et al. 1970; Simonsson and Björklund 1978). The data accumulated from these experiments demonstrate that as a result of the ingestion of fine particulate feed, the contents were more fluid, there was less dry matter in the stomach contents, and there was increased mixing of gastric contents resulting in increased acidity and pepsin activity in the pars oesophegea region. The rate of passage of contents from the stomach was also increased (Maxwell et al. 1970). The results substantiate the observations made earlier, i.e., that affected stomachs contained little solid food, were flaccid, and had a low pH. Maxwell et al. (1970) also indicate that although fineness of ground feed is a factor in precipitating ulcers, it is not solely responsible.

CHEESE WHEY. On farms where whey, a by-product of cheese manufacture, is fed ad libitum to pigs, ulceration occurs with greater frequency (Hannan and Nyhan 1962; Kinnard 1965; O'Brien 1966). The pH of the whey depends on the variety of cheese manufactured or whether the solids of skim milk are precipitated by HCl. The storage period of the whey also influences its final pH. O'Brien (1966) recorded a pH range of 3.50–6.05 for the by-products of seven varieties of cheese stored for 18 hours prior to consumption.

CORNSTARCH. Ulcers have been produced in pigs

fed diets high in cornstarch and low in protein (Wallin et al. 1968; Wesoloski et al. 1975). Wallin and his co-workers showed that pars oesophagea ulceration occurred in swine fed diets containing 48–89% cornstarch and 0–16% protein. High-cornstarch rations containing either raw cornstarch flour or partially heat-treated (gelatinized) cornstarch were equally ulcerogenic. Wesoloski and his colleagues, feeding a similar ulcerogenic diet, produced ulcers that were not alleviated significantly by the addition of such substances as corn oil, magnesium sulphate, or oat hulls.

Unsaturated Fatty Acids, Tocopherols, and Selenium.

Ulceration has been seen in association with toxic liver dystrophy or hepatosis dietetica (HD) (Obel 1953) and mulberry heart disease (MAP) (Grant 1961). O'Brien (1966) also noted the association of these conditions and muscular dystrophy (MD) with ulceration of the pars oesophagea. Obel and Grant incriminated dietary factors, chiefly polyunsaturated and oxidatively unstable fatty acids, and a relative inadequacy of tocopherols and selenium (Se) in the cause of these conditions. The work of Van Vleet et al. (1970, 1974) adds support to these views. Moir and Masters (1979) in western Australia showed an association of HD, MAP, and MD in pigs fed diets containing lupin seed as a protein and recommended Se supplementation of diets to prevent HD and MD. They suggest MAP is associated more with vitamin E. However, the interactions of vitamin E and Se in these conditions should be considered.

Experience with naturally occurring cases of these conditions in Sweden has led workers to suspect that the properties of natural cereal fat have an important place in the etiology of these diseases.

Swahn and Thafvelin (1962) showed that levels of unsaturated fatty acids and vitamin E in plants are governed by a number of factors and that the normal balance between vitamin E and polyunsaturated fatty acids can be easily disturbed. These workers showed that peroxidation of natural cereal fats occurs very rapidly—within a few hours—if grain is ground and stored in a moist atmosphere. Storage of cereals to the point of germination, a process that affects the vitamin E content, also seems to influence the biologic properties of the grain. Oxidative rancidity depends upon a great number of factors such as the degree of fat unsaturation and the structure of the fats, the presence of protein and of prooxidants or antioxidants, and the presence of lipoxidases. Moisture, access to oxygen, light, and temperature also influence the process of rancidity. Grain harvested after cold, wet summers contains fat with poor oxidative stability. The tocopherol content of such grain can be very easily depleted. Another point to be considered is the interaction between bad grain storage, fungal proliferation in the stored grain, and increase in fatty acids

(Christensen 1957). The yearly seasonal appearance or disappearance of the ulcer syndrome could perhaps be viewed in the light of these facts as well as the results of experiments and surveys where the chemical analyses may indicate the percentages of protein, carbohydrates, and fats as being similar. Since economic pressures have introduced the concept of low-cost formulation of feedstuffs with the attendant search for cheaper food substrates, especially protein, the biologic properties of those used may vary considerably.

EXPERIMENTAL PRODUCTION OF GASTRIC ULCERS.

It is now generally accepted that a spontaneous increase of gastric HCl and pepsin leads to the production of ulcers in the stomach or small intestine of humans (Dragstedt et al. 1969).

Certain substances such as histamine and reserpine are powerful gastric secretion stimulators. In endeavors to unravel the pathogenesis of ulceration of the pars oesophagea, several groups of workers induced ulceration by the use of such chemical stimulators. Huber and Wallin (1965, 1967) and Muggenburg et al. (1966b, 1967) induced pars oesophagea ulceration by the intramuscular (IM) injection of histamine in beeswax. The author has produced ulceration of the pars oesophagea by the IM injection of carbon tetrachloride (unpubl. data).

Muggenburg et al. (1966a) and Kokue et al. (1978) produced ulceration of the pars oesophagea by the IM injection of reserpine. Muggenburg et al. used 0.055 mg reserpine/kg body weight daily for up to 15 days, and Kokue et al. used reserpine at 0.02 mg/kg plus betazole at 50 mg/kg daily for 5 days.

Extensive ulceration of the pars oesophagea was produced in primary specific-pathogen-free (SPF) pigs by inoculations with embryonated *Ascaris suum* eggs (Gaafar and Keittevuti 1972; Rivera and Gaafar 1976). However, when this exercise was tried in secondary SPF pigs, ulceration was not produced (Nakamura et al. 1975).

In an endeavor to find a suitable experimental model for the development of liver transplantation techniques for humans, a group of workers in England (Terblancke et al. 1968) carried out liver homotransplantations in pigs. However, one of the problems encountered was the development of ulceration of the pars oesophagea in recipient pigs.

During studies on the toxicity and metabolism of ammonia compounds, ulceration of the pars oesophagea was noted after the ligation of the bile ducts (Bicknell et al. 1967).

In determining the effect of vagotomy on gastric ulcer production in pigs, Dragstedt et al. (1969) produced peptic ulcers in the glandular region and no ulceration of the pars oesophagea. They found that the experimental procedure resulted in decreased gastric tone and stasis. It should be noted that in swine the secretion of gastric juice appears to be a continuous process. The cause of this continuous secretion is unknown, but the rate increases when food is eaten (Muggenburg et al. 1966a,b).

Direct surgical and medical interferences to individual animals, field trials elucidating the role of stress factors, and clinical and laboratory observations incriminating the physical and chemical properties of feedstuffs point to the complexity of the influences leading to ulceration of the pars oesophagea. It seems that all three components of gastric secretion, namely, the cephalic and psychic, the extravagal via the pituitary-adrenal system, and the gastric phases, may contribute to ulceration. Of these it would appear that the most direct contribution is made by the gastric phase through stimulation by the fineness of the ground feedstuffs.

DIAGNOSIS.   Clinical diagnosis of stomach ulceration is difficult, since few clinical symptoms and no pathognomonic signs are associated with this condition. However, a few guidelines may be given.

Usually, single pigs in a pen are affected. Body temperature readings are normal or slightly subnormal. In peracute or acute cases the first indication of trouble may be finding a pig that has appeared to be in reasonably good condition dead overnight. The nonpigmented areas of the cadaver in such an instance are usually chalk white. In subacute cases pigs may pass dark, tarry, or even dark-pelleted feces for a few days. Such animals tend to suffer from anorexia and may grind their teeth as if in pain.

Many pigs suffering from various degrees of ulceration show no clinical symptoms during life; lesions are only detected at necropsy.

In differential diagnosis, swine dysentery (*Serpulina hyodysenteriae*), *Salmonella choleraesuis* infection, transmissible gastroenteritis, intestinal hemorrhagic syndrome, proliferative enteropathies, torsion of the intestines, MAP, warfarin poisoning, and copper poisoning should be considered. Bacterial or viral infections, however, usually manifest high temperatures and involve several or all pigs in a pen, as may copper poisoning. This latter condition should be considered when feed is mixed on the farm and a number of pigs appear pale and lose their appetites.

TREATMENT.   Because of difficulties of diagnosis, the early stages of ulceration are usually undetected. Treatment by drugs to aid clotting or enhance hemopoiesis have generally been ineffectual, since affected animals showing clinical symptoms usually have ulcers too far advanced to be influenced by medical treatment. However, in individual cases varying response has been reported by the use of nonabsorbable antacids such as aluminum hydroxide and magnesium silicate. The use of the combination of vitamin E and Se in the ration has in some instances afforded a

measure of protection (O'Brien 1968). Nafstad et al. (1967) used vitamin E alone in the feed and noted a partial and slight protective effect. Vitamin U (salts of S-methylmethionine sulfonium) found in certain vegetables has been claimed to ameliorate and accelerate the healing of ulcers (Hegedus et al. 1983).

Pigs suspected of being affected by this condition should be removed from their pen mates and kept separate so that they are not attacked, as this will exacerbate the condition. It has been noted on some farms that affected pigs being housed indoors return slowly to health if allowed access to pasture.

PREVENTION.   Since the weight of evidence seems to indicate that physical and chemical composition of feed is the most important factor causing ulcers of pigs, proper care must be given to ensure that grain in the feed is not ground too finely (not less than 3.5 mm screen size is suggested where ulceration is a problem) and that the grain used is mature, has been stored in a dry state, and is free from fungal growth that might tend to increase the unsaturated fatty acid content. The vitamin E and Se content of diets should be kept under review.

When copper is used in a diet as a growth promoter, the inclusion of zinc carbonate at 110 ppm to counteract the ulcerogenic effect should be considered.

Where cheese whey forms a large part of the diet, consideration should be given to increasing the meal or protein fraction for the buffering effects on gastric contents. However, such adjustments will depend on the economics of the prevailing situation.

A prophylactic effect on ulceration of the pars oesophagea has been noted by feeding, at 1.5%, dried algal biomass derived from cultures of *Scendesmus incrasatalus*, strain R-83 (Tsvetkov et al. 1989).

Since there is some evidence that genetic influences play a part in the increased susceptibility of certain bloodlines to ulcerogenic effects, it may be prudent to avoid breeding from such stock. This is especially true when selection is made for decreased backfat. Once again, economics will dictate the course of action.

Finally, stressful factors such as overcrowding of pens, dampness, and poor ventilation, which have been seen to be associated with the exacerbation of the condition, should be avoided.

ECONOMIC CONSEQUENCES.   In spite of its worldwide distribution and high level of occurrence in some producer units, the overall economic significance of ulceration is very difficult to assess. It is easy to determine the direct losses sustained by pigs that die from acute hemorrhage due to ulceration. It is more difficult to evaluate the effect of subacute and chronic ulcers. There appears to be a conflict between the earlier and more recent reports regarding the significance of ulcers on production and profitability.

Berruecos and Robinson (1972) in South Carolina reported that the presence of ulcers is not a cause of reduced growth rate and efficiency. Ehrensperger et al. (1976) in Switzerland reported that in an experiment with 80 SPF pigs, chronic ulcers had no effect on the fattening rate. Dobson et al. (1978) in Australia showed in their experiments that no significant difference in either the growth rate or food conversion occurred when SPF pigs balanced for weight, age, sex, and genetic background were fed finely ground food and other similar food coarsely ground, even though finely ground food produced more ulceration.

These findings would oppose those of Curtin et al. (1963) in conventional pigs; they observed that decreased weight gain and general unthriftiness accompanied progress of the syndrome. In a study carried out by the Ministry of Agriculture and Forestry in Japan, the loss for 1971 that was attributed to pars oesophagea ulceration on pig production was $15–20 million (U.S.).

REFERENCES

ALLEN, M. M., AND HARDING, J. D. 1962. Experimental copper poisoning in pigs. Vet Rec 74:173–179.

ANON. 1963. Ulcers in swine. Nutr Rev 21:118–120.

ARNOT, R. S.; TERBLANCHE, J.; VAN HICKMAN, R. H.; BARBEZAT, G. O.; AND LOUW, J. H. 1979. Acid secretion in the bile duct ligated pig. S Afr Med J 56:606.

ASDRUBALI, G., AND MUGHETTI, L. 1965. Study of haemorrhagic gastroesophageal ulcer in pigs. Atti Soc Ital Sci Vet 19:412–416.

BARZOI, D.; BARNURE, G. H.; ALEXANDRU, N.; AND STOICESCU, E. 1968. Data on the gastric-oesophageal ulcer in swine in Rumania. Rev Zootech Med Vet 18:59–69.

BERRUECOS, J. M., AND ROBINSON, O. W. 1972. Inheritance of gastric ulcers in swine. J Anim Sci 35:20–23.

BICKNELL, E. J.; BROOKS, B. S.; OSBORN, J. A.; AND WHITEHAIR, C. K. 1967. Extrahepatic biliary obstruction and gastric ulcers in pigs. Am J Vet Res 28:943–950.

BIVIN, W. S.; LOMBARDO DE BARROS, C.; SALLES DE BARROS, C.; AND NOGUEIRA DOS SANTOS, M. 1974. Gastric ulcers in Brazilian swine. J Am Vet Med Assoc 164:405–407.

BUNTAIN, D. 1961. Deaths in pigs on a high copper diet. Vet Rec 63:707–713.

CHAMBERLAIN, C. C.; MERRIMAN, G. M.; LIDVALL, E. R.; AND GAMBLE, C. T. 1967. Effects of feed processing method and diet form on the incidence of esophagogastric ulcers in swine. J Anim Sci 26:72–75.

CHRISTENSEN, C. M. 1957. Deterioration of stored grains by fungi. Bot Rev 23:108–134.

CURTIN, T. M.; GOETSCH, G. D.; AND HOLLANDBECK, R. 1963. Clinical and pathological characterization of esophagogastric ulcers in swine. J Am Vet Med Assoc 143:854–860.

DOBSON, D. J.; DAVIES, R. L.; AND CARGILL, C. F. 1978. Ulceration of the pars oesophagia. Aust Vet J 54:601–602.

DRAGSTEDT, L. R., AND WOODWARD, E. R. 1970. Gastric stasis, a cause of gastric ulcer. Scand J Gastroenterol [Suppl] 6:243–252.

DRAGSTEDT, L. R.; DOYLE, R. E.; AND WOODWARD, E. R. 1969. Gastric ulcers following vagotomy in swine.

Ann Surg 170:785–792.

DRIESEN, S. J.; FAHY, V. A.; AND SPICER, E. M. 1987. Oesophagogastric ulcers. Proc Pig Prod [Sydney Univ] 95:1007–1017.

EHRENSPERGER, F.; JUCKER, H.; PFIRTER, H. P.; POHLENZ, J.; AND SCHLATTER, C. 1976. Influence of food composition on the occurrence of esophagogastric ulcers and on fattening performance in pigs. Zentralbl Veterinaermed [A] 23:265–276.

GAAFAR, S. M., AND KEITTEVUTI, B. 1972. Experimental induction of oesophagogastric ulcers with inoculations of *Ascaris suum* eggs in swine. Gastroenterology 63:423–426.

GRANT, C. A. 1961. Dietetic microangiopathy in pigs. Acta Vet Scand [Suppl] 3:107.

GRIFFING, W. J. 1963. A study of etiology and pathology of gastric ulcers in swine. Diss Abstr 24:1581–1582.

GRONDALEN, T., AND VANGEN, O. 1974. Gastric ulcers in pigs selected for leanness or fatness. Nord Vet Med 25:50–53.

HALLORAN, P. O. 1955. A bibliography of references to diseases of wild mammals and birds. Am J Vet Res 16:1–465.

HANNAN, J., AND NYHAN, J. F. 1962. The use of some vitamins in the control of ulcerative gastric haemorrhage in pigs. Ir Vet J 16:196–197.

HEGEDUS, M.; BOKORI, J.; AND TAMAS, J. 1983. Oesophagogastric ulcer in swine and vitamin U. II. Nature of vitamin U. Acta Vet Hung 31:155–163.

HUBER, W. G., AND WALLIN, R. F. 1965. Experimental production of porcine gastric ulcers. Vet Med 60:551–558.

———. 1967. Gastric secretion and ulcer formation in the pig. Am J Vet Res 28:1455–1459.

ITO, T.; MIURA, S.; AND TANIMURA, J. 1974. Pathological studies on proventricular ulcer in swine. Jpn J Vet Sci 36:263–272.

JELINEK, O. 1957. Gastric ulcer syndrome in pigs. Veterinarstv 17:223.

JENSEN, L. B., AND FREDERICK, L. D. 1939. Spontaneous ulcer of the stomach in several domestic animals. J Am Vet Med Assoc 95:167.

JUBB, K. V. F.; KENNEDY, P. C.; AND PALMER, N. 1985. Pathology of Domestic Animals, 3d ed., vol. 2. New York: Academic Press, p. 44.

KASZUBKIEWICZ, C., AND BOCIANOWSKI, M. 1978. Wrzody stresowe motadka u swin (stress ulcers in the stomach of pigs). Med Weter 34:513–515.

KERNKAMP, H. C. H. 1945. Gastric ulcers in swine. Am J Pathol 21:111.

KINNARD, P. J. 1965. White pig disease. Victorian Vet Proc 23:45–46.

KOKUE, E. I.; NAKAMURA, T.; AND HAYAMA, T. 1978. Experimental production of porcine gastroesophageal ulcers by betazole and reserpine. J Vet Pharmacol Ther 1:217–224.

KOWÁCS, F. 1974. Occurrence of stomach ulcers in pigs in Hungary. Magy Allatorv Lap 29:226–229.

KOWALCZYK, T. 1975. Gastric ulcers. In Diseases of Swine, 4th ed. Ed. H. W. Dunne and A. D. Leman. Ames: Iowa State Univ Press, pp. 978–1010.

KOWALCZYK, T., AND MUGGENBURG, B. A. 1963. Recent developments in gastric ulcers in swine. Proc 17th World Vet Congr 2:1311–1314.

KOWALCZYK, T.; HOEKSTRA, W. G.; PUESTROW, K. L.; SMITH, I. D.; AND GRUMMER, R. H. 1960. Stomach ulcers in swine. J Am Vet Med Assoc 137:339–344.

KOWALCZYK, T.; MUGGENBURG, B. A.; SMITH, R. W.; HOEKSTRA, W. G.; FIRST, N. L.; AND GRUMMER, R. H. 1966. Stomach ulcers in farrowing gilts. J Am Vet Med Assoc 148:52–62.

KOWALCZYK, T.; TANAKA, Y.; MUGGENBURG, B. A.; OLSON, W. G.; AND MORRISSEY, J. F. 1968. Endoscopic examination of the swine's stomach. Am J Vet

Res 29:729–736.

LARENAUDIE, B. 1964. Le syndrome de l'ulcère gastro-oesophagien hemorragique du porc. Encycl Vet Period 21:110–112.

McERLEAN, B. A. 1962. Recently recognized clinical disease entities in pigs in Ireland. Ir Vet J 16:221–232.

McINTOSH, D. 1897. Diseases of Swine. Chicago: Donahue, p. 40.

MAHAN, D. C.; PICKETT, R. A.; PERRY, T. W.; CURTIS, T. M.; FEATHERSTON, W. R.; AND BEESON, W. M. 1966. Influence of various nutritional factors and physical form of feed on esophagogastric ulcers in swine. J Anim Sci 25:1019–1023.

MAXWELL, C. V. 1970. The relationship of several nutritional factors to the development of gastric ulcers in swine. Diss Abstr Int 31:777B.

MAXWELL, C. V.; REIMANN, E. M.; HOEKSTRA, W. G.; KOWALCZYK, T.; BENEVENGA, N. J.; AND GRUMMER, R. H. 1970. Effect of dietary particle size on lesion development and on the contents of various regions of the swine stomach. J Anim Sci 30:911–922.

MOIR, D. C., AND MASTERS, H. G. 1979. Hepatosis dietetica, nutritional myopathy, mulberry heart disease and associated hepatic selenium levels in pigs. Aust Vet J 55:360–364.

MUGGENBURG, B. A.; McNUTT, S. H.; AND KOWALCZYK, T. 1964. Pathology of gastric ulcers in swine. Am J Vet Res 25:1354–1365.

MUGGENBURG, B. A.; KOWALCZYK, T.; HOEKSTRA, W. G.; AND GRUMMER, R. H. 1966a. Experimental production of gastric ulcers in swine by reserpine. Am J Vet Res 27:1663–1669.

MUGGENBURG, B. A.; KOWALCZYK, T.; REESE, N. A.; HOEKSTRA, W. G.; AND GRUMMER, R. H. 1966b. Experimental production of gastric ulcers in swine by histamine in mineral oil–bees wax. Am J Vet Res 27:292–299.

MUGGENBURG, B. A.; REIMANN, E. M.; KOWALCZYK, T.; AND HOEKSTRA, W. G. 1967. Effect of reserpine and histamine in mineral oil–beeswax vehicle on gastric secretion in swine. Am J Vet Res 28:1427–1435.

NAFSTAD, I. 1967. Gastric ulcers in swine. Pathol Vet 4:1–14.

NAFSTAD, I.; TOLERSRUD, S.; AND BAUSTAD, B. 1967. Gastric ulcers in swine. Effects of different proteins and fats on their development. Pathol Vet 4:23–30.

NAKAMURA, T.; KOKUE, E.; AND HAYAMA, T. 1975. Can Ascaris infection be used for experimental induction of porcine esophagogastric ulcer? Gastroenterology 69:788–789.

OBEL, A. L. 1953. Studies on the morphology and etiology of so-called toxic liver dystrophy (hepatosis diaetetica) in swine. Acta Pathol Microbiol Scand [Suppl] 94:1–87.

O'BRIEN, J. J. 1966. Some aspects of gastric (pars oesophagea) ulceration in the pig. Ph.D. diss., National Univ of Ireland, Dublin.

———. 1968. Some dietary factors in gastric ulceration (pars oesophagea) of the pig. Ir Vet J 22:162–165.

———. 1969. Gastric ulceration (of the pars oesophagea) in the pig. Vet Bull 39:75–82.

O'CONNOR, D. 1958. Haemorrhage of unknown origin in pigs. Ir Vet J 12:28–30.

PERRY, T. W. 1962. Fifty per cent incidence of stomach ulcers in swine fed rations processed through a pelleting machine. Feedstuffs Minneap 34(47):54.

POCOCK, E. F. 1966. Gastric ulcers in swine. M.S. thesis, Univ. of Guelph.

POCOCK, E. F.; BAYLEY, H. S.; AND ROE, C. K. 1968. Relationship of pelleted, autoclaved and heat expanded corn or starvation to gastric ulcers in swine. J Anim Sci 27:1296–1302.

QURESHI, S. R.; OLANDER, H. J.; AND GAAFAR, S. M.

1978. Oesophagogastric ulcers associated with Ascaris suum infestation in swine. Vet Pathol 15:353–357.

REESE, N. A.; MUGGENBURG, B. A.; KOWALCZYK, T.; GRUMMER, R. H.; AND HOEKSTRA, W. G. 1966. Nutritional and environmental factors influencing gastric ulcers in swine. J Anim Sci 25:14–20.

REIMANN, E. M.; MAXWELL, C. V.; GRUMMER, R. H.; KOWALCZYK, T.; BENEVENGA, N. J.; AND HOEKSTRA, W. G. 1967. Differential effect of dietary particle size on the contents of various regions of the swine stomach. J Anim Sci 26:1498.

REMBOLD, G. 1965. Das Ulcera Gastrorrhagische Syndrom beim Schwein. Wien Tieraerztl Monatschr 52:851–857.

RICO LENZA, J. 1966. Incidence of gastric ulcer in pigs and its possible relationship with the ration. Rev Patron Biol Anim 10(1):7–18.

RIVERA, M. A., AND GAAFAR, S. M. 1976. Sequential development of esophagogastric ulcers induced in swine by infections with Ascaris suum (Geeze 1782). Vet Parasitol 2:341–353.

ROTHENBACHER, N.; NELSON, L. W.; AND ELLIS, D. J. 1963. The stomach ulcer gastrorrhagia syndrome in Michigan pigs. Vet Med 58:806–816.

ŠENK, L., AND ŠABEC, D. 1965. Ezofagogastrieai ulkus kod svinga u intenzivnom odgogu. Vet Glasn 19:595–602.

SHUGAM, N. A.; KOROBOV, A. V.; AND GLOTOVA, I. A. 1979. Izuchenie belkovogo i fermentnogo sostava syvorotki krovi i zheludochnogo soka. Sb Nauchn Trudov Mosk Vet Akad 106:21–25.

SIMONSSON, A., AND BJÖRKLUND, N. E. 1978. Some effects of the fineness of ground barley on gastric lesions and gastric contents in growing pigs. Vitam Horm 20:645–657.

SWAHN, O., AND THAFVELIN, B. 1962. Vitamin E and some metabolic diseases of pigs. Vitam Horm 20:645–657.

SZEMERÉDI, G., AND SOLÁ, A. 1979. Role of meteorological factors in the development of oesophageal gastric ulcers in pigs under tropical conditions. Magy Allatorv Lap 34:176–178.

TERBLANCKE, J.; PEACOCK, J. H.; HOBBS, D. E. F.; HUNT, A. C.; BOWES, J.; TIERRIS, E. J.; PALMER, D. B.; AND BLECHER, T. E. 1968. Orthotopic liver homotransplantation: An experimental study in the unmodified pig. S Afr Med J 42:486–497.

THOONEN, J., AND HOORENS, J. 1961. Meagulcera in de pars oesophagea big varkens. Vlaams Diergeneeskd Tidschr 30:79–92.

TSVETKOV, A.; PARVANOVA, L.; AND CHERKEZOV, L. 1989. Experiments for prophylaxis of ulcers in swine using algal biomass. Vet Sbir 87:40–42.

VAN VLEET, J. F.; CARLTON, W.; AND OLANDER, H. J. 1970. Hepatosis dietetica and mulberry heart disease associated with selenium deficiency in Indiana swine. J Am Vet Med Assoc 15:1208–1219.

VAN VLEET, J. F.; MEYER, K. B.; OLANDER, H. J.; AND RUTH, G. R. 1974. Efficacy and safety of selenium-vitamin E injections in newborn pigs to prevent subclinical deficiency in growing swine. Am J Vet Res 36:387–393.

WALLIN, R. F.; HUBER, W. G.; AND JENSEN, A. H. 1968. Esophagogastric ulcers in swine fed diets high in corn starch. Cornell Vet 59:561–569.

WALZL, M. L. 1964. Zwei Falle von "esophagogastric ulcers" beim Schwein. Schweiz Arch Tierheilkd 106:491–497.

WESOLOSKI, G. D.; JENSEN, A. H.; LADWIG, V. D.; AND GROSSER, H. 1975. Effects of different concentrations of corn oil, magnesium sulphate and oat hulls in a porcine ulcerogenic ration. Am J Vet Res 36:773–775.

56 Genetic, Developmental, and Neoplastic Diseases

M. J. Edwards

R. C. Mulley

Genetic and Developmental Diseases

DEVELOPMENTAL DISEASES or defects occur relatively frequently in swine. The defect might be anatomic (aplasia, hypoplasia, or dysplasia of an organ or part) or functional. Anatomic defects are also described as malformations, anomalies, and abnormalities; newborn animals with particularly bizarre malformations are often termed monsters. If present at birth it is termed a congenital defect or congenital abnormality. However, not all developmental defects are apparent at birth; e.g., an inguinal hernia might not develop until the pig is some weeks or months old. Some developmental abnormalities are more common in certain breeds or lines within breeds, indicating a heritable liability or tendency. Heritable defects are frequently apparent at birth; thus they can be classified also as congenital defects, but not all congenital defects are heritable.

Heritable conditions are quite common in swine and perhaps constitute the most economically important group of defects. There is an expanding list of agents known to be teratogenic for swine, but for many defects there are no immediately apparent heritable or environmental causes, and these are collectively termed spontaneous defects.

Developmental diseases are of economic significance, as they contribute to infertility by causing embryonic and fetal mortality; they also contribute to stillbirths, neonatal and preweaning deaths, and retarded growth rates of surviving piglets. Approximately 40–45% of pig embryos and fetuses do not survive to birth, and a further 5–7% are stillborn (Wrathall 1971). About 30–35% of embryos are lost during the embryonic period (up to 35 days) and 10% during the fetal period (35 days to term). Most of the embryonic loss occurs before the end of the third week and is heaviest during the second week when the blastocyst is forming (Perry and Rowlands 1962). Developmental abnormalities probably account for about one-third of the deaths, most being associated with abnormalities of fertilization resulting in chromosomal defects.

Although the occurrence of specific defects is reported quite frequently in swine, reliable figures for the overall prevalence of developmental disorders are not readily available. Priester et al. (1970), from a survey of the Veterinary Medical Data Program established by a number of North American veterinary clinics, found swine to have the highest proportion of congenital defects of all domestic species, mainly from cryptorchidism, umbilical and inguinal hernias, and anal atresia. Selby et al. (1971a, 1976), using survey data obtained from a mailed questionnaire to pig producers in the United States, estimated the occurrence of congenital defects in piglets as 0.67%. This is probably an underestimate, as approximately 75% of respondents reported no defects at all. The commonest malformations were conjoined twins, anal atresia, malformed limbs, cleft palate, hydrocephalus, and cranium bifida. Many piglets had multiple anomalies. Smidt (1972) found that anal atresia, paralysis of the backquarters (splayleg), myoclonia congenita, inguinal and scrotal hernias, and intersexes were the most common defects in the Netherlands; together they occurred in about 1.5% of piglets, mainly of the Dutch Landrace breed.

Deeble (1974) reported only 0.03% heritable defects in the progeny of the first 20 litters sired by artificial insemination by British Large White and Landrace boars. The record for progeny of Landrace boars was consistently worse than that of Large White; the most common conditions recorded in the piglets were splayleg, inguinal hernia, anal atresia, deformed tail, pityriasis rosea, and umbilical hernia. A herd-to-herd variation of 0.6–2.4% (mean 1.4%) of congenital malformations was found in piglets in the preweaning age at necropsy in Denmark (Bille and Nielsen 1977). The most common conditions were anal atresia, heart defects, and contracted hind limbs, but conditions such as splayleg or myoclonia congenita were not recorded. The incidence of defective piglets in a large commercial piggery in Eastern Australia recorded over 1 year was 2.9% among 14,535 piglets. The defects are listed in Table 56.1, which provides a population frequency. The breeding stock were mainly Large White and Landrace crosses; the most common defects were

Table 56.1. Congenital defects detected among 14,535 piglets between birth and 1 week

Site of Defect	Number of Piglets	Total	Proportion of all Malformations (%)
Nervous system		16	4.2
Micrencephaly	10		
Hydrocephalus	2		
Cyclopia	2		
Encephalocoele	1		
Spina bifida	1		
Head		25	6.5
Cleft palate	10		
Tongue hypertrophy	6		
Cranioschisis	4		
Ear defects	2		
Brachygnathia superior	2		
Anophthalmia	1		
Limbs		183	47.4
Myofibrillar hypoplasia	152		
Arthrogryposis	15		
Micromelia	14		
Polydactyly	1		
Club foot	1		
Circulatory		27	7.0
Anemia	20		
Cardiac hypertrophy	5		
Portal vessel atresia	2		
Body wall		14	3.6
Exomphalos	10		
Diaphragmatic hernia	3		
Inguinal hernia	1		
Gastrointestinal tract		43	11.1
Anal atresia	36		
Intestinal atresia	7		
Miscellaneous		78	20.2
Cryptorchidism	57		
Tail deformity	11		
Epitheliogenesis imperfecta	7		
Scoliosis	2		
Torticollis	1		
Total	386		

Source: Mulley and Edwards (1984).

splayleg, cryptorchidism, and anal atresia (Mulley and Edwards 1984).

It seems likely that congenital defects would occur in at least 2–3% of piglets if all abnormalities are taken into account and that certain breeds or lines within breeds might contribute more than others.

CAUSES OF DEVELOPMENTAL DEFECTS.

Huston et al. (1978) have published a comprehensive catalog of congenital defects in pigs that lists 4 conditions due to chromosomal abnormalities and 144 due to heritable, environmental, or unknown causes. In approximately 13% of defects the cause was known or believed to be heritable; a known environmental or teratogenic agent was identified as the cause in a similar number, and the cause was unknown or classified as possibly heritable in approximately 75% of conditions. Defects with dominant modes of inheritance are usu-

ally mild, since severe defects are lethal and carriers are easy to recognize and cull. Defects with recessive inheritance are more common and difficult to eliminate, and very few show simple modes of inheritance. Huston et al. (1978) made a positive statement on heritability in only 13 of 144 defects (hemophilia, abnormal tongue, hairlessness, wattles, dermatosis vegetans, inguinal hernia, rickets, hydrocephalus, cerebrospinal lipodystrophy, myoclonia congenita, cryptorchidism, and true and pseudohermaphrodism). Most embryos with defects resulting from heritable or chromosomal abnormalities die before implantation.

It has been suggested that a minority of malformations have a major genetic cause, a minority have a major environmental cause, and most malformations are due to multifactorial causes with complex interactions between a genetic liability and one or a number of environmental agents (Fraser 1959). This multifactorial causation makes it difficult to identify the agent responsible for most defects in pigs. The susceptibility to a teratogen can be characteristic to the species; e.g., hog cholera (HC) virus affects prenatal development only in pigs. There is frequently considerable variation also between embryos of a species in their response to a teratogenic agent, and part of this is due to differences in the genotype between embryos. Even within a litter there is often a wide range in the response of littermates to teratogenic agents. Littermates are not identical genetically; they can also vary considerably in their state of development at a given stage of gestation.

The reaction of embryos and fetuses to teratogenic agents varies with their developmental ages. Before differentiation of the germ layers (preimplantation), damaging agents may cause embryonic death but rarely produce malformations. Any that produce malformations are likely to do so by causing genetic mutations. Many factors, including those that do not cause malformations, can cause the death of undifferentiated embryos, which degenerate and are quickly resorbed.

The embryonic period in the pig extends from the time of uterine attachment on day 13 or 14 to about day 35 when organogenesis is more or less complete. This is the stage of development during which conceptuses are most easily and severely affected by teratogens. Within this period the developmental stages between 14 and 25 days are most at risk (Wrathall 1975). Certain organs or structures appear particularly susceptible to damage by one or a number of agents at quite well-defined stages (critical periods). Severely damaged embryos usually die and are resorbed more slowly than in the preimplantation period, or they may become mummified. When the majority of embryos die, abortion is common. Less severely damaged embryos may survive for varying periods before they die and become mummified or aborted, or they may survive to be born with malformations.

The susceptibility to damaging agents diminishes rapidly during the fetal stage (between 35 days and term) and decreases further with advancing age. The fetus, however, is not immune to teratogens; a number of cerebral, cerebellar, cardiac, and urologic malformations may be induced after the embryonic period. Again, severely damaged fetuses may die immediately and be mummified or aborted, while less severely damaged fetuses may die during later gestation or at birth or may be born as living, malformed piglets.

The reaction of the embryo or fetus also depends on the nature and dose of the teratogen. Many agents that do not cause malformation can cause maternal illness, which is often followed by general growth retardation or immediate or delayed death of the embryo, fetus, or neonate. Fewer agents are teratogenic; those that are will usually cause embryonic or fetal death if given in large doses, while smaller doses cause malformations and growth retardation. There is usually a threshold dose below which no effect is found, but a subthreshold dose might alter susceptibility so that very small doses of other agents acting additively produce a threshold effect. Many teratogens that produce severe embryonic damage are of very low virulence or toxicity to the dam. The vaccine strain of HC virus causes little or no maternal reaction but can be very damaging to the embryo and fetus. The maternal body, however, does insulate the conceptus against many teratogens by diluting, detoxifying, and excreting them before they reach an embryotoxic level. The placental barrier can further reduce the dose that reaches the embryo.

The general principles defining the nature of the susceptibility of mammalian embryos to teratogens are discussed in detail by Wilson (1973), who summarized the main categories of causes as radiation, chemicals, dietary imbalance, infection, hypoxia, hypercapnia, temperature extremes, metabolic or endocrine imbalance, physical trauma, and placental failure. These agents result in mutations or other changes in cellular function, and the pathogenic pathways lead to cell death, failure of cell interactions, reduced synthesis, impeded cell movements, tissue disruptions, or alterations of programmed differentiation. Malformation is the final result.

Many agents consistently cause characteristic patterns of defects, probably because they interfere with certain metabolic (enzymatic) processes. Although each of the many primary effects on enzymatic processes is specific, the subsequent pathogenic pathways are relatively few, as noted above. Thus diverse types of teratogens can cause similar defects; e.g., arthrogryposis, which is the fixation of a number of joints in the limbs and vertebral column, can be caused in many species of animals by a number of agents including genetic, viral, chemical, and physical agents; plant toxins; and drugs.

Thus if a teratogenic agent affects a group of sows at various stages of pregnancy, an epidemiologic study of the herd will often reveal a syndrome that includes recently mated sows returning to service (indicating heavy embryonic mortality), small litter size and an increase in the number of mummified fetuses (as a result of mortality in individual embryos and fetuses), an increase in stillbirths and neonatal mortality, and piglets of small birth weights as well as an increase in the number of malformed piglets born.

Genetic and heritable abnormalities contribute to early embryonic death mainly through chromosomal defects and also to a number of developmental malformations such as splayleg and anal atresia, which are important because of their relatively frequent occurrence and associated high neonatal mortality. Chromosomal defects might be visible microscopically as changes in numbers of chromosomes (an excess – polyploidy; a deficiency – aneuploidy) or in chromosomal morphology. Heritable translocation (aneuploid) abnormalities have been recorded (Vogt et al. 1972). Polyploidy is commonly attributed to aging of the gametes, particularly of the egg before fertilization, e.g., after delayed mating. McFeely (1967) found grossly detectable chromosomal defects in 10% of blastocysts and a further 2.3% of degenerating blastocysts from gilts at 10 days after mating.

Heritable defects are transmitted by the parents according to Mendelian principles, and mating of closely related animals carrying genetic defects increases the incidence of the defect in the offspring. The contribution of genotype to defects can be very complex. Wrathall (1988) gives a concise account of genetic transmission and liability and gene-environment interaction in causation. Diagnosis of a heritable defect requires pedigree analysis; this can be confirmed by test matings between suspected defective and normal parents.

There is evidence that the incidence of malformations increases with advancing parity (Mulley and Edwards 1984) and this probably contributes to the higher perinatal losses that occur in older sows. There is also evidence that litters containing one or more malformed piglets have higher preparturient, parturient, and preweaning death rates than normal litters, and malformation rates are higher following autumn and spring conceptions.

The known teratogens for swine that might be or have been met under field conditions include HC virus, Japanese B encephalitis, *Toxoplasma gondii,* methallibure, Neguvon (metrifonate, trichlorfon), tobacco (*Nicotiana tabacum, Nicotiana glauca*) stalks, poison hemlock (*Conium maculatum*), and deficiencies of iodine and vitamin A.

Under experimental conditions border disease virus, ionizing radiations, trypan blue, and hypervitaminosis A have produced malformations in swine.

Agents that are probable or possible but unproven teratogens include pseudorabies (PR) (Aujeszky's disease); mycotoxins; *Leucaena leucocephala*; jimsonweed or thorn apple (*Datura stramonium*); wild black cherries (*Prunus serotina*); blighted potatoes; dietary deficiencies of choline,

pantothenic acid, ascorbic acid, zinc, or manganese; and hyperthermia. These agents have been reviewed in detail by Wrathall (1975).

In this chapter only the more common developmental defects and teratogens of particular interest for swine will be considered. The review by Huston et al. (1978) provides an extensive bibliography of original publications on congenital defects in pigs. Table 56.2 outlines the common developmental defects of swine and their etiology.

Table 56.2. Common developmental defects of swine

Defect	Etiology	Diagnosis
Micrencephaly	Heat stress midpregnancy	History of heat stress
	Unknown (most cases)	An agent affecting development in early or mid-pregnancy
Microphthalmia	Vitamin A deficiency	Multiple defects in affected litters; heavy neonatal mortality; history; diet analysis; serum and liver vitamin A analysis
	HC infection	HC infection in herd; virus isolation; fluorescent antibody test; serology; congenital tremor A1 present in herd
	Heritable	Mode of inheritance uncertain; dominant gene?
	Unknown	An agent affecting embryos at 12–16 days development
Neural tube defects (anencephaly, encephalocele, hydrocephalus, spina bifida)	Unknown	An agent affecting embryos at 12–14 days development
	Vitamin A deficiency (hydrocephalus)	Multiple defects in affected litters; heavy neonatal mortality; history; diet analysis; serum and liver vitamin A analysis
Congenital tremor	HC virus (type AI)	HC infection in herd; virus isolation; fluorescent antibody test; serology; affects piglets of all breeds and both sexes; hypomyelinogenesis; cerebellar hypoplasia; neurochemical analysis of myelin lipids of spinal cord; small cross sectional area of the spinal cord
	Type AII (unidentified virus)	Hypomyelinogenesis of the spinal cord; analysis of the myelin lipids of the spinal cord; small cross sectional area of spinal cord
	Type AIII	Monogenic sex-linked gene in Landrace affecting male piglets only
	Type IV	Autosomal recessive gene in Saddleback affecting both sexes
	Pseudorabies virus	PR infection in herd; virus isolation; serology; transmission tests
	Neguvon (metrifonate, trichlorfon)	History of dosing sows in midpregnancy; hypoplasia of cerebrum and cerebellum; Purkinje-cell loss; changes in neurotransmitters
Arthrogryposis	Tobacco stalks, jimsonweed, poison hemlock, wild black cherry	History of exposure to plants in early to midpregnancy
	Vitamin A deficiency	Multiple defects; high neonatal mortality; history; diet analysis; serum and liver vitamin A analysis
	HC attenuated vaccine virus	History of vaccination during early pregnancy
	HC infection	HC infection in herd; virus isolation; fluorescent antibody test; serology; congenital tremor AI in herd
	Heritable	Recessive gene?; autosomal recessive in Yorkshire pigs
	Unknown (most cases)	An agent affecting development in early to midpregnancy
Micromelia	Unknown	Possibly caused by limb vascular defects in early pregnancy
Cleft palate/harelip	Heritable	Possibly a recessive gene; cleft palate in Poland China probably genetic
	Unknown (most cases)	An agent affecting development in early to midpregnancy

Table 56.2. *Continued*

Defect	Etiology	Diagnosis
Deformed tail	Possibly heritable	Mode of inheritance uncertain; occasionally urogenital defect associated
	Unknown	Often associated with motor defects in hind limbs; vertebral defects
Myofibrillar hypoplasia	Heritable	Most common in Landrace, less in Large White; probably polygenic mode of inheritance; incidence modified by maternal stress, slippery floors, birth weight, maternal nutrition
	Fusarium toxin	Higher mortalities than other forms; feed analysis
Inguinal hernia	Heritable	Mode of inheritance uncertain; incidence modified by environment
Umbilical hernia	Unknown	Possibly polygenic inheritance
Anal atresia	Heritable	Possibly polygenic inheritance or an autosomal recessive or autosomal dominant form of transmission
Hypotrichosis	Heritable in some breeds	Mode of inheritance uncertain
	Iodine deficiency	Stillbirths and high neonatal mortality; enlarged thyroids; skin edematous; feed analysis
Epitheliogenesis imperfecta	Heritable	Possibly autosomal recessive gene; hydronephrosis-associated
Dermatosis vegetans	Heritable	Autosomal recessive; associated with fatal giant-cell pneumonia
Pityriasis rosea	Probably heritable	Mode of inheritance uncertain; affects young pigs, especially Landrace; benign and self-limiting
Von Willebrand's disease	Heritable	Recessive gene in Poland China; excess bleeding from minor wounds; decrease in factor VIII and platelet retention time
Navel bleeding	Unknown	Cord is edematous
Cardiac defects	Unknown	Most cases recognized at 4–7 weeks; mostly males
Cryptorchidism	Probably heritable	Polygenic transmission; left testicle most commonly involved
Female genital hypoplasias, duplications	Probably a heritable component	Mode of inheritance uncertain; genital tract incomplete or duplicated
Male pseudo-hermaphroditism	Heritable	Mode of transmission uncertain; testicles in abdomen together with female tubular tract
True hermaphroditism	Heritable	Mode of inheritance uncertain; testicular and ovarian tissues usually with female tubular tract

DEFECTS OF THE NERVOUS SYSTEM AND EYES.

The survival of newborn piglets depends on their ability to walk and suck from the sow within a few minutes of birth. Although at birth there are some indications of immaturity of the central nervous system (CNS), it usually functions quite efficiently. Myelination is incomplete in the newborn piglet, but at this stage myelin deposition is taking place actively and the brain is in its most rapid growth phase (Dobbing 1974). In some piglets, however, myelination is deficient and these animals show clinical signs of congenital tremor, which can prejudice survival. Congenital tremor is the most common defect of the nervous system of pigs, but numerous less common and often bizarre conditions exist, most of which cause death at birth or soon after.

Done (1968) reviewed the congenital defects of the nervous system of pigs, which he classified as due to hereditary, toxic, or nutritional causes, transplacental infections, and unknown or accidental causes.

The heritable conditions include some forms of congenital tremor, failure of closure of the anterior neuropore leading to meningocele (Fig. 56.1), encephalocele or hydrocephalus, and paralysis.

Defects due to nutritional or toxic causes include microphthalmia (Fig. 56.2) associated with avitaminosis A up to 18 days of gestation, arthrogryposis and hydrocephalus associated with avitaminosis A throughout pregnancy, and congenital tremor and cerebellar hypoplasia due to Neguvon. Infections include HC virus, which causes congenital tremor, cerebellar and spinal hypoplasia, hydrocephalus, and arthrogryposis; Japanese B encephalitis, which causes congenital convulsions and weakness; and possibly PR as a cause of congenital tremor. A list of defects caused by unknown agents is very long and includes anencephaly, hydrocephalus, cyclopia (Fig. 56.3), cerebellar hypoplasia, spina bifida, duplication of parts of the spinal cord or brain, syringomyelia, and other forms of myelodysplasia.

Although congenital malformations due to prenatal infection with HC virus are now rare, they are still of considerable interest. Vaccination of pregnant sows with avirulent vaccine viruses or field viruses leads to a variety of malformations but little or no maternal illness. Certain strains, when injected in early pregnancy, produced deformed heads and noses, cyclopia, microphthalmia, and micrencephaly (Sautter et al. 1953).

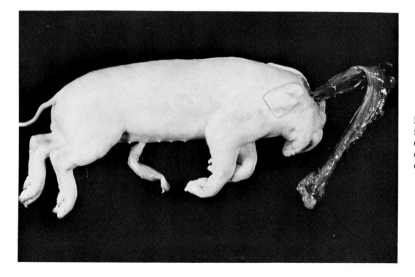

56.1. Meningocele in a newborn piglet. Defective development of the brain and other parts of the head and overgrowth of meninges.

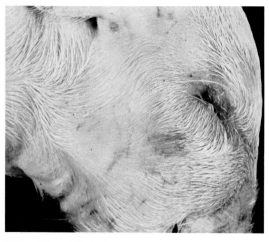

56.2. Microphthalmia.

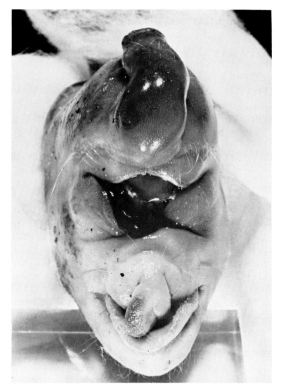

56.3. Cyclopia. Cause unknown.

Other defects produced by this virus are congenital tremor associated with hypomyelinogenesis and cerebellar hypoplasia (Harding et al. 1966), edema and ascites, and pulmonary hypoplasia (Emerson and Delez 1965). The cerebellar hypoplasia and hypomyelinogenesis are probably caused by inhibition of mitosis within the developing nervous system.

Congenital Tremor.   Many types of congenital tremor (CT) (myoclonia congenita, trembles, jumpy pig disease) can be differentiated etiologically and pathologically, and the clinical condition has been recorded in many countries. Smidt (1972) found it to affect 0.2% of piglets in the Netherlands. All types of the condition are characterized by a tremor of the head and limbs of newborn piglets. It has been proposed (Done 1976a) that the forms of congenital tremor in which morphologic lesions are found be designated type A and the rest type B. Within type A at least two infections (HC–AI and an unidentified virus–AII) and two heritable subtypes (AIII and AIV) have been identified. In addition, Maré and Kluge (1974) have isolated PR virus from piglets with tremors, suggesting that it might also have an etiologic role, but at present the position is uncertain. More recently an antiparasitic drug, Neguvon (metrifonate, trichlorfon), given to pregnant sows has been identified as another cause of the condition (Bölske et al. 1978; Knox et al. 1978; Berge et al. 1987), which has been designated as the AV subtype.

Types AI, AII, and AV affect piglets of all breeds and both sexes, type AIII affects Landrace male piglets (Harding et al. 1973), and type AIV affects British Saddleback piglets of both sexes (Patterson et al. 1973). All or part of the litter may be involved in the nonheritable forms, while about 25% of piglets are affected in the heritable forms (50% of males in type AIII).

Affected piglets show signs within a few hours of birth. The tremor may be fine or gross; it affects the muscles of the limbs and neck, producing rhythmic twitchings that abate when the piglet lies down and ceasing when it is asleep. The fore and hind limbs or head may be more severely affected than other parts. Animals affected with a fine tremor of the head and limbs are usually able to walk about and feed, but a gross tremor usually interferes seriously with these functions, often leading to death from starvation, cold, or crushing by the sow. The clonus can be severe enough to cause the hind limbs to be lifted clear of the ground. It is exacerbated by cold and excitement. Piglets with congenital tremor might also be affected with splayleg. In type AIII there is a lateral undulation of the hindquarters.

Mildly affected piglets usually recover spontaneously in a few days to several weeks. Mortality is high in all but the AII type, and death occurs usually within the first 3–4 days.

The tremor appears to result from hyperactivity of the spinal reflex arc, as it persists after cord section posterior to the site of the operation (Fletcher 1968).

Myelin deficiency is a feature of congenital tremor types AI–AIV and the types associated with Neguvon (AV) and PR virus. Tremor types AI–AIV can be differentiated by the epidemiologic features of outbreaks, the gross pathology of affected piglets, and a fairly simple neurochemical examination of the cord (Patterson and Done 1977). Congenital tremor AI, which results from transplacental infection apparently with both field (Done 1976a) and vaccine strains (Emerson and Delez 1965) of HC virus, is characterized by hypoplasia, dysgenesis, and cortical dysplasia of the cerebellum. The spinal cord is reduced in size and contains less than half the normal complement of myelin at birth (Done 1976a). Done et al. (1984, 1986) found smaller cross-sectional areas of the white and gray matters of the spinal cords of piglets after experimental infection of the sows both with the HC virus and with the (presumed) viral agent of CT AII. In type AII the lipid content of the cord is reduced by about one-third, with depressed and aberrant cerebroside synthesis and evidence of demyelination. Type AIII, due to a monogenic sex-linked factor in Landrace

sows, is characterized by a relative deficiency of oligodendrocytes leading to hypoplasia of the cord with reduced cellular and lipid contents. Type AIV is due to an autosomal recessive gene in Saddleback pigs. The cord is underdeveloped, and there is evidence of demyelination and marked deficiency of all myelin lipids. Demyelination of the white matter of the cerebellum was found in piglets from which PR virus was isolated. The condition produced by Neguvon during pregnancy is characterized by cerebral and cerebellar hypoplasia, hypoplasia of the spinal cord, myelin deficiency of the affected parts, and decrease in specific activity of neurotransmitter synthesizing enzymes (Berge et al. 1987).

Survival of piglets may be aided by warmth and assisting them to feed. Control of the condition depends on identification and elimination of the cause through disease control, breeding policy, and care in the use of drugs in pregnant sows. Until a firm diagnosis is made, empty females should be deliberately exposed to affected piglets to immunize them before they become pregnant. All affected pigs should be disposed of, and none from affected litters should be retained for breeding. The herd should be considered potentially infected until no further affected litters have been born over a period of 4 months (Done 1976b).

Anophthalmia and Microphthalmia. Hale (1933, 1935) showed for the first time that a nutritional deficiency during pregnancy could cause congenital malformation. Sows depleted of vitamin A during the first month of pregnancy, but later receiving supplements, gave birth to piglets with multiple defects, the most obvious being anophthalmia and microphthalmia. He showed that the defects were not hereditary. Severe and prolonged deprivation is required to deplete reserves of the vitamin. For instance, Hale (1935) maintained gilts on a vitamin A–free ration for about 160 days before mating and for the first 30 days of pregnancy, and Palludan (1961) maintained gilts on a vitamin A–free diet from 2 months of age but gave a number of supplements of vitamin A at various stages of early pregnancy. Neonatal mortality was very high; defects recorded included microphthalmia; hydrocephalus; compression of the spinal cord; arthrogryposis; edema; accessory ears; cleft palate and harelip; skin and hair defects; subcutaneous cysts; polydactylism; and defects of the heart, liver, lung, diaphragm, kidneys, colon, and genital organs. Bilateral renal agenesis and polycystic kidneys have also been reported.

It is unlikely that vitamin A deficiency of this severity would be common in commercial piggeries since most rations contain some vitamin, but there are reports of association between the birth of piglets with microphthalmia and sows being fed vitamin A–deficient diets (Watt and

Barlow 1956). Excessive amounts of vitamin A are also teratogenic (Wrathall 1975).

Microphthalmia has also been reported to be associated with HC virus (Harding and Done 1956), and a heritable form has been described (Maneely 1951).

DEFECTS OF THE MUSCULOSKELETAL SYSTEM.
There is an almost infinite variety of individual defects and possible combinations that involve the musculoskeletal system. Huston et al. (1978) list 32 identifiable individual and multiple abnormalities. Conditions such as syndactyly, polydactyly (Fig. 56.4), and tail deformities are of minor importance, but arthrogryposis, splayleg, micromelia (Fig. 56.5), and inguinal hernia are quite common and may cause appreciable losses. Conjoined twins (Fig. 56.6), congenital thick foreleg (congenital hyperostosis), and diaphragmatic hernia are uncommon but lethal conditions.

Congenital Splayleg.
Congenital splayleg (spraddleleg, myofibrillar hypoplasia) has been recognized as a clinical entity for at least 20 years and is probably the most important of the inherited defects of piglets. It was first described clinically by Thurley et al. (1967) and since then has been reported from other European countries, Australia, and North America. Ward (1978a,b) estimated that in Britain it affects about 0.4% of piglets of which about 50% die, mainly from starvation and crushing by the sow. The condition is particularly prevalent in Landrace and, to a lesser extent, Large White breeds. The cause of the functional defect is not known, but there is strong evidence that it is multifactorial, depending on a genetic liability to muscular weakness on which other factors such as birth weight, maternal stress, maternal nutrition, and slippery and sloping floors might act (Done and Wijeratne 1972). The histologic appearance of affected muscles re-

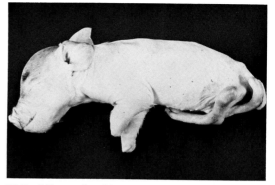

56.5. Micromelia of forelimbs with failure of proper development below the carpus. Arthrogryposis of the hind limbs.

sembles that of experimentally produced glucocorticoid myopathy (Jirmanová 1983; Jirmanová and Lojola 1985), suggesting that the condition could result from stress during pregnancy. Male and female piglets from gilts or sows may be affected, but male offspring are significantly more susceptible (Vogt et al. 1984). There are usually one to four splayed piglets in a litter, but occasionally the whole litter can be affected. The mean birth weight of affected piglets is average or slightly below average.

The trend toward smooth and sloping floors in farrowing pens appears to precipitate the condition in susceptible piglets. Kohler et al. (1969) produced splayleg experimentally by penning newborn piglets on a slippery surface for 18 hours. Littermates held on straw were unaffected. It has been suggested that a dietary deficiency of choline during pregnancy could cause splayleg and that supplementation with 3–4.5 g choline daily throughout pregnancy would reduce its incidence (Cunha 1972). However, Dobson (1971) failed to reduce the incidence of splayleg in

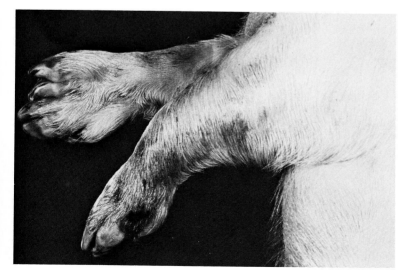

56.4. Polydactyly of a forelimb.

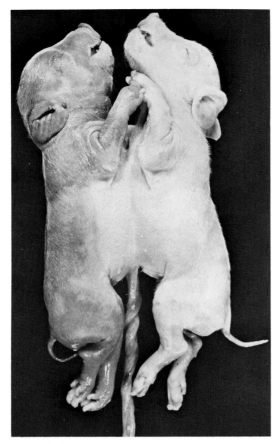

56.6. Conjoined twins.

piglets from susceptible sows with added daily dietary supplements of 3 g choline and 5 g methionine.

An atypical splayleg incoordination of the hind limbs of piglets was reported by Miller et al. (1973) following consumption by the sows of grain contaminated with *Fusarium* (F-2) toxin (zearalenone) in late pregnancy. The condition was also reproduced experimentally by the administration of purified F-2 toxin to pregnant sows. In addition to its estrogenic effects on the sow, increased stillbirths, neonatal mortality, small litters, and splayleg were recorded. The splayleg piglets did not show the classic histopathologic lesions as described by Thurley et al. (1967), and there was a higher morbidity and mortality than normally associated with the usual form of the condition.

Splayleg appears at or within a few hours of birth. It is characterized by a weakness of varying severity of the hind limbs and occasionally of the forelimbs also. Some piglets are able to move around with difficulty, while more severely affected piglets are unable to stand. The affected limbs tend to be abducted or splayed sideways, so that the animal commonly sits on its hindquarters (or forequarters) with its hind limbs (or forelimbs) splayed sideways (Fig. 56.7). The limbs are usually held straight out but can be flexed. Ataxia is not a feature of the condition. Affected piglets suffer greater abrasion of the skin; this, along with ulceration and infection, can lead to arthritis. Secondary traumatic damage to muscles and joints may exacerbate the condition and can lead to persistent weakness or lameness. Affected piglets are unable to compete as actively for food as unaffected littermates. If the piglet does not die from these causes or from crushing by the sow, spontaneous and complete recovery occurs within 1 week.

Histologic examination of affected muscle may show myofibrillar hypoplasia (Thurley et al. 1967), interpreted as an immaturity of the muscle (Thurley and Done 1969). Jirmanová (1983) considered the histologic features of affected muscle to resemble experimentally induced glucocorticoid myopathy. The muscle most affected in the hind limb is the semitendinosis; in the lumbar area it is the longissimus dorsi and in the forelimb it is the triceps. Myofibrillar hypoplasia can also be found in some normal piglets, but it is present in all splaylegged piglets.

Control of splaying might be possible through selection of breeding stock, as occurrence can be influenced markedly by breeding for or against the condition (Anon. 1971). Hobbling or tying together the hind limbs below the hocks with adhesive tape probably accelerates recovery and appears to assist affected piglets to stand and move around. If required, the tapes may also be applied to forelimbs. They should not occlude the circulation of the limbs and should be removed as soon as recovery occurs.

Arthrogryposis. Arthrogryposis (arthrogryposis multiplex congenita, amyoplasia congenita, multiple congenital articular rigidities) occurs in many species of animals, including humans. It is characterized by fixation or ankylosis of joints in various degrees of flexion or extension (Fig. 56.8). Usually a number of joints of the limbs and frequently also of the vertebral column are involved. Arthrogryposis of the vertebral joints results in lordosis, kyphosis, or scoliosis. If only the

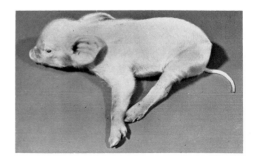

56.7. Splayleg affecting forelimbs and hind limbs.

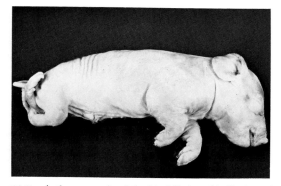

56.8. Arthrogryposis of the hind limbs with flexion of the stifle, hyperextension of the tarsus, and moulding of the limbs.

carpal or tarsal joints are involved, the condition is termed talipes or clubfoot. It is generally accepted that arthrogryposis has a number of causes and can be classified at least into neurogenic and myogenic forms (Adams et al. 1962). The neurogenic forms are more common and are usually associated with spinal cord dysplasias, including localized to widespread loss of ventral (motor) horn neurones, spina bifida, and syringomyelia with fibrofatty replacement of muscles typical of denervation atrophy (Edwards 1971). It is believed that prolonged prenatal immobilization due to any cause will lead to fixation of the joints of the immobilized parts (Whittem 1957).

Numerous causes have been demonstrated in various species, including prenatal viral infection, plant and chemical poisonings, hyperthermia, dietary deficiencies, and heredity.

A number of known or suspected causes of arthrogryposis in pigs have been recorded. Feeding on tobacco stalks between days 4–50 of pregnancy has caused the condition (Menges et al. 1970; Crowe 1978; Keeler et al. 1981). The succulent central pith appears attractive to some sows. The abnormality has been reproduced experimentally by feeding stalks and stalk juice to sows. In outbreaks some sows have shown signs of illness, but no signs were seen in experimental sows. In 15 outbreaks 1148 of 2358 piglets from 246 sows were affected with arthrogryposis of varying severity. Between 40 and 50% of piglets in affected litters were deformed. Affected piglets may have caused dystocia, as parturition was prolonged by several hours and neonatal deaths from asphyxia and hypoglycemia were common. Joints mainly of the fore and hind limbs but also of the spinal column and mandible were fixed in position. Limbs were in extension or flexion, and in some instances the forelimbs were folded over or parallel to the thorax. Vertebral involvement was associated with spinal curvatures. Some long bones of affected limbs showed curvatures or twisting. No other defects were found.

Poison hemlock also has caused the birth of piglets with arthrogryposis; 6 of 55 piglets from 4 sows were born with arthrogryposis of the hind limbs and all died within 4 days. The sows involved in the outbreak had access to hemlock, and some showed severe nervous signs after the 43rd to 61st day of gestation (Edmonds et al. 1972). Dyson and Wrathall (1977) recorded a high incidence of arthrogryposis affecting the limbs and vertebral column in two litters. The sows had access to hemlock but were not observed to be ill. In addition to arthrogryposis, the right kidney and testis were misshapen. Panter et al. (1985a,b) confirmed the teratogenicity of hemlock in feeding trials producing cleft palate when fed at 30–45 days and arthrogryposis when fed at 43–61 days of pregnancy.

Jimsonweed or thorn apple poisoning of sows in the second and third months of pregnancy was suspected as the cause of arthrogryposis (Leipold et al. 1973), which was the only defect found in an exposed litter. From one or two to all piglets in a litter were affected to a variable degree. Joints of fore and hind limbs were involved, and associated muscles were atrophic and pale, showing fibrous replacement of myofibrils. Some sows with access to the plant showed signs of intoxication (incoordination) during pregnancy.

Multiple anomalies including arthrogryposis were found in piglets from sows that had eaten leaves and bark of wild black cherry during pregnancy. Associated defects included aplasia of the tail, anal atresia, and rudimentary external genitalia (Selby et al. 1971b). Feeding trials with jimsonweed, and wild black cherry are needed before they can be confirmed as teratogens.

Other recorded known and possible causes of arthrogryposis in swine include feeding with methallibure (1 mg/kg body weight) between days 24 and 74 of pregnancy (Barker 1970), maternal vitamin A deficiency (Palludan 1961), manganese deficiency (Miller et al. 1940), and heredity. These conditions have been reviewed by Swatland (1974).

Hernias. Inguinal and umbilical hernias are among the most common developmental defects of swine. Priester et al. (1970), from the Veterinary Medical Data Program, found inguinal hernias to be more common than umbilical hernias; but their figures might not reflect the true proportions, as fewer cases of umbilical hernia might require surgical treatment (Hayes 1974). In the other species included in the survey, the incidence of umbilical hernia exceeded that of inguinal hernia. However, Bille and Nielsen (1977), from a postmortem survey of piglets, found inguinal hernias to be twice as common as the umbilical type. Smidt (1972) estimated the incidence of inguinal hernia in Holland to be 0.4–0.5%.

Inguinal hernia rarely affects the female pig. It might not be apparent at birth but can develop some weeks later. Smidt (1972) found the incidence to more than double between birth and 5 weeks of age. It may affect one (usually the left) or both inguinal canals. The major economic consequence of the condition is death due to intestinal or omental eventration after castration, although intestinal strangulation may also occasionally cause death. The condition is of less significance where male pigs are not castrated and are slaughtered at under 6 months of age so that boar odor or taint is not a problem. The testicles have normally descended to the scrotum at birth, and the inguinal canal begins to close some 14–16 days earlier, after the testicles have passed through the external inguinal ring. Inguinal hernia is thought to be caused by an abnormally large inguinal ring or weakness of the tunica vaginalis (Warwick 1926), which allows the abdominal contents to be forced into the inguinal canal by the increased intraabdominal pressures at or after birth. The number of cases that occur can be modified strongly by environmental influences, which increase pressure at or after the time of birth (Wrathall 1988). It is believed that the condition is inherited polygenically. Warwick (1926) studied a herd with an incidence of 1.68% in male pigs. By mating pigs with inguinal hernias to related sows the incidence was increased within two generations to 42%. Control of the condition is by culling affected and related animals.

Umbilical hernia is of less importance economically than inguinal hernia. Its incidence has been estimated at over 1% in females and 0.6% in males (Warwick 1926). Occasionally the hernia becomes so large that surgery or early slaughter is necessary. Umbilical hernia is also thought to be a polygenically inherited condition (Wrathall 1975).

DEFECTS OF THE DIGESTIVE SYSTEM.

Harelip, cleft palate, and anal atresia are the most common defects of the digestive system. Harelip may be unilateral or bilateral and is frequently associated with cleft palate (Fig. 56.9). Cleft palate may involve the soft palate only, but more frequently both the soft and hard palates are affected. Additional malformations of the head, tongue, and other structures may be found. Affected piglets appear sporadically in litters. They have difficulty feeding and usually die within a few days. The cause is unknown but is possibly genetic.

Anal Atresia. Bille and Nielsen (1977) found anal atresia in approximately 0.4% of pigs in Denmark, and in their survey it was the most common single defect. Smidt (1972) found a similar incidence in Dutch Landrace pigs. Mulley and Edwards (1984) found 36 in 14,535 pigs in Australia (0.25%), and Norrish and Rennie (1968) found it in 35 of 5531 pigs (0.6%) in Canada. The rectum ends blindly at a variable distance from the skin of the perineum and no anus has formed.

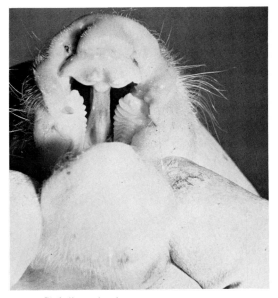

56.9. Cleft lip and palate.

The incidence (Norrish and Rennie 1968) and extent of the deficit is greater in males than in females. The condition is almost invariably fatal within 2–3 weeks in males. A fistula may form between the rectum and the vagina, which accounts for the reduced but still substantial mortality in females. Surgical repair is possible but is rarely justifiable on genetic or economic grounds. The cause is accepted generally as heritable, but the mode of transmission is uncertain. Norrish and Rennie (1968) believed it to be polygenic. Mating of surgically corrected boars and sows increased the ratio of normal to affected piglets from 227:1 in normal parents to 3:1 from parents with atresia. In another experimental study on heritability of the condition, Ohkawa et al. (1985) found both an autosomal recessive and an autosomal dominant mode of transmission. Atresia of the small intestine is rare; Mulley and Edwards (1984) found an incidence of 0.05%. Megacolon (Hirschsprung's disease) is rarely reported.

DEFECTS OF THE SKIN. A number of rare congenital conditions of the skin have been reported, many of which were reviewed by Parish and Done (1962). Hypotrichosis (hairlessness) has been shown to be a heritable condition (Meyer and Drommer 1968). It is also associated with iodine deficiency during pregnancy. Pregnancy is prolonged, often up to 7 days, and affected piglets are usually weak at birth and die within a few hours. The thyroid is usually enlarged, colloid is absent, and the parenchyma appears hypertrophied on histologic examination. The skin is shiny and edematous, particularly over the head, neck, and shoulders. Patent foramen ovale is usually found when the heart is examined

(Smith 1917). Most commercial rations have adequate iodine to prevent deficiency.

Epitheliogenesis imperfecta is a heritable defect of skin growth, possibly with an autosomal recessive mode of inheritance, consisting of round areas 2–10 cm in diameter or larger and occurring usually over the back, loins, or hind legs (Bentinck-Smith 1951). Hydronephrosis is frequently associated with this condition and the mortality is high. Other rare skin conditions include wattles or skin tags on the neck, hemangiomas, and dermatosis vegetans. In the latter condition wartlike lesions develop on the feet and belly at 1–3 weeks of age. It is a heritable condition due to a recessive autosomal gene and associated with a giant cell pneumonitis that is usually fatal (Jericho 1974). Pityriasis rosea is a benign, self-limiting disease of young pigs that appears to be heritable, as some Landrace families appear to be more frequently affected (Corcoran 1964).

DEFECTS OF THE CARDIOVASCULAR SYSTEM AND BLOOD.
Huston et al. (1978) list 19 recorded defects of the heart and great vessels, all being rare except patent foramen ovale, persistent atrioventricular canal, and subaortic or subpulmonary arterial stenosis. Another review of congenital cardiac diseases of swine at necropsy categorized 122 cases (Hsu and Du 1982). Most were recognized between 29 and 56 days of age, a majority were male, and dysplasia of the tricuspid valve, atrial septal and ventricular septal defects, and subaortic stenosis were the most common anomalies. The causes were not established.

A severe bleeding disorder in a strain of inbred male and female Poland China pigs commonly results in death from hemorrhage from minor wounds such as castration or ear notching and after farrowing. It was labelled porcine Von Willebrand's disease (hemophilia) due to a recessive gene transmitted by nonbleeding carrier parents that can be identified by a number of tests. Compared with normal animals, a decreased concentration of factor VIII, decreased platelet retention time, and increase in ear-bleeding times are found (Owen et al. 1974).

Continued excess bleeding from the umbilicus of newborn pigs (navel bleeding) can cause losses of up to 2.1% of all pigs born (Bille et al. 1976). It can be treated by ligating the cord, but this requires constant attention throughout the day and night. The cords of affected pigs remain large and fleshy and fail to shrivel. Some pigs may also bleed excessively from ear notching. Sandholm et al. (1979) found markedly decreased platelet aggregation in bleeders and completely prevented the condition by giving sows 1 g ascorbic acid daily for at least 6 days before farrowing.

Congenital porphyria has been described by Jorgensen (1959) in Denmark as a heritable defect with one or more dominant genes. Yamashita

et al. (1980) in Japan found evidence of a recessive mode of inheritance in offspring of a Duroc boar. Subcutaneous edema and serous accumulations of fluid in the pericardial sac and peritoneal cavity are associated with prenatal infection with HC virus in later pregnancy (Emerson and Delez 1965). A thrombocytopenic purpura has been described in piglets following isoimmunization of the sow by antigenically different platelets from their fetuses. The piglets had normal platelet counts at birth but developed thrombocytopenia and purpura within a few hours of receiving colostrum (Linklater 1975).

DEFECTS OF THE REPRODUCTIVE SYSTEM.
Anomalous development of the reproductive system occurs frequently in swine. Cryptorchidism is the most frequently encountered genital defect of male piglets. Mulley (1982) found an incidence of 8% in a series of 700 male piglets presented for postmortem examination. Unilateral cryptorchidism, usually affecting the left testicle, is more common than the bilateral condition. The undescended testicle may be located between the caudal pole of the kidney and the external ring of the inguinal canal. If the condition is bilateral, the boar will be sterile. The carcasses of uncastrated cryptorchid pigs may be graded down due to boar taint or odor, but this is not a problem if the pigs are slaughtered before six months of age. It is generally accepted that cryptorchidism is usually an inherited defect (Bishop 1972) with a polygenic mode of transmission, and control would depend on detection of carriers and their elimination from the breeding stock. The methods used are discussed by Wrathall (1975). Other less common defects of the male genitalia include aplasias and hypoplasias of the testicles, penis, and epididymis; persistent frenulum; and seminal defects (Huston et al. 1978).

Defects of the female genital system are also common. Einarsson and Gustafsson (1970) found an incidence of 22.1% in gilts at slaughter in Sweden. About one-third were cysts of the mesosalpinx, usually of minor importance, while 4% showed partial duplication of the vagina. Segmental or complete aplasia of the uterine horns was found in 0.8% and intersexuality in 0.3%. Wiggins et al. (1950) examined over 5000 genitalia from sows and gilts at slaughter in the United States. Gross genital abnormalities affected approximately 5% of the subjects. Segmental or complete aplasia of the uterus, cervix, vagina, or vulva was found in 0.68%, duplications of the cervix or uterine horns in 0.06%, and tubal abnormalities in 1.5%. The aplasias, hypoplasias, and duplications appear to have genetic components that can be expressed in varying degrees in different individuals (Wrathall 1975) and may contribute to infertility and perhaps dystocia.

Intersexuality is an important defect. True intersexes or hermaphrodites have both testicular and ovarian tissues, while pseudohermaphrodites have gonads of one sex and other genital organs of the opposite sex. The incidence varies between 0.2 and 0.6% in slaughter pigs (Bäckström and Henricson 1971; Pfeffer and Winter 1977). While at least six phenotypic expressions of swine intersexes have been described (Halina et al. 1984), four varieties of male and one type of female pseudohermaphrodite and a true hermaphrodite, the external genitalia of intersex pigs are usually female in type. In most instances the vulva appears normal with a variable enlargement of the clitoris, but in some the clitoris is greatly enlarged and the vulva is underdeveloped or prepucelike. Some affected individuals may show male behavior, while others may show estrus and even become pregnant (Hulland 1964; O'Reilly 1979). An inguinal hernia may develop and at times contains a testicle.

Most intersexes in swine have a female (XX) karyotype. Bäckström and Henricson (1971) reported that testicles were present in each of the 45 intersex pigs found in an extensive survey. Of the 45 pigs, 13 (29%) were true hermaphrodites and the other 32 were male pseudohermaphrodites; of 42 examined cytologically, all had a normal female karyotype. Litters with intersex piglets had a deficit of males and a higher incidence of other defects compared with normal litters.

Male pseudohermaphrodites have testicles that are commonly retained in the abdominal cavity. They usually have a recognizable uterus, cervix, and vagina, which might end blindly. Some development of the male accessory glands, epididymis, and vas deferens may also be found. True hermaphrodites have both ovarian and testicular tissues, and the development of the female tubular tract is usually typically female. Estrus, ovulation, and pregnancy are possible. Reports of female pseudohermaphrodites in pigs are rare.

Bruere et al. (1968) and Basrur and Kanagawa (1971) have found XX/XY mosaics in lymphocyte cultures from pigs with male pseudohermaphroditic characteristics, which suggests that vascular anastomoses in adjoining placentas may allow sharing of circulations of male and female piglets, producing a freemartin type of intersex in the female piglet. Breeuwsma (1968) found an intersex Dutch Landrace pig with the XXY karyotype, and Toyama (1974) has found four cases of XX/XY mosaicism in hemopoietic cells, one of which had a normal female karyotype in skin and kidney cells, and a fifth case with XX/XXY mosaicism in hemopoietic and other tissues. True hermaphrodism, male pseudohermaphrodism, and segmental aplasia and hypoplasia of the male and female tubular genital tracts have all been reported to be inherited conditions.

Other defects of the female genital system include persistence of the hymen; duplications of the cervix, vagina, and uterine horns; ovarian aplasia and other ovarian defects; and hypoplasia or malformation of the nipples (Done 1980; Clayton et al. 1981). The incidence of these conditions is low, and in most instances the cause is unknown or suspected to be heritable.

RECOGNITION AND CONTROL OF DEVELOPMENTAL DEFECTS. Detection of environmental teratogens can be extremely difficult. In most instances these agents act on embryos in early gestation and their effects are not apparent until the piglets are born many weeks or months later, by which time the teratogen has usually disappeared. In many cases teratogens are recognized by chance observations and by keeping good records of the environmental management of pregnant females. Wilson (1973) listed criteria for the recognition of a new teratogenic agent in humans, and these have been adopted for animals. They are (1) an abrupt increase in the incidence of a particular defect or association of defects (syndrome) and coincidence of this increase with a known environmental change, e.g., use of a new drug or occurrence of an infectious disease; (2) known exposure early in pregnancy to an environmental change that yields characteristically defective offspring; and (3) absence of other factors common to all pregnancies that yield young with the characteristic defect(s).

Control depends upon the recognition of the cause—heritable, infectious, drug, toxin, or physical agent—and its elimination, if this is economically feasible, by breeding policy; disease control; and protection from teratogenic physical agents, drugs, and toxins.

Neoplastic Diseases

NEOPLASMS have not been studied intensively in pigs, and it is generally believed that the incidence is less than in most other species. The current efficiency of swine production depends largely on high growth rates and high fecundity, resulting in a large proportion of the population being slaughtered before reaching the "cancer age" (Ramsay and Migaki 1975). Also, the proportion of young to parent stock is much higher than in all other domestic species. The commonly reported tumors are those affecting young pigs.

The prevalence of neoplasia in swine at slaughter has been studied in a number of countries. Monlux et al. (1956) found 23 and 34 tumors/million swine slaughtered in the United States during 1953 and 1954 respectively, the most common being embryonal nephroma, lymphosarcoma, and melanoma in that order. In the Netherlands, Misdorp (1967) found 40/million in pigs at abattoirs between 1960 and 1965. Anderson and Jarrett (1968) examined tumors in slaughtered pigs in England during 1965 and 1966 and found 38/million, of which 25/million were lymphosarcoma.

The most common tumors appear to be lymphosarcoma, embryonal nephroma, and melanoma. Bostock and Owen (1973) found lymphosarcoma to be the most common tumor of pigs in England, and the incidence in the United States and some European countries to range between 3 and 25/million. Cotchin (1960) also found lymphosarcoma to be the most common porcine tumor in England; in the United States it was embryonal nephroma. Migaki et al. (1971) in a survey of embryonal nephroma found a prevalence approaching 200/million in some areas. Fisher and Olander (1978) over a period of 11 years found 31 neoplasms (0.2%) among 15,782 biopsy and necropsy specimens at Purdue University. Over 25% were lymphosarcomas; 23% were melanomas; 16% were hemangiomas and hemangiosarcomas; about 10% were papillomas; and the rest were embryonal nephromas, an angioblastoma, an ameloblastoma, a lipoma, a chondroma, and a leiomyoma.

EMBRYONAL NEPHROMA.

Embryonal nephromas affect pigs mostly under 1 year of age of both sexes but with a marked excess of females (Hayashi et al. 1986). Affected pigs usually show no clinical signs, but a few may be unthrifty. The origin is in the parenchyma of the kidney, and most have unilateral involvement (Monlux et al. 1956; Hayashi et al. 1986). The lesions are fleshy, solid, and attached firmly to the kidney and vary in size from 1 to 40 cm, weighing up to 34 kg (Migaki et al. 1971). Metastases are uncommon but may affect the lungs and liver. The tumors can be classified histologically into four types. Nephroblastic and epithelial types are the most common and mesenchymal and miscellaneous (mixed elements) are much less common (Hayashi et al. 1986).

LYMPHOSARCOMA.

Lymphosarcomas affect pigs of both sexes, primarily in the young animal before maturity but also in mature animals (Bostock and Owen 1973). Anderson and Jarrett (1968) considered the condition in Britain to be a sporadic disease, occurring only as isolated cases. A possible viral etiology has been considered, but attempts to transmit the condition to young swine or fetuses in utero have been unsuccessful (Bostock and Owen 1973). Head et al. (1974), however, have studied a Large White herd, described

by McTaggart et al. (1971), in which multiple cases of lymphosarcoma occurred, apparently associated with an autosomal recessive gene. This mode of inheritance was confirmed by test matings of carrier animals (McTaggart et al. 1979). Clinical signs include ataxia or paralysis, enlargement of superficial lymph nodes (particularly submandibular and prescapular), anorexia, emaciation, dyspnea, tachycardia, and sudden death. A leukemic phase is common in the terminal stages, but the hematology may be normal at other stages. Pigs with the condition (Imlah et al. 1979) showed an increase in serum gamma globulin over the period 10–24 weeks of life. In the later stages of the disease, IgG heavy- and light-chain components were detected in the serum and urine of all cases.

Anderson and Jarrett (1968) classified lymphosarcomas of animals into three clinicopathologic types: (1) multicentric, in which there is enlargement of superficial lymph nodes and variable infiltration of internal organs; (2) thymic, which is usually also a disseminated form, but the tumor appears to start or grow most rapidly in the area of the thymus, producing an obvious mass at the thoracic inlet; (3) skin, which is also a disseminated lymphosarcoma in which infiltration of the skin and subcutaneous tissues produces nodular thickening and loss of hair. In pigs most cases are the multicentric type and the rest are thymic (especially in young pigs). In the multicentric and thymic types, besides the lymph node or thymic involvement, infiltration of the liver, spleen, and kidney were most common; but tumor infiltration into lung, pleura, peritoneum, pancreas, ovaries, heart, skeletal muscle, vertebrae, and bone marrow also occurred.

Affected lymph nodes are very enlarged and bulge from the cut surface. They contain densely packed homogeneous sheets of cells within the capsule, or sometimes tumor cells infiltrate surrounding tissues and destroy the usual architecture of the nodes. Lesions in the liver may consist of numerous pale nodules scattered throughout its substance or a massive selective infiltration of the portal connective tissue, which gives an accentuated lobular pattern (marbling). The affected spleen is enlarged, grayish red, and friable and contains numerous spherical, pale nodules a few millimeters in diameter, which are Malpighian corpuscles infiltrated by tumor cells (Bostock and Owen 1973). Kidney involvement usually consists of large, bulging, gray, soft nodules, especially in the cortex, which produce irregularities in the capsule.

Migaki (1968) classified lymphosarcomas of pigs into three main types by histologic means: the lymphocytic (most common), lymphoblastic, and histiocytic. A small proportion of lesions were of mixed types. Some reports have shown marked reductions of blood mononuclear cell counts from corticosteroid treatment (Brownlie et al. 1978), but these changes reversed rapidly in the posttreatment period.

MELANOMA. Melanomas occur in young pigs, especially of the Duroc breed (Hjerpe and Theilen 1964), and may be present at birth. They primarily affect the skin and may be malignant. Fisher and Olander (1978) described seven cases, including a 2-week-old black pig that had posterior paralysis from birth. There were widespread metastases. The other six tumors were from cutaneous sites, and recurrence or metastases were not reported in any of these pigs. The Sinclair strain of miniature swine shows a high incidence (54%) of malignant melanomas in newborn piglets and the incidence increases to 85% by 1 year of age (Hook et al. 1982). Cutaneous lesions show nearly 100% incidence of spontaneous regression (Oxenhandler et al. 1982).

Monlux et al. (1956) reported only 3 benign melanomas in 28 tumors of swine, and Case (1964) gave a detailed account of a malignant melanoma that had been noted at birth with widespread dissemination in a 5-week-old black pig. On histologic examination the malignant tumors consisted of plump, spindle- or polygonal-shaped cells arranged in broad sheets or whorls. The cells contained hyperchromatic oval nuclei with mitotic figures in certain areas of the tumor. The amount of pigment varied from cell to cell.

REFERENCES

Genetic and Developmental Diseases

ADAMS, R. D.; DENNY-BROWN, D.; AND Pearson, C. M. 1962. Diseases of Muscle: A Study in Pathology, 2d ed. New York: Harper & Row.

ANON. 1971. Report of the chief veterinary officer. Ministry of Agriculture, Fisheries and Food. Her Majesty's Stationery Office, London.

BÄCKSTRÖM, L., AND HENRICSON, B. 1971. Intersexuality in the pig. Acta Vet Scand 12:257–273.

BARKER, C. A. V. 1970. Anti-gestation and teratogenic effects of Aimax (methallibure) in gilts. Can Vet J 11:39–40.

BASRUR, P. K., AND KANAGAWA, H. 1971. Sex anomalies in pigs. J Reprod Fertil 26:369–371.

BENTINCK-SMITH, J. 1951. A congenital epithelial defect in a herd of Berkshire swine. Cornell Vet 41:47–51.

BERGE, G. N.; FONNUM, F.; AND BRODAL, P. 1987. Neurotoxic effects of prenatal trichlorfon administration in pigs. Acta Vet Scand 28:321–332.

BILLE, N., AND NIELSEN, N. C. 1977. Congenital malformations in pigs in a post-mortem material. Nord Vet Med 29:128–136.

BILLE, N.; NIELSEN, N. C.; SVENDSEN, J.; AND RIISING, H. J. 1976. Piglet mortality in the early neonatal period. Proc 4th Int Congr Pig Vet Soc, Ames, p. Z12.

BISHOP, M. W. H. 1972. Genetically determined abnormalities of the reproductive system. J Reprod Fertil [Suppl] 15:51–78.

BÖLSKE, G.; KRONEVI, T.; AND LINDGREN, N. O. 1978. Congenital tremor in pigs in Sweden. Nord Vet Med 30:534–537.

BREEUWSMA, A. J. 1968. A case of XXY sex chromosome constitution in an intersex pig. J Reprod Fertil 16:119–120.

BRUERE, A. N.; FIELDEN, E. D.; AND HUTCHINGS, H. 1968. XX/XY mosaicism in lymphocyte cultures from a pig with freemartin characteristics. NZ Vet J 16:31–38.

CLAYTON, G. A.; POWELL, J. C.; AND HILEY, P. G. 1981. Inheritance of teat number and teat inversion in pigs. Anim Prod 33:299–304.

CORCORAN, C. J. 1964. Pityriasis rosea in pigs. Vet Rec 76:1407–1409.

CROWE, M. W. 1978. Tobacco—a cause of congenital arthrogryposis. In Effects of Poisonous Plants on Livestock. New York: Academic Press, p. 419.

CUNHA, T. J. 1972. Vitamins for swine feeding and nutrition. Vet Med Small Anim Clin 67:263–268.

DEEBLE, K. 1974. New look at heritable defects. Pig Farming 22:60–63.

DOBBING, J. 1974. The later development of the brain and its vulnerability. In Scientific Foundations of Paediatrics. London: Heinemann, p. 565.

DOBSON, K. J. 1971. Failure of choline and methionine to prevent splayleg in piglets. Aust Vet J 47:587–590.

DONE, J. T. 1968. Congenital nervous diseases of pigs: A review. Lab Anim 2:207–217.

_____. 1976a. Developmental disorders of the nervous system in animals. In Advances in Veterinary Science and Comparative Medicine, vol 20. Ed. C. H. Brandly and E. L. Jungherr. New York: Academic Press, pp. 69–114.

_____. 1976b. The congenital tremor syndrome in pigs. Vet Annu 16:98–102.

_____. 1980. Teat deficiencies in pigs. Vet Annu 20:246–254.

DONE, J. T., AND WIJERATNE, W. V. S. 1972. Genetic disease in pigs. In Pig Production. London: Butterworth, p. 53.

DONE, J. T.; WOOLLEY, J.; UPCOTT, D. H.; AND HEBERT, C. N. 1984. Porcine congenital tremor type AI: Spinal cord morphometry. Zentralbl Veterinaermed [A] 31:81–90.

_____. 1986. Porcine congenital tremor type AII: Spinal cord morphometry. Br Vet J 142:145–150.

DYSON, D. A., AND WRATHALL, A. E. 1977. Congenital deformities in pigs possibly associated with exposure to hemlock (*Conium maculatum*). Vet Rec 100:241–242.

EDMONDS, L. D.; SELBY, L. A.; AND CASE, A. A. 1972. Poisoning and congenital malformations associated with consumption of poison hemlock by sows. J Am Vet Med Assoc 160:1319–1324.

EDWARDS, M. J. 1971. The experimental production of arthrogryposis multiplex congenita in guinea-pigs by maternal hyperthermia during gestation. J Pathol 104:221–229.

EINARSSON, S., AND GUSTAFSSON, B. 1970. Developmental abnormalities of female sexual organs in swine. Acta Vet Scand 11:427–442.

EMERSON, J. L., AND DELEZ, A. L. 1965. Cerebellar hypoplasia, hypomyelinogenesis, and congenital tremors of pigs associated with prenatal hog cholera vaccination of sows. J Am Vet Med Assoc 147:47–54.

FLETCHER, T. F. 1968. Ablation and histopathologic studies on myoclonia congenita in swine. Am J Vet Res 29:2255–2262.

FRASER, F. C. 1959. Causes of congenital malformations in man. J Chronic Dis 10:97–110.

HALE, F. 1933. Pigs born without eyeballs. J Hered 24:105–106.

_____. 1935. The relation of vitamin A to anophthalmos in pigs. Am J Ophthalmol 18:1087–1093.

HALINA, W. G.; BARRALES, D. W.; PARTLOW, G. D.;

AND FISHER, K. R. S. 1984. Intersexes in swine: A problem of descriptive anatomy. Can J Comp Med 48:313–321.

HARDING, J. D. J., AND DONE, J. T. 1956. Microphthalmia in piglets. Vet Rec 68:865–866.

HARDING, J. D. J.; DONE, J. T.; AND DERBYSHIRE, J. H. 1966. Congenital tremors in piglets and their relation to swine fever. Vet Rec 79:388–390.

HARDING, J. D. J.; DONE, J. T.; HARBOURNE, J. F.; RANDALL, C. J.; AND GILBERT, F. R. 1973. Congenital tremor type AIII in pigs: An hereditary sex-linked cerebrospinal hypomyelinogenesis. Vet Rec 92:527–529.

HAYES, H. M. 1974. Congenital umbilical and inguinal hernias in cattle, horses, swine, dogs, and cats: Risk by breed and sex among hospital patients. Am J Vet Res 35:839–842.

HSU, F. S., AND DU, S. J. 1982. Congenital heart diseases in swine. Vet Pathol 19:676–686.

HULLAND, T. J. 1964. Pregnancy in a hermaphrodite sow. Can Vet J 5:39–41.

HUSTON, R.; SAPERSTEIN, G.; SCHONEWEIS, D.; AND LEIPOLD, H. W. 1978. Congenital defects in pigs. Vet Bull 48:645–675.

JERICHO, K. W. F. 1974. Dermatosis vegetans – giant cell pneumonitis in pigs: Further observations and interpretations. Res Vet Sci 16:176–181.

JIRMANOVÁ, I. 1983. The splayleg disease: A form of glucocorticoid myopathy? Vet Res Commun 6:91–101.

JIRMANOVÁ, I., AND LOJDA, L. 1985. Dexamethasone applied to pregnant minisows induces spayleg in minipigs. Zentralbl Veterinaermed [A] 32:445–458.

JORGENSEN, S. K. 1959. Congenital porphyria in pigs. Br Vet J 115:160–175.

KEELER, R. F.; BALLS, L. D.; AND PANTER, K. 1981. Teratogenic effects of Nicotiana glauca and concentration of Arabasine, the suspect teratogen in plant parts. Cornell Vet 71:47–53.

KNOX, B.; ASKAA, J.; BASSE, A.; BITSCH, V.; ESKILDSEN, M.; MANDRUP, M.; OTTOSEN, H. E.; OVERBY, E.; PEDERSEN, K. B.; AND RASMUSSEN, F. 1978. Congenital ataxia and tremor with cerebellar hypoplasia in piglets borne by sows treated with Neguvon vet. (metrifonate, trichlorfon) during pregnancy. Nord Vet Med 30:538–545.

KOHLER, E. M.; CROSS, R. F.; AND FERGUSON, L. C. 1969. Experimental induction of spraddled-legs in newborn pigs. J Am Vet Med Assoc 155:139–142.

LEIPOLD, H. W.; OEHME, F. W.; AND COOK, J. E. 1973. Congenital arthrogryposis associated with ingestion of jimsonweed by pregnant sows. J Am Vet Med Assoc 162:1059–1060.

LINKLATER, K. A. 1975. The experimental reproduction of thrombocytopenic purpura in piglets. Res Vet Sci 18:127–133.

McFEELY, R. A. 1967. Chromosome abnormalities in early embryos of the pig. J Reprod Fertil 13:579–581.

MANEELY, R. B. 1951. Blindness in new-born pigs. Vet Rec 63:398.

MARÉ, C. J., AND KLUGE, J. P. 1974. Pseudorabies virus and myoclonia congenita in pigs. J Am Vet Med Assoc 164:309–310.

MENGES, R. W.; SELBY, L. A.; MARIENFELD, C. J.; AUE, W. A.; AND GREER, D. L. 1970. A tobacco related epidemic of congenital limb deformities in swine. Environ Res 3:285–302.

MEYER, H., AND DROMMER, W. 1968. Inherited hypotrichosis in pigs. Dtsch Tieraerztl Wochenschr 75:13.

MILLER, J. K.; HACKING, A.; HARRISON, J.; AND GROSS, V. J. 1973. Stillbirths, neonatal mortality and small litters in pigs associated with the ingestion of Fusarium toxin by pregnant sows. Vet Rec 93:555–559.

MILLER, R. C.; KEITH, T. B.; McCARTY, M. A.; AND THORP, W. T. S. 1940. Manganese as a possible factor influencing the occurrence of lameness in pigs. Proc Soc Exp Biol Med 45:50–51.

MULLEY, R. C. 1982. Congenital malformations in pigs. M.S. thesis, Univ of Sydney, Australia.

MULLEY, R. C., AND EDWARDS, M. J. 1984. Prevalence of congenital abnormalities in pigs. Aust Vet J 61:116–120.

NORRISH, J. G., AND RENNIE, J. C. 1968. Observations on the inheritance of atresia ani in swine. J Hered 59:186–187.

OHKAWA, H.; SAWAGUCHI, S.; KANEKO, M.; KONDO, I.; AND FURUKAWA, T. 1985. Experimental studies on the heredity of congenital anorectal malformations in the pig. Teratology 32:46B.

O'REILLY, P. J. 1979. Oestrous cycles and fertility in porcine hermaphrodites. Vet Rec 104:196.

OWEN, C. A.; BOWIE, E. J. W.; ZOLLMAN, P. E.; FASS, D. N.; AND GORDON, H. 1974. Carrier of porcine von Willebrand's disease. Am J Vet Res 35:245–248.

PALLUDAN, B. 1961. The teratogenic effect of vitamin A deficiency in pigs. Acta Vet Scand 2:32–59.

PANTER, K. E.; KEELER, R. F.; AND BUCK, W. B. 1985a. Induction of cleft palate in newborn pigs by material ingestion of poison hemlock (Conium maculatum) Am J Vet Res 46:1368–1371.

———. 1985b. Congenital skeletal malformations induced by maternal ingestion of Conium maculatum (poison hemlock) in newborn pigs. Am J Vet Res 46:2064–2066.

PARISH, W. E., AND DONE, J. T. 1962. Seven apparently congenital non-infectious conditions of the skin resembling congenital defects in man. J Comp Pathol 72:286–298.

PATTERSON, D. S. P., AND DONE, J. T. 1977. Neurochemistry as a diagnostic aid in the congenital tremor syndrome of piglets. Br Vet J 33:111–119.

PATTERSON, D. S. P.; SWEASEY, D.; BRUSH, P. J.; AND HARDING, J. D. J. 1973. Neurochemistry of the spinal cord in British Saddleback piglets affected with congenital tremor, type A-IV, a second form of hereditary cerebrospinal myelinogenesis. J Neurochem 21:397–406.

PERRY, J. S., AND ROWLANDS, I. W. 1962. Early pregnancy in the pig. J Reprod Fertil 4:175–188.

PFEFFER, A., AND WINTER, H. 1977. Hermaphrodites in Australian pigs. Occurrence and morphology in an abattoir survey. Aust Vet J 53:153–162.

PRIESTER, W. A.; GLASS, A. G.; AND WAGGONER, N. S. 1970. Congenital defects in domesticated animals: General considerations. Am J Vet Res 31:1871–1879.

SANDHOLM, M.; HONKANEN-BUZALSKI, T.; AND RASI, V. 1979. Prevention of navel bleeding in piglets by preparturient administration of ascorbic acid. Vet Rec 104:337–338.

SAUTTER, J. H.; YOUNG, G. A.; LEUDKE, A. J.; AND KITCHELL, R. L. 1953. The experimental production of malformations and other abnormalities in fetal pigs by means of attenuated hog cholera virus. Proc 90th Annu Meet Am Vet Med Assoc 23:146–150.

SELBY, L. A.; HOPPS, H. C.; AND EDMONDS, L. D. 1971a. Comparative aspects of congenital malformations in man and swine. J Am Vet Med Assoc 159:1485–1490.

SELBY, L. A.; MENGES, R. W.; HOUSER, E. C.; FLATT, R. E.; AND CASE, A. A. 1971b. Outbreak of swine malformations associated with the wild black cherry, Prunus serotina. Arch Environ Health 22:496–501.

SELBY, L. A.; EDMONDS, L. D.; AND HYDE, L. D. 1976. Epidemiological field studies of animal populations. Can J Comp Med 40:135–141.

SMIDT, W. J. 1972. Congenital defects in pigs. 7th Int

Congr on Animal Reproduction and Artificial Insemination, Munich, pp. 1145–1148.

SMITH, G. E. 1917. Fetal athyreosis: A study of the iodine requirement of the pregnant sow. J Biol Chem 29:215–225.

SWATLAND, H. J. 1974. Developmental disorders of skeletal muscle in cattle, pigs and sheep. Vet Bull 44:179–202.

THURLEY, D. C., AND DONE, J. T. 1969. The histology of myofibrillar hypoplasia of newborn pigs. Zentralbl Veterinaermed [A] 16:732–740.

THURLEY, D. C.; GILBERT, F. R.; AND DONE, J. T. 1967. Congenital splayleg of piglets: Myofibrillar hypoplasia. Vet Rec 80:302–304.

TOYAMA, Y. 1974. Sex chromosome mosaicisms in five swine intersexes. Jpn J Zootech Sci 45:551–557.

VOGT, D. W.; AROKAKI, D. T.; AND BROOKS, C. C. 1972. Aneuploidy and reduced litter size in swine. J Anim Sci 35:184.

VOGT, D. W.; GIPSON, T. A.; AKREMI, B.; DOVER, S.; AND ELLERSIECK, M. R. 1984. Associations of sire, breed, birth weight, and sex in pigs with congenital splayleg. Am J Vet Res 45:2408–2409.

WARD, P. S. 1978a. The splayleg syndrome in new-born pigs: A review. I. Vet Bull 48:279–295.

———. 1978b. The splayleg syndrome in new-born pigs: A review. II. Vet Bull 48:381–399.

WARWICK, B. L. 1926. A study of hernia in swine. Res Bull Wis Agric Exp Stn 69.

WATT, J. A., AND BARLOW, R. M. 1956. Microphthalmia in piglets with avitaminosis A as the probable cause. Vet Rec 68:780–783.

WHITTEM, J. H. 1957. Congenital abnormalities in calves: Arthrogryposis and hydranencephaly. J Pathol 73:375–387.

WIGGINS, E. L.; CASIDA, L. E.; AND GRUMMER, R. H. 1950. The incidence of female genital abnormalities in swine. J Anim Sci 9:269–276.

WILSON, J. G. 1973. Environment and Birth Defects. New York: Academic Press.

WRATHALL, A. E. 1971. Prenatal survival in pigs. I. Ovulation rate and its influence on prenatal survival and litter size in pigs. Rev Ser 9. Commonw Agric Bur, Farnham Royal, England.

———. 1975. Reproductive disorders in pigs. Rev Ser 11. Commonw Agric Bur, Farnham Royal, England.

———. 1988. The boar and congenital problems. Proc Pig Vet Soc, p. 116.

YAMASHITA, C.; SHIMAZAKI, H.; MIYAKE, T.; SAITOH, M.; SAKEHI, Y.; AND ISHITANI, R. 1980. Congenital porphyria in swine. Jpn J Vet Sci 42:353–359.

Neoplastic Diseases

ANDERSON, L. J., AND JARRETT, W. F. H. 1968. Lymphosarcoma (leukaemia) in cattle, sheep and pigs in Great Britain. Cancer 22:398–405.

BOSTOCK, D. E., AND OWEN, L. N. 1973. Porcine and ovine lymphosarcoma: A review. J Natl Cancer Inst 50:933–939.

BROWNLIE, S. A.; CAMPBELL, J. G.; HEAD, K. W.; IMLAH, P.; MCTAGGART, H. S.; AND MCVIE, J. G. 1978. Prednisolone treatment of hereditary pig lymphoma. Eur J Cancer 14:983–994.

CASE, M. T. 1964. Malignant melanoma in a pig. J Am Vet Med Assoc 144:254–256.

COTCHIN, E. 1960. Tumours of farm animals: A survey of tumours examined at the Royal Veterinary College, London, during 1950–60. Vet Rec 72:816–822.

FISHER, L. F., AND OLANDER, H. J. 1978. Spontaneous neoplasms of pigs—a study of 31 cases. J Comp Pathol 88:505–517.

HAYASHI, M.; TSUDA, H.; OKUMURA, M.; HIROSE, M.; AND ITO, N. 1986. Histopathological classification of nephroblastomas in slaughtered swine. J Comp Pathol 96:35–46.

HEAD, K. W.; CAMPBELL, J. G.; IMLAH, P.; LAING, A. H.; LINKLATER, K. A.; AND MCTAGGART, H. S. 1974. Hereditary lymphosarcoma in a herd of pigs. Vet Rec 95:523–526.

HJERPE, C. A., AND THEILEN, G. H. 1964. Malignant melanomas in porcine littermates. J Am Vet Med Assoc 144:1129–1131.

HOOK, R. R.; BERKELHAMMER, J.; AND OXENHANDLER, R. W. 1982. Animal model of human disease. Melanoma. Sinclair swine melanoma. Am J Pathol 108:130–133.

IMLAH, P.; BROWNLIE, S. E.; HEAD, K. W.; MCTAGGART, H. S.; AND MCVIE, J. G. 1979. Serum gammaglobulin levels and the detection of IgG heavy chain and light chain in the serum and urine in cases of pig hereditary lymphosarcoma. Eur J Cancer 15:1337–1349.

MCTAGGART, H. S.; HEAD, K. W.; AND LAING, A. H. 1971. Evidence for a genetic factor in the transmission of spontaneous lymphosarcoma (leukaemia) of young pigs. Nature 232:557–558.

MCTAGGART, H. S.; LAING, A. H.; IMLAH, P.; HEAD, K. W.; AND BROWNLIE, S. E. 1979. The genetics of hereditary lymphosarcoma of pigs. Vet Rec 105:36.

MIGAKI, G. 1968. Hematopoietic neoplasms of slaughter animals. Natl Cancer Inst Monogr 32:121–151.

MIGAKI, G.; NELSON, L. W.; AND TODD, G. C. 1971. Prevalence of embryonal nephroma in slaughtered swine. J Am Vet Med Assoc 159:441–442.

MISDORP, W. 1967. Tumours in large domestic animals in the Netherlands. J Comp Pathol 77:211–216.

MONLUX, A. W.; ANDERSON, A. W.; AND DAVIS, C. L. 1956. A survey of tumors occurring in cattle, sheep and swine. Am J Vet Res 17:646–677.

OXENHANDLER, R. W.; BERKELHAMMER, J.; SMITH, G. D.; AND HOOK, R. R. 1982. Growth and regression of cutaneous melanomas in Sinclair miniature swine. Am J Pathol 109:259–269.

RAMSAY, F. K., AND MIGAKI, G. 1975. Tumors, intestinal emphysema, and fat necrosis. In Diseases of Swine, 4th ed. Ed. H. W. Dunne and A. D. Leman. Ames: Iowa State Univ Press, p. 1032.

57 Genetic Influences on Liability to Acquired Disease

B. E. Straw
M. F. Rothschild

GENETIC resistance to disease involves many facets of the body's defense system and their interactions and is extremely complex. The concept of genetic resistance to disease in animals as an alternative to other disease prevention approaches is not a new concept. In the 1930s and 1940s the idea of breeding animals with superior resistance to disease had many strong supporters and considerable research and numerous breeding trials were completed with a number of domestic species. The results of these studies demonstrated the possibility of such an approach to disease control. However, with the rapid expansion in the number of antibiotics and vaccines available, the concept of increasing the innate ability of livestock to resist disease was replaced in favor of a more direct attack on the causative organisms. The advent of modern molecular biology has enhanced our understanding of the intricacies of immunology and has rekindled interest in the possibilities of selection for disease resistance.

HISTORY. Genetic resistance to disease has been extensively used in the production of cultivated crops (Walker 1953). Results of breeding animals for resistance to disease have not been as impressive as in plants. Because of the longer generation interval and the comparatively limited number of progeny, genetic progress through traditional methods of selection has been unavoidably slower and less effective in animals than in plants. However, there is still an impressive list of diseases to which animals have been demonstrated to have genetic resistance (Gavora and Spencer 1983; Warner et al. 1987; Rothschild 1989). Strains of mice with resistance to piliformis disease, mouse typhoid, *Salmonella enteritidis,* louping ill, St. Louis encephalitis, pseudorabies, and yellow fever have been developed (Gowen and Schott 1933; Gowen 1948). Similarly, strains of chickens have been developed that were resistant to pullorum disease, fowl typhoid, avian leukosis complex, blue comb disease, aspergillosis, coccidiosis, Newcastle disease, infectious bronchitis, and Marek's disease (Hutt 1958; Payne 1973; Freeman and Bumstead 1987). Sheep resistant to infectious pulmonary adenomatosis (Dungal et al. 1938), trichostrongylosis

(Stewart et al. 1937), parasite infestation (Albers et al. 1987), and foot rot (Bulgin et al. 1988) have been reported. In cattle, mastitis and ketosis (Ward 1938; Legates and Grinnells 1952; Philipsson et al. 1980; Solbu 1982), babesiosis, anaplasmosis (Stewart 1951), and Johne's disease (Matthews 1947) appear to have a genetic component. In addition to resistance to infectious disease, certain animals appear to have a genetically determined ability to cope with the environment (Hutt 1958).

GENETIC RESISTANCE TO INFECTIOUS DISEASE. Przytulski and Porzeczkowska (1980a) reported that the ability to resist infection from leptospirosis was inherited in a herd of Large White pigs. Boars and sows were classified as susceptible if 25% or more of their progeny were positive to the microscopic agglutination test and were classified as negative if less than 10% of their progeny were positive. Matings of susceptible sows and boars produced 67% positive offspring. Matings of resistant sows and boars produced 2.2% positive progeny. The heritability (h^2) of resistance to leptospirosis was calculated to be 0.20. Pigs that were resistant to leptospirosis had low antibody levels, while susceptible pigs had high levels. Lack of an antibody titer was presumed to be associated with the inability of the organism to invade and multiply in the host. Earlier, a relationship had been found between the phenotypes and alleles (A and B) of blood serum amylase (Am) and the level of leptospiral antibodies (Przytulski and Porzeczkowska 1976, 1980b). The Am[A] allele was associated with high antibody titer and Am[B] allele was associated with low antibody titer.

While attempting to experimentally induce erysipelas, Fortner (1949) observed great variation between pigs in their response to *Erysipelothrix rhusiopathiae* inoculated through scarified skin. Pigs that showed no reaction were considered to have passive immunity. However, among pigs that lacked passive protection there was a wide range of signs after inoculation, ranging from a small localized reaction at the site to generalized lesions and death. By breeding the most resistant pigs and their offspring, Fortner developed a line of pigs that reacted to the skin inoculation with only a small localized skin lesion, while an unselected control population reacted with generalized skin lesions, septicemia, or death.

During a 5-month period in which pigs on one farm were affected by hog cholera, Manresa and Mondonedo (1936) reported lower mortality rates in Berkjala pigs (48%) than in Poland China (59%) or Duroc (80%) pigs. Prior to the outbreak, these three breeds had shown much lower mortality rates, but corresponding differences among breeds had been recorded. Therefore, it could not be determined whether the Berkjala pigs had specific resistance to hog cholera or a superior general ability to resist disease. Other studies (Lambert et al. 1928) specifically designed to increase resistance to hog cholera in pigs were not successful.

In a series of papers Cameron et al. (1940, 1941, 1942, 1943) reported findings on inherited resistance to brucellosis in inbred Berkshire swine. All resistant animals failed to develop agglutination titers after repeated inoculation with *Brucella suis,* while control animals developed positive titers of 1:50 or greater. Lack of agglutinating antibodies in resistant swine was due to the failure of organisms to survive. After oral inoculation, *B. suis* could be recovered from the liver, spleen, and lymph nodes of control animals but not from the resistant ones. Breeding trials with resistant and susceptible pigs suggested that resistance to infection with *B. suis* was inherited as a recessive trait.

Resistance to infection with *Bacillus anthracis* was reported in a strain of miniature swine (Walker et al. 1967). After either aerosol or intraperitoneal inoculation, *B. anthracis* spores could be found in the tissues of the injected animals, but they failed to germinate. Also there was rapid clearance of organisms from lymph nodes and other points of localization.

Duroc, Hampshire, and crossbred pigs showed differential response to experimental infestation with *Strongyloides ransomi* (Johnson et al. 1975). Results of fecal egg counts, daily gains, and feed efficiency indicated that the Duroc breed had a low threshold of response to *S. ransomi* exposure and quickly overcame any deleterious effects of infestation. The Hampshire breed appeared to have a higher threshold of response than the Duroc breed, and once response was elicited, compensation was very slow. The F_1 crossbreds of these two breeds showed an intermediate response to *S. ransomi* exposure, indicating that the response phenomenon is additive in nature.

A genetic basis for resistance to enteric disease has been demonstrated for colibacillosis caused by strains carrying the K88 antigen (Sellwood et al. 1974; Rutter et al. 1975). Whether the K88 enteropathogenic *Escherichia coli* establish in the gut and proliferate depends on the adhesive/nonadhesive phenotype of the pig. In the susceptible animals, the *E. coli* strains producing K88ab, K88ac, and K88ad adhesions attach and multiply to reach large numbers in the small intestine, whereas in the resistant animals, these strains are unable to attach and thus rapidly disappear from the gut. Resistance is recessive and most likely results from two alleles at a single locus, inherited in a simple Mendelian manner. Phenotypes of the progeny from selected matings support the conclusion that the susceptibility is dominant over resistance, but susceptible animals remain in the population because maternal antibodies allow some protection.

In a study of epidemiologic factors in piglet diarrhea, piglets of certain breed combinations appeared to be more frequently affected than others. The greatest risk of diarrhea was found in purebred Landrace piglets, followed by offspring from the cross between Landrace/Yorkshire sows and Hampshire boars. Hampshire boars were highly and significantly associated with the risk of piglet diarrhea in their offspring while piglets sired by Yorkshire boars had the lowest risk (Halgaard 1981).

Numerous investigators have examined genetic aspects of atrophic rhinitis (AR). Comparisons of degree of turbinate atrophy between parents and offspring, and between siblings have been used to estimate the h^2 of AR (Table 57.1).

Table 57.1. Heritability estimates for atrophic rhinitis

Investigators		h^2
Schonmuth et al. 1970		0.45–0.62
Bäckström et al. 1976		0.13, 0.14
Elias and Hamori 1976		0.42
Planchenault et al. 1978		0.09, 0.21
Lundeheim 1979		0.16
Kennedy and Moxley 1980	Incidence:	0.10
	Severity:	0.03

Breed differences in prevalence of AR have been observed. Kennedy and Moxley (1980) found a tendency for a lower incidence of turbinate atrophy in Landrace than in Yorkshire pigs. They also noted a trend for lesions of AR to be less severe in Landrace pigs than in Yorkshires. Crossbreds of the two breeds were less affected. Eikelenboom et al. (1978) also found turbinate atrophy to be more common in Yorkshires than in the Landrace breed. Conversely, Landrace pigs were found to be more affected by AR than Yorkshires (Bjorklund and Henricson 1965; Lundeheim 1979). Mean turbinate space measurements of four breeds of specific-pathogen-free pigs showed little difference (Hampshires 2.53 mm, Yorkshires 2.59 mm, Durocs 2.64 mm, and crossbreds 2.83 mm); a slight tendency for a higher incidence of severe lesions (turbinate measurement > 6 mm) in crossbred than purebred pigs was seen (Socha 1980). In two groups of pigs comparisons of turbinate space measurements graded on a 0–5 scale showed large and significant differences among breeds. In the first group, Hampshire, Yorkshire, Duroc, and Spot pigs had more turbinate atrophy than Landrace, Chester White, and Berkshire pigs (Straw et al. 1983a). In the second group, Hampshire, Yorkshire, and Poland China pigs had more turbinate atrophy than Landrace pigs (Straw et al. 1984a). This was also confirmed by Meeker et al. (1985) who showed that Hampshire pigs had significantly greater turbinate damage than Chester White pigs.

Heritability estimates and breed prevalences have also been reported for pneumonia in pigs; h^2 estimates of 0.13 (Lundeheim 1979) and 0.14 (Smith et al. 1962) have been reported. Researchers generally agree that Yorkshires have a higher prevalence and severity of pneumonia lesions than Landrace pigs (Bjorklund and Henricson 1965; Lundeheim 1979; Straw 1982). When pigs of nine American breeds were compared at two different times, there was a consistent pattern of severely affected and minimally affected breeds. In both studies, pneumonia lesions in Yorkshire and Hampshire pigs were nearly twice as extensive as lesions in Berkshire, Spotted, Poland China, and Chester White pigs (Straw et al. 1983a, 1984a).

Puerperal disease was studied in a herd of breeding swine comprising Landrace and Large White breeds and crossbreds. Mastitis was not found more frequently in any specific breed combination. However, farrowing fever had a significant association (about 33% risk) with the breed composition of the sow (Halgaard 1983). A regression analysis showed a high association between susceptibility and the proportion of Yorkshire genes in the genome. Ringarp (1960) also reported a genetic susceptibility to puerperal disease.

GENETIC RESISTANCE TO NONINFECTIOUS DISEASE.

Gastric ulceration is more prevalent in some breeds than others. The incidence of gastric ulcers was found to be greater in Hampshires and Yorkshires than in Landrace, Spot, Berkshire, or Poland China pigs (40% and 36% vs. 11%, 5%, 2%, and 1% respectively) (Curtin et al. 1963). Conley et al. (1967) calculated a h^2 of 0.04 for gastric ulcers. Berruecos and Robison (1972) reported a much higher h^2 (0.52) and found a significantly higher prevalence of ulcers in Durocs (29%) than in Yorkshires (12%).

Locomotor disorders are another area in which inheritance has been shown to be an important predisposing factor. Smith (1966) reported a low h^2 for leg weakness in pigs, while Teuscher et al. (1972) found a fairly high h^2 of 0.5. Bereskin (1979) reported h^2 estimates of 0.27 ± 0.21 for front legs and 0.15 ± 0.24 for hind legs. When Johansson (1981) calculated the h^2 for various leg defects individually, they ranged from 0.16 to 0.30. Most investigations of breed effects on leg weakness have been done by European research-

ers, so comparisons were limited to Landrace and Large White pigs; most researchers agree that the Landrace breed had a higher incidence of leg weakness and bone abnormalities than the Large White breed. Results with U.S. breeds revealed that Durocs and Hampshires appear to have a higher frequency of front leg disorders. In a five-generation divergent-selection experiment for front leg structure in Durocs, Rothschild and Christian (1988) found that the heritability for improved leg soundness was 0.29 ± 0.06, while the h^2 for increased leg weakness was 0.42 ± 0.04.

Grondalen (1974) found Yorkshires to have a lower incidence and a less severe degree of osteochondrosis and arthrosis than Landrace pigs. Johansson (1981) also found a higher incidence of leg weakness in Landrace pigs: 13.5% for the Landrace as compared with 7.0% for the Yorkshire. Much larger differences were found when osteochondrotic (OCD) lesions were compared; 57% percent of Yorkshires and 59% of Hampshires were not affected with OCD lesions compared with only 10% of unaffected Landrace pigs. In Australia the tendency for Landrace pigs to be less sound than Large Whites was reversed. At the Queensland Testing Station, Large White boars had significantly more front leg faults, but not hind leg faults, than Landrace boars (McPhee and Laws 1976). Goedegebuure et al. (1988), using Durocs from the selection experiment of Rothschild and Christian (1988) found no relationship between leg weakness and OCD.

Pityriasis rosea has been shown to have a genetic component. Lesions are seen especially in the Landrace breed and more frequently in the offspring of certain individuals. In a total of 120 litters in 30 herds that had been sired by a specific Landrace boar, 72 litters were reported to contain pigs affected with pityriasis rosea (Corcoran 1964).

Mortality has been used as a rough estimate of the pigs' ability to cope with their environment. Differences among breeds and offspring of different individuals in the inability to cope with infections, social stress, and climatic effects have been reported.

Preweaning mortality appears to be influenced by genetics. In 134 litters sired by five Landrace boars and five Large White boars in one herd, both breed of sire and individual within the breed significantly affected total piglet production. Preweaning mortality in Large White offspring was 18.9% compared with 12.5% for Landrace offspring (Scofield and Penny 1969). A similar relation between preweaning mortality rates was seen in Indian breeding stations where mortality in Landrace piglets was 13.9% compared with 16.8% in Large White/Landrace piglets. Congenital tremors were seen only in the Landrace piglets and accounted for 4.5% of deaths (Rao and Rao 1981). Wijeratne et al. (1970) and Crossman et al. (1973) studied the sire effect on preweaning piglet mortality by examining litters produced by heterospermic matings. They found a significant difference in mortality between the offspring of different boars. As an explanation of the sire effect, they postulated polygenic inheritance, in which liability to mortality depended on the genetic constitution and environmental factors. Toelle and Robison (1982) used cross-fostering to eliminate maternal effects and found a higher mortality rate for Yorkshire piglets than for Durocs. In one study, preweaning mortality was recorded during a 6-month period in 200 litters sired by six boars. Significantly different mortality rates of 12.2, 16.0, 17.5, 22.0, 25.4, and 28.2% in the offspring of the six boars were noted (Straw et al. 1984b).

Postweaning mortality rates have also shown variation among breeds and sires. In a study of boars at a test station over a 7-year period, mortality rates were in Yorkshires, 3.1%; Hampshires, 1.3%; Durocs, 0.7%; Poland Chinas, 0.7%; Spots, 0%; and Chester Whites, 0% (Seykora 1981). A study of two groups of barrows in successive years at a test station reported mortality rates for Yorkshires, 13.6 and 8.6%; Berkshires, 6.7 and 11.6%; Spots, 3.8 and 11.9%; Chester Whites, 8.4 and 7.0%; Landraces, 7.9 and 3.6%; crossbreds, 2.4 and 7.2%; Poland Chinas, 5.0 and 3.2%; Hampshires, 1.9 and 2.9%; and Durocs, 1.3 and 3.1% (Straw et al. 1983b). A 7-year study of 5617 test station pigs reported overall breed mortality rates: Durocs, 1.9%; Hampshires, 2.1%; Poland Chinas, 3.1%; Spots, 3.1%; crossbreds, 2.8%; Landraces, 3.3%; Chester Whites, 4.5%; Berkshires, 4.8%; and Yorkshires, 6.6% (Straw et al. 1984c). Nursery and finishing-house deaths in the offspring of 13 boars of three breeds were recorded over a 1-year period. According to the breed of sire, pigs had significantly different mortality rates of 1.8, 3.1, and 3.5% (Straw et al. 1984b). Differences in the working life span of different breeds have been reported. The average age at culling was 27.5 months for Swedish Landrace boars compared with 23.6 months for Yorkshire boars. More Swedish Landrace boars were culled for leg weakness and malformed piglets than were Yorkshire boars (Einarsson and Larsson 1977).

CLIMATIC TOLERANCE.

Landrace pigs were found to be less capable of homeostatic adjustment than Duroc pigs (Balbo and Macari 1979). Pigs carrying the gene responsible for porcine stress syndrome (PSS) were less able to tolerate high environmental temperatures. Eight stress-prone pigs and eight controls were exposed at two different times to a 3-hour period of 35°C temperature and 65% relative humidity, resulting in the death of two of the stress-prone pigs. Blood gases and blood pH values of the heat-exposed, stress-prone pigs suggested another mechanism of death rather than metabolic acidosis produced by an acute PSS episode (Aberle et al. 1974). A clinical case in which sows were experiencing mortality rates of 15% was attributed to the inability of PSS carrier sows to tolerate high environmental temperatures (Straw 1984). Comparison of histomorphometric measurements of the adrenal glands of Large White pigs, West African indigenous pigs, and crossbred pigs maintained in hot, humid climatic conditions indicated that Large White pigs were more susceptible to thermal stress than West African indigenous pigs or crossbred pigs (Egbunike 1980). Results also suggest that some Chinese breeds may be more tolerant to certain environmental conditions (Zhilong 1990).

IMMUNOLOGY.

Ollivier and Sellier (1982) have provided a review of the genetics of swine immunology. The major histocompatibility complex (SLA) of pigs was first described by Vaiman et al. (1970). The SLA complex is found on chromosome 7 and is composed of three major regions, coding for class I, class II, and class III genes. The class I genes code for serologically defined antigens and are involved in T-cell recognition of virally infected target cells. The class II genes control the interaction of T cells, B cells, and macrophages in the generation of the humoral immune response and participate in aspects of cellular immunity. The class III genes are involved with the complement cascade, which ends with the lysis of the cell or virus particle to which antibody is formed. The number of genes, their order, and methods of determining SLA type have been reviewed by Warner and Rothschild (1991).

Warner et al. (1987) and Rothschild (1989) reviewed the breed differences in response to vaccination with various antigens. Radzikowski et al. (1974) examined variation of the immune response to sheep erythrocytes in pigs of seven breeds and two crossbreeds by measuring plaque-forming cells of the spleen and the amounts of hemagglutinins and hemolysins in the serum. Among the several breeds and hybrids there were significant differences in the immune response. Buschmann et al. (1974) immunized pigs of eight breeds with dinitrophenol–bovine serum albumin. No antibody was detected in 49% of the pigs, while 38% had low titers and 13% had high titers. Breed-specific differences in the frequencies of reactors and nonreactors appeared. This frequency distribution could in some instances be correlated with the phenotype distribution of the lymphocyte antigenic system of the pigs as revealed by cytotoxicity tests. Peak levels of antibodies produced in response to vaccination with human and bovine albumin ranged from 0.25 to 2.48 mg/ml serum, indicating substantial differences in individual response. Variation in response was much less within litters than between litters, suggesting that ability to produce antibody is both under genetic control and influenced by the maternal environment. In a separate series of experiments, the h^2 of secondary and peak immune response to bovine serum albumin was estimated to be 0.51 and 0.42, respectively (Huang 1977). No difference was detected between Duroc and Yorkshire pigs in the response to vaccination with bovine albumin (Straw et al. 1984c).

Immune responses to vaccines containing *E. coli* antigens were shown to be under moderate control, with h^2 estimates ranging from 0.29 to 0.45 (Edfors-Lilja et al. 1984, 1985). Rothschild et al. (1984a) reported breed differences in antibody titers produced in response to vaccination with a commercial *Bordetella bronchiseptica* bacterin. Using an agglutination test, the breeds were ranked from highest to lowest titer as follows: Chester Whites, Yorkshires, Landraces, Hampshires, and Durocs. Significant differences among sire progeny were also detected. Small but significant breed differences were found in immune response to vaccination with a modified live-virus pseudorabies vaccine with Yorkshire and Chester White pigs having the highest response and Duroc and Landrace pigs the lowest (Rothschild et al. 1984b). Meeker et al. (1987a,b) used commercial vaccines for *B. bronchiseptica* and a modified pseudorabies virus in a cross-breeding and cross-fostering experiment designed to estimate heritability of immune response, the extent of maternal influence, and the amount of heterosis for immune response. Maternal influence was high early in life while genetic control of immune response was moderate later in life. No heterosis appeared to exist.

Genetic control of cell-mediated responses in vitro has been demonstrated by a number of researchers (Jensen and Christensen 1980; Mallard et al. 1989a; Edfors-Lilja et al. 1990). Response to mitogen stimulation by phytohemagglutinin, pokeweed mitogen, and concanavalin A (Con A) has been reported. Genetic variation in time course and magnitude of interleukin 2 induced by Con A was also seen in progeny of several Swedish Yorkshire boars (Edfors-Lilja et al. 1991). Efforts to create an immunocompetence index in pigs have been only moderately successful (Buschmann et al. 1985).

SLA-complex control of immune response has been reported for hen egg-white lysozyme, synthetic antigens, *B. bronchiseptica* bacterin, and sheep red blood cells (Vaiman et al. 1978b; Rothschild et al. 1984a; Lunney et al. 1986; Mallard et al. 1989a). The SLA complex also affects level of complement (Vaiman et al. 1978a; Mallard et al. 1989c).

GENETIC MARKERS.

One of the major problems in development of disease-resistant animals is finding effective methods for measuring such resistance in the laboratory. Methods of direct conventional selection for disease resistance have been described by Gavora and Spencer (1983),

Warner et al. (1987), and Rothschild (1989). The program of mass inoculation and hunting for survivors that has been effective with plants is not as practical with animals. The quest for easily measured indicators of disease resistance or performance (genetic markers) is an old one. Indicators of resistance are not necessarily the factors involved in repelling the pathogen. They may be a gene or genes that are easily detectable and are linked to the resistance factor(s) on the chromosome(s). Specific genetic markers for disease resistance have been reported in some species. Chickens lacking the blood antigen R_1 are susceptible to avian leukosis (Crittenden et al. 1970). Sheep with AB blood types were more resistant to inoculation with *Leptospira pomona* than sheep with either type A or type B blood (Hodges et al. 1976). Coat color, especially white, has been associated with susceptibility to certain diseases; two-thirds of all pleiotropic conditions associated with the lack of pigment show homozygous lethality or sublethality, but only one-third of other coat color pleiotropisms do so (Searle 1968).

In swine, genetic markers have been found for resistance to some diseases and have been associated with certain production traits. Genotypes and phenotypes in the H blood-group system were related to reproductive performance in pigs as a result of both incompatibility for the H_a factor and differences in fitness among genotypes for H-system alleles (Rasmusen and Hagen 1973). Serum cholesterol was correlated positively with average daily gain and backfat and negatively with loin-eye area (Heidenreich et al. 1964).

Glutathione peroxidase (GSH-Px) activity in swine blood may be an indicator of general resistance. Supplementation with selenium or vitamin E has been shown to enhance the immune response in swine inoculated with an *E. coli* bacterin (Ellis and Vorhies 1976) and sheep red blood cells (Peplowski et al. 1980). Vitamin E and selenium supplementation was also shown to enhance the hemagglutinin response of peripheral lymphocytes (Larsen and Tollersrud 1981). While supplementation can increase the GSH-Px level, the basal level appears to be under genetic control. In animals fed a diet adequate in selenium and vitamin E, there was a wide range of individual differences in GSH-Px levels, indicating that such differences in selenium requirement exist in pigs (Jorgensen and Wegger 1979). This difference may result from genetic variation among pigs in their ability to either absorb selenium, incorporate it into GSH-Px, or synthesize the apoenzyme (Jorgensen and Wegger 1979). Clearly, breed and strain differences have been shown to exist in the requirement for selenium. Duroc pigs were more susceptible to selenium toxicity than crossbred pigs (Goehring et al. 1984). Porcine red cell GSH-Px has been shown to be under genetic control (Jorgenson et al. 1977), and matings between identified relatively hyposelenic gilts and boars and relatively hyperselenic gilts and boars (as determined by blood GSH-Px levels) produced similarly affected offspring (Stowe and Miller 1985).

Evidence of direct control of disease resistance by genes of the SLA complex is limited. Early pig mortality was found to be associated with one SLA haplotype (Renard et al. 1982, 1985). The SLA complex has been shown to be associated with cutaneous malignant melanoma in Sinclair miniature swine (Tissot et al. 1989). Researchers suggest that one SLA haplotype is associated with the ability of the tumor locus to be fully penetrant and that tumor expression from birth to weaning involves different mechanisms but is also SLA-haplotype-dependent. Using miniature pigs, Lunney and Murrel (1988) found some association between SLA haplotype and infection to *Trichinella spiralis.*

The complexity of disease and the problems of unravelling the effects of different genotypes on disease in a natural setting have encouraged other approaches. Given the expense of disease-challenge approaches, in vitro tests have been suggested as indicators of disease resistance. In addition to results that have been discussed concerning the SLA-complex effects on immune response, evidence exists that the SLA complex is associated with phagocytic and bactericidal actions of peripheral blood monocytes against *Salmonella typhimurium* and *Staphylococcus aureus* in National Institutes of Health (NIH) miniature pigs (Lacey et al. 1989). Better-responding SLA genotypes to the bactericidal challenges were not the same as those that were good-responding haplotypes to challenges with sheep red blood cells, hen egg-white lysozyme, or synthetic antigens (Mallard et al. 1989a,b,c). These results suggest that the mechanisms of resistance are under different genetic control.

The SLA complex is known to control or influence a number of production and reproduction traits in swine. These traits include litter size, embryo survival, backfat, and growth rate (as reviewed in Warner and Rothschild 1991). Further research to determine the exact alleles of the SLA complex that are markers or have direct effects on both disease resistance and production traits is still needed.

PRACTICAL APPLICATION. Real progress in genetic resistance will come when it is possible to insert the desired gene(s) into the genome of a pig. Before this is possible, the gene(s) responsible for resistance must be identified, then recombinant DNA techniques could be used to isolate, clone, and insert the gene(s) into the host genome. Breeding for disease resistance should be done in nucleus breeding herds because of the high degree of technical expertise required. Selection for resistance will be a continuing process, since strains of animals selected for their disease resistance are not likely to remain so without continued selection.

Genetically resistant animals would have an advantage over conventional animals in geographic locations affected by enzootic disease in which the causative organism is not likely to be eliminated. Animals of known resistance or susceptibility to a certain disease would be superior research subjects for the testing of new drugs or biologics.

In the future, herd health monitoring may include the use of new technology developed to assess the genetic composition of individual herds in regard to innate disease susceptibility and nutrient requirements, and the recommendation for appropriate genetic or nutritional changes in the breeding program.

REFERENCES

ABERLE, E. D.; MERKEL, R. A.; FORREST, J. C.; AND ALLISTON, C. W. 1974. Physiological responses in susceptible and stress-resistant pigs to heat stress. J Anim Sci 38:954–959.

ALBERS, G. A.; GRAY, G. D.; PIPER, L. R.; BARKER, J. S. F.; LE JAMBRE, L. F.; AND BARGER, I. A. 1987. The genetics of resistance and resilience to *Haemonchus contortus* in young Merino sheep. Int J Parasitol 17:1355–1363.

BÄCKSTRÖM, L.; BREMER, H.; DYRENDAHL, I.; AND OLSSON, H. 1976. Nyssjuka hos svin. Sven Vet Tidn 28:449–555.

BALBO, J. C., AND MACARI, M. 1979. Effect of prolonged exposure of swine to heat on thermal insulation and on plasma proteins, sodium and potassium. Comparison of Duroc and Landrace breeds. Cientifica (Brazil) 6:65–69.

BERESKIN, B. 1979. Genetic aspects of feet and legs soundness in swine. J Anim Sci 48:1322–1328.

BERRUECOS, J. M., AND ROBISON, O. W. 1972. Inheritance of gastric ulcers in swine. J Anim Sci 35:20–23.

BJORKLUND, N. E., AND HENRICSON, B. 1965. Studier over pneumoni och kronisk atrofisk rinit svin. Nord Vet Med 17:137–146.

BULGIN, M. S.; LINCOLN, S. D.; PARKER, C. F.; SOWTH, P. J.; DAHMEN, J. J.; AND LANE, V. M. 1988. Genetic-associated resistance to foot rot in selected Targhee sheep. J Am Vet Med Assoc 192:512–515.

BUSCHMANN, H.; RADZIKOWSKI, A.; KRAUSSLICH, H.; SCHMID, D. O.; AND CWIK, S. 1974. Studies on the immune response to DNP hapten in various pig breeds. Zentralbl Veterinaermed 22:155–161.

BUSCHMANN, H.; KRAUSSLICH, H.; HERRMANN, H.; MEYER, J.; AND KLEINSCHMIDT, A. 1985. Quantitative immunological parameters in pigs – experience with the evaluation of an immunocompetence profile. Z Tierz Zuchtsbiol 102:189–199.

CAMERON, H. S.; HUGHES, E. H.; AND GREGORY, P. W. 1940. Studies on genetic resistance in swine to *Brucella* infection. Preliminary report. Cornell Vet 30:218–222.

CAMERON, H. S.; GREGORY, P. W.; AND HUGHES, E. H. 1941. Studies on genetic resistance in swine to *Brucella* infection. II. A bacteriological examination of resistant stock. Cornell Vet 31:21–24.

CAMERON, H. S.; HUGHES, E. H.; AND GREGORY, P. W. 1942. Genetic resistance to brucellosis in swine. J Anim Sci 1:106–110.

CAMERON, H. S.; GREGORY, P. W.; AND HUGHES, E. H. 1943. Inherited resistance to brucellosis in inbred Berkshire swine. Am J Vet Res 2:387–389.

CONLEY, G. O.; DAL KRATZER, D.; AND BICKNELL, E. J.

1967. Genetic analysis of gastric ulceration in swine. J Anim Sci 26:884.

CORCORAN, C. J. 1964. Pityriasis rosea in pigs. Vet Rec 76:1407–1409.

CRITTENDEN, L. B.; BRILES, W. E.; AND STONE, H. A. 1970. Susceptibility to an avian leukosis-sarcoma virus: Close association with an erythrocyte isoantigen. Science 169:1324–1325.

CROSSMAN, P. J.; WIJERATNE, W. V. S.; IMLAH, P.; BUCKNER, D. R. P.; AND GOULD, C. M. 1973. Experimental evidence of sire effect on piglet mortality. Br Vet J 129:58–62.

CURTIN, T. M.; GOETSCH, G. D.; AND HOLLANDBECK, R. 1963. Clinical and pathologic characterization of esophagogastric ulcers in swine. J Am Vet Med Assoc 143:854–859.

DUNGAL, N.; GISLASON, G.; AND TAYLOR, E. L. 1938. Epizootic adenomatosis in the lungs of sheep – comparisons with jaagsiekel, verminous pneumonia and progressive pneumonia. J Comp Pathol Ther 51:46–63.

EDFORS-LILJA, I.; GAHNE, B.; JOHNSON, C.; AND MOREN, B. 1984. Genetic influence on antibody response to two *Escherichia coli* antigens in pigs. I. Standardization of immunization procedure. Z Tierz Zuchtsbiol 101:367–379.

EDFORS-LILJA, I.; GAHNE, B.; AND PETERSSON, H. 1985. Genetic influence on antibody response to two *Escherichia coli* antigens in pigs. II. Difference in response between paternal half sibs. Z Tierz Zuchtsbiol 102:308–317.

EDFORS-LILJA, I.; WATTRANG, E.; MAGNUSSON, U.; AND FOSSUM, C. 1990. Differences between paternal half sib pigs in various immune response traits. Proc 4th World Congr Genet Appl Livest Prod 16:411–414.

EDFORS-LILJA, I.; BERGSTROM, J.; GUSTAFSSON, U.; MAGNUSSON, A.; AND FOSSUM, C. 1991. Genetic variation in Con A induced proliferation of interleukin 2 by porcine peripheral blood mononuclear cells. Vet Immunol Immunopathol 27:351–363.

EGBUNIKE, E. G. N. 1980. Genetic and sex influences on the histomorphometric characteristics of porcine adrenals under hot humid climatic condition. Acta Anat 107:324–329.

EIKELENBOOM, G.; DIK, K. J.; AND JONG, M. F. 1978. Use of radiography in the diagnosis of atrophic rhinitis. Tijdschr Diergeneeskd 103:1002–1008.

EINARSSON, S., AND LARSSON, K. l977. Length of time in service and reasons for culling boars in a production herd. Sven Vet Tidn 29:595–597.

ELIAS, B., AND HAMORI, D. 1976. Data on the aetiology of swine atrophic rhinitis. V. The role of genetic factors. Acta Vet Acad Sci Hung 26:13–19.

ELLIS, R. P., AND VORHIES, M. W. 1976. Effect of supplementary dietary vitamin E on the serologic response of swine to an *Escherichia coli* bacterin. J Am Vet Med Assoc 168:231–232.

FORTNER, J. 1949. Uber Konstitutionell und erblich bedingte Resistenz gegen den Schweinerotlauf. Berl Muench Tieraerztl Wochenschr 37:37–39.

FREEMAN, B. M., AND BUMSTEAD, N. 1987. Breeding for disease resistance – the prospective role of genetic manipulation. Avian Pathol 16:353–365.

GAVORA, J. S., AND SPENCER, J. L. 1983. Breeding for immune responsiveness and disease resistance. Anim Blood Groups Biochem Genet 14:159–180.

GOEDEGEBUURE, S. A.; ROTHSCHILD, M. F.; CHRISTIAN, L. L.; AND ROSS, R. 1988. Severity of osteochondrosis in genetic lines of Duroc swine divergently selected for front leg weakness. Livest Prod Sci 19:487–498.

GOEHRING, T. B.; PALMER, I. S.; OLSON, O. E.; LIBAL, G. W.; AND WAHLSTROM, R. C. 1984. Toxic effects of selenium on growing swine fed corn-soybean meal diets. J Anim Sci 59:733–737.

GOWEN, J. W. 1948. Inheritance of immunity in animals. Annu Rev Microbiol 2:215–254.

GOWEN, J. W., AND SCHOTT, R. G. 1933. Genetic constitution in mice as differentiated by 2 diseases, pseudorabies and mouse typhoid. Am J Hyg 18:674–687.

GRONDALEN, T. 1974. Osteochondrosis and arthrosis in pigs. II. Incidence in breeding animals. Acta Vet Scand 15:26–42.

HALGAARD, C. 1981. Epidemiologic factors in piglet diarrhea. Nord Vet Med 33:403–412.

———. 1983. Epidemiologic factors in puerperal diseases of sows. Nord Vet Med 35:161–174.

HEIDENREICH, C. J.; GARWOOD, V. A.; AND HARRINGTON, R. B. 1964. Swine growth and composition as associated with total serum cholesterol. J Anim Sci 23:496–498.

HODGES, R. T.; MILLAR, K. R.; AND REVFEIN, K. J. A. 1976. The effects of *Leptospira* serotype *pomona* in sheep of different haemoglobin types. NZ Vet J 24:163–166.

HUANG, J. 1977. Quantitative inheritance of immunological response in swine. Ph.D. diss., Univ of Hawaii.

HUTT, F. B. 1958. Resistant birds. In Genetic Resistance to Disease in Domestic Animals. Ithaca: Comstock, pp. 100–123.

JENSEN, P. T., AND CHRISTENSEN, K. 1980. Genetic studies on the in vitro PRA transformation of porcine blood lymphocytes. Vet Immunol Immunopathol 2:133–143.

JOHANSSON, K. 1981. Personal communication.

JOHNSON, Jr., J. C.; STEWART, T. B.; AND HALE, O. M. 1975. Differential responses of Duroc, Hampshire and crossbred pigs to a superimposed experimental infection with the intestinal threadworm, *Strongyloides ransomi*. J Parasitol 61:517–524.

JORGENSEN, P. F., AND WEGGER, I. 1979. Glutathione peroxidase and health in swine. Acta Vet Scand 20:610–612.

JORGENSEN, P. F.; HYLDGAARD-JENSEN, J.; AND MOUSTGAARD, J. 1977. Glutathione peroxidase activity in porcine blood. Acta Vet Scand 18:323–334.

KENNEDY, B. W., AND MOXLEY, J. E. 1980. Genetic factors influencing atrophic rhinitis in the pig. Anim Prod 30:277–283.

LACEY, C.; WILKIE, B. N.; KENNEDY, B. W.; AND MALLARD, B. A. 1989. Genetic and other effects on bacterial phagocytosis and killing by cultured peripheral blood monocytes of SLA-defined miniature pigs. Anim Genet 20:371–382.

LAMBERT, W. V.; MURRAY, C.; AND SHEARER, P. S. 1928. Selection for natural resistance to cholera in swine. Proc Am Soc Anim Prod, pp. 33–39.

LARSEN, H. J., AND TOLLERSRUD, S. 1981. Effect of dietary vitamin E and selenium on the phytohaemagglutin response of pig lymphocytes. Res Vet Sci 31:301–305.

LEGATES, J. E., AND GRINNELLS, C. D. 1952. Genetic relationships in resistance to mastitis in dairy cattle. J Dairy Sci 35:829–833.

LUNDEHEIM, N. 1979. Genetic analysis of respiratory diseases in pigs. Acta Agric Scand 29:209–215.

LUNNEY, J. K., AND MURRELL, K. D. 1988. Immunogenetic analysis of *Trichinella spiralis* infections in swine. Vet Parasitol 29:179–193.

LUNNEY, J. K.; PESCOVITZ, M. D.; AND SACHS, D. H. 1986. The swine major histocompatibility complex: Its structure and function. In Swine in Biomedical Research, vol. 3. New York: Plenum Press, pp. 1821–1836.

McPHEE, C. P., AND LAWS, L. 1976. An analysis of leg

abnormalities of boars in the Queensland Performance Testing Station. Aust Vet J 52:123–125.

MALLARD, B. A.; WILKIE, B. N.; AND KENNEDY, B. 1989a. Genetic and other effects on antibody and cell-mediated immune response in swine leucocyte antigen (SLA)-defined miniature pigs. Anim Genet 20:167–178.

———. 1989b. The influence of the swine major histocompatibility genes (SLA) on variation in serum immunoglobulin (Ig) concentration. Vet Immunol Immunopathol 21:139–151.

———. 1989c. Influence of major histocompatibility genes on serum hemolytic complement activity in miniature swine. Am J Vet Res 50:359–363.

MANRESA, M., AND MONDONEDO, M. 1936. Resistance of the Berkjala breed of swine to hog cholera. Philipp Agric 25:214.

MATTHEWS, H. T. 1947. On Johne's disease. Vet Rec 59:397–399.

MEEKER, D. L.; LI, J.; ROTHSCHILD, M. F.; CHRISTIAN, L. L.; AND WARNER, C. M. 1985. Response to selection for immune response following vaccination with atrophic rhinitis vaccine. ISU Swine Res Rep. AS-570-H. Ames: Iowa State Univ.

MEEKER, D. L.; ROTHSCHILD, M. F.; CHRISTIAN, L. L.; WARNER, C. M.; AND HILL, H. T. 1987a. Genetic control of immune response to pseudorabies and atrophic rhinitis vaccines. I. Heterosis, general combining ability and relationship to growth and backfat. J Anim Sci 64:407–413.

———. 1987b. Genetic control of immune response to pseudorabies and atrophic rhinitis vaccines. II. Comparison of additive direct and maternal genetic effects. J Anim Sci 64:414–419.

OLLIVIER, L., AND SELLIER, P. 1982. Pig genetics: A review. Ann Genet Sel Anim 14:481–544.

PAYNE, L. N. 1973. Genetics and control of avian diseases. Avian Pathol 2:237–250.

PEPLOWSKI, M. A.; MAHAN, D. C.; MURRAY, F. A.; MOXON, A. L.; CANTOR, A. H.; AND EKSTROM, K. E. 1980. Effect of dietary and injectable vitamin E and selenium in weaning swine antigenically challenged with sheep red blood cells. J Anim Sci 51:244–351.

PHILIPSSON, J.; THAFVELIN, G.; HEDEBROVELANDER, I. 1980. Genetic studies on disease recordings in first lactation cows of Swedish dairy breeds. Acta Agric Scand 30:327–335.

PLANCHENAULT, D.; SELLIER, P.; AND OLLIVIER, L. 1978. Le développement des cornets nasaux chez le porc, son appréciation, aspects génétiques. Ann Biol Anim Biochem Biophys 18:211–218.

PRZYTULSKI, T., AND PORZECZKOWSKA. D. 1976. Polymorphism of blood serum amylase and leptospirosis of pigs of Large White Polish breed. Theor Appl Genet 48:237.

———. 1980a. Studies on genetic resistance to leptospirosis in pigs. Br Vet J 136:25–32.

———. 1980b. Serum protein and enzyme polymorphism and leptospirosis of pigs of Polish Large White breed. Ann Genet Sel Anim 11:121–125.

RADZIKOWSKI, A.; MEYER, J.; BUSCHMANN, H.; AVERDUNK, G.; BLENDL, H. M.; AND OSTERKORN, K. 1974. Zur Variation der immunantwort bei mehreren Schweinerassen. I. Mitteilung: Variation der immunantwort gegenuber Schaferythrozylen. Z Tierz Zuchtsbiol 91:59–74.

RAO, A. V. N., AND RAO, C. R. 1981. Pre-weaning piglet mortality in pig breeding stations in Andhra Pradesh. Livest Advis (Bangalore, India) 6:53–55.

RASMUSEN, B. A., AND HAGEN, K. L. 1973. The H blood group system and reproduction in pigs. J Anim Sci 37:568–573.

RENARD, C.; VAIMAN, M.; CAPY, P.; AND SELLIER, P.

1982. SLA markers and characters of production in the pig. Proc 2d World Congr Genet Appl Livest Prod 8:570–583.

RENARD, C.; BOLET, G.; DANDO, P.; AND VAIMAN, M. 1985. Relations d'un marqueur génétique, le complexe majeur d'histocompatibilité, avec la prolificité des truies et la mortalité des porcelets. J Rech Porcine France 17:105–112.

RINGARP, N. 1960. Clinical and experimental investigation into post-parturient syndrome with agalactia in sows. Acta Agric Scand [Suppl] 7.

ROTHSCHILD, M. F. 1989. Selective breeding for immune responsiveness and disease resistance in livestock. AgBiotech News Inf 3(1):355–360.

ROTHSCHILD, M. F., AND CHRISTIAN, L. L. 1988. Genetic control of front leg weakness in Duroc swine. I. Direct response to five generations of divergent selection. Livest Prod Sci 19:459–471.

ROTHSCHILD, M. F.; CHEN, H. L.; WARNER, C. M.; CHRISTIAN, L. L.; LIE, W. R.; VENIER, L.; COOPER, M.; AND BRIGGS, C. 1984a. Breed and SLA haplotype differences in agglutination titers following vaccination with B. bronchiseptica. J Anim Sci 59:643–649.

ROTHSCHILD, M. F.; HILL, H. T.; CHRISTIAN, L. L.; AND WARNER, C. M. 1984b. Genetic differences in serum neutralization titers of pigs after vaccination with pseudorabies modified live-virus vaccine. Am J Vet Res 45:1216–1218.

RUTTER, J. M.; BURROWS, M. R.; SELLWOOD, R.; AND GIBBONS, R. A. 1975. A genetic basis for resistance to enteric disease caused by E. coli. Nature 257:135–136.

SCHONMUTH, G.; SEIFERT, H.; AND NAGEL, E. 1970. Experimentelle Untersuchungen zur Vererbung der Rhinitis atrophicans suum ("Schnuffelkrankheit") mit Hilfe des Rontgentestes. Arch Tierz 13:345–360.

SCOFIELD, A. M., AND PENNY, R. H. C. 1969. Sire effect on piglet production. Br Vet J 125:36–45.

SEARLE, A. G. 1968. Comparative pathology of coat color mutants. In Comparative Genetics of Coat Color in Mammals. London: Logos Press, pp. 230–239.

SELLWOOD, R.; GIBBONS, R. A.; JONES, G. W.; AND RUTTER, J. M. 1974. A possible basis for breeding pigs relatively resistant to neonatal diarrhea. Vet Rec 95:574–575.

SEYKORA, A. J. 1981. Performance of boars in the North Carolina swine evaluation station 1973–1979. M.S. thesis, NC State Univ.

SMITH, C. 1966. A note on the heritability of leg weakness scores in pigs. Anim Prod 32:345–348.

SMITH, C.; KING, J. W. B.; AND GILBERT, N. 1962. Genetic parameters of British Large White bacon pigs. Anim Prod 4:128–145.

SOCHA, T. E. 1980. Influence of breed and season on pneumonia and atrophic rhinitis lesions. Proc George A. Young Conf, Lincoln, Nebr., pp. 77–93.

SOLBU, H. 1982. Heritability estimates and progeny testing for mastitis, ketosis and all diseases. Z Tierz Zuchtsbiol 101:210–219.

STEWART, J. L. 1951. The West African shorthorn cattle. Their value to Africa as trypanosomiasis-resistant animals. Vet Rec 63:454–457.

STEWART, M. A.; MILLER, R. F.; AND DOUGLAS, J. R. 1937. Resistance of sheep of different breeds to infestation by Ostertagia circumcinta. J Agric Res 55:923–930.

STOWE, H. D., AND MILLER, E. R. 1985. Genetic predisposition of pigs to hypo- and hyper-selenemia. J Anim Sci 60:200–211.

STRAW, B. 1982. Studies on pneumonia, atrophic rhinitis, and their interactions in finishing pigs. Proc 7th Int Congr Pig Vet Soc, Mexico City, p. 115.

———. 1984. A previously undescribed clinical expression of porcine stress syndrome in adult swine. Proc Am Assoc Swine Pract Annu Meet, Kansas City, Mo., p. 188.

STRAW, B. E.; BURGI, E. J.; HILLEY, H. D.; AND LEMAN, A. D. 1983a. Pneumonia and atrophic rhinitis in pigs from a test station. J Am Vet Med Assoc 182:607–611.

STRAW, B. E.; NEUBAUER, G. D.; AND LEMAN, A. D. 1983b. Factors affecting mortality in finishing pigs. J Am Vet Med Assoc 189:452–455.

STRAW, B. E.; LEMAN, A. D.; AND ROBINSON, R. A. 1984a. Pneumonia and atrophic rhinitis in pigs from a test station – a follow-up study. J Am Vet Med Assoc 185:1544–1546.

STRAW, B. E.; LEMAN, A. D.; WILSON, M. R.; AND DICK, J. E. 1984b. Sire and breed effects on mortality in the offspring of swine. Prev Vet Med 2:707–713.

STRAW, B. E.; ROBISON, O. W.; CARTER, P.; TOELLE, V. D.; AND KOTT, B. 1984c. Mortality rates in different breeds and a comparison of antibody production by Yorkshire and Duroc pigs. Proc 8th Int Congr Pig Vet Soc, Ghent, p. 224.

TEUSCHER, T.; WENIGER, J. H.; AND STEINHAUF, D. 1972. Leg weakness in pigs. Breeding and production importance. Schweinezucht und Schweinemast. Z Schweineprod 20:292–296.

TISSOT, R. G.; BEATTIE, C. W.; AND AMOSS, JR., M. S. 1989. The swine leucocyte antigen (SLA) complex and Sinclair swine cutaneous malignant melanoma. Anim Genet 20:51–57.

TOELLE, V. D., AND ROBISON, O. W. 1982. Breed prenatal, breed postnatal and heterosis effects for preweaning traits in swine. J Anim Sci 2:263–273.

VAIMAN, M.; RENARD, C.; LA FAGE, P.; AMETEAU, J.; AND NIZZA, P. 1970. Evidence for a histocompatibility system in swine (SL-A). Transplantation 10:155–164.

VAIMAN, M.; HAUPTMAN, G.; AND MAYER, S. 1978a. Influence of the major histocompatibility complex in the pig (SLA) on hemolytic complement levels. Immunogenetics 5:59–63.

VAIMAN, M.; METZGER, J. J.; RENARD, C.; AND VILA, J. P. 1978b. Immune response gene(s) controlling the humoral anti-lysozyme response (Ir-Lys) linked to the major histocompatibility complex SLA in the pig. Immunogenetics 7:231–238.

WALKER, J. C. 1953. Disease resistance in the vegetable crops. II. Bot Rev 19:606–643.

WALKER, J. S.; KLEIN, F.; LINCOLN, R. E.; AND FERNELIUS, A. L. 1967. A unique defense mechanism against anthrax demonstrated in dwarf swine. J Bacteriol 93:2031–2032.

WARD, A. H. 1938. Preliminary report on inheritance of "susceptibility" to severe udder infection (mastitis). NZ J Sci Technol 20:109a.

WARNER, C. M., AND ROTHSCHILD, M. F. 1991. The swine major histocompatibility complex (SLA). In Immunogenetics of the Major Histocompatiblity Complex, vol. 2. Ed. R. Srivastava, B. Ram, and P. Tyle. New York: Verlag Cherme Int Publ, pp. 368–397.

WARNER, C. M.; MEEKER, D. L.; AND ROTHSCHILD, M. F. 1987. Genetic control of immune responsiveness: A review of its use as a tool for selection for disease resistance. J Anim Sci 64:394–406.

WIJERATNE, W. V. S.; CROSSMAN, P. J.; AND GOULD, C. M. 1970. Evidence of a sire effect on piglet mortality. Br Vet J 126:94–98.

ZHILONG, Z. 1990. The characteristics of Chinese pig breeds. Proc Chinese Pig Symp, Toulouse, France, pp. 55–65.

58 Internal Parasites

R. M. Corwin

T. B. Stewart

INTERNAL PARASITES are ever present and must be considered in the economic production of pork. Losses caused by parasites of up to $3 per pig produced in the United States were estimated by Batte (1977). Losses vary greatly in relation to geographic regions, types of housing, management, nutrition, breed and strain of pigs, and species of parasites. Cross-discipline knowledge is important in understanding the effects of the independent factors and their interactions that are involved. The impact of swine parasites and the need for research were recently reviewed (Stewart et al. 1985a), as well as the economic losses in production (Stewart and Hale 1988). Condemnation of parts of and even entire carcasses due to parasites can be dramatic and easily documented; however, probably the more important losses come from insidious depressant effects of parasites on feed intake, daily gain, and feed conversion. Controlled experimental single infections at different levels with the ubiquitous *Ascaris suum* have shown that low levels of infection depress feed intake and daily gain with a concomitant increase in maintenance cost; at higher levels of infection depression in feed conversion also occurs. Periodic analyses of metabolic function during the prepatent period showed a significant effect on nitrogen (N) metabolism on days 33–37, coincident with rapid growth of the immature worms in the small intestine (Hale et al. 1985). The average number of worms recovered at slaughter ranged from 13 to 18, although the infecting doses in the studies ranged from 600 to 60,000. Such lack in correlation between infecting numbers and establishment of adults has been observed many times (Schwartz 1959; Andersen et al. 1973).

Most schemes for parasite control have been aimed at reducing condemnation of livers caused by *A. suum* or *Stephanurus dentatus;* e.g., the "McLean County" system developed in the midwest (Raffensperger and Connely 1927), the "Profit" program in North Carolina (Behlow and Batte 1974), and the "Gilt-only" system developed in Georgia (Stewart et al. 1964). These systems incorporated sanitation, anthelmintics, and management, singly or in combination to reduce condemnation and production losses. All anthelmintics introduced for swine since the 1950s have

been highly efficacious against *A. suum,* yet it is still the most prevalent swine worm parasite in the world. Incidentally, this is also true of *A. lumbricoides* of humans.

The organization of this chapter is by anatomic system infected by the important cosmopolitan parasites, beginning with the anterior alimentary tract. Other parasites are included as miscellaneous or incidental parasites. The distribution, morphology, life cycle, pathology, and diagnosis of each parasite are discussed and, where appropriate, other special effects such as immune response, public health significance, and economic importance. The location, occurrence, intermediate host, mode of infection, and treatment for internal parasites of pigs are summarized in Table 58.1. A separate section is included on control and on anthelmintic compounds currently being used and those under development.

STOMACH

Hyostrongylus rubidus. The trichostrongyloid nematode, *H. rubidus,* the red stomach worm of pigs is concentrated in the lesser curvature in the fundic area of the stomach of pigs. The adult worms are less than 10 mm in length and are bright red when first removed from the host. Of cosmopolitan distribution, they are essentially parasites of pastured animals.

MORPHOLOGY. These slender red worms have cuticular striations (Fig. 58.2). Males are 4–7 mm and females 5–9 mm in length. Males have a pair of short spicules and a bursa. The female vulva is located on the midposterior half of the body. Cervical papillae are present. The eggs are typical strongyle type and are in the 16- to 32-cell stage when passed in the feces. They are thin-shelled and measure 60–76 by 30–38 μm (Fig. 58.1F).

LIFE CYCLE. Eggs develop on the ground into infective larvae (L₃) in about 7 days. After ingestion, infection becomes patent in about 3 weeks. The L₃ enter pits of the gastric glands where they remain for about 2 weeks as they go through two molts and return to the lumen as L₅, young adults. Larvae can remain in the mucosa for several months in a histotrophic stage similar to *Osterta-*

Table 58.1. Location, occurrence, intermediate host, mode of infection, and treatment for helminth parasites of pigs

Location	Common Name	Scientific Name	Occurrence[a]	Host	Mode of Infection	Treatment[b]
Lungs	Lungworm	*Metastrongylus apri, M. pudendotectus, M. salmi*	+++	Earthworm	Eating earthworm with encysted larvae	FBZ, IVE, LVM
Gullet	Gullet worm	*Gongylonema pulchrum*	+	Dung beetle	Eating beetle with encysted larvae	None
Stomach	Red stomach worm	*Hyostrongylus rubidus*	++	None	Swallowing infective larvae	DCV, FBZ, IVE, TBZ
	Thick stomach worm	*Ascarops strongylina*	++	Dung beetle	Eating beetle with encysted larvae	FBZ, DCV
		Physocephalus sexalatus	++			
	Large roundworm	*Ascaris suum*	++++	None	Swallowing infective eggs	DCV, FBZ, IVE, LVM, PIP, PRT
Small intestine	Intestinal threadworm	*Strongyloides ransomi*	++++	None	Through milk, prenatal, larvae boring into skin	LVM, IVE, TBZ
	Hookworm	*Globocephalus urosubulatus*	+	None	Larvae boring into skin	None
	Thorny-headed worm	*Macracanthorhynchus hirudinaceus*	++	May beetle grub	Eating grub with encysted larvae	LVM
Large intestine	Nodular worm	*Oesophagostomum dentatum*	++++	None	Swallowing infective larvae	DCV, FBZ, IVE, PIP, PRT
		O. quadrispinulatum	+++			
		O. brevicaudum	++			
	Whipworm	*Trichuris suis*	+++	None	Swallowing infective eggs	FBZ
Kidney area	Kidneyworm	*Stephanurus dentatus*	+++	None	Larvae boring into skin, oral, prenatal	FBZ, LVM
Liver	Liver fluke	*Fasciola hepatica*	+	Snail	Eating encysted metacercariae on grass	None
Muscle	Trichina	*Trichinella spiralis*	+	None	Eating muscle with encysted larvae	FBZ (?)
	Measles	*Taenia solium*	+	Pig	Eating human excrement	None

[a]Relative incidence shown by +'s. Reported, +; up to 30% on surveys, ++; up to 60%, +++; greater than 60%, ++++.
[b]DCV = dichlorvos; FBZ = fenbendazole; IVE = ivermectin; LVM = levamisole; PIP = piperazine; PRT = pyrantel; TBZ = thiabendazole.

58.1. (A) *Strongyloides* egg, thin-shelled, lacking one of three layers, and larvated; (B) *Ascarops* egg, larvated and similar morphologically to those of *Physocephalus* and *Gongylonema;* (C) *Ascaris* egg has an outer proteinaceous layer, often missing; (D) *Metastrongylus* egg, morphologically similar to *Ascaris* but is larvated; (E, F, G) *Oesophagostomum-Hyostrongylus-Globocephalus*-type eggs; (H) *Stephanurus dentatus* egg passed in the urine; (I) *Trichuris* egg; (J) *Macracanthorhynchus* egg. (All eggs photographed and printed at the same magnification.)

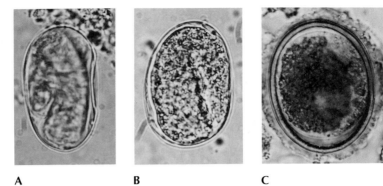

A

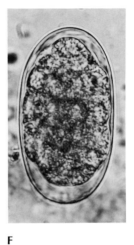

B

C

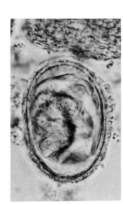

D

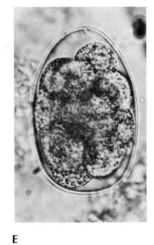

E

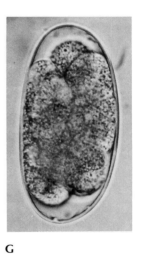

F

G

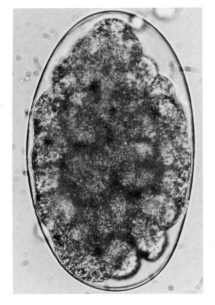

H

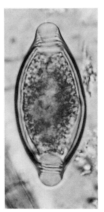

I

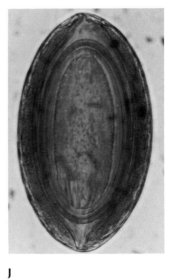

J

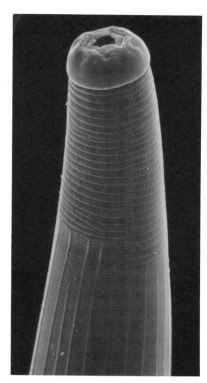

58.2. Scanning electron micrograph of anterior of *Hyostrongylus rubidus* showing cuticular striations.

gia of cattle and sheep and cause formation of small nodules.

PATHOLOGY. Infections usually are not pathogenic, but if enough worms are present, hyperemia, catarrhal gastritis, submucosal edema, hyperplasia of the gastric gland area, erosion of the mucosa, and ulcer formation may result (Porter 1940; Kendall et al. 1969; Stockdale et al. 1973; Stockdale 1974). *H. rubidus* is a blood sucker, and in herds with clinical hyostrongylosis, emaciation and pallor of the skin and mucous membranes may be apparent in adult animals (Davidson et al. 1968; Appert and Taranchon 1969). Clinically inapparent infections can lead to reduced weight gains, feed conversion, and N balance (Dey-Hazra et al. 1972; Stewart et al. 1985b).

DIAGNOSIS. The eggs are almost indistinguishable from those of *Oesophagostomum* spp. in both size and morphology, although, *H. rubidus* eggs are more advanced in development. Larval culture is a better method of differentiation (Honer 1967).

SMALL INTESTINE

Strongyloides ransomi. *Strongyloides ransomi,* the small intestinal threadworm is a rhabditoid nematode of cosmopolitan distribution. Its prevalence and importance are greater in the warmer climatic regions where it is an important parasite of suckling pigs.

MORPHOLOGY. Only parthenogenetic females are present in the parasitic generation. Adults are practically microscopic, measuring 3.3–4.5 mm in length. The filariform esophagus occupies about a third of the total body length. The vulva is located near the middle of the body. Males and females, quite different from the parasitic female, are present in the free-living generation, which occurs outside of the host. The free-living stages are difficult to differentiate from other nematodes found in the environment, except for the L_3 infective larva, which lacks a sheath and has a digitiform tail. The thin-shelled eggs passed in the feces contain larvae and measure 45–55 by 26–35 μm (Figs. 58.1A, 58.3).

LIFE CYCLE. Larvated eggs that pass in the feces hatch in a few hours into L_1 rhabditiform larvae. These may develop either directly into infective larvae (homogonic cycle) or into males and females (heterogonic cycle), which in turn will produce infective larvae. In the homogonic cycle, infective larvae can appear in a little more than a day. In the heterogonic cycle, infective larvae can appear in 2½ days. Different routes of infection have been proven for *S. ransomi*: percutaneous, oral, transcolostral, and prenatal.

Percutaneous penetration by larvae produces patency in 6–10 days after infection. Larvae enter the bloodstream, proceed to the lungs, undergo tracheal migration, and are swallowed. Oral infections are possible when the ingested larvae penetrate the mucous membranes and migrate to the lungs, L_3 being killed by gastric juices.

Transcolostral infection may also occur, resulting in patency by 4 days after birth. This is considered the primary means of infection in neonates in the southeastern United States. Larvae in the sow colostrum differ physiologically from L_3 and pass through the stomach and develop into adults in the small intestine without migration. Larvae responsible for infection for the neonates are sequestered in the mammary fat of the sow and apparently are mobilized and included in the colostrum (Moncol 1975; Stewart et al. 1976).

Prenatal infection producing patency in suckling pigs as early as 2–3 days after birth can occur. Larvae from the sow accumulate in various tissues of the fetus during the latter part of pregnancy and complete migration to the small intestine of the newborn very rapidly after birth.

PATHOLOGY. Diarrhea followed by progressive dehydration are the usual signs. In heavy infections, death generally occurs before pigs are 10–14 days old, but stunting and unthriftiness are the more usual sequelae of *S. ransomi* infection. No pathognomonic lesions are associated with field

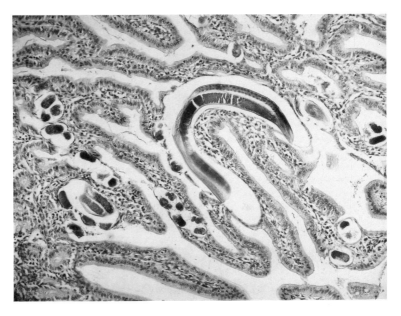

58.3. Histosection of pig small intestine infected with *Strongyloides ransomi.* Sections of worms and eggs are present.

cases of strongyloidosis (Stewart et al. 1968). Larvae apparently can be distributed widely in most tissues of the body and lesions are dependent on the number of larvae and host response (Stone 1964; Stone and Simpson 1967).

IMMUNE RESPONSE. Breed differences in susceptibility to *S. ransomi,* which appeared to be genetic (Johnson et al. 1975), have been reported. Duroc pigs were less susceptible to effects of infection than Hampshire pigs and the F_1 cross of the two breeds was intermediate in response. Murrell and Urban (1983) showed that enteral exposure of pigs infected with milk larvae produced protective immunity to subsequent subcutaneous inoculation with *S. ransomi* L_3.

DIAGNOSIS. Identification of the eggs in feces or finding the adults in the small intestine at necropsy, with a history of diarrhea and unthriftiness, confirms a diagnosis of strongyloidosis; however, care must be taken because clinical disease can be confused with colibacillosis and coccidiosis.

Ascaris suum. *Ascaris suum,* the large roundworm of swine is an ascaridoid (ascarid) nematode of cosmopolitan distribution. It is the most common gastrointestinal worm parasite in pigs with a prevalence of 50–75%. It is more common in growing pigs than in mature pigs. Although now recognized as a separate species, the large roundworm of humans, *A. lumbricoides,* was thought to be the same as that in pigs.

MORPHOLOGY. Ascarids are large, stout-bodied nematodes, pinkish-yellow with three prominent lips surrounding the mouth (Fig. 58.4). Females

are 20–40 cm long, males 15–25 cm. The male tail is conical and bent ventrad. Males have two stout spicules. The female vulva is anterior to the middle of the body. Eggs are thick-shelled, brownish yellow with a mammillated proteinaceous coating on the exterior and measure 50–80 by 40–60 μm. The eggs are unsegmented when passed in the feces (Fig. 58.1C).

LIFE CYCLE. The life cycle is direct. A hepato-tracheal migration route occurs. Eggs are layed in the intestine of the pigs and pass out in the feces. Under optimum conditions the L_1 is reached in about 10 days and the L_2 in 13–18 days; additional time is required for maturation of the L_2. Eggs become infective in about 21–30 days and may remain infective for 7 years or longer in protected areas of lots and pastures.

When ingested, infective eggs hatch in the digestive tract. The liberated L_2 penetrate the intestinal wall and generally pass by the hepatic portal system to the liver. A few, however, may pass via the lacteals to the mesenteric lymph nodes; others may even be found in the peritoneal cavity and other locations. Most larvae are in the liver by the second to third day after ingestion, where they molt to L_3 (Douvres et al. 1969), and in the lungs by days 4–7. From days 8–10 after infection, L_3 leave the lungs by penetrating the bronchioles, are coughed up into the trachea, and swallowed. By 10–15 days after infection, L_3 have returned to the small intestine and molted to L_4. At this time, some L_4 are spontaneously eliminated from the small intestine into the cecum and colon. L_4 molt to young adults (L_5) 21–30 days after ingestion of eggs. Worms are again eliminated at this time. The prepatent period is 40–53

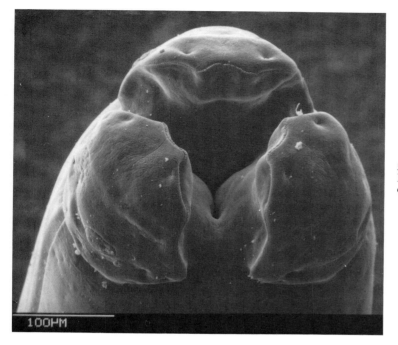

58.4. Three lips of *Ascaris suum.* Note sensory papillae and denticles on edges of lips.

days. Female ascarids are phenomenal egg producers capable of laying hundreds of thousands to nearly 2 million eggs per day. The eggs are sticky and are easily transported by cockroaches and other arthropods, birds, workers' boots, etc. Most disinfectants have no effect on the eggs, but heat (steam) and direct sunlight are effective in destroying their viability.

Most adults live in pigs only about 6 months, at which time they begin to be expelled; but pigs may continue to carry a light infection for a year or longer. In foreign hosts, as in humans or domesticated and laboratory animals, larvae may migrate but are generally unable to develop to adults in the intestine and are expelled in the feces if they reach the digestive system.

PATHOLOGY. The larvae migrate through the liver and cause hemorrhagic foci, which microscopically show mild eosinophilic infiltration and a few, small lymphoid nodules in portal areas. On repeated exposure to larvae, there is an increase in connective tissue, infiltrating eosinophils, and dilation of lymphatics, which grossly appear as whitish spots, commonly referred to as "milk spots." Such lesions disappear within 25 days. In the lungs, migrating larvae cause a verminous pneumonia, which may result in death if large numbers of larvae are involved. Clinical signs are those of pneumonia. Pigs have an asthmatic cough ("thumps") and may breathe with difficulty. Hemorrhagic foci of various sizes are present. There may be an exudate, edema, and emphysema with secondary bacterial pneumonia. Migra-

tion of *A. suum* larvae markedly enhances the pathogenicity of swine influenza as well as viral pneumonia.

Adult worms compete with the host for nutrients and interfere with absorption of nutrients by the host. They may occlude and rupture the small intestine (Fig. 58.5). In addition, adults may migrate into the common bile duct and occlude it resulting in icterus.

IMMUNE RESPONSE. Embryonated eggs fed to naive or immunized pigs by previous exposure to *A. suum* larvae hatch (Rhodes et al. 1977). Acquired resistance can be induced in pigs by oral inoculation with infective eggs or L₃ pulmonary larvae (Eriksen 1982; Stewart et al. 1985c). The presence of adults or late larval ascarids can prevent development of additional larval stages (Stewart and Rowell 1986). High levels of protective immunity based on the number of lung larvae recovered after challenge with 10,000 larvae following repeated experimental or natural exposure was shown by Urban et al. (1989). Protective immunity was not altered by strategic anthelmintic treatment that prevented growth retardation of pigs constantly exposed to natural infection. Sterilizing immunity is transitory, and periodic boosting or anthelmintic treatment is necessary to eliminate both intestinal worms and lesions during the growing/finishing period (Urban et al. 1988, 1989). The intestine is considered important as a defense mechanism in preventing larval penetration of the gut mucosa (Bindseil 1970), and it has been shown that the intestinal phase of

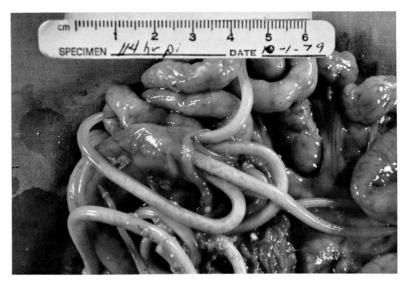

58.5. *Ascaris* emerging from a tear in the gut wall. (Photo by Mark Martinez.)

ascarids can induce circulating antibodies without prior somatic migration (Leigh-Brown and Harpur 1974). Protective immunity is characterized by antibody in serum and in intestinal washings (Urban et al. 1984).

ECONOMIC IMPORTANCE. Ascariasis is undoubtedly the most important parasitism of pigs worldwide. The effects of ascarids on the performance of pigs were detailed by Spindler in 1947 and by many others since then. Losses from condemnation of parts and lowered performance of pigs in the United States were calculated at more than $385 million annually (Levine 1980). More recently, losses due solely to lowered feed conversion from low-level *A. suum* infections were estimated at $155 million for 1987 in the United States (Stewart and Hale 1988). There are no estimates of the value of losses incurred from the potentiation or exacerbation of other diseases by migrating ascarid larvae, or the effect of different management practices or nutritional levels on pathogenicity of ascarid infection (Underdahl and Kelley 1957; Underdahl 1958; Zimmerman et al. 1973).

DIAGNOSIS. Typical eggs in fecal flotation or "milk spot" liver lesions at necropsy are diagnostic. In heavy infections the adult worms can be seen and felt in the intact small intestine. In areas where the kidney worm is endemic, liver lesions must be differentiated because early *S. dentatus* lesions can be confused with those produced by *A. suum.*

Trichinella spiralis.   All mammalian species are probably susceptible to *Trichinella spiralis* infection, although natural cycles seem climatically based. In the temperate zone the usual cycle has swine and bears as natural hosts (Schad et al.

1984), and in the arctic zone the polar and grizzly bears (Kim 1983) and walrus (MacLean et al. 1989) are natural hosts. Other species, including humans, are involved incidentally. Trichinellosis is found less frequently in the tropics. Regulation of feeding garbage to swine, public health programs, and recently improved trichinoscopic and serodiagnostic techniques have reduced the incidence of this infection.

MORPHOLOGY. The life stage most frequently observed is the encysted larvae (L_1) in skeletal muscle fibers (Fig. 58.6); these cysts are 400–600 μm long and 250 μm in diameter. Prior to skeletal muscle fiber penetration, L_1 may be found in the circulatory system. Adult females are in the lamina propria of the small intestine, have a stichoform-type esophagus, produce larvated eggs in utero, and are 3–4 mm long and 60 μm in diameter. Adult males are rarely seen but are about one-half the size of females.

LIFE CYCLE. Muscle cysts are ingested, digested in the stomach and small intestine, and L_1 are liberated into the small intestine. Molting from L_1 to L_4 then occurs in 2–6 days. Intracellar infection of enterocytes with adults was demonstrated in mice by electron microscopy (Wright 1979). Males die soon after mating and females burrow into lymph spaces, depositing larvae. Larvae are numerous in the blood from 8 to 25 days postinfection; these L_1 penetrate the sarcolemma of skeletal muscle fibers throughout the body and become encysted by 3 months. Although calcification of cysts begins at 6–9 months, L_1 remain viable for up to 11 years, demonstrating the symbiotic relationship between L_1 and its host muscle fiber, the "nurse cell" (Despommier 1990). Modes of transmission in swine herds include cannibalism, tail biting, scavenging on carcasses of dead

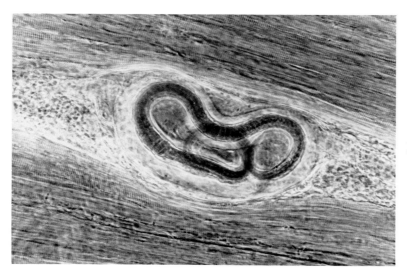

58.6. *Trichinella* larvated cyst. (Photo by Blaise Brazos.)

farm cats (Hanbury et al. 1986), feeding of raw garbage and the presence of hog lots on covered garbage dumps (Zimmerman et al. 1962), and eating wild animal carcasses such as raccoon and fox (Kazacos 1986; Campbell 1988).

PATHOLOGY. *Trichinella* is much less pathogenic for swine than for rats and humans. Experimental infections in pigs caused decreased weight gains and intense muscle pain, but most of these infected pigs recovered with rapid weight gain (Scholtens et al. 1966); in experimentally infected miniature pigs, eosinophilia and hypergammaglobulinemia were observed (Beck and Anfinson 1965). Clinical illness has not been described for natural infections with the muscle fiber cyst, and infiltration of eosinophils is often the only lesion observed.

IMMUNE RESPONSE. Intraperitoneal inoculation of pigs with *T. spiralis* excretory-secretory products induced moderate but variable degrees of immunity to subsequent challenge per os with doses of 2500–2700 L_1. These pigs harbored fewer adult worms, and the fecundity of female worms recovered (measured by shedding of newborn larvae) was significantly lower than that of females recovered from control pigs (Gamble et al. 1986). Prospects for potential use of a targeted vaccine in an integrated control program for swine trichinosis is being investigated (Murrell 1985).

DIAGNOSIS. Federal, and until recently state, meat inspection regulations have not included examination for *Trichinella*, but procedures for diagnosis would be by digestion of muscle at slaughter or by enzyme-linked immunosorbent assay (ELISA) for serologic detection of *Trichinella*-specific antibodies (Gamble et al. 1983). A pooled sample/digestion method using 5–6 g diaphragm samples from lots of 20 pig carcasses has been adopted by several European countries but not by USDA (Zimmerman 1967). These pooled samples are digested and homogenized using 1% pepsin/1% HCl and a mixing action, which simulates peristaltic motion of the stomach (using a stomacher device). Analysis of pooled samples can be accomplished in 1½ hours (Oliver et al. 1985).

An ELISA test using an excretory antigen for diagnosis of trichinosis was evaluated in the field with sera from herds with ongoing transmission of *T. spiralis* (Murrell et al. 1986). Results showed a high sensitivity of 93–96% with sera from infected pigs. Of those that were false-negative, five-sixths had < 5.0 larvae per gram (LPG). This should prove to be a major technique for antemortem diagnosis in herd screening.

PUBLIC HEALTH. In Europe, trichinoscopic examination of pork appears to have practically eliminated *T. spiralis* from domestic swine. Incidence for swine trichiniasis in the United States was 0.125% in 1966–70 (Zimmerman and Zinter 1971). Pork, mainly prepared as sausage, apparently is the major source of human trichinellosis with 73.2% of 254 cases for which a source was identified (U.S. Dep. Health and Human Services [USDHHS] 1976). There are close to 40 million potential exposures each year based on the estimated number of infected pigs; the estimated number of human cases is 300,000, the majority of which cause no symptoms of infection (Leighty 1974). Non-pork products included meat from walrus and blackbear, horse meat and ground beef (James 1989), with beef likely adulterated with pork. Small custom slaughterhouses are important epidemiologically, for these often prepare fresh, whole, dressed pork for social occasions where one animal is consumed by many persons (Schad et al. 1985). There have been several recent small epidemics among Indo-Chinese immigrants in the United States (US-DHHS 1982); an update on trichinosis surveillance in the United States appeared in 1988 (USDHHS 1988).

In the United States, educating the public to recognize the hazard and to cook pork adequately to kill the organisms, and control of manufactured pork products eaten without adequate cooking have been the two principal patterns used by federal and state meat inspection programs (Leighty 1974). A more concerted effort to identify herds with active infections in order to provide a "safe" product was initiated by the state of Illinois with the introduction of a Trichinosis Control Act in 1986. The pooled-digestion and ELISA techniques are employed to identify and subsequently to quarantine, depopulate, and indemnify those herds found infected. Other states such as North Carolina are following suit with use of a semiautomatic ELISA used to screen hogs in a packing plant at the rate of 400/hour; all recorded positives then are screened by the diaphragm-digestion technique.

For chemotherapy, ivermectin was confirmed as having no antiparasitic activity, while excellent efficacy was reported for albendazole. Calf thymus extract, cyclosporin A, and the experimental compound luxabendazole have also been proved efficacious (James 1989).

CECUM, COLON

Trichuris suis. Pigs and wild boars are considered the natural hosts, although primates including humans may be infected with *T. suis*. Whipworms are distributed widely and represent a fairly common problem in swine.

MORPHOLOGY. Adult females measure 6–8 cm long and males half that length. This trichuroid has a unique morphology with the anterior or esophageal portion ≤ 0.5mm in diameter and extending two-thirds of the body length. The esophagus is a stichosome-type consisting of a column of spiralling stichocytes, one-cell layer in thickness. A microscopic lancet has been described protruding from the stoma in all stages. Glandular and muscular components are interspersed along the esophagus. The posterior third of the body is thicker, 0.65 mm; protrudes into the gut lumen; and it contains the midgut of the worm and its reproductive tract. Bipolar thick-shelled eggs may be seen in the uterus of the female and a single copulatory spicule in the male. Eggs are 60 by 25 μm, yellow to brown, and in the one-cell stage (Fig. 58.1I).

LIFE CYCLE. Eggs passed in the feces require 3–4 weeks to reach infectivity, still in the L_1 stage, and can remain infective for as long as 6 years. Infective eggs hatch in the small intestine and ce-

cum, with the released L_1 penetrating cells lining the crypts. A histotrophic phase persists for 2 weeks with gradual larval migration from the deeper lamina propria to the submucosa. Luminal development begins the third week postinfection with the posterior body coming into view and the anterior end remaining buried in the mucosa (Fig. 58.7). Meanwhile four molts have occurred, prepatency is 6–7 weeks, and life span is 4–5 months (Beer 1973).

PATHOLOGY. *Trichuris* infections cause enterocyte destruction, ulceration of the mucosal lining, loss of capillary blood, and probable secondary bacterial and *Balantidium coli* infection. Thus, trichuriosis must be considered in the differential diagnosis of swine dysentery complex that does not respond to antibiotic therapy. The spectrum of gross lesions may be edema with formation of nodules containing exudates surrounding portions of worms to formation of a fibrinonecrotic membrane. Erosion of capillary beds and vasodilatation result in hemorrhage, anemia, and hypoalbuminemia. Clinical signs include anorexia, mucoid to bloody diarrhea, dehydration, and death.

IMMUNE RESPONSE. Susceptibility with accompanying clinical signs is up to 6 months although mature hogs may show clinical infection when stressed. Light infections persist allowing intermittent shedding of eggs.

DIAGNOSIS. Clinical signs, including bloody scouring, are presumptive. Eggs in stools and whipworms at necropsy are confirmative. Trichurids are sporadic egg layers, therefore little significance can be made to eggs per gram (EPG).

***Oesophagostomum* spp.** These are strongyloid nematodes of which *O. dentatum* and *O. quadrispinulatum* are most common in occurrence. *O. brevicaudum* occurs in the southeastern United States and other areas with similar climates. Two other species, *O. granatensis* in Europe and *O. georgianum* in southeastern United States, are probably morphovariants of *O. dentatum* (Raynaud et al. 1974; Stewart and Gasbarre 1989).

MORPHOLOGY. Adult *Oesophagostomum* have stout, white, slightly curved bodies with females 1–2 cm long and males slightly shorter. Species differentiation is by shape of esophagus, width of buccal capsules, and length of tail and spicules (Figs. 58.8, 58.9). Eggs are 70 by 40 μm, morulated when passed, thin shelled, and typically strongylid (Fig. 58.1E).

LIFE CYCLE. The preparasitic cycle is of the strongylid type, with L_1 emerging from eggs and ensheathed L_3 appearing by 1 week. Larvae can survive on pastures up to 12 months. Swine are

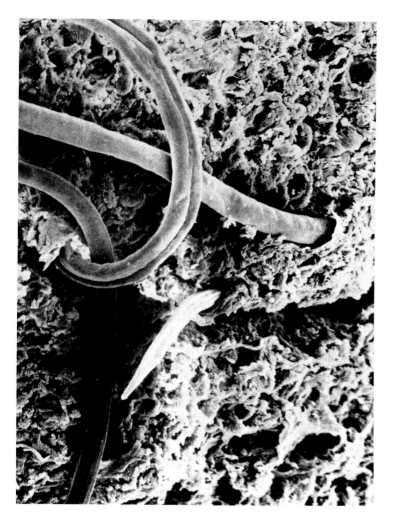

58.7. *Trichuris* worm. Note intracellular penetration. (Batte et al. 1977.)

infected by ingesting L₃ from contaminated pasture, by mechanical transmission by psychodid flies (midges), or from rats with encysted larvae (Jacobs and Dunn 1968). The L₃ enter the mucosa of the cecum and colon and molt to L₄, remain for 2 weeks causing small nodules, and emerge into the lumen where patency is reached in 3 weeks.

PATHOLOGY. Formation of nodules from the cecum to the rectum is the major change (Taffs 1966). The sequela is petechiation at the point of entry of the L₃ (Jacobs 1969); focal thickening of the mucosa consisting of lymphocytes, macrophages, and eosinophils; and then presence of luminal nodules by day 4. Encysted larvae may be found in the muscularis mucosa (McCracken and Ross 1970). By 1 week, nodules are up to 8 mm in diameter and plugged with yellow to black necrotic debris. Walls of the cecum and colon become edematous from extensive thrombosis of the lymphatics; there is possibly a localized fibrinonecrotic membrane. Resolution begins the

second week with some remnants of nodules and scarring. Secondary infection may occur and enhance clinical signs of depression, anorexia, and scouring.

IMMUNITY. There is no apparent age immunity (Taffs 1966), but pigs over 3 months of age seem more susceptible (Hass et al. 1972). Periparturient rise of EPG is maintained through lactation with a subsequent expulsion of worms (Connan 1967; Hass et al. 1972).

DIAGNOSIS. Eggs are typically strongylid and therefore may be confused with *Hyostrongylus*. Larval culture to L₃ does aid in differentiation, but necropsy is the most reliable means.

RESPIRATORY TRACT

***Metastrongylus* spp.** Species include *M. elongatus (apri), M. pudendotectus,* and *M. salmi,* which occur in the bronchi and bronchioles, espe-

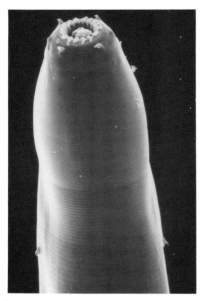

58.8. Scanning electron micrograph of anterior of *Oesophagostomum brevicaudum.*

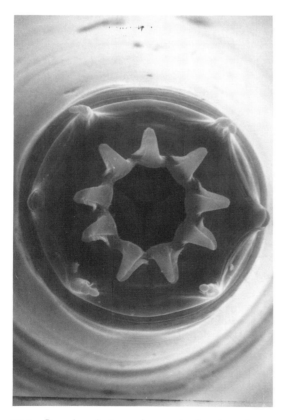

58.9. Scanning electron micrograph of en face view of *Oesophagostomum dentatum.* The nine elements of the corona radiata surround the mouth opening and the triradiate lumen of the esophagus is distinct. Two dorsal and two ventral cephalic papillae and two lateral amphids are present.

cially in the diaphragmatic lobes, and exclusively in swine. Although *M. elongatus* is the most common, all occur worldwide and natural infections occur with one to three species present.

MORPHOLOGY. Adults are slender and white, with females 50 mm in length and males 25 mm; males have paired spicules. Mucoid deposits around these adults make it difficult to separate individuals. Eggs are larvated, thick shelled, and measure 40 by 50 μm (Fig. 58.1D).

LIFE CYCLE. Larvated eggs are coughed up, swallowed, and passed in feces. Earthworms ingest these eggs, which then hatch, and L_1 migrate to the heart. Infective larvae appear in 10 days and are then available for hogs rooting in the soil and eating infected earthworms. These L_3 penetrate the small intestine and are transported to the mesenteric lymph nodes where they molt to the L_4. These L_4 are then swept through the right heart to the lungs (Fig. 58.10) and molt to L_5, with patency in 4 weeks.

PATHOLOGY. Dissecting the bronchioles reveals mucoid plugs in the diaphragmatic lobes of the lungs; these are filled with adults and eggs. Parasites, mucus, and cellular exudate cause occlusion and induce atelectasis observed as coughing or "thumps." Apparently *Mycoplasma hyopneumoniae* is not transmitted with *Metastrongylus* via earthworms (Preston and Switzer 1976). There does seem to be a lessened number of these parasites in breeding stock.

DIAGNOSIS. It is difficult to find *Metastrongylus* eggs in a fecal exam, but it is important to look for "fuzzy" areas in which eggs are held in mucus. At necropsy, lungworm can be extruded by clipping the posteroventral margins of the diaphragmatic lobes of the lungs.

URINARY TRACT

Stephanurus dentatus. The kidney worm is a strongyloid nematode of swine. Domestic and feral pigs raised on soil in wooded areas with warm climates are most often infected. In the United States, endemicity is from the Carolinas to southern Missouri with interstate transport accounting for its appearance as far north as Canada (Smith and Hawkes 1978).

MORPHOLOGY. Adults are thick bodied with a black and white mottling from contents of the reproductive and intestinal tracts showing through the cuticle; they are 2–3 cm long by 2 mm in diameter. The strongylid eggs are ellipsoidal, thin walled, morulated, and measure 120 by 70 μm (Fig. 58.1H).

LIFE CYCLE. Kidney worms are found in cysts in

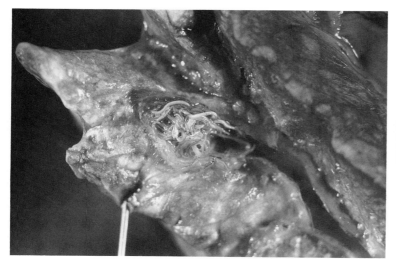

58.10. Cluster of *Metastrongylus* worms in a terminal bronchiole of the diaphragmatic lobe of the lung. (Photo by Blaise Brazos.)

perirenal fat with fistulous openings into the ureters, in the kidney, and in ectopic sites such as the pancreas, lumbar muscles, spinal cord, and lungs. Eggs are voided, with greatest numbers found at first urination because of overnight accumulation in the bladder. Eggs may hatch in 1–2 days on urine-soaked wooded lots and shaded farrowing pens; larvae may survive several months in warm, moist, shaded conditions. L_3 may be infective in 3–5 days and are invasive by ingestion, skin penetration, and infected earthworms (Tromba 1955; Batte et al. 1960). Prenatal infection also has been reported (Batte et al. 1966).

Infective L_3 migrate from the small intestine to the mesenteric lymph nodes and molt to L_4, which move through the portal veins to the liver (Lichtenfels and Tromba 1972). Bronchiole lymph nodes, lungs, pancreas, and spleen also may be infected by L_3 (Waddell 1969). In the liver, L_4 increase from 0.4 to 6.0 mm and then molt to L_5 (Lichtenfels and Tromba 1972). At 2–4 months, L_5 leave the liver and migrate through the body cavity to perirenal and mesenteric fat. Patency is uncommon before 9 months to a year and eggs are shed for 3 years following initial infection (Batte et al. 1966). Patent kidney worm infection is more common in breeding stock 2 years old and older, although liver lesions are seen in young market-weight pigs in endemic areas.

PATHOLOGY. Gross pathologic changes may be found where there is migration. Mesenteric lymph nodes are edematous and swollen; liver changes include inflammation, eosinophilia, abscessation, and extensive fibrosis, making this infection easily differentiated from ascarid migration. Similar lesions can be seen in other organs. Nodules are formed in perirenal fat and fistulous tracts are present along the ureters. Posterior paralysis has been associated with larval migration around the spinal cord.

DIAGNOSIS. Worms, abscessation, and liver scarring can be seen at the postmortem exam. Eggs in urine may be confirmatory antemortem.

ECONOMIC CONSIDERATIONS. At least 95% of liver condemnations are due to kidney worms and ascarids in hogs in the southeastern United States (Batte et al. 1975). Marked reduction in growth rate and feed efficiency were shown in pigs infected experimentally with 72–842 L_3/kg body weight (Hale and Marti 1983).

MISCELLANEOUS PARASITES. Three spiruroid parasites that require dung beetles as intermediate hosts can be found in pigs: *Ascarops strongylina* and *Physocephalus sexalatus* in the stomach and *Gongylonema pulchrum* under the epithelial layer of the esophagus and tongue. The two thick stomach worms may cause a gastritis if present in large numbers. Tongues for human consumption may have to be scalded and the skin peeled off to remove *G. pulchrum* for esthetic reasons. Eggs of these spiruroids are thick shelled and measure 34–40 by 18–22 μm, *Ascarops* (Fig. 58.1B); 31–39 by 12–17 μm, *Physocephalus;* and 57–59 by 30–34 μm, *Gongylonema.*

Two trichostrongylid nematodes, commonly parasites of ruminants, can also be found in pigs: *Trichostrongylus axei* in the stomach and *T. colubriformis* in the small intestine.

The hookworm of swine, *Globocephalus urosubulatus,* of cosmopolitan distribution, is more common in the southern part of the United States in feral and pastured swine. It apparently is not as common or pathogenic as hookworms of carnivores and has received little attention. The eggs are typically strongylid and measure 52–56 by 26–35 μm (Fig. 58.1G).

Macracanthorhynchus hirudinaceus, the thorny-headed worm of swine, is an acanthocephalan. It attaches to the ileal portion of the small intestine and causes nodular lesions, which are sometimes invaded by secondary organisms. Occasionally the gut wall is perforated by the proboscis and peritonitis results. Eggs measure 110 by 65 μm, are brown, and have a thick three-layered shell (Fig. 58.1J). A beetle is the required intermediate host.

Of public health importance, *Taenia solium* (*Cysticercus cellulosae*) has humans as the host for the adult tapeworm and as the potential intermediate host for the cysticercus. Swine are the natural intermediate hosts and are an integral part of the life cycle. Adult tapeworms are 3–5 m long with an armed rostellum; humans are usually infected with a single worm. Gravid proglottids are 12 by 6 mm; have a single, lateral genital pore; and contain taeniid eggs of 42 μm in diameter. Following ingestion of eggs by swine, cysticerci later develop in skeletal and cardiac muscle, measuring up to 18 mm in diameter. These are infective by 2–3 months and remain so for 2 years; prepatency in humans is 2 months. Cysticercosis in swine and adult tapeworms in humans are usually of no clinical significance, but cysticercosis in humans is life threatening, for cysticerci become space-occupying lesions in the central nervous system and have unrestricted growth with no outer limiting membrane (racemose). Diagnosis for humans is made by finding segments in the stool and for swine, cysticerci in muscle.

Swine may also be infected with *Fasciola hepatica* and *Echinococcus granulosus* in the liver but with no apparent clinical problems. These infected swine are found in endemic areas where there is common pasture use with sheep.

The ciliated protozoan *Balantidium coli* is harbored primarily in the cecum and anterior colon of swine, in which it appears to be a commensal. The motile form is pleomorphic, 30–150 μm by 25–120 μm, and ciliary action is in longitudinal waves. The cyst is spherical and 45–65 μm in diameter. Reproduction is by binary fission; resistant cysts are formed. Transmission is by ingestion of cysts or trophozoites passed in feces. Under usual conditions, *B. coli* feeds on starch, bacteria, and ingesta including nematode eggs. Although it cannot initiate penetration, it is a secondary invader to other invaders of the mucosa and produces hyaluronidase, which enlarges lesions. Diagnosis is based on appearance of ciliated trophozoites, and presence of cysts and flask-shaped ulcers. Humans, other primates, and dogs have been found clinically affected in zoos and in areas surrounding hog farms. *B. coli* may cause an explosive bloody diarrhea in these species.

PREVENTION. Control of parasites can be achieved at several different levels that may be broadly categorized as prevention and treatment. Infection by parasites requiring an intermediate host can usually be successfully prevented by re-moving pigs from contact with the intermediate hosts, nominally, dung beetles and earthworms that inhabit pastures and lots. Therefore, by maintaining pigs on concrete, infection with the spiruroids, acanthocephalans, and metastrongyloids can be prevented. An added benefit would also be the reduction or prevention of other parasites, such as *Hyostrongylus*, *Globocephalus*, and *Trichostrongylus*, that also require pasture conditions for transmission.

Good sanitation and adequate nutrition are very important in controlling infections and reducing the adverse effects of parasites. The major mode of transmission of worm parasites is through contamination of food, soil, or bedding with feces or urine. Worm eggs need moisture and warmth to develop and survive. They cannot live in direct sunlight or under dry conditions very long. The usual disinfectants used on the farm do not kill eggs of worms such as ascarids. Thorough cleaning of buildings, pens, and equipment with detergent and steam is the best way of killing worm eggs and larvae. Worms in the gut compete with the pig for available nutrients. Research has shown that levels of protein and vitamins in the feed affect the performance of parasitized pigs. Average daily gain and feed efficiency of infected pigs tend to improve with each increase in protein and vitamins in the feed.

A management system in which only gilts are used as breeders has been shown to be effective in eradicating kidney worms. This is possible because of the lengthy prepatent period of 6 months or longer and the fact that only animals 2 years old or older pass kidney worm eggs in numbers. By selling breeders as soon as first litters are weaned and maintaining boars separately or replacing them as with the gilts, will prevent contamination of the premises. Eradication can be achieved in 2 years or less by using the "gilt-only" system (Stewart et al. 1964).

TREATMENT. Therapeutic treatment of pigs with anthelmintics may present only a temporary solution, unless the conditions under which the parasites were acquired are altered. No drug is effective against all parasites and certainly the damage done by developing worms or migrating larvae prior to patency cannot be cured. A good management system will incorporate practices aimed at prevention of infections and will not use treatment as the sole method of controlling parasites. The choice of dewormer is dependent on the species of parasites present and the relative cost of the products. Routine, strategic treatment for worms is advisable on farms with previous history of clinical parasitism. Treatment reduces the number of egg-producing worms and keeps further contamination of premises to a minimum.

The use of chemical agents such as hygromycin or pyrantel tartrate fed for several weeks can be helpful under lot or pasture conditions to control infections and reduce lesions from ascarids and nodular worms. Prophylactic use of pyrantel or repetitive treatments with fenbendazole reduces worm populations and also appears to stimulate immunity against *A. suum* (Southern et al. 1989; Stankiewicz and Jeska 1990).

Treatment of sows 10–14 days before farrowing with ivermectin has been shown to be effective in preventing transmission of *S. ransomi* from sows to their pigs. Such treatment of sows is also beneficial in preventing transmission of *Sarcoptes scabiei.*

Anthelmintics. The period of 1960–90 has been one in which new classes of anthelmintic compounds have been developed, approved by FDA for use in swine, and marketed in formulations for administration in water, feed, and by injection. Spectrum of activity varies by compound, with some most effective against a few target species and others broader in effect.

AVERMECTINS. These are derived from fermentation products of *Streptomyces avermitilis.* Only one compound, ivermectin, was approved by FDA in the mid-1980s and is marketed for swine in an injectable formulation. Mode of action is to stimulate the release of inhibitory neurotransmitter gamma-aminobutyric acid (GABA) in target organisms. This inhibits neuromuscular transmission leading to paralysis and death. Spectrum of activity includes internal and external parasites including *Ascaris, Oesophagostomum,* and *Metastrongylus,* with less effect for *Trichuris* and excellent effect for *Haematopinus* (sucking lice) and *Sarcoptes.* Formulations to be added to the feed and several new anthelmintics of similar sources were under development in 1991.

BENZIMIDAZOLE CARBAMATES. There are several efficacious compounds among the benzimidazole carbamates, but only thiabendazole (TBZ) and fenbendazole (FBZ) are approved for use in swine in the United States. The progenitor of this class of anthelmintics is TBZ, which has been available since the early 1960s. At 50 mg/kg body weight TBZ has a greater than 95% efficacy against *Hyostrongylus, Strongyloides,* and *Oesophagostomum* but much less activity against ascarids and whipworms. Commercially, it is used in a paste form given therapeutically in a single oral dose for *Strongyloides* infections in baby pigs. Its pharmacologic action is to block nematode fumarate reductase activity. Absorption is a passive diffusion through the cuticle of the worm. Thiabendazole has little solubility in water; therefore, only a small amount is rapidly absorbed from the intestinal tract. Its metabolites are excreted completely in feces and urine within 3 days. There is negligible mammalian toxicity, with 20 times the therapeutic dose producing no adverse effects.

Fenbendazole was approved for use in swine in the United States in 1984. It is known to be effective against ascarids, whipworms, nodular worms, lungworms, and larval and adult kidney worms (Batte 1978). It is more potent than TBZ, especially against ascarids. Pharmacologic activity is known to be inhibition of glucose uptake from luminal fluid of the nematode gut, which results in an inability of the worm to produce adenosine triphosphate (ATP). Worms are expelled over a 2- to 3-day period following treatment. Fenbendazole may also affect fumarate reductase. It is administered in feed over a 3-day period (Corwin et al. 1984).

IMIDAZOTHIAZOLES. Levamisole was introduced in the late 1960s and demonstrates a broad range of activity in the removal of gastrointestinal, respiratory, and urinary tract nematodes. It removes 90–100% of *Ascaris, Strongyloides,* and *Metastrongylus* and 72–99% of *Oesophagostomum, Trichuris,* and mature *Stephanurus.*

Levamisole has a paralyzing effect (blocking of ganglionic transmission), with a rapid expulsion of living worms. It also blocks the metabolic pathway responsible for formation of ATP at the site of fumarate reduction and succinate oxidation. Worms expelled later are decomposed and may not be apparent in the feces.

Only the hydrochloride form is approved for use in swine and is administered in the feed or water at 8 mg/kg body weight. Levamisole hydrochloride is marketed in a pelleted ready-to-use form with a dehydrated alfalfa carrier or as a powder for use in drinking water. It is intended to be consumed within a 24-hour period. It is highly soluble in water and is rapidly absorbed from the gastrointestinal tract, with 40% excreted in the urine in 12 hours and 41% in the feces over 8 days. It should not be administered within 72 hours of slaughter, although tissue residues are not appreciable.

ORGANOPHOSPHATE COMPOUNDS. Dichlorvos is the only organophosphate compound approved for use as a swine anthelmintic. It was the first broad-spectrum compound for use in swine with greater than 90% efficacy against the L_4 and immature and mature adult *Ascaris* and mature *Oesophagostomum, Trichuris, Hyostrongylus,* and *Ascarops.* Its additional advantage is its efficacy against whipworms.

Dichlorvos inhibits nematode cholinesterase, leading to interference with neuromuscular transmission (Knowles and Cassida 1966). Nematode cholinesterase is removed by complexing with the organophosphate, whereas host cholinesterase may fail to complex, thus providing a margin of safety for the treated host. Dichlorvos is rapidly absorbed from the gastrointestinal tract and detoxified by the liver. Metabolites do not persist as tissue residues. Dichlorvos should not be given within a few days of other organophosphates, other anthelmintics, or modified live virus vaccines. There apparently are no adverse effects upon conception or gestation. The compound causes increased intestinal peristalsis. A withdrawal time of at least 7 days is required prior to slaughter.

Dichlorvos is a unique organophosphate in that it is incorporated into polyvinyl chloride pellets, which allow for slow release of the volatile active ingredient from these undigestible units during passage along the intestinal tract. Slow release allows for continued effect in the cecum, thereby producing the desired removal of whipworms. This also provides greater safety for an otherwise toxic compound, since the host can then detoxify dichlorvos as it is absorbed over a 2- to 3-day period. Dichlorvos is administered in the feed, mixed with one-third the regular ration. The recommended dose is 11.2–21.6 mg/kg body weight.

TETRAHYDROPYRIMIDINES. Pyrantel tartrate is the only tetrahydropyrimidine approved for swine and was introduced as a broad-spectrum anthelmintic compound in 1966. It is efficacious in the removal of adult and infective larval stages of *Ascaris, Oesophagostomum,* and *Hyostrongylus.*

Pyrantel acts as a neuromuscular blocking agent by depolarization of synapses. The musculature contracts irreversibly. The powdered premix is given at a single therapeutic dose level of 22 mg/kg body weight with an overnight fast or as a prophylactic measure at 96 g/ton of feed. For maximum effect against luminal forms, it is administered dry in the feed to minimize absorption. It is most commonly used as a continuous dewormer in feed for starter and growing pigs and is given in combination with carbadox, which promotes growth. It has a great margin of safety and can be used concurrently with organophosphate insecticides. It is not recommended for use in severely debilitated animals because of more pronounced nicotinic activity.

PIPERAZINE SALTS. An older generation of antiparasitic drugs includes piperazine salts. Piperazine compounds are still widely used, being efficacious in removal of ascarids and nodular worms. Up to 100% of the lumen-dwelling stages may be eliminated with a single treatment, but mature worms are more susceptible than earlier stages. A second treatment is recommended 2 months later to remove emerging larval stages.

Piperazine is a diethylenediamine, with the hexahydrate formed in water. It is readily absorbed from the proximal region of the gastrointestinal tract. Some of the base is metabolized in tissues, with 30–40% excreted in the urine. The pharmacologic effect is an anticholinergic action at the myoneural junction, producing a neuromuscular block. In addition, succinic acid production is inhibited with an overall narcotic effect because of these combined activities. Affected worms are passively removed by intestinal peristalsis and voided live in the host feces. There are no known contraindications, and the compound can be given to animals with gastrointestinal distress.

Piperazine salts are administered in the feed or water. For example, piperazine citrate is given as a 1-day medication in feed, and the hexahydrate form is used in drinking water because of its suitability for storage in solution. Medicated feed or water should be consumed in an 8- to 12-hour period; therefore, withholding feed or water the previous night is beneficial. The recommended dosage is 275–440 mg/kg body weight.

HYGROMYCIN B. This is another older generation antiparasitic drug and is a fermentation product of *Streptomyces hygroscopicus.* It proved efficacious against mature stages of *Ascaris* and *Oesophagostomum* when administered as a powder in feed for several weeks (Goldsby and Todd 1957). It was recommended that it be fed at 12 g/ton to sows for 6 weeks prior to farrowing and during nursing, and to weaned pigs until market weight. It is no longer marketed in the United States.

REFERENCES

ANDERSEN, S.; JORGENSEN, R. J.; NANSEN, P. V.; AND NIELSEN, K. 1973. Experimental *Ascaris suum* infection in piglets. Inverse relationship between the numbers of inoculated eggs and the numbers of worms established in the intestine. Acta Pathol Microbiol Scand [B] 81:650–656.

APPERT, A., AND TARANCHON, P. 1969. Existence et fréquence en France de *Hyostrongylus rubidus* (Hassal et Stiles 1892) chez le porc. Bull Acad Vét 42:249–253.

BATTE, E. G. 1977. A review and update of swine parasite control. J Am Vet Med Assoc 170:343–344.

———. 1978. Evaluation of fenbendazole as a swine anthelmintic. Vet Med Small Anim Clin 73:1183–1186.

BATTE, E. G.; HARKEMA, R.; AND OSBORNE, J. C. 1960. Observations on the life cycle, and pathogenicity of the swine kidney worm (*Stephanurus dentatus*). J Am Vet Med Assoc 136:622–625.

BATTE, E. G.; MONCOL, D. J.; AND BARBER, C. W. 1966. Prenatal infection with the swine kidney worm (*Stephanurus dentatus*) and associated lesions. J Am Vet Med Assoc 149:758–765.

BATTE, E. G.; MCLAMB, R. D.; AND VESTAL, T. J. 1975. Swine parasites: Causes of liver condemnations. Vet Med Small Anim Clin 70:809–812.

BATTE, E. G.; MCLAMB, R. D.; MUSE, K. E.; TALLY, S. D.; AND VESTAL, T. J. 1977. Pathophysiology of swine trichuriasis. Am J Vet Res 38:1075–1079.

BECK, J. W., AND ANFINSON, T. A., JR. 1965. Some host responses of miniature pigs to infection with *Trichinella spiralis*. J Parasitol 51:60–62.

BEER, R. J. S. 1973. Studies on the biology of the life cycle of *Trichuris suis* Schrank 1788. Parasitology 67:253–262.

BEHLOW, R. F., AND BATTE, E. G. 1974. North Carolina Swine Parasite Control Program. Ext Folder 259. NC Agric Ext Serv, Raleigh.

BINDSEIL, E. 1970. Immunity to *Ascaris suum*. 3. The importance of the gut for immunity in mice. Acta Pathol Microbiol Scand [B] 78:183–190.

CAMPBELL, W. C. 1988. Trichinosis revisited—another

look at modes of transmission. Parasitol Today 4:83–86.

CONNAN, R. M. 1967. Observations on the epidemiology of parasitic gastroenteritis due to *Oesophagostomum* spp. and *Hyostrongylus rubidus* in the pig. Vet Rec 80:424–429.

CORWIN, R. M.; PRATT, S. E.; AND MUSER, R. K. 1984. Evaluation of fenbendazole as an extended anthelmintic treatment regimen for swine. J Am Vet Med Assoc 185:58–59.

DAVIDSON, J. B.; MURRAY, M.; AND SUTHERLAN, I. H. 1968. *Hyostrongylus rubidus:* A field study of its pathogenesis, diagnosis and treatment. Vet Rec 23:582–588.

DESPOMMIER, D. D. 1990. *Trichinella spiralis:* The worm that would be virus. Parasitol Today 6:193–196.

DEY-HAZRA, A.; KOLM, H. P.; ENIGK, K.; AND GIESE, W. 1972. Gastrointestinal loss of plasma proteins in *Hyostrongylus* infected pigs. Z Parasitenkd 38:14–20.

DOUVRES, F. W.; TROMBA, F. G.; AND MALAKATIS, G. M. 1969. Morphogenesis and migration of *Ascaris suum* larva developing to fourth stage in swine. J Parasitol 55:689–712.

ERIKSEN, L. 1982. Experimentally induced resistance to *Ascaris suum* in pigs. Nord Vet Med 34:177–187.

GAMBLE, H. R.; ANDERSON, W. R.; GRAHAM, C. E.; AND MURRELL, K. D. 1983. Diagnosis of swine trichinosis by enzyme-linked immunosorbent assay (ELISA) using an excretory-secretory antigen. Vet Parasitol 13:349–361.

GAMBLE, H. R.; MURRELL, K. D.; AND MARTI, H. P. 1986. Inoculation of pigs against *Trichinella spiralis*, using larval excretory-secretory antigens. Am J Vet Res 47:2396–2399.

GOLDSBY, A. I., AND TODD, A. C. 1957. Hygromycin, a broad-spectrum anthelmintic for swine. J Am Vet Med Assoc 131:471.

HALE, O. M., AND MARTI, O. G. 1983. Influence of an experimental infection of swine kidney worm (*Stephanurus dentatus*) on performance of pigs. J Anim Sci 56:616–620.

HALE, O. M.; STEWART, T. B.; AND MARTI, O. G. 1985. Influence of an experimental infection of *Ascaris suum* on performance of pigs. J Anim Sci 60:220–225.

HANBURY, R. D.; DOBY, P. B.; MILLER, H. O.; AND MURRELL, K. D. 1986. Trichinosis in a herd of swine: Cannibalism as a major mode of transmission. J Am Vet Med Assoc 188:1155–1159.

HASS, D. K.; BROWN, L. J.; AND YOUNG, R., JR. 1972. Infectivity of *Oesophagostomum dentatum* larvae in swine. Am J Vet Res 33:2527–2534.

HONER, M. R. 1967. The routine differentiation of the ova and larvae of two parasites of swine, *Hyostrongylus rubidus* (Hassall and Stiles 1892) and *Oesophagostomum dentatum* (Rud 1803). Z Parasitenkd 29:40.

JACOBS, D. E. 1969. Experimental infections of guinea pigs with *Oesophagostomum* spp. of porcine origin: Pathogenesis and parasitology of a single infection. In Pathology of Parasitic Diseases. Purdue Univ Studies, p. 231.

JACOBS, D. E., AND DUNN, A. M. 1968. The epidemiology of porcine oesophagostomiasis. Nord Vet Med 20:258–266.

JAMES, E. R. 1989. ICT7: The 1988 *Trichinella* Olympics. Parasitol Today 5:66–67.

JOHNSON, J. C., JR., STEWART, T. B.; AND HALE, O. M. 1975. Differential responses of Duroc, Hampshire, and cross-bred pigs to a superimposed experimental infection with the intestinal threadworm, *Strongyloides ransomi.* J Parasitol 61:517–524.

KAZACOS, K. R. 1986. Trichinosis. J Am Vet Med Assoc 188:1272–1275.

KENDALL, S. B.; THURLEY, D. C.; AND PEIRCE, M. A.

1969. The biology of *Hyostrongylus rubidus.* I. Primary infection in young pigs. J Comp Pathol 79:87–95.

KIM, W. C. 1983. Geographical distribution and prevalence. In Trichinella and Trichinosis. Ed. W. C. Campbell. New York: Plenum Press, pp. 445–500.

KNOWLES, C. O., AND CASSIDA, J. E. 1966. Mode of action of organophosphate anthelmintics. Cholinesterase inhibition in *Ascaris lumbricoides.* J Agric Food Chem 14:566.

LEIGH-BROWN, G., AND HARPUR, R. P. 1974. Repeated precise infection with adult *Ascaris suum* by per fistulam implantation in miniature swine. J Parasitol 60:298–301.

LEIGHTY, J. C. 1974. The role of meat inspection in preventing trichinosis in man. J Am Vet Med Assoc 165:994–995.

LEVINE, N. D. 1980. Nematode Parasites of Domestic Animals and of Man, 2d ed. Minneapolis, Minn.: Burgess Publishing Co. p. 477.

LICHTENFELS, J. R., AND TROMBA, F. G. 1972. The morphogenesis of *Stephanurus dentatus* (Nematoda: Strongylina) in swine with observations on larval migration. J Parasitol 58:757–766.

McCRACKEN, R. M., AND ROSS, J. G. 1970. The histopathology of *Oesophagostomum dentatum* infections in pigs. J Comp Pathol 80:619–623.

MacLEAN, J. P.; VIALLET, J.; LAW, C.; AND STAUDT, M. 1989. Trichinosis in the Canadian Arctic: Report of five outbreaks and a new clinical syndrome. J Infect Dis 160:513–520.

MONCOL, D. J. 1975. Supplement to the life history of *Strongyloides ransomi* Schwartz and Alicata, 1930 (Nematoda:Strongyloididae) of pigs. Proc Helminthol Soc Wash 42:86–92.

MURRELL, K. D. 1985. Strategies for the control of human trichinosis transmitted by pork. Food Technol 39:65–68, 110–111.

MURRELL, K. D., AND URBAN, J. F., JR. 1983. Induction of immunity by transcolostrally-passed *Strongyloides ransomi* larvae in neonatal pigs. J Parasitol 69:74–77.

MURRELL, K. D.; ANDERSON, W. R.; SCHAD, G. A.; HANBURY, R. D.; KAZACOS, K. R.; GAMBLE, H. R.; AND BROWN, J. 1986. Field evaluation of the enzyme-linked immunosorbent assay for swine trichinosis: Efficacy of the excretory-secretory antigen. Am J Vet Res 47:1046–1049.

OLIVER, D. G.; HANBURY, R. D.; AND VAN HOUWELING, C. D. 1985. Proc 89th Annu Meet US Anim Health Assoc, Milwaukee, Wisconsin.

PORTER, D. A. 1940. Experimental infections of swine with the red stomach worm, *Hyostrongylus rubidus.* Proc Helminthol Soc Wash 7:20–27.

PRESTON, K. S., AND SWITZER, W. P. 1976. Failure of lungworm-larvae-infected earthworms to transmit mycoplasmal pneumonia in swine. Vet Microbiol 1:15–18.

RAFFESPERGER, H. B., AND CONNELY, J. W. 1927. The swine sanitation system as developed by the Bureau of Animal Industry in McLean County, Ill. Tech Bull 44. US Dep Agric, Washington, D.C.

RAYNAUD, J-P; GRABER, M.; AND EUZÉBY, J. 1974. Experiments in the biology of 3 species of *Oesophagostomum: quadrispinulatum, granatensis* or *dentatum.* Attempts to validate those 3 species. Proc 3d Int Congr Pig Vet Soc, Lyons, Sec P, p. 5.

RHODES, M. B.; McCULLOUGH, R. A.; MEBUS, C. A.; KLUCAS, C. A.; FERGUSON, D. L.; AND TWIEHAUS, M. J. 1977. *Ascaris suum:* Hatching of embryonated eggs in swine. Exp Parasitol 42:356–362.

SCHAD, G. A.; LEIBY, D. A.; AND MURRELL, K. D. 1984. Distribution, prevalence and intensity of *Trichinella spiralis* infection in furbearing mammals of Pennsylvania. J Parasitol 70:372–377.

SCHAD, G. A.; LEIBY, D. A.; DUFFY, C. H.; AND MURRELL, K. D. 1985. Swine trichinosis in New England slaughterhouses. Am J Vet Res 46:2008–2010.

SCHOLTENS, R. G.; KAGAN, I. G.; QUIST, K. D.; AND NORMAN, L. G. 1966. An evaluation of tests of the diagnosis of trichinosis in swine and observations. Am J Epidemiol 83:489–500.

SCHWARTZ, B. 1959. Experimental infection of pigs with *Ascaris suum*. Am J Vet Res 20:7–13.

SMITH, H. J., AND HAWKES, A. B. 1978. Kidney worm infection in feral pigs in Canada with transmission to domestic swine. Can Vet J 19:30–43.

SOUTHERN, L. L.; STEWART, T. B.; BODAK-KOSZALKA, E.; LEON, D. L.; HOYT, P. G.; AND BESSETTE, M. E. 1989. Effect of fenbendazole and pyrantel tartrate on the induction of protective immunity in pigs naturally or experimentally infected with *Ascaris suum*. J Anim Sci 67:628–634.

SPINDLER, L. A. 1947. The effect of experimental infection with ascarids on the growth of pigs. Proc Helminthol Soc Wash 14:58–63.

STANKIEWICZ, M., AND JESKA, E. L. 1990. Evaluation of pyrantel-tartrate abbreviated *Ascaris suum* infections for development of resistance in young pigs against migrating larvae. Int J Parasitol 20:77–81.

STEWART, T. B., AND GASBARRE, L. C. 1989. The veterinary importance of nodular worms (*Oesophagostomum* spp.). Parasitol Today 5:209–213.

STEWART, T. B., AND HALE, O. M. 1988. Losses to internal parasites in swine production. J Anim Sci 66:1548–1554.

STEWART, T. B., AND ROWELL, T. J. 1986. Susceptibility of fourth-stage *Ascaris suum* larvae to fenbendazole and to host response in the pig. Am J Vet Res 47:1671–1673.

STEWART, T. B.; HALE, O. M.; AND ANDREWS, J. S. 1964. Eradication of the swine kidney worm, *Stephanurus dentatus,* from experimental pastures by herd management. Am J Vet Res 25:1141–1150.

STEWART, T. B.; SCHROEDER, W. F.; SHALKOP, W. T.; AND STONE, W. M. 1968. Strongyloidosis: Natural infection of suckling pigs with *Strongyloides ransomi.* Vet Med Small Anim Clin 63:1145–1150.

STEWART, T. B.; STONE, W. M.; AND MARTI, O. G. 1976. *Strongyloides ransomi:* Prenatal and transmammary infection of pigs of sequential litters from dams experimentally exposed as weanlings. Am J Vet Res 37:541–544.

STEWART, T. B.; BATTE, E. G.; CONNELL, H. E.; CORWIN, R. M.; FERGUSON, D. L.; GAMBLE, H. R.; MURRELL, K. D.; PRESTWOOD, A. K.; STUART, B. P.; TROMBA, F. G.; AND WHEAT, B. E. 1985a. Research needs and priorities for swine internal parasites in the United States. Am J Vet Res 46:1029–1033.

STEWART, T. B.; HALE, O. M.; AND MARTI, O. G. 1985b. Experimental infections with *Hyostrongylus rubidus* and the effects of performance of growing pigs. Vet Parasitol 17:219–227.

STEWART, T. B.; SOUTHERN, L. L.; GIBSON, R. B.; AND SIMMONS, L. A. 1985c. Immunization of pigs against *Ascaris suum* by sequential experimental infections terminated with fenbendazole during larval migration. Vet Parasitol 17:319–326.

STOCKDALE, P. H. G. 1974. Pathogenesis of *Hyostrongy-*

lus rubidus in growing pigs. Br Vet J 130:366–373.

STOCKDALE, P. H. G.; ASHTON, G. K.; HOWES, M. A.; AND EWERT, E. 1973. Hyostrongylosis in Ontario. Can Vet J 14:265–268.

STONE, W. M. 1964. *Strongyloides ransomi* prenatal infection in swine. J Parasitol 50:568.

STONE, W. M., AND SIMPSON, C. F. 1967. Larval distribution and histopathology of experimental *Strongyloides ransomi* infection in young swine. Can J Comp Med Vet Sci 31:197–202.

TAFFS, L. F. 1966. Helminths in the pig. Vet Rec 79:671.

TROMBA, F. G. 1955. The role of the earthworm, *Eisenia foetida,* in the transmission of *Stephanurus dentatus.* J Parasitol 41:157–161.

UNDERDAHL, N. R. 1958. The affect of *Ascaris suum* migration on the severity of swine influenza. J Am Vet Med Assoc 133:380–383.

UNDERDAHL, N. R., AND KELLEY, G. W. 1957. The enhancement of virus pneumonia of pigs by the migration of *Ascaris suum* larvae. J Am Vet Med Assoc 130:173–176.

U.S. Dep. Health and Human Services. 1976. Public Health Services, Centers for Disease Control, Atlanta, Georgia. Morb Mortal Wkly Rep 25:393.

———. 1982. Public Health Services, Centers for Disease Control, Atlanta, Georgia. Morb Mortal Wkly Rep 31:61.

———. 1988. Public Health Services, Centers for Disease Control, Atlanta, Georgia. Morb Mortal Wkly Rep 37:1–8.

URBAN, J. F., JR.; ALIZADEH, H.; AND ROMANOWSKI, R. 1984. Acquired gut immunity to the large roundworm (*Ascaris suum*) of swine. Proc Int Pig Vet Soc 8:200.

URBAN, J. F., JR.; ALIZADEH, H. A.; AND ROMANOWSKI, R. D. 1988. *Ascaris suum:* Development of intestinal immunity to infective second-stage larvae in swine. Exp Parasitol 66:66.

URBAN, J. F., JR.; ROMANOWSKI, R. D.; AND STEELE, N. C. 1989. Influence of helminth parasite exposure and strategic application of anthelmintics on the development of immunity and growth of swine. J Anim Sci 67:1668–1677.

WADDELL, A. H. 1969. The parasitic life cycle of the swine kidney worm *Stephanurus dentatus.* Diesing Aust Vet J Zool 17:607–618.

WRIGHT, K. A. 1979. *Trichinella spiralis:* An intracellular parasite in the intestinal phase. J Parasitol 65:441–445.

ZIMMERMAN, D. R.; SPEAR, M. L.; AND SWITZER, W. P. 1973. Effect of *Mycoplasma hyopneumoniae* infection, pyrantel treatment and protein nutrition on performance of pigs exposed to soil containing *Ascaris suum* ova. J Anim Sci 36:894–897.

ZIMMERMAN, W. J. 1967. A pooled sample method for post slaughter detection of trichiniasis in swine. Proc US Livest Sanit Assoc 72:358–366.

ZIMMERMAN, W. J., AND ZINTER, D. E. 1971. The prevalence of trichinosis in swine in the United States, 1966–70. Health Serv Mental Health Adm Health Rep 86:937–945.

ZIMMERMAN, W. J.; HUBBARD, E. D.; SCHWARTE, L. H.; AND BIESTER, H. E. 1962. Trichinosis in Iowa swine with further studies on modes of transmission. Cornell Vet 52:156–163.

59 Mycotoxins

G. D. Osweiler

OCCURRENCE OF MYCOTOXINS IN GRAINS AND FEEDS. Mycotoxins are chemicals produced by mold growth in grains or forages. Mold growth results from a variety of plant and environmental factors affecting the ability of fungi to invade and colonize plant parts. Most susceptible are the feed grains such as corn, wheat, and milo as well as cottonseed. Basic needs for fungal growth in grains include a proper substrate, usually a readily available carbohydrate, and adequate moisture and oxygen to support growth. In addition, temperatures ranging from somewhat below freezing up to approximately 50°C will support mold growth, although optimal temperatures are often 12–25°C (Carson 1986). An appropriate combination of conditions may allow proliferation and metabolism of fungus resulting in production of a mycotoxin (Richard and Cole 1989).

Mycotoxins are defined as secondary metabolites of mold growth, and their occurrence is influenced by factors of the plant, environment, and fungus. Secondary metabolites are generally believed to be produced in response to stress factors acting on the fungus. Different strains of a toxigenic fungus can vary in virulence, growth rate, competitiveness, ability to produce toxins, and type and quantity of toxin produced. Water stress, high-temperature stress, insect damage, and reduced plant vigor often predispose crop plants to infestation, colonization, and contamination by toxigenic fungi and are major determinants in mold infestation and toxin production (Richard and Cole 1989). In many instances, environmental and stress factors are used by plant pathologists to predict mold infestations and probable mycotoxin production.

Although presence of a specific fungal infestation correlated with environmental conditions conducive to mycotoxin formation may be suggestive of a problem, simple visual or cultural examination of grain or feed cannot be used to determine safety for animals. Many toxigenic strains of molds can occur in grains without the production of mycotoxins. There is little correlation between spore counts and presence of known mycotoxins. Conversely, absence of molds does not mean that a feed is safe from mycotoxins. High temperature and pressure during milling may reduce fungal populations so that mold growth is not apparent. However, common mycotoxins are resistant to the temperatures that kill molds and may persist in feeds when there is no evidence of fungal contamination (Osweiler et al. 1985).

Field fungi grow in crops prior to harvest. Those generally recognized as a source of common mycotoxins are in the genus *Fusarium*. Fusaria require high relative humidity (>90%) and grain moisture (>23%) for growth. Field fungi often cause death of ovules, shriveling of seeds or kernels, and weakening or death of embryos. The grading term for this effect is "weathering." They rarely grow after harvest because storage to prevent spoilage precludes these conditions, and growth and toxin production appears not to occur if dry grain is remoistened (Christensen and Kaufmann 1965). In recent years, *Aspergillus flavus,* normally considered a storage fungus, has produced significant concentrations of aflatoxin in crops prior to harvest.

Storage fungi include the genera *Aspergillus* and *Penicillium,* which account for several mycotoxins important in swine production. These fungi may grow and produce mycotoxins even when moisture content ranges from 14 to 18% and at temperatures that vary from 10 to 50°C.

Mycotoxins have traditionally been considered to occur sporadically both seasonally and geographically (Pier 1981). Certain geographic regions are considered at high risk for specific mycotoxins. This regional predilection may be strongly influenced, however, by local conditions such as early frost, drought, and insect damage. In addition, movement of grains and finished feeds long distances, as well as blending of grains, damage in transit, and improper storage can obscure regional differences.

INTOXICATION BY MYCOTOXINS. Several circumstances may increase the chance of intoxication by mycotoxins. Higher concentrations are found in damaged, light, or broken grain such as occur in screenings. When screenings are fed on the farm or sold locally at harvest time, there may be increased exposure to high concentrations of mycotoxins; grain producers who also have a farrowing operation may give lower-quality grain to sows for short periods of time during harvest. Grain that is slightly above optimum moisture for storage may continue to respire and produce water; eventually a portion of the storage bin will

735

achieve free-moisture levels supportive of mold growth and toxin production. Alternating warm and cool temperatures during fall and spring may favor moisture migration and condensation within a storage bin. Each time a fungal-contaminated grain is cracked or ground the protective seed coat is broken and the grain is susceptible to molding. Feed stored in warm, humid conditions such as a nursery may mold and produce mycotoxins within only a few days.

Dietary deficiencies of protein as well as selenium and vitamins have been implicated as predisposing factors in mycotoxicosis. Drugs that reduce or enhance foreign-compound metabolism could influence response to mycotoxins, since most common mycotoxins are metabolized to intermediate or final products that are different in toxicity from the parent mycotoxin (Osweiler et al. 1985; Beasley et al. 1986).

Combinations of mycotoxins may potentiate the action of one another, or at least exert an additive effect. One example of this is the combination of aflatoxin and ochratoxin (Huff et al. 1988; Harvey et al. 1989c). Currently there is little information on the effects of common mycotoxins acting together. Fortunately, conditions for production of several mycotoxins concurrently in the same grain appear relatively uncommon.

Mycotoxins may alter immune function. Aflatoxins, some trichothecenes, and ochratoxin A have been demonstrated to be immunosuppressive in domestic or laboratory animals. Common diseases influenced by aflatoxin under experimental conditions include swine erysipelas, swine dysentery, and salmonellosis. Generally, immunosuppressive effects of aflatoxins and trichothecenes are seen at concentrations that cause subtle or chronic changes characteristic of the mycotoxin. Because the interaction is usually expressed as the infectious disease, mycotoxin-facilitated disease is difficult to detect or confirm. Normal immune function is expected to return after exposure to toxin is ended (Pier 1981; Panangala et al. 1986; Richard and Cole 1989).

Effects of Mycotoxins. Swine are susceptible to the basic mechanisms of action of mycotoxins. An appreciation of these mechanisms is important to the understanding of subtle clinical effects of mycotoxins and those metabolic, endocrine, and nutritional interactions that impact swine health and productivity.

Carbohydrate metabolism is altered by aflatoxins, ochratoxin A, and rubratoxin B. There is decreased activity of glycogenic enzymes and increased activity of enzymes that deplete glycogen precursors, resulting in reduced incorporation of glucose into glycogen. Inhibition of mitochondrial enzymes in the tricarboxylic acid cycle results in reduced oxygen consumption and altered adenosine diphosphate to oxygen ratios. Electron transport is inhibited and oxidative phosphorylation may be uncoupled (Hsieh 1979).

Trichothecenes and aflatoxin alter nucleic acid function and protein biosynthesis. Aflatoxin modifies the DNA template and inhibits RNA polymerase thus reducing transcription. Increased RNA destruction is associated with altered lysosomal membranes and release of ribonuclease from lysosomes. Trichothecenes inhibit protein synthesis by binding to ribosomal subunits and inhibiting peptidyl transferase. Aflatoxin inhibits protein formation by depressing messenger RNA synthesis (McLaughlin et al. 1977; Hsieh 1979).

Endocrine and neurohumoral changes induced by mycotoxins may significantly affect productivity without causing traditional disease or lesions in swine. Zearalenone and ergot alkaloids exert profound endocrine and hormonal changes that alter the reproductive cycle of gilts and sows (Whitacre and Threlfall 1981; Edwards et al. 1987). Trichothecenes such as T-2 and deoxynivalenol may cause imbalances of brain neurotransmitters and affect appetite and feed intake (MacDonald et al. 1988).

CLINICAL MYCOTOXICOSES. Clinical response of swine to mycotoxins may be acute, subacute, or chronic and is both dose and time dependent, similar to other chemical toxins. For known mycotoxins of clinical importance, response is usually subacute or chronic and the presenting signs are often subtle and vague. Many times problems are only expressed as alterations of the reproductive cycle, reduced feed intake, slow growth, or impaired feed efficiency. Nevertheless, an understanding of the range of effects for specific mycotoxins is important in differential diagnosis and evaluation of clinical prognosis for mycotoxin diseases. Common mycotoxins affecting swine are summarized in Table 59.1.

Aflatoxins. *Aspergillus flavus* and *A. parasiticus* produce aflatoxins in grains and oilseeds in storage and occasionally before harvest. While many areas of North America have conditions supportive of aflatoxin production, the southeastern United States often have conditions leading to aflatoxin production (Richard and Cole 1989).

Aflatoxins B_1, B_2, G_1, and G_2 occur in grains; when metabolized by mammals they occur in milk or urine as aflatoxin M_1. Aflatoxin B_1 is the most abundant and most toxic fraction under natural contamination (Jelinik et al. 1989; Richard and Cole 1989).

Aflatoxin B_1 is metabolized by liver microsomal mixed-function oxidases to form at least seven metabolites. The major metabolite of aflatoxin is an epoxide, which binds covalently to nucleic acids and proteins and is believed responsible for causing hepatic cancer as well as toxic signs and lesions. Impairment of protein synthesis and related ability to mobilize fats result in characteristic early lesions of hepatic fatty change and necro-

Table 59.1. Clinical guide to mycotoxins in swine

Toxin	Category of Swine	Dietary Level[a]	Clinical Effects
Aflatoxins	Growing/finishing	<100 ppb	No clinical effect; residues in liver
		200–400 ppb	Reduced growth and feed efficiency; possible immunosuppression
		400–800 ppb	Microscopic liver lesions, cholangiohepatitis; increased serum liver enzymes; immunosuppression
		800–1200 ppb	Reduced growth; decreased feed consumption; rough hair coat; icterus; hypoproteinemia
		1200–2000 ppb	Icterus; coagulopathy; depression; anorexia; some deaths
		>2000 ppb	Acute hepatosis and coagulopathy; deaths in 3–10 days
	Brood sows/gilts	500–750 ppb	No effect on conception; deliver normal piglets that grow slowly due to aflatoxin in milk
Ochratoxin and citrinin	Finishing	200 ppb	Mild renal lesions seen at slaughter; reduced weight gain
		1000 ppb	Polydipsia; reduced growth; azotemia and glycosuria
		4000 ppb	Polyuria and polydipsia
	Sows/gilts	3-9 ppm	Normal pregnancy when fed first month
Trichothecenes T-2 toxin and DAS	Growing/finishing		
		1 ppm	No effect
		3 ppm	Decreased feed consumption
		10 ppm	Decreased feed consumption; oral/dermal irritation; immunosuppression
		20 ppm	Complete refusal, vomiting
Deoxynivalenol		1 ppm	No clinical effect, minimal reduction in feed consumption
		5–10 ppm	25–50% reduction in feed consumption
		20 ppm	Complete refusal
Zearalenone F-2 toxin	Prepuberal gilts	1–3 ppm	Estrogenic; vulvovaginitis, prolapse
	Cycling sows/gilts	3–10 ppm	Retained corpora lutea, anestrus, pseudopregnancy
	Pregnant sows	>30 ppm	Early embryonic death when fed 1–3 weeks postmating
Ergot	All swine	0.1%[b]	Reduced gain
	Sows, last trimester	0.3%	Reduced piglet birth weight; agalactia
	All swine	0.3%	Gangrene
	All swine	3.0%	Decreased feed consumption
Fumonisins	All swine	50–100 ppm (estimated)	Acute pulmonary edema; hepatosis; impaired lymphoblastogenesis; decreased feed consumption

[a]Estimated toxic concentrations are based on literature values and the author's experiences.
[b]Concentration of ergot sclerotia in diet.

sis, as well as reduced growth rate. Animals on protein-deficient diets are more susceptible to aflatoxin, and increased dietary protein will protect against aflatoxin effects on weight gain (Osweiler et al. 1985; Coffey et al. 1989).

Toxicity of aflatoxin is both time and dose related, and age is an important factor in susceptibility. Young swine are more susceptible to afla-

toxins than are finishing hogs or adults. Exposure to low or moderate concentrations in feed for a period of several weeks is a common circumstance of exposure. Acute toxicosis is uncommon. The single oral dose LD50 for swine is 0.62 mg/kg body weight; dietary levels of 2–4 ppm are associated with acute fatal toxicosis, while rations containing 260 ppb for several weeks were associated only with reduced growth rate (Carson 1986). Combined evidence from experimental reports, field cases, and the author's personal experience indicate that concentrations of naturally occurring aflatoxins above 300 ppb fed for a period of several weeks will likely cause reduced growth and feed efficiency. The threshold dose for clinical signs varies widely, but subtle effects could be expected at concentrations above 600 ppb. Liver lesions are reported to be caused by concentrations as low as 140 ppb fed for 12 weeks in 18- to 64-kg swine, while 690 ppb was associated with mild liver lesions in 64- to 91-kg finishing hogs (Allcroft 1969). In the author's experience, prolonged feeding of aflatoxin at concentrations above 400 ppb could cause microscopic liver lesions.

In acute to subacute toxicosis, affected animals are depressed and anorectic. Anemia, ascites, icterus, and hemorrhagic diarrhea may develop. Coagulopathy characterized by hypoprothrombinemia may occur. Several enzymes associated with hepatocellular damage are elevated, including aspartate aminotransferase, alanine aminotransferase, alkaline phosphatase, and gammaglutamyltransferase. Other serum clinical chemistry changes observed have been decreases in serum total iron-binding capacity, total protein, albumin, cholesterol, blood urea nitrogen, and glucose (Harvey et al. 1989a). Total bilirubin, icterus index, sulfobromophthalein clearance, prothrombin time, and partial thromboplastin time are also elevated in clinical aflatoxicosis (Osweiler et al. 1985; Panangala et al. 1986).

Gross lesions associated with porcine aflatoxicosis include pale tan or clay-colored liver with centrilobular hemorrhages, subserosal petechial to ecchymotic hemorrhages, and intestinal and colonic hemorrhages. As the course of aflatoxicosis progresses, liver becomes yellow and fibrosis develops, characterized by firm, hard liver with accentuated lobular pattern. The yellow discoloration of icterus occurs at serosal and mucosal surfaces (Cook et al. 1989; Harvey et al. 1989b).

Microscopic alterations are useful for diagnostic confirmation and generally include hepatocyte vacuolization, necrosis, and fatty change, which is more predominant around central veins. As disease progresses to subacute or chronic, hepatomegalocytosis, including multiple nuclei, are seen. Interlobular fibrosis and characteristic biliary hyperplasia develop in chronic cases (Osweiler et al. 1985; Harvey et al. 1988). Full evaluation and diagnosis of aflatoxicosis should include a search for the characteristic lesions.

Significant reproductive effects of aflatoxin in swine have not been documented. Sows fed aflatoxin have maintained normal reproduction through four successive gestations; sows fed aflatoxin at dietary concentrations of 500 and 700 ppb had normal pregnancies and litters, but piglets nursing these sows had reduced growth

rate due to aflatoxin excretion in the milk (Armbrecht et al. 1972; McKnight et al. 1983).

Residues of aflatoxin M_1 occur in tissues, milk, and urine of swine, but are not persistent. Concentrations of 400 ppm in the diet resulted in tissue residues of 0.05 ppb or less and these rapidly disappeared when aflatoxin feeding stopped (Trucksess et al. 1982).

Diagnosis of aflatoxicosis should be considered when acute icterus, hemorrhages, or coagulopathy are not explained by other causes. Chronic signs of slow growth, malnutrition, and persistent low-grade infectious diseases should also suggest investigation for aflatoxicosis. Characteristic liver lesions and clinical chemistry changes would strongly suggest aflatoxicosis. Chemical analysis of the ration and grain supply may identify aflatoxin, but sometimes the grain that initiated a chronic problem is no longer available or representative. Any grain sampling should be representative (see **PREVENTION AND MANAGEMENT OF MOLD AND MYCOTOXIN PROBLEMS** for sampling procedure).

Aflatoxicosis is generally a herd problem and not amenable to individual animal treatment. Specific practical antidotes for affected animals are not available. Work in poultry has shown some benefit from increased dietary selenium. Increased dietary levels of high-quality protein and supplementation with vitamins (A, D, E, K, and B complex) are recommended (Coppock and Swanson 1986; Coffey et al. 1989). Hydrated sodium calcium aluminosilicate (HSCAS) at 0.5% in the diet provided substantial protection against loss of gain and occurrence of lesions induced by dietary aflatoxin in swine (Harvey et al. 1989a). Treatment of grain with anhydrous ammonia for 10–14 days has reduced aflatoxin concentration in grain. Swine accepted ammoniated grain and their growth was comparable to the group fed untreated control grain. Presently, this method of treatment has not been cleared by the U.S. Food and Drug Administration.

Since aflatoxin may compromise the immune system, animals with concurrent infectious diseases should be aggressively treated with appropriate antimicrobial therapy and passive immunization if appropriate.

Ochratoxin and Citrinin. Ochratoxin is a fungal nephrotoxin produced by *Aspergillus ochraceus* and *Penicillium viridicatum*. Citrinin, also a nephrotoxin, is produced by *P. citrinum.* Based on clinical and pathologic effects in swine, both toxins can be considered together. Toxins are associated with corn, barley, rye, and wheat, most commonly from northern Europe, Canada, and the northern United States. Significant concentrations of ochratoxin can occur at temperatures as low as 4°C. Ochratoxin A has been prevalent in Denmark and is associated with the feeding of barley and oats (Carlton and Krogh 1979; Carson

1986). In the United States, at least one case has been documented in swine fed contaminated corn (Cook et al. 1986).

Ochratoxin A at 1 mg/kg body weight is lethal in 5–6 days. Concentrations of 1 ppm in the diet for 3 months caused polydipsia, polyuria, reduced growth, and lowered feed efficiency. Levels as low as 200 ppb for several weeks will induce detectable renal lesions (Carson 1986). Additional clinical signs are diarrhea, anorexia, and dehydration. Sometimes no clinical signs are noted and the only effect observed is the appearance of pale, firm kidneys at slaughter, commonly associated with ochratoxin in endemic areas such as Denmark or Sweden.

Clinical pathology changes include increases in blood urea nitrogen, plasma protein, packed-cell volume, aspartate aminotransferase, and isocitric dehydrogenase, as well as increased urinary glucose and protein. Citrinin, ochratoxin, and penicillic acid are synergistic and primarily produce nephroses characterized by necrosis of the proximal convoluted tubules followed by interstitial fibrosis. Liver damage, characterized by fatty change and necrosis, may be present but is less severe than for other primary hepatoses. Gastric ulceration is a characteristic and consistent lesion in prolonged clinical cases (Szczech et al. 1973; Carlton and Krogh 1979).

Diagnosis should include demonstration of the toxin and/or its metabolite, ochratoxin alpha, in feed or fresh kidney. The approximate half-life for ochratoxin A in swine tissue is 3–5 days, and little or no ochratoxin can be found in kidneys 30 days after ochratoxin exposure ceases (Carlton and Krogh 1979). Mildly affected animals may recover if removed promptly from the contaminated feed. However, if the clinical course is prolonged, recovery is slow.

Trichothecenes. The trichothecenes include at least 148 structurally related compounds. Those of known veterinary importance are produced by *Fusaria,* especially *F. graminearum* and *F. sporotrichioides.* This group of sesquiterpene toxins has an epoxide group that is responsible for most toxic effects. The three receiving most attention in North America are T-2 toxin, diacetoxyscirpenol (DAS), and deoxynivalenol (DON, vomitoxin). Even though much work has been done with T-2 and DAS in swine, there is little evidence that these two agents occur at toxic concentrations more than occasionally in North American grains. They are well known to cause direct skin irritation and necrosis, profound lymphoid depletion, gastroenteritis, diarrhea, shock, cardiovascular failure, and death from experimental direct dosing. Chronic administration causes hematopoietic suppression and eventual pancytopenia. In addition, they are strong immunosuppressants (Coppock et al. 1985; Beasley 1986; Lundeen et al. 1986). Although T-2 and DAS are potent toxins,

their strong tendency to induce feed refusal and/or vomiting in swine makes them somewhat self-limiting as toxins, except as potential causes of reduced feed consumption.

Vomitoxin has great economic importance in North America because it is established as a common mycotoxin of corn and wheat and is well documented as a cause of feed refusal or reduced feed intake in swine (Trenholm et al. 1984). Swine will begin to reduce voluntary feed consumption at concentrations of vomitoxin of 1 ppm or more, and feed refusal may be complete at concentrations in excess of 10 ppm (Young et al. 1983; Pollman et al. 1985). Vomitoxin in corn occurs at low levels during some harvest seasons with an incidence as high as 50%. Available studies have demonstrated only feed refusal. Any concurrent health effects in swine have been consistent with effects of reduced nutrient intake (Lun et al. 1985). Recent work has shown that vomitoxin in swine causes conditioned taste aversion, meaning that flavoring agents will be ineffective in inducing swine to consume contaminated grain (Osweiler et al. 1990). Others have shown that T-2 toxin, closely related to vomitoxin, may affect brain neurotransmitters, such as serotonin or dopamine, contributing to feed refusal and lethargy (MacDonald et al. 1988).

Diagnosis of mycotoxin-related feed refusal presents a difficult problem to the clinician. Other toxins, drugs, concurrent disease, inclement weather, and reduced water intake may contribute to feed refusal. Often the vomitoxin concentration detected chemically is insufficient to fully explain feed refusal. One should remember that feed concentrations are approximations, that sampling is never completely representative, and that many factors in the herd and environment may not be apparent to either the clinician or producer.

Zearalenone (F-2 Toxin). *Fusarium graminearum* (*F. roseum*) produces zearalenone, an estrogenic mycotoxin in corn, milo, and wheat. High moisture (23–25%) is required for growth. Poorly dried ear corn and alternating high and low ambient temperatures favor zearalenone production (Christensen and Kaufman 1965). Often it is produced in the field prior to harvest. Zearalenone is a substituted resorcyclic acid lactone similar in structure to the anabolic agent zearanol used in cattle. Zearalenone is an estrogen and will cause hypertrophy of the uterus and cornification of vaginal epithelium.

Clinical signs vary with age of swine exposed. In prepuberal gilts, concentrations as low as 1–5 ppm in the ration cause vulvovaginitis characterized by tumescence and edema of the vulva and vagina and precocious mammary development. Tenesmus is common, occasionally with resultant rectal prolapses (Carson 1986). Prepuberal gilts fed as little zearalenone as 2 ppm for up to 90 days attained normal sexual maturity with no adverse effects on subsequent reproductive function (Green et al. 1990; Rainey et al. 1990).

Reproductive effects of zearalenone on mature cycling sows are quite different than the effects seen in prepuberal gilts. As with other estrogens, zearalenone is luteotropic in swine, and dietary concentrations of 3–10 ppm can induce anestrus in sows, if consumed during the middle portion of the estrous cycle. Since estrogens are luteotropic in swine, the probability of abortion in the last two trimesters of gestation appears very unlikely. Anestrus and elevated serum progesterone persist for several months, long after exposure to zearalenone has stopped (Edwards et al. 1987). Fewer pigs per litter are seen in sows given zearalenone. The susceptible period for reduced litter size appears to be in the preimplantation stage during days 7–10 postmating, and viability of individual embryos is apparently not maintained beyond 21 days (Long et al. 1983; Diekman and Long 1989). Piglets born to sows receiving zearalenone may have enlarged external genitalia and uteri. Zearalenone and its metabolites, alpha and beta zearalenol, are present in milk of exposed sows and may contribute to estrogenic effects in piglets (Palyusik et al. 1980).

Preputial enlargement may occur in boars exposed to zearalenone. Young boars may have reduced libido and decreased testicular size, but mature boars are unaffected by concentrations of zearalenone as high as 200 ppm (Ruhr et al. 1983; Young and King 1983).

Differential diagnosis of zearalenone toxicosis should include estrogenic feed additives and natural estrogens such as coumestrol in mature alfalfa. Suspect rations or corn should first be analyzed for presence of zearalenone, then for other estrogens. Feed samples available at the time of anestrus or return to service may not represent the contaminated feed that initiated the problem.

Treatment of zearalenone depends on the nature of the effect and the age and reproductive status of swine. Removal of the feed from prepuberal gilts will allow regression of signs within 3–7 days. Medical and surgical treatment of vaginal and rectal prolapse may be necessary. For mature, nongravid sows with anestrus, administration of one 10-mg dose of prostaglandin $F_{2\alpha}$ or two 5-mg doses on successive days is useful in eliminating retained corpora lutea (Day 1982, personal communication). Dehydrated alfalfa has experimentally shown some protection from zearalenone-induced enlargement of the uterus of gilts (James and Smith 1982).

Ergot. Ergot, *Claviceps purpurea,* is a parasitic fungus that affects cereal grains, especially rye, oats, and wheat. The fungus invades the grass ovary, forming a dark, elongated body called a sclerotium. The toxic alkaloids may affect animals and humans in various ways but commonly cause gangrene and reproductive interference. Major toxic alkaloids include ergotamine, ergotoxine, and ergometrine; total ergot alkaloid content commonly ranges from 0.2 to 0.6% of sclerotia weight. USDA has set a tolerance of 0.3% ergot in grain (Christensen and Kaufmann 1965; Carson 1986).

Gangrenous ergotism is the result of a combination of vasoconstriction and endothelial damage, leading to prolonged ischemia of appendages and eventually gangrene. Because venous and lymphatic drainage remains intact, the gangrene is "dry" in nature. Signs occur over a period of days or weeks and include depression, reduced feed intake, rapid pulse and respiration, and general unthriftiness. Lameness may occur, most commonly in rear limbs, and in advanced cases necrosis and sloughing of the tail, ears, and hooves can occur. Signs may be exacerbated by cold weather.

Ergot alkaloids affect reproduction indirectly by causing agalactia. Pregnant gilts fed either 0.3% or 1% sclerotia during gestation had low piglet birth weights, low piglet survival, and poor piglet weight gains. Agalactia occurred in 50% of gilts fed 0.3% sclerotia in the gestation and lactation rations (Nordskog and Clark 1945; Wiernusz and Schneider 1984). The agalactia induced is noninflammatory and results from the well-known ability of ergot to inhibit prolactin release in late gestation (Whitacre and Threlfall 1981). Both experimental and clinical evidence indicates that ergot in rations of pregnant sows is not generally a cause of abortion, and swine exposed to ergot during late gestation routinely suffer agalactia but rarely abortion (Osweiler et al. 1985).

As little as 0.1% ergot in the ration of feeder pigs is associated with reduced weight gain. Higher levels (3.0%) have been implicated in feed wastage and slow growth (Roers et al. 1974).

Differential diagnosis should include zearalenone or other estrogenic factors, bacterial infections, and mastitis-metritis-agalactia syndrome. If the clinical signs suggest ergotism, grains should be examined for the presence of significant amounts of ergot sclerotia. In the case of ground or processed feeds, feed microscopy or chemical analysis for ergot alkaloids may be necessary to confirm the diagnosis.

Treatment of ergotism is general and supportive. Gangrenous areas should be cleaned and treated locally and secondary infections controlled with broad-spectrum antibiotics. Removal of the feed is followed by improvement within 2 weeks for gangrenous effects. When agalactia has occurred, milk production returns 3–7 days after feed is changed. In the interim, supplemental nutrition and milk replacers may be used to save the piglets.

Fumonisins. Recently, a class of mycotoxins produced by *Fusarium moniliforme* has been recognized (Gelderblom et al. 1988). The principal toxins, fumonisin B$_1$ and fumonisin B$_2$, are linear hydrocarbon chains substituted with alcohols and an amine. A clinical syndrome of acute pulmonary edema has been associated with and experimentally reproduced by feeding corn screenings heavily contaminated with fumonisins and infected only with *F. moniliforme*. An epizootic of this condition occurred primarily in the midwestern United States in 1989. Clinical features included acute onset of labored breathing, cyanosis, and weakness commencing from 4 to 10 days after initial consumption of contaminated grain. Morbidity ranged from 5 to 50% and mortality was from 50 to 90%. Clinical course from onset to death was typically 1–2 days. Pregnant sows that recovered aborted 2–3 days later. Gross lesions at postmortem included cyanosis, hydrothorax, and extensive diffuse pulmonary edema, which was primarily interstitial. Interlobular pulmonary edema was a prominent lesion. Microscopically there was severe subpleural and interlobular edema. Some pigs that survived the acute pulmonary edema syndrome experienced subacute hepatotoxicosis with elevated hepatic enzymes and bilirubin in serum. Gross lesions were icterus of the mucosal and serosal surfaces and orange- to yellow-colored livers. Microscopically, affected livers had individual hepatocellular necrosis, hepatomegalocytosis, and increased numbers of mitotic figures (Harrison et al. 1990; Osweiler 1990).

Presently the toxic dose and pathogenesis of this condition are under investigation.

PREVENTION AND MANAGEMENT OF MOLD AND MYCOTOXIN PROBLEMS.
When mycotoxicosis occurs or is suspected, the first action should be to change the source of feed. This may be beneficial, even when a specific mycotoxin cannot be identified. A thorough inspection of the grain storage bins, mixing equipment, and feeders may reveal caking, molding, or musty odors. All contaminated feed should be removed and the equipment cleaned. Additionally, walls and containers should be washed with a dilute solution of hypochlorite (laundry bleach) to reduce contaminating fungi. All equipment should be completely dry before fresh feed is added.

Any suspect feed should be analyzed to determine if known mycotoxins were present. Although spore counts or fungal cultures alone do not confirm a diagnosis, they may give some indication of the potential for mycotoxin production. With this information, the swine producer can better formulate a preventive program.

If storage conditions are adverse or if grain moisture is too high, use of a mold inhibitor may be advisable. Most commercial mold inhibitors are based on an organic acid such as propionic acid and are effective in reducing or delaying mold growth. Mold inhibitors do not destroy preformed toxins, which commonly may have formed in the field prior to harvest. Except for ammoniation (not yet approved by FDA) to destroy aflatoxin, there are no practical commercial treatments that effectively destroy preformed mycotoxins.

Dilution of contaminated grain with clean grain is commonly used to reduce mycotoxin effects; this is not an approved procedure for aflatoxin. For any mycotoxin problem, dilution may reduce exposure initially, but care must be taken that wet or contaminated grain does not introduce new fungi and conditions that eventually lead to the entire mixture being contaminated.

Mycotoxin contamination may not be suspected until most or all of a contaminated feed is consumed. A prudent practice is to save a representative sample of all grains and feeds purchased and hold them in stable condition until swine are marketed or at least a month past when the feed was consumed. When questions about feed quality arise later, these samples may be valuable in documenting if specific feeds were involved in a problem.

Sampling feeds or grain should be representative of the entire supply. Representative sampling can best be done after feed is ground and mixed by passing a cup through the moving auger stream at frequent intervals, mixing these samples thoroughly, and saving a 4.5-kg (10-pound) sample for analysis (Davis et al. 1980). Alternatively, probe sampling of large bins may give some idea of contamination levels. Bins should be probed in at least 6–10 perimeter locations and 2–4 central locations for each 1.8 m (6 feet) of bin height. High-moisture samples should be either dried to 12% moisture or stored frozen. Long-term storage is recommended in paper bags permanently marked with the date and source of the feed or grain, and samples should be held in a dry, clean location.

Mycotoxins present formidable challenges to the swine producer and veterinarian. Diagnosis is sometimes difficult and effective therapy is virtually lacking. A sound and practical preventive program should be a part of every swine management system.

REFERENCES
ALLCROFT, R. 1969. Aflatoxicosis in farm animals. In Aflatoxin. Ed. L. A. Goldblatt. New York: Academic Press.
ARMBRECHT, B. H.; WISEMAN, H. G.; AND SHALKOP, W. T. 1972. Swine aflatoxicosis. II. The chronic response in brood sows fed sublethal amounts of aflatoxin and the reaction in their piglets. Environ Physiol Biochem 2:77–85.
BEASLEY, V. R. 1986. Trichothecenes. In Current Veterinary Therapy 2: Food Animal Practice, 2d ed. Philadelphia: W. B. Saunders, pp. 372–373.
BEASLEY, V. R.; SWANSON, S. P.; CORLEY, R. A.; BUCK, W. B.; KORITZ, G. D.; AND BURMEISTER, H. R. 1986. Pharmacokinetics of the trichothecene mycotoxin, T-2 toxin in swine and cattle. Toxicon 24:13–23.
CARLTON, W. W., AND KROGH, P. 1979. Ochratoxins: A

review. Conference on Mycotoxins in Animal Feeds and Grains Related to Animal Health. Springfield, Virginia: National Technical Information Service, pp. 165–287.

CARSON, T. C. 1986. Toxic chemicals, plants, metals and mycotoxins. In Diseases of Swine, 6th ed. Ed. A. D. Leman, B. Straw, R. D. Glock, W. L. Mengeling, R. H. C. Penny, and E. Scholl. Ames: Iowa State Univ Press, pp. 696–701.

CHRISTENSEN, C. M., AND KAUFMANN, H. H. 1965. Deterioration of stored grains by fungi. Annu Rev Phytopathol 3:69–84.

COFFEY, M. T.; HAGLER, W. M.; AND CULLEN, J. M. 1989. Influence of dietary protein, fat and amino acids on the response of weanling swine to aflatoxin B₁. J Anim Sci 67:465–472.

COOK, W. O.; OSWEILER, G. D.; ANDERSON, T. D.; AND RICHARD, J. L. 1986. Ochratoxicosis in Iowa swine. J Am Vet Med Assoc 188:1399–1402.

COOK, W. O.; VAN ALSTINE, W. G.; AND OSWEILER, G. D. 1989. Aflatoxicosis in Iowa swine: Eight cases (1983–1985). J Am Vet Med Assoc 194:554–558.

COPPOCK, R. W., AND SWANSON, S. P. 1986. Aflatoxins. In Current Veterinary Therapy 2: Food Animal Practice, 2d ed. Philadelphia: W. B. Saunders, pp. 363–366.

COPPOCK, R. W.; GELBERG, H. B.; HOFFMAN, W. E.; AND BUCK, W. B. 1985. The acute toxicopathy of intravenous diacetoxyscirpenol (Anguidine) administration in swine. Fund Am Appl Toxicol 5:1034–1049.

DAVIS, N. D.; DICKENS, J. W.; FREIE, J. W.; HAMILTON, P. B.; SHOTWELL, O. L.; WILEY, T. D.; AND FULKERSON, J. F. 1980. Protocols for surveys, sampling, postcollection handling and analysis of grain samples involved in mycotoxin problems. J Assoc Off Anal Chem 63:95–102.

DIEKMAN, M. A., AND LONG, G. G. 1989. Blastocyst development on days 10 or 14 after consumption of zearalenone by sows on days 7 to 10 after breeding. Am J Vet Res 50:1224–1227.

EDWARDS, S.; CANTLEY, T. C.; ROTTINGHAUS, G. E.; OSWEILER, G. D.; AND DAY, B. N. 1987. The effects of zearalenone on reproduction in swine. I. The relationship between ingested zearalenone dose and anestrus in non-pregnant, sexually mature gilts. Theriogenology 28:43–57.

GELDERBLOM, W. C. A.; JASKIEWICZ, K.; MARASAS, W. F. O.; THIEL, P. G.; HORAK, R. M.; VLEGGAAR, R.; AND KRIEK, N. P. J. 1988. Fumonisins—novel mycotoxins with cancer-promoting activity produced by *Fusarium moniliforme*. Appl Environ Microbiol 54:1806–1811.

GREEN, M. L.; DIEKMAN, M. A.; MALAYER, J. R.; SCHEIDT, A. B.; AND LONG, G. G. 1990. Effect of prepubertal consumption of zearalenone on puberty and subsequent reproduction of gilts. J Anim Sci 68:171–178.

HARRISON, L. R.; COLVIN, B. M.; GREEN, J. T.; NEWMAN, L. E.; AND COLE, J. R., Jr. 1990. Pulmonary edema and hydrothorax in swine produced by fumonisin B₁, a toxic metabolite of *Fusarium moniliforme*. J Vet Diagn Invest 2:217–221.

HARVEY, R. B.; HUFF, W. E.; KUBENA, L. F.; CORRIER, D. E.; AND PHILLIPS, T. D. 1988. Progression of aflatoxicosis in growing barrows. Am J Vet Res 49:482–487.

HARVEY, R. B.; KUBENA, L. F.; PHILLIPS, T. D.; HUFF, W. E.; AND CORRIER, D. E. 1989a. Prevention of aflatoxicosis by addition of hydrated sodium calcium aluminosilicate to the diets of growing barrows. Am J Vet Res 50:416–420.

HARVEY, R. B.; KUBENA, L. F.; HUFF, W. E.; CORRIER, D. E.; CLARK, D. E.; AND PHILLIPS, T. D. 1989b. Ef-

fects of aflatoxin, deoxynivalenol, and their combinations in the diets of growing pigs. Am J Vet Res 50:602–607.

HARVEY, R. B.; HUFF, W. E.; KUBENA, L. F.; AND PHILLIPS, T. D. 1989c. Evaluation of diets cocontaminated with aflatoxin and ochratoxin fed to growing pigs. Am J Vet Res 50:1400–1404.

HSIEH, D. P. H. 1979. Basic metabolic effects of mycotoxins. In Interactions of Mycotoxins in Animal Production. Washington, D.C.: National Academy Press, pp. 43–45.

HUFF, W. E.; KUBENA, L. F.; HARVEY, R. B.; AND DOERR, J. A. 1988. Mycotoxin interactions in poultry and swine. J Anim Sci 66:2351–2355.

JAMES, L. J., AND SMITH, T. K. 1982. Effect of dietary alfalfa on zearalenone toxicity and metabolism in rats and swine. J Anim Sci 55:110–117.

JELINIK, C. F.; POHLAND, A. E.; AND WOOD, G. E. 1989. Worldwide occurrence of mycotoxins in foods and feeds—an update. J Assoc Off Anal Chem 71:1176–1179.

LONG, G. G.; DIEKMAN, M. A.; TUITE, J. F.; SHANNAN, G. M.; AND VESONDER, R. F. 1983. Effect of *Fusarium roseum* (*Giberella zea*) on pregnancy and the estrous cycle in gilts fed molded corn on days 7–17 postestrus. Vet Res Commun 6:199–204.

LUN, A. K.; YOUNG, L. G.; AND LUMSDEN, J. H. 1985. The effects of vomitoxin and feed intake on the performance and blood characteristics of young pigs. J Anim Sci 61:1178–1185.

LUNDEEN, G. R.; POPPENGA, R. H.; BEASLEY, V. R.; BUCK, W. B.; TRANQUILLI, W. J.; AND LAMBERT, R. J. 1986. Systemic distribution of blood flow during T-2 toxin induced shock in swine. Fundam Appl Toxicol 7:309–323.

MACDONALD, E. J.; CAVAN, D. R.; AND SMITH, T. K. 1988. Effect of acute oral doses of T-2 toxin on tissue concentrations of biogenic amines in the rat. J Anim Sci 66:434–441.

MCKNIGHT, C. R.; ARMSTRONG, W. D.; HAGLER, W. M.; AND JONES, E. E. 1983. The effects of aflatoxin on brood sows and the newborn pigs. J Anim Sci 55 [Suppl 1]:104.

MCLAUGHLIN, C. S.; VAUGHN, M. H.; CAMPBELL, I. M.; WEI, C. M.; STAFFORD, M. E.; AND HANSEN, B. S. 1977. Inhibition of protein synthesis by trichothecenes. In Mycotoxins in Human and Animal Health. Ed. J. V. Rodericks, C. W. Hesseltine, and M. A. Mehlman. Park Forest, Ill.: Pathotox Publishers, pp. 263–273.

NORDSKOG, A. W., AND CLARK, R. T. 1945. Ergotism in pregnant sows, female rats, and guinea pigs. Am J Vet Res 6:107–116.

OSWEILER, G. D. 1990. Mycotoxins and livestock: What role do fungal toxins play in illness and production losses? Vet Med 85:89–94.

OSWEILER, G. D.; CARSON, T. L.; BUCK, W. B.; AND VAN GELDER, G. A. 1985. Mycotoxicoses. Clinical and Diagnostic Veterinary Toxicology, 3d ed. Dubuque, Iowa: Kendall Hunt, pp. 409–442.

OSWEILER, G. D.; HOPPER, D. L.; AND DEBEY, B. M. 1990. Taste aversion in swine induced by deoxynivalenol. J Anim Sci 68[Suppl 1]:403.

PALYUSIK, M.; HARRACH, B.; MIROCHA, C. J.; AND PATHRE, S. V. 1980. Transmission of zearalenone into porcine milk. Acta Vet Acad Sci Hung 28:217–222.

PANANGALA, V. S.; GIAMBRONE, J. J.; DIENER, U. L.; DAVIS, N. D.; HOERR, F. J.; MITRA, A.; SCHULTZ, R. D.; AND WILT, G. R. 1986. Effects of aflatoxin on the growth, performance and immune responses of weanling swine. Am J Vet Res 47:2062–2067.

PIER, A. C. 1981. Mycotoxins and animal health. Adv Vet Sci Comp Med 25:185–243.

POLLMAN, D. S.; KOCH, B. A.; AND SEITZ, L. M. 1985. Deoxynivalenol-contaminated wheat in swine diets. J Anim Sci 60:239–247.

RAINEY, M. R.; TUBBS, R. C.; BENNETT, L. W.; AND COX, N. M. 1990. Prepubertal exposure to dietary zearalenone alters hypothalamohypophyseal function but does not impair postpubertal reproductive function of gilts. J Anim Sci 68:2015–2022.

RICHARD, J. L., AND COLE, R. J., eds. 1989. Mycotoxins: Economic and health risks. Task Force Report No. 116, Council for Agricultural Science and Technology, Ames, Iowa, pp. 1–99.

ROERS, J. E.; HARROLD, R. L.; HAUGSE, C. N.; AND VINUSSON, W. E. 1974. Barley rations for baby pigs. Farm Research Nov-Dec, North Dakota Agriculture Experiment Station.

RUHR, L. P.; OSWEILER, G. D.; AND FOLEY, C. W. 1983. Effect of the estrogenic mycotoxin zearalenone on reproductive potential in the boar. Am J Vet Res 44:483–485.

SZCZECH, G. M.; CARLTON, W. W.; TUITE, J.; AND CALDWELL, R. 1973. Ochratoxin A toxicosis in swine. Vet Pathol 10:347–364.

TRENHOLM, H. L.; HAMILTON, R. M. G.; FRIEND, D. W.; THOMPSON, B. K.; AND HARTIN, K. E. 1984. Feeding trials with vomitoxin (deoxynivalenol)-contaminated wheat: Effects on swine, poultry, and dairy cattle. J Am Vet Med Assoc 185:527–531.

TRUCKSESS, M. W.; STOLOFF, L.; BRUMLEY, W. C.; WILSON, D. M.; HALE, O. M.; SANGSTER, T.; AND MILLER, D. M. 1982. Aflatoxicol and aflatoxins B_1 and M_1 in the tissues of pigs receiving aflatoxin. J Assoc Off Anal Chem 65:884–887.

WHITACRE, M. D., AND THRELFALL, W. R. 1981. Effects of ergocryptine on plasma prolactin, luteinizing hormone, and progesterone in the periparturient sow. Am J Vet Res 42:1538–1541.

WIERNUSZ, M. L., AND SCHNEIDER, N. 1984. Effects of feeding ergot-contaminated rye diets on swine gestation and lactation. Proc 1984 George A. Young Conf, Lincoln, Nebr.

YOUNG, L. G., AND KING, G. J. 1983. Prolonged feeding of low levels of zearalenone to young boars. J Anim Sci 57[Suppl 1]:313–314.

YOUNG, L. G.; MCGIRR, L.; VALLI, V. E.; LUMSDEN, J. H.; AND LUN, A. 1983. Vomitoxin in corn fed to young pigs. J Anim Sci 57:655–664.

60 Nutrition, Deficiencies and Dietetics

J. L. Nelssen

E. R. Miller

S. C. Henry

ATTEMPTS TO simplify diet and disease interactions into cause and effect relationships are rarely satisfactory. Traditionally, suboptimal performance in swine has been met with a search for some "bad disease" or a "deficient diet." Neither approach has proven itself appropriate to understanding or solving most problems of poor performance. A more proactive effort toward specific, optimal diets and feeding practices is becoming the contemporary standard in swine feeding. Thus, consideration of nutrition and pig health is wide in scope and goes beyond the relative adequacy or inadequacy of specific nutrients in the diet. Increasingly rapid rates of lean tissue gain are being attained through genetic selection, environmental improvement, and health optimization measures. Detailed information on diet contents, ingredient quality, and nutrient levels is available to the producer. These advances decrease the acceptable margin of error in swine diet formulations.

Historically, the concept of "average" diets, with a single diet recognized as adequate for a broad weight and age range that included both sexes and all seasons, has been the common practice. Increased understanding of necessary dietary intake for optimum performance by sex, age, season, and genotype is now being applied at the farm level. Technologic advancement in feed-milling and feed-handling equipment has made on-farm feed manufacturing dietarily and economically attractive to producers, thus rapidly replacing centralized feed mills.

Nutritional requirements are not set points. Rather, needs of pigs are met only when the consumption and content match maintenance requirements and growth potential. Dietary insufficiency is often a qualitative, temporary event and results from the many interactions possible in diet content, environment, feed availability, diet palatability, group size, and endemic disease. While the result may be reflected merely in diminished growth rate or less-efficient feed utilization, at times augmentation of subclinical pathogen-tissue interactions results in overt signs of illness.

Within a herd, group, or pen of pigs a dynamic state of infection, pathology, and recovery exists.

Diet represents a controllable input and is the economically most important input in swine production. A constant, positive effort to optimize diet quality, content, and applicability for the type of animals being fed allows goals of economy, performance, and health to be realized. This chapter provides an overview of many specific features involved in maintaining high-quality, appropriate diets in pig feeders. Definitions of specific requirements for classes of pigs are constantly being refined and readers are referred to regional university publications and National Research Council guidelines for specific, appropriate dietary recommendations.

A knowledge of diet and disease interactions has a scope much broader than a relative or absolute lack of nutrients. Clinically, an assessment of feeding and disease interrelationships must encompass not only diet contents but the physical form, availability, palatability, economy, rates of feed intake, and ration variations over time. Such a broad view, appropriately considered swine dietetics, is necessary in clinical efforts to define and solve diet-related problems.

There are no "secrets" regarding optimal nutrition for pigs. Feed-product merchandizers that depend on "secret" ingredients or have unavailable nutrient profiles delude the swine producer. Unless a producer has a compelling, nonnutritional reason to use a feedstuff for which nutrient content is not documented, it should be avoided. Swine producers and their advisors should know what swine diets contain and what they cost. Knowledge of existing diets is necessary in evaluating and comparing alternatives. The difference in ration costs from farm to farm is surprisingly great. These cost differences are rarely justified by performance differences.

Rations, feed systems, and feed mills are not static; they change with time. Reevaluation of systems and rations, with consideration of costs, contents, preparation quality, and wastage must be a regular discipline.

ALTERNATIVE PREPARATION SYSTEMS FOR SWINE RATIONS.

There are four general systems for swine ration preparation commonly in use on farms. Which one or which combinations are applied depends on labor, equipment, grain storage, and the interests of the producer. Each farm is different and there is a need to determine which systems best apply and what improvements are possible. The priorities are to provide the proper ration quantity and quality to the pig and to optimize the costs of diets for best returns.

Complete Feed. Rations are prepared and delivered by a commercial mill as ready-to-feed products. While convenient, complete feeds are the most expensive in most cases. Additionally, flexibility is limited when specific ration changes are required. If producers have the capability to manufacture quality rations on the farm they generally cannot afford complete feeds.

Supplement and Grain, On-Farm Ration Preparation. Mixing farm grain and commercial supplement has long been popular. In most cases a basic 40% protein supplement containing all ingredients except the grain portion is added to grain to prepare major diets. For special diets additional packages may be included with this supplement, for example, mineral additions to sow diets, that bring rations more nearly into line with requirements. This system offers few positive advantages over the base-mix system in ration accuracy and is more expensive and less sensitive to changes in nutritional requirements than base-mix systems.

Base-Mix Systems, On-Farm Ration Preparation. Base mixes contain all needed ingredients except grain, protein, and antibiotics and account for 3–5% of the completed ration by weight. Base mix fits well with many portable farm feed mills. For most portable farm mill systems, base mix affords the best compromise between cost and convenience. It is also best with volumetric, stationary mills. The term "premix" is often used erroneously to describe base-mix products.

Premix System, On-Farm Ration Preparation. Premixes offer the greatest opportunity for specifically tailored rations at the best cost. Accuracy in preparation and ingredient care are critical to good premix ration formulation. They require time and discipline in quality control yet provide the best performance for cost. Premixes of vitamins and trace minerals are added to calcium, phosphorus, salt, protein, and grain in a basic premix system. Seven or more ingredients are needed for premix constructed diets.

NUTRIENT DEFICIENCIES AND DIETARY EXCESSES.

Most diets of U.S. and Canadian swine are composed of one or more grains, together with soybean meal or other protein sources that complement the indispensable amino acids lacking in the grains. These major ingredients of the diet should be supplemented with vitamins and essential mineral elements to provide all the known nutrient requirements. Diets formulated in this manner should prevent any signs of nutrient deficiencies or excesses when fed to swine reared under suitable environmental conditions and free from infectious diseases. Overt clinical signs and subclinical changes associated with nutrient deficiencies are presented in Table 60.1.

Dietary excesses, with readily recognizable clinical signs, seldom occur. They are nevertheless a potential problem, particularly with micronutrients such as the trace minerals and some nonnutrients. A toxicity of copper would not likely occur unless copper were added at a high level (250 ppm or more), and with low dietary iron or zinc or high levels of calcium. Iron toxicity is less likely unless there is a vitamin E–selenium deficiency. Sodium chloride toxicity is avoided if adequate water is provided. Fluorosis is seldom seen unless all supplemental phosphorus is from a nondefluorinated raw rock phosphate source, but high levels of fluoride will reduce rate and efficiency of gain. Because of an interference with zinc absorption, an excess of calcium may be manifested by the skin condition, parakeratosis. Thus, signs of dietary excess are commonly conditioned by the interrelationship of two or more factors. Signs of these and other dietary excesses are presented in Table 60.2. The toxic dietary levels listed are those which experimentally produced signs indicated and are not necessarily minimum toxic or maximum tolerant levels (NRC 1980).

FEEDING: FROM WEANING TO MARKET.

In the United States, pigs are allowed to consume feed ad libitum from weaning until they have reached market weight. The control of voluntary feed intake is influenced by (1) dietary factors, including deficiencies or excesses of nutrients, energy density, antibiotics, flavors, feed processing, and water; (2) environmental factors, including temperature, humidity, air movement, number of pigs per pen, and available space per pig; (3) physiological factors, including neural and hormonal (responses) mechanisms; (4) disease factors, including respiratory, enteric, and other diseases; and (5) genetics (NRC 1988).

Within any population of pigs, voluntary feed intake may be highly variable, which results in uneven growth rates. In the swine industry, uniform and rapid growth is essential for profitability. To evaluate a swine production unit, swine producers, veterinarians, and consultants to the swine industry must have a knowledge of performance standards (Table 60.3).

In swine, lean gain per day and feed cost per unit of lean gain are important biological response

Table 60.1. Signs of nutrient deficiences

	Signs of Nutrient Deficiency	
Nutrient	Clinical	Subclinical
Energy	Weakness Low body temperature Loss of weight Coma Death	Hypoglycemia Loss of subcutaneous fat Elevated hematocrit and serum cholesterol Reduced blood glucose, calcium, and sodium

Protein: amino acid	Impaired growth
	Unthriftiness
	Reduced resistance to bacterial infection
		Kwashiorkorlike signs in baby pigs, includ-
		  ing reduced serum protein and albumin,
		  anemia, gross edema, and increased liver
		  lipid concentration

Fat: linoleic acid	Scaly dermatitis may appear	Small gallbladder Elevated triene/tetraene in tissue lipids
Vitamin A	Incoordination Lordosis Paralysis of rear limbs Night blindness Congenital defects	Retarded bone growth Increase in cerebrospinal fluid pressure Degeneration of sciatic and femoral nerves Minimal visual purple Atrophy of epithelial layers of genital tract

Vitamin D	Rickets
	Osteomalacia
	Low calcium tetany
		Lack of bone calcification and proliferation
		  of epiphyseal cartilage
		Rib and vertebra fracture
		Low plasma calcium, magnesium, and
		  inorganic phosphorus levels
		Elevated serum alkaline phosphatase levels

Vitamin E-selenium	Edema Sudden death	Generalized edema Liver necrosis (hepatosis dietetica) Microangiopathy Cardiac muscle degeneration (mulberry heart) Pale, dystrophic muscle
Vitamin K	Pale newborn pigs with loss of blood from umbilical cord Sudden death following dicoumarin intake	Increased prothrombin time Increased blood-clotting time Internal hemorrhage Anemia due to blood loss
Thiamin	Poor appetite Poor growth Sudden death	Cardiac hypertrophy Bradycardia First and second degree auriculoventricu- lar block Elevated plasma pyruvate
Riboflavin	Slow growth Seborrhea Impaired sow reproductivity	Lens cataracts Increase in neutrophilic leukocytes Birth of weak pigs with skeletal anomalies
Niacin	Poor appetite Poor growth Severe diarrhea Dermatitis	Necrotic lesions of intestine
Pantothenic acid	Poor appetite Poor growth Diarrhea Unusual gait (goose-stepping) Impaired sow reproductivity	Inflammation of colon Degeneration of sciatic and peripheral nerves Reduced blood pantothenic acid level Reduced free pantothenic acid level in milk
Vitamin B$_6$	Poor growth Epileptic seizures	Microcytic hypochromic anemia Elevated serum iron Fatty infiltration of liver Elevated urinary xanthurenic acid Elevated gamma globulinlike blood protein fraction
Vitamin B$_{12}$	Depressed growth Hypersensitivity Reduced sow reproductivity	Reduced serum and tissue B$_{12}$ levels
Choline	Slow growth Reduced litter size	Fatty infiltration of liver Reduced conception rate
Biotin	Dermatosis Spasticity of hind legs	Reduced urinary biotin excretion

Table 60.1. *Continued*

Nutrient	Signs of Nutrient Deficiency — Clinical	Signs of Nutrient Deficiency — Subclinical
Folacin	Poor growth Weakness	Normocytic anemia
Calcium	Rickets Osteomalacia Low calcium tetany	Lack of bone calcification Bones easily fractured Low plasma calcium level Elevated serum inorganic phosphorus and alkaline phosphatase
Phosphorus	Poor growth Rickets Osteomalacia	Lack of bone calcification Bones easily fractured Low serum inorganic phosphorus Elevated serum calcium and alkaline phosphatase Enlarged costochondral junction (beading)
Magnesium	Poor growth Stepping syndrome Weakening carpo-metacarpo-phalangeal and tarso-metatarso-phalangeal joints	Low serum magnesium and calcium Reduced bone magnesium
Potassium	Anorexia Rough hair coat Emaciation Ataxia	Reduced heart rate Increased PR, QRS, and QT intervals on electrocardiogram Reduced serum potassium
Sodium	Poor appetite Low water consumption Unthriftiness	Negative sodium balance Elevated serum potassium Elevated plasma urea nitrogen Reduced chlorine retention
Chlorine	Poor growth	Reduced plasma chlorine Reduced sodium and potassium retention
Iron	Poor growth Rough hair coat Pallor Anoxia	Hypochromic microcytic anemia Enlarged heart and spleen Enlarged fatty liver Ascities Clumping of erythroblastic cells in bone marrow Reduced serum iron and percent transferrin saturation
Copper	Leg weakness Ataxia	Microcytic hypochromic anemia Reduced serum copper and ceruloplasmin Aortic rupture Cardiac hypertrophy
Zinc	Poor growth Poor appetite Parakeratosis	Reduced serum, tissue, and milk zinc Reduced serum albumin-globulin ratio Reduced serum alkaline phosphatase Reduced thymus weight Retarded testicular development Impaired reproductivity of sows
Iodine	Goiter Myxedema Sows farrow weak, hairless pigs	Enlarged hemorrhagic thyroid Hyperplasia of follicular epithelium of thyroid Reduced plasma protein-bound iodine
Manganese	Lameness in growing pigs Increased fat deposition in pregnant gilts with birth of weak pigs with poor sense of balance	Replacement of cancellous bone with fibrous tissue Early closure of distal epiphyseal plate Low serum manganese and alkaline phosphatase Negative manganese balance
Water	Poor appetite Dehydration Loss of body weight Possible salt poisoning Death	Elevated hematocrit Elevated plasma electrolytes Loss of temperature regulation Tissue dehydration

Source: NRC. 1979. The Nutrient Requirements of Swine, 8th rev ed. Washington, D.C.: National Academy Press, with permission.

Table 60.2. Signs of dietary excesses

Nutrient	Toxic Dietary Level[a]	Age	Signs of Dietary Excess
Calcium	1% (with limited zinc)	Immature	Depressed appetite, reduced rate of gain, parakeratosis
	1% (with adequate zinc and limited phosphorus)	Immature	Reduced rate of gain, reduced bone strength
Copper	300–500 mg/kg (in absence of higher levels of dietary iron and zinc[b])	Immature	Reduced growth, lower hemoglobin, icterus, death[c]
Iodine	800 mg/kg	Immature	Depressed feed intake and rate of gain, lowered hemoglobin[d], eye lesions
Iron	5000 mg/kg	Immature	Depressed feed intake and rate of gain, reduced serum inorganic phosphorus and femur ash, rickets[e]
Manganese	4000 mg/kg	Immature	Depressed feed intake, reduced growth rate, stiffness, stilted gait
Selenium	5–8 mg/kg[f]	Immature	Anorexia, hair loss, separation of hoof and skin at coronary band, degenerative changes in liver and kidney
	10 mg/kg (sows)	Breeding	Reduced conception, pigs small, weak or dead at birth
Sodium chloride and other sodium salts	1–8% (with severe water restriction)	All ages	Nervousness, weakness, staggering, epileptic seizures, paralysis, death
Zinc	2000 mg/kg	Immature	Growth depression, arthritis, hemorrhage in axillary spaces, gastritis, enteritis
Arsenic	990 mg/kg	Immature	Poor growth, erythema, ataxia, posterior paralysis, quadraplegia, blindness, myelin degeneration of optic and peripheral nerves
Cadmium	50 mg/kg	Immature	Reduced gain and hematocrit
	150 mg/kg	Immature	Severe depression of gain and hematocrit
	450 mg/kg	Immature	Severe depression of gain and hematocrit and appearance of dermatitis
Cobalt	400 mg/kg	Immature	Anorexia, growth depression, stiff-legged, humped back, incoordination, muscle tremors, anemia[g]
Fluorine			
Soluble fluorides	100 mg/kg	Mature	Mottled enamel, enamel hypoplasia, softening of teeth, osteomalacia, excessive loss of weight by lactating sows
Rock phosphate F	200 mg/kg	Mature	
Gossypol[h]	200 mg/kg	Immature	Muscular weakness, dyspnea, generalized edema, death; myocarditis, hepatitis, nephritis
Lead	660 mg/kg	Immature	Squealing as if in pain, diarrhea, salivation, grinding of teeth, depressed appetite, reduced growth rate, muscular tremors, ataxia, increased respiratory rate, decreased heart rate, enlarged carpal joints, impaired vision, clonic seizures, death
Mercury	Single oral dose of 5–15 mg methyl mercury or mercury dicyandiamide/kg body weight	Immature	Anorexia, bodyweight loss, central nervous system depression, weakness, gagging, vomiting, diarrhea, ataxia, cyanosis, muscular tremors, postural and gait abnormalities, polyuria
Nitrate	1800 mg NO_3/kg	Immature	Growth depression, dyspnea, cyanosis, elevated methemoglobin, lymphocytosis, reduced serum vitamin A and E levels
Nitrite	400 mg NO_2/kg	Immature	
Urea	2.5%	Immature	Reduced feed intake and growth rate, increased plasma urea nitrogen level

Source: NRC. 1979. The Nutrient Requirements of Swine, 8th rev ed. Washington D.C.: National Academy Press, with permission.

[a]The toxic dietary levels listed are those that have experimentally produced the signs indicated and are not necessarily minimum toxic or maximum tolerant levels (NRC 1980).

[b]In a few instances, a dietary level of 250 mg/kg has resulted in signs of excess.

[c]In some instances, 500 mg/kg of copper has been fed without icterus or death occurring.

[d]Anemia of iodine toxicity alleviated with supplemental iron.

[e]Rickets from excessive dietary iron alleviated by increasing dietary phosphorus.

[f]Selenium toxicity partially alleviated with arsenic.

[g]Cobalt toxicity alleviated by supplemental methionine, iron, zinc, and manganese.

[h]Gossypol toxicity alleviated by increasing dietary iron to equal the weight of free gossypol.

Table 60.3. Pig performance standards

Phase	Wt. Range (kg)	Daily Gain (kg) Actual[a]	Daily Gain (kg) Goal	Feed Intake (kg) Actual[a]	Feed Intake (kg) Goal
Hot nursery	5.5–11.5	0.21	0.23	0.32	0.34
Cold nursery	11.5–22.0	0.37	0.45	0.71	0.86
Grower	22.0–55.0	0.57	0.66	1.57	1.70
Finisher	55.0–110.0	0.70	0.91	2.49	2.73

[a]Swine Graphics, Inc., Webster City, Iowa.

criteria for both the consumer and producer. Diets and feeding practices that result in optimum lean tissue growth are increasingly important as the pork industry moves toward marketing of boneless retail cuts. Daily amino acid intake and energy density of diets are the key nutritional factors affecting lean tissue growth in swine.

Feeding a properly formulated diet to exactly meet the nutrient needs for optimum daily lean gain in the growing pig is essential. The concept of "phase feeding" has been introduced to describe this nutritional plan.

Phase feeding is a management practice that limits large changes in diet composition as a pig moves through the various growth phases. Traditionally, swine producers often applied only three different diets from weaning to market weight, which resulted in dramatic over- and underformulation of diets in relation to actual requirements. Phase feeding incorporates up to seven different diets from weaning through market weight. Additionally, split-sex feeding and diets of different nutrient density in the summer, as compared to the winter, are increasingly employed in the swine industry. These nutrition management practices provide cost-effective diets and meet the goal of optimizing lean gain.

Weanling Pigs

DIETARY CONSIDERATIONS. Pigs are most often weaned at four weeks of age or less to increase sow productivity. Such early weaning often results in a lag in performance that includes decreased gain and feed intake with increased disease morbidity and mortality. Nutritionists are presented with an obvious challenge to devise an economical, nutritional regimen to eliminate this postweaning lag performance.

Three- to 4-week-old weanling pigs have very immature digestive and immune systems. The predominant gastrointestinal enzymes at this stage are most appropriate for digestion of milk products instead of the plant products, which are normally fed. Feed intake is also very low the first 2 weeks after weaning. Thus, a highly digestible and nutritious diet is essential to maximize performance during this critical period. Research at Kansas State University resulted in the formulation of a high–nutrient density diet for early weaned pigs in 1985. This was followed by the development of a three-phase starter program for early weaned pigs as a management practice to optimize pig performance and minimize product costs (Nelssen 1986) (Table 60.4). Phase 1 involves feeding a high–nutrient density diet (40% milk product, dry diet) until pigs reach 7.0 kg body weight. From 7.0 to 11.5 kg (Phase 2), a grain-soybean meal diet containing dried whey and fish meal is fed. The last phase (Phase 3) is a grain-soybean meal diet to be fed from 11.5 to 22.0 kg.

PROTEIN SOURCES. Conventional high–nutrient density diets for nursery pigs are based largely on milk products that are not only costly, but are likely to be used for human consumption. There is considerable economic incentive, therefore, to seek alternative protein sources for starter diets. In recent years the use of soybean products as potential protein sources have been intensively examined. Traditional soybean products are known to have antigenic properties that induce transient hypersensitivity in calves (Seegraber

Table 60.4. Characteristics of a three-phase starter program

Item	Phase 1: to 7 kg	Phase 2: to 11.5 kg	Phase 3: to 22 kg
Protein, %	20–25	18–20	18
Lysine, %	1.4–1.5	1.25	1.10
Added fat, %	4–6	3	3
Dried edible whey, %	15–20	10–15	0–5
Dried skim milk, %	15–25	– – –	– – –
Fish meal, %	0–3	3–5	– – –
Copper, ppm	190–260	190–260	190–260
Vitamin E, IU/ton	40,000	40,000	40,000
Selenium, ppm	0.3	0.3	0.3
Antibacterial or antibiotic	+	+	+
Physical form	1/8″ pellet	1/8″ pellet or meal	Meal form

and Morrill 1979, 1982, 1986; Dawson et al. 1988), in pigs (Giesting et al. 1986; Stokes et al. 1986), in chickens (Klasing et al. 1988), and in mice (Mowat and Ferguson 1981).

The "transient hypersensitivity theory" of soy protein has been tested in weanling pigs fed a diet containing soybean meal (Newby et al. 1984). Piglets nursing a sow can be exposed or "sensitized" to soybean proteins by consuming sow feed or creep feed containing soybean meal. "Sensitization" with soybean meal and then feeding diets containing soybean meal postweaning can lead to abnormalities in digestive processes, including disorders in digesta movement and inflammatory responses in the intestinal mucosa of pigs. Transient hypersensitivity response to soybean proteins appeared to be caused by certain antigenic proteins present in the soybeans, such as glycinin and beta-conglycinin.

A recent study (Li et al. 1990) was conducted to determine if further processing of soybean protein products would lower their antigenic properties, thus reducing or eliminating the transient hypersensitivity response commonly seen in the early weaned pig. Particular attention was given to ethanol extraction and heat treatment encountered in commercial processing of soybean products. Additionally, the effect of moist extrusion of soy protein concentrate on immunological criteria and growth performance was also evaluated.

Pigs infused with soybean meal or soy protein concentrate preweaning and then fed diets containing soybean meal or soy protein concentrate after weaning showed poorer growth performance at 2 weeks postweaning compared to those fed extruded soy protein concentrate or dried skim milk as the primary dietary protein source. It is postulated that antigenic materials remaining in the soybean meal or soy protein concentrate cause gastrointestinal disorders, which, in turn, influence the digestive process and depress apparent nitrogen digestibility in pigs (Li et al. 1990). In these trials, both extruded soy protein concentrate and dried skim milk resulted in similar growth performance and nitrogen digestibility at 2 weeks postweaning.

Pigs fed soy protein concentrate or extruded soy protein concentrate had longer villi compared to those fed soybean meal, yet, all villi were shorter than those of pigs fed dried skim milk. Moist extrusion processing of alcohol-extracted soy protein concentrate may have reduced antigenic materials and other antinutritional factors, such as trypsin inhibitors. Pigs fed dried skim milk had longer villi and a larger villus area and perimeter than pigs fed any of the soybean products.

Consistent with other research (Kilshaw and Sissons 1979; Li et al. 1990), pigs dosed with soybean meal and then fed soybean meal showed high titers of IgG antibodies against dietary soybean protein. Stimulation of the systemic immune system by undenatured glycinin and beta-congly-

cinin absorbed from digesta in the gut lumen could account for these circulating antibodies.

In summary, baby pigs dosed with soybean meal and then fed a diet containing soybean meal processed by conventional methods showed decreased growth performance, lowered villus height, and increased serum anti-soy IgG titers. Pigs fed soy protein concentrate showed decreased average daily gain (ADG) and nitrogen digestibility and poorer feed conversion at 2 weeks postweaning compared with those fed dried skim milk and extruded soy protein concentrate. This research demonstrates that processing methods significantly affect the utilization of soy protein for nursery pigs.

FAT LEVELS AND SOURCES. Fat is often included in starter diets to increase the energy density of the diet in an attempt to increase caloric intake of the early weaned pig. Many studies have been conducted to determine the young pig's ability to utilize fat. The high–nutrient density diet consists of 40% milk products with some added fat (Nelssen 1986). Fat is added for two reasons: to increase dietary energy density and to improve pellet quality and efficiency in the feed mill. Diets containing high levels of milk products are extremely difficult to pellet, and pellet scorching may reduce the milk product quality in diets containing low or no added fat. The consequence is reduced pig performance.

Recent studies conducted at the University of Minnesota (Tokach et al. 1989a) and Kansas State University have found that, based on growth performance, the level of fat can be reduced in the Phase 1 diets. Tokach et al. (1989a) found that increasing the level of fat in a Phase 1 starter diet had no effect on ADG. However, feed efficiency was improved through 6% added fat, during the initial 14 days postweaning. Other experiments conducted by Tokach et al. (1989b) and Li et al. (1989) have found no improvement in ADG or feed efficiency with high levels of added fat in dry diets with a high milk content. Thus, a level of 4–6% supplemental fat may be warranted in high–nutrient density diets to improve pelleting efficiency and to increase the energy density of the diet.

The source of fat affects lipid utilization in the young pig. Cera et al. (1988) found corn oil to be more digestible than lard or tallow by the early weaned pig. Turlington et al. (1987) reported that 21-day-old pigs fed soybean oil, choice white grease, or coconut oil had higher growth rates than those fed tallow during the first 5 weeks postweaning. Tallow is the least desirable fat source to use in formulating starter pig diets.

Many factors influence the ability of pigs to utilize fat including age of pigs, fatty acid chain length and degree of saturation, fat level in the diet, fatty acid–binding protein activity, and pH of the small intestine. Therefore, a series of experiments were conducted to evaluate if combinations of various fat sources would improve fat utilization by the 21-day-old pig (Thaler et al. 1988; Li et al. 1989). Results demonstrated that ADG and feed efficiency were improved by adding fat to starter diets, with 50% soybean oil and 50% coconut oil maximizing performance. Pigs fed a combination of soybean oil and coconut oil had increased villus height and slightly higher ileal digestibility of medium-chain fatty acids compared to those fed soybean oil or coconut oil alone (Li et al. 1989). These results indicate that a mixture of soybean oil and coconut oil is a superior fat product for the early weaned pig.

When fat is added to a high–nutrient density diet, a high-quality, stabilized fat source must be used. Obviously, a constant ratio of nutrients to energy is important for efficient utilization of the energy from fat. The importance of fat as an adjunct to the pelleting process in a high-milk, dry diet should not be underestimated.

CARBOHYDRATE SOURCES. Lactose is the carbohydrate fraction of milk. Dried skim milk and dried whey are extremely high in lactose, 50% and 70% respectively. Since the addition of dried skim milk or dried whey to starter diets improves pig performance, pigs would be expected to respond favorably to lactose additions.

Giesting et al. (1985) reported that lactose promoted a greater daily gain and feed intake than other carbohydrate sources, suggesting that lactose stimulates early acceptance of dry diets by the weaning pig. Turlington et al. (1989) also suggested that lactose will improve nutrient digestibility and slow digesta flow rate as compared to dextrose as a carbohydrate source for 21- to 35-day-old pigs.

The literature suggests that the addition of lactose to corn-soybean meal starter diets will improve performance of pigs weaned earlier than 35 days of age. The mode of action may be an increased nutrient digestibility due to slower digesta flow and (or) an improvement in feed intake.

Early weaning of pigs has brought a series of new challenges to the swine industry, including nutritional concerns. The transition from a high-fat, high-energy, liquid (sow's milk) diet to a low-fat, high-carbohydrate diet results in metabolic, physiologic, and compositional changes in weaned pigs. Several researchers have demonstrated that the inclusion of proteins and carbohydrates similar to those found in milk improves performance of early weaned pigs.

Recent research has focused on evaluating feed ingredients that will result in comparable performance to the high–nutrient density, high–milk produce diets, at a lower cost. In evaluating a diet program for the early weaned pig, consideration must be given both to the improvements in nursery growth performance and subsequent performance, from 22 kg to market weight.

Growing-Finishing Pigs.   The swine industry is placing greater emphasis on production of lean meat desired by modern consumers. Pork processors are increasing the production of lean products such as boneless loins or 95% fat-free hams in response to consumer willingness to pay a premium for low-fat products. New methods of measuring the amount of lean pork in carcasses are being developed rapidly, allowing accurate, predictable price differentials for lean compared to fat pigs. Pork producers will adjust production systems to meet consumer demands for lean pork when monetary differentials are offered by the packer for high-percentage lean carcasses.

Recent studies have shown that there are different dietary amino acid concentrations necessary to achieve various production goals. Lysine is one of the most important nutrients in swine diet formulation. Diet formulations low in lysine limit daily lysine intake and reduce lean tissue growth in growing pigs. Amino acid levels currently recommended by the National Research Council (1988) may not be adequate for optimum lean tissue growth.

Nutritional manipulation of lean growth in pigs is not difficult. The basic principles of lean growth have been summarized:

1. Maximum lean tissue growth can occur only when the daily intake of all essential nutrients is sufficient, particularly amino acids and energy.
2. Shortages of protein intake will reduce daily live-weight gain, feed-conversion efficiency, and carcass lean content.
3. An oversupply of dietary protein may improve the percentage lean in the carcass, but may result in slightly poorer feed efficiency.
4. Limited daily energy supplied to pigs may improve carcass leanness, but growth rate will deteriorate.
5. Energy supplied over and above that needed for maintenance and maximum lean-tissue gain will be used for fat deposition.

The commercial swine industry historically pens barrows and gilts together, and they are fed one grower diet, beginning at 22 kg, of approximately 16% crude protein until it is changed to a 14% crude protein finishing diet at about 55 kg live weight fed to market. This practice is changing as segregation by sex, diet formulation for environmental and seasonal variation, and multiple diet stages optimize lean growth most economically.

SPLIT-SEX FEEDING. There are large differences in lean gain potential between barrows and gilts. Split-sex feeding involves sorting gilts from barrows and feeding each a separate diet. As gilts consume 200–250 gm less feed per day than barrows, gilts require higher concentrations of dietary amino acids to meet requirements for lean growth. Also, gilts may be selectively fed higher levels of other nutrients, such as calcium and phosphorus, if they will be retained for the breeding herd.

Barrows eat 10–14% more feed daily and grow more rapidly than do gilts. Feeding barrows separately provides opportunity to benefit from the relatively high feed intake of barrows compared to gilts. Less dietary nutrient density is needed for barrows, resulting in more economical diets.

Split-sex feeding may also offer tremendous opportunities at marketing. Because of less backfat and larger loin-eyes compared to barrows, gilts may command premiums on "lean value" marketing systems. Also, gilts fed to heavier weights (≥ 115 kg) have some advantages in production efficiency (feed utilization, etc.) when compared to barrows that must be considered in swine-feeding practices.

GENOTYPE DIFFERENCES. In the swine industry, there is currently great variation in the lean growth potential of the various genetic lines. There is an erroneous but popular concept that genotype differences in lean growth are due to breed differences alone. However, within-breed differences in lean growth potential are greater than are between-breed differences. Little if any improvement in lean growth performance has been made in some genetic lines during the last decade, whereas tremendous progress has been made with others.

The option to formulate diets differently for various genetic lines may be practically applicable. A recent experiment, conducted at the University of Kentucky, evaluated the effects of various lysine levels in diets for growing-finishing pigs of different genotypes (Stahly et al. 1989). Based on genotype, pigs were placed in high or low lean-tissue growth potential groups. Pigs were fed ad libitum a corn-soybean meal diet from 22 to 110 kg. Littermate barrows were randomly allotted to four dietary lysine levels (0.50, 0.65, 0.80, or 0.95%). Daily gain and lean-tissue gain were maximized with a dietary lysine level of 0.65% in the "low lean" genotype. However, the "high lean" genotype required a much higher lysine level (0.80–0.95%) to maximize daily gain and carcass leanness.

Lean growth rate and lean-tissue feed conversion can be improved through consistent performance testing and selection. Pigs with low lean-gain potential only require low amino acid inputs to achieve their maximum daily lean deposition. Pigs with high lean-gain potential respond to higher nutrient inputs by increasing lean growth rate. In fact, with higher lysine levels, the high-lean genotypes had larger loin-eye areas, less backfat, and greater lean gain than the low-lean genotypes in the Kentucky experiment. This research indicates that the relatively unimproved pig will not respond to increases in protein or ly-

sine levels and, therefore, will perform satisfactorily on conventional grain-soybean meal diets containing 16% crude protein during the growing phase and 14% crude protein during the finishing phase.

FEED INTAKE AND LEAN GROWTH. The nutritional program needed to realize the genetic capacity for maximum lean growth of pigs depends on feed intake, as well as digestibility and efficiency of nutrient use. As the pig grows, changes in voluntary feed intake and in maintenance requirement reduce energy efficiency in conversion of feed to tissue or product. Pigs that have high lean-growth potential possess a higher maintenance requirement but efficiently utilize energy for body protein accretion. In fact, in pigs selected for high lean-tissue accretion, feed intake may be the upper ceiling limiting further improvements in lean growth.

It is generally considered that the growing-finishing pig regulates feed intake within the environmental "comfort zone" to maintain a constant daily intake of energy. The amount of feed consumed is determined by the energy density of the diet fed. As the energy density of the diet increases, for example, with the addition of fat, the amount of feed consumed decreases to maintain a constant energy intake. Diets that do not adequately provide the required amounts of essential nutrients, such as amino acids, in relation to energy intake fail to allow maximum lean growth.

Feed intake and maintenance requirements of finishing pigs are greatly influenced by the effective temperature of the environment. Table 60.5 illustrates the influence of air temperature on feed intake, gain, and feed efficiency. Feed intake is greatly influenced at temperatures above and below the comfort zone. Pigs exposed to freezing temperatures consume excessive quantities of feed in an effort to offset heat loss. At the other extreme, during heat stress, feed intake is extremely low, which is a major production problem. Swine diet formulations should be adjusted to account for variation in feed intake related to environmental temperature changes.

BIOTECHNOLOGY AND GROWTH. In recent years

Table 60.5. Effect of temperature on finishing pig performance

Temperature (°C)	Daily Intake (kg)	Daily Gain (kg)	Feed Conversion
0	5.07	1.18	9.45
5	3.76	1.17	7.10
10	3.50	1.76	4.34
15	3.15	1.74	3.99
20	3.22	1.87	3.79
25	2.63	1.58	3.65
30	2.21	0.98	4.91
35	1.51	0.68	4.87

several researchers have demonstrated the beneficial effects of parenteral administration of natural or recombinant porcine somatotropin (PST) in increasing rate of body weight gain and efficiency of feed utilization for gain. Equally important is the increased accretion of body protein and decreased body fat of finishing pigs administered PST. Walton et al. (1986) have shown that PST antagonizes insulin action and depresses lipogenesis in porcine adipose tissue culture. Porcine somatotropin can increase daily gains up to 19%, improve feed efficiency up to 28%, and reduce backfat thickness up to 33%.

Porcine Somatotropin. Since growing-finishing pigs administered PST grow faster on less feed intake, it is evident that the dietary concentration of the structural nutrients (amino acids for muscle growth and Ca and P for skeletal growth) as well as energy for protein and bone synthesis must be increased to realize optimum benefits. Steele et al. (1987) have demonstrated that, when treated with PST, the inherent differences in sex effect (boar vs. barrow vs. gilt) are negated with respect to nutrient partitioning; all sexes respond as intact males on deposition rates of protein, water, fat, and ash. Thus, when proper levels of PST are administered to barrows and gilts, they need to be fed a diet in which nutrient and energy concentrations are similar to the diet that is appropriate for the ad libitum–fed boar. A typical diet for ad libi-

tum–fed boars that are reared for slaughter market is presented in Table 60.6. This is similar to diets utilized by Goodband et al. (1988) and Schricker (1989). Schricker (1989) demonstrated that if lysine is not increased above NRC (1988) requirement levels when PST is administered, performance of finishing barrows is suppressed. Thus, unless nutrient and energy density of diets are adjusted, the benefits of PST will not be realized.

A recent trial conducted at Kansas State University evaluated the influence of dietary lysine on growth performance and carcass characteristics of finishing swine (Goodband et al. 1990). Treatments included either a daily injection of 4 mg PST or a placebo, in combination with a diet containing 0.6% lysine (NRC requirement) or diets containing 0.8, 1.0, 1.2, or 1.4% lysine provided by synthetic lysine. Average daily gain was maximized at the 1.2% dietary lysine level, with those pigs gaining approximately 35% faster than untreated controls or the somatotropin-treated pigs receiving the 0.6% lysine diet. PST-treated pigs fed either a 1.2 or 1.4% lysine diet were 33% more efficient than control or somatotropin-treated pigs fed the 0.6% lysine diet. It would appear that the lysine requirement of PST-treated pigs is at least double the present recommendations for finishing swine. Table 60.7 lists the recommended lysine levels useful in formulating diets that optimize lean tissue growth in swine.

Table 60.6. Diet designed to result in optimum performance of ad libitum–fed finishing gilts or barrows administered porcine somatotropin

Diet formulation		
Corn, ground shelled	66.85	
Soybean meal	25.00	
Soybean oil	5.00	
Dicalcium phosphate	1.50	
Calcium carbonate	1.00	
Vitamins and trace minerals	0.35	
L-lysine · HC1	0.30	
	100.00	
Calculated analyses		Level relative to NRC (1988)
ME, kcal/kg	3500.0	107%
Crude protein, %	16.8	129%
Lysine, %	1.10	183%
Tryptophan, %	0.17	170%
Threonine, %	0.64	160%
Calcium, %	0.70	140%
Phosphorus, %	0.60	150%

Note: ME = metabolizable energy.

Table 60.7. Percentage dietary lysine recommendations

	Winter		Summer	
Weight in kg (lb)	Gilts	Barrows	Gilts	Barrows
22–55 (50–120)	0.90	0.80	1.00	0.90
55–77 (120–170)	0.85	0.75	0.90	0.80
77–market (170–market)	0.75	0.65	0.85	0.75

Note: These recommended nutrient allowances are only useful if split-sex feeding is employed as a management practice.

Beta-adrenergic Agonists. Beta-adrenergic agonists (BAA) are chemical analogs of naturally occurring catecholamines, epinephrine and norepinephrine. These compounds are active when given orally and may be incorporated at low levels (1–20 ppm) in the diet of growing-finishing pigs (Convey 1987). Anderson et al. (1987) obtained a significant improvement in rate of weight gain, efficiency of feed utilization for weight gain, and improved carcass characteristics of growing-finishing pigs fed a diet containing 20 ppm of ractopamine, a phenethanolamine, but only when the diet protein level was elevated to 16 or 18%. Thus, it is important to give attention to higher levels of nutrients and energy of diets when either PST or BAA are used with growing-finishing pigs.

The swine industry must optimize lean accretion and improve the efficiency of lean meat production to meet future packer and consumer demands for pork. Swine diets that do not adequately provide essential nutrients, match the genotype, or accommodate consumption variations fail to allow maximum lean tissue growth. Many factors influence the nutrient requirements of pigs, including sex, genotype, feed intake, housing, etc. It is evident that the advantages offered by enhancing the growing pigs' capacity for lean growth can only be fully realized when dietary nutrient levels are adjusted with a phase feeding strategy.

REFERENCES

Anderson, D. B.; Weenhuizen, E. L.; Waitt, W. P.; Paxton, R. E.; and Young, S. S. 1987. The effect of dietary protein on nitrogen metabolism, growth performance and carcass composition of finishing pigs fed ractopamine. Fed Proc 46:1021.

Cera, K. R.; Mahan, D. C.; and Reinhart, G. A. 1988. Weekly digestibilities of diets supplemented with corn oil, lard or tallow by weanling swine. J Anim Sci 66:1430–1437.

Convey, E. M. 1987. Advances in animal science: Potential for improving meat animal production. Proc Cornell Nutr Conf, Cornell Univ, Ithaca, N.Y., p. 1.

Dawson, D. P.; Morrill, J. L.; Reddy, P. G.; and Minocha, H. C. 1988. Soy protein concentrate and heated soy flours as protein sources in milk replacer for preruminant calves. J Dairy Sci 71:1301–1309.

Giesting, D. W.; Easter, R. A.; and Roe, B. A. 1985. A comparison of protein and carbohydrate sources of milk and plant origin for starter pigs. J Anim Sci 61[Suppl 1]:299. Abstr.

Giesting, D. W.; Kelley, K. W.; and Easter, R. A. 1986. Evaluation of early exposure to soy protein on pre- and postweaning performance and immunological characteristics of young pigs. J Anim Sci 63[Suppl 1]:278. Abstr.

Goodband, R. D.; Nelssen, J. L.; Hines, R. H.; Kropf, D. H.; Thaler, R. C.; Schricker, B. R.; and Fitzner, G. E. 1988. The effect of porcine somatotropin and dietary lysine level on growth performance and carcass characteristics of finishing swine. J Anim Sci 66[Suppl 1]:95.

Goodband, R. D.; Nelssen, J. L.; Hines, R. H.; Kropf, D. H.; Thaler, R. C.; Schricker, B. R.; Fitzner, G. E.; and Lewis, A. J. 1990. The effects of

porcine somatotropin and dietary lysine on growth performance and carcass characteristics of finishing swine. J Anim Sci 68:3261–3276.

Kilshaw, P. J., and Sissons, J. W. 1979. Gastrointestinal allergy to soybean protein in preruminant calves. Allergenic constituents of soybean products. Res Vet Sci 27:366–371.

Klasing, K. K.; Maynard, P. M.; and Laurin, D. E. 1988. Hypersensitivity to dietary soy protein. Poult Sci 67[Suppl 1]:104. Abstr.

Li, D. F.; Thaler, R. C.; Nelssen, J. L; Harmon, D. Allee, G. L.; Weeden, T.; Stoner, G.; Fitzner, G.; Hines, R.; and Nichols, D. 1989. Effect of fat source and fat combinations on starter pigs. J Anim Sci 67[Suppl 1]:230. Abstr.

Li, D. F.; Nelssen, J. L.; Reddy, P. G.; Blecha, F.; Hancock, J. D.; Allee, G. L.; Goodband, R. D.; and Klemm, R. D. 1990. Hypersensitivity to soybean meal in early weaned pigs. J Anim Sci 68:1790–1799.

Mowat, A. M., and Ferguson, A. 1981. Hypersensitivity in the small intestine. V. Induction of cell-mediated immunity to a dietary antigen. Clin Exp Immunol 43:574.

National Research Council. 1979. Nutrient Requirements of Swine, 8th rev ed. Washington, D.C.: National Academy Press.

———. 1980. Mineral Tolerance of Domestic Animals. Washington, D.C.: National Academy Press.

———. 1988. Nutrient Requirements of Swine, 9th rev ed. Washington, D.C.: National Academy Press.

Nelssen, J. L. 1986. High nutrient-density diets for weaning pigs. Kansas State Univ Res Rep 306, Manhattan, p. 35.

Newby, T. J.; Miller, B.; Stokes, C. R.; Hampson, D.; and Bourne, F. J. 1984. Local hypersensitivity responses to dietary antigens in early weaned pigs. In Recent Advances in Animal Nutrition. Ed. W. Haresign and D. J. A. Cole. London: Butterworth, pp. 49–59.

Schricker, B. R. 1989. PST administeration may influence swine nutrient requirements. Feedstuffs 61(18):13.

Seegraber, F. J., and Morrill, J. L. 1979. Effect of soy protein on intestinal absorptive ability of calves by the xylose absorption test. J Dairy Sci 62:972–977.

———. 1982. Effect of soy protein on calves' intestinal absorptive ability and morphology determined by scanning electron microscopy. J Dairy Sci 65:1962–1970.

———. 1986. Effect of protein source in calf milk replacers on morphology and absorptive ability of small intestine. J Dairy Sci 69:460–469.

Stahly, T. S.; Cromwell, G. L.; Terhune, D.; Bark, L. J.; and Schenck, B. C. 1989. Influence of genetic capacity for lean tissue growth on the amino acid needs of pigs. Univ of Kentucky Swine Res Rep Prog 321:21–23.

Steele, N. C.; Campbell, R. G.; and Caperna, T. J. 1987. Update of porcine growth hormone research: Practical and biological implications. Proc Cornell Nutr Conf, Cornell Univ, Ithaca, N.Y., p. 15.

Stokes, C. R.; Mill, B. G.; Bailey, M.; and Bource, F. J. 1986. The immune response to dietary antigens and its significance in animal production. Proc 6th Int Conf Prod Dis Farm Anim, Belfast, Northern Ireland.

Thaler, R. C.; Nelssen, J. L.; and Allee, G. L. 1988. Effect of fat source and fat combinations on starter pig performance. Kansas State Univ Res Rep 556, Manhattan, p. 38.

Tokach, M. D.; Cornelius, S. G.; Rust, J. W.; and Pettigrew, J. E. 1989a. The appropriate level of fat addition to high milk product diets for the early weaned pig. J Anim Sci 67[Suppl 1]:231. Abstr.

TOKACH, M. D.; CORNELIUS, S. G.; AND RUST, J. W. 1989b. An evaluation of fat in high milk product diets for the early weaned pig. Univ of Minnesota Res Rep, St. Paul, p. 65.

TURLINGTON, W. H.; ALLEE, G. L.; AND NELSSEN, J. L. 1987. Effects of fat source on performance of weaned pigs. Kansas State Univ Res Rep 528, Manhattan, p. 35.

_____. 1989. Effects of protein and carbohydrate sources on digestibility and digesta flow rate in weaned pigs fed a high-fat, dry diet. J Anim Sci 67:2333–2340.

WALTON, P. E.; ETHERTON, T. D.; AND EVOCK, C. M. 1986. Antagonism of insulin action in cultured pig adipose tissue by pituitary and recombinant porcine growth hormone: Potentiation by hydrocortisone. Endocrinology 118:2577–2581.

61

Porcine Reproductive and Respiratory Syndrome

D. A. Benfield

J. E. Collins

A. L. Jenny

T. J. Loula

A MYSTERY SWINE DISEASE was first recognized in 1987–88 in herds in North Carolina, Iowa, and Minnesota. Surprisingly, this disease syndrome was relatively unknown until reports of several outbreaks of the disease in Indiana swine herds (Quaife 1989, 1990). The "mystery" disease is characterized by reproductive disorders (late-term abortions, premature farrowings, stillborns, mummification, and weak liveborn pigs), high piglet mortality, and respiratory disease in neonates to market pigs (Keffaber 1989; Loula 1991). The predominant reproductive and respiratory clinical signs associated with this syndrome have resulted in the descriptive term "Swine Infertility and Respiratory Syndrome" (SIRS), which has become the most commonly used name for mystery swine disease in the United States.

A disease similar to SIRS has been reported in Canada (Dea et al. 1990), Germany (Lindhaus and Lindhaus 1991), the Netherlands (Wensvoort et al. 1991), Belgium (Pensaert 1991), and Spain and England (White 1991). The disease described in Europe is clinically similar to SIRS in the United States, except disease has spread much more rapidly throughout the European swine community, and cutaneous cyanosis of the ears, vulva, and abdomen is more frequently observed as a clinical sign in swine in Europe. Hence, the European veterinary community has given various names to this syndrome: new pig disease, blue ear disease, porcine epidemic abortion and respiratory syndrome (PEARS), and the official name porcine reproductive and respiratory syndrome (PRRS).

In North America, swine herds have experienced two emerging respiratory syndromes in recent years. One is a component of SIRS and the other one is a separate syndrome for which an atypical influenza A virus is believed to be the etiologic agent (Girard et al. 1991). In this latter syndrome, respiratory disease is the most obvious feature, but it can be accompanied by some reproductive disorders that are usually less severe than those observed in SIRS. The lesion is a proliferative and necrotizing pneumonia (PNP) (Morin et al. 1990). Since the two syndromes appeared approximately at the same time and the etiologies were unknown until recently, both syndromes have often been considered as part of mystery swine disease. At this time, it seems appropriate to consider SIRS and PNP as two separate and distinct entities causing the so-called mystery swine disease (Collins 1991; Morin and Robinson 1991).

ETIOLOGY. Epidemiologic and other observations prompted speculation that PRRS/SIRS was a transmissible disease caused by an infectious agent. Porcine parvovirus (PPV), encephalomyocarditis virus (EMCV), porcine enteroviruses (PEV), pseudorabies virus (PRV), porcine cytomegalovirus, hemagglutinating encephalomyelitis virus (HEV), classical swine influenza virus (SIV), transmissible gastroenteritis virus (TGEV), bovine viral diarrhea virus, border disease virus, Japanese B encephalitis virus, hog cholera virus (HCV), *Leptospira interrogans* serovar *bratislava, Chlamydia psittaci,* and mycotoxins were at one time considered potential etiologic agents (Bane and Hall 1990; Bolin and Cassels 1990; Mengeling and Lager 1990; Van Alstine 1990; Woollen et al. 1990). These infectious agents are not likely the primary cause of PRRS/SIRS, due to the following reasons: (1) none of these agents produced spontaneous or experimental respiratory and reproductive disorders similar to PRRS/SIRS; (2) these agents could not be isolated with any consistency from acutely ill pigs, stillborn fetuses, or liveborn pigs from farms with PRRS/SIRS; and (3) seroconversion or increased antibody titers to the above agents could not be demonstrated with any consistency in serum collected from sows affected with PRRS/SIRS. In fact, an early serologic survey conducted by the National Veterinary Services Laboratories on sera collected from sows in SIRS-affected herds in four midwestern states found no evidence of antibodies to African swine fever virus or HCV, and did not clearly implicate HEV, PPV, classical SIV, EMCV, PRV, PEV, or TGEV as the primary cause of this disease in these herds (Boyt 1989).

The general consensus indicates that an "unidentified virus" is the causative agent of PRRS in the Netherlands (Wensvoort et al. 1991) and Germany (Ohlinger 1991), and SIRS in the United States (Collins et al. 1991). In 1991, the causative agent of PRRS in the Netherlands was isolated and designated the Lelystad virus (Wensvoort et al. 1991). Shortly thereafter, independent isolations of a similar virus were reported in Germany (Ohlinger 1991) and the United States (Benfield et al. 1991; Collins et al. 1991). The Netherlands PRRS virus was isolated in porcine alveolar macrophage cultures from tissues of 2- to 10-day-old piglets and blood samples of sows affected with PRRS. The German isolate of PRRS was also isolated on porcine alveolar macrophages using tissue homogenates from pigs with PRRS, whereas the U.S. isolate of SIRS was isolated on the permanent cell line 2621 using a lung homogenate from a gnotobiotic pig, which had been previously inoculated with tissue homogenates collected from pigs with the respiratory form of SIRS.

Each of these PRRS and SIRS cell culture-propagated viruses has been reported to induce clinical signs and lesions resembling those of the reproductive form of the disease in sows (Collins et al. 1991; Ohlinger 1991; Terpstra et al. 1991; Christianson et al. 1992), and of the respiratory form of the disease in piglets (Collins et al. 1991; Ohlinger 1991; Pol et al. 1991). Virus was reisolated from lungs, spleen, or other lymphoid organs after intranasal inoculation of either gnotobiotic, specific-pathogen-free (SPF), or conventional piglets. The PRRS/SIRS viruses were also reisolated from tissues of stillborn or liveborn fetuses after intranasal inoculation of pregnant sows. In addition, 75% (123/165) of sows with clinical signs of PRRS seroconverted to the Netherlands PRRS isolate, whereas less than 10% converted to EMCV and PEV types 2 and 7, which were also isolated from pigs and sows with PRRS (Wensvoort et al. 1991). Limited seroepidemiologic data indicated that 17/31 piglets (55%) and 24/30 sows (80%) affected with SIRS seroconverted to the U.S. isolate of SIRS, whereas 8 pigs and 22 sows on a farm with no history of SIRS had no antibody to the SIRS virus (Collins et al. 1991).

The above studies indicate that an "unidentified virus" is the etiologic agent of PRRS in Europe and SIRS in the United States. Successful isolation of three separate virus isolates from three distinct geographic locations, together with the reproduction of both the respiratory and reproductive syndrome of PRRS/SIRS and reisolation of the virus, fulfill Koch's postulates. It should be noted that each of these three PRRS/SIRS isolates were extensively tested to rule out adventitious virus and mycoplasma contaminaton of the inoculum.

Properties of the PRRS/SIRS Agents. The Netherlands and German isolates of PRRS and the U.S. isolate of SIRS have not been completely characterized and classified into an appropriate virus family. The PRRS/SIRS viruses are antigenically similar. Antisera to the Netherlands isolate of PRRS strongly neutralize the German isolate of PRRS (Ohlinger 1991), and antisera from

pigs experimentally inoculated with tissue homogenate containing the U.S. SIRS isolate also neutralize the Netherlands isolate of PRRS (Collins et al. 1991). The PRRS/SIRS viruses appear to be an unidentified enveloped RNA virus approximately 50–100 nm in diameter. Ohlinger (1991) has tentatively classified the German isolate of PRRS as a member of the family Togaviridae. Additional evidence is needed to definitively classify the PRRS and SIRS viruses and to determine if these viruses are the same or different isolates.

The PRRS/SIRS viruses are fastidious and appear to replicate in only a few cell lines: porcine alveolar macrophages and the stable cell lines PS-EK and 2621. Each of the three virus isolates is inactivated by lipid solvents (chloroform) or detergents (sodium deoxycholate, Triton X-100, and NP-40). Replication of the German and U.S. PRRS/SIRS viruses is not inhibited by actinomycin D, mitomycin C, and BUDR, which interfere with the replication of DNA, but not the nononcogenic RNA viruses. This indicates that the German and U.S. PRRS/SIRS viruses have an RNA genome. The U.S. isolate of SIRS is very stable when stored at $-70°C$ for at least 1 year and at $4°C$ for at least 1 month without loss of titer. Heating to $56°C$ destroys infectivity after 30–90 minutes. The PRRS/SIRS viruses do not hemagglutinate erythrocytes of chickens, ducks, guinea pigs, mice, rats, rabbits, pigs, sheep, cattle, and humans (type O).

Antisera directed to PRV, TGEV, porcine epidemic diarrhea virus, HEV, African swine fever virus, HCV, SIV, PI-3, respiratory syncytial virus, avian leukemia virus and infectious bronchitis virus, EMCV, and PPV do not neutralize the SIRS or PRRS virus isolates (Benfield et al. 1991; Wensvoort et al. 1991).

EPIDEMIOLOGY. Since the etiologic agent of PRRS/SIRS has only recently been identified, there is little information on the epidemiology of this syndrome. The mode of transmission of the disease is also unknown, but rapid spread of PRRS/SIRS between farms in some localities has been reported (Keffaber 1990; Lindhaus and Lindhaus 1991; Terpstra et al. 1991), suggesting airborne spread. Also, aerosol spread may be the most likely route of transmission because the disease can be readily reproduced in pigs and sows by intranasal inoculation (Collins et al. 1991; Ohlinger 1991; Pol et al. 1991; Terpstra et al. 1991; Christianson et al. 1992). Sows apparently shed the virus, for sentinel pigs in contact with clinically ill sows become infected with the PRRS/SIRS virus and seroconversion can be demonstrated (Ohlinger 1991; Wensvoort et al. 1991; Christianson et al. 1992). Pig movement is also suspected in the transmission of the disease.

The spread of the disease on individual farms can be quite rapid, or it may progress over a period of 2–4 weeks. The disease has been reported from total confinement facilities, premises with a mixture of confinement and open pens, and premises with total outside production facilities. Genetics, health status, size of farm, and parity distribution seem to play no role in determining the incidence of this disease syndrome. Some herds have experienced the problem shortly after the introduction of new swine onto the premise, whereas other herds that have been affected have not introduced new stock in the recent past.

No concurrent disease problems in other domestic livestock or pet animals have been associated with outbreaks of PRRS/SIRS. Wildlife, birds, and rodents have been suggested as possible sources of the causative agent, but additional studies are needed to confirm this.

CLINICAL SIGNS. Initially, the disease was described as acute, with clinical signs occurring in sows or gilts during gestation, sows and their suckling pigs at farrowing, or older pigs in the nursery or finishing units. A chronic form of the disease syndrome, usually manifested by continued poor performance in the nursery and decreased farrowing rates, has recently been reported. Initially, the magnitude and duration of clinical illness and mortality appeared to differentiate this disease syndrome from other common swine diseases. However, subclinical disease seems to become more frequent and considerable variations in clinical signs are observed.

Breeding/Gestation. Severe drops are seen in number bred, conception rate, and farrowing rate (Fig. 61.1). Clinical signs during gestation include prolonged anorexia, pyrexia (body temperature of 40–41°C, 104–106°F), lethargy, depression, respiratory distress, occasional vomiting, late-term abortion, premature farrowing (usually occurring day 107–113), and sometimes death. Many cases of PRRS/SIRS in breeding swine are characterized by a high incidence and severity of clinical signs.

Farrowing. Clinical signs observed in individual animals are similar to those listed above. Affected sows may deliver a combination of stillborn pigs, partially macerated stillborn pigs, weak pigs, or mummified fetuses. The number of stillborn pigs in each litter is variable. Some litters will contain no stillborn pigs, but some litters will be composed of 80–100% stillborn pigs (Keffaber 1989). The percentage of stillborn pigs delivered begins to rise shortly after the abortions subside, will be high (12–30%) for a 2- to 3-week period (Fig. 61.1), and then will usually slowly regress to normal limits (7–8%). In some instances, stillborn rates do not return to normal until 4–5 months after the initial episode. An increase in mummified fetuses (20%) usually follows the rise in abortions and stillborns (Schultz 1989).

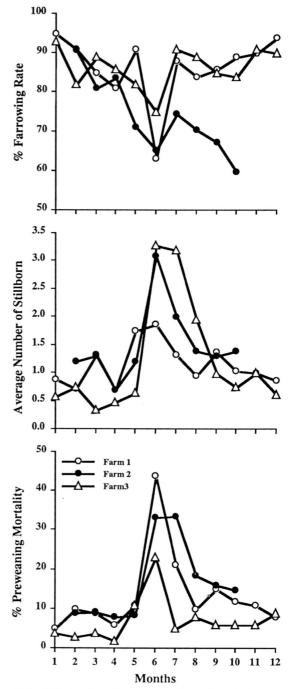

61.1. Effects of porcine reproductive and respiratory syndrome on some parameters of three midwestern swine breeding herds.

Suckling Pigs. Rapid abdominal breathing, lethargy, depression, and inability to nurse are observed. Average preweaning mortality may increase to 30–50%, with some individual litters experiencing 80–100% mortality (Fig. 61.1). Surviving baby pigs often have an increased incidence of secondary disease problems.

Nursery Pigs. Clinical signs include rapid abnormal breathing, sneezing, partial anorexia, rough hair coat, poor performance, and occasional death. The initial phase is often followed by secondary disease problems, resulting in additional clinical signs related to respiratory and enteric diseases.

Finishing Pigs. Clinical signs include anorexia, pyrexia (40–41°C, 104–106°F), depression, lethargy, cough, and rapid abnormal breathing. As in the nursery, the initial phase is also often followed by secondary disease problems resulting in additional clinical signs related to respiratory and enteric diseases.

Slight differences in clinical signs are observed between SIRS and PRRS. The disease has spread much more rapidly through the European than the U.S. swine community. Cutaneous cyanosis of the ears, vulva, and abdomen, although uncommon, is seen more frequently in sows affected by PRRS than by SIRS. Since several of the clinical signs reported with SIRS have also been observed with PNP in North America, the clinical aspect of these diseases might have been confounded.

PATHOGENESIS. The pathogenesis of PRRS/SIRS has been studied in sows that were experimentally inoculated with cell culture–propagated PRRS/SIRS virus (Terpstra et al. 1991; Christianson et al. 1992). Sows intranasally inoculated at either 84 or 93 days of gestation become anorectic and listless and sometimes develop a transient fever (39–40°C) of 1–2 days duration. Clinical signs appear 4–7 days postinfection (PI). Sows may develop cutaneous erythema of the ears after inoculation with the Netherlands isolate, but this has not been observed in sows inoculated with the U.S. isolate.

The PRRS virus has been isolated from serum, plasma, and leukocyte samples from sows in field cases (Wensvoort et al. 1991), which suggests that the virus may be transmitted to placenta via the blood. Transplacental infection has been documented by isolating the SIRS agent from fetuses as early as 14 days after intranasal infection of pregnant sows (Christianson et al. 1992), but the mechanisms by which the virus crosses the placenta are unknown. Migration of infected macrophages across the placenta may be an important means of fetal infection because the virus has been isolated from peripheral white blood cells and is readily cultivated in alveolar macrophages (Terpstra et al. 1991).

The SIRS/PRRS virus also causes fetal death and neonatal weakness by unknown mechanisms. The virus has been isolated from fetal organ homogenates (Collins et al. 1991; Wensvoort et al. 1991), blood, and ascitic fluids (Wensvoort et al. 1991), but microscopic lesions are seldom evident in fetal tissues (Collins et al. 1991). Multiplication of the virus to a high titer may damage vital tissues, causing fetal disease in the absence of microscopic lesions.

The pathogenesis of PRRS/SIRS has also been studied using gnotobiotic (Collins et al. 1990), colostrum-deprived (Pol et al. 1991), and conventionally reared pigs (Ohlinger 1991). Pigs become listless and anorectic 2–4 days after intranasal infection with the PRRS/SIRS virus. Colostrum-deprived and conventional pigs but not gnotobiotic pigs develop fevers (41.4°C) by 5 days PI. Virus can be reisolated from many organs including peripheral white blood cells, thymus, spleen, bone marrow, peribronchial lymph nodes, lung, and brain. Colostrum-deprived pigs have gross and microscopic lung lesions by 1 day PI, but gnotobiotic pigs do not have gross pulmonary lesions at necropsy 7 days PI, although microscopic lung lesions (interstitial pneumonitis) are well developed by 7 days.

The PRRS virus is shed in sufficient quantity to be infectious for contact-exposed animals. Four of 12 SPF pigs placed in contact with sows from herds with PRRS became infected and virus was recovered from nasal secretions, lung, or tonsil of the contact-exposed pigs (Wensvoort et al. 1991).

Speculation about the immunosuppressive effects of the PRRS/SIRS virus has occurred because secondary bacterial infections appear to increase in herds following a PRRS/SIRS outbreak. Experimental studies to document the potential immunosuppressive properties of PRRS/SIRS virus have not been done, but Pol et al. (1991) have reported microscopic evidence of lymphoid depletion in the spleen, thymus, tonsil, and mesenteric lymph node in pigs inoculated with the Netherlands isolate of PRRS. Hyperplasia of lymph nodes and thymic lymphoid depletion have also been described in pigs inoculated with the German isolate of PRRS (Ohlinger 1991).

LESIONS

Fetuses and Stillborn Pigs. Fetuses and stillborn pigs in field or experimental infections do not have specific gross lesions. Late-term abortions and premature farrowings containing weakborn, stillborn, and partially mummified fetuses of approximately the same size are typically seen in the early stages of PRRS/SIRS outbreaks. Partially mummified fetuses have brownish tan discoloration of the skin and increased amounts of straw-colored fluid in abdominal cavities. Microscopic lesions are seldom seen in fetuses or stillborn pigs.

Piglets and Growing/Finishing Pigs. Results of field investigations and experimental studies indicate that lung is a major target organ of the PRRS/SIRS virus. Microscopic examination of lung from field cases reveals multifocal to diffuse interstitial pneumonitis, characterized by thickening of alveolar septae by many large macrophages (Fig. 61.2). Alveolar spaces and alveolar septae contain proteinaceous debris and degenerating cells with pyknotic nuclei. Cranial, middle, and caudal lung lobes are equally affected. Secondary infection by bacterial pathogens is common in field cases and may obscure pulmonary lesions.

Gross and microscopic lung lesions of PRRS/SIRS should be distinguished from those of proliferative and necrotizing pneumonia (PNP), another emerging respiratory disease recognized in Quebec, Canada, in the fall of 1988 (Morin et al. 1990). In contrast to PRRS/SIRS, the lungs of pigs affected by PNP have prominent gross pulmonary lesions, with the entire lung being reddened and "meaty" in consistency. Microscopically, PNP is characterized by hypertrophy and hyperplasia of pneumocytes type II, coagulates of necrotic cells in alveoli, syncytial cells, and necrosis of epithelium in respiratory ducts and terminal bronchioles. An atypical strain of influenza A is considered the most likely cause of PNP. At this time, this disease should be considered as a separate entity from PRRS/SIRS.

DIAGNOSIS. The ability to cultivate the PRRS and SIRS viruses on cell culture will allow for the future development of standard reagents and procedures for laboratory diagnosis of this syndrome. Currently, the best approach is to collect the proper specimens for diagnosis of the other diseases that must be considered in the differential diagnosis. When possible, acutely affected live animals, including neonatal pigs, sows or gilts, and growing/finishing pigs, should be submitted to the local diagnostic laboratory. Submissions should also include fetal serum or fetal thoracic fluid, intact aborted or stillborn fetuses from affected litters, mummified fetuses, and fresh and formalin-fixed tissues (brain, heart, kidney, liver, spleen, and lung) collected from aborted fetuses and stillborn pigs. Paired serum samples (acute and convalescent) should be taken from affected sows/gilts when possible.

Although diagnostic methodology for the diagnosis of PRRS/SIRS is still in development, histopathology, virus isolation, and detection of neutralizing antibodies can be used to render a tentative diagnosis of the disease.

Histopathology. Lesions have not been detected in stillborn and mummified pigs from sows affected with PRRS/SIRS. Interstitial pneumonia is the most consistent lesion in pigs with the respiratory form of PRRS/SIRS.

Virus Isolation. The best samples for isolation of PRRS/SIRS virus include pooled tissue (brain, heart, kidney, liver, spleen, and lung) homogenate from stillborn or liveborn pigs. The virus has not been isolated from mummified fetuses obtained from naturally or experimentally infected sows. Although some virus, such as PPV antigens, can be detected in mummified fetuses, the PRRS/SIRS virus is apparently inactivated by the decomposition of tissue in these fetuses (Collins et al. 1991). In suckling, weaned, or fattening pigs, lung appears to be the choice tissue for virus iso-

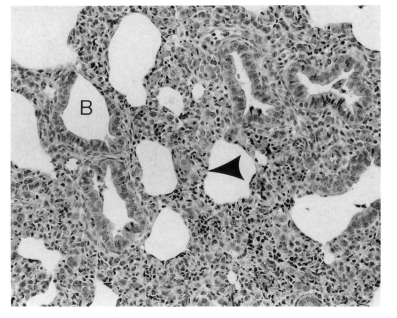

61.2. Lung of a 14-day-old pig from a field case of porcine reproductive and respiratory syndrome has marked thickening of alveolar septae (arrow). Many small dark spots in the interstitium represent nuclei of degenerating and necrotic cells. Epithelial cells lining terminal brochioles (*B*) do not have lesions. H & E.

lation, but virus has also been isolated from spleen, brain, tonsil, peripheral white blood cells, peribronchial lymph nodes, and thymus (Collins et al. 1991; Ohlinger 1991; Pol et al. 1991; Wensvoort et al. 1991). The virus has also been isolated from serum, plasma, and peripheral blood leukocytes of sows (Wensvoort et al. 1991). Virus isolation can be done using porcine alveolar macrophages, and detection of virus in macrophage cultures can be enhanced by using antisera to virus antigens by the immunoperoxidase technique (Pol et al. 1991; Terpstra et al. 1991).

Serology. Currently, serologic diagnosis of PRRS/SIRS is done in a few laboratories. This situation will change in the immediate future as additional isolates of the PRRS/SIRS virus become available and the characterization of the virus is completed. Neutralizing antibodies (low titers) can be detected in precolostral blood of liveborn pigs and thoracic fluids of stillborn pigs (Wensvoort et al. 1991). Pigs and sows that survive infection with PRRS/SIRS do seroconvert. Nonneutralizing antibodies have been detected in a 4-week-old conventional pig at 7 days PI. These antibodies were detected using an immunoperoxidase macrophage assay (Ohlinger 1991). In sows, neutralizing antibodies can be demonstrated at 19 days PI, and these antibodies were detected at least 18 months after the outbreak (Collins et al. 1991; Christianson et al. 1992). Sera collected from sows at abortion may be seronegative, but these animals usually seroconvert within 2–4 days after abortion (Ohlinger 1991).

TREATMENT. There is no specific treatment for PRRS/SIRS. Supportive therapy, such as supplemental concentrated energy sources and vitamins, may be required in some adults that fail to regain their appetite. Other drugs to stimulate appetite and control fever have also been used. Parenteral antibiotics, as well as medicated feed and water, have been used in a variety of ways with mixed results. The antibiotics are used primarily to control concurrent or secondary bacterial infections that often follow the acute phase of the disease.

Because of the possible implication of mycotoxins, attempts have been made to counteract the effects of contaminated feedstuffs. Feed sources have been switched and Novasil, a sodium calcium aluminosilicate product reported to ameliorate the effects of aflatoxicosis (Harvey et al. 1989), has been added. Since vitamin E deficiency has been shown to result in decreased antibody production (Van Vleet 1980), feed-grade and injectable forms of vitamin E have been used by practitioners.

PREVENTION. Vaccines to control PRRS/SIRS are not commercially available; however, the successful adaptation of the virus to cell culture improves the chances that a commercial vaccine will be available in the future. Currently, the best means of prevention are not known. Producers should be advised to follow management procedures that will minimize the introduction of any new disease into their herds. Suggested precautions include obtaining new breeding stock from farms with no history of PRRS/SIRS and isolation of new stock for at least 30 days. Strict rodent control measures and prevention of contact between swine and wildlife, feral animals, or free-flying birds is recommended. Limiting the on-farm traffic, requiring visitors to change into clean coveralls and boots, and strict precautions when loading pigs off the farm or when returning vehicles after taking pigs to market all decrease the possible introduction of any infectious agent.

REFERENCES
BANE, D. P., AND HALL, W. F. 1990. Fumonisin as a predisposing factor for "mystery swine disease." Proc Mystery Swine Dis Comm Meet. Livest Conserv Inst, Denver, Colo., pp. 77–79.
BENFIELD, D. A.; COLLINS, J. E.; HARRIS, L.; CHLADEK, D. W.; NELSON, E. A.; CHRISTIANSON, W. T.; AND MORRISON, R. B. 1991. Etiologic agent of swine infertility and respiratory syndrome in the United States. Proc Conf Res Workers Anim Dis.
BOLIN, C. A., AND CASSELLS, J. A. 1990. Isolation of *Leptospira interrogans* serovar *bratislava* from stillborn and weak pigs in Iowa. J Am Vet Med Assoc 196:1601–1604.
BOYT, P. A. 1989. Personal communication.
CHRISTIANSON, W. T.; COLLINS, J. E.; BENFIELD, D. A.; HARRIS, L.; JOO, H. S.; AND MORRISON, R. B. 1992. Experimental reproduction of swine infertility and respiratory syndrome in pregnant sows. Vet Rec. Submitted.
COLLINS, J. E. 1991. Newly recognized respiratory syndromes in North American swine herds. Am Assoc Swine Pract Newsl 3(5):7–11.
COLLINS, J. E.; BENFIELD, D. A.; GOYAL, S. M.; AND SHAW, D. P. 1990. Experimental transmission of swine reproductive failure syndrome (mystery swine disease) in gnotobiotic pigs. Proc Conf Res Workers Anim Dis, No. 2.
COLLINS, J. E.; BENFIELD, D. A.; CHRISTIANSON, W. T.; HARRIS, L.; GORCYCA, D. E.; CHLADEK, D. W.; AND MORRISON, R. B. 1991. Swine infertility and respiratory syndrome (mystery swine disease). Proc Minn Swine Conf Vet, pp. 200–205.
DEA, S.; BILODEAU, R.; SAUVAGEAU, R.; AND MARTINEAU, G. P. 1990. Virus isolations from farms in Quebec experiencing severe outbreaks of respiratory and reproductive problems. Proc Mystery Swine Dis Comm Meet. Livest Conserv Inst, Denver, Colo., pp. 67–72.
GIRARD, C.; MORIN, M.; AND ELAZHARY, Y. 1991. Experimentally induced porcine proliferative and necrotizing pneumonia with an influenza A virus. Vet Rec 129. In press.
HARVEY, R. B.; KUBENA, L. F.; PHILLIPS, T. D.; HUFF, W. E.; AND CORRIER, D. E. 1989. Prevention of aflatoxicosis by addition of hydrated sodium calcium aluminosilicate to the diets of growing barrows. Am J Vet Res 50:416–420.
KEFFABER, K. K. 1989. Reproductive failure of unknown etiology. Am Assoc Swine Pract Newsl 1:1, 4–5, 8–10.

———. 1990. Swine reproductive failure of unknown etiology. Proc George A. Young Swine Conf and Annu SPF Swine Conf. Lincoln, Nebr.

LINDHAUS, W., AND LINDHAUS, B. 1991. Ratselhafte schweinekrankheit. Prakt Tieraerztl 5:423–425.

LOULA, T. 1991. Mystery pig disease. Agri-Practice 12:23–34.

MENGELING, W. L., AND LAGER, K. M. 1990. Mystery pig disease: Evidence and considerations for its etiology. Proc Mystery Swine Dis Comm Meet. Livest Conserv Inst, Denver, Colo., pp. 88–90.

MORIN, M., AND ROBINSON, Y. 1991. Letter to the editor. Vet Rec. 129:367–368.

MORIN, M.; GIRARD, C.; ELAZHARY, Y.; FAJARDO, R.; DROLET, R.; AND LAGACÉ, A. 1990. A severe proliferative and necrotizing pneumonia in pigs: A newly recognized disease. Can Vet J 31:837–839.

OHLINGER, V. F. 1991. Personal communication.

PENSAERT, M. 1991. Personal communication.

POL, J. M. A.; VAN DIJK, J. E.; AND TERPSTRA, C. 1991. Pathological, ultrastructural, and immunohistochemical changes caused by Lelystad virus in experimentally induced infections of mystery swine disease (synonym: Porcine epidemic abortion and respiratory syndrome [PEARS]). Vet Q 13:137–143.

QUAIFE, T. 1989. Scramble is on to solve mystery disease. Swine Pract (July):5–10.

———. 1990. Helping labs to solve a "mystery" disease. Swine Pract (February):8–12.

SCHULTZ, R. 1989. Mystery disease. Hog Farm Manag, Nov 1989, p. 42.

TERPSTRA, C.; WENSVOORT, G.; AND POL, J. M. A. 1991. Experimental reproduction of porcine epidemic abortion and respiratory syndrome (mystery swine disease) by infection with Lelystad virus: Koch's postulates fulfilled. Vet Q 13:131–136.

VAN ALSTINE, W. 1990. Past diagnostic approaches and findings and potentially useful diagnostic strategies. Proc Mystery Swine Dis Comm Meet. Livest Conserv Inst, Denver, Colo., pp. 52–58.

VAN VLEET, J. F. 1980. Current knowledge of selenium-vitamin E deficiency in domestic animals. J Am Vet Med Assoc 176:321–325.

WENSVOORT, G.; TERPSTRA, C.; POL, J. M. A.; TER LAAK, E. A.; BLOEMRAAD, M.; DE KLUYVER, E. P.; KRAGTEN, C.; VAN BUITEN, L; DEN BESTEN, A.; WAGENAAR, F.; BROEKHUIJSEN, J. M.; MOONEN, P. L. J. M.; ZETSTRA, T.; DE BOER, E. A.; TIBBEN, H. J.; DE JONG, M. F.; VAN'T VELD, P.; GROENLAND, G. J. R.; VAN GENNEP, J. A.; VOETS, M. T.; VERHEIJDEN, J. H. M.; AND BRAAMSKAMP, J. 1991. Mystery swine disease in the Netherlands: The isolation of Lelystad virus. Vet Q 13:121–130.

WHITE, M. 1991. Blue ear disease of pigs. Vet Rec 128:574.

WOOLLEN, N.; DANIELS, E. K.; YEARY, T.; LIEPOLD, H. W.; AND PHILLIPS, R. M. 1990. Chlamydial infection and perinatal mortality in swine herd. J Am Vet Med Assoc 197:600–601.

62 Porcine Stress Syndrome

L. L. CHRISTIAN

K. LUNDSTROM

STRESS develops from an animal's response to noxious environmental stimuli. The importance to the field of veterinary medicine of stress encountered from the environment or husbandry systems is now realized. The interaction between stress and the disease state of animals is evident. Since limited information is available on stress adaptation in farm animals, a much greater research effort is needed to expand our knowledge of this most-complicated area of study.

Extreme stress susceptibility of pigs is an abnormality that must be described as a syndrome rather than a single abnormal characteristic. When stress-susceptible pigs are subjected to extreme excitement such as fighting during marketing or when they show resistance to normal management practices, a series of signs often de-velop. These have been reported as the porcine stress syndrome (PSS) (Topel et al. 1968).

Early signs of stress susceptibility in the pig are muscle and tail tremors. Further stress can result in marked dyspnea, irregular breathing, alternating blanched and reddened areas of the skin, rapid increase in body temperature, cyanosis, and development of an extreme acidosis condition. The next stage in the syndrome results in a total collapse, marked muscle rigidity, and hyperthermia; death occurs in a shocklike state (Fig. 62.1).

INCIDENCE. Reports from Denmark, Germany, France, the Netherlands, England, Poland, Japan, Mexico, and South Africa indicate that this stress-adaptation problem exists throughout

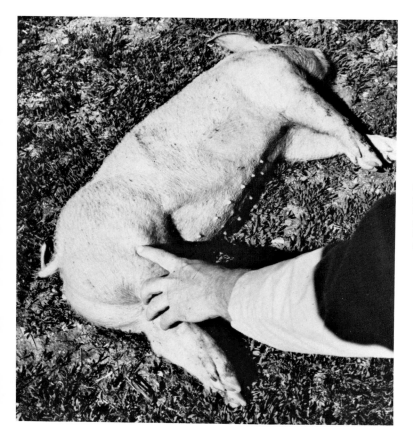

62.1. Stress-susceptible pig in the terminal stages of the stress syndrome. The skin shows alternating blanched and reddened areas. Muscle rigidity can be seen prior to death.

the world. Prior to 1971, approximately 35% of the hog producers in the United States encountered the condition. Less than 1% of the swine population in the United States, however, expresses the condition to the point where death occurs under normal marketing or management situations. A survey conducted by Webb (1982) revealed that the frequency of PSS varied from 0 to 89% among the world's breeds. The Pietrain and Belgian Landrace breeds had the highest incidence and the Duroc and Large White the lowest. The incidence was highest among producers utilizing confinement systems and those who have used intensive genetic selection for extreme muscle deposition (Fig. 62.2) and improved growth rate and feed efficiency. The stress syndrome has, however, been observed in pigs grown on pasture, and certainly not all extremely muscular swine show signs when subjected to severe excitement. After slaughter, problems with pale, watery muscle (or pale, soft, exudative, PSE muscle) are common in stress-prone pigs. The incidence of PSE in ham and loin muscles of the carcasses marketed in the United States has been reduced from 18–20% in the early 1970s to levels of 12% or less in the 1980s. The Pork Challenge Tests evaluated over 2400 carcasses and revealed incidences of 11.4, 8.5, and 8.9%, respectively in 1988, 1989, and 1990 (Goodwin 1990). It has also been shown that reproductive traits are influenced negatively in stress-susceptible pigs. (For a review of the influence of PSS on performance, reproductive and carcass traits, see Webb et al. 1982).

The same symptoms as in PSS occur after the use of some anesthetic agents such as halothane (Hall et al. 1966; Sybesma and Eikelenboom 1969; Allen et al. 1970; Jones et al. 1972), and also after succinylcholine chloride (Hall et al. 1966; Harrison et al. 1969). Due to the rapid and progressive rise in the core temperature to 42–45°C (107.6–113°F) or higher, the syndrome is called malignant hyperthermia (MH), and is probably identical to PSS.

INHERITANCE. Autosomal recessive inheritance with variable penetrance as the mode of inheritance of PSS was first proposed by Christian (1972). This hypothesis was later supported by results of Ollivier et al. (1975), Minkema et al. (1976), Webb and Smith (1976), Smith and Bampton (1977), and Mabry et al. (1981). Results of test matings at the Iowa Experiment Station (Table 62.1) are consistent with those expected with autosomal recessive inheritance. These studies also revealed the frequency of affected offspring to be similar in purebred and crossbred litters. In humans, an autosomal dominant in-

Table 62.1. Stress classification of offspring from various mating types

Mating Type	Litters	Stress Classification	
		Positive	Negative
Stress × stress	33	194	4
Stress × carrier	73	230	309
Carrier × carrier	40	67	224
Stress × control	15	0	85

Note: Stress classification is based on response to halothane anesthetic at 8–12 weeks of age.

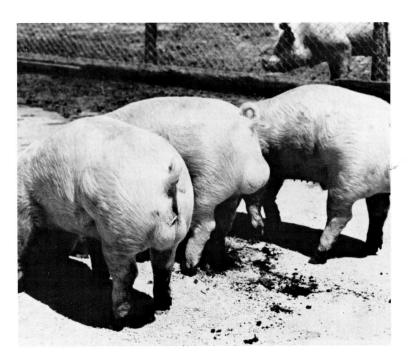

62.2. An example of the ham and body conformation in three stress-susceptible boars. Note the extreme bulge and round musculature of the hams.

heritance has been suggested by Britt and Kalow (1970a,b) for MH.

Rasmusen and Christian (1976) discovered an association between genotypes of the H blood group system and PSS. Jensen et al. (1976) revealed a relationship between H blood type and meat color score. Jorgensen et al. (1976) discovered a relationship between variants of the blood enzyme of phosphohexose isomerase (PHI) and PSS. Andresen (1971) had shown previously that the PHI and H blood-type loci and the locus for another enzyme, 6-phosphogluconate dehydrogenase, are all closely linked on the same chromosome. Because of knowledge concerning genetic factors closely linked to the stress gene, blood typing offers a means of indirectly determining the stress genotype of a pig.

Several studies during the last three decades have indicated that genetic predisposition to develop the drug-induced malignant hyperthermia (MH) in pigs and humans represents an identical (homologous) disease in these species. This is a very rare disease in humans, estimated to affect 1 out of 20,000 individuals. MH has been implicated to result from some disorder in calcium regulation. With the recent discovery and characterization of the calcium release channel protein (ryanodine receptor, RYR), it has been suggested that some mutation(s) in this protein may be the primary cause for MH susceptibility. Supporting evidence includes the fact that, first, the RYR gene has been mapped to the same chromosomal location as the MH gene, both in humans (MacLennan et al. 1990) and in pigs (Harbitz et al. 1990). Second, the three different electrophoretic phenotypes of the Ca^{++} release channel protein observed in pigs correspond to the HAL (MH) genotype (NN, Nn, or nn) of the individual pig (Knudson et al. 1990). It is thus very probable that the RYR gene is the long-sought MH gene.

PATHOPHYSIOLOGY

Body Temperature and Muscle Metabolism.
When pigs are subjected to stress conditions, they utilize muscle glycogen as a primary source of readily available energy. It appears that the stress-susceptible pig overresponds to stressful stimuli with excessive beta-adrenergic receptor stimulation from epinephrine. The response results in a rapid muscle glycogenolysis, rapid breakdown of adenosine triphosphate (ATP), and an excessive formation of muscle lactate. This metabolic activity is associated with a rapid increase in muscle temperature (42.5°C or 108.5°F in the center of the semimembranosus) when the pigs die from the disease. The combined abnormalities of a lactate acidosis and high body temperature are important contributory factors that cause death in swine when they develop the stress syndrome signs.

Harrison et al. (1969) and Nelson et al. (1972)

reported that halothane rapidly depletes skeletal muscle ATP in stress-susceptible pigs but not in normal pigs. The two major sources of ATP in skeletal muscle are glycolysis and oxidative phosphorylation. Oxidative phosphorylation is an aerobic system and glycolysis is an anaerobic system, but each may have an important, indirect influence on the other because the concentration of ATP determines, by means of a feedback mechanism, the activity of the oxidative phosphorylation or glycolysis pathway.

The oxidative phosphorylation process occurs in the mitochondria, and studies by Cheah and Cheah (1978) indicate that a difference exists in the structural or functional integrity of the mitochondria membranes of stress-susceptible pigs. This abnormality results in a much higher rate of mitochondria Ca^{++} efflux and a lower capacity to accumulate Ca^{++} under stress conditions. The excess Ca^{++} is free to activate the myofibrillar ATPase, and it could also activate the phosphorylase kinase so that glycogen is degraded to pyruvate. As the stress syndrome reaches the final phases, the skeletal muscle becomes more anaerobic and more of the pyruvate derived from the breakdown of glycogen is converted to lactate.

Nelson and Denborough (1977) proposed a theory that also involves excess Ca^{++} efflux into the sarcoplasm, except the release is from the sarcoplasmic reticulum. The Nelson-Denborough theory is based on the actions of the muscle relaxant dantrolene. Dantrolene has its main effect by blocking the mechanisms coupling the depolarization of the sarcolemma membrane to release calcium from the sarcoplasmic reticulum. This is commonly referred to as the excitation-contraction coupling mechanism, which can be regulated by at least two sites. The signal produced at site A is transmitted through site B. The signal released at site B causes calcium release from the sarcoplasmic reticulum for production of twitch tension response. Halothane is agonistic and dantrolene is antagonistic for site A.

Harrison (1975) and Gronert et al. (1976) have demonstrated the value of dantrolene in preventing the development of malignant hyperthermia in stress-susceptible pigs. Dantrolene apparently blocks the abnormal or excess signal from site A in halothane-sensitive pigs when they are given the anesthetic halothane. This reduces the release of Ca^{++} from the sarcoplasmic reticulum, the degree of contracture and rigidity of skeletal muscle, and stimulation for greater ATP depletion and lactate production by controlling the amount of Ca^{++} in the sarcoplasm. It appears that lack of proper Ca^{++} control of membranous portions (sarcoplasmic reticulum and mitochondria) is important in triggering the stress syndrome.

pH. The high levels of lactic acid produced in the skeletal muscle during the stress syndrome result in very low blood pH. Stress-susceptible pigs may have blood lactic acid levels as high as 425 mg/100 ml and a blood pH lower than 6.95 before the pig enters its terminal stages of the syndrome. Also, the stress-susceptible pig has a reduced ability to metabolize the acid waste produced from excessive and uncontrolled metabolism of glycogen.

Rates of lactate, alanine, and aspartate conversion to CO_2 in livers of stress-susceptible pigs were 61, 59, and 76% respectively of the rates observed in stress-resistant pigs in studies by Darrah et al. (1979). This is the result of an unknown metabolic lesion and apparently is another contributing factor in the development of PSS.

Plasma Electrolyte Levels.   The metabolic activity of the pig can alter the serum concentration of phosphorus, which in the stress-susceptible pig is increased from 2.6 mg/100 ml before exercise to 3.2 mg/100 ml after exercise but is virtually unchanged with exercise in controls (2.7 vs. 2.8). This indicates a possible abnormality in the intermediary metabolism where phosphorus is an end product. The research of Jones et al. (1972) suggesting an accelerated breakdown of ATP in stress-susceptible pigs following their exposure to stress conditions may explain the increased levels of blood phosphate.

Serum potassium levels are elevated to approximately 9.3 mEq/L when the blood pH drops below 7. Also, serum calcium is significantly increased in the stress-susceptible pigs after severe stress, but no major change in serum sodium concentration is evident.

Blood Enzyme Levels.   Lactate dehydrogenase (LDH), aldolase (ALD), and creatine kinase (CK) levels have been extensively studied in the pig. Variable relationships, however, have been reported between serum levels of LDH, ALD, and CK and stress susceptibility in swine (Addis et al. 1974; Schmidt et al. 1974). Irregularities in sample collection procedures or differing physiologic condition of the animal prior to taking samples may be responsible for the variation in the reported results. Diurnal variation, enzyme inactivation, hemolysis, organ-specific diseases and disorders not directly related to stress adaptation, excitement prior to sample collection, contamination of blood enzymes by needle puncture through muscle tissue, and difficulty involved in collecting blood from pigs without variation in the degree of stress are some variables that must be controlled for serum enzyme levels to be predictive of a pig's stress susceptibility.

When these conditions are controlled, a definite trend exists between the levels of these blood enzymes and the stress-adaptation traits in the pig.

Adrenal Glands.   The histologic characteristics of the adrenal cortex in stress-susceptible pigs were studied by Cassens et al. (1965). Large accumulations of lipid droplets in the zona reticularis were observed. Ball et al. (1972, 1973) verified these observations in a high percentage of stress-susceptible animals, but not all exhibited the abnormality. Ultrastructural examinations of these droplets suggest that they are mainly composed of morphologically normal lipids.

The adrenal cortex of stress-susceptible pigs has a greater residue of organelle remnants in the form of laminated membranous debris (myeline bodies). These may represent the result of a series of "spikes" or intermittent stress episodes caused by increased adrenal function and followed by depressed adrenal function and a consequent periodic increase in organelle turnover. The zona reticularis serves as the final zone of deposition of the membranous remnants.

Observations with the electron microscope indicated that the zona reticularis of stress-susceptible pigs often had large mitochondria with elaborate cristae and adjacent smooth-surfaced endoplasmic reticulum.

Hormones

ADRENAL CORTICOIDS.   Circulating levels of adrenal corticoids have been extensively studied in stress-susceptible and normal pigs (Topel et al. 1967; Judge et al. 1968; Steinhauf et al. 1969; Whipp et al. 1970; Staun et al. 1972; Marple and Cassens 1973). Considerable variation exists in plasma corticoid levels of both normal and stress-susceptible pigs; therefore, it is difficult to associate circulating levels of adrenal corticoids with stress-susceptibility traits in swine. Circulating levels of adrenal corticoids may not, however, reflect utilization. Therefore, Marple and Cassens (1973) studied the cortisol turnover rate and found it to be three times faster in stress-susceptible pigs than in normal pigs, and the former cleared plasma of cortisol approximately five times faster. The studies reported on adrenal function would suggest a major difference in the body metabolism of cortisol.

THYROXINE.   Levels of thyroxine seem to play a role in the stress syndrome. Halothane-sensitive swine had a significantly lower thyroxine half-life and plasma thyroxine concentration and a significantly greater thyroxine distribution space, thyroxine metabolic clearance rate, and triiodothyronine metabolic clearance rate. Thyroxine injections given to normal swine resulted in lower levels of muscle ATP, while thyroidectomized swine exhibited slower rates of postmortem glycolysis and a slower accumulation of muscle lactic acid (Marple et al. 1977). Also, administration of thyroxine to animals can reduce calcium uptake by the sarcoplasmic reticulum, and this may contribute to the calcium efflux from the sarcoplasmic reticulum during the stress syndrome.

CATECHOLAMINES. Little is known of catecholamine levels in stress-susceptible pigs. Research at the Iowa Experiment Station indicates that dopamine has an important role in stress adaptation in the pig (Draper et al. 1984). Urinary dopamine levels were significantly lower ($P < 0.01$) in the stress-susceptible pigs (22.9 μg/24 hour) as compared to the levels in the normal or control pigs (31.1 μg/24 hour). No significant differences were found in the urinary epinephrine or norepinephrine levels in the two types of pigs. The mean dopamine levels in the caudate nucleus of the brain were 6.0 μg/g of tissue in the stress-susceptible pigs and 10.9 μg/g of tissue in the normal pigs. The lower dopamine levels in the caudate nuclei suggest that an abnormality exists in the function of the striate body (caudate nuclei and putamen) when stress-susceptible pigs are subjected to extreme exercise or other types of physical stress. A lower dopamine concentration in this portion of the brain could reduce the inhibitory effect on acetylcholine stimulation under stress conditions and result in an overstimulation of the motor end plates of skeletal muscle. This would result in excessive calcium efflux into the sarcoplasm and could trigger PSS.

NUTRITIONAL RELATIONSHIPS. Signs of selenium (Se) and vitamin E deficiencies and those of PSS have been confused by some workers in the swine industry. Field cases have been reported where high levels of vitamin E were supplemented in the ration as a method of reducing deaths from PSS. Research studies have clearly shown that high supplementation of vitamin E has no major influence on reducing management problems or deaths of pigs when they possess the genetic abnormalities associated with PSS.

The symptoms that occur with a vitamin E–Se deficiency are liver necrosis, heart hemorrhages, pale areas in the heart and skeletal muscles, intestinal hemorrhages, yellowish brown discoloration of body fat, generalized edema of internal tissues, anemia, icterus, and a high mortality rate in young pigs. Of these symptoms, the only one in common with PSS is development of a pale, soft musculature postmortem. Histologic studies show that skeletal muscle from vitamin E– and Se-deficient pigs exhibits degeneration, a lesion not observed in pigs dying from the stress syndrome. This further indicates that the two conditions are separate problems.

Ullrey (1973) stated that symptoms associated with vitamin E or Se deficiency are most often expressed under extreme environmental stress. Excessive chilling or overheating causes the incidence of vitamin E–deficiency symptoms to increase. Similar symptoms have been reported when excessive fighting occurs among litters of pigs mixed at weaning. Apparently stressful events often produce death among pigs that are borderline in this deficiency. Supplementing deficient diets with Se or vitamin E is likely to prevent such deaths, thus avoiding the confusion of this condition with the genetic abnormality of PSS.

NECROPSY OBSERVATIONS. A typical necropsy of a pig that has died of PSS generally reveals nonspecific alterations. The viscera may be congested and frothy material evidently from terminal pulmonary edema is sometimes found in the bronchioles, but the most striking feature is the very rapid development of rigor mortis immediately after death. The latter is simply a continuation and accentuation of the muscle rigidity that is so characteristic of pigs that succumb to PSS.

Approximately 60–70% of stress-susceptible pigs develop a pale, soft, watery musculature (Fig. 62.3) within 15–30 minutes after death. This is caused by muscle protein denaturation from the combination of a high muscle temperature and a high muscle lactic acid content immediately postmortem. The pale, watery musculature can also develop in pigs slaughtered under normal conditions in packing plants. This problem has received wide publicity because of the deleterious economic effects associated with processing of this pork (Briskey 1964; Wismer-Pedersen 1968; Topel et al. 1972).

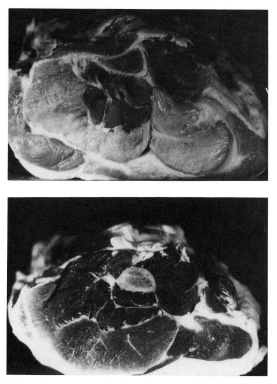

62.3. An example of pale, soft musculature (above) and normal musculature (below) in the hams of stress-susceptible pigs.

Examination of a large number of heart and longissimus muscle tissues with the light and electron microscopy has failed to reveal any evidence of inflammatory exudate or lesions indicative of antemortem necrosis. Heart weights of stress-susceptible pigs are smaller than those of normal pigs, yet the right ventricle weight as a ratio of total heart weight and total ventricle weight is significantly greater (Draper et al. 1989). This right ventricular hypertrophy may contribute to the physiological patterns and clinical signs observed under stress. Cassens et al. (1969) reported giant fibers in muscles of stress-prone pigs, however, Essen-Gustavsson et al. (1988) found similar fiber types between stress types but larger fiber areas and lower capillary density in the stress-susceptible group.

Most organs from pigs that have died from PSS have not received adequate study from the histologic viewpoint. Postmortem observations of these organs, however, show no pathologic complications.

In the PSS breeding herd maintained at Iowa State University, hysteria during farrowing and savaging attempts at the newborn are common among PSS-positive females. Death losses do occur among PSS-positive adult sows and boars during the normal production process but with few exceptions have occurred within 1/2 hour to 2 hours of a stressful activity such as mating, mixing, parturition, or weaning. Extremely high ambient temperatures and high relative humidity have produced a higher frequency of death loss among positive than negative herd mates, but the frequency of these deaths has been low.

TREATMENT. If the early signs (muscle and tail tremors and irregular, heavy breathing) of the syndrome are observed in specific individuals, remove them immediately from the impending stress and allow them to rest. If the syndrome has not advanced too far, the pigs will recover without further treatment. If blotchy cyanosis of the skin is observed and slight muscle rigidity starts to develop, intravenous administration of a tranquilizer, fast-reacting hydrocortisone, and a bicarbonate to reduce the lactate acidosis is sometimes helpful.

Dantrolene sodium administered to stress-susceptible pigs before halothane administration completely prevented the development of malignant hyperthermia when given in doses of 5 mg/kg or 7.5 mg/kg body weight. Also, dantrolene sodium reversed the signs of the malignant hyperthermia syndrome dramatically after it was triggered by halothane, except for lactate levels that returned toward control levels slowly (Harrison 1975; Gronert et al. 1976). Even though intravenous injection of dantrolene sodium is effective in the prevention and treatment of porcine malignant hyperthermia, dantrolene is relatively insoluble. Gronert et al. (1977) reported a simple and fast method to solubilize dantrolene sodium.

If it is known that specific pigs are stress susceptible, advanced tranquilization prior to subjecting them to stressful situations will help to reduce deaths from the PSS problem.

DETECTION. Elimination of or reduction in the incidence of this hereditary problem depends on identification of PSS animals and carriers of the defective gene and their subsequent elimination from the breeding herd. Although reliable means of detecting carriers are unknown, numerous techniques are successful in diagnosing the PSS animal.

Visual Appraisal. Classification of pigs based on their visual appearance by experienced evaluators provides an inexpensive and rapid means of detecting the PSS animal. Visual indicators include extreme muscling, small stature, and tight skin in the belly and jowl region. When physically stressed, the affected animals often show muscle and tail tremors, blotchy cyanosis of the skin, and dilated pupils. This technique requires experienced evaluators, lacks the objectivity desired for widespread use, and often leads to misdiagnosis of heavy-muscled, stress-resistant animals.

CK Levels. Whole blood or serum levels of CK have been shown to relate to PSS classification. The pitfalls of improper collection techniques have been discussed previously. When blood samples are carefully drawn from an ear vein 2–8 hours after severe physical stress has been uniformly imposed on all animals to be tested, CK measurements obtained by either the Sigma Chemical Company or Antonik laboratory procedures have produced accuracies varying from 60 to 90% (Mabry et al. 1983).

Halothane Screening. Exposure to halothane offers the most accurate means of detecting susceptibility. The procedure, as developed by Christian (1974) and Eikelenboom and Minkema (1974), involves exposure of 7- to 11-week-old pigs to 3–6% halothane anesthetic for 3–5 minutes or until evidence of muscle rigidity is apparent. Oxygen at 1–5 L/minute serves as the carrier, and the anesthetic is administered via a semiclosed system through a large-animal mask (Fig. 62.4). This procedure is lethal to 0–25% of the reactors, but losses are minimized when administration is stopped immediately upon observation of the first sign of progressive rigidity. The procedure is approximately 98% repeatable (Alva-Valdes 1979). False-negative responses of animals previously responding in a positive manner are generally preceded by periods of malnutrition or prolonged stress. McGrath et al. (1984) reported that halothane concentrations of 3% or more are necessary to eliminate false-negative responses and that this level will reduce reaction time. Only animals of the nn genotype respond to the halothane test. Carriers (genotype Nn) do not respond even in an intermediate manner. Carriers have, however, been observed to be intermediate for several muscle-quality traits, including 45-minute muscle pH, reflectance, and percent transmission, and for muscle-quantity traits of the loin muscle area and percent separable lean (Christian and Rothschild 1981).

Blood Typing.   Erythrocyte typing of the H and A-O systems offers potential for detecting not only the PSS animal but the carrier of the stress gene as well (Rasmusen and Christian 1976). It is now known that a number of other recognizable genes are located on the same chromosome as the halothane gene (HAL). These include loci that control variants of the enzyme phosphohexose isomerase (PHI^A and PHI^B), the enzyme 6-phosphogluconate dehydrogenase (PGD^A and PGD^B), the serum protein postalbumin-2 (PO-2^F and PO-2^S), the red cell antigens (H^a, H^c, and H$^-$), and the locus (designated S and s), which has a suppressing effect on the expression of the A-O blood type (Rasmusen et al. 1980; Juneja et al. 1983). Accumulated evidence suggests that these six loci are located in the order S, HAL, PHI, H, PO-2, and PGD (Van Zeveren et al. 1988) on chromosome 6 (Davies et al. 1988). Once the linkage relationship has been determined in a litter where PSS is thought to exist, knowledge of these blood types has proven valuable as a supplement to halothane screening and alone in identifying positive animals as well as carriers of the stress gene. This approach has been used in Sweden since 1982 on a nationwide scale encompassing about 100 elite breeding herds. The results show that the HAL genotypes (NN, Nn, or nn) of individual pigs are predicted with an accuracy of about 95%. Thus an effective selection against the HAL n allele could be practiced (Gahne and Juneja 1985, 1988). This method has subsequently been applied also on a large scale in some other countries in Europe including Norway, Finland, Switzerland, Poland, and Czechoslovakia.

PREVENTION

Genetic Measures.   Genetic selection offers the only sensible approach to reducing the incidence of PSS in problem herds. Herds encountering a high frequency of the disorder should consider halothane screening of all potential replacements. Blood typing of littermates to halothane-positive animals permits identification of those that are carriers. These along with their parents and positive littermates should be removed from the herd.

Environmental Measures.   Once identified, positive animals should be managed carefully until they attain acceptable market weight. Avoid mixing them with strange pigs. Plan marketings for dry, cool days and precede their movement to market with 12–24 hours of starvation. Do not mix pigs from different pens on the truck, but place them in compartments with pen mates only. With careful management, positive animals can reach the marketplace alive, thus minimizing a portion of the economic loss.

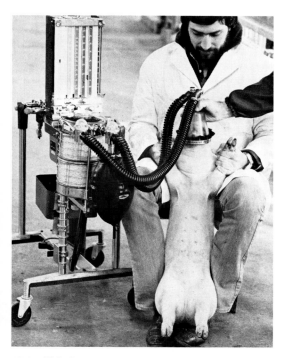

62.4. Halothane screening procedure. An oxygen-halothane mixture is delivered to the pig from the anesthetic machine via a face mask.

REFERENCES

Addis, P. B.; Nelson, D. A.; Ma, R. T. I.; and Burroughs, J. R. 1974. Blood enzymes in relation to porcine muscle properties. J Anim Sci 38:279–286.

Allen, W. M.; Berrett, S.; and Harding, J. D. J. 1970. Experimentally induced acute stress syndrome in Pietrain pigs. Vet Rec 87:64–69.

Alva-Valdes, R. 1979. Repeatability of halothane as a detector of porcine stress susceptible swine. M.S. thesis, Iowa State Univ.

Andresen, E. 1971. Linear sequence of the autosomal loci PHI, H and 6-PGD in pigs. Anim Blood Groups Biochem Genet 2:119–120.

Ball, R. A.; Topel, D. G.; Annis, C. L.; and Christian, L. L. 1972. Diagnostic aspects of the porcine stress syndrome. Proc 76th Annu Meet US Anim Health Assoc, Miami, pp. 517–530.

Ball, R. A.; Annis, C. L.; Topel, D. G.; and Christian, L. L. 1973. Clinical and laboratory diagnosis of the porcine stress syndrome. Vet Med Small Anim Clin 68:1156–1159.

Briskey, E. J. 1964. Etiological status and associated studies of pale, soft, exudative porcine musculature. Adv Food Res 13:89–178.

Britt, B. A., and Kalow, W. 1970a. Malignant hyperthermia: A statistical review. Can Anaesth Soc J 17:293–315.

———. 1970b. Malignant hyperthermia: Aetiology unknown. Can Anaesth Soc J 17:316–330.

CASSENS, R. G.; JUDGE, M. D.; SINK, J. D.; AND BRISKEY, E. J. 1965. Porcine adrenocortical lipid in relation to striated muscle characteristics. Proc Soc Exp Biol Med 120:854–856.

CASSENS, R. G.; COOPER, C. C.; AND BRISKEY, E. J. 1969. The occurrence and histochemical characteristics of giant fibers in the muscle of growing and adult animals. Acta Neuropathol (Berl) 12:300.

CHEAH, K. S., AND CHEAH, A. M. 1978. Calcium movements in skeletal muscle mitochondria of malignant hyperthermia pigs. FEBS Lett 95:307.

CHRISTIAN, L. L. 1972. A review of the role of genetics in animal stress susceptibility and meat quality. Proc Pork Qual Symp, Univ of Wisconsin, Madison, pp. 91–115.

———. 1974. Halothane test for PSS field application. Proc Am Assoc Swine Pract, p. 6.

CHRISTIAN, L. L., AND ROTHSCHILD, M. F. 1981. Performance and carcass characteristics of normal, stress-carrier and stress-susceptible swine. Anim Sci Res Rep AS-528 F, Iowa State Univ, Ames, pp. 1–3.

DARRAH, P. S.; DIMARCO, N. M.; BEITZ, D. C.; AND TOPEL, D. G. 1979. Conversion of alanine, aspartate and lactate to glucose and CO_2 in liver of stress-susceptible and stress-resistant pigs. J Nutr 109:1464–1468.

DAVIES, W.; HARBITZ, I.; FRIES, R.; STRANZINGER, G.; AND HAUGE, J. G. 1988. Porcine malignant hyperthermia carriers detection and chromosomal assignment using a linked probe. Anim Genet 19:203–212.

DRAPER, D. D.; BEITZ, D.; ROTHSCHILD, M. F.; AND CHRISTIAN, L. L. 1984. Age changes in striatal catecholamine concentrations in the stress-susceptible and normal pig. Exp Gerontol 19:377.

DRAPER, D. D.; BERG R.; CHRISTIAN, L. L.; AND SKAGGS, C. 1989. Strain differences in heart weights of stress positive and stress negative pigs. Swine Res Rep ASL-R653, Iowa State Univ, Ames, pp. 47–49.

EIKELENBOOM, G., AND MINKEMA, D. 1974. Prediction of pale, soft and exudative muscle with a non-lethal test for the halothane-induced porcine malignant hyperthermia syndrome. Neth J Vet Sci 99:421–426.

ESSEN-GUSTAVSSON, B.; KARLSTROM, K.; AND LUNDSTRÖM, K. 1988. Muscle metabolism and glycogen depletion within fibretypes at slaughter in pigs with different halothane genotypes: Relation to meat quality properties. Proc 34th Int Congr Meat Sci Tech. Ed. C. S. Chandler and R. F. Thornton. Brisbane, Australia, pp. 581–583.

GAHNE, B., AND JUNEJA, R. K. 1985. Prediction of the halothane (*hal*) genotypes of pigs by deducing *hal, phi, po2, pgd* haplotypes of parents and offspring: Results from a large-scale practice in Swedish breeds. Anim Blood Groups Biochem Genet 16:265–283.

———. 1988. In vivo prediction of meat quality in pigs by genetic markers. In Pig Carcass and Meat Quality. Ed. Reggio Emilia. Italy: Univ Bologna, pp. 113–125.

GOODWIN, R. N. 1990. World Pork Expo Challenge Tests. National Pork Producers, Des Moines, Iowa.

GRONERT, G. A.; MILDE, J. H.; AND THEYE, R. A. 1976. Dantrolene in porcine malignant hyperthermia. Anesthesiology 44:488–495.

GRONERT, G. A.; MANSFIELD, E.; AND THEYE, R. A. 1977. Rapid soluble dantrolene for intravenous use. In 2d International Symposium on Malignant Hyperthermia. Ed. J. A. Aldrete and B. A. Britt. New York: Grune and Stratton, p. 535.

HALL, L. W.; WOOLF, N.; BRADLEY, J. W. P.; AND JOLLY, D. W. 1966. Unusual reaction to suxamethonium chloride. Br Med J 2:1305.

HARBITZ, I.; DAVIES, W.; HAUGE, J. G.; CHOWDHARY, B. P.; GUSTANSSON, I.; AND THOMSEN, P. D. 1990.

Assignment of the porcine calcium release channel gene, a candidate for the malignant hyperthermia locus, to chromosome 6 p11-q21. Proc 22d Int Conf Anim Genet, Int Soc Anim Genet, Michigan State Univ, East Lansing, Abstr no. 6.2.5.

HARRISON, G. G. 1975. Control of malignant hyperthermia syndrome in MHS swine by dantrolene sodium. Br J Anaesth 47:62–65.

HARRISON, G. G.; SAUNDERS, S. J.; BIEBUYCK, J. F.; HICKMAN, R.; DENT, D. M.; WEAVER, U.; AND TERBLANCKE, J. 1969. Anaesthetic induced malignant hyperpyrexia and a method for its prediction. Br J Anaesth 41:844–854.

JENSEN, P.; STAUN, H.; BRAUNER-NIELSEN, P.; AND MOUSTGAARD, J. 1976. Undersogelse over sammengaengen mellen blood type system H og points for hodfarve has svin. Med Fra Statens Husdyrbrugsfors 83, Copenhagen.

JONES, E. W.; NELSON, T. E.; ANDERSON, I. L.; KERR, D. D.; AND BURNAP, T. K. 1972. Malignant hyperthermia of swine. Anesthesiology 36:42–51.

JORGENSEN, P. F.; HYLDGAARD-JENSEN, J.; MOUSTGAARD, J.; AND EIKELENBOOM, G. 1976. Phosphohexase isomerase (PHI) and porcine halothane sensitivity. Acta Vet Scand 17:370–372.

JUDGE, M. D.; BRISKEY, E. J.; CASSENS, R. G.; FORREST, J. C.; AND MEYER, R. K. 1968. Adrenal and thyroid function in stress susceptible pigs (*Sus domesticus*). Am J Physiol 214:146–151.

JUNEJA, R. K.; GAHNE, B.; EDFORS-LILJA, I.; AND ANDRESEN, E. 1983. Genetic variation at a pig serum protein locus, PO-2, and its assignment to the PHI, HAL, S, H, PGD linkage group. Anim Blood Groups Biochem Genet 14:27–36.

KNUDSON, C. M.; MICKELSON, J. R.; LOUIS, C. F.; AND CAMPBELL, K. P. 1990. Distinct immunopeptide maps of the sarcoplasmic reticulum Ca++ release channel in malignant hyperthermia. J Biol Chem 265:2421–2424.

MABRY, J. W.; CHRISTIAN, L. L.; AND KUHLERS, D. L. 1981. Inheritance of porcine stress syndrome. J Hered 72:429–430.

MABRY, J. W.; CHRISTIAN, L. L.; KUHLERS, D. L.; AND RASMUSEN, B. A. 1983. Prediction of susceptibility to the porcine stress syndrome. J Hered 74:23–26.

MCGRATH, C. J.; LEE, J. C.; AND REMPEL, W. E. 1984. Halothane testing for malignant hyperthermia in swine: Dose-response effects. Am J Vet Res 45:1734–1736.

MACLENNAN, D. H.; DUFF, C.; ZORZATO, F.; FUJILL, J.; PHILLIPS, M.; KORNELUK, R. G.; FRODIS, W.; BRITT, B.; AND WORTON, R. G. 1990. Ryanodine receptor gene is a candidate for predisposition to malignant hyperthermia. Nature 343:559–560.

MARPLE, D. N., AND CASSENS, R. G. 1973. Increased metabolic clearance of cortisol by stress-susceptible swine. J Anim Sci 36:1139–1142.

MARPLE, D. N.; NACHREINER, R. F.; PRITCHETT, J. F.; MILES, R. J.; BROWN, H. R.; AND NOE, L. S. 1977. Thyroid and sarcoplasmic reticulum function in halothane-sensitive swine. J Anim Sci 45:1375–1381.

MINKEMA, D.; EIKELENBOOM, G.; AND VAN ELDIK, P. 1976. Inheritance of M.H.S.-susceptibility in pigs. Proc 3d Int Conf on Production Diseases in Farm Animals, Wageningen, The Netherlands, pp. 203–207.

NELSON, T. E., AND DENBOROUGH, M. A. 1977. Studies on normal human skeletal muscle in relation to the pathopharmacology of malignant hyperpyrexia. Clin Exp Pharmacol Physiol 4:315.

NELSON, T. E.; JONES, E. W.; VENABLE, J. T.; AND KERR, D. D. 1972. Malignant hyperthermia of Poland China swine. Anesthesiology 36:52.

OLLIVIER, L.; SELLIER, P.; AND MONIN, G. 1975. Déterminisme génétique du syndrome d'hyperthermie maligne chez le porc de Pietrain. Ann Génét Sél Anim 7:139–166.

RASMUSEN, B. A., AND CHRISTIAN, L. L. 1976. H blood type in pigs as predictors of stress susceptibility. Science 191:947–948.

RASMUSEN, B. A.; BEECE, C. L.; AND CHRISTIAN, L. L. 1980. Halothane sensitivity and linkage of genes for H red blood cell antigens, phosphohexose isomerase (PHI) and 6-phosphodehydrogenase (6-PGD) variants in pigs. Anim Blood Groups Biochem Genet 11:93–107.

SCHMIDT, G. R.; CRIST, D. W.; AND WAX, J. E. 1974. Muscle G-6-P and serum CPK as related to pork quality. J Anim Sci 38:295–303.

SMITH, C., AND BAMPTON, P. R. 1977. Inheritance of reaction to halothane anesthesia in pigs. Genet Res 29:287–292.

STAUN, H.; TOPEL, D. G.; AND LAURSEN, B. 1972. Undersogelser over stress-resistens hos svin. Landoekon Forsoegslab Exter, p. 115.

STEINHAUF, D.; WENIGER, J. H.; AND AUGUSTINE, C. 1969. Stress resistance as a production character in the pig. Soderdr "Zuchlungskunde" 41:335.

SYBESMA, W., AND EIKELENBOOM, G. 1969. Malignant hyperthermia syndrome in pigs. Neth J Vet Sci 2:155–160.

TOPEL, D. G.; MERKEL, R. A.; AND WISMER-PEDERSEN, J. 1967. Relationship of plasma 17-hydroxy corticosteroid levels to some physical and biochemical properties of porcine muscle. J Anim Sci 26:311–315.

TOPEL, D. G.; BICKNELL, E. J.; PRESTON, K. S.; CHRIS-TIAN, L. L.; AND MATSUSHIMA, C. Y. 1968. Porcine stress syndrome. Mod Vet Pract 49:40.

TOPEL, D. G.; PARRISH, F. C., JR.; RUST, R. E.; AND WILSON, D. G. 1972. Certain chemical and physical properties of ham muscle portions after thermal processing. J Food Sci 37:907.

ULLREY, D. 1973. Selenium deficiency in swine production. Feedstuffs 47(45):30.

VAN ZEVEREN, A.; VAN DE WEGHE, A.; BONQUET, Y.; AND VAREWYCK, H. 1988. The porcine stress linkage group. J Anim Breed Genet 105:187.

WEBB, A. J. 1982. The halothane test for porcine stress syndrome. Anim Breed Res Organ Rep, Edinburgh, Scotland, p. 5.

WEBB, A. J., AND SMITH, C. 1976. Some preliminary observations on the inheritance and application of halothane-induced MHS in pigs. Proc 3d Int Conf on Production Diseases in Farm Animals, Wageningen, The Netherlands, p. 211.

WEBB, A. J.; CARDEN, A. E.; SMITH, C.; AND IMLAH, P. 1982. Porcine stress syndrome in pig breeding. Proc 2d World Congr Genet Appl Livest Prod, Madrid, vol 5, pp. 588–604.

WHIPP, S. C.; WORDLAND, R. L.; AND LYON, N. C. 1970. Diurnal variation in concentration of hydrocortisone in plasma of swine. Am J Vet Res 31:2105–2107.

WISMER-PEDERSEN, J. 1968. Modern production practices and their influence on stress conditions. In The Pork Industry: Problems and Progress. Ed. D. G. Topel. Ames: Iowa State Univ Press, p. 163.

63 Prolapses

W. J. Smith

THE RECTUM and vagina are held in place by a complex matrix of fascia, collagen fibers, muscles, and ligaments. This support mechanism may become heavily infiltrated with fat in some animals. In theory, rectal prolapses will occur if the support mechanism is either overcome by pressure or is weakened for some reason. Pressure on the support mechanism may be brought about by straining (proctitis, urethritis, constipation, coughing, and farrowing) or by physical pressure (excessive slope on the floor or weight of abdominal contents). Weakness of the support mechanism may be brought about by edema (including that due to mycotoxins), fat infiltration, tumor infiltration, certain drugs, and genetic susceptibility. In most animals, and especially growing pigs, rectal and/or vaginal prolapse is almost an all-or-nothing phenomenon with the early stages rarely being observed. The prolapse in the growing pig usually protrudes about 10–13 cm. This relatively constant degree of prolapse is probably due to anchorage by the short mesorectum and muscles of the pelvic diaphragm (Hindson 1958; Done 1990). Although the stockperson is usually presented with a complete rectal prolapse, some pigs have a temporary protrusion of a portion of the rectal mucosa on defecation. This phenomenon is also seen during coughing, and one might conjecture that such pigs might be prime candidates for complete rectal prolapse at a later stage.

The comparative anatomy of the pelvic and perineal regions of several species, including the pig, has been studied by Bassett (1971).

INCIDENCE. Most swine production units experience cases of rectal or vaginal prolapse in swine of various ages. These are nearly always sporadic in nature, and most often the cause is not determined. However, outbreaks do occur and may occasionally be prolonged. Kjar (1976) noted that the incidence of rectal prolapse was highest in pigs 6–12 weeks of age and came to the conclusion that the cause was unknown, but the incidence, which varied from 1 to 10%, increased during a change from cold to damp weather.

In a study of one finishing herd over 7 years (total throughput 56,363 pigs), Garden (1988) noted that the incidence varied from 0.7% to 4.7% on an annual basis. In another study in one herd over 6 months, Gardner et al. (1988) noted that 30 (1%) of 2862 pigs of 12–28 weeks of age

suffered from rectal prolapse with a peak incidence between 14–16 weeks of age. Becker and Van der Leek (1986) noted an estimated 10–15% prevalence of rectal prolapse over a 12-month period in pigs of 2–4 months of age, in a herd of 125 sows (farrow to finish).

Smith (1979) noted that rectal prolapse was most common in pigs 3–5 months of age; the incidence in three herds of 1000, 600, and 120 sows (all in confinement) was 0.7%, 0.9%, and 0.6% respectively. The affected pigs ranged from 45 to 180 days of age and from 10 to 90 kg in weight. Swine were not observed to be ill before prolapse occurred, and the only common factor was mild constipation. Straining was not observed in any of these pigs before prolapse of the rectum occurred, but this clinical sign may have been missed due to the intensity of confinement.

Daniel (1975) noted that rectal prolapse in sows could occur in all sizes of units and the incidence varied from 0.5 to 1%. Two-thirds of the cases occurred around the time of parturition. Although prolapse of the rectum and vagina and/or cervix was not mentioned as a specific reason for culling sows from U.K. pig herds (Anon. 1964), Jones (1967) reported an 8.9% frequency of culling for rectal prolapse in one herd. In Australia 7.1% of sows culled in a 2500-sow unit were cases of rectal or vaginal prolapse (Penny 1972).

Information regarding the incidence of vaginal and uterine prolapse is sparse, apart from outbreaks of vulvovaginitis associated with mycotoxins when vaginal prolapses might occur in 30% of affected females (McNutt et al. 1928).

CAUSES AND PREDISPOSING FACTORS

Inflammation. Vaginal prolapse is very rare in suckling swine. However, rectal prolapse is sometimes associated with enterocolitis caused by viral, bacterial, parasitic, or mycotic infection. In cases where the inflammation is severe and irritation of the rectum occurs, tenesmus results and rectal prolapse may be a sequel. Outbreaks of prolapse have been seen in association with swine fever, although less than 0.1% of piglets with diarrhea will suffer from rectal prolapse. In older swine, urethritis and vaginitis from any cause may lead to straining, which may in turn lead to prolapse of the rectum or vagina or both.

Nutritional Factors. Shanks (1955) observed an outbreak of rectal prolapse in a group of pigs that had been fed waste food material from the floor of a feed mill. He came to the conclusion that unusual constituents in the diet led to straining, with resultant prolapse. Morbidity was approximately 30%. More recently, Wood (1979) described an outbreak of rectal prolapse in early-weaned pigs between 2 and 6 weeks of age. Thirty-one of 235 piglets (13.2%) died during the outbreak and all were males. Subsequent investigation revealed the cause of death to be uremia from blockage of the urethra with calculi—a sequel to an unusually high level (2.25%) of calcium in the diet. Partial or complete obstruction of the urethra had caused excessive straining and subsequent prolapse of the rectum. During the outbreak the piglets fed for short periods only, making frequent visits to the automatic drinker. The food consisted of a mixture of denatured skim milk, dried whey, fish meal, and soya meal.

Sudden changes in the diet (e.g., from meal to whey) may lead to occasional cases of rectal prolapse. Chronic shortage of water will lead to constipation, with rectal prolapse as a sequel. Diets that are low in fiber, e.g., those without bran or wheat feed, may also lead to constipation. Constipation produced by this means may also be aggravated by lack of exercise, e.g., sows confined in farrowing crates or dry-sow stalls. A higher incidence of rectal prolapse is therefore to be expected in confinement, although the daily feeding of a little straw may help prevent the condition.

In a 250-sow, breeding-to-finishing unit, the number of rectal prolapses in the growing pigs decreased from five to one a week when the barley in the ration was replaced by a variety with a higher fiber content. Reintroduction of the lower-fiber barley and its removal repeatedly worsened or improved the situation respectively.

In a 300-sow, breeding-to-finishing unit, 15-kg weaners were randomly divided and placed into strawed kennels or second-stage flat decks, both units being contained in the same large general purpose building. The pigs were fed the same ration and the stocking density in both types of housing was almost identical. Prolapse of the rectum was a chronic problem only in the pigs in the strawed kennels. When the barley straw was changed for wheat straw from a neighboring farm, the prolapse problem disappeared during the time the wheat straw was used. As soon as the barley straw was reintroduced (three times), the prolapse problem reappeared (Anon. 1985). It was later postulated that the barley straw might have contained mycotoxins.

Prolapse of the rectum and vagina was a chronic problem in a 400-sow herd in Spain. The sows were housed in level, partly slatted stalls and fed brewers' grains as part of the ration. These were kept in an outside pit, which held enough to last about 3 weeks. Prolapses increased toward the end of the 3-week period, by which time the contents were heavily contaminated with fungi. No mycotoxin assays were carried out (Marco 1990).

Sudden outbreaks of rectal and vaginal prolapse were noted in pigs over 30 kg, every time whey feeding was reintroduced after a few days of absence. The pigs in this 2000-sow herd were normally fed a mixture of meal and whey without access to water. When whey was unavailable (e.g., Christmas holidays), the pigs were fed meal and water, which they did not like and intake dropped markedly. As soon as whey was reintroduced (on a restricted basis), the hungry pigs gorged themselves and the incidence of prolapse rapidly rose to about 1.5% for a short period. Deaths due to torsion also rose.

Muirhead (1989) investigated a chronic problem of rectal prolapse in finishing pigs. The incidence varied from 4 to 6% at 12–18 weeks of age. Reducing the density of the diet reduced the incidence of prolapse to less than 1%, but this measure also reduced growth rate significantly. In this particular herd most of the prolapses occurred within 1–2 hours of the lights being switched on at 7 A.M.; this observation might be of some significance.

It has to be admitted that many outbreaks of rectal prolapse respond to a change in diet, but the reason for this response is rarely found.

Physical Factors. Injury to the rectum or urethra from service by the boar may also lead to tenesmus and prolapse. In addition, gradual weakening of the pelvic diaphragm may arise as sows age or during pregnancy as the abdominal contents become heavier. Rupture of one or more of the supporting structures may then occur, with prolapse of either rectum or vagina or both as a sequel.

Outbreaks have been observed when sows are confined in stalls or in tethers with an excessive slope to the floor. When the fall is greater than 1 in 20, increased intraabdominal pressure may overcome the resistance of one or more structures of the pelvic diaphragm, especially as the abdominal contents increase in weight as pregnancy progresses (Richmond 1979). An outbreak of rectal and vaginal prolapse was also observed in a herd where the dry sows were tethered in stalls with solid floors that were shorter than usual and there was a 13-cm drop from the solid lying area to the dunging passage; the rear end of the sows hung over the dunging passage. Partial or complete rectal or vaginal prolapse was seen in 14%. Sometimes the rectum prolapsed, sometimes the vagina, and in a few cases both. When the sows were recumbent, the first clinical sign was an outward bulging of the vaginal mucous membrane (partial prolapse). In the upright or standing position the prolapse usually disappeared, but as pregnancy progressed and the uterine load increased, the prolapse became more evident when the sow was lying. Eventually, bacterial contamination occurred, inflammation gradually became more severe, and the partial prolapse became complete. Complete prolapse was prevented by removal of affected animals to a spacious pen with a level solid floor.

Physical damage to the vaginal tract may also occur during parturition, either by natural means or by human interference. This may damage some of the structures of the pelvic diaphragm or in turn may lead to inflammation that will cause excessive straining. In either case, vaginal prolapse may result.

Le Bret (1980) noted that sows in five herds from the same origin were more likely to suffer from rectal prolapse at farrowing. These sows were characterized by a particular pelvic conformation shown by measuring different pelvic angles. The larger the angle between the coccygeal vertebrae and the pelvis, the higher the risk of rectal prolapse.

Guise and Penny (1989) noted that rectal prolapses occurred when pigs were transported at high-stocking density; no prolapses were noted in the low-stocking density treatment groups. These authors also reported that haulers had observed prolapses occurring as pigs struggled up steep ramps.

Drugs. The repeated use of estrogens or any estrogenic substance to stimulate estrus in sows or gilts may lead to excessive swelling of the vulva, with vulvovaginitis and prolapse as a sequel. Rectal prolapse has been described in growing pigs with therapeutic levels of tylosin in the diet. It is not known why this should occur (Mackinnon 1979), but it has been suggested by Hogg (1979) that tylosin may alter the normal bacterial flora of the gut with overgrowth of fungi such as *Monilia* as a sequel. Moniliasis may cause proctitis and straining, leading to prolapse. Smith (1978) noted that when Tylasul (tylosin/sulfadimidine) was added to the diet (5 kg/ton) of 10 experimental feeder pigs, 3 suffered from rectal prolapse within 10 days. It was noticeable that the pigs in this group seemed to suffer from a form of anal irritation, manifested as frequent episodes of rapid tail shaking.

Rectal prolapse due to edema has been noted when pigs were medicated with Lincomycin. This reaction is frequently observed when swine are first placed on the drug, but symptoms usually subside within 72 hours (Kunesh 1981).

Genetic Factors. Hogg (1979) reported a severe problem characterized by vaginal and uterine prolapse in a large breeding herd in the United States; uterine prolapse occurred both before and after farrowing. Apparently inbreeding had emphasized a recessive genetic factor.

In a commercial swine herd in California, pigs sired by Yorkshire boars were 3.3 times more likely to suffer from rectal prolapse; one Yorkshire boar in particular was 9.4 times more likely to sire affected pigs. In the same herd, sows of low parity (1, 2, and 3) were likely to farrow pigs more susceptible to rectal prolapse, but it was not possible to determine if this was a genetic effect (Gardner et al. 1988). In their studies, Hindson (1958) and Saunders (1974) concluded that hereditary factors were involved. Becker and Van der Leek (1988) concluded that genetic factors were strongly implicated in an outbreak of rectal prolapse in a commercial 125-sow, farrow-to-finish herd.

Environmental Factors. It is generally agreed that rectal prolapse occurs more commonly during winter months and there is some evidence to support this (Kjar 1976; Wilson 1984; Gardner et al. 1988). However, in one study over 7 years in a finishing herd (throughput 56,363 pigs, average incidence 2.9%), Garden (1988) found no evidence of seasonal effect. It has been suggested that cold weather causes pigs to pile, thus increasing the likelihood of prolapses occurring; no objective data have been produced to support this hypothesis.

Muirhead (1989) reported a problem of rectal prolapse in recently weaned pigs on flat decks. The problem resolved when the climatic environment was improved, particularly temperature and ventilation.

Mycotoxicosis. Rectal and/or vaginal prolapse is a common sequel to vulvovaginitis caused by mycotoxicosis (see Chapter 59 for further details).

Other Factors. In a study in one commercial herd, Gardner et al. (1988) noted that male pigs were more likely to suffer from rectal prolapse than females. However, Garden (1988) in another study of one herd over a much longer period and with a higher incidence of prolapse could find no evidence of a sex effect. In another very small experimental study, Smith (1980) observed that 6 (32%) of 19 randomly acquired pigs with rectal prolapse were males.

Gardner et al. (1988) noted that pigs of low birth weight (less than 1000 g) were more likely to suffer from rectal prolapse later in life. It was hypothesized that low–birth weight pigs that have fewer muscle fibers at birth have an inherently weaker rectal support mechanism, which may fail when a period of rapid growth occurs.

When pigs cough, the rectal mucosa often protrudes temporarily. As with piling, it has been suggested that coughing may precipitate rectal prolapse, but again there is no objective data to support this hypothesis. Indeed, Gardner et al. (1988) could find no relationship between coughing and the prevalence of rectal prolapse. In another study the prevalence of rectal prolapse was dramatically reduced from 4.7 to 0.7% when weaners (30–35 kg) were placed in a strawed yard for 3 weeks between the second-stage flat decks and the fully slatted finishing accommodation (Garden 1985).

Diarrhea is not a common precursor of rectal prolapse, and in one herd studied by Gardner et al. (1988), an outbreak of transmissible gastroenteritis did not increase the prevalence.

Jennings (1984) noted that a significant number of sows with hypocalcemia suffered from uterine prolapse.

In a survey of sow mortality, Chagnon et al. (1990) noted that uterine prolapse was the cause of death of 6.6% of sows. The average parity was 6.0, and it is possible that some weakness of the support mechanism may have been the main determinant (see Chapter 69).

RECTAL STRICTURES. In the United States, rectal strictures were first reported in Illinois (Gibbons 1967); later outbreaks were observed in Indiana (Lillie et al. 1973). Outbreaks have also been noted in the United Kingdom (Taylor 1988). Rectal stricture is considered to be a sequel to rectal prolapse (Saunders 1974; Van der Gaag and Meyer 1974; Häni and Scholl 1976; Von Müller et al. 1980; Prange et al. 1987).

Smith (1980), in a more detailed study of 25 pigs with rectal prolapses that were allowed to heal naturally without treatment, noted that 3 developed complete rectal stricture and died; the remainder grew normally, but in every case there was evidence of partial rectal stricture at slaughter (Fig. 63.1).

Harkin et al. (1982) considered that a strong genetic component was implicated in the etiology of rectal stricture. However, Wilcock and Olander (1977a) noted that many cases of rectal stricture were preceded by severe enteric disease.

Salmonella typhimurium was frequently isolated and ulcerative proctitis, a possible precursor of rectal stricture, was also noted. In later studies Wilcock and Olander (1977b) produced rectal strictures experimentally by injecting chlorpromazine into the cranial hemorrhoidal artery, and suggested that rectal prolapses may be a sequel to ischemic proctitis induced by thrombosis associated with salmonellosis.

TREATMENT AND CONTROL. Apart from treatment and noting any factors peculiar to each case, it is not considered worthwhile taking any specific control or preventive measures for sporadic cases of rectal prolapse. If an outbreak occurs, however, attempts should be made to identify the causes and predisposing factors. Whatever conclusion is reached, measures taken must be cost effective; e.g., if the lack of exercise in farrowing sows is the main factor, the cost of providing that exercise in confinement may be greater than the cost of the disorder. Treatment should also be cost effective. In the United Kingdom it is now common practice to deal with rectal prolapse in feeder pigs by isolation only. No surgical treatment is carried out and the prolapse is simply left to resolve naturally in 10–14 days. However, this procedure could not be regarded as good welfare and a simple nonsurgical amputation technique such as described by Douglas (1985) should be considered. Many surgical procedures for treating rectal prolapse have been described (Hindson 1958; Chalmin 1960; Ivascu et al. 1976; Kjar 1976; Vonderfecht 1978).

It should be noted that amputation of the uterus often results in a high mortality rate, and the condition is best treated by surgical replacement; a laparotomy technique, which ensures that each horn of the womb can be properly repositioned, has been successful. Nonsurgical intervention is

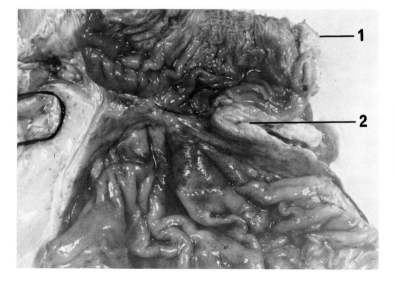

63.1. Longitudinal section of rectum and anus of a 140-kg pig 9 weeks after resolution of a prolapsed rectum, showing mucocutaneous junction (*1*) and scar tissue/partial stricture (*2*).

greatly assisted by general anesthesia and hoisting the hind quarters of the sow with a block and tackle or similar device.

Treatment of rectal stricture is rarely cost effective but a surgical technique has been described (Boyd et al. 1988).

REFERENCES

ANON. 1964. Sow wastage survey 1962–1963. Pig Industry Development Authority, London.

_____. 1985. Scottish Veterinary Investigation Service Report. Vet Rec 117:424.

BASSETT, E. G. 1971. The comparative anatomy of the pelvic and perineal regions of the cow, goat and sow. NZ Vet J 19:277–290.

BECKER, H. N., AND VAN DER LEEK, M. 1988. Possible genetic predisposition to rectal prolapse in swine: A case report. Proc Int Pig Vet Soc 10:395.

BOYD, J. S.; TAYLOR, D. J.; AND REID, J. 1988. Surgery in relieving the rectal stricture syndrome. Proc Int Pig Vet Soc 10:403.

CHAGNON, M.; DROLET, R.; AND D'ALLAIRE, S. 1990. A prospective study of sow mortality in commercial breeding herds. Proc Int Pig Vet Soc 11:383.

CHALMIN, R. 1960. Rectal prolapse in pigs and its surgical treatment. Thèse de Doctorat Vétérinaire, École Nationale Vétérinaire d'Alfort.

DANIEL, M. 1975. Study of prolapse of the rectum in breeding sows. Thèse de Doctorat Vétérinaire, École Nationale Vétérinaire d'Alfort.

DONE, S. H. 1990. Personal communication.

DOUGLAS, R. G. A. 1985. A simple method for correcting rectal prolapse in pigs. Vet Rec 117:129.

GARDEN, S. 1985. Mortality in feeding pigs. Proc Pig Vet Soc 15:100–107.

_____. 1988. Rectal prolapse in pigs. Vet Rec 123:654.

GARDNER, I. A.; HIRD, D. W.; FRANTI, C. E.; AND GLENN, J. 1988. Patterns and determinants of rectal prolapse in a herd of pigs. Vet Rec 123:222–225.

GIBBONS, W. J. 1967. Rectal constriction in swine. Mod Vet Pract 48:20.

GUISE, H. J., AND PENNY, R. H. C. 1990. Factors influencing the welfare and carcass and meat quality of pigs. 1. The effects of stocking density in transport and the use of electric goads. Anim Prod 49:511–515.

HÄNI, H., AND SCHOLL, E. 1976. Stricture of the rectum in pigs. Schweiz Arch Tierheilkd 118:325–328.

HARKIN, J. T.; JONES, R. T.; AND GILLICK, J. C. 1982. Rectal strictures in pigs. Aust Vet J 59:56–57.

HINDSON, J. C. 1958. Prolapse of the rectum in the pig. Vet Rec 70:214–216.

HOGG, A. 1979. Personal communication.

IVASCU, I.; CHRISTEA, I.; AND GATINA, L. 1976. Therapeutical research work on rectal prolapse in swine. Proc Int Pig Vet Soc 4:Z15.

JENNINGS, D. S. 1984. Hypocalcaemia in sows. Proc Pig Vet Soc 14:38–40.

JONES, J. E. T. 1967. An investigation of the causes of mortality and morbidity in sows in a commercial herd. Br Vet J 123:327–339.

KJAR, H. A. 1976. Amputation of prolapsed rectum in young pigs. Proc Int Pig Vet Soc 4:6.

KUNESH, J. P. 1981. Therapeutics. In Diseases of Swine, 5th ed. Ed. A. D. Leman, R. D. Glock, W. L. Mengeling, R. H. C. Penny, E. Scholl, and B. Straw. Ames: Iowa State Univ Press, p. 724.

LE BRET, M. V. 1980. Rectal prolapse in sows. Influence of pelvis conformation determined by goniometry. Ann Zootech 29:226–227.

LILLIE, L. E.; OLANDER, H. J.; AND GALLINA, A. M. 1973. Rectal stricture n swine. J Am Vet Med Assoc 163:358–361.

MACKINNON, J. D. 1979. Personal communication.

MCNUTT, S. H.; PURWIN, P.; AND MURRAY, C. 1928. Vulvovaginitis in swine. J Am Vet Med Assoc 73:484.

MARCO, E. 1990. Personal communication.

MUIRHEAD, M. R. 1989. Rectal prolapse. Int Pig Lett 9(1):3.

PENNY, R. H. C. 1972. Some current thoughts on lameness in the pig. Vet Annu 13:31–36.

PRANGE, H.; UHLEMANN, J.; SCHMIDT, A.; AND GERICKE, R. 1987. Aetiology and pathogenesis of acquired rectal stricture of swine. Monatsh Veterinaermed 42:425–428.

RICHMOND, S. M. 1979. Personal communication.

SAUNDERS, C. N. 1974. Rectal stricture syndrome in pigs: A case history. Vet Rec 94:61.

SHANKS, P. L. 1955. Personal communication.

SMITH, W. J. 1978. Unpublished data.

_____. 1979. Unpublished data.

_____. 1980. A study of prolapse of the rectum in swine with naturally occurring resolution. Proc Int Pig Vet Soc 6:356.

TAYLOR, D. J. 1988. Personal communication.

VAN DER GAAG, I., AND MEYER, P. 1974. Rectal strictures in pigs. Proc Int Pig Vet Soc 3:v–v3.

VONDERFECHT, H. E. 1978. Amputation of rectal prolapse in pigs. Vet Med Small Anim Clin 73:201–206.

VON MÜLLER, E.; SCHOON, H. A.; AND SCHULTZ, L. C. 1980. Rectal strictures in pigs. Dtsch Tieraerztl Wochenschr 87:196–199.

WILCOCK, B. P., AND OLANDER, H. J. 1977a. The pathogenesis of porcine rectal stricture. I. The naturally occurring disease and its association with salmonellosis. Vet Pathol 14:36–42.

_____. 1977b. The pathogenesis of porcine rectal stricture. II. Experimental salmonellosis and ischemic proctitis. Vet Pathol 14:43–55.

WILSON, M. R. 1984. More on rectal stricture. Int Pig Lett 4(5):4.

WOOD, E. N. 1979. Personal communication.

64 Toxic Minerals, Chemicals, Plants, and Gases

T. L. Carson

INCREASED UTILIZATION of confinement facilities, more accurately formulated rations, and improved management practices have resulted in swine having less opportunity to roam freely in large outdoor lots, with their feeds and feeding conditions being more carefully controlled. These management practices have been reflected in a decreased proportion of swine toxicology cases observed at the Iowa Veterinary Diagnostic Laboratory (Meerdink 1979). Nevertheless, the occurrence of swine toxicoses is frequent enough to warrant their inclusion in differential diagnostic considerations for swine health problems. The following discussion summarizes some of the major toxicology problems associated with swine production.

MINERALS

Trace Minerals. Most swine formula feeds are properly fortified with trace elements. However, some trace minerals have been deliberately added in excess for various reasons. They include copper (Cu), iron (Fe), iodine (I), and occasionally selenium (Se) and zinc (Zn) (Lloyd 1980).

COPPER. Dietary requirements of 5–6 ppm Cu have been established for swine. The maximum tolerable level (MTL) is approximately 250 ppm; levels ranging from 300 to 500 ppm cause reduced growth and anemia. The tolerance to Cu is related positively to dietary levels of Fe, Zn, molybdenum, and sulfate. Animals receiving 750 ppm are essentially normal if supplemented with 750 ppm Fe and 500 ppm Zn. A hemolytic crisis elicited by intravascular hemolysis, icterus, anemia, hemoglobinuria, and nephritis may be observed in swine, although not as commonly as in sheep. Diagnosis can be made from clinical signs and a history of feeding excess Cu. Liver and kidney Cu levels >250 and 60 ppm respectively on a wet weight basis are diagnostically supportive.

IODINE. The dietary requirement for I is 0.14 ppm in all classes of swine. Pigs are relatively resistant to I toxicosis. Levels of 400–800 ppm have resulted in depressed feed intake and rate of gain, lowered hemoglobin values, and depressed liver Fe levels in general and have caused skin and eye lesions in growing pigs. The same dietary I levels have failed to affect reproduction. The

clinical signs, history of feeding excess I (usually ethylenediamine dihydroiodide), and analysis of the feed can be used for a diagnosis.

IRON. The recommended dietary levels of Fe range from 40 to 150 ppm, the highest requirements being in the youngest pigs. Many factors influence Fe toxicity. Elemental Fe and iron oxides are relatively nontoxic, while iron salts are more toxic. Dietary phytate, phosphate, Co, Zn, Cu, manganese (Mn), and disaccharides competitively depress Fe absorption. Ascorbic acid, sorbitol, fructose, and several amino acids improve Fe absorption, which is facilitated by being chelated with citric, lactic, pyruvic, and succinic acids, while Fe chelated by desferrioxamine is poorly absorbed.

Pigs fed 1100 ppm Fe as a salt have had reduced weight gains. Animals fed 5000 ppm have displayed depressed feed intake and rates of gain as well as rickets characterized by hypophosphatemia and reduced bone ash. The condition has not been prevented by providing 0.92% dietary phosphorus (P). Injections of Fe, usually as the dextran, have caused intoxications characterized by cardiovascular shock and death within hours after administration as well as staining at injection sites and in regional lymph nodes, liver, and kidneys. The incidence of this acute toxicosis appears to be decreasing. High single doses of iron salts will cause gastroenteritis, followed by apparent recovery and then, frequently, collapse and death within 2 days. Diagnosis may be facilitated by consideration of history, clinical signs, and necropsy changes. Feed and serum should be analyzed for Fe. Normal serum Fe levels are approximately 100 mg/dl and will increase during toxicosis. Iron toxicosis should be differentiated from other forms of rickets. There is no practical individual treatment for Fe toxicosis. Desferrioxamine (Desferal) may be used in selected cases. Dietary imbalances should obviously be corrected.

MANGANESE. Dietary requirements of Mn for swine range from 2 to 10 ppm, with the highest being for breeding swine. Levels of 50 ppm and higher have retarded growth and depressed appetites in young swine, and a level of 4000 ppm also has caused stiffness and a stilted gait. More than normal dietary levels of Fe will decrease Mn toxicity, but the condition would not be commonly suspected.

SELENIUM. The recommended dietary level of Se varies from 0.1 to 0.3 ppm. Selenium, as the selenate or selenite, is approved for addition at 0.1 ppm in rations for swine weighing greater than 25 kg and at 0.3 ppm for swine less than 25 kg. Several dietary factors reduce the toxicity of Se in laboratory animals. They include sulfate, sulfur amino acids, arsenic (As), tungsten, cadmium (Cd), mercury (Hg), Cu, and linseed meal.

When Se levels of 5–8 ppm have been fed to growing swine, anorexia, alopecia, separation of hooves at the coronary band, and degenerative changes in the liver and kidney have occurred. Liver changes may look remarkably like those seen with vitamin E–Se deficiency. A level of 10 ppm fed to breeding sows has caused retarded conception and pigs dead or weak at birth. Misformulated feeds containing from 10 to 27 ppm Se produced a paralytic disease in growing swine characterized by quadriplegic or posterior paralysis while remaining mentally alert and continuing to eat and drink. Focal symmetrical poliomyelomalacia was found in affected swine (Harrison et el. 1983; Casteel et al. 1985).

Several injectable products containing varying concentrations of Se are currently available for treatment or prevention of Se-responsive diseases. Death losses have approached 100% when Se overdose occurred from the mistaken use of a more concentrated product or from miscalculation of the recommended dosage. The minimum lethal dose of injectable Se is about 0.9 mg/kg body weight, with pigs that are Se deficient being the most susceptible to toxicosis (Van Vleet et al. 1974). Weakness and dyspnea progressing to irregular gasps and death occur within 24 hours of the parenteral overdose.

Diagnosis of Se toxicosis in swine can be made by consideration of a history of Se supplementation, clinical signs, necropsy findings, and chemistry of tissues and feeds. When evaluating ration Se levels, it should be remembered that grains from seleniferous areas may have elevated Se levels. Liver and kidney Se concentrations greater than 3 ppm (wet weight) are seen with toxicosis.

ZINC. Recommended dietary levels of Zn for swine are 50–100 ppm, with the highest levels being in the youngest pigs. A level of 2000 ppm has caused growth depression, arthritis, intramuscular hemorrhage, gastritis, and enteritis. The MTL is probably less than 300 ppm, possibly because zinc salts in large concentration are unpalatable. Pigs fed 268 ppm Zn developed arthritis, bone and cartilage deformities, and internal hemorrhages. Zinc interacts competitively for absorption with Fe, Ca, and Cu. In addition to

dietary supplementation, Zn intake is increased by water fed through galvanized, copper, or plastic pipe. Diagnostic considerations should include clinical signs, history, and chemical analyses of feed and tissues. Normal kidney and liver levels of Zn are 25–75 ppm, wet weight, and may increase during toxicosis. However, excretion is quite rapid.

Nonessential Minerals

ANTIMONY. Antimony (Sb) is found in alloys, paints, and tartar emetic, but toxicosis in swine is rare. The clinical signs during toxicosis include vomiting, colic, diarrhea, collapse, and death. Smaller doses cause degeneration of the liver and kidneys. Analysis of hair and blood for Sb should be done to confirm a diagnosis.

ARSENIC. Inorganic arsenicals, which are distinctly different from the phenylarsonics discussed later under feed additives, are used in ant baits, antiquated crab-grass control products, herbicides, and insecticides. Monosodium methanearsonate (MSMA) and disodium methanearsonate (DSMA) are cotton defoliants in current use. Fowler's solution, an aqueous solution of potassium arsenite, has been used to treat anemias and eperythrozoonosis. Pigs are relatively resistant to inorganic arsenical poisoning, with 100–200 mg/kg body weight of sodium arsenite being the lethal dose. This is equivalent to 1000–2000 ppm in drinking water or 2000–4000 ppm in feed. However, pigs have refused to consume 1000 ppm in feed. Clinical signs of acute toxicosis are colic, vomiting, diarrhea, dehydration, collapse, convulsions, and death in hours to days. Prominent necropsy findings are dehydration and hemorrhagic gastritis and enteritis. The condition is entirely different from clinical signs of overdoses of phenylarsonic compounds. Diagnostic considerations should include history, clinical signs, necropsy findings, and chemical analysis. Liver and kidney levels of 10 ppm (wet weight) are significant in confirming a diagnosis of acute inorganic arsenic toxicosis. Although dimercaprol (BAL) has been used to treat As toxicosis, symptomatic treatment is relatively ineffective after clinical signs have been elicited. Prognosis is poor.

CADMIUM. Cadmium is used in paints, solders, batteries, and fungicides. Cadmium salts are relatively toxic. A level of 0.47 ppm has caused reduced liver Fe in growing pigs. Levels of 75 ppm may cause reduced gain and hematocrit values, renal tubular nephrosis, and infertility. When cadmium salts were employed as an ascaricide, 150 ppm Cd in the diet was tolerated, but larger doses caused vomiting with gastroenteritis. Increasing dietary Zn, Cu, Fe, Se, and vitamin C will reduce the incidence of Cd toxicosis. Diagnosis should be confirmed by chemical analysis of feed, kidney, and muscle. Kidney Cd levels can be expected to be concentrated at 10–20% of feed Cd levels. The treatment should be withdrawal and symptomatic therapy.

FLUORINE. Fluorosis may be observed in animals consuming water or forages contaminated by nearby industrial plants or eating crops raised on soils high in fluorine (F). A common source is consumption of minerals high in F. Feed-grade phosphates by law must contain no more than one part F to 100 parts P. It is recommended that swine be fed feeds containing no more than 70 ppm F during their lifetime to prevent the development of fluorosis. Sodium fluoride has been used as an ascaricide at levels of 500 ppm; higher levels have caused vomiting. Other signs of acute toxicosis are diarrhea, lameness, tetany, collapse, and death. A tentative diagnosis of chronic fluorosis may be difficult, since the lameness may appear similar to rickets, mycoplasmosis, and erysipelas. Normal bone F levels in swine are 3000–4000 ppm. Higher levels are associated with fluorosis. Normal urine F levels are 5–15 ppm; higher levels are diagnostically significant. Necropsy findings may reveal exostoses on the long bones and tooth mottling. Treatment should be aimed at reducing dietary F and feeding aluminum or calcium (Ca) mineral supplements.

LEAD. Swine are quite resistent to elevated lead (Pb) exposure. Consequently, field cases of lead poisoning in swine are extremely rare. Experimentally, pigs fed 35.2 mg lead (as the acetate)/kg body weight for 90 days did not die from lead poisoning despite blood lead concentrations observed up to 290 μg/dl (Lassen and Buck 1979). If toxicosis occurs, injections of Ca EDTA are recommended for the individual treatment of animals. Adding magnesium and sodium sulfates and Ca and Fe supplements to diets will reduce Pb absorption.

MERCURY. Mercury has been used in paints, batteries, paper, and fungicides, but use in the latter has been diminishing. All mercurial compounds are toxic, but organic forms are most toxic to all species. Mercury is cumulative, and toxicity depends on form, dose, and duration. Swine have frequently been poisoned after consuming seeds containing organic mercurial fungicides. Initially, signs of gastroenteritis may be evident, followed by uremia and central nervous system (CNS) disturbance, including ataxia, blindness, aimless wandering, paresis, coma, and death. Mercury toxicosis may be confused with erysipelas, cholera, or poisoning by pigweed or phenylarsonics. Clinical signs, history, necropsy findings, and chemistry should aid in the diagnosis. Kidney and liver normally contain less than 1 ppm Hg but will contain much higher levels following Hg toxicosis. Treatment is usually disappointing.

FEED ADDITIVES. Adverse effects of drug additives are rare except in cases of misuse or misformulation of rations (Lloyd 1978). Details of specific drug effects have been reviewed (Booth and McDonald 1988).

Phenylarsonic Compounds. The phenylarsonic compounds, occasionally referred to as organic arsenicals, have been used as growth promotants and to treat swine dysentery and eperythrozoonosis. Arsanilic acid and roxarsone (3-nitro-4-hydroxyphenylarsonic acid) are approved for use in swine rations, and their sodium salts are frequently used in drinking water. Arsanilic acid is approved for continuous use in complete swine rations at levels ranging from 50 to 100 ppm (45–90 g/ton) or for 5–6 days at levels of 250–400 ppm. Clinical signs of toxicosis in swine are ataxia, posterior paresis, blindness, and quadriplegia. Paralyzed animals will continue to live and grow if provided food and water.

Clinical signs of arsanilic acid toxicosis will start within a few days at levels of 1000 ppm, 2 weeks at 400 ppm, and 3–6 weeks at 250 ppm. Animals that receive lower doses for extended periods are prone to develop goose-stepping (a chronic posterior nerve affliction) and total blindness from optic nerve damage. Swine that receive very large doses, e.g., 10,000 ppm in the ration, will exhibit a gastroenteritis resembling poisoning by inorganic arsenic compounds. Roxarsone is approved for continuous use in swine rations at levels of 25–75 ppm and at 200 ppm for 5–6 days. Except for being more toxic, roxarsone causes the same effects as arsanilic acid.

Clinical signs and a history of administration of arsenicals in feed or water may be the best basis for diagnosing phenylarsonic toxicosis. Necropsy findings are generally nonproductive, but histopathologic examination of peripheral nerves, especially the sciatic, may reveal a demyelination.

Diagnosis of phenylarsonic acid poisoning by chemical analysis for the specific compound may be difficult, since the compounds are excreted within a few days after withdrawal. However, analysis of kidney, liver, muscle, and feed for As may assist in the diagnosis. Elemental arsenic levels (wet weight) greater than 2 ppm in kidney and liver and 0.5 ppm in muscle are illegal and indicative of excess As intake. Further analyses of feed for the specific phenylarsonic compound will provide more diagnostic evidence.

Deficiencies of B complex vitamins, especially pantothenic acid and pyridoxine, may cause a similar demyelination of peripheral nerves. Chronic phenylarsonic toxicosis may also resemble rickets. Although water deprivation, organic mercurial poisoning, and viral diseases affect the

CNS primarily, they may be confused with phenylarsonic compound toxicosis. Toxicoses are reversible if arsenicals are promptly removed from the feed and water.

Carbadox. Carbadox (Mecadox, Pfizer) is approved for use in swine weighing less than 34 kg and is incorporated in feed at 11–27.5 ppm as a growth promotant or at 55 ppm to control swine dysentery or enteritis. A feed level of 100 ppm has caused decreased feed consumption and growth retardation. Higher levels have caused feed refusal and emesis. Mild lesions in the glomerular zone of the adrenal cortex are reported with 50 ppm carbadox in the feed for 10 weeks, while more extensive lesions are seen at feed levels of 100–150 ppm after 5 weeks of consumption (Van der Molen 1988).

When fed a ration containing from 331 to 363 ppm carbadox, recently weaned pigs refused to eat and showed poor weight gains, posterior paresia, the passing of hard, pelleted feces, and death in 7–9 days (Power et al. 1989).

Dimetridazole. Dimetridazole is listed as an antihistomoniasis drug used in turkey rations and for treatment and prevention of swine dysentery in some countries. A level of 1500 ppm has caused no toxicosis, but 17,000 ppm have caused diarrhea in swine. Large overdoses of dimetridazole would cause ataxia, bradycardia, dyspnea, salivation, muscle spasms, prostration, and death. Death or recovery would be rapid.

Monensin. Monensin is marketed as Rumensin for cattle supplements or as Coban, a coccidiostat. Use levels range up to 120 ppm for poultry or to 1320 ppm in cattle supplements. Swine may be fed monensin by mistake, but the drug is not highly toxic for them. Pigs fed levels ranging from 11 to 120 ppm in the feed for 112 days were not affected as far as feed consumption and weight gains were concerned. Gilts fed 110–880 ppm had a transient anorexia for 14 days; thereafter, only weight gains were depressed.

The LD50 of monensin in swine is 16.8 mg/kg. Pigs suffering from monensin toxicosis showed open-mouth breathing, frothing around the mouth, ataxia, lethargy, muscle weakness, and diarrhea. These signs were visible within 1 day of exposure and persisted for about 3 days. Myocardial and skeletal muscle necrosis was present in pigs receiving 40 mg monensin/kg (Van Vleet et al. 1983). The toxicity of monensin in swine is potentiated by the concurrent administration of tiamulin, an antibiotic approved for use in treatment of swine dysentery (Van Vleet et al. 1987).

Lasalocid. Lasalocid is a polyether antibiotic marketed as Bovatec for feedlot cattle to improve feed efficiency and weight gains. Swine fed lasalocid at 2.78 mg/kg and 21 mg/kg showed no adverse effects. However, transient muscle weakness occurred at a dose of 35 mg/kg (equivalent to about 1000 ppm of lasalocid in the feed), and death occurred at 58 mg/kg when fed for 1 day.

Nitrofurans. Furazolidone and nitrofurazone have been used to treat porcine enteric diseases. Furazolidone is approved at levels ranging from 110 to 330 ppm for 10 days to 5 weeks. Nitrofurazone is approved in swine rations at 550 ppm for 5–7 days. Overdoses of the nitrofurans, especially nitrofurazone, cause CNS disturbances in swine. The condition must be distinguished from other CNS disturbances (including pseudorabies, water deprivation, and edema disease) largely from clinical signs and the history of nitrofuran administration. The clinical signs of toxicosis will reverse if the drug is withdrawn early.

Sulfonamides. The sulfonamide drugs are antibacterials commonly used in swine medicine. Overdoses will cause crystalluric nephroses. Pigs are not likely to be intoxicated from drinking water containing sulfonamides because of the lack of palatability, but overdosing in the feed, coupled with low water intake, may cause nephrosis and uremia. Nephrotoxic mycotoxicoses such as those caused by citrinin and ochratoxin will predispose sulfonamide toxicoses. The high incidence of sulfonamide residues in pork is related to persistence of the drugs in feed and excreta and is not a toxicosis.

Urea and Ammonium Salts. Swine frequently may be fed cattle feeds containing the nonprotein nitrogen compounds such as urea and ammonium salts. Urea is relatively nontoxic for swine, a level of 2.5% causing only reduced feed intake and growth rate, elevated blood urea nitrogen (BUN), polydypsia, and polyuria. Higher levels of urea should not cause signs of acute toxicosis. Ammonia and ammonium salts are toxic for swine, however, with individual doses of 0.25–0.5 g/kg body weight causing intoxication and doses of 0.54–1.5 g/kg being lethal. Considering that growing swine consume feed equal to 5–10% of their body weights, the expected toxic and lethal levels of ammonium salts are 0.25–1% and 1.5–3% respectively. Pigs poisoned with ammonia and ammonium salts would be expected to become depressed, have tonoclonic convulsions, and either die or recover within a few hours.

PESTICIDES

Insecticides. The concurrent production of both livestock and crops on the same premises provides a unique opportunity for exposure of swine to agricultural chemicals. Among the chemicals presenting the greatest potential hazard of poisoning are the organophosphorus (OP), carbamate, and chlorinated hydrocarbon insecticides.

Poisoning may occur when insecticides are accidently incorporated into swine feed. Discarded or unlabelled portions of granular insecticides can be mistaken for dry feed ingredients and mixed into animal feeds. When farm equipment used for feed handling is also used for insecticide transportation, contamination of this equipment may result in insecticides being inadvertently mixed into animal feeds. In addition, animals may have accidental access to insecticides when they are stored or spilled on the farm premises. Improperly operating back rubbers and oilers may provide an additional source of these insecticides for livestock.

Miscalculation of insecticide concentrations in spraying, dipping, and pour-on procedures may also result in toxicosis. Re-treating animals with OP or carbamate preparations within a few days time may result in poisoning.

ORGANOPHOSPHORUS AND CARBAMATE INSECTICIDES. The OP and carbamate insecticides will be discussed together because of their similar mechanisms of action. The use of these insecticides has increased dramatically as the more environmentally persistent chlorinated hydrocarbon insecticides have been restricted.

Cholinergic nerves utilize acetylcholine as a neurotransmitter substance. Under normal conditions, acetylcholine released at the synapses of parasympathetic nerves and myoneural junctions is quickly hydrolyzed by cholinesterase enzymes. When the hydrolyzing enzymes are inhibited, the continued presence of acetylcholine maintains a state of nerve stimulation and accounts for the clinical signs observed with poisoning from these insecticides. In general, inhibition of these enzymes by the OP insecticides tends to be irreversible, while inhibition by the carbamates is reversible.

Clinical Signs. The clinical syndrome produced by OP and carbamate insecticides is characterized by overstimulation of the parasympathetic nervous system and skeletal muscles. Earliest clinical signs of acute poisoning frequently include mild to profuse salivation, defecation, urination, emesis, stiff-legged or "sawhorse" gait, and general uneasiness. As the syndrome progresses, profuse salivation; gastrointestinal hypermotility resulting in severe colic, vomiting, and abdominal cramps; diarrhea; excessive lacrimation; sweating; miosis; dyspnea; cyanosis; urinary incontinence; and muscle tremors of the face, eyelids, and general body musculature can be observed. Hyperactivity of the skeletal muscles is generally followed by muscular paralysis as the muscles are unable to respond to continued stimulation.

Swine may exhibit increased CNS stimulation but rarely if ever convulsive seizures. More commonly, severe CNS depression occurs.

Death usually results from hypoxia caused by excessive respiratory tract secretions, bronchoconstriction, and erratic slowed heartbeat. The onset of clinical signs of acute poisoning may appear within a few minutes in severe cases to several hours in milder ones.

Lesions. Lesions associated with acute OP or carbamate toxicosis are usually nonspecific but may include excessive fluids in the respiratory tract as well as pulmonary edema.

Diagnosis. A history of exposure to OP or carbamate insecticides associated with clinical signs of parasympathetic stimulation warrants a tentative diagnosis of poisoning with these compounds.

Chemical analyses of animal tissues for the presence of insecticides are usually unrewarding because of the rapid degradation of OP and carbamate insecticides, resulting in low tissue residue levels. However, finding the insecticide in the stomach contents and the feed or suspect material can be quite valuable in establishing a diagnosis. In addition, the degree of inhibition of cholinesterase enzyme activity in the whole blood and tissue of the suspected animal should be assessed. A reduction of whole blood cholinesterase activity to less than 25% of normal is indicative of excessive exposure to these insecticides. The cholinesterase activity level in the brain tissue of animals dying from these insecticides will generally be less than 10% of normal brain activity. Depressed whole blood cholinesterase activity may not necessarily correlate with inhibition of cholinesterase at the parasympathetic synapses and myoneural junctions and therefore should be viewed as only an indicator of the status of the cholinesterase enzymes in the body.

Whole blood and brain samples should be well chilled but not frozen for best laboratory results. Samples of stomach contents as well as the suspect feed or material should be submitted to a laboratory for chemical analysis.

Treatment. Treatment of animals poisoned by OP or carbamate insecticides should be considered on an emergency basis because of the rapid progression of respiratory distress in the clinical syndrome.

Initial treatment for poisoned swine should be the intramuscular use of atropine sulfate at approximately 0.5 mg/kg body weight. One-quarter of this dose may be given intravenously for a quick response in especially severe cases. Atropine does not counteract the insecticide-enzyme bond but blocks the effects of accumulated acetylcholine at the nerve endings. Although a dramatic cessation of parasympathetic signs is generally observed within a few minutes after administration of atropine, it will not affect the skeletal muscle tremors. Atropine at approximately one-half the initial dose may be required but should be used only to control recurring parasympathetic signs. Although the use of atropine alone is generally adequate, especially if vomiting has occurred, specific cases may warrant the use of pralidoxime chloride (20 mg/kg) or activated charcoal given orally.

Oral activated charcoal is recommended for treatment of any ingested insecticide to reduce continued absorption of the insecticide from the gut. Although a useful treatment, the need for activated charcoal in swine may be reduced when vomiting helps emptying of the gut and thereby reduces further absorption of the insecticide.

The oximes (e.g., TMB-4, 2-PAM, pralidoxime chloride) are human drugs that act specifically on the organophosphorus-enzyme complex, freeing the enzyme. The use of the oximes in large animals, although efficacious, may be economically unfeasible. Pralidoxime chloride is recommended at a dose of 20 mg/kg body weight. The oximes are of no benefit in treating carbamate toxicoses.

Dermally exposed animals should be washed with soap and water to prevent continued absorption of these compounds.

Morphine, succinylcholine, and phenothiazine tranquilizers should be avoided in treating OP poisoning.

CHLORINATED HYDROCARBONS. The chlorinated hydrocarbon (CH) insecticides (e.g., toxaphene, chlordane, aldrin, dieldrin, and lindane) produce toxicosis in swine by acting as diffuse but powerful stimulants of the CNS.

Clinical Signs. Clinical signs often appear 12–24 hours after exposure. Initially, animals may appear apprehensive. A period of hyperexcitability and hyperesthesia characterized by exaggerated responses to stimuli and spontaneous muscle spasms is usually observed. The spontaneous tremors and fasciculation are usually in the facial region and involve lips, muscle, eyelids, and ears, progressing caudally to involve the heavy muscles of the shoulder, back, and rear quarters. These spasms may progress into a tonicoclonic convulsive seizure. Abnormal posturing, elevation of the head, and chewing movements may be observed. Varying degrees of respiratory paralysis occur during the seizures, with periods of depression and inactivity between successive seizures.

The rapidity of onset and severity of clinical signs provide a poor index of the prognosis of the episode in individual animals. Occasionally, animals will die during seizures, while others may completely recover following several severe episodes.

Lesions. Specific lesions other than those from the physical trauma of the seizures are generally not observed.

Diagnosis. Clinical signs of hyperexcitability and tonicoclonic convulsive seizures with a known exposure to CH insecticides should yield a tentative diagnosis of toxicosis.

The presence of significant levels of CH insecticide in liver, kidney, and brain tissue is essential for confirming a diagnosis. Samples of these tissues as well as stomach contents and suspect material such as feed or spray should be submitted to a laboratory. Avoid contamination of specimens with hair or gut contents to prevent erroneous analytic results.

Laboratory tests are usually required to differentiate this toxicosis from pseudorabies, water deprivation, or gut edema.

Treatment. Treatment is essentially symptomatic, since there is no specific antidote for the CH insecticides. Animals should be sedated with long-acting barbiturates to control convulsive seizures. Animals with dermal exposure should be washed with warm soapy water to remove the chemical and prevent continued contact. If the chemical is orally ingested, activated charcoal in a water slurry may be used to prevent further absorption. Oil-based cathartics should be avoided, as they may hasten absorption of the chemicals. Intravenous fluids plus glucose may be needed in protracted cases.

Residues. Because of the persistence of CH insecticides and their concentration in fat deposits of the body, the carcasses of animals dying from CH insecticide toxicosis are a source of contamination for feed ingredients such as tankage, meat and bone meal, and fats. Therefore, proper disposal of contaminated carcasses is vitally important. Enough tissue residues of these chemicals are often found in animals surviving an episode of insecticide exposure to have significant economic impact in market animals. The time required for excretion of these residues is frequently too long to make decontamination economically feasible.

SYNTHETIC PYRETHROIDS. Several synthetic pyrethroids (e.g., permethrin, fenvalerate) are commercially available for fly and external parasite control. As a class, the synthetic pyrethroids are relatively nontoxic to mammals and are unlikely to produce poisoning in swine.

FORMAMIDINES. Amitraz is a formamidine pesticide with insecticidal and acaricidal properties. It is available in the United States as Taktic for control of lice and mange on swine. This compound has low mammalian toxicity and is unlikely to produce toxicosis in swine.

Fungicides

CAPTAN. Captan is widely used as a seed treatment. Field corn seed produced commercially in the United States is generally treated with captan at a level of approximately 1000 ppm. Consumption of captan-treated seed corn represents little hazard of poisoning, as the acute lethal dose of captan for livestock is >250 mg/kg body weight.

ORGANOMERCURIALS. The organomercurials include phenyl mercuric chloride, phenyl mercuric acetate, various aliphatic compounds such as ethyl mercuric chloride, and complex aromatic derivatives like hydroxy mercuric cresol. These toxicoses associated with mercury-based seed treatments are discussed under Mercury.

PENTACHLOROPHENOL. Pentachlorophenol (PCP) has been employed for over 45 years as a wood preservative and fungicide. PCP- or "penta"-treated wood has found wide application in livestock handling and housing facilities where wood is in contact with soil, manure, or moisture. Acute poisoning is not a major problem from PCP-treated wood, although toxicosis, including stillborn pigs, may occur when livestock have contact with surfaces that have been freshly treated with PCP preparations (Schipper 1961). A single oral dose of 80 mg/kg was not fatal to a weanling pig. If toxicosis occurs, depression, emesis, muscular weakness, accelerated respiratory rate, and posterior paralysis are clinical signs that may be observed.

A problem of greater concern may be the recognition of blood and tissue residues of PCP in livestock that has been in contact with PCP-treated facilities. The finding of from 10 to 1000 ppb PCP in whole blood is apparently unrelated to manifestations of toxicosis.

Herbicides

PHENOXY HERBICIDES. 2,4-D; 2,4,5-T; MCPA; and silvex are selective herbicides widely used in crop production and pasture and range management. Because the toxic dose of 2,4-D and 2,4,5-T is greater than 300 mg/kg body weight for several days, the hazard of poisoning by these compounds under normal conditions of use is low. When large doses have been administered experimentally, depression, anorexia, weight loss, muscular weakness, and incoordination have been observed.

DIPYRIDAL HERBICIDES. Paraquat, a plant desiccant type of herbicide, has found widespread application in no-till farming technology. Accidental as well as malicious poisoning of swine with paraquat has resulted in toxicosis. An approximate lethal dose of paraquat for swine is 75 mg/kg.

Acute effects involving necrosis and erosion of the oral and gastric mucosa are attributed to the carrier solvent. The more classic effects, however, occur 7–10 days after ingestion and are characterized by pulmonary congestion and edema. The pulmonary lesions progress to a severe diffuse interstitial pulmonary fibrosis. Initial clinical signs include emesis and diarrhea, while the later stages are characterized by respiratory distress. Once clinical signs suggesting pulmonary involvement develop, therapeutic measures are usually futile.

Rodenticides. The rodenticides are a class of compounds used to control rat and mouse populations in or around farmsteads, feed storage areas, or swine production facilities. Accidental access to these compounds constitutes the usual route of exposure, although malicious poisoning of swine with rodenticides has also occurred.

ANTICOAGULANT RODENTICIDES. The anticoagulant rodenticides (e.g., warfarin, diphacinone, chlorophacinone, bromadiolone, brodifocoum, pindone) compose the largest group available through retail outlets. Swine are quite susceptible to this class of compound, as evidenced by toxicosis occurring after a single oral dose of warfarin at 3 mg/kg body weight. Repeated oral doses of only 0.05 mg/kg per day for 7 days also produced toxicosis in swine (Osweiler 1978). These rodenticides produce lowered prothrombin levels by interfering with vitamin K utilization. The physiologic result is increased blood clotting time, which is manifested clinically as mild to severe hemorrhage. The clinical signs—including lameness, stiffness, lethargy, recumbency, anorexia, and dark tarry feces—are related directly to extravasation of blood. Observed lesions include hematoma, articular swelling, epistaxis, intermuscular hemorrhage, anemia, and melena.

A diagnosis of anticoagulant rodenticide toxicosis should include demonstration of a defect in the clotting mechanism as evidenced by increases in clotting time, one-stage prothrombin time, or activated partial thromboplastin time. The chemical detection of the rodenticide in samples of blood, liver, or suspect baits is also helpful.

Injectable vitamin K_1 along with oral vitamin K supplements are included in a successful treatment regime. Whole blood transfusions may be utilized successfully in special cases.

STRYCHNINE. Strychnine, an indole alkaloid, is widely available commercially, often as either a green- or red-dyed pellet or grain or a white powder. This alkaloid acts by selectively antagonizing certain types of special inhibitory neurons, thereby allowing uncontrolled and relatively diffuse reflex activity to proceed unchecked. The approximate oral lethal dose of strychnine for swine varies from 0.5 to 1 mg/kg body weight. Clinical signs appear within 10 minutes to 2 hours after ingestion and are characterized by violent tetanic seizures that may occur spontaneously or in response to external stimuli such as touch, light, or sound. The intermittent seizures are usually separated by periods of relaxation. Death occurs from anoxia and exhaustion during the seizures, often in less than 1 hour. Diagnosis is best confirmed by detection of the strychnine alkaloid in either the stomach contents or urine. Treatment consists of controlling seizures with long-acting barbiturates and other muscle relaxants.

OTHER RODENTICIDES. Cholecalciferol (vitamin D₃) containing rodenticides are commercially available as Rampage, Quintox, or Ortho Rat-B-Gone. Toxic doses of these products produce vitamin D poisoning with hypercalcemia, mineralization of soft tissues, and clinical signs of depression, weakness, nausea, anorexia, polyuria, and polydipsia.

Bromethalin-based rodenticides, marketed as Assault, Vengeance, or Trounce produce cerebral edema and signs of rear leg ataxia and/or paresis and CNS depression. Hyperexcitability, muscle tremors, and seizures may be seen with higher doses of bromethalin in the dog (Dorman et al. 1990).

TOXIC PLANTS

Amaranthus **(Pigweed).** A distinct disease syndrome of swine called perirenal edema occurs during the summer and early fall months. Its onset is associated with sudden access to pastures, barn lots, or fence rows containing moderate amounts of *Amaranthus retroflexus* (redroot pigweed).

Clinical signs appear suddenly 5–10 days after access to the pigweed. Initial signs are weakness, trembling, and incoordination. The disease progresses rapidly to knuckling of the pastern joints and finally to almost complete paralysis of the rear legs. Affected pigs usually lie in sternal recumbency, and if disturbed, attempts to walk will be in a crouching gait or with the rear legs dragging. The body temperature is usually normal and the eyes are bright. Coma and death generally occur within 48 hours of the onset of clinical signs, but affected swine may live from 5 to 15 days, with progression from signs of acute nephrosis to those of chronic fibrosing nephritis. In affected herds, new cases may appear for as long as 10 days after removal from the source. Morbidity ranges from less than 5% in some herds to 50% in others, and the mortality is usually about 75–80% in those showing clinical signs.

Gross necropsy findings are dramatic and chracterized as edema of the connective tissue around the kidneys. The amount of fluid in the perirenal area varies, at times occupying the greater portion of the abdominal cavity. The edematous fluid may contain considerable blood, although the kidney itself is usually normal size and pale. Edema of the ventral body wall and perirectal areas as well as ascites and hydrothorax may be observed. Histologic lesions of affected swine are characterized by hydropic degeneration and coagulative necrosis of both proximal and distal convoluted tubules. Glomeruli may be shrunken, with dilation of Bowman's capsules. Proteinaceous casts are numerous in distal and collecting tubules.

As a consequence of severe renal disease, there are elevations in BUN, serum creatinine, and serum potassium. The electrocardiograph of affected swine is characteristic of hyperkalemic heart failure (Osweiler et al. 1969). The changes include bradycardia, a wide and slurred QRS complex, and an increase in magnitude and deviation of the T wave. The probable cause of death is hyperkalemic heart failure.

Immediate removal of affected pigs from the source of the weeds is the only definite therapeutic recommendation that can be made at this time.

Xanthium **(Cocklebur).** Cockleburs, including *Xanthium strumarium* and other species, are annual herbs that reproduce only from seed. They may be found throughout the world in cultivated fields, fence rows, and ditches and may heavily infest pastures as a result of being washed in from adjacent cropland.

The greatest potential for cocklebur poisoning arises when the more toxic two-leaf seedling stage or ground seeds are ingested. The unpalatable more mature plant contains less of the toxic principle, carboxyatractyloside. Within 8–24 hours after ingestion, swine develop signs of depression, nausea, weakness, ataxia, and subnormal temperature. Spasms of the cervical muscles, vomiting, and dyspnea may occur. Death occurs within several hours after the onset of symptoms. Lesions typically include ascites with large fibrin strands on the surface of the liver and other viscera and congestion and centrilobular accentuation of the liver. Microscopically acute centrilobular hepatic necrosis is observed (Stuart et al. 1981).

Treatment includes mineral oil per os to delay absorption of the carboxyatractyloside. Intramuscular injection of 5–30 mg physostigmine may produce a dramatic response in some cases (Link 1975).

Solanum nigrum **(Nightshade).** Nightshade is found in woods, permanent pastures, and fence rows. The leaves and green berries principally contain the alkaloid solanine. The plant is not palatable and is usually consumed under conditions of its abundant growth and lack of other suitable forage. Actual cases of poisoning are rare.

Affected animals display anorexia, constipation, depression, and incoordination. Poisoned swine may vomit. Dilation of the pupils and muscular trembling are neurologic signs observed. Animals may be seen lying on their sides and kicking with all feet, progressing then to coma and death. Necropsy may reveal some degree of gastrointestinal irritation. The toxic alkaloid is rapidly eliminated through the urine (Kingsbury 1964).

Nitrates and Nitrites. Nitrate or nitrite toxicosis occurs most commonly when these ions accumulate in either water and/or plant sources. However, fertilizers like ammonium nitrate or potassium nitrate may also be a source of nitrate for animals (Osweiler et al. 1985).

Several different species of plants may accumulate nitrate, depending on varying climatic and soil fertility conditions. Nitrate accumulates in the stalk and leaves of plants and not in the fruit or grain.

The nitrates from both water (see **WATER QUALITY, Toxic Elements**) and plant sources are additive and should be evaluated together in particular field cases. The nitrate ion (NO_3^-) itself is not particularly toxic and may produce no more than gastrointestinal irritation. However, nitrite (NO_2^-), the reduced form of nitrate, is quite toxic. The nitrite ion oxidizes ferrous iron in hemoglobin to the ferric state, forming methemoglobin, which cannot accept and transport molecular oxygen. The result is tissue hypoxia from poorly oxygenated blood.

Pigs given single oral doses of greater than 10–20 mg nitrite nitrogen (as potassium nitrite)/kg body weight developed clinical signs of poisoning but recovered, while those given doses greater than 20 mg nitrite nitrogen/kg body weight died within 90–150 minutes after ingestion (London et al. 1967). Clinical signs became apparent when approximately 20% of the total hemoglobin was present as methemoglobin, while death was associated with methemoglobin levels of approximately 80%. Clinical signs observed with acute nitrite toxicosis include increased respiratory rate, salivation, miosis, polyuria, weakness, ataxia, and terminal anoxic convulsive seizures. The blood and tissues are a chocolate brown color from the methemoglobin. Treatment of acute nitrite toxicosis consists of intravenous injection of 10 mg methylene blue/kg body weight in a 4% solution (Link 1975).

WATER QUALITY

Microbiologic Standards. Microbiologic examination of water samples determines the general sanitary quality of the sample and indicates the degree of contamination of the water with waste from human and animal sources.

In general, these examinations do not attempt to isolate pathogenic bacteria but detect the presence of indicator organisms. The coliform group of bacteria has traditionally been the indicator used to assess the degree of water pollution and thus the sanitary quality of the particular sample. As an advance in the microbiologic examination of water, the differentiation of fecal coliforms as a subgroup within the general category of coliforms is encouraging. The U.S. Environmental Protection Agency (1973) proposed that acceptable limitations for water to be used directly by livestock should not exceed 1000/100 ml. Many believe, however, that as long as animals are allowed to range freely and drink surface waters, these proposed limits would be unenforceable and of doubtful value.

The standard plate count, which enumerates the number of bacteria multiplying at 35°C, is of doubtful significance in evaluating livestock water sources other than helping to judge the efficiency of various water treatment processes.

Salinity. Salinity, or total dissolved solids (TDS), generally expressed in milligrams per liter, is an expression of the amount of soluble salts in a particular water sample. The ions most commonly involved in saline waters are Ca, Mg, and sodium (Na) in the bicarbonate, chloride, or sulphate form. Waters containing less than 1000 mg soluble salts/L should present no serious hazard to any class of swine. Waters containing between 1000 and 5000 mg soluble salts/L may cause mild temporary diarrhea or be refused at first by swine not accustomed to them, although health or performance should not be greatly affected (NRC 1974; Anderson and Strothers 1978; Paterson et al. 1979). Waters containing 5000–7000 mg soluble salts/L may present a health risk for pregnant, lactating, or stressed animals. Water containing >7000 mg soluble salts/L should be considered unsafe for swine.

Hardness is sometimes confused with salinity, but the two are not necessarily correlative. Hardness is expressed as the sum of Ca and Mg reported in equivalent amounts of calcium carbonate. Waters containing high levels of sodium salts, and therefore having high salinity, could be quite soft if they contain low levels of Ca and Mg.

Toxic Elements

NITRATES AND NITRITES. Nitrates and nitrites are water soluble and thus may be leached from the soil or soil surface into groundwater. Animal wastes, nitrogen fertilizers, decaying organic matter, silage juices, and soils high in nitrogen-fixing bacteria may be sources of contamination through surface water runoff to adjacent poorly cased, shallow, or low-lying wells or reservoirs.

The upper limit for nitrate in human drinking water is 45 mg nitrate/L (USEPA 1975). This level has the intent of preventing the methemoglobinemia of "blue baby" syndrome in human infants who receive formulas made from high nitrate waters. Although it has been suggested that neonatal swine are also quite susceptible to elevated nitrates, evidence to support this theory is unavailable. Emerick et al. (1965) have concluded, however, that 1-week-old pigs are no more susceptible to nitrite-induced methemoglobinemia than older growing swine. A review of water quality for livestock (NRC 1974) proposed 440 mg nitrate/L as the maximum nitrate that could safely be allowed in livestock water.

Reports of experimental production of a chronic or low-level nitrate-poisoning syndrome in livestock have been extensively reviewed (Turner and Kienholz 1972; Emerick 1974; Ridder and Oehme 1974). The bulk of the evidence indicates that sublethal or chronic effects are extremely rare and difficult to verify. London et al. (1967) fed growing pigs up to 18.3 mg nitrite nitrogen/kg body weight for 124 days without serious effects developing. No effect on the performance of growing/finishing swine or on reproductive performance of gilts was observed when the drinking water contained 1320 ppm nitrate (Seerley et al. 1965).

OTHER ELEMENTS. Water quality guidelines for livestock have been recently proposed and are listed in Table 64.1.

Table 64.1. Water quality guidelines for livestock

Item	Maximum Recommended Limit (ppm)
Major ions	
Calcium	1000
Nitrate + nitrite	100
Nitrite alone	10
Sulphate	1000
TDS	3000
Heavy metals and trace ions	
Aluminum	5.0
Arsenic	0.5[a]
Beryllium	0.1[b]
Boron	5.0
Cadmium	0.02
Chromium	1.0
Cobalt	1.0
Copper (swine)	5.0
Fluoride	2.0[c]
Iron	No guideline
Lead	0.1
Manganese	No guideline
Mercury	0.003
Molybdenum	0.5
Nickel	1.0
Selenium	0.05
Uranium	0.2
Vanadium	0.1
Zinc	50.0

Source: Canadian Task Force on Water Quality (1987).
[a]5.0 if not added to feed.
[b]Tentative guideline.
[c]1.0 if fluoride is present in feed.

MISCELLANEOUS TOXICANTS

Sodium Ion Toxicosis. Sodium ion toxicosis, also called water deprivation or salt poisoning, is very common in swine (Osweiler et al. 1985). The occurrence of sodium ion toxicosis is inversely related to water intake. The condition is almost invariably related to water deprivation caused by inadequate water supply or to changes in husbandry. The likelihood of toxicosis will increase with increased dietary salt, but the condition may occur when rations contain normal levels of added salt, e.g., 0.25–1%. It has also been associated with the feeding of whey and other milk by-products. Sodium ion toxicosis may occur after water deprivation of only a few hours, but in most cases the time exceeds 24 hours.

The initial clinical signs are thirst and constipation, followed by CNS involvement. Intermittent convulsions start within 1 to several days after water deprivation and may be exacerbated by rehydration. The frequency of characteristic tonoclonic convulsions with opisthotonus increases. Affected animals may also wander aimlessly and appear to be blind and deaf. Moribund pigs become comatose, often lying on their sides with continuous paddling. Most affected animals die within a few days. Some pigs that appear to be unaffected may succumb later to a subacute polioencephalomalacia. Salt poisoning, from eating excess salt or consuming brine, usually causes vomiting and diarrhea.

Diagnosis is best accomplished by establishing that water deprivation occurred, which may be difficult in some cases. If water deprivation is not evident, other means must be used to aid the diagnosis. Necropsy findings may reveal a gastritis, gastric ulcers, constipation, or enteritis. Chemical analysis of serum and cerebrospinal fluids may confirm a hypernatremia with levels of Na above 160 mEq/L (Osweiler and Hurd 1974). However, after rehydration, normal values of 140–145 mEq/L may exist. Histologic examination of brain tissue, especially cerebrum, will usually reveal the presence of a pathognomonic cuffing of meningeal and cerebral vessels with eosinophils. However, the eosinophils may disappear or be replaced by mononuclear cells when pigs live several days. Brains of pigs affected subacutely may have a laminar subcortical polioencephalomalacia. Analysis of feed for Na is not usually of any value. Differential diagnosis should include viral encephalitic diseases such as pseudorabies and hog cholera, chlorinated hydrocarbon insecticide poisoning, and edema disease. In known cases of water deprivation, rehydration should be gradual, but the prognosis is poor.

Coal Tar Pitch. Coal tars are a mixture of condensable volatile products formed during the destructive distillation of bituminous coal. The phenolic portions of these products have the greatest acute toxicity. Sources of these substances for swine are clay pigeons, lignite tar flooring slabs, tar paper, and tar used in waterproofing and sealing. Because of the rapid clinical course, sudden death is often the first physical sign observed. Weakness, depression, and increased respiratory rate can be observed in animals that may live for several hours or even days. Icterus and a secondary anemia may develop. Necropsy of pigs poisoned by coal tar pitch reveals a greatly enlarged friable liver. The hepatic lobules are very distinct grossly, with some being darkened in color, while others are yellowish orange. Microscopically, this lesion is observed as severe centrilobular necrosis with subsequent intralobular hemorrhage. Ascites and large turgid kidneys may also be observed.

There is no specific treatment for this condition. Removal of animals from the source of the coal tar is important to prevent recurrence of poisoning.

Ethylene Glycol.   Most permanent anti-freeze/coolant mixtures for liquid-cooled engines contain approximately 95% ethylene glycol. A hazard of poisoning exists when animals have accidental access to antifreeze solutions during periods of engine maintenance or when these solutions are used in plumbing systems to prevent freezing. Swine may be poisoned by ingesting 4–5 ml ethylene glycol/kg body weight. Ethylene glycol toxicosis is exhibited in two clinical phases. Initially the glycol may enter the cerebrospinal fluid, producing a narcotic or euphoric state of intoxication. Later clinical signs are associated with metabolism of the glycol to oxalic acid, with subsequent formation of calcium oxalate and nephrosis. Renal tubular blockage with development of uremia is observed 1–3 days after ingestion. Clinical signs generally include emesis, anorexia, dehydration, weakness, ataxia, convulsions, coma, and death. The entire course of illness may be as short as 12 hours following consumption of large quantities of ethylene glycol. Oxalate nephrosis can be demonstrated histopathologically and is characterized by finding pale yellow birefringent oxalate crystals in the convoluted tubules. Polarizing filters greatly aid in the detection of oxalate crystals in kidney sections or in impression smears of freshly incised kidney. Once clinical signs of renal failure are evident, treatment is usually of no avail. If treated within the first 6–12 hours after ingestion, reasonable response has been achieved in ethylene glycol–poisoned dogs by using 5.5 ml/kg body weight of 20% ethyl alcohol intravenously and 98 ml/kg body weight of 5% sodium bicarbonate intravenously.

Gossypol.   Cottonseed meal (CSM), a by-product of the cotton fiber and cottonseed oil industries, is an important protein supplement for livestock rations in cotton-producing regions. Its use

as a protein supplement for swine, however, is limited by gossypol content, which varies with the strain of the cotton plant, its geographic location, climatic conditions, and the oil extraction procedure used. Gossypol, a polyphenolic binaphthalene, is a yellow pigment in glands of decorticated cottonseed. The toxic "free" gossypol becomes partially inactivated (bound) during the extraction and milling processes, as well as spontaneously in the prepared meal. Toxicity of gossypol depends on the species and age of the animal, and on various components of the diet, particularly the protein, lysine, and iron concentrations (Eisele 1986).

Toxicosis only follows prolonged feeding (weeks to months) of CSM with a high content of free gossypol and may be manifested simply as ill thrift or as an acute respiratory problem followed by death. The main pathologic changes are cardiomyopathy, hepatic congestion and necrosis, skeletal muscle injury, and severe edematous changes throughout the animal. A decrease in hemoglobin total serum, protein concentration, and packed-cell volume is seen in pigs fed a diet containing ≥ 200 mg of free gossypol/kg (Haschek et al. 1989).

Recommendations for growing and fattening swine include feeding no more than 9% CSM in the diet, with less than 100 mg (0.01%) of free gossypol/kg, in a 15–16% protein diet. Tolerance to gossypol can be induced by adding $FeSO_4$ (≤ 400 mg/kg) at a 1:1 weight ratio with free gossypol. Increasing the amount of crude protein or supplementing with lysine can also induce tolerance (Pond and Maner 1984).

TOXIC GASES.   The most important gases released by the decomposition of urine and feces either in anaerobic underfloor waste pits or in deep litter or manure packs are (1) ammonia, (2) carbon dioxide, (3) methane, and (4) hydrogen sulfide (Table 64.2). A number of vapors responsible for the odors of manure decomposition are also produced. These include organic acids, amines, amides, alcohols, carbonyls, skatoles, sulfides, and mercaptans.

Confinement of swine in closed structures increases the hazard of potential gas toxicosis. Fortunately even at relatively low ventilation rates used during cold weather, concentrations of ammonia and hydrogen sulfide, the two most potentially dangerous gases associated with manure decomposition, usually remain below toxic levels. Unfortunately, however, accidents, poor design, and improper operation may result in insufficient ventilation and the concentration of poisonous gases may become higher.

Material on TOXIC GASES is modified, with permission, from Osweiler, G. D.; Carson, T. L.; Buck, W. B.; and Van Gelder, G. A. (1985). Toxic gases, pp. 369–377, Clinical and Diagnostic Veterinary Toxicology, 3d ed. © Kendall/Hunt Publishing Co.

Table 64.2. Characteristics of toxic gases associated with swine production

Agent	Odor and Weight[a]	Effect and Prominent Symptoms	Dangerous Working Conditions
Ammonia (NH_3)	Sharp, pungent, lighter than air (0.77 g/L)	Irritation of respiratory tract, asphyxiation at high concentrations	Agitation of manure pit, ventilation failure
Carbon dioxide (CO_2)	Odorless, heavier than air (1.98 g/L)	Trouble breathing, headaches, drowsiness, asphyxiation	Agitation of manure pit, combustion-engine exhaust, ventilation failure
Hydrogen sulfide (H_2S)	Rotten egg smell, heavier than air (1.54 g/L)	Irritation of eyes and nose, headaches, dizziness, nausea, unconsciousness, death	Agitation of manure pit, ventilation failure
Methane (CH_4)	Odorless, lighter than air (0.72 g/L)	Mild asphyxiant, primarily explosion hazard	Agitation of manure pit, ventilation failure
Carbon monoxide (CO)	Odorless, lighter than air (1.25 g/L)	Headaches, drowsiness, asphyxiation	Unvented heaters and engines

Source: Adapted from Osweiler et al. (1985), with permission.
[a]The density of dry air at 0°C and 760 mm Hg is 1.29 g/L.

Concentrations of toxic gases are usually expressed as parts of the gas per million parts of air (ppm) by volume.

Ammonia. Ammonia (NH_3) is the toxic air pollutant most frequently found in high concentrations in animal facilities, and production is especially common where excrement can decompose on a solid floor. This gas has a characteristic pungent odor that humans can detect at approximately 10 ppm or even lower. The NH_3 concentration in enclosed animal facilities usually remains below 30 ppm even with low ventilation rates, however, it may frequently reach 50 ppm or higher during long periods of normal facility operation.

Ammonia is highly soluble in water, and as such will react with the moist mucous membranes of the eye and respiratory passages. Consequently, excessive tearing, shallow breathing, and clear or purulent nasal discharge are common symptoms of aerial NH_3 toxicosis.

At concentrations usually found in practical animal environment (less than 100 ppm), the primary impact of this gas is as a chronic stressor that can affect the course of infectious disease as well as having a direct influence on the growth of healthy young pigs. The rate of gain in young pigs was reduced by 12% during exposure to aerial NH_3 at 50 ppm and by 30% at 100 or 150 ppm (Drummond et al. 1980). Aerial NH_3 at 50 or 75 ppm reduced the ability of healthy young pigs to clear bacteria from their lungs (Drummond et al. 1978). At 50 or 100 ppm aerial NH_3 exacerbated nasal-turbinate lesions in young pigs infected with *Bordetella bronchiseptica,* but did not add to the infection-induced reduction in the pigs' growth rate (Drummond et al. 1981a). In another study, aerial NH_3 at 100 ppm reduced the rate of gain by 32% and ascarid infection by 28%; however, effects of the NH_3 and infection, when imposed on the pigs at the same time, were additive

and the rate of gain was reduced by 61% (Drummond et al. 1981b). More extensive reviews of aerial NH_3 and its effect on animal production are provided by Curtis (1983) and the National Research Council (1979a).

Carbon Dioxide. Carbon dioxide (CO_2) is an odorless gas present in the atmosphere at 300 ppm. It is given off by swine as an end product of energy metabolism and by improperly vented, though properly adjusted, fuel-burning heaters. It is also the gas evolved in the greatest quantity by decomposing manure. Despite all this, CO_2 concentration in closed animal facilities rarely approaches levels that endanger animals health (Curtis 1983).

Methane. Methane (CH_4), a product of microbial degradation of carbonaceous materials, is not a poisonous gas. It is biologically rather inert and produces effects on animals only by displacing oxygen in a given atmosphere thereby producing asphyxiation. Under ordinary pressures a concentration of 87–90% CH_4 in a given atmosphere is required before irregularities of respiration and eventually respiratory arrest due to anoxia are produced.

The chief danger inherent in this material is its explosive hazard as concentrations of 5–15% by volume in air are reached (Osweiler et al. 1985).

Hydrogen Sulfide. Hydrogen sulfide (H_2S) is a potentially lethal gas produced by anaerobic bacterial decomposition of protein and other sulfur containing organic matter. The source of H_2S which presents the greatest hazard to livestock is liquid manure holding pits. Most of the continuously produced gas is retained within the liquid of the pit. However, when waste slurry is agitated to resuspend solids prior to being pumped out, it rapidly releases much of the H_2S that may have been retained within it. The concentration of H_2S

usually found in closed animal facilities (less than 10 ppm) is not toxic, but this release of gas upon agitation may produce concentrations of hydrogen sulfide up to 1000 ppm or higher within the facility.

Acute H_2S poisoning is directly responsible for more deaths in closed animal facilities than any other gas with the possible exception of carbon monoxide. Additionally, several human deaths are recorded each year from H_2S accidents associated with animal facilities.

Humans can detect the typical odor of H_2S at very low concentrations (0.025 ppm) in air. Exposures to these low concentrations have little or no importance to human health and thus the olfactory response is a safe and useful warning signal of its presence. However, at higher concentrations (greater than 200 ppm) H_2S presents a distinct hazard of a paralyzing effect on the olfactory apparatus, thus effectively neutralizing the warning signal (National Research Council 1979b).

Hydrogen sulfide is an irritant gas. Its direct action on tissues induces local inflammation of the moist membranes of the eye and respiratory tract. When inhaled, the irritant action of H_2S is more or less uniform throughout the respiratory tract, although the deeper pulmonary structures suffer the greatest damage. Inflammation of the deep lung structures may appear as pulmonary edema. If inhaled at sufficiently high concentrations, H_2S can also be readily absorbed through the lung and can produce fatal systemic intoxication.

At concentrations in air exceeding 500 ppm, H_2S must be considered a serious imminent threat to life; between 500 and 1000 ppm it produces permanent effects on the nervous system. If spontaneous recovery does not occur and artificial respiration is not immediately provided, death results from asphyxia. The effects of increasing concentrations of H_2S in swine are presented in Table 64.3.

Management is the most important part of preventing animal deaths from H_2S. When manure stored in a pit beneath a building is agitated, animals should be moved out of the building if at all possible. When movement of the animals is not possible, other steps should be taken to protect the animals during agitation. In mechanically ventilated buildings the fans should run at full capacity, even during the winter; in naturally ventilated buildings, manure pits should not be agitated unless there is a brisk breeze blowing. Immediate rescue of affected swine should not be attempted for the rescuer may quickly become a victim of H_2S toxicosis.

Carbon Monoxide. In addition to gases associated with decomposition of excreta, carbon monoxide (CO), which is produced from the inefficient combustion of carbonaceous fuel and is present in the exhaust fumes of gasoline-burning internal-combustion engines, is also potentially lethal to swine. Poisoning occurs when improperly adjusted and improperly vented space heaters or furnaces are operated in tight, poorly ventilated buildings such as farrowing houses.

Ambient background levels of CO are 0.02 ppm in fresh air, 13 ppm in city streets, and 40 ppm in areas with high vehicular traffic.

Carbon monoxide acts by competing with oxygen for binding sites on a variety of proteins, including hemoglobin, with which most of the compound is associated in the body. The affinity of hemoglobin for CO is some 250 times that for oxygen. When CO becomes bonded to the heme group, forming carboxyhemoglobin, the molecule's oxygen-carrying capacity is reduced. This results in tissue hypoxia.

High concentrations of CO (>250 ppm) in swine farrowing houses are capable of producing an increased number of stillborn piglets. Clinical history generally associated with these stillbirths reveals (1) nonexistent ventilation, (2) inadequate ventilation due to blocked apertures of natural systems or reduction to minimal winter rates for mechanical systems, (3) use of unvented or improperly vented LP gas–burning space heaters, (4) a high percentage of near-term sows delivering dead piglets within a few hours of being put in an artificially heated farrowing facility, (5) sows appear clinically normal although the whole litter is born dead, and (6) laboratory examinations for the detection of infectious causes of abortion are negative (Carson 1990).

Exposure to high levels of CO can be confirmed by actually measuring the CO level in the air or by measuring the percentage of carboxyhemoglobin in the blood of the affected animal. In addition to these two parameters, carboxyhemoglobin concentration of greater than 2% in fetal thoracic fluid may be used as an aid in diagnosing CO-induced stillbirth in swine (Dominick and Carson 1983).

Table 64.3. Clinical effects of increasing concentrations of hydrogen sulfide in swine

H_2S Concentration (ppm)	Effect
250	Discomfort, distress, eye irritation, salivation
400	Muscle spasms, shallow breathing
700	Semicoma
1000	Sudden cyanosis, convulsive spasms, death

Source: Modified from O'Donoghue (1961), as in Osweiler et al. (1985), with permission.

REFERENCES

ANDERSON, D. M., AND STROTHERS, S. C. 1978. Effects of saline water high in sulfates, chlorides, and nitrates on the performance of young weanling pigs. J Anim Sci 47:900–907.

BOOTH, N. H., AND MCDONALD, L. E. 1988. Veterinary Pharmacology and Therapeutics, 6th ed. Ames: Iowa State Univ Press.

CANADIAN TASK FORCE ON WATER QUALITY. 1987.

Task Force on Water Quality Guidelines. Prepared for the Canadian Council of Resource and Environment Ministers.

CARSON, T. L. 1990. Carbon monoxide–induced stillbirth. In Laboratory Diagnosis of Livestock Abortion, 3d ed. Ed. C. A. Kirkbride. Ames: Iowa State Univ Press, pp. 186–189.

CASTEEL S. W.; OSWEILER, G. D.; COOK, W. O.; DANIELS, G.; AND KADLEE, R. 1985. Selenium toxicosis in swine. J Am Vet Med Assoc 186:1084–1085.

CURTIS, S. E. 1983. Environmental Management in Animal Agriculture. Ames: Iowa State Univ Press.

DOMINICK, M. A., AND CARSON, T. L. 1983. Effects of carbon monoxide exposure on pregnant sows and their fetuses. Am J Vet Res 44:35–40.

DORMAN, D. C.; SIMON, J.; HARLIN, K. A.; AND BUCK, W. B. 1990. Diagnosis of bromethalin toxicosis in the dog. J Vet Diagn Invest 2:123–128.

DRUMMOND, J. G.; CURTIS, S. E.; AND SIMON, J. 1978. Effects of atmospheric ammonia on pulmonary bacterial clearance in the young pig. Am J Vet Res 39:211–212.

DRUMMOND, J. G.; CURTIS, S. E.; SIMON, J.; AND NORTON, H. W. 1980. Effects of aerial ammonia on growth and health of young pigs. J Anim Sci 50:1085–1091.

DRUMMOND, J. G.; CURTIS, S. E.; MEYER, R. C.; SIMON, J.; AND NORTON, H. W. 1981a. Effects of atmospheric ammonia on young pigs experimentally infected with *Bordetella bronchiseptica*. Am J Vet Res 42:963–968.

DRUMMOND, J. G.; CURTIS, S. E.; SIMON, J.; AND NORTON, H. W. 1981b. Effects of atmospheric ammonia on young pigs experimentally infected with *Ascaris suum*. Am J Vet Res 42:969–974.

EISELE, G. R. 1986. A perspective on gossypol ingestion in swine. Vet Hum Toxicol 28:118–122.

EMERICK, R. 1974. Consequences of high nitrate levels in feed and water supplies. Fed Proc 33:1183.

EMERICK, R.; EMBRY, L. B.; AND SEERLY, R. W. 1965. Rate of formation and reduction of nitrite induced methemoglobin in vitro and in vivo as influenced by diet of sheep and age of swine. J Anim Sci 24:221–230.

HARRISON, L. H.; COLVIN, B. M.; STUART, B. P.; SANGSTER, L. T.; GORGACZ, E. J.; AND GOSSER, H. S. 1983. Paralysis in swine due to focal symmetrical poliomalacia: Possible selenium toxicosis. Vet Pathol 20:265–273.

HASCHEK, W. M.; BEASLEY, V. R.; BUCK, W. B.; AND FINNELL, J. H. 1989. Cottonseed meal (gossypol) toxicosis in a swine herd. J Am Vet Med Assoc 195:613–615.

KINGSBURY, J. M. 1964. Poisonous Plants of the United States and Canada. Englewood Cliffs, N.J.: Prentice-Hall.

LASSEN, E. D., AND BUCK, W. B. 1979. Experimental lead toxicosis in swine. Am J Vet Res 40:1359–1364.

LINK, R. P. 1975. Toxic plants, rodenticides, herbicides, and yellow fat disease. In Diseases of Swine, 4th ed. Ed. H. W. Dunne and A. D. Leman. Ames: Iowa State Univ Press, p. 861.

LLOYD, W. E. 1978. Feed additives toxicology. Unpublished data. Iowa State Univ.

_____. 1980. Toxicology of heavy metals and trace elements. Unpublished data. Iowa State Univ.

LONDON, W. T.; HENDERSEN, W.; AND CROSS, R. F. 1967. An attempt to produce chronic nitrite toxicosis in swine. J Am Vet Med Assoc 150:398–402.

MEERDINK, G. L. 1979. Epidemiology of domestic animal toxicology in the state of Iowa. Final report. Environ Prot Agency CC71740-J, Vet Diagn Lab, Iowa State Univ.

NATIONAL RESEARCH COUNCIL (NRC). 1974. Nutrients and toxic substances in water for livestock and poultry. Washington, D.C.: National Academy Press.

_____. 1979a. (Committee on Medical and Biologic Effects of Environmental Pollutants, Subcommittee on Ammonia) Ammonia. Baltimore: Univ Park Press.

_____. 1979b. (Committee on Medical and Biologic Effects of Environmental Pollutants, Subcommittee on Hydrogen Sulfide) Hydrogen Sulfide. Baltimore: Univ Park Press.

O'DONOGHUE, J. G. 1961. Hydrogen sulfide poisoning in swine. Can J Comp Med Vet Sci 25:217–219.

OSWEILER, G. D. 1978. Hemostatic function in swine as influenced by warfarin and an oral-antibacterial combination. Am J Vet Res 39:633–638.

OSWEILER, G. D., AND HURD, J. W. 1974. Determination of sodium content in serum and cerebrospinal fluid as an adjunct to diagnosis of water deprivation in swine. J Am Vet Med Assoc 64:165–167.

OSWEILER, G. D.; BUCK, W. B.; AND BICKNELL, E. J. 1969. Experimental production of perirenal edema in swine with *Amaranthus retroflexus.* Am J Vet Res 30:557–577.

OSWEILER, G. D.; CARSON, T. L.; BUCK, W. B.; AND VAN GELDER, G. A. 1985. Clinical and Diagnostic Veterinary Toxicology, 3d ed. Dubuque, Iowa: Kendall/Hunt.

PATERSON, D. W.; WAHLSTROM, R. C.; LIBAL, G. W.; AND OLSON, O. E. 1979. Effects of sulfate in water on swine reproduction and young pig performance. J Anim Sci 49:664–667.

POND, W. G., AND MANER, J. H. 1984. Swine Production and Nutrition. Westport, Conn.: AVI Publishing Company, Inc.

POWER, S. B.; DONNELLY, W. J. C.; McLAUGHLIN, J. G.; WALSH, M. C.; AND DROMEY, M. F. 1989. Accidental carbadox overdosage in an Irish weaner-producing herd. Vet Rec 124:367–370.

RIDDER, W. E., AND OEHME, F. W. 1974. Nitrates as an environmental, animal, and human hazard. Clin Toxicol 7:145.

SCHIPPER, I. A. 1961. Toxicology of wood preservatives to swine. Am J Vet Res 22:401–405.

SEERLEY, R. W.; EMERICK, R. J.; EMBRY, L. B.; AND OLSON, O. E. 1965. Effect of nitrate and nitrite administration continuously in the drinking water for sheep and swine. J Anim Sci 24:1014–1019.

STUART, B. P.; COLE, R. J.; AND GOSSER, H. S. 1981. Cocklebur intoxication in swine: Review and redefinition of the toxic principle. Vet Pathol 18:368–383.

TURNER, C. A., AND KIENHOLZ, E. W. 1972. Nitrate toxicity. Feedstuffs 44:28–30.

U.S. ENVIRONMENTAL PROTECTION AGENCY (USEPA). 1973. Proposed criteria for water quality. Quality of water for livestock. Environ Rep 4(16):663.

_____. 1975. Primary drinking water proposed interim standards. F. R. 40(51)11990.

VAN DER MOLEN, E. J. 1988. Pathological effects of carbadox in pigs with special emphasis on the adrenal. J Comp Pathol 98:55–67.

VAN VLEET, J. F.; MEYER, K. B.; AND OLANDER, H. J. 1974. Acute selenium toxicosis induced in baby pigs by parenteral administration of selenium-vitamin E preparations. J Am Vet Med Assoc 165:543–547.

VAN VLEET, J. F.; AMSTUTS, H. E.; WEIRICH, W. E.; REBAR, A. H.; AND FERRANS, V. J. 1983. Clinical, clinicopathologic, and pathologic alterations of monensin toxicosis in swine. Am J Vet Res 44:1469–1475.

VAN VLEET, J. F.; RUNNELS, L. J.; COOK, J. R.; AND SCHEIDT, A. B. 1987. Monensin toxicosis in swine: Potentiation by tiamulin administration and ameliorative effect of treatment with selenium and/or vitamin E. Am J Vet Res 48:1520–1524.

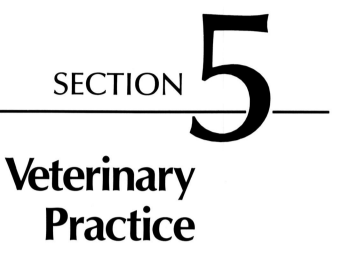

SECTION 5

Veterinary Practice

A. D. Leman, EDITOR

65 Physical Examination

B. E. Straw

D. J. Meuten

VETERINARIANS may be asked to perform examinations on swine in three general areas: the individual sick pig, a herd outbreak of disease, and herd health evaluation. Examination of only one animal is usually reserved for adult sows or boars, since they are of sufficient individual worth to warrant examination and care when ill. Investigations of disease outbreaks involve examinations of individuals that are showing typical signs of the disease as well as investigation of the epidemiologic aspects of the outbreak. In the absence of a specific disease outbreak, a herd may be examined to determine its overall level of health and productivity. Herd health evaluation includes assessment of population and environment interactions and comparisons between the biologic capacity of pigs and the performance being realized on the farm (Goodwin 1971; Heard 1981).

Regardless of which of the three types of examination is performed, it will include a history, physical examination of individual pigs, assessment of pig and environment interactions, and possibly necropsies. This chapter describes procedures for examination of individuals, assessment of herd interactions, necropsy, and collection of information regarding history.

EXAMINATION OF INDIVIDUAL PIGS. In general, swine are not accustomed to being handled or restrained. To avoid misleading physiologic changes caused by restraint or excitement, as much of the examination as possible should be done visually on the pig in its normal environment; it can be restrained later for further examination if necessary. Posture, behavior, nutritional status, and respiration should be observed prior to restraint.

Certain postures assumed by the pig when left to itself indicate the nature of its illness. Recumbent pigs lie in either a sternal or lateral position. Lateral recumbency is avoided by animals with heart disease, while it is favored by animals suffering from exhaustion or overheating. Cold pigs frequently assume sternal recumbency with all four legs tucked under their body to minimize contact with the cold floor (Fig. 65.1). Dog-sitting is associated with respiratory difficulty from pneumonia, cardiac insufficiency, pleuritis, or anemia. A pig standing with its head extended also indicates respiratory distress. Lame pigs frequently are reluctant to rise or will be seen leaning against the pen. Head tilt or circling in pigs is commonly associated with otitis media or interna, which may extend to a brain abscess or meningitis. The head tilt and circling are toward the side with the lesions (Sawaya et al. 1974).

The affected pig's behavior should be compared with that of the others in its pen to determine if it is listless or hyperkinetic. Changes in behavior are most likely a result of a systemic problem, while localized disorders such as lameness are usually accompanied by a normal degree of alertness. Healthy pigs hold their ears up or forward. Drooping ears or ears held flat against the head indicate despondency. Pigs that run into others or do not respond to noise may be deaf or blind.

Conformation and body shape reflect health. The nutritional status of the sick pig is compared to others in the pen. Growing pigs should not have observable bony structure in the body; they

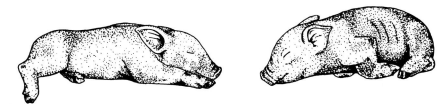

65.1. Postures adopted by warm and cold baby pigs. The pig on the right attempts to keep its thorax and abdomen out of contact with the cold floor, while the pig on the left lies in a relaxed position in full contact with the floor.

should have a slightly arched back and a rounded stomach. An excessive arch or hump in the back and visible vertebrae, ribs, or pelvis are abnormal. The belly should have a good degree of fill but not appear bloated. Adult animals should have a straight to slightly arched back and flat to slightly rounded sides while standing. The degree of fat cover can be estimated visually (Fig. 65.2) and by palpation over the ischium, ribs, verte-

brae, and tailhead. Table 65.1 lists the prominence of these bony landmarks in thin to fat pigs.

Because of the wide range of normal values the respiratory rate of the affected pig should be compared to others in the pen. General ranges of respiratory rates are given in Table 65.2. Rapid rates are associated with pneumonia, cardiac insufficiency, pleuritis, anemia, and pain. Abdominal breathing is seen with pneumonia and pleuritis,

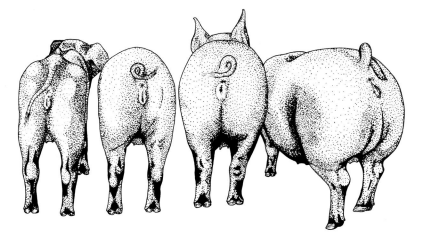

65.2. Sows just after weaning. Using the criteria in Table 12.1, from left to right their body condition scores are 1, 3, 4, and 6.

Table 65.1. Body condition evaluation

Pelvic Bones (ilium and ischium) and tailhead	Loin	Vertebrae	Ribs	Inches (mm) of Backfat	Numerical Score
Pelvic bones very prominent; deep cavity around tailhead	Loin very narrow; sharp edge on transverse spinal process; flank very hollow	Vertebrae prominent and sharp throughout length of backbone	Individual ribs very prominent	0.5 (13) or less	1
Pelvic bones obvious but some slight cover; cavity around tail	Loin narrow; only very slight cover to edge of transverse spinal processes; flank rather hollow	Vertebrae prominent	Rib cage less apparent; difficulty in seeing individual ribs	0.6 (15)	2
Pelvic bones covered	Edge of transverse spinal processes covered and rounded	Vertebrae visible over shoulder; some cover farther back	Ribs covered but can be felt	0.7 (17)	3
Pelvic bones only felt with firm pressure; no cavity around tail	Edge of transverse spinal processes felt only with firm pressure; flank full	Vertebrae felt only with firm pressure	Rib cage not visible; very difficult to feel any ribs	0.8 (20)	4
Pelvic bones impossible to feel; root of tail set deep in surrounding fat	Impossible to feel bones; flank full and rounded	Impossible to feel vertebrae	Ribs impossible to feel	0.9 (23)	5
Pelvic bones impossible to feel; folds of fat surrounding tail; folds of fat obscure vulva in sows	Thick fat cover	Midline appears as a slight hollow between rolls of fat	Thick fat cover	1.0 (25) or more	6

while increased rates from other causes are costal. Occasionally, respiratory disease produces vocal changes in which the voice becomes squeaky or persistent.

Pigs have a wide range of rectal temperatures, and the rapidity with which their temperature rises when excited frequently limits the usefulness of its determination. However, in recumbent animals that tolerate a rectal temperature determination, it is a useful adjunct to the physical exam. Ranges of normal rectal temperatures for swine are given in Table 65.2 (Elmore et al. 1979; Littledike et al. 1979).

After the initial visual examination, the pig can be restrained if necessary and a careful systemic examination performed.

The color of the skin in general and especially the snout, ears, lower belly, inner thighs, vulva, and anus should be observed. Natural light or in- candescent (not fluorescent) light gives the most accurate reflection of color. In white pigs, the color may be bluish (circulatory disturbance), red (hyperemia, pyrexia, infection), white (anemia), yellow (liver dysfunction or hemolysis), or grayish and crusted (parasites or nutritional imbalance). The hair should be smooth and flat. A rough hair coat indicates a cold, sick, or undernourished pig (Fig. 65.3). If skin lesions are seen, their distribution should be defined as to location and symmetry. Lesions should be determined to be flat or raised or with discrete or diffuse edges. The pig should be observed for scratching and rubbing. Skin scrapings in pigs suspected of mange should be taken from the ear canal. When specific skin lesions are present, the scrapings should be taken from the edge of the lesion. Scrapings are made with a scalpel blade deep enough into the skin to produce slight bleeding. Mineral oil, 10% potas-

Table 65.2. Temperature, respiration, and heart rate of pigs of different ages

Age of Pig	Rectal Temperature (range +0.3°C, 0.5°F)		Respiratory Rate (breaths/min)	Heart Rate (beats/min)
	°C	°F		
Newborn	39.0	102.2	50–60	200–250
1 hr	36.8	98.3		
12 hr	38.0	100.4		
24 hr	38.6	101.5		
Unweaned piglet	39.2	102.6		
Weaned piglet (20–40 lb)	39.3	102.7	25–40	90–100
(9–18 kg)				
Growing pig (60–100 lb)	39.0	102.3	30–40	80–90
(27–45 kg)				
Finishing pig (100–200 lb)	38.8	101.8	25–35	75–85
(45–90 kg)				
Sow in gestation	38.7	101.7	13–18	70–80
Sow				
24 hr prepartum	38.7	101.7	35–45	
12 hr prepartum	38.9	102.0	75–85	
6 hr prepartum	39.0	102.2	95–105	
Birth of 1st pig	39.4	102.9	35–45	
12 hr postpartum	39.7	103.5	20–30	
24 hr postpartum	40.0	104.0	15–22	
1 wk postpartum				
until weaning	39.3	102.7		
1 day postweaning	38.6	101.5		
Boar	38.4	101.1	13–18	70–80

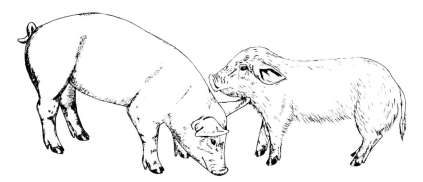

65.3. Two 9-week-old pigs. The one on the left is in good condition. The one on the right has failed to grow properly and shows the associated long rough hair coat, prominent spine, and relatively oversized head.

sium hydroxide, or glycerin may be used to facilitate transfer of the scraped material from the skin to a glass slide or tube (see Chapter 54).

In addition to skin color, the cardiovascular system is assessed by pulse rate and occasionally auscultation of the heart. The nature of the pig and its rough hair make auscultation difficult, but under quiet conditions the heart can be assessed using the same criteria as for other domestic animals.

In addition to the observations made on respiration during the initial visual exam, the respiratory system is also examined for discharges (serous, purulent, bloody) from the nares and for snout anatomy (straight, bent, shortened).

The eyes are examined for conjunctivitis, discharge, cataracts, and vision.

Examination of the gastrointestinal system may begin at the mouth by checking for condition of the teeth, damage or infection of the gums, or vesicle formation and ulcers. Baby pigs have extremely sharp canine teeth at birth, which should be clipped within 24 hours of age so that the points are removed and a flat smooth surface remains. The abdomen should be rounded, not tucked up or bloated. The patency of the rectum and anus should be verified in pigs that appear bloated. Hernias may occur at the umbilicus or inguinal ring. The normal color of manure ranges from brownish yellow or brownish green to dark brown, depending on the type of feed pigs are consuming. Reddish, black, or yellow feces (especially when associated with blood or mucus) indicate gastrointestinal disorder. Manure with normal consistency holds a formed shape with minimal spreading. Watery or extremely dry hard feces are seen in various disease states.

The mammary system should be inspected for color, consistency, heat, and pain. The behavior of the piglets reflects the quantity of milk being produced. Noisy piglets that are restless and make frequent nursing attempts are receiving an inadequate amount of milk. Diagnostic tests of milk in cases of suspected infectious mastitis include bacterial isolation and the California mastitis test for estimation of the leukocyte count. Teats should be prominent and not have blind ends. The mammary glands should be evenly spaced along the underline and well forward. (See Chapter 4 for an excellent description of the mammary system.)

The external examination of the genital system of sows is primarily restricted to inspection of the vulva. The vulva should be prominent and at an angle conducive to mating. The mucosa should be a healthy pink color. Swellings, lacerations, and hematomas may affect the vulva. Some postparturient vaginal discharge is normal unless the discharge is excessive, purulent, or foul smelling.

The boar's testicles are inspected visually for uniformity of size and color of scrotal skin. Palpation will reveal heat, pain, or abnormal consistency. The penis should be extended and examined for lacerations, ulcers, malformations, adhesions, or persistent frenulum. The preputial diverticulum is checked for ulcers or dilation with urine. Mating behavior including libido, aggressiveness, and ability to mount and copulate should be determined. Additional information regarding the male and female genital systems is given in Chapter 6.

If an animal is being examined for a locomotor problem, the limb(s) involved should be examined last, since there is usually pain involved and manipulation will produce excitement and disarrangement of other systems. The primary emphasis in examination for lameness centers on the foot, hock or knee, and the hip. Initially, the gait is observed. Locomotor abnormalities caused by neurologic deficits appear as weakness, paresis, ataxia, incoordination, spasticity, or dysmetria, while traumatic or infectious lesions appear as a shortening of stride and avoidance of weight bearing on the affected limb(s). The posture may differ from normal by a pronounced curve in the back, degree of flexion in the legs, and position of legs compared to body (whether drawn up under the body or spraddled out to the sides). Postural changes are primarily an attempt to relieve weight bearing from the affected limb(s). The feet are examined for bruising, cuts, cracks, infection, hardness of hoof, and overgrown or worn hooves. Joints are examined for comparative size with the complementary joint and for heat, pain, and crepitation. Chapter 8 contains additional information concerning examination of the skeletal system.

An individual pig may be examined because of its relative value (sow, boar) or more frequently because it is typical of a problem that has been occurring in a portion of the herd.

EXAMINATION OF GROUPS OF PIGS. Veterinarians are frequently asked to look at groups of pigs when the herd is experiencing a disease outbreak, or the examination is made on the herd in its usual state to identify areas of suboptimal performance. In either case, a herd examination is more than just the sum of many individual examinations. In addition to changes in physical condition, the population dynamics, environment, feed, and management must be assessed. A herd visit usually proceeds from the farrowing area to the weaned pigs and then to either the growing-finishing pigs or the breeding and gestation areas.

The area of population dynamics includes interactions between and among pigs and between people and pigs. Specific areas to be observed include pig density (pigs/pen, square footage/pig, and pigs/building or shared air space), pig uniformity (sizes and ages in the same pen or building), pig-to-pig social interactions (fighting, tail and ear biting), number of competitive situations (feeder, waterer, and sleeping space compared to number), and pig reaction to the presence of herders. Weights and ages should be determined and compared against those given in Figure 65.4.

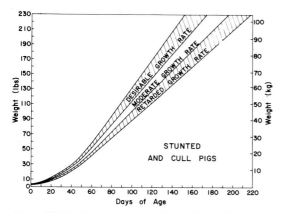

65.4. Weight for age of pigs with rapid, moderate, and slow growth rates.

Weights of pigs within one pen should not differ from each other by more than 10%.

The environment is examined for temperature appropriate to the age of the pigs, draftiness, and contamination with dust and gases. Floors are examined for appropriateness of surface material (slipperiness, abrasiveness, warmth), design (width of slots and slats, floor slope), condition of material (wear and tear), cleanliness, and dryness. Pens should contain feeders and waterers that are readily accessible and free of broken parts or sharp protruding corners. Dunging patterns are observed with particular attention to whether dunging is occurring in the sleeping or eating areas. The position of pigs in regard to each other (whether piled up in one spot or spread out over the pen) is determined. The presence and condition of footbaths is noted. Buildings are examined for evidence of rodent damage such as chewed insulation and rodent tracks or droppings in the feeders and along the top of the pen dividers. Bird and wild animal access to the building is assessed (Muirhead 1983).

Feed is considered for its nutrient analysis in regard to the intended concentration of nutrients and the actual composition of the diet. The physical form of the feed is examined for correctness of grind or integrity of pellets. The feed should be fresh and not contaminated with mold, rodent manure, or spoiled or rancid ingredients. The amount offered is monitored regarding daily allotment given to limit-fed animals and feeder adjustment for those fed ad libitum.

Finally, management practices are examined. Pig flow through buildings should be determined to be either all-in/all-out, or continuous. The amount of mixing, sorting, and moving and the stages at which it is done should be recorded. Breeding practices regarding estrus detection and timing and number of services should be observed or determined from records. Tables 65.3–65.5 list desirable and undesirable characteristics of groups of pigs of different ages.

Complete understanding of the situation on the farm requires a thorough examination of pigs and their environment coupled with careful questioning of the caretaker. A complete history of the pigs and farm can be collected, or information gathering may center on the area where problems are occurring. Areas of history to inquire into include the following.

Herd security: Were any animals brought onto the farm recently? What are the quarantine and isolation procedures for new stock? Is there one or more sources of breeding stock? What steps are taken to control human and animal traffic? How are animals loaded out of the farm?

Genetics: What is the genetic composition of the herd? What procedures are used to guarantee that proper matings will take place? What selection criteria are used for boars, gilts, and sows? Is there a family or breed relationship between animals experiencing the disease?

Breeding management: What is the boar-to-sow ratio? How frequently are individual boars used? Does mating occur in a pen or is hand mating used? With hand mating what sanitary precautions are taken between boars? How is estrus detection done? How frequently and at what times are sows and gilts mated? When and how is pregnancy diagnosis done? What is the conception rate for sows and gilts? What is the farrowing rate for sows and gilts? How many females return to estrus 21 days after mating and at other intervals? Have abortions been noted?

Farrowing performance: Are sows washed prior to entering the farrowing area? What is the size of litters and total born alive, mummies, and stillbirths? What do piglets weigh at birth? How frequently do sows require assistance to farrow? Is cross-fostering practiced?

Mortality: What are the mortality rates for unweaned pigs, nursery pigs, growing-finishing pigs, and sows and boars? Are there seasonal fluctuations in mortality rates?

Medications and immunizations: What vaccines are used routinely in the herd? What animals are vaccinated and at what time? Is there a routine worming program for sows, boars, and growing pigs? How are external parasites controlled? What medications are used in the feed? Are drugs used at a growth-promoting or therapeutic level? Is drug usage rotated? What injectable treatments are given to sick pigs?

Feed: Is feed grown on the farm or purchased? Where and how is feed mixing done? What nutrient composition is intended for each class of pig? How is feed stored, and delivered to the pigs? What quantity of feed is given to limit-fed pigs, and how is the feed measured?

Disease outbreak: What was the progression of signs within a pig? How old was the pig when signs started? How long did illness persist? Is recovery complete or is pig unthrifty? In the group affected, what is the morbidity and mortality? Has

Table 65.3. Examination of pigs in the farrowing area

Condition	Desirable	Undesirable
Sows		
Physical condition		
Body	Normal weight	Thin, fat, or obese
Cleanliness	Sows thoroughly washed	Sows dirty with caked mud and manure
Mammary glands	At least 12 prominent, evenly spaced nipples	Inverted, juvenile, or overcrowded teats; glands hot, red, swollen, painful; abnormal milk
Vulval discharges	Watery, clear to whitish fluid	Purulent, bloody, or foul smelling discharge
Skin	Unblemished, pink in unpigmented areas	Burns from heat lamp; abrasions or calluses; anemia
Feet and legs	Normal stance and movement	Splayleg; foot lesions; difficulty lying down and getting up
Feed		
Amount	4–6 lb (2–2.5 kg) plus 1 lb (0.5 kg) for each pig in litter	Less than desired level
Feeder	Clean, large capacity and easily accessible	Dirty, broken, containing old or moldy feed
Water	Unlimited supply of fresh water	Fouled water, inadequate flow, or inaccessible
Environment		
Temperature	Between 60 and 75°F (16–24°C)	Too hot or too cold
Floor design	Proper spacing between slats; good traction; nonabrasive	Slippery material, sharp edges, uneven slats; slots sized to trap teats and dewclaws
Floor	Clean and dry	Dirty, wet, cracked, or broken
Crate design	Right size for sow; permits good exposure of underline	Too large, allowing sow to flop over and crush pigs; bottom bar hinders nursing
Baby pigs		
Physical condition		
Piglet birthweight	Average, 3 lb (1.3 kg) or greater	Average less than 3 lb (1.3 kg)
Litter sizes	All litters uniform in size, 8–12 pigs	Wide variation in litter size, with 20% or more containing 8 pigs or less
Weights within the litter	Less than 1 lb (0.5 kg) difference between largest and smallest	More than 1 lb (0.5 kg) difference between largest and smallest
Skin	Unblemished; pink in unpigmented areas	Knee abrasions; facial lacerations; teat necrosis; anemia; greasy pig disease
Locomotor	Normal anatomy and gait	Splayleg; swollen joints; foot lesions; lameness
Infectious disease	None	Diarrhea; sneezing; unthriftiness
Teeth	Clipped on day-old pigs; gums healthy	Teeth not clipped; infected gums
Tails	Clipped neatly or left long	Clipped tails are swollen, red, infected
Feed		
Feed	Fresh creep feed given daily	None; or stale feed offered
Water	Fresh water easily accessible	None; inaccessible or foul water
Environment		
Temperature	Creep area with temperature of 85–90°F (29–32°C)	Piling or lying next to sow; pigs too hot and avoiding heat lamp
Drafts	Air evenly distributed through building	Incoming air moving directly onto litters
Floor design	Good traction for pigs in nursing area; uniform spacing of slats; nonabrasive	Slippery flooring material; slats laid so that slot length perpendicular to sow
Floor	Clean, dry, and bedded if appropriate	Dirty, wet, broken, or cracked
Management		
Flow		
Building use	All-in/all-out	Continuous farrowing
Farrowing schedule	All farrowings within a few days; pigs weaned at the same time	Farrowing spread out over 1 or 2 wk; weaning at various times and ages
Sanitation		
Cleanliness	Excess manure and afterbirths removed daily	Accumulation of manure; wet bedding
Downtime	Building empty for a few days between farrowing batches	New sows added the same day or day after previous sows weaned
Washing procedures	High-pressure washer to remove all organic material; porous surfaces sealed or disinfected	Manure left in corners and cracks; dust accumulation and cobwebs

Table 65.4. Examination of growing pigs

Condition	Desirable		Undesirable
	Nursery-weaner pigs	Growing-finishing pigs	
Physical condition			
Weight for age	3 wk, 9–12 lb (4–5.5 kg); 5 wk, 14–20 lb (6.3–9 kg)	8 wk, 40 lb (18 kg); 14 wk, 100 lb (45 kg); 24 wk, 220 lb (100 kg)	Low weight for age
Number of pigs/pen	Maximum, 15–25	Maximum, 30–40	Too many pigs per pen; Pig density too high
Space/pig on partial or total slats	15–30 lb (7–14 kg), 2.5 ft² (0.23m²); 30–60 lb (14–27 kg), 3.5 ft² (0.32m²)	60–100 lb (27–45 kg), 4 ft² (0.36 m²); 100–150 lb (45–68 kg), 6 ft² (0.54 m²); 150–220 lb (68–100 kg), 8 ft² (0.72 m²)	
Uniformity of size	Pen mates differ in weight by less than 10%		Large variation in weights; many runts and culls
Respiratory system	None or occasional coughing or sneezing		Frequent coughing or sneezing; bent snouts or discharge
Skin	Unblemished; pink in unpigmented areas		Frequent scratching; redness, keratinization, abrasions, anemia
Gastrointestinal	Normal		Diarrhea—hernias, prolapsed rectum; rectal stricture
Locomotor	Normal gait and anatomy		Swollen joints, foot lesions, lameness
Vices	None; dunging in proper area		Bitten tails, ears, flanks; umbilical sucking; dunging in eating/sleeping areas
Environment			
Temperature	85°F (29°C) at weaning and 5°F (3°C) less each week	55–75°F (13–24°C)	Too cold or drafty; pigs piling or panting
Floor	Wire or slatted floor; holes small enough not to trap feet	Total slats, partial slats, or solid	Solid floor; uneven slat spacing; broken, rough, or abrasive surface
Feed			
Feeder	15 cm feeder space/pig; fresh feed added several times daily	1 hole for every 4 pigs; feeder adjusted to reduce wastage	Inadequate feeder space; excessive fighting at feeder
Water	One waterer for every 10–15 pigs	One waterer for every 20–25 pigs	Not enough waterers or poor accessibility; inadequate water flow
Management			
Building use	All-in/all-out		Continuous flow
Sanitation	Few days of downtime when building is pressure washed		Inadequate cleaning; manure left in corners, cracks, and under feeder; dust and cobwebs; dirty fans

Table 65.5. Examination of sows in gestation

Condition	Desirable	Undesirable
Physical condition		
Body	Normal weight	Thin, fat, or obese
Skin	Unblemished; pink in unpigmented areas	Abrasions, lacerations, fight wounds; hygromas, calluses, pressure sores; thickened keratinized skin; scratching
Locomotor	Stands normally; able to lie down and get up easily	Shifting weight from leg to leg; foot lesions, overgrown hooves; splayleg
Vulva	Normal size; pink mucosa	Reddened, enlarged vulva; estrus; discharges; prolapse
Mammary glands	At least 12 prominent, evenly spaced nipples	Enlarged, reddened, or hard glands
Sows in groups	Sows grouped according to size; in competitive feeding situation, less than 6 sows/pen	Much size variation; sows and gilts penned together; fighting
Environment		
Temperature	Stalls – 68-75°F (20-24°C); pens – 60-75°F (16-24°C)	Too hot or too cold; sows lying in sternal recumbency or panting
Floor design	Good traction; smooth edge to slats	Uneven slat spacing; broken, rough, or abrasive surface
Floor condition	Clean and dry	Wet, dirty

treatment been used, and to what effect? What is the course of disease within the herd? Did the disease start with an explosive outbreak or was it insidious? What animals were originally affected? What animals has disease spread to? Did the initial disease picture differ from the later signs? Is disease becoming more or less severe? Are any other animals besides pigs affected? What is the distribution of affected animals? Is disease sporadic or endemic? Are affected animals grouped by litter, pen, or building? Is one sex affected to a greater extent than the other? Were any changes in management made prior to the outbreak of the disease?

Disease affecting pigs in litters: Are whole litters affected or is incidence sporadic within litters? Are the biggest or smallest pigs affected? Are litters of gilts or sows more frequently or severely affected?

NECROPSY. Necropsy of individual pigs that represent a herd problem is an excellent diagnostic tool (Williams and Perry 1978). The success of necropsy for diagnosis, however, is directly dependent on the animal selected (or found). When possible, choose a live animal that has become symptomatic within the last 24 hours and has developed a pattern of clinical signs similar to other members of the group. Do not accept an owner's selection of a dead animal or a chronic "poor-doer" when there are live pigs that clearly represent the problem being investigated.

With practice, a systematic approach, and the correct tools a complete necropsy should take only 15-20 minutes for a piglet and 30-45 minutes for an adult. For the time and money invested there is not a more complete diagnostic aid. Additionally, a proficient and complete necropsy procedure often improves the relationship

between practicing veterinarian and owner (Benbrook 1947).

Equipment. Necessary equipment includes rubber gloves and boots, knife with 5- to 7-inch blade, scalpel with blades, scissors, tissue forceps, large-mouth plastic or glass containers with formalin, plastic bags, string, and culture swabs. Other helpful equipment includes knife steel, rib cutters, glass microscope slides, labels, single-edge razor blades, ruler, sterile syringes, and needles. All necessary equipment for a necropsy must fit into a hand-carried holder.

Preservation. The only fixative necessary for histopathology in clinical practice is 10% neutral buffered (to prevent the formation of artifactual pigment and acid hematin) formalin. To prepare 1 L, mix 900 ml water with 100 ml 40% formaldehyde (9:1 solution) and add 6.5 g diphasic anhydrous sodium phosphate and 4 g monobasic sodium phosphate.

To ensure proper preservation, tissues for histology must be 5 mm or less in thickness (except brain, spinal cord, and eyes). Length and width of tissues saved for histology are not critical, but a 3 × 4 cm section is recommended. Correct ratio of tissue to formalin is 10:1.

Specimens for bacteriology and virology should be placed in plastic bags, refrigerated (not frozen), and labelled. To save time during necropsy and to avoid contamination, solid organs such as liver, lung, and lymph node should be submitted for culture as blocks of fresh tissue, approximately 3-4 cm². The laboratory technician will sterilize the surface and collect a sample aseptically from the center. Intestines are submitted as loops about 6 cm long, securely tied at both ends or folded into a U shape and tied with a single ligature at the top of the loop. Tissues for virology, other than gastrointestinal specimens, can be pooled in a single container.

When diseases caused by such organisms as *Salmonella, Haemophilus, Campylobacter, Serpulina, Brucella, Nocardia,* fungi, yeast, or anaerobes such as *Clostridium* spp. are suspected, the appropriate chapters of this book and the local laboratory should be consulted regarding pecific collection, storage, and transport considerations. Laboratory technicians must be informed of the possibility of these organisms for them to perform the appropriate testing.

Colonic contents and/or feces for electron microscopic examination for viruses should be refrigerated. Specimens for toxicology can be frozen. Depending on the suspected toxin, different tissues (5 cm²) may be more helpful than others (e.g., brain for organophosphate toxicity); however, a good general group of samples to save are stomach contents, liver, kidney, urine, serum, and feed.

General.   The necropsy procedure described here is a modification of several techniques (Roderick 1954; VanKruiningen 1971; King et al. 1979). The important principles are *consistency* and *thoroughness.* Although clinical evaluation may suggest a specific body system and disease, the prosector must do a thorough job to avoid overlooking lesions that may either be the primary problem or contributing to that problem.

Always dissect an organ completely. This includes gross observations of natural and cut surfaces and collection of samples for histology, bacteriology, virology, etc. Do not proceed to another organ until the last is completed.

External.   Much of the external exam may have been accomplished antemortem. Evaluate hydration, postmortem interval (if cornea is cloudy and abdomen is discolored green do not bother with a necropsy), skin lesions (distribution, color, shape, proliferative, flat, ulcerative), joints (swollen, ulcerated), and feet and ears (bite wounds, necrosis). Place the pig in left lateral recumbency.

Dissection.   Keep your knife *sharp.* Always insert the knife into the subcutis and cut outward. Avoid cutting into hair, skin, and bone, as these tissues will dull a knife rapidly. Table 65.6 is an outline of the necropsy procedure that follows, and Table 65.7 lists the specimens that should be submitted to ancillary laboratories.

Make a stab incision into the right axilla and extend the incision cranially to the point of the mandible and caudally to the anus following a path just right of the midline. Dissect through the muscles beneath the right scapula and adjacent subcutis and reflect the forelimb off the carcass. Examine the inguinal and axillary lymph nodes. Cut the muscles around the coxofemoral joint, ex-

Table 65.6.   Outline of necropsy procedure

1. Left lateral recumbency, external exam
2. Cut deep into right axilla, extend incision to point of mandible and to anus, reflect skin, cut right coxofemoral joint, open right stifle and reflect limb, examine inguinal lymph nodes
3. Open abdomen with a paracostal incision, extend to pelvis with a paralumbar cut, reflect abdominal wall ventrally
4. Stab diaphragm and incise, cut ribs and remove
5. Examine peritoneal and thoracic cavities; if exudates, adhesions, fibrin, etc., present, collect tissues for culture; if urine or blood needed, collect now
6. Open pericardium in situ, free and break one rib
7. Cut on medial side of both mandibles close to bone and free tongue; pull tongue caudally, cut hyoid bones, cut soft tissues along vertebrae, free cervical and thoracic viscera intact
8. Examine oral cavity, save tonsil for pseudorabies, examine regional lymph nodes, incise tongue, open esophagus
9. Palpate lungs, open trachea and major airways, cut bronchial lymph nodes, open heart
10. Squeeze gallbladder to test patency
11. Compress feces from rectum and cut; free entire intestinal tract with blunt and sharp dissection as intestines are pulled toward prosector
12. Remove both adrenals (cranial pole of kidneys), incise with scalpel
13. Remove kidneys by sharply pulling caudally, ureter will not break; peel capsules; cut to the pelvises, examine; open urinary bladder
14. Examine and remove reproductive tract
15. Remove spleen from stomach, make incisions
16. Remove skin and muscles from head; flex neck to locate atlantooccipital joint; cut to ventral surface of joint; collect cerebrospinal fluid if needed; insert knife through joint and into vertebral canal, severing spinal cord; cut neck muscles
17. Snap head into maximum extension, cut all attachments
18. Make transverse cut in skull, caudal to orbits; extend the lateral margins on a line medial to each occipital condyle; cut at a 45° angle
19. Pry skull cap off, sever attachments, tap condyles on table, sever olfactory tracts and cranial nerves as brain is slowly removed
20. Spread intestines and open stomach, duodenum, sections of jejunum, ileum, cecum, sections of spiral colon, descending colon, rectum; save appropriate areas[a]

[a]The gastrointestinal tract is examined last in most necropsies. If the clinical problem is referable to this system, examine it earlier in the necropsy, since it autolyzes rapidly.

Table 65.7.   Submission of necropsy specimens to ancillary laboratories

Histopathology (10% neutral buffered formalin)
  Gross lesions, 5 mm thick or less
  Important tissues – lung, kidney, liver, spleen, adrenal, lymph nodes, tonsil, heart .
  Gastrointestinal tract – stomach, duodenum with pancreas, proximal and distal jejunum, ileum with cecum, colon
  Central nervous system and eyes when indicated by clinical signs – brain, spinal cord, eyes; all in a separate
    container of 10% formalin
Bacteriology (refrigerate specimens)
  3–4 cm² blocks of tissue
  Individual containers
  Tied loops of intestine
  If you suspect any of the following organisms, be sure to inform the lab – *Haemophilus, Salmonella, Campylobacter,
    Serpulina, Brucella, Nocardia,* fungi, yeast or anaerobes (e.g., *Clostridium)*
Virology (refrigerate specimens)
  3–4 cm² blocks of tissue
  Specimens other than intestines may be pooled in one container
  Tied loops of intestine
Toxicology (freeze specimens)
  Stomach contents, kidney, liver, urine, serum, feed
Coccidia
  Glass slide with scraping of ileal mucosa
  Histologic section of intestines in formalin

amine the joint fluid, and reflect the limb. Remove skin and subcutis from the right stifle and open the joint by a horizontal cut made by inserting the knife medial to the patella and cutting outward as the knife is pushed proximally. Open the right shoulder joint and right hock. If changes suggestive of sepsis (increased fluid, cloudy fluid, fibrin, and prominent synovium) are present in a preceding joint, then open the next as cleanly as possible and collect a sample for culture (syringe or culture swab).

Enter the abdominal cavity via a paracostal incision and continue with a paralumbar cut that extends from the ribs to the right pelvic limb and across the abdomen cranial to the pubis. Reflect the abdominal wall toward you. Examine the peritoneum for lesions of sepsis (hydroperitoneum, cloudy fluid, fibrin). Incise the diaphragm from side to side, cutting muscles along the dorsal and central borders of the ribs. Cut the costal cartilage of ribs with rib cutters (knife for neonate), cut the ribs along their dorsal border, and remove the rib cage. Cut one rib free, dissect the muscle off, and break the rib for a crude estimate of bone strength.

At this point, examine the thoracic and peritoneal cavities closely. Do not try to examine them through small openings or without opening both. This is also a good time to assess the nutritional status of the animal. Obvious muscle wasting and absence of fat or presence of serous atrophy of fat (gelatinous) are associated with chronic problems. Generally, an adequate nutritional status is associated with acute problems. Examine the umbilicus of neonates at this time. If you suspect bacteremia, now is the proper time to collect blocks (3–4 cm²) of liver, spleen, and lung before there is gross contamination.

If clinical signs (e.g., neonatal diarrhea) indicate gastrointestinal involvement, proceed with this system first to avoid artifacts produced by rapid autolysis. Otherwise the gastrointestinal tract is usually the last system examined and the following description is for a nonintestinal problem.

Head, Neck, Thorax.   Incise the pericardium in situ and examine for excess fluid, fibrin, and adhesions. Cut along the medial side of both mandibles, hook a finger over the tongue, and pull caudoventrally, severing remaining attachments. Cut the hyoid cartilage with a knife or rib cutters and pull the tongue toward the thorax while dissecting the esophagus and trachea free of cervical muscles. Hold the esophagus and trachea near the thoracic inlet and pull caudally, cutting all attachments that secure the heart and lungs to the thoracic pleura. Remove the tongue and thoracic viscera intact and set aside. Examine the oral cavity for lesions (cleft palate, ulcers, erosions, vesicles) and collect the pharyngeal tonsil for pseudorabies examination if desired (virology laboratory, fluorescent antibody). Use scissors or a knife to open the esophagus.

Examine the lungs visually and palpate them. Pulmonary lesions are evaluated better by palpation than visual inspection. Open the trachea, bronchi, and major airways with scissors. Evaluate numerous cut surfaces. Depressed consolidated lesions of variable size at the tips of anteroventral lobes are relatively common in swine. They may be attributed to mycoplasma, mild resolving pneumonia, or regional atelectasis. More important than trying to make a definitive gross diagnosis is the recording of an accurate description of the lesions (distribution, extent, texture, color) and collection of specimens for histology and culture to correctly identify the disease.

Leave the heart attached to the lungs and examine the natural surfaces of the heart for hemorrhages, serous atrophy of fat, or enlarged chambers. Epicardial and endocardial petechiae are fairly common and usually not significant. However, if the hemorrhages are extensive and/or especially if they extend into the myocardium, they are likely to be significant. Open the right side of the heart like a flap, making a U-shaped cut from the pulmonary trunk into the right ventricle, following the interventricular septum, and the right atrium. Open the left side of the heart like a book, making a straight transmural incision from the left auricle, through the coronary groove, and to the tip of the left ventricle. Examine the chambers and left atrioventricular valve and then cut through this valve to visualize the aorta and left semilunar valves.

Abdomen. If there are discolored loops of intestine compatible with volvulus or markedly distended loops of colon as seen with atresia coli, then carefully palpate the lesion(s) and the mesentery. Evaluate displaced organs in situ; do not remove any organs until you have carefully dissected and identified the problem or established important anatomical landmarks. Compress the gallbladder to test patency. Squeeze feces from the rectum; cut the rectum and pull it out of the abdomen. With tension on the rectum, cut any attachments that secure the gastrointestinal tract and root of the mesentery to the dorsal body wall. Cutting the gastrohepatic ligaments and esophagus should free the intestines so they can be pulled from the abdomen and set aside.

Locate the adrenal glands at the cranial pole of each kidney, remove and incise them longitudinally, and save sections in formalin. Grasp the right kidney, cut the cranial attachments, and pull caudally. The ureter will remain attached. Repeat this procedure with the left kidney and dissect the urinary bladder free with ureters and kidneys attached. Cut each kidney longitudinally to the pelvis and peel the capsule. If no lesions are observed, submit a section (5 mm thick) that includes cortex, medulla, and pelvis. The pelvis is needed to evaluate pyelonephritis.

Remove the liver and examine the natural surface and numerous cut surfaces. Save any lesions or two randomly chosen 5-mm slices.

Remove and examine the reproductive tract.

Brain and Eyes. Many diseases affect the central nervous system of young swine. Generally, only microscopic lesions are produced, and it is therefore important to collect tissues for the ancillary laboratories.

Leave the head attached and remove the skin, ears, and muscles from the head and neck. Cut ventrally through the cervical muscles to expose the atlantooccipital joint. Insert the point of a knife, sever the spinal cord, and cut laterally and dorsally around the atlantooccipital joint, avoiding bone. Bend the head over the edge of a table and snap it downward as you stabilize the neck with your opposite hand. The joint will open

widely and remaining attachments can be cut.

To remove the calvarium of an adult, use a butcher's saw or a cast-cutting saw. The calvarium of a neonate is so thin that it can be removed with bone forceps or cutting pliers. Secure the head by grasping the mandibles with your fingers and inserting a thumb in an orbit. The first cut is made transversely through the frontal bones. Cut close to the orbits in a neonate and more caudally in an adult. Make a second cut from the medial angle of one occipital condyle to the lateral margin of the first cut. This cut is at an approximate 45° angle to the longitudinal axis of the skull. Repeat on the opposite side. The calvarium should pry free in one unit. It may be necessary to cut the tentorium cerebelli before the skull cap can be removed in its entirety. Two common errors are cutting so deeply that the brain is cut (usually not a significant problem) and misplacement of cuts too far laterally and too close to the orbits in an adult so that the cranial vault is not entered. If this latter situation occurs simply identify which cut(s) is incorrect and repeat.

To remove the brain, hold the skull vertically in one hand and tap the condyles on a hard surface. Sever the olfactory tracts, and as the brain slowly emerges sever each cranial nerve from the floor of the cranial vault. Examine the meninges for meningitis, usually visualized best over the cerebellum or on the ventral surface of the brain (white to yellow foci or mats and strands of fibrin). Submit pieces of brain with meninges for bacteriology and virology if clinical signs indicate a central nervous system problem. If rabies is a consideration, it may be best to submit the entire head (contact regional laboratory for information). Should you decide to remove the brain of a rabies suspect, use a manual saw to cut the bone (prevents the potential of an aerosol) and then cut the brain longitudinally, submitting one-half for rabies virus detection and one-half for histology.

Gastrointestinal System. Open the stomach along its greater curvature, then open the duodenum, various sections of jejunum that are straightened out, the ileum, and the cecum. Handle the intestines carefully, as it is easy to introduce artifacts. When a gross lesion is observed, submit it and a section of adjacent unaffected bowel. In the absence of gross lesions, submit a piece of stomach, duodenum with pancreas attached, proximal and distal jejunum, and ileum with cecum attached. These sections should be 3–6 cm long and only partially opened. This will permit the pathologist to collect longitudinal and circular cross sections. In neonatal diarrheas it is difficult for the pathologist to trim in sections of intestine that do not have a closed tubular portion. Submit a random section of colon if no gross lesions are seen. Examine the mesenteric lymph nodes.

Because of the importance of the gastrointestinal system in diseases of swine, the prosector should have a routine method to collect specimens.

Musculoskeletal System. The most important structures to evaluate in the musculoskeletal system of pigs are arthrodial joints. Joints to be examined and the general lesions of septic arthritis were discussed under **Dissection.** Atrophic rhinitis is common in swine. The most frequent lesion is atrophy of the inferior scroll of the ventral turbinates. The lesion is best visualized by cutting through the nose at the level of the first premolar.

Osteomyelitis is an uncommon problem but may result in lameness or pathologic fracture of vertebrae with compression of the spinal cord. The bones will need to be cut longitudinally on a table saw to visualize the lesions.

Osteochondrosis is an extremely common problem of pigs (up to 100% incidence) but may not be of major clinical significance, nor does it kill pigs. The best joint surfaces to examine are the distal femur and proximal and distal humerus.

Most myopathies will have macroscopic or microscopic lesions in cardiac muscle (vitamin E–selenium responsive problems, gossypol toxicity); therefore, careful examination of skeletal muscle is not needed. Porcine stress syndrome (PSS) may be the most important skeletal muscle disease of swine that will not have concurrent cardiac muscle lesions. However, in many cases there are no macroscopic lesions of skeletal muscle in PSS pigs either. Approximately 60% of stress-suceptible pigs will develop pale, watery, soft skeletal muscles (fishlike, parboiled, blanched).

Completion. Brief descriptions of all lesions should be recorded and a copy submitted with the tissues for histopathology. Be descriptive and avoid gross diagnoses or interpretations of lesions (Pritchard 1966). A good system is to describe the lesion, then if you choose to add your diagnosis or perhaps a question, do so in parentheses after the description, e.g., GI–blood-stained ingesta confined to colon, material adhered to mucosa, multiple 5-mm to 1-cm circular erosions and ulcers (salmonellosis, swine dysentery, coccidiosis).

BLOOD SAMPLING. Blood collection in swine is difficult because of the inaccessibility of good veins and arteries. Many different techniques using various sites have been described. Some of these techniques have some role in experimental work with pigs, but if the practicing veterinarian is to sample blood of any number of pigs with some degree of speed and collect a reasonable volume, the technique of sampling from the jugular vein or the anterior vena cava must be mastered (Brown 1979; Muirhead 1981). Appropriate blood collection techniques for various sizes of pig are given in Table 65.8.

Anterior Vena Cava. Depending on the size of the pig, it is restrained either standing by means of a hog snare (Fig. 65.5) or manually by holding the front legs (Fig. 65.6). The position of the standing pig is important; the head should be raised, the body straight, and the front legs well back. In the standing pig, the jugular groove is traced to its caudal limit just anterior to the thoracic inlet. The needle inserted at the caudal end of the jugular groove and directed dorsally and somewhat caudomedially along an imaginary line

Table 65.8. Blood collection in swine

Site	Type of Pig	Needle Size	Quantity	Comments
Anterior vena cava	Up to 100 lb (45 kg) 100–250 lb (45–113 kg) Adult	20 ga, 1½ in. (38 mm) 18 ga, 2½ in. (65 mm) 16 ga, 3½ in. (90 mm)	Unlimited	Danger of damaging vagus nerve; vacutainer usable
Jugular vein	Any age	20 ga, 1½ in. (38 mm)	Unlimited	More difficult to do; vacutainer usable
Ear veins	Adult	20 ga, 1 in. (25 mm) Scalpel blade	1–2 cm³	Possible hematoma; contaminated sample
Tail	Adult	20 ga, 1 in. (25 mm)	5–10 cm³	Requires practice; vacutainer usable
Orbital sinus	Up to 40 lb (18 kg) 40–120 lb (18–54 kg) Over 120, adult (over 54 kg)	20 ga, 1 in. (25 mm) 16 ga, 1½ in. (38 mm) 14 ga, 1½ in. (38 mm)	5–10 cm³	Slow; unesthetic; possibility of postcollection orbital hemorrhage and pressure on globe
Cephalic vein	20–50 lb (9–23 kg)	20 ga, 1½ in. (38 mm)	5–10 cm³	Restraint difficult to prevent movement; vacutainer usable

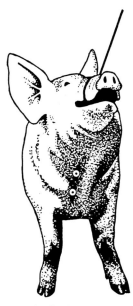

65.5. Proper restraint for blood sampling from a standing pig. The lower circle indicates the site for sampling from the anterior vena cava; the upper circle indicates the site for sampling from the jugular vein.

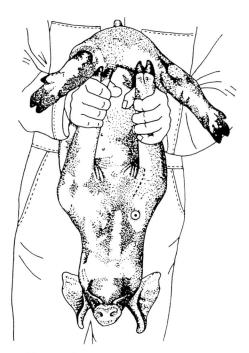

65.6. Method of restraining pigs weighing less than 20 kg for blood sampling from the anterior vena cava (circle). Location of the cephalic vein is indicated by the dashed line.

that passes through the top of the opposite shoulder. The location of some of the major veins are shown in Figure 65.7. When drawing blood samples from either the anterior vena cava or the jugular vein, the blood is taken from the right side, since the right vagus nerve provides less innervation to the heart and diaphragm than the left vagus. If the vagus nerve is accidentally punctured, the pig may show dyspnea, cyanosis, and convulsive struggling.

Jugular Vein. The pig is restrained in a standing position as for sampling from the anterior vena cava. The needle is inserted in the jugular

groove about 5 cm cranial to the thoracic inlet. The needle is directed dorsally and slightly medially.

Ear Veins. The ear veins are raised by slapping the ear and maintained by a rubber band around the base (Fig. 65.8). Venipuncture is done with a quick thrusting stab to prevent the vein from rolling away from the needle. A syringe should be used, since vacutainer collection usually results in collapse of the vein. Alternately, the ventral ear

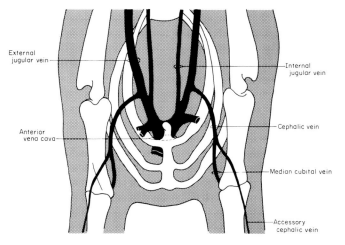

External jugular vein

Internal jugular vein

Cephalic vein

Anterior vena cava

Median cubital vein

Accessory cephalic vein

65.7. Location of some of the major veins in the pig in relation to the skeleton.

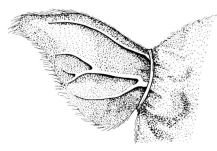

65.8. Ear veins of a pig raised by a rubber band placed at the base of the ear.

vein may be incised with a scalpel cut made into and parallel to the vein and the blood collected in a tube as it drips from the incision.

Tail Vessels. Collection from tail vessels is possible only in mature pigs whose tails have not been docked. The tail is held vertically and the needle directed toward the point of junction of the tail with the body (Muirhead 1981).

Orbital Venous Sinus. Large pigs are restrained by snare and smaller ones held manually, with care to securely restrain the snout. A needle is placed at the medial canthus of the eye just inside the nictitating membrane and advanced medially and slightly anterioventrally until it punctures the venous sinus. Blood is allowed to drip out of the needle and is collected in an open-top tube (Huhn et al. 1969).

Cephalic Vein. Blood may be withdrawn from the cephalic vein by restraining the pig on its back with the front legs stretched backward and a little outward from the body. The vein is visible under the skin (Figs. 65.6, 65.7) and is raised with digital pressure (Tumbleson et al. 1968; Sankari 1983).

Miscellaneous Methods. Cardiac puncture (Calvert et al. 1977) and femoral venipuncture techniques (Brown et al. 1978) have been described.

Indwelling Catheters. Indwelling catheters have been used for research that requires repeated blood sampling or minimal excitement of the pig. Investigators have described techniques for placing catheters in the femoral artery and vein (Weirich et al. 1970; Jackson et al. 1972), subcutaneous abdominal vein and middle sacral artery (Witzel et al. 1973), ear vein (Grün et al. 1973; Brussow et al. 1981), jugular vein (Brown et al. 1973; Wingfield et al. 1974; Ford and Maurer 1978), and uterine vein (Rodriquez and Kunavongkrit 1983).

REFERENCES

Benbrook, E. A. 1947. The value of the necropsy in veterinary medicine. J Am Vet Med Assoc 111:65.

Brown, C. M. 1979. A method for collecting blood from hogs using the thoracic inlet. Vet Med Small Anim Clin 74:361–363.

Brown, D. E.; King, G. J.; and Hacker, R. R. 1973. Polyurethane indwelling catheters for piglets. J Anim Sci 37:303–304.

Brown, J. R.; Tyeryar, E. A.; Harrington, D. G.; and Hilmas, D. E. 1978. Femoral venipuncture for repeated blood sampling in miniature swine. Lab Anim Sci 28:339–342.

Brussow, V. K.-P.; Bergfeld, J.; and Parchow, G. 1981. Über mehrjährige Erfahrungen zur Blutgewinnung durch intravenöse Dauerkatheter beim Schwein. Monatsh Veterinaermed 36:300–303.

Calvert, G. D.; Scott, P. J.; and Sharpe, D. N. 1977. Percutaneous cardiac puncture in domestic pigs. Aust Vet J 53:337–339.

Elmore, R. G.; Martin, C. E.; Riley, J. L.; and Littledike, T. 1979. Body temperatures of farrowing swine. J Am Vet Med Assoc 174:620–622.

Ford, J. J., and Maurer, R. R. 1978. Simple technique for chronic venous catheterization of swine. Lab Anim Sci 28:615–618.

Goodwin, R. F. 1971. A procedure for investigating the influence of disease status on productivity efficiency in a pig herd. Vet Rec 88:387.

Grün, E.; Hüller, G.; and Möckel, H.-G. 1973. Dauerkatheter am Schweineohr. Monatsh Veterinaermed 28:263–265.

Heard, T. W. 1981. Methods of approach to diagnosis and resolution of pig health problems. Br Vet J 137:337–347.

Huhn, R. G.; Osweiler, G. D.; and Switzer, W. P. 1969. Application of the orbital sinus bleeding technique to swine. Lab Anim Care 19:403–405.

Jackson, V. M. D.; Cook, D. B.; and Gill, G. 1972. Simultaneous intravenous infusion and arterial blood sampling in piglets. Lab Anim Sci 22:552–555.

King, J. M.; Dodd, D. C.; and Newsome, M. E. 1979. Gross Necropsy Technique for Animals. Ithaca, N.Y.: Arnold Printing.

Littledike, E. T.; Witzel, D. A.; and Riley, J. L. 1979. Body temperature changes in sows. Lab Anim Sci 29:621.

Muirhead, M. R. 1981. Blood sampling in pigs. In Pract 3:16–20.

———. 1983. Pig housing and environment. Vet Rec 113:587–595.

Pritchard, R. W. 1966. Descriptions in pathology. Avoiding pathological descriptions. Pathol Vet 3:169.

Roderick, L. M. 1954. Necropsy procedure for swine. In Veterinary Necropsy Procedures. Philadelphia: J. B. Lippincott, p. 38.

Rodriquez, H., and Kunavongkrit, A. 1983. Chronical venous catheterization for frequent blood sampling in unrestrained pigs. Acta Vet Scand 24:318–320.

Sankari, S. 1983. A practical method of taking blood samples from the pig. Acta Vet Scand 24:133–134.

Sawaya, H.; Nomura, Y.; Tsuchiya, T.; Saito, Y.; Ohtani, H.; and Nozawa, Y. 1974. Pathological findings in pigs with circling movements. Bull Azabu Vet Coll 28:63–76.

Tumbleson, M. E.; Dommert, A. R.; and Middleton, C. C. 1968. Techniques for handling miniature swine for laboratory procedures. Lab Anim Care 18:584–587.

VanKruiningen, H. J. 1971. Veterinary autopsy procedure. Vet Clin North Am 1:163.

Weirich, W. E.; Will, J. A.; and Crumpton, C. W. 1970. A technique for placing chronic indwelling catheters in swine. J Appl Physiol 28:117–119.

Williams, M. J., and Perry, T. 1978. The autopsy: A beginning not an end. Am J Clin Pathol 69:215.

Wingfield, W. E.; Tumbleson, M. E.; Hicklin, K. W.; and Mather, E. C. 1974. An exteriorized cranial vena caval catheter for serial blood sample collection from miniature swine. Lab Anim Sci 24:359–361.

Witzel, D. A.; Littledike, E. T.; and Cook, H. M. 1973. Implanted catheters for blood sampling in swine. Cornell Vet 63:432–435.

66 Methods of Disease Control

T. J. L. Alexander
D. L. Harris

DISEASE CONTROL is all embracing; nutrition, housing, and all aspects of swine management have a bearing on it. Treatment of the subject here must be selective and is confined to recent developments in disease control and in recent developments in swine production that affect disease control.

A very important development in swine production is a general increase in unit size, combined in some countries with greater intensification and sophistication. Two other relevant developments are the growth of large seedstock organizations and large weaner marketing groups.

Pig enterprises are so diverse and patterns of disease against which they operate are so varied that methods of disease control suitable for one are often inappropriate for others. The following measures should be regarded as guidelines that should be adapted to fit any particular case.

DISEASE CONTROL FOR LARGE-SCALE SLAUGHTER PIG PRODUCTION.
Russia and some of the countries bordering the Danube River, such as Yugoslavia, Hungary, and Bulgaria, were the first to build large production units, i.e., 2500–10,000 sows and their progeny on one site. Relatively large units were also built in Australia and parts of Southeast Asia. They were started from scratch in the 1950s and 1960s without going through an evolution in size. Elsewhere, the development of large units has been more gradual.

In parts of North America and some countries of Western Europe, full-confinement breeding herds of between 200 and 2000 sows and their progeny are now commonplace and are increasing in number. Some organizations own or manage over 50,000 sows and are enlarging rapidly.

The first example swine production program to be discussed concerns a 1000-sow unit and for convenience the breeding aspect of the enterprise is considered separately from the feeder pig operation. The second program represents a current trend in the United States in states such as Colorado, Nebraska, and North Carolina, i.e., toward production units containing 3000–5000 sows and the establishment of 3-site operations.

It is assumed in these considerations that there is freedom of choice of location, husbandry system, and source of pigs and also that adequate funds are available to set up the enterprise properly from the beginning. One point that will emerge is the compromise that must be made between the veterinary ideal and other conflicting demands.

Commercial 1000-Sow Breeding Unit. Disease is likely to be the greatest concern, since the bigger the unit, the greater the investment and loss if disease occurs. Outbreaks of infectious disease tend to be more serious, to persist longer, and to be more difficult to control in larger units.

A 1000-sow unit is more vulnerable than a 100-sow unit; there are 10 times as many susceptible pigs in one area, 10 times as much food to be delivered, 10 times as many pigs to be delivered and collected, etc. To offset this, there is an economy of scale that makes it relatively cheaper to incorporate measures for disease control.

In planning a 1000-sow unit, two aspects should be considered first: the source of breeding stock and the location of the site (Alexander 1973).

SOURCE OF BREEDING STOCK. A unit should be started with stock as free from infectious disease as possible. However, conflicting priorities place constraints upon choice.

For reasons of cash flow, the unit should be in full production as quickly as possible, which usually means acquiring more than 1000 maiden gilts (to allow for rejects) over a period of 5 months at the longest. This might be achieved by monthly deliveries of about 250, 210, 210, 210, and less than 200 gilts of serviceable age and weight. It would be better if the pigs in the last four deliveries were at least 6 weeks younger than serviceable age, which would allow them to adapt to the new buildings before they are required for service. A total of 50 young boars are required also, over half with the first batch of gilts so that they are not overworked. Since a 10–20% cull rate can be anticipated after the first farrowing and since in repopulations of older units (as distinct from primary populations of new units, which are often still being built when the first pigs enter), there will be many buildings empty for some time, it is sometimes feasible and economic to put 10–20% extra gilts in with each initial batch (Leman 1989). The need to obtain so many animals at prescribed times obviously limits choice of supply. Cash flow is improved still further if most of the gilts are delivered already pregnant. Movement is relatively safe during the second half of gestation but may cause fetal loss and reproductive problems during the first 8 weeks.

Ideally, the gilts and boars should possess the best available genetic potential for reproductive efficiency and lean-tissue growth. This again limits choice.

From the viewpoint of disease control, foundation gilts and boars and all subsequent replacements should come from the same herd. Depending on the pyramidal structure of the supplier, this may not be possible. The boars may have to come from one herd and the gilts from another, but both herds should be in the same closed pyramid.

Having found sources of stock that satisfy these criteria, how can the producer decide which is most suitable from the standpoint of disease? Two questions commonly arise. From which diseases should the pigs be free? What checks should be made to ensure freedom from these diseases? Neither can be answered comprehensively. In most but not all situations, it is advisable that stock be free from the viruses of hog cholera (HC), pseudorabies, transmissible gastroenteritis (TGE), and porcine epidemic diarrhea, and free from *Serpulina hyodysenteriae, Brucella suis, Leptospira pomona,* toxigenic *Pasteurella multocida,* virulent strains of *Actinobacillus (Haemophilus) pleuropneumoniae* and *Streptococcus suis* type 2, mange, and lice. Whether they should be free from *Mycoplasma hyopneumoniae* depends on the locality. In some countries, African swine fever (ASF) and perhaps foot-and-mouth disease (FMD) may have to be considered. Beyond these infections the list becomes vague. This may be misleading because there is a marked difference in performance between very high–health status pigs such as those derived from sources set up by surgical derivation (specific-pathogen-free [SPF] repopulation), medicated early weaning (MEW), or Isowean (discussed later) and those from long-standing conventional herds that are free from the above diseases. The SPF repopulation may be best for isolated locations but the Isowean may be more suitable for areas of high pig density, as in parts of Iowa, Japan, Belgium, the Netherlands, Germany, or Eastern England.

Having drawn up a list of diseases to be avoided, how best can the source be checked? Organizations such as the Danish SPF association favor laboratory tests (e.g., serology for *A. pleuropneumoniae* or *M. hyopneumoniae*). Unfortunately, there are as yet few reliable tests to ascertain freedom from disease that are not bedeviled by false-positive and false-negative results (Tyler 1989; Alexander 1991). This unsatisfactory situation may improve soon, due to the application of monoclonal antibodies to enzyme-linked immunologic serum assays (ELISAs) and other tests and possibly the use of gene probes. Even so, it must be remembered that where a reliable test is available, it may only be reliable for the period previous to the time it was carried out.

Another approach is to seek a source of supply that fulfills three broad criteria: the breeding organization should follow a sound program of disease control and monitoring, it should have a good history of supplying other herds, and there should be reasonable assurance that supplies to the purchaser will be stopped if a potentially damaging disease is suspected.

LOCATION OF SITE. Location is the most important factor for maintaining a high and stable health status. It would be foolish to build a new 1000-sow unit close to a source of serious contamination. It would be equally foolish to enlarge a unit from 200 to 1000 sows on an unsuitable site unless possibly by Isowean 3-site procedures (discussed later). The following factors should be considered.

Proximity of Other Pigs. The greatest danger is other pigs. Not only should the unit be as far away from other pig herds as possible but there should also be assurance that it will remain so in the foreseeable future. How far is far enough? Two to 5 miles (3–8 km) is commonly cited, but there is no absolute answer. It depends on the terrain, function of the herd, and local disease patterns.

Some windborne diseases can travel many miles, others survive only short distances, and others appear not to spread on wind at all. For example, FMD virus can be windblown at least 12 miles (20 km) over land and 190 miles (300 km) over sea (Sellers and Gloster 1980; Gloster et al. 1981, 1982). There is strong evidence that pseudorabies virus (PRV) can be windblown at least 6 miles (9 km) over land and 25 miles (40 km) over sea (Christensen et al. 1990). Bacterial diseases are unlikely to be carried so far on the wind. *Mycoplasma hyopneumoniae* is thought to be windborne for up to 2 miles (3 km) (Goodwin 1985). In addition to wind, flies and rats often travel about 2 miles (3–4 km) between pig units and can carry infections such as salmonellae, *Streptococcus suis,* and encephalomyocarditis virus. Swine dysentery (SD) and mange never appear to spread on wind, rats, flies, or other fomites, thus distance from other herds is not a major factor in excluding them.

Size of the neighboring herd is another factor; 2 miles (3 km) is the minimum distance from the nearest large herd to build a new 1000-sow herd, provided it is in rolling wooded countryside in an area of generally low pig density.

Proximity of Other Animals. Other livestock and poultry do not pose the same threat as other pigs, and there are not many veterinary reasons for situating the unit away from them. A few exceptions are pathogens such as *Erysipelothrix,* the avian tubercle bacillus; salmonella in the case of poultry; or *Pasteurella,* parainfluenza viruses, or salmonella in the case of sheep and calves. Field evidence is lacking on the danger these animals pose except where FMD is common.

Roads, Railroads, and Public Rights-of-Way. The unit should not be situated along a public road or railroad carrying livestock, or along a public right-of-way. It should be at the end of a farm road rather than at a junction. The unit should also be well away from slaughter and rendering plants and garbage dumps.

Urban Areas. The unit should not be situated near housing estates or where urban development is planned. There are a number of obvious reasons for this, of which disease control is only one.

Shelter or Exposure. In a windy, cold, or changeable climate, units should be relatively sheltered, e.g., in valleys rather than on hilltops; but in hotter climates, hilltops may be better. In hot countries where diseases such as FMD and ASF are prevalent, isolated sites high in hills or near the coast are desirable.

Other Limiting Factors. A number of other factors limit the choice of site. Chief among these is effluent disposal, which has some bearing on disease control. Other factors not related to disease control are suitability for construction; availability of labor, water, electricity, feed, and market outlets; and amenities such as public transport, schools, and stores for the personnel and their families. Finding a suitable site in areas of high pig density is not easy. It is usually better to seek sites away from pig-rearing areas.

PRECAUTIONS AGAINST CONTAMINATION. Having selected a suitable source of pigs and a good location and having drawn up a general plan of the layout, what measures should be taken to minimize chances of contamination?

The most disastrous contaminants are those that cause a total shutdown of the unit. Depending on the country, these might be FMD, ASF, HC, swine vesicular disease (SVD), and possibly pseudorabies, TGE, and SD. There may also be concern for respiratory infections and the numerous less-serious pathogens, such as agents that result in mild diarrhea or the stillbirths, mummified fetuses, embryonic death, infertility (SMEDI) syndrome, or new strains that might exacerbate respiratory and enteric problems already present and so disrupt productivity.

The aim is to establish a stable balance be-tween the herd and its potentially pathogenic microflora; this cannot be achieved if new pathogens are repeatedly introduced. The following precautions should therefore be considered (Fig. 66.1).

Compound Perimeter. There should be a clear demarcation between pig compound and noncompound. In isolated, relatively safe areas this may be no more than a simple fence, stout enough to keep out people and animals, including dogs, stray livestock, and wild animals, particularly wild pigs. In less law-abiding, more-diseased areas, a high double fence, perhaps with patrolling guards and dogs, may be necessary. Imposing "Keep Out" signs should also be erected. In countries such as Denmark where herds are in single, enclosed buildings, the walls of the buildings are sufficient barriers. Perhaps a short fence at a vulnerable place is all that is needed.

Pig-loading Bay. Pigs, pig transport vehicles, and drivers should be regarded as major risks. Vehicles that take pigs to slaughter are particularly dangerous. They should be washed and disinfected after each slaughter plant delivery and precautions taken about the drivers' boots and coveralls. Ideally, all pigs moved into and from the unit should be moved in transport controlled by the owner of the unit, but in many cases this is impractical and uneconomic.

It is essential to have a pig-loading bay situated on the perimeter fence close to the farm office. It should have pens to hold pigs prior to loading and be so designed that pigs can be loaded without the driver entering the compound. There should be one-way gates to prevent the re-entry of pigs into the production unit once they are placed on the transport vehicle. The bay and vehicles should be hosed down and disinfected after each use and the liquid drained away from the unit, not into it.

Personnel and Visitors. People entering the compound should be classified either as regular workers or as visitors. Regular workers are those employed in the unit daily. They should understand the principles of disease control and agree not to go near any pigs outside the unit. They should be provided with showers and a complete change of clothing in a dressing room on the compound perimeter. Whether they must shower each time they enter the compound depends on where they live, whether they have to leave the general area, what other work they do, and the current disease pattern in the region.

All visitors should be kept to a minimum and required to shower and change their clothes before entering the compound. Furthermore, they should not be allowed to enter the unit if they have been with other pigs during the previous 1–4 days, depending on the diseases in the region. The need for a shower and a 1–4 day rule have

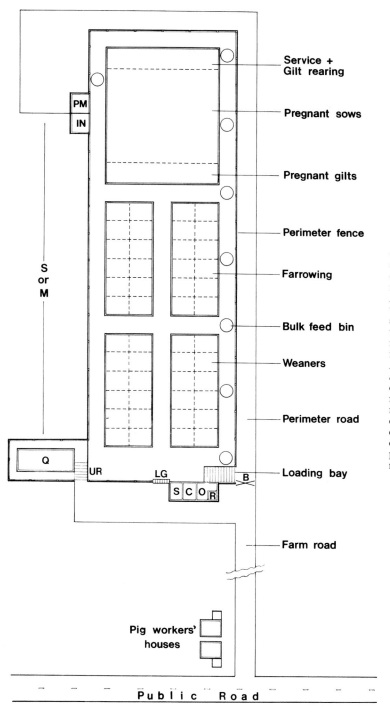

66.1. Layout of a large intensive farrowing and weaner production unit. *PM* = postmortem room for attending veterinarian; *IN* = incinerator or pig disposal unit; *S* or *M* = slurry storage or solid manure pads; *Q* = quarantine and adaptation pens for replacement stock; *UR* = unloading ramp for replacement stock; *LG* = locked main gate; *S* = showers, changing room, entrance; *C* = canteen and rest rooms; *O* and *R* = office with reception area for dealing with callers without them entering the compound (there should be a bell or siren to call workers from the pig buildings); *B* = simple barrier.

been challenged in Denmark and Germany. The purpose of a shower is to wash contamination from the hair and hands and force a complete change of clothes. If the showering and changing is done properly, then an overnight rule is probably sufficient in most cases. Both have a psychological effect, particularly if visitors are made to put in writing where they have been.

Feed and Other Deliveries. In practice, most good feed does not constitute a major risk (except perhaps for salmonella), but it is wise to arrange bulk bins and augers inside the fence and a perimeter road outside the fence so that feed trucks can deliver without entering the compound. Similarly, other materials should be delivered through the fence. Straw presents a small risk and its source should be known. Straw stacks open to birds, particularly starlings, may pose a risk of disease such as TGE when the straw is used as bedding. Spilled feed under feed bins carries a similar risk. In countries such as the United States where there may be a rapid turn around through the local mill, feed may be contaminated with TGE and pseudorabies from the trucks of farmers supplying grain. Storage of such feed before use reduces the risk.

Farm Office, Canteen, Toilets. The farm office should be situated on the perimeter fence, close to the pig-loading bay and parking lot, and at a point convenient for feed-delivery and other vehicles to stop. There should be a loud bell or siren to summon workers from inside the buildings and a hatch or counter so that documents may be exchanged without workers going out or callers entering.

No human food should be allowed into the compound beyond the office. It is convenient to have a small canteen adjacent to that location.

Toilets and washrooms should be provided and their use should be mandatory. It is usually convenient to have these, the canteen, the office, and the changing rooms all in the same block.

Effluent Disposal. Effluent disposal is a major consideration for a number of reasons, but it is also relevant to disease control. Trucks, manure wagons, or tractors should not go in and out of the compound. It is not difficult to build systems in which slurry can be removed by suction applied from outside the compound perimeter. Separators may be necessary in some areas. For solid manure it may be necessary to have adjacent to the unit two or more fenced pads, which can alternately be regarded as inside or outside the compound.

Isolation and Acclimatization. Many production units buy-in all replacement parent stock (boars and gilts used to produce pigs for slaughter) or grandparent stock (for production of replacement parents) rather than maintain a genetic selection program, which limits the introduction of live pigs. The number of replacement boars and gilts depends upon the breeding policy but 35% of the adult population may be replaced annually. Some producers isolate or quarantine all replacement breeding stock in a segregated area away from the main unit for 3–4 weeks prior to acclimatization or adaptation to the microflora of the farm. The isolation period allows for the occurrence of disease such as TGE, which may have been in the incubatory stage at delivery time; testing for diseases such as pseudorabies both in the source farm(s) and the replacement stock; the detection of any disease that may have been in the incubatory stage in the source farm(s); and/or the

elimination of infectious agents such as *Serpulina hyodysenteriae* by medication.

After entry into the herd, it is good practice to allow replacement stock 3–6 weeks to adapt to the herd gradually. Manure from the herd, particularly from the weaners and service area, should be placed in their pens during the second and third weeks of segregation. Some producers also move cull pigs to adjacent pens. When adapting pigs from a high–health status source to a conventional herd, it may be necessary to medicate the feed for incoming pigs at lower than therapeutic levels for 3–6 weeks with a drug such as chlortetracycline or spectinomycin. In any case, the incoming gilts should be moved to pens adjacent to young boars and left for at least one estrous cycle before being mated, to stimulate immunity to parvovirus by natural exposure and/or vaccination before gestation starts.

Dogs, Cats, Rats, Mice, Flies, Birds. Dogs should not be allowed in the compound except perhaps as guard dogs, in which case they should be tightly controlled. If cats are kept to control rodents, they should not leave the compound; if they do leave they should then be kept out.

Every effort should be made to control rats, mice, flies, and birds. This is not always easy in climates where open-sided buildings and natural ventilation are used. In areas where diseases such as ASF, TGE, or PRV are prevalent, control may be essential. Small harmless slurry flies are used in Eastern Germany to eat the larvae of pig-farm flies such as *Mustica domestica* (Blaha 1990).

Postmortem Facilities and Pig Disposal. The local veterinarian must obey the same regulations as everyone else. It is therefore convenient for postmortem examinations to be performed outside the perimeter fence. Depending on the climate, it may be necessary to provide some simple facility with water available. Disposal facilities for dead pigs should also be nearby.

GENERAL LAYOUT OF BUILDINGS. Personnel housing should not be within the compound or closely adjacent to it. If they are nearby, they should be situated on the access side of the compound, with separate arrangements for services and deliveries.

The offices, changing rooms, parking lot, and loading bay should all be on the side of the main access road; the manure disposal area should be on a different side from these and from feed delivery.

Gilt-rearing accommodations should be adjacent to the service area to ensure early exposure to SMEDI viruses. Sometime after the first 12 weeks of gestation, pregnant gilts should be exposed to effluent from the farrowing and nursery rooms.

Arrangements for moving pigs easily within the compound should be considered carefully. The flow should be from the service area and dry-sow houses, through the farrowing and weaner and feeder-pig accommodations, toward the loading ramp. The stress of moving and mixing not only affects growth rate adversely but triggers disease conditions such as porcine stress syndrome (PSS), pneumonia, dysentery, and streptococcal meningitis. Excessive movement is also expensive.

In a farrow-to-finish unit there should be a gap between the growing accommodation and the breeding herd. It is probably preferable with units of around 1000 sows to rear the slaughter pigs in grow-out units on different sites, with several being supplied from one large feeder-pig production unit, rather than the other way around.

Consideration should also be given to the direction of the buildings in relation to strong, cold winds in winter, which may reverse the airflow in the ventilation system and trigger diseases such as pneumonia, meningitis, or diarrhea or may cool the sides of buildings unilaterally, making it impossible to maintain even temperatures. In very hot climates, exposure to winds may be desirable in helping aeration and cooling, thus improving conception and growth rates.

The sequence in which buildings are to be erected and completed should also be planned in advance so that the buildings first completed can be used to house gilts for service and gestation. It may then be economical to build in several stages; but if so, the sections still under construction should be sealed off from those in use.

NUTRITION, HOUSING, MANAGEMENT. The design and management of the husbandry system are integral to disease control and play as big a role as any other factor. There is no such thing as a pathogen-free herd and no substitute for good management to suppress the pathogens that are present. The measures mentioned above serve to reduce the disruptions caused by infectious disease to profitable production. They do not eliminate infectious disease altogether.

In relation to noninfectious disease, nutrition, housing, and management usually represent both the cause and the cure. In relation to infectious disease, their role is to swing the balance in favor of the pigs' defenses against potential pathogens.

For example, piglet diarrhea is usually more effectively tackled in the long run if it is regarded primarily as a husbandry and environmental problem rather than one of infectious disease. Problems such as diarrhea, pneumonia, uneven growth, and unthrifty pigs, which commonly occur in large units following 3- or 5-week weaning, are more often the result of factors such as overcrowding, insufficient trough space or water supply, unsuitable or stale feed, dirty water, and poor temperature and ventilation control than they are

of disease. Reproductive problems are usually more a result of poor management, housing, and feeding than of SMEDI viruses, brucellosis, or leptospirosis.

The salient broad aims for a new unit can be summarized as follows: to provide pig comfort throughout and avoid stresses that result in lowered resistance; to reduce the concentration of infection in buildings and prevent the levels building up in any area; and to so design the systems that limited groups of pigs may be readily treated in water and feed or by injection so that outbreaks of infectious disease may be contained quickly and economically.

VETERINARY SERVICES. Hospital pens should also be included in the plans. Chapter 81 deals with veterinary services, and only a few points relevant to large intensive-breeding units need be made here.

A 1000-sow unit requires the regular services of a veterinarian who has a particular interest in pigs. If the enterprise is made up of several large units, it is helpful if they are all serviced by the same veterinarian.

Routine visits at regularly scheduled intervals are preferable to intermittent emergency calls. On such visits the veterinarian should look at each stage of the operation and advise the manager or pig handlers on what treatments and measures should be used and what modifications might be made to husbandry and management to suppress disease. The veterinarian should also examine the performance records regularly and attempt to identify where, if at all, disease is causing problems. This is easier with computerized recording systems. Records should also be kept of the postmortem examinations, laboratory tests, and diagnoses. It is useful if the veterinarian provides a written report after every visit.

When disease flares up, the veterinarian must not only act quickly and thoroughly, probably by comprehensive medication, but must also ensure that an accurate diagnosis is made, using laboratory services where necessary. Also needing consideration are the long-term implications in relation to medication, vaccination, and management systems. Drug costs and use should be closely monitored and not allowed to escalate. Vaccine use depends on the area, but vaccines should never be given within the period from 3 days before to 8 weeks after insemination. The views prevalent in some countries that vaccines should never be given at anytime during pregnancy is wrong for many vaccines. For some, the last 2–4 weeks of gestation is the best time to give them.

If the husbandry system does not provide adequate exposure of gilts to SMEDI virus and pregnant females to piglet enteric pathogens, so-called "feedback" is sometimes adopted as an adjunct to or instead of vaccination. In the case of SMEDI, this entails feeding a soup of mummified fetuses and their afterbirth and feces from the gilt service area to gilts several times 3–6 weeks prior to mating. In the case of piglet diarrhea, it entails feeding a soup of piglet feces (which may be picked up with paper towels), untreated piglet intestines, and weaner feces, along with a small amount of afterbirth as a vehicle, to pregnant females about twice a week for the last 4 weeks before they enter the farrowing house. The soups are prepared by passing the materials with an equal quantity of water through a sink waste disposal unit. They can be frozen in small quantities for storage. Note that feedback should be stopped and is dangerous when another clinical disease such as erysipelas, clostridial piglet dysentery, SD, or salmonellosis is present in the unit. Vaccines should then be used.

The veterinarian must understand the husbandry system and correlate it with any diseases that occur. It is equally important to understand the economics of the unit. If not, decisions may be made that are correct from a veterinary viewpoint but detrimental to overall profitability.

For example, a major controllable factor in the profitability of a commercial breeding unit is the number of pigs sold. The veterinarian in a praiseworthy desire to reduce the risk of contaminating the unit with new diseases may advise that the herd be closed and new genes be introduced only by artificial insemination (AI). While this advice may be correct from a disease-control and possibly from a genetic viewpoint, it may prove very costly if it results in lowered overall farrowing rates and litter sizes. A loss of 2 pigs sold/sow/year in a 1000-sow unit means a loss of profit equivalent to the difference between the feed cost and sale price of 2000 pigs.

Commercial Grow-out Units

ECONOMIC EFFECTS OF DISEASE. In a farrow-to-finish operation, the veterinary input tends to concentrate on the breeding animals and their offspring up to about 2 weeks postweaning. Sometimes older growing pigs are almost ignored, the breeding section being more complex and interesting and more demanding of veterinary attention. Furthermore, the capital investment in the breeding section is about twice that of the grow-out section. Yet the bulk of the profit usually comes from the latter. In most circumstances the overall profitability of a farrow-to-finish operation is affected far more by the efficiency with which the weaned pigs are grown to slaughter weight (e.g., factors such as pen utilization, speed of throughput, efficiency of feed to lean meat conversion, and carcass grading) than by reproductive performance provided that sufficient numbers of good-quality feeder pigs are produced to fill the finishing places. Concentrating only on increasing the reproductive performance of the

sow herd may result in overcrowding in the nursery and finisher pens, leading to a downward spiral in feeder pig health and performance.

It could therefore be argued that the veterinarian should concentrate more on the growing pigs. The difficulty is that the scope for expertise of a specifically veterinary nature is limited. Diseases that increase mortality above an acceptable level of, say, 1–2% require veterinary attention, as do diseases that obviously affect growth rate, such as overt SD, severe atrophic rhinitis (AR), and clinical pneumonia. Medication of individual pigs and blanket feed medication is also a veterinary matter. (The cost of feed medication has a direct effect on profitability and must be balanced against benefits gained. The cost is often overlooked because in most accounting systems it is hidden in feed costs.) However, for the most part alterable factors that affect the economic efficiency of growing pigs (e.g., ventilation, pig comfort, avoidance of stress, effluent removal, stocking density, feed purchase, ration formulation, feeding method, slaughter-pig marketing) are peripheral to veterinary medicine and not obviously related to disease. It would be argued, therefore, that disease control is unimportant in grow-out units. This is not so. As stated above, diseases that affect mortality rates, the speed and evenness of throughput or feed conversion, or that require routine medication and extra labor to suppress them obviously affect profitability. Furthermore, there is a positive relationship between health in its broadest sense and economy of gain.

ALL-IN/ALL-OUT VERSUS CONTINUOUS SYSTEMS. Pigs in small units that operate on an all-in/all-out policy, particularly if the pens are washed thoroughly between batches, tend to grow better and have better feed conversion than those in larger units that operate a continuous system. The precise reasons for this are not clear. One may be that there is not a continuous buildup of infection, and each batch of pigs starts fresh.

Another obvious advantage is that if a serious disease breaks out, it affects only the one batch of pigs and can usually be eliminated following slaughter. It is also easier to deal with disease during the critical early period, i.e., the first 2 weeks after arrival when pigs are stressed by loading, transport, mixing, and adapting to a new environment. In all-in/all-out systems the total pig density is at its lowest during this period, thus reducing the concentration of organisms in the air and feces and the challenge to the recently arrived pigs. Prophylactic medication can be carried out thoroughly on a whole-unit basis. Also during this period labor can be organized to give maximum attention to individuals.

In contrast, although pens can be cleaned prior to entry (which often has a noticeable beneficial effect) and medication administered on a pen basis in continuous systems, cross-infection, carryover of infection, initial challenge, and buildup of infection are more difficult to prevent. Furthermore, it may be more expensive to slaughter all the pigs in a unit when serious disease occurs. However, the disadvantages of a large continuous system that accrue from disease and poorer performance may be offset financially by some economies of scale, more consistency of slaughter at optimum weights, and better use of pen space.

SOURCE OF PIGS. It is much better for one large breeding unit to supply several grow-out units than it is for several small breeding units to supply one large grow-out (Fig. 66.2). Even if no disease is present, there is a demonstrable effect on efficiency of gain and consequently on profitability. If diseases are present, the effects are obviously greater.

If all pigs entering a grow-out unit are from the same source, it is possible in some circumstances for them to remain completely free of damaging outbreaks of enteric and respiratory diseases. Even if potentially damaging diseases are present in the herd of origin, it is usually easier to suppress and control them if the pigs are not mixed with those from other sources.

If each new intake comes from different breeding units, the mixing of infections and challenge of new infections are considerable; pigs newly introduced during the critical period of adaptation and those already present are threatened. In the extreme case where feeder pigs for a continuous grow-out unit are derived from many unknown breeding units, having been marketed through dealers and/or auctions, it is likely that all the major diseases of the collection areas eventually will become endemic. Infections such as TGE, which normally establish a herd immunity and disappear, tend to be kept going by being passed down to each successive batch of newly introduced susceptible pigs. The effect is not only cumulative but also synergistic; e.g., newly introduced enteric viruses and bacteria may exacerbate SD. Also, newly introduced respiratory pathogens, which may be mild or subclinical, may exacerbate pneumonia and AR.

In many feeder-pig operations, however, the undoubted health advantages of a single source of supply or a limited number of controlled sources of supply are outweighed by other economic, social, or logistic factors. If this is so and the feeder pigs must be derived from a variety of sources, often of unknown disease status, the inevitability of disease should be recognized from the outset and measures taken to minimize its effect.

The most obvious measure is to adopt an all-in/all-out system with rigorous washing and disinfecting between batches and a prophylactic medication regime operating for at least the first 2 weeks after entry. Mechanisms should be established for prompt and thorough treatment of disease whenever it occurs. Inevitably, drug use and veterinary costs will be high. A less obvious measure would be to procure, move, and mix the pigs immediately after weaning as in Isowean procedures (see **3-Site Production**).

LOCATION. From the viewpoint of disease control, the choice of the location of a grow-out unit in most cases is less critical than that of a breeding unit. Other factors such as effluent disposal, market outlet, feed source, environmental pollution, and odor are usually of greater importance. If pigs are purchased from dealers or a variety of sources, the location in relation to contamination from other herds is of little importance. If all the pigs are derived from one breeding unit that is free of diseases potentially damaging to feeder pigs, location in relation to other pigs may be important. This is particularly true if the breeding unit is free of serious respiratory disease. In grow-out units in which freedom from contamination is deemed important (i.e., in which the pigs are relatively free from disease and in the rearing of breeding animals), the factors affecting the suitability of a location are similar to those mentioned above for feeder-pig production units.

PRECAUTIONS AGAINST CONTAMINATION. There may be little point in taking any precautions against contamination in a unit that receives feeder pigs from a wide variety of sources. Where pigs are received from one healthy source, max-

DISTRIBUTION OF WEANERS

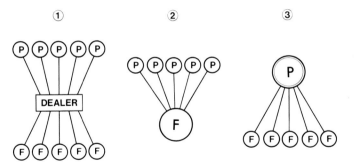

66.2.   Distribution of feeder pigs: P = breeding herd nursery-grower unit, F = feeder-pig grow-out finisher unit. From the viewpoint of disease control, (3) is preferable to (2), which is preferable to (1).

imum precautions may be indicated, particularly where serious diseases are prevalent. Precautions that should be considered are the same as those listed for breeding units, and only a few relevant points will be made here.

Although housing, nutrition, and management may appear less critical to the health of pigs in a grow-out than a breeding unit, they are important to economy of gain and to disease control.

Movement of pigs for weighing, loading or unloading, and mixing can trigger overt diseases or increase mortality, and arrangements for movement without undue stress should be considered. The fewer moves a pig makes, the healthier it remains and the better it grows.

Ventilation, including the removal of noxious gases, and temperature control are important to the suppression of respiratory diseases and vices such as tail biting. Reducing airborne dust containing endotoxins and allergens is also important but cannot be achieved primarily by ventilation. Removal or dilution of feces and changes in nutrition are relevant in the control of enteric diseases such as SD. Overcrowding and discomfort also exacerbate disease as well as slowing growth, by lowering the pigs' resistance and raising the concentration of pathogens.

VETERINARY SERVICES. A grow-out unit receiving pigs from numerous sources requires veterinary help to devise prophylactic medication and prescribe treatment. Organizations that operate numerous grow-out units in a limited area should probably employ one veterinarian to advise on standardized methods for all.

3-Site Production. Very large producers may want to build breeding herds of 3000–5000 sows. Conventional veterinary advice would probably be to build three to five 1000-sow farrow-to-finish units short distances apart. However, Harris (1988a,b, 1990a,b) proposed a new system, namely Isowean 3-site production (Fig. 66.3), in which the various stages of production are separated onto multiple sites.

Site 1 is composed of the breeding, gestation, and farrowing facilities. Pigs are weaned at up to 21 days of age and moved to site 2, where they remain until approximately 20–35 kg body weight. Site 3 is either grower-finisher or finisher facilities. All three sites are well isolated from one another and strict health control precautions are adhered to regarding personnel movement and animal transport. For example, when the herds are running smoothly personnel may move freely from site 2 to site 3 to site 1, but movement from site 1 to 2 may be restricted. Farrowing, prenursery, nursery, and grower-finisher facilities are constructed and managed utilizing strict all-in/all-out principles in order to maximize pig performance and to allow for partial depopulation if disease occurs. If a farmer asks a veterinarian for advice on setting up a 3000-sow herd, the conventional veterinary advice is likely to be that for safety and insurance, he should set up three 1000-sow farrow-to-finish units. However, it would be safer, on the basis of Isowean, to set up one 3000-sow herd and wean the piglets at up to 3 weeks of age to a nursery on another site (Fig. 66.4). All the pigs could then be finished for slaughter on a third site or on several sites. In some European countries and possibly other areas of the world, it may not be possible, or not allowed, to have 3000 sows in one site, but the Isowean principle could still be used as shown in Figure 66.5. In fact, smaller producers in the United States have recently expanded their 1-site farrow-to-finish operations by applying Isowean 3-site principles. The original site is utilized for breeding, gestation, and farrowing, with conversion of the finishing accommodation to gestation and of nursery accommodation to farrowing. Harris (1988a, 1990a) suggests that if comingling of feeder pigs from many farrowing operations is done, then the preferable age for comingling is 3 weeks of age or less, when the passive immune status of the piglet is still high and the infection status is minimal. The need for two separate sites (sites 2 and 3) after weaning is debatable. The advantages of two versus three sites for production of breeding stock are discussed later.

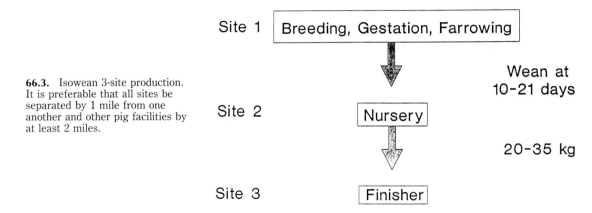

66.3. Isowean 3-site production. It is preferable that all sites be separated by 1 mile from one another and other pig facilities by at least 2 miles.

Conventional Production Systems

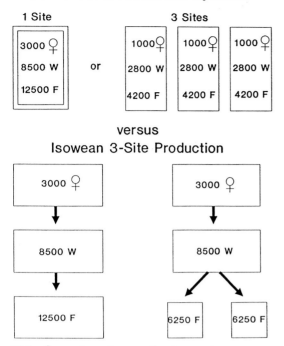

66.4. Comparison of conventional reasoning versus Isowean technology for a 3000-sow farrow-to-finish operation. W = number of nursery pigs; F = number of finisher pigs.

SUPPLY OF BREEDING STOCK. For many years, breed improvement was the prerogative of individual purebred breeders, and in some countries it still is. Their main function is the sale of boars to commercial producers, usually on a local or regional scale.

The 1960s saw the formation of multiple-herd breeding organizations in some countries. A few were set up as fairly large organizations from the start, but many grew from small beginnings. They sometimes began as groups of purebred breeders forming integrated breeding pyramids,

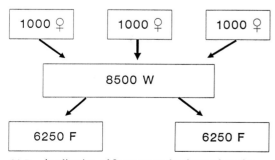

66.5. Application of Isowean technology when the breeding, gestation, and farrowing (site 1) is at more than one location. Pigs are moved to nurseries (W) (site 2) at 3 weeks of age or less and then to finishers (F) (site 2) at 20–35 kg body weight.

usually associated with central test stations. As these organizations became more successful, central testing diminished, being replaced by on-farm testing on premises owned by the group or company. This provides better controlled contemporary comparisons and selection and also has advantages for disease control. Rapid generation turnover is usually practiced, and considerable genetic progress is achieved.

Although the development is varied in different countries, multiple-herd breeding organizations and breeding companies are now established to a greater or lesser degree in North America, Western Europe, some countries of Eastern Europe, South America, and Australasia. As development continues to its logical conclusion, multiple-herd breeding organizations are becoming the dominant force in genetic improvement in most of the major pig-producing areas of the world. The advent of gene transfer is unlikely to radically modify this in the short term, although the application of partitioning agents may modify the evolution. Veterinarians who work mainly with pigs now often find themselves involved with breeding organizations, either directly or on behalf of commercial producers purchasing stock.

Breeding Organizations. To understand the methods of disease control appropriate to breeding organizations, it is necessary to appreciate their structure (Alexander 1970). To remain commercially viable, breeding organizations must respond to market forces and commercial opportunities. Consequently, the detailed structure that evolves as they grow is complex, varying within and between organizations. Nevertheless, a basic pyramidal structure is common to most; this is illustrated in its simple form in Figure 66.6.

At the apex of the pyramid is the nucleus herd in which intensive testing and selection is carried out. Some of the largest breeding companies now test several thousand boars and gilts per year within each nucleus unit. The very best boars and gilts are retained within the nucleus herds. Extensive AI is used in some organizations to reduce genetic lag and broaden the genetic base. Many organizations now produce prolific dam lines and meaty sire lines, which may result in dual pyramids. The methods of testing differ among breeding organizations.

Many of the traits that seem desirable from a veterinary standpoint – strong legs, robust constitution, neonatal vigor, farrowing ability, mothering ability, quiet temperament, resistance to disease – are not measurable, are too difficult to measure, possess too low a heritability, or are too low in economic priorities. This limitation is partly compensated by culling animals with undesirable characteristics at both the nucleus and the multiplier levels and crossing at the multiplier level to obtain hybrid vigor.

The main function of multiplier herds is to in-

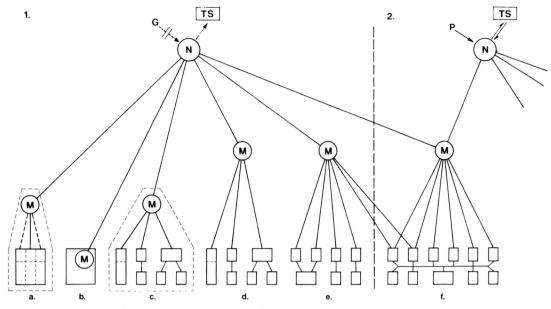

66.6. Diagram of a simple breeding pyramid: N = nucleus herd and M = multiplier herd—commercial breeding and growout units (there would be many more commercial units than depicted here); TS = central test station; P = live pigs introduced; G = genes introduced by AI, surgery, and fostering, or embryo transplant; (a) commercial operation of over 1000 sows and progeny on one or more sites possessing its own separate multiplier unit; (b) commercial unit containing grandparent as well as parent stock; (c) cooperating group of commercial producers jointly owning a multiplier herd; (d) multiplier supplying stock to independent producers by straight-line distribution; (e) same as (d) but by both mixed and straight-line distribution; (f) mixed distribution, including distribution of feeder pigs through markets or dealers; (1) closed pyramid; (2) open pyramid.

crease the improved stock derived from the nucleus. Some units may be boar multipliers; others may be gilt multipliers; some may be both.

The simplest and most economic system is shown in Figure 66.7. Two breeds or lines are tested. Boars are sold to commercial producers along with first-cross gilts from multiplier herds. The slaughter pigs are therefore back-crosses. Now, four or more breeds or lines more commonly may be used, and both hybrid sire and dam lines are sold to the commercial producer. In some countries where testing is carried out in several nucleus herds, the multiplication struc-

ture is then complex, sometimes involving extensive use of AI and statistical equalization of test results.

In Figure 66.7 the slaughter pigs at the base of the pyramid are the final generation. The sows and boars in commercial herds are therefore regarded as parents, those in multiplier herds as grandparents, and those in the nucleus as great-grandparents. In many breeding pyramids there are one or more additional layers, so the nucleus may contain great-great-grandparents, and so on.

Figure 66.6 greatly oversimplifies the distribution of stock, for even within one organization

66.7. Number of pigs in a simple breeding pyramid.

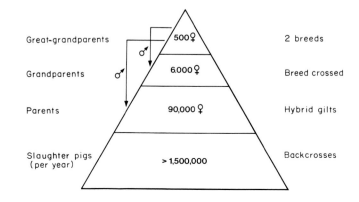

variations may be complex. A number of arrangements are represented at the base of the figure and are explained in the legend.

The arrangement labelled "a" represents a multiplier supplying one very large commercial breeder who operates one or more commercial unit(s). To give some indication of the size of such enterprises, one multiplier herd of 100 sows can supply all the replacements required for one 1200- to 1500-sow unit or three 400- to 500-sow units.

The arrangement labelled "c" represents what may be termed a "group multiplier." In its simplest form it consists of a central multiplier supplying a cooperative group of perhaps 20–30 commercial producers. The group gains the advantages of scale activities such as joint marketing, joint purchase of feed, joint purchase and maintenance of vehicles, a single veterinary service, etc.

More often the arrangement is as depicted in "d," "e," and "f," i.e., a number of multipliers supplying a large number of independent producers. The distribution is usually controlled by the parent organization, but feed companies or large farm cooperatives that frequently operate locally or nationally and perhaps own one or more of the multipliers distribute the stock.

The presence of boar multipliers may complicate the pyramid still further, particularly if customers use rotational crosses as in the United States, or where sire lines and dam lines are reared separately.

The financial structure of the leading pig-breeding organizations is complex. Some are composed entirely of independent breeders and pig farmers integrated by an outside agency or cooperative into a breeding network. Others are companies originating from one or more purebred breeders who banded together. Some are owned partly or completely by larger industrial companies, which include feed manufacturers, meat-packers, agricultural investment and finance companies, and drug companies. In these cases the parent company usually owns most of the nucleus herds and either owns, partly owns, or has contractual control over the multiplying herds. At present, few have any great financial control over the commercial herds they supply. Antimonopoly laws or anticorporation farming laws may prevent integrated developments such as feed and breeding or breeding and meat-packing in some countries or regions.

SPREAD OF INFECTIOUS DISEASE. To understand the responsibilities of breeding organizations toward controlling spread of disease, the number of pigs at different levels of the breeding pyramid must be appreciated.

Theoretically (Fig. 66.7), a 500-sow nucleus herd could provide all the replacements for 6000 grandparent sows at the multiplier level, which in turn could provide all the replacements for a total of 90,000 parent sows at the commercial level; together, these would produce 1,400,000–1,700,000 slaughter pigs per year. The possibility of disease spread is in fact much wider than this because only a portion of producers purchase all their replacement gilts; many buy only boars. Furthermore, the multiplier herds and customers of a single company are not usually confined to one area but are spread across the country.

Testing of a large gene pool in the nucleus herds, combined with rapid generation turnover, should limit the possible spread of genetic defects, including those of conformation or reproduction. If breeding records are accurate and computerized, it should be relatively easy to cull whole segments of a pyramid if a serious defect is noted.

A breeding organization has a responsibility to control disease, particularly if it is infectious. The design of a comprehensive disease control program is difficult in organizations composed of numerous independent breeders. It is somewhat easier in a breeding company because all the herds are under one management. However, from a strictly veterinary viewpoint, the perfect disease control program can never be achieved because many of the control measures a veterinarian would like to impose are too expensive or conflict with the requirements of management, marketing, and sales or with the demands of the geneticist to move genes freely between herds. Practical disease control programs must inevitably be based on compromises.

Disease Control in a Breeding Company. Breeding organizations vary so widely in structure and function that the rest of this section will be concerned only with aspects of disease control appropriate to one hypothetical type of expanding breeding company, but the discussion will apply in varying degrees to other types or organization.

The successful growth of a breeding company depends on many factors other than health. These include flexibility of management, marketing ability, technical expertise, ancillary services, company image, and genetic potential of the stock and its suitability for market and customer satisfaction. In the early stages of growth, when the number of herds are few and the movement of stock is relatively simple, these factors appear more important to success than a sound disease control program. When they occur, diseases can be readily controlled. But as a company grows and becomes more complicated, the risk of disease increases and controlling it becomes more difficult. If a company begins without a sound control program, disease may eventually limit expansion and even threaten company survival.

EFFECTS OF DISEASE. Disease affects the internal economy of a breeding company in a least three ways. First is the direct damage done to production; more than 60% of pigs produced by a breeding organization are slaughtered for meat. Second is the effect of disease on the efficiency of genetic selection. Disease has an unknown and variable effect on traits being tested and therefore on the reliability of test results. Any disease that affects the growth of the pig before testing affects its performance in the test, again to an unknown and variable degree. The third effect is much more serious—the disruption of supply. One of the biggest influences on the profitability of a breeding company is its ability to match supply with demand. Once a boar multiplier is in full production with a complete set of customers, the introduction of a disease that forces temporary or permanent closure is disproportionately damaging to the profitability of the company overall. The position is much worse if a nucleus herd becomes contaminated.

Disease also has a major effect on sales. Although a company may put great effort into genetic improvement, the purchaser cannot readily assess it. For example, few producers readily or accurately measure growth rate or feed conversion, but they are quickly aware of the appearance of a new disease in their herds following the purchase of new breeding stock. Even if the disease is relatively mild, they may never purchase stock from the company again. No company can afford to get a bad reputation for spreading disease.

AIMS AND METHODS. In planning a disease control program the breeding company should strive for the following aims: (1) to protect the customers' herds against disease and, in so doing, protect the company's reputation, remembering that the disease status of every customer's herd is different; (2) to reduce the disruption to supply caused by outbreaks of disease (i.e., to protect the nucleus and multiplier herds against contamination); (3) to prevent disease from causing the productivity of all the units to drop or become unpredictable; and (4) to remove the unknown variable of disease from testing and selection. Some people argue a fifth aim, namely, to improve the national production by setting up herds of exceptionally high health status. Note that the first two are much more important than the third. This contrasts with commercial production in which the third is the main objective. Methods for disease control are (1) establishing herds relatively free from infectious disease, (2) taking precautions against contamination and suppressing effects of certain types of potentially damaging infection, (3) exercising constant disease surveillance across a broad front to provide an early warning system, and (4) implementing mechanisms for immediate action as soon as a disease is suspected.

THE INITIAL NUCLEUS HERD

Foundation Stock. There are two extreme points of view with regard to the foundation stock in the initial nucleus herd. One is that it should be assembled from the best sows and boars available regardless of the diseases they may carry. Thereafter, rapid generation turnover and large-scale intense selection should be practiced in the face of disease, so that the pigs selected are those that will perform well in whatever conditions they or their progeny find themselves. The other is that as many infectious diseases as possible should be excluded at the outset and every effort made thereafter to keep infection out of the nucleus herd and the multipliers established from it. Experiences of established breeding companies leave no doubt that the second viewpoint is the correct one.

One reliable way of establishing the initial healthy nucleus herd is by the classic specific-pathogen-free (SPF) procedure of primary swine repopulation. This allows the nucleus to be formed from the offspring of sows and boars that have the best genetic potential available.

If no facilities are available for artificially rearing surgically derived piglets, alternative means may have to be sought. One possibility is to purchase a very healthy herd or the offspring from it, regardless of its genetic potential, and to foster onto the healthy farrowing sows surgically derived piglets obtained from the best bred sows available. AI and/or embryo transplants can also be used to introduce genes. The difficulty is in determining how healthy the originally purchased herd is. To do so may require detailed knowledge of its history, including drugs used, along with detailed laboratory and postmortem investigations. Another possibility is to use medicated early weaning or Isowean. These options are discussed later.

Introduction of New Genes. Whatever method is used for establishing the first nucleus herd and whatever diseases are found to be present, it should be closed to the introduction of more pigs. This will certainly conflict with the requirements of the geneticist, and a compromise will have to be found.

The least dangerous option is the introduction of surgically derived pigs fostered by recently farrowed sows. The foster sows should be held in isolation from the main herd. The isolation or quarantine unit should consist of a small farrowing complex outside but adjacent to the nucleus perimeter. It should have the same barriers to contamination as the main nucleus. The foster piglets stay in the quarantine unit after weaning and are then mixed with sentinel pigs of similar age taken from the nucleus. The checks carried out on the pigs prior to entry to the nucleus and on the donor sows prior to surgery depend on the diseases prevalent in the locality.

An alternative to fostering is surgery and artificial rearing, followed by mixing with sentinel pigs in quarantine. Another is embryo transplant. Both require more sophisticated techniques than hysterectomy and fostering.

AI may also be used to introduce genes. This, however, only introduces half the genes required and presupposes that there are suitable recipient breeds or strains in the nucleus already. It is also much less safe than hysterectomy. The donor boars should be held in an isolated secure unit, should undergo quarantine and testing before entry, and be regularly checked by a veterinarian. Recipient sows may also be held in isolation as a quarantine measure and suitable tests for antibodies to various diseases (e.g., *Brucella suis, Leptospira pomona,* or pseudorabies) carried out.

The most dangerous option is the introduction of conventional pigs, particularly from a number of different sources or from a central test station. Quarantine alone provides a totally inadequate safeguard. This option should be avoided if possible (Fig. 66.6).

Precautions against Contamination. The precautions against contamination are the same as those described earlier for large commercial units. They should be of the highest standard and adhered to strictly. The suitability of the location is of crucial importance and should be away from areas of high pig density and in the securest terrain obtainable. Visitors should be excluded altogether, and the minimum of a three-night rule should be applied; i.e., anyone entering should have been away from pigs and sources of infection for at least three nights (e.g., one weekend). Perimeter fencing, changing rooms, showers, feed delivery systems, offices, canteens, and pig-loading bays should be the best available. Necropsy facilities and pig disposal units should be located outside the perimeter. Bird, fly, and rodent control should be carried out conscientiously, depending on the diseases in the region.

Husbandry and Prophylactic Measures. It is preferable to keep drug use to a minimum. Prophylactic use of drugs on a routine basis should be avoided, and antibiotic growth promoters should be restricted to low levels and to those not used for therapeutic purposes. The routine use of drugs commonly used for the control of diseases such as SD should be avoided. Outbreaks of diseases such as neonatal coliform scours, metritis-mastitis-agalactia syndrome, and postweaning scours must be diagnosed accurately and treated promptly. Worms should be kept to a minimum. Routine vaccination against ubiquitous diseases such as coliform scours and erysipelas can be used, but its use against diseases such as pseudorabies and HC

should be considered carefully. Vaccination tends to mask newly introduced infection, which may then spread throughout the pyramid before it is recognized. The newer gene-deleted vaccines plus selective serology may avoid this.

MULTIPLIER HERDS. The consequences of outbreaks of infectious disease in multiplier herds are less far-reaching than those in nucleus herds. Nevertheless, for the reputation and profitability of the organization at large, it is best to ensure that sound disease prevention and control measures are practiced at the multiplier level.

Multiplier herds are best set up on isolated "green-field" sites in new buildings, but this is not always possible. Sometimes units that have housed pigs before must be used, but total depopulation, cleaning, and disinfection is recommended prior to repopulation from the nucleus herd.

Multiplier units are populated and subsequently kept filled with selected gilts and boars direct from the nucleus herd. The precautions against infection and factors such as drug use should be similar to those of the nucleus.

It would be wrong to try to standardize methods of disease control too rigidly throughout a multiplication network. In a large organization the multiplier herds may be widely separated in different types of locations with different local diseases, and roles may differ. For example, precautions adopted in a multiplier (Fig. 66.6) that is wholly owned by one large producer or group of producers should be tailored to their needs; whereas precaution adopted in a multiplier supplying widely dissociated individual producers may have to be of a higher standard.

In the case of small multiplier herds (less than 150 sows), it is probably best if the gilts or boars are grown out on the same premises. In larger multiplier herds (500 sows), separate grow-out facilities may be advisable. If carefully planned, they can provide a small added measure of security. However, it may be necessary to vaccinate gilts and boars against parvovirus and/or expose them to effluent from the breeding unit's service area (and possibly also the farrowing and weaner rooms) around the time of selection to reduce the chances of SMEDI problems when they are sold into commercial production units.

Very large multiplication herds (over 1000 sows) have several advantages (e.g., the supply of large customers from one source) but they have a major disadvantage. If such a herd becomes contaminated by a disease such as TGE, PRV, or AR, it has to be closed, causing a major reduction in supply. Furthermore, before being reopened it may have to be depopulated, cleaned and disinfected, left empty, and then repopulated. The most costly part of this expensive procedure is the long gap in production resulting from the sows' reproductive cycle. In contrast, repopulation of a grow-out unit is much quicker and cheaper. For this reason Isowean 3-site production is now being adopted in large multipliers in the United States (Fig. 66.8).

Isowean 3-site systems utilizing all-in/all-out principles in each stage of production allows for the elimination of disease without the need for total depopulation (Table 66.1). PRV and AR have been eliminated from Isowean 3-site herds of 1000–2000 sows (Harris 1990b; Harris et al. 1990b,c). The point of entry of an infectious agent into the facilities, the nature of the infectious disease, and the facility design and lay-out determine the steps necessary to eliminate disease from such a system. The placement of animals from each 1–2 weeks of production in an isolated location for sites 2 and 3 greatly enhances elimination protocols but increases initial capital and operating costs (Fig. 66.3).

Facilities constructed and situated in this manner decrease the chance of vertical disease transmission and allow for elimination of disease more readily. Nursery facilities should be constructed to accommodate pigs weaned as early as 10 days should the need arise to eliminate an agent that enters site 1 (Fig. 66.8). Although construction on three sites increases initial costs, certain advantages may decrease operating costs such as pig performance and labor utilization. In addition, less space per pig may be required because of improved rate of gain and faster throughput. It is conceivable that only two sites be utilized with site 1 being as described above and site 2 containing facilities for pigs from weaning through finishing. However, three sites seem preferable and may be necessary for disease elimination purposes (Table 66.1).

ESTABLISHMENT OF SUBSEQUENT NUCLEUS HERDS. When the first multiplier units of the first pyramid are in operation, it is advisable to set up a second nucleus as insurance against a serious disease permanently or temporarily disrupting supplies from the first. As the organization grows, it may be advisable to have a third

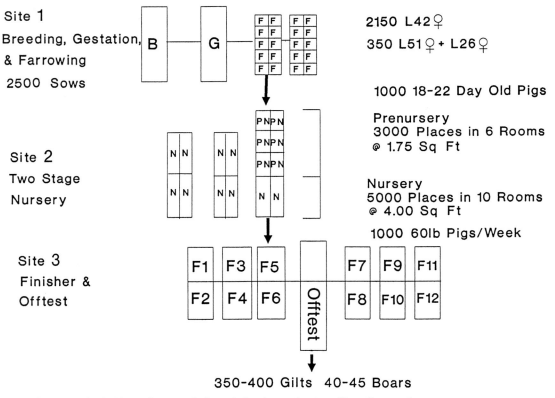

66.8. Diagram of a 2500-sow Isowean 3-site unit for the production of breeding stock. Prenursery accommodations are constructed in case it becomes necessary to wean at 5–10 days of age to eliminate an infectious agent. Off-test building is for increasing the body weight of selected boars and females to be sold as breeding stock as compared to pigs being sold to slaughter.

Table 66.1.   Action to be taken if a high-health status herd becomes diseased in Isowean 3-site production

Disease	Site 1	Age at Weaning (days)	Site 2	Site 3
Severe pneumonia	Vaccinate/R_x[b]	10	All-in/all-out	Depopulate[a]
Atrophic rhinitis	Vaccinate/R_x	10	All-in/all-out	Depopulate
Aujeszky's disease	Vaccinate	21	All-in/all-out	Depopulate
Transmissible gastroenteritis	Virus exposure[c]	21	Virus exposure	Virus exposure
Swine dysentery	Vaccinate/R_x	21	R_x	Depopulate

Source: Harris (1990a).
[a]May not be necessary to depopulate if all-in/all-out.
[b]R_x treat with drugs.
[c]Exposure to virulent virus from sick pigs on farm itself.

nucleus herd (and possibly more) in different regions.

If these nucleus herds are to act as full insurance for each other, each must have a complete genetic spectrum. If the second nucleus is set up soon after the first and the first has suffered no serious disease, the easiest and cheapest method is to use a cross section of breeding stock direct from the first. It may be possible to set up the third in a similar manner. However, with time the health status of the first nucleus may decline. If it does, acting on the guiding principle that all new nucleus herds should start as free from infectious disease as possible, it may be advisable to consider the use of primary SPF pig production, medicated early weaning (MEW), or Isowean.

If all nucleus herds are to remain at an equivalent genetic level, there must be considerable movement of genes between them. This can be done by surgery and fostering, embryo transplantation, AI, MEW, or Isowean with quarantine, or a combination of these. Although it should be avoided whenever possible, sometimes it may be necessary in exceptional circumstances to move a batch of normally reared pigs from one nucleus to another. In this case strict quarantine and testing should be carried out.

The movement of genes between nucleus herds is simplified if only one of the nucleus herds carries out the major part of testing and selection, particularly with regard to research and development of new lines. Facilities and technicians can then be concentrated at one site.

For further assurance of supply in case one whole pyramid becomes infected, it may be helpful to maintain surplus production in each nucleus, possibly by devoting part of the nucleus unit to multiplication.

MOVEMENT OF PIGS DOWN A PYRAMID

Direction of Movement. All movements of pigs should be in one direction only, i.e., down the pyramid from nucleus to multipliers to customers. Under no circumstances should the flow be upward or horizontal.

Vehicles and Drivers. Vehicles carrying breeding stock between herds must be owned or strictly controlled by the parent organization. Cleaning and disinfection between loads is important, and so is the order in which journeys are arranged, e.g., collecting stock from the nucleus first and multipliers second and delivery to the abattoir last.

The drivers of the vehicles should be trained in simple disease precautions; they should not enter pig-rearing facilities and should avoid proximity to other livestock vehicles, etc.

No customers should be allowed to collect breeding stock directly from nucleus or multiplier herds. In some regions where the customers are scattered and sales are small, this may present difficulties and unacceptably high transport costs. One way to overcome this is to set up collection depots, preferably on an all-in/all-out batch basis. It may be possible to allow farmers visiting these depots to view their prospective purchases safely through windows.

Straight-Line Distribution. One of the most important control measures is straight-line distribution. It is a common fallacy to believe that a standard health status can exist throughout all the herds of a multiple-herd company, however strictly the rules of isolation and hygiene are enforced. Because the function and size of multiplier units vary and locations of premises differ, the spectrum of potential pathogens in each will vary and differ also. Each herd develops its own herd immunity to agents endemic to it. This delicate balance can be drastically upset by introduction of new agents.

For these reasons, the lines of distribution from the nucleus herd through the multipliers to the commercial producers should not overlap (Fig. 66.6, pyramid 1); i.e., each herd from the customer level up should receive all its foundation and replacement gilts from the same supply herd. It is usually necessary in most companies to supply boars from one unit and gilts from another but, ideally, this should be the maximum degree of mixing.

As in other aspects of disease control, the ideal from a veterinary viewpoint cannot be achieved in practice. There is a natural tendency for even the most disease-conscious breeding company to move toward a policy of mixed distribution; i.e., individual customers receive replacement stock from a variety of sources. It is impossible to avoid this completely. No one multiplier can consistently supply exactly the right number of replacement animals to fulfill the requirements of a given number of commercial herds. Another reason is sudden and unexpected changes in demand in relation to supply or transport difficulties. Also, when multiplier herds become contaminated, sources have to be changed. The more complicated a pyramid becomes, the more difficult straight-line distribution becomes. In extreme cases, where there are numerous small nucleus herds each with only one breed of pig and both hybrid boar and hybrid gilt lines are produced for final crossing, it may become impossible to avoid extensive mixing throughout.

Nevertheless, the trend toward mixed distribution in a company should never be accepted without prior consideration of options. One such option is the use of Isowean 3-site procedures to elevate the health status of multiplier herds. Locating the second and third sites of production isolated from the breeding, gestation, and farrowing stages results in the production of breeding stock with less variation in the spectrum of pathogens present, especially if all-in/all-out procedures are utilized. In the future, new technologic advances in testing and immunization may allow for standardization of health status among pigs produced by Isowean in varied locations.

Isolation. No matter what precautions are taken, mistakes will be made. Occasionally, stock will be moved from a herd that is in the incubation stages of a disease, and this may spread through a whole section of a pyramid before it is recognized. Or perhaps stock becomes contaminated en route by aerosol or dust from another pig vehicle.

For these reasons, it is highly recommended that replacement stock be quarantined for a minimum of 3 weeks prior to entry into the herd. The quarantine area should be well isolated and precautions taken to avoid contamination. This period of time allows for medications to be administered for elimination of asymptomatic carrier pigs, e.g., SD; clinical outbreaks or serologic test results indicating disease occurrence in the source herd; and for selective testing of the pigs in quarantine. Tests chosen for screening pigs in quarantine should be chosen carefully with full knowledge of previous test results in the recipient herd. Testing for a wide variety of disease agents may only lead to confusion due to false-positive reactions (see above).

Acclimatization. After quarantine, gilts and boars should be allowed to adapt to new premises for a minimum of 3 weeks before they are used for breeding. This includes recovery from the psychophysiologic trauma of being moved from an accustomed environment into a strange one, as well as adaptation to the new husbandry system, feed, and potential pathogens. The climate may also be different.

Adaptation problems are most common and severe when pigs from different sources are mixed together, when pigs from one system (full confinement) are put into an entirely different system (semiextensive), when pigs are moved from a healthy herd into a very diseased herd, or when pigs are moved from one climate to a totally different one.

Where straight-line distribution is practiced, adaptation problems are usually minimal. However, in most cases it is wise to carry out a routine adaptation program similar to that described earlier for commercial herds. In some cases it may be necessary to move potential breeding stock at a younger weight and age. This must be decided on the basis of circumstances.

DISEASE SURVEILLANCE. All preventive measures serve to reduce the risks of disease; they do not eliminate them altogether. A breeding company must be constantly alert for the appearance of disease anywhere in its pyramid; the closer to the top of a pyramid a disease occurs, the wider its implications are likely to be.

Disease Surveillance in the Nucleus. Surveillance in the nucleus should include regular herd inspections by the veterinarian, necropsy examinations by the veterinarian and the local diagnostic laboratory, and examination on the slaughter line. Detailed performance records that are kept by nucleus herds should be monitored for indications of disease. Regular checking for specific pathogens may be carried out. However, careful consideration should be given to each test employed and its implications, since the majority of tests produce occasional false-positive results, which cause disruption of supply and sometimes serious embarrassment with customers (Plonait 1979). For example, in the large Danish SPF program, herds are checked routinely by blood testing for certain serotypes of *Actinobacillus pleuropneumoniae* and for *Mycoplasma hyopneumoniae*. The high incidence of false-positive results leads to herd closures, which are subsequently found to be unnecessary. It is hoped that with the adoption of monoclonal antibodies and more sophisticated ELISAs this problem will diminish. In some cases, routine blood testing before moving from one state or country to another is mandatory; e.g., for PRV in the United States, Germany, or Denmark, or for brucellosis in the European community. Routine culturing (e.g., of the tonsils for toxigenic *Pasteurella multocida* or *Streptococcus suis* type 2) can also be misleading because of the occurrence of strains of low pathogenicity.

All manifestations of disease should be investigated thoroughly to reach an accurate diagnosis. Laboratory support is essential. All diagnoses should be recorded so that the disease spectrum of the herd becomes increasingly well documented.

Disease Surveillance in Multiplier Herds. Surveillance in the multiplier unit should include regular herd inspections by veterinarians and trained nonveterinary technicians who visit the herds to select boars and gilts. It should also include random postmortem examinations and slaughter checks, veterinary examination of performance data, and accurate diagnosis of diseases before they are masked by therapy. Routine checks for specific pathogens in most multipliers are usually ill-advised for the reasons given above, but may be indicated in special circumstances.

The type and degree of surveillance depends on the role of the multiplier and the nature of the herds it is supplying. However, regular inspection reports by the local or regional veterinarians and selection technicians should be examined and filed in central company veterinary offices.

Investigation of Complaints. A useful check on nucleus and multiplier herds is the prompt and conscientious investigation and central documentation of customer complaints that appear to have disease implications.

Veterinary Services. Regardless of whether the company employs a veterinarian full-time, each multiplier should have access to a local practicing veterinarian. It may be advantageous to employ practicing veterinarians on a regional basis to cover several multipliers and any veterinary complaints that arise in the region. A company may also need university, government laboratory, or institute backing to help with difficult issues and general policy.

ACTIONS TAKEN. Continuous disease surveillance acts as an early-warning system, but it is also essential to have a standby mechanism for rapid confirmation of diagnosis when disease occurs, as well as the availability of authoritative advice. This should include an evaluation of all the options, which must be weighted against other constraints (economic, genetic, management) before acting. It is generally advisable where serious disease is suspected to stop the movement of pigs from the suspect herd until a decision is made. This is costly to the breeding company and its customers, which is one reason why action must be prompt. The other reason is to halt the spread of disease. It is clearly essential for an expanding breeding company to have sound veterinary support that is not only knowledgeable about pig production and disease but familiar with the function and economics of the company.

Actions to be taken can rarely be standardized or prescribed in advance. Disease outbreaks are almost always unexpected and take a different form than anticipated. Understanding of disease and disease patterns is constantly evolving. The roles of each multiplier in relation to the herds they supply are often so different that an action appropriate to a given disease in one herd may be different to that taken for the same disease in another.

ESTABLISHING HERDS FREE FROM SERIOUS ENDEMIC DISEASE

Repopulation Directly from Another Herd.
Sometimes herds become so severely affected by intractable disease that the best option may be to depopulate and start again with healthy stock. Several questions should be answered before a decision is made: (1) Why did the herd become so diseased? If the causes still persist, will the herd be reinfected? Can any measures be taken to reduce the risk of reinfection? (2) Is there a supply of reliably healthy pigs available for restocking and subsequent replacements? (3) Are the premises amenable to thorough cleaning and disinfection? If they are not, will any of the disease carry over to the new herd? (4) How long should the premises remain empty to ensure that the diseases do not carry over?

The answers depend on the diseases present and the climate. Many infections can remain viable for long periods in freezing weather but are inactivated rapidly in hot weather. Therefore, repopulation should be carried out in late spring, summer, or early fall, when many infections such as *Mycoplasma hyopneumoniae* (Whittlestone 1976) or *Serpulina hyodysenteriae* (Glock et al. 1975; Chia and Taylor 1978) are inactivated within a few hours or days. Thus enzootic pneumonia (EP) never carries over, and SD does so only if pools of slurry are not drained or infected mouse colonies are not exterminated. Except in freezing weather, most infectious diseases will not carry over if premises are left empty for 6 weeks and cleaning and rodent extermination have been thorough. A notable exception is SVD (Herniman et al. 1973; Callender 1978).

If it is decided to proceed with repopulation, the cost may be reduced if it is timed to coincide with the economic pig cycle. It will probably be cheaper to depopulate over a short period rather than wait for all sows to farrow and all pigs to reach slaughter weight. In the case of breeding units, some replacement gilts can be served in advance of repopulation so that farrowings start soon after their arrival on the unit.

During depopulation some buildings may become empty and available for cleaning before others and some are repopulated long before others. It is tempting to allow depopulation and repopulation to overlap. This is a dangerous policy. However, depending on the diseases present, climate, layout, and type of buildings, it may be safe in some circumstances to shorten the time during which the entire unit is empty of pigs to about 2 weeks provided no building is restocked in less than 6 weeks after it has been cleaned and each empty building is sealed off.

Cleaning should be carried out twice at 2-week intervals and should be thorough, with use of pressure washer, detergents, and disinfectants appropriate to the disease(s). All porous materials, straw, and feed should be removed. A blow torch may be useful for some areas. A thorough rodent extermination campaign should be carried out.

Eradication of Individual Diseases. Numerous attempts have been made to eradicate specified diseases from herds without resorting to total depopulation. One of the earliest methods was that of isolated farrowing (Waldman and Radtke 1937; Barber et al. 1955; Whittlestone and Betts 1955; Pullar 1958; Roe and Alexander 1961; Goodwin 1965). This was directed at the eradication of respiratory disease, principally EP but also AR in some cases. The method was based on the assumption that older sows become immune to the respiratory diseases endemic in a herd and stop excreting the causal agents. Older sows are farrowed in isolation, usually in temporary huts. They are kept with their offspring until a proportion of each litter is slaughtered and the lungs and snouts examined. If lesions are found, the sows and the rest of the litters are slaughtered. If lesions are not found, the sows and remainder of the litters are used as the future breeding herd.

Early results were promising, but later attempts met with mixed success. For example, Roe and Alexander (1961) succeeded in eradicating EP from six small herds, but when the next generation were born, AR was worse in some herds than it had been previously. Goodwin (1965) attempted to eradicate EP from two herds, but when the gilts from the litters that were thought to be pneumonia free farrowed, EP appeared in their litters. Whether these failures were due to the inaccuracy of the slaughter tests, to carryover of subclinical infection, or to reinfection is not known. It may also have been due to cross-infection between the litters in isolation because they were often relatively close. The method has not gained wide acceptance and would not be applicable to large herds.

Various attempts have been made to eradicate other single infections from herds without depopulation. Examples are bordetella rhinitis (Farrington and Switzer 1977), SD (Windsor 1979; Harris 1984; Wood and Lysons 1988), TGE (Gray et al. 1982; Harris et al. 1987), *A. pleuropneumoniae* (Larivière et al. 1990; Larsen et al. 1990), and PRV (Basinger 1979).

Methods have been based on strategic medication, blanket vaccination, and/or testing for freedom from infection, with culling of individual reactors. Testing may be serologic, as in PRV, or cultural, as in bordetella infection. Results have been variable. In general, elimination without depopulation has been most successful with TGE and SD, and also more recently PRV. Failure to eliminate TGE and SD probably is due to survival of the infectious agents in the environment or, in the case of *Serpulina hyodysenteriae,* in mice or slurry. The introduction of gene-deleted vaccines against PRV, with selective tests to distinguish antibodies to natural infection with wild virus from those induced by vaccine, has facilitated the elimination of PRV. Blanket vaccination of all the sows four times per year for 3 years with the gene-deleted vaccine, plus incoming gilts before and after entry, plus all growing pigs either with gene-deleted vaccine or conventional inactivated vaccine can result in the replacement of carrier sows by seronegative sows and elimination of the virus from the herd. This is being done extensively in the United States, Holland, and Germany.

Medicated Early Weaning. A new method of eliminating a wide spectrum of infectious disease was introduced in 1979. It combined some of the features mentioned above with medicated early weaning (MEW) (Alexander et al. 1980a,b, 1981; Alexander 1982; Lysons et al. 1982). It is an alternative to SPF swine repopulation, particularly for large herds and areas of the world where facilities for artificially rearing surgically derived piglets on a large scale are not readily available. It was devised specifically for setting up new high–health status nucleus herds from older established ones.

PRINCIPLES. In a closed herd in which reasonable precautions are taken, mature sows become immune to most of the endemic infectious pathogens. With few exceptions, piglets are microbiologically sterile before birth and take several weeks to develop a complex microflora equivalent to that of the mature pig. They are not immediately infected by all the infections present in a herd. For the first week of life at least, the biggest, thriftiest piglets in a litter are strongly protected against many of the endemic pathogens by colostral and lactogenic immunity.

If older sows in a closed herd are removed from the cross-contamination of other pigs and from the contaminated environment of the unit and are farrowed in small synchronized groups in isolation, and if their biggest, thriftiest piglets are weaned to an isolated rearing unit at 4–5 days of age, the piglets escape infection by most of the pathogenic organisms present in the herd. Medication of sows from 5 days before until 5 days after farrowing and of piglets from birth until 10–20 days of age provides an added safeguard.

METHOD. Sows with at least one previous litter are bred in small groups at regular intervals. They are removed from the herd on day 110 of gestation to farrowing crates in an isolated far-rowing unit of small rooms, each sufficient for one group and operated on an all-in/all-out basis. Medication of the sows starts immediately prior to leaving the herd and is continued until 5 days postfarrowing. The sows are injected intramuscu-larly with prostaglandins at midday on day 113 or day 114 of gestation, depending on the average gestation length in the herd, to induce parturition on the following day. Farrowings are attended so that piglets can be medicated soon after birth and regularly thereafter.

Pigs in each litter that weigh over 2 kg are weaned from the sow at about 5 days of age. They are moved in an insulated container to an isolated nursery, where they are reared to be-tween 5 and 8 weeks of age on expanded metal floors. They are initially fed milk pellets, then creep feed. They are then moved to simple iso-lated grow-out units or to the recipient herd (Fig. 66.9).

EFFECTIVENESS. This method has now been ap-plied on a large enough scale in the United Kingdom, West Germany, the United States, Canada, Brazil, and Hungary to establish its effec-tiveness against a range of infections. These in-clude *M. hyopneumoniae, M. hyosynoviae,* tox-igenic *P. multocida, A. pleuropneumoniae, H. parasuis, B. bronchiseptica, S. hyodysenteriae,* TGE, and PRV. Relatively large, primary MEW herds have been set up from old diseased herds, the new being free from unwanted infections present in the old. Numerous secondary MEW herds have been set up by direct repopulation from the primary herds and have provided added proof of the effectiveness of the method. Their high level of freedom from potential pathogens has not been entirely without drawbacks. Pigs sold from these herds have proved to be immuno-logically naive and some, particularly when they have been moved in large groups, have suffered serious adaptation problems. For example, severe outbreaks of Glasser's disease have occurred,

similar to those reported for SPF herds (Madsen 1984). Paradoxically, this immunologic naivete provides further evidence of the effectiveness of this method. Various modifications have been made to the above technique by different workers. For example, first-litter gilts have been used without detriment, and the dams' immunity has been boosted by vaccination. Major modifica-tions were suggested by Harris (1988a,b).

MODIFICATIONS OF MEW (ISOWEAN). In a series of trials, Harris et al. (1988a,b, 1990a,b,c) tested the principles underlying MEW to simplify the technique and to give it wider application. In Iso-wean, sows farrow on the source farm and the piglets are weaned to an isolated nursery at 5–21 days of age. The age at weaning and the vaccines and medications used are based on the infectious disease agents present on the source farm (Table 66.1). After weaning, the pigs are reared as origi-nally described in the MEW procedure (Fig. 66.9).

Isowean has been used successfully to elimi-nate *M. hyopneumoniae* (Connor 1990), toxigenic *P. multocida,* TGE, and PRV (Harris et al. 1988a,b, 1990a,b,c).

Repopulation with SPF Pigs. Repopulation with SPF pigs is a well-tried method for establish-ing new healthy herds from diseased herds while maintaining a similar genetic spectrum.

TERMINOLOGY. The term "specific-pathogen-free" was introduced in about 1960 by pioneers of SPF pig production in Nebraska to replace their original term "disease-free" (Caldwell et al. 1959, 1961; Young et al. 1959; Young 1964). At about the same time workers in Britain introduced the term "minimal disease" (Betts et al. 1960; Betts 1961). Although in some contexts the two terms are synonymous, in others they have slightly dif-ferent connotations.

The terminology used by the Nebraska workers is adopted here. "Primary SPF pigs" are

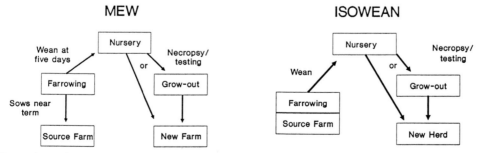

66.9. Comparison of medicated early weaning (MEW) and Isowean. In MEW, the pregnant sows are removed from the source farm near term and placed in isolated farrowing accom-modations. Piglets are weaned at 5 days of age. By contrast, in Isowean, piglets are simply removed from the source farm at weaning. In Isowean, the weaning age is variable depend-ing upon the disease agent to be eliminated.

those that have been removed aseptically from their dams at birth and reared away from direct contact, and, as far as possible, indirect contact with conventional pigs. An "SPF laboratory" is a unit for obtaining primary SPF piglets and rearing them away from their conventional dams. "Secondary SPF pigs" are subsequent generations of naturally farrowed and reared pigs derived originally from the primary SPF group.

"Swine repopulation" or "farm repopulation" is the process of totally populating farms with SPF pigs. A "primary SPF herd" is one set up with surgically derived pigs. A "secondary SPF herd" is one set up with pigs from a primary or another secondary SPF herd. SPF implies that appropriate precautions have been taken throughout to reduce the opportunities for contamination with certain pathogenic organisms. It implies that although SPF pigs inevitably develop a complex normal flora that may include potential pathogens such as coliform bacteria, streptococci, and staphylococci, they can be kept free of certain other pathogens that tend to occur in conventional herds.

PRINCIPLES. The concept of swine repopulation starts from the assumption that unborn fetuses near term are free from infectious organisms. Although some organisms (e.g., parvovirus, *Leptospira bratislava*) may cross the placental barrier, this concept holds true for the majority of viable fetuses and the majority of infectious organisms.

The aim of swine repopulation is to remove piglets from their dams as aseptically as possible, rear them to maturity away from other non-SPF pigs, and breed them naturally to produce SPF herds.

APPLICATION. SPF swine repopulation was developed and applied in the United States mainly in the midwestern states (Young et al. 1955b, 1959; Shuman et al. 1956; Whitehair and Thompson 1956). Of the different groups involved, Young, Underdahl, and their coworkers appear to have been most influential in the early developments.

Extensive swine repopulation programs were launched in Switzerland in 1962 and in Denmark in 1970 (Mandrup 1974). These are now the biggest SPF programs in the world. Primary SPF pigs have also been produced and swine repopulation carried out in numerous other countries, including Canada (Alexander 1960; Alexander and Roe 1962), England (Betts et al. 1960), Germany, France, the Netherlands, Czechoslovakia, Yugoslavia, Australia, Japan, and Taiwan (Twiehaus and Underdahl 1975; Forest 1978).

METHODS. The methods originally developed for procuring and rearing primary SPF pigs by Young and coworkers (Young and Underdahl 1951, 1953; Young et al. 1955a; Young 1964) were adopted widely during the 1960s. However, numerous

modifications have been made, including the adoption of gnotobiotic techniques (Trexler and Reynolds 1957; Coates 1968; Trexler 1971).

Procurement of Primary SPF Piglets. Primary SPF piglets have been obtained by snatching them from the vagina during natural birth (Young and Underdahl 1951, 1953; Bauriedel et al. 1954; Done 1955; Johnson et al. 1955; Shuman et al. 1956). The difficulty of forecasting parturition accurately (now partly overcome by prostaglandins) and the disturbance in parturition caused by the attendants' interference make this method unreliable and impracticable on a large scale. More important, it is impossible to catch the piglets without contaminating them. Since the establishment of a primary SPF herd is expensive and the crucial point in the whole procedure is to make a clean break between conventional pigs and SPF piglets, this method is not recommended.

Removal of the piglets from the sow is better accomplished by surgery. Basically, there are two methods, both of which can be carried out using germ-free techniques (Meyer et al. 1963, 1964; Whitehair and Waxler 1963; Bahr et al. 1968; Alexander et al. 1969; Trexler 1971; Twiehaus and Underdahl 1975): hysterotomy (Hoerlein et al. 1956; Whitehair and Thompson 1956; Roe and Alexander 1961) and hysterectomy (Young et al. 1955a; Underdahl and Young 1957a,b; Betts et al. 1960). In hysterotomy the sow is anesthetized, the piglets are removed from the uterus through an abdominal incision, and the sow is allowed to recover. In hysterectomy the sow is killed by asphyxiation with carbon dioxide (Underdahl and Young 1957a) or simply shot (Keller 1971), and the uterus containing the piglets is removed. The sow may be hung by her hind legs or left lying down. The gravid uterus is removed immediately in the case of asphyxiation or after 2 minutes in the case of shooting, passed through a disinfectant lock into a hysterectomy hood (Underdahl and Young 1957a; Meyer et al. 1964) or into another room (Abelseth 1962), or carried some distance away in a tub of disinfectant. The piglets are then ripped from the uterus and resuscitated.

Care of the pregnant sow prior to surgery is sometimes overlooked. To reduce the danger of congenital virus infections, the sow should not be moved to a new environment within 3 weeks prior to or at least 8 weeks after service. It is better if she is not moved at all until the time of surgery. In general, sows are less prone to congenital infections than gilts.

As a precaution against transient bacteremias at the time of hysterectomy, the sow should not be stressed preceding surgery. Some workers inject the sows with antibiotics at surgery to guard against bacterial contamination of the piglets. Surgery is usually carried out at 112 or 113 days of gestation. Bahr et al. (1968) described a procedure by which parturition could be delayed for as long as 8–10 days. Such procedures are useful for coordinating surgery with foster rearing.

Rearing Primary SPF Piglets. The easiest way to rear primary SPF piglets is by suckling them on foster sows (Koch 1978); if done properly, the primary SPF piglets grow and develop like naturally reared pigs and adapt quickly to farm conditions. Several potential recipient foster sows should be bred about a day before the donor. Synchronized service dates can be achieved by weaning all the sows involved at the same time or by hormone therapy. If necessary, surgery may be delayed in the donor sow as described by Bahr et al. (1968). Synchronized farrowings may be helped with prostaglandins. The naturally born litter(s) of the recipient foster sow(s) should be prevented from suckling at all and removed until the primary SPF piglets are introduced.

The surgically derived piglets should be suckled by the foster sow as soon as they are strong enough to walk. If a delay is inevitable, they should be held in an insulated, dark, comfortable box at 32–38°C. Cleanliness and warmth are essential. The temptation to feed them artificially should be resisted so that stimulation of digestive enzymes may be delayed. Surgically derived litters have been flown or driven long distances without unduly bad effects.

The most hazardous part of primary SPF piglet production is artificial rearing from birth. These difficulties can be reduced by using flexible-film isolators and gnotobiotic techniques for up to the first 4 weeks of life (Trexler and Reynolds 1957; Meyer et al. 1963, 1964; Bahr et al. 1968; Coates 1968; Alexander et al. 1969; Trexler 1971). Even then there is difficulty in adapting the pigs to a normal flora when they are removed from the isolators. It is possible to rear them in simple individual cages instead of germ-free conditions. High standards of hygiene, constant high temperature, freedom from dampness and drafts, and regular small feedings with a fortified sow milk replacer are essential. Porcine immunoglobulin can only be given orally in the first day of life, while parenteral administration is possible at older ages. Bovine colostrum given orally is usually ineffective.

It is not difficult to rear small numbers of primary SPF piglets artificially, but when rearing them for large herd repopulation, the hazards and problems tend to increase.

Adaptation of artificially reared pigs to farm conditions sometimes poses problems (Underdahl et al. 1963). They may undergo a setback in growth that may last several weeks. Ailments such as fever, anorexia, polyarthritis, meningitis, and diarrhea may occur sporadically. Fortunately, most respond to prompt antibiotic therapy. To reduce these problems, the pigs should be allowed to adapt gradually. Later, because of the relatively narrow spectrum of immunity that primary SPF

gilts acquire, there may be farrowing problems and the first litters may be more susceptible to neonatal infection. All these problems disappear, however, when a new primary SPF herd is established and in full production.

APPLICATION OF SWINE REPOPULATION. Not only is the establishment of a large primary SPF herd a difficult and somewhat hazardous procedure, it is also expensive. It is easier to establish a small primary SPF herd (30–60 sows) than a large one (200–600 sows), and there is greater assurance of success. It may be best in some circumstances to establish a large herd in two stages, i.e., to establish a small herd first and then build it up from itself by natural reproduction assisted by AI, surgery, and fostering.

It is much easier, quicker, cheaper, and more reliable to establish a secondary SPF herd from a primary one. This means that in modern breeding pyramids and commercial pig production, the main application of primary SPF repopulation is in setting up new nucleus herds. All the multipliers and some of the commercial units can then be set up as secondary and tertiary herds by total swine repopulation. Secondary, nucleus herds can also be set up in this way. The classic pyramid structure lends itself admirably to swine repopulation. The benefits derived from primary SPF repopulation of the initial nucleus herd are disseminated throughout the network.

MOVING GENES BETWEEN HERDS. In a herd kept completely closed and in which precautions are taken against contamination from other pigs, potential pathogens reach a relatively stable balance with herd immunity; if the herd is small, some pathogens may disappear altogether. To a veterinarian, who properly focuses attention on disease prevention, and to the producer, who is worried by disease problems, the maintenance of a closed herd may appear to be an attractive way of achieving and maintaining a high health status. However, as a permanent measure it is usually untenable. Different methods by which genes can be moved safely between herds have been reviewed by Reed (1976, 1978) and Bichard (1978).

Naturally Reared Replacement Stock. The best and easiest means for a large, highly geared commercial breeding unit to achieve maximum productivity is the introduction of all replacement parent gilts and boars from another genetically improved source. But this policy is the worst from the viewpoint of disease risk. Criteria for safe choice of replacement stock and control measures to be adopted in supplying such stock have been discussed.

Some producers attempt to reduce risk by introducing purebred grandparent boars and gilts and crossing them in the unit to produce their own hybrid replacements. The advantage here is that the number of animals brought into the unit is reduced; e.g., in a 500-sow unit, gilt replacements are reduced from around 200/year to about 15/year. However, there are disadvantages to this management: ensuring correct matings of grandparent boars and gilts, supplying adequate numbers of replacement gilts when required, and maintaining maximum productivity.

These disadvantages can be largely overcome if the unit or group of units includes over 1000 sows. The grandparents can then be removed to a separate weaner production unit of 65 sows or more, depending on the supply required (Fig. 66.6).

Many producers buy only boars and select replacement gilts from their own slaughter pigs. While this fails to take full advantage of genetic gains, it obviously reduces the disease risk if all the boars come from one safe source. However, if they come from a number of sources and from communal test stations, the risk is increased.

Other Methods for Moving Genes. Other possibilities for moving genes are AI, hysterectomy and fostering, embryo transfer, and MEW or Isowean.

ARTIFICIAL INSEMINATION. AI is the easiest and most readily available method for transferring genes, but it has two major disadvantages: AI carries only half the genetic complement, it tends to result in lower reproductive performance, i.e., lower farrowing rate and smaller litter size except in the most skilled hands, and it carries disease risk. Furthermore, during episodes of reproductive inefficiency the performance of artificially inseminated sows tends to drop more than those naturally served. Even where AI is being applied expertly, it can rarely be used for all services; some boars must be present. Generally, in commercial units no more than half the services should be by AI, in which case boars still must be purchased.

The lack of productivity that usually results from wide-scale use of AI in commercial production is partly offset by the genetic merit of the donor boars. It is usually impossible to purchase sufficient boars of equivalent merit. Productivity is such an important factor in commercial profitability that the value of AI must be carefully balanced economically.

Disease risks of AI have been assessed by Reed (1976, 1978) and Larsen et al. (1978). Some serious infections are known to enter the semen of infected boars, either directly or by urine contamination (HC virus, PRV, parvovirus, *Brucella suis, Leptospira bratislava, Leptospira pomona*) and could be introduced to herds via AI. Semen is also readily contaminated from the urogenital tract and environment; e.g., the preputial sac contains large numbers of bacteria. Theoretically, in the early bacteremic or viremic phase of any infec-

tion, the pathogen might contaminate the semen. Semen should always be regarded as a heavily contaminated body fluid containing 10^2-10^6 bacteria/ml. Antibiotics will eliminate most of the bacteria (e.g., penicillin and streptomycin will kill *L. pomona* and *L. bratislava*) but will not inactivate virus. To reduce these risks, it is essential that AI boars are thoroughly screened for infectious disease and housed away from other pigs and livestock; high standards of hygiene should be maintained throughout the AI process. Boars entering an AI station should be quarantined for a month and blood-tested for appropriate diseases.

Most AI stations routinely add antibiotics to the semen, usually penicillin and streptomycin, thus reducing the risks from bacterial infections. Schulman and Estola (1974) reported the presence of mycoplasmas in boar semen, so some AI centers also include tylosin. Unfortunately, this is thought to have a deleterious effect on semen quality (Reed 1978).

The use of frozen semen not only helps to overcome distributive storage problems of fresh semen but helps to reduce disease risk by allowing a quarantine time before use. One main value of frozen semen is likely to be in the relaxing of import restriction, thus allowing freer international exchange of genes. Unfortunately, while the semen from some boars survives freezing well, that from others does not, so overall, frozen semen seems much less effective than fresh.

SURGERY AND FOSTERING. Surgery and fostering is most valuable for introducing a full complement of genes into nucleus herds. In practice, it seems to be relatively safe. The main dangers are pseudorabies, HC, *Leptospira bratislava,* and the possibility that the sow was in the prodromal or subclinical septicemic phase of an infectious disease. For these reasons, litters containing mummified fetuses should be discarded and fostering should be done in quarantine. In practice, surgery and fostering has been done extensively from herds with subclinical endemic PRV without transfer of the virus. However, *L. bratislava* appears to have been transmitted from one herd to another in this way.

Surgically derived piglets can be transported long distances by road or air if they are in suitable containers. Some laboratories use portable germ-free isolators for added security, but most use simple, insulated, heated boxes. Piglets require humidity and cannot withstand very dry heat for long periods.

EMBRYO TRANSFER. Embryo transfer (ET) has not been as widely applied as AI or hysterectomy and fostering. For reviews of its methods and possible applications, see Betteridge (1977) and Polge (1982a,b). Disease risks appear to be low, and James et al. (1983) suggest that vertical transmission of pseudorabies can be stopped by embryo transfer techniques.

Although the method has been used to transfer genes into SPF herds (Curnock et al. 1975), it is difficult to see what advantages it may have over surgery and fostering, except perhaps for ease of transport (Baker and Dziuk 1970). One disadvantage is that it requires a relatively high level of technical expertise at both the donor and recipient ends. Also, for transfers to be successful, the estrous cycles of donor and recipient sows must be synchronous. If they are more than 24 hours out of phase, the number of transferred embryos to survive is likely to be low. In practice, ET has proved less reliable and slower (small litter sizes) than surgery and fostering.

The technique has been used successfully to transfer genes between countries (Wrathall et al. 1970; James et al. 1980), and thus it probably has a marked advantage over both surgery and fostering and AI. Its value for this and for interherd movement within a country would be greatly enhanced if embryos could be stored deep frozen. This would overcome importation objections of some countries, give greater flexibility of transport, and help synchronization. With current techniques, fresh embryos remain fully viable for only 24 hours and degenerate rapidly over the next 24.

DISEASE CONTROL PROGRAMS.
Disease control programs fall into three categories: (1) compulsory government-run programs; (2) voluntary programs run by government agencies, statutory authorities, private associations, or cooperatives; and (3) private programs for individual units, small groups of related units, or multiple-herd companies. The first two will be dealt with briefly here. The third has been discussed earlier.

Compulsory Government Programs.
Compulsory government programs operate at international, national, state, provincial, or local levels. They are concerned with the complete eradication and/or exclusion of individual specified infections or their suppression. Examples of infections included in government regulations are FMD, ASF, HC, SVD, Teschen disease, vesicular exanthema, PRV, and brucellosis. Further information on these can be found in other chapters.

Exclusion of specified infections is brought about by import controls, not only of animals but also of animal products. The complexity of international trade in pig products combined with the increased speed and volume of international travel makes all countries more vulnerable to the introduction of new infections, e.g., the introduction of SVD to Western Europe and ASF to Portugal, Spain, Italy, Cuba, Malta, Brazil, Haiti, and the Dominican Republic.

Eradication of individual diseases is achieved mainly by detection, notification, and slaughter combined with ancillary measures such as re-

stricting movement, boiling garbage, disinfecting premises and trucks, etc. The classic example is FMD (Anon. 1978; Henderson 1978). All countries in FMD-free and FMD-fringe areas of the world (Australia, New Zealand, North America, Mexico, and most of Western Europe) attempt to exclude FMD by import regulations. When these fail and FMD gains entry, rigorous stamping-out policies are adopted, sometimes with ring vaccination. Praiseworthy examples of national eradication programs were those against HC in the United States and United Kingdom (Beynon 1971; Foreign Animal Disease Report 1978) and more recently against PRV in the United Kingdom and Denmark (Andersen et al. 1989; Basinger 1989; Christensen et al. 1990). The virus was eradicated from most of Denmark by 1986, but unfortunately outbreaks continued to occur in the South of Jutland bordering Germany and on the Danish islands off the coast of Germany. There is strong evidence that these were windborne infections from Germany where the disease was widespread. In Holland and parts of Germany attempts are being made to eradicate PRV by blanket vaccination of all herds for 5 years with the gene-deleted vaccine followed by selective blood tests, which detect wild virus, followed presumably by elimination of infected herds. All such attempts may be frustrated in the countries of the European community after 1992 when national barriers to trade are removed.

Suppression of infection, as distinct from eradication, is usually based on vaccination, notification of clinical cases, restriction on pig movements, and regulations governing the cooking of garbage fed to pigs. Examples of this are programs covering the control of HC in countries from which the disease has not been eradicated (Terpstra and Robijns 1977).

Programs such as those concerned with ASF and HC are of direct benefit to the pig industry (Ellis 1972; McDaniel 1976), whereas those concerned with SVD are of more benefit to cattle. Regrettably, some control programs are based on technically unsound assumptions and are of little benefit. A notable example is Teschen disease. The Teschen virus is subclinically endemic in most national pig populations, yet most governments persist with regulations for its exclusion or eradication.

Voluntary Programs

CHECKING AND ACCREDITATIONS.
Classic examples of checking and accreditation programs are those run by SPF associations. The first of these was in Nebraska. Its early history was outlined by Underdahl et al. (1968). Various SPF associations soon followed in other states, the biggest being in Iowa. In 1964 most of these were united under a parent organization, the National SPF Swine Accrediting Agency, Inc. In 1990 the agency had

144 members with 161 herds comprising 17,107 sows (Anon. 1990). Also in that year, the agency began dividing its herds into two categories, accredited and health controlled, based on health status. An accredited herd was defined as one being "free of symptoms of pneumonic lesions, turbinate atrophy, brucellosis, pseudorabies, mange, lice, swine dysentery, and leptospirosis." A health-controlled herd was defined as "a herd showing minor respiratory problems at the time of its last slaughter inspection."

In Canada the government-sponsored Ontario Certified Herd Programme was started in 1960 to designate herds free from EP and AR (Roe and Alexander 1961; Alexander and Roe 1962). This was not exclusively for SPF herds, but in practice it became so. Dual certification was introduced to cover EP and/or AR because of the difficulty of determining freedom from rhinitis at slaughter. The Ontario program remained relatively small, consisting in 1979 of 23 herds, and was later merged with a general swine health program.

Some of the SPF associations in other countries, notably Switzerland and Denmark, have expanded considerably. In Switzerland a swine-repopulation program similar to the one in Nebraska was launched privately in 1962. In 1965 it was integrated with the Swiss Federal Pig Health Service and subsidized by the state. Six primary SPF herds were established initially, and by 1970 more than 400 secondary SPF herds had been established from them, representing a sow population of more than 13,000 (Keller 1968, 1971; Koch 1973, 1978). By 1989 there were about 1821 SPF herds with about 47,051 sows (Keller 1990). The SPF herds now represent 6.5% of the national herd.

In Denmark an ambitious program of swine repopulation was started between 1968 and 1970. By 1979 approximately 500 hysterotomies had been performed in a central SPF laboratory using germ-free techniques. The pigs are moved to a 200-sow primary SPF herd at about 3 weeks of age. From this herd an SPF breeding network has been established, composed of nucleus breeding herds, candidate herds, multiplying herds, supplying herds, and commercial production units. In 1982 there were 1768 SPF herds containing 98,000 sows. In the next 2 years the national slaughter policy for the eradication of pseudorabies boosted the number of commercial herds repopulated with SPF pigs (Svineavl og-produktion i Danmark 1982). By 1990 there were 1100 SPF breeding herds, 1000 *Mycoplasma* status (MS) breeding herds, 365 SPF feeder pig herds, and 565 MS feeder pig herds. MS herds are SPF herds that had become reinfected with EP only. The total number of SPF and MS slaughter pigs was about 3.75 million, which represented 25% of the total pigs slaughtered in Denmark. The breakdown rate has been 14% with *Mycoplasma hyopneumoniae*, 3% with *Actinobacillus pleuro-*

pneumoniae, and 3% with other diseases (Madsen 1990).

SPF associations generally require all herds to have been repopulated with primary or secondary SPF pigs. Other accreditation programs, which are based on freedom from specified diseases, do not necessarily require this, although SPF herds are not barred from membership. A notable example of such a program is that run by the Pig Health Control Association (1984) in the United Kingdom, which monitors herds for freedom from EP, SD, AR, PRV, mange, and *Streptococcus suis* type 2 meningitis.

Checking programs involve regular tests for the specified pathogens or diseases. These tests may include slaughter checks and laboratory tests for EP and AR; serologic tests for EP, PRV, brucellosis, leptospirosis, and *Actinobacillus pleuropneumoniae;* composite tests for SD; checks for mange and lice; and tests for bacteria. The trouble with laboratory checks, particularly serology, is the uncertainty arising from false-positive results. Membership requirements vary between associations and tend to change from time to time. A common requirement is that members should take precautions against contamination with the diseases specified.

Checking associations are of greatest benefit to individual purebred breeders and small breeding companies. Membership confers a number of advantages, the most obvious providing an objective evaluation of the presence or absence of the diseases specified. This provides some reassurance to the prospective purchaser of breeding stock and enhances the customers' trust in the breeder. Membership often has other advantages such as joint advertising and increased awareness of matters relating to disease control.

Most associations do not guarantee freedom from the specified infections; this would be open to litigation. They usually record that on the basis of the tests carried out the herd appeared to be free of the infections at the time of the tests. The herd might have become infected in the interim, or tests may not have been sufficiently sensitive to detect low levels of infection. One drawback of membership is the reinfection rate. With some diseases, (e.g., SD) the breakdown rate is usually very low, but with others, notably EP, the annual breakdown rate may average about 2–6% of herds per year, particularly in pig-dense areas (Jensen and Madsen 1980; Keller 1980; Madsen 1982; Goodwin 1984). In some pig-dense areas it is virtually impossible to keep herds free of EP, presumably caused by aerosol infection on windy, cold, damp nights. Because it may undergo long periods of subclinical infection, EP may spread through the movement of subclinical carriers to other units before a breakdown is diagnosed (Keller 1980; Madsen 1982).

GENERAL HEALTH PROGRAMS. The broad aim of

general health programs is to pool the resources available (expertise, research and development, diagnostic facilities, ancillary services) to provide a comprehensive disease control policy covering husbandry factors as well as infectious disease. The emphasis is more on suppression of disease than on eradication.

The classic example of these is the Swedish Pig Health Scheme. This is a nationwide program started over 30 years ago, which by 1979 covered 21,000 herds and 220,000 sows (92% of the national sow herd). The scheme aims to control all disease of economic importance by the eradication of some and the suppression of others, resulting in optimum health and productivity (Melrose 1975; Smith 1978; Thavelin 1980).

Numerous other health schemes have been modeled on the Swedish scheme (Melrose 1975). For example, a Swedish-type program was adopted in Switzerland in 1962 to run in parallel with the SPF program mentioned above. By 1979 this scheme covered 478 herds and 10,000 sows (Keller 1980). A somewhat similar program was set up by the United Kingdom in 1967, mainly for breeders submitting pigs to central test stations (Anon. 1972, 1979). By 1984 it covered 247 herds comprising 46,480 sows. By 1990, however, due to various pressures, the number of herds had dropped to 97 and a new category was introduced. The aim of this was not directly concerned with health control but was to reassure pig meat retailers that the registered herds met certain standards of welfare, salmonella control, and drug usage. Similar consumer-orientated schemes were also started in other countries.

Health programs have also been reported in Denmark, Finland, France, Alberta, Ontario, Nova Scotia, the Netherlands, and South Africa (Loveday 1976; Stone 1976; Truijen and Tielen 1976; Smith 1978). These generally include regular herd inspections, postmortem examinations, laboratory diagnoses, and centralized recording and documentation. Some monitor individual diseases as well. The Finnish scheme is directed primarily at control of respiratory diseases.

It is difficult to evaluate the benefits or effectiveness of such programs. Initially, the main benefit in small herds is usually the upgrading of management and husbandry and the tightening of disease control measures. Later, and with larger herds and breeding companies, the benefits are likely to be related mainly to ancillary services such as laboratory diagnoses.

REFERENCES

ABELSETH, M. K. 1962. The application of specific pathogen-free animals to research and production. Can Vet J 3:48–56.

ALEXANDER, T. J. L. 1960. The establishment of isolation units for newborn pigs and studies on an encephalomyelitis of nursing pigs. Ph.D. diss., Univ of Toronto.

_____. 1970. Disease control in multiple-herd breeding organisations. Vet Annu 11:83–93.

_____. 1973. Veterinary aspects of planning large pig units. Vet Annu 14:61–64.

_____. 1982. The establishment of new herds by medicated early weaning. Proc 7th Int Congr Pig Vet Soc, Mexico City, p. Z64.

_____. 1991. Necrotic pleuropneumonia in pigs caused by *Actinobacillus* (*Haemophilus*) *pleuropneumoniae.* Vet Annu. In press.

ALEXANDER, T. J. L., AND ROE, C. K. 1962. Attempts at establishing swine herds free from atrophic rhinitis and virus pneumonia. II. Repopulation with specific pathogen-free pigs. Can Vet J 3:299–306.

ALEXANDER, T. J. L; MINIATS, O. P.; INGRAM, D. G.; THOMSON, R. G.; AND THACKERAY, E. L. 1969. Gnotobiotic pigs: Procurement, microbial flora, serum proteins, and lymphatic tissues. Can Vet J 10:98–105.

ALEXANDER, T. J. L.; BOON, G.; LYSONS, R. J.; and NELSON, E. P. 1980a. Medicated early weaning: A method of breaking the cycle of endemic infection. Proc 6th Int Congr Pig Vet Soc, Copenhagen.

ALEXANDER, T. J. L.; THORNTON, K.; BOON, G.; LYSONS, R. J.; AND GUSH, A. F. 1980b. Medicated early weaning to obtain pigs free from pathogens endemic in the herd of origin. Vet Rec 106:114.

ALEXANDER, T. J. L.; BOON, G. I.; AND THORNTON, K. 1981. The establishment of a new nucleus herd by medicated early weaning. Proc Pig Vet Soc (UK) 8(Pt 3):74–81.

ANDERSEN, J. B.; BITSCH, V.; CHRISTENSEN, L. S.; HOFF-JORGENSEN, R.; AND KIRKEGAARD PETERSEN, B. 1979. The government pig health scheme. Pig Breeders Gaz (UK) 161:30–32.

_____. 1989. The control and eradication of Aujeszky's disease in Denmark – epidemiological aspects. In Vaccination and Control of Aujeszky's disease. Ed. J. Van Oirschot. Curr Top Vet Med Anim Sci 49:175–183.

ANON. 1972. Ministry of Agriculture, Fisheries and Food. Her Majesty's Stationery Office, London.

ANON. 1978. Foot and mouth disease. Vet Rec 102:184–198.

ANON. 1990. What is SPF? Hog Health Today 9:1–2.

BAHR, VON K. H.; RICHTER, L.; AND PLONAIT, G. 1968. Versuche zur Gewinnung und Aufzucht spezifisch-pathogen-freien Ferkel mit dem Isolator Hannover II. DTW 75(3):55–64.

BAKER, R. D., AND DZIUK, P. J. 1970. Aerial transport of fertilized pig ova. Can J Anim Sci 50:215–216.

BARBER, R. S.; BRAUDE, R.; MITCHELL, K. G.; AND BETTS, A. O. 1955. The eradication of virus pneumonia from a herd of Large White pigs at a research station. Vet Rec 67:690–692.

BASINGER, D. 1979. A brief description of Aujesky's disease in Great Britain and its relative importance. Br Vet J 135:216–224.

_____. 1989. The politico-economic aspects of Aujeszky's disease control in Great Britain from 1953–1989. Pig Vet J (formerly Proc Pig Vet Soc [UK]) 24:102.

BAURIEDEL, W. R.; HOERLEIN, A. B.; PICKEN, J. C., JR.; AND UNDERKOPLER, L. A. 1954. Selection of diet for studies of vitamin B12 depletion using unsuckled baby pigs. J Agric Food Chem 2:468–472.

BETTERIDGE, K. J., ed. 1977. Embryo transfer in farm animals. A review of techniques and applications. Can Dep Agric Monogr 16.

BETTS, A. O. 1961. "Pathogen-free" pigs for research and practical control of pig diseases. Vet Rec 73:1349–1363.

BETTS, A. O.; LAMONT, P. H.; AND LITTLEWORT, M. C. G. 1960. The production by hysterectomy of pathogen-free colostrum-deprived pigs and the foundation of a minimal-disease herd. Vet Rec 72:461–468.

BEYNON, A. G. 1971. The eradication of swine fever from Great Britain. Proc 19th Int Vet Congr, Mexico, pp. 516–519.

BICHARD, M. 1978. Is genetic movement worthwhile? Proc Pig Vet Soc (UK) 3:57–65.

BLAHA, T. 1990. Personal communication.

CALDWELL, J. D.; SUMPTION, L. J.; AND YOUNG, G. A. 1959. Swine repopulation. II. Performance of "disease-free" boars on farms with diseased pigs. J Am Vet Med Assoc 135:504–505.

———. 1961. Swine repopulation. III. Performance of primary specific pathogen-free pigs on farms. J Am Vet Med Assoc 138:141–145.

CALLENDER, D. E. 1978. Swine vesicular disease. State Vet J (UK) 33:145–163.

CHIA, S. P., AND TAYLOR, D. J. 1978. Factors affecting the survival of *Treponema hyodysenteriae* in dysenteric pig faeces. Vet Rec 103:68–70.

CHRISTENSEN, L. S.; SORENSEN, K. J.; STRANDBYGAARD, B. S.; HENRIKSEN, C. A.; AND ANDERSEN, J. B. 1990. Evidence of long distance airborne transmission of Aujeszky's disease virus. 1. Identification of emerging strains. Proc 11th Int Congr Pig Vet Soc, Lausanne, p. 206.

COATES, M. E., ed. 1968. The Germ-free Animal in Research. New York: Academic Press.

CONNOR, J. 1990. Modified medicated early weaning. Proc Am Assoc Swine Prod, Denver, Colo., pp. 261–265.

CURNOCK, R. M.; DAY, B. N.; AND DZIUK, P. J. 1975. Embryo transfer in pigs: A method for introducing genetic material into primary specific-pathogen-free herds. Am J Vet Res 37:97–98.

DONE, J. T. 1955. Aseptic delivery and artificial rearing: A technique for disease control in pigs. Vet Res 67:623–625.

ELLIS, P. R. 1972. An economic evaluation of the swine fever eradication programme in Britain, using cost benefit analysis techniques. Univ Reading (England) Dep Agric Study 11.

FARRINGTON, D. O., AND SWITZER, W. P. 1977. Evaluation of nasal culturing procedures for the control of atrophic rhinitis caused by *Bordetella bronchiseptica* in swine. J Am Vet Med Assoc 170:34–36.

FOREIGN ANIMAL DISEASE REPORT. 1978. USDA Emergency Programs Publ (Jan-Feb).

FOREST, J. 1978. The SPF swine programme in France. Proc 5th Int Congr Pig Vet Soc, Zagreb, p. KA38.

GLOCK, R. D.; VANDERLOO, K. J; AND KINYON, J. M. 1975. Survival of certain pathogenic organisms in swine lagoon effluent. J Am Vet Med Assoc 166:273–275.

GLOSTER, J.; BLACKALL, R. M.; SELLERS, R. F.; AND DONALDSON, A. I. 1981. Forecasting the airborne spread of foot-and-mouth disease. Vet Rec 108:376.

GLOSTER, J.; SELLERS, R. F.; AND DONALDSON, A. I. 1982. Long distance transport of foot-and-mouth disease virus over sea. Vet Rec 100:47–52.

GOODWIN, R. F. W. 1965. The phenomenon of suppressed respiratory disease in litters of older sows. Vet Rec 77:383–387.

———. 1984. Apparent reinfection of enzootic pneumonia-free pig herds: Early signs and incubation period. Vet Rec 115:320–324.

———. 1985. Apparent reinfection of enzootic-pneumonia-free pig herds: Search for possible causes. Vet Rec 116:690–694.

GRAY, J.; DOUGLAS, R. G. A.; AND SUTHERLAND, D. J. B. 1982. Field experience of transmissible gastroenteritis in a pig breeding pyramid. Proc 7th Int Congr Pig Vet Soc, Mexico City, p. 5.

HARRIS, D. L. 1984. The epidemiology of the disease as it relates to the eradication of the disease. Comp Cont Educ 6:683–688.

———. 1988a. Alternative approaches to eliminating endemic diseases and improving performance of pigs. Vet Rec 123:422–423.

———. 1988b. New approaches for the elimination of infectious diseases from swine. Proc US Animal Health Assoc, Little Rock, Ark., pp. 416–426.

———. 1990a. Isolated weaning–eliminating disease and improving performance. Large Anim Vet (May/June):10–12.

———. 1990b. The use of Isowean 3-site production to upgrade health status. Proc 11th Int Congr Pig Vet Soc, Lausanne, p. 377.

HARRIS, D. L.; BEVIER, G. W.; AND WISEMAN, B. W. 1987. Eradication of transmissible gastroenteritis virus without depopulation. Proc Am Assoc Swine Prod, Indianapolis, Ind., pp. 555–561.

HARRIS, D. L.; WISEMAN, B. S.; PLATT, K. B.; HILL, H. T.; ARMBRECHT, P. J.; AND ANDERSON, L. A. 1988a. Continuous-flow procedure for deriving PRV free pigs from a PRV infected herd. 69th Annu CRWAD:69. Abstr.

HARRIS, D. L.; EDGERTON, S. L.; WILSON, E. R.; WISEMAN, E. W.; WOOLLEY, K. W.; CROCKER, D. B.; KINYON, J. M.; HILL, H. T.; ROSS, R. F.; AND GLOCK, R. D. 1988b. Modifications of medicated early weaning. 69th Annu CRWAD:69. Abstr.

HARRIS, D. L.; EDGERTON, S. L.; WILSON, E. R.; KINYON, J. M.; ROSS, R. F.; AND GLOCK, R. D. 1990a. Large thymus glands and improved weight gains in pigs reared in isolation after weaning. In preparation.

HARRIS, D. L.; EDGERTON, S. L.; AND WILSON, E. R. 1990b. Large thymus glands in Isowean pigs. Proc 11th Int Congr Pig Vet Soc, Lausanne, p. 377.

HARRIS, D. L.; ARMBRECHT, P. J.; WISEMAN, B. S.; PLATT, K. B.; HILL, H. T.; AND ANDERSON, L. A. 1990c. Production of pseudorabies virus free breeding stock from a pseudorabies virus infected vaccinated herd by Isowean 3-site production. In preparation.

HENDERSON, W. M. 1978. Quality control and field use of foot-and-mouth disease vaccine. Br Vet J 134(1):3–82.

HERNIMAN, K. A. J.; MEDHURST, P. M.; WILSON, J. N.; AND SELLERS, R. F. 1973. The action of heat, chemicals and disinfectants on swine vesicular disease virus. Vet Rec 93:620–624.

HOERLEIN, A. B.; ADAMS, C. H.; AND MEADE, R. J. 1956. Hysterotomy to obtain "disease-free" baby pigs. J Am Vet Med Assoc 128:127–130.

JAMES, J. E.; REESER, P. D.; DAVIES, D. L.; STRAITON, E. C.; TALBOT, A. C.; AND POLGE, C. 1980. Culture and long-distance shipment of swine embryos. Theriogenology 14:463–469.

JAMES, J. E.; JAMES, D. M.; MARTIN, P. A.; REED, D. E.; AND DAVIES, D. L. 1983. Embryo transfer for conserving valuable genetic material from swine herds with pseudorabies. J Am Vet Med Assoc 183:525–528.

JENSEN, H. K., AND MADSEN, K. S. 1980. Insignificant reinfection risk in Danish SPF swine production. Dansk Vet Tidsskr 63:229–232.

JOHNSON, T. K.; BONE, J. R.; AND OLDFIELD, J. E. 1955. Atrophic rhinitis in swine. I. Methods of control in a purebred herd. North Am Vet 36:191–195.

KELLER, H. 1968. Der schweizerische Beratungs und Gesundheitsdienst in der Schweinezucht (SGD) unter besonderer Berucksichtigung der Verhaltnisse im Zentrum Zurich. Grune 36:1339–1355.

———. 1971. Die Gesundheit als Rentabilitaetsfaktor in der Schweinproduktion. Schweiz Arch Tierheilkd 113:130–138.

———. 1980. Aktuelle Probleme des schweizerischen SPF-Programmes. DTW 87:449–451.

———. 1990. Personal communication.

KOCH, W. 1973. Der Aufwand fur die SPF-Sanierung und der Ertrag im Vergleich zu den Kosten. Ph.D. Diss., Univ Zurich.

———. 1978. Foster-rearing of hysterectomy-produced piglets to prevent the health risks in introducing new stock in SPF herds. Proc 5th Int Congr Pig Vet Soc, Zagreb, p. KA39.

LARIVIÈRE, S; D'ALLAIRE, S.; DELASALLE, F.; NADEAU, M.; MOORE, C.; AND ETHIER, R. 1990. Eradication of Actinobacillus pleuropneumoniae serotypes 1 and 5 infections in four herds. Proc 11th Int Congr Pig Vet Soc, Lausanne, p. 17.

LARSEN, H.; HOGEDAHL JORGENSEN, P.; AND SZANCER, J. 1990. Eradication of Actinobacillus pleuropneumoniae from a breeding herd. Proc 11th Int Congr Pig Vet Soc, Lausanne, p. 18.

LARSEN, R. E.; HURTGEN, J. P.; HILLEY, H. D.; AND LEMAN, A. D. 1978. Diseases transmissible with artificial insemination. Proc 19th Annu George A. Young Conf, Lincoln, Nebr., pp. 59–69.

LEMAN, A. D. 1989. Personal communication.

LOVEDAY, R. K. 1976. Pig health scheme in South Africa. Proc 4th Int Congr Pig Vet Soc, Ames, p. X1.

LYSONS, R. J.; LEMCKE, R. M.; BEW, J.; BURROWS, M. R.; AND ALEXANDER, T. J. L. 1982. An avirulent strain of Treponema hyodysenteriae isolated from herds free of swine dysentery. Proc 7th Int Congr Pig Vet Soc, Mexico City, p. 40.

McDANIEL, H. A. 1976. Highlights of hog cholera eradication in the United States, seminar on hog cholera and African swine fever. Comm Eur Communities (EEC), Hannover, Germany, pp. 441–447.

MADSEN, K. S. 1990. Personal communication.

MADSEN, P. 1982. A reevaluation of the role of Mycoplasma suipneumoniae s. hyopneumoniae in swine herd health. Proc 7th Int Congr Pig Vet Soc, Mexico City, p. 97.

———. 1984. Atypical outbreak of Glasser's disease in Danish pig herds. Proc 8th Int Congr Pig Vet Soc, Ghent, p. 107.

MANDRUP, M. 1974. SPF-pig production in Denmark. 12th Nord Vet Kongr, Reykjavik, pp. 75–76.

MELROSE, D. R. 1975. Report on pig health control in relation to pig improvement programmes in different countries and future development. Comm Pig Prod, Eur Assoc Anim Prod, Warsaw.

MEYER, R. C.; BOHL, E. H.; HENTHORNE, R. D.; THARP, V. L.; AND BALDWIN, D. E. 1963. The procurement and rearing of gnotobiotic swine. Lab Anim Care [Suppl] 13:655–663.

MEYER, R. C.; BOHL, E. H.; AND KOHLER, E. M. 1964. Procurement and maintenance of germ-free swine for microbiological investigations. Appl Microbiol 12:295–300.

PIG HEALTH CONTROL ASSOCIATION. 1984. Annual report, abstracts of publications and herd lists. Madingley, Cambridge, England.

PLONAIT, H. 1979. Konsequenzen falsch-positiver Befunde bei der Gesundheitsuberwachung von Zuchtbestanden. 30th Annu Meet, Eur Assoc Anim Prod, Harrogate, England, Pap M3.6.

POLGE, C. 1982a. Embryo transplantation and preservation. In Control of Pig Reproduction. Ed. O. Cole and G. Foxcroft. London: Butterworth, pp. 277–291.

———. 1982b. Embryo transplantation in the pig. 2d World Conf on Embryo Transfer and In Vitro Fert.

PULLAR, E. M. 1958. The establishment of disease-free pig herds with particular reference to infectious pneumonia. I. General principles and method. Aust Vet J 34:305–315.

REED, H. C. B. 1976. Pig artificial insemination and its future. Proc Pig Vet Soc (UK) 1:67–75.

———. 1978. Genetic movement and health. Proc Pig Vet Soc (UK) 3:45–55.

ROE, C. K., AND ALEXANDER, T. J. L. 1961. Attempts at establishing swine herds free from atrophic rhinitis and virus pneumonia. I. Review of initial work at the Ontario Veterinary College. Can Vet J 2:139–146.

SCHULMAN, A., AND ESTOLA, T. 1974. Isolation of mycoplasmas from boar semen. Vet Rec 94:330–331.

SELLERS, R. F., AND GLOSTER, J. 1980. The Nothumberland epidemic of foot-and-mouth disease, 1966. J Hyg (Camb) 85:129–140.

SHUMAN, R. D.; EARL, F. D.; AND STEVENSON, J. S. 1956. Atrophic rhinitis. VI. The establishment of an atrophic-rhinitis-free herd of pigs. J Am Vet Med Assoc 128:189–192.

SMITH, D. H. 1978. Report on European pig production. Comm Prod Eur Assoc Anim Prod.

STONE, M. W. 1976. The Alberta swine herd health program. Proc 4th Int Congr Pig Vet Soc, Ames, p. X7.

SVINEAVL OG-PRODUKTION I DANMARK. 1982. Landsudvalget for Svineavl og-produktion.

TERPSTRA, C., AND ROBIJNS, K. G. 1977. Experiences with regional vaccination against swine fever. Tijdschr Diergeneeskd 102(2):106.

THAVELIN, B. 1980. Personal communication.

TREXLER, P. C. 1971. Microbiological isolation of large animals. Vet Rec 88:15.

TREXLER, P. C., AND REYNOLDS, L. I. 1957. Flexible film apparatus for the rearing and use of germ-free animals. Appl Microbiol 5:406–412.

TRUIJEN, W. T., AND TIELEN, M. J. M. 1976. Experiences with two new developments in pig health control programmes. Proc 4th Int Congr Pig Vet Soc, Ames, p. X2.

TWIEHAUS, M. J., AND UNDERDAHL, N. R. 1975. Control and elimination of swine disease through repopulation with specific pathogen-free (SPF) stock. In Diseases of Swine, 4th ed. Ed. H. W. Dunne and A. D. Leman. Ames: Iowa State Univ Press, pp. 1163–1179.

TYLER, J. W. 1989. Titers, tests and truisms: Rational interpretation of diagnostic serologic testing. J Am Vet Med Assoc 194:1550–1558.

UNDERDAHL, N. R., AND YOUNG, G. A. 1957a. An improved hood for swine hysterectomies. J Am Vet Med Assoc 131:222–224.

———. 1957b. An isolation brooder for raising disease-free pigs. J Am Vet Med Assoc 131:279–283.

UNDERDAHL, N. R.; WELCH, L. C.; AND YOUNG, G. A. 1963. Evaluation of problems related to introduction of secondary specific pathogen-free (SPF) boars into SPF and non-SPF herds. J Am Vet Med Assoc 142:634–638.

UNDERDAHL, N. R.; COUPE, R. E.; FERGUSON, D. L.; PEO, E. R.; AND TWIEHAUS, M. J. 1968. Nebraska's specific pathogen-free (SPF) swine program: Tenth year report. Univ Nebraska Publ SB499.

WALDMAN, O., AND RADTKE, G. 1937. Erster Bericht uber Erfolge der Bekampfung der Ferkelgrippe durch die Riemser Einzelhuttenanlage. Berl Tieraerztl Wochenschr 53:241–246.

WHITEHAIR, C. K., AND THOMPSON, C. M. 1956. Observations on raising disease-free swine. J Am Vet Med Assoc 128:94–98.

WHITEHAIR, C. K., AND WAXLER, G. L. 1963. Rearing caesarotomy-derived swine in controlled environments—present status. Lab Anim Care 13:655–672.

WHITTLESTONE, P. 1976. Effect of climate conditions on enzootic pneumonia of pigs. Int J Biometeorol 20:42–48.

WHITTLESTONE, P., AND BETTS, A. O. 1955. The eradication of virus pneumonia of pigs from a commercial herd. Vet Rec 67:692–693.

WINDSOR, R. S. 1979. Swine dysentery. Vet Annu 19:89–96.

WOOD, E. N., AND LYSONS, R. J. 1988. Financial benefit from the eradication of swine dysentery. Vet Rec 122:277–279.

WRATHALL, A. E.; DONE, J. T.; STUART, P.; MITCHELL, D.; BETTERIDGE, K. J.; AND RANDALL, G. C. B. 1970. Successful inter-continental pig conceptus transfer. Vet Rec 87:226–228.

YOUNG, G. A. 1964. SPF swine. Adv Vet Sci 9:61–112.

YOUNG, G. A., AND UNDERDAHL, N. R. 1951. A diet and technique for starting pigs without colostrum. Arch Biochem Biophys 32:449–450.

_____. 1953. Isolation units for growing baby pigs without colostrum. J Vet Res 14:571–574.

YOUNG, G. A.; UNDERDAHL, N. R.; AND HINZ, R. W. 1955a. Procurement of baby pigs by hysterectomy. Am J Vet Res 16:123–131.

YOUNG, G. A.; HINZ, R. W.; AND UNDERDAHL, N. R. 1955b. Some characteristics of transmissible gastroenteritis (T.G.E.) in disease-free antibody-devoid pigs. Am J Vet Res 16:529–535.

YOUNG, G. A.; UNDERDAHL, N. R.; SUMPTION, L. J.; PEO, E. R.; OLSEN, L. S.; KELLY, S. W.; HUDMAN, D. B.; CALDWELL, J. D.; AND ADAMS, C. H. 1959. Swine repopulation. I. Performance within a disease-free experiment station herd. J Am Vet Med Assoc 134:491–496.

67 Therapeutics

S. C. Henry

D. W. Upson

THERAPEUTIC CONSIDERATIONS. Development and implementation of a therapeutic regimen has long been a major responsibility for veterinarians in food animal practice. Because a majority of swine production problems are manifest as infectious disease, most therapy is antibacterial. Until recent years, in fact, infectious disease therapeutics consumed much of the time and energy of practitioners. Recent changes in the swine production industry and societal sensitivity to food safety are altering this long-standing veterinary role in livestock therapeutics. Swine producers desire less dependence on chemical intervention as a response to disease. They are readily adapting to disease-prevention procedures and production systems that maintain health. Repopulation of herds with high–health status animals, use of group-segregation methods, and various disease elimination programs reduce the need for repeated or continuous therapy.

Use and application of drugs approved for swine vary from country to country. This chapter deals with medications used for swine in the United States and emphasizes those most used, the antimicrobial compounds. It should be noted that global standards for drug use in food-producing animals are being developed. Efforts of the Codex Alimentarius Committee, an arm of the World Health Organization, are underway to standardize recommendations on food-animal drug use that will impact therapeutic options on an international basis.

It is likely that human food safety concerns over potential chemical residues will lead to increasingly restrictive policies on medication and therapy in food animals. The challenge in establishing a therapeutic regimen is one of selecting approved drugs to give a "best fit" of therapeutic efficacy, food safety, and economy.

For regulatory purposes pharmaceutical compounds are categorized by law as over-the-counter (OTC) or prescription drugs; these categories relate to the intended distribution and use of a drug and are part of that preparation's official approval, granted by government agencies.

Over-the-Counter Drugs. OTC drugs are available to the general public and are sold for application by the purchaser only in accordance with the directions included in the label.

Prescription Drugs. Prescription drugs are for use by or on the order of the veterinarian and are always identified by the following statement included on the drug label. "Caution: Federal law restricts this drug to use by or on the order of a licensed veterinarian."

Extra-Label Drug Use. This category is not a part of the law or regulations but is recognized in discretionary privileges granted to veterinarians. Use of OTC drugs in therapies or dosages not approved in the labelling constitutes extra-label drug use. Only in a carefully defined set of circumstances may veterinarians employ a therapy that includes drugs, dosages, duration of therapy, or routes of administration not specifically approved for swine. These circumstances are detailed in the Food and Drug Administration Center for Veterinary Medicine Compliance Guide.

The extra-label use of any veterinary drug in or on a food-producing animal by any person other than a veterinarian or a person working under the control of a veterinarian is prohibited. Extra-label use of such drugs by or on the order of a veterinarian is not prohibited provided all the following conditions are met:

1. A careful medical diagnosis is made by the veterinarian within the context of a valid veterinary/client/patient relationship.
2. A determination is made that there is no marketed drug specifically labelled to treat the condition diagnosed, or that drug therapy as recommended by the labelling has been found to be clinically ineffective in the animal(s) to be treated.
3. Procedures are instituted to assure that the identity of the treated animal is carefully maintained.
4. A significantly extended time period is assigned for drug withdrawal prior to marketing meat, milk, or eggs; steps are taken to assure that the recommended withdrawal times are met; and no illegal residues occur.

Government restrictions, in response to consumer food safety concerns, may increasingly limit therapeutic alternatives. Therapeutic decisions must be formulated with these restrictions on drug use in mind. While a specific therapy is the ultimate goal, it is not always possible.

Documentation of therapy, with written prescriptions and specific labels, is recommended when therapy must differ from manufacturers' recommendations. Some common pharmacology abbreviations and standardized prescription format are presented in Table 67.1 and Figure 67.1.

THERAPEUTIC RESPONSIBILITIES AND DECISIONS.
Therapeutic decisions and applications must satisfy many parties to whom the vet-

Table 67.1. Pharmacology abbreviations

Abbreviation	Latin	English
ad lib.	*ad libitum*	As desired
b.i.d.	*bis in die*	Twice a day
ft.	*fiat*	Make
h.	*hora*	Hour
m.	*misce*	Mix
q.i.d.	*quater in die*	Four times a day
q.s.	*quantum sufficit*	As much as needed
sig. or S.	*signa*	Label
sol.	*solutio*	Solution
tab.	*tabella*	Tablet
t.i.d.	*ter in die*	Three times a day
o.d.	*omnie die*	Daily
s.i.d.	*semel die*	Once a day
cap		Capsule

erinarian and livestock producer are responsible:

1. Animal. The goal is to provide a specific, targeted, efficacious therapy that is delivered in a humane manner.

2. Producer/owner of livestock. The producer/owner expects a practical, applicable therapy that is cost effective and does not pose undue risk to the personnel administering the medication.

3. Government regulators. The government requires adherence to state, federal, and international constraints on medication of animals intended for human food, including responsibility for documentation of therapy.

4. Pharmaceutical manufacturers. Manufacturers expect application of products within their established envelope of safety and in a manner allowing efficacy at demonstrated potency.

5. Consuming public. Responsibility for therapeutic decisions is expected of livestock producers and veterinarians. While the law broadly suggests limits of proper therapeutics, the universally appreciated dual concern for the well-being of animals and for safe food encourages a diligence in food animal therapeutics.

Pharmacotherapy must be based upon (1) a thorough evaluation of the animals with a specific diagnosis if possible; (2) an understanding of pathophysiology of the diseased animal; (3) a thorough understanding of and ability to apply

67.1. Standardized prescription format. DEA = Drug Enforcement Agency.

Telephone 123-456-7890   Date_____

DAN W. UPSON, D.V.M.

201 Cedar Drive   Manhattan, KS 66502

Client's Name_____   Address_____

Species_____   Description_____

Rx

Sig.

Refill_____times

_____   _____D.V.M.

DEA No.

the principles of pharmacology in establishing the treatment regimen; and (4) a consideration of precautions, warnings, side effects, drug interactions, and ultimately, human food safety associated with the therapy selected.

DRUGS AVAILABLE FOR SWINE THERAPY.

Compared with the number of medications available for other species, a relatively small number of pharmaceutical compounds are approved for use in swine (Table 67.2). Though limited in number these compounds are available in a wide array of dosage forms, trade names, concentrations, and in various combinations with one another. Formulations for in-feed use, oral therapy in water, and for injection are generally available for most antibacterial compounds listed. Drugs available for swine are best considered in two broad categories, the feed-additive drugs and the unit-dose drugs.

Feed-Additive Drugs. Feed additives make up by far the greatest volume of chemotherapeutic agents administered to swine. Most feed additives are antimicrobial or anthelminthic drugs, used to enhance production or for disease therapy. Thus, the practice of feeding antimicrobial compounds serves the dual purposes of disease control and improvement in growth rate and feed efficiency. At low, often subtherapeutic, doses, most antimicrobial compounds exert a protein-sparing effect and produce an acceleration in daily weight gain. Certain drugs, for example bambermycin, are exclusively production-enhancing drugs and are marketed without any disease control claims. Others may be solely for therapeutic purposes, but most are labelled for both production and therapeutic applications (Table 67.3).

FEED-ADDITIVE EFFECTS ON PRODUCTION. As observed, the growth response to antimicrobial

Table 67.2. Compounds approved for use in the United States for swine

A. Antimicrobial Compounds

Aminoglycoside group	Sulfonamide group	Other antimicrobial compounds
Apramycin	Sulfachlorpyridazine	Bacitracin
Dihydrostreptomycin	Sulfadimethoxine	Bambermycin
Gentamicin	Sulfaethoxypyridazine	Carbadox
Neomycin	Sulfamethazine	Erythromycin
Streptomycin	Sulfathiazole	Lincomycin
Arsenical compounds	Tetracycline group	Oleandomycin
Arsanilic acid	Chlortetracycline	Spectinomycin
Roxarsone	Oxytetracycline	Tiamulin
Sodium arsanilate	Tetracycline	Tylosin
Penicillin group		Virginiamycin
Amoxicillin		
Ampicillin		
Procaine penicillin G		

B. Anthelmintic Compounds

Compound	Method of Administration
Dichlorvos	In-feed
Fenbendazole	In-feed
Hygromycin B	In-feed
Ivermectin	Parenteral
Levamisole	In-feed, water
Piperazine	Water
Pyrantel tartrate	In-feed
Thiabendazole	In-feed, per orum paste

C. Other Pharmaceutical Compounds

Compound	Route of Administration	Usage
Azaperone	Parenteral	R_x, tranquilizer
Colloidal ferric sulfate	Oral	Iron supplement
Dinoprost tromethamine	Parenteral	R_x, prostaglandin
Fenprostalene	Parenteral	R_x, prostaglandin
Ferrous hydroxide	Oral	Iron supplement
Gleptoferran	Parenteral	Iron supplement
Iron dextran	Parenteral	Iron supplement
Isoflupredone acetate	Parenteral	Glucocorticosteroid
Oxytocin	Parenteral	R_x, aid to parturition
Pregnant mare serum/human chorionic gonadotropin (P.G. 600)	Parenteral	Estrous cycle stimulation/ synchronization
Thiamylal sodium	Intravenous	R_x, barbiturate anesthetic
Vitamin E/selenium	Parenteral	R_x, supplement

Table 67.3. Feed additives for swine feeds

Feed Additive and Use	Approved Levels (g/ton)	Withdrawal Period
Apramycin	150	28 days
ASP-250 (combination)	(250 total)	15 days
Chlortetracycline	(100)	
Sulfamethazine	(100)	
Penicillin	(50)	
Arsanilic acid or sodium arsanilate	45–90	5 days
Swine dysentery therapy	225–360	5 days
Bacitracin	10–250	None
Growth performance	10–30	None
Bacterial enteritis therapy	250	None
Bambermycins	2–4	None
Carbadox	10–50	10 weeks
Growth performance	10–25	10 weeks
Swine dysentery control	50	10 weeks
Chlortetracycline	10–400	Varies
Growth and feed efficiency	10–50	None
Diarrhea and rhinitis	50–100	None
Bacterial enteritis	100–200	None
Leptospirosis therapy	200–400	14 days
Dichlorvos	334–500	None
Fenbendazole	3 mg/kg body weight	None
Hygromycin B	12	15 days
Levamisole	720	None
Lincomycin hydrochloride	20–200	Varies
Growth performance	20	6 days
Swine dysentery control	40	6 days
Swine dysentery therapy	100	6 days
Mycoplasmal pneumonia control	200	6 days
Neo-terramycin (combination)	(120–290 total)	Varies
Neomycin	(70–140)	5–10 days
Oxytetracycline	(50–150)	5–10 days
Oxytetracycline	7.5–500	Varies
Growth performance	7.5–50	None
Bacterial enteritis control	50–100	None
Atrophic rhinitis control	50–150	None
Leptospirosis therapy	500	5 days
Penicillin (growth performance)	10–50	None
Penicillin-streptomycin (combination)	9–270	None
Growth performance	9–50	None
Bacterial enteritis control	50–90	None
Bacterial enteritis therapy	90–270	None
Pyrantel tartrate (continuous)	96	1 day
Single therapeutic treatment	800	1 day
Roxarsone	22.7–24	5 days
Tiamulin	10 or 35	Varies
Growth performance	10	None
Swine dysentery control	35	2 days
Thiabendazole	45.4–90.8	30 days
Tylosin	10–100	None
Growth performance	10–100	None
Swine dysentery therapy	100	None

Table 67.3. *(Continued)*

Feed Additive and Use	Approved Levels (g/ton)	Withdrawal Period
Tylan-sulfa (combination)	(200 total)	15 days
Tylosin	(100)	
Sulfamethazine	(100)	
Virginiamycin	5–100	None
Growth performance	5–10	None
Bacterial enteritis control	25	None
Swine dysentery therapy	100	None

feeding is closely related to the size and age of pig being medicated. The greatest response, a 10% improvement in rate of gain and a 5% improvement in feed efficiency, is observed in pigs from 5 to 40 kg body weight. Response declines with age and size until, at weights >100 kg, only a 2–3% response is expected. Diet cost, drug cost, and the expected pig response for a given compound are necessarily considered in these growth promotion applications of pharmaceutical compounds. When costs and the expected percentage improvement is known, the formula *Price* $1 \times F.E.$ $1 / Price$ $2 = F.E.$ 2 can be used to estimate the relative cost:benefit of applying a particular growth promoter. It should be noted that this formula does not account for the indirect benefits of enhanced rate of gain; thus, applying antimicrobial compounds is often a dietary and economic decision as well as one in which therapeutic effects are considered.

IN-FEED THERAPY. By law, therapeutic application of feed-additive compounds is allowed only within the strict confines of the product label. Specific disease conditions, dose ranges, and class of animal to be treated are required on such labels. All feed-additive drugs are OTC products and do not require a prescription or veterinary order for use. In fact, regulations on feed-additive use do not recognize such orders. Nevertheless, veterinary counsel is often sought regarding the pharmacologic and economic considerations of in-feed antimicrobial therapy. These are not simple decisions, for uses of a drug for therapeutic or production purposes can overlap. Also, swine producers, the feed industry, and veterinarians recognize and apply many compounds at approved levels for other than label indications. The use of tetracycline compounds, at levels approved only for leptospirosis therapy, in respiratory disease control is one common example. The Feed Additive Compendium (1990), published annually, is a valuable resource reference on approved feed additives, indications, and withdrawal times.

Unit-Dose Drugs. Unit-dose drugs are those packaged for parenteral, oral, or topical use. Included are OTC drugs and those with a veterinary prescription label. Only a few drugs, primarily hormones, steroids, and anesthetics, have a veter-

inary prescription label. Package inserts and labelling provided with unit-dose drugs are an underappreciated source of information on the pharmacology and approved uses of these products. Therapeutic doses for common unit-dose drugs are presented in Table 67.4.

PHARMACOLOGIC CONSIDERATIONS OF ANTIBACTERIAL COMPOUNDS. Antibacterial medications comprise the majority of pharmaceutical compounds used in swine practice. Pharmacokinetic information on absorption, tissue distribution, elimination, bacteriostatic or bacteriocidal effects, spectrum of activity, and possible adverse effects is necessary to establish the most appropriate therapy. While Table 67.4 presents guidelines for some doses, readers are encouraged to review drug labels for guidelines for specific doses.

Sulfonamides

ABSORPTION. Most sulfonamides are readily absorbed when administered orally.

ELIMINATION. Sulfonamides are eliminated through the liver and kidney; one-half the total ($t_{1/2}$) sulfamethazine is eliminated in 16 hours and $t_{1/2}$ sulfathiazole is eliminated in 1 hour.

STATIC/CIDAL. Sulfonamides used alone are bacteriostatic; sulfonamides plus trimethoprin are bacteriocidal.

SPECTRUM. Sulfonamides are broad spectrum but are of questionable value in treatment of chronic infections.

ADVERSE EFFECTS. Acute toxicity is unlikely; bacterial resistance may develop rapidly and persist over many generations.

DRUG FORMS AVAILABLE. Sulfonamides are available as an in-feed additive in combination with penicillin, tetracycline, and tylosin or as water-soluble preparations.

SULFONAMIDES AND HUMAN FOOD SAFETY. Low-level feeding, 110 ppm, of sulfamethazine or sulfathiazole has long been a standard therapy in

Table 67.4. Antimicrobial regimens for unit-dose drugs

Drug	Daily Dose[a] (mg/kg)	Interval[b]	Route[c]
Amoxicillin	11–13	SID	Oral
Ampicillin sodium	20	TID	SC, IM
Apramycin	13	SID	Oral
Dihydrostreptomycin sulfate	11	BID	IM
Erythromycin	11–22	SID	IM
Lincomycin hydrochloride	11	SID	IM
Neomycin	11	SID	oral
Oxytetracycline-LA200	20–33	q 72 hr	IM
Oxytetracycline	7–11	SID	IM
	44–55	SID	Oral
Procaine penicillin G	22–45,000 IU/kg	SID	SC, IM
Sulfachlorpyridazine	77–110	SID	Oral
Sulfaethoxypyridazine	110	SID	Oral
Sulfamethazine	240	SID	Oral
Sulfathiazole	220	SID	Oral
Tiamulin	9	SID	Oral
Tylosin	18–22	BID	IM
Ceftiofur	3	SID	IM
Enrofloxacin	2.5	SID	IM

[a]Doses noted are upper limits and most are extra-label; such doses may not be necessary and label doses may be proper.
[b]SID = once a day; BID = twice a day; TID = three times a day; q = every.
[c]SC = subcutaneous; IM = intramuscular.

control of atrophic rhinitis and enzootic pneumonia in swine. Due to continuing instances of violative residues in swine tissues in the United States, regulatory procedures are in process to withdraw approval of sulfamethazine for use in swine. Presently, use of sulfamethazine is approved only in combination with chlortetracycline and penicillin or tylosin for in-feed use. Persistence of sulfamethazine in feed systems and cross-contamination of nonmedicated feeds results in inadvertent tissue residues. Failure to withdraw all sources of the drug for an adequate time prior to slaughter is the primary cause of these residues. Sulfathiazole, like sulfamethazine, is approved for feed use only in combination products. Violative residue has not been a problem with sulfathiazole because of the more rapid rate of elimination.

Penicillins

ABSORPTION. All penicillins are well absorbed following parenteral administration; oral penicillin G is degraded by stomach acid.

DISTRIBUTION. All penicillin compounds are protein bound in plasma. High concentrations are in lung, skin, liver, kidney, and intestine; low concentrations are in joints, pleural fluid, and milk.

ELIMINATION. Pencillins are eliminated rapidly by way of the kidney; $t_{1/2}$ is 1–2 hours.

STATIC/CIDAL. Pencillins are bacteriocidal at low and high doses and low and high concentrations.

SPECTRUM. Penicillin G is used mainly against gram-positive organisms; ampicillin and amoxicillin are broad-spectrum drugs.

ADVERSE EFFECTS. Allergy, but rarely anaphylaxis, is a common adverse effect to the penicillins.

DRUG FORMS AVAILABLE. Only procaine penicillin G, ampicillin, and amoxicillin are approved for swine use. They are available as in-feed additives and intramuscular injections; amoxicillin is available as oral suspension for neonates. Benzathine penicillin is not approved for swine and can only be applied under extra-label use guidelines.

Tetracyclines

ABSORPTION. Oxytetracycline is well absorbed following parenteral administration. Orally, all are relatively well absorbed. Chlortetracycline has a higher bioavailability than oxytetracycline. Effective blood levels are attained 2–4 hours after oral administration. Food, calcium, iron, magnesium, and aluminum salts inhibit absorption.

DISTRIBUTION. Large concentrations are present in liver, kidney, urine, bone, and lung; tetracyclines pass from plasma into milk and readily cross into fetal circulation.

ELIMINATION. Elimination is through kidney, and liver; $t_{1/2}$ for chlortetracycline is 6 hours, for oxytetracycline, 10–12 hours.

STATIC/CIDAL. Low doses and low concentrations are bacteriostatic; high doses and high concentrations are bacteriocidal.

SPECTRUM. Tetracyclines are broad spectrum and are used against gram-positive and gram-negative bacteria, coccidia, rickettsias, large viruses, and mycoplasmas.

ADVERSE EFFECTS. Tetracyclines are nephrotoxic.

DRUG FORMS AVAILABLE. Tetracycline and chlortetracycline are available as in-feed additives alone and in combination with other antimicrobial compounds; oxytetracycline is available as intramuscular injection; and tetracycline and chlortetracycline are available as oral water-soluble powders.

Tylosin

ABSORPTION. Tylosin is well absorbed rapidly following parenteral administration. Orally, there is approximately 50% absorption; with intramuscular application, the duration of action is 12–24 hours.

DISTRIBUTION. Tylosin is not well distributed to the central nervous system but is well distributed to other tissues. It passes readily into milk in greater concentrations than into plasma.

ELIMINATION. Elimination is through liver and kidney; $t_{1/2}$ is 2–3 hours.

STATIC/CIDAL. Tylosin is bacteriostatic.

SPECTRUM. Tylosin is used primarily against gram-positive and some gram-negative bacteria, *Leptospira, Mycoplasma, Campylobacter,* and large viruses; resistance to tylosin develops rather slowly.

CAUTIONS. Tylosin should not be mixed with other drugs that are administered by parenteral routes.

ADVERSE EFFECTS. Basically, there should be no adverse affects; however, edema and erythema of rectal mucosa, anal protrusion, diarrhea, and pruritus have been reported in swine.

DRUG FORMS AVAILABLE. Tylosin is available as an in-feed additive, alone and in combination with other antimicrobial compounds; orally as a water-soluble powder; and as an intramuscular injectable solution.

Aminoglycosides: Streptomycin, Neomycin, Gentamicin, Apramycin

ABSORPTION. When these drugs are administered parenterally, absorption is good. When administered orally, absorption is poor, 3–8%; apramycin, 10%; all remain active in the gastrointestinal tract.

ELIMINATION. These drugs are eliminated rapidly by the kidney; $t_{1/2}$ is 2–3 hours; for gentamicin, $t_{1/2}$ is <6 hours. Residues may persist for extended periods in the kidney.

STATIC/CIDAL. Aminoglycosides are bacteriocidal at all concentrations; resistance develops rapidly and cross-resistance among aminoglycoside antibiotics is common.

SPECTRUM. These drugs are used primarily against gram-positive bacteria.

ADVERSE EFFECTS. These drugs are nephrotoxic.

DRUG FORMS AVAILABLE. Apramycin is available as in-feed or as a water-soluble powder; streptomycin as in-feed or as a parenteral injectable solution in combination with penicillin; gentamicin as an injectable solution for piglets less than 3 days of age and as an oral solution for swine dysentery therapy; neomycin in combination with tetracycline and as an oral solution.

Lincomycin

ABSORPTION. When lincomycin is administered orally, absorption is rapid with peak plasma levels reached in 2–4 hours; duration of action is 8 hours. When drug is administered intramuscularly, absorption is rapid with peak plasma levels reached in 10 minutes; duration of action is 12 hours (with intravenous administration, 12 hours).

DISTRIBUTION. Large concentrations are found in bone, heart, pericardial fluid, skin, and bile; there is poor distribution to the central nervous system.

ELIMINATION. Lincomycin is eliminated through liver, kidney, and milk; $t_{1/2}$ is 4 hours.

STATIC/CIDAL. Low doses and low concentrations are bacteriostatic. Lincomycin is bacteriocidal if high doses are administered and if organisms are quite sensitive; presence of erythromycin in body reduces or eliminates the action of lincomycin and vice versa.

SPECTRUM. Lincomycin is used mainly against gram-positive bacteria.

ADVERSE EFFECTS. When lincomycin is used, loose stools are reported; there is rectal protrusion with edema and transient erythema soon after pigs are placed on the drug.

DRUG FORMS AVAILABLE. Lincomycin is available as an in-feed additive, intramuscular injection, and oral water-soluble powder.

Erythromycin

ABSORPTION. Following parenteral administration, absorption is very good; after oral administration, absorption is variable.

DISTRIBUTION. Large concentrations can be found in lung, liver, kidney, and salivary gland; there is poor central nervous system distribution; and duration of action is 8–12 hours.

ELIMINATION. Erythromycin is eliminated primarily through the liver; $t_{1/2}$ is 4–6 hours; large concentrations are present and active in urine.

STATIC/CIDAL. Erythromycin is bacteriostatic.

SPECTRUM. The spectrum resembles that of penicillins, i.e., it is used primarily against gram-positive bacteria.

ADVERSE EFFECTS. There are minimal adverse effects.

DRUG FORMS AVAILABLE. Erythromycin is available as an injectable intramuscular solution and as an in-feed additive.

Tiamulin

ABSORPTION. Absorption is very good after oral administration.

ELIMINATION. Elimination is primarily through liver, some renal; $t_{1/2}$ is 8 hours with initial dose, 16 hours with later doses.

STATIC/CIDAL. Low doses and low concentrations are bacteriostatic; high doses and high concentrations are bacteriocidal.

SPECTRUM. The spectrum is for gram-positive bacteria; there are claims in labelling for *Actinobacillus* and *Treponema.*

ADVERSE EFFECTS. There are acute fatalities if pigs are concurrently consuming ionophore compounds.

DRUG FORMS AVAILABLE. Tiamulin is available as an in-feed additive and as an oral water-soluble powder.

Spectinomycin

ABSORPTION. After oral administration, absorption is very poor, approximately 7%; after parenteral administration, good. Spectinomycin remains active in the gastrointestinal tract.

ELIMINATION. Elimination is through kidney; $t_{1/2}$ is 2–3 hours.

STATIC/CIDAL. Low doses and low concentrations are bacteriostatic; high doses and high concentrations are bacteriocidal.

SPECTRUM. Spectinomycin is a broad-spectrum drug.

ADVERSE EFFECTS. There are no adverse effects likely.

DRUG FORMS AVAILABLE. Spectinomycin is available as an oral solution for administration to pigs less than 4 weeks of age.

NUTRIENT SUPPLEMENTATION.
Parenteral forms of iron, vitamin E, and selenium are approved for use in the prevention or treatment of dietary insufficiencies. Rapidly growing nursing piglets have a physiologic need for iron that exceeds the amount they obtain orally under contemporary production methods. The administration of 100–200 mg of iron by injection is a standard production practice.

ANESTHETICS AND TRANQUILIZERS.
Only three products, azaperone, thiamylal sodium, and methoxyflurane, are approved for analgesia, tranquilization, and anesthesia in swine. Other compounds approved for use in other species are perhaps more widely used. While an effective anesthetic, thiamylal sodium is difficult to administer and has a rather narrow margin of safety in the pig. Methoxyflurane must be administered with an anesthetic machine, a feature that greatly limits field application.

HORMONES.
Oxytocin is widely used as an aid in stimulating parturition and milk let-down. The synthetic form, available as 20 IU/ml of injectable solution, is perhaps overused by swine producers in attempts to maximize sow milk production. Inhibition of posterior pituitary release of endogenous oxytocin is possible with excessive, repetitive administration.

Prostaglandin compounds are approved for the induction of parturition in sows and gilts. While several are available in the U.S. market, only dinoprost tromethamine is labelled for swine use. Administration in late gestation allows scheduling of parturition. Animal caretakers may thus assist the delivery, a practice that reduces perinatal death loss.

Follicle-stimulating hormone and luteinizing hormone are available in a combination product for stimulating estrus. Marketed as an aid in synchronization of estrous cycles of puberal gilts, this hormone is also applied in attempts to return anestrous sows to cyclicity.

THERAPEUTIC METHODS.
Swine therapy is generally delivered through a carrier such as feed or the water supply. Individual treatment by parenteral injection or mass treatment is recommended in septicemic or acute respiratory conditions; for example, swine erysipelas or *Actinobacillus pleuropneumonia.* Per orum dosing is limited to small, nursing pigs. Medication delivery systems affect therapeutic decisions and efficacy of treatment.

In-feed medication is preferred by producers for mass treatment because of simplicity and economy. Disadvantages, especially in acute illnesses, are that depressed feed intake due to illness results in a less than desired therapeutic dosage. Approved in-feed dose limits do not account for subnormal feed intake associated with illness. Therapeutic response time in acute conditions is often delayed unless the nonmedicated feeds are completely removed from the system and replaced with medicated feeds. Cleaning and emptying feed systems is a difficult task on most farms and the general practice is to wait for existing feed supplies to be exhausted before medication is begun, often resulting in a therapeutic delay of a few days to a week. For these reasons, in-feed medication is most appropriate as ongoing therapy for existing endemic or chronic diseases and is less valuable in acute disease outbreaks.

Medication via water has the advantage of rapidly delivering medication to large groups of animals. Disadvantages include the limited control over dose due to variation in intake and wastage of medication. Additionally, poor solubility of many medications at concentrations needed for metering equipment, depressed water intake due to season, and the poor palatability of medications often limit therapy through the water supply. In certain types of water some medications lead to sedimentation and restriction of water flow through watering devices and pumps. If any other source of water is present, for example, that used to flush a gutter or to spray for cooling, pigs often will refuse to drink the medicated water. Water medication is used most often for an interim few days to allow time to prepare in-feed medication. Long-term medication through water is only rarely attempted. While estimates of daily water consumption may be utilized to calculate therapeutic doses based on intake, one must be aware of these substantial variations in intake that can exist (Table 67.5). Most soluble formulations of medication are also available in in-feed form.

Parenteral therapy, generally by intramuscular injection, is labor intensive and adds to the stress of already ill animals if careful handling is not practiced. However, it remains the preferred method of treatment in acute illnesses. The control over dose, timing, and animals selected for treatment provides the most rapid and efficacious disease intervention and therapeutic response. Penicillin, ampicillin, tetracycline, tylosin, linco-

mycin, erythromycin, and streptomycin are approved for parenteral treatment of nonsuckling swine. Gentamicin has approval for use in pigs less than 3 days of age.

Preslaughter withdrawal times are clearly stated on drug packaging and should be observed when medicating animals (Table 67.6). Certain

Table 67.6.   Preslaughter withdrawal time from drugs

Drugs	Days
Parenteral unit-dose	
Dihydrostreptomycin	30
Erythromycin	2
Lincomycin	2
Oxytetracycline	20
Oxytetracycline	22
Oxytetracycline	18
Oxytetracycline-LA200	28
Procaine penicillin G	7
Procaine penicillin G and	30
dihydrostreptomycin	
Tylosin	4
Parenteral unit-dose: neonatal pigs	
Lincomycin	2
Erythromycin	2
Gentamicin	40
Oral unit-dose	
Ampicillin trihydrate (water)	1
Arsanilic acid	5
Bacitracin methylene disalicylate	0
Carbadox	70
Chlortetracycline (water)	5
Chlortetracycline bisulfate and	15
sulfamethazine (water)	
Chlortetracycline, sulfathiazole, and	15
procaine penicillin (feed)	
Chlortetracycline, sulfamethazole, and	7
procaine penicillin (feed)	
Hygromycin B	15
Levamisole (feed or water)	3
Levamisole HCl	3
Lincomycin (feed or water)	6
Neomycin base	20
Roxarsone	5
Sodium arsanilate	5
Sodium sulfachlorpyridazine	4
Sodium sulfamethazine (feed)	15
Tetracycline hydrochloride (water)	4
Tiamulin	3
Tylosin (with vitamins, water)	2
Tylosin and sulfamethazine	15
Tylosin plus Hygromycin B	15
Oral unit-dose: neonatal pigs	
Chlortetracycline	1
Gentamicin	10
Spectinomycin dihydrochloride	
pentahydrate	21
Thiabendazole	20

Table 67.5.   Average daily water consumption

Size of Animal	Amount	
	(Liters/head/day)	(Gallons/head/day)
15–40 lb body weight	2–4	0.5–1
40–110 lb body weight	4–6	1–1.5
110–240 lb body weight	6–8	1.5–2
Pregnant sows	8–12	2–3
Lactating sows	16–20	4–5

products such as tylosin, oxytetracycline, erythromycin, and lincomycin may produce tissue irritation at the site of subcutaneous or intramuscular injections. Evidence of tissue inflammation and drug residues at the injection site may persist beyond the slaughter withdrawal time for that compound. Because of the possible need for carcass trimming at slaughter, it is advised that these compounds be used cautiously in pigs nearing slaughter weight and that the volume of drug per injection site be administered per label recommendations. The label literature accompanying each drug should always be reviewed, for withdrawal times may be changed or may vary with dose.

For further information see Upson (1981), Kunesh (1986), and Ensmenger et al. (1990).

REFERENCES

ENSMINGER, M. E.; OLDFIELD, J. E.; AND HEINEMANN, W. W. 1990. Feeding Swine. In Feeds and Nutrition. Clovis, Calif.: Ensminger Publishing Co., pp. 974–976.

FEED ADDITIVE COMPENDIUM. 1990. Minnetonka, Minn.: Miller Publishing Co.

KUNESH, J. P. 1986. Therapeutics. In Diseases of Swine, 6th ed. Ed. A. D. Leman, B. Straw, R. D. Glock, W. L. Mengeling, R. H. C. Penny, and E. Scholl. Ames: Iowa State Univ Press, pp. 803–812.

UPSON, D. W. 1981. Clinical Veterinary Pharmacology. Bonner Springs, Kans.: V. M. Publishing, Inc.

68 Preweaning Mortality

R. S. Cutler
V. A. Fahy
E. M. Spicer

PREWEANING MORTALITY is a major cause of wastage in pig production. Throughout the world, 4–10% of pigs born die during parturition and, depending on the farm, as many as a further 20–30% die before weaning. Recorded data collated from studies in different countries between 1985 and 1990 indicate that preweaning mortality rates are between 11.0 and 19% (Table 68.1). The best 20 herds in the Cambridge University Pig Management Scheme (Ridgeon 1989) had preweaning mortality rates of 11–12%; however, overall, herd performances depended more on total pigs born per year than preweaning mortality rates. While these data are representative of herds recorded, they likely underestimate mortality on other farms.

In Britain, Meat and Livestock Commission data indicate that preweaning rates have improved gradually over the years from 20.5% in 1961 to 11.0% in 1989. Further industrywide improvement in performance is possible and already has been achieved on many farms.

Over half of the preweaning deaths occur in the first 3–4 days of life and most of these occur in the first 36 hours. The majority of sows successfully rear their litters, but aged sows, sows with large litters, litters with uneven-sized pigs, and sick sows have disproportionately high preweaning mortality rates (Friendship et al. 1986; Pettigrew et al. 1986; Spicer et al. 1986a).

The key issue in the resolution of preweaning mortality problems relates to the attitude, diligence, and skill of the farrowing-house staff. Major contributing factors also include the distribution of creep heat, farrowing-crate and -pen design, disease control, and sow nutrition.

FACTORS AFFECTING PREWEANING MORTALITY RATE

Sow Feed Intake during Gestation. Birth weight in pigs is directly correlated with the energy intake of the sow during pregnancy. Feeding levels that increase sow body weight by about 30 kg during gestation will be sufficient to sustain acceptable birth weights. As a guide, for sows of weights 120 kg, 140 kg, 160 kg, and 180 kg, daily energy intakes of 23.6, 25.5, 27.4, and 29.4 megajoules of digestible energy (MJDE) are required. Additional energy allowances are required as environmental temperature falls below the lower critical temperature (LCT) (19°C for sows in stalls, 15°C for sows in groups). For every 1°C below the LCT, group-housed sows require an additional 3 MJDE/day. Individually stalled sows require a further 2.5 MJDE/day to allow for higher activity levels. Baker et al. (1969) and Libal and Wahlstrom (1977) found that weights of newborn pigs increased as sow gestation energy intake increased but plateaued at about 26.4 MJDE/day. Henry and Etienne (1978) concluded that over the range of 13–53 MJDE/day, average pig birth

Table 68.1. Preweaning mortality rates from published studies 1985–90

Country	Author	Number of Litters Studied	Number Weaned per Litter	Preweaning Mortality Rate (%)
Australia	Spicer et al. (1986a)	293	8.3	11.3
Brazil	Fonseca et al. (1988)	1043	NA	15.4
Canada	Friendship et al. (1986)	30 farms	8.2	18.6
France	Anon. (1985)	8825 farms (national survey)	9.0	13.5
Netherlands	Anon. (1986)	36,000 farms (national survey)	8.7	14.2
United Kingdom	Ridgeon (1989)	142 farms	9.3	12.3
United States	Cromwell et al. (1989)	1080	8.2	16.8
Venezuela	Gonzalez et al. (1987)	461	8.0	12.1
West Germany	Kunz and Ernst (1987)	7866	9.0	11.1
Yugoslavia	Radoc et al. (1985)	1375	9.12	16.3

weight increased by 15 g in gilt litters and 37 g in sow litters for each additional 4.4 MJDE fed per day during gestation (about 300 g of a 15% protein dry sow diet).

Fetal weight gain is most rapid in the last 10 days of pregnancy. Indeed, more than 50% of fetal energy reserves are deposited in the last month. Moser and Lewis (1981) concluded that supplemental fat in sow diets increased the fat content of milk and colostrum and decreased the preweaning mortality rate from 18 to 15.4%. Pettigrew (1981) indicated that it was necessary to feed 1 kg of fat to the sow in the last 10 days of gestation to demonstrate an effect on the piglets, and improvement in survival is unlikely if the average piglet birth weight is normal (i.e., 1.3–1.4 kg) and preweaning survival is >85%.

While the value of feeding fat in the last 10 days of gestation is perhaps equivocal, higher energy intakes for longer periods may be worthwhile. Cromwell et al. (1989) demonstrated that feeding an extra 1.36 kg/day of a maize or sorghum diet (14% protein) from day 90 of gestation resulted in greater sow weight gain to term, more piglets born alive, and as a consequence, more pigs alive at 21 days. Pigs born to high-feeding-level sows were heavier both at birth and at 21 days of age.

The key factor in piglet performance is likely to be birth weight in relation to the pigs' ability to withstand cold stress. Heavier pigs at birth have a LCT and can more readily mobilize their fat or glycogen reserves. Pettigrew et al. (1986) were unable to increase survival solely by feeding corn oil, indicating that the survival is due more to environmental factors than individual pig nutrition.

Farrowing-Crate Design. Where sows are closely confined, neonatal mortality rates from trauma are reduced compared to sows farrowing in unconfined conditions. The farrowing crate is that portion of the pen that confines the sow. Refinements have been added, which aim to slow the descent of the sow and which contribute to reduced losses from trauma. These include farrowing "cradles" (English et al. 1982) or narrow (500-mm) crates with vertically movable restraining bars (Muirhead 1987). The farrowing cradles are essentially hinged bars placed parallel to the sides of the farrowing crate. As the sow rises she pushes the bars upward, but as her body passes the bars, they fall back to the original position. When the sow lies down again, the position of the bars forces her to slow her descent and gives piglets in the lying area a chance to move to safety. The mortality rate from birth to 3 days of age was reduced from 11.1% for controls to 6.2% for the crates fitted with cradles. These refinements, however, do not prevent the sow from lying on her piglets when she moves from a sitting to a lying position.

Crate designs involving hydraulically controlled lower restraining bars reduce the risk of overlain pigs by supporting the sow as she descends. Once recumbent, the sow's pressure on the hydraulically controlled bottom bar keeps the bars wide apart and usually permits excellent access to the udder. When the sow stands she releases pressure on the bars and they return to the resting position, narrowing the internal crate width, ready to support the sow again when she descends.

Spatial Arrangements. Environmental factors clearly influence neonatal mortality. In farrowing pens, two spatial zones can be identified: a safe zone for the piglets where they can rest, free from the sow, and an interaction zone where the sow and the piglets occupy a common space. The safe zone (creep area) must be attractive, large enough for suckling pigs of all ages, and the piglets must find it comfortable (and prefer it) for resting.

The space requirements of pigs are relative to the thermal environment. In cool conditions piglets huddle and use about 60% of the space they would in warm conditions. Under hot conditions, rectangular creep areas of about 1.3 m² will provide adequate space for about 10 pigs 3 weeks of age (Baxter 1989).

The interaction zone is the most dangerous area in the farrowing pen. For the piglet, the greatest risk occurs when the sow changes position (to stand, sit, lie down, or move about), during feeding, or when the pen is being cleaned (Svendsen et al. 1986). The danger is compounded by the fact that piglets prefer lying against walls or close to the sow even when the temperatures in the pen are very high.

Danger increases if the sow acts suddenly; gentle, deliberate movements are readily tolerated, provided there is enough space within the crate for the sow to change position. However, movement is often restricted due to the length of the crate, in which case sows adapt their posture or movement but often at the risk of injury to themselves or their piglets (Baxter 1989).

The "blowaway unit" (Medata) is a device designed to attract piglets away from the danger zone. When the sow stands an electric cell is triggered and the device blows cold air under the sow, ideally causing any piglets in its path to seek the warmer (safer) environment of the crib. The units appear to be effective in reducing overlays but not necessarily overall preweaning mortality rate (Thacker and Barber 1987).

Heating. Curtis (1970) demonstrated that although newborn piglets can mobilize carbohydrate energy reserves in response to cold stress, they utilize it poorly due to physiologic immaturity. However, by 2 days of age the pig can mobilize and use efficiently both glycogen and lipids in response to cold. Thus, the 2-day-old pig has a much better response to cold stress. Protecting the newborn pig is the key priority.

Sows and piglets have different heat requirements. The newborn pig has a LCT of about 30–34°C, while the sow's LCT is closer to 15°C (Baxter 1989). When the deep body temperature is 39°C, at the LCT (34°C) the piglet can generate heat through increased metabolism and conserve heat to a limited degree by piloerection and vasoconstriction. When the environmental temperature falls below 34°C, the single newborn pig is subjected to cold stress and must utilize glycogen to maintain body temperature. In farrowing rooms maintained at 17°C, as many as 72% of newborn pigs have rectal temperatures below 37°C (Table 68.2). If deep body temperature is reduced by 2°C, piglet vigor is severely reduced. Sucking is less vigorous, and, hence, less colostrum is consumed. As a result serum IgG levels are lower than in piglets kept warm (Le Dividich and Noblet 1981; Kelly et al. 1982).

Due to their higher surface area to mass ratio, light pigs experience a larger body temperature decrease soon after farrowing than do heavier pigs, further emphasizing the importance of warmth for neonates (Ahlmann et al. 1983).

The electric or gas heater is the most common method of providing warmth for young pigs, but additional comfort factors are required to attract the neonate away from the sow toward the creep area. Large amounts of straw bedding have been the traditional method, but heated floors or heat pads, covered creeps, insulated or heated creep boxes, and carpet have replaced straw on many farms for convenience and safety. Good-quality, deep bedding (sawdust, wood shavings) raises the effective environmental temperature (relative to concrete floors) by 8°C and is attractive to piglets (Welch and Baxter 1986).

THE IMPORTANCE OF PROPERLY APPLIED HEAT. Following birth the piglet has an instinctive desire to remain close to the udder for the first 24–48 hours of life. Hence, an extra heat source needs to be provided for this period (Morrison et al. 1983).

With creep areas on both sides of the sow, piglets spent less time lying in the danger zone and mortality rate was reduced from 19.3% to 6.9% in the first 7 days of life (Table 68.3). Svendsen et al. (1986) reduced mortality rate in the first week of life from 7.0% to 1.1% by providing a movable heat source.

Morrison et al. (1983) also demonstrated the effect of farrowing-house temperature on survival. As farrowing-house temperature was increased from 13.6 to 20.5°C, live-weight gain to 7 days increased (135 g/day vs. 169 g/day) and 7-day mortality rate fell (15.1% vs. 10.7%).

Interaction of People and Pigs.
Hemsworth et al. (1986) studied the interactions between pigs

Table 68.2. Rectal temperature of piglets in farrowing houses maintained at 24°C and 17°C

Age (hours)	24°C (room temp.)	17°C (room temp.)
	Mean Rectal Temperature (°C)	
1	37.2	36
24	38.2	36.9
48	38.4	37.6
	Percentage of pigs with rectal temperatures below 37°C	
1	23	72
24	3	59
48	0	6

Source: English (1989).

Table 68.3. Effect of providing greater warmth for piglets from the moment of birth

	Basic Treatment[a]	Luxury Treatment[b]
Number of litters	15	15
Live-born pigs/litter	11.4	11.4
Live pigs at 7 days	9.2	10.6
Mortality %	19.3	6.9
Proportion of total resting time on day 1		
Against udder	54	22
In heated creeps	24	60

Source: Morrison et al. (1983).
[a]Heat lamp in corner of pen.
[b]Basic treatment plus heat lamps adjacent to place of birth during farrowing and in both side creeps for the first 48 hours.

and their handlers. The attitude of the handlers affects their behavior and when pigs were afraid of their handlers, a range of production characteristics (especially growth and reproductive performance) was affected.

Segundo et al. (1990) interviewed farm workers and asked them to rank job-related factors in order of importance and then express the degree to which they were satisfied or dissatisfied with these factors in their present job. Almost half of the respondents were dissatisfied because of a lack of bonus or incentive schemes together with the failure to hold formal meetings and discuss the physical performance of the farm. In more than 50% of cases the most dissatisfying aspects of employment were related to human behavior and human management. Dissatisfaction runs the risk of affecting the attitudes of farm workers and their interaction with the pigs.

Prime et al. (1989) demonstrated how training staff had a positive effect on pigs weaned and how it reduced neonatal mortality rate. Widespread extension campaigns failed to have the same effect because they failed to address specific issues.

Spicer et al. (1987) described how the successful operation of a crib care system for neonates depended heavily on the diligence of the individual operator. Two operators supervised the care of 600 farrowing sows and their progeny over a 4-week period. Operator A obtained 6.1% mortality rate (range 5.5–7.0%) in the first week of life, whereas operator B achieved a piglet mortality rate of 1.3% (range 0.95–1.63%) over the same period.

Vaillancourt et al. (1990) in a study to validate producer diagnosis of preweaning mortality against laboratory autopsy showed farms with lower preweaning mortality generally had a greater accuracy in diagnosing the cause of death, indicating that animal attendants with a sound knowledge of their job can apply strategies to reduce preweaning mortality.

Fostering. Effective fostering of piglets has a marked effect on preweaning mortality. For piglets to survive to weaning, they must be able to compete with littermates for heat and milk. To reduce competition each sow should only have a number of piglets equal to or less than her number of functioning teats. If large and small piglets are mixed within the same litter the smaller piglets suffer. English and Smith (1975) showed that the major factor affecting preweaning mortality was the degree of variation in birth weight. They showed that piglets of average birth weight were not competitive if mixed with larger piglets. Increased mortality is even more pronounced when small piglets are mixed randomly with large piglets. Marcatti Neto (1986) showed that piglets with a birth weight of 800 g had a preweaning mortality rate of 62.5% if left on their dam compared with 15.4% if fostered into groups with

equivalent birth weights. Piglets fostered according to birth weight also grew faster and had half the mortality rate of piglets fostered without regard to weight.

Several practical fostering strategies can be followed. Where only a few sows have farrowed and the number of piglets is in excess of functional teats, larger piglets can be removed from the sow for up to 4 hours to ensure that small piglets gain adequate colostrum. This is called split suckling and can be carried out for 2–3 days until more sows have farrowed and additional fostering opportunities are presented. Small piglets (800 g or less) can be removed from the sow, placed in a heated crib, and fed either colostrum milked from the sow or a colostrum substitute. Later, these piglets can be fostered to a sow selected for a low teat line and small nipples. Parity 1 sows make good foster mothers. Some larger farms collect all newborn piglets daily and then redistribute them according to piglet size and available teats on each sow.

Fostering should continue up to weaning. Any individuals that fall back can be transferred to a younger or smaller litter. If an entire litter is not thriving and the sow appears not to be milking well, swapping the unthrifty litter with a litter of vigorously sucking older piglets will stimulate greater milk production.

Hygiene. Good shed hygiene is important in reducing preweaning mortality. It may spell the difference between a microbial challenge that the piglet can cope with and an overwhelming infection. Thorough cleaning and disinfecting of empty sow crates helps to reduce environmental microbial burdens and more specifically to reduce pathogens that may be exclusive to newborn piglets. Svendsen et al. (1975) demonstrated that both morbidity and mortality rates associated with gastrointestinal disease were higher in herds with poor hygiene standards. The prevalence of diarrhea fell from 28 to 5% during the year an organized hygiene program was developed.

Field data on litters of unvaccinated gilts indicate that piglets born early in the week take 3–4 days before commencing to scour, whereas piglets born later in the week, when the environmental microbiological load is heavy, may show profuse diarrhea within 24 hours of life (Fahy, unpublished).

Studies with coccidiosis in pigs indicate that as hygiene measures lessen in intensity, coccidiosis emerges in herds where it had earlier been controlled, indicating that the severity of disease reflects the intensity of the challenge dose (Stuart and Lindsay 1985).

Sanitation programs based on thorough cleaning followed by disinfectants effective in the presence of organic matter are preferred.

SOW FACTORS AFFECTING PREWEANING MORTALITY

Litter Size.   Litter size increases with parity. Although preweaning mortality rate increases in numerical terms, more pigs are weaned from the larger litters, including those of older sows, until a plateau is reached between four and six litters. As litter size increases, the number of deaths during parturition increases. Also, birth weight decreases and the number of small pigs per litter increases (Table 68.4) (Spicer et al. 1986a).

Sow Health.   Spicer et al. (1986a) indicated that of overlain pigs that died 15% were associated with sow illness.

An assessment of sow health using the checklist below is an important part of farrowing-house management.

1. Assess water availability. Sows require up to 50 L/day during hot summer days. To consume this amount they need a drinker flow rate of 1.5–2.0 L/minute.

2. Assess feed intake. There should be a target of 6–7 kg/day (80 MJDE/day) average between farrowing and weaning.

3. Observe fecal consistency, urine (color and pus), vulval discharge, vomition, skin pallor, skin wounds, udder condition, abdominal bloat, and lameness.

4. Rectal temperatures may exceed 40°C during hot weather.

5. The normal resting respiratory rate is 12–30 breaths per minute. Observers should allow for a physiologic increase during hot weather.

6. Past history including genetic susceptibility to stress.

Stillbirths.   Stillborn pigs represent about one-quarter of all deaths between parturition and weaning and are the major cause of mortality in the pig production cycle. The percentage of pigs born dead varies from 4 to 10%; veterinary intervention is suggested when stillbirths exceed 8%. Approximately 70% of pigs classified stillborn are actually alive at birth. Although the heart is beating the pigs are severely anoxic and die within minutes of birth. The anoxia can be related to compression or premature rupture of the umbilical cord during farrowing (Randall 1978). In general, stillborn pigs weigh less than normal pigs and are born after a longer interpig interval (Spicer et al. 1986a) (Table 68.5).

Pigs are relatively neurologically mature at birth, hence a period of anoxia can be serious. As the duration of farrowing increases beyond 4–5 hours, or after 80% of the pigs have been born, the number of stillbirths increases. Most stillbirths occur in the last three pigs born. Svendsen and Andreasson (1980) found that sows kept in stalls during gestation had higher stillbirth rates than sows kept in pens, the difference due to longer farrowing time in stalls. In fact the duration of farrowing has a greater impact on stillbirths than parity. Long farrowing times also reduce neonatal survival.

Cutler and Prime (1988) found that parity, litter

Table 68.4.   Effects of litter size on preweaning mortality

Litter Size	Number of Litters	Total Born	Preparturient Deaths	Parturient Deaths	Number Weaned	Birth Weight (kg)	Piglets/Litter <0.8 kg	% Litters with Pigs <0.8 kg	Length of Parturition (min)
2, 3	3	2.7±0.3	0	0	1.4±0.3	1.60±0.22	0.0	0.0	53±23
4, 5	15	4.4±0.1	0.07±0.2	0.27±0.6	3.9±0.2	1.56±0.05	0.1	11.1	144±34
6, 7	25	6.7±0.1	0.08±0.3	0.16±0.5	6.1±0.1	1.51±0.04	0.1	8.3	117±18
8, 9	45	8.6±0.1	0.27±0.6	0.31±0.9	7.2±0.2	1.44±0.03	0.2	17.8	179±49
10, 11	69	10.6±0.1	0.41±0.9	1.93±5.9	8.8±0.1	1.35±0.02	0.4	25.0	154±14
12, 13	51	12.4±0.1	0.14±0.4	1.02±1.5	9.7±0.2	1.33±0.02	0.7	45.1	207±40
14, 15	24	14.3±0.1	0.46±0.7	1.08±1.1	11.0±0.3	1.29±0.04	1.1	66.7	158±18
16, 17	6	16.3±0.1	1.50±1.1	0.66±0.8	11.8±0.7	1.26±0.06	1.0	66.7	131±35

Source: Spicer et al. (1986a).

Table 68.5.   Number of stillbirths, mummies, and small weak pigs relative to their littermates in 238 litters

	Average Position in Litter	Average Interpig Interval (min)	Average Birth Weight (kg)	Time: Birth to First Suck (min)
All pigs	5.9±0.1	21±2	1.36±0.01	55±2
Stillbirths (SB)	7.9±0.4	70±26	1.17±0.04	
Littermates of SB	6.3±0.2	16±2	1.30±0.01	54±3
Mummies	6.3±0.6	16±4		
Littermates of mummies	6.5±0.2	16±1	1.35±0.01	48±3
Small weak (SW) pigs	5.8±0.7	9±2	0.82±0.07	133±35
Littermates of SW pigs	6.3±0.3	34±15	1.29±0.03	65±5

Source: Spicer et al. (1986a).

size, season, and the occurrence of stillborn pigs in previous litters influenced the number of stillborn pigs farrowed. About 60% of the sows farrowed litters without stillborn pigs; a small percentage of the sows farrowed most of the stillborn pigs. Sows farrowing two or more stillborn pigs per litter delivered 70% of the total number of stillborn pigs while comprising only 17.5% of the farrowings.

PARITY. As sows age, the duration of parturition increases and, consequently, the percent of stillborn pigs farrowed increases. An exception occurs for parity 1 sows, which have a higher percent of stillbirths than might be expected if the relationship between parity and stillbirths was truly linear. Parity 1 sows and aged sows (parity 7–10) have the greatest risk of farrowing multiple stillbirths.

PREVIOUS HISTORY OF STILLBIRTH. It is unusual for a sow to repeatedly farrow stillborn pigs. However, sows that had multiple stillbirths at the previous farrowing have an increased chance of farrowing multiple stillbirths at the next.

SEASON. The percent of stillbirths is higher for sows farrowing during summer (7.3%) than winter (6.4%), although the number of affected sows remains the same.

Strategies available to farrowing-house staff to reduce stillbirths include cooling sows in summer, inducing parturition in old sows, and providing close supervision of high-risk sows including manual assistance after the seventh pig has been delivered and interpig intervals exceed 30 minutes. Attempting to influence stillbirth rates by chemotherapy is generally unrewarding.

Induction of Parturition. Effective supervision of farrowing can reduce stillbirths and preweaning mortality on farm. For example, where savaging of newborn piglets is a problem, planned supervision of gilt farrowings may be necessary to reduce these losses (Spicer et al. 1986a).

Several techniques exist for manipulating the timing and duration of parturition. For greatest piglet vigor, induction of parturition should target farrowing sows 3 days on either side of the average gestation length for the herd. Farrowing sows earlier than day 111 or greater than 118 generally results in increased numbers of stillbirths. Piglet survival is highest when farrowing is induced on the due date for the sow, i.e., 115 days after service.

If the producer wishes to synchronize or to avoid weekend farrowings, early farrowings can be prevented by daily injections of progesterone (100 mg) from day 112 to 114. Meclophenamic acid, which causes an irreversible inhibition of prostaglandin synthetase, can be fed orally to achieve similar results (Hartmann and Whitely

1987). Farrowing is most commonly initiated with a 10-mg intramuscular injection of prostaglandin $F_{2\alpha}$ (PGF$_{2\alpha}$) or a synthetic analog (Dial et al. 1987). Sows farrow 2–44 hours following injection of PGF$_{2\alpha}$, with a mean time of 22–26 hours. This technique has proved valuable where all-in/all-out systems are practiced to ensure that all farrowing occurs within a current week.

Several authors have used PGF$_{2\alpha}$ injection followed by 20–30 IU oxytocin 18–24 hours later in an attempt to more closely control the time of parturition (Welp et al. 1984; Wilson 1984). This amount of oxytocin can induce uterine spasms in some sows, which increases the number of stillbirths and the number of manual interventions required (Welp et al. 1984). Holtz and Welp (1984) achieved reliable induction of parturition by combining 5 IU oxytocin with 1.5 mg of carazolol, a beta blocker that effectively blocks adrenalin receptors in the uterus and allows a lower level of oxytocin to initiate parturition. Carazolol shortens farrowing time and can reduce stillbirths, especially in older sows (Bostedt and Rudloff 1983).

Despite attempts to control the time of parturition with PGF$_{2\alpha}$ many sows still farrow overnight, making supervision impractical. To overcome this, Zerobin and Kundig (1980) injected 150 μg of clenbuterol, a beta-sympathomimetic agent, during labor but before the birth of the first piglet and delayed parturition for up to 15 hours. Zerobin (1980) showed that clenbuterol-induced uterine relaxation could be overridden with higher doses of oxytocin (20–40 IU) without uterine spasms. The following schedule using PGF$_{2\alpha}$ to initiate parturition followed by clenbuterol and carazolol/oxytocin has been successful for farrowings needing special supervision (Spicer et al. 1986b): 9:00 A.M., the sows are dosed with 10 mg PGF$_{2\alpha}$; sows not farrowed by 4:00 P.M. are injected with 150 μg clenbuterol to reduce the chance of overnight farrowing; parturition is reinitiated the following morning using 10 IU oxytocin plus 1.5 mg carazolol.

It is clear that several strategies for manipulating parturition are available. However, the success of these regimes in improving piglet survival relies heavily on the quality and assistance of the staff during and soon after farrowing.

CAUSES OF PREWEANING MORTALITY ON INTENSIVE PIG FARMS. Several papers have been published documenting the causes of piglet mortality (Nielsen et al. 1974; English and Smith 1975; Glastonbury 1976). These studies have been based mainly on the autopsy of dead piglets. However, English and Smith (1975) and Spicer et al. (1986a) supplemented autopsy findings with case histories so that factors predisposing to illness and death could be documented. The causes of preweaning mortality (Table 68.6) are therefore discussed in the light of the authors' experience, from veterinary diagnostic laboratory submis-

Table 68.6. Causes of preweaning mortality

Cause of Death	Number of Piglets	Deaths (percent) of Pigs Born	Age at Death[a] (days)	Birth Weight (kg)
Preparturient deaths	70	2.9		
Parturient deaths	132	5.4		1.15 ± 0.01[b]
Scours	42	1.7	6.5 ± 0.9	1.27 ± 0.04[b]
Overlay	50	2.1	4.2 ± 0.8	1.31 ± 0.5
Small, weak	22	0.9	2.3 ± 0.8	0.82 ± 0.07[b]
Anemia	30	1.2	2.5 ± 0.9	1.24 ± 0.05[b]
Splayleg	11	0.5	2.6 ± 0.4	1.20 ± 0.07[b]
Savaged	27	1.1	0.9 ± 0.3	1.14 ± 0.05[b]
Pneumonia	12	0.5	4.5 ± 0.9	1.30 ± 0.1
Other infections	23	1.0	9.1 ± 1.2	1.39 ± 0.07
Noninfectious	27	1.1	7.7 ± 1.8	1.24 ± 0.07
Nil diagnosis	8	0.3	7.2 ± 2.5	1.33 ± 0.06
Total deaths	454	18.7	4.7 ± 0.4	1.21 ± 0.02[b]
% deaths	18.7			

Source: Spicer et al. (1986a).
[a]Mean $\pm$ SE.
[b]Significantly ($p < 0.05$) less than the average birth weight of all piglets that survived to weaning (1.39 ± 0.01 kg).

sions, and from the documentation of other investigators.

Enteritis. Enteritis is the most common infectious cause of mortality in suckling pigs. While Glastonbury (1977) found that 5% of all deaths were due to enteritis, the Veterinary Investigation Service (Anon. 1959), Svendsen et al. (1975), and Spicer et al. (1986a) put the figure at 15%. The causative agents of enteritis in suckling pigs are transmissible gastroenteritis virus, porcine adenovirus, porcine epidemic diarrhea virus (*Coronavirus*), *Rotavirus, Calicivirus,* Aujesky's disease, Enterotoxigenic *E. coli, Clostridium perfringens* types A and C, *Salmonella* sp., *Coccidia* sp., *Campylobacter* sp., *Candida* sp., and *Strongyloides ransomi.* The reader is referred to specific chapters on each agent in this text. On a worldwide basis the organisms most commonly causing diarrhea are *E. coli, Coccidia* sp., and *Rotavirus. Clostridium perfringens* and transmissible gastroenteritis, while not cosmopolitan, are nonetheless important causes of enteritis, also.

ENTERITIS RISK FACTORS. The following factors associated with an increasing risk of enteritis are drawn from Svendsen et al. (1975).

1. Parity. Diarrhea was more prevalent in gilt litters, suggesting a lack of specific antibodies.
2. Litter Size. The incidence of diarrhea increased with litter size, suggesting lack of access to protective milk antibodies. Similarly, there was an increase in enteritis in litters where the sow was ill and/or dysgalactic.
3. Season. There was a higher incidence in winter, probably due to the effect of cold stress, particularly on small piglets.
4. Hygiene. There was a significantly higher level of mortality associated with a low level of hygiene.
5. Age. More than 60% of deaths occurred during the first week of life, with 10.5% occurring in the second week and 1.3% each week thereafter until weaning. The mortality rate is invariably proportional to age at onset and directly proportional to the duration of diarrhea (Table 68.7).

Table 68.7. The association between age at onset and duration of diarrhea and preweaning mortality

Duration of Diarrhea (days)	Number of Piglets	Number of Deaths[a]	% Deaths
No diarrhea[b]	1648	103	6.3
1	275	24	8.7
2	90	11	12.2[c]
3[c]	93	15	16.1[c]
Age at Onset of Diarrhea (days)			
1	125	7	5.6
2–4	123	27	22.8[c]
5–7	77	12	15.6[c]
8–11	64	4	6.3
12	64	2	3.1

[a]Includes deaths from all causes.
[b]Excludes piglets that died before 2 days of age.
[c]Significantly ($p < 0.05$) different from no diarrhea.

6. Intercurrent Disease. Fifty-three percent of animals that died of enteritis had intercurrent disease or disabilities, such as polyarthritis, respiratory disease, were small or starved pigs, or had been overlain.

PREVENTION. Immunity to enteric infections is achieved primarily from passive antibodies, which bathe the intestine and prevent attachment and multiplication of pathogens. It is imperative that piglets receive adequate antibodies from colostrum and milk. Vaccination is extremely effective against neonatal colibacillosis. Fostering of piglets to equalize litter size and supplementary feeding of little pigs with colostrum will prevent them from scouring and contaminating the environment. Both warmth and hygiene play pivotal roles in the prophylaxis of neonatal diarrhea.

TREATMENT. Piglets with diarrhea die when they lose approximately 10% of their total body fluid. In addition to specific antimicrobial therapy, based on known susceptibility patterns, piglets should be rehydrated. Although parenteral rehydration can be given by subcutaneous or intraperitoneal injection, oral rehydration via a stomach tube is the preferred method. The volume to be given daily is 10% of total body water (which is 75% of body weight); thus, a 1-kg pig requires 75 ml/day.

Overlay/Trauma. Overlay, the most common noninfectious cause of mortality of suckling pigs, accounts for the death of up to 20% of all pigs born alive. Most of the deaths occur within 72 hours of birth (Table 68.6).

Overlays occur more often in larger litters and more frequently in sow than gilt litters (Svendsen et al. 1986). Up to 30% of deaths occur around feeding time. It is obvious that the risk of overlay is directly proportional to the number of times a sow stands or sits; therefore, factors that cause sows to be restless increase the chance of overlay. These factors include inadequate water supply, sore teats, too many piglets for the number of active teats, annoying piglets, etc. Spicer et al. (1986a) reported that 44% of deaths due to overlay were secondary to illness in the sow or piglet. Sow illness was associated with overlay in 15% of cases. The illnesses included mastitis, agalactia, purulent vulval discharge, rectal prolapse, and inappetence.

Piglet illness or defect was associated with 26% of overlays. These included enteritis, anemia, splayleg, weakness, and pneumonia. Hungry piglets (agalactia or piglets in excess of active teats) will be constantly at the teats. This annoys the sow and leads to increased restlessness. Excessive or sudden noise may upset or startle sows causing them to stand; thus, there may be merit in providing continuous background noise (music). Also, staff should enter and leave sheds quietly. Inadequate creep heating is a common risk factor for overlays. Creep heaters that are too hot or too cold result in the piglets lying next to the sow with consequent risks.

NECROPSY FINDINGS. Overlays are usually not hard to diagnose at postmortem; often there is gross deformity. The pigs are described as flat-sided, with the tongue protruding. Death is caused by suffocation or exsanguination. In the former case there is often extensive bruising and edema of the subcutaneous tissue and muscles, particularly of the head and neck. The lungs are usually edematous and petechial, hemorrhages may be present in the upper respiratory tract. In those animals that die of exsanguination, the former lesions may be present in addition to the thoracic and/or abdominal cavities containing extravasated blood. The skull should be checked for fractures.

PREVENTION. Sows should be monitored closely for the first 48–72 hours after farrowing for signs of illness or restlessness, evidence of mastitis, udder edema, and vulval discharge. Check to determine if the sow is eating feed and passing feces. If there is inappetence, make sure that the water supply is adequate.

Since a highly disproportionate number of traumatic injuries occur during feeding, particular diligence should be applied at these times. Where splayed pigs are fostered, the foster mother should be a gilt for they seem more attentive to the shrieking sounds of an overlain piglet and will stand up to release it; thus, the incidence of overlay is less.

Small Nonviable Pigs. The newborn pig is very susceptible to cold stress and hypoglycemia. Piglets have no brown fat for thermogenesis (Le Dividich and Noblet 1983), thus rely first on increased metabolic rate and then shivering to maintain warmth (Mellor and Cockburn 1986). In the shivering process muscles initially utilize muscle glycogen stores. Once these are depleted they utilize blood glucose, which in turn is replenished from liver glycogen. However, the liver contains a limited supply of glycogen. In addition, glucogenolysis and glycolysis are poorly developed and cannot keep pace with the demand. To avoid hypoglycemia and hypothermia, the piglet needs an exogenous source of energy, i.e., colostral lactose. Normally the average piglet feeds 15 times in the first 12 hours of life; it takes in 15 ml feed (Werhahn et al. 1981) and consumes 6.75 g of lactose, 15.75 g of fat, and 18.75 g of immunoglobulin. Not only does colostrum provide lactose but it also has an enhancing effect on the hormonal and metabolic mechanisms controlling blood-glucose levels. A fasting newborn piglet can resist hypoglycemia for 18 hours under favorable conditions (28–32°C). However, this is reduced to 12 hours if the temperature is low (18–26°C) (Mellor and Cockburn 1986). Cold stress of the neonate reduces its acquisition of colostral immunoglobulins and results in an increased mortality rate (Blecha and Kelley 1981). Additionally, a delay in the intake of colostrum after birth will affect the absorption of immunoglobulins: a 4-hour delay in access to colostrum resulted in 15% of piglets having very low levels of serum immunoglobulin (Coalson and Lecce 1973). Low serum immunoglobulin resulted in higher mortality rates when compared with littermates with normal levels (Werhahn et al. 1981).

It is against this background that the fate of small pigs weighing less than 800 g is considered. There are two basic problems: there is a tendency for them to be born weak and they find it difficult to compete with larger littermates. In the study of Spicer et al. (1986a) pigs less than 800 g had a higher stillbirth rate (25% vs. total stillborn rate of 8.3%) and 62% of those born alive perished compared with the average of 11.3%. These pigs were assessed as being unable to survive under standard husbandry conditions because they were too weak and/or small. There was a relationship between birth weight and vitality as determined by the time taken to achieve an adequate first suck (Table 68.5). The number of small piglets increased markedly in litters with greater than 11 piglets; in litters of more than 13 piglets, 66% of the piglets weighed less than 800 g (Table 68.4). This may reflect a degree of fetal growth retardation due to a small placenta for some of the piglets (Mellor and Cockburn 1986).

The number of mammary glands per pig varies between 8 and 18, with an average of 12. However, 95% of sows have between 10–14 glands (Schmidt 1971). Therefore, the small pig born in a large litter will be the one most likely to miss out. Even assuming there are enough teats, in older parity sows with large udders, the top row of teats tend to point upwards when the sow is lying. The small piglet is often unable to reach such teats and will starve to death in the midst of plenty. Because the little pig may be hungry, it is continually at the teat and therefore at a significantly greater risk of being overlain.

NECROPSY FINDINGS. In the study of Spicer et al. (1986a) the average age of these small weak pigs at death was 2.3 days; those pigs that survived to that time appeared emaciated and dehydrated. At autopsy there was little if any food in the stomach. Glastonbury (1977) found that 17% of 538 dead sucking pigs had empty alimentary tracts. Bille et al. (1974) described a characteristic mahogany brown color of the striated muscle, which they considered almost pathognomonic for pigs dying of starvation. Often in pigs less than 24 hours of age there are no gross abnormalities, but the size of the pig and absence of food in the stomach prompts a diagnosis of hypoglycemia/hy-

pothermia. Nielsen et al. (1975) reported that 63% of 589 cases of death from septicemia were secondary to low birth weight and starvation.

PREVENTION AND TREATMENT. Small pigs need to be transferred to sows that have farrowed around the same time. Ideally, the foster sow should have an entire litter made up of small pigs. The foster dam also should have a teat line that is accessible to small piglets, hence gilts are favored as foster dams. If a piglet is splayed as well as small, a special crate or crib may be required where extra heating is provided. The crib is essentially a temperature-controlled box (30–32°C) where ill or disadvantaged neonatal piglets are kept for a limited period of time (usually less than 24 hours) to prevent them being overlain, or dying from hypothermia/hypoglycemia. While they are in the crib, piglets are fed colostrum milked from a sow during farrowing, or an artificial colostrum composed of hyperimmune sow serum and milk powder.

The piglets are fed 20 ml of colostrum every 1.5–2 hours using a standard human baby bottle and teat during the period staff are available. An electrolyte solution is available for the piglet to drink overnight. If they do not have a swallowing reflex (or will not drink), they can be fed using a human infant nasogastric tube (French Gauge 8, 40 cm in length). Colostrum can be obtained from the sow by injecting 1–2 ml of oxytocin intramuscularly after one or two pigs have been born; after a few minutes colostrum can be milked into a wide-necked container and stored at 4°C or frozen until needed.

Piglets selected to be placed in the crib are those with a high risk of perishing, e.g., the small, weak, or splayleg pigs. Piglets that have survived overlay also respond well to a period in the crib. The rule is, "if in doubt, place them in the crib." Piglets suffering from hypothermia should be warmed in a bucket of warm water (43°C) for 5–10 minutes, dried, given 20 ml of colostrum via a stomach tube, and placed in the crib.

After receiving nourishment and warmth for 24–48 hours, most piglets can be fostered back to a sow selected for having small nipples and a low teat line to ensure they can readily gain access to milk. Using these approaches small, weak piglet mortality rate can be reduced to 10–20% compared with 40–60% under normal husbandry practices.

Neonatal Hemorrhagic Anemia. Spicer et al. (1986a) reported that of 2224 live-born piglets from 238 litters, 4.8% were born anemic (as determined clinically by skin pallor) or became anemic shortly after birth as a result of bleeding from the navel cord. This syndrome has been reviewed by Penny (1980). The preweaning mortality rate of anemic piglets was 35% compared with 10% for the remainder of the population. Anemia was the primary cause of death in 75% of cases, and a major predisposing factor in the death of the remainder. In subsequent studies using packed-cell volume (PCV) as an indicator, it was found that 6.8% of piglets were anemic (PCV <20%) and 30% of litters had at least one anemic piglet. Statistical analysis indicated that there was a familial effect (Connaughton, personal communication; Spicer et al. 1986a).

Factors contributing to piglet anemia include deficiency of vitamins K or C; toxicity due to mycotoxins, pentachlorophenol, and warfarin; isoimmune thrombocytopenic purpura and isoimmune hemolytic anemia; *Eperythrozoon suis* infection; and anemia in the sow. Martelli et al. (1989) reported that the propensity to bleed is due to a hypofibrinogenemia. Penny (1980) cites data showing that some of these pale pigs have below-normal levels of platelets. These effects may follow blood loss and the consequent platelet dilution, from movement of extracellular fluid into the vascular compartment.

NECROPSY FINDINGS. Often the umbilical cord is large and fleshy. The skin, muscles, mucous membranes, and internal organs are pale. There is no evidence of internal bleeding, which allows differentiation from pale overlain pigs. PCVs as low as 5% have been recorded.

TREATMENT. Piglets at risk of bleeding can be identified by their large fleshy umbilical cords; there is also excessive blood on the floor of the farrowing pen. The umbilical cord should be ligated as soon as possible in these pigs. Because they appear to bleed for longer than normal pigs, tail docking and ear notching should be left until 10–14 days of age. Iron is best given orally or in drinking water because excessive bleeding from the injection site follows intramuscular injection. Physical stress of handling should be avoided for this may greatly increase the tissue demand for oxygen and acute cardiac failure may ensue.

Splayleg. Splayleg appears in newborn pigs as a severe but transient paresis in the hind limbs, and less frequently, in the forelimbs, which characteristically results in postural collapse with a failure of limb adduction. Piglets with splayleg assume a posture in which the hind limbs or all four legs are laterally extended (Ward 1978). (See also Chapter 5, Nervous and Muscular Systems.) Splayleg is usually evident within 2–4 hours of birth and the problem has resolved in piglets that survive to 5 days of age. Often one or several pigs in a litter are affected. However, on occasions the whole litter may be affected.

Spicer et al. (1986a) demonstrated that splayleg occurred in 5.5% of piglets born alive and 24% of these died. This is higher than the 0.5% incidence reported by Ward (1978). In the former study afflicted piglets were unable to compete with litter-mates and died of starvation, hypoglycemia, hypothermia, or were overlain. The death rate was higher (66%) in pigs with both fore- and hind limbs affected. The average age at death (2.6 days) was similar to that of small weak pigs (2.3 days). There was a greater incidence of splayleg from older sows (0.8/litter) than gilts (0.1/litter).

Splayleg piglets were generally lighter than average (1.20 ± 0.07 kg) and took longer than average to obtain a first suck. Those that survived to weaning had a reduced growth rate to weaning. Offspring from Landrace boars had a 13.7% incidence of splayleg compared with 4.5% for Large White boars and 3.4% for hybrid boars (p<0.01). Ward (1978) states that in Britain the disease is particularly prevalent within the Landrace and Large White breeds. Identical matings do not always result in splayleg piglets being born (Dobson 1968). The etiology of splayleg is multifactorial, comprising genetic and environmental components (Ward 1978). Slippery floors are an important predisposing environmental factor in the development of splayleg (Kohler et al. 1969). Deficiencies of choline and thiamine may result in splayleg as does the presence of zearalenone mycotoxin in sow feed, but correction of these problems does not universally eliminate the abnormality.

There is still confusion over the lesion present in splayleg piglets. The basic defect is thought to be hypoplasia of the myofibrils of individual muscle fibers. However, this lesion is often seen in clinically normal piglets as well as affected ones (Thurley and Done 1969). Dobson (1968) was unable to detect myofibrillar hypoplasia in splayed pigs. Bergmann (1976) proposes that hypoplastic, dystrophic, and metabolic insufficiencies occur in the skeletal muscles of splayleg pigs.

TREATMENT AND PREVENTION. The standard treatment for splayleg is to tape the legs so that they cannot abduct further than in the normal standing position. Where the hind limbs extend forward beneath the animal after taping, a strip of tape is attached to the middle of the first tape and taken back over the tail to join to a third strip encircling the body in the flank region. If an animal can move adequately after taping it can be left with the sow. If, however, they still have difficulty in walking, as is often the case with small piglets that are splayed or piglets splayed in both front and back legs, they need to be transferred to a crib to avoid starvation and crushing. By 3–4 days of age the problem has usually resolved. This also coincides with disappearance of histologic signs of myofibrillar hypoplasia. Massaging the affected limbs has been advocated as a treatment for splayleg (Blackburn, personal communication). Where slippery floors are a risk factor old mats or carpets in the farrowing crate for the first 48–72 hours of life are worthwhile.

Savaging. Spicer et al. (1986a) found that savaging accounted for 11% of mortalities and was confined predominantly to gilt litters. This is consistent with the findings that a high proportion of gilts attempt to savage at least their first piglet (English et al. 1977). Pomeroy (1960) suggested that pain and fear predisposed gilts to savage their piglets. Some gilts savage the entire litter. Savaging was responsible for increased mortality in piglets born outside the working hours of the piggery staff (13.7% compared with 9.7%) and was the only significant factor in this mortality difference; only 2 of the 27 piglets savaged were born during working hours (Spicer et al. 1986a). During savaging the gilt will snap at any piglet that wanders into reach, behavior similar to that of savage sows toward stockpeople. Cronin (1989) found that the level of savaging in gilt litters was higher when animals farrowed in a large pen bedded with straw compared with those farrowed in a standard farrowing crate. Therefore, it seems that the farrowing crate, in addition to minimizing overlay, also protects (in part) piglets and attendants from savage sows.

NECROPSY FINDINGS. The lesions of savaging are essentially caused by the crushing effect of the sow's teeth and jaw. In some cases savaged piglets may be difficult to distinguish from overlain pigs. However, the lesions are more focal and the skin is often broken.

PREVENTION. Nothing can be done to prevent savaging in the absence of staff. Therefore, if savaging is a problem, induced farrowing will ensure that the majority of gilts farrow when staff are present. Savage gilts may be tranquillized (1–2 mg/kg of azaperone). Piglets can be placed in a small cage in the creep area as they are born. Once farrowing is over the piglets can be removed from the cage and the gilt usually makes no further attempt to savage. The birth weight of savaged piglets was significantly lower than the average birth weight of pigs that survived to weaning (Table 68.6). Gilts that savage their litters were likely to be those mated at lower body weights (Spicer et al. 1985). The lower weights at mating were due to inadequate feed intake between selection and mating of submissive pigs penned in groups of 20. The problem was overcome by periodically drafting off those animals that appeared to be losing weight. It is unusual for dams to savage more than one of their litters, therefore there is no valid reason to cull them.

Pneumonia. Pneumonia is responsible for the death of around 1% of all live-born piglets (Fahmy and Bernard 1971; Bille et al. 1975; Spicer et al. 1986a). The pneumonia is primarily a bronchopneumonia, and gilt litters are more often affected than sow litters. Bille et al. (1975) found a higher incidence in winter, but the pneumonia was unrelated to the indoor climate or level of hygiene. In the majority of cases, only one pig per litter was affected, with an average incidence of 10% per litter. Organisms responsible included *Streptococcus* spp., *Bordetella bronchiseptica*, *Pasteurella* spp., *Moraxella* spp., *Escherichia coli*, *Actinomyces pyogenes* (Bille et al. 1975), and *Staphylococcus aureus*, *Pasteurella multocida*, *Pseudomonas aeruginosa*, and *Citrobacter freundii* (Spicer et al. 1986a).

In a study of pneumonia in 55 baby pigs, Kott (1983) isolated *Hemophilus parasuis*, *Mycoplasma hyorhinis*, and *Bordetella bronchiseptica*. Pleuropneumonia due to *Actinobacillus pleuropneumoniae* has been reported by Bille et al. (1975) and Cameron and Kelly (1979). Septicemia due to the same organism has been reported in suckling pigs (Thomson and Rhunke 1963).

Although *Mycoplasma hyopneumoniae* infections are commonly thought to begin in weaned pigs, the organism has been reported from pneumonic suckling pigs; however, microbiologic evidence that it is common in such lesions has not been forthcoming (Ross 1986).

TREATMENT AND PREVENTION. With the above mortality level treatment is probably not a practical procedure due to the difficulty of identifying the affected animals. However, where the problem exceeds the 1% level of mortality, injecting gilts at farrowing with an appropriate antibiotic to lower excretion rate may be warranted. Ensuring piglets adequate access to colostrum is recommended, for the low incidence of the disease and its occurrence in predominantly gilt litters suggests that lack of specific antibody is a major contributing factor.

Generalized Infections and Septicemia.

Field data indicate that as many as 2% of the population die of septicemia (Driesen 1990). Affected piglets were all less than 48 hours of age. Nielsen et al. (1975) surveyed 28,000 live-born pigs and found that 2.1% died from septicemia, 37% of which were a primary septicemia and the remainder were secondary to low birth weight, starvation, or preceding illness; 44% of mortalities occurred before 3 days of age. In the survey by Spicer et al. (1986a), septicemias in the first week of life were a secondary manifestation of other causes of mortalities. However, generalized infection was responsible for most deaths in the second and third week of life. Organisms isolated and diseases produced included *Actinobacillus suis*: septicemia, arthritis, peritonitis, and meningitis; *Citrobacter freundii*: septicemia, meningitis, alpha-hemolytic streptococci-septicemia, arthritis, and meningitis; *E. coli*: septicemia and peritonitis. Glastonbury (1977) and Nielsen et al. (1975) found *E. coli* and beta-hemolytic streptococci were the most common causes of septicemia in dead suckling pigs.

A major predisposing factor in generalized infection would appear to be the quantity and specificity of maternal antibodies absorbed by piglets. In this regard Nielsen et al. (1975) found (1) a significantly higher incidence in piglets of sows with mastitis and agalactia, (2) mortality rate from septicemia increased with litter size, (3) a higher incidence in open versus closed herds, and (4) a higher incidence in winter.

NECROPSY FINDINGS. Often there is excess fluid and small amounts of fibrin in the serous cavities. Lungs may be edematous and fail to collapse. Jaundice, subserosal petechial hemorrhage, and mild dehydration may be seen.

TREATMENT AND PREVENTION. The most common isolates are *Streptococcus* spp. and *E. coli,* thus broad-spectrum antibiotics may be of use therapeutically, but the success rate is low (Driesen 1990). Prevention should be aimed at ensuring adequate intake of colostrum for all piglets and providing adequate heating.

Miscellaneous Causes of Death. This group includes anal atresia, cleft palate, renal hypoplasia, hydrocephalus, and accidental death and accounts for 1.2% of all pigs born alive (Spicer et al. 1986a).

REDUCING PREWEANING MORTALITY RATE.

Cutler et al. (1989) reported farm studies where preweaning mortality rates were reduced by 5–7%, largely due to a reduction in overlain pigs. This response followed recognition that lack of attention to detail on the part of farm staff was a major factor contributing to high preweaning mortality rate. After an intensive period of "hands on" staff training and demonstration, farrowing-house performance was monitored. In addition to increasing the intensity of staff training and staff awareness, the following measures were considered to be instrumental in decreasing neonatal mortality:

1. PVC pipes (100 mm diameter) were installed to reduce internal farrowing-crate width and to slow the descent of the sow. The pipes ran the length of the crate, were suspended by light chains from the top bar of the farrowing crate, and rested about 350 mm above the floor, just above the udder. When the sow rose she easily displaced them.

2. Creep areas were made draught free and comfortable. Washable carpet was glued to heavy galvanized metal (350 × 600 mm) and installed in the creep area to improve comfort. The carpet was comfortable, attracted the pigs, and did not become excessively hot. The carpet was disinfected between litters. In the studies of Cutler et al. (1989), excessively high creep temperatures associated with poor heating adjustment or black flooring material that absorbed heat were just as detrimental as inadequate heating. Sawdust, wood shavings, or straw would also be suitable.

3. An additional heat lamp was provided toward the rear of the sow during the farrowing period and the immediate 24 hours afterward to reduce the chance of chilling newborn pigs and to provide an extra (lateral) creep area.

4. A heated crib was made available for the care of sick pigs and to house small or supernumerary pigs during split suckling sessions.

5. Small or weak pigs were fed by bottle or stomach tube. Supplementary milk feeding was available when the pigs in large litters were split suckled and required extra feeding. Pigs were supervised to ensure access to colostrum, or they were dosed with hyperimmunized sow serum mixed with milk to supplement colostrum.

6. Thorough hygiene programs were followed for the farrowing house and processing equipment.

7. An active and expert fostering program was introduced. It was based on cross-fostering early in lactation and equalizing piglet weights within the litter. Foster mothers were carefully selected on the basis of temperament and udder conformation. Fostering became an ongoing process, and pigs that slipped behind were moved to more compatible litters.

8. Sows were regularly inspected and promptly treated if they were sick. A health check list was followed.

9. A vaccination program against neonatal colibacillosis was implemented.

REFERENCES

AHLMANN, K.; SVENDSEN, J.; AND BENGTSSON, A. C. 1983. Rectal temperature of the newborn pig. Rep 31. Swedish Univ of Agriculture, Lund.

Anon. 1959. A survey of the incidence and causes of mortality in the pigs. 1. Sows survey. Vet Rec 71:777–786.

BAKER, D. H.; BECKER, D. E.; NORTON, H. W.; SASSE, C. E.; JENSEN, A. H.; AND HARMON, B. G. 1969. Reproductive performance and pregnancy development in swine as influenced by feed intake during gestation. J Nutr 97:489–498.

BAXTER, S. H. 1989. Neonatal mortality: The influence of the structural environment. In Manipulating Pig Production, 2d ed. Ed. J. L. Barnett and D. P. Hennessy. Werribee, Aust.: Australasian Pig Science Association, pp. 102–109.

BERGMANN, V. 1976. Elektronenmikroskopische Befunde an der Skelettmuskulatur von Neugeborenen Ferkeln Mit Gratschstellung. Arch Exp Vet Med 30:239–260.

BILLE, N.; NIELSEN, N. C.; LARSEN, J. L.; AND SVENDSEN, J. 1974. Preweaning mortality in pigs. 1. The perinatal period. Nord Vet Med 26:294–313.

BILLE, N.; LARSEN, J. L.; SVENDSEN, J.; AND NIELSEN, N. C. 1975. Preweaning mortality in pigs. 6. Incidence and cause of pneumonia. Nord Vet Med 27:482–495.

BLECHA, F., AND KELLEY, K. W. 1981. Cold stress reduces the acquisition of colostral immunoglobulin in piglets. J Anim Sci 52:595–600.

BOSTEDT, H., AND RUDLOFF, P. R. 1983. Prophylactic

administration of the beta-blocker carazolol to influence the duration of parturition in sows. Theriogenology 20(2):191–196.

CAMERON, R. D. A., AND KELLY, N. R. 1979. An outbreak of porcine pleuropneumonia due to *Haemophilus parahaemolyticus*. Aust Vet J 55:389–390.

COALSON, J. A., AND LECCE, J. G. 1973. Influence of nursing intervals on changes in serum proteins (immunoglobulins) in neonatal pigs. J Anim Sci 36:381–385.

CROMWELL, G. L.; HALL, D. D.; CLAWSON, A. J.; COMBS, G. E.; KNABE, D. A.; MAXWELL, C. V.; NOLAND, P. R.; ORR, D. E.; AND PRINCE, T. J. 1989. Effects of additional feed during late gestation on reproductive performance of sows: A cooperative study. J Anim Sci 67:3–14.

CRONIN, G. M. 1989. Neonatal mortality: The influence of maternal behaviour. In Manipulating Pig Production, 2d ed. Ed. J. L. Barnett and D. P. Hennessy. Werribee, Aust.: Australasian Pig Science Association, pp. 110–115.

CURTIS, S. E. 1970. Environmental-thermoregulatory interactions and neonatal pig survival. J Anim Sci 31:576–587.

CUTLER, R. S., AND PRIME, R. W. 1988. Reducing stillbirths in pigs. Aust Adv Vet Sci, pp. 111–113.

CUTLER, R. S.; SPICER, E. M.; AND PRIME, R. W. 1989. Neonatal mortality: The influence of management. In Manipulating Pig Production, 2d ed. Ed. J. L. Barnett and D. P. Hennessy. Werribee, Aust.; Australasian Pig Science Association, pp. 122–126.

DIAL, G.; ALMOND, G. W.; HILLEY, H. D.; REPASKY, R. R.; AND HAGEN, J. 1987. Oxytocin precipitation of prostaglandin-induced farrowing in swine: Determination of the optimal dose of oxytocin and optimal interval between prostaglandin F$_{2\alpha}$ and oxytocin. Am J Vet Res 48:966–970.

DOBSON, K. J. 1968. Congenital splayleg of piglets. Aust Vet J 44:26–28.

DRIESEN, S. J. 1990. Intensive care systems for weak piglets: Colostrum substitute and crib system. Rep PRDC. Dep Primary Industries and Energy, Canberra, Australia.

ENGLISH, P. R., AND SMITH, W. J. 1975. Some causes of death in neonatal pigs. Vet Annu 15:95–104.

ENGLISH, P. R.; SMITH, W. J.; AND MacLEAN, A. 1977. The Sow-Improving Her Efficiency. Ipswich, Eng.: Farming Press Ltd.

ENGLISH, P. R.; DIAS, M. F. M.; AND BAMPTON, P. R. 1982. Evaluation of an improved design of farrowing crate. Proc Int Congr Pig Vet Soc, Mexico City, p. 289.

FAHMY, M. H., AND BERNARD, C. 1971. Causes of mortality in Yorkshire pigs from birth to 20 weeks of age. Can J Anim Sci 51:351–359.

FRIENDSHIP, R. M.; WILSON, M. R.; AND McMILLAN, I. 1986. Management and housing factors associated with piglet preweaning mortality. Can Vet J 27:307–311.

GLASTONBURY, J. R. W. 1976. A survey of preweaning mortality in the pig. Aust Vet J 52:272–276.

————. 1977. Preweaning mortality in the pig: Pathological findings in piglets dying between birth and weaning. Aust Vet J 53:310–314.

GONZALEZ, A. C.; NECCHINACCE, H.; AND DIAZ, I. 1987. A comparison of some production traits in gilts and sows. In Informe Anual. Inst Prod Anim, Univ Cent Vennez, pp. 127–128.

HARTMANN, P. E., AND WHITELY, J. L. 1987. Farrowing. Univ Sydney, Post Grad Comm Vet Sci Proc 95(1):937–941.

HEMSWORTH, P. H.; BARNETT, J. L.; AND HANSEN, C. 1986. The influence of handling by humans on the behaviour, reproduction and corticosteriods of male and female pigs. Appl Anim Behav Sci 15:303–314.

HENRY, Y., AND ETIENNE, J. 1978. Alimentation energetique du porc. J Res Porc Fr, p. 119.

HOLTZ, W., AND WELP, C. 1984. Induction of parturition in sows by prostaglandin-oxytocin programs. Proc Int Congr Pig Vet Soc, Ghent, p. 378.

KELLY, K. W.; BLECHA, F.; AND REGNIER, J. A. 1982. Cold exposure and absorption of colostral immunoglobulins by neonatal piglets. J Anim Sci 55:363–368.

KOHLER, E. M.; CROSS, R. F.; AND FERGUSON, L. C. 1969. Experimental induction of spraddled-legs in newborn pigs. J Am Vet Med Assoc 155:139–142.

KOTT, B. E. 1983. Chronological studies of respiratory disease in baby pigs. M.S. thesis. Iowa State Univ.

LE DIVIDICH, J., AND NOBLET, J. 1981. Colostrum intake and thermoregulation in the neonatal pig. Biol Neonate 40:167–174.

————. 1983. Thermoregulation and energy metabolism in the neonatal pig. Ann Rech Vet 14:375–381.

LIBAL, G. W., AND WAHLSTROM, R. C. 1977. Effect of gestation metabolizable energy levels on sow productivity. J Anim Sci 45:286.

MARCATTI NETO, A. 1986. Effect of crossfostering on piglet preweaning performance. Arq Brasil Med Vet Zootec 38:413–417.

MARTELLI, P.; MANOTTI, C.; AND ROSSI, L. 1989. Haemorrhagic syndrome (Hypofibrinogenaemia) in piglets: preliminary note. Sel Vet 30:1673–1677.

MELLOR, D. J., AND COCKBURN, F. 1986. A comparison of energy metabolism in the newborn infant, piglet and lamb. Q J Exp Physiol 71:361–379.

MORRISON, V.; ENGLISH, P. R.; AND LODGE, O. A. 1983. The effect of alternative creep heating arrangements at two house temperatures on piglet lying behaviour and mortality in the neonatal period. Anim Prod 36:530–531.

MOSER, B. D., AND LEWIS, A. J. 1981. Fat additives to sow diets—a review. Pig News Inf 2:265–269.

MUIRHEAD, M. R. 1987. Mortality. Univ Sydney, Post Grad Comm Vet Sci Proc 95(1):525–558.

NIELSEN, N. C.; CHRISTENSEN, K.; BILLE, N.; AND LARSEN, J. L. 1974. Preweaning mortality in pigs. 1. Herd investigations. Nord Vet Med 26:137–150.

NIELSEN, N. C.; RIISING, H. J.; LARSEN, J. L.; BILLE, N.; AND SVENDSEN, J. 1975. Preweaning mortality in pigs. 5. Acute septicaemia. Nord Vet Med 27:129–139.

PENNY, R. H. C. 1980. Navel bleeding and the pale pig syndrome. Vet Annu 20:281–290.

PETTIGREW, J. E. 1981. Supplemental dietary fat for peripartal sows: A review. J Anim Sci 53:107.

PETTIGREW, J. E.; CORNELIUS, S. G.; AND MOSER, R. L. 1986. Effects of oral doses of corn oil and other factors on preweaning survival and growth of piglets. J Anim Sci 62:601–612.

POMEROY, R. W. 1960. Infertility and neonatal mortality in the sow. Neonatal mortality and foetal development. J Agric Sci (UK) 54:31–56.

PRIME, R. W.; FAHY, V. A.; RAY, W.; CUTLER, R. S.; AND SPICER, E. M. 1989. On farm validation of research—lowering preweaning mortality in pigs. Rep PRDC. Dep. Primary Industries and Energy, Canberra, Australia.

RANDALL, G. C. B. 1978. Perinatal Mortality: Some problems of adaption at birth. Adv Vet Sci Comp Med 22:53–81.

RIDGEON, R. F. 1989. Pig management scheme results. In Special Studies in Agricultural Economics No. 7. Dep Land Economy, Univ of Cambridge, England.

ROSS, R. F. 1986. Mycoplasmal diseases. In Diseases of Swine, 6th ed. Ed. A. D. Leman, B. Straw, R. D. Glock, W. L. Mengeling, R. H. C. Penny, and E.

Scholl. Ames: Iowa State Univ Press, pp. 978–1010.

SCHMIDT, G. H. 1971. Biology of Lactation. San Francisco: W. H. Freeman.

SEGUNDO, R. C.; ENGLISH, P. R.; AND BURGESS, G. 1990. Factors affecting the job satisfaction of pig stockpeople. Proc Int Congr Pig Vet Soc, Lausanne, p. 407.

SPICER, E. M.; DRIESEN, S. J.; FAHY, V. A.; AND HORTON, B. J. 1985. Trauma–overlay and savaging of baby pigs. Aust Adv Vet Sci, p. 122.

SPICER, E. M.; DRIESEN, S. J.; AND FAHY, V. A. 1986a. Causes of preweaning mortality on a large intensive piggery. Aust Vet J 63:71–75.

SPICER, E. M.; PRIME, R. W.; AND FAHY, V. A. 1986b. Controlled induction of parturition in swine. Aust Adv Vet Sci.

SPICER, E. M.; DRIESEN, S. J.; FAHY, V. A.; WILLIAMSON, P. L.; AND CONNAUGHTON, I. D. 1987. Preweaning mortality in pigs. Univ of Sydney, Post Grad Comm Vet Sci Proc 95(1):979–985.

STUART, B. P., AND LINDSAY, D. S. 1985. Coccidiosis. In Swine Consultant. Veterinary Learning Systems.

SVENDSEN, J.; AND ANDREASSON, B. 1980. Perinatal mortality in pigs: Influence of housing. Proc Int Congr Pig Vet Soc, Copenhagen, p. 83.

SVENDSEN, J.; BILLE, N.; NIELSEN, N. C.; LARSEN, J. L.; AND RIISING, H. J. 1975. Preweaning mortality in pigs. 4. Diseases of the gastrointestinal tract in pigs. Nord Vet Med 27:85–101.

SVENDSEN, J.; BENGTSSON, A. C.; AND SVENDSEN, L. S. 1986. Occurrence and causes of traumatic injuries in neonatal pigs. Pig News Inf 7:159–170.

THACKER, P. A., AND BARBER, E. M. 1987. Use of planned drafts in an attempt to reduce preweaning mortality in baby pigs. Can Agric Eng 29:197–200.

THOMSON, R. G., AND RUHNKE, L. 1963. *Haemophilus septicaemia* in piglets. Can Vet J 4:271–275.

THURLEY, D. C., AND DONE, J. T. 1969. The history of myofibrillar hypoplasia of newborn pigs. Zentralbl Vet Med 16[A]:732–740.

VAILLANCOURT, J. P.; STEIN, T. E.; MARSH, W. E.; LEMAN, A. D.; AND DIAL, G. D. 1990. Validation of producer-recorded causes of preweaning mortality in swine. Proc Int Congr Pig Vet Soc, Lausanne, p. 386.

WARD, P. S. 1978. The splayleg syndrome in new born pigs: A review. Vet Bull 4:279–295.

WELCH, A. R., AND BAXTER, M. R. 1986. Responses of newborn pigs to thermal and tactile properties of their environment. Appl Anim Behav Sci 15:203–215.

WELP, C.; JOCHLE, W.; AND HOLTZ, W. 1984. Induction of parturition in swine with a prostaglandin analog and oxytocin: A trial involving dose of oxytocin and parity. Theriogenology 22:509–520.

WERHAHN, E.; KLOBASA, F.; AND BUTLER, J. E. 1981. Investigation of some factors which influence the absorption of IgG by the neonatal piglet. Vet Immunol Immunopathol 2:35–51.

WILSON, M. R. 1984. Synchronisation of farrowing using a combination of oxytocin and prostaglandin administration: An aid to piglet survival rates. Proc Int Congr Pig Vet Soc, Ghent, p. 279.

ZEROBIN, K. 1980. Possibilities to influence the motility of the uterus during parturition and during puerperium in swine. Proc Int Congr Pig Vet Soc, Copenhagen, p. 26.

ZEROBIN, K., AND KUNDIG, P. 1980. The control of myometrial function during parturition with a B2 mimetic compound Planipart (clenbuterol). Theriogenology 14(1):21–35.

69 Culling and Mortality in Breeding Animals

S. D'Allaire

R. Drolet

EFFECTIVE culling strategies are an essential part of herd health management, since culling policies influence herd economic performances in many different ways. Removal rates influence the herd age distribution: an excessively low removal rate is often associated with a higher proportion of older sows, which are more prone to certain diseases and may have lower production levels. A high removal rate is generally associated with a shift toward younger females, which are less productive, and with an increase in the number of nonproductive sow days (Dijkhuizen et al. 1986). These factors contribute to decrease both litters per sow per year and pigs weaned per sow per year, and to increase the cost per weaner (Dagorn and Aumaitre 1979; Kroes and Van Male 1979; Pattison et al. 1980a). A high removal rate requires many replacement animals, which will increase disease risks and the cost of production. Difficulty in supplying replacement animals may also lead to a suboptimum population that will decrease the herd output (Kroes and Van Male 1979).

Boar culling is a part of breeding-herd management that is often neglected by producers. Good boar culling policies are also important for they facilitate the replacement program. Planning problems associated with boar introduction are considerable, taking into account that boars should be kept in quarantine for a month and that their full workload will be attained only at 1 year of age.

Evaluation of a culling program should include determination of the annual removal rate, mean parity or age at removal, reasons for culling and death, and for females, the interval between the last production event and removal.

ANNUAL REMOVAL RATE. Determining the annual removal rate is the first step in assessing a herd culling program. This rate is defined as the number of animals removed from the herd during a year divided by the average inventory, multiplied by 100%. The number of animals removed should include deaths; however, culling and death rates should be analyzed separately. Annual removal rates of 35–55% for sows have been reported in different surveys (Svendsen et al. 1975; Dagorn and Aumaitre 1979; Kroes and Van Male

1979; Pattison et al. 1980a; Friendship et al. 1986; D'Allaire et al. 1987). Because these values represent an average rate, higher or lower rates may be found on individual farms; however, high removal rates seem to be more frequent than excessively low rates. Muirhead (1976) suggested a removal rate target of 39% (i.e., 36% for culling plus 3% for death).

High boar removal rates seem to be more frequent than excessively low rates. In a study involving 84 commercial herds, the annual removal rate for boars averaged 59% (D'Allaire and Leman 1990). Higher rates are to be expected for seedstock herds to ensure genetic improvement and to reduce the genetic lag for commercial producers.

Comparisons of sow removal rates between herds or studies are often difficult because the definition of "average female inventory" may be different. The inventory may refer to sows only or to sows and gilts, with gilts being introduced at different times of their production cycle. It has been suggested for a better standardization of terms to consider only mated females in the calculation of the annual removal rate. On some farms, however, culling of gilts introduced into the breeding herd but not yet mated is very high and may require more investigation.

The annual removal rate for the herd is also influenced by specific circumstances, such as a change in the inventory, a change in the culling policies, and the average length of the lactation period. A decrease in the inventory will increase the culling rate for the corresponding year; conversely, an increase in the inventory may decrease the rate if the producer culls less extensively in order to increase the number of females. On some farms, an involuntary cycle is established in culling patterns. For example, a producer realizes that the herd is getting older and reacts by culling more extensively that year. The following year, the rate may be lower because a large proportion of the herd is now very young. This is not counterproductive in itself but it makes production planning more difficult and herd output less constant. Information on such changes in culling policies is needed to evaluate a program. A cycle in culling patterns may also occur in newly established or repopulated herds.

861

The average length of lactation for the herd may also influence the annual removal rate. Herds with shorter lactation periods tend to have higher removal rates even though the mean parity at culling is similar (D'Allaire et al. 1989). A reasonable explanation is that the number of litters per sow per year is higher when the lactation period is shorter. Because a sow has a certain probability of being culled during each farrow-to-farrow interval, more farrowings per year result in a higher annual probability of being removed.

The productive lifetime of a sow can also be evaluated by the replacement rate, which is defined as the total number of animals entering the herd divided by the average inventory, multiplied by 100%. The removal rate and replacement rate should be similar in a stable herd if the inventory remains constant. However, in a herd undergoing expansion, the replacement rate may be higher than the removal rate. Conversely, when reduction in herd size occurs, the replacement rate may be lower than the removal rate. Therefore, population dynamics should be considered when analyzing these rates.

PARITY OR AGE AT REMOVAL. The second step in evaluating a culling program is to determine the mean parity of sows at removal. This parameter will indicate the average length of time that sows stay in the herd; however, because the mean can be influenced by extreme values, a parity distribution of removed sows is usually more informative. Breeding-life expectancy is low in most swine breeding herds. Several studies reveal that the average parity at removal lies between 2 and 4, but it can vary from 2 to 8 for a particular herd (Pomeroy 1960; Einarsson and Settergren 1974; Svendsen et al. 1975; Dagorn and Aumaitre 1979; Arganosa et al. 1981b; D'Allaire et al. 1987; Stein et al. 1990).

A high proportion of females are removed in their early parities. First-parity females often represent a large proportion of the cullings, with percentages of up to 40%. Considerable losses are involved with such high removal rates of young females. Kroes and Van Male (1979) reported that the cost per weaner is highest in the first litter and decreases over the next two litters. Many authors reported that from 50% to 69% of the removals occur before the fourth litter (Pomeroy 1960; Dagorn and Aumaitre 1979; Arganosa et al. 1981b; D'Allaire et al. 1987); however, this range is merely a reflection of the parity distribution of all females in the herd, as the risk of being removed is usually similar among parity groups 1–5, increases slightly in parity groups 6–8, and increases substantially in parities 9 and over (Stein et al. 1990).

The lifetime breeding expectancy for boars is estimated at 15–20 months but varies considerably between 0.3 and 38.5 months (Le Denmat et al. 1980; Arganosa et al. 1981a; D'Allaire and Leman 1990).

REASONS FOR CULLING SOWS. Sows are culled when they are considered unsuitable for further production. A knowledge of the reasons for removal can be beneficial in identifying underlying diseases or management problems. The list of reasons can be as complete as desired, but for the purpose of data analysis, the reasons should be summarized according to a few categories. Data from different studies reveal a general pattern of removal in which reproductive failure is the main reason for culling, followed by old age, inadequate performance, locomotor problems, death, and milking problems. The culling pattern, however, varies considerably among herds and among parities (D'Allaire et al. 1987).

Reasons for removal can be analyzed according to two rates: a proportionate rate, which is the percentage of all removals attributable to a specific reason, and a reason-specific removal rate (D'Allaire 1987). The proportionate rate is useful in indicating the relative importance of a given reason in the total culling picture and helps in determining priorities for improving the herd. The reason-specific removal rate is defined as the number of animals removed for a specific reason divided by the average inventory, multiplied by 100%, and measures the annual probability of an animal being removed for that specific reason and indicates the extent of a problem. This latter rate is more informative and is not influenced as much by the number of animals removed for other reasons as is the proportionate rate. Unfortunately, in most of the literature, only the proportionate rate is used. Table 69.1 outlines the proportionate rate for six reasons for removal; results were obtained from 12 studies involving more than one herd. In Table 69.2, proportionate rate, reason-specific removal rate, and mean parity at culling or death are reported for nine reasons for removal.

Reproductive Failure. Reproductive failure is used to define a variety of conditions: no observed puberty in gilts, no observed postweaning estrus, regular and irregular returns to estrus, negative pregnancy diagnosis, failure to farrow, and abortion. Reproductive failure is the main reason for culling, representing between 13% and 49% of all removals. Thus, good reproductive management with an increased awareness of the reproductive state of each sow at all times should be emphasized.

Young females are more likely than older sows to be culled for reproductive failure (Dagorn and Aumaitre 1979; D'Allaire et al. 1987; Stein et al. 1990). The average number of litters produced by these culled sows is between two and four. Inefficient estrous detection, mating at an early age, improper male stimulation, use of young boars that are less mature and can more easily be over-used, improper nutrition, infectious or toxic agents, management practices, and environment may be responsible for these high levels of culling for reproductive failure in young females. Older sows that have stayed in the herd also have undergone a selection process and may be less prone to reproductive failure.

Failure to conceive or to maintain pregnancy after a successful mating is the major problem reported, accounting for 21–37% of the animals removed. Females that did not conceive are often found late into their presumed gestation. Sows culled for return to estrus stayed in the herd for an average of 79 days, whereas sows removed because they failed to farrow remained for 121 days after the first service (Pattison et al. 1980a). It is important to decrease this period of nonproductive days, for it is very costly because of the extra feed and labor required as well as the underutilized production facilities. To decrease this period, management must differentiate between late loss of pregnancy and late detection of nonpregnant females; these two variables indicate different problems that necessitate different solutions on a farm.

The proportion of females culled because they do not exhibit estrus either at puberty or weaning is low, ranging from 3% to 8%. The acceptable period between introduction or weaning and mating differs among farms and may be partly responsible for the variation in proportion of animals culled. The length of the period allowed is worth investigating; on some farms it might be too short, especially for younger females, which usually have a longer interval from weaning to breeding, thus unnecessarily increasing the number culled. Abortions do not seem to be a major reason for removal, generally representing less than 2% of all cullings.

When the proportion of culling for reproductive failure is high, a slaughter check may be useful to compare the reasons given by the producer and the physiologic status of reproductive tracts. Josse et al. (1980) examined 338 reproductive tracts and compared the findings with the reasons for culling reported by producers. The reason for removal could not be substantiated in 36% of the cases. Einarsson et al. (1974) found similar results in a study of genital organs in gilts: of 54 gilts culled for anestrus, 23 had apparently active corpora lutea and 2 were pregnant. Possible explanations for these discrepancies are inefficient estrous detection or pregnancy testing, silent heat, or physiologic changes occurring between the decision of culling and slaughtering.

Old Age. Old age is often the second most likely reason for removal, accounting for 3–33% of all removals; the average parity at culling varies between 7 and 9. As the proportion of sows

Table 69.1.   Percentage of sows removed from herds for each of six reasons

Number of Herds or Sows	Reproductive Failure	Old Age	Inadequate Performance	Locomotor Problems	Death	Other	Country	Source
5118 herds	39.2	27.2	8.4	8.8	6.5	9.9	France	Dagorn and Aumaitre (1979)
7242 sows	32.4	16.8	14.0	8.9	11.6	16.3	United States	D'Allaire et al. (1987)
7 herds	28.8	3.9	10.0	15.0	NA[a]	42.3	Sweden	Einarsson and Settergren (1974)
6 herds	32.6	16.7	15.7	9.7	NA	25.3	Korea	Joo and Kang (1981)
593 sows	49.1	13.8	4.2	10.6	NA	22.2	France	Josse et al. (1980)
75 herds	31.3	10.1	8.0	19.7	3.8	27.1	Norway	Karlberg (1979)
60 herds	37.5	24.4	13.8	11.8	NA	12.5	England	Pattison et al. (1980a)
468 herds	21.4	17.1	32.5	NA	NA	29.0	England	Pomeroy (1960)
774 sows	29.6	11.1	9.4	11.0	10.7	28.2	United States	Stein et al. (1990)
140 herds	12.9	33.4	20.6	14.0	NA	19.1	Canada	Stone (1981)
9 herds	41.4	2.9	16.7	9.7	11.9	17.4	Denmark	Svendsen et al. (1975)
1657 sows	33.7	14.5	12.4	4.3	20.3	14.8	Belgium	Van Snick et al. (1965)

Source: Chagnon et al. (1991). Can J Vet Res 55:180–184.
Note: Results based on 12 studies.
[a]NA = not available.

Table 69.2. Reasons for removal and average parity at removal in 7242 females

Reasons for Removal	Percentage of All Removals	Reason-specific Removal Rate	Average Parity at Removal
Reproductive failure	32.4	16.1	2.37
Inadequate performance	16.8	8.4	5.11
Old age	14.0	6.9	7.11
Death	11.6	5.7	3.40
Locomotor problems	8.9	4.4	2.93
Peripartum problems	7.2	3.6	4.18
Transfer	2.9	1.4	0.34
Other diseases	1.6	0.8	2.76
Miscellaneous	4.6	2.3	3.18
Total	100.0	49.6	3.77

Source: D'Allaire et al. (1987). Can J Vet Res 51:506–512.

removed for other reasons decreases, the percentage of sows culled because of old age increases. Overlappings between old age and inadequate performance are likely to occur, for old sows may experience a decrease in productivity. Old age is a relative term; some producers routinely cull sows as soon as the fifth or sixth parity and others only after the tenth litter. Some researchers suggest culling older sows when productivity in terms of live-born pigs is comparable with that of gilts. This method, however, only takes into account the number of live-born pigs. According to a model developed by Dijkhuizen et al. (1986), the economic optimal herd life for average-producing sows is generally 10 parities. Rarely is it economically beneficial to cull sows before parity 8, considering the economic losses associated with the cost of replacement, the lower litter size and farrowing rate, and the longer interval from weaning to mating in younger sows. Their model took into account the annual replacement rate, the average parity of farrowed and removed sows, the average slaughter price of culled sows, and the cost of replacement gilts.

Inadequate Performance. This category includes a variety of reasons: small litter size at farrowing or weaning, high preweaning mortality, and low piglet birth or weaning weights. Inadequate performance is usually ranked as the second or third most common reason for culling sows, with a range of 4–21% of removals attributable to this category. Pomeroy (1960) reported that inadequate performance was the main reason for removal, accounting for 33% of all cullings. However, management was different in those years; herds were smaller, usually less than 10 sows, and were farrowing outside. The preweaning mortality was also high, up to 48% during certain months of the year.

In a herd with a high level of culling for inadequate performance, a parity analysis is useful. If too many young animals are culled for this reason, action should be taken because it is well known that litter size increases with parity until the third litter. In such a herd, the benefit of culling sows for the purpose of improving productivity might be lost because of a decrease in herd productivity associated with a high proportion of young sows. Culled females will have to be replaced by gilts that are not very predictable. Dijkhuizen et al. (1986) reported that parity 1 sows with a litter size of even 50% below average should not be culled on economic grounds. Moreover, the repeatability of litter size is low, which means that predicting the next production from the previous one is very inaccurate.

Locomotor Problems. Locomotor problems refer to a variety of conditions, including lameness, injury, posterior paralysis, fracture, and downer sow syndrome. The proportion of sows removed for locomotor disorders varies between 9% and 20%; some reports, however, have indicated a percentage as high as 45%. In these sporadic cases of high removal for locomotor disorders, housing and flooring types have often been incriminated (Jones 1967; Smith and Robertson 1971). In general, group housing is associated with more injuries, presumably because several animals of different ages are kept together; whereas individual housing is related to a higher incidence of joint, foot, and leg problems, possibly because of a lower frequency of movement.

In swine breeding herds, flooring and housing are closely related and thus it is often difficult to separate the effects of one from the other. Certain types of housing will rarely be found with a specific type of flooring; for example, crates will rarely, if ever, be seen on an earthen floor. There may also be an interaction between the flooring type and the housing type. Moreover, flooring can vary in many respects, including design, material used, quality and characteristics, and hygienic conditions associated with it. All these variables should be considered when analyzing a problem of high culling for locomotor problems.

The adverse effects of slatted floors have often been associated with foot and leg problems, but most of these reports have pertained to faulty slats that were damaged, poorly designed with rough edges, or too wide apart (MAFF 1981;

Muirhead 1981). Injuries are frequently recorded for sows tethered or kept in stalls, and often the only reason for injury is the faulty distribution of nonslippery and nonabrasive materials included in the concrete (MAFF 1981).

The likelihood of a sow being culled for lameness decreases as her age increases (Jović et al. 1975; Dagorn and Aumaitre 1979; D'Allaire et al. 1987). Sows culled for locomotor problems produce, on average, only three litters. The reasons that culling for locomotor problems is more frequent in young females are unclear; among possibilities are marginal nutritional problems, management or environment differing for young females compared with older sows, or a selection process by which sows less prone to problems are kept in the herd. Another possibility is an abrupt change in the environment that could trigger locomotor problems. Gilts are often kept in a type of housing or on flooring that differs from the housing or flooring used for sows; then, after farrowing, the sows have to adapt to a new environment. The same is often true when moving from the growing to the breeding period.

Milking Problems. Milking problems include mastitis, agalactia, low milk production, and poor mothering abilities. This category may overlap with inadequate performance, for milk failure can influence weaning weights and preweaning mortality. The proportion of sows culled for these reasons ranges from less than 1% up to 15%. In some reports, milking problems are included with peripartum problems. In a study from Minnesota (United States), sows culled because of milking problems produced an average of 4.6 litters (D'Allaire et al. 1987). Svendsen et al. (1975) reported that parity 2 sows were more prone to culling for mastitis. Halgaard (1983) observed that the risk of mastitis increased with increasing age up to the third or fourth litter; however, for farrowing fever the trend was opposite, with a marked fall in relative risk as age increased.

Death. Sow mortality may represent important losses to the herd, yet it is often neglected by those intervening in swine production. In fact, many producers are not aware of the extent or causes of death in their herds. Knowledge of the main causes of death can help reduce high mortality rate in severely affected herds.

The proportion of sows removed because of death ranges from 4% to 20%, giving a herd death rate of 3–8%. On some farms, however, the death rate is as high as 14% (Svendsen et al. 1975; D'Allaire et al. 1987). Straw (1984) suggested a target death rate of 3% for herds of 150 sows or less, and 5% for herds of 200 or more sows. Variation in death rates can be attributed to differences in management, nutrition, environment, and culling policies; some producers preferably cull their sick sows quickly, hence, reducing

the death rate. It is important to know whether the producer includes sows euthanized for humane reasons in the death category or in a category specific to each cause of euthanasia, because the rates in each category will be influenced accordingly. In most studies, euthanasia is included in the death category. The cause of death, if known, is useful and can reveal underlying problems.

Information on seasonality of sow losses is limited. A higher incidence of mortality during hot summer months was reported from a Canadian study, in which all herds were kept in total confinement year round (Chagnon et al. 1991). In the United Kingdom, however, Jones (1967, 1968) observed that more than 55% of the sows died during the winter months. In these latter reports, sows were kept inside during winter and outside during summer.

Sows appear to be at risk most during the peripartum period (Madec 1984). In a study of sow mortality, 42% of all deaths occurred during this short period of the reproductive cycle (Chagnon et al. 1991) (Table 69.3).

The mean parity at death varies between 3.4 and 4.2; the variation among studies and possibly among herds may be a reflection of the relative incidence of certain causes of sow losses, as some of them appear to be age related. Cystitis-pyelonephritis occurs more frequently in older sows (Madec 1984), whereas some locomotor problems seem to be more prevalent in young breeding stock (Spencer 1979; Doige 1982; D'Allaire et al. 1987).

CAUSES OF DEATH. Assessing the reasons for death is the first step in understanding and controlling the factors influencing sow losses due to mortality. Many conditions responsible for death in sows are often reported by the producers as sudden or rapid deaths associated with some rather nonspecific premonitory clinical signs. It appears then imperative when trying to ascertain the causes of death in a particular herd, to have a significant number of sows necropsied during the year to identify the general pattern of causes of death. Sows die from a variety of causes; some, however, seem to have a greater incidence. Relevant data from studies on sow mortality are shown in Table 69.4.

Table 69.3. Stages of reproductive cycle for mated gilts and 133 dead sows

Stages	Number of females	Percentage
Peripartum[a]	56	42.1
Lactation[b]	22	16.5
Postweaning	8	6.0
Gestation	47	35.4

Source: Chagnon et al. (1991).

[a]From 3 days before the predicted farrowing date to 3 days after farrowing inclusively.

[b]From 3 days after farrowing until weaning.

Table 69.4. Main causes of death in sows

Causes of Death			Number of Herds	Total Sow Inventory (duration of study)	Number of Dead Sows	Number of Sows Necropsied	Death Rate (%)	Country	Source
First	Second	Third							
Cystitis-pyelonephritis	Peritonitis	Septicemia	1	457 (1 year)	46	36	10.1	England	Jones (1967)
Complication at parturition	Cystitis-pyelonephritis	Endocarditis	106	2488 (1 year)	96	81	3.9	England	Jones (1968)
Heart failure problems	Locomotor problems	Urogenital	NA	NA[a]	NA	1002	NA	Yugoslavia	Senk and Sabek (1970)
Locomotor problems	Heart failure	Cystitis-pyelonephritis	9	436 (4 years)	114	109	6.4	Denmark	Svendsen et al. (1975)
Torsion abd. organs[b] metritis	Cystitis-pyelonephritis	Gastric ulcer	1	565 (2 years)	69	69	6.1	England	Ward and Walton (1980)
Cystitis-pyelonephritis	Metritis	?	52	3600 (1 year)	132	88	3.7	France	Madec (1984)
Cystitis-pyelonephritis	Torsions abd. organs	Heart failure	6	4260 (NA)	NA	102	NA	Scotland	Smith (1984)
Postparturient bleeding and uterine prolapse	Torsions abd. organs	Gastric ulcer	3	3575 (2 years)	NA	131	NA	Taiwan	Hsu et al. (1985)
Heart failure	Torsions abd. organs	Cystitis-pyelonephritis	24	3755 (1 year)	137	116	3.3	Canada	Chagnon et al. (1991)
Heart failure	Torsions abd. organs	Cystitis-pyelonephritis	NA	NA (7 years)	NA	426	NA	Canada	D'Allaire et al. (1991)

Note: Results based on 10 studies.
[a]NA = not available.
[b]Torsions abd. organs = torsions and other accidents involving abdominal organs.

Torsions and Accidents Involving Abdominal Organs.
Torsions and accidents involving abdominal organs are among the major causes of death in breeding stock; gastric, splenic, and hepatic lobe torsions are the most common conditions reported within this category. Gastric dilation can also occur without concurrent torsion (Ward and Walton 1980). Intestinal accidents such as volvulus are also observed in breeding animals but are less frequent than in growing pigs. In studies on sow mortality published before 1980, torsions of abdominal organs are not reported as significant causes of death. The emergence of these problems, recognized in the early 1980s (Ward and Walton 1980; Morin et al. 1984; Sanford et al. 1984), might have been concurrent with the intensification of swine production and the associated changes in management practices. In some herds, these conditions may represent a serious problem.

Torsions of abdominal organs are found mostly in old sows (Morin et al. 1984; Sanford et al. 1984; Chagnon et al. 1991). Although affected sows are usually pregnant, sows may die at any stage of the reproductive cycle. Rough movements and manipulations, noise, and excitement among sows have been incriminated in the pathogenesis of torsion of abdominal organs (Morin et al. 1984). Feeding management and possibly housing type can influence the incidence of these conditions. It has been suggested that any factors that provoke a rapid intake of food and water in excited animals predispose to gastric dilation or torsion; such factors include the number of meals per day, omitting a meal, as often occurs during the weekend; and possibly the fineness of the ground feedstuffs. Gastric contents in these cases are generally abundant and fluid.

Heart Failure. Heart failure has been reported as being among the three main causes of death in sows (Senk and Sabec 1970; Svendsen et al. 1975; Smith 1984; Chagnon et al. 1991; D'Allaire et al. 1991), accounting for up to 31% of the mortalities. However, in several other studies, heart failure per se is either not even reported among the causes of death or is considered of negligible incidence in sows (Jones 1967, 1968; Ward and Walton 1980; Madec 1984; Hsu et al. 1985). The diagnosis of heart failure can be difficult to make, particularly in acute cases. Diagnosis should be based on the presence of lesions indicative of heart failure, such as cutaneous cyanosis; transudate in the pericardial, thoracic, and abdominal cavities; cardiac chamber changes; pulmonary edema; and passive congestion of lungs and liver, along with the absence of other gross, microscopic, and microbiological findings, to carefully exclude other diseases.

Some of the predisposing factors for this condition have to be regarded in light of the ways pigs often overreact to exogenous factors and, proba-

bly more importantly, of their particularly delicate cardiovascular system. The pig's heart has many anatomic and physiologic peculiarities, namely, low volume and small weight, abnormal systolic to diastolic ratio, and exceptional myocardial sensitivity to oxygen deficiency. This precarious situation may easily lead to irreversible overload of the circulation and to acute heart failure (Thielscher 1987). Thus, any factor that requires effort from the cardiovascular system may be considered as predisposing for this condition: high ambient temperature, stress, exercise, parturition, obesity, etc. In a study involving 137 dead sows, of which 43 had heart failure, more than 60% of these deaths occurred during the peripartum period, suggesting that parturition is a demanding event for the sow's cardiovascular system (Chagnon et al. 1991). Sows dead from heart failure also were significantly heavier and fatter than sows dead from other causes, the average parity being similar in the two groups. The ratio of their heart weight to body weight was significantly smaller; this was associated with an increased body weight since the heart weights were similar in the two groups (Drolet et al. 1992).

Cystitis-Pyelonephritis. The proportion of all deaths attributable to cystitis-pyelonephritis generally varies between 3% and 15% (Jones 1968; Senk and Sabec 1970; Svendsen et al. 1975; Ward and Walton 1980; Hsu et al. 1985; Chagnon et al. 1991; D'Allaire et al. 1991). However, in some studies, urinary tract infection represented the major cause of mortality, accounting for up to 40% of all deaths (Jones 1967; Madec 1984; Smith 1984).

Bacteria most commonly isolated from cases of cystitis-pyelonephritis are *Escherichia coli* and *Eubacterium suis* (formerly *Corynebacterium suis*) (Madec and David 1983; Smith 1984; D'Allaire et al. 1991). Other bacteria commonly associated with urinary tract infection include *Proteus* spp., streptococci, klebsiellae, and *Actinomyces pyogenes*.

Determination of urea concentration in ocular fluids can be a useful aid in diagnosing cystitis-pyelonephritis in dead sows, particularly when a complete necropsy is not possible (Drolet et al. 1990). A significantly higher aqueous humor urea concentration was found in sows dead of cystitis-pyelonephritis (52.3 mmol/L ± 19.0 standard error of mean) compared to those dead of other causes (9.9 mmol/L ± 1.5) (Chagnon et al. 1991).

The risk of cystitis-pyelonephritis increases with age (Jones 1967; Madec 1984; Chagnon et al. 1991; D'Allaire et al. 1991). The underlying reasons for this age-related susceptibility have not yet been fully investigated. Lack of exercise, limb injuries (Madec and David 1983), and obesity (Smith 1983), appear to be more frequent in old sows and predispose to urinary tract infection. These factors are associated with a decreased frequency of micturition, hence leading to a change in the pH of urine and a decreased flushing of bacteria (Smith 1983). It has also been reported that restricted water intake is a risk factor for cystitis-pyelonephritis, suggesting that the type of waterer can influence the incidence of urinary problems. These problems are also more common when sows are tethered or kept in stalls, possibly due to hygiene conditions, i.e., confined sows often having to lie in their own feces and urine (Madec and David 1983; Muirhead 1983). A flooring type that does not allow easy cleaning and good elimination of urine and feces can also lead to urogenital diseases and serious reproductive problems (Madec and David 1983; Muirhead 1983). For detailed information on cystitis-pyelonephritis, see Chapter 10.

Locomotor Problems. Sow mortality due to locomotor problems is generally low. However, on certain farms, these conditions account for a high proportion of sow losses (Senk and Sabec 1970; Svendsen et al. 1975). When investigating the extent of locomotor problems on a farm, it is important to assess both the death rate and the culling rate associated with these conditions, since culling policies influence both rates, especially for these problems.

Endometritis. In most studies, endometritis represents less than 9% of all deaths. This condition can be associated with concurrent urinary tract infection or, less frequently, with mastitis, this latter being an uncommon cause of death in sows.

Uterine Prolapse. Uterine prolapses are generally responsible for less than 7% of all deaths. This condition is mostly observed in old sows and the reasons for this increased frequency are unclear. Among possibilities are large pelvic inlet, long and flaccid uterus, and excessive relaxation of the pelvic and perineal region, which are probably mostly encountered in full-grown females (Roberts 1986).

Pneumonia. Pneumonia is not a major cause of mortality; it rarely represents more than 5% of all deaths. Pneumonia is often more severe in young growing pigs, compared to full-grown pigs (Pijoan 1986). This could partly explain why pneumonia is not a frequent cause of death in adult sows, and is likely to affect younger females (Chagnon et al. 1991).

Other Causes. Other causes of death can be encountered but with a generally low incidence except in some sporadic cases. They include lethal gastric ulcers various enteropathies such as swine dysentery and hemorrhagic proliferative enteropathy, septicemia, endocarditis, porcine stress syndrome, and some contagious diseases. Although dystocia or complications at parturition

are occasionally reported as causes of death, we must be careful not to ascribe every death occurring in the peripartum period to these latter causes. As mentioned previously, sows are most at risk of dying during the peripartum period, due to various causes.

The general pattern of causes of death varies among studies. Several factors may be responsible for these differences. The size and the number of herds vary considerably among the studies, and range from an average of 23 to more than 1000 sows per herd, and from 1 to 106 herds. The years in which the studies were conducted may have influenced the results; problems such as torsions and accidents of abdominal organs have been increasingly reported in recent years. Environment, management practices, and geographic areas also influence the occurrence of certain diseases and may explain some of the variation among herds. Nevertheless, torsion and other accidents involving abdominal organs, heart failure, and cystitis-pyelonephritis are the overall major causes of death in sows.

REASONS FOR CULLING BOARS. Overweight and old age, reproductive problems, and locomotor problems are the major reasons for culling boars. Le Denmat et al. (1980) in their study on 246 boars reported the following reasons for removal: old age or being overweight, 31%; reproductive problems, 20%; locomotor problems, 20%; and other reasons, 29%. From a different survey involving 98 boars, Le Denmat and Runavot (1980) concluded that reproductive problems (32%) and leg disorders (32%) were the two main reasons for removal, followed by overweight and old age (23%). However, in their study, the general pattern of removal varied according to the breed of the boars: culling for reproductive or leg problems was higher in purebred than in crossbred boars, whereas culling for old age and overweight was more frequent in crossbred than purebred boars. In a study involving 440 boars, removal was the result of being overweight (34%), reproductive problems (18%), old age (13%), leg problems (12%), death (7%), other diseases (4%), and miscellaneous conditions (12%) (D'Allaire and Leman 1990).

Overweight and Old Age. Since overweight and old age are not always easily distinguishable, they are often grouped into one category to avoid the risk of misclassification. Indeed, some producers use these two reasons interchangeably, because older boars are frequently considered too heavy to appropriately serve younger sows without the risk of injurying them. Both overweight and old age are often in relation to the sow herd. The introduction of many replacement gilts into the herd and the necessary introduction of young boars may require culling older or large boars, which are not necessarily aged. This aspect of culling is peculiar to commercial herds; overweight and old age are rarely reported as causes of culling in testing stations or artificial insemination centers (Melrose 1966; Navratil and Forejtek 1978). High rates of removal caused by overweight may also reflect a feeding-management problem, in which cases feeding management on the farm should be reviewed and corrected to improve boar longevity.

Reproductive Problems. The proportion of boars culled for reproductive problems is considerably lower in commercial herds than in artificial insemination stations (Melrose 1966; Navratil and Forejtek 1978). These differences may be attributed partly to the fact that semen quality is regularly evaluated for boars from artificial insemination centers. Consequently, boars may be removed more quickly and at a higher rate; culling rate for poor semen quality can be as high as 23% in these stations (Navratil and Forejtek 1978). In two French studies conducted in commercial breeding herds, reproductive problems represented 20% and 32% of all removals, and were considered one of the two major causes of culling (Le Denmat and Runavot 1980; Le Denmat et al. 1980). Breed difference may also be responsible for the variations in the proportion of boars culled for reproductive problems; purebred boars are more likely to be culled for this reason than crossbred boars (Le Denmat and Runavot 1980).

In commercial herds, the reason most frequently reported by producers in this culling category is poor libido or behavioral problems, which preclude efficient mating. Culling for low reproductive performance is also reported but to a lesser extent. Low reproductive performance is difficult to confirm for boars in commercial herds. A high amount of information is required to make a valid decision; it takes approximately 50 litters to show a one pig per litter difference from the herd average. Therefore, culling for that reason without sufficient data is rarely justified. On the other hand, by the time this information is available, the boar has often completed his productive life in the herd.

Locomotor Problems. Although locomotor problems are rarely the main cause of culling, the percentage of removal can be very high on certain farms (Einarsson and Larsson 1977; D'Allaire and Leman 1990). In herds with high culling for locomotor disorders, environment of the boars, such as housing and flooring types, should be evaluated carefully. Misclassification between locomotor and reproductive problems may also occur, for locomotor problems often result in poor libido or inability to mate.

Death. Death generally accounts for less than 7% of all removals, giving a herd death rate of lower than 4% (D'Allaire and Leman 1990). In a study by Senk and Sabec (1970), the causes of death in 30 boars were found to be heart failure (50%), locomotor problems (23%), splenic torsions (10%), gastric ulcer (7%), endocarditis (3%), and others (7%).

EFFECTS OF REMOVAL ON HERD PRODUCTIVITY. High removal rates can affect herd productivity by causing a shift in the herd age distribution toward younger females, which usually have fewer pigs born alive per litter, a lower conception rate, and a longer interval from weaning to first service. They are also more likely to be culled for reproductive failure.

The interval between a production event and the removal of a breeding female affects the number of nonproductive days in a herd, which is one of the best biologic predictors of litters per sow per year (Wilson et al. 1986; Duffy and Stein 1988). A high removal rate is generally associated with an increase in the number of nonproductive sow days. Target values for intervals between different production events and removal have been proposed by Polson et al. (1990). The interval between a production event and culling is determined by two factors: the interval from the production event to the decision to cull, and the period between when the decision to cull is made and the actual culling. An excessively long interval may be due to the manager's inefficiency in identifying animals that will eventually have to be culled or to the manager holding animals to be removed too long after the decision to cull is made.

Intervals from weaning to culling varying between 47 and 61 days have been reported (Dagorn and Aumaitre 1979; Pattison et al. 1980a; Stein et al. 1990). Pattison et al. (1980a) observed an 88-day interval from first service to culling; however, for sows found to be not pregnant, this interval was 121 days. The time lost from cullings, deaths, and abortions was found to add the equivalent of 11 days to the farrowing interval and to result in a decrease of 0.16 in the number of litters per sow per year (Pattison et al. 1980b). Kroes and Van Male (1979) observed an increase of 6–8 days in the farrowing interval for each increase of 12% over an annual removal rate of 31%, which was considered to be the base value.

High annual removal rates contribute to decrease the herd productivity by influencing the herd age distribution and the number of nonproductive sow days. Many authors have documented that high removal rates are associated with a decrease in litters per sow per year and pigs weaned per sow per year (Dagorn and Aumaitre 1979; Kroes and Van Male 1979; Pattison et al. 1980a). However, others have found that productivity is not influenced by removal rates (Svendsen et al. 1975; Parsons et al. 1990; Stein et al. 1990). A study by Duffy and Stein

(1988) has contributed to the understanding of these conflicting results; they found that, although the annual removal rate was not associated with either litters per sow per year or pigs weaned per sow per year, removal rate per litter farrowed was negatively correlated with both variables. Therefore, when comparing the effects of removal rates on productivity between herds, controlling for the number of litters per sow per year seems necessary.

Determination of the annual removal rate is the first step in evaluating a culling program. Rates that are too high seem to be more common than excessively low rates. Unusual circumstances, such as a change in inventory or culling policy, may temporarily increase the removal rate. The mean parity at removal is also useful, but a parity distribution of culled females may be more informative. The removal rate for each category of reasons can indicate the extent of a problem. Analysis of reasons by parity may reveal which group of females is more susceptible or whether some cullings are unjustified, either physiologically or economically. An assessment of the interval between a production event and removal is important because it influences the number of litters per sow per year and pigs weaned per sow per year, which can result in economic loss. Clearly the failure to identify and remove nonproductive sows at an early stage will increase the number of nonproductive sow days. Management decisions regarding sow culling should be based on economic grounds.

Culling policies for both sows and boars should be evaluated, since sow and boar removal rates are correlated (r = 0.52) (D'Allaire and Leman 1990). This relationship is due either to a direct association between boar and sow culling or to common factors influencing boar and sow removal. These factors might include management, environment, nutrition, and managers' attitudes. It has been reported that management practices and environment influence sow culling (D'Allaire et al. 1989). To improve breeding-life expectancy of sows and boars in commercial herds, greater attention to the environment, nutrition, and management should be emphasized.

REFERENCES

ARGANOSA, V. G.; ACDA, S. P.; AND BANDIAN, M. M. 1981a. Lifetime breeding and reproductive performance of boars. Philipp Agric 64:41–47.

ARGANOSA, V. G.; ACDA, S. P.; AND DE GUZMAN, A. L. 1981b. Lifetime reproductive performance of sows in selected piggeries in the Philippines. Philipp Agric 64:1–20.

CHAGNON, M.; D'ALLAIRE, S.; AND DROLET, R. 1991. A prospective study of sow mortality in breeding herds. Can J Vet Res 55:180–184.

DAGORN, J., AND AUMAITRE, A. 1979. Sow culling: Reasons for and effect on productivity. Livest Prod Sci 6:167–177.

D'ALLAIRE, S. 1987. Assessment of culling programs in swine breeding herds. Compend Cont Educ Pract Vet 9:F187–F191.

D'ALLAIRE, S., AND LEMAN, A. D. 1990. Boar culling in swine breeding herds in Minnesota. Can Vet J 31:581–583.

D'ALLAIRE, S.; STEIN, T. E.; AND LEMAN, A. D. 1987. Culling patterns in selected Minnesota swine breeding herds. Can J Vet Res 51:506–512.

D'ALLAIRE, S.; MORRIS, R. S.; MARTIN, F. B.; ROBINSON, R. A.; AND LEMAN, A. D. 1989. Management and environmental factors associated with annual sow culling rate: A path analysis. Prev Vet Med 7:255–265.

D'ALLAIRE, S.; DROLET, R.; AND CHAGNON, M. 1991. The causes of sow mortality: A retrospective study. Can Vet J 32:241–243.

DIJKHUIZEN, A. A.; MORRIS, R. S.; AND MORROW, M. 1986. Economic optimization of culling strategies in swine breeding herds, using the "PorkCHOP" computer program. Prev Vet Med 4:341–353.

DOIGE, C. E. 1982. Pathological findings associated with locomotory disturbances in lactating and recently weaned sows. Can J Comp Med 46:1–6.

DROLET, R.; D'ALLAIRE, S.; AND CHAGNON, M. 1990. The evaluation of postmortem ocular fluid analysis as a diagnostic aid in sows. J Vet Diagn Invest 2:9–13.

———. 1992. Some observations on cardiac failure in sows. Can Vet J. In press.

DUFFY, S. J., AND STEIN, T. E. 1988. Correlations between production, productivity, and population factors in swine breeding herds. Proc Int Pig Vet Soc 10:345.

EINARSSON, S., AND LARSSON, K. 1977. Hallbarhet och utslagsorsaker hos galtar i en bruksbesattning. Sven Vet Tidn 29:595–597.

EINARSSON, S., AND SETTERGREN, I. 1974. Fruktsamhet och utslagsorsaker i ett antal mellansvenska suggbesattningar. Nord Vet Med 26:576–584.

EINARSSON, S.; LINDE, C.; AND SETTERGREN, I. 1974. Studies of the genital organs of gilts culled for anoestrus. Theriogenology 2:109–113.

FRIENDSHIP, R. M.; WILSON, M. R.; ALMOND, G. W.; MCMILLAN, R. R.; HACKER, R. R.; PIEPER, R.; AND SWAMINATHAN, S. S. 1986. Sow wastage: Reasons for and effect on productivity. Can J Vet Res 50:205–208.

HALGAARD, C. 1983. Epidemiologic factors in puerperal diseases of swine. Nord Vet Med 35:161–174.

HSU, F. S.; CHUNG, W. B.; HU, D. K.; YANG, P. C.; AND SHEN, Y. M. 1985. Incidence and causes of mortality in growing-finishing pigs and sows on the large-scale intensive pig farms. J Chin Soc Vet Sci 11:93–101.

JONES, J. E. T. 1967. An investigation of the causes of mortality and morbidity in sows in a commercial herd. Br Vet J 123:327–339.

———. 1968. The cause of death in sows: A one-year survey of 106 herds in Essex. Br Vet J 124:45–54.

JOO, H. S., AND KANG, B. J. 1981. Reproductive performance on intensive swine farms in Korea. J Korean Vet Med Assoc 17:40–43.

JOSSE, J.; LE DENMAT, M.; MARTINAT-BOTTÉ, F.; VANIER, P.; AND VAUDELET, J. C. 1980. A propos d'une enquête sur les causes de réforme des truies. Schweiz Arch Tierheilkd 122:341–349.

JOVIĆ, M.; VARADIN, M.; AND NIKOLIC, P. 1975. The length of reproduction of breeding sows at intensive piglet production and the chief reasons of their elimination from the breeding herd. Veterinaria (Yugoslavia) 24:17–23.

KARLBERG, K. 1979. Utrangeringsarsaker hos avlspurker. Norsk Vet Tidsskr 91:423–426.

KROES, Y., AND VAN MALE, J. P. 1979. Reproductive lifetime of sows in relation to economy of production.

Livest Prod Sci 6:179–183.

Le Denmat, M., and Runavot, J. P. 1980. Premiers résultats d'une enquête sur l'âge, la durée d'utilisation et les causes de réforme des verrats en service dans les élevages de production. J Rech Porcine Fr 12:149–156.

Le Denmat, M.; Runavot, J. P.; and Albar, J. 1980. Les caractéristiques de la population des verrats en service dans les élevage de production. Résultats d'une enquête sur 293 troupeaux. Techni-Porc 3:41–48.

Madec, F. 1984. Analyse des causes de mortalité des truies en cours de période d'élevage. Rec Méd Vét 160:329–335.

Madec, F., and David, F. 1983. Les troubles urinaires des troupeaux de truies: Diagnostic, incidence et circonstances d'apparition. J Rech Porcine Fr 15:431–446.

Melrose, D. R. 1966. A review of progress and of possible developments in artificial insemination of pigs. Vet Rec 78:159–168.

Ministry of Agriculture, Food, and Fisheries (MAFF). 1981. Injuries caused by flooring: A survey in pig health scheme herds. Proc Pig Vet Soc 8:119–125.

Morin, M.; Sauvageau, R.; Phaneuf, J.-B.; Teuscher, E.; Beauregard, M.; and Lagace, A. 1984. Torsion of abdominal organs in sows: A report of 36 cases. Can Vet J 25:440–442.

Muirhead, M. R. 1976. Veterinary problems of intensive pig husbandry. Vet Rec 99:288–292.

———. 1981. A comparison of different systems of sow housing and management. Proc Pig Vet Soc 8:18–28.

———. 1983. Pig housing and environment. Vet Rec 113:587–593.

Navratil, S., and Forejtek, P. 1978. The reasons for culling boars from artificial insemination centers. Veterinarstvi 28:354–355.

Parsons, T. D.; Johnstone, C.; and Dial, G. D. 1990. On the economic significance of parity distribution in swine herds. Proc Int Pig Vet Soc 11:380.

Pattison, H. D.; Cook, G. L.; and MacKenzie, S. 1980a. A study of culling patterns in commercial pig breeding herds. Proc Br Soc Anim Prod, Harrogate, pp. 462–463.

———. 1980b. A study of natural service, farrowing rates and associated fertility parameters. Proc Br Soc Anim Prod, Harrogate, p. 452.

Pijoan, C. 1986. Respiratory system. In Diseases of Swine, 6th ed. Ed. A. D. Leman, B. Straw, R. D. Glock, W. L. Mengeling, R. H. C. Penny, and E. Scholl. Ames: Iowa State Univ Press, pp. 152–162.

Polson, D. D.; Dial, G. D.; Marsh, W. E.; and Nimis, G. 1990. The influence of nonproductive days on breeding herd productivity and profitability. Proc Am Assoc Swine Pract, Denver, Colo., pp. 61–67.

Pomeroy, R. W. 1960. Infertility and neonatal mortality in the sow. 1. Lifetime performance and reasons for disposal of sows. J Agric Sci (Camb) 54:1–17.

Roberts, S. J. 1986. Veterinary Obstetrics and Genital Diseases (Theriogenology), 3d ed. Woodstock, Vt: S. J. Roberts.

Sanford, S. E.; Waters, E. H.; and Josephson, G. K. A. 1984. Gastrosplenic torsions in sows. Can Vet J 25:364.

Senk, L., and Sabec, D. 1970. Todesursachen bei Schweinen aus Grobbetrieben. Zentralbl Veterinaermed [B] 17:164–174.

Smith, W. J. 1983. Cystitis in sows. Pig News Inf 4:279–281.

———. 1984. Sow mortality–limited survey. Proc Int Pig Vet Soc 8:368.

Smith, W. J., and Robertson, A. M. 1971. Observations on injuries to sows confined in part slatted stalls. Vet Rec 89:531–533.

Spencer, G. R. 1979. Animal model: Porcine lactational osteoporosis. Am J Pathol 95:277–280.

Stein, T. E.; Dijkhuizen, A.; D'Allaire, S.; and Morris, R. S. 1990. Sow culling and mortality in commercial swine breeding herds. Prev Vet Med 9:85–94.

Stone, M. W. 1981. Sow culling survey in Alberta. Can Vet J 22:363.

Straw, B. 1984. Causes and control of sow losses. Mod Vet Pract 65:349–353.

Svendsen, J.; Nielsen, N. C.; Bille, N.; and Riising, H.-J. 1975. Causes of culling and death in sows. Nord Vet Med 27:604–615.

Thielscher, H.-H. 1987. The pig's heart–a problem of pathophysiology. Pro Vet 3:12.

Van Snick, G.; Vergote de Lantsheere, W.; and LeJeune, A. 1965. Les causes de réforme des truies d'élevage. Rev Agri 18:289–309.

Ward, W. R., and Walton, J. R. 1980. Gastric distension and torsion and other causes of death in sows. Proc Pig Vet Soc 6:72–74.

Wilson, M. R.; Friendship, R. M.; McMillan, I.; Hacker, R. R.; Pieper, R.; and Swaminathan, S. 1986. A survey of productivity and its component interrelationships in Canadian swine herds. J Anim Sci 62:576–582.

70 Control of Pseudorabies (Aujeszky's Disease) Virus

R. B. Morrison

PSEUDORABIES VIRUS (PRV) may be found in swine herds around the world (Fig. 70.1) and control policies vary among countries. Countries that are free of the virus strive to prevent its entry; where the virus is already present, a control program may be directed at reducing the prevalence of infected herds to a level that is biologically and/or economically justifiable. An eradication program may be in effect with the goal of eliminating the virus from a specified area by means of a time-limited campaign. Alternatively, a country may choose to ignore the presence of PRV and have no formal policy.

The decision whether to ignore, control, or eradicate PRV is often controversial. Since PRV vaccines reduce the clinical severity in swine, many veterinarians advocate no formal policy imposed on producers. However, recent experience indicates that in the absence of an effective control program, PRV will increase in prevalence in areas of high swine concentration where herds are relatively large, intensively managed, and housed in partial or total confinement. Under these intensive conditions, the implications of having no formal policy will be ongoing spread of PRV among swine herds, vaccine expenditures for an indefinite time, reduced productivity due to the absence or failure of a vaccination program, and fatalities in certain other domestic species

that may become infected. Benefit-cost analyses indicate that under certain circumstances a successful eradication program is less expensive than no formal policy or one of long-term control (Hallam 1987; Le Foll 1988).

Whether the policy is to control or eradicate PRV, there are three components that are common to both: it must be established whether PRV is present in a region/country, and if so, how prevalent it is; if PRV is detected, guidelines must be established to control the spread among herds; the prevalence of existing infected herds must be reduced. In a control or eradication program, these procedures usually occur simultaneously.

DETECTION OF PRV AND ESTIMATION OF PREVALENCE

Surveillance. Surveillance involves the collection and interpretation of data for use in PRV prevention, control, or eradication programs. Data may be assembled passively by monitoring clinical and diagnostic reports. More frequently, data are actively collected by serologic surveys of individual pigs at a slaughter facility, at the first point of sale, or at the herd of origin. Two different observations may be made from actively collected surveillance data. First, one can detect with a specific level of confidence if PRV is present in the

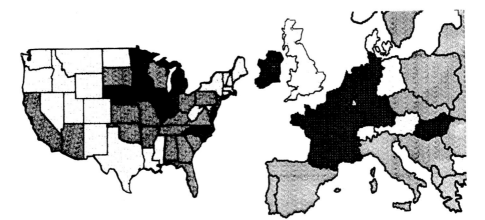

70.1. Prevalence of pseudorabies within the United States and Europe. Dark shade denotes area with high prevalence; light shade denotes area with low prevalence; dotted area denotes area with no pseudorabies. Map of the United States is not drawn to the same scale as Europe.

population to which the sample of pigs refers. Second, if PRV is detected, the prevalence in the population can be estimated. The accuracy of this latter estimate is extremely important, since prevalence within a specified area is a major factor influencing the decision to control or eradicate the virus.

An important part of establishing a reliable surveillance program is to sample the appropriate pigs. To have absolute proof that PRV is not present in a population, particularly if it could be at a low prevalence, all pigs in the population need to be tested. One must weigh the cost of having absolute proof versus the risk involved in not having 100% confidence in the interpretation. Surveying 100% of the population is usually not economically feasible, nor practical, and one of various sampling procedures may be performed. A simple random sample provides each pig in a population an equal opportunity of being included. Thus, results can be validly extrapolated to the population from which it came. Most commonly, a sample is chosen haphazardly without employing formal randomizing techniques. Although there may have been an attempt to have a truly representative sample, this procedure is often biased in some fashion and the results should be viewed with caution.

The number of pigs in the sample also will determine the likelihood of detecting PRV in the herd. As the sample size increases, the probability of detection increases. Tables are available that give sample sizes required to meet the conditions desired (Cannon and Roe 1982). A practical and effective decision is to select a sample size such that the investigator is 95% confident of detecting PRV if the prevalence of PRV is at least 10% in that section of the herd. For example, a random sample of 25 sows in a 100-sow herd with a prevalence of 10% in the sows, will detect at least 1 positive sow 95% of the time.

The investigator must also choose whether sows, boars, and/or finishing pigs should be tested. Testing only finishing pigs will grossly underestimate the prevalence of herds infected with PRV. Testing only boars at slaughter may be more convenient than sows, since fewer boars are sold per herd than sows. However, this will also underestimate the prevalence, since boars are negative in many infected herds (Anderson et al. 1989). A representative sample of sows from each herd will most accurately reflect the prevalence of infected herds in the population.

Although simple random sampling is superior to haphazard sampling, it may also be biased. A random sample of pigs at a slaughter facility will underrepresent small herds because large herds market a higher proportion of the pigs sold. Conversely, a random sample of herds will underrepresent large herds, since they make up a smaller proportion of the total population of swine herds. Stratified sampling ensures that all seg-

ments of a population are represented appropriately. All herds must be identified and allocated to the appropriate size category. The correct number of herds from each category is then selected, preferably by simple random selection. Although this system is more inconvenient, it is considerably more accurate.

Another variable that can influence the accuracy of the surveillance program is the sensitivity and specificity of test employed. No tests are 100% accurate and there is an inverse relationship between sensitivity and specificity. Ideally, a highly sensitive test such as the enzyme-linked immunosorbent assay (ELISA) is used to screen sera, and then a less-sensitive but more specific test such as serum neutralization (SN) is used as confirmation. The prevalence of PRV in the population being sampled will also influence the predictive value of the serologic results. For example, as the prevalence of PRV declines in an area as a result of a control program, one can expect an increasing proportion of false-positive reactors (Martin et al. 1987).

Case Finding.   There are several methods of identifying infected herds; no single method provides all the information required and each varies in complexity (Schnurrenberger et al. 1987). Reporting clinical evidence of PRV in a herd and having confirmatory diagnoses is the most uncomplicated method of identifying infected herds.

Traceback is a procedure that begins with a known infected pig or herd and traces all possible exposures back toward the source and forward to other contacts. The effectiveness depends on having a pig identification system, owners' cooperation and access to their records, and investigative skills. If a slaughter surveillance program is in effect, seropositive pigs can be retrospectively traced to their herd of origin. This is very cost effective, especially if the prevalence of PRV is low in the population. Once a herd is located, blood should be collected from the appropriate number of representative sows and tested to confirm the PRV status of the herd.

Once a herd becomes infected with PRV, herds in proximity are more likely to become infected also. Therefore, testing herds that surround the known infected herd, referred to as circle testing, will often reveal other infected herds. Although available resources will influence the radius of the circle, approximately 1.5 miles is thought to be sufficient (Taylor 1989). As new herds are located, circle testing is also conducted around these herds.

CONTROL OF SPREAD AMONG HERDS. The fact that countries such as Canada and Australia with significant swine industries have remained free of PRV indicates that programs can be established to effectively prevent the introduction of the virus into an area. In England, after 8 years of monitoring over 100 herds that were registered in a health control association, none had become infected with PRV despite the presence of PRV in the country (Goodwin and Whittlestone 1986). Danish experiences suggest that the proximity of infected herds plays a strong role in influencing the success of a prevention program (Andersen et al. 1989).

Herds can become infected with PRV by being exposed to infected pigs, wildlife, or contaminated fomites, or aerosol (see Chapter 24). The source of a herd infection is usually determined by investigating recent pig purchases, herd security measures, and the PRV status of neighboring herds. In the absence of evidence indicating that infected pigs were introduced to the herd, it is often difficult to determine the source of virus. New techniques, including geographic information systems (Damrongwatanapokin et al. 1990) and restriction endonuclease analysis (REA) patterns of viral DNA (Lomniczi et al. 1989), are being used to further elucidate transmission among herds. With this latter technique, if an isolate from a newly infected herd has a different restriction fragment pattern than the suspected source herd, the investigator can conclude that the source is likely elsewhere. If the two REA patterns are similar, then the originally infected herd may have been the source for the newly infected herd. The method of transmission between the herds must still be defined.

Pig Movement. A very high proportion of pigs infected with PRV become latently infected (Sabo 1985). Any pig that is latently infected with PRV has the potential to reactivate and shed virus. Therefore, when attempting to control the spread of PRV among herds, any pig that has been infected must still be considered as a potential source of virus.

Two steps have the greatest impact on reducing the spread of PRV. First, the movement of pigs from infected herds should be restricted only to slaughter or other known infected herds. Herds with such restrictions are commonly referred to as being quarantined. Second, all introductions of breeding stock or feeder pigs to noninfected herds should be required to originate from known noninfected herds. This includes a requirement that where communal boars are used, they should test negative for PRV (Andersen et al. 1989). Such controls can impose substantial financial hardship on owners of infected herds, especially when a protracted control program is in place.

Although PRV has been reported to be capable of infecting embryos (Bolin et al. 1982), embryo transfer has been successfully used to derive PRV-negative embryos from infected sows (James et al. 1983; Haraszti et al. 1989), and there are no documented reports of herds becoming infected from this procedure. Similarly, PRV has

been isolated from semen of naturally infected boars. Although no reports exist documenting the infection of a herd by contaminated semen, the risk exists and one should avoid using semen from infected boars in PRV-negative herds.

Circumstantial evidence suggests that pigs may be latently infected and yet be undetected by conventional serologic tests. In one experimental study, piglets having passive antibodies to PRV were experimentally infected and did not seroconvert as detected by SN (Zimmerman et al. 1988). Three field studies provide circumstantial evidence that PRV-seronegative, latently infected pigs occur (Thawley et al. 1984; Bognar et al. 1986; Komaniwa et al. 1986). One clinical report suggested that seronegative latently infected pigs may have been the source of PRV for four swine herds (Annelli et al. 1991). The frequency of undetected latently infected swine is unknown, but the impact on a control-eradication program is probably relatively low.

Fomites and Wildlife. It has been well documented that PRV can survive for several days on some materials and can infect many other species of domestic animals and wildlife (see Chapter 24). Moreover, PRV infection has been experimentally reproduced by exposing pigs to contaminated feed, flies, carcasses, manure, and infected sheep (Mocsari et al. 1989). However, there are surprisingly few documented cases of herds becoming infected with PRV by exposure to infected wildlife or fomites, including contaminated equipment, feed, boots, coveralls, or people. This is due, in part, to the difficulty of having conclusive evidence of the source of infection in the absence of exposure to infected pigs. More importantly, however, the dose of virus necessary to infect pigs orally is higher than via the intranasal route (Wittmann and Rziha 1989), which makes infection by oral exposure less likely.

Airborne. There is an accumulating body of evidence indicating that airborne transmission of PRV occurs between swine herds and in sufficient quantity to infect a previously negative herd. The first clinical report of airborne transmission involved cattle becoming infected (Bitsch 1975). In a typical case, cattle were housed 10–20 m away from infected pigs and were close to a fan exhausting air from the pigs (Bitsch and Andersen 1982). These same workers also speculated that two pig herds that were 120 and 500 m away from known infected herds had become infected by airborne transmission. Subsequently, airborne transmission was experimentally reproduced when susceptible pigs that were ventilated by a 10 m/second airflow originating from a pen containing recently infected pigs housed 15 m away became infected (Donaldson et al. 1983). Since then, investigators have reported airborne transmission between herds separated by 1.2 miles (Bitsch 1984), 5.6 miles (Gloster et al. 1984), 1.9 miles (Andersen et al. 1989), and 2.4 miles (Rueff 1990). Most recently, Danish investigators have suggested that airborne transmission of PRV can occur over long distances, that is, up to 25 miles if meteorological conditions are appropriate (Christensen et al. 1989).

Although these conditions have not been defined, the following requirements are likely. First, a sufficient quantity of virus must be generated from the infected herd. It has been reported that a susceptible pig can excrete up to $10^{5.2}$–$10^{5.8}$ tissue culture infective dose (TCID)50 of PRV during a 24-hour period (Donaldson et al. 1983; Wittmann 1984). While most of the excreted virus stays in oronasal secretions, some is aerosolized and can be readily detected within barns (Mack et al. 1986). Since spread of PRV within a susceptible herd can be rapid, the amount of virus generated during an epidemic could be $10^{5.8}$ TCID50 multiplied by the number of pigs in the herd. That is, large herds will generate more virus than small herds and therefore represent a more likely source of airborne transmission. One would expect the amount of virus generated to be reduced in PRV-vaccinated herds. The second factor affecting the likelihood of airborne transmission may be the strain of PRV involved. Some strains may generate more virus by having a propensity to affect the respiratory system with consequently more sneezing, coughing, and nasal discharge (Donaldson et al. 1983). Concomitant respiratory bacterial infections may also irritate the respiratory tract and increase these signs further. Since PRV strains differ in virulence and minimum infective dose (McCullough 1989), some strains are more likely to be in sufficient quantity to infect pigs at the new herd. A third prerequisite is to have appropriate environmental conditions for survival of the viral droplet during airborne transmission. In one study maximum droplet survival was observed at 4°C and 55% relative humidity. Under these conditions, the viral half-life was approximately 45 minutes (Schoenbaum et al. 1990), which is more than enough to be carried between herds. A fourth prerequisite proposed for airborne transmission is suitable meteorological conditions to avoid complete dispersion of the virus. This might involve wind of constant direc-

tion for many hours (Gloster et al. 1984), and possibly a certain barometric pressure or change in pressure. Fifth, certain topographical features, such as over water or through valleys, may be more conducive to airborne transmission than others. Finally, pig herds need to be of sufficient proximity that if all the above conditions are met, susceptible pigs are available to exposure to the contaminated aerosol. If PRV behaves like other infectious agents that exhibit airborne transmission, a herd's risk of becoming infected will be a function of the square of the distance from the source infected herd (Rumney 1986). That is, the closer the herds, the greater is the risk of airborne transmission.

Given the unique conditions that are needed for airborne transmission to occur between herds, it is difficult to estimate how common this is. However, after controls are imposed on the movement of infected pigs, and herd owners are practicing herd security measures, airborne transmission will be an increasingly likely source of infection.

ELIMINATION OF EXISTING HERD INFECTIONS. Three basic plans to eliminate PRV that have been described in the literature and conducted in many herds are test and removal, offspring segregation, and depopulation-repopulation (Thawley et al. 1982). In one study involving 119 herds, these methods were employed to eliminate PRV from 116 (97.5%) of the herds that were involved with the project for at least 18 months (Thawley et al. 1987). Each plan has its advantages and appropriate applications (Table 70.1). Three major factors influence the decision of which plan to choose. First, the PRV prevalence in the herd dictates the current options. Test and removal is the method of choice if the prevalence is relatively low. Second is whether there is a financial need to eliminate PRV as quickly as possible. For example, herd owners who sell breeding stock or feeder pigs are most affected by sales restrictions and may wish to eliminate PRV very rapidly. Conversely, a farrow-to-finish producer may suffer minimal or no financial impact due to sales restrictions and therefore may want to adopt a conservative elimination program. Third, the cost of elimination plans vary substantially (Zimmerman et al. 1989). Other influential factors include risk of the herd becoming rein-

Table 70.1. Comparison of advantages of PRV elimination programs

	Test and Removal	Offspring Segregation	Depopulation-Repopulation
Cost	Least	Intermediate	Most
Time to achieve	Slow	Intermediate	Intermediate
Genetics	Maintain	Maintain	Replaced
Disruption to management	Minor	Intermediate	Major
Concomitant diseases	Same	Some improvement	Major improvement
Likely to succeed	Least	Intermediate	Most

fected, disease profile of the herd, value of the herd genetics, and the commitment and management ability of farm personnel.

Determine Prevalence. The first steps in choosing an elimination program are to determine if the growing/finishing pigs are infected and to estimate the PRV seroprevalence in the breeding herd (Thawley and Morrison 1988). If growing pigs are moved in a continuous flow, then only a single group needs to be tested. If pigs move in all-in/all-out groups, then each group should be tested. Testing only pigs over 4 months of age will avoid misinterpretation due to passive antibodies. A sample of 9 representative pigs per group will detect PRV with 95% confidence if the prevalence is at least 30%. This detection level is appropriate, since the prevalence is rarely below this in finishing pigs. In estimating the seroprevalence in the breeding herd, one is more confident that the prevalence in the sample accurately reflects that in the breeding herd as the number in the sample increases. For example, if 30 adults are tested and 15 are positive, one is 95% confident that the prevalence in the breeding herd is 50% ± 17.5%. If the sample is increased to 100 adults and 50% are positive, the 95% confidence interval narrows to ±10%. In most cases 30 representative adults give a reasonable estimate of the prevalence. A more accurate reflection of the breeding herd PRV status can be achieved by sampling 5–10 representative females per parity.

Test and Removal. Under favorable conditions this program is the least disruptive to management and least expensive to conduct. In this program, noninfected breeding stock are introduced into the existing infected herd and gradually replace all infected sows and boars. In a best-case scenario, PRV may be eliminated from a herd with no premature culling of infected breeding stock. There are three steps to conduct a test and removal program: (1) noninfected breeding stock must be available, which usually involves ensuring that PRV is not spreading among the growing/finishing pigs within this herd; (2) PRV spread within the existing breeding herd must be slow or nonexistent; (3) all infected sows and boars must be detected and removed from the herd, and the herd must be officially recognized as virus free.

STOP SPREAD IN GROW/FINISH. During a PRV epidemic, virus usually spreads rapidly throughout the herd, so that the seroprevalence approaches 100% (Van Aarle et al. 1978). Subsequently, virus spontaneously stops spreading within the grow/finish section in the majority of herds (Morrison and Thawley 1989; Anderson et al. 1990). Three factors associated with PRV continuing to spread within a grow/finish unit include housing pigs in complete confinement, having a

clinical problem with *Actinobacillus pleuropneumoniae* and, a short period of time since the epidemic occurred (Anderson et al. 1990). Virus usually spreads continuously among growing pigs in large herds. This tendency reflects the increased likelihood of being completely confined and the increased number of susceptible pigs being continuously introduced. Considering these factors, one can formulate a program to stop spread in growing/finishing pigs.

The most powerful management change is to move pigs in an all-in/all-out flow. This change alone will usually stop the spread of PRV and coincidentally improve performance. In practice, all-in/all-out management is a matter of degree. Ideally, each group of pigs should have less than 400 pigs with a 1- to 2-week age spread, 4 weeks maximum. Additionally, rooms should be cleaned before introducing pigs and contact (physical or aerosol) between groups should be eliminated. While this is ideal, PRV often stops spreading when groups are separated by a wall and no other changes are made.

The decision whether to vaccinate must consider the anticipated economic benefit of vaccinating versus the cost of the vaccination program. Vaccination for PRV will prevent neither infection nor latency, nor will it eliminate viral shedding after infection. However, there is ample experimental (see Chapter 24) and some field evidence to suggest that vaccination will inhibit spread within a herd (De Waele et al. 1990). A dilemma exists when considering the vaccination program in growing pigs versus the breeding swine; i.e., there is a negative association between the concentration of passively acquired anti-PRV antibody and the pigs' response to vaccination. Therefore, a program that stimulates a high degree of immunity in the breeding herd will also evoke high passive antibody in the pigs and, consequently, there will be more inhibition of the growing pigs' response to vaccination. To overcome this problem, vaccination is commonly delayed until the pigs are approximately 8–10 weeks of age when passive immunity may have waned sufficiently. Vaccination is commonly repeated 2–4 weeks later with the goal that all growing pigs will acquire some degree of active immunity. Two problems with vaccinating at this age are that some inhibition still occurs (De Waele et al. 1990) and PRV infection may have already occurred. A second approach to overcoming passive immunity is intranasal administration of modified live virus (MLV) vaccine. By stimulating local immunity, the duration of viral shedding has been reported to be less after infection than intramuscular vaccination (Van Oirschot 1986).

At present, there is no consensus on the most effective age at which to vaccinate or the route of administration. Ideally, vaccination would be delayed until 2–4 weeks prior to when infection takes place. This age appears to vary among herds and therefore the age and route of vaccination may need to be a herd-specific decision. Similarly, there is no consensus concerning what type of vaccine (MLV, killed, or subunit) or in the case of MLV vaccines, which deletion (gI, gX, or gIII), is most efficacious under field conditions. The decision must take into account the cost of the vaccine, availability of a companion diagnostic test to differentiate between vaccinated and infected pigs, clinical experiences, and reported efficacy.

STOP SPREAD IN THE BREEDING HERD. As PRV-negative gilts are introduced into the existing breeding herd, they become exposed to infected breeding stock. The prevalence of infection in the breeding herd will depend upon the proportion of the herd that has been replaced by negative stock and the incidence of new infections. In a year-long study of 17 PRV endemically infected herds in Minnesota, spread was detected in the breeding section in only 9 of the herds and when it occurred, it was very slow and irregular (Duffy et al. 1990a). This occurred in the absence of any intervention, other than biannual PRV vaccination. A similar observation was made in 2 herds in the Netherlands (Van Oirschot et al. 1990).

If gilts and sows tend to become infected more in one stage of production than another, then control measures might be emphasized in this area. The first documented case of spontaneous reactivation and shedding was recorded at farrowing (Davies and Beran 1980). However, in a study of seven endemically infected Belgian herds, no evidence of reactivation and shedding could be detected from 172 sows that were monitored at farrowing (Maes and Pensaert 1984). In one herd in Hungary, infection occurred predominantly in the breeding area (Medveczky et al. 1990). In the Minnesota study described above, an effect of location within the farm (gilt pool, breeding, gestation, farrowing) on the incidence of infection was evident in only one of the herds (Duffy et al. 1990b). Overall, the gestation barn was the location in which more females became infected with PRV than any other location. However, the greater number of females infected in gestation appeared to be a consequence of a longer period at risk rather than a higher incidence rate. Considering these four field studies, although the incidence of infection may vary with location within selected herds, gilts and sows may become infected at any location or stage of production within a herd. Therefore, control measures to reduce spread should be applied throughout the breeding section of a herd.

The vaccination program in the breeding herd is critical, since it is the main method of control that exists at present. The goal is to (1) inhibit shedding if reactivation of latent PRV occurs, (2) decrease new infections if a gilt or sow is exposed to virus, and (3) decrease the incidence of latency if infection occurs. The frequency of administra-tion has an effect on the immune response but no data exist on the optimum interval. Currently, most herds are vaccinated biannually or prefar-rowing. A more intensive program would be quarterly, or prefarrowing and again at weaning. Most herd owners will use the same deletion of the vaccine in the breeding herd as in the growing pigs. This will avoid the possibility of serologic false-positive reactions if gilts are selected from within the herd.

An additional general recommendation is to reduce stress whenever possible. Stressed sows have lower productivity, but more important in the case of PRV is that stress suppresses the immune response. This is thought to predispose these individuals to recrudescence of latent PRV and possible shedding. Known stressors include fighting, extreme environmental temperatures, housing changes, and rough handling. Although it will be exceedingly difficult to document, managers' attitudes toward the pigs and their husbandry skills may have a critical effect on the sows' immune system and, consequently, may be the most important determinant in a herd's chance of eliminating PRV.

DETECT AND REMOVE INFECTED ADULTS. As negative gilts are continually introduced, the PRV prevalence will decline if infected adults are removed at a faster rate than new infections occur. Annual serologic sampling, stratified by parity if possible, can be used to monitor this process. Simultaneously, or instead, a cohort of negative females can be serologically monitored (quarterly) to ensure that increased spread has not occurred. In general, a convenient time to cull infected sows is at weaning. New diagnostic tests are being developed that require little equipment and can be used in the field (Annelli et al. 1990). Such tests will give results rapidly (within hours) to the producer and will make it more feasible to cull infected sows at weaning.

As the prevalence in a herd declines, the major issue is the degree to which PRV infection status should influence the herd owner's culling policy. A temptation is to cull based in part on PRV status to hasten the decline in prevalence; that is, cull PRV-infected individuals before they would be culled normally. There is a cost to the producer for having such a policy, which needs to be weighed against the probability that one of those individuals would have reactivated and shed virus. Since the latter is unknown, the culling policy will depend upon current prevalence, risk of the herd being reinfected, cost of replacements, and the producer's aversion to risk.

The only way to have absolute proof that PRV has been eliminated from the herd is to obtain a blood sample from all pigs and find them all PRV negative. This is a formidable and costly task; therefore, one of two options may be employed. In both options, blood should be collected from a representative sample of finishing pigs (older than 4 months) from each separate group (if managed all-in/all-out) or from each barn (if managed continuous flow). As described previously, the sample size will depend on the level of confidence desired to detect a specified prevalence. The first option is to require a negative test on all individuals in the breeding herd. A second, somewhat controversial, option is to require a negative test on a representative sample of individuals in the breeding herd with a predetermined level of confidence and a minimum prevalence that can be detected. This latter method is obviously less accurate and has the risk that infected individuals may go undetected. Reports show that herds with a very low prevalence of infected adults are relatively common, and many would not be detected with representative sampling (Annelli and Morrison 1990). Although unlikely, these individuals may reactivate and shed virus and be the source of another epidemic within the herd. Representative sampling may still be practical and effective in very large herds if the owner is aware of the risk. Herds declared free of PRV by this method should remain in a higher risk category and have periodic monitoring to improve the chance of rapid detection if another epidemic does occur within the herd.

A problem that may occur when attempting to declare a herd free of PRV is that of false serologic reactions. Since no test is 100% sensitive and 100% specific, false reactions will occur. False-negative reactions may cause problems by failing to detect infected individuals, and thereby allowing the premature declaration that a herd is free of PRV. However, these will be extremely difficult to detect in the field and one must rely on experimental data generated in the development of the test to indicate how commonly this will occur. False-positive reactions will cause problems by incorrectly identifying individuals as infected and thereby preventing the declaration that the virus has been eliminated. For example, if a test is 99% specific, one can expect 1 false-positive reaction in every 100 samples tested. One way to pursue these tentative false-positive reactions is to retest only the suspicious sera (serial testing). This should preferably be done with a more specific test, but in the absence of such a test, the same test may be used. Occasionally, these sera retest positive, and a second sample should be collected from the pig at least 2 weeks later and tested (Duffy et al. 1990c). If the second sample is still positive, the pig may be culled and the herd retested. If it is negative, the sample of pigs is declared free of PRV. A second way to manage apparent false-positive reactions is to utilize the known specificity of the test to interpret the apparent prevalence of PRV that was determined in the herd sample. For example, if the specificity is 99% and 1 sow in a test of 100 sows was positive,

the sample of sows could be declared free of PRV by the following formula:

$$\text{True prevalence} = \frac{(\text{apparent prevalence} + \text{specificity} - 100\%)}{(\text{specificity} + \text{sensitivity} - 100\%)}$$

The probability of successfully eliminating PRV from a herd by a test and removal program depends upon several factors: herd size, facility design, management practices, commitment of the owner/manager. Additionally, some viral strains are less infectious than others (McCullough 1989) and may be easier to eliminate. However, this method has been successfully used in large intensively housed herds in the United States and the Netherlands (Van Oirschot et al. 1990). Furthermore, there has been some speculation that recurrent epidemics may have occurred in some herds because of reintroduction of virus from an outside source, rather than from reactivation and shedding of a latently infected individual within the herd (Andersen et al. 1989).

Offspring Segregation. In this procedure, the female offspring of PRV-infected sows are weaned at 3–4 weeks of age and raised in a facility segregated from the infected herd. A sufficient number of gilts are raised so that the infected herd can be completely replaced over a 3-month period. This method is effective for eliminating PRV because pigs receive passive immunity, which affords considerable protection against infection. It is difficult to specify the distance between the infected and segregated facility, but the farther apart, the better. All isolated gilts are tested at 16 weeks of age, when maternally derived antibodies should not be detected. These segregated pigs should be vaccinated with a vaccine having a companion diagnostic test, if regulations permit. All gilts that test positive for PRV must be considered as infected and removed with all their pen mates. Upon maturity, the gilts may be bred to newly acquired PRV-negative boars and maintained through gestation in isolation from the infected herd. When breeding starts in the segregated facility, breeding is generally halted in the infected herd and sows are culled at weaning. As gilts become due to farrow, they are moved to the original facility, which should be depopulated by this time. The herd owner may elect to reduce costs by attempting to replace the infected breeding and growing/finishing pigs with the negative pigs as they are produced, hoping that a PRV epidemic does not occur. The success of this option will depend upon the degree of segregation between infected and susceptible pigs that can be maintained.

The major disadvantage of the traditional PRV offspring segregation program is the disruption to herd management with the only benefit being the elimination of PRV. Recent innovations that involve weaning at a relatively early age have permitted the elimination of other infectious agents simultaneously (see Chapter 65). If offspring segregation is being considered to eliminate PRV, weaning pigs at 5–10 days of age may also eliminate *Actinobacillus pleuropneumoniae, Haemophilus parasuis, Streptococcus suis, Serpulina hyodysenteriae,* and *Leptospira* spp. This modified segregation of offspring should be even more successful for eliminating PRV, since the chance of infection occurring prior to segregation will be lower.

Depopulation-Repopulation. Although this option has the highest probability of success, the prolonged time during which the facilities are nonproductive is extremely costly (Hoblet et al. 1987). However, depopulation may be the option of choice if there is a high PRV seroprevalence within the herd, there are multiple disease problems, the genetic strains are of little value, the facility is completely confined, and the owner has a strong financial base.

The most common method is to depopulate over a period of months as the pigs reach market weight. Alternatively, the entire facility may be depopulated by selling all market-weight pigs and breeding swine to slaughter, and moving the growing pigs to alternative facilities. For decontamination, the best time to depopulate is during warm months, since heat and drying inactivate PRV quickly. After depopulation, the entire facility, including feeders and pits, should be cleaned and disinfected (Thawley and Morrison 1988). After this is completed, a general guideline is to leave the buildings vacant for at least 30 days. The facility is then repopulated with known PRV-negative pigs.

The facility may be restocked with pregnant gilts due to farrow to reduce the cost of nonproductive time of the facility. Additionally, off-site finishing may be available. If the facility is to be vacant for a period of time, reducing the downtime to less than 30 days might be considered. The increased risk of doing so is impossible to quantify; however, the reduction in cost to the program can be substantial. An even more risky innovation involves replacing the breeding herd with no whole-herd downtime (Kislingbury 1987); i.e., the infected herd is gradually replaced as noninfected bred gilts are introduced. If PRV is spreading in the herd, contact between the infected and new stock must be minimized, if not eliminated. The infected herd should be vaccinated to decrease the amount of virus being shed by recently infected swine. Additionally, vaccinating the noninfected herd should be considered, since it may decrease the chance of infection.

NATIONAL PROGRAMS FOR PRV ERADICATION

United States. Serologic surveys conducted in 1974, 1977, 1980, and 1984 at slaughter facilities across the United States estimated the prevalence of PRV at 0.6%, 3.7%, 8.4%, and 8.8% respectively (Schnurrenberger 1984). In 1989, with the support of the National Pork Producers Association and various livestock associations, a national program was initiated, with a goal of eradicating PRV from all domestic swine herds by the year 2000. As of December 31, 1989, there were 5886 of 327,569 (1.8%) swine herds in the country known to be infected with PRV and the status of 85.4% of the herds was unknown. Most infected herds are concentrated in areas of intensive pig production in the Midwest and Southeast (Fig. 70.1).

A national database has been established to collate data collected from all states and to monitor progress. Observations include the current prevalence of quarantined herds, number of newly identified infected herds and suspected sources of infections, number of herds where PRV has been eliminated, progress reports on quarantined herds, and surveillance and traceback findings.

The program has been designed around five stages: 1, preparation; 2, control; 3, mandatory PRV elimination; 4, continued surveillance; and 5, PRV free. Each state is responsible for establishing an advisory committee, composed primarily of producers who will oversee that state's progress. A National Pseudorabies Control Board was formed that, in conjunction with the U.S. Department of Agriculture Veterinary Service Division, defined the requirements for each stage. This board also evaluates applications from states to proceed through the five stages.

Surveillance is primarily conducted at slaughter, although first point-of-sale and on-farm testing is also performed. A prerequisite for advancing to stage 3 is that a system be in place to randomly sample and test 10% of the breeding swine annually. If positive sera are detected, at least 80% must be successfully traced back to the herd of origin. Several states have elected to select a random sample of herds stratified by herd size. The use of PRV vaccines is regulated at the state level. Where vaccination is permitted, gene-altered PRV vaccines that have complimentary differential diagnostic tests are encouraged. Currently available modified live and killed PRV vaccines include those having no differential capability and those having differential capability based on deletions in the genome encoding for glycoprotein I (gI^-), $gIII^-$, and gX^-.

In the first year of the PRV eradication program, quarantine was removed from 1805 herds after PRV was eliminated by one of the methods described above. To be released from quarantine, herd owners who wish to sell breeding stock must have an initial negative test of all breeding stock, followed by monthly testing of 10% of the breeding herd. Herd owners wishing to sell feeder pigs must have a representative sample of the breeding herd tested annually. The regulations for farrow-to-finish herds are less restrictive. Some states require a test on a representative sample of the breeding herd to establish a herd's PRV status. In states in stages 1 or 2, these herds may be released from quarantine by sampling a representative group of the finishing and breeding herd. Herds removed from quarantine in such a manner remain in a high-risk category for 1 year when another sample of the breeding herd must be obtained.

A consideration in the national program is the PRV status of feral pigs. Pseudorabies is endemic in the feral pig population in many of the 22 states where they are present, and there are no effective means to prevent transmission among them. The impact that this will have on the national eradication program in domestic swine herds is unknown.

The U.S. program appears to be progressing on schedule. The general mood of producers and veterinarians is optimistic, especially since the advent of tests that can differentiate between infected and vaccinated pigs. It appears relatively uncomplicated to eliminate PRV from most herds. A more complex problem is to ensure that a herd does not become reinfected, especially in endemically infected areas.

Europe. In 1992 the European Community (EC) proposes to have free agricultural trade among member countries. England and Denmark have instituted programs to eradicate PRV, and appear to have succeeded. Other countries in the EC are implementing control/eradication programs to avoid inhibiting free trade of pigs. Where vaccine is used, most countries have permitted only products with a gI deletion.

COUNTRIES FREE OF PRV. Although PRV was present in England since at least 1953, it was not until the late 1970s, early 1980s, that the incidence in pig herds appeared to rise dramatically (Taylor 1989). Vaccination for PRV has not been permitted. An eradication program, funded in part by a producer check-off program, was initiated in 1983 when there were 220 known infected herds. Retesting these 220 herds revealed that 118 were still infected. Circle testing 2 km around these 220 herds, traceback, and clinical reporting revealed another 316 herds. Infected herds were depopulated with compensation. Slaughter surveillance was established in 1983 and approximately 10% of the culled sows were tested annually. In 1988, a decision was made to survey all boars at slaughter instead of sows. In 1989, after depopulating 520 herds and 430,000 pigs, the eradication program was announced successful and the check-off was terminated.

In Denmark, as in England, the epidemiologic picture of PRV changed in the late 1970s (Andersen et al. 1989). Clinical signs appeared to become more severe and incidence increased. Vaccination was not permitted. In 1980, a control/eradication program was initiated when PRV was made a notifiable disease. Herd owners were encouraged to have their herds accredited for PRV, and virus was eliminated from low-prevalence areas. This program was extended to include surveillance of all culled boars at slaughter, compulsory testing of a representative sample from all herds every other year, and monthly testing of communal boars. A range of 62–105 newly infected herds was identified annually from 1978–83. Starting in 1983, high-prevalence herds were depopulated and test and removal was practiced in low-prevalence herds with the herd owner being compensated by a producer-funded check-off. In 1986, 32 of 47,814 (0.07%) herds were known to be infected and PRV was eliminated from these by test and removal. Considering that on December 1, 1986, all herds in Denmark had been tested and no new herd epidemics had been detected for the previous year, it was concluded that PRV had been eliminated from the country. Since then, epidemics have occurred repeatedly in the southern districts, close to the border with Germany. Epidemiologic investigations and restriction enzyme analysis of isolates indicate that these epidemics are due to new introductions rather than reactivation of latent virus. The source of virus is speculated as being airborne transmission from Germany, which, if true, emphasizes the need for cooperation between regions and countries.

The occurrence of PRV in Switzerland was sporadic from 1973–83. In 1981–82, a survey of all swine herds (669) was conducted, regulations were imposed, and the virus was apparently eliminated in 1983 (Ehrensperger et al. 1984). In Austria, the prevalence has been very low, and the last case was reported in 1983. There is no evidence of rampant spread among herds and it has been speculated that ecologic conditions in Austria may not be conducive for PRV transmission (Kubin 1984). Bulgaria reported its last case in 1985.

LOW-PREVALENCE COUNTRIES. Luxembourg, Spain, Portugal, Italy, Greece, Yugoslavia, Albania, Czechoslovakia, Poland, and Romania are reported to have a low prevalence of PRV-infected herds (FAO 1988). Programs vary among these countries.

HIGH-PREVALENCE COUNTRIES. Germany, France, Netherlands, Belgium, Hungary, Republic of Ireland, and Northern Ireland have a relatively high prevalence of PRV in areas where swine are concentrated. In a serologic survey of 97 herds conducted in 1987 in the Netherlands, all were found to be positive for PRV. Vaccination for PRV is estimated to be practiced in 95% of the breeding herds and 65% of the fattening herds. In the province of Brittany, France, where pigs are most concentrated, 23 of 128 (18%) farrow-to-finish herds were estimated to be infected in one survey (Vannier 1989). While PRV was reported to be eliminated from what was then East Germany in 1985, approximately 1500 newly infected herds are identified annually in then West Germany. The current policy in these countries is to control movement of pigs originating from infected herds and to apply a blanket vaccination of all herds in endemically infected areas. This vaccination program is an attempt to suppress the circulation of virus within herds so that the incidence of new herd infections is reduced, and so that test and removal can be performed. If these large-scale vaccination programs are deemed successful, then these countries may opt to proceed toward national eradication programs.

Pacific Rim. Most countries in Southeast Asia are reported to be free of PRV. Hong Kong and Thailand appear to have a high prevalence, while Laos, Philippines, Malaysia, Singapore, and Viet Nam have a low prevalence (FAO 1988; Ninh 1990, personal communication). The status in China is unreported. Korea, Taiwan (Sung 1990, personal communication), and Japan are reported to be experiencing an increasing incidence of herd infections. Although some of these countries permit only killed PRV vaccine, there is no uniform policy on gene-altered vaccines or on which deletions may be used.

Other Countries with PRV. In Central and South America, only Venezuela has a relatively high prevalence of PRV. Cuba, Mexico, Guatemala, Brazil, and Argentina all have a low prevalence. Elsewhere, Sweden, Soviet Union, and New Zealand are reported to have a low prevalence.

CONCLUSION. Epidemiclike spread of PRV occurred in many countries in the late 1970s, early 1980s. It has been postulated that more virulent strains have evolved and are responsible for this increased spread. It also has been suggested that the coincidental increased intensification and concentration of the swine industry may provide an environment more conducive for PRV. Regardless of the reason, in the absence of controls, PRV has increased in prevalence in many countries around the world. The three components of a control/eradication program are to (1) estimate the prevalence of infected herds, (2) decrease the incidence of new herd infections, and (3) decrease the prevalence of existing herd infections. Effec-

tive methods have been developed and successfully implemented in several countries for each of these steps, and new techniques are continually being devised and adopted.

REFERENCES

ANDERSEN, J. B.; BITSCH, V.; CHRISTENSEN, L. S.; HOFF-JORGENSEN, R.; AND KIRKEGAARD PETERSEN, B. 1989. The control and eradication of Aujeszky's disease in Denmark: Epidemiological aspects. In Vaccination and Control of Aujeszky's Disease. Ed. J. T. Van Oirschot. Boston: Kluwer Academic Publishers, pp. 175–183.

ANDERSON, P. L.; MORRISON, R. B.; THAWLEY, D. G.; AND MOLITOR, T. W. 1989. Identification of pseudorabies virus–infected swine herds by evaluating the serostatus of boars or finishing pigs. J Am Vet Med Assoc 195:1709–1711.

ANDERSON, P. L.; MORRISON, R. B.; MOLITOR, T. W.; AND THAWLEY, D. G. 1990. Factors associated with circulation of pseudorabies virus within swine herds. J Am Vet Med Assoc 196:877–880.

ANNELLI, J. F., AND MORRISON, R. B. 1990. Estimation of pseudorabies seroprevalence in the breeding herd and its application in representative sample testing for monitoring herd status. Proc Int Congr Pig Vet Soc, Lausanne, p. 200.

ANNELLI, J. F.; JOO, H. S.; AND MORRISON, R. B. 1990. The use of dried whole blood collected on filter paper in ELISA and gel-ELISA for detection of pseudorabies antibodies. Proc Int Congr Pig Vet Soc, Lausanne, p. 216.

ANNELLI, J. F.; MORRISON, R. B.; GOYAL, S. M.; BERGELAND, M. E.; MACKEY, W. J.; AND THAWLEY, D. G. 1991. Swine herds having a single reactor to serum antibody tests for Aujeszky's disease virus. Vet Rec 128:49–53.

BITSCH, V. 1975. A study of outbreaks of Aujeszky's disease in cattle: II. Further investigations on the route of infection. Acta Vet Scand 16:434–448.

––––––. 1984. The main epidemiologic features of Aujeszky's disease. Proc Off Int Epizoot, Aujeszky's Disease, Vienna, pp. 381–391.

BITSCH, V., AND ANDERSEN, J. B. 1982. On the epidemiology of Aujeszky's disease in Denmark and the possibilities of its control. In Aujeszky's Disease. Boston: Martinus Nijhoff Publishers, pp. 227–236.

BOGNAR, K.; HASSAN, H. B.; ANTAL, T.; KUCSERA, L.; RACS, C.; REVAI, R.; AND SZABO, I. 1986. Active immunization against infectious bovine rhinotracheitis and Aujeszky's disease. Magy Ao Lapja 11:647–657.

BOLIN, S. R.; RUNNELS, L. J.; SAWYER, C. A.; AND GUSTAFSON, D. P. 1982. Experimental transmission of pseudorabies virus in swine by embryo transfer. Am J Vet Res 43:278–280.

CANNON, R. M., AND ROE, R. T. 1982. Livestock disease surveys: A field manual for veterinarians. Canberra: Australian Government Publishing Service, pp. 1–35.

CHRISTENSEN, L. S.; STRANDBYGAARD, S. B.; HENRIKSEN, C. A.; AND ANDERSEN, A. B. 1989. Aujeszky's disease in Denmark: The epidemiologic situation in winter 1987–88 studied by restriction fragment pattern analysis. Dansk Vet Tidsskr 72:322–325.

DAMRONGWATANAPOKIN, T.; MARSH, W. E.; ANDERSON, P. L.; MORRISON, R. B. 1990. Development of a geographic information system to assess spread of pseudorabies virus (Aujeszky's virus) between swine herds. Proc Int Congr Pig Vet Soc, Lausanne, p. 373.

DAVIES, E. B., AND BERAN, G. W. 1980. Spontaneous shedding of pseudorabies virus from a clinically recovered postparturient sow. J Am Vet Med Assoc 176:1345–1347.

DE WAELE, K.; DE SMET, K.; AND PENSAERT, M. 1990. Attempts to eradicate Aujeszky's disease virus on closed farms by intensive vaccination under field circumstances. Proc Int Congr Pig Vet Soc, Lausanne, p. 256.

DONALDSON, A. I.; WARDLEY, R. C.; MARTIN, S.; AND FERRIS, N. P. 1983. Experimental Aujeszky's disease in pigs: Excretion, survival and transmission of the virus. Vet Rec 113:490–494.

DUFFY, S. J.; MORRISON, R. B.; AND THAWLEY, D. G. 1990a. Spread of pseudorabies virus within quarantined swine breeding herds. J Am Vet Med Assoc. Submitted for review.

———. 1990b. Factors associated with the spread of pseudorabies virus within the breeding section of quarantined swine herds. J Am Vet Med Assoc. Submitted for review.

DUFFY, S. J.; MORRISON, R. B.; AND GOYAL, S. M. 1990c. Use of a differential ELISA for the detection of antibodies to pseudorabies virus at the herd level. J Am Vet Med Assoc. Submitted for review.

EHRENSPERGER, F.; KIHM, U.; PROBST, U.; AND IRRALL, B. 1984. Epidemiology of Aujeszky's disease in Switzerland. Schweiz Arch Tierheilkd 126:429–439.

FAO-WHO-OIE. 1988. Animal Health Yearbook. Rome: FAO.

GLOSTER, J.; DONALDSON, A. I.; AND HOUGH, M. N. 1984. Analysis of a series of outbreaks of Aujeszky's disease in Yorkshire in 1981–82: The possibility of airborne disease spread. Vet Rec 114:234–239.

GOODWIN, R. F. W., AND WHITTLESTONE, P. 1986. Eight years' experience with a register of pig herds monitored for Aujeszky's disease. Vet Rec 119:493–494.

HALLAM, J. 1987. A preliminary cost-benefit analysis of the proposed national pseudorabies eradication program. Proc Livest Conserv Inst, pp. 84–96.

HARASZTI, J.; MEDVECZKY, I.; RONAY, G.; SEREGI, J.; SOLTI, L.; AND VARGA, J. 1989. Transfer as a possibility for the eradication of Aujeszky's disease in swine. Magy Ao Lapja 44:325–327.

HOBLET, K. H.; MILLER, G. Y.; AND BARTTER, N. G. 1987. Economic assessment of a pseudorabies epizootic, breeding herd removal and downtime in a commercial swine herd. J Am Vet Med Assoc 190:405–409.

JAMES, J. E.; JAMES, D. M.; MARTIN, P. A.; REED, D. E.; AND DAVIS, D. L. 1983. Embryo transfer for conserving valuable genetic material from swine herds with pseudorabies. J Am Vet Med Assoc 183:525–528.

KISLINGBURY, C. K. 1987. Assisting clients with cash flow analysis. Comp Food Anim 9:F285–F292.

KOMANIWA, H.; MAKABE, T.; FUKUDA, M.; OGAWA, T.; AND HATAKEYAMA, H. 1986. Levels of passive antibodies against Aujeszky's disease virus in piglets derived from infected sows. Jpn J Vet Sci 48:633–635.

KUBIN, G. 1984. Aujeszky's disease in Austria. Proc Off Int Epizoot, Paris, pp. 29–33.

LE FOLL, P. 1988. Analysis of cost/benefits of the French Aujeszky's disease control program. Rec Med Vet 164:929–937.

LOMNICZI, B.; NAGY, E.; KUKEDI, A.; AND ZSAK, L. 1989. Molecular epidemiology of Aujeszky's disease in Hungary. In Vaccination and Control of Aujeszky's Disease. Ed. J. T. Van Oirschot. Boston: Kluwer Academic Publishers, pp. 93–102.

McCULLOUGH, S. J. 1989. Vaccination and control of Aujeszky's disease in Northern Ireland. In Vaccination and Control of Aujeszky's Disease. Ed. J. T. Van

Oirschot. Boston: Kluwer Academic Publishers, pp. 231–238.

MACK, H.; WEKERLE, J.; AND STRAUCH, D. 1986. Isolation of Aujeszky virus from pig faeces, slurry and piggery air samples. Tierarztl Umsch 41:32–38. Abstracted in Vet Bull 7:1776.

MAES, L., AND PENSAERT, M. 1984. Examination for virus persistence on swine fattening and breeding farms after an outbreak of Aujeszky's disease. Tijdschr Diergeneeskd 109:439–445.

MARTIN, W. S.; MEEK, A. H.; AND WILLEBERG, P. 1987. Veterinary Epidemiology, 1st ed. Ames: Iowa State Univ Press, pp. 67–71.

MEDVECZKY, I.; MAYER, G.; OVARY, L.; BODRI, G.; BALINT, J.; AND NAGY, J. 1990. Epizootiological investigations and eradication by the selection (test and cull) method in a piggery latently infected with Aujeszky's virus (PRV-1). Proc Int Congr Pig Vet Soc, Lausanne, p. 226.

MOCSARI, E.; SZOLNOKI, J.; GLAVITS, R.; AND ZSAK, L. 1989. Horizontal transmission of Aujeszky's disease virus from sheep to pigs. Vet Microbiol 19:245–252.

MORRISON, R. B., AND THAWLEY, D. G. 1989. Serologic status of pseudorabies virus in growing-finishing pigs in quarantined herds. J Am Vet Med Assoc 195:1577–1579.

RUEFF, L. 1990. Epidemiologic study of pseudorabies within a naive county. Proc Am Assoc Swine Pract, Denver, pp. 201–206.

RUMNEY, R. P. 1986. Meteorological influences on the spread of foot-and-mouth disease. J Appl Bacteriol [Suppl]:105S–114S.

SABO, A. 1985. Analysis of reactivation of latent pseudorabies virus infection in tonsils and gasserian ganglia of pigs. Acta Virol 29:393–402.

SCHNURRENBERGER, L. W. 1984. Slaughter serum surveys. Proc Livest Conserv Inst, Madison, pp. 170–171.

SCHNURRENBERGER, P. R.; SHARMAN, R. S.; AND WISE, G. H. 1987. Attacking Animal Diseases: Concepts and Strategies for Control and Eradication. Ames: Iowa State Univ Press, pp. 96–114.

SCHOENBAUM, M. A.; ZIMMERMAN, J. J.; BERAN, G. W.; AND MURPHY, D. P. 1990. Survival of pseudorabies virus in aerosol. Am J Vet Res 51:331–333.

TAYLOR, K. C. 1989. Epidemiologic aspects of Aujeszky's disease control in Great Britain. In Vaccination and Control of Aujeszky's Disease. Ed. J. T. Van Oirschot. Boston: Kluwer Academic Publishers, pp. 185–196.

THAWLEY, D. G., AND MORRISON, R. B. 1988. Programs for the elimination of pseudorabies virus from large herds of swine. J Am Vet Med Assoc 193:184–190.

THAWLEY, D. G.; GUSTAFSON, D. P.; AND BERAN, G. W. 1982. Procedures for the elimination of pseudorabies virus from herds of swine. J Am Vet Med Assoc 181:1513–1518.

THAWLEY, D. G.; SOLORZANO, R. F.; AND JOHNSON, M. E. 1984. Confirmation of pseudorabies virus infection, using virus recrudescence by dexamethasone treatment and *in vitro* lymphocyte stimulation. Am J Vet Res 45:981–983.

THAWLEY, D. G.; BERAN, G.; HOGG, A.; GUSTAFSON, D. P.; AND VINSON, R. 1987. Summary report of pilot projects for eradication of pseudorabies in swine. J Am Vet Med Assoc 191:1386–1390.

VAN AARLE, P. A. M.; TRUIJEN, W. T.; AND TIELEN, M. J. M. 1978. Aujeszky's disease. Studies on the possibility of differentiating between contaminated pig-breeding farms on which the pigs have been inoculated with the Bartha vaccine. Tijdschr Diergeneeskd 103:213–219.

VANNIER, P. 1989. The control program of Aujeszky's disease in France: Main results and difficulties. In Vaccination and Control of Aujeszky's Disease. Ed. J. T. Van Oirschot. Boston: Kluwer Academic Publishers, pp. 215–226.

VAN OIRSCHOT, J. T. 1986. Intranasal vaccination of pigs against Aujeszky's disease: Comparison with one or two doses of attenuated vaccines in pigs with high maternal antibody titres. Res Vet Sci 42:12–16.

VAN OIRSCHOT, J. T.; WIJSMULLER, J. M.; DE WAAL, C. A. H.; AND VAN LITH, P. M. 1990. A novel concept for the control of Aujeszky's disease: Experiences in two vaccinated pig herds. Vet Rec 126:159–163.

WITTMANN, G. 1984. Aujeszky's disease: Factors important for epizootiology and control. Proc Off Int Epizoot, Aujeszky's Disease, Vienna, pp. 3–28.

WITTMANN, G., AND RZIHA, H. J. 1989. Aujeszky's disease (Pseudorabies) in pigs. In Herpesvirus Diseases of Cattle, Horses, and Pigs. Boston: Kluwer Academic Publishers, pp. 233.

ZIMMERMAN, J. J.; BERAN, G. W.; AND PLATT, K. B. 1988. Pigs can be infected with pseudorabies virus by the conjunctival route without seroconversion. Proc Conf Res Workers Anim Dis, p. 56.

ZIMMERMAN, J. J.; HALLAM, J. A.; AND BERAN, G. W. 1989. The cost of eliminating pseudorabies from swine herds in Iowa. Prev Vet Med 7:187–199.

71 Housing and Environmental Influences on Production

S. E. Curtis

L. Backstrom

ENVIRONMENT influences every aspect of the pig's life. It includes all elements of the pig's surroundings, but in this chapter nutritional elements are not considered (see Chapter 60).

Swine can adapt to a wide range of environments. They can be produced successfully in a variety of facilities and climates, including even some that provide suboptimal conditions. Pigs respond quickly to environmental stresses to survive and reproduce in adverse surroundings. These adaptive responses take the form of changes in body functions and structures and behavior, which may be counterproductive in terms of health and performance and may affect the pig's well-being (Curtis 1987; Duncan 1987).

The environments in which most swine are now raised differ greatly from those prevalent even in the 1960s. The several systems of pork production in use include low- and high-investment feeder-pig production operations, a variety of farrow-to-finish options (one- and two-litter pasture systems and low- and high-investment confinement systems), and low- and high-investment feeder-pig finishing enterprises (Bache and Foster 1976).

Choice of production system traditionally has been based on several factors, including farm size and type, management ability, capital position, labor supply, and business organization. Now, environmental protection regulations and animal welfare concerns have been added to this list. In general, low- and high-investment confinement production systems generate the highest returns on investment per hour of labor (Bache and Foster 1976), so for some time there has been a marked trend away from more extensive production systems to those involving continuous farrowing schedules and space-intensive facilities. This means management ability has become more crucial.

The decision as to which production system to use is thus based on several factors in addition to the health and productivity of the pigs. Fundamental defects of the feeder-pig finishing system (mixing pigs from several sources) and the continuous farrow-to-finish system (the temptation to use facilities continuously with no sanitation breaks) are reflected to some extent in economic analyses. However, the nature of different techno-logic requirements of various production systems is not addressed adequately in such an approach. This is especially so for environmental and disease management. For a given operation, management ability is a fixed factor, and variation in productivity among operations using the same system owes more to variation in management than to any other single factor (Backstrom 1973). Another important element of the intensification trend is the control the pig has over its environment. Given the opportunity, pigs will seek shelter and alter their microenvironments and schedules to achieve comfort. The more intensive the production system, the fewer options and resources the pig has; thus, it is imperative that the manager know the pigs' needs and how to meet them.

Equipment design has become more critical, too. Sow and piglet behavior vary markedly in farrowing crates of different design, and this is reflected in sow and piglet performance (Curtis et al. 1989; Rohde Parfet et al. 1989). Similarly, sow feeders of various designs are quite different in terms of feed wastage, sow injury, and other traits (Taylor 1990).

Intensification of swine production has been followed by new challenges in environmental and disease management (Backstrom 1973; Lindqvist 1974; Curtis 1983). Deficiencies of some operations are immediately apparent. However, evidence that first appearances can be deceiving is the healthy and productive environment for pigs provided by the poorly ventilated, crowded sweat house (Gordon 1963).

Direct effects of the environment on the performance of healthy swine has been well-recognized (Sorensen 1961; Meyer and Van Fossen 1971; Sainsbury 1974). Much attention has been paid to effects of the thermal environment on growth and feed-conversion efficiency. Some direct pathologic consequences of stresses such as the porcine stress syndrome (Marple and Judge 1976), cardiac infarcts (Johansson et al. 1974), and fundic gastric ulceration (Backstrom and Bjorklund 1974) have been studied.

A new class of diseases has also arisen. They are the syndromes of multiple etiology, known variously as production or factorial diseases. They may be exemplified by the finding of Kalich

(1970) that piglets born to specific-pathogen-free (SPF) sows and kept under poor, fair, or optimal environmental conditions developed histopathologic signs of pneumonia, the severity of which depended on environmental quality (Table 71.1). Thus clinical manifestations of some infectious diseases clearly can be affected by the environment in which the pig resides.

Further evidence in support of this arises from air pollution in closed facilities. For example, effects of atmospheric ammonia stress and early ascarid infection on the growth of young pigs are additive (Drummond et al. 1981a). Either condition alone depressed body weight gain by around 30%; when combined, growth was reduced by 60%, even though the air pollutant did not intensify liver and lung lesions left by migrating ascarid larvae. Severity of turbinate and lung lesions due to *Bordetella bronchiseptica* infection in young pigs was directly related to aerial concentration of ammonia, while growth rate, depressed by the infection alone, was unaffected by additional stress from ammonia (Drummond et al. 1982b). Hence, environmental stressors can affect performance of swine not only directly but indirectly via influences on health as well.

ASSESSING SWINE ENVIRONMENTS.
While the environment in a swine facility is complex, most of its elements can be measured. Interpreting results of such measurements in terms of pig health and performance remains the dilemma. Environmental factors interact with one another; the effect of one stressful factor often depends on the nature of the rest of the environment. Also, the ability of the pig to successfully resist environmental challenges changes from time to time and varies among individuals.

Advances have been made as experience has been gained, but often the troubleshooter still must engage in trial and error to identify the problem. Following are some points to be considered when assessing swine environments (Curtis 1983).

Consider all environmental factors. Environment results from all external conditions the pig experiences. Even elements that cannot be readily measured or controlled influence the health, well-being, and performance, so these should also

be considered to the extent possible.

Remember interactions. The environmental complex acts as a whole on the pig. Combined effects of two or more environmental components may be difficult to evaluate, but nonetheless they should be considered.

Environmental factors vary over space at a given time. Values obtained at one place in a facility may not hold for other locations. It is important to measure environmental variables where all the pigs experience them—in all the microenvironments throughout the unit.

These factors also change with time at a given place. Swine facilities may be occupied continuously. Because environmental factors and occupancy vary with time, needed control measures do also. This is especially so when days are warm and nights cool. Environmental assessments and control schemes should consider daily and seasonal environmental cycles and variations due to short-term weather events. The pig can readily adjust to many environmental cycles as long as extremes are not unduly stressful.

The rate of environmental change is critical. Abrupt changes tend to be more stressful than those occurring over a longer period. For example, preconditioning young pigs to a cool environment before moving them from a closed nursery to an open-front unit during cold weather reduces stress.

Pigs modify their own environments. They give off heat, water vapor, urine, and feces and shed pathogenic organisms. Thus the animals' own processes help determine the nature of their environments. Changes in age or number of pigs in a facility alter animal impacts and therefore the control measures required.

Manage swine environments with the pigs' needs in mind. There is a tendency to assume that if a human is comfortable in a certain environment, a pig would be also. Beware of this pitfall. Pigs may be more or less sensitive to a certain stressor than humans.

INFECTIOUS AGENTS.
The ultimate source of an infectious agent is an infected animal. The environment serves as the transport medium between hosts and also determines the agent's survival time outside the host. Crowding increases

Table 71.1. Effect of environmental quality on incidence and severity of pneumonia lesions in 4- to 12-week-old piglets born to SPF sows

	Environment of Farrowing House					Incidence of Pneumonia of Various Grades				
	Air Temperature (°C)		Percent Relative Humidity	Airspeed (m/sec)	Piglets	−	±	+	+ +	+ + +
Group	House	Nest								
A	6–9	12–14	90–95	0.2–0.3	18	0	0	4	10	4
B	9–12	20	70–85	0.2	18	0	4	11	3	0
C	16	30	70	0.1	18	16	2	0	0	0

Source: Kalich (1970).

the contact spread of infectious agents, but environmental management is equally crucial in indirect transmission, during which the agent is exposed to the environment and must survive this excursion with intact virulence to remain a threat.

Pathogen Survival. Pathogenic agents rarely grow or multiply outside a host, although some multicellular parasites have necessary periods of development outside the host. Each form has an optimal range of certain environmental factors for survival away from the host.

PATHOGENS FROM FECAL SOURCES. Slotted floors reduce infections by gastrointestinal parasites but do not eliminate them (Gaafar and Jones 1965). Even in closed facilities equipped with underfloor waste-holding pits, the excreta remains close to the swine, moist, and shielded from sunlight. Hence the chance of transmission remains, especially for agents that can be made airborne or carried by a vector.

Several pathogenic microbes survive at least a few months in underfloor waste (Burrows and Rankin 1970). Salmonellae are particularly persistent. When the solid content of waste is 5% or more and the temperature is below 10°C (P. W. Jones 1976), such microbes can be carried into the pigs' microenvironments. Various pathogenic coliforms, streptococci, and staphylococci have been found in considerable quantities in fresh sawdust, shavings, and straw (Rendos et al. 1975; Natzke and LeClair 1976).

Pigs can contaminate their feed. In one study as many as 5000 enterobacteria were found per gram of dry diet (Hill and Kentworthy 1970). A sow's fecal flora can contain new enteropathogenic strains of *Escherichia coli* within a week after exposure to the microbes (Arbuckle 1968). These eventually contaminate the udder and teats, so susceptible piglets might be challenged by bacteria shed by their resistant carrier dams.

PATHOGENS IN THE AIR. Microbes can travel from host to host in airborne droplets, droplet nuclei, and particles. If animals are close together, the droplet route may be almost as effective as direct contact (Wells 1955). For some diseases, airborne transmission is virtually the only natural way the agent effectively challenges a susceptible host. In fact, when dead and thus nonbreathing and nonsneezing pigs that had suffered from mycoplasmal pneumonia were placed in a pen with susceptible pigs, none of the latter became infected (Lannek and Wesslen 1957). Airborne transmission is also involved in a number of diseases that ordinarily travel by other means. Even transmissible gastroenteritis virus (TGEV) and *E. coli* can move from pig to pig in the air (Reber 1956; Wathes 1988a).

Pathogens in droplets and droplet nuclei are susceptible to changes of temperature and vapor pressure and to ultraviolet radiation (Cox 1987). Only because they are generated in such huge quantities, as during sneezing, do enough survive to constitute an effective dose. For both airborne bacteria and viruses, the higher the air temperature the more quickly they die, primarily due to desiccation.

Effects of vapor pressure are more complex. Lipid-containing viruses seem to survive better at low humidities, whereas those composed only of protein and nucleic acids are less vulnerable to higher vapor pressures (Buckland and Tyrrell 1962). Airborne bacteria survive better at relative humidities either above or below a range of 50–80%; this range is most lethal (Dunklin and Puck 1948; Jones and Webster 1981; Jones et al. 1982; Wathes 1988b). Change in humidity, as commonly occurs when air leaves a facility or space occupied by an animal, is also a critical factor. When the relative humidity was abruptly switched from either high or low to the lethal midrange, over 90% of the airborne mycoplasmal organisms present died within 8 minutes (Wright et al. 1968; Hatch et al. 1970).

Ultraviolet rays in the wavelength range of 0.25–0.28 μm, as found in solar radiation, are bactericidal and virucidal (Kundsin 1968), but an organic-matter coating may protect microbes from the radiation. Most infectious microbes in the air of a swine facility are transported as part of a particulate vector. These dustborne microbes have three sources: droplets or droplet nuclei settling onto dust particles, contamination of particles with parasite-laden excretions or secretions, and dried excretions or secretions themselves.

Vectors and Carrier Animals. Animate vectors of infectious microbes may be of the same species as or a different species from the host. In a commercial swine-production setting it is a difficult task to eliminate all animate vectors, which may include—in addition to the pigs themselves—cats; dogs (Haelterman 1962); birds (Pilchard 1965); rodents (Schnurrenberger et al. 1970); and perhaps the most flagrant nonporcine vector of all, humans. Nevertheless, their elimination must be the goal, because a disease-barrier system is only as strong as its weakest link.

Oddly enough, the vector overlooked most frequently is the pig itself. In one study almost 90% of the healthy pigs 4 months or older harbored beta-hemolytic streptococci (J. E. T. Jones 1976). The carrier pig is usually an unrecognized source of infection, and its presence makes all other efforts at herd isolation useless. Older animals are often immune carriers of forms pathogenic to younger animals; e.g., sows often shed TGEV in the feces.

BATCH OR ALL-IN/ALL-OUT SYSTEM. Carrier newcomers are the most common means of introducing a pathogen into a group of swine. The newcomers may have originated in a different facility at the same operation or at another. Hence, though often tempting at first in terms of economical use of facilities, there can be serious problems associated with mixing animals of different origins in the same facility.

Even at large-volume operations there has been a trend away from continuous occupation of large farrowing and nursery facilities in favor of smaller units that can be occupied by series of batches of animals. Usually a sanitation break between groups is applied as well. This scheme has returned substantial dividends in terms of the health of the young pigs leaving such units.

Young pigs in farrowing and nursery units are the most susceptible of any age group to infectious disease, since their immune systems are still developing. These young pigs are also more vulnerable to various debilitating stressors that are often present and can affect several elements of resistance negatively. Thus it is in these areas that environmental and disease management must be accomplished most scrupulously. A healthy pig at weaning has a better chance to stay healthy and perform well in the nursery, just as the prospects for a healthy pig leaving the nursery are brighter than for a sickly one.

Swine in feeder-pig finishing operations generally have healthier respiratory tracts and grow faster when the facilities are operated according to the batch system as compared to continuous occupancy (Backstrom and Larsson 1971; Backstrom and Bremer 1978; Martinsson 1979).

QUARANTINE. When new stock must be added to a herd, it should be quarantined for 3 or 4 weeks before being mixed into the existing group. While being held in the isolated area, the newcomer should be observed frequently for symptoms of acute disease; treated for external and internal macroparasites; and (if it is to be used in breeding) tested for leptospirosis, brucellosis, and pseudorabies and possibly for swine influenza, parvoviruses, and enteroviruses.

When introducing boars into a herd it is a good practice to add a few gilts on their way to market to the boar's pen at the end of the quarantine period. By this method the gilts serve to test the boar for the presence of any agents of acute disease he may be carrying; the boar can adjust (or succumb) to acute diseases in the herd. He also has a chance to demonstrate his mating ability.

HERD SIZE. Most studies have revealed a direct relationship between herd size and disease problems (Backstrom and Larsson 1971; Lindqvist 1974; Backstrom and Bremer 1976, 1978). Some of this undoubtedly can be attributed to limited management ability, but there are biologic components as well. For example, when a carrier pig is introduced into a large group, the pathogenic microbes it harbors can be transmitted throughout

more readily than in a small group. The relation between the number of animals in the group (n) and the possible number of transmissions of microbes from one pig to another (N) is given by the equation $N = n^2 - n$. For example, in a group of 4 there are 12 such avenues, and in a group of 100 there are 9900.

Another factor is the increasing virulence a microbe can attain by serial passage through a group of pigs. Even ordinarily innocuous or opportunistic microbes can become pathogenic in this way. As herd size increases, so do the chances of this happening. Older animals may carry microbe strains of relatively high virulence to which they have become immune. Hence younger, more susceptible pigs should be isolated from growing-finishing swine and the breeding herd.

OPERATION ISOLATION. A pork-production operation should take as much advantage as possible of the least expensive and most useful natural barrier to disease transmission among operations, i.e., distance.

Sanitation. By reducing the concentration of pathogenic agents in the environment between occupancy periods, these agents' challenges to the next group of swine to reside in the facility are reduced. The rational level of sanitation depends on the health of the previous occupants. A true sanitation break can be accomplished only when the room is completely emptied of animals, for they constitute the ultimate source of most of the disease-causing agents. Thorough removal of manure and other biologic residues, including that in or on underfloor waste-handling equipment, eliminates most but not all parasitic forms. Terminal chemical disinfection is a necessary sequel to manure removal and power (water) or steam washing in most operations.

The effectiveness of chemical disinfectant agents varies with the microbe or other parasite (Sykes 1965; Harry 1967; Curtis 1983). Formaldehyde gas is the most effective all-around choice, but it is a deadly poison and must be used very carefully (Graham and Michael 1932; Graham and Brandly 1937). The fumigant can be generated either by aerosolizing a 20% formalin (i.e., 8% formaldehyde) solution at the rate of 10 L/1000 m³ space or by reacting potassium permanganate with formalin (40% aqueous solution of formaldehyde) at the rate of 620 g of the compound to 1240 ml formalin for each 100 m³ space. Formaldehyde fumigation is most effective when all surfaces are wet down prior to fumigation and the air's relative humidity is 80–90%.

Other major types of disinfectants are cresols, phenols, quaternary ammonium compounds, chlorhexidine, iodophors, hypochlorite (bleach), and sodium hydroxide (lye) (Biehl 1983). These generally have excellent effects against bacteria (chlorhexidine is less effective against pus-forming bacteria and pseudomonads), while efficacy against viruses varies. Hypochlorite, lye, and formaldehyde are most effective against viruses. Presence of organic debris tends to inactivate chemical disinfectants, especially iodophors, quaternary ammonium compounds, and bleach. Previous mechanical cleaning is crucial to obtaining maximal effects of these disinfectants. Cresols and phenols have good effects even in the presence of organic materials, but a negative side effect is their irritating effect on skin.

Feed Additives. Antibiotics, chemotherapeutics, and anthelmintics constitute an important part of the environmental complex in modern pork production. These drugs must be available to treat specific diseases and in certain cases to prevent diseases as well. However, it is likely that the drugs are being used more extensively than would be necessary if more effective environmental management were being practiced. With continued use of certain drugs, many microbe strains become resistant to the growth-inhibiting effects of those drugs, so they become useless for either growth-promotant or therapeutic applications (N. C. Nielsen et al. 1976).

AGE AT WEANING. Feed additives are most efficacious in young pigs at the ages they are naturally most susceptible to microbial challenges and most vulnerable to other environmental rigors (Whiteker et al. 1978).

If the pigs are reasonably healthy, they should be weaned as soon after 4 weeks of age as possible. At an earlier age the pig is simply unequipped physiologically and immunologically. It is extremely sensitive to its thermal environment during the first 4 weeks after birth and requires the very warm environment that is most readily maintained in the farrowing house. At 3 weeks of age or so, the passive immunity the pig gained from the sow's colostrum shortly after birth has very often dropped below the protective level, before the pig's own active immunity mechanisms are completely developed. So during the third and fourth weeks after birth, the pig is highly vulnerable to certain diseases. In addition, there are nutritional and sociobehavioral considerations. Weaning age is a compromise between waiting long enough for the pigs to be ready and getting the pigs out of expensive farrowing facilities as soon as feasible. The compromise works out to be weaning at around 4 weeks of age in most commercial situations.

Many of the problems against which feed additives are most effective have their roots, directly or indirectly, in early weaning. The environmental and social requirements as well as the immune status of the 3-week-old pig argue against its being weaned at this age. Successful early weaning requires a strictly controlled environment with re-

gard to temperature (29°C the first week and 24°C the second); low-intensity light; dry pens; and restricted, high-quality diet during the first 2 weeks (H. E. Nielsen et al. 1976). With increasing age, the piglets' environmental needs are reduced. Waiting until 4 weeks of age or even older has resulted in excellent productivity and is commonly recommended in herds with persistent pig health problems. However, litter space requirement in the farrowing area increases rapidly as the pigs grow older. A minimum of 5 m² of pen area is required for optimal development of the litter when pigs are weaned at 6 weeks (Simensen 1971; Backstrom 1973).

STRESS AND RESISTANCE. A variety of environmental stressors – including cold and hot environments, crowding, mixing, weaning, limit-feeding, noise, and movement restraint – are known to alter animals' immunity and other defenses against infections (Kelley 1980). The pig's disease resistance is also affected by the environment (Curtis and Kelley 1983).

The vulnerability of the pig's pulmonary bacterial clearance mechanisms to several stressors will be detailed later. Cold stress has also been found to increase newborn and young pigs' susceptibility to TGEV (Furuuchi and Shimizu 1976; Shimizu et al. 1978). Acquisition of colostral immunoglobulins by newborn piglets is impeded by cold stress (Blecha and Kelley 1981), perhaps because cold-stressed piglets nurse less vigorously (Kelley et al. 1982; LeDividich and Noblet 1981). There doubtless are many other such effects.

The nature of these stress-induced changes in disease-resistance processes in pigs is not yet understood (Dantzer and Kelley 1989), but the secretion of glucocorticoid hormones in nonspecific response to the impingements of most stressors is likely to be involved (Hudson et al. 1974). The breadth of the effects already ascertained in pigs emphasizes the crucial role the environment plays in the balance between microbic challenge and pig resistance.

THERMAL ENVIRONMENT. The pig regulates its body temperature by balancing heat loss against metabolic heat and heat gain from the environment (Mount 1968; Curtis 1983). As the difference between body and environmental temperatures become greater, heat-loss rate increases.

Effective Environmental Temperature. The environment's demand of heat from the pig is determined largely by air temperature, the temperatures of radiant environmental surfaces (walls, ceilings, equipment), air speed in the pig's microenvironment, and floor characteristics. Mount (1975) has shown that, in a house with walls and ceiling 3°C cooler than the air and a 0.3 m/second draft across the animals, effective temperature is more than 8°C lower than air temperature as registered by a common thermometer. Further, if the pigs are on a concrete-slat floor, effective temperature drops another 6°C, but with straw bedding the adjustment is to add 4°C.

Straw provides a huge amount of thermal comfort for young pigs, and this is reflected by their health and performance (Backstrom and Fagerberg 1972; Backstrom 1973). Its use has been abandoned by many producers because of its scarcity in some areas and its alleged incompatibility with comtemporary waste-management systems. However, modern farrowing systems incorporating straw bedding have been devised and used with success (Curtis 1978). Growing/finishing swine also respond positively to straw bedding during cold periods (Moustgaard et al. 1959). Moreover, in older pigs straw has recreational and dietary value in addition to insulative, radiation-shield, and draft-breaking effects (Fraser 1975), and peripartal sows may have a need to use straw or some other manipulable environmental feature (Widowski and Curtis 1990).

Thus air temperature, as measured by a common thermometer, is an insufficient parameter of a pig's thermal microenvironment. Management decisions must be based on the more complete assessment of effective environmental temperature.

Lower Critical Temperature. Age and body size, thermal insulation, feed-intake rate, and group size determine the effective temperature below which pigs must increase their heat-production rate to keep their bodies warm — the point called the lower critical temperature (LCT) (Mount 1975; Holmes and Close 1977; Verstegen et al. 1978; Verstegen and Curtis 1988). Not only are younger, smaller pigs more sensitive to cool quarters but their zone of thermal indifference is narrower.

When consuming 1.5 kg of feed daily in a group of four, the LCT of 36-kg pigs is 17°C, but when taking in 1.8 kg daily and in a group of nine, it is 10°C. In large groups, 21-kg pigs fed to maintenance at thermoneutrality have a LCT of 24°C, but when fed ad libitum (around 1 kg/day) it is 13°C. Dry sows in individual stalls limit-fed 1.8 kg feed/day have a lower critical effective temperature of around 17°C.

Feed and/or Fuel. During cold weather, a pig's heat balance can be achieved by raising environmental temperature to reduce environmental heat demand, increasing the pig's heat gain by such means as a radiant heater, or letting the pig raise its metabolic rate to produce more heat for itself. The first two options require more fuel or power, the third more feed.

How much extra feed is required to keep the body warm? For example, when effective environmental temperature is 11°C below the LCT, the 21-kg pig would need to consume around 0.15 kg

additional feed daily just to keep body temperature up to normal. A dry sow's feed allowance should be increased when effective environmental temperature falls below 18°C, as it often does when she is held singly on bare concrete. At an effective 10°C, for example, such a sow should be fed almost 0.5 kg of extra feed each day.

Water Vapor. Swine rely less on evaporative heat loss than many species, so high vapor pressure that suppresses evaporation is less critical for them. Vapor pressure has little influence on the well-being or performance of swine unless air temperature exceeds 32°C. Moisture control is nonetheless necessary in swine facilities because damp surroundings favor survival of pathogens outside a host and lead to structural deterioration of the building.

Air Distribution. Effective ventilation of a swine house depends on uniform air distribution and an adequate ventilation rate (Brugger and Brooks 1977; Curtis 1983; Midwest Plan Service 1983; Esmay and Dixon 1986; Albright 1990). Drafts may cold-stress animals, while stagnant areas may lead to heat stress as well as high concentrations of air pollutants. Thus knowledge of air-flow patterns is essential to an understanding of the pigs' thermal environment.

Regardless of whether natural or mechanical ventilation is employed, air flows as it does inside an animal house largely because of its density and velocity when it enters the house. Warm air entering through an inlet under the eave or in the ceiling is buoyant and tends to continue moving along the ceiling to the outlet. It mixes with the building air before reaching the animals; but when incoming air is much cooler and denser than building air, it tends to drop to pig level before mixing with it. This is the major source of drafts inside a swine house. Characteristic rotary air flows are set up, and these may also lead to drafts at animal level (Randall 1975). In some places during the seasons of change, incoming air is warm during the day but cool at night. On such days, airflow patterns within the facility change at least twice daily. As this reversal occurs in the evening, the pigs may experience sudden environmental changes as air temperature drops and air-speed picks up. Airflow patterns in swine facilities are controlled mainly by inlet position, assuming adequate fan capacity is present. Inlet-opening size influences the air's speed as it enters the house, and this in turn has a great effect on air distribution. Velocity should be in the range of 180–360 m/minute for adequate control of distribution (Randall 1975). Air may be directed to a certain extent by inlet baffles. When an exhaust-fan system is used during winter, cracks and gaps in the building may become inlets for small jets of cold air, which may cold-stress nearby pigs.

Even in environments in which the air is normally still, application of radiant heat sets into motion convective eddies that partially erase any beneficial effect of the radiant heat itself. This is especially harmful when the draft so created carries to the pig cold air that has just dropped into the building from the outside.

Newborn Piglets. The individual piglet's LCT is around 35°C the first or second week after birth (Mount 1968; Curtis 1974). The piglet's thermoregulatory ability improves markedly during the first postnatal day (Curtis et al. 1967). Its total heat-loss rate is two-thirds higher in a 21°C environment than at 29°C. Evaporation from skin and respiratory passages amounts to less than 10% of its heat loss, regardless of effective environmental temperature. No more than 15% of the piglet's heat loss is to the floor, so floor temperature has relatively little effect on total heat balance. Nevertheless, heat-loss rate is twice as great to concrete as to wood. The remaining 75% of the piglet's heat loss flows by either radiation or convection. Thus environmental conditions that affect these flows are important determiners of the piglet's thermal comfort.

Wall and ceiling temperatures are major factors in radiant heat loss, whereas air temperature and speed largely influence convective heat loss. Dropping wall and ceiling temperatures by 11°C even when air temperature remains the same increases the piglet's total heat-loss rate by around 20%, which emphasizes the need for well-insulated farrowing houses.

A practical problem is providing comfortable areas for both piglets and the sow at the same time, since their thermal-comfort ranges are at least 10°C apart. When able to do so, the sow makes a warm, dry, draft-free nest for her young and ordinarily lies close to it. When an artificial nest is provided for newborn piglets too far away from the sow's udder, the piglets prefer to stay near the sow during the crucial first few days, even though they may be under cold stress (Titterington and Fraser 1975).

AIR ENVIRONMENT. The pig's respiratory tract is in intimate contact with the air and consequently, in closed facilities, with air pollutants. Those of major concern include microbes, dust, gases, and odorous vapors—all arising from the pigs and their activities. Air pollutants can affect pig performance directly by altering metabolic reactions or indirectly by influencing health (Lillie 1970; Curtis 1972). Caretakers may also be affected (Donham et al. 1984).

Bacteria. Concentration of airborne bacterial particles in a closed swine facility ranges from around 15,000/m³ during warm weather to around 350,000/m³ during cold, the variation being due mainly to ventilation rate (Curtis et al. 1975a). In modified open-front units, the range is lower

(3500–175,000/m³) but still considerably higher than the 300/m³ found in outdoor air. Vapor pressure and airborne bacterial concentration are generally related inversely; moister, heavier particles settle faster.

Most of the airborne bacteria in swine facilities are staphylococci or fecal streptococci; coliforms are scarce. Roughly 20% of the coccal particles and 10% of the coliform particles are small enough (less than 5 μm in aerodynamic diameter) to be drawn all the way down into the lungs (Curtis et al. 1975b). In addition to bacteria that arise from the pigs' skin and excreta, respiratory pathogens can also be present in the air. Each sneeze aerosolizes around 40,000 microbe-laden droplets.

The pig normally can clear bacteria and keep its lungs relatively sterile. However, exposure to various stressors, e.g., cold exposure (Curtis et al. 1976), atmospheric ammonia (Drummond et al. 1978), and migration of ascarid larvae (Curtis et al. 1987), depress pulmonary bacterial clearance processes, predisposing the pigs to respiratory tract infections.

Dust. Most of the aerial dust in facilities where pigs are fed meal diets originates in the feed. Some is skin and hair debris. When the ventilation rate is low, dust concentration in many such units approaches the threshold limit (10 mg/m³) for human industrial occupancy. But even at this concentration, airborne dust has little direct influence on the healthy pig's growth (Curtis et al. 1975c).

Gases and Odorous Vapors. Swine-facility air is polluted by several dozen fixed gases and odorous organic vapors given off as manure decomposes (Day et al. 1965; Hammond et al. 1974). It appears that the most important of these that are related to pig health and performance are hydrogen sulfide and ammonia (Curtis 1986).

At concentrations normally present in closed units (less than 10 ppm), pigs tolerate hydrogen sulfide well. But when underfloor waste is agitated prior to its removal, hydrogen sulfide concentration above the floor can reach over 1000 ppm, which is lethal within seconds to pigs as well as humans (Buck et al. 1976). Ammonia sometimes is present in swine-facility air at concentrations exceeding 100 ppm. At 50 ppm, atmospheric ammonia hinders the young pig's ability to clear bacteria from its lungs and depresses growth of even healthy pigs (Drummond et al. 1980).

Carbon monoxide may arise from incomplete combustion of fuel in a heater. When the proportion of blood hemoglobin present as carboxyhemoglobin reaches 30%, pigs become lethargic; they die when it exceeds 60%. Fetal hemoglobin has a greater affinity for oxygen and carbon monoxide than adult hemoglobin (Buck et al.

1976); thus carboxyhemoglobin percentage in perinatal piglets, which are also more sensitive than adults, may be several times higher than that in an adult in the same environment. High but sublethal concentrations of carbon monoxide in air (e.g., 200 ppm for newborns, 300 ppm for weanlings) make newborn piglets behave sluggishly and weanling pigs grow slowly.

Control of air pollution can aim at prevention or elimination. Prevention centers on waste management and feed distribution. Biologic and chemical preparations for odor control in swine facilities may be beneficial in some cases. Eliminating air pollutants still depends mainly on dilution by ventilation. The threshold sanitary ventilation rate is the air-change rate that eliminates airborne transmission of infectious agents (Wells 1955), and ordinarily it is higher than economically feasible in swine facilities.

SOCIAL ENVIRONMENT AND BEHAVIOR.

Behavioral reactions by pigs to environmental stimuli are numerous and varied (Signoret et al. 1975; Pond and Houpt 1978; Fraser 1984). Behavioral maladjustments are often at the root of unthriftiness (showing up as a high frequency of stragglers), injuries, and other unproductive factors.

Social Environment

GROUP SIZE AND SPACE ALLOWANCE. Many studies have been conducted on the effect of group size on the performance of finishing pigs, and the results have been mixed. In general, performance is not much affected in groups up to at least 40. In most closed or semiclosed facilities where ad libitum feeding is employed, it is convenient and practical to keep pigs in groups of 20–30, while groups are often larger when the animals have access to an outside lot or apron (Fritschen and Muehling 1978a). In limit-feeding systems, group size is usually kept to around 10; otherwise social discord arises and performance is affected negatively.

Pigs grouped together organize themselves in a dominance order (Meese and Ewbank 1973). The resulting social stability is an advantage, since little energy is spent in further combat and injuries are minimized. But there are also drawbacks. Competition for feed spurs intake somewhat, but some of the variation in growth among pigs is due to dominance-order rank.

Under poor husbandry, especially when access to feed is marginal, the connection is more marked. When restricted feeding is used, it is important that all pigs in the group be able to eat at the same time. It is generally recommended that the ratio of feeding places to pigs be at least 1:4 in multiple-place self-feeding situations. In either situation, it is advisable to provide, on the average, 35 cm of trough width per nominal feed-

ing place for finishing swine, 25 cm for growing pigs, and 15 cm for nursery pigs (Taylor 1990, personal communication).

The dominance order seems less able to control aggression when space allowance is reduced (Ewbank and Bryant 1972). At high density, pigs are more active and aggressive, thus the sizeable effect space allowance has on growth and feed-conversion efficiency (Gehlbach et al. 1966; Backstrom and Anderson 1984). Fritschen and Muehling (1978a) recommended space allowances for swine as given in Table 71.2. These recommendations are in harmony with those of Hogsved (1973).

MIXING. The fights that result when strange pigs are grouped have little direct long-term effect on growth unless other stresses such as inadequate floor or feeder space are present (Sherritt et al. 1974). Short-term growth depression can be reduced sometimes by administering a tranquilizing drug (Symoens 1970). Fighting can alter disease resistance or cause injury (even death) and thus affect growth indirectly. Pigs should be mixed only when absolutely necessary and then in a pen that is new to all; they can become extremely aggressive toward intruders on home territory. Hiding areas to which submissive pigs can retreat reduce the fighting and injuries (McGlone and Curtis 1985).

Once a dominance order has been established, it remains more or less stable indefinitely. It is ordinarily not disrupted by moving an intact group of pigs to a new area of its own (Scheel et al. 1977).

Anomalous Behavior. Especially when confined, swine exhibit several anomalous behaviors,

Table 71.2. Recommended space allowances for swine

Pig Weight or Class	m²/pig[a]
Partially or totally slotted floor	
Weanlings on deck	0.14–0.19
7- to 14-kg pigs	0.16–0.23
14- to 27-kg pigs	0.28–0.37
27- to 45-kg pigs	0.46
45- to 68-kg pigs	0.56
68-kg pigs to market	0.74
Gestating sows or gilts	1.30–1.49
Developing boars	1.86
Mature boars	3.72
Housing with outside apron	
Growing/finishing pigs	0.56 in, 0.56 out
Sows	1.02–1.11 in, 1.02–1.11 out
Boars	3.72 in, 3.72 out
Pasture with shade	
Sows (10/acre)	1.39–1.86 shade
Sows and litters (7/acre)	1.86–2.79 shade
Boars (0.25 acre each)	3.72–5.57 shade

Source: Fritschen and Muehling (1978a).
[a]Adjusting pig number per pen seasonally may result in improved performance; e.g., increasing group size by 1 or 2 during cold weather may be desirable.

some of which are vicious and lead to injury of groupmates. Tail biting and ear chewing are common examples. While routine practices such as tail docking shortly after birth reduce such vices as tail biting, they do not attack the basic causes of such behaviors.

To a large extent the triggers of anomalous behaviors are still unknown (Fraser 1987). Frustration, the interference with any goal-oriented behavior by any means, increases aggressive activities as well as circulating glucocorticoid concentration in pigs (Arnone and Dantzer 1980; Dantzer et al. 1980). Frustration is generally recognized as a precursor of anomalous behavior in animals. Confined swine are frustrated in some respects.

Movement restraint of sows by being crated or tethered during gestation and the peripartal period leads to sterotyped behaviors such as bar biting in pregnant sows (Fraser 1975; Ekesbo et al. 1979; Jensen 1983; Cronin 1985) and to a higher frequency of standing-sitting-lying activity during the 48-hour period before delivery begins (Hansen and Curtis 1980). The incidence of peripartal diseases, including the mastitis-metritis-agalactia (MMA) complex, and piglet stillbirths and postnatal mortality are also related to restraint of the sow around farrowing time (Backstrom 1973; N. C. Nielsen et al. 1976; Backstrom et al. 1984). The sow kept in a crate prior to farrowing cannot fulfill her strong instinct to build a nest for her young, and this interference may contribute to farrowing and lactation problems (Widowski and Curtis 1990; Widowski et al. 1990). Tethering gilts before puberty can have untoward consequences because the reproductive tracts of many never mature (Jensen et al. 1970). England and Spurr (1969) found poorer results in individually crated sows in terms of heat signs and farrowing results.

Restlessness in gestating sows was reduced by access to straw for recreational use (Fraser 1975), but this was not so in the peripartal period (Hansen and Curtis 1980; Widowski and Curtis 1990). Some attempts to reduce tail biting and other anomalous behavior patterns in swine by providing recreational straw or suspending playthings in the pens have been successful (Van Putten 1968; Hogsved et al. 1970; Mowitz 1971; Madsen et al. 1978; Grandin 1989). Also the incidence of tail injuries was 29% in pigs on slotted floors but only 2% on solid floors (Madsen et al. 1978). Attempts to change tail-biting behavior by dietary alterations or air pollutants have been unsuccessful (Ewbank 1973; Krider et al. 1975).

Sows sometimes savage their newborn young for no apparent reason. Sows that kill their piglets have been observed to sit and stand during the 48 hours before delivery begins (Hansen and Curtis 1980) more than sows that do not, suggesting that the savage-sow syndrome is a manifestation of environmental maladjustment.

Pigs prefer comfortable surroundings, and they learn to operate devices such as a waterer that provide reward. There are possibilities for pigs to exercise more control over their own environments; e.g., pigs will operate a supplemental heater in response to a cool environment (Baldwin 1979; Curtis and Morris 1982). This may also serve to reduce some of the pigs' frustration.

Reproductive Behavior. The social environment in which young boars and gilts are kept influences their reproductive function and behavior. Much sexual behavior is learned around the time of puberty (Signoret et al. 1975). Young boars in homosexual groups cannot gain heterosexual experience when they are ready to learn at 3–6 months of age. Often, failure to "get boars to work" is due to lack of such social experience (Dziuk 1985, personal communication). Confinement per se does not impede sexual development in boars (Esbenshade et al. 1979).

Gilts raised in confinement frequently reach puberty late or not at all. Sometimes a move outdoors triggers the onset of estrus. Group size is also a factor. Gilts in groups of around six show heat more readily than those in larger groups, regardless of space allowance (Dziuk 1985, personal communication). Solid partitions between groups help in this regard, as pigs count in their group any other pigs they can touch. Although estrous gilts seek out boars by using olfactory cues (Signoret 1967), keeping a boar near gilts supports their reproductive development and achievement of first estrus.

LIGHT. Relatively little attention has been paid to light as an environmental factor in pork production. With intensification of the industry and movement of animals into lightproof facilities, knowledge of light requirements has become more important in designing appropriate systems.

Young pigs permitted to operate lights for themselves keep them on around three-fourths of the time, with some dark period called for each hour of the day (Baldwin and Meese 1977). However, growing pigs kept in continuous darkness usually perform similarly to those given periodic or constant illumination (Comberg and Doenen 1968). In some studies, however, pigs under continuous darkness were socially maladjusted and became somewhat photophobic (Van Putten 1968).

Reproductive phenomena in many species are closely linked with photoperiod. It appears that a daily photoperiod of at least 9 hours is sufficient to ensure normal attainment of puberty in gilts (Ntunde et al. 1979). Boars provided a 15-hour daily photoperiod had greater overall seminal sperm concentration and total viable sperm output than those raised under natural short-day photoperiods (Mahone et al. 1979). Also, by 8 months of age semen had been collected from all the supplementally lighted boars but from only half of those raised under the natural photoperiod regimen.

SOUND. Little study has been made of the pig's reactions to sound or any of its effects on health and productivity. What evidence is available indicates sound has little or no effect on swine (Bond et al. 1963). In particular, sounds of various frequencies or of jet aircraft chronically reproduced at intensities of 120–130 decibels in the animals' environment did not interfere with mating, parturition, lactation, growth, or feed-conversion efficiency. However, piglets' nursing behavior might be atypical when extraneous noise, as from a fan, is louder than the sow's grunts (Jensen 1983).

FLOORS. The nature of the floor required in a swine facility is dictated partly by the waste-management system employed (Fritschen and Muehling 1978b). If wastes are handled as solids or semisolids, the floor is usually without slots or perforations. Liquid-waste systems are generally used with partly or totally slotted or perforated floors.

Injuries to foot claws tend to be less severe in pigs on soil and most severe on totally slotted or perforated floors (Fritschen 1976). They also tend to be more severe on aluminum and concrete slats than on steel and least severe on plastic slats. Wider slats (up to 20 cm) lead to less claw injury. Smooth, clean floors are preferable to rough, dirty ones. Claw lesions seem to have little effect on the performance of growing/finishing swine (Fritschen 1976). However, mating activity of breeding animals can be severely hampered by sore feet.

Newborn pigs on unbedded floors commonly develop abrasions on feet and legs and other areas of the body that are often entry portals for pathogenic microbes, particularly those associated with streptococcal arthritis and abscesses (Nielsen et al. 1975). Various means of providing better footing and less abrasive floor surface for swine have been devised, but most have proved to have drawbacks as well as advantages (Christison and Farmer 1983; Applegate et al. 1988). Some cleaning procedures, especially those involving high-pressure solutions on concrete, tend to make the surface more abrasive.

PARTITIONS. A variety of materials are used to construct pen dividers. From the point of view of environmental and disease management, partitions can be classified as solid or perforated. The solid type have advantages in terms of controlling transmission of infections, limiting social contact to a pig's own group, and reducing drafts. Perforated partitions are sometimes recommended because they permit freer flow of air throughout the animal space, but air-distribution systems can be built that permit adequate ventilation quality even when solid partitions are employed.

The disease-management benefits mentioned above have a corollary in unit size, i.e., the number of pens in the same air space. In this latter context the walls are analogous to the partitions in the former. Viewed from the opposite perspective, solid partitions between pens are extensions of the walls that make an all-in/all-out scheduling scheme effective (Backstrom et al. 1978). Especially with large-volume units, it is essential that basic design planning take disease transmission into account. Some such means of managing disease are relatively inexpensive, one-time costs.

PRACTICAL SITUATIONS. The environmental complex in a swine facility involves many highly variable, interacting factors. Webster (1970) diagrammed one view of general interrelationships among environmental elements and infectious disease (Fig. 71.1), from which it is clear that a holistic approach to disease management is a necessity in situations where other production factors may be affecting the delicate balances between the infectious challenges on the one hand and the animals' defenses on the other. Muirhead (1976) outlined the more important factors that must be kept in mind when assessing the etiology of one particular syndrome, mastitis, in the sow (Fig. 71.2). A review of the findings in several field studies will be instructive.

In a study of finishing units, Tielen (1978) found that both a temperature-fluctuation index and a draftiness index were clearly related to the percentage of severely affected lungs at the time of slaughter (Table 71.3). Vapor pressure and ammonia and carbon dioxide concentrations were unrelated to lung disease in swine in this study.

From results of another study of over 500 growing/finishing operations, it was found that the quality of housing and management was strongly related to the incidence of pulmonary lesions at slaughter (Table 71.4). The lowest incidence would thus be expected in operations where there is only one source of pigs, facilities are operated on an all-in/all-out basis, and pigs are not moved from unit to unit during the growing-finishing period.

The relationship between the size of operation and lung disease (Table 71.4) was ascribed to microenvironmental differences related to operation size. In particular, data show that width of the building and floor type during the growing period are related to lung-lesion incidence at slaughter weight, and the number of pigs per room and floor type during the finishing period is therefore related to lung disease (Table 71.5).

In a somewhat different approach, Backstrom and Bremer (1978) selected from 150 swine herds the 10 with the lowest and the 10 with the highest incidence of moderately or more severe pneumonia at slaughter time. These two groups were

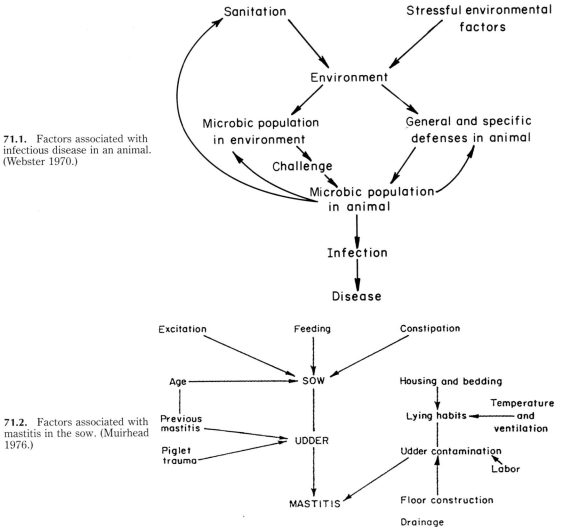

71.1. Factors associated with infectious disease in an animal. (Webster 1970.)

71.2. Factors associated with mastitis in the sow. (Muirhead 1976.)

Table 71.3. Environmental conditions over 10 months inside a finishing unit as related to percentage of lungs with severe lesions at slaughter

Percentage severely affected lungs			
Range	>20	10–20	<10
Actual average	26	14	6
Temperature-fluctuation index[a]	0.78	0.60	0.48
Draftiness index[b]			
Winter	188	187	155
All 10 months	137	130	114

Source: Tielen (1978).

[a]Daily temperature range in unit per daily temperature range outside.

[b]Average airspeed inside (m/min) × temperature difference between inside and outside (°C).

Table 71.4. Relationship between housing-management systems and incidence of lung lesions in pigs at slaughter time

System Factor	Percent
Source of pigs	
Same farm	16
One outside farm	16
Two outside farms	25
More than two outside farms	23
House operation	
All-in/all-out	14
Continuous	19
Moving among houses	
None	16
Once	19
More than once	22
Size of operation[a]	
<100	8
100–200	16
200–300	19
>300	23

Source: Tielen (1978).

[a]Number of places for a 100-kg pig.

Table 71.5. Relationship between housing factors and incidence of lung lesions in pigs at slaughter time

Housing Factor	Percent	Housing Factor	Percent
Growing period		*Finishing period*	
Width of house		Size of room[a]	
One row of pens	17	<100	15
Two rows of pens	19	100–200	18
Four rows of pens	32	200–300	21
Floor type		<300	29
Solid	16	Floor type	
Half-slotted	20	Solid	13
Fully slotted	23	Half-slotted	18
		Fully slotted	22

Source: Tielen (1978).
[a]Number of places for a 100-kg pig.

then compared with respect to a number of environmental factors (Table 71.6). Their results show that several factors merit further study, since they might be related to the etiology of chronic pneumonia in swine. These include floor-space allowance, waste-management method, and ventilation efficiency.

Backstrom (1973) also studied the health of sows and litters as related to whether the females were isolated from the farrowing facilities during pregnancy (Table 71.7). The notion is that sows that spend at least the end of the gestation period

Table 71.6. Comparison of several environmental factors in swine herds with high or low incidence of moderately severe pneumonia at slaughter

Factor	Incidence of Moderately Severe Pneumonia	
	Low (%)	High (%)
Incidence of moderately severe pneumonia	3.1 (0–3.4)	24.6 (15.0–25.1)
Hygiene and husbandry[a]	1.7	2.2
Producer interest in disease prevention[a]	1.5	2.3
Pigs medicated individually[b]	8	4
High antibiotic use for 2 weeks after weaning[b]	3	1
Finished pigs farrowed on same farm[b]	5	0
All-in/all-out only[b]	5	2
Continuous operation of facilities[b]	5	7
Water available ad libitum[b]	8	4
Floorspace allowance >0.5 m²/pig[b]	9	6
Slotted floor in dunging alley[b]	3	2
Liquid manure in unit[b]	2	5
Underfloor fan in dunging alley	3	2
Ventilation efficacy[a]	1.6	2.8

Source: Backstrom and Bremer (1978).
[a]Subjective grade: 1 = excellent, 4 = poor.
[b]Number of herds.

Table 71.7. Comparison of sow and piglet health in swine herds in which pregnant sows are kept in or away from farrowing facilities

Health Factor	Pregnant Sows in Farrowing Facilities	Pregnant Sows Away from Farrowing Facilities
Sows		
MMA syndrome[a]	6	9
Total morbidity[a]	17	20
Piglets		
Alive per litter	11.0	11.0
Weaned per litter	9.1	8.8
Stillbirths[a]	5	6
Infectious diseases[a]	3	4
Other mortality[a]	10	10
Litters		
Diarrhea, < 1 week old[a]	4	8
Diarrhea, 1–5 weeks old[a]	12	11
Respiratory diseases[a]	10	10
Unthriftiness[a]	18	16
Total morbidity[a]	55	53

Source: Backstrom (1973).
[a]Percent incidence.

in the same environment in which they farrow and lactate can build up immunity within 1 week to the microbes prevalent there and then pass this on to their offspring via colostrum and milk (Arbuckle 1968). Backstrom results on nearly 5000 litters suggest there might be health advantages for both sow and piglets in keeping pregnant sows near farrowing-lactating facilities.

Here again the sow's and piglets' needs are at odds. It is important for the sow to be exposed widely to potential piglet pathogens, but the challenge in the piglets' environments must be low (Coalson and Lecce 1973). N. C. Nielsen et al. (1976) generated striking evidence in favor of a sanitation break in farrowing rooms. During the 6 months preceding such a break, the incidence of neonatal diarrhea was 33% and deaths from it almost 4%; during the first 6 months after the sanitation break the incidence had fallen to 11% and less than 1% respectively. Pepper and Taylor (1977) depopulated and thoroughly disinfected a farrowing house after collecting data on the last 30 litters in a continuous series of farrowings. They then collected data on the first and second 30 litters farrowed in the facility after the sanitation break. Depopulation and disinfection clearly led to improved piglet performance, but there was evidence also that disease buildup started immediately after the break (Table 71.8), suggesting that sanitation breaks should be imposed as frequently as feasible.

HEALTH-ENVIRONMENT RELATIONS IN PRACTICAL SITUATIONS. Comprehensive studies of relations between practical environmental complexes and the health and performance of piglets (Backstrom 1973) and finishing swine (Lindqvist 1974) have been reported. In

Table 71.8. Results in terms of piglet performance of a depopulation disinfection break in a farrowing house

Factor	30 Litters Preceding Break	First 30 Litters after Break	Second 30 Litters after Break
Average litter size (8 weeks)	7.6	8.2	8.0
Average pig weight (kg at 8 weeks)	11.2	13.9	12.3
Mortality (percent at 8 weeks)	18.3	13.7	15.2

Source: Pepper and Taylor (1977).

such field surveys, qualitative and quantitative observations are made on both the environment and the animals, and correlations are calculated. Evidence of strong relationships from empirical investigations of this sort can complement results of controlled studies as well as identify relationships that merit more detailed experimental inquiry.

A review of the categories of animal and environmental traits studied by Backstrom (1973) and Lindqvist (1974) will serve to delineate the scope of their investigations as well as provide a guide to the holistic diagnosis of factorial diseases in modern systems of swine production. The original publications should be consulted for a full appreciation of the scope and results of these studies.

Piglet Production. Inspections of animals and facilities and interviews with producers took many factors into account (Backstrom 1973).

SOWS. Based on inspections and interviews, the following were observed and recorded for lactating sows and those separated from their still identifiable litters: breed; parity; origin (born in operation or purchased); health at farrowing (1 week before till 1 week after); health at time of inspection; medical treatment or prophylactic measures administered at farrowing and up to time of inspection; all cases of illness and farrowing difficulties resulting in death of all piglets recorded 2 months retroactively from inspection, including cases where the sow died or was culled.

PIGLETS. Piglets in individual litters, present in the herd at the time of inspection, were observed for the following: number born into the litter; number alive at time of inspection; number stillborn; number lost by accidents; number dead from a sow ailment (including mastitis, savage sow syndrome, and piglet disease considered resulting from sow disease); number that were splaylegged; number that were weak (dead plus recovered); number dead from specific primary diseases; number with congenital deformities; number seriously ill or retarded at time of inspection; number placed in other litters and alive at

time of inspection; health of the litter at time of inspection; health of the litter between birth and inspection; medical treatment or prophylactic measures employed; litter age in weeks; and weaning status at time of inspection.

HERD ENVIRONMENT. The swine herd environment was assessed at the time of inspection and the following traits were recorded: number of sows in production; number in different life-cycle categories; boar used (owned or rented); pregnant sow environment (pen, crate, or tether design and flooring under hindquarters); exercise program for sows; days before farrowing that sows were placed in farrowing house; design and equipment in farrowing and rearing areas (including pen size, crate design, sow and piglet access to dunging area, floor slope, nature of floor, farrowing rails, creep area); nature of bedding in farrowing and rearing areas; method of waste management (liquid vs. solid); method of feeding; type of water supply; ventilation (air inlets, natural ventilation facilities, fans); heating (lamps, floor heating, other heat sources); air temperature and vapor pressure inside and outside the house; hygiene and husbandry level; other details of construction.

Finishing Operations. Lindqvist (1974) made observations on numerous factors, recorded them, and analyzed the data in search of correlations. The animals were inspected at the time of slaughter; the facilities were inspected at regular intervals during the course of the study.

OBSERVATIONS AT SLAUGHTER. Animals inspected at slaughter revealed the following: lung lesions; serous membrane lesions (pleurisy and pericarditis); livers ("white spots" and "other"); abscesses; arthritides; pale, soft, exudative muscle; injured tails; deaths in transit.

INSPECTIONS OF OPERATIONS. Inspections of swine operations resulted in the following observations: source of feeder pigs (same operation, other, or both); if from the same operation, number of sows, number of farrowing and rearing pens, weaning age, weight on arrival at the finishing unit; production system (continuous, continuous in batches, batches with unit empty less than 7 days, 7–14 days, or more than 14 days); size of facility (number of pigs per section, number of pens, year of construction); management of pigs at arrival; pen environments (length, width, number of pigs per pen, lying area per pig—for each stage of production); pen wall construction, including height; abrasiveness of floor; nature of floor insulation; slope of floor; difference in level from pen floor to dunging area floor; drainage from pen floor to dunging area; dunging habits; means of waste disposal; type of dunging area; total area per pig (pen plus dunging area); presence of reflushing; quality of fluid drainage in dunging area; waste management outside the unit; presence of water trap; quality of water trap function; year of construction of waste container; nature of waste container, including presence of cover; waste-storage capacity; separate or common container for each unit; presence of leaks in waste container; nature of bedding; control of feeding level; source of feed; feed-mixing equipment; feedstuff storage; special feed processing; means of feed delivery; wet feeding versus dry feeding; trough length per pig; access to drinking water; means of delivering water; presence of risks of infection in feeding system; nature of ventilation inlets; ventilation system category; presence of circulation fans; presence of underfloor ventilation; volume of inside unit per pig; ceiling height; ventilation rate per pig; nature of supplementary heating system; odors in unit during waste-pit emptying; odors in unit at other times; light conditions (windows, painted windows, no windows); if no windows, hours of illumination daily; unit cleaned before arrival of present batch of pigs; quality of cleaning job; latest arrival of pigs; number of pigs in facility at time of inspection; amount of variation in pig density in pens; nature of medical treatment (drugs, vitamins, anthelmintics); hygiene standard; husbandry standard; overall ventilation quality assessment; dust formation; respiratory health; presence of diarrhea; incidence of tail biting; signs of foot or leg lesions; visible swellings; number of pens with mange; number of pens with impetigo; number of pens with other skin diseases; other disease problems.

REFERENCES

ALBRIGHT, L. D. 1990. Environmental Control for Animals and Plants. St. Joseph, Mich.: Am Soc Agric Engl.

APPLEGATE, A. L.; CURTIS, S. E.; GROPPEL, J. L.; MC-FARLANE, J. M.; AND WIDOWSKI, T. M. 1988. Footing and gait of pigs on different concrete surfaces. J Anim Sci 66:334–341.

ARBUCKLE, J. B. R. 1968. The distribution of certain *Escherichia coli* strains in pigs and their environment. Br Vet J 124:152–159.

ARNONE, M., AND DANTZER, R. 1980. Does frustration induce aggression in pigs? Appl Anim Ethol 6:351–362.

BACHE, D. H., AND FOSTER, J. R. 1976. Pork production systems with business analysis: Selecting the "right" system. Pork Ind Handb, p. P1H-48.

BACKSTROM, L. 1973. Environment and animal health in piglet production: A field study of incidences and correlations. Acta Vet Scand [Suppl] 41.

BACKSTROM, L., AND ANDERSON, K. L. 1984. Influence of crowding on economics and production in growing swine. Agri-Practice 5(2):33–37.

BACKSTROM, L., AND BJORKLUND, N.-E. 1974. Gastric ulcers in swine: A study of incidences under different environmental conditions at abattoir before slaughter. Proc 11th Nord Vet Congr, Reykjavik, p. 262.

BACKSTROM, L., AND BREMER, H. 1976. Disease recordings on pigs at slaughter as a method of preventive and therapeutic veterinary medicine in swine production. Sven Veterinaertidn 28:312–336.

———. 1978. The relationship between disease incidence of fatteners recorded at slaughter and environmental factors in herds. Nord Vet Med 30:526–533.

BACKSTROM, L., AND FAGERBERG, R. 1972. The effect of different pen beddings in piglet production. Sven Veterinaertidn 24:749–752.

BACKSTROM, L., AND LARSSON, K. 1971. Disease statistics recorded at swine slaughter related to environmental factors in confinement hog production. Sven Veterinaertidn 23:294–306.

BACKSTROM, L.; HELLSTON, C.; HULTGREN, L.-E.; HOGSVED, O.; KRANTZ, G.; OHLEN, P.; OLSSON, O.; PETTERSSON, B.; AND SANDBERG, C. 1978. Partitioning of farrowing units in piglet production. Swed Dep Agric Vet Med.

BACKSTROM, L.; MORKOC, A. C.; CONNER, J.; LARSON, R.; AND PRICE, W. 1984. Clinical study of mastitis-metritis-agalactia in sows in Illinois. J Am Vet Med Assoc 185:70–73.

BALDWIN, B. A. 1979. Operant studies on the behavior of pigs and sheep in relation to the physical environment. J Anim Sci 49:1125–1134.

BALDWIN, B. A., AND MEESE, G. B. 1977. Sensory reinforcement and illumination preference in the domesticated pig. Anim Behav 25:497–507.

BIEHL, L. G. 1983. Breaking the disease and parasite cycle: Cleaning and disinfecting hog facilities. Univ Ill Coop Ext Serv Swine Semin, p. 67.

BLECHA, F., AND KELLEY, K. W. 1981. Cold stress reduces the acquisition of colostral immunoglobulin in piglets. J Anim Sci 52:594–600.

BOND, J.; WINCHESTER, C. F.; CAMPBELL, L. E.; AND WEBB, J. C. 1963. Effects of loud sounds on the physiology and behavior of swine. USDA Tech Bull 1280.

BRUGGER, M. F., AND BROOKS, L. A. 1977. Ventilation of dairy and other livestock buildings—design, operation, and equipment. Univ Wis Ext Bull A2812.

BUCK, W. B.; OSWEILER, G. D.; AND VANGELDER, G. A. 1976. Clinical and Diagnostic Veterinary Toxicology. Dubuque, Iowa: Kendall/Hunt.

BUCKLAND, F. E., AND TYRRELL, D. A. J. 1962. Loss of infectivity on drying various viruses. Nature 195:1063–1064.

BURROWS, M. R., AND RANKIN, J. D. 1970. A further examination of the survival of pathogenic bacteria in cattle slurry. Br Vet J 126:32–34.

CHRISTISON, G. I., AND FARMER, C. 1983. Physical characteristics of perforated floors for young pigs. Can Agric Eng 25:75.

COALSON, J. A., AND LECCE, J. G. 1973. Herd differences in the expression of fatal diarrhea in artificially reared piglets weaned after 12 hr vs 36 hr of nursing. J Anim Sci 36:1114–1121.

COMBERG, G., AND DOENEN, H.-D. 1968. Der Einfluss von fensterlosen, kunstlich beleuchteten Stallen auf die Mast von Schweinen. Schweinezucht Schweinemast 16:209–211.

COX, C. S. 1987. The Aerobiological Pathway of Microorganisms. New York: John Wiley and Sons.

CRONIN, G. M. 1985. The development and significance of abnormal stereotyped behaviors in tethered sows. Ph.D. diss., Dutch Agric Univ, Wageningen, The Netherlands.

CURTIS, S. E. 1972. Air environment and animal performance. J Anim Sci 35:628–634.

———. 1974. Responses of the piglet to perinatal stressors. J Anim Sci 38:1031–1036.

———. 1978. Saving baby pigs. Proc Univ Ill Pork Ind Conf, p. 1.

———. 1983. Environmental Management in Animal Agriculture. Ames: Iowa State Univ Press.

———. 1986. Toxic gases. In Current Veterinary Therapy in Food Animal Practice, vol. 2. Philadelphia: W. B. Saunders.

_____. 1987. Animal well-being and animal care. In Farm Animal Behavior. Philadelphia: W. B. Saunders.

CURTIS, S. E., AND KELLEY, K. W. 1983. Environment and health in the hog house. Proc Univ Ill Pork Ind Conf, p. 56.

CURTIS, S. E., AND MORRIS, G. L. 1982. Operant supplemental heat in swine nurseries. Proc 2d Int Livest Environ Symp, Am Soc Agric Eng, p. 295.

CURTIS, S. E.; HEIDENREICH, C. J.; AND HARRINGTON, R. B. 1967. Age dependent changes of thermostability in neonatal pigs. Am J Vet Res 28:1887–1890.

CURTIS, S. E.; GRUNLOH, D. J.; KELLEY, K. W.; DRUMMOND, J. G.; MEARES, V. J.; JENSEN, A. H.; AND NORTON, H. W. 1975a. Diurnal and annual fluctuations of aerial bacterial and dust levels in enclosed swine houses. J Anim Sci 41:1502–1511.

CURTIS, S. E.; GRUNLOH, D. J.; DRUMMOND, J. G.; LYNCH, P. B.; AND JENSEN, A. H. 1975b. Relative and qualitative aspects of aerial bacteria and dust in swine houses. J Anim Sci 41:1512–1520.

CURTIS, S. E.; ANDERSON, C. R.; SIMON, J.; JENSEN, A. H.; DAY, D. L.; AND KELLEY, K. W. 1975c. Effects of aerial ammonia, hydrogen sulfide and swine-house dust on rate of body-weight gain and respiratory-tract structure in swine. J Anim Sci 41:735–739.

CURTIS, S. E.; KINGDON, D. A.; DRUMMOND, J. G.; AND SIMON, J. 1976. Effects of cold stress and age on pulmonary bacterial clearance in young pigs. Am J Vet Res 37:299–301.

CURTIS, S. E.; TISCH, D. A.; TODD, K. R.; AND SIMON, J. 1987. Pulmonary bacterial deposition and clearance during ascarid larval migration in weanling pigs. Can J Vet Res 51:525–527.

CURTIS, S. E.; HURST, R. J.; WIDOWSKI, T. M.; SHANKS, R. D.; JENSEN, A. H.; GONYOU, H. W.; BANE, D. P.; MUEHLING, A. J.; AND KESLER, R. P. 1989. Effects of sow-crate design on health and performance of sows and piglets. J Anim Sci 67:80–93.

DANTZER, R., AND KELLEY, K. W. 1989. Stress and immunity: An integrated view of relationships between the brain and the immune system. Life Sci 44:1995–2008.

DANTZER, R.; ARNONE, M.; AND MORMEDE, P. 1980. Effects of frustration on behavior and plasma corticosteroid levels in pigs. Physiol Behav 24:1.

DAY, D. L.; HANSEN, E. L.; AND ANDERSON, S. 1965. Gases and odors in confinement swine buildings. Trans Am Soc Agric Eng 8:118–121.

DONHAM, K. J.; ZAVALA, D. C.; AND MERCHANT, J. A. 1984. Acute effects of the work environment on pulmonary function of swine confinement workers. Am J Ind Med 5:367–376.

DRUMMOND, J. G.; CURTIS, S. E.; AND SIMON, J. 1978. Effects of atmospheric ammonia on pulmonary bacterial clearance in young pigs. Am J Vet Res 39:211–212.

DRUMMOND, J. G.; CURTIS, S. E.; SIMON, J.; AND NORTON, H. W. 1980. Effects of aerial ammonia on growth and health of young pigs. J Anim Sci 50:1085–1091.

_____. 1981a. Effects of atmospheric ammonia on young pigs experimentally infected with *Ascaris suum*. Am J Vet Res 42:969–974.

DRUMMOND, J. G.; CURTIS, S. E.; MEYER, R. C.; SIMON, J.; AND NORTON, H. W. 1981b. Effects of atmospheric ammonia on young pigs experimentally infected with *Bordetella bronchiseptica*. Am J Vet Res 42:963–968.

DUNCAN, I. J. H. 1987. The welfare of farm animals: An ethological approach. Sci Prog (Oxf) 71:317–326.

DUNKLIN, E. W., AND PUCK, T. T. 1948. The lethal effect of relative humidity on air-borne bacteria. J Exp Med 87:87–101.

EKESBO, I.; JENSEN, P.; AND LOCK, R. 1979. Behavioral changes in crated dry sows. Sven Veterinaertidn 31:315–319.

ENGLAND, D. C., AND SPURR, D. T. 1969. Litter size of swine confined during gestation. J Anim Sci 28:220–223.

ESBENSHADE, K. L.; SINGLETON, W. L.; CLEGG, E. D.; AND JONES, H. W. 1979. Effect of housing management on reproductive development and performance of young boars. J Anim Sci 48:246–250.

ESMAY, M. L., AND DIXON, J. E. 1986. Environmental Control for Agricultural Buildings. Westport, Conn.: Avi.

EWBANK, R. 1973. An unsuccessful attempt to induce tail biting by feeding a high energy, low fibre vegetable protein ration. Br Vet J 129:366–369.

EWBANK, R., AND BRYANT, M. J. 1972. Agressive behavior amongst groups of domesticated pigs kept at various stocking rates. Anim Behav 20:21–28.

FRASER, D. 1975. The effect of straw on the behavior of sows in tether stalls. Anim Prod 21:59–68.

_____. 1984. The role of behavior in swine production: A review of research. Appl Anim Ethol 11:317–339.

_____. 1987. Mineral-deficient diets and the pig's attraction to blood: Implications for tail-biting. Can J Anim Sci 67:909–918.

FRITSCHEN, R. D. 1976. Housing and its effect on feet and leg problems. Proc Am Assoc Swine Pract, p. 4.

FRITSCHEN, R. D., AND MUEHLING, A. J. 1978a. Space requirements for swine. Pork Handb, p. PIH-55.

_____. 1978b. Slotted floors for swine. Pork Ind Handb, p. PIH-53.

FURUUCHI, S., AND SHIMIZU, Y. 1976. Effect of ambient temperatures on multiplication of attenuated transmissible gastroenteritis virus in the bodies of newborn piglets. Infect Immun 13:990–992.

GAAFAR, S. M., AND JONES, H. W. 1965. Effect of housing on ascariasis in growing-finishing swine. J Am Vet Med Assoc 146:358–360.

GEHLBACH, G. D.; BECKER, D. E.; COX, J. L.; HARMON, B. G.; AND JENSEN, A. H. 1966. Effects of floor space allowance and number per group on performance of growing-finishing swine. J Anim Sci 25:386–391.

GRAHAM, R., AND BRANDLY, C. A. 1937. The disinfecting properties of formaldehyde for demophilic bacteria associated with avian coryza, the filtrable viruses of infectious laryngotracheitis and infectious bronchitis. Poult Sci 16:428–433.

GRAHAM, R., AND MICHAEL, V. M. 1932. Germicidal effects of formaldehyde, released by potassium permanganate and cheesecloth. Poult Sci 11:197–207.

GRANDIN, T. 1989. Effect of rearing environment and environmental enrichment on behavior and neural development in young pigs. Ph.D. diss., Univ of Illinois, Urbana-Champaign.

HAELTERMAN, E. O. 1962. Epidemiological studies of transmissible gastroenteritis of swine. Proc US Livest Sanit Assoc 66:305–315.

HAMMOND, E. G.; KUCZOLA, P.; JUNK, G. A.; AND KOZEL, J. 1974. Constituents of swine house odors. Proc Int Livest Environ Symp, Am Soc Agric Eng, p. 364.

HANSEN, K. E., AND CURTIS, S. E. 1980. Prepartal activity of sows in stall or pen. J Anim Sci 51:456–460.

HARRY, E. G. 1967. Disinfection and hygiene of buildings. In Environmental Control in Poultry Production. Edinburgh: Oliver and Boyd, p. 153.

HATCH, M. T.; WRIGHT, D. N.; AND BAILEY, G. D. 1970. Reponse of airborne *Mycoplasma pneumoniae* to abrupt changes in relative humidity. Appl Microbiol 19:232–238.

HILL, I. R., AND KENWORTHY, R. 1970. Microbiology of pigs and their environment in relation to weaning. J Appl Bacteriol 33:299–316.

HOGSVED, O. 1973. Swine confinement and health relations: Recommendations. Sven Veterinaertidn 25:185–188.

HOGSVED, O.; BACKSTROM, L.; LUNDBERG, R.; AND PETTERSSON, H. 1970. Tailbiting reduced by dietary straw. Proc NJF Symp 52:82–83.

HOLMES, C. W., AND CLOSE, W. H. 1977. The influence of climatic variables on energy metabolism and associated aspects of productivity in the pig. In Nutrition and the Climatic Environment. Boston: Butterworth, p. 51.

HUDSON, R. J.; SAKEN, H. S.; AND EMSLIE, D. 1974. Physiological and environmental influences on immunity. Vet Bull 44:119–128.

JENSEN, A. H.; YEN, J. T.; GEHRING, M. M.; BAKER, D. H.; BECKER, D. E.; AND HARMON, B. G. 1970. Effects of space restriction and management on pre- and postpuberal response of female swine. J Anim Sci 31:745–750.

JENSEN, P. 1983. Confinement and continuous noise as environmental factors affecting communication in domestic pig. Ph.D. diss. Swedish Univ Agric Sci, Skara.

JOHANSSON, G.; JONSSON, L.; LANNER, N.; BLOMGREN, L.; LINDBERG, P.; AND POUPA, O. 1974. Severe stress-cardiopathy in pigs. Am Heart J 87:451–457.

JONES, C. R., AND WEBSTER, A. J. F. 1981. Weather induced changes in airborne bacteria within a calf house. Vet Rec 109:493–494.

JONES, C.; WATHES, C. M.; AND WEBSTER, A. J. F. 1982. Release and clearance rates of airborne bacteria within a controlled climate calf house. Proc 2d Int Livest Environ Symp, Am Soc Agric Eng, p. 529.

JONES, J. E. T. 1976. The carriage of beta-hemolytic streptococci by healthy pigs. Br Vet J 132:276–283.

JONES, P. W. 1976. The effect of temperature, solids content and pH on the survival of salmonellas in cattle slurry. Br Vet J 132:284–293.

KALICH, J. 1970. Untersuchungen uber die Beziehungen zwischen enzootischer Pneumonie (Ferkelgrippe) und Umwelt Perl. Berl Muench Tieraerztl Wochenschr 83:289–292, 309–313.

KELLEY, K. W. 1980. Stress and immune function: A bibliographical review. Ann Vet Res 11:445–478.

KELLEY, K. W.; BLECHA, F.; AND REGNIER, J. A. 1982. Cold exposure and absorption of colostrol immunoglobulins by neonatal pigs. J Anim Sci 55:363–368.

KRIDER, J. L.; ALBRIGHT, J. L.; PLUMLEE, M. P.; CONRAD, J. H.; SINCLAIR, C. L.; UNDERWOOD, L.; JONES, R. G.; AND HARRINGTON, R. B. 1975. Magnesium supplementation, space and docking effects on swine performance and behavior. J Anim Sci 40:1027–1033.

KUNDSIN, R. B. 1968. Aerosols of mycoplasmas, L forms and bacteria: Comparison of particle size, viability, and lethality of ultraviolet radiation. Appl Microbiol 16:143–146.

LANNEK, N., AND WESSLEN, T. 1957. Evidence that the SEP agent is an etiological factor in enzootic pneumonia in swine. Nord Vet Med 9:177–190.

LEDIVIDICH, J., AND NOBLET, J. 1981. Colostrum intake and thermoregulation in the neonatal pig in relation to environmental temperature. Biol Neonate 40:167–174.

LILLIE, R. J. 1970. Air pollutants affecting the performance of domestic animals. USDA Handb, p. 380.

LINDQVIST, J. O. 1974. Animal health and environment in the production of fattening pigs. Acta Vet Scand 51:1–78.

McGLONE, J. J., AND CURTIS, S. E. 1985. Behavior and performance of weanling pigs in pens equipped with hide areas. J Anim Sci 60:20–24.

MADSEN, A.; NIELSEN, E. K.; AND SOGAARD, A. 1978. Environmental Influence on Health of Bacon Pigs. Beret Statens Husdyrbrugsfors Kbh, p. 472.

MAHONE, J. P.; BERGER, T.; CLEGG, E. D.; AND SINGLETON, W. L. 1979. Photoinduction of puberty in boars during naturally occurring short day lengths. J Anim Sci 48:1159–1164.

MARPLE, D. N., AND JUDGE, M. D. 1976. Porcine stress syndrome. Pork Ind Handb, p. PIH-26.

MARTINSSON, K. 1979. Study of methods in herd health programs for finishing swine. Swed Meat Mark Assoc.

MEESE, G. B., AND EWBANK, R. 1973. The establishment and nature of the dominance hierarchy in the domesticated pig. Anim Behav 21:326–334.

MEYER, V. M., AND VAN FOSSEN, L. 1971. Effects of environment on pork production. Iowa State Univ Coop Ext Serv, AE-1063.

MIDWEST PLAN SERVICE. 1983. Structures and environment Handbook. MWPS-1.

MOUNT, L. E. 1968. The Climatic Physiology of the Pig. London: Edward Arnold.

———. 1975. The assessment of thermal environment in relation to pig production. Livest Prod Sci 2:381–392.

MOUSTGAARD, J.; SORENSEN, P. H.; AND NIELSEN, P. B. 1959. Staldkimaets indfly delse pa vaekst, foderudnyttelse og slagtekvalitet hos svin. Arsberet, Inst Steril Kbh, p. 173.

MOWITZ, H. 1971. Effects of group size and straw on growth and tail biting in finishing pigs. Inst Anim Sci, Coll Agric (Uppsala) Publ 6.

MUIRHEAD, M. R. 1976. Veterinary problems of intensive pig husbandry. Vet Rec 99:288–292.

NATZKE, R. P., AND LeCLAIR, B. J. 1976. Coliform contaminated bedding and new infections. J Dairy Sci 59:2152–2154.

NIELSEN, H. E.; DANIELSON, F.; LAURSEN, B.; LINNEMAN, F.; AND RUBY, V. 1976. Nutritional experiments with early weaned pigs. Beret Husdyrbrugsfors.

NIELSEN, N. C.; BILLIE, N.; LARSEN, J. L.; AND SVENDSEN, J. 1975. Preweaning mortality in pigs. VII. Polyarthritis. Nord Vet Med 27:529–543.

NIELSEN, N. C.; BILLIE, N.; SVENDSEN, J.; AND RUSING, H.-J. 1976. Prevention and Therapy of Swine Diseases. Royal Veterinary and Agricultural Univ, Copenhagen.

NTUNDE, B. N.; HACKER, R. R.; AND KING, G. J. 1979. Influence of photoperiod on growth, puberty, and plasma LH levels in gilts. J Anim Sci 48:1401–1406.

PEPPER, T. A., AND TAYLOR, D. J. 1977. Breeding record analysis in pig herds and its veterinary applications: Experience with a large commercial unit. Vet Rec 101:196–199.

PILCHARD, E. I. 1965. Experimental transmission of transmissible gastroenteritis virus by starlings. Am J Vet Res 26:1177–1179.

POND, W. G., AND HOUPT, K. A. 1978. The Biology of the Pig. Ithaca, N.Y.: Cornell Univ Press.

RANDALL, J. M. 1975. The prediction of airflow patterns in livestock buildings. J Agric Eng Res 20:199–215.

REBER, E. F. 1956. Airborne transmissible gastroenteritis. Am J Vet Res 17:194–195.

RENDOS, J. J.; EBERHART, R. J.; AND KESLER, E. M. 1975. Microbial populations of teat ends of dairy cows and bedding materials. J Dairy Sci 58:1492–1500.

ROHDE PARFET, K. A.; GONYOU, H. W.; CURTIS, S. E.; HURST, R. J.; JENSEN, A. H.; AND MUEHLING, A. J. 1989. Effects of sow-crate design on sow and piglet behavior. J Anim Sci 67:94–104.

SAINSBURY, D. W. B. 1974. The influence of environmental factors on the health of livestock. Proc Int Livest Environ Symp, Am Soc Agric Eng, p. 4.

SCHEEL, D. E.; GRAVES, H. B.; AND SHERRITT, G. W. 1977. Nursing order, social dominance and growth in swine. J Anim Sci 45:219–230.

SCHNURRENBERGER, P. R.; HANSON, L. E.; AND MARTIN, R. J. 1970. Long term surveillance of leptospirosis on an Illinois farm. Am J Epidemiol 92:223–239.

SHERRITT, G. W.; GRAVES, H. B.; GOBBLE, J. L.; AND HAZLETT, V. E. 1974. Effects of mixing pigs during the growing-finishing period. J Anim Sci 39:834–837.

SHIMIZU, M.; SHIMIZU, Y; AND KODAMA, Y. 1978. Effects of ambient temperatures on induction of transmissible gastroenteritis in feeder pigs. Infect Immun 21:747–752.

SIGNORET, J. P. 1967. Attraction de la femelle en oestrus par la male chez les porcins. Rev Comp Anim 4:10–22.

SIGNORET, J. P.; BALDWIN, B. A.; FRASER, D.; AND HAFEZ, E. S. E. 1975. The behavior of swine. In The Behavior of Domestic Animals, 3d ed. Baltimore: Williams & Wilkins, p. 295.

SIMENSEN, E. 1971. Environmental factors in pig production. A survey. Inst Agric Struct, Agric Coll (Oslo) Rep 6.

SORENSEN, P. H. 1961. Influence of climatic environment on pig performance. In Nutrition of Pigs and Poultry. London: Butterworth, p. 88.

SYKES, G. 1965. Disinfection and Sterilization. Philadelphia: Lippincott.

SYMOENS, J. 1970. Influence of a Stresnil-treatment on feed conversion and weight gain after mixing. Proc Symp Stress in the Pig. Janssen Pharmaceutica, Beerse, p. 45.

TAYLOR, I. A. 1990. Design of the Sow Feeder. Ph.D. diss., Univ of Illinois, Urbana-Champaign.

TIELEN, M. J. M. 1978. Buildings, environmental conditions and diseases. Proc 29th Annu Meet Eur Assoc

Anim Prod M-P/4.05/1.

TITTERINGTON, R. W., AND FRASER, D. 1975. The lying behavior of sows and piglets during early lactation in relation to the position of the creep heater. Appl Anim Ethol 2:47–53.

VAN PUTTEN, G. 1968. An investigation into tailbiting in fattening pigs. Ph.D. diss., Univ of Amsterdam.

VERSTEGEN, M. W. A., AND CURTIS, S. E. 1988. Energetics of dry sows and gilts in gestation crates in the cold. J Anim Sci 66:2865–2875.

VERSTEGEN, M. W. A.; BRASCAMP, E. W.; AND VAN DER HEL, W. 1978. Growing and fattening of pigs in relation to temperature of housing and feeding level. Can J Anim Sci 58:1–13.

WATHES, C. M. 1988a. Airborne transmission of enteric pathogens in farm livestock. Proc 6th Int Congr Anim Hyg, Swedish Univ of Agric Sci, Skara, p. 421.

———. 1988b. Survival of *P. haemolytica* and *S. typhimurium* in air. Proc 6th Int Congr Anim Hyg, Swedish Univ Agric Sci, Skara, p. 428.

WEBSTER, A. J. F. 1970. Environmental and physiological interactions influencing resistance to infectious disease. In Resistance to Infectious Disease. Saskatoon: Modern Press.

WELLS, W. F. 1955. Airborne Contagion and Air Hygiene. Cambridge: Harvard Univ Press.

WHITEKER, M. D.; HAYS, V. W.; AND PARKER, G. R. 1978. Feed additives for swine. Pork Ind Handb, p. PIH-31.

WIDOWSKI, T. M., AND CURTIS, S. E. 1990. The influence of straw, cloth tassel, or both on the prepartum behavior of sows. Appl Anim Behav Sci 27:53–72.

WIDOWSKI, T. M.; CURTIS, S. E.; DZIUK, P. J.; WAGNER, W. C.; AND SHERWOOD, O. D. 1990. Behavioral and endocrine responses of sows to prostaglandin F2a and cloprostenol. Biol Reprod 43:290–297.

WRIGHT, D. N.; BAILEY, G. D.; AND HATCH, M. T. 1968. Role of relative humidity in the survival of airborne *Mycoplasma pneumoniae*. J Bacteriol 96:970–974.

72 Animal Welfare

P. R. English

S. A. Edwards

THE BASIC OBJECTIVE of the pig producer is to meet customer demand. Until recently, consumer demand appeared to be a simple one, i.e., for meat of satisfactory quality at an acceptable price. However, with increased public concern in many countries about animal welfare within production systems, consumer demand may be changing. Producers have to monitor this demand situation carefully and respond appropriately. During this transitional period there is much doubt, thinking, debate, research, advice, and speculation about welfare. Rumors abound about welfare legislation, which might result in the immediate or eventual banning of some current production methods that have developed for good reasons over many years.

In all the major pig-producing countries there has been a marked reduction in the number of pig herds over the past 20–30 years and a steady increase in herd size on those farms remaining in production. Concurrently, there have been major changes in production systems aimed at simplifying management, reducing cost, and increasing production efficiency. In Britain, and probably also in most other European countries, against an unfavorable trend in product prices in relation to input costs, pig meat prices have risen considerably less than sheep meat and beef prices. At the same time, consumption of pig meat has increased slightly while that of beef and sheep meat has tended to decrease. These trends would indicate that pig producers have succeeded in meeting the demand for meat of satisfactory quality at an acceptable price.

However, the increasing size of production units, the increased intensiveness, and the nature of some of the systems in use have become matters of public concern in recent years. Greatest concern has been expressed about the close confinement of the breeding sow. Stall and tether systems for the dry sow and farrowing crates for the lactating sow have been developed to provide ease of management and high performance levels at low cost. However, the restriction of movement, the barren environment, and the incidence of stereotyped behaviors seen in some of these systems have led to public questions on whether they are able to provide acceptable animal welfare. Similarly, the widespread adoption of un-bedded, slatted pens for growing pigs to provide large-scale, hygienic housing with low labor costs has led to questions about the lack of variety and whether outbreaks of vice are indicative of a fundamental deficiency in these environments. Earlier weaning has enabled producers to achieve major improvements in annual sow productivity but has been questioned on the basis of welfare because of the greater susceptibility to disease of such piglets and the abnormal social interactions that they sometimes show.

In the interests of improving the welfare of the pig, meeting the desires of the consumer, and clarifying the production objectives of the producer, urgent action must be taken to reduce the present confusion and uncertainty. It is therefore vital to address such questions as, what is pig welfare and how can we measure it? When these questions can be answered, current systems can be evaluated and improved in terms of pig welfare and new improved systems can be developed.

DEFINING WELFARE. In discussing the relationship of welfare to the health of the pig and the economy of production, the first major challenge is to attempt to define the welfare needs of the pig.

Hughes (1976) defined farm animal welfare on a general level as "a state of complete mental and physical health where the animal is in harmony with its environment." It must be emphasized that welfare is not a simple entity but is made up of many interacting elements. There is great danger in ignoring this fact and neglecting some basic elements because of overemphasis on other, more currently fashionable aspects of welfare.

For simplicity, welfare can be divided into two categories of physical and psychological welfare, although it must be recognized that there are many complex interactions between these, which are discussed later.

Physical welfare is easier to deal with, since most aspects can be easily quantified and abuses are readily apparant to the producer and veterinary surgeon. Many of the requirements for good physical welfare correspond closely with those for good biologic and economic performance, including such factors as good health (the absence of disease and parasites), adequate feeding (the absence of nutritional deficiencies and the maintenance of good body condition), and good housing. This latter category includes not only providing an environment that causes no visible injuries (from pen fittings or from the unwanted attentions of other animals) but also providing adequate physical comfort in terms of such elements as flooring, temperature, and airspeed.

Psychological welfare is less easily measured. This incorporates concepts such as absence of fear (whether arising from elements of the physical environment, from humans, or from other pigs), a need for control or choice of environment, and the widely discussed idea that a pig has an innate requirement to carry out certain patterns of behavior (i.e., that it has not only physical but also behavioral needs). When framing the codes of practice and legislation relating to farm animal welfare in many European countries, both physical and psychological welfare are being considered.

Webster (1987) described the essential principles behind the Farm Animal Welfare Codes in Britain as being governed by the "5 freedoms" as follows:

1. Freedom from malnutrition; i.e., the diet should be sufficient in both quantity and quality to promote normal health and vigor.
2. Freedom from thermal and physical discomfort, which means that the environment (e.g., housing) should be neither excessively hot nor cold, nor should it impair normal rest or activity.
3. Freedom from injury or disease; i.e., the husbandry system should minimize the risk of injury or disease and any cases that do occur should be recognized and treated without delay.
4. Freedom to express most normal patterns of behavior.
5. Freedom from fear and stress.

The requirements to provide for the first 3 freedoms are well documented and the adequacy of provision of these can be assessed fairly readily. The requirements to satisfy freedoms 4 and 5, on the other hand, cannot be specified accurately in our present state of knowledge. Among the reasons for this are the difficulty of defining what constitutes "normal" behavior, the problems of diagnosing mental as well as sometimes physical illness, and the complications involved in measuring fear and stress. Several approaches are being used to measure welfare.

ASSESSING WELFARE

Productivity. It can be argued that the level and efficiency of production of the group, herd, or flock, and of the individual animal in particular, representing as it does the degree of harmony of the animal with its environment, constitutes a reliable measure of welfare in most situations. While support can be forwarded to uphold this view, several reasons can also be cited to indicate why productivity cannot be used as a valid measure of welfare in all situations. This aspect will be further developed later in this chapter.

Mortality and Health. Mortality is the ultimate objective measure of welfare but generally requires too great a degree of abuse to differentiate between alternative systems. Poor health is unquestionably an indication of impaired welfare, but the converse may not necessarily be true. Thus, health measures such as the incidence of infectious disease, lameness, or skin lesions (Backstrom 1973; De Koning 1985; Edwards et al. 1985) may be useful ways of assessing welfare in many circumstances. However, the absence of poor health does not necessarily imply that welfare is good, since the detrimental effects of inadequate systems may be obscured by the routine use of antibiotics. It must also be recognized that impaired welfare arising from psychological stress may exist without apparent impairment of physical health, the only signs being changes in behavior patterns.

Ethological Measures. Recognition of subtle changes in behavior has always been one of the ways in which a good service worker or veterinarian identifies the onset of a problem with health or environment. Simple examples are the apathy of a sick pig or the huddling of a group of pigs that are too cold. In this context, animal behavior is a widely recognized practical method of measuring welfare. Similarly, behavior patterns that result in direct injury to an animal itself (such as rooting on inappropriate surfaces) or inflict injury on others (such as the vices of tail, ear, and flank biting) are simple and generally accepted measures of impaired welfare.

However, more complex use of ethological measurements in the assessment of welfare is now receiving scientific attention because of the increasing demand for understanding such concepts as mental suffering and behavioral needs. Behavior patterns can be readily recorded and quantified, but assessing the significance of such data is still fraught with difficulty. Interpretation is generally based on the incidence of abnormal behaviors, necessitating both a qualitative and quantitative definition of normality. Following an international survey of expert opinion, a list of behaviors widely accepted as "abnormal" has been published (CEC 1983). However, the frequency at which such behaviors must occur before being indicative of unacceptable welfare is still a subject for opinion rather than objective decision making.

One approach is to quantify the behavior patterns of animals in seminatural or enriched environments (Van Putten 1977; Stolba 1981). However, while providing a useful starting point, the use of such reference systems to provide definitions of normality can be criticized on many grounds, including lack of understanding of the motivational basis for performance of behavior patterns and of the psychological consequences of failing to perform them (Baxter 1983). Behavior patterns are essentially adaptive responses to the environment in which the animal is placed. The fact that a pig in intensive housing behaves differently from one in the wild is not in itself an indication of impaired welfare. It is necessary to demonstrate that newly observed behaviors really are a reflection of mental suffering or neural pathology, e.g., stereotyped bar biting (Cronin 1985), or that the inability to perform certain innate behavior patterns because of an inadequate environment is stressful to the animal, as may be the case for nest building in the farrowing sow. Such indications require more detailed investigation of the relationships between behavior and physiology in the pig.

Physiological Measures. Acute stress activates both the sympathetic nervous system and the hypothalamo-pituitary-adrenal axis. Sympathetic stimulation results in release of noradrenaline at the nerve endings and secretion of adrenaline and noradrenaline into circulation from the adrenal medulla. This is an immediate, short-term response and is accompanied by release of a corticotrophin-releasing factor from the hypothalamus, which causes release of adrenocorticotrophic hormone (ACTH) from the anterior pituitary. This causes the adrenal cortex to secrete corticosteroid hormones into the circulation. A negative feedback of plasma corticosteroid on the hypothalamus restores normal conditions when the stressor is removed (Stephens 1980).

Plasma cortisol or ACTH levels have been used as a measure of stress, and it has been shown that psychologic stress is as effective as physical stress in activating this system. However, there are a number of problems in using this technique. Taking a blood sample to assess hormone levels may induce a greater adrenal response than any environmental treatment difference (Moss 1981). Moreover, a single blood sample taken at any given point in time is an unreliable measure of chronic stress. When response to stress is reduced, corticosteroid release is also pulsatile with refractory periods.

Therefore, it is necessary to find a more integrated measure of chronic stress that is relatively insensitive to transient environmental conditions. The weight of the adrenal glands is a relatively simple measure but can only be obtained postmortem. The activity of the enzymes controlling catecholamine synthesis in the adrenals and sympathetic ganglia has been used as a parameter (Stanton and Mueller 1976), but this again requires sacrificing the animal. The most useful current test is an adrenal function test based on the principle that adrenal response to an acute stressor is altered by long-term, chronic stress. Controlled acute stress is applied by injecting a standard amount of ACTH; the resulting blood level of corticosteroid is measured (Ladewig 1986). Ideally the response is measured by serial sampling, requiring catheterization, although a single sample may give some indication. However, it has been noted that acute stress immediately prior to the test, such as might result from the sampling procedures, can influence the test result (Ladewig 1986). A pretreatment with dexamethasone has been used to overcome this problem. However, interpretation of the result is still difficult because of genetic differences between animals in adrenal response to ACTH challenge and the fact that some animals in adverse conditions appear to cease adrenal responsiveness after a period.

Immunological Measures. It has been recognized for many years that environmental stress may increase the susceptibility of pigs to disease. Accumulated evidence indicates that this is mediated by effects of stress on the immune system (Kelley 1980). Elevated blood levels of corticosteroids can reduce proliferation of lymphocytes (Kelley 1988), decrease the number of antibodies produced, and reduce the size of the lymph nodes (Martin 1977). Chronic stress resulting in sustained high levels of corticosteroid hormones in the blood can therefore impair the ability of the pig to resist infection. The fact that both physical and psychological aspects of environmental stress may be reflected in immune responsiveness provides the basis for measuring a parameter that reflects the integrated effects of chronic stress without being influenced by short-term effects of the measuring process. It has been demonstrated that sows tethered in a barren environment show a poorer immune response when challenged with a novel antigen, and that after farrowing, their piglets also have lower antibody levels (Metz and Osterlee 1981). This is an important new field in the study of animal welfare, since it provides a meeting place for physical and psychological welfare assessment and is of real significance to the biologic and economic success of the pig enterprise.

Thus, there are several approaches for assessing the standard of welfare in any situation. Each approach has its own strengths as well as associated difficulties and a sensible combination of some or all of the methods outlined is likely to provide a better overall measure of welfare in a given system than the use of any one approach alone.

RELATIONSHIP BETWEEN ANIMAL WELFARE AND PRODUCTIVITY. Some indications of the close relationship between animal productivity and welfare have already been mentioned. Kelley (1988) demonstrated an important relationship between stressors resulting in high blood corticosteroid levels and lower immune status, resulting in greater liability to disease. Moreover, Spencer (1985) has drawn attention to the effect of high corticosteroid levels in reducing protein synthesis and lean-tissue growth rate. In breeding animals, higher corticosteroid levels induced by unpleasant, relative to kindly, handling by humans resulted in both a lower pregnancy rate in gilts and delayed reproductive development in young boars (Hemsworth et al. 1986). Thus, systems that are more stressful and induce higher corticosteroid levels would be expected to be associated with poorer health status, higher mortality levels, poorer growth and food conversion efficiency, and depressed reproductive performance.

Other signs of a stressful or faulty situation that are detrimental to productivity and efficiency in a given system include lesions resulting in infections and lameness associated with such factors as faulty floors, inadequate pen design, poor hygiene, or bullying behavior in group-housed animals. Vices such as ear, flank, and tail biting can sometimes be caused by a specific nutrient deficiency, such as salt (Fraser 1987), or by overcrowding (Blackshaw 1981); but, more often such vices are of more complex etiology, being induced by a combination of inadequate provisions for the pig (English and MacDonald 1986). Stereotypic behavior such as bar and chain biting, which is frequently observed in individually stalled or tethered sows, while possibly helping the animal to cope with a stressful situation, has been found to be associated with higher energy expenditure and, therefore, with a higher food requirement and poorer food conversion efficiency (Cronin et al. 1986).

There are many examples of the effects of inadequacies in climatic environment and nutrition on the welfare and performance of the pig. Close (1987) has documented the penalties imposed on the pig if it is kept either below its lower critical temperature (LCT) or above its upper critical temperature (UCT). These can influence general comfort, food intake, growth, food conversion efficiency, health, and viability. Welfare problems associated with dropping below the LCT or exceeding the UCT constitute one of the main reasons for the much greater popularity of intensive (i.e., housed) relative to extensive or outdoor production systems in world pig production.

Nutritional deficiency can predispose to vices such as tail biting (Fraser 1987), depressed feed intake, growth, feed efficiency, and survival. The effect of dietary inadequacy on pig welfare is probably best exemplified in the early weaned pig. A diet formulated with undue emphasis on reducing the cost of ingredients can cause severe depressions in intake and growth and greatly increase incidence of scouring and mortality, relative to a diet using ingredients that are acceptable and highly digestible to the young pig (English et al. 1988). However, nutrition is not only important in relation to satisfying basic metabolic needs for health but can also influence behavior. For example, the provision of higher feed levels (Appleby and Lawrence 1987) to individually stalled sows resulted in a significant reduction in bar biting, while higher feed levels resulted in newly farrowed sows being less restless with an increase in survival of their piglets (English 1970).

These are some examples of provisions made for the pig that are equally in the interests of its welfare and also necessary for the attainment of a high level of productivity.

However, attainment of high productivity is not always synonymous with providing a high standard of welfare. For example, while mortality is the ultimate measure of welfare, the worst effects of an intrinsically inadequate system on mortality can be masked by the routine use of antibiotics. Moreover, poor growth rate in a system may not necessarily indicate poor welfare, for such a level of performance may be the result of feeding a low-density diet, which is nevertheless both nutritionally adequate and cost effective in a particular situation. Webster (1987) cites the case of the very high-yielding dairy cow that is more prone to metabolic disease problems. Curtis (1987) places the pig treated with growth hormone or repartitioning agents, yet is depositing lean meat very quickly, in the same high-risk category from metabolic diseases while at the same time being more prone to cold stress.

There are also difficult situations in which the animal can maintain a high level of productivity only by major adaptations from so-called normal to abnormal behavior, which may involve development of stereotypes. Although this change in behavior may help the animal to adapt to its difficult circumstances with impunity in terms of either any obvious physiological signs of stress or of productivity, the change in behavior may be disturbing to human observers and therefore be considered by some to be an unacceptable price to pay for perpetuating the system in question. Thus productivity can on occasions be misleading if used as a measure of welfare. Nevertheless, in many situations, the average productivity of a group of animals combined with the range in productivity of individuals within the group can be used as a simple but fairly useful index of welfare.

THE NEED TO EVALUATE SYSTEMS AND FORMULATE WELFARE LEGISLATION.
There are many difficulties in assessing both welfare in a given system and the welfare implications of a component of a system.

Deciding on Priorities. When considering the overall welfare of animals within a system, it is essential to recognize that in some circumstances the welfare of some animals may be improved while the welfare of others may deteriorate. The system that has received most criticism to date in terms of welfare has been individual confinement of the dry sow in a stall or tethered system, The sow in this situation has little opportunity for exercise and cannot socialize freely with pen mates. Therefore, the preferred system is to have dry sows in groups in a less barren and more interesting environment where the animal has greater freedom to move around, to explore, and to socialize. However, since dry sows are offered very limited levels of conventional diets in order to avoid overfatness, there can be excessive competition for feed when group feeding is practiced; this is a situation in which the dominant sows in the social hierarchy can obtain much more than their share of the ration and the timid (and younger) sows much less, if any at all. The group system can be improved by providing individual feeders to protect the timid sows during feeding; however, in a group situation, aggression toward the timid sow can occur at times other than during feeding (Carter and English 1983; Petherick 1989). It remains to be seen how well the timid sow in the group is provided for in terms of its physical and psychological needs in group-housing systems, which incorporate computerized feeding of the individual sow (Edwards and Riley 1986).

The farrowing sow and her newborn litter constitute another delicate situation. The sow in most situations is confined to a crate during and after farrowing to minimize the risk of piglets being overlain by the sow; specially warmed areas are arranged adjacent to the crate to provide the very high temperature required by the newborn piglet to minimize the high risk of hypothermia and resulting problems such as starvation, overlying, and diseases (e.g., scouring) (English 1989). The main criticism of this system to date has been that by confining the farrowing sow, she is unable to engage in the normal farrowing behavior that is demonstrated in the wild, especially that of nesting. When deprived of this opportunity to practice nesting behavior, some workers have suggested that sows in this situation show stress, exhibited by stereotyped behavior such as floor nosing and bar chewing and symptoms indicative of raised adrenalin levels, which depress oxytocin production (Baxter and Petherick 1980). In turn, this may reduce the speed and efficiency of parturition and lead to a higher incidence of intrapartum stillbirths and higher anoxia levels in live-born piglets (English 1969). Confinement of the sow in a crate creates the dilemma of imposing difficulties on the sow while being advantageous to the piglet in terms of its protection from overlying by the sow and organizing perfect creep areas to eliminate the risk of hypothermia and its ensuing problems. Therefore, research and development studies are necessary to establish if the provision of bedding or bedding substitute can satisfy the basic motivational desires of the sow to make a bed prior to farrowing and thus reduce or eliminate stress of the sow confined in the farrowing crate. Studies also need to determine if so-called "voluntary" farrowing systems (in which the sow is not confined at farrowing but can choose at farrowing to use facilities provided for her and her newborn piglets) can provide for the welfare needs of the newborn piglet as effectively as well-designed so-called "intensive" systems involving a crate for the sow and strategically placed warmed and comfortable creep areas for the newborn piglets.

When the relevant knowledge on the above is eventually obtained, it may show that what is conducive to normal behavior and what is best in the "wild" is not necessarily best in commercial practice. In terms of evolution, in the wild there is merit in a "survival of the fittest" strategy with the weak individuals dying very soon after birth from a combination of hypothermia, starvation, and overlying, whereas in a commercial situation there are obviously severe disadvantages to the weaker piglets and to the pig producer in allowing a "survival of the fittest" situation to prevail.

In a practical situation where decisions have to be made about welfare priorities for different individuals within a group, the emphasis should be in catering for the needs of the most underprivileged individuals. Thus emphasis should be on the individuals of lowest social status within the group of adult pigs and on the newborn piglets in the farrowing facility.

The Role of Bedding. The provision of adequate, good-quality bedding at all stages is frequently cited as contributing to the welfare of the pig, since it provides for such needs as physical comfort, insulation, and recreation. Although bedding provides these and other potential advantages, there may be more convenient and cost-effective alternatives to achieve the same attributes that bedding provides.

It has been postulated that providing a small amount of straw or bedding substitute in the farrowing pen might satisfy the nesting instincts of a sow prior to farrowing, and that providing strategically placed creep areas that incorporate bedding below and heat sources above might be more beneficial to the piglet than a bed made by a sow in the wild. Such possibilities have still to be resolved.

Fraser (1985) examined the use of straw bedding by 4- to 8-week-old pigs in an experimental pen that was bedded on one side but had a bare concrete floor on the other side. The side selected by the pigs for resting depended on pen temperature; when the temperature was 18–21°C, pigs showed a strong preference for the straw bedding, but at a temperature of 25–27°C pigs showed an equally strong preference for the bare concrete. There was no real preference between the sides for feeding and general activity. However, when fresh straw was provided, the animals generally chewed and rooted in the straw, causing a temporary preponderance of activity on the bedded side. Thus, the usefulness of straw in terms of its insulation value was dependent on the environmental temperature. If the recreational opportunity associated with introducing straw to the pen is considered important, either relatively small quantities of straw or perhaps straw substitutes that evoke chewing and rooting can be provided (Fraser 1985).

Petherick et al. (1987) examined the usefulness of straw bedding in relation to the incidence of agonistic behavior in groups of dry sows in Queensland, Australia. It was hoped that the sows on limited-feed would satisfy their appetite by eating straw, which would keep them more contented and make them less aggressive. Sows were in groups of four and had partial barriers along the food trough. Sows were offered 1 kg of feed twice daily and on one treatment had ad libitum access to straw. The partial barriers in the feed trough appeared to be associated with minimal conflict at feeding. However, agonistic encounters took place at times other than at feeding; severe fights occurred on the day of grouping. Straw appeared to have no effect on agonistic encounters because the sows largely ignored it. While environmental temperatures are not quoted in this work, it can be assumed that in Queensland sows would not be below their LCT and, therefore, straw used for bedding would confer no advantage in terms of thermal comfort. However, neither was it used to any extent to achieve satiety or for recreational purposes.

Thus, in situations where environmental temperature is adequate for the pig in the absence of bedding, the importance of the other attributes conferred by bedding or bedding substitutes must be more clearly evaluated relative to costs.

The Role of the Stockperson. There is a prevalent belief that the quality of care by the stockperson has a much more important influence on pig welfare than the choice of system (Brambell 1965; Curtis 1980; House of Commons Committee 1981; English and MacDonald 1986). There is increasing scientific evidence that the empathy between the stockperson and the animals is a major factor contributing to the positive welfare of those animals and to the enhancement of their performance (Seabrook 1983). It has been shown that pigs that receive frequent and sympathetic handling from the stockperson are easier to manage and have lower levels of circulating corticosteroid hormones, faster growth rates, and better reproductive performance than those that receive minimal or unpleasant handling (Hemsworth et al. 1981a, 1986, 1987; Gonyou et

al. 1986). In a comparison of otherwise similar farms, reproductive performance of the unit showed a negative correlation with the level of fear of humans that was shown by the sows (Hemsworth et al. 1981b). Thus, when comparing systems in terms of their welfare, it is important to control the quality of care between the systems and, perhaps even more importantly, to evaluate alternative systems under the wide range of quality of care experienced in commercial practice.

The Problems in Comparing Systems. In terms of providing appropriate scientific information that will result in the improved welfare through either legislation or persuasion, it is important to avoid certain potentially dangerous pitfalls.

Attention is often focussed on contentious systems of keeping pigs. However, it must be recognized that a system comprises many parts, including the physical building structures, the type of animal, the management practices, and the stockperson. No two examples of a supposed system are identical in practice, and it is important that generalizations should not be made on the basis of a small number of bad examples arising from deficiencies in perhaps only one of the component parts. Therefore, it is essential that when alternative systems, or preferably components of systems, are being evaluated that there is adequate replication in such comparisons; replication of animals within a system is not enough. The system itself also must be replicated in different situations. This need is partly influenced by the varying quality of care available, since, to a large extent, the system can only be as good as the person looking after it. It is widely recognized that well-designed group-housing systems for dry sows, including electronic feeding systems, require a higher standard of management than that required in well-designed individual stall and tether systems to achieve the same level of performance (Edwards and Riley 1986; English and MacDonald 1986). It could be argued that the simpler the system is to operate, the easier it will be to manage and to look after the well-being of all the animals involved. Thus, before novel systems that have been designed to improve welfare are fully launched into commercial practice, it is imperative that they be evaluated with existing systems under a wide range of conditions already in commercial practice, including variable qualities of management and care. Likewise, no existing system should be banned by legislation until an alternative system has been proven superior following comprehensive comparative evaluation. At the same time, it is imperative to upgrade the level of management and care. Such improvement will not only directly enhance pig welfare, but the improved quality of farm animal attendants will better enable them to look after the interests of stock on so-called "improved welfare" systems if these systems, in fact, turn out to be more difficult to manage than the systems they are to replace.

THE WELFARE ISSUE AND THE PIG PRODUCER.

Pig producers are concerned about the so-called welfare movement for obvious reasons. One of these reasons already referred to is that their clear objective in the past of producing pig meat of acceptable quality at a competitive price in conditions of good husbandry is no longer clear. This is because the acceptability of the conditions in which much pig meat is produced has been called into question by members of the consuming public. The initial questioning has lead to a gathering debate and considerable investment in research and development to determine the problems in existing systems and to attempt to develop new approaches that will reduce the problems of present systems without introducing too many new problems. The objectives of pig producers, in terms of the conditions under which they should be operating, will not become clear until the advantages and disadvantages of alternative production systems are clarified and until consumers make their judgments regarding the relative acceptability of these alternative systems. When this picture becomes clearer, pig producers will again be in a sound position to make commercial decisions as to whether or not they should remain in business and, if so, what sector of the market they should supply.

However, it is likely to take some considerable time before the demands of the consumer and therefore the objectives of the producer are clarified. Meanwhile, producers of pig meat are naturally concerned about the security of their present business investments. Mention of legislation that might ban the use of certain systems of production that are presently in operation arouse the greatest fears. Various estimates have been made, for example, of the cost of changing from the use of individual confinement systems for dry sows, such as stall and tethered systems, to group-housing systems (Sandiford 1985; Thow 1989).

The estimated cost to change a system (while varying according to how recently present buildings were erected and the length of any maximum phasing-out period for a system imposed by legislation) is very considerable. When this situation becomes clearer, pig producers will be in a better position to make a commercial decision regarding whether or not they can afford to remain in business. Of course, while there is an obligation on the part of the producer to comply with any impending legislation on pig welfare, there is an equal obligation on those responsible for framing such legislation. Such legislation must be based on comprehensive, sound scientific evidence about the merits, in terms of pig welfare, of alternative production systems. This information must be placed before the consuming public and, hopefully, the well-informed consumer will make objective rather than emotional decisions on the production systems of the future.

Curtis (1990) has pointed out the great dangers of framing welfare legislation on pig-production systems and practices based on emotion rather than on sound scientific evidence: "Swine welfare is based on swine biology. It is not based on the emotions, the opinions, the whims of people who are not well versed in the biology of the pig. The potential for harm to the animals that could result from perhaps well intentioned but naive regulations is alarming. . . . Perhaps the biggest danger is that a dissatisfied public may demand changes that eliminate what is disliked but result in no improvement or even a reduction in the welfare of the animals involved." Such an outcome will not only be detrimental to the pig but will cause confusion in the pig industry and higher prices for the consumer.

On the other hand, if future changes in the production systems or in components of the systems are guided by legislation based on sound scientific evidence, the well-being of the pig will be improved and the objectives of the producers will be clarified. Moreover, in view of the apparently close relationship between pig welfare and pig productivity, it is likely that production efficiency can be at least maintained at prelegislation levels; product prices can be more effectively controlled; and the pig, the pig producer, and the consumer are all likely to benefit in the long term.

THE ROLE OF VETERINARIANS AND EXTENSION SPECIALISTS.

Curtis (1990) emphasized the importance of educating pig farmers and stockpersons in terms of improving pig welfare. Management and care have such an important influence on the well-being of the pig in any system that continuing guidance and education from experts serving the pig industry has a most important part to play in the progressive improvement of pig well-being. It is highly likely, of course, that many of the efforts that are successful in improving the well-being of the pig will also be reflected in increased efficiency of production and higher profit margins.

REFERENCES

Appleby, M. C., and Lawrence, A. B. 1987. Food restriction as a cause of stereotyped behaviour in tethered gilts. Anim Prod 45:103–110.

Backstrom, L. 1973. Environment and animal health in piglet production. Acta Vet Scand Suppl 41.

Baxter, M. R. 1983. Ethology in environmental design for animal production. Appl Anim Ethol 9:207–220.

Baxter, M. R., and Petherick, J. C. 1980. The effect of restraint on parturition in the sow. Proc Int Congr Pig Vet Soc, Copenhagen, p. 84.

Blackshaw, J. K. 1981. Some behavioural deviations in weaned domestic pigs: Persistent inguinal nose thrusting and tail and ear biting. Anim Prod 33:325–332.

BRAMBELL, F. W. R. 1965. Report of the Technical Committee to Enquire into the Welfare of Animals kept under intensive livestock husbandry systems. Cmnd 2836. Her Majesty's Stationary Office, London.

CARTER, A. J., AND ENGLISH, P. R. 1983. A comparison of the activity and behaviour of dry sows in different housing and penning systems. Anim Prod 36:531–532.

CLOSE, W. H. 1987. Pig Housing and the Environment. Ed. A. T. Smith and T. L. J. Lawrence. British Society of Animal Production, Occasional Publication No. 11, pp. 9–24.

COMMISSION OF THE EUROPEAN COMMUNITIES. 1983. Abnormal behaviours in farm animals. CEC report 16 pp.

CRONIN, G. M. 1985. The development and significance of abnormal stereotyped behaviours in tethered sows. Ph.D. diss., Univ of Wageningen, Netherlands.

CRONIN, G. M.; VAN TARTWIJK, J.; VAN DER HEL, W.; AND VERSTEGEN, M. W. A. 1986. The influence of degree of adaptation to tether housing by sows in relation to behaviour and energy metabolism. Anim Prod 42:257–268.

CURTIS, S.E. 1980. Animal Welfare concerns in modern pork production. In Animal Welfare Committee of the US Animal Health Association at Louisville, Ky. National Pork Producers Council, Des Moines, Iowa, p. 19.

_____. 1987. Proc Univ of Illinois Pork Ind Conf. Dec 10–11, pp. 64–68.

_____. 1990. Swine welfare: Biology as the basis. Proc 21st Annu Meet Assoc Swine Pract, Denver, Colo., pp. 165–179.

DE KONING, R. 1985. On the well-being of dry sows. Thesis, Utrecht.

EDWARDS, S. A., AND RILEY, J. E. 1986. The application of the electronic identification and computerised feed dispensing system in dry sow housing. Pig News Inf 7:295–298.

EDWARDS, S. A.; LIGHTFOOT, A. L.; AND SPECHTER, H. H. 1985. Effects of farrowing crate design and floor type on pig performance and leg and teat damage. Anim Prod 40:540.

ENGLISH, P. R. 1969. Mortality and variation in growth in piglets. Ph.D. diss., Univ of Aberdeen, Scotland.

_____. 1970. A comparison of two sow feeding systems from 5 days before to 7 days after farrowing. Anim Prod 12:375.

_____. 1989. Reducing piglet losses by management and climatic control. Irish Pig Health Soc Proc, 17th Annu Symp. Co. Dublin, pp. 41–52.

ENGLISH, P. R., AND MACDONALD, D. C. 1986. Animal Behaviour and Welfare. In Bioindustrial Ecosystems. Ed. D. J. A. Cole and G. C. Brander. Amsterdam: Elsevier Science Publ, pp. 89–105.

ENGLISH, P. R.; FOWLER, V. R.; BAXTER, S. H.; AND SMITH, W. J. 1988. The growing and finishing pig: Improving efficiency. Ipswich, Engl: Farming Press, Chap. 12.

FRASER, D. 1985. Selection of bedded and unbedded areas by pigs in relation to environmental temperature and behaviour. Appl Anim Behav Sci 14:117–126.

_____. 1987. Mineral-deficient diets and the pig's attraction to blood: Implications for tail-biting. Can J Anim Sci 67:909–918.

GONYOU, H. W.; HEMSWORTH, P. H.; AND BARNETT, J. L. 1986. Effects of frequent interactions with humans on growing pigs. Appl Anim Behav Sci 16:269–278.

HEMSWORTH, P. H.; BARNETT, J. L.; AND HANSEN, C. 1981a. The influence of handling by humans on the behaviour, growth and corticosteroids in the juvenile

female pig. Horm Behav 15:396–403.

HEMSWORTH, P. H.; BRAND, A.; AND WILLENS, P. J. 1981b. The behavioural response of sows to the presence of human beings and its relation to productivity. Livest Prod Sci 8:67–74.

HEMSWORTH, P. H.; BARNETT, J. L.; AND HANSEN, C. 1986. The influence of handling by humans on the behaviour, reproduction and corticosteroids of male and female pigs. Appl Anim Behav Sci 15:303–311.

_____. 1987. The influence of inconsistent handling by humans on the behaviour, growth and corticosteroids of young pigs. Anim Behav Sci 17:245–252.

HOUSE OF COMMONS COMMITTEE. 1981. House of Commons First Report from the Agriculture Committee, Session 1980–81. Animal welfare in poultry, pig and veal calf production. Her Majesty's Stationary Office, London, vol. 1, pp. 26–35.

HUGHES, B. O. 1976. Behaviour as an index of welfare. Proc 5th Eur Poult Conf, Malta, pp. 1005–1012.

KELLEY, K. W. 1980. Stress and immune function: A bibliographic review. Ann Rech Vet 11:445–478.

_____. 1988. Cross-talk between the immune and endocrine systems. J Anim Sci 66:2095–2108.

LADEWIG, J., et al. 1985. Physiological aspects of social space in heifers and pigs. In Social Space in Domestic Animals. Ed. R. Zayan. The Hague: Martinus Nijhoff, pp. 151–159.

MARTIN, P. 1987. Psychology and the immune system. New Sci 9:46–50.

METZ, J. H. M., AND OSTERLEE, C. C. 1981. Immunologische und ethologische Kritorien fur die artgemasse Haltung von Sauen und Ferkeln. Kuratorium Tech Bauwesen Landwirtschaft Schr 264:39–50.

MOSS, B. W. 1981. The development of a blood profile for stress assessment. In The Welfare of Pigs. Ed. W. Sybesma. The Hague: Martinus Nijhoff, pp. 112–125.

PETHERICK, C. 1989. Feeding regime and the behaviour of group housed nonlactating sows. Appl Anim Behav Sci 22:90.

PETHERICK, C.; BODERO, D.; AND BLACKSHAW, J. 1987. The effect of feeding regime on agonistic interactions in group-housed sows. Proc 13th Conf Aust Soc Anim Behav.

SANDIFORD, F. 1985. An economic analysis of the introduction of legislation governing the welfare of farm animals. 2. Animal Welfare in Pig Production. Bull 201, Dep of Agric Econ, Univ of Manchester, England.

SEABROOK, M. F. 1983. Stockmanship on the farm. Univ Fed Anim Welfare, pp. 7–18.

SPENCER, G. S. G. 1985. Hormonal systems regulating growth. A review. Livest Prod Sci 12:31–46.

STANTON, H. C., AND MUELLER, R. L. 1976. Sympathoadrenal neurochemistry and early weaning of swine. Am J Vet Res 37:779–783.

STEPHENS, D. B. 1980. Stress and its measurement in domestic animals: A review of behavioural and physiological studies under field and laboratory situations. Adv Vet Sci Comp Med 24:179–209.

STOLBA, A. 1981. A family system in enriched pens as a novel method of pig housing. In Alternatives to Intensive Husbandry Systems. Univ Fed Anim Welfare, pp. 52–67.

THOW, D. 1989. What welfare changes could cost the industry. Pig Farming, April, p. 25.

VAN PUTTEN, G. 1977. Reference systems in applied ethology and the demands they have to meet. Comm Int Génie Rural seminar, Norway 1:40–48.

WEBSTER, J. F. 1987. Meat and right: Farming as if the animals mattered. In New Perspectives in Pig Production. Ed. A. M. Petchey, 9th Lawson Lecture. North of Scotland College of Agriculture, Aberdeen, pp. 5–10.

73 Manipulation of Body Composition

R. D. Boyd

D. H. Beermann

THE MISSION of animal science research is to provide management and biotechnological "tools" to animal agriculture that facilitate efficient animal production and product quality. Productive efficiency of growing swine is largely determined by the proportion of nutrients partitioned to fat relative to muscle and by the rate at which tissue deposition occurs (i.e., dilution of total maintenance cost). Acceptability of the meat product is influenced markedly by fat content. A report from the National Research Council (1988a) cites medical recommendations that urge reduced consumption of dietary fat; particularly that of animal origin. Furthermore, consumers are becoming more health conscious with a growing preference for leaner meat. Thus, efforts by animal scientists to alter the rate and composition of gain simultaneously address the issues of productive efficiency and product acceptability.

Traditional techniques for altering the balance between muscle and fat growth in swine have involved genetic selection and various management strategies (e.g., intact males and limit feeding).

Technological advances have given rise to new possibilities that permit dramatic alteration growth and development through metabolic regulation. These metabolism modifiers (e.g., porcine somatotropin and beta-adrenergic agonists) enable scientists to better regulate the use of absorbed nutrients for muscle growth. Unprecedented responses have accordingly been achieved, with increased levels of protein deposition and decreased levels of lipid deposition. Achievements are beyond those previously expressed for any genotype or sex (Campbell et al. 1988; Evock et al. 1988; Boyd et al. 1991). Normally, 10–20 years of intense genetic selection would be required to accomplish changes of this magnitude.

IMPACT AND BIOLOGIC POTENTIAL FOR LEAN TISSUE DEPOSITION

Composition of Gain in Modern Genotypes. Data in Table 73.1 provide an opportunity for evaluation of compositional growth in pigs

Table 73.1. Assessment of the composition of gain and approximation of the biologic capacity for lean growth in growing pigs fed al libitum from 50 to 100 kg

Item	Control Females	Control Castrate Males	Control Intact Males	Somatotropin Intact Males
Growth data				
Daily gain, kg/day	1.15	1.12	1.31	1.36
Feed efficiency, F:G	2.99	3.08	2.37	1.82
Energy intake, Mcal DE/day	12.1	12.3	11.0	8.8
Protein deposition, g/day[a]	145	128	186	240
Lipid deposition, g/day[a]	318	357	219	30
Carcass data				
Backfat (rib 10), mm	22	29	18	12[b]
Loin eye area, cm²	35	31	36	40
Estimated muscle, kg/carcass[c]	– –	34.0	– –	49
Estimated fat, kg/carcass[c]	– –	25.5	– –	6.9
Protein, kg/carcass	12.34	11.42	13.17	14.38
Lipid, kg/carcass	22.08	25.02	15.39	9.81

Source: Data for control female and castrated male pigs (eight per group) were acquired over the 50- to 100-kg phase of growth (Krick and Boyd, unpublished data); Intact male pigs were half-sib contemporaries but evaluated over the 60- to 100-kg phase (four per group; dose optimum for porcine somatotropin, 150 μg pST/kg body weight) (Boyd and Roneker, unpublished data).

Note: F:G = feed:gain; DE = digestible energy.

[a]Whole-body deposition rates were determined by comparative slaughter.

[b]Inherent error of over estimation due to characteristic increase in skin thickness with pST.

[c]Dissectable muscle and fat estimated from the data of Thiel et al. (1990). The yield of muscle and fat for intact males receiving ST and killed at 90 kg was 42.8 and 6.0 kg respectively.

fed ad libitum. The genotype selected is believed to be typical for relatively progressive producers in North America. Measures include both qualitative (commercial) and quantitative measures of body composition. Rates of deposition for both protein (indexes of lean mass) and lipid are particularly revealing and suggestive of the extent to which body composition could be altered.

The data show that male castrates and females deposit an inordinate amount of lipid (23 kg). The intact male is sometimes used in preference to the castrate because of the advantages observed for fat and muscle deposition. The intact male also represents a sensible standard for commercial production with the benefits of greatly reduced fat or lipid deposition concurrent with increased protein deposition, reflected in the efficiency of gain. Although the rate and extent of lipid deposition is significantly less for the intact male (219 g/day and 15.4 kg) as compared to castrate males and females (337 g/day and 23.5 kg), deposition is considerably greater than justifiable for either productive efficiency or nutrient composition of the meat.

Relationship between Lean Body Mass and Growth Efficiency.

The impact of lean growth on the efficiency of gain is further illustrated in Table 73.2. In this study, the efficiency was determined for two groups of pigs in which the rate of gain (from 60 to 90 kg) was similar, but where composition of gain differed markedly. This is important, since the confounding effects of differential growth rates have been eliminated (i.e., increased rates could dilute maintenance energy cost). Porcine somatotropin (pST) was used to alter the rates of protein and lipid deposition. Protein deposition was increased sufficiently to compensate for the reduction in lipid but constrained from maximal expression by restricting dietary protein input.

The compositional shift shown in Table 73.2 resulted in a 27% improvement in the efficiency of growth. However, this was not due to an energetic advantage conferred by the protein component (+53%) per se, as compared to lipid (−69%). In fact, deposition and maintenance of protein is energetically less efficient than lipid (Boyd and Bauman 1989) and tends to increase maintenance energy expenditure. The advantage is due to an associated increase in the water component and thus reduced energy density of gain.

Biologic Potential for Growth and Lean Deposition.

Attempts have been made to estimate the biologic potential for muscle (or protein) deposition in order to establish production targets. The task of estimating the "ceiling" or genetic limit for such is not presently achievable, since the biologic principles are not entirely clear. Data in Table 73.1 show that earlier projections are realistic for accomplishment in the near future (English et al. 1988) and, in fact, underestimate the capacity based on the results of recent studies in which pST was administered to growing swine (50–100 kg). These data also illustrate that the expressed level for protein deposition is considerably below the inherent capacity and that endogenous secretion of somatotropin is limiting gene expression.

The potential for protein deposition is at least 250–280 g/day based on individual data from the experiment in Table 73.1 (Krick, personal communication). These estimates exceed previous reports for intact males by at least 30%. The net effect of this dramatic change in protein and lipid deposition was an unprecedented efficiency of gain (feed:gain [F:G] ratio, 1.8), coincident with a high rate of growth (>1300 g/day). However, even more impressive results were obtained with intact males from a genotype that had been intensively selected for lean growth. They were administered a near optimum dose of pST from 60 to 90 kg and gained approximately 1500 g/day with a F:G ratio of 1.6. Thus, the biologic potential for the efficiency of gain is comparable to commercial broiler chickens.

STRATEGIES FOR MANIPULATING LEAN DEPOSITION.

A variety of strategies have been used to alter the balance between muscle and fat growth. Traditional methods include (1) genetic selection, (2) exploiting the endocrine advantages of the intact male (vs. castrate or female), (3) constraining fat (or lipid deposition) by restricting energy intake, and (4) slaughtering earlier in the growth phase. Recent advances in growth biology will, if approved, permit animal scientists to employ a powerful new tool to alter the pattern of tissue growth. This technology involves using metabolism modifiers, which alter nutrient metabolism so that a greater proportion of nutritional constituents are diverted toward muscle growth. The basis and merit for each of the strategies are discussed below. Attention will

Table 73.2. Effect of similar rates of growth but altered composition on the efficiency of live-weight gain in swine

| | Accretion Rate (g/day) | | Growth | |
Treatment	Protein	Lipid	Rate (kg/day)	Efficiency (feed:gain, FG)
Conventional	135	450	1.13	3.13
Lean enhanced[a]	207	138	1.16	2.27 (−27%)

Source: Krick, unpublished data.

[a]Rate of lean growth manipulated by administration of somatotropin (150 μg/kg body weight) with dietary protein increased sufficiently to offset the loss in fat accretion.

also be given to nutritional constraints that restrict expression of the inherent capacity for protein deposition.

Genetic Capacity. Genetic selection represents an attempt at gene optimization. Marked differences in genetic capacity are known to exist for protein and lipid deposition. An example of differences for two strains in Australia is summarized in Table 73.3 (see also Yen 1979; Bark 1990). Intact males from strain A were derived from a herd of 6000 sows in which strict methods of selection and quantitative assessment for lean content were practiced. Strain B represents pigs from a herd with a different genotype but which were maintained genotypically "constant." Marked differences in protein deposition rates are evident and representative of the expected range in practice. The castrated male (strain B) might be contrasted to the strain cited in Table 73.1, which exhibited a protein deposition rate of 130 g/day. The differences observed between and within genotypes are important to document, since protein deposition rate is a determinant of the dietary amino acid requirement.

The rate of progress for lean tissue deposition has been documented by a number of authors. There are striking examples of the benefits derived from national improvement schemes involving disciplined use of selection principles (e.g., United Kingdom, Finland; see Fowler et al. 1988). Data compiled by the Meat and Livestock Commission were used by Mitchell et al. (1982) to illustrate the rate of progress achievable through selection (Table 73.4). This paper was used because selection objectives and traits for simultaneous emphasis were most relevant to commercial production. These data quantitate the rate of progress achievable for various criteria and justify the conclusion that improvements of the order observed with pST would require a minimum of 10–20 years to accomplish (Boyd and Wray-Cahen 1989). This strategy nevertheless remains very relevant to animal production, since considerable progress can be made with time and because it establishes the genetic base from which other strategies effect further improvement (Krick et al. 1991; Nossaman et al. 1991).

Techniques for genetic improvement will become more sophisticated and specific for gene identification, controlled expression, or gene insertion (Wagner and Jöchle 1986). The emergence of recombinant genetic technology and embryo manipulation have provided the facility for alteration of the genome (transgenesis). Genes coding for somatotropin or its releasing factor have recently been inserted into the genome of farm animals. The first report of transgenesis in swine was by Hammer et al. (1985). However, Pursel et al. (1989) were the first to produce a sufficient number of pigs with somatotropin transgenes to document the potential for improved growth and carcass composition of transgenic pigs.

The remarkable accomplishments of transgenesis must not overshadow the fact that critical biological questions must be addressed before application to farm animals can occur. For example, the basic mechanisms responsible for regulation of gene expression in mammalian cells are not yet understood. It is conceivable that existing genes can be regulated for greater (or lesser) expression. Also, the process of insertion into the genome of the germ line is largely random, with

Table 73.3. Genotype and gender effects on lean deposition and growth performance from 45 to 90 kg

Criteria	Strain A Intact Male	Strain B Intact Male	Castrate
Protein deposition, g/day	188	129	84
Carcass fat, %	25	33	43
Growth rate, g/day	1249	844	728
Growth efficiency, F:G	2.3	3.10	3.40

Source: Adapted from Campbell (1987).
Note: F:G = feed:gain.

Table 73.4. Comparison of relative responses to genetic selection and somatotropin administration

Item	Genetic Selection[a] Change per Generation	Change %
Lean growth, g/day	+ 6.0	+2.1
Growth rate, g/day	+ 5.0	+0.7
Growth efficiency, F:G	− .03	−1.0
Diet intake, g/day	− 7.3	−0.4
Loin eye area, mm²	+27	+0.8
Backfat depth, mm	− 1.8[a]	−5.5

Source: Adapted from Mitchell et al. (1982), using data derived from the Meat and Livestock Commission (1970–77) data set.
Note: F:G = feed:gain.
[a]Cleveland et al. (1982) (five generations of selection).

generalized incorporation across tissues and uncertainty relative to the determination of gene placement. The integrity of associated genomic sequences are possibly in question. Finally, the specific approach to transgenesis will undoubtedly evolve and have multiple approaches for a given end point as we learn more about the biology of growth, recognize specific points of regulation, and determine how amenable they are to regulation at the gene level.

Gender. There are well-established differences in the expressed capacity for lean tissue deposition between the intact male, castrate, and female pigs. The effect of gender does not manifest itself until the 20- to 50-kg phase of growth and although distinct differences exist, they are slight (Yen 1979; Campbell et al. 1983). Thereafter, differences are decidedly more manifest (Campbell et al. 1985; Campbell 1987) with the rate and proportion of lean deposition being greatest for the boar, intermediate for the female, and least for the castrated male. For example, protein deposition rates for the strain B genotype (Table 73.3) were estimated to be 129, 100, and 84 g/day respectively, with lipid deposition being inversely related to protein deposition (Campbell 1987). This illustrates that the expressed capacity for protein deposition is a function of the endocrine environment (Table 73.3).

The reason that sex differences in protein deposition are not manifested earlier in the growth phase are not clear but two possibilities exist. First, Campbell (1988) proposed that differences are not manifested earlier because the potential for protein deposition exceeds the energy intake required to accommodate the relatively high rate of deposition (Carr et al. 1977). Beyond 50 kg, energy intake exceeds that required for maximum lean deposition, which allows sex differences for protein deposition to be manifest (Campbell 1988). Another important consideration, however, is that the intact male and female, prior to 50 kg, are prepubertal and thus would not have the endocrine environment characteristic of the sex. Thus, differences in energy partition between protein and lipid would not be anticipated, since sex steroids appear to play an important role.

Nutritional Considerations. Nutritional considerations are twofold and the ultimate determinant of whether the capacity for protein vs. fat deposition can be expressed. First, sufficient protein (amino acids) must be provided to accommodate the potential for protein deposition; the requirement is a function of gender and genotype and both factors should be considered when designing diets. Second, fat deposition may be constrained by restricting energy intake. The latter has been traditionally accomplished through feeding management but may occur indirectly with

the use of metabolism modifiers. The latter alters fat tissue metabolism so that less dietary energy (as glucose) is deposited as lipid. Intake is accordingly reduced, since the caloric density of the gain is less.

RESTRICTED FEEDING. Restricted feeding is an effective means for altering the proportion of muscle to fat in pigs beyond 50 kg. In principle, this strategy attempts to match energy intake with the potential for muscle growth or protein deposition. The pattern of muscle and fat deposition in relation to energy intake is portrayed in Figure 73.1. During the linear phase for lean growth, fat deposition will be constrained to an "obligatory" minimum characteristic for the genotype and sex. Fat deposition continues beyond the energy intake required for maximum muscle deposition (Fig. 73.1 A,B; point *A*) with the extent being a function of energy consumed (Whittemore 1986; Campbell 1988).

The net effect of incremental changes in energy intake (from restriction to ad libitum) on rate and efficiency of growth are likewise illustrated (Fig. 73.1C,D). Restriction of energy intake to the point of maximum muscle deposition yields the highest proportion of muscle to fat, with efficiency of gain being optimized. Rate of gain is compromised slightly when restricted to point *A*, but the proportion of lean gain is optimized. Intact males and genotypes that have been highly selected for muscle deposition exhibit a higher potential for such (plateau) and, accordingly, shift the energy intake needed for maximum protein deposition (Campbell 1988; Bark 1990). There is also evidence that highly selected strains of intact males have a capacity for muscle deposition that cannot be exhibited within the limits of intake (e.g., strain A, Table 73.3; Campbell 1988). It is clear from the above data that the rate and efficiency of growth in pigs are a direct reflection of their expressed capacity for muscle growth and thus caloric density of the gain. Although restricted feeding reduces growth rate, profitability is greatest provided that payment is a function of meat yield.

NUTRITIONAL CONSTRAINTS. It is well known that the capacity for protein (or muscle) deposition may ultimately be constrained by inadequate intake of protein (see reviews by Australian Animal Nutrition Subcommittee 1987; Campbell 1988; Boyd et al. 1991a). The interrelationship between protein (amino acid) intake and protein deposition and the rate and efficiency of growth were illustrated by Krick et al. (1990a) in a recent study with a genotype selected for high rates of muscle deposition (Fig. 73.2). Protein and lysine equivalent dose–response curves were established for pigs over the 20- to 60-kg phase of growth. The amino acid lysine was computed to be first-limiting in the protein component. It was

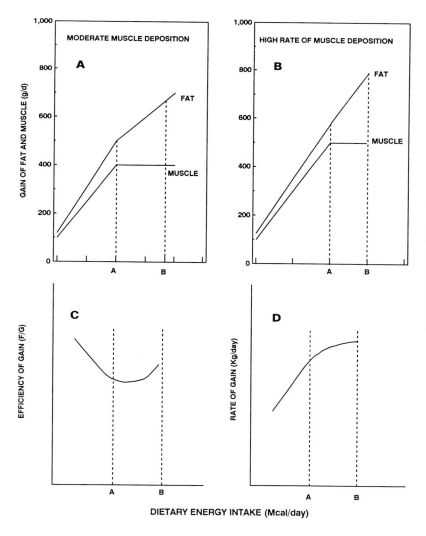

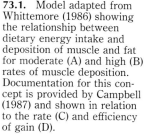

73.1. Model adapted from Whittemore (1986) showing the relationship between dietary energy intake and deposition of muscle and fat for moderate (A) and high (B) rates of muscle deposition. Documentation for this concept is provided by Campbell (1987) and shown in relation to the rate (C) and efficiency of gain (D).

selected for emphasis since it is generally the first to be limiting to growth in practical pig diets.

Increasing increments of protein resulted in a corresponding increase in protein deposition to an apparent maximum (Fig. 73.2). The effect on rate and efficiency of gain are likewise shown. This data illustrates how an inadvertant deficiency in dietary protein can constrain performance. In this regard, the estimate for the dietary lysine requirement for this improved genotype is considerably higher (+38%, 22 g/day) than the NRC (1988; 16 g/day at 0.75% of 2145 g/day, actual feed intake). We are unable to account for this disparity, since nutrition subcommittees are almost never provided the information required to adequately characterize the animal for which the estimate is appropriate. However, the higher estimate is in good agreement with both ARC (1981) and Australian subcommittee (1987) estimates (21 g/day at 0.67 g lysine/MJ digestible energy intake). Of particular relevance to this discussion is that our calculations suggest that the NRC estimate is ap-

propriate for pigs depositing approximately 80 g protein/day and gaining 760 g/day with an estimated efficiency of gain of 2.85 g/day (NRC estimated 700 g/day and 2.71 respectively). Thus, adherence to the NRC estimate for this genotype would have had a marked impact on days and feed required for this genotype to gain 30 kg body weight (Table 73.5). A similar conclusion and magnitude of difference was observed for this genotype over the 50- to 100-kg phase of growth (Krick et al. 1990b). In each case, however, failure to accommodate dietary protein needs would result in reciprocal increases in fat deposition, which has been nicely illustrated by Campbell (1988).

STAGE OF GROWTH. Electing to slaughter earlier in the growth phase takes advantage of knowledge that deposition of fat relative to muscle accelerates as the pig grows. Choice of a specific point requires knowledge of the allometric pattern of tissue growth, so that slaughter occurs at

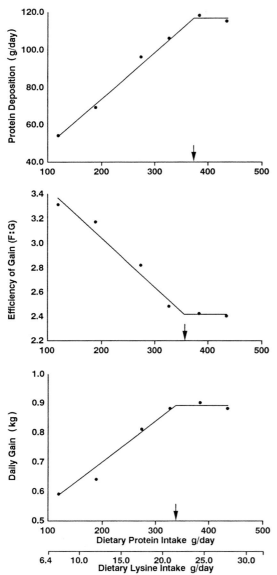

73.2. Relationship between dietary intake of protein (and equivalent lysine) and the rate of protein deposition, rate of gain, and efficiency of gain for the 20- to 55-kg phase of growth in pigs (Krick et al. 1990a). Dietary protein approximates the dietary ideal pattern of amino acids as estimated by the ARC (1981) with each point being the mean of six pigs. Arrows indicate the approximate requirement for dietary protein (or lysine) for each criterion.

an appropriate fatness or prior to the inflection in lipid deposition. The temporal pattern of tissue deposition for a given genotype is shown in Figure 73.3.

BIOLOGY AND POTENTIAL IMPACT OF METABOLISM REGULATORS

Biology of Somatotropin. Growth is a highly orchestrated process involving a number of hor-

mones and growth factors. The hormone somatotropin (ST) has been shown to exhibit regulatory effects on metabolism and to occupy a central role in determining how absorbed nutrients are partitioned postnatally. Exogenous administration of ST increases the blood concentration, which alters the rate and pattern of tissue growth in growing swine by directing nutrients toward or diverting them from specific tissues in a highly coordinated manner (Boyd and Bauman 1989).

ST is a protein synthesized and secreted by the anterior pituitary gland. ST from farm animal species contains 191 amino acids, which share a high degree of homology. However, pituitary preparations from farm animals are not biologically active in humans, since they are unable to effectively bind to the ST receptor of human cells (NRC 1992a). An overview of the controls on ST secretion and its direct and indirect involvement in tissue metabolism is portrayed in Figure 73.4. Any strategy that increases the blood concentration of ST would potentially be a feasible approach for manipulating animal growth. For example, manipulation of endogenous ST secretion can occur by overriding the inhibitory effects of somatostatin or by increasing the secretory stimulant–growth hormone–releasing factor (GRF). Given the present technologies and our understanding of the biology, there are at least four conceivable targets or approaches to manipulation of the ST pathway. These have been discussed in recent reviews (Boyd and Wray-Cahen 1989; Campion and Novakofski 1990).

The specific effects of ST are discussed elsewhere (Boyd and Bauman 1989; Beermann et al. 1990; Etherton and Smith 1991; NRC 1992c), but a brief overview is provided here. The precipitous decrease in the rate of fat deposition of growing swine administered exogenous ST is the most graphic illustration of nutrient redirection (i.e., glucose) from adipose growth in support of muscle deposition. This effect is due almost exclusively to a reduction in lipid synthesis, which occurs because the stimulatory effect of insulin is severely antagonized. This redirection of glucose, the main carbohydrate constituent of grain, is required for, but in excess of, the needs for muscle deposition. Less is known about the specific metabolic mechanisms by which the profound changes in muscle deposition occur, but one of the characteristic responses to exogenous pST is a dose-dependent decrease in blood urea nitrogen concentration. This suggests that whole-body oxidation of amino acids is reduced. These adaptations in amino acid metabolism are consistent with an increased use of amino acids for protein synthesis.

Thus, it is possible that scientists have discovered a biologic mechanism by which genetically superior and intact male pigs partition nutrients toward greater muscle deposition. The limiting step in administering ST to farm animals, how-

Table 73.5. Predicted difference in performance if a high muscle deposition genotype were fed the NRC recommended level for lysine vs. the experimentally determined level

Item	Dietary Lysine Concentration		
	Predicted NRC[a]	Actual[b]	Difference[c]
Performance			
Protein deposition, g/day	80	115	− 35
Daily gain, g/day	760	890	−130
Feed efficiency, F:G	2.85	2.41	+ 44
Predicted for 30 kg gain			
Time required, days	39.5	33.7	+ 5.8
Feed required, kg	85.5	72.3	+ 13.2

Note: F:G = feed:gain.
[a]NRC (1988) minimum recommendation for lysine = 0.75%. Data were predicted from Figure 73.2 assuming the NRC daily lysine intake (0.75% × 2145 g feed intake/day for this test group).
[b]Experimentally determined requirement based on rate and efficiency of gain was approximately 22 g lysine/day or 1.09% at 2014 g intake/day.
[c]Difference = actual − NRC predicted.

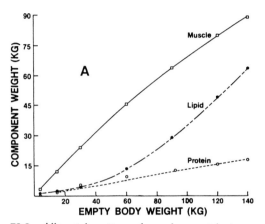

73.3. Allometric pattern of muscle or nutrient deposition for pigs from birth to 145 kg body weight. (From Shields et al. 1983.)

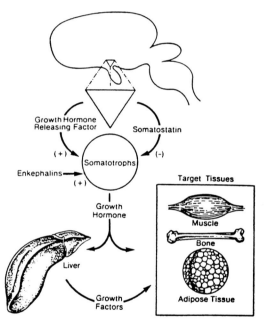

73.4. Synthesis and secretion of the anterior pituitary hormone, somatotropin (or growth hormone), is determined by the hypothalamic hormones, growth hormone–releasing factor (stimulatory) and somatostatin (inhibitory). (From Convey 1987.)

ever, is in the development of a suitable delivery system, since this molecule is not orally active.

Biology of Beta-Adrenergic Agonists. Since the early 1980s, several synthetic analogues of the naturally occurring catecholamines, norepinephrine and epinephrine, have been investigated for their ability to alter the growth patterns for muscle and fat in growing farm animals. These compounds are known as phenethanolamine derivatives and are classified as beta-adrenergic agonists, or more commonly "beta-agonists" because they bind to the beta-receptors present on cell membranes and produce effects consistent with beta-adrenergic activity. While it is convenient to discuss beta-agonists collectively, one should appreciate that they differ structurally; thus, differences in mode of action and efficacy in promoting lean deposition are to be expected. Some of the compounds that have been reported in the literature are shown in Figure 73.5. This area was the subject of recent reviews (Reeds and Mersmann 1991; NRC 1992c).

Unlike somatotropin, the beta-agonists studied thus far are orally active and efficacious at relatively low concentrations (2–20 ppm). Their general effect is to increase the rate of skeletal muscle growth, concurrent with a reduction in the rate of lipid deposition. Rate and efficiency of growth are generally improved, but responses are quite variable and possibly related to differences in phases of growth, diet, and genotype (Dunshea 1991). In general the magnitude of the response appears to be greater in cattle and sheep than in pigs. The magnitude of response to the beta-agonist cimaterol has been shown to be greatest

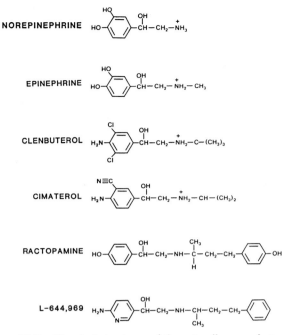

73.5. Chemical structures of the naturally occurring catecholamines, epinephrine and norepinephrine, and selected synthetic beta-adrenergic agonists.

when administered during the latter phase of growth (e.g., >50 kg vs. 25 kg) (Jones et al. 1985; Mersmann et al. 1987). The lack of response in very young pigs (and ruminants) may be related to fewer receptors, lesser binding affinity, or more rapid development of refractoriness to these compounds. Responses are dose dependent with exemplary data for the beta-agonist ractopamine, presented in Table 73.5.

At the present time, we do not know enough about the mechanism of action to discuss how metabolism is altered. However, it is believed that the increase in skeletal muscle growth and the reduction of adipose tissue accretion is achieved through the interaction of the synthetic compounds with beta receptors on the specific tissue

site (vs. indirect means), but this has not been unequivocally demonstrated. Administration of hormone causes muscle hypertrophy rather than hyperplasia (consistent with somatotropin), but it is noteworthy that a differential growth response is observed. For example, skeletal muscle mass increases while visceral wieght does not. This appears to be in contrast with what is observed for somatotropin. The mechanism by which lipid content is reduced is uncertain, but Liu et al. (1989) have shown that for at least clenbuterol and ractopamine, insulin binding to porcine adipocytes is reduced, thereby antagonizing insulin action toward lipid deposition.

Anticipated Field Response to Metabolism Modifiers. The expected growth responses to pST and the beta-adrenergic agonist ractopamine, in practice, are summarized in Table 73.6. We anticipate that the first-generation pST product will approximate the effectiveness of a 50-μg/kg/day dose. Results from a recent dose-titration study suggest that this would yield approximately 70% of the response at dose optimum (Krick et al. 1991). The potential for manipulating growth with beta-agonists is likewise impressive but relative changes, to date, have been less than those observed with pST. The dose anticipated for beta-adrenergic agonists is specified and achievable in practice, since it is orally active.

NET YIELD OF MEAT AND ORGANOLEPTICS. The effect of metabolism modifiers on net yield of meat has recently been addressed in the context of pST-treated swine. It is important to note that swine exhibit a dose-dependent decrease (small) in dressing percent because organs increase simultaneously with skeletal muscle growth. However, these variety meats are also of value and should not reflect a decreased value of the live animal. In addition, yield of skeletal muscle is increased dramatically, but the inept expression of dressing percent is unable to reflect it. Recent dissection work by Thiel et al. (1990) demon-

Table 73.6. Expected field responses to porcine somatotropin and the beta-agonist ractopamine

	Metabolism Modifier – Relative Response	
Criteria	Somatotropin[a]	Ractopamine[b,c]
Growth rate	+12%	+ 9%
Growth efficiency	−25%	−12%
Diet intake	−16%	− 4%
Backfat (rib 10)	−35%	−14%
Loin eye area	+28%	+15%
Dissected tissue mass		
Skeletal muscle	+25%	+12%
Adipose	−30%	−14%

   [a]Computed from Krick et al. (1991); tissue mass data derived from Thiel et al. (1990); dose level used was 50 μg/kg of body weight.
   [b]Adapted from Veenhuizen and Anderson (1990).
   [c]Growth performance data are summarized for 12 trials; dissection data represent 24 animals.

strated that at constant live-weight, total skeletal muscle mass increased by 28–38% with an increasing dose of pST (Fig. 73.6). Coincident with the skeletal muscle mass increase is a 35–74% reduction in separable adipose tissue mass and a 10–17% increase in bone. Thus, for a 105-kg pig (76-kg carcass) a practical dose of pST would increase the yield of muscle by 10 kg and reduce separable fat by 11 kg.

The effects of porcine somatotropin, its releasing factor, or beta-adrenergic agonists on meat quality have been addressed in recent papers (summarized by Beermann 1990). One of the consistent effects of these metabolism modifiers is to reduce carcass and intramuscular lipid concentration. The latter is linked to sensory perception of juiciness and overall acceptability. Porcine somatotropin reduces intramuscular lipid concentration in a dose-dependent manner (to 20% of control) coincident with a small but significant increase in protein concentration. A practical dose of pST on the basis of the dose response study of Thiel et al. (1990), would be expected to decrease lipid concentration in skeletal muscle by approximately 35–40%. Although lipid concentration in muscles is reduced, cholesterol concentration in muscle is not altered and fatty-acid composition of lipid is affected very little. A cross section of loins (with associated side) for conventional and pST-treated pigs is displayed in Figure 73.7.

Despite these changes in proximate and nutritional composition, sensory characterization of fresh pork is only influenced at very high doses of pST, and these changes are small. Thus, consumer acceptance of pork derived from pST-treated pigs is anticipated to be equal to or greater than pork from untreated animals. Likewise, the beta-adrenergic agonist, ractopamine, apparently has no significant effect on indexes of pork quality or on objective or subjective assess-ment of sensory measures (Cole et al. 1987; Merkel 1988).

NUTRITIONAL MANAGEMENT OF METABOLISM-MODIFIED PIGS

Implications. The challenge presented with the anticipated introduction of one or more metabolism modifiers is potentially one or both altered nutrient requirements and introduction of a more dynamic nutritional situation. The latter is anticipated, since it is conceivable that different doses and types of nutrient-partitioning agents will be used. This will result in an enlarged spectrum of protein deposition rates and suggests that nutritional approaches must be more dynamic. Thus, experimental attempts to estimate the requirement for a particular nutrient should contribute, where possible, to clarification of biologic principles and mathematic relationships that may be subsequently used in a dynamic model to derive estimates. Recent reviews attempt to address the impact of metabolic regulators on protein and energy (or intake) requirements (Boyd et al. 1991; Campbell et al. 1991; Reeds and Mersmann 1991). Information, to date, almost exclusively addresses amino acids and energy.

There are several nutritional implications for which definitive statements can be made. First, a markedly different nutrient-to-energy (or intake) relationship will be needed, due to the effects of pST on both intake and the rate and proportion of protein (or lean) deposition. A consistent effect of both pST and beta-agonists is reduced energy intake (Table 73.6), but the extent to which intake is altered depends on the energy density of gain allowable by the dose of a particular modifier. This is dynamic and has been documented for pST (Boyd and Krick 1989). Thus, nutrient concentration in the diet would need to be increased in or-

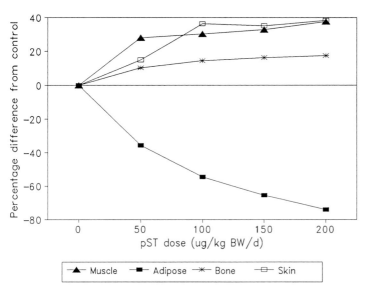

73.6. Dose response effects of porcine somatotropin on yield of tissues in pork carcasses. Somatotropin was administered to 30- to 90-kg male castrates (10 per dose) by intramuscular injection.

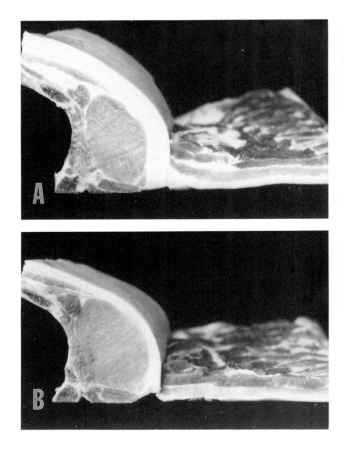

73.7. Cross section of loins (rib 10) and associated side for conventional (A) and porcine somatotropin–treated pigs (B) (at dose optimum, 120 µg/kg body weight). The control pig was representative of its contemporaries and had 1.05 inches of backfat with a 5.5 in.² loin eye area.

der to keep nutrient intake constant. Second, an increase in the rate and extent of protein deposition suggests that both the daily amino acid intake and total quantity of amino acids needed to reach a given body weight must be increased. However, the extent to which this is true depends on whether pST or beta-agonists such as ractopamine alter digestibility and/or the efficiency with which absorbed amino acids are used for protein deposition. Third, the question of whether nutrient requirements will be altered is more encompassing than for amino acids alone, since dramatic changes were observed for mineral deposition when pST is administered (Boyd and Krick 1989; +63% g/day and +31% total kg at dose optimum).

Protein or Amino Acids. The effects of pST on protein deposition cannot be realized without some increase in protein (or amino acid) intake, but a striking difference exists in the extent to which the requirement might be increased for different phases of growth (e.g., 20–50 kg vs. 50–100 kg). For example, an increase in protein deposition of approximately 24% occurred with pST administration during the 20- to 50-kg phase, but this was achievable with only a small increase (3–5%) in the daily requirement for dietary protein (Krick et al. 1990a). All studies to date are in

agreement on this for this phase of growth (Campbell et al. 1990; Caperna et al. 1991), suggesting that the mechanism involves an improvement in the efficiency of amino acid use for protein deposition (Fig. 73.8). Results just cited conform to panel B where the ceiling for protein deposition was increased (middle dotted line) coincident with an improvement in the efficiency of amino acid use (i.e., increased line slope). Consequently, little or no increase in dietary protein was required. Alternatively, less dietary protein would have been required to achieve the level of protein deposition observed for the conventional counterparts.

At present, the effect of pST on the requirement for protein during the 50- to 100-kg phase of growth in pigs is less clear despite the fact that a number of experiments have been conducted (Newcomb et al. 1988; Goodband et al. 1990; Boyd et al. 1991; Campbell et al. 1991). This is a concern, since this growth phase will be the target for initial implementation. The extent to which protein deposition can be increased when pST (at dose optimum) is administered during this phase, as compared to either control counterparts or 20- to 50-kg pigs (administered pST) is portrayed in Figure 73.8 (upper dotted line, panel B). It is not yet clear whether the requirement for dietary protein is directly proportional to the in-

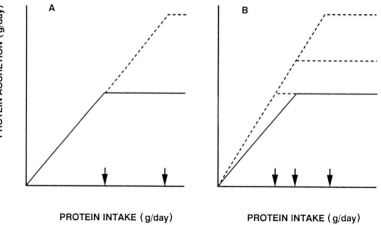

73.8. Conceptual model of potential relationships between protein (amino acid) intake and protein deposition for conventional or metabolism-modified pigs. (A) The relationship when a metabolism modifier raises the ceiling for protein deposition (dotted line) but does not alter the efficiency of amino acid use. (B) The protein-sparing effect that can occur when the efficiency of amino acid use is increased by a metabolism modifier or some other mechanism. The arrows indicate the effect on the requirement for dietary protein.

crease in protein deposition (panel A) or if an increase in the efficiency of amino acid use occurs, as observed in the earlier phase of growth (panel B) and with growing cattle and sheep (Houseknecht et al. 1990; Beermann et al. 1991). Two quantitative studies were conducted to determine if the efficiency is altered and ultimately how the requirement is affected at various pST doses, but different results were obtained (Boyd et al. 1991; Campbell et al. 1991).

All studies to date agree, however, that the dietary protein requirement must be significantly increased or the response to pST will be compromised for this phase. A preliminary recommendation for barrows and gilts given a commercially anticipated dose of pST is 1.10–1.20% dietary lysine, which is equivalent to 20–22% dietary protein (lysine supplemented) (Newcomb et al. 1988; Goodband et al. 1990; Boyd and Krick 1992). This corrects for the pST-induced decline in intake and provides additional amino acids for increased muscle deposition (+25%, Table 73.6).

The effects of ractopamine on protein deposition and consequently the rate and efficiency of gain also appear to be dependent upon additional dietary protein intake (Anderson et al. 1987; Dunshea 1991). We anticipate that an absolute increase in nutrient requirement will be less because the effect on protein deposition appears to be less than observed for pST (Table 73.6; Dunshea 1991). Furthermore, very little correction in the dietary concentration will be needed because of effects on intake, which appears to be reduced but only slightly. Until recently, a sufficiently quantitative study was not available to give specific recommendations as to the protein requirement in ractopamine-treated pigs. Dunshea (1991) established separate protein dose–response curves with growing female pigs in the 60- to 90-kg phase of growth, and the data suggests that the efficiency of amino acid use is not improved and that a 20% increase in the dietary protein requirement was required (17% vs. 14%) for

ractopamine-treated pigs to deposit 23% more protein.

Since beta-agonists cause differential rather than generalized muscle growth (as shown for pST), the pattern of amino acids needed for tissue growth would appear to be different. Thus, the relative importance of lysine to protein deposition is expected to be greater relative to other essential amino acids, since intestinal growth is conserved, coincident with enhanced muscle growth (Reeds and Mersmann 1991). We anticipate that lysine would be the first limiting amino acid, for the relative requirement is expected to increase in relation to others.

Minerals and Vitamins. Research shows that the rate of bone deposition is markedly increased in pigs receiving pST (Table 73.1; Bark 1990), but not by the beta-agonist ractopamine (Bark 1990). The rate of deposition for pST-treated pigs appears to be a function of dose, with an approximate increase of 35–40% occurring with a dose anticipated for commercial use (Bark 1990; Krick et al. 1992). This suggests that an increase in the requirement for calcium, phosphorus, magnesium, and other minerals may be required, but it is not known if pST improves digestibility and/or the efficiency of absorbed mineral use as observed for amino acids. Thus, only a tentative recommendation can be given. In so doing, one cannot overstate the need to characterize and correct for reductions in intake, since the latter is dramatically affected and dose dependent. Accordingly, at least 0.60% calcium and 0.48% phosphorus is needed just to compensate for the decline in intake with a commercially anticipated pST dose (−16%, Table 73.6). This assumes the NRC-recommended minimum of 0.50% and 0.40% respectively. Carter et al. (1991) demonstrated that a further increase to at least 0.70% and 65% for calcium and phosphorus, respectively, is required. Thus, a quantitative increase in the requirement is apparent.

Little information is available for other minerals, but Caperna et al. (1989) showed that hematocrits and serum iron were reduced by pST treatment. These results presumably reflect the marked decrease in dietary-nutrient intake.

There is virtually no information relative to the impact of pST or ractopamine on vitamin requirements. It is advisable if not imperative to compensate for the reduction in intake for both vitamins and trace minerals. A tentative recommendation would be to increase intake-corrected concentrations by 30–40%. However, balanced formulations typically contain sufficient fortification (e.g., 50–100%) to easily satisfy this, so correction for intake may prove sufficient even in practice.

Health Considerations. As stated, this type of technology will require greater input of amino acids and recognition that intake (and accordingly nutrients) is reduced. Failure to accommodate the increased needs for amino acids will not compromise health, but the potential benefits on muscle deposition, growth rate, and efficiency will be partially eliminated. However, adverse effects could be manifested if vitamin and in particular macromineral concentrations are not increased to at least compensate for the reduced feed intake. The potential impact of vitamin and mineral deficiency is considerable, since approximately 50% of the nutrients are represented by these two classes.

PERSPECTIVES AND SUMMARY. Production efficiency of growing swine is greatly limited by the proportion of body fat relative to muscle. A number of strategies have been used to alter tissue growth, but none, with exception of the intact male, have the impact that is potentially available through metabolism modifiers. It is also crucial to understand that performance and body composition responses are a function of diet adequacy. Failure to feed a nutritionally appropriate diet will result in a diminished or adverse response.

The net impact of any technology that improves production efficiency and lean composition will likely be to improve the market share of meat consumption. Swine producers probably will not earn more per marketed pig in the long run but will observe a significant reduction in cost per unit of meat produced, which will narrow the price margin with poultry. This effect combined with improved consumer perception (due to a visible difference in product fat content) should be major factors in the quest for increased market share. A further and important possibility is that pigs could be marketed at heavier weights without fear of overfatness.

REFERENCES

AGRICULTURAL RESEARCH COUNCIL (ARC). 1981. Commonwealth Agricultural Bureaux. Slough, England.

ANDERSON, D. B.; VEENHUIZEN, E. L.; WAITT, W. P.; PAXTON, R. E.; MOWREY, D. H. 1987. The effect of dietary protein on nitrogen metabolism, growth performance and carcass composition of finisher pigs fed ractopamine. Fed Proc 46:1021. Abstr.

AUSTRALIAN SUBCOMMITTEE ON ANIMAL NUTRITION. 1987. Pigs: Feeding standards for Australian livestock.

BARK, L. J. 1990. Influence of genetic capacity for lean tissue growth on responses of pigs to metabolic regulators. Ph.D. diss., Univ of Kentucky.

BEERMANN, D. H. 1990. Implications of biotechnologies for control of meat animal growth. Proc 43rd Annu Recip Meats Conf, pp. 87–96.

BEERMANN, D. H.; ROBINSON, T. F.; BYREM, T. M.; BELL, A. W.; HOGUE, D. E.; AND McLAUGHLIN, C. L. 1991. Effects of abomasal casein infusion on nitrogen utilization and blood metabolites in growing lambs treated with exogenous somatotropin. Fed Am Soc Exp Biol J 5(5):A1295.

BOYD, R. D., AND BAUMAN, D. E. 1989. Mechanisms of action for somatotropin in growth. In Animal Growth Regulation. Ed. D. R. Campion, G. J. Hausman, and R. J. Martin, New York: Plenum Press.

BOYD, R. D., AND KRICK, B. 1989. Relationship between amino acid intake and protein accretion in growing swine receiving somatotropin: Theoretical versus empirical estimates. Proc Cornell Nutr Conf, p. 149.

————. 1991. Impact of metabolism modifiers on protein and energy requirements of growing pigs. Feedstuffs. In press.

————. 1992. Impact of metabolism modifiers on protein and energy requirements of growing pigs. Feedstuffs. In press.

BOYD, R. D., AND WRAY-CAHEN, D. 1989. Biotechnological 'tools' to regulate growth in swine. In Biotechnology for Control of Growth and Product Quality in Swine: Implications and Acceptability Ed. P. Van Der Wal, G. J. Nieuwhof, and R. D. Politiek. Wageningen Agricultural Univ, Netherlands, p. 21.

BOYD, R. D.; BAUMAN, D. E.; FOX, D. G.; AND SCANES, C. G. 1991. Impact of metabolism modifiers on protein accretion and protein and energy requirements of livestock. J Anim Sci [Suppl]69:56–75.

CAMPBELL, R. G. 1987. The effects of genotype and sex on the performance and nutrient requirements of growing pigs. Proc Maryland Nutr Conf, pp. 90–94.

————. 1988. Nutritional constraints to lean tissue accretion in farm animals. Nutr Res Rev 1:1–21.

CAMPBELL, R. G.; TAVERNER, M. R.; AND CURIC, D. M. 1983. The influence of feeding level from 20 to 45 kg live weight on the performance and body composition of female and entire male pigs. Anim Prod 40:193–199.

————. 1985. Effect of sex and energy intake between 48 and 90 kg live weight on protein deposition in growing pigs. Anim Prod 40:497–503.

CAMPBELL, R. D.; STEELE, N. C.; CAPERNA, T. J.; McMURTRY, J. P.; SOLOMON, M. B.; AND MITCHELL, A. D. 1988. Interrelationships between energy intake and exogenous porcine growth hormone administration on the performance, body composition and protein and energy metabolism of growing pigs weighing 25 to 55 kilograms body weight. J Anim Sci 66:1643–1655.

CAMPBELL, R. G.; JOHNSON, R. J.; KING, R. H.; TAVERNER, M. R.; AND MEISINGER, D. 1990. Interaction of dietary protein content and exogenous porcine growth hormone administration on protein and lipid accretion rates in growing pigs. J Anim Sci 68:3217–3225.

CAMPBELL, R. G.; JOHNSON, R. J.; TAVERNER, M. R.;

AND KING, R. H. 1991. Interrelationships between exogenous porcine somatotropin (PST) administration and dietary protein and energy intake on protein deposition capacity and energy metabolism of pigs. J Anim Sci 69:1522–1531.

CAMPION, D. R., AND NOVAKOFSKI, J. 1990. Technical perspective of biotechnology for control of growth and product quality in meat producton. In Biotechnology for Control of Growth and Product Quality in Meat Production. Implications and Acceptability (Provisional). Wageningen Agricultural Univ, Netherlands, pp. 2.1–2.12.

CAPERNA, T. J.; CAMPBELL, R. J.; AND STEELE, N. C. 1989. Interrelationships of exogenous growth hormone administration and feed intake level affecting various tissue levels of iron, copper, zinc and bone calcium of growing pigs. J Anim Sci 67:334–338.

CAPERNA, T. J.; STEELE, N. C.; KOMAREK, D. R.; McMURTRY, J. P.; ROSEBROUGH, R. W.; SOLOMON, M. B.; AND MITCHELL, A. D. 1991. Influence of dietary protein and recombinant porcine somatotropin administration in young pigs: Growth, body composition and hormonal status. J Anim Sci 68:4243–4252.

CARR, J. R.; BOORMAN, K. N.; AND COLE, D. J. A. 1977. Nitrogen retention in the pig. Br J Nutr 37:143–155.

CARTER, S. D.; CROMWELL, G. L.; AND STAHLY, T. S. 1991. Effect of pST administration on the calcium and phosphorus requirements of finishing pigs. J Anim Sci 69[Suppl 1]:384.

COLE, D. J. A.; WOOD, J. D.; KILPATRICK, M. J. 1987. Effects of the beta-agonist GAH/034 on growth, carcass quality and meat quality in pigs. In Beta-Agonists and Their Effects on Animal Growth and Carcass Quality. Ed. J. P. Hanrahan. London: Elsevier Applied Science, p. 137.

CONVEY, E. M. 1987. Advances in animal science: Potential for improving meat animal production. Proc Cornell Nutr Conf, p. 1.

DUNSHEA, F. R. 1991. Factors affecting efficacy of β-agonists for pigs. Pig News Inf 12(2):227–231.

ENGLISH, P. R.; FOWLER, V. R.; BAXTER, S.; AND SMITH, B. 1988. The growing and finishing pig: Improving efficiency. Ipswich, Engl: Farming Press Books, p. 18.

ETHERTON, T. D., 1989. The mechanisms by which porcine growth hormone improves pig growth performance. In Proceedings of the International Symposium on Biotechnology in Growth Regulation. Ed. R. B. Heap, C. G. Prosser, and G. E. Lamming. London: Butterworth, pp. 97–106.

ETHERTON, T. D., AND SMITH, S. B. 1991. Somatotropin and β-adrenergic agonists: Their efficacy and mechanisms of action. J Anim Sci [Suppl 2]69:2–26.

EVOCK, C. M.; ETHERTON, T. D.; CHUNG, C. S.; AND IVY, R. E. 1988. Pituitary growth hormone (pGH) and a recombinant pGH analog stimulate pig growth performance in a similar manner. J Anim Sci 66:1928.

GOODBAND, R. D.; NELSSEN, J. L.; HINES, R. H.; KROPF, D. H.; THALER, R. C.; SCHRICKER, B. R.; FITZNER, G. E.; AND LEWIS, A. J. 1990. The effects of porcine somatotropin and dietary lysine on growth performance and carcass characteristics of finishing swine. J Anim Sci 68:3261–3276.

HAMMER, R. E.; PURSEL, V. G.; REXROAD,C. E., JR.; WALL, R. J.; BOLT, D. J.; EBERT, K. M.; PALMITER, R. D.; BRINSTER, R. L. 1985. Production of transgenic rabbits, sheep and pigs by microinjection. Nature 315:680.

HOUSEKNECHT, K. L.; BAUMAN, D. E.; FOX, D. G.; SMITH, D. F.; AND MUSSO, T. M. 1990. Effect of abomasal casein infusion on nitrogen retention of growing steers treated with exogenous bovine somatotropin (bST). J Anim Sci [Suppl]68:272. Abstr.

JONES, R. W.; EASTER, R. A.; McKEITH, F. K.; DALRYMPLE, R. H.; MADDOCK H. M.; AND BECHTEL, P. J. 1985. Effect of the beta-adrenergic agonist cimaterol (CL 263,780) on the growth and carcass characteristics of finishing swine. J Anim Sci 61:905–913.

KRICK, B. J.; RONEKER, K. R.; HARRELL, R. J.; BOYD, R. D.; BEERMANN, D. H.; AND KUNTZ, H. T. 1990a. Impact of porcine somatotropin on the lysine requirement of growing pigs from 20–60 kg liveweight. J Anim Sci [Suppl 1] 68:383.

KRICK, B. J.; RONEKER, K. R.; BOYD, R. D.; BEERMANN, D. H.; AND ROSS, D. A. 1990b. Impact of porcine somatotropin on the lysine requirement of growing pigs from 55–100 kg liveweight. J Anim Sci [Suppl 1] 68:384.

KRICK, B. J.; RONEKER, K. R.; BOYD, R. D.; BEERMANN, D. H.; DAVID, P. J.; AND MEISINGER, D. J. 1992. Influence of genotype and sex on the response of growing pigs to recombinant porcine somatotropin. J Anim Sci. Submitted for review.

LIU, C. Y.; BOYER, J.; AND MILLS, S. E. 1989. Acute effects of beta-adrenergic agonists on porcine adipocyte metabolism in vitro. J Anim Sci 67:2930–2936.

MERKEL, R. A. 1988. Is meat quality affected by the use of repartitioning agents? Proc 41st Annu Recip Meats Conf, p. 101.

MERSMANN, H. J.; HU, C. Y.; POND, W. G.; RULE, D. C.; NOVAKOFSKI, J. E.; AND SMITH, S. B. 1987. Growth and adipose tissue metabolism in young pigs fed cimaterol with adequate or low dietary protein intake. J Anim Sci 64:1384–1394.

MITCHELL, G.; SMITH, C.; MAKOWER, M.; AND BIRD, P. J. W. N. 1982. An economic appraisal of pig improvement in Great Britain. Anim Prod 35:215.

NATIONAL RESEARCH COUNCIL (NRC). 1988a. Designing Foods–Animal Product Options in the Marketplace. Washington, D.C.: National Academy Press.

———. 1988b. Nutrient Requirements of Swine, 9th ed. rev. Washington, D.C.: National Academy Press.

———. 1992a. Metabolism Modifiers: Mechanism of Action and Impact on Nutrient Requirements. Washington, D. C.: National Academy Press, Chap. 1. In press.

———. 1992b. Metabolism Modifiers: Mechanism of Action and Impact on Nutrient Requirements. Washington, D.C.: National Academy Press, Chap. 3. In press.

———. 1992c. Metabolism Modifiers: Mechanism of Action and Impact on Nutrient Requirements. Washington, D.C.: National Academy Press, Chap. 4. In press.

NEWCOMB, M. D.; GREBNER, G. L.; BECHTEL, P. J.; McKEITH, F. K.; NOVAKOFSKI, J.; McCLAREN, D. G.; EASTER, R. A.; AND JONES, R. W. 1988. Response of 60–100 kg pigs treated with porcine somatotropin to different levels of dietary crude protein. J Anim Sci [Suppl 1]66:281.

NOSSAMAN, D. A.; SCHINCKEL, A. P.; MILLER, L. F.; AND MILLS, S. E. 1991. Interaction of sematotropin and genotype on the requirement for energy in two lines of finishing pigs. J Nutr 121:223–230.

PURSEL, V. G.; MILLER, K. F.; BOLT, D. J.; PINKERT, C. A.; HAMMER, R. E.; PALMITER, R. D.; AND BRINSTER, R. L. 1989. Insertion of growth hormone genes into pig embryos. In Biotechnology in Growth Regulation. Ed. R. B. Heap, C. G. Prosser, and G. E. Lamming. London: Butterworth, p. 181.

REEDS, P. J., AND MERSMANN, H. J. 1991. Protein and energy requirements of animals treated with β-adrenergic agonists: A discussion. J Anim Sci 69:1532–1550.

SHIELDS, R. G.; MAHAN, D. C.; AND GRAHAM, P. L. 1983. changes in swine body composition from birth to 145 kg. J Anim Sci 57:43.

THIEL, L. F.; BEERMANN, D. H.; AND BOYD, R. D. 1990. The effect of exogenous somatotropin treatment on dissectable tissue yield in market hogs. J Anim Sci [Suppl 1] 68:340. Abstr.

VEENHUIZEN, E. L., AND ANDERSON, D. B. 1990. Emerging agricultural technology: Issues for the 1990's. An assessment of the effects of beta-agonists on the food industry. Prepared for the Office of Technology Assessment, Congress, United States, pp. 1–40.

WAGNER, T. E., AND JÖCHLE, W. 1986. Recombinant gene transfer in animals: The potential for improving growth in livestock. In Control and manipulation of Animal Growth. Ed. P. J. Buttery, D. B. Lindsay, and N. B. Haynes. London: Butterworth, p. 293.

WHITTEMORE, C. T. 1986. An approach to pig growth modeling. J Anim Sci 63:615–621.

YEN, H. T. 1979. Ph.D. diss., Univ of Nottingham, England.

74 Veterinary Responsibility for Meat Hygiene

M. M. Pullen

VETERINARIANS are the authority figures on animal health and welfare and on zoonotic diseases. They are on-the-farm point-persons who can influence livestock production, education, and sanitary practices. Furthermore, because of their unique comprehensive background in animal microbiology, parasitology, pathology, and pharmacology, veterinarians are traditional leaders and implementors of meat hygiene programs (Kahrs 1989).

Because veterinarians are involved in diagnostic and prognostic decisions, they are asked to provide advice on the moving and sorting of animals prior to marketing. Often they are asked to assist in making salvage decisions, such as to forego any chemotherapy that requires a withdrawal time and to send the animal directly to slaughter. The determination of food safety and wholesomeness is then transferred to the veterinarian at the federal/state slaughter facility. Another option is custom slaughter, wherein inspection usually is more lenient about salvage decisions and is more compliant with the owner's preference. The third option is on-the-farm slaughter.

The impacts of veterinary clinicians on the wholesomeness of meat include (1) providing instruction on the proper use of biologic and therapeutic agents; (2) advising the livestock producer on the appropriate use and cost effectiveness of feed additives; (3) providing instructions for animal management techniques; and (4) providing both diagnostic and prognostic decisions for the treatment, marketing, or slaughter of food animals (Leman and Pullen 1985).

The Hazard Analysis Critical Control Point (HACCP) system was introduced in 1971. HACCP provides a more specific and critical approach to the control of microbiologic and chemical hazards in foods than that provided by traditional inspection and quality-control approaches. The HACCP system has three procedures: (1) identification and assessment of hazards associated with growing, harvesting, processing, marketing, preparation, and use of a given raw material or food product; (2) determination of critical control points to control any identifiable hazard; and (3) establishment of systems to monitor critical control points. HACCP, when properly applied, separates the essential from the superfluous aspects of hazard control by focusing atten-tion on those points that directly affect safety and quality and by monitoring to determine whether or not these points are under control (Pullen 1989).

In a 1985 National Academy of Sciences report, HACCP system was identified as a comprehensive approach applicable to the range of operations from production of animals to slaughter, processing and handling in retail outlets, food-service establishments, and homes; the system is concerned with criteria relevant to public health (NRC 1985).

Practicing veterinarians, as part of the pork industry, play a significant role and share a continuing obligation in educating pork producers about safe and effective antimicrobial usage and residue-avoidance management techniques. Under current management systems, some chemical usage is necessary for efficient, cost-competitive pork production. These compounds reduce disease levels, improve growth efficiencies, and improve animal well-being. A goal of veterinarians and pork producers is to manage the use of these compounds so as to deliver a residue-safe, cost-competitive pork supply to consumers. Veterinarians are in a unique position to offer assistance in the development and administration of quality-assurance programs. Veterinarians possess the knowledge of pharmacodynamics of compounds used and of available residue-testing procedures; the familiarity with the management style, the equipment, and the production facilities; and the ability to weave the interaction of these variables into a comprehensive and effective on-farm quality-assurance program.

Quality-assurance programs can be subdivided into an output, an input, or a combination of testing protocols. In all programs, appropriate product-usage directions, adherence to withdrawal times, and good manufacturing practices for feed production must be followed. Output testing concentrates on evaluating the finished swine prior to sale to ensure that a residue-safe status has been achieved. Input-testing protocols require that ingredient quality be monitored at a point after which contamination is unlikely to occur. Therefore, a combination of input and output testing may assure that residue-safe pork is produced (McKean 1989).

In April 1989 the Illinois Pork Producers Association in cooperation with the federal agencies,

923

Animal and Plant Health Inspection Service (APHIS), Food Safety Inspection Service (FSIS), Food and Drug Administration (FDA), and Cooperative Extension Service (CES), developed a pilot Producer Self-Certification Program (PSCP). The program is voluntary and permits producers to certify sulfa-safe pork. The program requires the producer to develop a farm plan in conjunction with an approved accredited veterinarian, and to periodically test a portion of his/her finishing pigs for possible sulfamethazine (SMZ) residues prior to marketing. Swine producers enlisting in the PSCP do not need to have their pigs tested further at slaughter except for standard quality-assurance testing.

The objective of the PSCP is to market swine free of violative SMZ residues. The PSCP is a voluntary program for swine producers in which they agree to take specific management steps and testing procedures in their swine-production units to prevent SMZ residues. Swine producers in the program enjoy certain privileges, and there is no penalty for withdrawing from the program (Biehl 1988).

The program was designed (1) to assure the public that SMZ residue–free pork can be produced, (2) to obtain higher prices for swine marketed by participating producers, and (3) to eliminate the need for testing slaughter swine from participating producers for SMZ residues.

During the first year of the program eight Illinois swine producers and five veterinarians participated. Five of the producers used SMZ routinely; the other three did not use it routinely, but one of them resorted to it for therapeutic emergencies. During the producer approval process, two pigs tested on producers' farms were discovered to have violative SMZ residue levels. Both swine producers, with the assistance of their respective veterinarians, were able to make the necessary management changes to correct the residue problem.

During the course of the program, 7,032 pigs in 116 lots were marketed at three slaughter establishments. One animal at each of 69 of these lots was tested for SMZ residues by the FSIS at the receiving plants. All slaughter animals tested were found negative for SMZ residues.

To date only one of the three objectives has been attained; the swine producers, with the help of veterinarians, can assure that produced pork is free from violative SMZ residues. The other two goals, higher prices for slaughter pigs and eliminating the necessity for residue testing at slaughter, were not attained (Raef 1990).

Recently, FSIS has developed a Residue Violation Information System (RVIS), which is a nationwide, interagency computer information system designed to handle pertinent regulatory information related to residue violations in domestically slaughtered livestock. For the first time, both FSIS and FDA have the on-line ability to simultaneously trace back and link an individual or series of individuals involved in a residue problem (Blair 1988). The RVIS should provide an additional incentive for swine producers to voluntarily participate in a program such as the Illinois PSCP.

The dramatic reduction in swine SMZ violative levels due to the in-plant implementation of the sulfa-on-site (SOS) test has set the regulatory framework for both FSIS and FDA, relative to residue problems. Mandatory animal identification, in-plant/on-farm tests, and strict regulatory enforcement are three key ingredients in future residue activities.

Veterinary medicine plays a major role in the quantity, quality, and safety of the supply of feeds of animal origin, an essential part of public health. Animal breeding, nutrition, and health care for greater individual productivity; concentration and integration of animal production into large environmentally controlled units and increasingly the use of more by-products for feed; and the raising of livestock in marginal agricultural areas not suited to direct production of human foods all accentuate veterinary problems and require greater expertise. Drugs and biologics used in veterinary medicine have potent effects, both desired and adverse. Drugs and biologics must be used so that no residues harmful to the public health may be in edible products of animal origin, and the use of antimicrobials in animals must not result directly or indirectly in human infections (Beran 1986).

REFERENCES

Beran, G. W. 1986. Teaching public health in veterinary medical curriculums. In Practices in Veterinary Public Health and Preventive Medicine in the United States. Ed. G. T. Woods. Ames: Iowa State Univ Press, p. 75.

Biehl, L. G. 1988. Sulfamethazine producer self-certification pilot program. In Food Animal Professional Topics, vol. 14, no. 3, Urbana-Champaign: Cooperative Extension Service, Univ of Illinois, p. 1–3.

Blair, J. L. 1988. A residue violation information system that works. Proc 92d Annu Meet U.S. Anim Health Assoc. Little Rock, Arkansas, p. 324–337.

Kahrs, R. F. 1989. Food safety opportunities for veterinary medical education for the 21st century. Proc Vet Perspect Safety Foods Anim Origin Symp. Washington, D.C.: Am Vet Med Assoc, p. 51.

Leman, A. D., and Pullen, M. M. 1985. The clinician's impact on meat safety. J Vet Med Educ [Special Issue] 11(3):97–98.

McKean, J. D. 1989. Safe food from healthy swine. Proc Vet Perspect Safety Foods Anim Origin Symp. Washington, D.C.: Am Vet Med Assoc, p. 31.

National Research Council. 1985. Meat and Poultry Inspection: The Scientific Basis of the Nation's Program. Washington, D.C.: National Academy Press, 209 pp.

Pullen, M. M. 1989. Perspectives on the hazard analysis critical control point (HACCP) approach. Proc Vet Perspect Safety Foods Anim Origin Symp. Washington, D.C.: Am Vet Med Assoc, p. 43.

Raef, T. A. 1990. Pilot program produces residue-free pork. Regulatory front. J Am Vet Med Assoc 197(3): 307.

75 Obstetrics

L. J. Runnels

L. K. Clark

THE OBJECTIVE of manipulative and surgical swine obstetrics is to deliver a maximal number of viable pigs while preserving the strength and health of the sow so that she can effectively nurse and care for the live pigs and maintain her reproductive capacity. The broadest application of obstetrics includes complete management of the reproductive process from selection and development of animals for the breeding herd to breeding, gestation, parturition, lactation, and weaning — thus satisfying the demands of modern swine production to achieve maximal production for each breeding female maintained in the herd.

NORMAL PARTURITION. Knowledge of the normal process of parturition in swine is essential if the need for obstetrical assistance is to be recognized. Direct supervision of farrowing is desirable, but the amount of effort and time allotted must be compatible with the value returned. Thus, supervision time expended will vary among herds. Observations made at intervals of 30–60 minutes are necessary to optimize production. Too much supervision and manipulative intervention may lead to complications; therefore, good judgment must be exercised by both the farrowing manager and the veterinarian in making decisions as to the need for intervention.

Induction techniques are available to provide for more efficient management of parturition (First and Bose 1979; Cutler et al. 1981; Arthur et al. 1982; Dial 1984).

Preparturient Behavior. Prepartum sows exhibit conspicuous signs of the approach of parturition (Jones 1966a). Swelling of the vulval lips occurs about 4 days before parturition. The vaginal and vulval mucosa remains rather dry until shortly before the first birth when the passage of a little amniotic fluid moistens it. The mammary glands may remain flaccid until 3–4 hours of birth, but they usually become enlarged and sometimes edematous a few days before parturition (Jones 1966a; Diehl et al. 1974; Coggins et al. 1977). The distal extremities of the glands become cone shaped, turgid, and tense during the last 2 days before farrowing. Generally, a serous secretion is present 48 hours prepartum; once this secretion becomes milky, parturition occurs within 24 hours. When milk secretion becomes abundant, parturition commonly occurs within 6 hours.

Rectal temperature is not a reliable indicator of the time of farrowing, but postfarrowing body temperatures are higher than prefarrowing temperatures (King et al. 1972; Elmore et al. 1979). A general rise in respiratory rate from an average of 54 breaths/minute during the 24- to 12-hour period before parturition to an average of 91 breaths/minute at about 6 hours before parturition, with a gradual fall to 72 breaths/minute during the period just preceding the birth of the first pig, is a reliable indicator of impending parturition (Hendrix et al. 1978; Kelley and Curtis 1978). When considered together, behavioral changes are a very reliable indication of the onset of parturition (Jones 1966a). These usually begin at some point during the preceding 24 hours and consist of "bed making" and restlessness manifested by changes in position, either from side to side in recumbency or from recumbency to the standing position. Phases of activity are followed by short periods of resting until 60–15 minutes before birth of the first pig; then the sow becomes quieter and settles into lateral recumbency. Immediately after this phase, some straining will occur, and the hind legs may be drawn toward the abdomen. A small amount of slightly blood-stained, viscid fluid is passed from the vulva, often containing pellets of meconium, and the first pig is usually delivered within the next 15–20 minutes (Randall 1972).

Intrapartum Behavior. Piglets are usually delivered while the sow is in lateral recumbency, and most sows remain in this position for the duration of farrowing. Intermittent abdominal straining is common before the birth of the first pig, but is less so before the expulsion of the remaining pigs, although mild straining usually coincides with the moment of expulsion. Perhaps the most outstanding feature of parturition in the sow is the apparent ease with which fetuses are expelled (Jones 1966b). There is considerable variation in the time taken for delivery, ranging from 30 minutes to 10 hours and 30 minutes (Randall 1972). Mean duration of second-stage labor was 2 hours and 36 minutes in one study (Randall 1972) and 2 hours and 53 minutes in another (Jones 1966b). Intervals between individual births range from 1 minute to almost 4 hours; however, the average time between births is usually 15–16 minutes. Limited studies indicate that the type of housing and farrowing accommodations may influence duration of farrowing and viability of the litter (Foster 1982). The interval between the first and second piglet and between the next to last and last piglet is commonly longer than the interval between other piglets in the litter.

Presentation of Piglets. The percentage of piglets presented cranially is 55.4% and caudally is 44.6%, respectively. The dorsoventral position with the forelimbs extended caudally along the thorax is normal for cranial presentations. The dorsoventral position with hind legs extended caudally is normal for caudal presentations (Randall 1972). Others have made similar observations (Jones 1966b; Dziuk and Harmon 1969; Reimers et al. 1973).

Expulsion of the Fetal Membranes. The average time for expulsion of the fetal membranes has been reported as being 4 hours, with variations of 21 minutes to 12 hours and 30 minutes after birth of the last piglet (Jones 1966b). The passing of placenta is not a reliable indicator of completion of farrowing; portions of placenta are often passed during the farrowing period. Retained placenta is rare for the pig; if placenta is retained, it is an indication that at least one more pig is present in the reproductive tract.

DYSTOCIA. Dystocia occurred in 2.9% of 103 farrowings observed by Randall (1972) and 0.25% of 772 farrowings observed by Jones (1966b). Jackson (1976) observed that dystocia in which assistance was needed occurs in 0.25–1% of all farrowings. Among the purebreds, Welsh sows are particularly prone to dystocia, whereas Landrace sows seldom encounter difficulty (Jackson 1976). Generally, dystocia in swine represents only a small portion of the problems and potential losses in swine production.

Signs. Signs of dystocia are prolonged gestation (more than 116 days); anorexia; appearance of blood-tinged vulvar discharges and meconium without signs of straining; straining without delivery of one or more piglets; cessation of labor after previous straining and delivery of one or more piglets; and foul-smelling and discolored (brown, gray) vulval discharge, depression, weakness, and exhaustion after prolonged labor.

Causes

MATERNAL. Uterine inertia is one of the most common causes of dystocia in the sow (Arthur 1964). Jackson (1976) reported the incidence of

uterine inertia to be 37%. Primary uterine inertia (failure of induction of parturition) results from interactions between hormonal factors, nutritional insufficiency, illness of the sow, and sometimes heat exhaustion. The interactions are complex, and some of the mechanisms and intermediate factors through which changes occur have not been determined (First and Bose 1979). Secondary uterine inertia is the result of uterine and maternal exhaustion subsequent to prolonged labor as the result of fetal malpresentations and maternal obstructions. Idiopathic uterine inertia is described by Jackson (1976) as a cessation of farrowing for no apparent reason other than cessation of uterine contractions, but the causes are probably linked to those of primary inertia.

Once the cervix is dilated, uterine inertia in the sow can be treated by intramuscular administration of 20–40 units of oxytocin every 15–30 minutes. Overdosage of oxytocin may cause excessive contraction of smooth muscle followed by occasional vomiting and extreme uterine contraction, resulting in delay or cessation of parturition (Ladwig 1975). Oxytocin should be injected only after examination of the sow to determine that the cervix is dilated and mechanical obstruction is not present. Urging sows to their feet and forcing them to mild exercise for a short time outside the farrowing quarters is useful in the treatment of uterine inertia. Use of a parasympathomimetic drug such as 5 mg of neostigmine bromide to stimulate mild prolonged uterine contraction has been reported by Sprecher et al. (1975). Overheating, resulting from high environmental temperature and humidity, can be corrected by providing extra air movement, or mist or drip cooling systems over the sow. Manual delivery of one or more pigs may initiate uterine contraction after primary uterine inertia. Secondary uterine inertia nearly always requires manipulative delivery or cesarean section.

Uterine deviation occasionally occurs in the sow and can include such conditions as partial torsion or folding of the uterus just cranial to the pelvic brim or at the junction of the horns and body. It is observed almost exclusively in older sows carrying very large litters that drag the uterus ventrally below the brim of the pelvis. When pressure from straining is exerted, the uterus projects caudally beneath the pelvic brim, making progression into the birth canal impossible. Manipulative intervention is nearly always required in these cases and is usually possible in the large older sow with a large pelvic opening. The condition usually corrects itself after one or two pigs are manually delivered.

Varying degrees of obstruction of the birth canal can be caused by a distended bladder; constipation; persistent hymen; vulval hematoma; trauma and edema of the soft tissues of the birth canal due to repeated manipulative intervention;

vaginal prolapse; previous maternal pelvic bone fracture; small, underdeveloped, immature pelvis and birth canal; and by crowding of the birth canal by excessive pelvic and perineal fat.

A distended bladder results when a sow has been in labor and recumbent for extended periods. Relief can usually be effected by administering 20–40 USP units of oxytocin and by urging the sow to her feet and out of her farrowing quarters for 5–10 minutes. Emptying the bladder nearly always occurs, and the sow can be returned to her quarters to complete a normal farrowing. Catheterization may occasionally be required. This may be accomplished with a bovine catheter or a porcine plastic insemination rod with bent tip. Lubricate either instrument with K-Y jelly, locate the urethral orifice by palpation, and direct the instrument into the urethra and bladder, using a slight twisting motion if resistance is encountered.

Persistent hymen is corrected by manual dilation or by severing the hymen with scissors, thus allowing farrowing to proceed normally. Constipation is relieved by manually emptying the rectum after first softening the fecal material with mineral oil or a warm soapy enema.

Vulvar hematomas are common but rarely completely obstruct passage of the fetus. Hematomas that bleed excessively must be controlled by ligation of the bleeding vessel or by packing and suturing the vaginal wall (Railsback 1950; Ladwig 1975). Careful manual delivery of some pigs may be necessary to avoid further trauma to the hematoma.

Swelling, edema, and laceration of the soft tissues of the birth canal are due to rough and unskilled manipulative efforts. Occasionally, a fetal toe or canine tooth may inflict trauma on the tissues during passage through the birth canal. Accessible tears can be sutured. Rarely, the bladder may prolapse through a vaginal tear. Bladder prolapse is corrected by draining the bladder with a 14-gauge needle, replacement, and suturing of the laceration in the vaginal wall. Suitable local and systemic therapy should follow these procedures.

Vaginal prolapse is a serious complication if all or some of the piglets remain in the uterus. The prolapsed tissues are commonly traumatized and edematous, making manual delivery difficult or impossible. Cesarotomy may be the treatment of choice if the sow is in good condition and there is reasonable assurance that the pigs are still alive. Whether the pigs are delivered manually or by cesarotomy, the postpartum vaginal prolapse must be treated by debriding and replacing the exposed tissues, followed by vulval suturing and appropriate topical and parenteral antibiotic therapy.

All sows with major maternal reproductive problems should be culled after their pigs are weaned.

FETAL. Oversize fetus has been reported to be one of the more common causes of dystocia in the sow (Arthur 1964). Large fetuses are more likely to be present in small litters and gilt litters, and to be the first or last pigs farrowed.

Malpresentations of the fetus are involved in about 33.5% of all dystocias. Breech and simultaneous presentation of two or more piglets were the two principal malpresentations encountered by Jackson (1976). Transverse presentations were a cause of dystocia in two cases noted by Randall (1972).

Fetal anomalies such as hydrocephalus and conjoined twins can produce dystocia, although studies have shown that malformations of all types have a low incidence varying from 0.5 to 0.6% of all pigs born (Wrathall 1975).

Remedy. A preliminary vaginal examination is indicated when the normal pattern of farrowing is disrupted. Attention to cleanliness is important. A thorough washing of the sow's hind parts prior to entering the birth canal is required (Fig. 75.1). Fingernails must be cut short and hands and arms washed and lubricated. The vagina must also be lubricated. A cleansed plastic or rubber sleeve should be worn to reduce friction and contamination. If at all possible, the sow should be in lateral recumbency. The operator should use the hand that corresponds with the side the sow is lying on. The hand is cupped in the shape of a cone, and the lips of the vulva are carefully separated and the coned hand is inserted gently into the birth canal (Figs. 75.2, 75.3). Older sows seldom resist manipulation, but gilts are less amenable. After entering the vulva the hand passes into the vagina, which is confluent with the uterus, and the bony pelvis can be felt below and to the sides of the vagina. The hand can usually be passed through the pelvic opening of sows, but in some gilts this is impossible. The birth canal should be explored for evidence of trauma such as tears and bruises. Piglets encountered will fill the whole diameter of the birth canal, making determination of position relatively easy. If in cranial presentation, the head, lower jaw, or feet may be grasped. If in caudal presentation, the feet are grasped. A great amount of force is usually not necessary; gentle, steady traction is effective to accomplish delivery of most pigs.

Several instruments are available for use in dystocias. Familiarity and experience will dictate a choice of swine obstetrical instruments. Some instruments of simple design and proven effectiveness are the Knowles forceps, lamb and pig cable snare, and sharp or blunt hooks (Fig. 75.4). A very effective wire snare has been described by Railsback (1950). The cable snare is probably one of the most useful instruments for swine obstetrics because it can be used on live pigs without injuring them. If a nose or foot can be touched, the snare can be passed over these parts

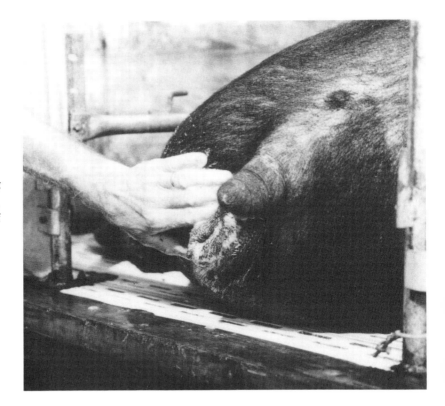

75.1. Thorough washing of the perineum is essential to decrease the possibilities for introduction of infection.

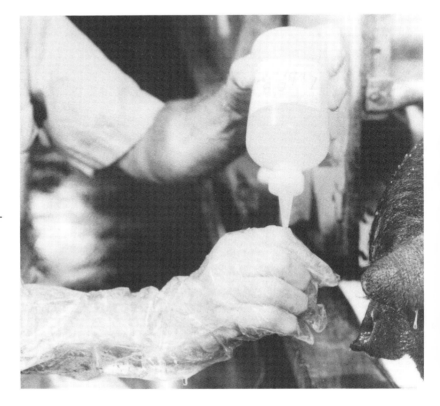

75.2. Lubrication of hands and arms reduces friction and irritation to delicate tissues of the birth canal during manipulation.

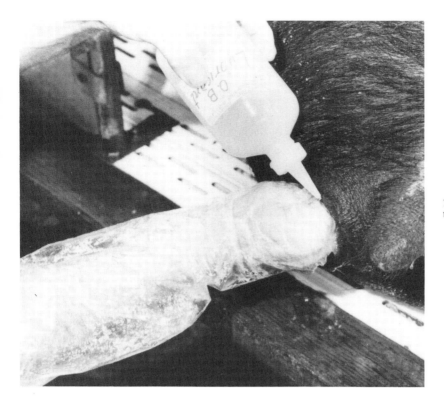

75.3. Gentle entry, with the hand coned.

and set in position for traction. Care must be taken not to lose the position of the snare on the fetus or to damage the part. Alternatively, the sharp or blunt hooks can be used on dead fetuses by placing one in each eye socket or by inserting one into the mouth with the hook directed dorsally and placed caudal to the hard palate. Either hold with the hooks can be lost with hard traction, especially in attempts to deliver fetuses undergoing autolysis. Knowles forceps can be used to grasp any part presented, but they are traumatic and must be used carefully to avoid destruction of parts grasped. Breech presentations are often the most difficult. If the fetus can be reached, the index finger is hooked under the hock of each hind leg. The legs are extended caudally and the fetus is delivered with mild traction. The cable snare can be used successfully to assist delivery of pigs in breech presentations by directing the loop ventrally over the brim of the pelvis and slid-

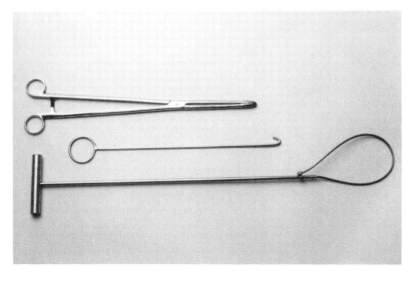

75.4. Useful swine obstetrical instruments: Knowles forceps (top), blunt hook (center), pig and lamb snare (bottom).

ing it over one or both hind legs. The legs are then extended for normal caudal delivery. In large sows, pigs can sometimes be delivered in the breech position by placing the snare around the hind parts of the fetus just cranial to the wings of the ilium.

Immediately after delivery, live pigs must have the membranes and mucus cleared from the air passages. Gentle shaking and massaging of the piglet in head-down position is helpful to drain fluids from the mouth and nose and to stimulate respiration. Routine ligation of the navel cord is not necessary, but may be done if there is excessive hemorrhage. Disinfection of the cord is a generally accepted practice to prevent entry of infection.

Once the dystocia is relieved, the birth canal should be reexamined for additional fetuses, and all easily accessible fetuses should be delivered. It is impossible to determine with certainty that parturition has been completed because the greater part of the horns of the uterus are not accessible by vaginal examination. A reasonable judgment can be made, however, based on visual appraisal of the distention of the sow's abdomen, the number of piglets previously delivered, the quantity of placenta passed, and the character of the vaginal mucus. Primary retention of the placenta is rare in the sow. If placenta is observed at the vulval opening, it must be assumed that at least one piglet remains in the uterus. Sows that have had manual intervention of farrowing should be injected with oxytocin and antibiotic at completion, and observed closely for further problems.

CESAREAN SECTION. Indications for cesarean operation in the sow are primary inertia; secondary inertia; juvenile or damaged pelvis; oversize fetuses; fetal monsters; injured or swollen birth canal; emphysematous fetuses; vaginal, cervical, uterine, rectal, or bladder prolapse; obese gilts; and uterine torsion. The frequency of indication for cesarotomy may be greater for an obstetrician with large hands, which limit the possibilities for efficient application of manipulation and traction (Arthur 1964; Frank 1964; Bouters and Vandeplassche 1975). The operation is most advantageously performed on sows that are not suffering from exhaustion, toxemia, and shock, and with the expectation that a majority of the piglets will be delivered alive. Although there is no data on risk of death from cesarotomy, the authors would not recommend this procedure for delivery of emphysematous fetuses.

Cesarean section can be performed in most modern farrowing facilities with only minor adjustments. The sow can be transported to a surgery if the farm facilities are not satisfactory, but generally it is better to avoid the additional stress and time required for transport.

The anesthesia used should suit the preference and experience of the surgeon and the conditions of surgery. Suggested procedures usually include combinations of tranquillizers and local infiltration along the line of incision, epidural anesthesia, general anesthesia employing barbiturates intravenously, or gas anesthesia. A procedure that has been most useful is epidural anesthesia (Getty 1963; Runnels 1974). It is inexpensive, requires minimal equipment, needs no monitoring, and causes no depression of sow or fetuses. Procaine or lidocaine (2%) is administered in amounts varying from 8 to 20 ml depending on the condition, size, and temperament of the sow. The lower dosage should be used for sows suffering from shock and exhaustion. For additional restraint, thiamylal may be given in 5% or 10% solution in the marginal vein of the ear, especially after the surgical delivery of all live pigs. A dose of 6.6–11 mg/kg, depending on sow condition, will give satisfactory results. Another quite satisfactory procedure for restraint following epidural anesthesia is the administration of 1.1 mg/kg ketamine and 1.1 mg/kg xylazine via the marginal vein of the ear immediately prior to surgery. Live piglets are only slightly depressed, and it has been used safely in a number of sows. Epidural anesthesia is maintained as far cranially as the umbilicus, rendering the hindquarters immobile. All legs and the snout must be tied down to prevent excessive movement that would interfere with surgery. In toxic animals, general anesthesia should be used with reduced dosage and caution, if used at all. Frank (1964) states that if the sow is suffering from toxemia and shock, only a local infiltration anesthesia should be used. If fetuses are alive, general anesthesia usually causes an undesirable depression of the piglets at delivery.

Standard aseptic preoperative preparation is used commensurate with the conditions under which the surgery is to be performed. Operative procedures should be performed in a manner that provides the least opportunity for contamination.

Several different operative sites have been used. A vertical incision starting just below the transverse processes of the lumbar vertebrae and halfway between the last rib and the external angle of the ilium and extending ventrally a distance of 15–20 cm is satisfactory but has some disadvantages in presenting considerable fat in the incision along with the necessity for incising through heavy muscle tissue. A ventral incision on the linea alba has disadvantages that require the sow to be placed on her back; additionally, there is interference from mammary gland tissue, possibility of incising mammary tissue with subsequent contamination of the surgical site, and irritation from the postoperative nursing of piglets. The preferred site allows the sow to be placed in lateral recumbency on either side; the incision is made 7.5–10 cm dorsal and parallel to the base of the mammary glands, extending 20–25 cm cranially from just caudal and ventral to the cranial part of the fold of the flank. A site somewhat lower, extending below and caudal to the fold of the flank, is said to offer excellent accessibility. The preferred site requires that the uppermost leg be tied back (Mather 1966). The incision is made through the skin, subcutaneous tissues, and muscle layers down to the peritoneum, which is usually overlaid with fat. Some of the branches of the subcutaneous abdominal vein may require ligation before entry into the abdominal cavity. After hemostasis is established, the peritoneum is incised, using care not to damage the distended uterus. The incision opening should be just large enough to allow the uterus to be brought to the outside with minimal traction. Care needs to be exercised to prevent transverse tearing, especially in uteruses that are friable or distended with a large number of fetuses.

A sterile plastic or rubberized sheet is fastened just below the incision. The abdominal cavity is examined and the location of piglets in one or both horns is determined. The most accessible portion of the horn containing fetuses is brought through the incision and allowed to lie on the sterile sheet. If the horn contains a large number of fetuses and it is obvious that the contralateral horn is similarly filled, it is best to attempt to make the incision in the uterus over a fetus at a midpoint between the ovarian end and the bifurcation. Pigs can be delivered from both directions with a minimum of manipulation. The incision in the uterus must be of sufficient length to allow easy delivery of the pigs, and is made on the side of the uterus opposite the attachment of the broad ligament, avoiding as much of the vascular supply as possible. Usually, some fetuses must be delivered by entering the lumen of the uterus, grasping the accessible fetus, and withdrawing it with gentle traction. Occasionally, multiple incisions are indicated because fetuses cannot be moved to one incision site due to lack of intrauterine fluid and uterine contraction. No attempt is made to remove the placenta unless it comes away easily.

After all pigs are delivered from a horn, the external surface is rinsed with warm saline and all but the incision site is replaced in the abdominal cavity. The incision is sutured with No. 1 or 2 chromic catgut with a continuous right-angle Cushing pattern. Just prior to final closure of the uterine incision, antibiotic boluses or a solution of choice is placed in the uterine lumen, especially if decomposition of the fetuses has occurred. The sutured horn is then replaced and the contralateral horn is withdrawn and the procedure is repeated.

If the initial examination reveals only a few fetuses in each horn, an incision may be made through the uterine wall near the bifurcation, thus delivering all pigs from both horns through one incision. Care must be exercised in locating this incision because tearing can easily occur if it becomes necessary to enter the uterine lumen to extract pigs from the ovarian end. A torn incision will usually bleed profusely and will present difficulties in suturing. Before closure of the final uterine incision, both horns and the body of the uterus must be examined for any fetuses that might have been overlooked.

The abdominal incision is closed in standard fashion using appropriate suture material, placing one layer in the peritoneum and aponeurosis of the transverse abdominal and internal oblique muscles and another layer in the external oblique muscles. The skin incision is closed with a nonabsorbable suture that is removed in 10 days. As an alternative, a subcuticular suture may be placed for skin closure using appropriate absorbable suture material, thus eliminating the need for suture removal.

Postoperatively, an injection of oxytocin is given to enhance uterine contraction; in cases in which there was a contaminating environment or decomposed pigs, an antibiotic is administered parenterally for 3–5 days.

The time required for cesarotomy will depend on the availability of assistance. In most field circumstances the surgeon has minimal help other than the producer or the farrowing barn manager and must perform preoperative, operative, and postoperative tasks as well as administering the anesthesia, thus extending total operating time.

For further information see Pond and Houpt (1978) and Leman and Dziuk (1975).

REFERENCES

ARTHUR, G. H. 1964. Cesarean section in the sow. In Wright's Veterinary Obstetrics, 3d ed. Baltimore: Williams & Wilkins, pp. 301–304.

ARTHUR, G. H.; NOAKES, D. E.; AND PEARSON, H. 1982. Pregnancy and parturition: Dystocia and other parturition problems. In Veterinary Reproduction and Obstetrics. London: Baillière Tindall, p. 314.

BOUTERS, R., AND VANDEPLASSCHE, M. 1975. Committee for the control of infertility at Ghent, Belgium. Diergeneeskd Tijdschr 44(2):56–72.

COGGINS, E. G.; VAN HORN, D.; AND FIRST, N. L. 1977. Influence of prostaglandin F2 alpha, dexamethasone, progesterone and induced CL on porcine parturition. J Anim Sci 46:754.

CUTLER, R.; HURTGEN, J. P.; AND LEMAN, A. D. 1981. Reproductive system. In Diseases of Swine, 5th ed. Ed. A. D. Leman, R. D. Glock, W. L. Mengeling, R. H. C. Penny, E. Scholl, and B. Straw. Ames: Iowa State Univ Press, p. 117.

DIAL, G. D. 1984. Clinical applications of prostaglandins in swine. J Am Vet Med Assoc 185:1523–1530.

DIEHL, J. R.; GODKE, R. A.; KILLIAN, D. B.; AND DAY, B. N. 1974. Induction of parturition in swine with prostaglandin F2 alpha. J Anim Sci 38:1229.

DZIUK, P. J., AND HARMON, B. G. 1969. Succession of fetuses at parturition in the pig. Am J Vet Res 30:419–421.

ELMORE, R. G.; MARTIN, C. E.; RILEY, J. L.; AND LITTLEDIKE, T. 1979. Body temperatures of farrowing swine. J Am Vet Med Assoc 174:620–622.

FIRST, N. L., AND BOSE, M. J. 1979. Proposed mechanisms controlling parturition and the induction of parturition in swine. J Anim Sci 48(6):1407–1421.

FOSTER, J. 1982. Farrowing: More freedom, fewer

problems? Pig Farming (Oct):24–27.

FRANK, E. R. 1964. Cesarean section in the sow. In Veterinary Surgery, 7th ed. Minneapolis: Burgess, p. 243.

GETTY, R. 1963. Epidural anesthesia in the hog—its technique and applications. Proc 100th Annu Meet Am Vet Med Assoc, pp. 88–98.

HENDRIX, W. F.; KELLEY, K. W.; GASKINS, C. T.; AND BENDEL, R. B. 1978. Changes in respiratory rate and rectal temperature of swine near parturition. J Anim Sci 47:188–191.

JACKSON, P. 1976. When things go wrong at farrowing. Pig Farming (Jan):43–47.

JONES, J. E. T. 1966a. Observations on parturition in the sow. The prepartum phase. Br Vet J 122:420–426.

———. 1966b. Observations on parturition in the sow. The parturient and post-parturient phases. Br Vet J 122:471–478.

KELLEY, K. W., AND CURTIS, S. E. 1978. Effects of heat stress on rectal temperature, respiratory rate and activity rates in prepartal sows and gilts. J Anim Sci 46:356.

KING, G. J.; WILLOUGHBY, R. A.; AND HACKER, R. R. 1972. Fluctuations in rectal temperature of swine at parturition. Can Vet J 13:72.

LADWIG, V. D. 1975. Surgical procedure to control hemorrhage of the porcine vulva. J Am Vet Med Assoc 166:598–599.

LEMAN, A. D., AND DZIUK, P. J. 1975. Reproductive efficiency and artificial insemination. In Diseases of Swine, 4th ed. Ed. H. W. Dunne and A. D. Leman. Ames: Iowa State Univ Press, pp. 911–912.

MATHER, C. E. 1966. Lower flank incision for swine cesarean. Vet Med 61:890–891.

POND, W. G., AND HOUPT, K. A. 1978. The Biology of the Pig. Ithaca, N.Y.: Cornell Univ Press, pp. 73, 155.

RAILSBACK, L. T. 1950. Dystocia in the sow. J Am Vet Med Assoc (Jan):27–30.

RANDALL, G. C. B. 1972. Observations on parturition in the sow. Vet Rec 90:178–186.

RIEMERS, T. J.; DZIUK, P. J.; BAHR, J.; SPRECHER, D. J.; WEBEL, S. K.; AND HARMON, B. G. 1973. Transuterine embryonal migration in sheep, anterio-posterior orientation of pig and sheep fetuses and presentations of piglets at birth. J Anim Sci 37:1212–1217.

RUNNELS, L. J. 1974. Epidural anesthesia in swine. Am Assoc Swine Pract Newsl 1 (9).

SPRECHER, D. J.; LEMAN, A. D.; AND CARLISLE, S. 1975. Effects of parasympathomimetics on porcine stillbirth. J Am Vet Med Assoc 36:1331–1332.

WRATHALL, A. E. 1975. Reproductive disorders in pigs. Commonw Bur Anim Health, Rev Ser 11, Farnham Royal, England, pp. 79–80, 216–217.

76 Chemical Restraint and Anesthesia

S. R. Bolin

L. J. Runnels

D. P. Bane

CHEMICAL RESTRAINT. The primary objectives of chemical restraint are to reduce apprehension and eliminate struggling. Economic influences dictate that most minor surgical procedures in swine (castration, ear notching, teeth clipping, tail docking) be conducted without anesthetizing animals. Done quickly and skillfully in young pigs by trained and experienced personnel, these procedures are less traumatic without an anesthetic than with one. When procedures are to be performed on older animals, anesthesia should be considered. Tranquillizers, sedative-analgesics, hypnotics, dissociative anesthetics, and anesthetic steroids are the pharmacologic classifications for the agents used to accomplish this. Relatively few anesthetic and anesthetic-related agents are currently approved for use in swine.

Preanesthetic Medications. Preanesthetic agents facilitate the induction of anesthesia, reduce the amount of general anesthetic needed, and frequently promote a smooth recovery following anesthesia. Table 76.1 lists some of these drugs by generic name, trade name, and dosage. Atropine sulfate, a parasympatholytic agent, is given to decrease saliva production and alleviate bradycardia. When inhalation anesthesia is to be used, atropine should be given intramuscularly (IM) 10–20 minutes prior to induction.

The phenothiazine derivative tranquillizers (chlorpromazine, promazine, triflupromazine, acepromazine, and propiopromazine) decrease spontaneous motor activity and produce sedation. The results obtained from using these drugs in swine are inconsistent. Tranquillizers should be given under circumstances that cause the least possible distress to the animal. The animal should be in a quiet place and left undisturbed until maximal drug response occurs. Stimulation of the animal prior to this time will produce less than a desirable response (Thurmon and Benson 1986). Chlorpromazine will sedate swine when given intravenously (IV), but general anesthesia or excitement may also occur (Ritchie 1957). Sedation is produced 5–10 minutes after administration, with the peak effect occurring in 10–20 minutes. An increased respiratory rate lasting about 15 minutes occurs immediately following IV administration of chlorpromazine. The sedation produced following IM administration is less reliable; 30–45 minutes are required before maximum effect is obtained. Promazine and acepromazine are routinely used for nervous sows during parturition; however, it is important to note that all tranquillizers cross the placenta, causing fetal depression. Phenothiazine tranquillizers should be avoided in ill or debilitated animals because of their tendency to complicate such existing conditions as hypovolemia, anemia, hypothermia, shock, and hepatic dysfunction (Thurmon and Benson 1986). Acepromazine (0.39 mg/kg IM) followed in 30 minutes by ketamine (15 mg/kg IM) has been an effective combination for immobilization of miniature swine (Gray et al. 1978). This combination will provide 20 minutes of immobilization.

Azaperone and droperidol are neuroleptic agents of the butyrophenone group used to sedate swine and are of considerable value as preanesthetics. Azaperone has a dose-dependent range of effects and is therefore indicated for use in a variety of circumstances (prevention of aggressiveness, treatment of stress, savaging of newborn pigs by sows, and minor surgical procedures). The first effects of IM administration of 2.2 mg/kg in young feeder pigs are ataxia and recumbency after 4–5 minutes (Thurmon and Benson 1986); fighting after intermingling is then reduced. At a higher dose (4–8 mg/kg IM) azaperone will produce sedation sufficient for minor surgical procedures (Anderson 1977), but the sedation is without analgesia; therefore, local anesthesia is indicated. Maximum sedation occurs after 5–15 minutes, and the animal should be left undisturbed until the full effect is obtained. Excessive salivation, a drop in body temperature (Greene 1979), sensitivity to noise, and a slight decrease in blood pressure (Clarke 1969) occur in pigs given azaperone, which has been shown to be compatible with organophosphate anthelmintics and insecticides (Porter and Slussor 1984).

The hypnotic agent metomidate is combined with azaperone to produce a light plane of surgi-

933

Table 76.1. Preanesthetic medications for swine

Generic Name	Trade Name (Manufacturer)	Dose (mg/kg) IV	IM	References
Atropine sulfate	Atropine sulfate (Tech America Group, Inc., Elswood, KS 66024)	NA	0.04	Thurmon and Benson (1986)
Chlorpromazine hydrochloride	Thorazine (Pitman-Moore, Inc., Mundelein, IL 60060)	0.55–3.3	2.0–4.0	Ritchie (1957); Vaughn (1961); Regan and Gillis (1975)
Promazine hydrochloride	Sparine (Wyeth Laboratories, Division of American Home Products Corp., Philadelphia, PA 19101)	0.44–1.0	0.44–1.0	Thurmon and Benson (1986)
Triflupromazine hydrochloride	Vetame (E. R. Squibb and Sons, Inc., Princeton, NJ 08540)	0.88	1.3	Thurmon and Benson (1986)
Acepromazine maleate	Acepromazine maleate injectable (Ayerst Laboratories, Divison of American Home Products Corp., New York, NY 10017)	NA	0.03–0.1	Thurmon and Benson (1986)
Propiopromazine hydrochloride	Tranvet (Diamond Laboratories, Inc., Des Moines, IA 50304)	0.55–1.0	0.55–1.0	Lumb and Jones (1973)
Ethyl isobutrazine	Diquel (Jensen-Salsbery Laboratories, Division of Richardson-Merell, Inc., Kansas City, MO 64141)	1.25	2.2–4.4	Lumb and Jones (1973)
Azaperone	Stresnil (Pitman-Moore, Inc., Mundelein, IL 60060)	NA	4.0–8.0 (small swine) 2.0 (large swine)	Ferguson (1971); Callear and VanGestel (1973)
Diazepam	Valium (Hoffman-LaRoche, Inc., Nutley, NJ 07110)	NA	5.5–8.5	Regan and Gillis (1975)
Chlorprothixene	Taractan (Hoffman-LaRoche, Inc., Nutley, NJ 07110)	0.3–1.0	NA	Jones (1972)
Fetanyl citrate and droperidol	Innovar-Vet (Pitman-Moore, Inc., Mundelein, IL 60060)	NA	1 ml/12–25 kg body weight	Thurmon and Benson (1986)

Note: Read package insert for approval of use in food-producing animals and for slaughter withdrawal times. NA = not appropriate.

cal anesthesia. Azaperone is given first at a dose of 2 mg/kg IM. This is followed immediately with 10–15 mg/kg of metomidate intraperitoneally (IP) or alternatively at 2.5–5 mg/kg IV, 10–20 minutes after injecting the azaperone (Jones 1972; Callear and VanGestel 1973). The 5-mg/kg level of metomidate given IV following azaperone will allow endotracheal intubation (Jones 1972). A decrease in cardiac and pulmonary function occurs with the use of azaperone and metomidate; but this is insignificant when compared to the decrease caused by barbiturate or inhalant anesthetics (Orr et al. 1976).

Droperidol can be combined with the synthetic opioid fentanyl to produce sedation. The droperidol-fentanyl combination (Innovar) is used as a preanesthetic for halothane general anesthesia (DeYoung et al. 1970; Piermattei and Swan 1970). The recommended dose for Innovar in swine is 1

ml/14 kg IM; however, in miniature swine, Innovar may cause central nervous stimulation instead of sedation (Regan and Gillis 1975). A combination of 0.05 mg/kg atropine sulfate IM and 1 ml/13.7 kg Innovar IM, followed in 10 minutes by 11 mg/kg ketamine hydrochloride IM, and 3% pentobarbital solution IV produced a safe, reliable surgical anesthesia of 45 minutes' duration (Bauck 1984).

Cantor et al. (1981) compared and evaluated four short-acting anesthetic combinations: (1) acepromazine maleate, 0.5 mg/kg IM, followed in 20 minutes with a 3% solution of sodium thiamylal, 11 mg/kg IV; (2) Innovar, 1 ml/13.6 kg IM, followed in 10–15 minutes with ketamine, 11 mg/kg IM; (3) acepromazine, 0.5 mg/kg IM, followed in 30 minutes with ketamine, 15 mg/kg IM; and (4) xylazine, 0.2 mg/kg IM, followed in 10 minutes with ketamine, 11 mg/kg IM. The Innovar/ketamine combination provided a statistically significant longer time until pigs responded to toe-pinch stimulus. The acepromazine/sodium thiamylal combination provided a significantly longer period of muscle relaxation. Pigs given xylazine/ketamine and acepromazine/ketamine exhibited spontaneous, sharp, involuntary movements during anesthesia. Pigs given Innovar/ketamine exhibited slow, smooth movements.

Chloral hydrate has been given IP in pigs for sedation and general anesthesia at a dose of 4–6 ml of a 5% solution/kg body weight (Thurmon and Benson 1986). The incidence of peritonitis following IP chloral hydrate administration appears to be high; therefore, this route cannot be recommended. Oral administration of chloral hydrate by stomach tube will produce successful anesthesia about 80% of the time in 20–30 minutes, following administration of a dose of 13 g/50 kg (Bemis et al. 1924). Chloral hydrate is seldom used because many superior agents are available.

GENERAL ANESTHESIA. Injectable anesthetic agents are commonly used to induce general anesthesia in older swine when surgical procedures are to be performed that require immobilization, muscle relaxation, and good analgesia. Feed should be removed 24–36 hours before induction of general anesthesia in swine. Failure to do so may result in vomition or severe gaseous gastrointestinal distension, which may interfere with ventilation and venous return, predisposing the animal to acute cardiovascular failure. Water should be made available until 2 hours before anesthesia as a precaution against sodium chloride toxicity. Pretreatment of the animal with atropine will control salivation and bronchiolar secretions. Barbiturates, thiobarbiturates, cyclohexylamines, and various xylazine combinations have been ef-

fectively used for general anesthesia in swine (Table 76.2); IV, IM, and IP routes of administration may be used depending on the characteristics of the drug used. The most accessible veins for IV injections are the anterior vena cava and auricular veins (Figs. 76.1, 76.2) (Hall and Clarke 1983).

Injectable Anesthetic Agents. Pentobarbital will provide 20–30 minutes of relatively safe anesthesia in adult swine (Thurmon and Benson 1986). Supplemental injections to prolong anesthesia are not recommended because of respiratory suppression and increased likelihood of apnea. Analgesia and muscle relaxation are poor, except in deep planes of anesthesia. Recovery is prolonged (60–90 minutes) and requires close patient surveillance if satisfactory results are to be achieved.

Intratesticular injections of pentobarbital can be used to induce anesthesia for castration of mature boars. The site for injection is below the tail of the epididymis in the upper third of the testicle. A 4-cm needle is directed into the testicle at an angle of 30° above horizontal. When this method is used, a 30% solution of pentobarbital is given at the rate of 1 ml/7 kg, dividing the dose between the testicles and not exceeding 20 ml each (Henry 1968). The castration should be completed immediately once the boar becomes recumbent and sensation is lost to the scrotum. This is necessary to prevent a barbiturate overdose from continued absorption of pentobarbital from the testicles. Pentobarbital can also be given IM as a 3% solution to sedate swine (Benson and Thurmon 1979); the dose given is 2.2–6.6 mg/kg. IP injections of pentobarbital are unreliable (Kernkamp 1939) and should only be used as a last resort.

Thiobarbiturates (thiopental sodium, thiamylal

Table 76.2. Injectable anesthetic agents for swine

Generic Name	Trade Name (Manufacturer)	Dose (mg/kg)		References
		IV	IM	
Pentobarbital sodium	Pentobarbital	15–30	NA	Thurmon and Benson (1986)
Thiopental sodium	Penthothal (Abbott Laboratories, North Chicago, IL 60064)	10–20	NA	Thurmon and Benson (1986)
Thiamylal sodium	Surital (Parke-Davis and Company, Detroit, MI 48232)	6–18	NA	Thurmon and Benson (1986)
Ketamine hydrochloride	Ketaset (Bristol Laboratories, Division of Bristol-Myers Co., Syracuse, NY 13201	2–4	11–20	Thurmon and Benson (1986); Thurmon et al. (1972)
Tiletamine and zolazapam	Telazol (A. H. Robins Co., Richmond, VA 23261	2.0	4.4–6.0	Thurmon et al. (1988)
Alphaxalone and alphadolone	Saffan (Glaxo Laboratories, Greenford, Middlesex, England)	4–6	6–8	Hall and Clarke (1983); Cox et al. (1975)
Xylazine hydrochloride	Rompun (Haver-Diamond Scientific, Mobay Corp., Shawnee, KS 66201)	1–2	0.2–2.2	Thurmon et al. (1986, 1988); Bolin and Runnels (1979, unpublished data)

Note: Read package insert for approval of use in food-producing animals and for slaughter withdrawal times. NA = not appropriate.

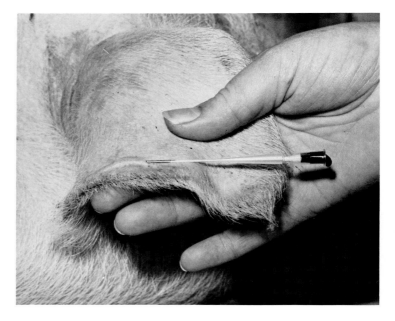

76.1. Intravenous anesthesia can be established and maintained by insertion of a catheter in the auricular vein, which is usually located along the caudal margin of the ear. Vigorous massage followed by placement of a rubber band around the base of the ear results in distension of the vein for easier visualization and needle insertion.

sodium) are used more extensively in swine, primarily as induction agents when inhalation anesthetics are to be used to maintain anesthesia. These drugs should be administered only until the desired effect is achieved and should not be given in set dosages. Extravascular injection of thiobarbiturates produces severe phlebitis, which may lead to ear necrosis and sloughing; therefore, dilute concentrations (5% or less) of these drugs are recommended. Surgical anesthesia from initial injection of appropriate doses will last for 10–15 minutes, with recovery requiring approximately 1 hour (Thurmon and Benson 1986). Adequate time for tracheal intubation is usually available. Extending anesthesia time with supplemental injections of thiobarbiturates may result in apnea and is not recommended.

Ketamine, a nonbarbiturate anesthetic, induces a peculiar state of unconsciousness often referred to as "cataleptoid" or dissociative anesthesia. This anesthetic state differs markedly from that induced by barbiturates. Endotracheal intubation is difficult because protective reflexes (cough, swallowing, etc.) remain intact to a degree. Somatic analgesia is profound, but visceral analgesia is poor. Patient movement during anesthesia is common and does not necessarily indicate pain perception. Immobilization following IM injection occurs in 3–5 minutes. To increase the degree of analgesia and prolong the duration of surgical anesthesia, small increments (2–4 mg/kg) may be given intravenously (Thurmon and Benson 1986). Injection of 2% lidocaine at the surgical site can be used to enhance analgesia. Intratesticular (3–5

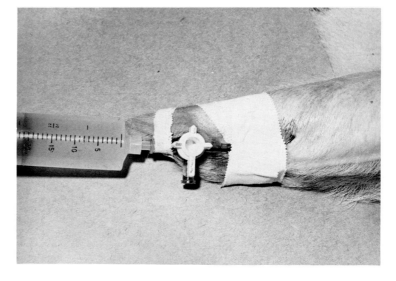

76.2. A three-way valve has been attached to a catheter placed in an auricular vein. This allows the anesthetist to administer fluids or inject additional anesthetic solution without having to disturb the catheter. The catheter and valve are held in place with strips of adhesive tape wrapped around the ear.

mg/kg) injection of ketamine has been used to immobilize large boars for castration (Thurmon and Benson 1986). A ketamine-xylazine combination, each dosed at 2.2 mg/kg IV, will produce anesthesia in 2–3 minutes sufficient for minor surgery or endotracheal intubation (Bolin and Runnels 1979, unpublished data).

Induction and maintenance of surgical anesthesia in mature swine has been obtained with a combination of glyceryl guaiacolate (a 5% solution in 5% dextrose and water) containing 1 mg/ml of ketamine and 1 mg/ml of xylazine (Thurmon et al. 1986). This mixture is initially given rapidly IV at a dose of 0.5–1.0 ml/kg to induce anesthesia. Thereafter, the infusion is continued at a rate of 2 ml/kg/hour. The combination of drugs has been used to maintain surgical anesthesia for 2.5 hours and has produced profound muscle relaxation and analgesia. Recovery has been rapid (30–40 minutes) once infusion is discontinued.

A combination of ketamine (2 mg/kg), xylazine (2 mg/kg), and oxymorphone (0.075 mg/kg) mixed in the same syringe and given IV has been used to induce and maintain surgical anesthesia (Breese and Dodman 1984). IM administration required that the dose of each drug be doubled.

Tiletamine, an anesthetic agent similar to ketamine, has been combined with zolazepam and xylazine to produce effective anesthesia in swine (Thurmon et al. 1988). This mixture (2–6 mg/kg tiletamine-zolazepam with 1.1–2.2 mg/kg xylazine) has been used both IM and IV. Recumbency occurred in 1–2 minutes following administration, anesthesia was maintained for 30–60 minutes, and recovery occurred in approximately 100 minutes following injection of this combination.

The semisynthetic opiate derivative etorphine, in combination with acetylpromazine, is very effective for immobilization of swine. This combination (Immobilon) is dosed at 0.5–1.0 ml/45 kg IM. Lateral recumbency is produced about 5 minutes after administration (Cox et al. 1973). Analgesia accompanies sedation, allowing minor surgical procedures to be performed without additional anesthetics. Cardiopulmonary depression, muscular rigidity, and hind leg tremors are frequently encountered side effects; therefore, it is recommended that pigs given Immobilon not be left unattended (Greene 1979). Diprenorphine and nalorphine are antagonists for etorphine and can be given to reverse the untoward side effects.

Alphaxalone and alphadolone are pregnanediones that are combined to form an anesthetic steroid preparation (Saffan) available in the United Kingdom. When given at 6–8 mg/kg IM, sedation is produced within 10 minutes; if given at 2–3 mg/kg IV, a loss of consciousness occurs within 10–20 seconds (Cox et al. 1975). The anesthesia obtained is of short duration, with the peak effect lasting 4–10 minutes; however, it is possible to prolong the duration by administering further increments of Saffan at 10-minute intervals (Greene

1979). Saffan should not be used with barbiturates, and a large volume of the mixture is needed to attain the recommended dose in swine heavier than 10 kg.

Inhalation Anesthesia. The use of inhalation agents is the safest and most satisfactory means of maintaining general anesthesia in swine (Thurmon and Benson 1986). Although equipment cost, the economic value of the average animal, and the inconvenience of transporting equipment to the field are major disadvantages of the use of inhalation anesthesia in swine, it should be emphasized that there is no satisfactory substitute for inhalation anesthesia when valuable animals require general anesthesia for major surgical procedures.

Inhalation anesthesia is usually administered to small pigs by open or semiopen methods; however, in larger swine, the semiclosed and closed systems are preferred. Inhalant anesthetics are delivered to larger swine through an endotracheal tube, nose tubes, or with a face mask. Small animal endotracheal tubes of 5–12 mm outside diameter are used for nose tubes. These are lubricated and inserted about 4–5 cm into the nares. They are held in place with the aid of a 4-cm-wide strip of rubber tied securely around the soft tip of the snout (Fig. 76.3). Face masks are simply applied to the snout and, if necessary, kept in place with adhesive tape (Fig. 76.4). Endotracheal intubation is slightly more complicated (Hall and Clarke 1983).

The facial, pharyngeal, and laryngeal structure of swine makes endotracheal intubation more challenging than in other species. It is difficult to open the jaws wide enough for good laryngeal exposure, and there is considerable distance from the oral opening to the larynx, especially in adult swine. Additional problems encountered are the narrow lateral boundaries of the throat and a long, mobile, narrow larynx with the arch of the cricoid cartilage set at an oblique angle to the trachea. Finally, laryngeal spasms occur frequently and are easily induced. Despite these problems, the use of proper equipment and adequate preintubation sedation and relaxation will allow efficient and successful endotracheal intubation in all sizes of swine.

A laryngoscope and blades of different lengths are needed. For mature swine, the blade length must be at least 250 mm. Cuffed endotracheal tube sizes should range from 5 to 20 mm outside diameter, with lengths from 25 to 50 cm. A malleable metal rod stylet, with the first 5 cm bent at a 30° angle, is required for placement inside the endotracheal tube. A length of gauze or small rope for spreading the jaws and a small wooden block to be placed between the teeth to prevent mouth closure must be available.

After suitable preinduction medication, the pig is placed in ventral recumbency, the upper and lower jaws are held open, and the tongue is

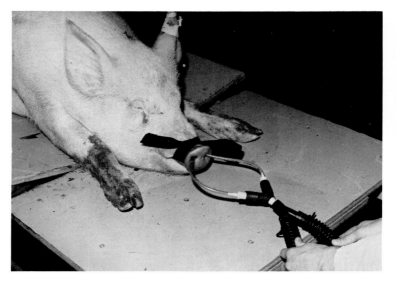

76.3. Nose tubes are inserted with tips directed medially toward the septum, then gently pushed 4–5 cm into the nostril. Note that the inflatable cuffs have been removed from the tubes and that a Y piece is needed to connect the nose tubes to the anesthetic machine. Basal anesthesia is required for insertion of nose tubes in swine.

grasped and pulled forward. A topical anesthetic is sprayed over the larynx. The laryngoscope is inserted, the soft palate is elevated, and then the epiglottis is depressed. The laryngeal opening is visualized and the endotracheal tube, with stylet extending slightly beyond the tip, is placed into the laryngeal opening. The stylet acts as a guide for the endotracheal tube (Fig. 76.5). The lubricated endotracheal tube is then pushed over the tip of the stylet and, with a twisting motion, is passed through the larynx into the trachea (Fig. 76.6). If the endotracheal tube cannot be passed, a smaller size is selected and the procedure repeated. The cuff is then inflated. Proper placement of the endotracheal tube in the trachea (it should not be in the esophagus) is confirmed by passage of expired air through the tube.

Inhalant Anesthetic Agents. Chloroform is a nonflammable, volatile anesthetic that is economical and very potent. It has largely been replaced by newer and safer inhalant anesthetics and is seldom used in swine. Induction of anesthesia with chloroform is rapid and does not require additional chemical agents. However, chloroform is directly toxic to the heart and causes central necrosis and fatty degeneration of the liver lobules. Because chloroform is so potent and relatively toxic, its use should probably be restricted to short periods of anesthesia not exceeding 30 minutes, and if possible, it should be used in combination with another agent such as nitrous oxide, which will reduce the level of chloroform needed to maintain anesthesia (Garner and Coffman 1974).

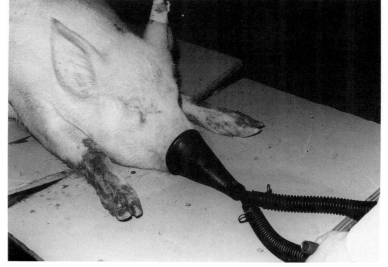

76.4. A nose cone or face mask can be used to deliver anesthetic vapors to swine. When compared to endotracheal intubation, face masks or nose tubes are simpler to apply, but they are also wasteful of anesthetic and do not allow efficient artificial respiration if it is indicated.

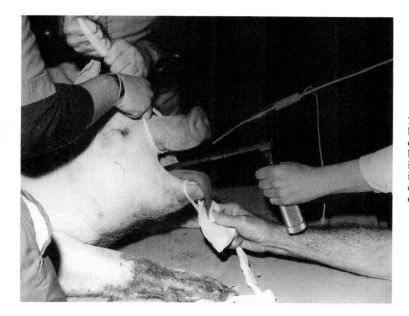

76.5. Endotracheal intubation can be accomplished with the pig in either ventral or lateral recumbency. When the larynx is visualized the bent tip of the metal rod is inserted between the vocal cords to serve as a guide for the endotracheal tube.

Ether is a fairly safe, volatile anesthetic, but it is also flammable and very irritating to mucous membranes. Induction of anesthesia with ether is prolonged and characterized by excitement. In addition, when administered to conscious pigs, copious salivation and bronchial secretion occur even after prior administration of atropine (Hall and Clarke 1983). It is therefore recommended that ether be used with a preanesthetic that produces basal anesthesia. Closed or semiclosed techniques are preferred for ether anesthesia in large pigs; in small pigs, the open-drop method can be used.

Cyclopropane is a potent inhalant anesthetic that is nonirritating and relatively free of toxicity at proper doses. It is flammable when mixed with air and expensive. Cyclopropane produces satisfactory anesthesia in pigs when administered by the closed-circuit method (Hill and Perry 1959). Recovery is prompt and occasionally accompanied by vomiting (Hall and Clarke 1983). In small pigs, anesthesia can be induced with cyclopropane with use of a face mask, but in large pigs, it is advisable to use a preanesthetic that will allow endotracheal intubation.

Halothane is the most widely used inhalant anesthetic in swine. Depth of anesthesia is readily controlled, induction is rapid, and recovery is prompt and smooth. Because halothane is expensive, the closed-circuit technique is usually used in swine weighing more than 20 kg. The minimum alveolar concentration for halothane for pigs

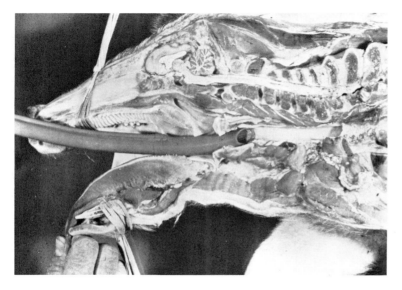

76.6. The tip of the endotracheal tube has passed through the larynx and is entering the trachea.

is 0.91 ± 0.3 as determined by lack of response to a standard stimulus consisting of a large Kelly hemostat applied to the tail for 1 minute (Tranquilli et al. 1983). Disadvantages associated with halothane are cardiopulmonary depression, hypotension, hepatotoxicity, and the initiation of malignant hyperthermia in susceptible animals. Nitrous oxide can be used with halothane to lower the level needed to maintain anesthesia and to reduce its adverse effects. Substitution of 50% nitrous oxide for halothane to maintain equipotent anesthesia results in a marked increase in regional brain blood flow, while myocardial perfusion is maintained near awake values (Manohar and Parks 1984).

Methoxyflurane is an excellent anesthetic agent that is superior to halothane for muscle relaxation and postoperative analgesia. Its main disadvantage for use in swine is its low vaporization rate. At room temperature, it is not possible to obtain an anesthetic concentration high enough for rapid induction of anesthesia. Methoxyflurane should be used only after anesthesia is induced by other agents. Cardiopulmonary depression, hypotension, and hepatotoxicity are adverse effects associated with its use. Recovery following methoxyflurane anesthesia is smooth and somewhat prolonged.

Nitrous oxide is a nonflammable gas used in combination with other inhalant anesthetics to maintain anesthesia. This agent is considered the safest inhalant anesthetic, having no ill effect on any body organ if used with adequate oxygen. Nitrous oxide lacks the potency required for induction and maintenance of anesthesia without concomitant use of other anesthetic agents. It is most frequently used in swine as an adjunct to methoxyflurane or halothane. Diffusion anoxia may occur following its use. This is caused by diffusion of nitrous oxide into the alveoli of the lung, which results in a dilution of the alveolar oxygen concentration, thus producing hypoxia. This can be avoided by flushing the lungs with oxygen for 5–10 minutes after nitrous oxide administration has stopped.

LOCAL ANESTHESIA.
Local anesthetics produce a reversible loss of sensation in a circumscribed area of the body by preventing the initiation and transmission of sensory impulses. Contact of a local anesthetic with a nerve trunk results in both sensory and motor paralysis to the area of the body supplied by the nerve. In general, local anesthesia is easy to perform, requires only minimal assistance or equipment, and is less toxic than general anesthesia. Local anesthesia is contraindicated when there is infection or induration of the area to be anesthetized and when hypersensitivity of the individual to the anesthetic agent exists. The use of local anesthesia without additional chemical restraint is limited in swine

because the pig, even in the absence of pain, will resist physical restraint by continuing to struggle and squeal.

Percutaneous infiltration and epidural injection are the two most frequently used techniques for local anesthesia in swine. The most commonly available and utilized agents are procaine and lidocaine, which are available or can be prepared in 1 or 2% solutions with or without epinephrine, as indicated. The addition of epinephrine usually extends the effective time of anesthesia. Duration of anesthesia by percutaneous infiltration of procaine with epinephrine at 1:200,000 ranges from 15 to 120 minutes. Lidocaine with epinephrine at 1:200,000, similarly infiltrated, has an anesthesia duration range of 60–435 minutes (Covino and Vassalo 1976). Excessive tissue concentrations of infiltrated anesthetic solutions containing epinephrine should be avoided because of potential tissue ischemia and subsequent local necrosis.

Percutaneous Anesthesia. Anesthesia by infiltration of anesthetic agents directly into and around the surgical site is sufficient for minor surgical procedures involving the skin and superficial underlying tissues. It is useful in scrotal hernia repair, scirrhous cord removal, and suturing in the perineal area after prolapse replacement. Infiltration of the skin and deeper tissues along the line of incision or cesarean section is used in lieu of regional or general anesthesia in sows suffering from the exhaustion and shock of prolonged labor and manipulation.

Epidural Anesthesia. Epidural anesthesia in swine is useful in any surgery caudal to the umbilicus. It is contraindicated in patients in shock because of sympathetic blockade and consequent depression of blood pressure (Benson and Thurmon 1979). Minimal equipment and expense, simplicity of application, and safety for the patient are definite advantages. The necessity to forcefully restrain the foreparts and the struggling that occurs are disadvantages in extensive and delicate surgery. The problems of restraint and struggling can be overcome by using tranquillizers, sedatives, and a light plane of general anesthesia in combination with the epidural injection.

The site for injection for epidural anesthesia in the pig is the lumbosacral space. The conus medullaris of the cauda equina of the pig terminates in the region of the first or second sacral vertebra. The filum terminale terminates at the sixth or seventh coccygeal vertebra. Although the meninges extend beyond the conus medullaris and thus beyond the lumbosacral articulation anatomically, there is, in practice, only a very slight probability of entering the subarachnoid space; the cord is extremely small at this site, even in large animals. However, an anesthetic injection made in error between the last two lumbar vertebrae can be placed in the subarachnoid space, resulting in possible death if large amounts are deposited (Getty 1963).

The pig is restrained in a standing position, snubbed by a rope or snare. The landmark for determining the site for needle placement is found by drawing an imaginary line from the fold of the flank vertically over the tuber coxae, horizontally across the back, extending over the contralateral tuber coxae, and down to the opposite flank fold. This line passes across the location of the dorsal spinous processes of the next-to-last or last lumbar vertebra, depending on the age and size of the pig. A region on the midline of the back, 6 inches caudal to and including the imaginary line, is prepared for aseptic insertion of the needle. The point for insertion is precisely on the midline and caudal to the imaginary transverse line, 1–1.5 cm for pigs 9–36 kg and 5–8 cm for pigs 45 kg and over (Fig. 76.7). The location is infiltrated with a local anesthetic agent prior to needle insertion. Needle lengths used are 6–8 cm for pigs 9–36 kg, 10 cm for pigs 45–90 kg, and 12–16 cm for pigs over 90 kg. Needle sizes range from 20 to 17 gauge depending on the age and weight of the pig.

The needle is inserted with the bevel directed cranially and at an angle 10° caudal to perpendicular. The depth of insertion varies according to the size and condition of the subject. Depth for pigs 9–36 kg is 2–5.2 cm, and for pigs 45–90 kg, it is 5.2–9 cm. Penetration will be as deep as 10–13 cm for heavy sows and boars. The lumbosacral aperture is 1–2 cm cranial to caudal and 1.5–3.5 cm transversely, depending on the size of the pig (Getty 1963; Hall and Clarke 1983). The needle passes easily through the back fat and muscle before encountering resistance at the interarticular ligament. After passage through the ligament, the needle drops to the floor of the spinal canal with

little or no resistance. Aspiration should be attempted before injection of the anesthetic to ensure that the subarachnoid space has not been entered. Little resistance to injection will be encountered if the needle is properly located in the epidural space.

The anesthetic agents most useful are 2% procaine and 2% lidocaine. Procaine usually will produce anesthesia of 30–90 minutes duration, while lidocaine results in a somewhat longer period, varying from 60 to 180 minutes. The initial onset is observed in 5–10 minutes, and anesthesia is complete in 10–20 minutes. The addition of epinephrine, 1:100,000, will enhance the effectiveness and lengthen the time of anesthesia by causing local vasoconstriction, resulting in decreased systemic absorption of the anesthetic compound. Thus, more of the agent is available for diffusion into neural tissue (Getty 1963; Covino and Vassalo 1976).

The dose varies according to age, size, amount of body fat, weight, stage of pregnancy, and clinical status of the patient. Generally, a dose of 1 ml/9 kg body weight is proper for 2% lidocaine, and a dose of 1 ml/4.5 kg body weight is satisfactory for 2% procaine. The maximum dose of either should not exceed 20 ml (Getty 1963; Benson and Thurmon 1979; Hall and Clarke 1983). Clinical use has shown that it is seldom necessary to administer more than 15 ml of lidocaine to achieve the desired results, especially if epinephrine is included.

Supportive Fluid Therapy during Anesthesia. In the healthy patient subjected to short-term, light surgical anesthesia, administration of supportive fluids is not considered to be absolutely necessary unless the animal has been starved of food and water for over 24 hours. Prolonged deep surgical anesthesia, on the other hand, is best managed with intravenous fluid support (Thurmon and Benson 1986).

Fluid-loading is essential in sows that are hypotensive or demonstrate other signs of shock. With a 16-gauge, over-the-needle catheter placed in a large central ear vein, 2–3 L of fluid can be given rather rapidly by pressurizing the fluid vial. This procedure is often the single most important measure that can be taken to promote safe anesthesia in a sow presented for cesarean section; this is particularly true if the sow is toxic from dead piglets in utero and epidural anesthesia is to be employed.

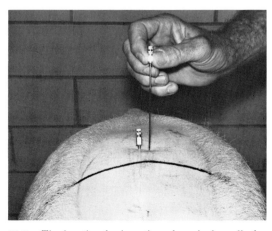

76.7. The location for insertion of a spinal needle for epidural anesthesia in the pig. Note the needle length and depth of insertion.

REFERENCES

ANDERSON, I. L. 1977. Anesthesia of swine. NZ Vet J 25:319–321.

BAUCK, S. W. 1984. An evaluation of a combination of injectable anesthetic agents for use in pigs. Can Vet J 25:162–165.

BEMIS, H. E.; GUARD, W. F.; AND COVAULT, C. H. 1924. Anesthesia, general and local. J Am Vet Med Assoc 17:407–439.

BENSON, G. J., AND THURMON, J. C. 1979. Anesthesia of swine under field conditions. J Am Vet Med Assoc 174:594–596.

BOOTH, N. H. 1977. Intravenous and other parenteral anesthetics. In Veterinary Pharmacology and Therapeutics, 4th ed. Ed. L. M. Jones, N. H. Booth, and L. E. McDonald. Ames: Iowa State Univ Press, p. 241.

BREESE, C. E., AND DODMAN, N. H. 1984. Xylazine-ketamine-oxymorphone: An injectable anesthetic combination in swine. J Am Vet Med Assoc 184:182–183.

CALLEAR, J. F. F., AND VANGESTEL, J. F. E. 1973. An analysis of the results of field experiments in pigs in the U. K. and Eire with the combination anaesthetic azaperone and metomidate. Vet Rec 92:284–287.

CANTOR, G. H.; BRUNSON, D. B.; AND REIBOLD, T. W. 1981. A comparison of four short-acting anesthetic combinations for swine. Vet Med Small Anim Clinic 76:715–720.

CLARKE, K. W. 1969. Effect of azaperone on the blood pressure and pulmonary ventilation in pigs. Vet Rec 85:649–651.

COVINO, B. G., AND VASSALO, H. G. 1976. Local anesthetics. Mechanisms of action and clinical use. In The Scientific Basis of Clinical Anesthesia. New York, San Francisco, London: Grune and Stratton, p. 50.

COX, J. E.; MEESE, G. B.; AND EWBANK, R. 1973. The use of large animal Immobilon in pigs. Vet Rec 93:354–358.

COX, J. E.; DONE, S. H.; LEES, P.; AND WALTON, J. R. 1975. Preliminary studies of the actions of alphaxalone and alphadolone in the pig. Vet Rec 97:497–498.

DEYOUNG, D. W.; LUMB, W. V.; AND SAWYER, D. C. 1970. An inhalation anesthetic technic for miniature swine. Vet Med 65:339–340.

FERGUSON, A. R. 1971. The use of azaperone in pig practice. Ir Vet J 25:61–64.

GARNER, H. E., AND COFFMAN, J. R. 1974. Anesthesia. Textbook of Large Animal Surgery. Baltimore: Williams & Wilkins, pp. 120–123.

GETTY, R. 1963. Epidural anesthesia in the hog—its technique and applications. Proc 100th Annu Meet Am Vet Med Assoc, p. 88.

GRAY, K. N.; RAULSTON, G. L.; FLOW, B. L.; JARDINE, J. H.; AND HUCHTON, J. I. 1978. Repeated immobilization of miniature swine with an acepromazine-ketamine combination. Southwest Vet 31:27–30.

GREENE, C. J. 1979. Animal anaesthesia. In Laboratory Animal Handbook. Middlesex, Engl.: MRC Clinical Research Centres, pp. 187–197.

HALL, L. W., AND CLARKE, K. W. 1983. Anesthesia of the pig. In Veterinary Anesthesia, 8th ed. London: Baillière Tindall, pp. 287–304.

HENRY, D. P. 1968. Anaesthesia of boars by intratesticular injection. Aust Vet J 44:418–419.

HILL, K. J., AND PERRY, J. S. 1959. A method for closed-circuit anaesthesia in the pig. Vet Rec 71:296–299.

JONES, R. S. 1972. A review of tranquilization and sedation in large animals. Vet Rec 90:613–617.

KERNKAMP, H. C. H. 1939. Narcosis and anesthesia in swine produced by pentobarbital sodium. J Am Vet Med Assoc 94:207–208.

LUMB, W. V., AND JONES, E. W. 1973. Veterinary Anesthesia. Philadelphia: Lea and Febiger.

MANOHAR, M., AND PARKS, C. 1984. Porcine regional brain and myocardial blood flows during halothane-O_2 and halothane-nitrous oxide anesthesia: Comparisons with equipotent isoflurane anesthesia. Am J Vet Res 45:465–473.

ORR, J. A.; MANOHAR, M.; AND WILL, J. A. 1976. Cardiopulmonary effects of the combination of neuroleptic azaperone and hypnotic metomidate in swine. Am J Vet Res 37:1305–1308.

PIERMATTEI, D. L., AND SWAN, H. 1970. Techniques for general anesthesia in miniature pigs. J Surg Res 10:587–592.

PORTER, D. B., AND SLUSSOR, C. A. 1984. Stresnil (azaperone), a new neuroleptic for swine. Proc Am Assoc Swine Prod Annu Meet, Kansas City, pp. 15–23.

REGAN, H. A., AND GILLIS, M. F. 1975. Restraint, venipuncture, endotracheal intubation, and anesthesia of miniature swine. Lab Anim Sci 25:409–419.

RITCHIE, H. E. 1957. Chlorpromazine sedation in the pig. Vet Rec 69:895–900.

THURMON, J. C., AND BENSON, G. J. 1986. Anesthesia in ruminants and swine. In Current Veterinary Therapy: Food Animal Practice. Philadelphia: W. B. Saunders, pp. 51–71.

THURMON, J. C.; NELSON, D. R.; AND CHRISTIE, G. J. 1972. Ketamine anesthesia in swine. J Am Vet Med Assoc 160:1325–1330.

THURMON, J. C.; TRANQUILLI, W. J.; AND BENSON, G. J. 1986. Cardiopulmonary responses of swine to intravenous infusion of guaifenesin, ketamine, and xylazine. Am J Vet Res 47(10):2138–2140.

THURMON, J. C.; BENSON, G. J.; TRANQUILLI, W. J.; AND OLSON, W. A. 1988. The anesthetic and analgesic effects of Telazol and xylazine in pigs: Evaluating clinical trials. Vet Med 83:841–845.

TRANQUILLI, W. J.; THURMON, J. C.; BENSON, G. J.; AND STEFFEY, E. P. 1983. Halothane potency in pigs (*Sus scrofa*). Am J Vet Res 44:1106–1107.

VAUGHAN, L. C. 1961. Anaesthesia in the pig. Br Vet J 117:383–391.

77 Castration, Vasectomy, Hernia Repair, and Baby Pig Processing

H. N. Becker

CASTRATION. Surgical castration of male pigs will undoubtedly continue to be a procedure that pork producers and veterinarians are required to do. It has been customary to castrate pigs at or after weaning, often when some other procedure such as vaccination is done.

Chemical castration with various compounds is being studied but is not presently approved or being used in the United States. When pigs are grown to market weight (90–110 kg) in relatively close confinement, there is little justification for castration, but federal regulations prohibit the sale of "boar" meat.

Two castration techniques are applicable to pigs less than 2 weeks of age. Castration using either of these methods is usually done at the same time iron injections are given, ears are notched, tails are docked, and needle teeth are clipped.

Knife Blade Method. In the knife blade method (Becker 1979), a surgical scalpel handle is required that accepts a hooked blade, such as a Bard-Parker No. 3 handle and a No. 12 blade. Producers often drill a hole in the end of the handle and attach a leather thong or cord that will wrap around the wrist, which helps prevent dropping the instrument. The pig may be held by the rear legs in either of two positions. In one position the thumb is used to push up the testicles (Fig. 77.1A), while the first finger is used in the other position. After the testicles are pushed up and the scrotal skin is tensed, the tip of the hooked blade is pushed through the scrotum and the blade is directed forward and upward toward the tail (Fig. 77.1B). This procedure is repeated over the other testicle. If the tunic surrounding the testicles is incised, the testicles will pop out through the incision. If this does not occur, the exposed testicles may be pushed out through the skin incisions (Fig. 77.1C). Each testicle is then grasped separately, pulled upward, and removed (Fig. 77.1D). The cord and as much loose tissue as possible should also be removed. When done properly, very little bleeding occurs and two small, clean incisions remain (Fig. 77.1E).

Even though inguinal hernias are difficult to detect in pigs this young, very few problems of post-castration herniation occur. Swelling begins very quickly in the surgical area and almost always prevents the intestines from coming through the scrotal incisions. In ruptured pigs the usual occur-rence after castration is for the intestines to fill the inguinal canal and scrotum. This will become visible as a swollen scrotum any time after castration but usually is seen during the first 2 weeks after surgery. The intestines will become adhered to the scrotum very quickly, so surgical correction should be done as soon as possible after detection of the rupture if it is to be done at all. It is the author's experience that very few of these pigs are adversely affected, and surgical correction is usually not worth the time, effort, and expense required.

Side-cutter Method. A procedure similar to the knife blade method uses side cutters (medium-sized wire cutters) (Mahan 1979). This same instrument is commonly used to cut needle teeth. The pig is held by one back leg with the belly outward, and the testicles are elevated within the scrotum by pressure from the middle finger (Fig. 77.2A). An incision is made into the

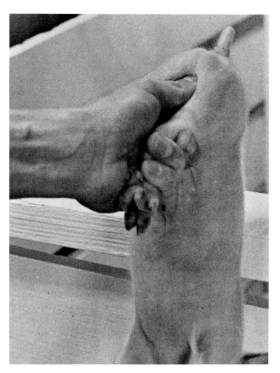

77.1. Knife blade method of castration for piglets under 2 weeks of age.

943

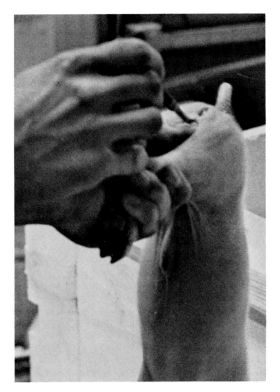

B

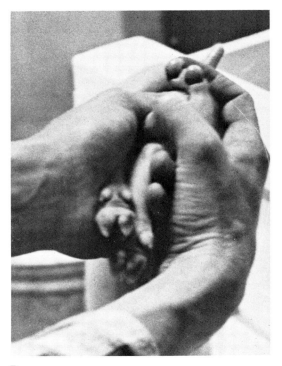

D

77.1. (*continued*)

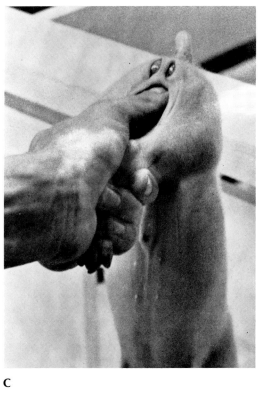

C

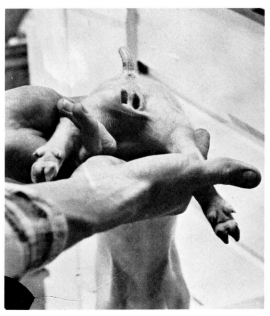

E

scrotum over each testicle (Fig. 77.2B), which is "popped" through the incision by pinching with the thumb and forefinger (Fig. 77.2C). After the testicles are exposed they are grasped, pulled upward, and removed (Fig. 77.2D). An attempt should be made to remove all loose tissue. Mild iodine or other disinfectant may be applied to the wound area.

Older Piglets. Pigs more than 2 weeks of age and younger than 16 weeks and weighing 4–30 kg may be castrated by incisions into the scrotum (high approach) or into the abdominal area (low or belly approach). A description of the scrotal technique is given by Bullard (1975) and involves the pig being restrained on its side. Two incisions are

made over the testicles, which are then removed.

The low or belly approach is preferred by the author. The pig is restrained by being held by the back legs, with the belly toward the operator. The back of the pig is cradled between and squeezed by the legs of the holder. Two incisions are made over the testicles that have been forced downward by the operator. If the hook-blade knife is used properly and the tunic is incised, the testicles will drop through the incisions readily (Fig. 77.3A). The testicles are then grasped and pulled upward out of the incisions (Fig. 77.3B). The tunic may be separated from the testicle (Fig. 77.3C) or removed with it. If the cords do not pull out easily, they may be cut or scraped with the knife blade with little resultant bleeding

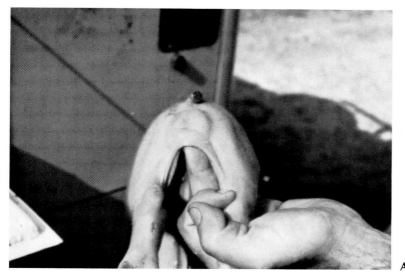

77.2. Side-cutter method of castration for piglets under 2 weeks of age.

A

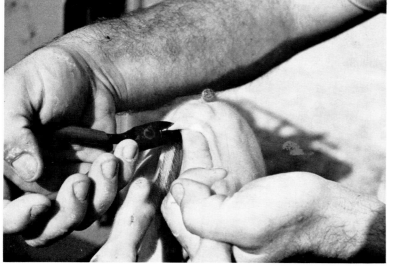

B

77.2. (*continued*)

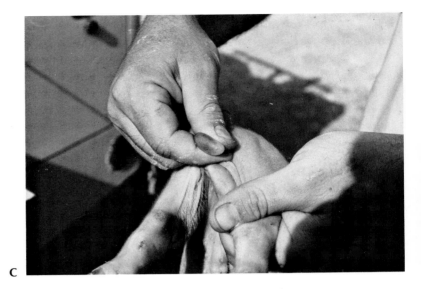

C

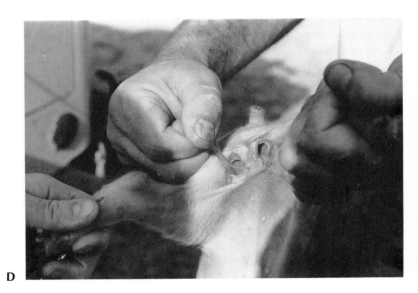

D

(Fig. 77.3D). The incisions should be liberal to allow for adequate drainage and prevention of serum pooling.

Subadults and Adults. Young boars and large adult boars may occasionally need to be castrated. This usually depends on individual owner preference, market acceptance or rejection of intact boars, and local custom or tradition. Very few adult boars are castrated in the Midwest, but this procedure is still common in the Southeast.

Methods of physical and chemical restraint are described by Bullard (1975) and in Chapter 76. The author's choice of anesthesia is intravenous injection of thiamylal (Surital) into the anterior vena cava or marginal ear vein. From 0.5 to 1.5 g

are used depending on size (see Chapter 76).

The surgical technique described by Bullard (1975) involves one midline incision in the scrotum through which both testicles are delivered. The tunic is quite thick, and much dissection must be done to deliver the testicles within an intact tunic (closed method).

The author prefers to make two bold incisions through the scrotum over each testicle, through the tunic, and into the testicle. This allows the testicles to fall from within the tunic. The tunic attachment at the tail of the epididymis is then cut, and the cord is clamped and cut with an emasculator. As much of the loose tissue and tunic is removed as is easily possible and the skin over the midline between the incisions is re-

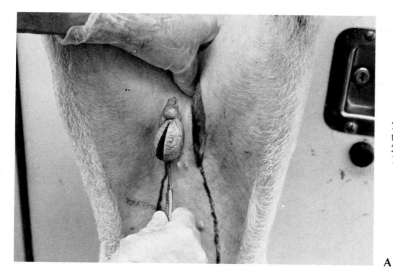

77.3. Low approach to castration of piglets that are more than 2 weeks of age and younger than 16 weeks.

A

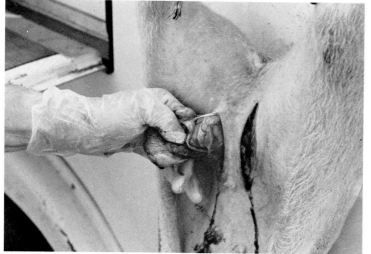

B

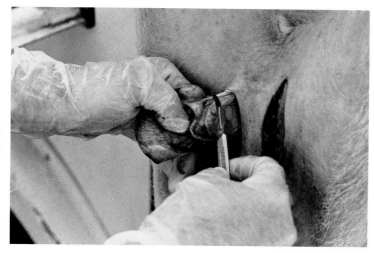

C

77.3. (*continued*)

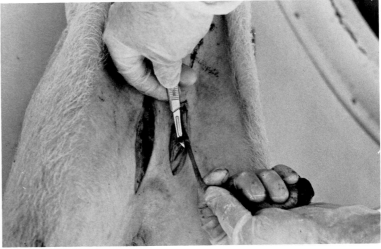

D

moved. The wound is sprayed with mild disinfectant or antibiotic powder, and a therapeutic dose of antibiotics is injected intramuscularly.

Complications. Postcastration infection rarely occurs in pigs less than 2 weeks of age. Infections are most common when pigs are castrated between the ages of 3–6 weeks. This time corresponds to the low point of colostral antibodies (passive) and acquired (active) antibodies. If pigs are dirty, are wet, or have diarrhea, infections will be more frequent.

VASECTOMY. Vasectomized boars may be used advantageously to promote the onset of estrus in young confined gilts or to detect standing heat in gilts/sows, particularly when artificial insemination or very valuable boars are being used for breeding.

Anesthesia is induced and the boar is placed in D-V recumbency and restrained with leg ties. The surgical area, located 2–4 cm laterally on either side of the penis and 5–10 cm cranially from the base of the scrotum, is prepared. The initial incision should extend 4–6 cm and is made down to the tunic (Fig. 77.4). The tunic containing the spermatic cord is freed by blunt dissection and is elevated from the incision (Fig. 77.5). A small incision is made through the tunic, being careful not to incise the veins or artery. The ductus deferens is a small, firm, white, round cord located adjacent to the spermatic artery; a 3–4 cm section is clamped on each end and the section between the clamps is cut and removed. The ends of the ductus are ligated with medium gut (Fig. 77.6). The clamps are removed, the ends of the ductus are replaced in the tunic, and the tunic is sutured with light gut (Fig. 77.7). After the procedure is repeated on the opposite side, the wounds are sprayed with mild antiseptic or antibiotic powder and the skin is loosely sutured. Healing

should be complete 1–2 weeks prior to using the boar as a teaser.

HERNIA REPAIR

Inguinal Hernia. Occasionally, herniation will occur after castration. When this happens, it is best to manually enlarge the inguinal ring, replace the prolapsed intestines, and suture the external inguinal ring.

When a hernia is detected before castration, it is much easier to repair. In the author's experience the majority of inguinal hernias occur in

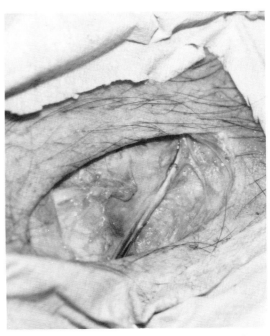

77.4. Incision through the skin, exposing the tunic.

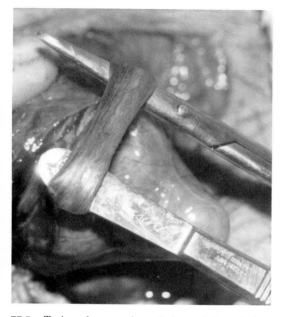

77.5. Tunic and spermatic cord elevated through the skin incision.

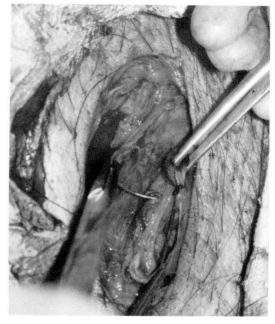

77.7. Suturing of tunic after replacing ligated ends of the ductus deferens.

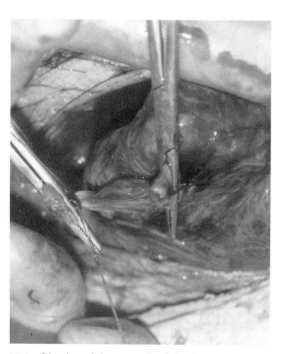

77.6. Ligation of the cut ends of the ductus deferens.

surrounding the testicles is removed from the scrotum (Fig. 77.8B) and twisted, forcing the intestines down into the abdomen. The twisted tunic is clamped close to the incision (Fig. 77.8C), and the tissue is ligated with the suture of choice (e.g., 6-mm umbilical tape) (Fig. 77.8D). The tunic and cord are then detached, and the external inguinal ring is sutured with gut (Fig. 77.8E). The opposite testicle may then be removed through the same incision. The wound is sprayed with mild disinfectant or antibiotic powder, and one suture is placed in the skin (Fig. 77.8F).

Occasionally, an undescended testicle is detected. These may be operated on in the manner described by Bullard (1975). Most of these will descend as the pig ages and may be removed then.

If operating on undescended testicles, the abdominal approach is preferred by the author. With the pig suspended by its rear legs, an incision is made over the external inguinal ring as in the hernia operation. Blunt dissection and probing will usually locate the testicle close to the internal inguinal ring. Occasionally, the testicle will be located quite forward. A spay hook may be used to advantage in such a situation.

Umbilical Hernia. Most umbilical hernias are due to navel infection that prevents the umbilical cord from shrinking to normal size after birth. The enlarged cord and/or attending abscess spreads the abdominal muscles at the navel.

the left inguinal canal. Bullard (1975) has adequately described the technique. The incision is made over the external inguinal ring (Fig. 77.8A), and by blunt dissection the tunic is isolated and freed from surrounding tissues. The intact tunic

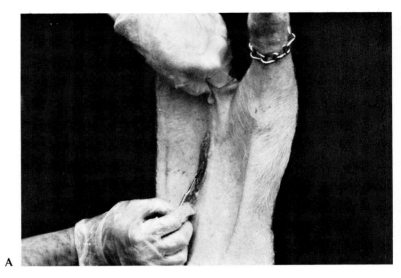

77.8. Repair of inguinal hernia.

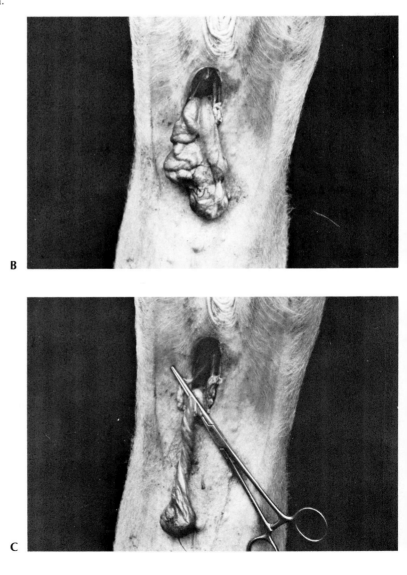

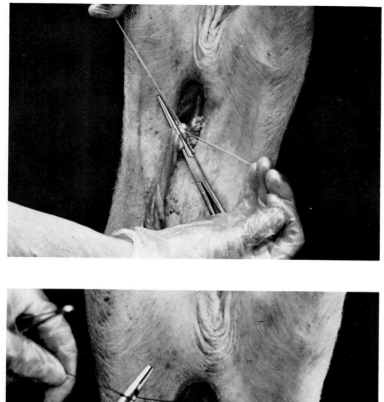

77.8. (*continued*)

D

E

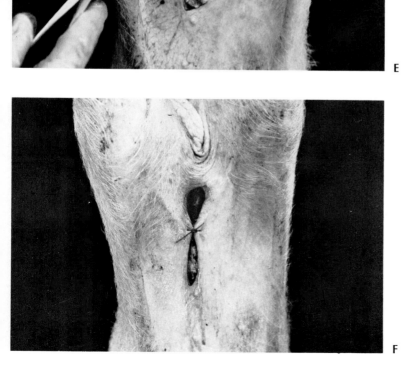

F

Omentum or intestines then fill the void and continue to enlarge the hernial ring. These herniated masses may become very large and nearly drag the ground on occasion. Depending on size and operator preference, these hernias may be repaired by the closed or open technique.

In closed reduction, abdominal relaxation is necessary, so general anesthesia is required (Chapter 76). Restraint is best accomplished by placing the pig on its back in a V-shaped trough (Fig. 77.9A). It is best if the trough is tilted so that the pig's head is lower than the body. The surgical area should be prepared and draped. In male pigs care should be taken to reflect the penis and prepuce (Fig. 77.9B). The skin at the base of the hernia is then incised and dissected from the underlying hernial tissue (Fig. 77.9C). If the hernia is easily reduced and few adhesions are present, the intact hernia may be replaced into the abdominal cavity. The abdominal musculature

and tissue forming the edge of the hernial ring may then be drawn together and sutured. Any excess skin is then removed, the prepuce is positioned, and the skin incisions are sutured.

In open reduction, preparation and skin incision are begun as in the closed technique. The skin is dissected from the underlying tissue. If the hernia is not easily reduced because of a small ring or if numerous adhesions and/or abscesses are present, the hernia sac is incised (Fig. 77.10A). The adhesions are separated, abscesses removed if present, and intestines replaced into the abdomen (Fig. 77.10B). Occasionally, such severe adhesions are present that a section of intestine must be removed and an anastomosis performed. The sac is then removed to the edges of the hernial ring. The edges of the ring are then sutured and drawn together and the skin is closed (Fig. 77.10C).

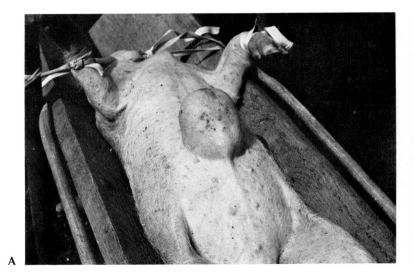

A

77.9. Closed reduction of umbilical hernia.

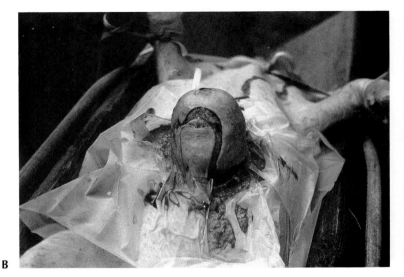

B

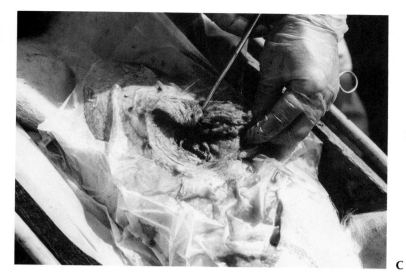

77.9. *(continued)*

C

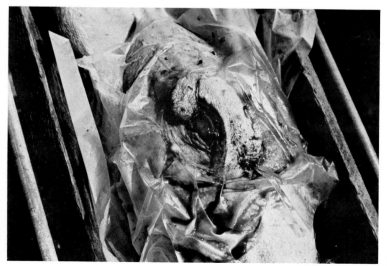

77.10. Open reduction of umbilical hernia.

A

B

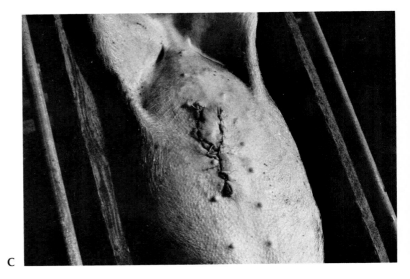

77.10. (continued)

C

BABY PIG PROCESSING.

It has become customary to routinely process newborn piglets between 1 and 3 days of age. Restraint and manipulation at this age seem to be less stressful than at a later time. The necessity of giving iron injections by 3–4 days of age to prevent anemia also provides good reason to perform the additional tasks of clipping needle teeth, ear notching for identification, tail docking, and castrating.

Clipping Needle Teeth.

The needle teeth (canines) are very sharp in piglets and are often routinely clipped with side-cutter pliers (Fig. 77.11). This prevents damage to the facial skin of littermates in the event of fighting among piglets. It also prevents damage to the sow's udder. If the volume of sow's milk is adequate for the number of piglets in the litter, clipping needle teeth is probably unnecessary; however, it is usually done as part of the processing procedure in anticipation of trouble.

The top teeth only or both top and bottom teeth may be clipped, based on owner preference and experience. It is important that only the sharp tip of the tooth be cut. If the tooth is cut too close to the gum, the tooth may be shattered and gum infection may occur. The sharp edges of shattered teeth may also traumatize the tongue and impede successful nursing by the piglet (Calderwood 1979).

Ear Notching.

Several numbering systems

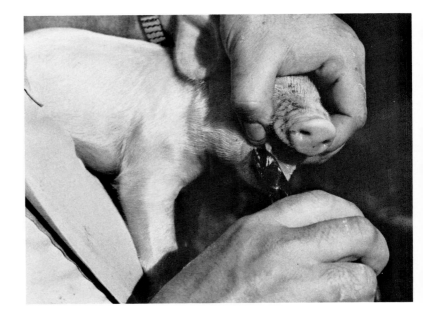

77.11. Clipping needle teeth.

have been devised whereby notches placed in the margins and tips of the ears enable identification of pigs individually. This allows for accurate recording of litter number and date of birth. Several breed associations recognize specific notching systems and should be consulted for accuracy. Examples of different notching systems are shown in Fig. 77.12.

Tail Docking.   Because of the trend toward confinement rearing of swine and the increasing incidence of tail biting in growing-finishing pigs, more pork producers are routinely docking (amputating) tails in newborn piglets. The procedure is simple and is performed using the same side-cutter pliers used to clip needle teeth.The usual location is 12–18 mm from the base of the tail (Berthelsen 1973). Caution must be used not to cut the tail too close to the body. This increases the chance of infection and may also contribute to rectal prolapse. Side-cutter pliers with dull edges work better for tail docking because they crush the tissues rather than cut them, thereby minimizing hemorrhage.

Iron Injection.   The use of injectable iron compounds to prevent piglet anemia is widespread. Although oral iron products have been shown to prevent anemia, most pork producers and veterinarians still rely on injectable iron. Certain antibiotics are often mixed with the iron to prevent the entrance and spread of infection in newborn piglets.

Iron and other products may be injected into piglets in several locations, but the author prefers the neck muscle technique (Becker 1977). The piglet is held between the left elbow and body, and the right ear is grasped and pulled firmly forward. The skin is pricked with the needle and pushed upward, and the needle is inserted to the hub (Fig. 77.13). The injection is made, the needle is withdrawn, and the ear is released simultaneously. Pushing the skin upward prior to injection prevents leakage. The best needle for most injectables is 18-gauge and 12 mm, but a 20-gauge needle may be used for thin liquids. The neck injection site is preferred over the ham area (Fig. 77.13).

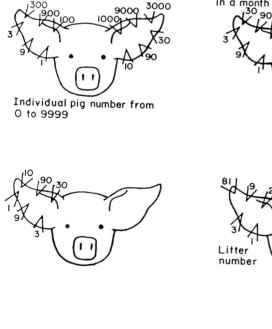

Individual pig number from 0 to 9999

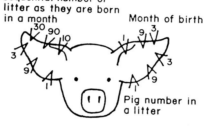

Sequential number of litter as they are born in a month

Month of birth

Pig number in a litter

Individual pig number

Litter number

77.12. Ear-notching systems.

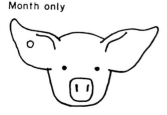

Month only

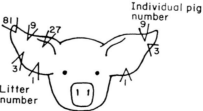

Month	Right	Left
1 or 7	0	–
2 or 8	–	0
3 or 9	–	–
4 or 10	00	–
5 or 11	–	00
6 or 12	0	0

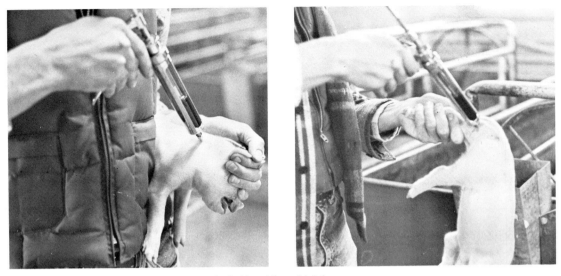

77.13.   Injection of iron into the neck muscle (left) and ham (right).

REFERENCES

BECKER, H. N. 1977. Stick it in the neck. Natl Hog Farmer (Oct):88–89.

——. 1979. Day-old piglet castration. Natl Hog Farmer (Sept):50.

BERTHELSEN, J. D. 1973. Baby pig management procedures. Iowa State Univ Coop Ext Serv.

BULLARD, J. F. 1975. Operations involving the testicle and inguinal canal. In Diseases of Swine, 4th ed. Ed. H. W. Dunne and A. D. Leman. Ames: Iowa State Univ Press, p. 1065.

CALDERWOOD, M. 1979. Personal communication.

MAHAN, D. C. 1979. Side cut castration for pigs 4–10 days old. Natl Hog Farmer (Dec):94.

78 Surgical Procedures in Boars and Sows

W. Bollwahn

ANESTHESIA AND SEDATION IN BREEDING PIGS. Surgical procedures on the genital organs should be done under general anesthesia as a matter of principle to avoid secondary lesions caused by irritation or trauma (e.g., acute cardiac insufficiency, acute necrosis of the back muscles, injuries). The depth of the anesthesia must be adapted to the general condition of the animal. When there has been loss of blood (e.g., vulval hemorrhage, prolapsed uterus) or intoxication (e.g., emphysematous fetuses, endometritis), the general anesthesia should be as shallow as possible (stage III, 1). The required analgesic is given by local or spinal anesthesia.

Spinal anesthesia in swine is administered in the form of extra- or subdural lumbosacral anesthesia. A 2% local anesthetic is injected through the lumbosacral foramen, which is located between the two highest points of the iliac prominences (Fig. 78.1). As soon as the 10- to 14-cm long mandrin cannula has penetrated into the vertebral canal, the mandrin is removed and about 1–2 ml of air injected to check the permeability of the cannula and make sure that the tip is in fact inside the vertebral canal. Aspiration is then attempted with the same syringe. Depending on the position of the tip of the cannula, it is possible to

aspirate fluid from the subdural space, blood from a vein on the floor of the spinal canal, or nothing at all if the cannula is in the extradural space. If blood has been aspirated, the cannula is withdrawn slightly, and its position is checked once more.

The dosage of 2% local anesthetic depends on the distance from the crown of the head to the base of the spine and is 0.5 ml/10 cm distance for a subdural injection and 0.7 ml/10 cm for an extradural injection. This dosage is sufficient to perform operations caudal to the costal arch. The full effects of the anesthetic develop within 4–10 minutes.

For general anesthesia, short-acting barbiturates or the combination of azaperone and methomidate is equally effective. Neuroleptics derived from phenothiazines (tranquillizers) should not be used to increase the potency of the barbiturate anesthesia, since they have a vasodepressive effect that is difficult to control (alpha blockage). In operations cranial to the umbilicus, spinal anesthesia can no longer be used. In such cases (e.g., amputation of claws on the forelimbs, mammectomy) a deep and long-acting anesthesia should be given, using pentobarbital that is intensified by the additional local subcutaneous appli-

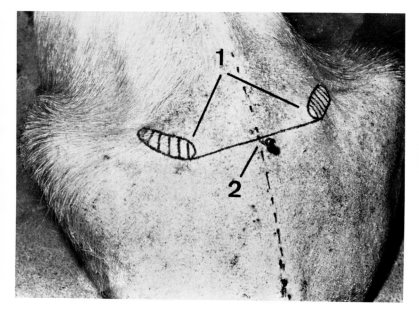

78.1. Spinal anesthesia: (*1*) tuber sacrale, (*2*) position for puncture of the lumbosacral foramen.

95

cation of a 2% local anesthetic. In a mammectomy a rhombic operative field is infiltrated; for a claw amputation a circular infiltration anesthesia is applied proximal to the fetlock.

SURGICAL TREATMENT IN SOWS. Operations on gravid sows are associated with the risk of abortion or fetal damage. This risk can be avoided only by inducing anesthesia without excitation, keeping blood losses to a minimum, and suppressing excitations conditioned by pain in the postoperative phase by means of drugs such as analgesics or neuroleptics. Maternal blood losses during the last 4 weeks of gestation lead to congenital anemia of baby pigs and should therefore be offset by iron substitution (1–2 g iron/injection or ferrous fumarate orally). The barbiturates and neuroleptics that enter the fetal circulation do not reach life-threatening concentrations as long as the respiration and circulation of the brood animal are intact.

Animals with acute loss of blood (e.g., vulval hemorrhage, amputation of the uterus, mammectomy) and clinically identifiable circulatory stress (i.e., tachycardia greater than 140 beats/minute, pale conjunctiva, cyanotic snout tip, lowered body surface temperature) must be protected from circulatory failure (shock) by intravenous volume substitution (0.9% saline solution, 6% glucose solution, plasma expander) and by the application of heat (straw, infrared light). In surviving pigs, erythropoiesis should be reinforced by iron substitution.

Reposition of the Prolapsed Uterus

DEFINITION. Inversion and prolapse of the uterus occur chiefly during parturition or up to day 3 postpartum. The prolapse may have been complete or partial. In a complete prolapse, there is the danger of rupturing blood vessels in the mesovarium. Delayed involution and painful lesions in the soft birth canal that stimulate straining are considered to be causes of prolapse.

The attempt to perform a reposition is appropriate only when the general condition of the animal still permits the use of anesthesia. In cases of severe injuries to the uterus, extended necrosis of the mucosa, and high-grade congestion, the reposition should not be attempted.

TREATMENT. After a general examination, the sow is anesthetized using shallow general anesthesia and spinal anesthesia. The prolapsed uterus is cleaned with cold water and placed on a clean cloth. The anesthetized sow is immobilized on her right side on a plank or ladder, so that the pelvis can be kept elevated.

Every reposition, including that of a partial prolapse, should be undertaken starting from the peritoneal cavity by pulling in the top of the horn and exerting pressure on the mucosa from the outside. Moreover, the opening of the peritoneal cavity makes it possible to determine if all the baby pigs have been born and if the inverted parts of the uterus have been completely everted.

If it proves impossible to reach the tip of the horn from the peritoneal cavity, the mesentery should not be pulled. Instead, the prolapsed horn must be opened in the vicinity of the bifurcation by a longitudinal incision, so that the operating surgeon can grasp the tip of the horn with the right hand and pull it into the pelvis. When the reposition has been completed, this incision is positioned forward through the laparotomy incision and is sutured.

The laparotomy is done from the left flank. The surgeon places the left arm in the peritoneal cavity and locates one tip of the horn. This is carefully repositioned by pulling from the inside and exerting pressure from the outside upward as far as the bifurcation. The same procedure is followed for the second horn. The body of the uterus and the cervix are repositioned mainly by pressure from the outside. Fetuses that have not yet been expelled are extracted only when the reposition has been completed. The abdominal and uterine cavities are prophylactically treated with a suspension of antibiotics. The laparotomy incision is closed either in two stages (peritoneal suture plus cutaneous-muscle suture) or three stages (peritoneal suture plus muscle suture plus cutaneous suture).

To prevent a recurrence, contraction of the uterus is stimulated by administering 20–30 IU of oxytocin intramuscularly, and the vagina is narrowed to an opening of approximately 4 cm by means of a Bühner closing, which is a deep subcutaneous suture around the vulva (Figs. 78.2, 78.3). A 10-cm long needle enters the skin lateral to the distal commissure, and a strong silk or synthetic thread is drawn along the base of the labium to the dorsal commissure, at which point the skin is pierced by the needle in the medial line of the perineum. Through this exit opening, the thread is then taken along the base of the other labium to a point lateral to the distal commissure, so that the beginning and end of the suture lie opposite each other there and can be tied together in a bow. The exit of the vagina is narrowed by tightly drawing the Bühner suture to approximately two finger breadths so that urination and expulsion of fetal membranes can occur without interruption. Placing the Bühner suture is digitally controlled from the vagina so neither the mucosa nor the rectum is perforated in the process.

On postoperative day 3 or 4 the Bühner suture can be loosened. It should not be removed before postoperative day 6, so that it can be closed again if the prolapse tends to recur. Following a prolapse, a catarrhal, purulent endometritis develops, which may negatively affect the chances of conception. Depending on the duration and de-

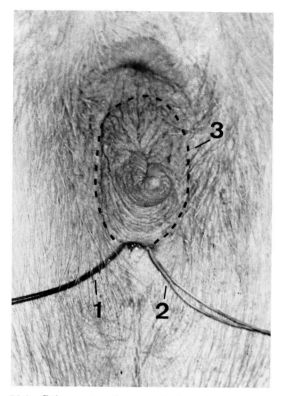

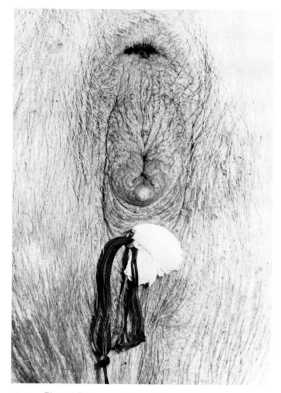

78.2. Bühner suture for prophylaxis against recurrence of vaginal prolapse: (*1*) entry of needle, (*2*) exit of needle, (*3*) subcutaneous suture.

78.3. Closed Bühner suture with gauze.

gree of the prolapse, the success rate for this operation ranges from 30 to 80%.

Reposition of the Prolapsed Vagina

DEFINITION. Vaginal prolapse occurs predominantly during the last days of gestation. A complete prolapse in such cases is mostly associated with a severe edema of the vulva. As a result of continuous straining, a prolapse of the rectal mucosa frequently develops as well. In addition to causing local lesions of the mucosa, this results in cervicitis and impeded urination. The latter conditions, in many cases, make it impossible to open the soft birth canal normally, so a cesarean section is called for. Vaginal prolapse that occurs early also involves the danger of uterine infection accompanied by fetal death. Because the etiology of vaginal prolapse is unknown, only symptomatic treatment can be carried out.

TREATMENT. To avoid further complications such as lesions or prolapse of the rectum, the sow is anesthetized and the pelvis elevated. The prolapse is cleaned with cold water and coated with a viscous suspension of antibiotics. The prolapse must be pushed back toward the sacrum. Because of the danger of perforation, one works with the palm or fist, not with the fingertips. As soon as

the prolapse has been repositioned as far as the pudendal cleft, it is pushed with the fist through the opening of the pelvis until it is in front of the pubic bone. The hand is then pulled back slowly to avoid creating a negative pressure in the vagina, for this could lead to a renewed inversion.

Before the vagina is closed to prevent a recurrence of the prolapse, the urinary bladder is emptied with a catheter. The vagina is closed with a Bühner suture, as previously described. When farrowing begins, the Bühner suture must be opened. An imminent farrowing should be expected as soon as a continuous stream of milk comes when the sow is milked.

Reposition of the Prolapsed Rectum

DEFINITION. Prolapse of the rectal mucosa occurs as a result of straining, when excretion has become difficult, and during a bout of proctitis (diarrhea, ulcer). It also appears as a secondary disorder in vaginal prolapse. The dark red mucosa quickly becomes edematous and often shows bleeding lesions. In contrast to rectal prolapse in fattened hogs, which mostly represents an invagination of the rectal wall and must be corrected by resection, the prolapsed rectal mucosa in sows can be repositioned. The prognosis is good even for severe lesions and necroses of the mucosa.

TREATMENT. The reposition is performed on the anesthetized animal with the pelvis elevated. Small prolapses are pushed back in toto with the arched inner surface of the palm. For larger prolapses the mucosa is rolled and pushed back with both thumbs. To prevent a renewed prolapse, the anus is narrowed by a circular purse-string suture. A strong silk or synthetic thread is passed in and out through the skin around the anal opening at a distance of 1 cm from the rim of the anus. The ends of the thread are pulled until the anus is tightly closed. The feces that collect in the ampulla of the rectum must be removed at least once a day. To do this, the closing of the purse-string suture is opened and then closed tightly once more. Before the suture is removed completely, it is left open for 1 or 2 days so that it can be closed again if necessary.

To assist in the treatment, the sow should receive no solid food for the first 2 days after the rectal prolapse appears and should only be given water ad libitum.

Amputation of the Prolapsed Uterus

DEFINITION. In most cases, amputation of the prolapsed uterus leads to circulatory failure. Amputation is indicated when prolapses cannot be repositioned and there are severe lesions. The procedure should be performed only if the sow still appears to be in relatively good general condition. Before the amputation, it must be ascertained that the nonprolapsed parts of the uterus contain no additional fetuses and that the urinary bladder or loops of intestine have not entered the prolapse.

TREATMENT. Before the amputation, the animal is anesthetized with thiobarbiturate and the pelvis is elevated. The wall of one prolapsed horn of the uterus is opened longitudinally near the bifurcation, using a control incision, so that one hand can be placed in the pelvis to check for retained fetuses or prolapsed abdominal organs such as the urinary bladder or intestinal loops. Unborn baby pigs must first be removed by extraction or cesarean section and the prolapsed organs repositioned. Next, a ligature of elastic material is placed around the prolapse at a distance of 10–15 cm from the vulva and tied very tightly.

The prolapse is then resectioned in the shape of a wedge so that a 5- to 10-cm long stump remains (Fig. 78.4) and the arteries located in its center cannot be retracted. It is not necessary to suture the stump. The prolapsed vagina with the amputated stump is repositioned, and the vulva is closed with a Bühner suture, as previously described. The elastic ligature must not be removed; it will be sloughed off spontaneously after 10–14 days. The amputation of the uterus results in severe loss of blood, which must be replaced intra- and postoperatively by volume substitution, as described earlier.

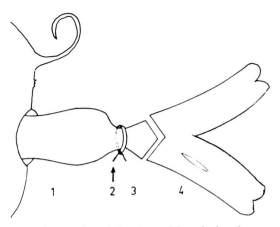

78.4. Amputation of the uterus: (*1*) vaginal prolapse, (*2*) ligature, (*3*) stump of amputation, (*4*) control incision.

Treatment of Vulval Hemorrhage

DEFINITION. As a rule, hemorrhages resulting from vulval lesions that are hard to arrest or threaten to be fatal occur only in connection with parturition. Initially, a primary vulval hematoma occurs, which increases the fragility of the labia. Lesions of the labia are then incapable of spontaneous coagulation of hemorrhages.

TREATMENT. The sow is anesthetized and placed with the bleeding labium facing upward. Both the considerable enlargement of the labium and the fact that the tissue is saturated with blood make regulated hemostasis impossible. The bleeding is therefore arrested by means of one to three U-shaped mass ligatures at the base of the labia, i.e., the area where the labia merge into the area of the thigh and the perineum. A round needle and silk or synthetic suture material are used. For each ligature the wall of the labium is pierced from the inside going outward, beginning in the dorsal commissure. The thread must be long enough (about 120 cm) so that it can be cut off on the outside after perforating the labium; thus with each perforation the beginning and end of a U suture are formed (Fig. 78.5). To keep the thread from cutting into the skin or the mucosa of the labium, rolls of gauze are placed under it before knotting. The sutures remain in place for 2 days. To accelerate the resorption of the vulval hematoma, lead or aluminum acetate is applied to the vulva and its surrounding area twice a day.

Catheterization of the Lateroflexed Bladder

DEFINITION. In older gravid sows in the last stage of gestation, lateroflexion of the urinary bladder into the space between the vagina and the pelvic wall occasionally occurs. The result is a unilateral forward arching of the vaginal mucosa and the vulva that looks deceptively like a vaginal prolapse (Fig. 78.6). The lateroflexion obstructs

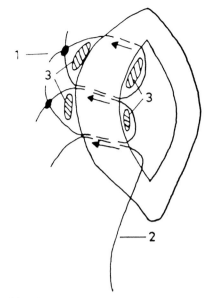

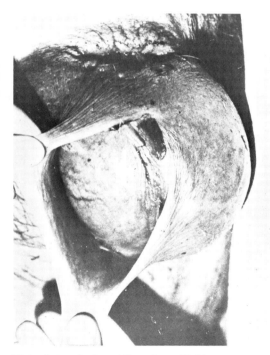

78.5. Mass ligature in bleeding vulval hematoma: (*1*) beginning, (*2*) end of thread, (*3*) gauze.

78.6. Lateroflexion of the urinary bladder.

urination and provokes straining, so a partial or complete vulval prolapse may result.

TREATMENT. The reposition of the displaced urinary bladder by exerting pressure on the vulva or the perineum is usually unsuccessful. Only when the bladder is emptied by a catheter does a spontaneous reposition occur within several hours. To bring about a permanent emptying of

the bladder and retraction of the bladder wall, a self-retaining permanent catheter (Foley-type balloon catheter) is introduced and taped to the skin of the thigh (Fig. 78.7).

Surgical Removal of the Mammae

DEFINITION. Chronic infection of the mammae with *Actinomyces suis* results in the tumorous alteration of the mammary parenchyma by granulomas, abscesses, and fistulas. As soon as the actinomycomas have become larger than a hen's egg, their conservative treatment becomes problematic, and a mammectomy is indicated. The operation should not be performed during the first and last 4 weeks of gestation to prevent the risk of abortion or congenital anemia of baby pigs.

This operation is contraindicated if there are fewer than 12 intact mammary complexes or if problems can be expected when the incision is sutured because of the size of the actinomycoma.

TREATMENT. For operations caudal to the umbilicus, the combination of general and spinal anesthesia is recommended. Operations in the anterior mammary region necessitate a deep general anesthesia (pentobarbital) as well as a circular infiltration of the complex to be resected, using a 2% local anesthetic without an adrenergic. This injection is given subcutaneously in rhombic form.

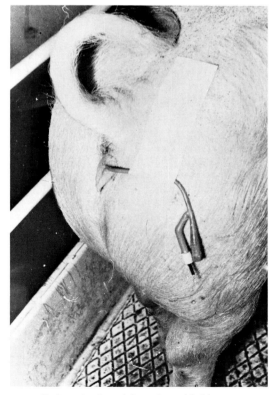

78.7. Catheterization of the urinary bladder.

Bleeding that occurs during the operation is at first temporarily arrested with artery clamps; on the average 12 clamps are required.

The operation begins with a circular incision in the skin at the base of the actinomycoma. The tissue that lies below the tumor is separated either by blunt dissection or with scissors to reduce the tendency to bleed (avoid the subcutaneous abdominal vein). On the lateral side of the actinomycoma, the surgeon first penetrates at a single point into the retromammary tissue (connective and fatty tissue) and enucleates the actinomycoma from this point, proceeding medially. Before the definitive hemostasis is performed by means of vessel and mass ligatures, the floor of the incision is carefully checked for isolated microactinomycomas (as small as pea-sized nodules).

The extirpation of an actinomycotic mammary complex unavoidably causes an extensive deep incision. The closing of this wound must therefore be performed in such a way that no cavity remains that could promote the formation of a seroma. The suture that is suitable for this purpose at first undulates through the floor of the incision and then returns in the opposite direction to catch the rims of the incision (external skin). In this way the floor of the incision and the external skin are brought into apposition when the thread is tied (Fig. 78.8). Gauze is placed under the extracutaneous part of the suture to protect the skin.

When the sutures have been tied, an aqueous suspension of penicillin or 5–10 ml of tincture of iodine is infiltrated in the area of the incision with a blunt cannula. The sutures are removed on the eighth postoperative day.

SURGICAL TREATMENT IN BOARS

Exposure and Examination of the Penis

DEFINITION. A passive exposure is performed on the anesthetized boar to examine and treat the penis. The most frequent indications for an exposure are bleeding on erection or urination, surgical treatment of injuries of the penis, and collection of sperm by electroejaculation.

TREATMENT. The boar is placed under shallow thiobarbiturate anesthesia. For the right-handed surgeon, the animal should be placed on its right side. During the early stage of anesthesia, there is a medium-grade intrapreputial erection that facilitates the exposure of the penis.

With the right hand, the surgeon grasps the erect shaft of the penis about 10 cm caudal to the tip. The thumb and forefinger of the left hand lie near the opening of the prepuce. While the penis is pushed cranially with the right hand, the prepuce is drawn back with the left. In this way the mucosa of the prepuce is everted forward through the opening of the prepuce so that a funnel-shaped orifice is formed, within which the tip of the penis becomes visible (Fig. 78.9). An assistant (wearing a cloth glove) must immobilize the penis and pull it upward.

In a complete exteriorization of the penis and retraction of the prepuce, the following should be examined primarily: the tip of the penis, the penal crest, the urethral fold, and the urethral orifice as well as the base of the penis. Near the base, extensive adhesions are occasionally found; in the area of the tip, lesions and abnormalities occur.

Reposition of the Prolapsed Penis

DEFINITION. After treatment with neuroleptics, a complete or partial prolapse of the penis and of the preputial mucosa occasionally develops (Fig. 78.10). Depending on the duration of the prolapse, the penis not only increases in volume because of congestion but lesions and contamination also appear. These may be significant causes of a later balanoposthitis.

TREATMENT. Until a veterinarian begins treatment, the prolapsed penis should be protected from injuries by being wrapped in a damp towel.

The reposition is performed on the anesthetized animal. First, the mucosa is cleaned with cold water and then covered with an oily antibiotic suspension. During the reposition the mucosa and penis must be pushed back through the ring-shaped opening that lies between the cranial and caudal sections of the preputial cavity (Fig.

78.8. Suturing technique to prevent a seroma: (*1*) entry of needle, (*2*) exit of needle, (*3*) gauze, (*4*) outside skin, (*5*) floor of incision.

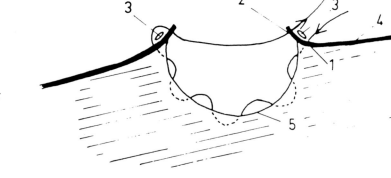

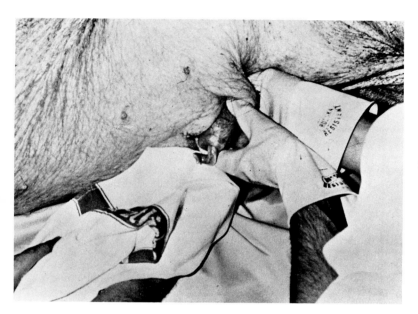

78.9. Exposure of the penis.

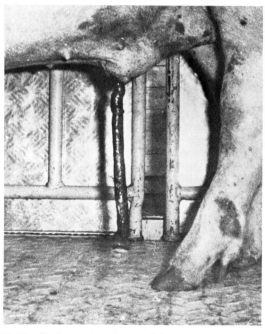

78.10. Prolapse of penis after injection of neuroleptic.

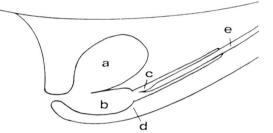

78.11. Prepuce of the boar: (*a*) preputial diverticulum, (*b*) cranial, (*c*) caudal section of preputial cavity, (*d*) ring-shaped bulge between *b* and *c*, (*e*) penis.

78.11D). The closing of the preputial opening with a purse-string suture should be undertaken only if another prolapse occurs, as this provides for prophylaxis against recurrence.

To avoid sexual excitation, the boar must be isolated for the first few days after the reposition. The risk of balanoposthitis can be minimized by repeated intrapreputial instillation of an antibiotic suspension. The drug, e.g., 5–10 ml of chlortetracycline (Aureomycin) suspension, is given by a catheter in the caudal section of the preputial cavity and thoroughly distributed by massage from the outside. Mating can resume 2 weeks postoperatively.

Surgical Removal of the Prolapsed Prepuce

DEFINITION. The prolapsed mucosa of the prepuce can develop severe swelling and rigidity as a result of injury and infection. This makes it impossible for reposition into the prepuce. The resection of this part of the mucosa is possible as long as the entrance into the preputial diverticulum has remained intact (Fig. 78.12).

TREATMENT. The operation is done with the animal under general anesthesia. First, the hairs at the opening of the prepuce are removed. The prolapse is pulled forward slightly and the skin of the prepuce pulled back somewhat so that intact mucosa becomes visible. At this point the prolapse is immobilized with a padded artery clamp or a gauze bandage so that the stump will not be re-

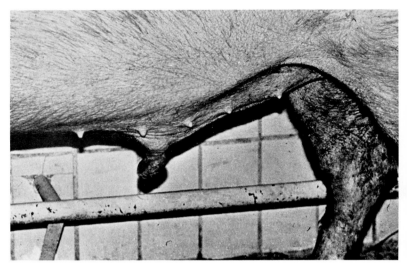

78.12. Prolapse of the preputial mucosa.

tracted into the prepuce after the resection.

Two catgut threads (Fig. 78.13), each 40 cm long, are run crosswise through the prolapsed tube of mucosa. The threads are pulled tight and the prolapse is cut off 5 mm in front of them. Now the threads are pulled upward from the middle of the tube of mucosa and are cut through so that four separate stay sutures can be tied. Between these four sutures, at least two more stay sutures are then placed. Now the immobilizing clamp or bandage is removed, and the stump is pushed back into the prepuce. Mating can resume 2 weeks postoperatively.

Resection of the Preputial Diverticulum

DEFINITION. The preputial diverticulum is dorsal to the anterior section of the preputial cavity. Its function is not known. The following diseases of the preputial diverticulum may result in impotentia coeundi: (1) dilatation with urine retention—in this condition the preputial opening is displaced and the erect penis is introduced into the preputial diverticulum, where ejaculation then takes place; (2) peridiverticulitis with constriction of the preputial opening, resulting in a mechanical obstruction of erection (functional phimosis); and (3) bleeding ulcers of the diverticulum (Fig. 78.14), resulting in loss of libido caused by anemia. Diverticular ulcers are caused by infected leukoplakias. The extirpation of the affected preputial diverticulum restores procreative capacity.

TREATMENT. To remove the preputial diverticulum, a general anesthesia of about 20 minutes is necessary; thus pentobarbital should be given. A blunt instrument, e.g., an artery clamp or catheter, is introduced into the diverticulum before the operation so that the wall of the diverticulum can be located at all times.

The operation begins with a 10-cm incision a little above and 5 cm caudal to the preputial opening. This area has much fatty and connective tissue. The incision is carefully deepened until the preputial musculature, whose coarse fibers surround the diverticulum, is reached. To avoid injuring the very thin wall of the diverticulum, the muscle fibers are pushed apart by blunt dissec-

78.13. Suture in resection of prolapse of the preputial mucosa: (A) threads crossing the mucosal tube, (B) button stay sutures made out of the threads in A, (*1*) mucosa, (*2*) catgut. (Modified from Berge and Westhues 1969.)

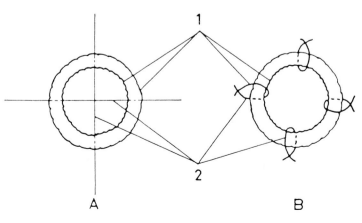

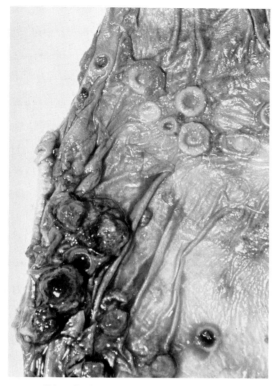

78.14. Diverticular mucosa with circular ulcers: bleeding ulcers (below) and nonbleeding ulcers (above) have a diameter of 3–10 mm.

tion. The diverticulum that lies below the fibers is also dissected bluntly from the area surrounding it. This dissection is continued to the point at which the diverticulum merges into the preputial cavity (Fig. 78.15). Now both halves of the diverticulum, which are palm-sized and linked with the preputial cavity over a short collum, can be recog-

nized. An artery clamp is placed over this collum and the diverticulum is cut off. The stump is closed with an inverting catgut suture (Fig. 78.16). An alternative possibility for diverticulum resection is to invert the dissected (mobilized) diverticulum and guide it through the preputium to the outside. The neck of the diverticulum is then closed with a purse-string suture. The diverticulum, which has been drawn through the preputial orifice, is tied off with a mass ligature and cut off near the orifice. The cavity that the extirpation of the diverticulum creates between the abdominal wall and the prepuce is drawn together with a few catgut sutures. The skin incision is closed with a suture so that the epidermis and floor of the wound are brought into close apposition. The sutures are removed on the eighth postoperative day. Mating can resume 14 days postoperatively.

Injuries to the Penis and Associated Hematuria

DEFINITION. The most frequent injuries to the penis are abrasions on the penal crest, lacerations in the course of the urethral fold, and loss of the tip of the penis. The injuries are caused for the most part by biting or masturbation. Acute hematuria appears after flexion of the erect penis as a result of a lesion of the corpus cavernosum or in association with urolithiasis. Bleeding from the urethra as well as from the injuries is especially intensive during ejaculation, so the fertility of these boars decreases or disappears because of hemospermia. This type of injury-related bleeding should be distinguished by differential diagnosis from bleeding caused by ulcers of the diverticulum.

The prognosis is poor and treatment is not available for fistulae of the urethra, injuries to the tip of the penis accompanied by loss of tissue, and

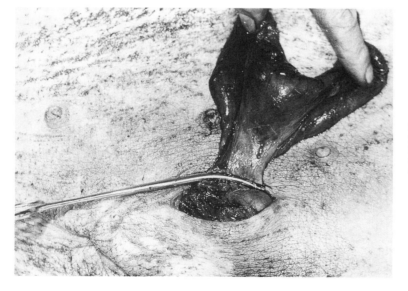

78.15. Resection of the preputial diverticulum. Artery clamp placed near transition to preputial cavity. Both halves of the diverticulum are exposed by dissection.

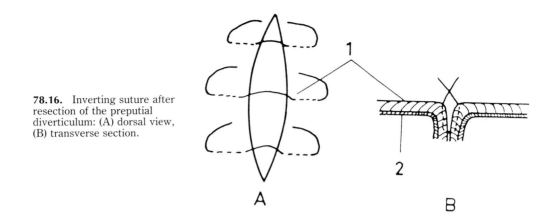

78.16. Inverting suture after resection of the preputial diverticulum: (A) dorsal view, (B) transverse section.

abnormalities such as hypospadia or persistent ligamentum penis.

TREATMENT. If surgical treatment of the injuries (sutures, regeneration of the wound) is required, it is undertaken in connection with the examination of the passively exteriorized penis discussed previously. However, suppression of the tendency to bleed that accompanies the erection of the penis is much more important, so that the wound can form a scab and epithelialize. For this it is necessary to keep the boar in isolation; reduce his reflex excitability by giving neuroleptics, e.g., diazepam (Valium), with food; promote the coagulation of blood by administering calcium solution and vitamin K; and interrupt mating for 4 weeks.

Amputation of the Claw

DEFINITION. Infection of claw wounds caused by pyogenic bacteria often turns into a purulent arthritis of the pedal joint with osteomyelitis of the distal and middle phalanges. The disease involves primarily the outer claws of the posterior limbs and causes an impotentia coeundi. As a rule, conservative attempts to treat this condition cause its protraction and deterioration. Therefore, amputation should be performed as soon as possible to prevent the formation of extensive necroses of the soft parts and enable primary healing by suturing the wound. The mating capacity of the boar returns after amputation of the claw.

TREATMENT. The amputation is a very painful procedure. It necessitates general anesthesia as well as a local infiltration anesthesia (forelimbs) or a spinal anesthesia (posterior limbs) as described earlier.

Preparation of the operative field (washing and shaving, removal of fat, disinfection) should reach as far as the tarsus or carpus so that the bandage can later be attached there with tape. To suppress bleeding during the operation, an elastic ligature (Esmarch's bandage) is placed immediately distal to the tarsus or carpus.

The operation begins by making a circular incision at the edge of the horny capsule and extending it diagonally across the heel. In this way the pedal joint is opened and the distal phalanx is disarticulated. The next step is the exarticulation of the second phalanx. A 5- to 6-cm incision (Fig. 78.17) is made across the outside surface of the second phalanx, extending across the pastern joint into the distal region of the first phalanx. Using this incision, the second phalanx is excised from the soft parts and exarticulated in the pastern joint. The cartilage of the distal articular surface of the first phalanx is removed with a curette.

After the exarticulation of both distal phalanges, all necrotic and discolored tissue is removed from the incision cavity and the navicular bone located in the heel is excised. With tweezers, the stumps of the sinews of the extensor tendon and the deep flexor tendon are then pulled up from their synovial sheaths and resected as far proximally as possible. After this, the incision is ready for suturing, which is done with thick silk. The sutures should bring the walls of the wound cavity into apposition over the entire breadth of the surface. An oily chlortetracycline suspension is instilled in the closed wound, and the stump is covered with gauze saturated with chlortetracycline.

Before the bandage is applied, the accessory digits must be specially padded with absorbent cotton. The bandage consists of three layers: cotton, gauze, and adhesive tape. The cotton should cover the stump up to the fetlock, including the accessory digits. The gauze bandage should be tight to have a compression effect. The adhesive tapes that are finally placed over the bandage act as mechanical protection and keep the gauze and cotton in place; they should reach as far as the metatarsus or metacarpus. The healthy claw remains outside the bandage. The elastic ligature is removed after the bandage has been put in place. If there is heavy bleeding from the stump, the ligature can be applied for another 20 minutes.

If the affected limb is knocked violently against

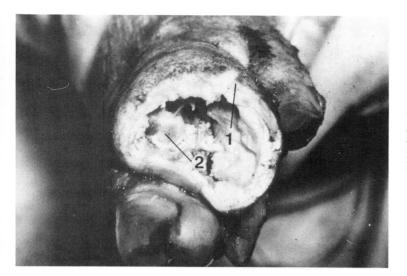

78.17. Amputation of the claw: (*1*) lateral incision for exarticulation of the second phalanx, (*2*) distal end of first phalanx.

the floor or wall during the awakening stage, the pig must be anesthetized or sedated once more.

The bandage is removed 8 days postoperatively under general anesthesia, the sutures are taken out, and a new bandage is applied after dressing the wound. On the 16th postoperative day, the wound is examined again. The rims should now be epithelialized, and the center should show signs of granulation. If this is the case, a new bandage is appied. This can be removed after another 8 days without veterinary supervision. If the healing has not yet reached this stage, super-vision should be continued.

Resection of the Canine Teeth

DEFINITION. Starting with the eighth month of life, the mandibular canine teeth of the boar have grown so long that they are a dangerous weapon. The boar uses them when he thrusts sideways or upward with his head. Attacks on human beings often produce injuries to the knee. To make deal-ing with boars less dangerous, the mandibular canines are sawed off. Pinching them off makes the teeth splinter and injures the gums.

TREATMENT. The boar is anesthetized with a short-acting barbiturate or a combination of aza-perone and methomidate and is placed on his side. With a wire saw 60–80 cm long, such as the one used for embryotomy, the canines are sawed off from the oral to buccal direction. The cut is made a few millimeters from the gums so that no soft parts are injured. Since the canines grow con-tinually, they must be shortened again a few months later. The resection of the maxillary canines is usually not necessary.

For further information on surgical procedures see Bühner 1958, Schulze and Bollwahn 1962, Bollwahn 1974, Evans and West 1976, and Bollwahn and Schoon 1980.

REFERENCES

Berge, E., and Westhues, M. 1969. Tieraerztliche Operationslehre 29. Auflage. Berlin, Hamburg: Paul Parey.
Bollwahn, W. 1974. Die Untersuchung des Eberpenis. DTW 81:235.
Bollwahn, W., and Schoon, H. 1980. Clinical and pathohistological findings in preputial ulcers of boars. DTW 87.
Bühner, F. 1958. Eine einfache chirurgische Ver-schlussmethode fur alle Scheiden- und Uterusvor-falle. Tieraerztl Umsch 13:183.
Evans, L. E., and West, J. K. 1976. Resection of the preputial diverticulum in the boar. Proc 4th Int Congr Pig Vet Soc, Iowa State Univ.
Schulze, W., and Bollwahn, W. 1962. Zu den Erkrankungen der Sauen vor, wahrend und nach der Geburt. DTW 69:641.

79 Disease Surveillance at Slaughter

A. M. Pointon

A. R. Mercy

L. Backstrom

G. D. Dial

RECORDING DISEASE data at slaughter defines herd health status for subclinical conditions, enabling veterinarians to link disease rates associated with certain environmental conditions and husbandry practices with biologic and financial performance. The health status of pigs can be quantified during their most costly phase of production, the grow/finish phase, by monitoring a range of organ systems from a representative sample of pigs taken from the grow/finish population.

The national slaughter surveillance schemes developed in Scandinavia contributed significantly to the ongoing international trend away from individual animal health management to a herd- and industry-based approach (Biering-Sorensen 1965; Backstrom and Bremer 1976; Willeberg et al. 1984–85). Surveillance schemes have been used by researchers to define interactions between animals, agents, environmental conditions, and management practices (Backstrom 1973; Lindqvist 1974; Aalund et al. 1976; Backstrom and Bremer 1978; Flesja et al. 1984; Martinsson and Lundeheim 1986). Through surveillance schemes, researchers have identified "risk factors" associated with disease complexes enabling them to manipulate management practices to maximize profit while minimizing disease. The increasing intensification of production systems and rising social pressures for assurances on animal welfare and product safety will likely make disease surveillance at slaughter an essential component of effective pig herd health management.

While the European schemes vary in design, they each have the same basic objectives (Pointon et al. 1987). In general, the primary objective has been to improve the diagnosis of subclinical diseases, so action can be taken to decrease disease on a herd basis. Secondary objectives have been to provide a cost-effective mechanism for reducing losses during growth and processing and to decrease the herd-to-herd spread of diseases via the ongoing monitoring of breeding stock source herds. European surveillance schemes also have

been aimed at minimizing the use of antibiotics and reducing the risk of residues. In addition, the schemes have been used to define industry problems and provide a basis for case-control studies to quantify the determinants of disease, so that economically sound management practices can be implemented. Slaughter-monitoring data is also of value in formulating extension messages for producers.

The slaughter check approach used in Scandinavia, where lesions are recorded in all stock, has been modified for use in the Pig Health Monitoring Schemes (PHMS) of Australia (Pointon et al. 1987; Mercy and Brennan 1988) and the United States (Pointon and Hueston 1990) to accommodate limited staff resources and fast-chain speeds (>500 pigs/hour). Inspections are performed on a sample of stock for participating producers who pay a fee for checks. In addition to providing reports for use as an individual herd health management tool, the data are collated centrally for use by industry. However, since producers participate voluntarily in the PHMS, the data do not represent a random sample of all herds, thus, caution is needed in extrapolating these data to the industry as a whole.

Fourteen production-limiting and zoonotic conditions are recorded in Australia (Pointon et al. 1987), including ileitis, nephritis, and sarcoptic mange, which have not been regularly included in previous schemes. All lesions are recorded irrespective of severity; however, severity scores are reported where appropriate. The recording of all lesions prevents the underestimation of diseases, such as pneumonia (Wallgren et al. 1990), pleurisy, and ascariasis (Wallgren, personal communication), that occurs when meat inspectors only record moderate to severe lesions. Severity scoring and disease prevalence estimates must be accurate and repeatable in order to provide reliable information on emerging disease and to detect changes in the prevalence of disease following the implementation of control programs. Quality control is achieved, in part, by using a small core of inspectors trained in veterinary pathology or by using veterinarians funded by the industry specifically for conducting surveillance. Also, careful consideration is given to sample size before conducting this slaughter surveillance. Data integrity is monitored routinely at the centralized data management bureau.

All data is sent to a bureau where it is immediately tabulated and summarized to facilitate timely management decisions. A detailed report on disease prevalence and severity in all individual groups monitored is then sent to the owner/manager and consultant of the herd. This contrasts with other systems (Willeberg et al. 1984–85) where data is only provided to producers when disease rates exceed programmed tolerance levels. Data is also summarized by herd size and region to facilitate development of target levels and to define localized research and extension priorities. Practicing veterinarians rather than state-employed specialists are responsible for on-farm follow-up. Farm visits can be timed so that results are used in a timely fashion to reinforce or encourage the implementation of health control measures. Immediate exposure of producers to the results of health surveillance helps to improve the utility of the information provided and increases support for the scheme.

FREQUENCY AND TIMING OF INSPECTIONS.
Inspections should be performed quarterly to coincide with predicted seasonal peaks of lesions at slaughter (Table 79.1) (Straw et al. 1986a). Additional checks can be strategically timed to allow the monitoring of the efficacy of disease preventive measures. Less frequent checks may miss peaks of disease but may be useful diagnostically to identify causes of disease epidemics. Inspections also can be done according to the disease history of the grow/finish herd to diagnostically investigate suspected problems and to determine what control measures need implementing.

In contrast to the United States, pneumonia was most prevalent during the summer, and liver spots were least common during the spring in the mediterranean climate of southwest Western Australia (Mercy and Brennan 1988). Some variation in seasonal patterns, therefore, may be anticipated in different climatic zones where differing production methods and facility types are used.

The inspection frequency selected by producers and their veterinarians participating in the Australian PHMS varies with herd size (Table 79.2). In herds with >500 sows, more frequent checks are used in order to detect emerging herd problems and to monitor prevalence fluctuations. Herds with <200 sows more commonly utilize the service for the diagnosis of problems and for disease detection than for monitoring herd trends.

GUIDELINES FOR SAMPLE SELECTION.
Monitoring the prevalence of pigs with gross lesions at slaughter provides an assessment of disease spread within herds. Prevalence monitoring for subclinical diseases is the only mechanism for quantifying disease within a herd and is useful for assessing conditions where severity scoring is not feasible or warranted, such as pericarditis and ileitis. Prevalence monitoring also provides supplementary information on the level of a disease such as pneumonia within a herd when severity scores do not consistently predict the impact of a disease

Table 79.1.   The seasonal pattern of diseases found in slaughter pigs

Disease	Summer	Autumn	Winter	Spring
Pneumonia[a]	+	+ + +	+	
Pleurisy[a]	+ + +	+ + +	+	+ + +
Atrophic rhinitis[a]	+ + +	+	+	+
Ascarids[a]	+ + +	+	+	
Mange[b]	+		+ + +	+ + +

Note: + + + = peak prevalence; + = least prevalence.
[a]Extracted from Straw et al. (1986a).
[b]Flesja and Ulvesaeter (1979); Mercy and Brennan (1988).

Table 79.2.   Average number of groups of pigs monitored at slaughter per year according to herd size in the South and Western Australian slaughter surveillance schemes (1987–90)

Number of Sows	Number of Inspections/year		Average Interval between Inspections (months)[a]
	South Australia	Western Australia	
1–25	0.9 (8)	1.13 (5)	12.1
26–50	1.23 (42)	1.36 (46)	9.2
51–100	1.90 (55)	1.77 (61)	6.5
101–200	2.42 (19)	2.09 (24)	5.3
201–500	3.94 (6)	3.36 (10)	3.4
>500	6.52 (9)	4.14 (6)	2.2
Finishing herds	(0)	1.95 (8)	6.2

Note: ( ) = number of herds.
[a]Based on the total number of inspections performed in both schemes.

on herd performance (see Table 79.9). It has previously been suggested that a minimum sample of 30 lungs should be monitored to predict the severity of respiratory disease within herds (Straw et al. 1986a). However, failure to relate sample size of the group to be monitored to farm and herd size limits the accuracy of prevalence estimates. Sample size must be defined to allow an assessment of data reliability and enable practitioners to determine if changes in estimates have been significant. In the United States, prevalence estimates are often so inaccurate that the data provided is worthless, since only a sample of 20–30 pigs is commonly inspected, irrespective of herd size (Pointon et al.1990).

Population Sampled. Lesions monitored at slaughter should be related directly to the "at risk" population. Interpretation of lesions recorded in market pigs is dependent on the rate of lesion resolution. Guidelines for determining the ages that pigs have experienced a disease based upon slaughter data have been developed using literature reports of lesion healing times (Table 79.3). A 16-week premarket population should be used as the basis for selecting the sample, since this incorporates pigs infected with the slowest resolving conditions, atrophic rhinitis and pneumonia (if infected early with subsequent secondary infections). For conditions that resolve at faster rates, slaughter results can reliably be related only to older growing pigs. Samples based on the 16-week population will allow detection of a low prevalence of disease and estimation of prevalence with greater accuracy for faster resolving conditions, such as liver spots and ileitis (Table 79.3). Relating slaughter data to stock younger than that indicated in Table 79.3 should be done only if indicated clinically and if the age pattern of disease occurrence is known.

Animals Sampled. A knowledge of the source, age, and performance of stock to be inspected is helpful in the interpretation of slaughter results. The population size to be represented by the sample must be determined to allow selection of the appropriate sample to be inspected. Sample size must also be considered in relation to the number of pigs normally marketed together. In general, pigs from more than 1 week of production need to be pooled in herds having less than 175 sows, to ensure that a sufficient number are inspected to achieve the proposed targets for disease detection and accuracy of prevalence estimates.

Selecting Sample Size

DETECTION OF DISEASE. In order to be confident of an assessment of absence of specific gross lesions in a herd, the sample size must be adequate to detect at least one positive pig in herds where disease is present at a low prevalence (Table 79.4). In practice, this is determined by the lowest expected prevalence, if in fact the disease is present. When calculating the sample size, the herd population used is determined by the condition that resolves at the slowest rate. In most herds, this will be atrophic rhinitis (Table 79.3), where the population to which results are to be related are within 16 weeks of slaughter. Using a typical market group size as the sample monitored, detection of one positive case given a 10% herd prevalence with 95% confidence is generally achievable for herds with more than 50 sows. A market group sample size is usually a sufficient size for most conditions. The numbers of pigs that must be examined to detect diseases varies with percentage of diseased animals in the population, herd size, and desired accuracy of the estimate (Table 79.4).

To detect enzootic pneumonia given a 10% herd prevalence with 95% confidence, a sample of 28 is required. This sample would be produced on a weekly basis by an 80-sow herd producing 18 pigs/sow/year. To detect a 5% prevalence with 95% confidence, a sample of 54 would be required, which is equivalent to the weekly production of a 156-sow herd producing 18 pigs/sow/year.

Table 79.3. Guidelines for defining populations to which slaughter lesions can be reliably related

Condition	"At risk" Population (before market)	Reference
Enzootic pneumonia	8–16 weeks	Backstrom and Bremer (1976); Wallgren et al. (1990); Noyes et al. (1990)
Pleurisy	8–12 weeks	Martinsson and Lundheim (1985); Mousing (1988)
Ascarid liver lesions		
Mild: first exposure	3 weeks	Copeman and Gaafar (1972); Jorgensen et al. (1975)
Moderately severe reinfection	6–12 weeks	Eriksen (1982); Bernardo et al. (1990a)
Atrophic rhinitis	4–5 months	Straw et al. (1986a); Scheidt et al. (1990)
Pleuropneumonia	10–12 weeks	Thacker, Clark (personal communication)
Ileitis–proliferative enteropathy	4–6 weeks	Rowland and Lawson (1986)
Necrotic enteritis	>4 weeks?	Emsbo (1951); Rowland and Hutchings (1978)
Regional ileitis	>4 weeks?	
Mange, high average score	4–5 months	Davies et al. (1990)
Leptospirosis-nephritis	4 months	Jones et al. (1987)

Table 79.4.   Sample sizes necessary to detect disease at low prevalence in different populations

Preslaughter Population	Percentage of Diseased Animals in Population					
	5%		10%		20%	
	90%[a]	95%[a]	90%	95%	90%	95%
100	36	44	20	25	10	13
125	38	47	20	25	10	13
150	39	48	20	26	10	13
175	39	49	21	26	10	13
200	40	50	21	26	10	13
250	41	52	21	27	10	13
300	42	53	21	27	10	13
450	43	55	22	28	10	13
650	43	56	22	28	10	13
750	44	56	22	28	10	13
3000	45	58	22	28	10	13

Source: Adapted from Cannon and Roe (1982).
[a]Confidence level.

ESTIMATING PREVALENCE. Besides detecting disease, the other principal reason for monitoring disease at slaughter is to estimate the prevalence of a condition with a desired level of confidence and accuracy (Table 79.5). Accuracy refers to the allowable error for estimating prevalence. For example, one may want to be 95% confident of being within 10% of the "true" prevalence of a disease. The sample size needed for determining the prevalence of a disease depends on the expected prevalence of the condition, the desired confidence level, the desired accuracy of the estimate, and size of the population represented (Cannon and Roe 1982). For a given level of accuracy and statistical confidence, the largest sample size for a population is required at prevalence estimates of 50%. The variance (i.e., a measure indicative of the fluctuations in repeated disease prevalence estimates on that herd) will be greatest for mid-prevalence estimates. Therefore, more animals must be sampled to reduce the variance (Fig. 79.1).

In practice the sample size must be adjusted for small populations to allow for nonreplacement of those sampled; e.g., when estimating prevalence at an accuracy of 10% with 90% confidence, the sample size must be reduced for populations <700 pigs (Fig. 79.2). Assuming a 16-week population of 700 pigs in a herd of 125 sows producing 18 pigs/sow/year, approximately 1½ weeks production would be required for the sample of 68 needed to provide an accuracy of 10% at 90% confidence (Table 79.5). A smaller sample from the same population will result in a reduced level of accuracy, with diseases having about 50% prevalence; smaller sample sizes will have less effect on the accuracy of prevalence estimates for diseases occurring at high or low prevalence. The extremes of prevalence require smaller sample sizes for accuracies similar to that sought for mid-prevalance estimates (Pointon et al. 1990). The target accuracy should be 10% with 90% or 95% confidence. In herds with >500 sows, an accuracy of 5% with 90% confidence is achievable using the weekly market pigs as the sample.

The sample required to achieve 10% accuracy with 90% and 95% confidence for a prevalence estimate is larger than that required to detect the presence of disease at a 5% or 10% prevalence (95% confidence level) for all population sizes. Therefore, if slaughter monitoring is being used to both detect the presence of a disease and to estimate prevalence, sample size should be calculated based on estimating prevalence.

MONITORING PROCEDURES

Conditions Monitored. Gross lesions monitored include those conditions commonly associated with economically significant subclinical herd infections: sarcoptic mange, ascarid liver spots, pneumonia, pleurisy, pericarditis, peritonitis, pleuropneumonia, ileitis, and atrophic rhinitis. The lesions and scoring systems used for conditions routinely monitored have been described previously (Straw et al. 1986b). Monitoring procedures for conditions not described previously (e.g., ileitis and nephritis) and conditions where new severity scoring systems have been developed (e.g., sarcoptic mange, nephritis, or liver spots) are provided in the interpretation of slaughter data section of this chapter. Other conditions potentially considered when establishing a surveillance system include lungworm, abscessation, tuberculosis, hernia, erysipelas, esophogastric ulcer, arthritis, foot lesions, kidney worm, nephritis, and pale soft exudative pork. These latter conditions are relatively uncommon, require additional staff to perform, or are recorded only if a problem is suspected. Meat inspectors may be asked to provide data on tuberculosis and abscessation/pyaemia. In the Australian scheme (Pointon et al. 1987; Mercy and Brennan 1988), where between 150 and 250 pigs are slaughtered/hour, it is feasible to routinely score kidneys and check the carcasses for trimming damaged tissue resulting from abcessation/pyaemia and arthritis.

Table 79.5. Guide to selecting sample size to estimate prevalence and to assist in interpreting results

Population Size	Estimated Prevalence[a] (%)	Accuracy[b] (90% confidence level)				Accuracy (95% confidence level)			
		±5%	10%	15%	20%	±5%	10%	15%	20%
		(Number of Animals to be Sampled)							
200	10	66	22	11	6	82	30	15	9
	20	93	36	19	11	111	47	24	15
	30	107	44	23	14	124	58	31	18
	40	113	49	25	16	130	63	34	21
	50	115	51	26	17	132	65	35	22
	60	113	49	25	16	130	63	34	21
	70	107	44	23	14	124	58	31	18
	80	93	36	19	11	111	47	24	15
	90	66	22	11	6	82	30	15	9
500	10	82	24	11	6	109	35	15	9
	20	129	43	19	11	165	55	27	15
	30	156	51	25	14	196	70	36	20
	40	171	58	29	16	212	78	41	23
	50	176	60	30	17	217	81	43	24
	60	171	58	29	16	212	78	41	23
	70	156	51	25	14	196	70	36	20
	80	129	43	19	11	165	55	27	15
	90	82	24	11	6	109	35	15	9
700	10	86	24	11	6	116	35	15	9
	20	139	43	19	11	182	61	27	15
	30	172	57	25	14	221	72	36	20
	40	190	65	29	16	242	82	41	23
	50	195	68	30	17	248	85	43	24
	60	190	65	29	16	242	82	41	23
	70	172	57	25	14	221	72	36	20
	80	139	43	19	11	182	61	27	15
	90	86	24	11	6	116	35	15	9
1000	10	97	24	11	6	122	35	15	9
	20	148	43	19	11	198	61	27	15
	30	185	57	25	14	244	81	36	20
	40	206	65	29	16	270	92	41	23
	50	213	68	30	17	278	96	43	24
	60	206	65	29	16	270	92	41	23
	70	185	57	25	14	244	81	36	20
	80	148	43	19	11	198	61	27	15
	90	97	24	11	6	122	35	15	9
>3000	10	97	24	11	6	138	35	15	9
	20	173	43	19	11	246	61	27	15
	30	227	57	25	14	291	81	36	20
	40	260	65	29	16	329	92	41	23
	50	271	68	30	17	341	96	43	24
	60	260	65	29	16	329	92	41	23
	70	227	57	25	14	291	81	36	20
	80	173	43	19	11	246	61	27	15
	90	97	24	11	6	138	35	15	9

Source: Extracted from Cannon and Roe (1982) and Pointon et al. (1990).
[a]Proportion of pigs with lesions in the population sampled.
[b]Range of prevalences in which the true population prevalence falls.

Monitoring Condemned Viscera. In a survey of condemnations in a processing plant in Minnesota (slaughtering 650–950 pigs/hour), approximately 10% of viscera sets were condemned for fluid/fecal contamination, generally involving both abdominal and thoracic organs (Pointon 1990, unpublished). An additional 10% of viscera sets were condemned for disease, with about 75% of those for diseases of thoracic organs alone. Because condemned viscera could not be handled, due to the potential for inadvertent contamination of clean viscera, these could only be scored visually. The specificity and sensitivity of such visually scored viscera were compared to the "gold standard," where organs were handled during inspection (Table 79.6). A moderate underestimate of all conditions occurred when lesions were scored only visually. Misclassification of lesions (i.e., reduced specificity) was greatest for pneumonia, where 88% of animals classified as positive actually had lesions.

As a result of these findings, it is suggested

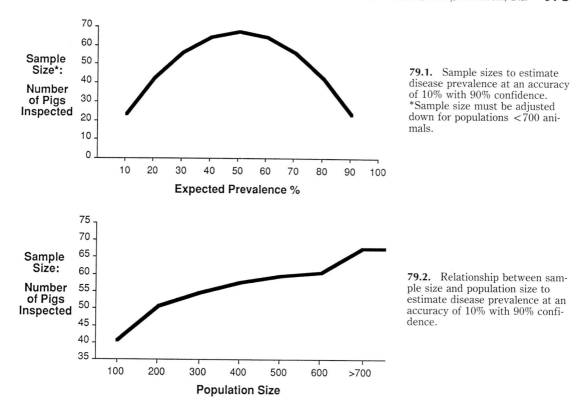

79.1. Sample sizes to estimate disease prevalence at an accuracy of 10% with 90% confidence. *Sample size must be adjusted down for populations <700 animals.

79.2. Relationship between sample size and population size to estimate disease prevalence at an accuracy of 10% with 90% confidence.

Table 79.6.   Specificity and sensitivity of recording lesions at slaughter by visual and manual inspection

Condition	Prevalence ("Gold Standard") Visual and Manual (%)	Specificity (%)	Sensitivity (%)	Predictive Value[a] Positive (%)	Negative (%)
Pneumonia	69	73	85	88	69
Pleurisy	33	97	81	93	91
Pericarditis	33	94	63	83	84
Pleuropneumonia	14	100	86	100	98
Ascariasis	41	86	70	78	81

Note: Calculations based on results of monitoring 49 sets of viscera condemned due to disease.
[a]Predictive value = the predictive value of a positive result is the proportion of the test-positive animals that really have the disease.

that all viscera condemned due to disease be inspected, but that they be inspected by visual means alone. These condemned viscera should not be omitted, for this may bias the prevalence estimate. To minimize errors in visual scoring, viscera condemned due to contamination are scored only for peritonitis. Whereas peritonitis may be associated with fecal contamination, the presence of other lesions may be assumed to occur independent of contamination. The omission of contaminated organs from a slaughter examination requires the inclusion of additional animals in the sample group to ensure that a sufficient number of animals are inspected. To avoid misclassification of lesions present in viscera condemned for conditions such as pleuropneumonia, some condemned viscera will have to be handled

so that tissue samples can be submitted for laboratory testing.

Procedures for Conducting Surveillance. A standardized data entry sheet should be used at the abattoir (Fig. 79.3). Disease conditions are monitored at several sites along the processing chain and different procedures are used for each. Examine carcasses as they hang on the rail before the evisceration table and determine presence of hypersensitivity lesions, such as mange, using a grading system with numerical scores 0, 1, 2, or 3 (Fig. 79.4).

Viscera are placed on trays and are passed or condemned by meat inspection staff on the basis of either disease or contamination. In fast plants (>500 pigs processed/hour), the following ap-

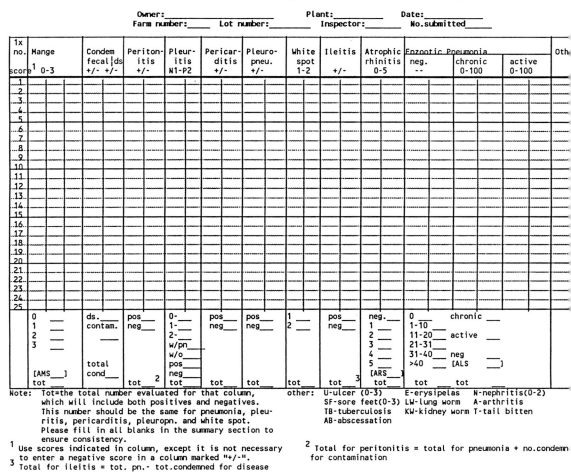

Swine Slaughter Surveillence Program

Owner:_____   Plant:_____   Date:_____
Farm number:_____   Lot number:_____   Inspector:_____   No.submitted_____

1x no. score[1]	Mange 0-3	Condem fecal⋮ds +/- +/-	Periton- itis +/-	Pleur- itis N1-P2	Pericar- ditis +/-	Pleuro- pneu. +/-	White spot 1-2	Ileitis +/-	Atrophic rhinitis 0-5	Enzootic Pneumonia neg. --	chronic 0-100	active 0-100	Oth
1													
2													
3													
4													
5													
6													
7													
8													
9													
10													
11													
12													
13													
14													
15													
16													
17													
18													
19													
20													
21													
22													
23													
24													
25													

Summary section:

Mange	Condem	Periton itis	Pleur itis	Pericar ditis	Pleuro pneu	White spot	Ileitis	Atrophic rhinitis	Enzootic Pneumonia		
0 ___	ds. ___	pos___	0- ___	pos___	pos___	1 ___	pos___	neg. ___	0 ___	chronic ___	
1 ___	contam. ___	neg___	1- ___	neg___	neg___	2 ___	neg___	1 ___	1-10 ___	active ___	
2 ___	___		2- ___					2 ___	11-20 ___		
3 ___			w/pn___					3 ___	21-31 ___		
			w/o___					4 ___	31-40 ___	neg ___	
	total		pos___					5 ___	>40 ___	[ALS ___]	
[AMS ___]	cond___		neg___					[ARS ___]			
tot ___		tot___[2]	tot___	tot ___	tot ___	tot ___	tot ___[3]	tot ___	tot ___	tot ___	

Note: Tot=the total number evaluated for that column, which will include both positives and negatives. This number should be the same for pneumonia, pleuritis, pericarditis, pleuropn. and white spot. Please fill in all blanks in the summary section to ensure consistency.

other: U-ulcer (0-3) E-erysipelas N-nephritis(0-2)
SF-sore feet(0-3) LW-lung worm A-arthritis
TB-tuberculosis KW-kidney worm T-tail bitten
AB-abscessation

[1] Use scores indicated in column, except it is not necessary to enter a negative score in a column marked "+/-".
[2] Total for peritonitis = total for pneumonia + no.condemn for contamination
[3] Total for ileitis = tot. pn.- tot.condemned for disease

79.3. Disease lesion record sheet for use at high-speed (>500 pigs/hour) abattoirs.

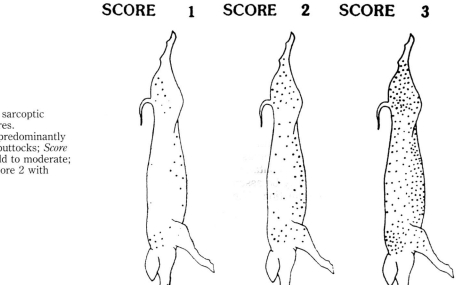

SCORE 1   SCORE 2   SCORE 3

79.4. Examples of sarcoptic mange severity scores.
Score 1 = localized predominantly to head, belly, and buttocks; *Score 2* = generalized, mild to moderate; *Score 3* = severe, score 2 with intense areas.

proach is recommended. On trays that pass inspection, score liver spots and palpate and inspect ileum as the trays pass. Check to ensure that meat inspectors have not missed peritonitis or abscessation. A technical assistant should remove lungs with the heart attached for scoring later. In slower abattoirs, it may be feasible to inspect all organs, including lungs, as they pass on the trays. Regardless of speed, lesion scores of all viscera in all trays should be recorded, even those having no lesions. The total number of trays acts as the denominator for calculations of prevalence of visceral lesions.

Trays containing viscera condemned due to disease (either partially or totally) should be inspected visually only. The presence of visible lesions and the fact that viscera were condemned for disease should be noted. Viscera lesions need to be recorded only if they occur; however, an entry should be made for all lungs irrespective of lesion status, to enable calculation of the denominator. Ilea cannot be inspected on trays containing condemned viscera.

Only peritonitis should be monitored on trays containing viscera condemned for contamination to minimize biasing results for other diseases. The occurrence of contaminated viscera should also be noted on the data sheet. Similar monitoring of condemned viscera is recommended in both large and small plants to avoid bias. Recording the number and reason for condemnation and the total trays inspected is required so that denominators can be calculated.

ILEITIS. Palpate and inspect the terminal ileum as the trays pass by. A thickened wall is indicative of ileitis. Careful palpation can be used to distinguish postmortem smooth-muscle contraction from disease. In the United States, only the presence of lesions is noted whereas in Australia an attempt is made to distinguish lesion severity (Pointon et al. 1987); thickened ilea are differentiated from ilea with both thickening and edema and congestion of the mesentery.

LIVERS. As viscera trays pass by, examine livers, scoring them according to the number of white spots: grade 0, no lesions; grade 1, <10 spots; and grade 2, 10 or more lesions.

HEARTS. Inspect hearts on the tray if viscera are condemned due to disease, otherwise evaluate hearts later, after they have been removed from the trays along with the lungs.

LUNGS. As needed (plants operating at >500 pigs per hour), label lungs with herd identification and arrange separate storage by herd. The volume of lung with cranio-ventral pneumonia should be severity scored (Fig. 79.5) and evaluated as to whether lesions are acute or chronic. The proportion of missing lung should be estimated in chronic cases. Pleuropneumonia should be recorded separately.

PLEUROPNEUMONIA. The dorsal aspect of the diaphragmatic lobes of the lungs should be carefully inspected, along with the other lobes for the presence of pleuropneumonia lesions.

PLEURISY. When present, pleurisy should be recorded as grade 1 (adhesions between lobes of lungs) or grade 2 (adhesions of lungs to chest wall). It should also be determined if pleurisy is in association with normal (N1, N2) or pneumonic (P1, P2) lungs.

KIDNEYS. If time and labor permit, while kidneys are on the tray or while they are still in the carcass, they should be inspected for the presence of scars visible through the capsule. When lesions are present, they should be scored grades 1 or 2, as described in the section on NEPHRITIS.

ESOPHOGASTRIC ULCERS. In order to assess the stomach for esophogastric ulcer, it must be removed from the trays. Stomachs should be incised along the greater curvature, turned inside out, and washed before scoring.

ATROPHIC RHINITIS. Snouts are scored for severity, grades 0–5 (Fig. 79.6). An appropriate sample of heads that are transversely sectioned with a saw at the second premolar teeth should be ex-

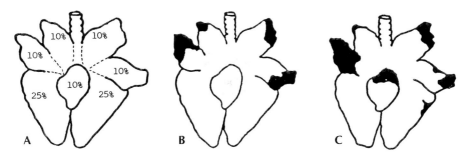

79.5. Examples of pneumonia scores (Straw et al. 1986b). (A) Normal lung and percent of whole for each lobe. (B) Lesioned lung with lobe score of 12%. (C) Lesioned lung with lobe score of 20%.

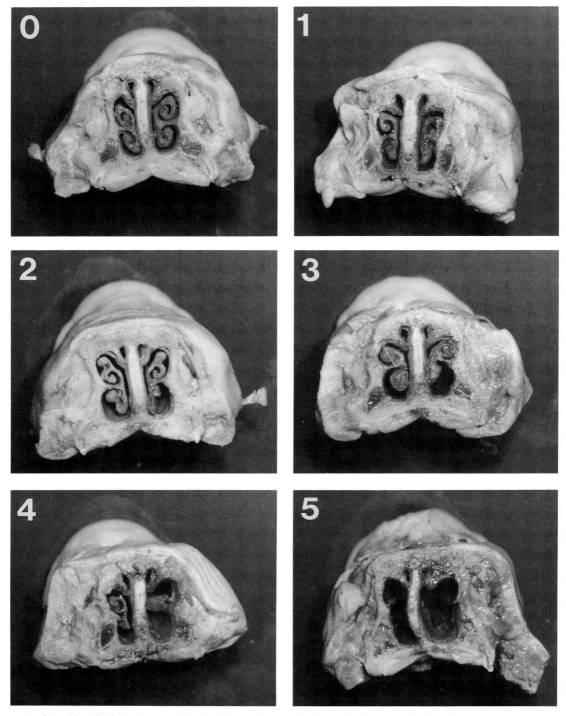

79.6. Atrophic rhinitis lesions showing typical severity grades from 0 to 5 (Done et al. 1964; Runnels 1982; Straw et al. 1983). (Courtesy of Dr. Barbara Straw.)

amined to detect the presence of significant lesions (i.e., grade 3, 4, or 5 at 10% prevalence with 95% confidence). In most instances, approximately 30 snouts will need examining. If a significant lesion is detected, additional snouts should be examined to improve the accuracy of the estimated prevalence.

OTHER CONDITIONS. Arthritis and abscessation/pyaemia can be more easily checked in the low-speed abattoirs, for there is sufficient time to observe, check, and record observations made by meat inspectors. In higher-speed plants, additional technical assistance may be needed if accurate assessments are to be made.

INTERPRETATION OF SLAUGHTER REPORTS.
The interpretation of slaughter surveillance reports requires consideration of the statistical accuracy and level of confidence of the data, the clinical history of the slaughtered stock including duration of lesions, the growth performance of the group, the age of stock, and the environment/management conditions to which stock was exposed during growth.

Statistical Interpretation

SAMPLE SIZE RELATIVE TO STATISTICAL ADEQUACY.
The sample size of slaughtered stock monitored determines the prevalence of detectable gross lesions and the accuracy of each prevalence estimate in the slaughter check report (Tables 79.4 and 79.5). The average size of groups monitored increases with herd size in voluntary schemes funded by producers (Table 79.7).

In the South Australian scheme, most groups of pigs inspected from farrow-to-finish herds over 50 sows are adequate to detect a 10% prevalence with 95% confidence. However, there is the potential that small sample sizes may lead to an underestimate of the number of herds affected with diseases occurring at a low within-herd prevalence. At normal slaughter group sizes, sample sizes will be sufficient to estimate prevalence at an accuracy of 10% with 90% confidence. For large herds (>300 sows), prevalence estimates will be accurate at 10% with 95% confidence. Populations used for these evaluations are represented by stock within 16 weeks of slaughter.

STATISTICAL INTERPRETATION OF HERD REPORTS.
Since lesion resolution rates vary for different conditions, the population to be sampled must be considered independently for each condition when determining the accuracy of data for each disease. For example, if 25 animals were inspected from a herd marketing 62 pigs/week, the accuracy would vary with prevalence estimates for different conditions (Table 79.8). If all 62 pigs were inspected, the accuracy of midrange prevalence would be substantially improved.

Clinical Association.
To assist in the interpretation of slaughter surveillance data, practitioners should encourage producers to keep a record of clinical observations and treatments. The duration of infections, e.g., pneumonia, determines the degree of growth depression (Noyes et al. 1990; Wallgren et al. 1990). Therefore, on-farm recording systems devised to identify peaks in infection will assist practitioners in relating morbidity and mortality information to lesions observed at slaughter. This can be achieved by establishing clinical indices for conditions of interest to determine the time of onset of peak infections and duration of lesions. Rubbing indices (rubbing episodes/pig/15 minutes) have been used as a basis of relating high-average mange score at slaughter to infestation of weaners with sarcoptic mange (Davies et al. 1990). Similar indices have been designed for pneumonia (Gardner and Hird 1990), atrophic rhinitis (coughing-sneezing episodes/pig/ 15 minutes), and ileitis (total pen scour days/ week).

Together with treatment and culling/mortality records, clinical indices add an important historic perspective to disease episodes and allows much more accurate interpretation of monitoring re-

Table 79.7. Average number of pigs monitored per inspection according to herd size in the South Australian and Minnesota slaughter surveillance schemes

	Average Sample Size[a]	
Number of Sows	South Australia (1987–90)[b]	Minnesota (1990)
1–25	15 (22)	(0)
26–50	24 (155)	20 (1)
51–100	37 (313)	19 (18)
101–200	50 (138)	27 (12)
201–500	59 (71)	37 (26)
>500	80 (176)	37 (10)
Finishing operation	. . .	30 (8)
Finish-off farm	. . .	44 (6)

Note: ( ) = number of inspections.
[a]Samples taken from the normal market lot.
[b]Davies and Moore, personal communication.

Table 79.8.   Accuracy of prevalence estimates for different conditions in a slaughter check of pigs from a herd of 180 sows producing 18 pigs/sow/year.

		Population Represented	Accuracy (90% confidence level)	
Condition	Estimated Prevalence	Premarket	25 Sampled	62 Sampled
Ileitis	10%	240 (4 weeks)	±10%	±10%
Pneumonia	80%	480 (8 weeks)	±15%	±10%
Liver Spots	50%	480 (8 weeks)	±20%	±10%
Atrophic rhinitis (severity grades 3, 4, and 5)	50%	960 (16 weeks)	±20%	±15%
Mange	95%	960 (16 weeks)	±10%	±10%

Note: ( ) = age of premarket population to which lesion data can be related; defined by rate of lesion resolution (Table 79.3).

sults. Each age group should be monitored when they will most likely be showing clinical signs. For example, pigs might be examined for indications of pneumonia or atrophic rhinitis when first disturbed in the morning. Clinical indices should be recorded approximately once per week. A more definitive approach for determining the age at which clinical disease occurs in a group of pigs would be to perform cross-sectional serologic profiles for each age group. Serologic profiling has been suggested as a useful adjunct for slaughter surveillance for pneumonia (Wallgren et al. 1990) and pleuropneumonia (Pijoan 1990, personal communication).

Slaughtering pigs at a standard age (e.g., 180 days), rather than according to weight, will provide a reference point for comparing the influence of disease on performance between animals with varying lesion severity (Dumas et al. 1990). While slaughtering at a set age is impractical under field conditions, knowledge of age at slaughter provides essential information for the interpretation of lesions monitored (Backstrom and Bremer 1976).

Consideration of the environmental and management conditions under which the stock were reared will also assist interpretation. For example, atrophic rhinitis is more likely to depress performance in pigs raised under adverse environmental conditions (Straw et al. 1983; Martinsson and Lundeheim 1986). In all instances, the confounding effect of seasonal fluctuations in prevalence should be considered when interpreting results (Table 79.1).

Significance of Lesions

PNEUMONIA. A description of lesions and a scoring system has been previously proposed (Straw et al. 1986b). Pneumonic lesions typically appear as cranioventral consolidation, consistent with *Mycoplasma hyopneumoniae* and secondary bacterial infections. The proportions of affected lobes are recorded (Fig. 79.5) and in the case of chronic lesions, the amount of contraction must be estimated. The average lung score is calculated over all lungs inspected. Lesions are classified as acute or chronic. When both types of lesions are present in the same lung, the lesion is

classified as acute. Lesions of uncomplicated mycoplasma infection may resolve over 8 weeks, while lesions complicated by secondary infections may last 16 weeks (Table 79.4).

Pneumonia has been found to impair production in approximately half of the published studies (Morrison et al. 1986). It has been speculated that variation in results among studies in the growth effects of pneumonia may be attributed to differences in management and environmental conditions and differences in study design. One reason for the increased risk of severe lesions with increasing age may be the increased probability of effective exposure (Gardner and Hird 1990). In environmentally controlled performance trials it was demonstrated that pigs grew slower because of pneumonia, rather than slow-growing pigs being more susceptible to pneumonia (Pointon et al. 1985).

The impact of pneumonia has been critically appraised in 13 reports (Straw et al. 1989), in which a consistent relationship was found between impaired growth rate and feed efficiency in pigs infected with pneumonia. If reduced growth rate can be measured, then depressed feed conversion can be calculated and disease costs estimated. Table 79.9 provides references for studies showing the relationship between lesion severity at slaughter and growth performance, which appears to be less consistent and requires clinical and performance data to assist interpretation.

Slaughter data must be related to the pattern of disease within the herd to predict its biologic and financial significance. Studies that recorded the time of infection (Noyes et al. 1990; Wallgren et al. 1990) show that resolution of lesions occurs when pigs are infected at younger ages. The degree of growth depression was related to duration of infection. Consequently, the significance of chronic, mild lesions at slaughter is greater if infection is contracted early. A coughing index was used as an effective means of establishing the time of lesion onset (Gardner and Hird 1990). Increased coughing occurs at an average of 31 days after natural exposure (Pointon et al. 1985).

Growth rate is affected relatively more by clinical episodes than by subclinical disease (Willeberg et al. 1978). This result was supported in experimental studies that reported peak coughing

Table 79.9. Studies that show the relationship between severity of pneumonia at slaughter and depressed growth performance

Association Established	No Association
Lindqvist (1974)	Shuman and Earl (1956)
Pichler (1980)	Bjorklund and Henricson (1965)
Straw et al. (1983)	Jericho et al. (1975)
Burch (1984)	Morrison et al. (1985)
Straw et al. (1984)	Scheidt et al. (1990)
Cowart et al. (1990)	Wallgren et al. (1990)[a]
Gardner and Hird (1990)[a]	Noyes et al. (1990)[a]
Bernardo et al. (1990b)	

[a]Duration of infection or lesions defined.

postweaning when the greatest depression in performance occurred (Pointon et al. 1985). Slower growth rates in these herds was due primarily to reduced daily feed intake. Recording daily feed intake may also assist timing the onset and spread of infection.

In studies where the extent of lesions are associated with reduced performance (Table 79.9), the onset of infection and lesions are generally not recorded. In these trials, it may be assumed that environmental and management conditions were not conducive to resolution of lesions that may have become established at an early age, and that subsequent secondary infections maintained or extended lesions. The observation of more severe lesions in faster growing pigs at slaughter (Scheidt et al. 1990) suggests a later onset of infection, allowing insufficient time for resolution of lesions and a substantial detrimental effect on growth performance.

The additive influences of other diseases and secondary infections must be considered when assessing the significance of pneumonia in pig herds. Reductions in the prevalence of atrophic rhinitis is likely to be associated with a concomitant reduction in pneumonia (Bernardo et al. 1990b). Similarly, a reduction in ascariasis results in improved pneumonia scores (Underdahl and Kelley 1957). There is a significant positive correlation between pneumonia and pleuritis, indicating that control of pneumonia is likely to reduce the incidence of pleuritis (Backstrom and Bremer 1976). Recording the prevalence and severity of pneumonia is also a means of detecting adverse housing conditions, such as poor ventilation, that may in turn directly reduce daily feed intake.

PLEURITIS. Pleuritic lesions (Straw et al. 1986a) are classified as grade 1 (between lung lobes) and grade 2 (between lobes and thoracic pleura). Scoring of pleuritic lesions ensures that all cases of thoracic serositis are recorded and that the proportion of carcasses requiring pleura stripping or trimming of the carcass are recorded. Pleurisy has also been recorded as occurring in association with normal or pneumonic lungs. While one study demonstrated a strong association between pleurisy and pneumonia in individual pigs (Pointon and Sloane 1984), another reported that some herds had a low prevalence of pneumonia with a relatively high prevalence of pleurisy (Backstrom and Bremer 1976). When pleurisy and pneumonia are not related, it is unlikely that pneumonia control will lead to a reduction in pleuritis, especially when primary pleuritic agents are involved (e.g., *Mycoplasma hyorhinis, Haemophilus parasuis,* or *Streptococcus suis*). Pleuritis found in association with lesions typical of *Actinobacillus pleuropneumoniae* infection is not classified separately but recorded as pleuropneumonia.

Lesions of pleuritis heal slowly. Nonetheless, the prevalence of pleuritis at slaughter may be a remnant of far wider herd infection (Backstrom and Bremer 1976; Hartley et al. 1988; Mousing 1988). Backstrom and Bremer (1976) found the prevalence of pleuritis increases from 4% in pigs of 30-kg carcass weight to 10% in 60-kg pigs and then declines to 2–3% in pigs >100 kg. Mousing (1988) suggested that pleuritis found at slaughter does not develop prior to 3–4 months of age and cites a study by Martinsson and Lundheim (1985) who found very low levels at 2½ months. The greatest odds of having pleurisy were found to be at 5 months (Mousing 1988). The doubling in the prevalence of pleurisy observed in Danish fatteners, whose average age at slaughter has dropped from approximately 200 to 180 days over the past 10 years, has been attributed to the reduced time for resolution. Because of lesion resolution, the population to which pleuritic lesions at slaughter should be related are pigs within the last 8–12 weeks of production.

Pigs with pleurisy at slaughter have reduced growth rate (Lindqvist 1974). Pigs with severe lesions at slaughter may, therefore, suffer two economic costs: hand trimming of adhesions in some cases and an additional 8 days to reach slaughter (Hartley et al. 1988). The proportion of pigs requiring pleura stripping increased as days to slaughter lengthened. This observation highlights the need to know the age of pigs monitored relative to the herd average when interpreting slaughter data.

PLEUROPNEUMONIA (*ACTINOBACILLUS PLEURO-PNEUMONIAE*). There are numerous descriptions of lesions typical of *A. pleuropneumoniae* infection (Brandreth and Smith 1985; Nicolet 1986; Straw et al. 1986a). Chronic lesions with abscessation, a fibrotic capsule, and overlying pleuritis located on the dorsal aspect of the diaphragmatic lobes are considered typical. Early, friable, hemorrhagic lesions are less typical and may yield "minor taxon" haemophili (Done et al. 1990). *A. pleuropneumoniae* lesions resolve over 12 weeks in both clinical outbreaks and experimental studies (Clark 1990, personal communication; Thacker 1990, personal communication). After 12 weeks, the remaining lesion may be a cavitation of lung parenchyma in place of the healed abscess. Lesions detected at slaughter may, therefore, only reflect the presence of disease during the last 12 weeks of production.

The sensitivity of monitoring pleuropneumonia lesions at slaughter as an indication of herd infection is low. However, a high prevalence of pleuritis in slaughtered pigs in the absence of typical pneumonic lesions is often associated with serologic evidence of *A. pleuropneumoniae* infections (Backstrom and Gunnarsson 1976). Serologic profiles of breeding sows are also likely to be a more sensitive method of detecting infected herds (Nicolet 1986). Nonetheless, monitoring at slaughter is an easy and inexpensive method of ongoing disease surveillance. In large herds prone to pleuropneumonia disease, inspections should be timed to detect early cases at times of greatest risk. Pleuropneumonia depresses both average daily gain and feed efficiency. The association between depressed feed efficiency and daily gain reduction is not as great for pleuropneumonia as for pneumonia (Straw et al. 1989).

ATROPHIC RHINITIS. A subjective scoring system (Done et al. 1964; Runnels 1982) has been found to be more successful in predicting growth rate (Cowart et al. 1990) than linear measurement (millimeter) scores (Backstrom et al. 1982). Grade 3 and above scores are considered indicative of atrophic rhinitis. This method is practical and may be performed at all abattoirs with minimal cost. However, inspectors should be subjected to regular quality control checks to assure validity of data when comparing results between checks (D'Allaire et al. 1988).

A review of studies shows conflicting results on the reliability of severity scores for atrophic rhinitis as indicators of performance losses (Table 79.10). Thus, clinicians should collect herd performance data to determine whether lesions are associated with reduced performance. Pneumonia status should also be considered in light of rhinitis scores in order to evaluate the indirect effects of atrophic rhinitis (Morrison et al. 1985; Bernardo et al. 1990b).

The inconsistent results obtained from performance studies involving atrophic rhinitis (Straw et al. 1983) may be due to there being no effect of rhinitis under good production conditions compared with a severe effect under poor conditions with concomitant disease. The observations of milder lesions in older pigs (Scheidt et al. 1990) suggests partial resolution as animals get older (Nielsen et al. 1976). Consequently, age at slaughter is needed to assist interpretation of slaughter data on atrophic rhinitis. While infection with atrophic rhinitis pathogens likely occurs 16–20 weeks before slaughter (Straw et al. 1986a), the use of a sneezing index may assist in determining the time of peak infection and, thus, define the population to which slaughter data applies.

PERICARDITIS AND PERITONITIS. It is likely that lesions of pericarditis and peritonitis will resolve in a similar manner to pleurisy; however, there is no specific information confirming this. While not reducing the value of the carcass at slaughter, pericarditis will lead to condemnation of the thoracic organs and possibly livers, resulting in loss to the processor. Peritonitis is likely to cause partial trimming and, in some cases, condemnation of the entire carcass. The occurrence of peritonitis and pericarditis should be recorded to provide information on condemnations. Both conditions are an indicator of polyserositis infections, possibly resulting from severe *A. pleuropneumoniae* infections; other primary polyserositis agents; or secondary pneumonic infections. There is an association between pleurisy, pericarditis, and peritonitis but not with arthritis (Flesja and Ulvesaeter 1980). Since *Mycoplasma hyorhinis* and *Haemophilus parasuis* have a strong affinity for joints, it was concluded that these agents were not the main cause of the polyserositis complex.

Pigs with these lesions are most likely to have been clinically ill. In response to the detection of a herd problem at slaughter, there should be increased clinical surveillance, and records of treatments (dates, age, clinical signs, and responses to treatment) should be maintained to further define the problem and assist in the development of preventive strategies.

SARCOPTIC MANGE. Hypersensitivity lesions indicative of sarcoptic mange were recorded in 12% of slaughtered hogs in Norway (Flesja and Ulvesaeter 1979). On histologic examination, these red papules were consistent with mite infestation, though mites were not observed, presumably because they had been removed with the outer layers during scalding. Smeets et al. (1989) also reported that these gross lesions are consistent with the allergic reactions produced by sarcoptic mites. These lesions are seasonally related with a peak prevalence in winter (Flesja and Ulvesaeter 1979; Mercy and Brennan 1988; Smeets et al. 1989), which is likely to be related to increased winter survival of mites and increased transmission (Martineau et al. 1987). The prevalence of lesions also decreases in response to treatment for mange (Flesja and Ulvesaeter 1979).

The contention that sarcoptic mange hypersensitivity is the predominant cause of erythematous papules in the skin of slaughtered pigs is supported by the reproduction of characteristic lesions in experimentally infected pigs, the low-average herd mange score (AMS) observed in inspections of mange-free pigs, and by the pres-

Table 79.10. Studies that show the relationship between the severity of atrophic rhinitis scores and depressed growth performance

Associated	Not Associated
Giles et al. (1980)	Bjorklund and Henricson (1965)
Backstrom et al. (1975, 1976, 1982)	Backstrom et al. (1982)
Bernardo et al. (1990b)	Straw et al. (1983, 1984)
Cowart et al. (1990)	Morrison et al. (1985)
	Scheidt et al. (1990)

ence of greater levels of rubbing on farms with high lesion scores (Davies et al. 1990).These observations complement findings of Hollanders and Vercruysse (1990) that pigs with lesions have a higher prevalence of *Sarcoptes scabiei* in ear scrapings. While the duration of lesions has not been defined, Davies et al. (1990) found that infection of weaners was indicated in herds with high AMS (Table 79.3).

A severity scoring system for mangelike allergy lesions has been described by Pointon et al. (1987) (Fig. 79.4). Pigs classified as mild or grade 1 have localized clusters of papules, generally 2–5 mm in diameter, located behind the ears and on the thinner skin of the belly and thighs. Grade 2 carcasses have generalized lesions, which should be differentiated from grade 3 carcasses, which have generalized lesions with intense papular areas. Central craters or bite sites left by lice, pox, or fleas are not observed with sarcoptic mite hypersensitivity. The specificity of grade 1 lesions were found to be 78%; grade 2 and grade 3 lesions were >98% (Davies and Moore 1990). A low proportion of grade 1 mangelike lesions can be expected in cesarean-derived stock inspected at slaughter. However, generalized lesions (grades 2 and 3) are highly specific for mange.

Depressed growth rate and feed conversion of up to 10% occurs as a result of hypersensitivity to the mites, and poorer performance was associated with increasing severity of rubbing (Cargill and Dobson 1979). In two similar trials, AMS of 1.5 and 1.6 were associated with a reduction in growth rate of 6% (Davies and Moore 1990). Herds with high AMS are likely to have considerable rubbing and performance losses occurring from weaning to slaughter. Skin lesions, in conjunction with evaluation of pruritus, should be used in assessing treatment programs. An AMS of <0.5 is suggested as a target level for infected herds. The scoring system provides a method to diagnose both the presence and severity of mange on a herd basis, as well as providing an objective method of evaluating the efficacy of control measures.

Due to the specifity of 78% for grade 1 lesions, the predictive value of a low prevalence of grade 1 lesions is poor; i.e., slaughter surveillance cannot be used to prove absence or eradication. As it may also be difficult to demonstrate mites in mildly affected herds, the continued absence of generalized grade 2 and 3 lesions in slaughtered stock from herds using no mange treatments will increase the assurance of freedom from infection. When implementing this scoring system the specificity should be evaluated on a regional basis to assess the role of other agents that may cause skin lesions in mange-free pigs.

LIVER WHITE SPOTS (ASCARIASIS). The classification described for liver white spots (Flesja et al. 1982) has been adopted for use in Australia (Poin-

ton et al. 1987; Mercy and Brennan 1988). Less than 10 spots are classified as grade 1, and 10 or more spots are classified as grade 2. Monitoring for liver spots is a more sensitive indicator of infestation than the intestinal presence of adult ascarids (Bernardo et al. 1990a). The absence of milk spots was also found to be a reliable indicator that pigs do not have established ascarid infections. However, intestinal ascarids may be present in a low proportion of pigs with negative livers. As ascarid liver lesions resolve, limitations are placed on relating slaughter results to stock other than grow/finish pigs. Lesions resolve quickly after first exposure (Table 79.3), but severe lesions following repeated challenge may be related to infection 12 weeks earlier (Bernardo et al. 1990a). The absence of liver spots in slaughtered stock may not indicate that younger pigs or sows are free of parasitism. Ascarid eggs have been observed in weaners from 2 of 15 herds, which had been free of liver white spots at quarterly checks over 18 months (Pointon, unpublished). Bulk fecal egg counts should supplement slaughter checks to confirm the absence or presence of these and other intestinal parasites. In addition, fecal egg counts will be necessary for determining the age group(s) responsible for contaminating the environment and for tailoring hygiene and treatment programs.

The presence of liver white spots at slaughter confirms egg exposure during the grow/finish phase of production. Once grow/finish exposure has been determined at slaughter, bulk fecal egg counts should be performed to identify groups responsible for spreading the infection and these groups targeted for medication and improved hygiene, such as cleaning pens between batches of pigs (Mercy et al. 1989). The identification and subsequent prompt treatment of groups shedding eggs will reduce the prevalence of lesions at minimal cost. Repeat slaughter checks can then be used to monitor control program efficacy. On the basis of repeated negative results, anthelmintic programs may be reduced, thus providing direct savings for the producer. While the direct cost of ascarid infection may be small (Bernardo et al. 1990b), there is the potential for an indirect effect of ascariasis through the exacerbation of respiratory disease.

Nematode infections have been shown to be widespread in Australia (Mercy and Brennan 1988; Mercy et al. 1989) and in the United States (Kennedy et al. 1988). Increased rearing intensity (Mercy et al. 1989) and the use of all-in/all-out production (Flesja and Solberg 1981) have both failed to eliminate nematodes. Case control studies to identify risk factors in intensively managed herds are required to define the epidemiology of intestinal parasitism in fully intensive units.

ABSCESSATION. Lung abscesses from causes other than *A. pleuropneumoniae* can be distinguished by using location and color of exudate. For example, the exudate of *Actinomyces pyogenes* is often green. Abscesses in the meat and/or lungs are commonly associated with infections secondary to tail biting or other cutaneous wounds (Backstrom and Bremer 1976).

ILEITIS. The proliferative enteropathies form a complex of gross lesions typified by thickening of the mucous membrane of the small intestine, and sometimes the mucosa of the large intestine (Rowland and Lawson 1986). Lesions are most commonly restricted to the terminal 50 cm of the ileum (Kubo et al. 1984; Rowland and Lawson 1986). Lesions of proliferative intestinal adenomatosis (PIA), necrotic enteritis (NE), and regional ileitis (RI) have been observed in stock at slaughter (Emsbo 1951; Rowland and Hutchings 1978; Kubo et al. 1984; Mercy and Brennan 1988; Pointon 1989), making slaughter monitoring a valuable technique for diagnosing these conditions, which may cause diarrhea and ill thrift in growing stock (Roberts et al. 1979).

Approximately 15% of 106 South Australian herds were found to have ileal lesions upon inspection (Pointon 1989). Based on 4-monthly inspections over the next year, one-third of herds had intestinal lesions. Classification of these lesions was based on gross thickening of the ileum and edema and congestion of the mesentery and serosa. Confirmation was made by histologic examination using special stains (Pointon et al. 1987). The lesions can be differentiated from normal postmortem contractions of the muscularis by firm palpation, which overcomes the apparent thickening, and lack of edema. The prevalence of ileitis within affected herds was commonly between 5 and 20%. Further studies (1985–87) revealed 18% of 196 herds at their first slaughter inspection had lesions (Table 79.11). In a 200-sow herd a maximum herd prevalence of 70% ± 10% at 90% confidence was detected.

Relying on clinical cases of proliferative hemorrhagic enteropathy to flag herd infection may lead to diagnosing the problem after it has caused a significant depression in the herd's growth performance. Since uncomplicated proliferative lesions resolve over a month, slaughter surveillance may be insensitive to detecting infection that occurs during earlier growth stages. Lesions of NE and RI, however, are likely to be more persistent. In the absence of specific tests for use in diagnosing proliferative ileitis in clinically affected animals, slaughter surveillance offers a practical tool for early detection of emerging problems in endemically infected herds.

NEPHRITIS. Kidney lesions represent a major zoonotic threat to meat and piggery staff (Peet et al. 1983), who isolated *Leptospira* from 83% of 42 selected kidneys condemned by meat inspectors. Thus, detection of lesions at slaughter has zoonotic implications for all producers and meat processors. Grade 1 lesions detected at slaughter are characterized by multiple grayish white areas, 2–5 mm in diameter, and visible on the cortical surface (Peet et al. 1983). Generalized grayish mottling of the cortical surface, with hypertrophy and possible adhesion of the capsule to the cortex are classified as grade 2 (Pointon et al. 1987).

Measures to control and eliminate infection should be implemented, especially in herds supplying breeding stock. Since gross lesions have been observed to persist for up to 4 months postinfection (Jones et al. 1987), investigation of the epidemiology of herd infection should consider all

Table 79.11. Initial herd prevalence and within-herd prevalence of diseases of pigs examined in Australian and Minnesota slaughter surveillance schemes

Disease	(1985–87) 196 South Australian Herds		(1986–89) 240 Western Australian Herds		(1990) 128 Minnesota, U.S., Herds	
	% Herds Affected[a]	% Av. Prev. Affected[b]	% Herds Affected[a]	% Av. Prev. Affected[b]	% Herds Affected[a]	% Av. Prev. Affected[b]
Atrophic rhinitis[c]	NA	NA	5 (56)	16	33	13
Abscessation	12	5	13	4	NA	NA
Arthritis	6	8	11	4	NA	NA
Pericarditis	28	9	25	6	25	7
Peritonitis	23	7	20	5	6	10
Pleuropneumonia	0	0	6	7	13	7
Pleurisy	58	13	86	18	72	15
Nephritis	65	24	53	16	NA	NA
Ileitis	18	7	7	11	30[d]	12
Pneumonia	87	45	82	41	100	75
Roundworms	37	27	49	45	49	37
Sarcoptic mange	93	66	93	49	77	33

Note: Australian slaughter live weight 85–90 kg compared with 105–110 kg in Minnesota. NA = not available.
[a]Herds with lesions.
[b]Average prevalence within affected herds.
[c]Total of grade 4 and 5 lesions.
[d]Not submitted for validation.

age groups of growing stock in attempts to identify times of peak infection and predisposing factors.

ESOPHOGASTRIC ULCERS. Esophogastric lesions have been described and the epidemiologic significance reviewed (Straw et al. 1986b). A severity scoring has been developed (Pointon et al. 1987), wherein lesions are scored from grade 0 (normal) to grade 3. Grade 1 lesions show hyperkeratinization of the squamous epithelium, which is often corrugated and stained yellow. Grade 2 lesions are typified by erosion of the epithelium, typically most severe at the junction of the squamous-glandular mucosal junction. Lesions classified as grade 3 are active ulcers. Cicatrization of the esophogastric junction of grade 3 lesions is due to the granulation that occurs during healing.

Prevalence of Lesions

PREVALENCE OF DISEASES IN PARTICIPATING HERDS. Herd data may be collated to provide a perspective of industry disease rates and problems (Table 79.11). This perspective is considered to be a biased estimate, since it has been observed that the majority of participating herds are large (>200 sows) breeding-stock suppliers and self-selected progressive producers. In the Australian scheme, data is collected from approximately 40–50% of stock marketed in the states where the scheme operates. In Minnesota, the majority of participating herds represented have >100 sows and use practicing veterinarians on a regular basis.

While comparisons between slaughter data from Australia and the United States may be confounded due to differences between years and production conditions, common disease and regional problems are apparent. In Australia, nephritis due to *Leptospira pomona* (Mercy et al. 1988) poses a serious zoonotic threat to piggery and abattoir workers. Respiratory complexes are endemic in all areas and are more severe in Minnesota than South and Western Australia. In Minnesota, 20% of herds have more than 97% of pigs with pneumonia and 31% with pleurisy. Pleurisy rates in the Australian and Minnesota herds indicate widespread serositis infection among grow/finish stock. Parasite infections were also found to be widespread among grow/finish stock, indicating either underdiagnosis or ineffective treatment programs.

ACCURACY OF SLAUGHTER DATA. A random survey of slaughtered stock in Minnesota has been performed (Pointon, unpublished) to determine if data collected from farms voluntarily participating in slaughter surveillance (Table 79.11) is representative of the industry in general (Table 79.12). Preliminary results indicate little difference with respiratory diseases, while ascarids

Table 79.12. Evaluation of lesion prevalence in randomly monitored pigs in Minnesota (preliminary data)

Disease	"Random" Prevalence[a] (95% confidence level)
Pneumonia	69 ± 4(605)
Pleurisy	15 ± 3(605)
Pericarditis	4.6 ± 2(605)
Pleuropneumonia	1.7 ± 1(605)
Roundworms	32 ± 4(605)
Peritonitis	2.6 ± 1(248)
Arthritis	1.6 ± 1(428)
Atrophic rhinitis (4 + 5)	NT
Ileitis	1.2 ± 1(428)
Sarcoptic mange	81 ± 5(252)

Note: NT = not tested; ( ) = number inspected for each condition.

[a]Represents a total population of 30,000 hogs slaughtered in 5 days (sample taken once/week).

and sarcoptic mange appear to be less in herds participating in the slaughter check program in Minnesota.

Overall, parasite infestations, mange, and roundworm, as well as respiratory diseases appear to be widespread in industry. Pigs with evidence of serositis or polyserositis at slaughter (Table 79.12) are likely to have on-farm performance losses and processing losses. Pleuritis may reflect environmental and management conditions predisposing pigs to infections, an important welfare consideration. The high prevalence of pneumonia is also likely to require substantial medication in many herds. As food safety is of paramount importance, the industry disease rates found should encourage development of higher health herds, thereby reducing the need for medication.

INDUSTRY TRENDS. Herd data compiled from herd samples in Western Australia has been analyzed (Mercy and Brennan 1988) to evaluate disease trends in industry. Even though the monitored herds comprise a biased herd sample, disease trends for respiratory disease support the observation that there is an association between increasing herd size and respiratory disease (Aalund et al. 1976). There is an increased proportion of pigs affected with liver white spots in herds with <50 sows than in larger herds. A similar trend in the relationship between herd size and prevalence of ascariasis has been observed in 196 herds in South Australia (Pointon, unpublished; Table 79.11). The odds of herds being affected with pneumonia, pleurisy, and ileitis increase with herd size; the odds decrease for liver white spots. Similarly, the proportion of affected animals in these herds is correlated with herd size.

There is growing evidence that herd data compiled by the modified Scandinavian approach, which uses only a sample of stock to define herd disease status, can be used to monitor disease trends in industry. For example, the emergence of *A. pleuropneumoniae* infections in the South Australian industry (Davies and Moore 1990, personal communication) was identified by the slaughter monitoring program. In the 11 months prior to June 1988, no lesions of pleuropneumonia were detected at slaughter (23 herd checks per month). Lesions were first detected in June, 1988, with a peak of 22% of 23 herds having lesions in November, 1988. Serotyping of isolates from these cases supported the view that infection had been introduced via imported stock from Canada. A similar trend has been observed in Western Australia, where the prevalence of herds with lesions of pleuropneumonia in 1987, 1988, and 1989 was 15%, 13%, and 34%, respectively (Mercy 1990, personal communication).

IMPACT OF SURVEILLANCE DATA. The impact of providing slaughter data is probably best evaluated in cost-benefit analysis of control programs implemented in response to information generated at slaughter. An indirect assessment can be obtained from the decisions of Scandinavian producers to maintain the large cooperative schemes, and Australian producers representing a large market share to maintain schemes on a user-pays basis. In Canada, 89% of producers felt slaughter checks were useful on a regular basis (Shadbolt et al. 1987).

Because no change in the health status of the more severely affected herds was observed, doubts about the value of surveillance programs and questions about the success of control programs initiated in response to slaughter reports have been raised (Backstrom and Bremer 1976). Similarly, concerns have been voiced because of the high proportion of producers "flagged" as having herd problems who declined the offer of a visit by a specialist veterinarian (Willeberg 1984–85). There is no doubt that the long-term effects and viability of these schemes rests on the problem-solving abilities of the field veterinarians and their ability to design changes that are practical and cost-effective for producers to implement. In a recently completed questionnaire survey of 120 producers participating in the Western Australian scheme, 84% of respondents had used the scheme to diagnose one or more diseases in their herd; 87% of respondents found the scheme either useful or very useful in the health management of their herds (Mercy 1990, personal communication).

MANAGEMENT CONSIDERATIONS

Reporting. Data collected at the abattoir is entered onto the software program PigMON (Western Australian Department of Agriculture), and herd reports are promptly sent to the herd owners and attending veterinarians. Full interpretation of slaughter reports requires a comprehensive understanding of the epidemiology of disease, which is best provided by a veterinarian. By operating through practicing veterinarians the value of the information generated is optimized for producers and supports the self-funding nature of the program. Reports are also available from the program covering the overall prevalence of each disease and comparing the best and worst 20% of herds. Summary reports for each disease may be produced for each region, abattoir, season, and herd size. Reports are also available that allow comparisons to be drawn between herds, regions, seasons, herd sizes, and groups within herds. Since PigMON collates data, the anonymity of herds is preserved.

Implementing the Program. Since the program is not implemented in the United States as a direct result of the management policies of pork processors, as in Scandinavian countries, cooperation must be obtained from plant management. Matters that should be clarified when making arrangements include (1) preservation of product hygiene and integrity; (2) avoidance of interference with processing speed; (3) simplification of pig group management in the yards by handling large samples; (4) identification of carcasses, lungs, and snouts with edible ink to ensure that product quality is unaltered and abattoir anonymity is guaranteed in summary reports; and (5) provision of clear instructions by processors on how checks are to be arranged and conducted.

It should be explained that the program defines herd disease problems that cause financial losses to the clients. Because many of these problems also interfere with processing and lead to condemnation, similar discussions regarding the value of the program in improving product quality should be held concurrently with the meat inspection service. It should be emphasized to processing-plant personnel that the monitoring team makes evaluations after viscera are routinely inspected and that condemned material is not handled. Viscera removed after inspection must be stored in approved containers and disposed of appropriately.

Quality Control. The standardized and accurate recording of lesions at slaughter in disease surveillance is paramount. In fast plants, lungs are removed to facilitate the accurate scoring and classification of several conditions. This also provides additional time to facilitate recording lesions present in viscera not removed from the trays. The implementation of a sound quality control program ensures that accumulating data from different inspectors is valid and useful to individual producers, industry, and abattoirs. For use as a herd health management tool, methods and standards of data collection must be reliable and repeatable.

Consist diagnosis and recording between inspectors is essential for making valid interpretations of the health status of breeding herds. Misclassification of lesions such as pleuropneumonia, ascarids, or leptospirosis can quickly lead to reduced confidence and support.

Components of a quality control program that should be implemented include: provision of (1) clear descriptions of lesions, (2) concise severity scoring methods with examples, and (3) a step-by-step description of how to perform the check (i.e., the sequence and sites where lesions are recorded). On-going quality control includes checking all slaughter inspection sheets for correct classifications and scores and totals of pigs inspected. Inspectors should be periodically checked at the abattoir to ensure that they are performing the check according to published protocols. Experienced inspectors should conduct "blind" severity scoring comparisons for mange, pneumonia, and atrophic rhinitis; comparisons can be supplemented by circulating photocopied snout profiles for atrophic rhinitis.

FUTURE PROSPECTS. It is likely that the swine industry will increasingly be held accountable for the husbandry standards (welfare) practiced and the safety of pork products (residues). Monitoring the prevalence of subclinical disease at slaughter provides an indirect assessment of the adequacy of the environmental and management practices. A reduction in the level of medication used in grow/finish stock should result from industry and veterinary efforts rather than from being forced by legislation. Disease surveillance on a herd basis provides the mechanism to detect problems and evaluate new technologies that are cost-effective in controlling endemic diseases. The meat-processing industry will place increasing pressure on producers to provide a wholesome product and carcasses that are easily processed. Control of disease, therefore, will play an increasing role in production management systems. Systems devised to provide an objective assessment of herd health will be an important part of this program. Slaughter surveillance will also play an integral role in evaluating the efficacy and durability of new high-health technologies.

Development of this program depends on collaboration between government agencies, practicing veterinarians, and university researchers. Reporting data on a regional basis will attract industry interest and serve as preliminary information for use in funding applications. Quality control programs will be an essential component to assure data validity. The meat inspection service should adopt a policy that facilitates the role of practicing veterinarians in performing standardized checks in plants. Researchers should use regularly monitored herds for case-control studies aimed at identifying risk factors predisposing to problems and providing information to assist interpretation of slaughter data.

REFERENCES

AALUND, O.; WILLEBERG, P.; AND RIEMANN, H. 1976. Lung lesions at slaughter: Association to factors in the pig herd. Nord Vet Med 28:487–495.

BACKSTROM, L. 1973. Environment and animal health in piglet production. A field study of incidences and correlations. Acta Vet Scand [Suppl] 41:1–240.

BACKSTROM, L., AND BREMER, H. 1976. Disease registrations on pigs at slaughter as a method of preventive and therapeutic veterinary medicine in swine production. Svensk Vet Tidn 28:312–336.

_____. 1978. The relationship between disease incidence of fatteners registered at slaughter and environmental factors in herds. Nord Vet Med 30:526–533.

BACKSTROM, L., AND GUNNARSSON, A. 1976. Serological studies of *Haemophilus parahaemolyticus* (now *A. plueropneumoniae*) in fattener herds, with, respectively, low and high prevalence of pleurisy at slaughter. Swedish Pig Health Conf, 3 pp.

BACKSTROM, L.; BREMER, H.; DYREUDAHL, I.; AND OLSSON, H. 1975. A study of respiratory diseases in fatteners from a herd with a high prevalence of atrophic rhinitis, enzootic pneumonia and pleurisy. Svensk Vet Tidn 27:1028–1040.

_____. 1976. The relationship between atrophic rhinitis, weight gain, age of the dam and the genetic disposition in a swine pedigree herd with a high prevalence of disease. Svensk Vet Tidn 28:449–455.

BACKSTROM, L.; HOEFLING, D.; MORKOC, A.; VINSON, R.; AND SMITH, A. R. 1982. Atrophic rhinitis in swine. I. Clinical signs, slaughter lesions, daily weight gain, disease transmissions. Proc Int Congr Pig Vet Soc, Mexico City, p. 102.

BERNARDO, T. M.; DOHOO, I. R.; DONALD, A.; OGILVIE, T.; AND CAWTHORN, R. 1990a. Ascariasis, respiratory disease and production indices in selected Prince Edward Island swine herds. Can J Vet Res 54:267–273.

BERNARDO, T. M.; DOHOO, I. R.; AND DONALD, A. 1990b. Effect of ascariasis and respiratory diseases on growth rates in swine. Can J Vet Res 54:278–284.

BIERING-SORENSEN, U. 1965. The value of recording disease conditions observed at slaughter houses and disposal plants. Veterinarian (Oxf) 3:87–97.

BJORKLUND, N. E., AND HENRICSON, B. 1965. Studies on pneumonia and atrophic rhinitis in pigs. Nord Vet Med 17:137–146.

BRANDRETH, S. R., AND SMITH, I. M. 1985. Prevalence of pig herds affected by pleuropneumonia associated with *Haemophilus pleuropneumoniae* in eastern England. Vet Rec 117:143–147.

BURCH, D. G. S. 1984. Tiamulin feed premix in the improvement of growth performance of pigs in herds severely affected with enzootic pneumonia. Vet Rec 112:209–211.

CANNON, R. M., AND ROE, R. T. 1982. Livestock Disease Surveys: A Field Manual for Veterinarians. Canberra: Australian Bur Anim Health.

CARGILL, C. F., AND DOBSON, K. J. 1979. Experimental *Sarcoptes scabei* infestation of pigs. II. Effects on production. Vet Rec 104:33–36.

COPEMAN, D. B., AND GAAFAR, S. M. 1972. Sequential development of hepatic lesions of ascaridosis in colostrum-deprived pigs. Aust Vet J 48:263–268.

COWART, R. P.; LIPSEY, R. J.; AND HEDRICK, H. B. 1990. Measurement of conchal atrophy and pneumonic lesions and their association with growth rate in comingled feeder pigs. J Am Vet Med Assoc 196:1262–1264.

D'ALLAIRE, S.; BIGRAS-POULIN, M.; PORRADIS, M. A.; AND MARTINEAU, C. P. 1988. Evaluation of atrophic rhinitis: Are the results repeatable? Proc Int Congr Pig Vet Soc, Rio de Janeiro, p. 38.

DAVIES, P. R., AND MOORE, M. J. 1990. Sarcoptic mite hypersensitivity and skin lesions in slaughtered pigs. Aust Adv Vet Sci, pp. 161–163.

DAVIES, P. R.; MOORE, M. J.; AND POINTON, A. M. 1990. Sarcoptic mite hypersensitivity and skin lesions in slaughtered pigs. Vet Rec. Submitted.

DONE, J. T.; RICHARDSON, M. D.; AND HERBERT, G. N. 1964. Animal Disease Survey, no. 3, MAFF, United Kingdom.

DONE, S. H.; GRIFFITH, I.; AND HEATH, P. 1990. Acute pleuropneumonia lesions in pigs. Proc Int Congr Pig Vet Soc, Lausanne, p. 48.

DUMAS, A.; DENICOURT, M.; D'ALLAIRE, S.; BIGRAS-POULIN, M.; AND MARTINEAU, A. P. 1990. Atrophic rhinitis and growth rate: A potential confounding effect related to slaughter weight. Proc Int Congr Pig Vet Soc, Lausanne, p. 385.

EMSBO, P. 1951. Terminal or regional ileitis in swine. Nord Vet Med 3:1–28.

ERIKSEN, L. 1982. Experimentally induced resistance to *Ascaris suum* in pigs. Nord Vet Med 34:177–187.

FLESJA, K. I., AND SOLBERG, I. 1981. Pathological lesions in swine at slaughter. IV. Pathological lesions in relation to rearing system and herd size. Acta Vet Scand 22:272–282.

FLESJA, K. I., AND ULVESAETER, H. D. 1979. Pathological lesions in swine at slaughter 1 baconers. Acta Vet Scand 20:498–514.

————. 1980. Pathological lesions in swine at slaughter. III. Inter-relationships between pathological lesions and (1) carcass quality and (2) carcass weight. Acta Vet Scand [Suppl] 74:1–22.

FLESJA, K. I.; FORUS, I. B.; AND SOLBERG, I. 1982. Pathological lesions in swine at slaughter. V. Pathological lesions in relation to some environmental factors in herds. Acta Vet Scand 23:169–183.

FLESJA, K. I.; FORUS, I. B.; AND SOLBERG, I. 1984. Pathological lesions in swine at slaughter. VI. The relationship between some mainly non-environmental factors, disease, weight gain and carcass quality. Acta Vet Scand 25:309–321.

GARDNER, I. A., AND HIRD, D. W. 1990. Host determinants of pneumonia in slaughterweight swine. Am J Vet Res 51:1306–1311.

GILES, C. J.; SMITH, I. M.; AND BASKERVILLE, A. J. 1980. Clinical, bacteriological and epidemiological observations on infectious atrophic rhinitis of pigs in southern England. Vet Rec 106:25–28.

HARTLEY, P. E.; WILESMITH, J. W.; AND BRADLEY, R. 1988. The influence of pleural lesions in the pig at slaughter on the duration of the fattening period: An on-farm study. Vet Rec 123:208.

HOLLANDERS, W., AND VERCRUYSSE, J. 1990. Sarcoptic mite hypersensitivity: A cause of dermatitis in fattening pigs at slaughter. Vet Rec 126:308–310.

JERICHO, K. W. F.; DONE, S. H.; AND SAUNDERS, R. W. 1975. Pneumonia and efficiency of pig production. Can Vet J 16:44–49.

JONES, R. T.; MILLAR, B. D.; CHAPPEL, R. J.; AND ADLER, B. 1987. Macroscopic kidney lesions in slaughtered pigs are an inadequate indicator of current leptospiral infection. Aust Vet J 64:258–259.

JORGENSEN, R. J.; NANSEN, P.; NEILSEN, K.; ERIKSEN, L.; AND ANDERSEN, S. 1975. Experimental *Ascaris suum* infection in the pig: Population kinetics following low and high levels of primary infection in piglets. Vet Parasitol 1:151–157.

KENNEDY, T. J.; BRUER, D. J.; MARCHIONDO, A. A.; AND WILLIAMS, J. A. 1988. Prevalence of swine parasites in major hog producing areas of the United States. Agri-Pract 9:25–32.

KUBO, M.; OHYA, T.; AND WATASE, H. 1984. Proliferative haemorrhagic enteropathy at abattoir in Kagoshima. Jpn J Vet Sci 46:413–417.

LINDQVIST, J. O. 1974. Animal health and environment in fattening pigs: A study of disease incidence in relation to certain environmental factors, daily weight gain and carcass classification. Acta Vet Scand [Suppl] 51:1–78.

MARTINEAU, A. P.; VAN NESTE, D.; AND CHARETTE, R. 1987. Pathophysiology of sarcoptic mange in swine. Compend Contin Educ Pract Vet 951–57.

MARTINSSON, K., AND LUNDHEIM, N. 1986. Prevalens av olika sjukanmarkningar hos slaktade formedlingsgrisar. Svensk Vet Tidn 37:815–820.

MERCY, A. R., AND BRENNAN, C. M. 1988. The Western Australian pig health monitoring scheme. Acta Vet Scand [Suppl] 84:212–214.

MERCY, A. R.; PEET, R. L.; AND HUSTAS, L. 1988. The significance of *Leptospira* isolated from the kidneys of slaughtered pigs. Aust Vet J 65:35–36.

MERCY, A. R.; DE CHANEET, G.; AND EMMS, Y. 1989. Survey of internal parasites in Western Australia pig herds. 2. Relationship to anthelmintic usage and parasite control practices. Aust Vet J 66:6–9.

MORRISON, R. B.; HILLEY, H. D.; AND LEMAN, A. D. 1985. The association between pneumonia and atrophic rhinitis in slaughter weight swine. Can Vet J 26:95–97.

MORRISON, R. B.; PIJOAN, C.; AND LEMAN, A. D. 1986. Association between enzootic pneumonia and performance. Pig News Inf 1:23–31.

MOUSING, J. 1988. Chronic pleurisy in pigs: The relationship between weight, age and frequency in 3 conventional herds. Acta Vet Scand [Suppl] 84:253–255.

NICOLET, J. 1986. Haemophilus infections. In Diseases of Swine, 6th ed. Ed. A. D. Leman, B. Straw, R. D. Glock, W. L. Mengeling, R. H. C. Penny, and E. Scholl. Ames: Iowa State Univ Press, pp. 426–436.

NIELSEN, N. C.; RIISING, H. J.; AND BILLE, N. 1976. Experimental reproduction of atrophic rhinitis in pigs reared to slaughter weight. Proc Int Congr Pig Vet Soc, Ames, p. 1.

NOYES, E. P.; FEENEY, D. A.; AND PIJOAN, C. 1990. A comparison of antemortem and postmortem pneumonic lesions in swine using a noninvasive radiographic technique and slaughter examinations. J Am Vet Med Assoc 197:1025–1029.

PEET, R. L.; MERCY, A. R.; HUSTAS, L.; AND SPEED, C. 1983. The significance of *Leptospira* isolated from kidneys of slaughtered pigs. Aust Vet J 60:226.

PICHLER, W. A. 1980. Zusammenhange zwischen der Zuwachsleitung und dem schlachtkerperwert von maskschweinen und dem post mortem ermittelten gesundheitlichen zustand von schweineinaneveien. Wien Tah Mon 67:167–172.

POINTON, A. M. 1989. Campylobacter associated intestinal pathology in pigs. Aust Vet J 66:90–91.

POINTON, A. M., AND HUESTON, W. D. 1990. The national animal health monitoring system (NAHMS): Evolution of an animal health information database system. Proc Vet Epi Prev Med 70–83.

POINTON, A. M., AND SLOANE, M. 1984. An abattoir survey of the prevalence of lesions of enzootic pneumonia of pigs in South Australia. Aust Vet J 61:408–409.

POINTON, A. M.; BYRT, D.; AND HEAP, P. 1985. Effect of enzootic pneumonia of pigs on growth performance. Aust Vet J 62:13–18.

POINTON, A. M.; FARRELL, M.; CARGILL, C. F.; AND HEAP, P. 1987. A pilot pig health scheme for Australian conditions. Univ of Sydney Post-Grad Comm Vet Sci Proc No. 95:743–777.

POINTON, A. M.; MORRISON, R. B.; HILL, G.; DARGATZ,

D.; AND DIAL, G. 1990. Monitoring pathology in slaughtered stock: Guidelines for selecting sample size and interpreting results. Proc Int Congr Pig Vet Soc, Lausanne, p. 393.

ROBERTS, L.; LAWSON, G. H. K.; ROWLAND, A. C.; AND LAING, A. H. 1979. Porcine intestinal adenomatosis and its detection in a closed pig herd. Vet Rec 104:366–388.

ROWLAND, A. C., AND HUTCHINGS, D. A. 1978. Necrotic enteritis and regional ileitis in pigs at slaughter. Vet Rec 103:338–339.

ROWLAND, A. C., AND LAWSON, A. H. K. 1986. Intestinal adenomatosis complex. In Diseases of Swine, 6th ed. Ed. A. D. Leman, B. Straw, R. D. Glock, W. L. Mengeling, R. H. C. Penny, and E. Scholl. Ames: Iowa State Univ Press, pp. 547–556.

RUNNELS, L. J. 1982. Infectious atrophic rhinitis of swine. Vet Clin North Am Large Anim Pract 2:301–319.

SCHEIDT, A. B.; MAYROSE, V. B.; HILL, M. A.; CLARK, L. K.; CLINE, T. R.; KNOX, K. E.; RUNNELS, L. J.; FRANZT, S.; AND EINSTEIN, M. E. 1990. Relationship of growth performance with pneumonia and atrophic rhinitis detected in pigs at slaughter. J Am Vet Med Assoc 196:881–884.

SHADBOLT, P. V.; MITCHELL, W. R.; BLACKBURN, D. J.; MEEK, A. H.; AND FRIENDSHIP, R. M. 1987. Perceived usefulness of the collection of subclinical and other disease entities detected at slaughter. Can Vet J 28:439–445.

SHUMAN, R. D., AND EARL, F. L. 1956. Atrophic rhinitis. VII. A study of the economic effect in a swine herd. J Am Vet Med Assoc 129:220–224.

SMEETS, J. F. M.; SMJDERS, J. M. A.; AND GRUYS, EN E. 1989. Dermatitis in slaughtered pigs. Studies on the prevalence, pathology and economic significance. Tijdschr Diergeneeskd 114:603–610.

STRAW, B. E.; BURGI, E. J.; HILLEY, H. D.; AND LEMAN, A. D. 1983. Pneumonia and atrophic rhinitis in pigs from a test station. J Am Vet Med Assoc 182:607–611.

STRAW, B. E.; LEMAN, A. D.; AND ROBINSON, R. A. 1984. Pneumonia and atrophic rhinitis in pigs from a test station–a follow-up study. J Am Vet Med Assoc 185:1544–1546.

STRAW, B. E.; BACKSTROM, L.; AND LEMAN, A. D. 1986a. Evaluation of swine at slaughter. I. The mechanics of examination, and epidemiologic considerations. Compend Contin Educ Pract Vet 8:541–548.

_____. 1986b. Examination of swine at slaughter. II. Findings at slaughter and their significance. Compend Contin Educ Pract Vet 8:106–112.

STRAW, B. E.; TUOVINEN, V. K.; AND BIGRAS-POULIN, M. 1989. Estimation of the cost of pneumonia in swine herds. J Am Vet Med Assoc 195:1702–1706.

UNDERDAHL, N. R., AND KELLEY, G. W. 1957. The enchancement of virus pneumonia of pigs by the migration of *Ascaris suum* larvae. J Am Vet Med Assoc 130:173–176.

WALLGREN, P.; MATTSON, S.; ARTURSSON, K.; AND BOLSKE, G. 1990. The relationship between *Mycoplasma hyopneumoniae* infection, age at slaughter and lung lesions at slaughter. Proc Int Congr Pig Vet Soc, Lausanne, p. 82.

WILLEBERG, P.; GERBOLA, M.-A.; MADSEN, A.; MANDRUP, M.; NIELSEN, E. K.; RIEMANN, H. P.; AND AALUND, O. 1978. A retrospective study of respiratory disease in a cohort of bacon pigs. 1. Clincico-epidemiological analyses. Nord Vet Med 30:513–525.

WILLEBERG, P.; GERBOLA, M.-A.; KIRKEGAARD PETERSEN, B.; AND ANDERSEN, J. B. 1984–85. The Danish pig health scheme: Nation-wide computer-based abattoir surveillance and follow-up at the herd level. Prev Vet Med 3:79–91.

80 Disease Transfer from Wild to Domestic Pigs

D. C. Roberts

PIGS BELONG to two families in the order Artiodactyla: Old World pigs (family Suidae) and New World pigs, or peccaries (family Tayassuidae). The family Suidae consists of five genera containing eight species, while the family Tayassuidae consists of two genera containing three species.

The domestic pig stems from the wild boar (*Sus scrofa*), which was originally distributed throughout Europe and Asia. Wild boars were extensively hunted by ancient man for use as food and because they were destructive to crops. This hunting and the ever-increasing population of the wild boar's habitat by humans has left only a few pockets of these animals in their original range. The wild boar was completely exterminated in the British Isles, Scandinavia, and Egypt but has been reintroduced in the wild form to Britain. Domestication of *Sus scrofa* probably occurred as early as 10,000 B.C. in Thailand and China, and since that time domestic pigs have become distributed throughout the world as humans travelled and populated new territories. However,

there is hardly another domestic animal more inclined to revert back to the wild state than *Sus scrofa*. Within a very short time it behaves like its ancestor, the wild boar, and will easily integrate and breed with free-ranging wild conspecifics. Hence, large feral populations have developed in many regions of the world, including North America, parts of Europe and Asia, the Pacific Islands, Australia, and New Zealand.

For the purposes of this chapter wild pigs are taken to mean all pigs excluding the domestic pig; therefore, feral *Sus scrofa* are taken to be wild. Details of the geographic distribution of wild pig populations throughout the world are shown in Table 80.1.

DISEASES OF WILD PIGS. The wild boar, the domestic pig, and the feral pig all belong to the same species (*Sus scrofa*), and therefore the wild boar and the feral pig are susceptible to all of the viral, bacterial, fungal, protozoal, helminth- and arthropod-derived diseases of the domestic pig (Fowler and Boever 1986). Other members of the

Table 80.1. Geographical distribution of wild pig populations

Species	Common Name	Distribution
Family Suidae		
Babyrousa babyrussa	Babirussa	Celebes, Togian and Sula Islands, Buru Island (Moluccas): swamp forests, reed thickets[a]
Hylochoerus meinertzhageni	Giant forest hog	Liberia to SW Ethiopia, N Tanzania: forest
Phacochoerus aethiopicus	Warthog	Africa south of Sahara: steppe, savanna
Potamochoerus porcus	Bushpig/Red River hog	Africa south of Sahara, Madagascar, Mayotte Island (comoros): forest, savanna
Sus barbatus	Bearded pig	Malay peninsula, Sumatra, Bangka, Borneo, Rhio archipelago, Palawan and Balabac Islands (Philippines): forest, jungle
Sus salvanius	Pygmy hog	Nepal, Sikkim, Bhutan, Assam, NE India: forest[a]
Sus scrofa	Wild boar/domestic pig/ feral pig	Domestic and feral: worldwide; originally in area from S Scandinavia and Portugal to SE Siberia and Malay peninsula, from W Sahara to Egypt, Britain, Ireland, Corsica, Sardinia, Sri Lanka, Andaman Islands, Japan, Taiwan, Hainan, Sumatra, Java, and E Indies Islands: steppe, savanna, forest
Sus verrucosus	Javan pig	Java, Celebes, Moluccas, Philippines: swamps, grasslands
Family Tayassuidae		
Tayassu pecari	White-lipped peccary/ javelina	S Mexico to NE Argentina, Cuba: forest
Tayassu tajacu	Collared peccary/ javelina	Arizona and Texas to N Argentina, Cuba: desert to forest[a]
Catagonus wagneri	Chacoan peccary	Gran Chaco region of SE Bolivia, Paraguay, N Argentina: thorn forest[a]

Source: Corbet and Hill 1986, Fradrich 1972, Nowak and Paradiso 1983.
[a]Endangered, vulnerable, or rare.

family Suidae are closely related to the domestic pig, and these eight species can therefore be expected to have similar, or slightly different, disease susceptibilities. For example, while the domestic pig is highly susceptible to the effects of the African swine fever virus, the giant forest hog (*Hylochoerus meinertzhageni*), the warthog (*Phacochoerus aethiopicus*), and the bushpig (*Potamochoerus porcus*) are asymptomatic carriers of the virus. The peccaries of the family Tayassuidae are more distantly related to the domestic pig, and thus larger differences in disease susceptibility can be expected when comparing these New World pigs to domestic swine. This is exemplified by the fact that peccaries (*Tayassu pecari, Tayassu tajacu,* and *Catagonus wagneri*) are not susceptible to African swine fever at all, while domestic swine are highly susceptible.

Wild pig populations are therefore a potential reservoir for many diseases of the domestic pig. Tables 80.2–80.4 list many of the documented diseases that affect wild pigs, and which could, under favorable epidemiologic conditions, be transmitted to and manifest as clinical disease in domestic swine.

TRANSMISSION OF DISEASE FROM WILD TO DOMESTIC PIGS. Although the wild pig is a potential source of disease for the domestic pig, few instances of proven transfer have actually been recorded. Often there are many larger and more obvious reservoirs of an infection than the

Table 80.2.   Viral diseases documented in wild pigs

Disease	Wild Pigs Affected	References
Pseudorabies	Feral pig	Beran (1989)
	Wild boar	Clark et al. (1983)
	Giant forest hog	Corn et al. (1986)
	Bushpig	Crandall et al. (1986)
	Warthog	Evtushevskii (1975)
	Peccary	Fowler and Boever (1986)
Hog cholera	All	Firnu and Scarano (1988)
	Peccary, mildly affected	Fowler and Boever (1986), Kohm (1982), Wallach and Boever (1983)
African swine fever	Wild boar	Firnu and Scarano (1988)
	Giant forest hog	Fowler and Boever (1986)
	Bushpig	Kohm (1982)
	Warthog	Thomson (1985)
	Peccary, not susceptible	Wallach and Boever (1983)
Foot-and-mouth disease	Feral pig, wild boar	Fletch (1970)
	Giant forest hog	Fowler and Boever (1986)
	Bushpig, warthog	Kohm (1982)
	Babirussa	Pech and Hone (1988)
	Peccary, mildly affected	Pech and McIlroy (1990)
Vesicular stomatitis	Feral pig, wild boar	Fowler and Boever (1986)
	Peccary, not susceptible	Nettles (1988)
Vesicular exanthema	Feral pig, wild boar	Fowler and Boever (1986)
	Peccary, not susceptible	Smith and Madin (1986)
Rabies	Wild boar, peccary	Fowler and Boever (1986)
	Giant forest hog	Hetrick et al. (1986)
	Bushpig, warthog	Schneider et al. (1989)
Rinderpest	All	Anon. (1979b)
	Feral pig and wild boar, mild transient fever only	Fowler and Boever (1986), Plowright (1982), Wallach and Boever (1983)

Table 80.3.   Bacterial diseases documented in wild pigs

Disease	Wild Pigs Affected	References
Pneumonic pasteurellosis	All	Wallach and Boever (1983)
Bordetellosis	All	Wallach and Boever (1983)
Tuberculosis	Feral pig	Clark et al. (1983)
	Wild boar	Essey et al. (1981)
	Peccaries	Kohm (1982), Scott (1986)
Salmonellosis	Bushpig	Kohm (1982)
Clostridial infections	All	Wallach and Boever (1983)
Erysipelas	All	Wallach and Boever (1983)
Leptospirosis	Feral pigs	Clark et al. (1983), Corn et al. (1986)
Brucellosis	Feral pig	Becker et al. (1978)
	Wild boar	Clark et al. (1983), Corn et al. (1986), Giovannini et al. (1988), Kohm (1982), Wallach and Boever (1983), Wood et al. (1976)
Actinomyces infections	All	Wallach and Boever (1983)
Yersiniosis	All	Clark et al. (1983), Evtushevskii (1975), Wallach and Boever (1983)

Table 80.4. Miscellaneous parasites documented in wild pigs

Parasite	Wild Pigs Affected	References
Ascaris sp.	Warthog	Horak et al. (1983)
Trichinella spiralis	Bushpig, peccaries, not susceptible	Fowler and Boever (1986), Nelson (1982)
Trichuris suis	Wild boar	Corwin et al. (1986)
Echinococcus granulosus	Feral pig	Thompson et al. (1988)
Stephanurus dentatus	Feral pig	Jinshu (1990)
	Wild boar	Smith and Hawkes (1978)
Sarcoptes scabei	Peccaries	Fowler and Boever (1986)
Haematopinus sp.	Warthog	Horak et al. (1983)
Ornithodorus moubata	Giant forest hog, bushpig, warthog	Thomson (1985)
Rhipicephalus sanguineus	Warthog, bushpig	Anon. (1979a)
Eimeria spp.	Wild boar	Jinshu and Choajun (1990)
Babesia trautmanni	Wild boar, warthog, bushpig	Anon. (1979a)
Trypanosoma spp.	Warthog, bushpig	Anon. (1979c)

wild pig population. This is particularly so with diseases having a wide host spectrum; e.g., cattle, sheep, and other domestic pigs are more likely to be the main source of pasteurellosis in a piggery than a herd of roaming wild pigs.

Furthermore, infectious agents must be directly or indirectly transferred from the diseased wild pig to the susceptible domestic pig. Close contact between wild and domestic swine is not usually possible in modern piggeries except for pig-production units that employ an extensive or free-range system. Many common diseases, such as sarcoptic mange, cannot be transmitted under conditions where close contact does not exist. In most cases of effective transmission between wild and domestic swine, fomites that can travel over long distances, mechanical vectors, and especially biologic vectors are involved. These biologic vectors are usually arthropods in which the infectious agent undergoes either a necessary part of its life cycle (e.g., *Babesia* spp. in the hard tick) or multiplication (e.g., African swine fever virus in the soft tick) before transmission to a susceptible host. Some important disease conditions where wild swine are implicated as reservoirs are discussed below.

Viral Diseases. Many of the viral diseases to which pigs are susceptible have a broad host range: pseudorabies, foot-and-mouth disease, vesicular stomatitis, vesicular exanthema, rabies. Wild pig populations certainly play a role in the epidemiology of these diseases but are probably only minor sources of infection for domestic pigs.

Hog cholera virus affects all wild pigs, but peccaries only develop a mild disease form. In some countries wild swine pose a threat of communicating hog cholera to domestic swine (Van Oirschot 1986). The most probable means of transmission other than by direct contact would be by a mechanical vector such as other animals or birds.

African swine fever is a serious disease of domestic swine in Africa, Portugal, Spain, Italy, and France. In Africa the warthog, bushpig, and giant forest hog are asymptomatic carriers of the causative virus and only develop a low level of vire-

mia. The biologic vector is the soft tick *Ornithodorus moubata,* which parasitizes wild and domestic swine. Infected domestic swine develop a high level of viremia and are severely affected. In Europe the virus spreads between domestic pigs by means of direct or indirect contact (e.g., people, horseflies, mosquitoes, garbage, etc.) and by means of the tick *Ornithodorus erraticus* in Spain and Portugal. There is considerable pressure to prevent accidental introduction of the disease into nonaffected countries. For example, no wild African swine are permitted into the United States where the ticks *Ornithodorus turicata* and *Ornithodorus coriaceous* could act as biologic vectors. In South Africa stringent regulations are in force to prevent African swine fever from spreading out of endemic areas populated by warthogs and bushpigs. All pig-production units within an endemic area must be enclosed by a double 1.6-m-high fence with at least a 1-m walkway separating the two fences (Henderson 1982). Pigs cannot cross either fence, and a soft tick cannot traverse the distance between the fences on its own. Removal of any pig or pig product from an African swine fever area is strictly controlled.

Another arthropod-borne disease affecting pigs is Japanese encephalitis. The vector is the mosquito *Culex tritaeniorhynchus,* and the disease manifests in many mammalian and avian hosts (Joo 1986). However, there are no reported cases of wild pigs acting as the source of disease for domestic pigs, probably because of the large reservoir of the virus in many other mammals and birds.

Rinderpest is caused by a virus belonging to the morbilli group of the Paramyxoviridae. It is the most lethal and potentially dangerous infectious disease affecting wild artiodactyls (Plowright 1982). Morbidity and mortality often exceeds 90%. The disease is transmitted by direct or indirect contact and is endemic in equatorial Africa and parts of Asia. Wild swine of Africa and Asia as well as peccaries are severely affected, but domestic pigs only show a mild transient fever resulting in a temporary loss of production.

Bacterial Diseases. Many bacterial diseases affecting wild pigs have a wide host spectrum; therefore, wild pigs only play a minor role in the spread of these infections to domestic pigs. An exception is brucellosis, where it has been established that feral swine are a significant reservoir of *Brucella suis.* Transmission is by means of direct or sexual contact, or by the ingestion of food and water contaminated with feces or urine of infected pigs. This requires close contact between feral and domestic pigs, which efficient swine management systems can avoid (Deyoe 1986).

Miscellaneous Parasites. Swine babesiosis is caused by the protozoan *Babesia trautmanni* and occurs in central and southern Africa, southern Europe, Russia, and South America. The vector involved is the hard tick *Rhipicephalus sanguineus* and possibly other hard ticks. Bushpigs and warthogs only develop subclinical disease, but domestic pigs suffer fever, anemia, and hemglobinuria and pregnant sows may abort. The disease is often diagnosed in free-ranging domestic pigs. Babesiosis in Europe, Indochina, and the Sudan can also be caused by *Babesia perronictoi,* in which case the vector is unknown but is suspected to be a tick.

Swine trypanosomiasis in Africa is caused by the protozoans *Trypanosoma simiae, T. congolense, T. brucei,* and *T. suis.* The latter three trypanosomes only cause mild symptoms in domestic pigs, but *T. simiae* causes pyrexia, apathy, ataxia, and respiratory distress. Bushpigs and warthogs act as asymptomatic carriers of the disease and the vector is the tsetse fly (*Glossina* spp.). The disease can be transmitted over large distances because the tsetse fly can fly of its own accord and can also be carried in wind currents. Pig-production units in endemic trypanosomiasis areas employ gauze netting and insecticides in an attempt to prevent domestic pigs being stung by the tsetse fly and subsequently developing trypanosomiasis.

REFERENCES

Anon. 1979a. Babesiosis. In The Merck Veterinary Manual, 5th ed. Ed. O. H. Siegmund, Rahway, N. J.: Merck & Co., pp. 426–431.

Anon. 1979b. Rinderpest. In The Merck Veterinary Manual, 5th ed. Ed. O. H. Siegmund, Rahway, N. J.: Merck & Co., pp. 262–263.

Anon. 1979c. The trypanosomiases. In The Merck Veterinary Manual, 5th ed. Ed. O. H. Siegmund, Rahway, N. J.: Merck & Co., pp. 420–426.

BECKER, H. N.; BELDEN, R. C.; BREAULT, T.; BURRIDGE, M. J.; FRANKENBERGER, W. B.; AND NICOLETTI, P. 1978. Brucellosis in feral swine in Florida. J Am Vet Med Assoc 173:1181–1182.

BERAN, G. W. 1989. Feral swine and disease (Aujesky's disease and brucellosis). Proc Annu Meet U.S. Anim Health Assoc 93:435–440.

CLARK, R. K.; JESSUP, A.; HIRD, D. W.; RUPPANNER, R.; AND MEYER, M. E. 1983. Serologic survey of California wild hogs for antibodies against selected zoonotic disease agents. J Am Vet Med Assoc 183:1248–1251.

CORBET, G. B., AND HILL, J. E. 1986. A World List of Mammalian Species, 2d ed. New York: Facts on File Publications, pp. 131–132.

CORN, J. L.; SWIDEREK, P. K.; BLACKBURN, B. O.; ERICKSON, G. A.; THIERMAN, A. B.; AND NETTLES, V. F. 1986. Survey of selected diseases in wild swine in Texas. J Am Vet Med Assoc 189:1029–1032.

CORWIN, R. M.; DIMARCO, N. K.; McDOWELL, A. E.; AND PRATT, S. E. 1986. Internal parasites. In Diseases of Swine, 6th ed. Ed. A. D. Leman, B. Straw, R. D. Glock, W. L. Mengeling, R. H. C. Penny, and E. Scholl. Ames: Iowa State Univ Press, pp. 646–664.

CRANDALL, R. A.; ROBINSON, R. M.; AND HANNON, P. G. 1986. Pseudorabies infection in collared peccaries (*Tayassu tajacu*). Southwest Vet 37:193–195.

DEYOE, B. L. 1986. Brucellosis. In Diseases of Swine, 6th ed. Ed. A. D. Leman, B. Straw, R. D. Glock, W. L. Mengeling, R. H. C. Penny, and E. Scholl. Ames: Iowa State Univ Press, pp. 599–607.

ESSEY, M. A.; PAYNE, R. L.; HIMES, E. M.; AND LUCHSINGER, D. W. 1981. Bovine tuberculosis surveys of axis deer and feral swine on the Hawaiian island of Molokai. Proc Annu Meet U.S. Anim Health Assoc 85:538–549.

EVTUSHEVKII, N. N. 1975. Causes of death of wild ungulates in the central Dnieper region, Russian–SFSR USSR. Vestn Zool 5:77–79.

FIRNU, A., AND SCARANO, C. 1988. African swine fever and classical swine fever (hog cholera) among wild boar in Sardinia. Rev Sci Techn, Off Int Epizoot 7:901–915.

FLETCH, A. L. 1970. Foot and mouth disease. In Infectious Diseases of Wild Mammals. Ed. J. W. Davis, L. H. Karstad, and D. O. Trainer. Ames: Iowa State Univ Press, pp. 68–75.

FOWLER, M. E., AND BOEVER, W. J. 1986. Superfamily Suidoidea. In Zoo & Wild Animal Medicine, 2d ed. Ed. M. E. Fowler. Philadelphia: W. B. Saunders, pp. 964–967.

FRADRICH, H. 1972. Swine and Peccaries. In Grzimek's Animal Life Encyclopedia, vol. 13, Mammals IV. Ed. B. Grzimek. New York: Van Nostrand Rheinhold Co., pp. 76–107.

GIOVANNINI, A.; CANCELLOTTI, F. M.; TURILLI, C.; AND RANDI, E. 1988. Serological investigations for some bacterial and viral pathogens in fallow deer (*Cervus dama*) and wild boar (*Sus scrofa*) of the San Rossore Preserve, Tuscany, Italy. J Wildl Dis 24:127–132.

HENDERSON, W. M. 1982. The control of disease in wildlife when a threat to man and farm livestock — general discussion. In Animal Disease in Relation to Animal Conservation. Ed. M. A. Edwards and U. McDonnell. London: Academic Press, p. 305.

HETRICK, M.; GOODMAN, H.; AND WRIGHT, M. 1986. Rabies in a javelina. USA Morb Mort Wkly Rep 35:555–561.

HORAK, I. G.; BIGGS, H. C.; HANSSEN, T. S.; AND HANSSEN, R. E. 1983. The prevalence of helminth and arthropod parasites of warthog, *Phacochoerus aethiopicus,* in South West Africa/Namibia. Onderstepoort J Vet Res 50:145–148.

JINSHU, J. 1990. The distribution of kidney worm disease of swine in China. Proc Int Congr Pig Vet Soc, Lausanne, p. 312.

JINSHU, J., AND CHAOJUN, L. 1990. Preliminary studies on the species of coccidia of swine and boar in Beijing district. Proc Int Congr Pig Vet Soc, Lausanne, p. 324.

JOO, H. S. 1986. Japanese encephalitis virus infection. In Diseases of Swine, 6th ed. Eds. A. D. Leman, B. Straw, R. D. Glock, W. L. Mengeling, R. H. C. Penny, and E. Scholl. Ames: Iowa State Univ Press, pp. 407–411.

KOHM, A. 1982. Pigs. In Handbook of Zoo Medicine. Ed. H. G. Klos and E. M. Lang. New York: Van Nostrand Rheinhold Co., pp. 205–216.

NELSON, G. S. 1982. Carrion feeding cannabalistic carnivores and human disease in Africa with special reference to trichinosis and hydatid disease in Kenya. In Animal Disease in Relation to Animal Conservation. Ed. M. H. Edwards and U. McDonnell. London: Academic Press, pp. 181–198.

NETTLES, V. 1988. Vesicular stomatitis on Ossabaw Island, USA. Foreign Anim Dis Rep 16:1–2.

NOWAK, R. M., AND PARADISO, J. L. 1983. Walker's Mammals of the World, 4th ed. Baltimore, London: The Johns Hopkins Univ Press, pp. 1175–1185.

PECH, R. P., AND HONE, J. 1988. A model of the dynamics and control of an outbreak of foot and mouth disease in feral pigs in Australia. J Appl Ecol 25:63–77.

PECH, R. P., AND McILROY, J. C. 1990. A model of the velocity of advance of foot and mouth disease in feral pigs. J Appl Ecol 27:635–650.

PLOWRIGHT, W. 1982. The effects of rinderpest and rinderpest control on wildlife in Africa. In Animal Disease in Relation to Animal Conservation. Ed. M. H. Edwards and U. McDonnell. London: Academic Press, pp. 1–28.

SCHNEIDER, L. G.; MULLER, W. W.; AND HOHNSBEEN, K. P. 1989. Rabies in Europe 1st quarter 1989. Rabies Bull Eur 13:1–9.

SCOTT, R. M. 1986. Status of tuberculosis in zoo animals. Proc Annu Meet Am Assoc Zoo Vet, Michigan State Univ, pp. 19–22.

SMITH, A. W., AND MADIN, S. H. 1986. Vesicular exanthema. In Diseases of Swine, 6th ed. Ed. A. D. Leman, B. Straw, R. D. GLock, W. L. Mengeling, R. H. C. Penny, and E. Scholl. Ames: Iowa State Univ Press, pp. 358–368.

SMITH, H. J., AND HAWKES, A. B. 1978. Kidney worm infection in feral pigs in Canada with transmission to domestic swine. Can Vet J 19:30–43.

THOMPSON, R. C. A.; LYMBERY, A. J.; HOBBS, R. P.; AND ELLIOT, A. D. 1988. Hydatid disease in urban areas of Western Australia: An unusual cycle involving western grey kangaroos (*Macropus fuliginosus*), feral pigs and domestic dogs. Aust Vet J 65:188–190.

THOMSON, G. R. 1985. The Epidemiology of African swine fever: The role of free-living hosts in Africa. Onderstepoort J Vet Res 52:201–209.

VAN OIRSCHOT, J. T. 1986. Hog cholera. In Diseases of Swine, 6th ed. Ed. A. D. Leman, B. Straw, R. D. Glock, W. L. Mengeling, R. H. C. Penny, and E. Scholl. Ames: Iowa State Univ Press, pp. 289–300.

WALLACH, J. D., AND BOEVER, W. J. 1983. Diseases of Exotic Animals – Medical and Surgical Management. Philadelphia: W. B. Saunders, pp. 631–639.

WOOD, G. W.; HENDRICKS, J. B.; AND GOODMAN, D. E. 1976. Brucellosis in feral swine. J Wildl Dis 12:579–582.

81 Veterinary Services

R. A. Vinson

THE LIVESTOCK industry in the United States has undergone tremendous change since the 1930s. Production of livestock has become highly industrialized or factorylike, exemplified most in the poultry industry, where large, mechanized production units are the rule. Cattle feeding is a similarly industrialized part of the U.S. livestock industry. The swine industry is rapidly patterning itself after the poultry and cattle-feeding industries. Many large swine production complexes have been built in the 1980s, particularly in the Southeast. An ever-changing swine industry has revolutionized swine veterinary practice.

In the early part of the twentieth-century veterinarians were almost exclusively horse doctors. Beginning in the 1930s the veterinarian's role changed from that of horse doctor to the care and treatment of other species as well. Small animal or pet veterinary medicine began then as well as the development of livestock practice. As the horse began to lose its economic value for farming, the veterinarian found it necessary to develop other areas of expertise.

During the 1930s most of the farms producing swine in the United States were located in the Corn Belt. Practitioners in this area became increasingly interested in the practice of swine veterinary medicine. Hog cholera (HC) was the leading hazard of the swine industry. HC vaccine was developed, and many practitioners administered it to large numbers of swine during the 1930s and 1940s. During that time veterinarians treated most diseases symptomatically. For example, scours in grow/finish pigs, caused primarily by salmonellosis, was treated with such crude substances as lye and soaked oats. External parasite infestation was treated with sulfur compounds. Gradually, more and more productive disease research for the swine industry took place. Many new, effective drugs became available and diagnostic services were improved. These changes enabled the practicing veterinarian to provide more sophisticated service.

During the 1950s, modified live virus vaccine was developed for HC control. Diseases such as erysipelas, leptospirosis, brucellosis, transmissible gastroenteritis (TGE), and swine influenza became more easily diagnosed and controlled. Antibiotics were beginning to be used in feed rations for both growth promotion and treatment. Swine-feeding practices changed from free choice to complete rations, and soybean meal became the main source of protein. During the 1950s the transition from field- or lot-raised swine to enclosed confinement production was begun. Most swine practitioners depended on fees from HC vaccination as their main source of practice revenue. Some veterinarians who were regularly vaccinating pigs for clients pioneered the first "herd health programs," and they were generally very familiar with the disease problems unique to the individual swine complexes they served. The age of pigs being vaccinated facilitated individual inspection of each pig at a critical stage of production.

With the advent of antibiotics and development of vaccines, swine practitioners were better able to control infectious diseases. Some veterinarians began offering more detailed and formal herd health programs for their clients. This type of service usually involved a flat-rate fee for vaccination for such diseases as leptospirosis, erysipelas, and HC, as well as for iron dextran injections and internal and external parasite control. Veterinarians continued to work more closely with producers, not only to handle disease problems but also to become involved in nutritional counseling as corn-soy rations came into vogue. Many swine practitioners developed a premix dispensing business as an adjunct to their herd health programs.

In the 1960s the role of swine practitioners changed markedly. The HC eradication program became a reality. Fees charged for herd health programs through the administration of vaccines became unrealistic, since many production units required no vaccination program. Confinement rearing was rapidly evolving as the common method of pig production. Veterinarians were called only when sickness occurred. Managing swine in confinement was new for both veterinarians and producers and many new types of diseases developed. Baby pig diarrhea rose in prominence, and chronic TGE developed in many confined midwestern herds. Anestrus became a problem in gilts, and viruses played an increasing role in reproductive diseases. Since veterinarians were not administering vaccine, regular visits were not made to many large confinement herds as had been the norm prior to that time. The result was that when disease occurred, it was often extremely difficult for practitioners to make a diagnosis and understand the role that management and environment were playing. Because of the chaotic health control of the 1960s many veterinarians saw a need for the development of more sophisticated programs for preventing disease. Formal herd health programs came into existence. Producers began using veterinarians as consultants or advisers for their units rather than as treaters of sickness or administrators of vaccines.

During the 1980s until now, the complexity of swine production has increased at an ever faster rate. This has made it necessary for swine practitioners to be knowledgeable not only in disease control but in all aspects of swine production. This includes genetics, nutrition, environment, personnel management, and financial management. With the advent of multiperson practices, specialization has become possible. One or more members of the practicing group may specialize in swine, dairy cattle, horses, or feedlot cattle. Until recently there has been no formal education preparing veterinarians for specialized swine practice. Education has been acquired mainly by trial and error, research publications, and attendance at university and other continuing education programs. Undergraduates attending veterinary colleges in the United States receive some training in swine veterinary medicine, but certainly not enough to really be called swine specialists upon graduation. For this reason, many veterinary colleges are developing postgraduate training for those desiring to become swine veterinary specialists.

An understanding of the economics of swine production has become of utmost importance for swine practitioners. Knowledge in this area enables practitioners to weigh the cost of disease control or management schemes against expected economic benefits. In recent years a high percentage of continuing education time has had to do with the relationship of disease control to economics of swine production.

As the swine industry continues to pattern itself more closely to the poultry industry, the role of the swine practitioner in the United States will change ever more rapidly. The percentage of self-employed veterinarians practicing swine veterinary medicine likely will go down. Many swine practitioners will become full-time employees of large corporate-structured swine production businesses or groups of independent producers. Others will work for companies selling seedstock, feed, and animal health products. Whether self-employed or not, the swine practitioner's basic job will still be to advise and consult regarding improving production efficiency. This is why an understanding of the economics of production is vital for the swine practitioner.

HERD HEALTH PROGRAM. To be effective, the swine practitioner must develop some sort of "herd health program" with the manager or owner

of the swine production unit. This necessitates regular farm visits by the veterinarian or in some cases people trained by the veterinarian. Because of changing seasonal patterns visits should occur at least quarterly or more often depending on the distance from practice headquarters and the number of problems the unit is experiencing. In the midst of a disastrous health problem, it may be necessary to visit the unit every day for awhile. Regular visits create familiarization with the herd and the people operating the unit, enabling the practitioner to maintain an effective health program.

A second important aspect of an effective program is a good production record–keeping system, preferably computerized, which should provide the practitioner and caretaker with accurate information for determining where problems are occurring, measuring the economic impact of problems, and for monitoring the effectiveness of disease control programs. Production record–keeping is especially important for large swine production units.

The Farm Visit. Prior to a visit, the practitioner should examine the records of the farm, including the last visit report, latest production reports, recent laboratory reports, latest slaughter check report, and ration and nutrition information. A problem agenda for the farm visit should be developed.

While at the farm, the practitioner and caretaker should examine and discuss the last farm visit report. Special emphasis should be placed on determining whether recommendations made at the last visit were properly carried through and if they proved effective. Aspects of the production records relating to recent recommendations should be examined at the same time. The records will aid in measuring the effectiveness of recommendations. Ideally, many of the problems noted during the last farm visit will now be under control. However, after examining the production records it may appear that new problems are occurring or the solution to one or more old problems has not yet been found. In this case the farm visit agenda should be revised, making sure to give attention to all problems.

After the preliminary discussion, a general examination and walk-through may reveal additional problems not anticipated in the preliminary agenda. These should be noted and strategy developed to handle them. During the walk-through the particular feed additive being used for each group of pigs should be noted. The drug inventory should be checked, making sure proper drugs and vaccines are available. The proper use, dosage level, and withdrawal times of drugs, vaccines, and feed additives being used should be reviewed, with special emphasis on any revisions in the protocol.

Following the walk-through any special testing,

necropsies, boar examinations, or other procedures needed for diagnosing disease or improving overall production efficiency should be performed. Before leaving the farm, the veterinarian should have a meeting with all personnel of the swine unit involved in production to sum up the results of the visit. At this time any strategy problems can be worked out. Finally, an appointment for the next farm visit should be made.

Upon return to practice headquarters, the veterinarian should make any necessary follow-up phone calls and recommend and/or carry out any special studies necessary to solve the current problems of the unit. A written report summarizing the recommendations and conclusions of the farm visit should be prepared and sent to the production unit as soon as possible.

The farm visit should accomplish four things. It should familiarize the practitioner with specific herd disease problems; help the practitioner understand the management scheme and goals of the owner or manager; result in specific recommendations being made by the practitioner to solve inefficiencies and disease problems of the unit; provide a written record of those recommendations along with a description of the status of the herd at the time of the farm visit and expected prognoses should the recommendations be adopted.

The most important part of a professional farm visit is the written report, which includes a summary of the problems found and the various recommendations to be used in attempting to solve those problems. A written report is necessary, because it is not always possible for all persons involved to be present at the time oral recommendations are made. A written communication guarantees that everyone understands what was suggested. It also provides the manager with a reference to check back for details on specific recommendations. Additionally, it provides a good record so that other colleagues in the practice may see what was accomplished at the visit; most importantly, it helps the practicing veterinarian to review what was discussed at the last visit while preparing for the next.

COMPUTERIZED PRODUCTION RECORD–KEEPING SYSTEM. An easy-to-use computerized record-keeping system is necessary to help pinpoint problems and measure the effectiveness of programs to solve them. The veterinarian and producer should agree as to which of the many computer software programs available will provide the most useful information.

SOURCE DOCUMENTS. For a record-keeping system to be useful it is necessary to have easy-to-use source documents for gathering needed data. For convenience and accuracy the documents being used should be located in the areas where the actual reported occurrence is happening; e.g., farrowing data source documents should be located and used in the farrowing room. The source documents should be such that entering data is as simple as possible; documents requiring filling in blanks or simple check marks are best. The documents should be made of durable material, since they are often dropped onto a wet floor. Stiff cardboard is the best. Several colors may be used so that categories of information can be separated at a glance. There should be no more source documents than absolutely necessary; too many records often reduce accuracy. For ease of entering data into the computer program the format of the source documents should be tailored to the particular software program being used. Figures 81.1–81.6 show examples of source documents.

KEYING IN AND AUDITING INFORMATION. The attending veterinarian should emphasize the importance of accuracy to those persons entering data onto the source documents and to the person actually keying in the computer information. This is necessary if proper conclusions for problem solving are to be made from the processed data. The person keying in the information must understand what to do when inconsistent or missing data is shown on the source documents. One advantage of having the data entered into the computer at the farm level is better communications between the person keying in and the person entering the data on source documents.

Reports generated by the computer software program are extremely valuable, if the data is accurate and the information is easily accessible. Computer reports should help the veterinarian and producer evaluate trends, diagnose disease, set priorities, measure effectiveness of the genetic program, determine the most efficient nutrition program, etc. If the data is inaccurate, conclusions may be incorrect.

Simple audits of the computer information should be made. A typical error is computer-calculated inventories not agreeing with actual pig counts. Another is pig marketings recorded on the bank deposit records not agreeing with production marketing records. If these items are not correctly recorded in the computer, important production parameters such as mortality rate, average daily gain, and feed efficiency will be inaccurate. The first thing to look for in computer reports is data that appears to be inconsistent.

LINKING PRODUCTION AND FINANCIAL RECORDS. As previously stated the swine practitioner must understand the economics of swine production, particularly changes in production results and their effect on profitability. Figure 81.7 shows an example of linking production records to financial records. This is a page from a "what-if" computer spreadsheet program. Various current production figures are listed under the column "Figs. Used." The column just to the right,

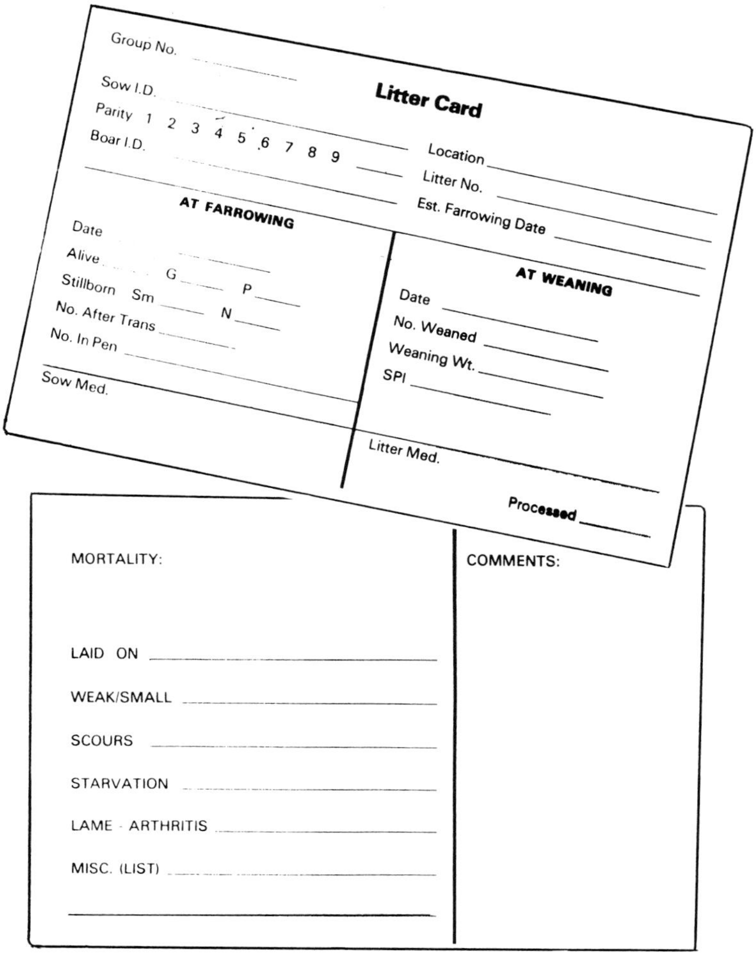

Group No.

Sow I.D.

Litter Card

Parity 1 2 3 4 5 6 7 8 9

Boar I.D.

Location

Litter No.

Est. Farrowing Date

AT FARROWING

Date

Alive G P

Stillborn Sm N

No. After Trans

No. In Pen

Sow Med.

AT WEANING

Date

No. Weaned

Weaning Wt.

SPI

Litter Med.

Processed

MORTALITY:

LAID ON

WEAK/SMALL

SCOURS

STARVATION

LAME - ARTHRITIS

MISC. (LIST)

COMMENTS:

81.1. Litter card.

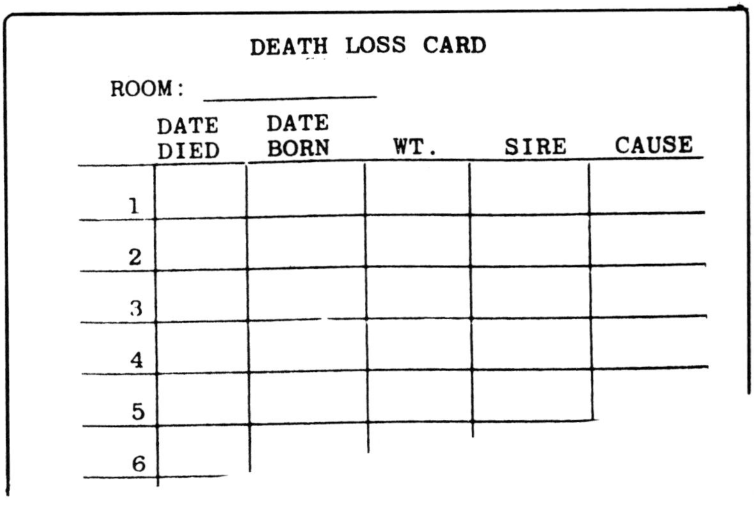

DEATH LOSS CARD

ROOM:

	DATE DIED	DATE BORN	WT.	SIRE	CAUSE
1					
2					
3					
4					
5					
6					

81.2. Death loss card.

WEEKLY SALES RECORD

Week Ending _____

DATE	NUMBER	MARKETS			CULLS	
		WEEK BORN	WEIGHT	NUMBER	WEIGHT	

W719

81.3. Weekly sales record.

WEEKLY SERVICE REGISTER

	TAG NO.	DATE WEANED	BOAR NO.	SERVICE DATE	RETURN DATE	P or O	DUE DATE	COMMENTS
1								
2								
3								
4								
5								
6								

81.4. Weekly service register.

"Figs. Used Last Visit," shows four production figures that have changed since the last farm visit. The two columns further right, "Dollars/Cwt" effect and "Net Dollars," show the effect on total annualized profits.

For example, the "Litters Born/Week" rate averaged only 38.00/week at the time the report was written compared to 40.00/week at the last farm visit. This change alone lowered profits on the example farrow-to-finish farm by $1.26 cwt of pork produced. The total annualized dollar effect was $48,174. "Pigs Born Live/Litter" and "Pre-Weaning Mortality, %" also made adverse changes, $38,754 and $33,144 respectively. While, for illustration purposes, these changes are rather severe in magnitude, one can see that small changes in production efficiency can have profound effects on profits in large units. This type of linking financial records to production records helps the swine practitioner set priorities and develop a general idea of cost-benefit of any proposed changes. Understanding how to gather accurate records and make use of them is an important challenge for swine practitioners.

Diagnostic Procedures. The consulting swine practitioner requires access to good veterinary diagnostic laboratory services. Accurate diagnoses must be made to solve disease problems. This is impossible with herd observation alone. The consulting swine practitioner must work closely with laboratory personnel and should understand what types of samples are needed for diagnosing particular problems. The laboratory in turn must run tests quickly and accurately, promptly sending reports to the attending veterinarian. Using a fax machine and telephone messages helps improve communication efficiency. On routine farm visits laboratory reports should be reviewed. The results will often dictate the course of action that should be taken to solve a particular problem.

A general diagnosis of a disease problem should pursue the following format: (1) observe symptoms exhibited by the pigs; (2) study the effects of symptoms on production parameters and profits; (3) analyze possible specific causes of the symptoms; (4) test live animals, e.g., serology, hematology, rectal temperatures, skin scrapings; (5) necropsy pigs that have died or are dying and appear to be representative of the problem; (6) deliver live pigs or tissues from necropsied pigs to the laboratory for virology, bacteriology, parasitology, and histopathology; (7) assess environmental conditions that may be contributing to the problem; (8) study possible genetic contributions to the problem, e.g., sows in a herd sired by a particular genetic line may have a greater incidence of agalactia than those of another line; (9) assess the management procedures contributing to the disease problem.

If the foregoing steps are carefully followed, it should be possible to determine the root causes of a disease problem. The most important aspect of diagnosis is to relate economics to the actual situation. An assessment of economic losses, the cost

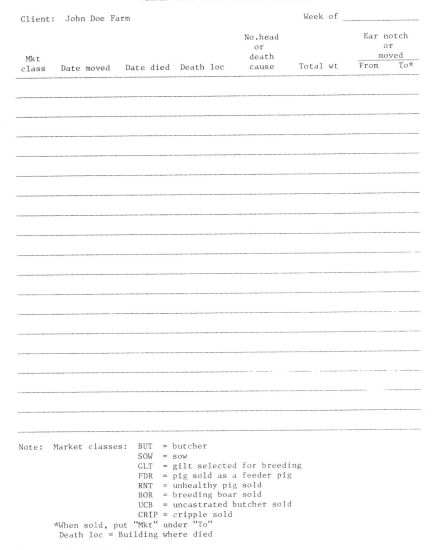

81.5. Weekly pigs moved and died register.

of options to solve the problem, and the relationship of the cost of the problem to the cost of rectifying it need careful scrutiny by the practitioner.

Nutritional Counselling. Nutritional counselling has become an important part of many herd health programs. The practitioner must have a good working knowledge of swine nutrition, since problems of nutrition and disease are often closely associated. The veterinarian or consulting nutritionist should adopt a nutritional program specifically tailored to the production unit, including recommendations for types of feedstuffs, nutrient levels, and feed additives. Feed additives have three primary functions: promote more efficient growth, prevent disease, and treat disease. The use of feed additives is one of those impor-

WEEKLY FEED USED FORM

Client: _____ Week of _____

Date Mixed or Purchased	Building or Bulk Bin	Ration	Batch Size

81.6. Weekly feed used form.

```
                    PORK PRODUCTION ANALYSIS SPREADSHEET
                            JOHN DOE, DVM
                 SWINE PRODUCTION MANAGEMENT CONSULTANT
                            HOG CITY, USA
      Client: EFFICIENT PORK PRODUCERS, INC.
        Date: August 31,1990          NOTE:    EXPECTED PRODUCTION 1991

      Section A:   Production Levels and Capacities              Effect
      ==========   ==================================  Figs.Used   of Changes
      Breeding Herd:                       Figs.Used Last Visit  $$ Cwt    Net $$
      --------------                       =========  =========  ========  ========
      No. Purchased Gilts/Week                1.4     --------
      Avg.Wt.Purchased Gilts, Lbs             230     --------
      Avg.Premium/Head Over Mkt.Value, $     $443     --------
      No.Home Raised Gilts/Week              10.4     --------
      Avg.Wt.Home Raised Gilts, Lbs           275     --------
      Avg.Gilt Pool Inventory                  44     --------
      GILT POOL RATION/Gilt/Day, Lbs          5.8     --------

      No.Purchased Boars/Year                  12     --------
      Avg.Wt.Purchased Boars, Lbs             312     --------
      Avg.Premium/Head Over Mkt.Value, $     $850     --------
      No.Home Raised Boars/Year                 0     --------
      Avg.Wt.Home Raised Boars, Lbs             0     --------
      No.Boars in Herd                         31     --------

      Avg.Working Sow Inventory               878     --------
      Avg.Cull Sow & Boar Inventory            20     --------
      GESTATION RATION/Sow/Day, Lbs           4.5     --------
      Annual Seedstock Death Loss              27     --------
      Avg.Seedstock Selling Wt., Lbs          404     --------

      Farrowing Production:
      ---------------------
      LACTATION RATION/Sow/Day, Lbs          11.7     --------
      Litters Born/Week                     38.00      40.00   ($1.26)    (48,174)
      Piglet Birth Wt., Lbs                   3.4     --------
      Weaning Age, Days                      20.7     --------
      Weaning Wt., Lbs                        12.5     --------
      No.Farrowing Crates                     140     --------
      Pigs Born Live/Litter                   9.7      10.1    ($1.01)    (38,754)
      Pre-Weaning Mortality, %              12.1%       9.0%   ($0.87)    (33,144)
      Weaning Avg.                           8.53       9.19  <--Calculated
      CREEP FEED/Pig, Lbs                    1.23     --------

      Nursery Production:
      -------------------
      Capacity                               1740     --------
      Avg.Inventory                          1646  <--Calculated
      STARTER 2/Pig, Lbs                      5.0     --------
      STARTER 3/Pig, Lbs                     37.4     --------
            Starter2:                         0.0     --------
      Mortality, %                          1.90%     --------
      Wt.Out                                   36     --------
      Days in Nursery                          36     --------

      Age Out, Days                            57     Cwt
      ADF(Avg.Daily Feed), Lbs               1.18  Cost Of Gain
      ADG(Avg.Daily Gain), Lbs               0.64  ============
      F/G(Feed Efficiency)                   1.84     $26.05
```

81.7. Spreadsheet for breeding production analysis.

tant aspects of herd health programming that requires an understanding of the economics of disease prevention and treatment.

The formulation of rations by hand calculation is a slow and inaccurate process, especially if a detailed study of all the important nutrients in the rations is needed. Using the computer for formulating and analyzing rations should be routine practice. Excellent computer software programs are available.

SUPPORT NEEDS FOR SWINE PRACTICE. The producer depends on the swine veterinary practitioner to be an expert. To accomplish this and to be effective in day-by-day counselling the swine specialist needs support from several groups. The practitioner needs good continuing education and the help of experts in other fields related to pork production. A good lay staff is necessary. The support of modern diagnostic laboratories is essential for making accurate diagnoses of disease problems.

Publications. Textbooks and trade journals provide current, detailed new information for practicing veterinarians. Trade journals are especially useful, because they tend to be most current. Many excellent trade journals are published and should be read regularly by veterinarians serving the swine industry. In recent years information services using personal computer modems have come into existence. This is a source of information, and news relating to the swine industry is disseminated quickest of all. Textbooks on diseases of swine and nutrition are essential as reference sources and as a complete review of any particular aspect of the swine industry.

Universities. Since it is the business of universities to educate, the practicing veterinarian is dependent upon them for help with continuing education. It is the task of universities to review current research and make specific recommendations for specific on-farm problems. Professional short courses have been effective in providing good continuing education for practicing veterinarians. University extension short courses and publications are quite useful in helping swine practitioners keep up with rapid changes in the field.

Organizations. Organizations such as the American Association of Swine Practitioners (AASP), International Pig Veterinary Society (IPVS), American Veterinary Medical Association (AVMA), state veterinary societies, and the National Pork Producers Council (NPPC) regularly conduct continuing education seminars and print publications relating to swine veterinary medicine and husbandry. The AASP, organized in the mid-1960s, has been the leader in providing high-quality continuing education seminars for swine prac-

titioners. IPVS has provided a forum for excellent international exchange of research, practice, and management techniques.

Private and Industrial Professional Seminars. Companies specializing in news and continuing education in the agricultural field have become an important source of information for swine practitioners. Generally, companies such as this run seminars, publish newsletters, and may also provide a personal computer modem news and electronic mail service. Professional seminars organized and presented by vendors of products or services are also an important support group for swine practitioners. Even though vendor seminars may be specifically attempting to sell their products or services, they provide good continuing education. It is important that private industry familiarize the veterinarian with their products and services so as to make most effective use of such. The practitioner is then in a position to provide good counsel for clients when it comes to using the products or services of a particular company.

Other Experts. For the practicing veterinarian to be effective, help should be sought from experts in related fields. Consulting agricultural engineers may provide valuable help in planning, remodelling, or construction of new buildings. Agricultural financial advisors can help the veterinarian understand the overall financial situation of a swine unit. Nutritionists can provide support with the latest nutritional technology. A team effort approach of experts will increase efficiency and profits of pork production units.

Perhaps advice and support of colleagues are the most valuable aids. Fellow practitioners generally are attempting to accomplish the same goals. Colleagues can relate well to each other with their problems. One practitioner may have more experience in the field with a particular disease than another because of location and everyday experience. Some may have more experience with types of management systems unfamiliar to others. Many swine practitioners have direct communication to colleagues available via computer electronic mail, which allows quick exchange of information.

Lay Staff. In modern veterinary practice, secretaries and laboratory technicians have become increasingly important as support for the practitioner. Since communication with clients is so important, good secretarial help is necessary for efficient operation. Availability of laboratory technicians to produce bacterins, perform simple diagnostic procedures, and properly dispense medicines is also important.

Diagnostic Laboratories. Availability and use of good diagnostic laboratories are necessary for modern swine practice. Veterinarians cannot effectively control disease without accurate diagnoses for which sophisticated equipment and expertise is needed. The midwestern United States is blessed with a wealth of good animal disease diagnostic laboratories.

COMMUNICATIONS WITH CLIENTELE.

The client and practitioner must be able to communicate with one another if effective solutions to problems are to be found. This requires good rapport between them. Honesty and sincerity by both are important. The practitioner can help gain this rapport if patient, yet firm, with recommendations. The practitioner must also recognize that at times suggestions are difficult for the client to implement. For example, in solving a particular problem the practitioner might recommend individual injections of a drug to many groups of pigs. Getting this job done may be a tremendous burden for both client and employees. In this type of situation the practitioner must test the solution of a problem to make sure it is the simplest yet effective. This helps the client gain confidence in the practitioner's recommendations.

Many disease and management problems are personnel rather than technical problems. Serious mistakes often are made through ignorance of the importance of following a particular protocol. The practitioner must make sure the client understands the priorities of the recommendations; must be able to perceive what is most important; and must also recognize it is sometimes impossible to solve all problems simultaneously. Again, this is an area where knowledge of the economic impact of a problem is important. The practitioner must decide which recommendations are feasible and which are not.

Since providing recommendations or advice are major parts of swine consultants' business, they must be able to help with the continuing education of the client, or more importantly, help the client or manager of the unit train employees. This is important because on-the-spot recognition of disease symptoms must be made by the farm workers themselves. Practitioners should train workers to recognize disease problems and should see to it that they are using good techniques for such routine tasks as castration, injections, hernia repair, obstetrics, etc. "How-to seminars" given at the farm by the practitioner are useful. Medication regimens and vaccination programs will fail if drugs are not administered properly. Disease problems may go unrecognized if workers are unable to recognize abnormal conditions.

Special meetings held for groups of clients and their employees are useful. Some practitioners provide programs with guest speakers for their clientele. During question-and-answer sessions it is possible to exchange ideas not only from the speaker but from their colleagues as the questions are discussed.

The importance of the written farm visit report has already been emphasized. The last item of business of the farm visit should be an oral summary of observations and recommendations. Upon return to the office the practitioner should mail the written report as quickly as possible. This procedure places a double emphasis on recommendations by presenting them orally and in writing; thus they are more likely to be carried out. In addition to the written report to the manager, copies may be sent to key employees. This ensures that all people will be following exactly the same instructions.

Written instructions may be posted on a bulletin board or in the actual area where a new procedure is being carried out, allowing the worker to use them on the spot. Written recommendations should be as short and to the point as possible. When making farm visits, the practitioner should be satisfied that communications among employees are good and that each understands what the recommendations are.

CONSULTATION FEES. As indicated above, as the industry becomes operated more similarly to the poultry industry, many, if not most, swine practitioners will be full- or part-time employees of large companies or production groups. Consultation fees as such will not exist for these practitioners, because they will be working on a salary basis. However, there is a period when most swine practitioners or consultants will be self-employed, working on a fee basis. Recognizing the consultation fee is part of the overhead of the production unit, the practitioner must make sure that services are delivered as efficiently as possible. Any procedure saving time for the practitioner or the client helps to increase efficiency for both. On the other hand the practitioner must be certain to take enough time to obtain a thorough understanding of the herd and its problems.

The consulting veterinarian must be careful to avoid conflict of interest. As swine farms become larger and larger, there is a trend toward purchase of premixes, drugs, and vaccines directly from the manufacturer rather than from a veterinarian or other retail outlet. This helps to increase efficiency by avoiding the middleman. A part of the practitioner's responsibility is to make sure these products are correct for the intended purpose and that quality products are being used. Many times it is still efficient for the practitioner to sell these products to clients. However, to avoid conflict of interest, the sale of products must not subsidize the consulting fee, which should carry itself with or without sales of health products.

In the past many practitioners have charged a consulting fee based on a per-pig-weaned or per-pig-sold basis. With this system regular visits were made to the unit at no extra cost. In a manner of speaking, this was a type of contingency fee—the more production, the higher the fee. With this arrangement, the fee per visit per unit of time is higher if problems are rather easy to solve; conversely, the fee per unit of time is lower if there are unusual difficulties.

The advantage of this system was that the producer could budget veterinary costs. The disadvantage is the fee is quite high if there are not many problems. Also with this type of arrangement there was some tendency to be inefficient in using the veterinarian's time, while on other occasions the producer would think the veterinarian was not spending enough time on his unit.

With the advent of much larger production units, a more equitable method of charging for consulting services is a fee per unit of time, i.e., so much per day or hour. The client pays only for actual time the veterinarian spends at the unit and in the office solving problems. This method of charging is the most commonly used by consulting swine practitioners today. The fee must be high enough to cover overhead expenses, including continuing education, secretarial help, laboratory technicians, office expense, etc. Transportation, lodging, meals away from home, etc., should be charged at actual cost. The disadvantage of a daily or hourly fee is the client may become so conscious of time being spent for services that the veterinarian is not allowed enough time to become properly familiarized with the herd. The practitioner should make the client aware of this.

Fee schedules will present no problem if the producer feels value is received. Difficulties can arise if efficiency of the unit is on a downward trend and the unit is losing money in spite of the services of a consulting veterinarian.

Index

Boldface numbers represent chapter opening pages for a topic or major discussions of a topic.